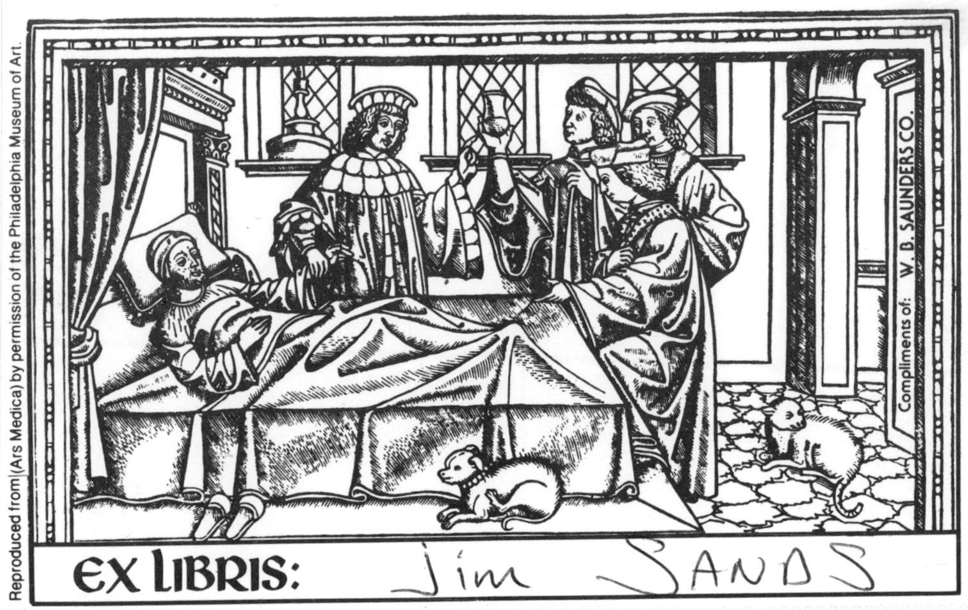
Reproduced from (Ars Medica) by permission of the Philadelphia Museum of Art.
Compliments of: W. B. SAUNDERS CO.
EX LIBRIS: Jim SANDS

Drug Treatment

Drug Treatment

Principles and Practice of Clinical Pharmacology and Therapeutics

Second Edition

EDITED BY

Graeme S. Avery

Editor-in-Chief
Australasian Drug Information Services
division of ADIS Press
Sydney · Auckland

Editor
Drugs · Clinical Pharmacokinetics
Current Therapeutics

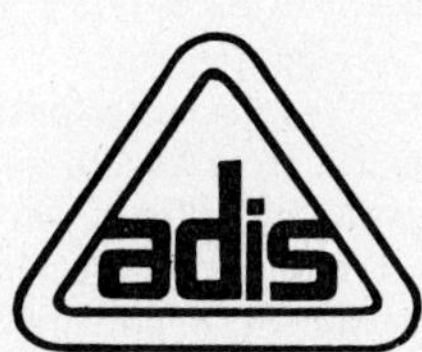

ADIS PRESS Sydney and New York

Drug Treatment

ADIS Press
404 Sydney Road, Balgowlah, NSW 2093, Australia
515 Madison Ave, New York, NY 10022, USA

ISBN 0-909337-08-X

To my wife, Gaby
and children, Simon, Nigel and Monique

Preface to Second Edition

The aim of the second edition of *Drug Treatment* has been to keep the disease orientated approach and level of the book the same as that of the first edition, but to extend its scope by giving more emphasis to descriptions of the clinical pharmacological properties of drugs. This information has been greatly expanded and reorganised and brought together in the one place most appropriate to the description of the clinical use of the drug. All chapters have been enlarged and have undergone thorough revision to include new concepts and those on therapeutics have been up-dated to include the role and effects of new drugs and changes in approach to treatment, as well as newly recognised adverse reactions and diseases caused by older drugs.

Throughout the text attempts have been made to provide more than just 'the facts' and where controversy or uncertainty exists about whether or not to use a certain drug or treatment, the arguments have been summarised. Diseases or conditions not included in the first edition have been added to virtually all chapters on therapeutics. Two new chapters have been included — 'Drug Overdosage and Poisoning' and 'Diseases of a Tropical Environment'. Both these chapters reflect the increasing importance of clinical pharmacology in these areas.

Reference citations have been added to the text itself rather than as a list of recommended reading at the end of each chapter. The decision not to include references in the text of the first edition was misconceived. It is important that readers have the wherewithal to assess the facts given as well as the uncertain issues. References have been selected very carefully and it is hoped that their inclusion in the text will enhance the reference and scholarly value of the book. The appendices have been up-dated and those on pharmacokinetic data greatly enlarged.

Descriptions of the pharmacological actions and pharmacokinetic characteristics of the more important drugs now appear in all chapters on therapeutics with particular consideration being given to the properties of the drugs as they relate to the disease(s) under discussion. The descriptions of the pharmacological actions of the drugs have been kept to a minimum and are intended only to provide information on fundamental pharmacodynamic properties. Standard reference texts on pharmacology should be consulted for more detailed or academic aspects of the pharmacological actions of drugs.

At the possible risk, in some cases, of overemphasis of the clinical importance of alteration in kinetics in disease states and pathophysiological conditions, much additional information has been included on the absorption and disposition of drugs in sick patients. This has been included not only to define principles and concepts and to assist in individualisation of dosage, but also for reference purposes, as in some cases knowledge is incomplete and therapeutic implications are yet to be clarified. In this regard much greater investigational emphasis needs to be placed in the correlation of the clinical effects of drugs with kinetic changes in sick patients. Until the clinical importance of such changes are elucidated practising clinicians will not be sufficiently interested in these apparent finer points. This is a pity. Good therapeutics depends on a firm knowledge of clinical pharmacological principles which at times means an understanding of the finer points involved. Acquisition and application of such knowledge should be no more difficult than that required to make an accurate diagnosis. It is hoped that the additional pharmacological information, apart from conveying the concept of multiple actions of drugs will also better emphasise that drugs, like patients, have their individual characteristics, and that within a class of drugs clinically important differences in pharmacodynamic and pharmacokinetic properties between individual compounds can exist.

All revisions have been made very carefully and with a defined purpose to keep the book to its original aim. *Drug Treatment* remains a general level text about treatment of diseases by drugs and the effect of diseases on the response to drugs, with major emphasis on practical clinical pharmacological concepts and principles. It is hoped that the revisions will extend its scope for those wishing to acquire fundamental knowledge about the clinically relevant pharmacological properties of drugs and up-to-date information on therapeutics. It is also hoped that this new edition will be more useful than its predecessor for both undergraduate students and practitioners alike.

Many of my colleagues at ADIS Press have assisted in the production of this new and enlarged edition. It has been a major secretarial, editorial and publishing task and their support, and that of contributors, was the continual stimulus to keep at it. In particular, I would like to thank Keith Groves, my secretary Judy Snelling (both of whom worked with me on the first edition) and editorial associate Rennie Heel for their outstanding assistance and major contribution in bringing to fruition a new edition. I would also like to thank my other editorial associates Rex Brogden and Trevor Speight for their valued discussions and Diane Torrance and Cushla Goode for their undivided attention to typesetting and proofs. My thanks also to Neal Benowitz, Bob Branch, Terry Blaschke, Pamela Davies, Alex Gallus, Peter Meffin, Trefor Morgan, Lawrie Powell, Rod Roberts and David Shand for technical comments on certain sections of the book. Sadly, I must record the death of Alex Steigman, whose chapter on viral diseases had been revised at the time of his death and has been up-dated prior to publication.

Graeme S. Avery
Auckland

Preface to First Edition

The aim of this book is to discuss the use and effects of drugs within a disease orientated context and so assist clinicians in an understanding of drug response in disease states and in the selection of the most appropriate drug and dosage for a particular patient. The book has been highly structured to achieve this purpose and covers: (1) the clinical pharmacological basis of therapeutics, with particular emphasis on pharmacokinetics; (2) rational selection and individualised use of drugs; (3) the influence of associated disease or intercurrent illness on drug response; (4) diseases caused by drugs; and (5) summary tables and appendices to enable quick reference and correlation of data on individual drugs and classes of drugs. Such a wide scope has never before been attempted in a single book. It was felt however, than an integrated format describing the effects and response to drugs within the context of their clinical use was essential for a proper understanding of clinical pharmacology and therapeutics. Knowledge of what drugs can and can not achieve in a particular disease and how that disease can modify the response to a drug are a prerequisite to safe and effective drug therapy.

A discussion of pathophysiological principles and the mode of action of drugs has only been included where these are of particular importance in the selection of a drug or dose regimen. This is not to say that an understanding of these aspects is not important generally — *it is,* but the central aim of this book is to show that before selecting a drug or dose regimen, the clinician should think first about the patient and his disease(s) and how this might modify drug response. In this way it is hoped that the desired therapeutic effect with minimum adverse effects may be more easily attained. A number of standard texts are available which discuss the pathophysiological and pharmacological basis of therapeutics. Such texts, although extremely valuable and important, describe drugs from the viewpoint of their actions and various uses, which is not ideal for the prescribing clinician whose special primary need is to know how to select and use a drug for an individual patient with a particular disease. The starting point in the therapeutic decision-making process is the patient and his disease or pathophysiological condition and how this relates to the pharmacodynamic actions and characteristic pharmacokinetic properties of individual drugs. The purpose of the book is therefore to complement standard texts in pharmacology on the one hand and medicine on the other — a kind of 'bridge text'.

The teaching of therapeutics is difficult. Traditional teaching of medicine places an excessive emphasis on proficiency in diagnosis while teaching in pharmacology has until recently placed too much emphasis on the pharmacological action of drugs and too little emphasis on how they behave and what they achieve in sick patients. This book aims to bridge this gap by defining clinical pharmacological principles of therapy within a disease orientated context and by describing established approaches to therapy on the basis of drug availability and specialist clinical experience with drugs on a worldwide basis. (Certain indications given in the book for use of some drugs may not be those at present 'approved' for general use in some countries — e.g. in the USA, β-adrenoreceptor blocking drugs in hypertension and co-trimoxazole for other than urinary tract infections). A synopsis of important principles appears at the head of each chapter. These synopses might help in defining learning objectives by itemising that material which is of most general significance and importance, which should be read during skimming for high points and for review, and also that material which most students should master. The relatively young discipline of clinical pharmacology is an essential component of modern medical practice. Already, it has made a very important contribution to improvement in teaching of therapeutics, but academic clinical pharmacology is developing so rapidly that if not careful, it runs the risk of moving away from the present level of understanding of the clinicians whom it is trying to serve. Perhaps also, too much effort in clinical pharmacology has been placed on the evaluation of new drugs rather than on the better utilisation and understanding of existing drugs.

Clinicians use drugs to achieve a preconceived clinical endpoint. This having been decided upon, it remains to select the most appropriate drug and dose regimen for a particular patient. Since clinical drug effects are the result of complex interaction between the drug, the patient and his disease, much emphasis in this book has therefore been placed on individualisation of therapy — both in terms of the characteristic pharmacokinetic properties of individual drugs and the response to a particular drug in an individual patient with a particular disease. Individualised dosage is the heart of therapeutics. Doses discussed in this book are not necessarily those 'approved by a regulatory body' but rather those which competent clinicians have by experience found to be both effective and safe. There is no such thing as a standard dose for all patients, nor a maximum dose for all patients. Therapeutics deals with individuals, not groups of patients.

Drug Treatment is primarily aimed at the student and the clinician in practice, but it should also be of use as a starting point for those studying for higher exams. It is hoped too that the wide scope of information, particularly the many reference tables of drug data, will provide something of value for everyone involved in the study, use and provision of information on drugs. For the prescribing clinician, information on drugs needs to be practical and authoritative. Great care has been placed in the writing and editing to achieve this purpose, all the time keeping the scope of the book within the bounds of understanding of its intended primary audience. It is a book for those who wish to prescribe drugs rationally and with confidence that therapy will be likely to be both effective and safe. The various discussions have been kept as concise as possible with emphasis placed on principles and major aspects of therapy and drug related effects. Those diseases which are most common and those drugs which are most often used have received the greatest attention, as have common therapeutic dilemmas and areas which illustrate clinical pharmacological principles of therapy. The planning of the book coincided with the rapid development of research interest in the study of pharmacokinetics of drugs in sick patients. Much of this information is still poorly defined, particularly its application to therapeutics. Interpretation of this data and its implications to therapy was one of the most difficult tasks in writing and editing the material in the book. Further study will no doubt elucidate many of the uncertain areas. In the meantime, the material pertaining to pharmacokinetic concepts in sick patients therefore relates to the better established principles and those findings of most practical application to therapeutics.

In designing the format of the book it was decided not to include reference citations within the text since it would have become too cumbersome to support all statements made. Rather, references for further reading are grouped under the relevant section headings in each chapter, so making identification of the appropriate reference an easy matter. The references have been selected both for the purpose of supporting statements made in the text and also to act as a starting point for those who wish to study a particular aspect in more depth. Major review articles and specific text books have been included for this purpose. Source data given in tables and figures are acknowledged separately at the beginning of the book, rather than in the text itself.

Therapeutics can and should be an enjoyable experience and I can only hope that this book gives readers as much pleasure (and assistance) as I have had in compiling and editing it.

Graeme S. Avery
Auckland, January 29th 1976

Contributors

Abel, Robert, Jr.
Senior, Department of Ophthalmology, Wilmington Medical Center, Wilmington, Del.; Assistant Professor, Department of Ophthalmology, Thomas Jefferson University, Phil. PA.; Director Corneal Services, Department of Ophthalmology, Temple University Hospital, Phil. PA.; 1300 North Harrison Street, Wilmington, Del. 19806, USA.

Avery, Graeme, S.
Editor-in-Chief, Australasian Drug Information Services, P.O Box 34-030, Auckland 10, New Zealand.

Bank, Simmy
Professor of Medicine, State University of New York at Stony Brook; Head, Division of Gastroenterology, Long Island Jewish-Hillside Medical Center and Queens Hospital Center Affiliate, New Hyde Park, N.Y. 11040, USA.

Barbezat, Gilbert, O.
Senior Lecturer in Medicine (Gastroenterology), Department of Medicine, University of Otago Medical School, P.O. Box 913, Dunedin, New Zealand.

Borgå, Olof
Chemist, Department of Clinical Pharmacology, Karolinska Institute, Huddinge University Hospital, Huddinge S-141 86, Sweden.

Brogden, Rex, N.
Associate Editor, Australasian Drug Information Services, P.O. Box 34-030, Auckland 10, New Zealand.

Burson, J.H.
Chief Resident Otolaryngology, Emory University Clinic, 1365 Clifton Road, Atlanta 30322, USA.

Carter, Stephen, K.
Director, Northern California Cancer Program, 1801 Page Mill Road, Building B, Suite 200, Palo Alto, CA 94304, USA.

Crooks, James
Professor of Department of Pharmacology and Therapeutics, University of Dundee; Consultant Physician Department of Pharmacology and Therapeutics, Ninewells Hospital, Dundee DD1 9SY, Scotland.

Dluhy, Robert, G
Associate Professor of Medicine, Harvard Medical School; Senior Associate in Medicine, Peter Bent Brigham Hospital, Division Affiliated Hospitals Center, Inc., 721 Huntington Avenue, Boston, Mass. 02115, USA.

Dundee, John, W.
Consultant Anaesthetist, Belfast Teaching Hospitals; Professor in Anaesthetics, Department of Anaesthetics, Queen's University of Belfast, Whitla Medical Building, 97 Lisburn Road, Belfast BT9 7BL, Northern Ireland.

Garrod, Lawrence, P.
Emeritus Professor of Bacteriology, University of London; Stradbroke, Gipsy Lane, Wokingham, Berks RG11 2HP, England.

Hall, Marion, H.
Consultant Obstetrician and Gynaecologist, Aberdeen Teaching Hospitals; University of Aberdeen, Foresterhill, Aberdeen AB9 2ZD Scotland.

Hart, F. Dudley
Consulting Physician, Westminster Hospital; Physician, Hospital of S. John and S. Elizabeth, London; 24 Harmont House, 20 Harley Street, London W1N 1AN, England.

Heel, Rennie, C.
Associate Editor, Australasian Drug Information Services, P.O. Box 34-030, Auckland 10, New Zealand.

Hollister, Leo, E.
Professor of Medicine and Psychiatry, Stanford University; Medical Investigator, Veterans Administration Hospital, 3801 Miranda Avenue, Palo Alto, CA 94304, USA.

Jackson, Richard, T.
Professor and Research Director, Otolaryngology Division, Emory University School of Medicine, Atlanta, Georgia 30322, USA.

Judge, Tom, G.
Consultant Physician, Geriatric Assessment Unit, Longmore Hospital, Salisbury Place, Edinburgh, Scotland.

Krishnaswamy, Kamala
Assistant Director, National Institute of Nutrition, Indian Council of Medical Research, Jamai-Osmania P.O., Hyderabad 500 007 A.P., India.

Kutt, Henn
Associate Professor of Neurology, The New York Hospital; 411 East 69th Street, New York, NY 10021, USA.

Leopold, Irving, Henry
Professor and Chairman, Department of Ophthalmology, California College of Medicine, University of California, Irvine 927664, USA.

MacGillivray, Ian
Consultant Obstetrician and Gynaecologist, Aberdeen Teaching Hospitals; Regius Professor Obstetrics and Gynaecology, University of Aberdeen, Maternity Hospital, Foresterhill, Aberdeen AB9 2ZA, Scotland.

Manolas, Emmanuel
Cardiology Research Fellow, Royal Melbourne Hospital, Victoria 3050, Australia.

Marble, Alexander
Clinical Professor of Medicine Emeritus, Harvard Medical School; Physician, Joslin Clinic and New England Deaconess Hospital; President, Joslin Diabetes Foundation, Inc.; 15 Joslin Road, Boston, Mass. 02215, USA.

Marks, I.N.
Senior Specialist, Groote Schuur Hospital; Senior Lecturer, University of Cape Town, Department of Gastroenterology, Observatory, Cape Town, South Africa.

Marks, Janet, M.
Senior Lecturer in Dermatology, University of Newcastle-Upon-Tyne; Honorary Consultant Dermatology, Newcastle Area Health Authority (Teaching); Newcastle-Upon-Tyne NE1 4LP, England.

Mathé, George
Director Institute of Cancer and Immunogenetics, Hôpital Paul-Brousse, 14, Avenue P.V. Couturier, 94800 Villejuif, France.

McCaughey, W.
Consultant Anaesthetist, Craigavon Area Hospital, Department of Anaesthesia, Craigavon, Co. Armagh, BT63 5QQ, Northern Ireland.

McDowell, Fletcher, H.
Professor of Neurology, The Burke Rehabilitation Center, 785 Mamaroneck Avenue, White Plains, New York 10605, USA.

McQueen, E.G.
Professor of Clinical Pharmacology, University of Otago Medical School, P.O. Box 913, Dunedin, New Zealand.

Mirkin, Bernard, L.
Director, Division of Clinical Pharmacology; Professor of Pediatrics and Pharmacology, Department of Pediatrics and Pharmacology, University of Minnesota, Health Sciences Center, Minneapolis, Minn. 55455, USA.

Novis, B.H.
Chief of Gastroenterology, Meir Hospital, Kfar Saba, Israel.

O'Malley, Kevin
Professor of Clinical Pharmacology, Royal College of Surgeons in Ireland; Consultant Physician in St Laurence's Hospital and Charitable Infirmary, Jervis Street, Dublin, Ireland.

Orme, Michael, L'E.
Senior Lecturer in Clinical Pharmacology, Department of Clinical Pharmacology, University of Liverpool, New Medical Building, Ashton Street, P.O. Box 147, Liverpool L69 3BX, England.

Palmer, K.N.V.
Reader in Medicine, University of Aberdeen; Honorary Consultant Physician, Aberdeen Royal Infirmary, Department of Medicine, Foresterhill, Aberdeen AB9 2ZD, Scotland.

Per-Lee, J.H.
Associate Professor Otolaryngology, Emory University Clinic, 1365 Clifton Road, Atlanta, Georgia 30322, USA.

Petrie, J.C.
Honorary Consultant Physician, Aberdeen Teaching Hospitals; Senior Lecturer in Therapeutics and Clinical Pharmacology, University of Aberdeen, Medical Buildings, Foresterhill, Aberdeen AB9 2ZD, Scotland.

Platts, W.M.
Venereologist, Christchurch Hospital; Consultant Venereologist, Department of Health, Wellington, New Zealand; Consultant Venereologist, WHO; 69 Hansons Lane, Christchurch 4, New Zealand.

Prescott, L.F.
Reader in Clinical Pharmacology, Edinburgh University Department of Therapeutics; Consultant Physician, Regional Poisoning Treatment Centre and Royal Infirmary; University Department of Therapeutics and Clinical Pharmacology, The Royal Infirmary, Edinburgh EH3 9YW, Scotland.

Robson, J.S.
Professor, Department of Medicine, The Royal Infirmary, Edinburgh EH3 9YW, Scotland.

Rose, Leslie, I.
Professor of Medicine and Director, Division of Endocrinology and Metabolism; The Hahnemann Medical College and Hospital of Philadelphia, Two-Thirty North Broad Street, Philadelphia, Pennsylvania 19102, USA.

Saunders, Stuart, J.
Professor of Medicine and Head, Department of Medicine, University of Cape Town; Chief Physician, Groote Schuur Hospital, Observatory, Cape Town, South Africa.

Selenkow, Herbert, A.

Associate Professor of Medicine, Harvard Medical School; Director of Medical Education and Chief of Endocrinology, The Waltham Hospital, Hope Avenue, Waltham, MA 02154, USA.

Shirkey, Harry, C.

Clinical Professor of Pediatrics, The University of Cincinnati, College of Medicine, Department of Pediatrics, Clifton Avenue, Cincinnati, Ohio 45221, USA

Simpson, F.O.

Professor of Medicine, University of Otago Medical School; Physician in Charge, Hypertension Clinic, Dunedin Public Hospital; Wellcome Medical Research Institute, P.O. Box 913, Dunedin, New Zealand.

Singh, Sharanjeet

Assistant Professor, Division of Pediatric Cardiology, Departments of Pediatrics and Pharmacology, University of Minnesota, 105 Millard Hall, 435 Delaware Street SE, Minneapolis, Minnesota 55455, USA.

Sjöqvist, Folke

Professor and Chairman, Department of Clinical Pharmacology, Karolinska Institutet, Huddinge University Hospital, S-141 86 Huddinge, Sweden.

Sloman, Graeme

Director of Cardiology, The Royal Melbourne Hospital, Victoria 3050, Australia.

Speight, Trevor, M.

Associate Editor, Australasian Drug Information Services, P.O. Box 34-030, Auckland 10, New Zealand.

Steigman, Alex, J.†

Formerly Professor of Pediatrics, Mount Sinai School of Medicine; Attending Pediatrician, Mount Sinai Hospital Medical Center, One Gustave L. Levy Place, New York, NY 10029, USA.

Teoh, P.C.

Senior Lecturer in Medicine, Consultant Physician, Department of Medicine (I), University of Singapore, Singapore General Hospital, Outram Road, Singapore, 3.

Tuchmann-Duplessis, H.

Professor, Laboratoire d'Embryologie, Faculté de Médecine de Paris, et Biologiste des Hôpitaux de Paris — Chef de Service, Paris, France.

Turner, John, S. Jr.

Professor and Chief, Division of Otolaryngology, Emory University School of Medicine, Atlanta, 30322, USA.

Verstraete, Marc

Professor of Medicine, University of Leuven; Director Laboratory of Blood Coagulation, University of Leuven, Kapucynenvoer 35, B-3000 Leuven, Belgium.

Verwilghen, R.L.

Professor of Haematology, Department of Medical Research, University of Leuven, Kapucynenvoer 35, B-3000 Leuven, Belgium.

Wade, Denis, N.

Professor of Clinical Pharmacology, Department of Clinical Pharmacology, St. Vincent's Hospital, Darlinghurst, NSW 2010, Australia.

Ward, Robert, M.

Fellow, Neonatology and Clinical Pharmacology, Pennsylvania State University, M.S. Hershey Medical Center, Division of Newborn Medicine, Hershey, 17033, USA.

Williams, Gordon, H.

Associate Professor of Medicine, Harvard Medical School; Director, Endocrinology — Hypertension Unit, Peter Bent Brigham Hospital, Division Affiliated Hospitals Center, Inc., 721 Huntington Avenue, Boston, 02115, USA.

Wright, Noel

Consultant Physician, Dudley Road Hospital; Lecturer, Department of Clinical Pharmacology, Birmingham University; Post Graduate Centre, Dudley Road Hospital, Birmingham B18 7QH, England.

Zegarelli, Edward, V.

Edwin S. Robinson Professor of Dentistry; Director of Stomatology; Director of Dental Service, Columbia-Presbyterian Medical Center; Dean, School of Dental and Oral Surgery, Columbia University, New York, NY 10032, USA.

Contents

Section I: Clinical Pharmacology

Section III: Appendices

Chapter I
Fundamentals of Clinical Pharmacology

F. Sjöqvist, O. Borgå and M. L'E Orme

Synopsis of Important Principles

1) Drugs act by affecting biochemical or physiological processes in the body. Most drugs act at specific receptors. The action of a drug is characterised by two variables; the magnitude of the response and the concentration required to produce the response.

2) A specific drug acts only at one receptor but may produce multiple effects due to the location of the receptor in various organs. A selective drug acts on one receptor in a particular tissue at concentrations which produce little effect on the receptor in other organs. All drugs have multiple actions and it is usually preferable to use more specific or more selective drugs.

3) Drugs are molecules with characteristic physicochemical and pharmacokinetic properties. Knowledge of these properties helps to predict the behaviour of a drug in the body and is an important guide in the selection of appropriate doses and dosage intervals.

4) The special and simultaneously operating processes in pharmacokinetics are drug absorption, distribution, metabolism (biotransformation) and excretion. The rate at which these processes proceed and consequently the concentration of drug in the body, is influenced by many factors pertaining to the drug and its dosage form, to pathophysiological or genetic variables of the individual patient, and to effects of other drugs taken concurrently.

5) Many drugs are bound to plasma proteins. Changes in the binding of a drug due to drug interactions or diseases such as uraemia or chronic inflammation, affect its distribution and elimination in the body in a way which is predictable from its kinetic properties. When distribution equilibrium is obtained under steady-state conditions, the unbound concentration of pharmacologically active drug should be equal in plasma and in tissues, and at receptor and metabolic (excretory) sites.

6) Individual patients show a wide variation in response to the same dose of many drugs. Much of this variability in drug response between patients can be explained by individual kinetic factors, particularly genetically determined differences in drug metabolism, and by the effects of intercurrent illness or disease states on pharmacokinetics or tissue response.

7) Drug dosage must be individualised if the desired therapeutic response with minimum side effects is to be obtained. The response to some drugs is better correlated with steady-state plasma concentrations than to dosage.

8) Rational drug prescribing involves a decision on whether or not to use a drug, and if so, selection of a suitable drug and regimen, consideration of compatibility between the drug and patient or any other drugs being given, a legibly written prescription, appropriate instruction of the patient about use of the drug and expectations from treatment and follow-up.

The rational pharmacological treatment of any patient requires adequate knowledge about the disease process, the pharmacodynamic properties of the drug(s) selected and the individual's handling of the drug(s) (pharmacokinetics). The purpose of this chapter is to discuss clinical pharmacological principles which can be applied in any therapeutic situation, particularly as these relate to dose and dose interval. Assuming that the diagnosis and the selection of the drug are appropriate the remaining problem for the clinician is to find a dosage schedule which gives an optimum drug concentration in the diseased organ. The concentration must not be too low, nor too high. In the former case, therapeutic failure may occur, while in the latter, side effects may prove troublesome to the patient.

General principles in drug therapy should be based on the concept that drugs, besides being remedies for a particular disease, are molecules with characteristic physicochemical and pharmacokinetic properties. Many of these properties, even such a simple variable as the plasma half-life, are not readily available in the published literature (see appendix A). It is our hope that doctors reading this chapter will become motivated to request such information when appropriate from representatives of pharmaceutical firms, members of the hospital formulary committee or regulatory agencies.

1. Basic Concepts of Drug Action

Drug action is determined by a physicochemical interaction between the drug and functionally important molecules (usually a 'receptor') in the body. The magnitude of the response is related to the concentration of the drug at the appropriate site of action, which in turn depends on dosage and the time course of the drug in the body. Knowledge of the physicochemical and kinetic properties of drugs and how drugs act can help greatly in understanding why individual drugs produce particular effects.

1.1 Physicochemical Characteristics of Drugs

There are three important physicochemical properties of a drug molecule — its lipid solubility, the extent to which it is ionised, and its molecular size (see Garrett, 1971; Keberle, 1971).

Many therapeutic agents are highly soluble in lipids and this property allows them to cross the gastrointestinal wall, the placenta, blood-brain 'barrier' and cell membranes. Having been filtered through the glomerulus, lipid soluble drugs will be almost completely reabsorbed during their passage through the nephron. Such drugs would remain in the body for an indefinite period unless they were metabolised to more water soluble metabolites, which can be excreted in the urine.

To gain access to their site of action, drugs must cross one or more barriers — the surface and capillary endothelia, the plasma membranes of the cell and the intracellular membranes. This transfer is usually accomplished by passive diffusion, although other processes such as active transport may occur.

The process of passive diffusion is characterised by the movement of drug molecules down a concentration gradient with no expenditure of energy. The rate of diffusion depends on the physicochemical properties of the drug. Many drugs can be considered as weak electrolytes and exist in two forms — ionised and unionised — de-

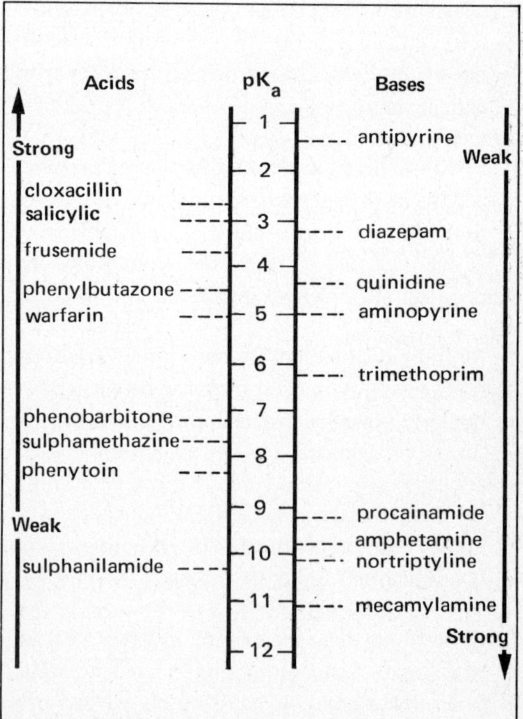

Fig. 1a. pK$_a$ values for some representative acidic and basic drugs.

pending on the pH of the medium (fig. 1a). It is usually assumed that only the unionised drug is sufficiently lipid soluble to diffuse through biological membranes, and that a highly ionised water soluble drug will only cross biological membranes if it is of small molecular size. Thus the passage of water soluble ions through the pores of the plasma membrane is sharply limited when the molecular weight is above 100, a notable exception being hepatic parenchymal cells. Almost all drugs have molecular weights well above 100 and thus can not pass through these pores, one exception being lithium ion with a molecular weight of 7.

In describing the lipid solubility of a drug it is understood that the various lipid:water partition coefficients used are crude indices of the diffusion process *in vivo*. It has nevertheless been shown that within the group of thiazide diuretics there is a close relationship between the chloroform/water partition coefficient, the uptake in renal tubular cells and the natriuretic activity (Duggan, 1966).

The extent to which ionisation takes place is dependent on the pK_a of the drug and the pH of the solution in which the drug is dissolved. The ionisation of a weak acidic drug (e.g. phenobarbitone) is an equilibrium reaction:

$$HA \rightleftharpoons H^+ + A^-$$

The following mathematic relationship exists:

$$K_a = \frac{(H^+)(A^-)}{(HA)}$$

where (HA) is the concentration of the unionised acidic drug and (H^+) and (A^-) represent the concentrations of the hydrogen ions and ionised drug respectively. The relationship between the ionisation of a weak acidic drug, its pK_a and the pH of the solution is given by the Henderson-Hasselbalch equation, which is obtained by logarithmic expression of the equation above:

$$pH = pK_a + \log \frac{(A^-)}{(HA)}$$

The pK_a of a drug is defined as the pH at which the drug is 50% ionised and if the equation above is rearranged such that

$$\log \frac{(A^-)}{(HA)} = pH - pK_a$$

it can be seen that small changes of pH near the pK_a of a weak acidic drug will markedly affect its

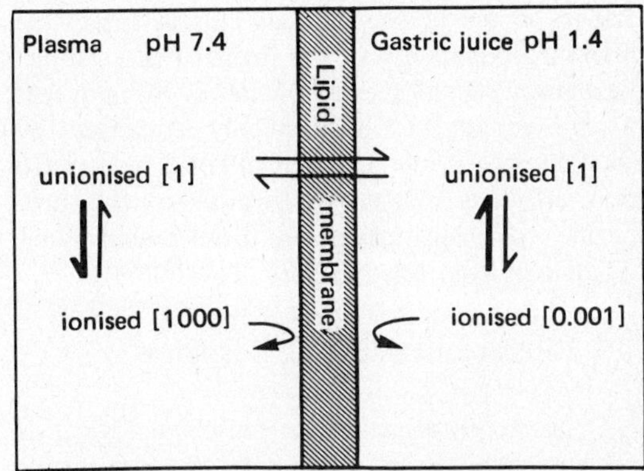

Fig. 1b. The distribution of a weak acid (e.g. warfarin pK_a 5.1) between plasma and gastric juice separated by a lipid membrane permeable only to the unionised form of the drug. The figures in square brackets refer to the approximate, relative concentrations of drug in arbitrary units [after Brodie; in Binns (Ed) Absorption and Distribution of Drugs, Livingstone, London 1964; by permission of author and publisher].

degree of ionisation and under certain conditions its distribution in the body.

For a base, the constants K_a and pK_a can be used, remembering that these terms now refer to the reaction:

$$BH^+ \rightleftharpoons B + H^+$$

The same equations thus apply if (B) and (BH^+) are exchanged for (A^-) and (HA) respectively.

The knowledge of the pK_a of a drug is useful in predicting its behaviour in various body fluids. Phenobarbitone, with a pK_a of 7.2 is largely unionised at acid pH and will be about 40% unionised in plasma.

$$\log \frac{(A^-)}{(HA)} = 7.4 - 7.2 = 0.2; \frac{(A^-)}{(HA)} = 1.58$$

On the other hand, phenobarbitone can be trapped in ionised form in the urine, a phenomenon which is utilised in management of acute phenobarbitone poisoning by forced alkaline diuresis. The principle is illustrated in figure 1b with warfarin, which has a pK_a of 5.1 and will thus be unionised in gastric fluid (pH 1.4), which will aid its absorption. The situation is reversed for basic drugs, such as amphetamine, which will be more ionised at an acidic pH. Such drugs will in fact diffuse from plasma into gastric fluid upon parenteral administration. Drugs with a similar pK_a may nevertheless be differently affected by changes in pH of body fluids. This is due to the different lipophilicity of the drugs. For example, the urinary excretion of amphetamine but not that of chlorpromazine, is markedly enhanced by acidifying the urine. This is explained by a much more effective tubular reabsorption of chlorpromazine, which in turn is due to its much higher lipophilicity (fig. 1c).

1.2 Receptors and Drug Response

Drugs act by affecting normal physiological or biochemical processes in the body, or by controlling changes in these processes brought about by disease. Whatever effects a drug produces they are a consequence of physicochemical interactions between the drug and functionally important molecules in the body. Some drugs act by combining with a small molecule or ion (e.g. neutralisation of gastric acid by antacids or chelation of ferrous ion by desferrioxamine in treatment of iron poisoning) or by a nonspecific effect on membrane function (e.g. local anaesthetics). However, in the

majority of cases drugs are presumed to interact with macromolecular components of tissues. Such elements with which a drug combines to produce its characteristic effects have been called receptors (see further Goldstein et al., 1974).

A receptor is not a readily identifiable physical entity. In many cases, receptors are areas of cell membranes with special structural features which result in the binding of endogenous compounds such as adrenaline (epinephrine), noradrenaline (norepinephrine), histamine, acetylcholine, etc. In other cases the functioning macromolecule may be an enzyme which is inhibited by a drug, or a nucleic acid molecule to which the drug binds. If the drug has an appropriate chemical structure it will also bind to these receptors and may produce a similar response to the endogenous transmitter or may block the response to the transmitter. The structural requirements for combining with a receptor site are specific, both molecular structure and stereochemistry playing an important role in determining the 'fit' of the drug to the receptor; for example, the *l*-form of a stereoisomer pair may be pharmacologically active while the *d*-form is less active (e.g. β-adrenoceptor blocking action of propranolol) or inactive (e.g. narcotic analgesics).

This section is intended as a very brief overview of how drugs act in normally responding tissues. It should be noted that receptor changes can play a part in altered sensitivity to some drugs, as is discussed elsewhere in this book (for review, see Snyder, 1979).

1.2.1 Drug-Receptor Interactions

A drug response is usually the result of a reversible combination between drug and receptor to form a drug-receptor complex; the response being assumed to be directly proportional to the amount of drug-receptor complex formed. A drug which 'fits' the receptor well, will bind strongly and is said to have a high affinity for the receptor. The graded dose-response relationship seen with most drugs (usually shown graphically as a plot of the logarithm of the drug concentration versus the response) is partially a reflection of the extent of occupancy of receptor sites by that drug, in which case the maximal response should correspond to occupancy of all receptor sites. However, this is an oversimplification since other steps involved between the interaction of a drug and receptor and the subsequent biological effect (e.g. 'second messenger' steps involving such agents as cyclic AMP) may be the limiting factors in production of

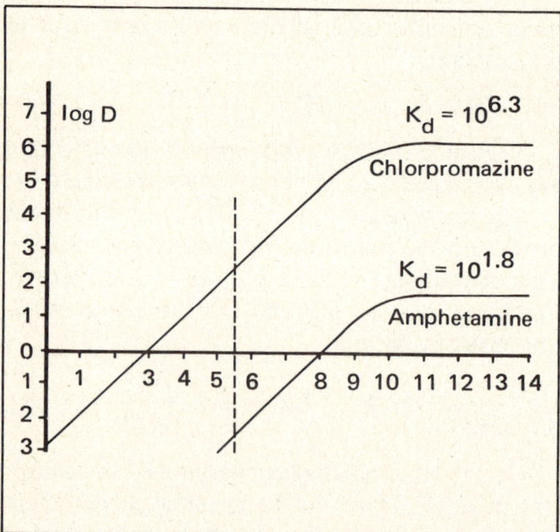

Fig. 1c. Logarithmic representation of the partition ratio (D) between dichloromethane and water at different pH values for two different basic drugs with similar pK_a, chlorpromazine (pK_a 9.3) and amphetamine (pK_a 9.8). Although both drugs are almost completely ionised at pH 5.5 (indicated by the broken line) the partition ratio of chlorpromazine is $10^{2.5} = 316$ but only $10^{-2.5} = 0.00316$ for amphetamine. This is due to the great difference in lipophilic properties of the drugs in unionised form. Thus, the partition coefficient (K_d) of unionised chlorpromazine is more than 30,000 x higher than that of amphetamine.

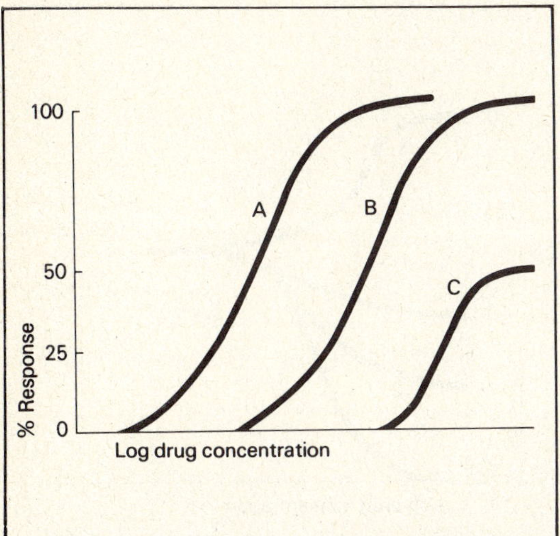

Fig. 2. Log concentration response curves for two full agonist drugs which produce the maximum response at high concentrations. Drug A has a higher affinity than drug B, as lower concentrations of drug A than B are required to produce the same degree of response. Drug C is a partial agonist. Very high concentrations of drug C produce a maximum response less than that produced by the two full agonist drugs A and B (after Meffin et al.: Curr. Ther. 20: 87, Apr. 1979; by permission of author and editor).

the maximal response. The relative affinity of a drug for the receptor can be defined as the concentration required to produce half maximal response (fig. 2).

To explain the different magnitude of response which may be seen between drugs which act on the same receptor site, and apparently have a similar affinity for the receptor, the property of intrinsic activity has been postulated. The intrinsic activity of a drug is a measure of the maximal response that the drug can produce when given in very high concentrations. Thus, two similarly acting drugs with the same affinity but differing intrinsic activities will require a different extent of receptor occupation to produce the same response. The drug with lower intrinsic activity will require a greater extent of receptor occupation, and so a larger dose. A drug with high affinity and high intrinsic activity is termed an agonist, while an agent with high affinity but no intrinsic activity is termed an antagonist since it prevents or tends to prevent a drug that does possess intrinsic activity from interacting with the receptor site. Falling between these two extremes are partial agonists; drugs which no matter how high their concentra-

tion will not produce the full response of which the tissue is capable (fig. 2).

Antagonists are of two main types. An antagonist is said to be competitive if it combines *reversibly* with the same receptor site as the agonist. Since the antagonist-receptor complex can be reversed, the maximum response to the agonist can still be obtained provided the concentration of agonist is high enough — i.e. the dose-response curve shifts to the right (fig. 3a). An antagonist is said to be non-competitive if it 'inactivates' the receptor so that an effective agonist-receptor complex cannot be formed. In this case, the effect of the antagonist on the receptor may be reversible or irreversible; the result is to reduce the intrinsic activity of the agonist without changing its affinity so that a maximal response cannot be obtained by increasing the concentration of the agonist (fig. 3b).

Partial agonists also have antagonist properties, since they occupy receptor sites, preventing access of full agonists to the receptor, but possess only relatively weak intrinsic activity of their own and do not elicit a maximal response of the tissue involved even at very high concentrations. The net effect of a combination of a partial agonist and a full agonist is dependent upon the concentrations

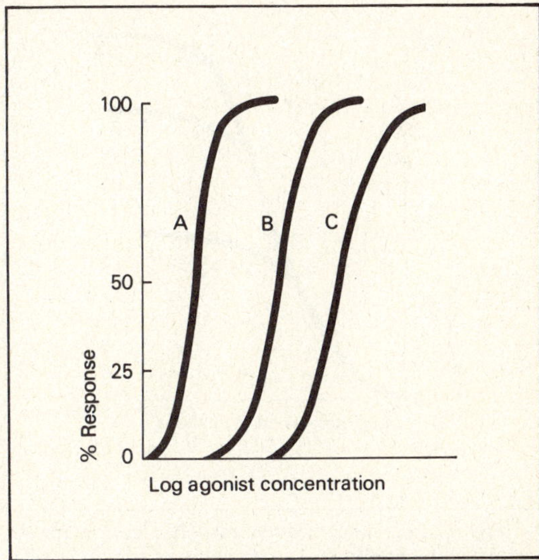

Fig. 3a. Log concentration response curves for an agonist in the presence of a competitive antagonist. Curve A shows the response of the agonist alone and curves B and C in the presence of increasing concentrations (C > B) of a competitive antagonist (after Meffin et al.: Curr. Ther. 20: 87, Apr. 1979; by permission of author and editor).

present. At low agonist concentrations, addition of a partial agonist will increase the response by occupying previously empty receptor sites, while at higher agonist concentrations the response may be decreased on addition of a partial agonist since receptor sites previously occupied by the full agonist may now become occupied by the less active (intrinsic activity) partial agonist (fig. 4).

Some drugs used therapeutically have this dual action. Strong analgesics such as pentazocine, butorphanol and buprenorphine have both narcotic agonist and lesser antagonist properties (see chapter X; sect. 8.4.3). Nalorphine on the other hand, has narcotic antagonist and lesser agonist properties and when used to reverse the effects of narcotics taken in overdosage, may potentiate respiratory depression due to any concomitantly ingested non-narcotic drugs such as barbiturates. Naloxone, a narcotic antagonist with no partial agonist activity avoids this potential problem. Some β-adrenoceptor blocking drugs have partial agonist activity, which is most marked with pindolol. This drug may produce significant agonist response as reflected in an increase in blood pressure in hypertensive patients when a ceiling

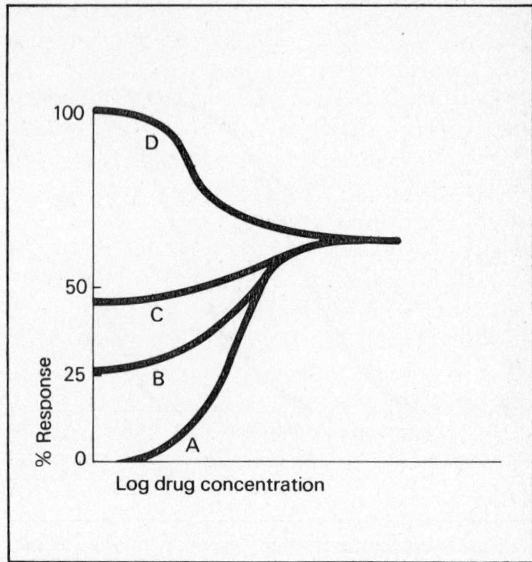

Fig. 4. Log concentration response curves for a partial agonist in the presence of a full agonist. Curve A: Partial agonist only. The relative concentrations of full agonist are B < C < D. In curves B and C, the concentrations of full agonist are less than that which will produce the maximum response of the partial agonist, and so the agonist effects are additive. In curve D the response due to the full agonist exceeds that of the partial agonist, and the response is antagonised to the maximum response of the partial agonist (after Meffin et al.: Curr. Ther. 20: 87, Apr. 1979; by permission of author and editor).

dosage is exceeded (see chapter XVIII; sect. 5.6.3, 5.6.9, table IIIa).

1.2.2 Specificity and Selectivity of Drug Action

Most drugs have multiple effects, some of which in varying degree may be undesirable, rather than the single one thought to be most important. It is therefore usually preferable to give more specific or more selective drugs. The phenothiazines as a class are relatively nonspecific drugs because they act on a variety of different receptors (see chapter XXVI; sect. 1.4.1, 3.5). Drugs may still act on a specific receptor but produce a number of pharmacological responses because of a wide distribution of this receptor in body tissues (e.g. atropine action on muscarinic receptors).

Some drugs can be both specific and selective, as is well illustrated by drugs acting on β-adrenoceptors. Selectivity however, is not absolute. Thus, β-adrenoceptor agonist bronchodila-

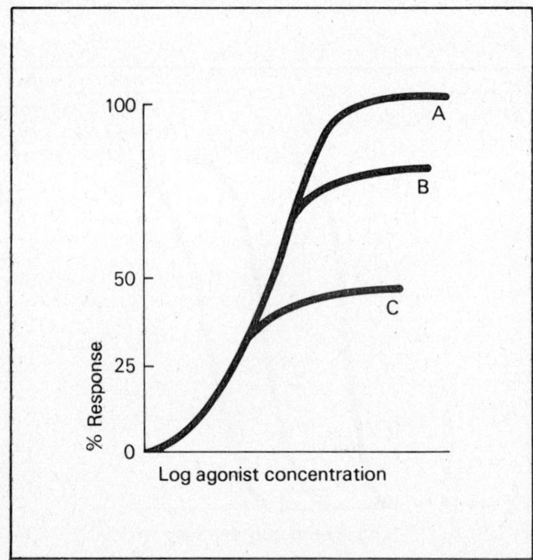

Fig. 3b. Log concentration response curves for an agonist in the presence of a non-competitive antagonist. Increasing concentrations of the antagonist (C > B) produce a reduced maximum effect with respect to that obtained with the agonist alone. In contrast to competitive antagonism (fig. 3a), increasing the concentration of the agonist fails to restore the maximum response (after Meffin et al.: Curr. Ther. 20: 87, Apr. 1979; by permission of author and editor).

tors such as salbutamol and terbutaline show relative selectivity for the β_2-adrenoceptors in bronchial smooth muscle, at doses which cause little stimulation of the β_1-adrenoceptors in the heart. Such relative selectivity is greater when these drugs are inhaled into the lungs than when given by oral or intravenous administration. Isoprenaline (isoproterenol) on the other hand is a specific but non-selective β-adrenoceptor agonist as it exerts an effect on both β_1 and β_2-adrenoceptors (see chapter XX; sect. 2.3.1). Similarly, the β-adrenoceptor antagonist drugs atenolol and metoprolol have a much greater selectivity for adrenoceptors in the heart than in the bronchioles and muscle blood vessels, whereas propranolol acts on both β_1 and β_2-adrenoceptors and is thus a specific but non-selective β-blocker (see chapter XVIII; sect. 5.6.2).

1.3 Potency and Drug Effect

Potency must not be confused with specificity and selectivity, nor used in a non-precise way to indicate clinical efficacy. Sometimes potency can be used to convey greater intrinsic activity. Thus, frusemide (furosemide) and other 'loop' diuretics produce a greater diuresis in renal failure than that from any dose of a thiazide diuretic. On the other hand, the different mg dose equivalents of the individual thiazides do not have clinical relevance, since the maximum diuretic effect produced by

each is the same when used at adequate dosage (see chapter XXI; sect. 7.1).

2. Basic Concepts of Pharmacokinetics

2.1 Simple Kinetic Characterisation of Drugs

Pharmacokinetics deals with the mathematical description of the biological processes which affect the time course of the absorption and fate of drugs and which are themselves affected by drugs (see Gibaldi, 1977). The description of the fate of drugs in the body can be simplified by the introduction of certain models. The mathematical formulas derived from these models make it possible to determine appropriate dosage regimens. The relevance of both the formulas and the derived dosage regimens can be tested by direct measurements of drug plasma levels. Usually the body is depicted as a system of compartments, even though these lack physiological or anatomical reality. The one compartment model depicts the body as a single homogeneous unit. The two compartment open model consists of a so called central compartment which includes plasma and a peripheral or 'tissue' compartment. It is assumed that absorption to and elimination from the system involve only the central compartment (fig. 5). Sometimes more complicated models are used.

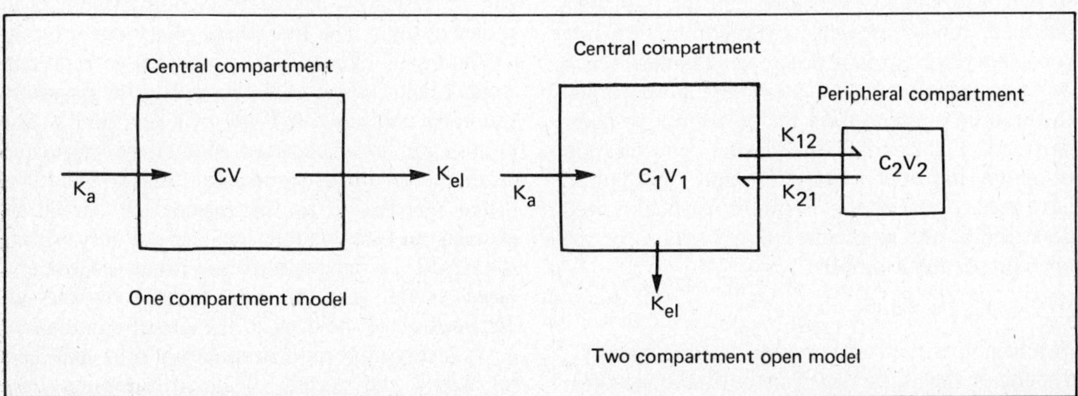

Fig. 5. Schematic diagram of the body (left) as a one compartment model, and (right) as a two compartment open model. K_a is the rate constant of absorption and K_{el} the rate constant of elimination (including both metabolism and excretion). K_{12} and K_{21} are transfer rate constants between the two compartments (i.e. from compartment one to compartment two and vice versa). The amount of drug in the body is given by the concentration of drug (C) times the apparent volume of distribution (V). V_1 and V_2 are the apparent volumes of distribution and C_1 and C_2 are the concentrations of drug in the two compartments respectively (see text). C and C_1 are assumed to be the same as the concentration of drug in plasma.

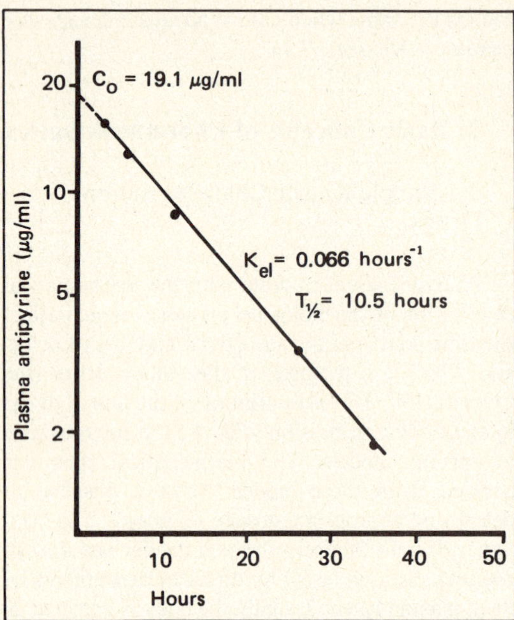

Fig. 6. An application of the one compartment model. Plasma concentration curve of antipyrine after a single oral dose (10mg/kg) given to a healthy volunteer. The drug is eliminated by an overall first order process, and thus the disappearance curve becomes linear if plotted on a log-lin paper.

2.1.1 Elimination Half-Life

Many processes in pharmacokinetics can be described satisfactorily by first order kinetics. This means that all rate constants for transport in and out of a compartment (e.g. from compartment one to two, K_{12}, and vice versa, K_{21}, in the two compartment model) as well as the elimination rate constants (K_{el}) are first order, i.e. changes which occur (transport or elimination) are proportional to the drug concentration in the respective compartment. For example, the plasma concentration of antipyrine after absorption and distribution have been completed (fig. 6) can be reasonably well described by the mathematical expression for the one compartment model:

$$C = C_o \cdot e^{-K_{el} \cdot t}$$

in which C is the concentration at time t and C_o designates the extrapolated zero time concentration. Therefore, by plotting the concentration data on a logarithmic scale against a linear time scale, a straight line describing the plasma fall off curve of antipyrine is obtained. This representation of the plasma concentration-time data is the one most often used.

The rate constant K_{el} is of first order. This means that the fraction of drug that is eliminated from the body in any given time period is constant, as with the decay of a radioisotope. For such a drug, it is meaningful to speak about the elimination or plasma half-life ($t_{1/2}$). This is the time required for any given drug concentration in plasma to decrease by half. The mathematical relationship between $t_{1/2}$ and K_{el} is as follows:

$$t_{1/2} = \frac{e_{\log 2}}{K_{el}} = \frac{0.693}{K_{el}}$$

In the example in figure 6, the half-life is 10.5 hours and thus K_{el} is 0.066 hours⁻¹. Since the extrapolated zero time concentration C_o was 19.1 mg/litre the equation that best fitted the experimental data was:

$$C = 19.1 \cdot e^{-0.066 \cdot t}$$

The elimination half-life of a drug varies among individuals. For drugs, that are excreted unchanged in the urine (e.g. digoxin and most antibiotics) the elimination half-life will depend on renal function. Many drugs are metabolised in the body and hence the half-lives will reflect their rate of metabolism, at least partly (see section 4.1). Some drugs, like procainamide and phenobarbitone are both metabolised and excreted unchanged.

The plot of log plasma concentration versus time sometimes yields two linear portions of the curve, rather than one (see fig. 7). Such a curve can be described by the two compartment open model system. The first phase of the curve (up to 10 hours in figure 7) is considered to represent mainly distribution of the drug into the tissues of the body and has a half-life of a few hours. The elimination rate constant should be calculated from the terminal exponential part of the curve (often referred to as the β-slope). It should be pointed out that this rate constant not only reflects the hepatic or renal elimination processes, but to a large extent may be rate limited by the redistribution of the drug to the site of elimination.

It is very important in studies of drug half-lives to extend the period of blood sampling long enough to get an adequate estimate of the β-slope. This point is illustrated by the following example. It has previously been reported that the elimination half-life of methaqualone is around 4 hours, which might be beneficial for a hypnotic drug, since most of the dose would be eliminated by the next morning. However, in this study the authors only followed the decline of plasma concentration during the initial part of the disappearance curve. Appropriate estimations (cf. fig. 7) reveal that the half-life of the β-slope is in the order of 40 hours with marked interindividual variations (Alvan et al., 1973), implying that any patient put on this drug once every evening will accumulate the drug until reaching a steady-state plasma concentration (see section 2.2).

Sometimes the metabolic process cannot be described by first order kinetics but by approximate zero order kinetics. Here, the rate of metabolism is proceeding at a constant rate, independent of the concentration of drug in the body. An intermediate between zero and first order kinetics is generally known as Michaelis-Menten kinetics. If such kinetics apply, the time required for an initial drug concentration to decrease by 50% increases with increasing dose (fig. 8). This is an example of dose (concentration) dependent elimination kinetics and has been documented for example, with salicylic acid, dicoumarol (bishydroxycoumarin) and phenytoin (diphenylhydantoin). The clinical use of such drugs is made more difficult because small increments of the dose may result in disproportionate increases of the plasma

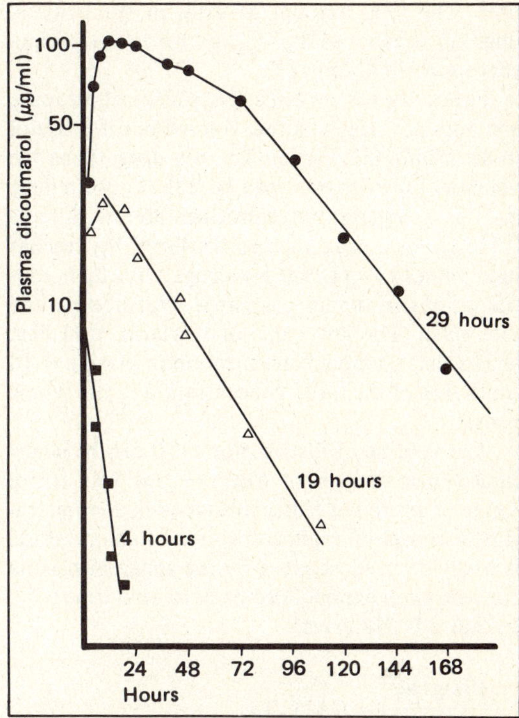

Fig. 8. Log plasma concentrations of dicoumarol (in µg/ml) versus time after varying oral doses of dicoumarol in man, 150mg (■) 450mg (Δ) and 2400mg (●). The plasma half-life is prolonged from 4 hours to 29 hours when the dose is increased. An example of dose dependent kinetics (after O'Reilly et al.: Thrombosis et Diathesis Haemorrhagica 11: 1 1964; by permission of author and editor).

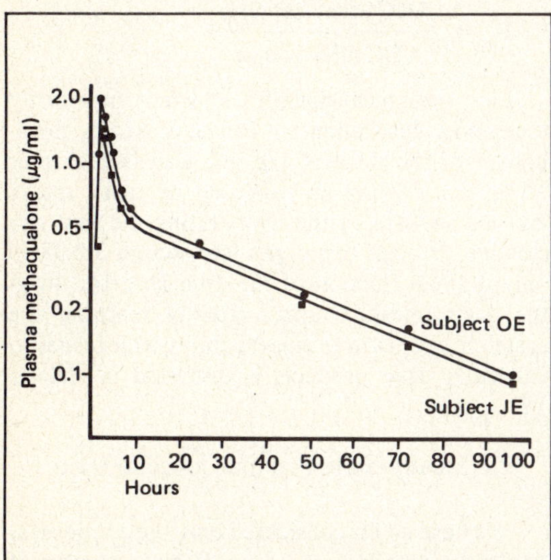

Fig. 7. Log plasma concentrations of methaqualone (in µg/ml) versus time after a single oral dose (4mg/kg) was given to two volunteers. Biphasic disappearance curve. The half-life of the β-phase is 36 hours. Compare text (after Alvan et al.: European Journal of Clinical Pharmacology 6: 187, 1973; by permission of author and editor).

concentrations, thereby resulting in toxicity.

The duration of effect of some drugs is much longer than can be predicted from their elimination half-life (e.g. corticosteroids; many antihypertensive drugs). In the case of corticosteroids, the term biological half-life is used to describe the time for a measured metabolic activity to decline by half of its initial level (see chapter XVI; sect. 9.1.2).

2.1.2 Volume of Distribution

The body is obviously not homogeneous, even if it can be treated as such in a mathematical model. Drug concentrations in the liver, kidneys, muscle, fat and other tissues will therefore differ from one another as well as from the concentration in the plasma. The term apparent volume of distribution (V_d) of a drug is a proportionality constant, which describes the amount of drug in the total body relative to that in plasma at any one time. The total amount of drug in the body A (mg/kg) is equal to V_d (L/kg), times the plasma concentration C (mg/L).

Factor V_d has no direct physiological meaning and does not refer to a real volume but it is useful in describing the distribution of a drug. Thus the volume of distribution may be $20L/kg$ for a drug such as a tricyclic antidepressant and as little as $0.1L/kg$ for a drug such as warfarin. V_d reaches high values ($> 1L/kg$) for drugs with high concentrations in tissues compared with plasma and vice versa. The low value of warfarin, $0.1L/kg$, shows that the drug concentration in plasma is 10 times that of the mean concentration in the whole body.

The volume of distribution (V_d) can be determined in a number of ways — one way (from figure 6, assuming either intravenous administration or complete, rapid absorption of an oral dose) is to divide the dose given by the apparent plasma concentration extrapolated back to zero time (C_o). In figure 6 this gives:

$$\frac{10mg/kg}{19.1mg/L} = 0.52L/kg$$

This figure is in agreement with the fact that antipyrine distributes in body water and actually has been used for measurement of body water content. A better way is to determine the area under the plasma concentration versus time curve (AUC) and to add the area beyond the last known plasma concentration up to the time when it approaches zero. This is accomplished by a simple calculation.

V_d then equals the dose (D) divided by the total area (AUC) times the elimination rate constant K_{el} thus:

$$V_d = \frac{D}{AUC \cdot K_{el}}$$

2.1.3 Plasma Clearance

The plasma clearance of a drug is given by:

$$Plasma\ clearance = V_d \cdot K_{el}$$

Thus from the relationship described above between K_{el} and $t_{1/2}$:

$$Plasma\ clearance = \frac{V_d \cdot 0.693}{t_{1/2}}$$

and from the relationship between V_d, D, AUC and K_{el} given above:

$$Plasma\ clearance = \frac{D}{AUC}$$

This term often gives a better idea of the elimination of a drug from the body than the half-life, since it incorporates changes in pool size. The clearance term is well known from nephrology, where it is used to describe the rate and mechanism of renal elimination of drugs. It can also be used to describe the rate of drug metabolism in the liver. In this case, hepatic clearance has an upper limit set by the blood flow through the organ (approximately $1.5L/min$). Using this term, some authors prefer to describe drugs as low, intermediate and high clearance drugs (see section 4.3.2).

2.1.4 Bioavailability

An important application of pharmacokinetics is in the determination of the proportion (fraction) of unchanged drug that reaches the systemic circulation — known as the bioavailability. This can be determined from plasma concentration (or urinary excretion) data. The bioavailability of an orally administered drug is often calculated by measuring AUC after oral and intravenous administration. The bioavailable fraction F of an oral dose is then simply expressed:

$$F = \frac{AUC\ after\ oral\ dose}{AUC\ after\ iv\ dose}$$

Low oral bioavailability may not necessarily mean poor absorption but can be caused by metabolism of the drug in the gut wall (see chapter XIX; sect. 1.2), or in particular by rapid uptake and metabolism in the liver during the first circulation through this organ (see section 3.3.3) — only a small fraction of the drug absorbed from the gastrointestinal tract actually reaching the systemic circulation. Bioavailability as it relates to particular drug products is discussed in chapter VI.

2.2 Steady-State Plasma Concentration

We have so far considered only the administration of a single dose of a drug. While a number of drugs such as analgesics or hypnotics may be given in this way, it is more common to give drugs on a regular basis. Let us take as an example digoxin, given without a loading dose, twice a day.

Digoxin has a half-life of about 30 hours (assuming normal renal function) and by the time

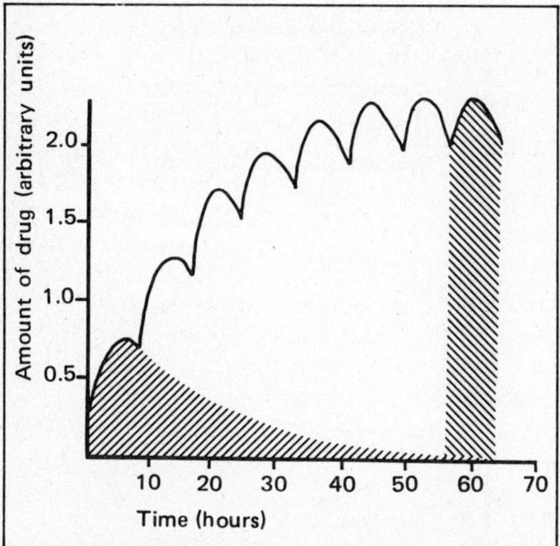

Fig. 9. Schematic representation of the accumulation of drug in the body (or plasma) after oral dosing. The drug is given every 8 hours and has a half-life of elimination of 12 hours. The area under the plasma concentration time curve after the first dose is equal to the area under the curve during the dosage interval, provided that plateau concentrations (steady-state) have been reached [after Rowland; in Melmon and Morelli (Eds) Clinical Pharmacology, p.53, Macmillan, New York 1972; by permission of author and publisher].

the second dose of digoxin is given at 12 hours the plasma concentration will still be more than half its peak value and thus the concentration of the second dose of digoxin will rise to higher levels than after the first dose and with each succeeding dose this pattern will be repeated until a steady-state concentration is reached. The elimination of digoxin from the plasma obeys first order kinetics so that as the concentration of drug in plasma increases, the amount of drug eliminated per unit of time increases.

The tendency for a drug to accumulate will therefore be balanced by the increased amount of drug being eliminated. As a result, a steady-state will be reached during which the amount of drug absorbed will equal the amount of drug being eliminated. The plasma concentration will then fluctuate around a mean or plateau concentration (fig. 9).

The rate at which the plateau or steady-state plasma concentration (C_{SS}) will be reached can be calculated (table I). Thus 50 % of the C_{SS} will be reached in one half-life, 75 % in two half-lives, 87.5 % in three half-lives, etc. Thus during oral

administration of digoxin once daily it will take 150 hours (5 x $t_{1/2}$) to reach 97 % of the steady-state concentration. This can be exemplified further (fig. 10) with data on nortriptyline and desipramine (desmethylimipramine). The time taken to reach the steady-state concentration is well illustrated and corresponds to about 4 to 5 half-lives. Clinically, a drug can be expected to have its full benefit when a therapeutic steady-state plasma concentration has been reached. A number of concepts follow from these observations.

Firstly, the shorter the elimination half-life of a drug the sooner the C_{SS} will be reached. (A drug with a half-life of 8 hours, given every 8 hours, will reach 90 % of the C_{SS} in 26 hours).

Secondly, the shorter the elimination half-life of a drug, the more the plasma concentration will fluctuate between doses and it is difficult in practice to dose more often than 4 times daily. Thus drugs like alprenolol and procainamide with half-lives between 2 to 3 hours will show marked variations in plasma concentration between doses when given every 6 hours. One way to avoid drastic fluctuations is to prepare such drugs in sustained release form. As an example, procainamide as sustained release tablets can be given 3 to 4 times daily while ordinary tablets have to be given every 3 hours to avoid marked fluctuation in plasma concentrations (Karlsson, 1978).

Thirdly, if the elimination half-life of a drug is prolonged above the normal value, as will happen with digoxin and with aminoglycoside antibiotics (e.g. gentamicin, kanamycin) in patients with renal failure, the time taken to reach a steady-state will

Table I. The plasma concentration at different time points as a percentage of the steady-state concentration[1]

Number of $t_{1/2}$[2]	Plasma level as % of steady-state level
1	50
2	75
3	88
4	94
5	97
6	98
7	99

1 Assuming continuous administration of the drug (intravenous infusion or frequent oral administration).

2 The time points are expressed as the number of half-lives elapsed from starting therapy.

be longer than before and concentrations reached will be considerably higher than under normal conditions. The dose must therefore be decreased and the dosage interval prolonged (see chapter XXI; section 2.1; 14). On the other hand, if a clinical effect is required quickly, it is possible to shorten the time taken to reach the steady-state concentration by giving a loading dose at the beginning, as is sometimes used for digoxin. The loading dose (L_D) can be calculated to be:

$$L_D = C_{SS} \cdot V_d$$

where C_{SS} is the required plasma concentration and V_d the apparent volume of distribution.

The maintenance dose is then half the loading dose given every half-life. In practice, particularly with a drug which has a long elimination half-life, this regimen is impracticable and even dangerous, and it is usually better to allow gradual accumulation following usual dose and dosage interval. The patient will reach his individual steady-state concentration in due course.

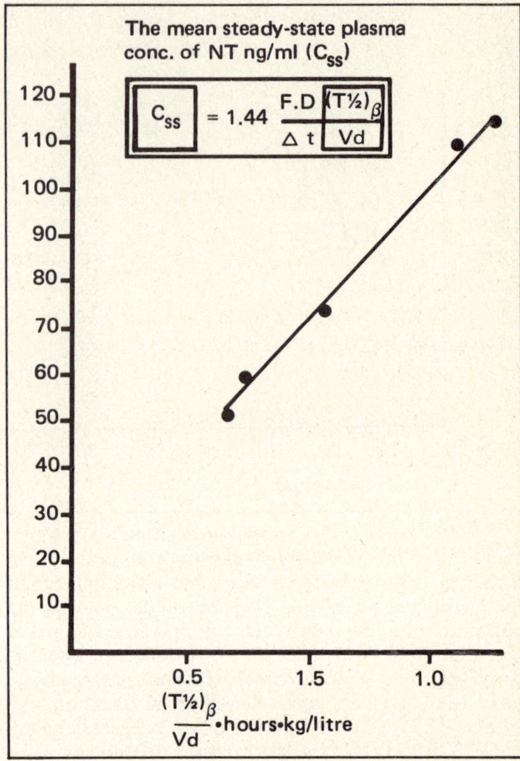

Fig. 11. Correlation between the steady-state plasma concentration (C_{SS}) of nortriptyline (NT) in 5 healthy humans given NT for 14 days and the ratio between the plasma half-life [β-slope = $(T_{1/2})\beta$] and apparent volume of distribution (V_d) of a single oral dose of NT in the same individuals. The plasma clearance of a drug is equal to [$V_d : 0.693/(T_{1/2})\beta$]. Hence the steady-state plasma concentration of NT will be proportional to the inverse plasma clearance of a single oral dose (cf fig. 14) [after Alexanderson and Sjoqvist: Annals of the New York Academy of Sciences 179: 739, 1971; by permission of authors and editor].

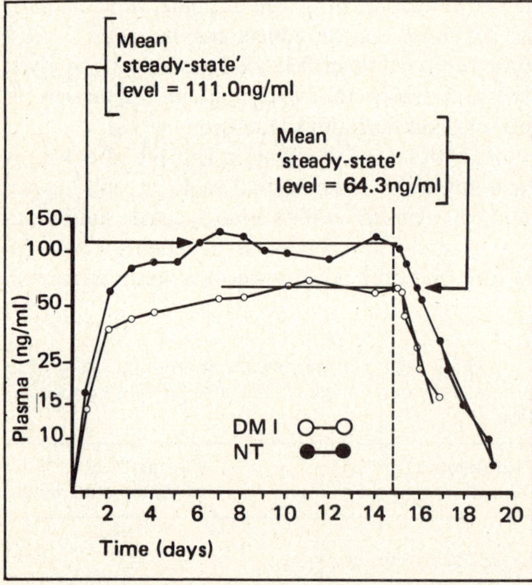

Fig. 10. Log plasma concentrations of desipramine or desmethylimipramine (DMI) and nortriptyline (NT) versus time during repetitive oral dosing. The drugs were given to the same volunteer several weeks apart in a daily dose of 0.4mg/kg administered every 8h for 15 days. Steady-state concentrations are reached within 4 to 5 days. When medication is stopped plasma concentrations decline monophasically with half-lives of 25 (NT) and 21 hours (DMI), respectively (after Alexanderson: European Journal of Clinical Pharmacology 5: 1, 1972; by permission of editor).

Fourthly, it is possible to predict the steady-state concentrations of a drug in plasma after multiple dosing from the kinetic behaviour of a single dose (fig. 11). This requires information about the elimination half-life (or K_{el}), apparent volume of distribution (V_d) and bioavailability (F). The formula is given:

$$C_{SS} = \frac{F \cdot D}{K_{el} \cdot V_d \cdot \Delta t}$$

where D is the dose and Δt the dosage interval. As pointed out in section 2.1.4, bioavailability (F) is dependent on both the fraction absorbed and the degree of metabolism during the first passage of the drug through the gut wall and/or liver. The formula implies first order kinetics. If $t_{1/2}$ is preferred rather than K_{el} the formula is as follows:

$$C_{SS} = \frac{1.44 \cdot F \cdot D \cdot t_{1/2}}{V_d \cdot \Delta t}$$

If the prediction does not hold, induction or inhibition of drug metabolism may operate. For example, predicted steady-state plasma concentrations of carbamazepine are always higher than those actually obtained since autoinduction of its metabolism occurs after a few doses (Bertilsson, 1978; see chapter XXV, sect. 3.4).

2.3 Drugs as Chemical Individuals — Conclusions

In summary, any drug can be characterised by several variables which will help to predict its behaviour in the body as well as guide the clinician in selecting appropriate doses and dosage intervals. These variables include:

a) pK value
b) Lipophilicity as measured, for example, by the oil/water partition coefficient
c) Bioavailability
d) Elimination half-life
e) Apparent volume of distribution
f) Plasma clearance.

We have also seen that the steady-state plasma concentration (C_{SS}) can be predicted from the above variables. This can be of great help in situations where the relationship between C_{SS} and clinical effects has been established (see section 5.1). In terms of the formula for C_{SS} it can be stated that the variable K_{el} (i.e. rate of elimination) is especially dependent on the individual, particularly for drugs that are metabolised. The relationship between doses and C_{SS} in different individuals can be used to distinguish between first order and saturation elimination kinetics.

3. Special Processes in Pharmacokinetics

3.1 Drug Absorption

3.1.1 Drug Absorption After Oral Administration

Before a drug can be absorbed after oral ingestion, a drug tablet or capsule must disintegrate and the drug must dissolve in the gastrointestinal fluids. Most studies of the process of absorption have been performed with the drug in solution. This has tended to emphasise the importance of factors such as lipid solubility for drug absorption and de-emphasise the many factors that can interfere with the dissolution of the drug product in the gastrointestinal tract. For the role of the dosage form for gastrointestinal absorption, see Gibaldi (1977).

There are four possible mechanisms of absorption: (1) passive diffusion; (2) active transport; (3) filtration through pores, and (4) pinocytosis (see Binns, 1971; Goldstein et al., 1974).

Passive Diffusion

This is by far the most important process. No energy is required for the absorption of the drug and the net transfer of the drug is directly proportional to the concentration gradient and to the lipid-water partition coefficient of the drug. Lipid soluble drugs are absorbed more rapidly than water soluble drugs and no competition for absorption will be seen between two drugs of similar chemical composition. The drug must initially be present in aqueous solution at the surface of the cell membrane, then dissolve in the lipid membrane and finally pass into the aqueous phase on the other side of the membrane. Drug absorption will depend on the physicochemical properties of the compound as illustrated in section 1.1, especially its degree of ionisation in the gastrointestinal lumen. The ionised forms of drugs are not appreciably lipid soluble and thus acids in theory should be better absorbed at acid pH (when they are relatively unionised) in the stomach than at the higher pH in the intestine. However, the short sojourn of the drug in the stomach and its limited surface area compared with that of the intestine outbalance the importance of this pH factor (see chapter XIX; sect. 1.1).

Active Transport

This term implies the utilisation of energy to convey a drug across a cell, often against a concentration gradient. This mechanism is highly specific and is used for the transport of naturally occurring substances, such as amino acids, sugars and some vitamins, but rarely for drugs unless they have close structural similarity to a naturally occurring compound. Methyldopa and levodopa are both absorbed by active transport via an amino acid transport mechanism.

Table II. Factors affecting drug absorption from the gastrointestinal tract

---

1. Formulation and characteristics of drug product
   a) Tablet disintegration time
   b) Dissolution time
   c) Presence of excipients in tablet or capsule formulation
   d) Stability in gastrointestinal tract

2. Patient characteristics
   a) pH of lumen
   b) Gastric emptying time
   c) Intestinal transit time
   d) Surface area of gastrointestinal tract
   e) Gastrointestinal disease
   f) Mesenteric blood flow

3. Presence of other substances in the gastrointestinal tract
   a) Interaction with other drugs, ions
   b) Food (large meal)

4. Pharmacokinetic characteristics of drug
   a) Drug metabolism by gut bacteria
   b) Drug metabolism in gut wall

Filtration Through Pores

In practice, these pores between cells are so small that only compounds with a molecular weight of less than 100 can be absorbed in this way. The total area of these pores is very small compared with the total lipoid cell membrane area.

Pinocytosis

This mechanism of absorption, whereby microscopic particles are engulfed by the cell membrane, is not of major importance for the absorption of drugs, although it may have some relevance to the uptake of macromolecules.

3.1.2 Factors Affecting Oral Absorption

Table II lists some factors known to affect the absorption of drugs.

The formulation of the drug product may have dramatic effects on its solubility and hence absorption (see chapter VI). Thus the acid form of phenytoin (diphenylhydantoin) is absorbed with rates which depend on its crystal size. An epidemic of phenytoin intoxication occurred in Australasia when the excipient was changed in the most commonly used product (Bochner et al., 1972). In Sweden, the most commonly used phenytoin product has been shown to have less than 50% bioavailability and instances of severe intoxication have occurred when patients were changed to other brands of phenytoin, which subsequently were found to have much higher bioavailability (Neuvonen, 1979). The sodium salt of tolbutamide is more rapidly absorbed than the acid form and might produce rapid changes in the blood sugar (see chapter VI; table III).

The presence of other drugs or even excipients believed to be inert may also modify drug absorption. The absorption of tetracycline is reduced by cations such as iron or calcium which produce insoluble chelates (Neuvonen, 1976; see chapter VIII, fig. 6). Bentonite, a constituent in for example, some PAS granules, is responsible for a marked impairment of the absorption of rifampicin when given together with some PAS products. This is due to adsorption of rifampicin onto bentonite (Boman et al., 1975). Drugs that are well absorbed are probably less affected by the presence of other drugs in the gut, compared with poorly absorbed drugs (see chapter VIII; sect. 2.3.1).

Gastric emptying and motility determine the rate of delivery of a drug to the small intestine where absorption of most drugs occurs. As a general rule, factors slowing gastric emptying will decrease the *rate* of absorption of most drugs (and vice versa) but for some drugs, such as those which are poorly soluble, erratically absorbed, or metabolised in the gut, the *amount* of drug absorbed may be increased when gastric emptying or intestinal motility is slowed (see section 4.3.1).

The presence of food might be expected to interfere with drug absorption by slowing gastric emptying or by altering the degree of ionisation of the drug in the stomach. It has been assumed that food will in general delay drug absorption by slowing the rate but not affecting the amount absorbed. However, this is too much of a generalisation (see Melander, 1978). Food intake may actually influence absorption of different drugs in different ways — increasing, decreasing or having no consistent effect on the amount absorbed. Improvement in absorption of some drugs might be due to alteration in tablet disintegration and drug dissolution and the variable effects of different types of meals on intestinal transit time. For drugs subject to extensive first-pass metabolism in the gut and/or liver (see section 3.3.3) such as hydrallazine and propranolol, food may enhance bioavailability; possibly by somehow decreasing the extent of first-pass metabolism. The effect of food intake on bioavailability should therefore be studied for each drug rather than predicted from general rules. A table showing the effect of food on the bioavailability of different drugs is given in chapter VI (sect. 5).

3.1.3 Alternative Sites of Drug Absorption

Although drugs are usually administered by mouth they may be given by a variety of other routes.

Intramuscular Absorption

Drugs may be administered by the parenteral route because they are destroyed in the stomach (e.g. benzylpenicillin), are subject to extensive and rapid hepatic first-pass metabolism (e.g. lignocaine/lidocaine), to aid compliance with therapy, or to ensure a more rapid onset of action. However, intramuscular administration of some drugs does not always assure rapid or complete absorption and some degree of local discomfort is probably inevitable with any intramuscular injection (Greenblatt and Koch-Weser, 1976).

Although lipid solubility favours absorption of drugs from an intramuscular injection, the water solubility of a drug is a major determinant of the rate and completeness of absorption. The drug must be sufficiently water soluble at physiological pH to remain in solution in the interstitial fluid of muscle tissue until absorption occurs. Drugs that are poorly soluble in water (e.g. diazepam) or soluble in water only at non-physiological pH (e.g. phenytoin, chlordiazepoxide) are most likely to have bioavailability problems after intramuscular injection. Such drugs precipitate at the injection site once the non-aqueous solvent diffuses away or buffering occurs. Absorption of phenytoin and digoxin can be very slow and erratic. Intramuscular injection is not a reliable means of administration of these drugs and should be avoided. Chlordiazepoxide and diazepam are slowly absorbed after intramuscular injection and diazepam may be incompletely absorbed. More rapid and reliable effects can be obtained by oral or intravenous administration of these drugs.

Absorption after intramuscular injection is also influenced by local blood flow. Thus, blood flow to skeletal muscle may be decreased by circulatory disturbances associated with reduced cardiac output. Morphine, for example, may be slowly absorbed after intramuscular injection in acute myocardial infarction. Differences in blood flow to specific muscle groups may explain different rates of absorption. Lignocaine (lidocaine) absorp-tion, for example, is more rapid after injection into the deltoid muscle than into the vastus lateralis and gluteus maximus (Meyer and Zelechowski, 1971).

Rectal Absorption

This route may be chosen to avoid direct gastric irritation or because of therapeutic customs in different countries. Absorption from the rectum is governed by the same processes which operate in other parts of the gastrointestinal tract. The absorptive surface area is however, small. In general, absorption is not as rapid but can be as complete as after oral administration. There are exceptions, such as incomplete and irregular absorption of certain dosage forms of diazepam and theophylline from the rectum (Mandelli et al., 1978; Ogilvie, 1978). Contrary to popular belief, most of the drug absorbed from the rectum passes via the hepatic portal vein to the liver and so the first-pass effect is not avoided (see section 3.3.3).

Pulmonary Absorption

Many drugs can be readily absorbed from the lungs by passive diffusion. This applies particularly to inhaled anaesthetic gases but also to drugs delivered either as aerosols or as particulate inhalations. Many drugs, initially produced in aerosol form to allow direct medication to the lung, are in fact absorbed into the body via this route. Dosage levels are usually small and thus little therapeutic effect is seen outside the lungs, but repetitive inhalation of isoprenaline (isoproterenol) aerosols was probably responsible for a number of deaths from cardiac arrhythmias in the 1960's (see chapter XX; sect. 3.1.2). The smaller the particle the more likely the drug is to be absorbed. Particles greater than 20μ in size are likely to be deposited on the bronchiolar epithelium and then the respiratory cilia will sweep the particles back to the larynx where they will be swallowed. Particles of 2μ in size are likely to reach the smallest bronchioles (see further chapter XX; sect. 1.4).

Percutaneous Absorption

It is often assumed that a drug applied to the skin surface has only a local effect but this has now been shown to be untrue. Most drugs are well absorbed when applied to the skin surface especially if the skin is occluded with polythene. Inflamed or diseased skin is more permeable to drugs than normal skin (see chapter XIV; sect.

1.3.1). The skin over the scrotum and behind the ear are particularly useful as a means of drug administration. Antimotion sickness drugs for example can be applied to the skin in a disc behind the ear and held in place by a plaster, whereupon the drug will be steadily absorbed until the disc is removed at the conclusion of the journey (Heilman, 1978). Application of an ointment of glyceryl trinitrate to an area of thin skin such as the forearm, has been used to provide sustained percutaneous absorption in patients with angina (see chapter XVII; sect. 4.2.1)

Conjunctival Absorption

The conjunctiva functions as a specialised skin surface, and drugs can be administered into the conjunctiva for local therapy to the eye or for more general therapy. Some success has been achieved with locally inserted sustained release preparations of drugs such as pilocarpine ocusert (see chapter XII; sect. 5.2).

3.2 Binding and Distribution of Drugs

After absorption, a number of factors influence the subsequent fate of a drug. Thus it will be distributed to receptors at its site of action, to silent or inactive receptors in other tissues, as well as to sites of metabolism and excretion (fig. 12). The process of distribution largely depends on the physicochemical properties of the drug such as lipid solubility and binding to macromolecules, but will also be affected by factors such as blood flow to various organs.

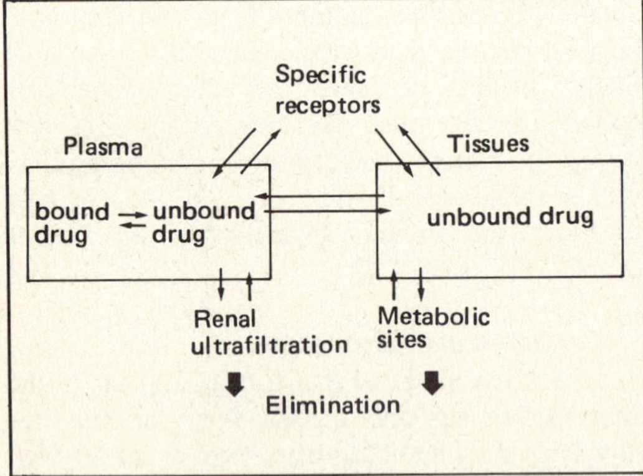

Fig. 12. Schematic representation of fate of a drug in the body. During distribution equilibrium the unbound concentration of drug is assumed to be the same in various parts of the body.

Drugs are transported from the site of administration to receptor sites by plasma proteins and red blood cells. Serum albumin can carry many types of drugs, but haemoglobin, lipoproteins, α_1-acid glycoprotein and certain other globulins are also important. The processes of distribution, metabolism and excretion operate simultaneously and thus a change in protein binding of a drug will affect its distribution and elimination, and hence steady-state plasma concentration, in the body in a way which is predictable from its kinetic properties (see Blaschke, 1977; Jusko and Gretch, 1976).

3.2.1 Protein Binding of Drugs

The exterior surface of a protein is composed principally of polar amino acids with the sidechains projecting into the surrounding environment. A given protein, e.g. serum albumin, may have several specific structures and reactive groups, permitting reversible binding of many structurally diverse small molecules. The forces involved in binding include ionic, hydrogen and hydrophobic bonds and weaker bonds called van der Waals forces.

Proteins are structures with clefts and holes that can also allow entry of small molecules into their interior areas. Once a small molecule is attached to a protein, it travels in the bloodstream until it dissociates from the protein and attaches to another macromolecule. Thiopentone for example is highly bound (75%) to plasma proteins but when the blood reaches brain or fat tissue the drug rapidly dissociates from the protein in blood and binds to lipids in the tissue.

Serum albumin (M = 66,400) probably exists in several closely related conformations and the location and number of binding sites may differ for different drugs. Albumin has a particularly high affinity for acidic drugs, such as warfarin, phenylbutazone, penicillins, sulphonamides and salicylic acid.

Two independent binding sites (I and II) for acidic drugs have been characterised on human serum albumin (Sjoholm 1978; Sjoholm et al., 1979; Sudlow et al., 1975, 1976). Site I, the less specific of the two sites, binds a variety of structurally diverse drugs such as warfarin, phenylbutazone, the antiepileptic drugs phenytoin and sodium valproate (valproic acid), and various sulphonamides (table III).

Warfarin is bound specifically to this site, and the ability of various drugs to displace warfarin

Table III. Binding sites of highly bound acidic drugs on human serum albumin (after Sjoholm et al., 1979; Sudlow, 1979)

Site I (warfarin site)	Site II (diazepam site)
Warfarin	Benzodiazepines
Ethylbiscoumacetate	
Nicoumalone	Ibuprofen
(acenocoumarol)	Flurbiprofen
Phenprocoumon	Ketoprofen
Dicoumarol	Naproxen
	Indomethacin
Chlorothiazide	Salicylic acid
Frusemide (furosemide)	Diflunisal
Bumetanide	Flufenamic acid
Several sulphonamides	Ethacrynic acid
Azidocillin	
Nalidixic acid	Clofibric acid[1]
Phenytoin	Cloxacillin
Valproic acid (valproate)	Dicloxacillin
Salicylamide	Probenecid
Salicylic acid	
Diflunisal	Sulphobromophthalein
Phenylbutazone	
Oxyphenbutazone	Tolazamide
Azapropazone	Glibenclamide
Sulphinpyrazone	Tolbutamide
Indomethacin	
Naproxen	Tryptophan
Chlorpropamide	
Glibenclamide	
Tolbutamide	
Bilirubin	

1　Active metabolite of clofibrate.

has been used as a criterion of site I binding. Similarly, diazepam has been used as a marker for the more specific site II. With the exception of the benzodiazepines, site II drugs are generally carboxylic acids (table III), among them the extremely strongly bound anti-inflammatory analgesic drugs naproxen and ibuprofen and their analogues. The latter drugs are also bound to site I, but in general with lower relative affinity. This means that they are less efficient in displacing type I drugs, unless in very high concentration, when binding to the less specific secondary site occurs.

Among endogenous compounds, it may be noted that tryptophan is bound to site II, while bilirubin is primarily bound to site I. This explains why bilirubin may be displaced by several sulphonamides (site I drugs) and salicylic acid (bound equally strong to sites I and II). It is a widespread misconception that compounds bound with very high affinity, such as bilirubin, cannot be displaced by compounds with lower affinity for the protein (e.g. sulphonamides). According to accepted theory, competitive displacement occurs when the product of the *free* concentration of displacer and its binding constant is high enough. This implies that important displacement will only occur with drugs used at plasma concentrations high enough to exceed the binding capacity of their own primary binding sites on albumin. This prerequisite makes salicylate, phenylbutazone, valproic acid, naproxen, dicloxacillin and several sulphonamides likely candidates for displacement of other drugs bound to the same site, but rules out warfarin, diazepam, indomethacin and phenytoin. This is because therapeutic plasma concentrations of the latter drugs are much below the saturation concentration of their albumin binding, and thus free drug levels are too low to exert any significant displacing effect.

Fatty acids have their own specific primary binding sites on albumin. By inducing conformational changes in the albumin molecule, fatty acids can affect the binding of other compounds to separate sites on albumin. Thus, high serum concentrations of free fatty acids released by heparin injection may cause either decreased or increased binding of drugs, as shown with digitoxin (Storstein, 1976) and warfarin (Nilsen et al., 1977) respectively. Normal physiological fluctuations in free fatty acid levels usually have little effect on drug binding.

There are qualitative differences between the binding of basic and acidic drugs. While acidic drugs bind mainly to albumin, many lipophilic basic drugs such as quinidine, imipramine, chlorpromazine, alprenolol, propranolol bind more avidly to other proteins in the plasma such as α_1-acid glycoproteins and lipoproteins (Borga et al., 1977; Fremstad et al., 1976).

3.2.2 Pharmacological Implications of Protein Binding

The interaction between protein and drug is reversible and obeys the law of mass action:

Drug + Protein $\rightleftharpoons$ Drug-Protein complex

The rate at which a drug-protein complex can

dissociate is very rapid (with a half-life of about 20 milliseconds) so that this is probably not a rate limiting factor in the removal of drug from plasma. Only unbound drug can diffuse into tissues because the drug-protein complex is unable to cross cell membranes. The drug-protein complex therefore acts as a store of drug and as unbound drug is removed from plasma, more of the complex dissociates.

The consequences of protein binding are quite different for drugs that are extensively bound in tissues compared with those which are not bound in the tissues. Much of the discussion in the literature concerning the importance of plasma protein binding has not taken this into account. It is also important to consider that the consequences of protein binding are different during the distributive phase after drug administration, compared with the distribution equilibrium that may occur during steady-state conditions. Also, in other non-equilibrium situations the plasma protein binding can have unexpected effects, as illustrated by the following examples.

For tissue bound drugs, the plasma can be completely cleared of drug during a single passage through an organ such as the brain (e.g. thiopentone), the kidney or the liver, irrespective of the extent of plasma protein binding. In such cases, the protein binding actually increases the concentration of drug available for diffusion into the tissues or the sites of elimination. For example, with some drugs having a high hepatic clearance, such as alprenolol, propranolol and hydrallazine, virtually all drug in blood, unbound and bound, is cleared during one passage through the liver. For these drugs, with this high 'hepatic extraction

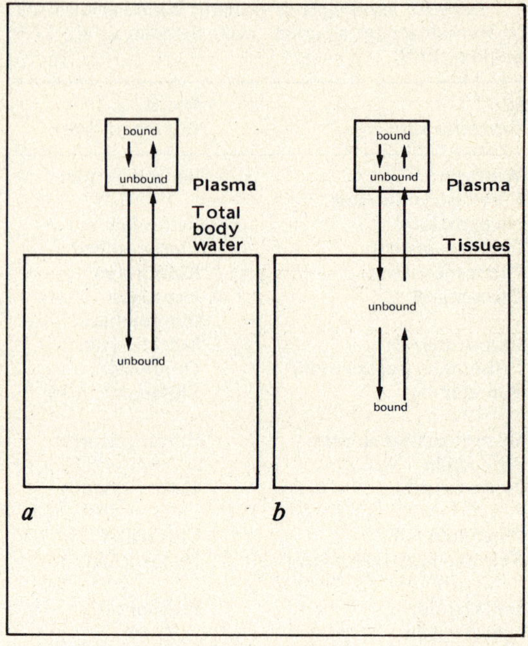

Fig. 13a. Schematic representation of the partitioning of a non-tissue bound drug between the plasma pool and total body water.

Fig. 13b. Schematic representation of the partitioning of a tissue and plasma bound drug between plasma and other tissues.

ratio' (see section 3.3.3), increased protein binding may increase rather than decrease the amount metabolised per unit of time, simply because increased binding to plasma protein results in elevated total drug concentrations in blood.

While the above examples concerned non-equilibrium situations, the following discussion will concern low clearance drugs only, and will be based on the assumption that distribution equilibrium has been obtained. That is the situation during the plateau concentration obtained during steady-state conditions. Under these circumstances, the unbound concentration of drug should be equal in plasma and in tissues, and at receptor and metabolic (excretory) sites. For example, during long term treatment with phenytoin the concentration of unbound drug in plasma during steady-state conditions is the same as the concentration in cerebrospinal fluid and saliva, which essentially can be considered as protein free solutions. Thus CSF and saliva concentrations are about 10 % of the total steady-state plasma concentration, corresponding to 90 % binding of phenytoin in plasma.

Table IV. Relationship between degree of binding to plasma proteins and total amount of drug in plasma (after Martin, 1965)

Binding to plasma proteins (%)	Drug in plasma as percentage of total amount in the body
0	6.7
50	12
60	15
70	19
80	26
90	42
95	59
98	78
99	88
100	100

Table V. Predicted increase in concentration of unbound drug *in vivo* resulting from drug displacement found *in vitro* (chosen as a doubling of the unbound percentage)

Displacement observed *in vitro*				Predicted[1] increase of unbound concentration *in vivo* by a factor of
% bound		% unbound		
before	after	before	after	
99	98	1	2	1.8
95	90	5	10	1.4
90	80	10	20	1.3
80	60	20	40	1.14
70	40	30	60	1.11
50	0	50	100	1.06

1 Based on the calculated total amount of drug in the plasma for a given degree of protein binding (see table IV). For example, displacement of a drug which is 90% protein bound to 80% *in vivo* results in a decrease in the total amount of drug in the plasma from 42 to 26% so that the concentration of unbound drug is increased by a factor of 1.3 — i.e.
$$\frac{100 - 26}{100 - 42} = 1.3;$$ rather than a factor of 2 as observed *in vitro*. Protein binding displacement leading to increases in the fraction of unbound drug becomes unimportant at binding degrees below 80%.

3.2.3 Displacement of Protein Bound Drugs

For a drug with negligible binding to tissues other than plasma, the model depicted in figure 13a can be used to describe some pharmacological consequences of a displacement interaction. Unbound drug in the plasma pool (4% of body weight) is in equilibrium with unbound drug in the 15 times bigger pool consisting of total body water (60% of body weight). Table IV shows that most of the total amount of drug (bound + unbound) in the body occurs in plasma at binding degrees above 90%. Table V is constructed in such a way that it shows the consequences *in vivo* of a displacement interaction observed *in vitro*. The model helps to show that the rise in unbound concentration as found *in vitro* never occurs to the same extent *in vivo*. In fact, protein binding displacement will affect the unbound concentration of drug in the body only at binding degrees above 80%. The model does not take extravascular albumin into account which might increase the quantitative importance of displacement.

In summary, if model 1 (fig. 13a) is applicable, a protein binding displacement interaction (i.e. in-

crease in fraction of unbound drug) may result in the following events if the initial binding exceeds 80 to 90%:

a) Increased unbound concentration in plasma and tissues
b) Increased rate of elimination (increase in amount of unbound drug available for metabolism or excretion)
c) Decreased concentration of total drug in plasma (small increase in V_d)
d) Increased pharmacological effects (if the concentration-effect curve is reasonably steep).

The increased rate of elimination will tend to counteract the events described in a, c and d above. Provided that the displacing agent is present in a constant concentration, a new steady-state will finally be established (after 4 to 5 half-lives) at which the unbound concentration has returned to its original (predisplacement) level. Therefore, if the displacing agent is given during continued administration of the displaced drug, the potentiation of the pharmacological effect should be greatest initially and then gradually diminish.

In model 2 (fig. 13b) the prerequisites are the same as in model 1, with the exception that the drug now binds considerably to tissue components as well. Table VI shows that with an increasing volume of distribution less and less drug occurs in plasma compared with tissues. One consequence of this is that induced changes in plasma protein binding (see also section 4.3.2) will be potentially important clinically only at small V_d values in the order of 0.15L/kg or less. At V_d values above this, less than 27% of the total drug in the body occurs in plasma.

Table VI. Relationship between apparent volume of distribution (V_d) and amount of drug in plasma (assuming a plasma volume equal to 4% of body weight)

V_d (L/kg)	% Drug in plasma of total amount in body
0.045	89
0.10	40
0.15	27
0.6	6.7
1.0	4.0
10	0.40

For highly bound drugs with a large V_d value, a displacement interaction at protein binding sites will lead to:

a) Negligible increase in the unbound concentration in plasma
b) Decreased concentration of total drug in plasma (increased V_d)
c) Little or no pharmacological consequences
d) Changed relationship between total drug concentration and clinical effects (i.e. effects will occur at a lower concentration of total drug).

These theoretical predictions have been validated by clinical studies. After adding the displacer valproic acid to maintenance therapy with phenytoin the unbound fraction of phenytoin in plasma increased, the total plasma concentration decreased, while the unbound concentration remained relatively stable (Mattson et al., 1978). The same phenomenon occurs with phenytoin in uraemia as a consequence of decreased protein binding (Odar-Cederlof and Borga, 1974). In both cases the therapeutic plasma concentration range of phenytoin was lowered (see also section 4.3.2; 5.1).

Hence by knowing the V_d of a drug and its degree of plasma protein binding we can predict the possible importance of a protein binding displacement interaction. Yet, V_d values are not easily available in the literature. Those for some drugs are listed in table VII and for many others in appendix A. It is seen that phenylbutazone and frusemide (furosemide) are characterised by low V_d values. Such drugs are potentially important displacers of other highly bound drugs with a low V_d such as warfarin and tolbutamide and the binding of these drugs may be affected to a clinically significant extent by conditions of hypoalbuminaemia (e.g. nephrotic syndrome, cirrhosis) and uraemia (section 4.3.2).

As discussed in section 3.2.1, displacement will only occur if the two drugs are bound to the same site on albumin. Ibuprofen has a low V_d value (table VII) and is highly protein bound (99 %) but binds to a different primary site on albumin than for example warfarin or tolbutamide (table III). Also, plasma concentrations of ibuprofen obtained with normal therapeutic doses are relatively low. This explains why a clinically important interaction does not occur between warfarin and ibuprofen (Penner and Abbrecht, 1975). Phenylbutazone, on the other hand, is bound to

Table VII. Apparent volume of distribution[1] of various drugs (approximate average values in normal subjects)

Drug	V_d (L/kg)
Frusemide (furosemide)	0.1
Phenylbutazone	0.1
Warfarin	0.1
Naproxen	0.1
Sulphamethoxazole	0.1
Ibuprofen	0.14
Tolbutamide	0.14
Valproic acid	0.15
Sulphafurazole (sulfisoxazole)	0.2
Dicloxacillin	0.2
Glibenclamide	0.3
Nalidixic acid	0.3
Penicillin G	0.3
Antipyrine (phenazone)	0.6
Phenytoin (diphenylhydantoin)	0.6
Diazepam	0.7
Pentobarbitone	0.7
Indomethacin	0.9
Carbamazepine	1
Lignocaine (lidocaine	1.3
Procainamide	2
Pentazocine	3
Methaqualone	6
Digoxin	6
Chlorpromazine	20
Nortriptyline	20

1 It should be noted that the V_d term is not unequivocally defined unless the pharmacokinetic model is defined. Even then there are several volume terms; e.g. $(V_d)_{area}$, $(V_d)_\beta$, $(V_d)_{ss}$, and $(V_d)_{extrap}$. For this table, $(V_d)_{extrap}$ has been used in most cases where the plasma fall off curve was essentially monoexponential. $(V_d)_\beta = (V_d)_{area}$ was used when there was a biphasic decline of plasma concentrations with time.

the same site on albumin as warfarin and tolbutamide and is a predictable cause of interaction with these drugs (see chapter XVI, sect. 3.3.5; XXIII, sect. 3.2.5). This is because phenylbutazone not only displaces warfarin and tolbutamide, but also inhibits the metabolism of these drugs (Aarbakke, 1978; Hansen and Christensen, 1977). It appears that most clinically important interactions due to protein binding displacement have involved inhibition of metabolism as well.

To summarise, the kinetic importance of drug protein binding, the rate-limiting factor for entry of a drug into tissue fluid, appears to be diffusion of unbound drug and not the rate of dissociation of drug-albumin complex. The best available indication of the concentration of unbound drug in tissue fluid is the unbound drug concentration in plasma. Displacement interactions of clinical importance only occur between highly albumin bound acidic drugs which are bound to the same site on the albumin molecule and which have small apparent volumes of distribution in the order of 0.15L/kg (for list see appendix A).

3.3 Drug Metabolism

3.3.1 General Principles

By an oversimplification, drugs can be divided into water soluble (polar) and lipid soluble compounds. Water soluble drugs are mainly excreted unchanged through the kidneys and will reach toxic concentrations in the body when kidney function deteriorates, unless the dose is reduced. Lipid soluble drugs are initially filtered in the glomeruli but may be fully reabsorbed further on in the distal portion of the nephron. Such drugs, therefore, have to be metabolised to more polar compounds before they can be excreted in the urine (Remmer, 1970). Their rate of metabolism will determine the duration of action of single doses and the intensity of action of multiple doses. This is because the steady-state concentration largely depends on the elimination rate constant (see section 2.2).

The metabolites formed are usually, but not always, less active than the parent compound (bioinactivation). Exceptions to this rule are drugs like the original sulphonamide Prontosil which had to be bioactivated by enzymatic reduction and the cytotoxic drug cyclophosphamide which has to be bioactivated by enzymatic hydroxylation (see chapter XXIV; sect. 2.3.1). Many other drugs like imipramine, alprenolol, propranolol, procainamide, diazepam and phenylbutazone are active *per se* but also have active metabolites, whose pharmacokinetic or pharmacodynamic (phenylbutazone) profile differs to some extent from that of the parent drug. The contribution of active metabolites to the therapeutic and/or toxic effects of a drug will be determined by their relative activity and quantitative importance (e.g. hydroxyhexamide, a major metabolite of acetohexamide, has 2.5 times the hypoglycaemic activity of acetohexamide but is present in plasma in only small amounts in patients with normal renal function; see chapter XVI, sect. 3.3.3) and whether they accumulate with repeated administration (e.g. desmethyldiazepam in the elderly) or in patients

with impaired renal function (e.g. procainamide; see chapter XXI, sect. 14.2.3).

Figure 14 shows the fate of a single oral dose of four drugs — isoniazid, oxazepam, nortriptyline and phenytoin. They have in common that they are extensively metabolised in the body and that the metabolites have weaker or no pharmacodynamic activity compared with the parent compound.

Isoniazid is rapidly absorbed and then disappears monophasically from plasma with a half-life of a few hours due to acetylation by a mitochondrial hepatic enzyme N-acetyltransferase (see section 4.2). Oxazepam and nortriptyline are much more slowly absorbed and their disappearance from plasma is biexponential. The second part of the disappearance curve reflects their rate of metabolism in the body. This has been shown

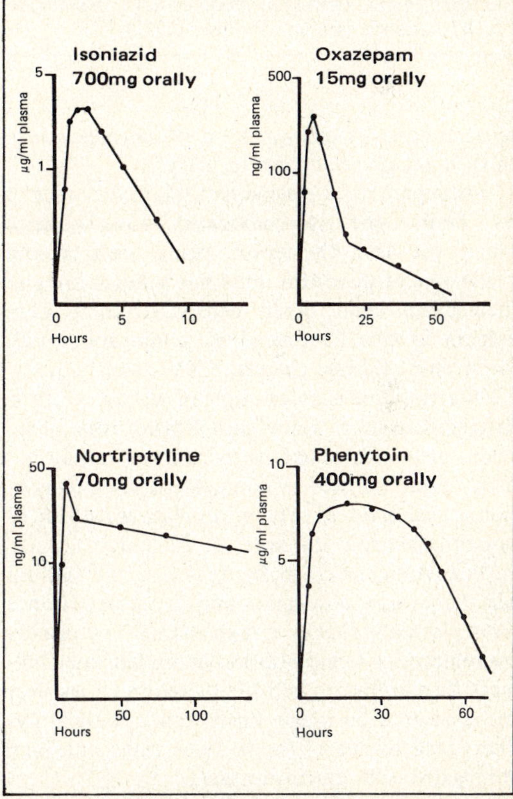

Fig. 14. Plasma concentration time curves after oral administration of single doses of isoniazid, oxazepam, nortriptyline and phenytoin (diphenylhydantoin). The drugs are metabolised by different pathways. The metabolites have little or no pharmacological activity and therefore the plasma disappearance curve (β-slope, see text) should reflect the duration of action.

Table VIII. Elimination half-lives of a few sedative-hypnotic drugs[1]

Drug	$t_{1/2}$ (h)
Hexobarbitone	3-7
Pentobarbitone	23-30
Phenobarbitone	2-6 days
Bromide	1 week
Glutethimide	5-22
Meprobamate	6-17
Methaqualone	20-60
Promethazine	Negative literature survey
Oxazepam	10-14
Nitrazepam	21-28
Diazepam	9-53
Desmethyldiazepam	42-96
Flurazepam	Very short but metabolised to desalkylflurazepam, see below
Desalkylflurazepam	47-100

1   Most data quoted from *D.D. Breimer,* Pharmacokinetics of hypnotic drugs, Ph.D thesis, University of Nijmegen, 1974, Drukkerij Brakkenstein, Nijmegen, The Netherlands (see also Breimer, 1977).

by simultaneous measurement of the appearance of their main metabolites in urine.

Oxazepam has a plasma half-life in the order of 12 hours and is conjugated directly with glucuronic acid. Oxazepam, being itself an end metabolite of diazepam, thus has a much simpler metabolism than other benzodiazepines. Lorazepam is also eliminated by conjugation with glucuronic acid (see chapter XXVI; sect. 1.5.3).

Nortriptyline is an example of a drug which is metabolised in a more complicated way. Two main metabolic reactions occur, an initial hydroxylation followed by conjugation. Desmethylation is also involved. The mean plasma half-life of nortriptyline is in the order of 24 hours.

Phenytoin, given in figure 14 as the sodium salt, has a slow absorption and the disappearance from plasma is slower at high than at low plasma concentrations (concentration-dependent metabolism). Its elimination half-life therefore varies over the concentration range. Phenytoin is initially hydroxylated in one of the benzene rings and then conjugated with glucuronic acid.

As discussed in section 4.2, it would be inappropriate to discuss the half-lives of these various drugs without giving the variation among individuals. But the average elimination half-life of a drug, whether long, intermediate or short, is nevertheless of great value to the practising clini-

cian. Inspection of table VIII raises a number of provocative questions. Why do we still call pentobarbitone short-acting? Why do we dose several of the drugs with half-lives above 24 hours tid? Why is the half-life of many drugs that we prescribe so liberally to our patients, such as promethazine, unknown?

3.3.2 Sites of Drug Metabolism

The main site of drug metabolism is the liver but other tissues may also metabolise drugs, such as lung, kidneys, blood and intestine. For example, isoprenaline (isoproterenol) is metabolised in the gut wall to inactive conjugates. This will reduce the bioavailability of the drug. The gut bacterial flora may also metabolise certain drugs (Goldman et al., 1974). See further section 3.3.1; chapter XIX (sect. 1.2); XX (sect. 1.4); XXI (sect. 1.3).

3.3.3 Hepatic First-pass Elimination

Orally administered drugs will traverse the hepatic portal system and the liver before reaching the systemic circulation (see fig. 2 chapter VI). If a drug is extensively cleared by the liver, only a small fraction of the administered unchanged drug will reach the systemic circulation and exert its pharmacodynamic effects. This so called extensive 'first-pass elimination' is seen for a number of drugs in common use. The fraction of drug removed from the blood during a single transit through the liver is referred to as the extraction ratio and drugs subject to extensive first-pass elimination in the liver therefore have a high hepatic extraction ratio (i.e. > 0.7).

Significant first-pass hepatic metabolism is one explanation of why an intravenous dose of such drugs is much smaller than an equipotent oral dose (Gibaldi et al., 1971). For example, the β-adrenoceptor blocking drugs propranolol and alprenolol are extensively removed by the liver on their first passage through this organ. This explains why the oral bioavailability of these drugs is in the order of a few per cent, in spite of complete absorption. However, the pharmacodynamic consequences of this kinetic behaviour after oral administration are diminished by the formation of an hydroxylated metabolite with β-blocking properties (Johnsson and Regardh, 1976; see also chapter XVII, sect. 6.1.5).

Some drugs (e.g. lignocaine) have such extensive and rapid first-pass metabolism that they cannot be used orally. Use of high doses orally has been complicated by toxicity due to metabolites which contributes to the need to give lignocaine parenterally (Benowitz and Meister, 1978).

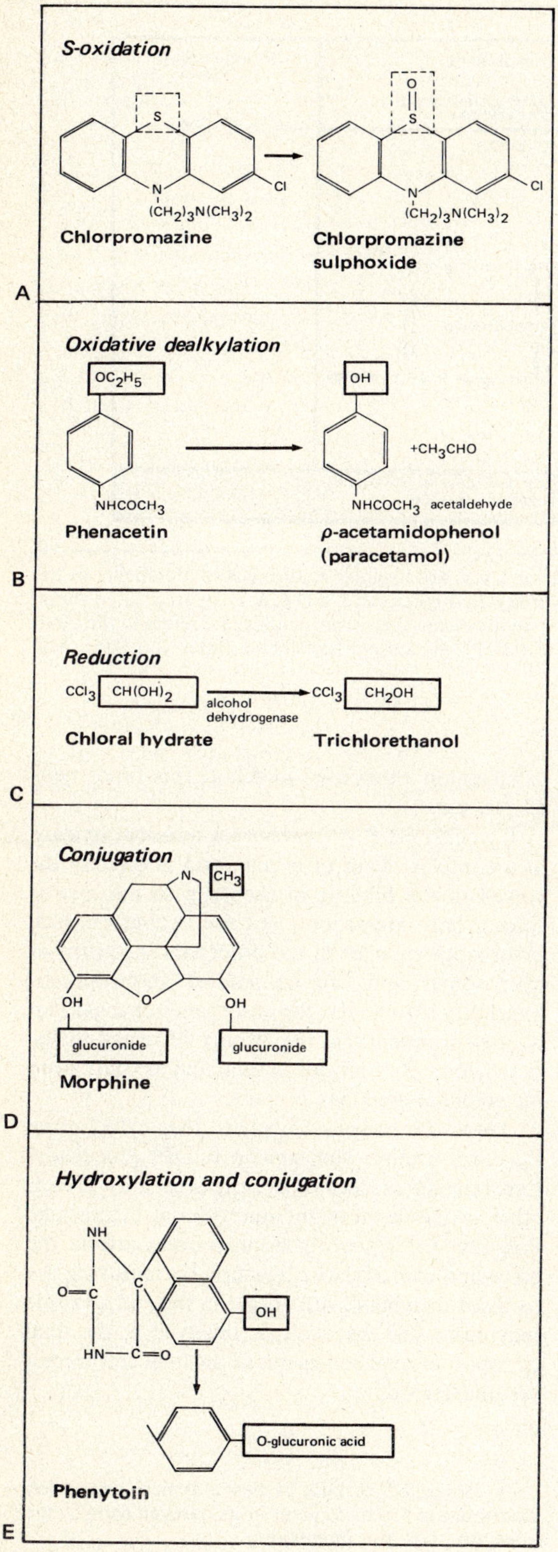

3.3.4 Pathways of Drug Metabolism

A wide variety of biochemical reactions can take place during the metabolism of a drug to more water soluble compounds (table IX). Considered simply, there are two basic types (Drayer, 1974; Glauser, 1974). In phase I reactions, polar groups are introduced into the drug molecule by, e.g. oxidation, reduction or hydrolysis, and of these, oxidation is by far the most important pathway. Phase II reactions are synthetic and involve conjugation with glucuronic acid, sulphate, glycine or other groups. Some drugs may pass through both phase I and phase II reactions before being excreted, while others only pass through phase I and others yet again only through phase II (fig. 15a). The metabolites produced are generally more water soluble than the parent compounds but as pointed out in section 3.3.1 are not necessarily pharmacologically inactive. Phenacetin, for example, is oxidised in the body to the active analgesic paracetamol (acetaminophen) and subsequently conjugated to form inactive glucuronides. Cyclophosphamide is inactive as such and it is only the oxidised metabolite that has antineoplastic activity. The metabolites produced are generally excreted in the urine, but some conjugates are excreted in the bile.

The enzymes that metabolise drugs in the liver are relatively nonspecific as compared with those involved in intermediary metabolism. Oxidation is by far the most important metabolic pathway and

Fig. 15a. Some examples of the metabolic transformation of drugs.

Reactions shown in frames. (A) Microsomal enzyme catalysed (cytochrome P$_{450}$) metabolism of chlorpromazine by S-oxidation (i.e. introduction of an oxygen group); one of the many metabolic pathways of chlorpromazine. (B) Microsomal enzyme catalysed (cytochrome P$_{450}$) metabolism of phenacetin by oxidative dealkylation (i.e. removal of an alkyl group). (C) Metabolism of chloral hydrate to an alcohol by the non-microsomal enzyme alcohol dehydrogenase (i.e. a reduction reaction). (D) Microsomal enzyme catalysed (transferase) metabolism of morphine by union of the endogenous substance glucuronic acid with the hydroxyl group of the molecule (i.e. conjugation by glucuronidation). A metabolic side reaction, oxidative desmethylation, also occurs. (E) Phenytoin is initially hydroxylated and then conjugated with glucuronic acid (after Crossland: Practitioner 206: 293, 1971; by permission of author and editor).

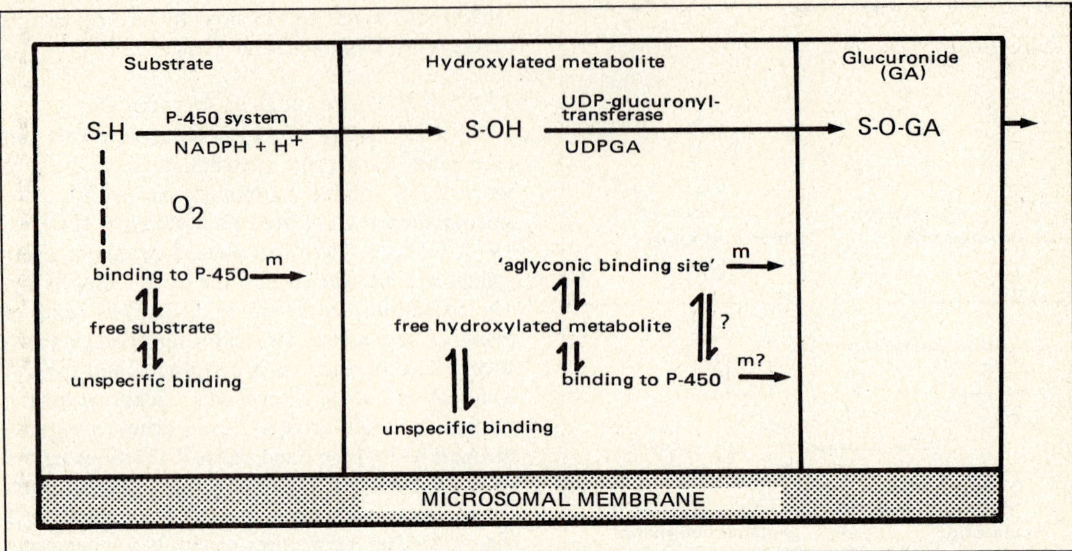

Fig. 15b. Hypothetical fate of a lipid soluble drug producing a less lipid soluble hydroxylated metabolite in the microsomal membrane. S-H = drug substrate. S-OH = hydroxylated metabolite. S-O-GA = hydroxylated metabolite. S-O-GA = the glucuronide conjugate of the latter. m = metabolism. Aglyconic binding site refers to the binding of the hydroxylated metabolite onto uridine diphosphate (UDP) glucuronyl transferase (after von Bahr: MD Thesis, Karolinska Institutet, 1972).

will therefore be considered in more depth (see Estabrook et al., 1972; Estabrook and Lindenlaub, 1979).

As schematically depicted in figure 15b, drug oxidation and conjugation with glucuronic acid are both catalysed by enzymes present in the endoplasmic reticulum which upon homogenisation and ultra centrifugation of the liver sample is recovered as membranes in the microsomal fraction. Drug oxidation in microsomal preparations has been studied intensely during the last 25 years with a variety of substrates and animal species including man, and under a variety of experimental conditions, particularly pretreatment *in vivo* with other drugs. Depending on the chemical structure of the drug substrate, the initial reaction may involve hydroxylation of an aromatic ring (phenytoin, imipramine) or hydrocarbon side chain (barbiturates), a dealkylation (e.g. demethylation of a variety of psychotherapeutic drugs), or sulphoxidation (chlorpromazine) etc (fig. 15a). All these reactions require nicotinamide adenine dinucleotide (NADPH) and molecular oxygen (fig. 15b). One of the oxygen atoms is incorporated into the substrate while the other is reduced to water. This dual destiny of the two oxygen atoms explains the terms 'mixed function oxidation' or 'mono-

oxygenation' often used to denote this fundamental process.

Cytochrome P_{450}[1] serves as a terminal oxidase in a complex chain of events, and is directly involved in the binding of the drug to the microsomes. This interaction gives rise to characteristic absorbance changes in the difference spectrum of microsomes and can be studied spectrophotometrically. Moreover, the absorbance changes can be used to quantitate the affinity of drugs to the cytochrome P_{450} enzyme system and to study drug metabolic interactions *in vitro*.

There are reasons to believe that cytochrome P_{450} and uridine diphosphate (UDP) glucuronyl transferase(s) are located in close proximity to each other in the depth of the microsomal membrane. Possibly, the glucuronidation process affects the preceding hydroxylation reaction by removing the oxidised metabolite still bound to the endoplasmic reticulum. The mechanisms involved in the final transport of metabolites out of the liver cell are not yet understood.

---

1 So called because it has a typical absorption maximum at 450 nanometer in its reduced form in the presence of carbon monoxide.

Table IX. Examples of important drug metabolic reactions

Reaction	Substrates (including drugs)
1. Cytochrome P_{450} mediated hydroxylation	Many drugs, carcinogens, insecticides, endogenous steroids and fatty acids
2. Oxidation of alcohols and aldehydes (dehydrogenases)	Chloral hydrate, ethyl alcohol
3. Oxidation of purines (xanthine oxidase)	6-Mercaptopurine and azathioprine
4. Oxidation by mono-amine oxidase (MAO)	Tyramine, catechol- and indolamines
5. Hydrolysis (serum cholinesterase)	Suxamethonium (succinylcholine)
6. Glucuronidation	Phenols, carboxylic acids, alcohols, aromatic amines
7. Acetylation	Isoniazid, hydrallazine, procainamide, dapsone, sulphonamides

There are three clinically important features of cytochrome P_{450} mediated oxidation: (1) unspecificity in relation to substrates; (2) high potential for drug interactions; particularly induction of metabolism; and (3) marked inter- and intraspecies variations. The latter two characteristics are vitally important for drug dosage and can be indirectly assessed by appropriate pharmacokinetic methods. There are multiple forms of cytochrome P_{450} with different inducibility and substrate specificity. This may explain the high intraindividual correlation coefficients between the rates of metabolism of certain drugs (Estabrook and Lindenlaub, 1979).

3.3.5 Factors Affecting Drug Metabolism

Many factors may affect the rate of drug metabolism and some are listed in table X. The influence of age on drug metabolism is now apparent although information is still incomplete. However, it appears that the ability to metabolise drugs, is reduced in the very young (neonates) and for some drugs in the elderly (see also chapters IV and V).

The concept that newborn babies cannot metabolise drugs has been derived largely from animal experiments showing poor development of the cytochrome P_{450} system prior to birth. There is however, a clear species difference between animals and man, since this enzyme is present early during human fetal development. Certain conjugation processes do however, seem to develop slowly in newborns (Pelkonen, 1979; Rane et al., 1973). Newborn babies are able to me-

Table X. Factors affecting drug metabolism

Factor	Response
Genetic influences	See table XI
Age Neonates Elderly	Reduced rate of drug metabolism (see also chapters IV, V)
Sex Pregnancy	Reduced rate of drug metabolism may be present in females[1], and an increased rate during pregnancy (see chapter XV; sect. 1.1.4)
Liver disease	Reduced rate of elimination with some drugs (depends on kinetics of drug and type and stage of liver disease); increased bioavailability and reduced elimination with orally administered high clearance drugs in cirrhosis (see section 4.3.3)
Environmental	Enhanced rate of metabolism with occupational exposure to chlorinated insecticides and benzpyrene (cigarette smoking, charcoal broiling)
Diet	Enhanced rate of metabolism (for certain drugs) by high protein/carbohydrate ratio and cruciferous vegetables (therapeutic implications not clear)
Malnutrition	Reduced rate of drug metabolism probable in severe malnutrition[1] (see chapter XXX; sect. 2.2.3)
Alcohol Acute ingestion	Inhibition of certain drug metabolising enzymes (sedatives)
Chronic long term intake	Induction of certain drug metabolising enzymes
Other drugs	Drug metabolism interaction (see chapter VIII)

1 Mainly based on animal work. More data therefore needed in man.

tabolise some transplacentally transferred drugs (phenytoin, carbamazepine) at adult rates (see chapter IV; sect. 2.3.1). This may be due partly to transplacental induction of the cytochrome P_{450} system.

A large variety of foreign compounds have the ability to increase the rate of drug metabolism (in particular drug oxidation) by enzyme induction. The induction process involves increased synthesis of cytochrome P_{450} and increased formation of liver cell membranes containing this enzyme (Estabrook and Lindenlaub, 1979).

Environmental factors such as heavy cigarette smoking (benzpyrene) and occupational exposure to chlorinated hydrocarbon insecticides may induce certain metabolic pathways and thereby modify the response to drugs (Alvares, 1978; Jusko, 1978). The metabolism of theophylline in particular is enhanced in heavy smokers who therefore may need higher average doses than non-smokers (Ogilvie, 1978). Similarly, the effectiveness of usual doses of analgesics such as pentazocine and dextropropoxyphene may be decreased in heavy cigarette smokers. A case of lack of response to usual dosage of warfarin has been observed following temporary intensive occupational exposure to chlorinated insecticides (Jeffery et al., 1976).

An extreme example of environmental influence on drug metabolism is the effect of charcoal broiled beef on the oral bioavailability of phenacetin/acetophenetidin (Conney et al., 1976; fig. 16). Probably benzpyrene and other polycyclic aromatic hydrocarbons contaminating the beef during broiling induce the first-pass dealkylation of phenacetin, resulting in lowered AUC's of the parent drug. A marked interindividual variation is seen in the induction. The ratio between the concentrations of the active metabolite paracetamol (acetaminophen) and phenacetin is increased markedly. A similar effect of charcoal broiled beef has been observed on the metabolism of theophylline and antipyrine. Presumably other drugs which are metabolised by the 'benzpyrene inducible' form of cytochrome P_{450} will also be affected (see Alvares, 1978).

It is possible that induction by food is particularly important for drugs subject to metabolism in the gut wall (see chapter XIX; sect. 1.2). For such drugs there may be substantial intraindividual differences in kinetics from time to time due to changes in dietary habits and life style. The effects of alcohol consumption on drug metabolism are far from being well understood at the present time (Sellers and Holloway, 1978).

It should be noted that hepatic enzyme inducing agents are of two major classes: (a) those such as phenobarbitone and rifampicin which in-

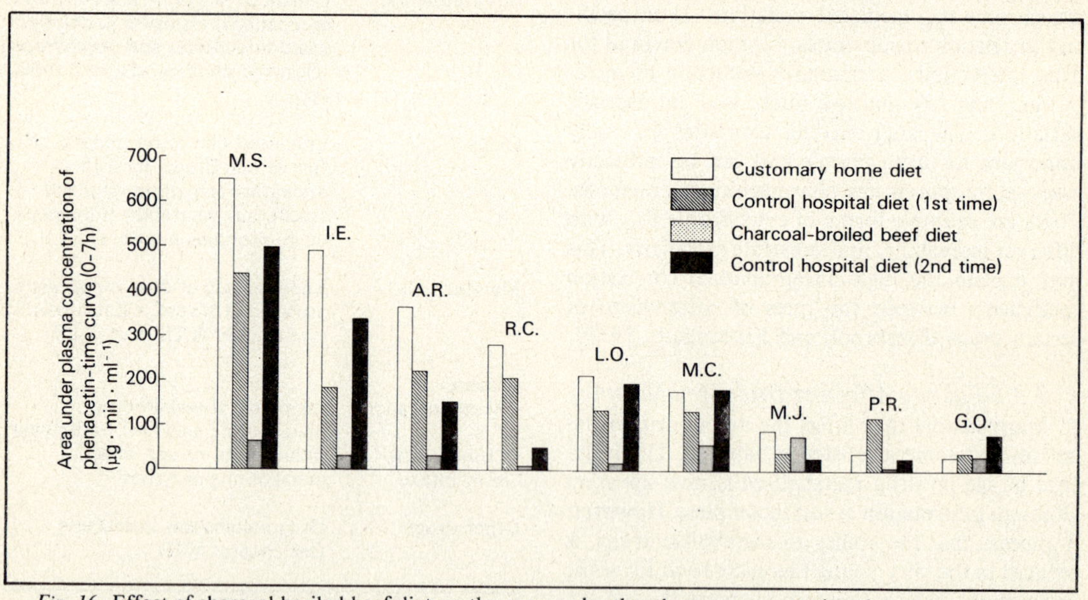

Fig. 16. Effect of charcoal broiled beef diet on the area under the plasma concentration-time curve of orally administered phenacetin. Note marked interindividual variation in the inducing effect on phenacetin metabolism (after Conney et al.: Clinical Pharmacology and Therapeutics 20: 633, 1976; by permission of author and editor).

crease the rate of metabolism of a wide variety of drugs, and (b) those comprised mainly of polycyclic hydrocarbons which increase the rate of metabolism of only a few drugs but also induce carcinogen metabolising enzymes.

More modest manipulation of the diet has also been found to affect the metabolism of a few drugs (theophylline, antipyrine, phenacetin), as evidenced by an increased rate of metabolism of these drugs the higher the protein/carbohydrate ratio in the diet (Alvares, 1978; Conney et al., 1979). Dietary intake of cruciferous vegetables such as brussels sprouts and cabbage can also increase the rate of metabolism of antipyrine and phenacetin (Pantuck et al., 1979). These effects of diet clearly add to the variability of drug metabolism in different individuals, but the clinical significance is not clear. On the other hand, severe malnutrition states may have a profound influence on drug metabolism and disposition (Krishnaswamy, 1978; see chapter XXX; sect. 2.2).

Many barbiturates and the antituberculosis drug rifampicin (rifampin) for example, increase the rate of oxidation of other drugs (Breckenridge et al., 1974; Zilly et al., 1977). Thus the rate of warfarin metabolism will be enhanced by phenobarbitone and rifampicin, causing a fall in the steady-state plasma concentration and a decrease of pharmacological effect (see chapter XXIII; sect. 3.2.5). If the pharmacological effect is mediated by an active metabolite such as with cyclophosphamide, then an increased pharmacological effect and toxicity might result from enzyme induction (see chapter XXIV; sect. 8). In the case of alprenolol, both the oxidation of the parent drug and the subsequent conjugation of the active metabolite 4-hydroxyalprenolol are induced by pentobarbitone leading to a measurable decrease in β-adrenoceptor blocking potency (von Bahr and Collste, 1979). Cessation of treatment with an inducing drug may result in decelerated metabolism of other drugs, i.e. the interaction now works the other way around.

Other drugs or foreign compounds may inhibit drug metabolism (Skovsted et al., 1974). This is not strictly the converse of enzyme induction since there is usually no effect on the enzyme protein. The most usual cause is a direct competition between two similar substrates for the metabolic site on the enzyme. In the therapeutic situation, enzyme inhibition is potentially more important than enzyme induction since it begins rapidly (within a few hours compared with a few days for

induction). Clinical examples of this type are relatively few compared with enzyme induction (Kristensen, 1976). However, some clinically important interactions of this type have been described, such as that between monoamine oxidase inhibitors and certain sympathomimetic amines, the inhibition of the metabolism of mercaptopurine and azathioprine by allopurinol, the inhibition of phenytoin metabolism by isoniazid (in slow acetylators), sulthiame and disulfiram, and the inhibition of warfarin and tolbutamide metabolism by phenylbutazone (see further chapter VIII; sect. 2.3.4).

3.4 Renal Excretion of Drugs

Comparatively few drugs are excreted unchanged by the kidney because of tubular reabsorption of lipid soluble drug. However, a number of important drugs are primarily excreted unchanged or as active metabolites by glomerular filtration and if renal function is impaired this will have important consequences for drug therapy. If usual dosage is not modified, the plasma concentration of such drugs or active metabolites will rise producing toxic symptoms (see section 4.3.4).

Active tubular secretion occurs for a few organic bases such as mecamylamine and for organic acids such as penicillin, probenecid and salicylates. It is envisaged that the organic acid is carried across the tubular cell by a carrier which liberates the drug into the tubule and returns to carry more drug (Caffruny, 1977). Competition for this carrier may occur and in this way probenecid impairs the excretion of penicillin by the kidney leading to higher plasma concentrations of penicillin. Saturable renal reabsorption of cephalosporins has been described (Arvidsson et al., 1979).

The renal clearance of many acidic and basic drugs varies over the urinary pH range (4.8 to 7.5) in accordance with the pH partition hypothesis. Strong acids (pK_a less than 2) and strong bases (pK_a greater than 12) are virtually completely ionised over the physiological range of urinary pH and their clearance is therefore unaffected by pH changes in urine. Weak organic bases (pK_a 7.5 to 10) and acids (pK_a 3.0 to 7.5) however, may be affected by urinary pH. Amphetamine, a weak organic base is excreted unchanged and is more ionised by acidic pH. Its rate of excretion may be increased by acidifying the urine with ammonium chloride. Phenobarbitone and salicylates, are excreted in part in the unchanged form and being weak organic acids are ionised by alkaline pH. Their excretion rate may be increased by the use of sodium bicarbonate to make the urine alkaline (see also section 1.1; chapter VIII, section 2.3.8). Renal excretion of drugs and modification of dosage in renal disease is discussed in more detail in section 4.3.4 and chapter XXI (sect. 2.1; 14).

3.5 Biliary Excretion of Drugs

Many drugs are actively transported by hepatic cells from blood to bile. Drugs and drug metabolites (particularly glucuronide conjugates) are likely to be excreted in bile if they are polar and if their molecular weight exceeds 400. Ampicillin and rifampicin for example, are excreted in high concentration in the bile and good use may be made of this information in the treatment of infections of the biliary tract.

Some drugs undergo an 'enterohepatic' circulation (e.g. digitoxin, oestrogens, indomethacin). A drug, or more usually a drug conjugate, is excreted into the bile and enters the gastrointestinal tract where, in the case of the metabolite, it may be broken down by enzymes in gut bacteria to liberate the unchanged drug (Plaa, 1975). Any drug appearing in this way may then be reabsorbed into the body as well as any drug which may have appeared in the gut from a recently taken oral dose. Theoretically, the enterohepatic circulation may be interfered with by drugs, such as broad spectrum antibiotics which will destroy any gut bacteria, and any drug conjugate now entering the gut from the bile will be excreted in the faeces. This would lead to a lowering of plasma concentrations of the drug in question and could be a possible cause of adverse drug interactions in certain situations. It has been suggested that the effectiveness of combined oral contraceptive steroids is reduced because of such an interaction with antibiotics like ampicillin (Roberton and Johnson, 1976; Tikkanen et al., 1973).

Biliary excretion may serve as an alternative route of elimination of some polar drugs in patients with renal impairment, but for drugs such as digoxin, the reduction in the rate of renal elimination is only partially compensated by biliary excretion (Bloom and Nelp, 1966). Oxazepam seems to have a more pronounced enterohepatic circulation in uraemic subjects compared with subjects with normal renal function (Odar-Cederlof et al., 1977).

4. Interindividual Differences in Pharmacokinetics

4.1 General and Methodological Aspects

Kinetic processes such as passive diffusion which are rate limited by the physicochemical characteristics of the drug, are not likely to vary significantly among patients unless pathophysiological factors exert an influence (see section 4.3). For example, buccal absorption of drugs seems to proceed at rates that differ markedly between drugs but not between subjects. In contrast, whenever enzymatic processes are involved in the fate of drugs in the body, biochemical individuality is to be expected. The extent of this variability has not been appreciated until recently.

Although active transport of drugs through biological membranes occurs and some interindividual variability has been documented in the binding and distribution of drugs, the quantitatively most important determinant of kinetic individuality is in the rate of drug metabolism (see Alvan, 1978). For example, steady-state plasma concentrations of tricyclic antidepressants vary 20 to 30-fold on a fixed maintenance dose, and most of this variability can be accounted for by differences in rate of hydroxylation (sect. 3.3.4), while interindividual differences in binding and distribution are approximately 2-fold (Alexanderson and Borga, 1972; Alexanderson and Sjoqvist, 1971).

It is important to use appropriate methods in assessing interindividual differences in drug metabolism. The clinically used laboratory procedures for liver function are of very little, if any, predictive value for the ability of an individual to metabolise a drug. Measurements of D-glucaric acid and 6-β-hydroxycortisol in urine may give an idea about the degree of induction of a patient's microsomal enzyme system. The correlation coefficients obtained between these two compounds in urine and the rate of metabolism of various drugs, are however, far too weak to have any clinical significance for a particular patient. The same holds true for the antipyrine half-life as a predictor of the rate of oxidation of another drug (Sjoqvist and von Bahr, 1973).

Therefore, the only accurate way to assess the rate of metabolism of a particular drug is to study it with appropriate chemical and kinetic methodology. Depending on the drug, different kinetic variables have to be used to assess rates of metabolism.

1) A drug which rapidly equilibrates between plasma and tissues after intravenous administration and does not have substantial first-pass elimination can usually be adequately described from the kinetic point of view by a one compartment model (see section 2.1). For such drugs, e.g. antipyrine, the elimination half-life is a good estimate of the rate of metabolism.

2) A large number of drugs confer on the body the characteristics of a two or multicompartment system. In the former situation, the liver is part of the central compartment, from where elimination occurs (see section 2.1). For such drugs, the elimination half-life will depend on metabolism and distribution, and therefore plasma clearance (see section 2.1.3) should be used to assess rates of elimination.

3) For drugs having substantial first-pass elimination in the liver (see section 3.3.3), kinetic models have been developed where the hepatoportal system is added as a separate compartment. For such high clearance drugs, the elimination half-life is a poor index of rates of metabolism and changes thereof (e.g. enzyme induction) and the most accurate term to use is the area under the plasma concentration time curve (AUC), or clearance.

As an example, treatment with pentobarbitone lowers the AUC (increases the first-pass metabolism) of orally administered alprenolol due to induction of cytochrome P_{450} (Grundin et al., 1974), but has little effect on the elimination half-life of alprenolol. This term will be determined mainly by distribution factors, particularly the rate at which the drug is delivered to the liver, which is determined by liver blood flow. Following intravenous doses of alprenolol there is little effect of pentobarbitone on its plasma concentration time curve (Alvan et al., 1977). This is because after intravenous administration the drug is distributed in the body before passing through the liver. Since virtually the whole amount of drug presented to the liver per unit of time will be metabolised in any case, induction of drug metabolising enzymes cannot be expected to enhance hepatic clearance more than marginally. After oral administration, only a small part of the drug will pass the liver without undergoing metabolic degradation. If the liver enzymes are induced, this fraction will be further substantially reduced. Thus, the amount of drug actually reaching the circulation will be relatively more affected after oral than after intravenous administration. These concepts have been elegantly described in mathematical terms by several authors (see Wilkinson and Shand, 1975; Nies et al., 1976). An important consequence is that drug metabolic interactions between high clearance drugs should be studied after oral administration.

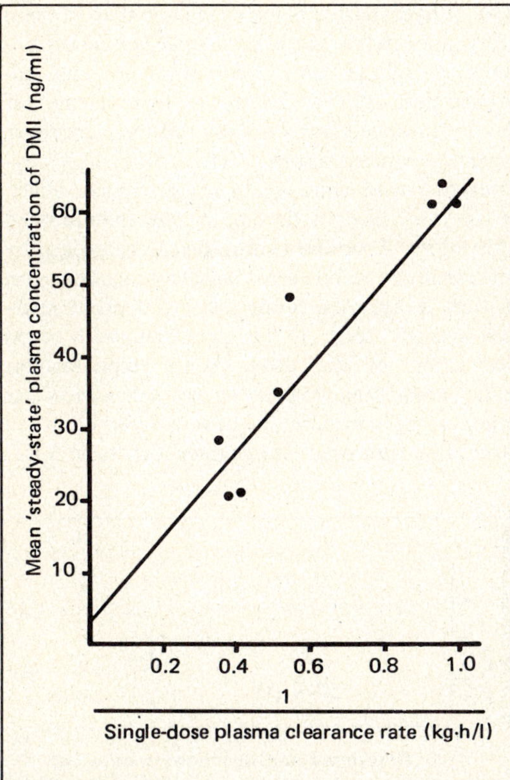

Fig. 17. The correlation between the reciprocal single dose plasma clearance rate of desmethylimipramine (desipramine) and the multiple dose mean steady-state plasma level in the same subjects (r = 0.94, p < 0.001) [after Alexanderson: European Journal of Clinical Pharmacology 5: 1, 1972; by permission of editor].

4) In clinical practice, drug metabolism usually has to be evaluated during continued therapy (items 1 to 3 above refer to single dose studies) and then the measurement of plasma clearance or steady-state plasma concentrations (section 2.2) as related to dose (supervised drug intake) give an accurate index of drug metabolism (fig. 17). With the use of tracer doses of stable radio-isotopes, the kinetic variables 1 to 3 above may be assessed without interrupting therapy.

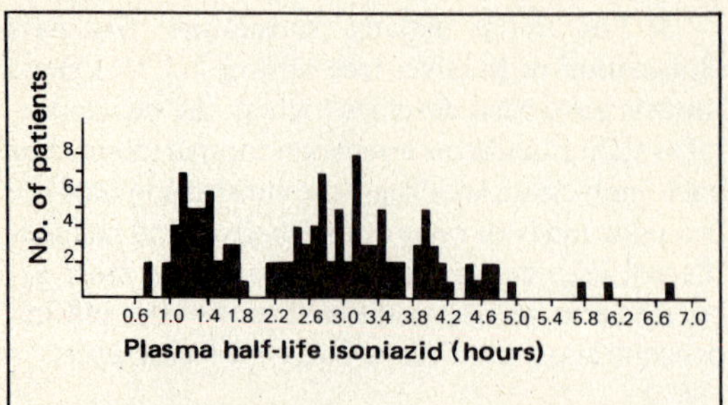

Fig. 18a. Bimodal distribution of the plasma half-lives of isoniazid (INH) in Swedish patients with tuberculosis. The antimode is at 2.1 hours (after Hanngren et al.: Scandinavian Journal of Respiratory Diseases 51: 61, 1970; by permission of author and editor).

4.2 Pharmacogenetics

Pharmacogenetics deals with the modification of drug responses by hereditary influences (Kalow, 1962, 1965; Vesell, 1975). Table XI gives some examples of genetically determined drug responses and it can be seen that all types of inheritance may occur. Not all of the variations in response involve drug metabolism (see chapter VII; sect. 4.2), but it is probably most convenient to discuss the topic in this context, especially since a developing area of pharmacogenetics concerns the interplay between environmental influences and those genes of an individual which control rates of drug metabolism (Vesell, 1977, 1979).

The importance to therapy of genetically controlled drug metabolism can be illustrated with one example — that of acetylator phenotype. Isoniazid (INH) has long been one of the first line drugs in the treatment of tuberculosis, its major route of metabolism being acetylation by the enzyme N-acetyltransferase in the liver. The ability to acetylate isoniazid is inherited as an autosomal recessive trait and distribution histograms of kinetic parameters are bimodal (fig. 18a), suggesting that patients are either slow or fast acetylators (example of monogenic control). The acetylator phenotype can be assessed from the isoniazid plasma half-life (antimode around 2 hours) or by measuring the ratio between acetylated and unchanged sulphapyridine in urine. The ratio of slow to fast acetylators varies from population to population (Lunde et al., 1977; Motulsky, 1964). Thus in most European groups about 40 %, and in the USA 45 %, of the population are fast acetylators, but 80 to 90 % of Asian

populations and nearly 100 % of Canadian Eskimos are fast acetylators (see chapter VII; table VII). It is now well established that with standard doses of the drugs mentioned in table XI, slow acetylators are much more likely to develop toxic effects than are fast acetylators (Drayer and Reidenberg, 1977; Lunde et al., 1977.

One might expect that treatment of tuberculosis with isoniazid regimens would be less effective among the rapid acetylators, but this appears to be true only when isoniazid is given intermittently on a once or possibly also on a twice weekly basis (Ellard, 1976; Ellard and Gammon, 1977). The inhibitory effect of isoniazid on the metabolism of phenytoin occurs predominantly in slow acetylators (see chapter XXV; sect. 3.1).

Hydrallazine, procainamide (fig. 18b), dapsone and some sulphonamides (e.g. sulphapyridine) are acetylated by the same N-acetyltransferase enzyme system as isoniazid. The effective antihypertensive dose of hydrallazine is lower in slow than in rapid acetylators, while the effective plasma concentrations are of the same order of magnitude. Administration of over 200mg of hydrallazine per day to slow acetylators usually results in excessive plasma concentrations. The lupus-like hydrallazine syndrome, which is a severe side effect, is also more likely to develop in slow than in rapid acetylators. A similar syndrome can be evoked by procainamide and it seems to have an earlier onset in slow acetylators. Some cases of dapsone resistant leprosy seem to be associated with rapid acetylation of the drug. With sulphasalazine (salicylazosulphapyridine), severe side effects are much more common in slow acetylators when large doses are used (see chapter VII; table VI).

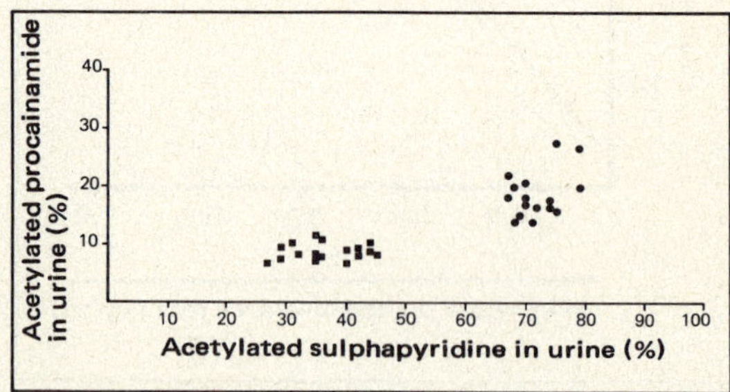

Fig. 18b. Relationship between percentage of acetylated sulphapyridine and acetylated procainamide in urine. Slow acetylators (■) of sulphapyridine excrete significantly less N-acetylprocainamide than rapid acetylators (●) [after Karlsson and Molin: Acta Medica Scandinavica 197: 299, 1975; by permission of author and editor].

Table XI. Genetically determined abnormal drug responses

Condition	Response	Mechanism	Inheritance	Frequency	Drug involved
Slow and fast acetylators[1]	Fast acetylators may respond poorly Slow acetylators more likely to show toxicity	Acetyl-transferase in liver	Autosomal recessive	40% of Caucasians are fast 80 to 90% of Asians are fast	Isoniazid Hydrallazine ? Phenelzine Procainamide Some sulphonamides Dapsone
Slow drug oxidation	Concentration dependent side effects	See text	See text	Rare	Phenytoin Nortriptyline Desipramine Tolbutamide Sparteine
			Autosomal recessive	5% of Caucasians	Debrisoquine
Suxa-methonium sensitivity[2]	Prolonged apnoea	Abnormal pseudo cholinesterase in plasma	Autosomal recessive	1 in 2,500 commonest type of allele	Suxamethonium (succinylcholine)
Porphyria[3]	Abdominal pain Paralysis	Abnormal inducibility of δ-amino levulinic acid synthetase	Autosomal dominant		Barbiturates
Warfarin resistance	Resistance to anticoagulation	Increased sensitivity to vitamin K in liver	Autosomal dominant	2 large pedigrees described	Warfarin
Favism, drug induced haemolysis[4]	Haemolysis on exposure to certain drugs or chemicals	Deficient glucose-6-phosphate-dehydrogenase	Sex linked incomplete dominant	Approx. 100 million affected in world	Many drugs, e.g. Primaquine Nitrofurantoin Aminopyrine Sulphonamides
Malignant hyperthermia[5]	Uncontrolled rise in body temperature	Unknown	Autosomal dominant	1 in 20,000	Certain drugs used in anaesthesia, especially halothane and suxamethonium
Glaucoma[6]	Glaucoma due to abnormal response to intraocular steroids	Unknown	Autosomal recessive	5% of USA population	Topical corticosteroids Systemic cortico-steroids (long term)
Chlorpropamide alcohol flushing[7]	Facial flushing after alcohol Non-insulin dependent diabetics	Unknown	Autosomal dominant	30% of Caucasians	Chlorpropamide

1　See further section 4.2; chapter VII (sect. 4.2.1).
2　See chapter VII (sect. 4.2.1), X (sect. 2.2.1).
3　See chapter VII (sect. 4.2.4).
4　See chapter VII (sect. 4.2.2), XXIII (sect. 8.4).
5　See chapter VII (sect. 4.2.2), X (sect. 5.6).
6　See chapter VII (sect. 4.2.2), XII (sect. 11.1.2).
7　See chapter XVI (sect. 3.3.5).

Table XII. Interindividual variations in elimination half-lives of some drugs metabolised by hepatic microsomal oxidation

Drug	Half-life (hours)	No. of individuals investigated
Antipyrine (phenazone)	5-35	33
Carbamazepine	18-55	6
Dicoumarol[1] (bis-hydroxycoumarin)	7-74	14 pairs of twins
Diazepam	9-53	22
Phenytoin[1]	10-42	
Indomethacin	4-12	15
Nortriptyline	15-90	25
Phenylbutazone[2]	1.2-7.3 days	14 pairs of twins
Primidone	3.3-12.5	
Tolbutamide	3-25	50
Warfarin	15-70	40

1   Dose dependent half-life due to zero order kinetics (see section 2.1.1, fig. 8).

2   Dose dependent half-life. Elimination half-life *decreases* with increasing dose due to saturation of plasma protein binding sites.

A possible exception is liver damage caused by isoniazid when used alone as chemoprophylaxis. In this case, some investigators reason that rapid acetylators are more sensitive because the toxicity is mediated by acetylhydrazine formed from acetylisoniazid. It has been suggested that this metabolite is particularly toxic in individuals with induced cytochrome P_{450} activity (Mitchell et al., 1973, 1975). However, acetylhydrazine is itself subject to polymorphic acetylation to diacetylhydrazine, a process which occurs more rapidly in rapid acetylators who excrete much more acetylhydrazine as diacetylhydrazine than do slow acetylators (Ellard and Gammon, 1976; Ellard et al., 1978). Metabolic activation of drugs and chemicals into reactive metabolites can cause tissue lesions by covalent binding (see below; Gillette, 1974). Such toxicity may be caused by minor drug metabolites trapped in tissues and can therefore not be avoided by, for example, monitoring of drug plasma concentrations (see section 5.2).

It is well known that the elimination half-lives of several drugs that are eliminated by oxidative

metabolism (table XII) vary many-fold among individuals. This is probably mainly due to corresponding differences in hepatic metabolism. For these and a variety of other drugs which are also oxidised in the body marked interindividual differences have been found in the steady-state plasma concentrations obtained on a fixed dose (fig. 19).

15 years ago Kutt et al. (1964) described an individual with unusually slow metabolism of phenytoin (excessive steady-state plasma concentrations), a feature also found in two of his family members. Although these observations were compatible with the assumption of dominant inheritance, it is still an open question whether a very rare phenotype exists with abnormally slow metabolism of phenytoin. The concentration dependent metabolism of phenytoin has complicated family studies. Studies with desmethylimipramine (desipramine) and nortriptyline also suggested the possibility of a rare slow hydroxylator phenotype (Hammer and Sjoqvist, 1967), but subsequent twin and family studies suggested that the variability between individuals in kinetic parameters

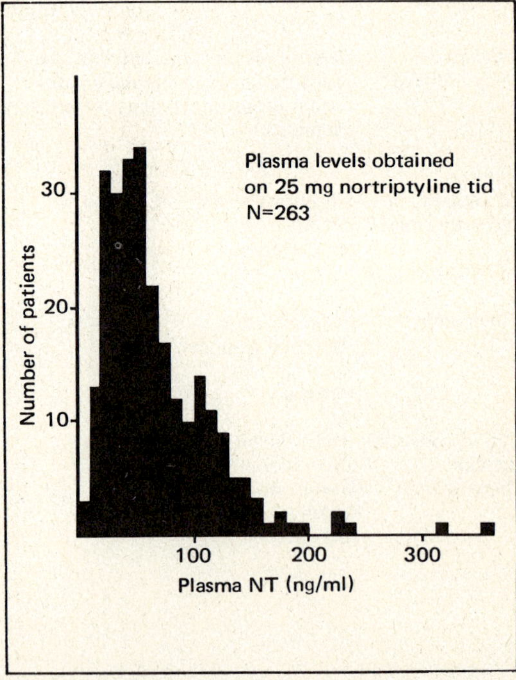

Fig. 19. Apparent unimodal distribution of steady-state plasma concentrations of nortriptyline (NT) in patients treated with 25mg tid. Note that the interindividual variability in plasma concentration is of a similar order of magnitude even if the dose is adjusted according to body weight.

was continuous rather than discontinuous (Alexanderson et al., 1969; Alexanderson, 1973; Alexanderson and Sjoqvist, 1973). This pattern is consistent with multifactorial (polygenic) inheritance. The urinary excretion pattern of the metabolites of nortriptyline is in keeping with this concept. Vesell (1975) suggests that the kinetics of a number of drugs is under polygenic control on the basis of observations in identical and non-identical twins. A complication in the interpretation of some of these studies is that the binding of drugs such as nortriptyline (Alexanderson and Borga, 1972) and warfarin (Wilding et al., 1977) to plasma proteins also seems to be governed by genetic factors.

Independent work with 4 drugs suggest the existence of a rare phenotype with distinctly different metabolism than the majority of the population. Kalow et al. (1977) described a case of deficiency of amylobarbitone (amobarbital) metabolism, later found to be an inability to conjugate on the nitrogen with glucose (Kalow et al., 1978). An apparent clear cut example of a polymorphism in drug oxidation has recently been shown with debrisoquine, an antihypertensive drug, which is metabolised by alicyclic hydroxylation at highly varying individual rates. Some individuals (about 5 % of a Caucasian population) have defective metabolism (Mahgoub et al., 1977). These observations agree well with the clinical notion that the dosage of this drug must be adjusted carefully in individual patients according to clinical response (see chapter XVIII; sect. 5.4.2). A deficiency of N-oxidation of sparteine has been identified as a new human pharmacogenetic defect (Eichelbaum et al., 1978). Finally, Scott and Poffenbarger (1979) found evidence for a trimodal distribution of plasma disappearance rates of tolbutamide. All these examples show that it may be rewarding to look for genetically determined abnormalities in drug metabolism in patients experiencing unusual drug responses.

The basic research on the so called Ah (arylhydrocarbon) locus in the mouse is clinically intriguing (Nebert and Bausserman, 1970). This dominant gene controls the induction of one type of cytochrome P_{450} and several associated mono-oxygenase activities. These enzyme systems metabolically activate or detoxify chemical carcinogens, environmental pollutants and drugs. Among conditions associated with the Ah allele, Thorgeirsson and Nebert (1977) list increased susceptibility to paracetamol (acetaminophen).

The genetically determined variability in drug metabolism seriously questions therapeutic tradition to give similar doses to all patients. Clearly, whenever drug response is abnormal (poor response, severe side effects) following an apparently therapeutic dose, an explanation should be sought in kinetic terms. Studies are now in progress in many laboratories on the possible interindividual variations in receptor response at a constant concentration of drug in the biophase surrounding tissue receptor sites (Snyder, 1979). If such significant differences are revealed, it will be even more important in the future to develop accurate and clinically applicable methods for measuring drug response (see also section 5.1; 7).

4.3 Effects of Disease States

Most pharmacokinetic drug studies are initially performed in volunteers and then the drug used in patients who may have a variety of diseases apart from the one for which the drug is given. Thus, recent attention has been paid to the effects that various disease states may have on the absorption, distribution, metabolism and excretion of drugs. In addition to altering the pharmacokinetics of drugs, certain disease states may alter their pharmacodynamic properties through an effect on the intrinsic sensitivity of receptors (Prescott, 1973; 1975). Thus, hypokalaemia enhances the toxicity of digitalis as well as potentiating the action of non-depolarising muscle relaxants. Such changes in tissue responsiveness in disease are discussed in other chapters.

4.3.1 Absorption in Disease

Gastrointestinal disease may alter both the rate of absorption of an orally administered drug as well as the amount of drug that may be absorbed (see chapter XIX; sect. 1.1). Further information is required before all the possible variations with particular drugs can be elucidated but some important concepts have emerged. It might be predicted that weak acids (which are largely unionised and lipid soluble in acid solution) would be poorly absorbed in elderly patients with achlorhydria. In practice, the studies that have been done in this field either show no difference from normal values, or a difference too small to be of clinical significance (Prescott, 1974).

The gastric emptying rate however, is an important factor in drug absorption, since this influences the rate of delivery of a drug from the stomach to the small intestine where most drugs are absorbed. In general, an increase in the rate of gastric emptying or in gastrointestinal motility increases the rate of drug absorption (and vice versa), but for poorly soluble drugs such as digoxin, the opposite holds (Nimmo, 1976). A change in the *rate* of absorption however, does not necessarily result in alteration of the *amount* of drug absorbed and depends on the clinical circumstances, the physicochemical and kinetic characteristics of the particular drug, and on formulation factors of the drug product (see chapter VI, sect. 5; XIX, sect. 1.1). If the drug is in solution by the time it reaches the small intestine, absorption will be rapid and may be complete, but if the drug dissolves relatively slowly delayed intestinal transit may increase the amount absorbed.

Delayed drug absorption due to slowed gastric emptying is most likely to be important when a rapid onset of effect is required, particularly if the drug has a short elimination half-life (e.g. procainamide), since therapeutic plasma concentrations may never be attained; or if the drug is metabolised in the stomach or gut wall. Therapeutic failure with levodopa may occur in patients with delayed gastric emptying time, partly because the drug is metabolised (decarboxylated) in the stomach wall, and partly because the drug is absorbed in the small intestine (by active transport); the amount of unchanged drug available for absorption thereby being reduced (see chapter VI; sect. 5).

Studies of drug absorption in malabsorption syndromes have yielded conflicting information (Parsons, 1977). However, for most drugs there is little evidence that absorption is significantly altered. Where incomplete absorption of drugs has occurred (e.g. penicillin in coeliac disease), treatment of the condition has restored absorption to normal (Bolme et al., 1977). These and other examples of altered absorption of particular drugs in various gastrointestinal diseases are fully discussed in chapter XIX (sect. 1.1; 1.2).

Other diseases or pathophysiological conditions may alter the absorption of some drugs, particularly as a result of altered gastric emptying (e.g. acute myocardial infarction, acute migraine, labour). Renal disease can also affect the bioavailability of certain drugs. These and other examples are discussed in the relevant chapters. Low cardiac output states might impair the absorption of some drugs after intramuscular injection (see section 3.1.3).

4.3.2 Drug Distribution in Disease

The onset and duration of action of a drug is dependent on its rate of distribution, which in turn depends on factors such as cardiac output, blood flow through tissues and cell membrane permeability. For drugs with pK_a values close to 7.4 (see appendix A) it has been shown that small changes in acid-base balance have a disproportionate effect on ionisation of weak organic acids and bases and may affect their uptake in tissues; for example, the myocardial uptake and efficacy of lignocaine (lidocaine; pK_a 7.85) might be reduced by severe acidosis (Hayes, 1971). In myocardial infarction, particularly that complicated by shock, or in heart failure, the apparent volumes of distribution of lignocaine and procainamide are reduced from normal — probably due to the reduced blood supply to peripheral tissues. This results in higher blood concentrations than expected and undue toxicity from usual doses. Clearance is also reduced, necessitating a decrease in both loading and maintenance intravenous dosage of lignocaine and procainamide (see chapter XVII; sect. 6.1.2, 6.1.3).

Protein binding too is affected by disease (Klotz, 1976; Tillement et al., 1978). In severe hypoalbuminaemia such as in the nephrotic syndrome and in cirrhosis, the degree of protein binding will be less than in normal subjects (see chapter XIX, sect. 1.3; XXI, sect. 1.2). In renal failure, the percentage binding of some acidic drugs (e.g. phenytoin, warfarin, sulphonamides, salicylate, phenylbutazone and certain barbiturates) to albumin is less than in patients with normal renal function (Reidenberg, 1976, 1977a; see chapter XXI, sect. 1.2). In the case of phenytoin (diphenylhydantoin), this will lead to a relatively larger volume of distribution of total drug. The unbound fraction of phenytoin in plasma is increased and the total plasma concentration is lower than in subjects with normal renal function, while the concentrations of unbound drug in plasma are similar (Odar-Cederlof and Borga, 1974). Since most analytical methods measure total phenytoin in plasma (i.e. unbound + bound) the therapeutic plasma concentration of phenytoin will therefore be lower in patients with renal failure than in patients with normal renal function (see section 5.1.2).

The impaired protein binding of acidic drugs in renal disease is at least partly due to the accumulation of endogenous compounds strongly attached to the plasma albumin, thereby acting as binding inhibitors (Sjoholm et al., 1976). The binding is

Table XIII. Binding of drugs to plasma proteins from patients with poor renal function (after Reidenberg, 1976, 1977a)

Drug	Acid (A) or basic (B)	Binding
Sulphonamides	A	Decreased
Phenytoin	A	Decreased
Tryptophan	A	Decreased
Clofibrate	A	Decreased
Salicylate	A	Decreased
Benzylpenicillin	A	Decreased
Dicloxacillin	A	Decreased
Cephalosporins	A	Decreased
Nitrofurantoin	A	Decreased
Doxycycline	A	Decreased
Barbiturates	A	Decreased
Diazoxide	A	Decreased
Phenylbutazone	A	Decreased
Warfarin	A	Decreased
Frusemide (furosemide)	A	Normal
Indomethacin	A	Normal
Desipramine	B	Normal
Quinidine	B	Normal
Dapsone	B	Normal
D-Tubocurarine	B	Normal
Propranolol	B	Normal
Triamterene	B	Decreased
Diazepam[1]	B	Decreased
Trimethoprim	B	Normal

---

1   This drug is bound to one of the main binding sites of albumin that normally binds acidic drugs.

---

partly restored a few days after kidney transplantation (Odar-Cederlof, 1977), suggesting that these inhibitors are reversibly bound to albumin. However, charcoal treatment at pH3 is necessary to fully restore the binding capacity of isolated albumin from uraemic subjects (Sjoholm et al., 1976).

Table XIII lists drugs whose binding has been investigated in uraemia. Basic drugs have normal binding in uraemia except when associated with inflammatory processes. During inflammation the plasma concentrations of α_1-acid glycoprotein increase and parallel with this, the binding of basic drugs such as propranolol, imipramine, quinidine and chlorpromazine increases. These drugs bind strongly to α_1-acid glycoprotein (Piafsky et al., 1978). The effect of certain inflammatory diseases

on propranolol binding relative to the concentration of this protein is seen in figure 20. For highly tissue localised drugs with avid hepatic elimination such as propranolol and chlorpromazine (high clearance drugs), a decrease in volume of distribution and reduced half-life would be predicted to result from increased plasma binding. With increased binding, for any given plasma concentration the free drug concentration will be less.

Drugs metabolised by the liver can be divided into two main types with respect to their hepatic clearance — high clearance (flow limited) and low clearance (capacity limited) [Blaschke, 1977]. For the former (e.g. propranolol, lignocaine) the extraction ratio in the liver is high and its ability to metabolise them is dependent upon the rate of transport of the drug (bound and unbound) to the organ; i.e. hepatic blood flow. The kinetics of such drugs will be altered by any disease that changes hepatic blood flow; e.g. certain liver diseases and congestive heart failure (see chapter XVII, sect. 1.1; XIX, sect. 1.4). For the low clearance or capacity limited drugs, hepatic clearance is depen-

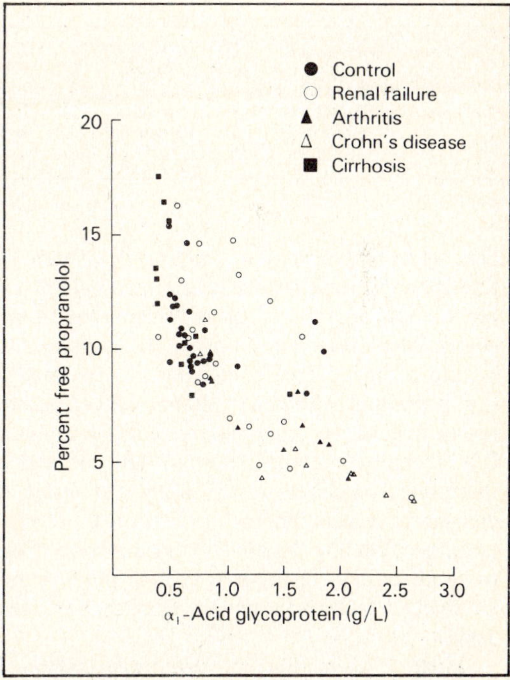

Fig. 20. Relationship between the binding of propranolol and the plasma concentration of α_1-acid glycoprotein. Note the decrease in free fraction of propranolol in arthritis and Crohn's disease (after Piafsky et al.: New Engl. J. Med. 299: 1435, 1978; by permission of author and editor).

Table XIV. Changes in bioavailability and clearance of high clearance (flow limited) drugs in patients with liver diseases

Drug	Hepatic extraction ratio	Disease[1] (route of administration)		Plasma clearance (% change)	Bioavailability (% change)	Reference[2]
Chlormethiazole	~ 0.9	C	(po)	− 94	+ > 1000	a
		C	(iv)	− 29		a
Labetalol	~ 0.7	C	(po)	− 62	+91	b
		C	(iv)	− 26		
Lignocaine	~ 0.7	C	(iv)	− 40		c
		AVH	(iv)	− 35		d
Pentazocine	~ 0.8	C	(po)	− 46	+278	e
Pethidine	~ 0.5	C	(po)	− 36	+81	e
		C	(po)	− 58	+40	f
		C	(iv)	− 50		g
		AVH	(iv)	− 49		h
Propranolol	~ 0.6	C	(po)	− 33	+42	i
		C	(iv)	− 52		j
		CAH	(iv)	− 46		j

1 C = cirrhosis, AVH = acute viral hepatitis, CAH = chronic active hepatitis.
2 a = Pentikainen et al.: Brit. Med. J. 2: 861 (1978)
   b = Homeida et al.: Brit. Med. J. 2: 1048 (1978)
   c = Thomson et al.: Ann. Int. Med. 78: 499 (1973)
   d = Williams et al.: Clin. Pharm. Ther. 20: 290 (1976)
   e = Neal et al.: Gastroent. 77: 55 (1979)
   f = Pond et al.: Clin. Pharm. Ther. 25: 242 (1979)
   g = Klotz et al.: Clin. Pharm. Ther. 16: 667 (1974)
   h = McHorse et al.: Gastroent. 68: 775 (1975)
   i = Wood et al.: Clin. Pharmacokin. 3: 478 (1978)
   j = Branch et al.: Brit. J. Clin. Pharm. 3: 243 (1976)

dent upon the capacity of the liver to metabolise the unbound drug available for metabolism and not on the amount of drug transported to this organ. Such drugs may be either binding sensitive, having a high degree of plasma protein binding (e.g. phenytoin, quinidine, tolbutamide) or binding insensitive, having a low degree of protein binding (e.g. theophylline, paracetamol). The kinetics of the latter is unlikely to be influenced much by changes in protein binding or blood flow. The low clearance, binding sensitive drugs are more likely to be affected by changes in protein binding than by changes in blood flow (see chapter XIX, sect. 1.4.1).

Further discussion on drug distribution in disease is given in other chapters in this book. Trauma and operation may also affect the binding of drugs to plasma proteins (Elfstrom, 1979; Fremstad et al., 1976). The extent of binding of phenytoin is decreased and that of quinidine in-creased after surgery, mostly due to changed concentration of plasma proteins; decreased albumin and increased α_1-acid glycoprotein concentrations respectively.

4.3.3 Drug Metabolism in Disease

A number of diseases and pathophysiological states are capable of altering the rate of drug metabolism as a consequence of changes in hepatic blood flow or hepatic microsomal drug metabolising enzyme activity (see Kato, 1977).

Liver Disease

The liver is the main organ of metabolism for many drugs and it would not be surprising if disease of the liver were to lead to impaired drug metabolism. In the early studies it appeared that liver disease needed to be very severe before the elimination of a drug became prolonged, but studies using various drugs with different pharma-

Table XV. Changes in protein binding and clearance of low clearance (capacity limited) drugs in patients with liver diseases

Drug	Disease[1] (route of administration)		Change in free fraction (%)	Plasma clearance (% change)	Reference[2]
Binding sensitive drugs					
Chlordiazepoxide	C	(iv)		− 50	a
	AVH	(iv)		− 66	a
Clindamycin	C	(iv)		− 59	b
	CAH	(iv)		− 26	b
	AVH	(iv)		− 2	b
Diazepam	C	(iv)	+210	− 50	c
	C	(iv)		− 51	d
	C	*(in vitro)*	+65		e
	CAH	(iv)		− 42	c
Lorazepam	C	(iv)	+68	+8	f
	AVH		+32	− 1	f
Oxazepam	C	(po)	+16	+14	g
	AVH	(po)	UNCH	+21	g
Phenytoin	AVH	(iv)	+27	+18[3]	h
Prednisone/prednisolone	C	(po)	↑	↓	i
Tolbutamide	AVH	(iv)	+28	+44[3]	j
Warfarin	AVH	(po)	UNCH	UNCH	k
Binding insensitive drugs					
Ampicillin	C	(iv)		− 18	l
Amylobarbitone	C[4]	(iv)	+77	− 55[4]	m
	C[5]	(iv)	UNCH	+29[5]	
Antipyrine	C	(iv)		− 69	n
	C	(po)		− 54	o
	CAH	(po)		− 59	o
	AVH	(po)		− 37	p
	AVH	(po)		− 33	q
Hexobarbitone	AVH	(iv)		− 46	r
	C[6]	(iv)		− 43	s
	C[7]	(iv)		− 62	
Theophylline	C	(iv)	+33	− 32	t
	C	(po)	+102	− 70	u

1   C = cirrhosis, CAH = chronic active hepatitis, AVH = acute viral hepatitis.
2   References

a = Roberts et al.: Gastroent. 75: 479 (1978)
b = Hinthorn et al.: Antimicrob. Agents Chemother. 9: 498 (1976)
c = Klotz et al.: J. Clin. Invest. 55: 347 (1975)
d = Andreasen et al.: Euro. J. Clin. Pharm. 10: 115 (1976)
e = Thiessen et al.: J. Clin. Pharm. 16: 345 (1976)
f = Kraus et al.: Clin. Pharm. Ther. 24: 411 (1978)
g = Shull et al.: Ann. Int. Med. 84: 420 (1976)
h = Blaschke et al.: Clin. Pharm. Ther. 17: 685 (1975)
i = Uribe et al.: Gastroent. 72: 1143 (1977); Uribe and Go: Clin. Pharmacokin. 4: 233 (1979)

j = Williams et al.: Clin. Pharm. Ther. 21: 301 (1977)
k = Williams et al.: Clin. Pharm. Ther. 20: 90 (1976)
l = Lewis and Jusko: Clin. Pharm. Ther. 18: 475 (1975)
m = Mawer et al.: Brit. J. Pharm. 44: 549 (1972)
n = Andreasen et al.: Euro. J. Clin. Invest. 4: 129 (1974)
o = Branch et al.: Clin. Pharm. Ther. 20: 81 (1976)
p = Williams et al.: Clin. Res. 24: 259A (1976)
q = Sorrell et al.: Clin. Pharm. Ther. 20: 365 (1976)
r = Breimer et al.: Clin. Pharm. Ther. 18: 433 (1975)
s = Zilly et al.: Clin. Pharm. Ther. 23: 525 (1978)
t = Piafsky et al.: New Engl. J. Med. 296: 1495 (1977)
u = Mangione et al.: Chest 73: 616 (1978)

3   The clearance of *unbound* drug was unchanged.
4   Hypoalbuminaemia.
5   Normal serum albumin concentration.
6   Compensated.
7   Uncompensated.

cokinetic characteristics have shown differences from normal, particularly when hepatic clearance is considered in terms of the classification of drugs discussed in section 4.3.2 (Blaschke, 1977).

Tables XIV and XV indicate the changes that can be expected in the pharmacokinetics of certain drugs in different types of liver disease. Viral hepatitis during the acute phase of the illness, will usually cause a diminution in the rate of drug elimination of high clearance (flow limited) and low clearance, binding insensitive drugs and as liver function returns to normal, so does the disposition of the drug. There is usually little or no change or an increase in clearance of low clearance, binding sensitive drugs in acute viral hepatitis.

In cirrhosis, there is a defect not only of liver function but also of the hepatic circulation. High clearance drugs in particular are subject to impaired elimination and increased bioavailability after oral administration. Drugs with the highest hepatic clearance will have the largest relative increase in bioavailability in cirrhosis (Neal et al., 1979) due to the presence of portal systemic vascular shunts through which the drug effectively bypasses the initial hepatic removal process. Elimination of intravenously administered high clearance drugs is also reduced in cirrhosis but the change is relatively small in some patients. Elimination of these drugs is more likely to be affected by the ability of the liver cell to metabolise the drug when hepatic blood flow is not significantly altered.

Low clearance drugs such as theophylline and diazepam are also subject to impaired metabolism in cirrhosis, reduced clearance being particularly important in the case of theophylline. When cirrhosis is severe enough to decrease the concentration of albumin, disposition of low clearance, binding sensitive acidic drugs such as phenytoin and tolbutamide will be affected since the free fraction will increase (table XV). Information on clearance is limited for such drugs in cirrhosis. However, the situation may well be the same as that in acute viral hepatitis in which clearance of total drug is increased but that of unbound drug is unaltered (e.g. tolbutamide).

A full discussion of disposition of various drugs in liver diseases and the clinicial significance of altered rates of elimination is given in chapter XIX (sect. 1.3, 1.4). This chapter also discusses abnormal responses to drugs in liver disease (sect. 13.4).

Thyroid Disease

The influence of thyroid disease on drug metabolism has been studied intensively in recent years, and controlled studies are relatively easy since the patient can be restudied when the thyroid status is restored to normal. In general, drug metabolism is accelerated in hyperthyroidism and reduced in hypothyroid states (Eichelbaum, 1976). See further, chapter XVI (sect. 1.4.2).

Renal Disease

It has always been assumed that the rate of metabolism of a drug will not be altered in patients with renal impairment, but this is not necessarily true. Thus, oxidation of some drugs may be enhanced, leading to a more rapid rate of drug metabolism, as has been shown for phenytoin, propranolol and antipyrine. Most glucuronide conjugation reactions are unaltered by renal disease but hydrolytic reactions may be slowed, as is seen with the hydrolysis of insulin, procaine and cephalothin. Reduction may also be slowed; e.g. cortisol (Reidenberg, 1977b). See further, chapter XXI (sect. 1.3).

Pulmonary Disease

The lungs are not only capable of metabolising drugs but disorders of lung function may also alter the disposition of drugs (du Souich et al., 1978). Clearance of theophylline is markedly reduced in patients with severe airways obstruction, especially when complicated by pneumonia or cor pulmonale (Ogilvie, 1978). Acute hypoxaemia appears to decrease metabolism of capacity limited drugs while chronic hypoxia appears to increase the rate of metabolism (see further chapter XX; sect. 1.4, 1.5).

Surgery and Trauma

Many factors exist which could alter the disposition of drugs after operation (Elfstrom, 1979). Apart from slowed gastric emptying and altered protein binding (see section 4.3.2), liver blood flow increases and hepatic microsomal drug metabolising enzyme activity increases. The increase in drug metabolic capacity, as reflected in an enhanced rate of elimination of antipyrine, may be due to altered secretion of hormones or concomitant use of enzyme inducing drugs. Impaired renal function is only likely after severe trauma with hypotension. The possible adverse effects of general anaesthetics on liver and kidney function must also be considered (see chapter X; sect. 5.4, 5.5). This area requires further study with drugs with different pharmacokinetic characteristics before the clinical implications are clear.

4.3.4 Drug Excretion in Disease

Those drugs which are largely cleared by renal excretion show a prolonged half-life in patients with age dependent (elderly and newborn) or pathological impairment of renal function. Thus, accumulation of the drug will occur and on normal doses toxicity will ensue (Fabre and Balant, 1976). Table XVI shows the expected elimination half-life of some of these drugs in anuric patients, with the inclusion of rifampicin and digitoxin for comparison, whose half-lives are not altered by renal failure, because they are metabolised. It has been advocated to use digitoxin rather than digoxin in uraemic subjects. This rests on the premise that digoxin formed by hydroxylation of digitoxin is a quantitatively unimportant metabolite, which usually seems to be the case (see chapter XVII; sect. 8.1.3).

It is generally assumed that drugs which are metabolised, can be safely given in the normal dose range to uraemic subjects. This assumption is only true if the polar metabolites, which accumulate in uraemia, are biologically inert. It is now well established that many drugs have active metabolites that will accumulate in the plasma of patients with impaired renal function and will lead to enhanced drug action or to unexpected drug toxicity (Drayer, 1976; 1977). For example, the main active metabolite of procainamide, N-acetylprocainamide, accumulates in patients with impaired renal function and has been associated with the presence of cardiac arrhythmias. Norpethidine (normeperidine) is an active metabolite of pethidine, the plasma concentration of which increases in renal impairment. It is less active as an analgesic but is more active as a convulsive agent than the parent drug and accumulation in patients with impaired renal function is associated with irritability and twitching. The toxicity associated with nitrofurantoin (peripheral neuritis), clofibrate (muscle weakness) and allopurinol (skin rash) is caused at least in part by the metabolites of these drugs which accumulate to high concentrations in the plasma of patients with impaired renal function (see chapter XXI, sect. 14; XXII, sect. 12.2.2).

It is therefore a *sine qua non* for scientifically sound drug therapy in uraemia to know the fate and plasma concentrations of such metabolites,

Table XVI. Elimination half-lives (hours) of some drugs in normal and impaired renal function

Drug	Normal	Anuria
Penicillin G	0.5	23
Erythromycin	1.4	5.5
Cephaloridine	1.7	23
Streptomycin	2.5	70
Gentamicin	2.5	35
Kanamycin	2.8	70
Vancomycin	5.8	230
Tetracycline	8.5	90
Digoxin	30-40	87-100
Digitoxin	170	170-200
Rifampicin	2.8	2.8
Doxycycline	23	23

and to adjust the dose in accordance with known pharmacokinetics of pharmacologically active compounds.

In order to achieve a required steady-state plasma concentration when the half-life of a drug is prolonged in renal failure, the following three facts should be understood:

1) The priming or loading dose will not need to be changed provided distribution volume does not change.
2) A smaller maintenance dose of the drug will be needed and/or that dose should be given less frequently than before.
3) The time taken to achieve the steady-state plasma concentration will be longer — since to achieve 90% of that concentration will take 3 times the half life (see section 2.2; table I).

During recent years a number of nomograms have been published to guide the clinician in the dosage of drugs in renal insufficiency, particularly those with a narrow therapeutic ratio such as gentamicin, kanamycin and digoxin (e.g. Dettli, 1976). These nomograms take into account creatinine clearance (or serum creatinine), body weight and age of the patient. When using such nomograms it must be remembered that the determination of creatinine may be inaccurate, that compensatory excretory routes such as faecal excretion may vary among individuals and that kidney function may change quickly. Such nomograms are thus poor replacements of longitudinal monitoring of steady-state plasma concentrations, which should be performed routinely when toxic drugs are used. This is particularly true in elderly patients, where kidney function may be impaired in spite of normal serum creatinine. Drug disposition and response and principles in the use of drugs in renal disease is discussed further in chapter XXI (sects. 1.4, 1.5, 2.1, 13).

4.4 Multiple Drug Therapy — Drug Interactions

Drugs are usually used in combination and it is often necessary to prescribe several potent drugs for the same individual. The initial tendency to overemphasise the clinical importance of drug interactions has been of little help to the practising clinician (Sjoqvist and Alexanderson, 1972). Drug interactions are discussed in perspective in chapters VII (sect. 7) and VIII. It should be emphasised that determinants of drug interactions are probably multifactorial and with drug metabolism interactions in particular, genetically determined differences are probably the most important single determinant (Kristensen, 1976; Vesell, 1977, 1979).

In order to clarify both mechanisms of interactions and their clinical importance, several points deserve consideration:

1) Specific drug analytical techniques must be used.

2) Pharmacokinetic data obtained must be correctly interpreted. Drug induced changes in measurements such as the elimination half-life of a drug may have several kinetic explanations. To distinguish between these it may be necessary to measure drug metabolites in body fluids, binding to plasma proteins etc.

3) Animal data cannot be extrapolated to man. Some tabulations of drug interactions contain both human and animal data. This may confuse the clinician when using the information in clinical practice.

4) *In vitro* data on for example synergism or antagonism between antibiotics and *in vitro* observations on drug binding displacement interactions are not always applicable to the conditions *in vivo* (see section 3.2.2). As an example, displacement of acidic drugs from plasma albumin might be of

clinical importance only in patients with slow elimination of such drugs.

5) The results of drug interaction experiments in healthy volunteers (often single dose experiments) may not be at all relevant for patients who are treated long term with drugs. Mechanisms like enzyme induction presumably vary in importance between individuals (evidence for genetic control).

6) Many interaction studies are based on rather small patient or volunteer samples and some are even 'case reports'. There are very few prospective studies aimed at documenting the incidence of clinically important drug interactions (see chapter VIII; sect. 1.4).

5. The Role of the Clinical Pharmacological Laboratory in Improving Drug Therapy

It is now realised that it may be clinically useful to monitor plasma concentrations of certain drugs in patients for whom therapy is essential (e.g. see Azarnoff, 1975; Davies and Prichard, 1973; Richens, 1979). For example, the effect of phenytoin (diphenylhydantoin) is much better correlated in patient populations to its steady-state plasma concentrations than to dosage (Lund, 1974). This may also be true for other drugs which are extensively metabolised in the body. As discussed in section 4, a fixed dose (x mg per kg) of such a drug may give a 10-fold interindividual range in the steady-state plasma concentrations due to the combined influence of genetic and environmental factors on drug metabolism.

It must be re-emphasised that there is no general biochemical test available to detect slow drug metabolisers. Thus in assessing drug metabolism, there is no alternative available but to study each compound separately, e.g. by measuring the steady-state plasma concentration. This is not only practical (it avoids stopping treatment and manipulation of dosage for half-life measurements) but also reveals important drug metabolic and psychological (drug compliance; see section 5.2.2) information about the patient.

The position with drugs that are excreted *unchanged* by the kidney is better, because laboratory tests such as serum creatinine or creatinine clearance are adequate rough guidelines for the modification of dosage when there is impairment of renal function (see further section 4.3.4).

Table XVII. A correlation between steady-state plasma concentration of a drug and clinical effect can be expected when the following criteria are fulfilled

---

1. The drug has a reversible action and acts per se (not through metabolites).

2. Development of tolerance at receptor sites does not occur.

3. The concentration of unbound drug in plasma should be equal to the concentration of unbound drug at receptor sites — i.e. plasma and tissue levels of unbound drug should be in equilibrium after some period of continued treatment.

4. The clinical effects of the drug are measured accurately.

5. Factors which modify the plasma concentration-clinical effect relationship are taken into account — e.g. other drugs, abnormal protein binding, stage of disease.

6. The pharmacokinetic properties of the drug are taken into account — e.g. time of sampling plasma, when to measure area under plasma concentration-time curve.

7. The chemical analytical method must be both sensitive and selective — NB take drug history as other drugs can interfere with the assay procedure.

5.1 Correlation Between Drug Plasma Concentrations and Clinical Effects?

The idea of using the plasma concentration of a drug as an objective means towards safer and more rational therapy in an individual patient is based on several prerequisites which are summarised in table XVII and discussed below (Sjoqvist, 1977).

5.1.1 Action at Receptor Sites

The drug should have a reversible action. For 'hit and run' drugs like monoamine oxidase inhibitors, the action may persist although the drug is no longer measurable in plasma. Most drugs in common use exert a reversible, concentration-dependent interaction with receptor sites (see section 1.2).

The development of tolerance at receptor sites should not be an important problem, as for example with barbiturates, ethyl alcohol and morphine (Snyder, 1979).

5.1.2 Distribution Equilibrium

The concentration of unbound drug in plasma should be equal to the concentration of unbound drug at receptor sites, and hence distribution equilibrium must exist. For drugs with a small apparent volume of distribution, it is easy to appreciate that the concentration of drug in plasma is a reasonable estimate of the amount of drug in the body (see table V; sect. 3.2.3). If the receptors are located in or close to the plasma pool, it is evident that the plasma concentration must have a relevant relationship to the drug's action.

Many drugs have a large apparent volume of distribution (appendix A) and for such compounds, attempts to relate effects and plasma concentration have been looked upon with scepticism, because so little drug is available in plasma compared with the tissues. The tissue concentration has been said to be more important for the pharmacological effect than the plasma concentration. Apart from the fact that there are few experimental studies on this point, and human studies are extremely difficult to perform, it should be realised that independently of the volume of distribution of the drug, plasma and tissue concentrations should be in equilibrium after some period of continued treatment. The length of this period will vary considerably between drugs.

Thus, there is little reason to believe that the ratio between the concentrations of unbound drug in plasma and in the biophase surrounding tissue receptor sites should differ markedly between patients, as long as we consider drug distribution as a passive process depending upon the physico-chemical properties of the drug rather than upon the genetic constitution of the individual.

An important question is whether total or unbound plasma concentrations should be measured or both. It appears quite clear that measurement of the total plasma concentration is usually appropriate. Under normal conditions the interindividual differences in plasma protein binding seem to be small compared with the marked interindividual differences in metabolism (see section 4). However, when the patient is treated simultaneously with two or more highly bound acidic drugs with a small apparent volume of distribution and which bind to the same site on albumin like warfarin and phenylbutazone, it is known that the pharmacological action of the displaced drug (warfarin) will increase because the unbound pharmacologically active concentration is increased (section 3.2.3). It has also been pointed out that the fraction of unbound drug increases in certain diseases and decreases in others (see section 4.3.2). For example, the unbound fraction of phenytoin (diphenylhydantoin) is increased markedly in patients with uraemia. These patients can therefore be expected to respond therapeutically or with side effects at much lower *total* plasma concentrations than epileptics with normal renal function. Hence monitoring of the *unbound* drug concentration is important in this and similar situations. For some drugs the unbound concentration in plasma and the total concentration in saliva are almost identical (Danhof and Breimer, 1978; Mucklow et al., 1978). This can be utilised in drug concentration monitoring.

In this context, it should be added that for example the diuretic chlorthalidone predominantly localises in the red cell, with ratios between red cell and plasma of 20 or more. In such cases the *whole blood concentration* may be important for the pharmacological effect.

5.1.3 Measurement of Clinical Effects

In many areas of pharmacology the ability to measure minute concentrations of drugs in biological fluids has become satisfactory. Drug analytical methods allow accurate measurement of concentrations down to 1 ng/ml or lower (1 ng = 10^{-9}g). The attempt to correlate plasma concentrations of drugs with their pharmacodynamic effect therefore, is dependent upon our ability to accurately detect and quantitate the therapeutic effect. In some areas of therapeutics this is relatively easy (e.g. cardiovascular drugs) and in others difficult (e.g. CNS active drugs), as discussed in section 7.

It is important that the variable being measured is relevant to the pharmacodynamic effect of the drug, otherwise no true relationship to drug plasma concentration can be expected. Even measuring such an apparently simple parameter as systemic arterial blood pressure imposes a number of questions: shall we measure it continuously or on a few occasions every day, in the sitting, standing or lying position, at rest or after exercise or both, in the clinic or at home?

At present, the accurate measurement of drug effects in patients is probably the most important area of endeavour in clinical pharmacology (see section 7).

5.1.4 Factors which Modify the Plasma Concentration-Effect Relationship

A number of factors may modify the plasma concentration-clinical effect relationship in an individual patient. Intercurrent illness, surgery or a change in environmental and dietary factors may

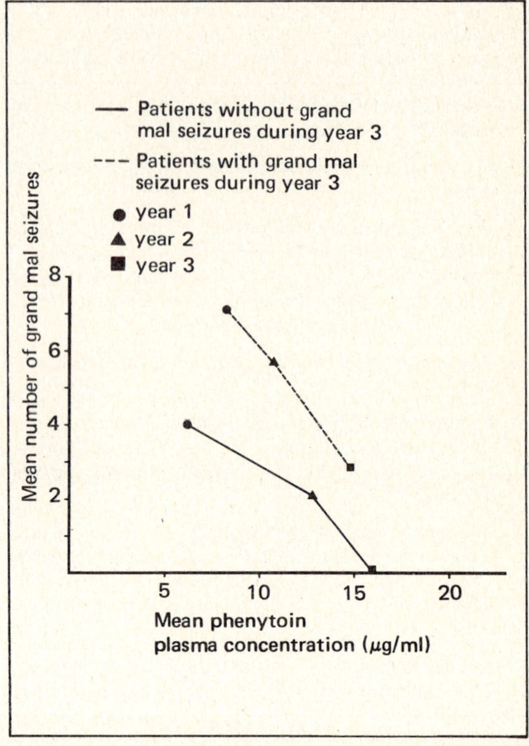

Fig. 21. The relationship between the annual mean number of grand mal seizures and the mean concentration of phenytoin (diphenylhydantoin) in two groups consisting of patients with or without seizures during the third year of a prospective study (after Lund: Archives of Neurology 31: 289, 1974; by permission of author and editor).

alter the usual absorption and disposition of a drug, as considered in sections 3.3.5 and 4.3. Concomitant drug therapy (section 4.4) is probably the most important factor and often impossible to control. The stage of the disease is also important, amply illustrated in the case of phenytoin (diphenylhydantoin) and grand mal epilepsy. With increasing severity of seizures, the plasma concentration needed for seizure control rises (fig. 21).

5.1.5 The Drug and its Chemical Assay

There are a number of points to take into consideration regarding the drug and its chemical assay. Ideally the drug is characterised by slow absorption and a long elimination half-life relative to the dosage interval such that only minor fluctuations of drug plasma concentrations occur during the day. In this case, the time for sampling plasma may be of little importance (e.g. phenytoin). For other drugs, very strict protocols have to be set up, the plasma concentration being measured at a specific time point in relation to dosage; e.g. 12 hours after the last dose with lithium and at least 6 to 8 hours with digoxin. For drugs with short half-lives (a few hours) and hence major fluctuations of plasma concentrations at conventional dosage intervals, the trough concentration obtained just before the next dose is to be administered, and the peak concentration obtained 1 to 2 hours after a dose, are appropriate times to obtain samples for evaluation (e.g. aminoglycoside antibiotics). Sometimes it may be desirable to measure the area under the plasma concentration-time curve (AUC) during the dosage interval.

In plasma concentration estimations, it is an advantage if the drug is active *per se*. However, with many drugs used in practice, the pharmacological effects of the metabolites are often unknown and the main metabolites may not even be identified. It becomes impractical and expensive to measure several compounds in plasma.

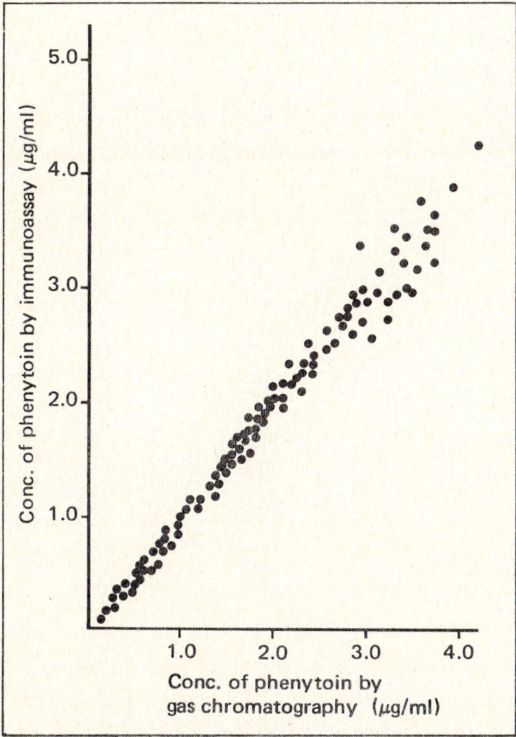

Fig. 22. Comparison between plasma phenytoin (diphenylhydantoin) concentrations as measured by gas chromatography and radioimmunoassay in 105 plasma samples drawn from 6 patients with impaired renal function (after Orme et al.: Clin. Chem. 22: 246, 1976; by permission of author and editor).

5.1.6 Chemical Analytical Methods

The chemical analytical methods must be both sensitive and selective. In many conventional analytical methods the drug history of the patient has importance for the choice of the procedure.

There are usually intellectual or organisational barriers between clinicians and pharmacologists on the one hand, and analytical chemists on the other. This may explain why many obsolete analytical methods have been and still are in use in clinical drug research.

The development of drug analysis has been particularly rapid during the last 15 years with methods such as conventional gas chromatography, mass fragmentography, radioimmunoassays and high pressure liquid chromatography.

How then can advancements in clinical pharmacokinetics be utilised in patient care when the research requires a team of professionals and expensive analytical methods. Two ways of utilising this expert knowledge are apparent: (a) to refer patients to regional centres for pharmacokinetic or drug metabolic work-ups in analogy with what now is being done in many countries with inborn errors of endogenous metabolism; and (b) to develop simpler analytical methods like the radioimmunoassay for digoxin, but only when rigorous control of specificity can be guaranteed. As an example, radioimmunoassay for phenytoin (diphenylhydantoin) has shown remarkable specificity in comparison with gas chromatography and mass fragmentography (Orme et al., 1976; fig. 22). With proper batch and product controls such an antiserum could become very valuable in routine laboratories. The position with the digoxin antibody is less satisfactory because there is as yet no easy back-up of the method with proper physical methods.

5.2 Main Indications for Measuring Drugs in Plasma (or other body fluids)

5.2.1 Therapeutic Monitoring

For the drugs listed in table XVIII the relationship between plasma concentration and clinical effects has been studied under relatively controlled conditions. Many of these drugs have a narrow therapeutic ratio (digoxin, lithium), others have dose dependent elimination kinetics (phenytoin) and others marked interindividual variability in elimination kinetics (nortriptyline). These factors strengthen the need to monitor plasma concentra-

Table XVIII. Drugs for which therapeutic and toxic ranges of plasma concentrations have been defined

Drug	Therapeutic range	Side effects	Further information	References
Antiepileptic Drugs				
Phenytoin (diphenylhydantoin)	10-20µg/ml	> 25µg/ml	See chapter XXV (sect. 3.1; 4.6)	Kutt (1974), Lund (1974), Hvidberg and Dam (1976)
Phenobarbitone	10-30µg/ml	> 35µg/ml	See chapter XXV (sect. 3.2; 4.6)	Buchtal and Lennox-Buchtal (1972), Hvidberg and Dam (1976)
Carbamazepine[2]	4-10(12)µg/ml	> 10µg/ml	See chapter XXV (sect. 3.4; 4.6)	Bertilsson (1978), Hvidberg and Dam (1976)
Ethosuximide	40-100µg/ml	> 100µg/ml	See chapter XXV (sect. 3.5; 4.6)	Penry (1975)
Cardiovascular Drugs				
Digoxin	1-2ng/ml	> 2ng/ml	See chapter XVII (sect. 8.1.3; 8.1.7)	Smith et al. (1969) Iisalo (1977), Weintraub (1977)
Digitoxin[2]	~ 15-25ng/ml	> 35ng/ml	See chapter XVII (sect. 8.1.3; 8.1.7)	Perrier et al. (1977)
Quinidine[3]	3-6µg/ml	> 6-9µg/ml	See chapter XVII (sect. 6.1.1)	Koch-Weser (1973)
Procainamide[4]	4-8µg/ml	> 8-12µg/ml	See chapter XVII (sect. 6.1.2)	Koch-Weser (1977), Karlsson (1978)
Lignocaine[5] (lidocaine)	2-5µg/ml	> 5µg/ml	See chapter XVII (sect. 6.1.3)	Benowitz and Meister (1978)
Psychotherapeutic Drugs				
Lithium	0.8-1.0mEq/L (0.5-1.2)	> 1.5mEq/L	See chapter XXVI (sect. 1.5.4; 5.3)	Amdisen (1977)
Nortriptyline[6]	50-180ng/ml	> 200ng/ml	See chapter XXVI (sect. 1.5.2; 1.6.3)	Kragh-Sorensen (1978), Asberg and Sjoqvist (1978)
Imipramine[6]	150-240ng/ml[7]		See chapter XXVI (sect. 1.5.2; 1.6.3)	Gram (1977), Perrel et al. (1978)
Miscellaneous				
Theophylline	(5)10-20µg/ml	> 20µg/ml	See chapter XX (sect. 2.3.1)	Ogilvie (1978)
Salicylate[2]	150-300µg/ml	> 300µg/ml	See chapter XXII (sect. 3.2.1)	Rumack (1978)

1   Antibiotics are excluded because the bioassay methods used seem to be less reliable than chemical procedures.
2   More clinical data needed.
3   Improved chemical methodology needed.
4   Has an active metabolite (see text).
5   Difficult to utilise in practice since acute determinations are needed.
6   Data concern endogenous depression.
7   Sum of imipramine and desipramine.

tions, but the prime reason for doing this should be that it is more difficult to assess the clinical effect of the drug objectively than to measure its concentration in plasma, especially if the drug is used prophylactically and has a low therapeutic ratio.

With this philosophy the monitoring of plasma concentrations of hypoglycaemic, antihypertensive and anticoagulant drugs is not justified, while an open mind according to individual circumstances has to be kept in relation to drugs affecting subjective variables such as mood and pain and drugs used prophylactically such as antiarrhythmics. For only a few drugs is routine monitoring justified (Richens, 1979). Monitoring the plasma concentrations of antiepileptic drugs has increased the efficacy and safety of drug therapy in epilepsy (see chapter XXV; sect. 2.3.5), while monitoring of lithium in plasma is necessary to avoid toxicity in long term prophylaxis of manic-depressive disorder (see chapter XXVI; sect. 5.3). The list of drugs for which a desirable therapeutic plasma concentration range has been defined is at present short but in many countries drug control agencies will require that new drugs are introduced to the market with this knowledge in the documentation file.

It must be emphasised that the measurement of drugs in plasma does not replace sound clinical judgement (Gugler and Azarnoff, 1976). On the contrary, this is a prerequisite for proper utilisation of the service, which should be part of a consultation in clinical pharmacology to be used mainly when patients are responding abnormally to a drug or when routine monitoring is justified to guide safe and effective use of a drug. It should also be appreciated that estimation of drug concentrations from a given plasma sample (as with antibacterial sensitivity testing) can vary between laboratories, as shown with antiepileptic drugs (Pippenger et al., 1976; Richens, 1978). This fact must always be borne in mind when plasma concentration estimations are requested. Contrary to the general belief, many more patients are under-medicated than overtreated when based upon drug concentrations obtained in plasma (e.g. Mucklow and Dollery, 1978). This phenomenon has been little published compared with side effects of drugs.

5.2.2 To Check Drug Compliance

It follows from the above that it is often justified to question whether the patient complies

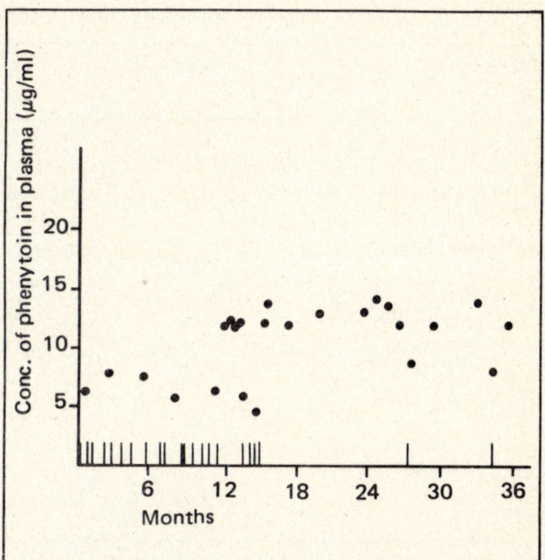

Fig. 23. Plasma concentrations of phenytoin (diphenylhydantoin) and seizure frequency in long term therapy. The patient was a 44-year-old woman with generalised epileptic seizures of unknown aetiology of 15 years' duration. A constant dose of phenytoin (6.8 mg/kg/day) was prescribed over a 3 year period. Too little attention was paid to the low plasma concentrations during the first year, and other anticonvulsant drugs were tried with unsatisfactory results. During hospitalisation in month 12, it was found that plasma concentrations rose (unreliable drug intake). After that time, plasma concentration remained between 12 and 15µg/ml, and the number of seizures diminished markedly. Only two seizures occurred during the last 2 years; on both occasions, the plasma concentration had dropped because of interruptions in drug intake. Seizures are shown by the event markers of the abscissa (after Lund: Lakartidningen 68: 73, 1971; by permission of author and editor).

with the prescription or not (see Blackwell, 1972, 1973, 1976; Mazullo, 1972). Experience with many years monitoring of phenytoin in plasma shows that many epileptic patients forget to take their medication. This is not only due to kinetically inappropriate dosage schedules such as 3 to 4 times daily, when once or twice daily will suffice, but is probably also due to the failure of the clinician to explain the benefit/risk equation (fig. 23).

It is easy to distinguish between poor drug compliance and rapid metabolism of drugs known to be completely absorbed. If the patient is in the steady-state then one should be able to account for a defined amount of the drug in a 24 hour urinary specimen as the main metabolite. For example, p-hydroxyphenytoin in conjugated and unconjugated

Table XIX. Choice of an oral anticoagulant with emphasis on pharmacokinetic considerations

Property	Warfarin	Dicoumarol (bishydroxycoumarin)	Phenindione
Absorption	Good	Poor and erratic[1]	Probably fair
Bioavailability	100%[2]	40-70%	? About 90%
Metabolism			
Half-life	30-40 hours	60-100 hours	5-10 hours
Kinetics	First order	Dose dependent	First order
Metabolites active?	Yes	?	Probably not
Toxic effects	Rare[3]	Rare[3]	Unacceptably frequent (tubular necrosis of kidney; severe skin rashes)

1   But may be improved by pharmaceutical reformulation.
2   Unless tablet size is greater than 10mg.
3   Apart from complications of overdosage.

form should amount to about 80% of the daily ingested dose of phenytoin. Therefore a pharmacokinetic service laboratory should have methods available for the main metabolite(s) of drugs.

5.2.3 In At-Risk Patients and Special Situations

These include patients with poor and rapidly changing kidney function, where even short term treatment with ordinary doses of drugs such as digoxin or aminoglycoside antibiotics may result in toxic concentrations and, in the latter case, irreversible damage of the inner ear (see chapter XI; sect. 7.1.1). Other indications may include suspicion of toxicity or malabsorption of drugs (e.g. digoxin).

5.2.4 In the Management of Certain Drug Intoxications

Since most treatment of drug overdosage and poisoning is symptomatic and unspecific there is usually no urgency in these measurements (see chapter IX). They are, however, an important guide to management of poisoning with some drugs (e.g. paracetamol/acetaminophen) and are a *sine qua non* for a correct evaluation of new treatments. As an example, in most studies of the efficacy of gastric lavage no drug measurements have been included. No wonder, that there are different opinions about its efficacy.

6. Pharmacokinetics in Drug Selection

It is useful now to consider whether the various theoretical factors discussed in the preceding sections can assist in drug selection. This can be best illustrated by thinking about a therapeutic situation and considering what the clinician should ask himself about the drug when selecting the best agent of a particular drug class. A good example is in the selection of an oral anticoagulant for a patient, say, with deep vein thrombosis.

Let us assume that the choice lies between three drugs, warfarin, dicoumarol (bishydroxycoumarin) and phenindione. Table XIX summarises some of the points of difference. Dicoumarol is poorly and erratically absorbed due to low lipid solubility. The other disadvantage is that it shows concentration dependent elimination kinetics and this makes the initial anticoagulant control more difficult, as small dose increments may result in large increases in the plasma concentration. Phenindione has a short half-life, which means that the dose must be given twice daily and its incidence of severe side effects, although small, is unacceptable to most clinicians. Warfarin has none of these disadvantages and may thus be the preferred oral anticoagulant in most countries. Although some of the metabolites of warfarin (the warfarin alcohols) possess pharmacological activity, this is not a problem in clinical practice (see

Table XX. Check list on clinical documentation of drugs

---

1. Structural formula — relationship to other drugs on the market

2. Mechanism(s) of action

3. Indications based on acceptable evidence of therapeutic efficacy in controlled clinical trials (see also section 8; 9.2)

4. Pharmacokinetics
   a) Pharmaceutical aspects
   b) Bioavailability
   c) Binding and distribution
   d) Metabolism (pathways, rates, active metabolites, interindividual variations)
   e) Excretion
   f) Pharmacokinetic and/or pharmacodynamic rationale for dose regimens. Interindividual variability of kinetic parameters
   g) Effects of disease on pharmacokinetics
   h) Anticipated or documented drug interactions

5. Contraindications and side effects (kinetic basis). Care with which side effects have been sought

6. Comparative clinical pharmacology and therapeutic efficacy in relation to other drugs used for the same indication

7. Comparative drug price

---

chapter XXIII; sect. 3.2.2). Table XX contains a check list on kinetic and clinical documentation of drugs which is used in our hospital when drugs are compared.

To the academic clinical pharmacologist, the overwhelming therapeutic problem is the inappropriate or suboptimal use of drugs that are already on the market (Boethius, 1977; Balter et al., 1974). Studies of the mechanisms involved in interindividual variations in pharmacokinetics and pharmacodynamics will, in the long term, help to define the properties of ideal drugs. This research will provide an important feedback to the chemists in the drug industry concerned with drug design. Any new, highly effective drug which represents a novel pharmacodynamic principle will be welcomed in clinical medicine. However, many drugs that are offered to the clinical academic community for trials do not belong to this category but are rather modifications of existing drugs. Usually, a number of derivatives are tried in animals and the most effective one is selected for clinical trial. For such drugs the following

characteristics may represent kinetic improvements:

1) The drug acts *per se* rather than through metabolites (simplified monitoring of plasma concentrations).
2) The drug does not have dose dependent elimination kinetics (upon 'saturation' of the metabolic pathways disproportionate increases in plasma concentrations may occur after small dose increases), nor a first-pass hepatic elimination — see sections 2.1.1; 3.3.3.
3) The drug does not have variable absorption or bioavailability problems.
4) The drug does not exhibit interindividual differences in protein binding.
5) The plasma concentrations should be relatively constant during conventional dosage intervals and proportional to dosage.
6) The relationship between steady-state plasma concentration and the clinical effects (including side effects) should be known.
7) A simple method should be available for specific measurement of the drug in plasma.

Very few drugs fulfil these criteria; lithium is close to doing so but it has a low therapeutic ratio (Amdisen, 1977). The best way for clinicians to cope with interindividual variations in kinetics may be to use drugs whose pharmacological effects are easy to measure or which have such a large therapeutic ratio that fixed doses can be used without complications.

7. Clinical Assessment of Drug Effects

Reliable and accurate methods of assessing the clinical response to drugs is essential, not only to determine if the desired therapeutic goal has been achieved but also to control measurement of drug response in therapeutic trials and for study of the correlation between plasma concentrations of drugs and their pharmacodynamic effect.

7.1 Cardiovascular Drugs

Much clinical pharmacological information arose initially in the field of cardiovascular medicine since it is easy to measure the blood pressure and pulse rate and to relate changes to the drugs given. Use of simple apparatus, such as the muddled zero sphygmomanometer enables the blood pressure to be measured relatively free of observer bias. The therapeutic effect can be measured in more sophisticated ways and the effect of β-adrenoceptor blocking drugs is commonly measured by the effect on submaximal exercise induced heart rate. The exercise needs to be submaximal to eliminate as far as possible the effects of vagal activity on the heart rate. Without resorting to invasive methods, other cardiac drugs can be monitored fairly accurately either for therapeutic benefit to the patient or for use in clinical trials. Thus, an antianginal drug may be monitored in the laboratory by assessing the work done by the patient (e.g. on a treadmill or bicycle ergometer) before the onset of chest pain. More simply, the patient can keep a diary card, recording every anginal attack and then relate these to the use or dosage of the drug concerned.

Antiarrhythmic drugs can be monitored by the use of a halter electrocardiogram (Clarke et al., 1976). An ECG lead is attached to the chest wall, and is connected to a small transmitter, powered by a battery, which can be easily carried by the patient for days on end if necessary. The ECG is transmitted to a tape recording device which can be several miles away and the tape can be rapidly analysed by computer for the presence of cardiac arrhythmias and related to the drug used. This is often used in clinical trial work.

7.2 Antiasthmatic and Hypoglycaemic Drugs

Outside the cardiovascular field, it is more difficult to quantitate the therapeutic action of drugs but progress is being made. In asthmatic patients, it is common practice to measure the vital capacity (VC) and forced expiratory volume in one second (FEV_1) in the clinic, while airways resistance can be measured more specifically by non-invasive methods. This is useful to assess the response of patients to their drugs (see chapter XX; sect. 2; 3). It is now possible to equip patients with a simple device for use at home to measure their peak expiratory flow rate. This will enable day to day or even hour to hour changes to be quantitated and there is some evidence that the peak expiratory flow rate starts to fall some time before the patient experiences wheezing, thus enabling changes in drug therapy to be made before an asthmatic attack develops (Clark and Hetzel, 1977).

In diabetes mellitus, it has been common practice to monitor therapeutic progress and drug effect by the measurement of urine glucose. It has however, been recognised for some time, that this method is insensitive and changes seen in the urine sugar occur too late for any effective preventive measures to be taken with the drug therapy (Holman and Turner, 1978). Monitoring of blood glucose, while ideal in theory, has not been practicable because of the apparatus required. There are now available simple and relatively cheap machines that, working on the reflectance principle, can accurately and reliably measure the concentration of glucose in a finger prick sample of blood. While these machines are not yet in routine use, some clinics are experimenting with their use by the patient in his own home (Howe-Davies et al., 1978). There is no doubt that in difficult cases of diabetes, control is much easier to achieve by monitoring of blood glucose and there is considerable potential for clinical trial use.

7.3 CNS Active Drugs

It is in the field of pain states and psychiatric or neurological disease that it is most difficult to measure the clinical effect of drugs with any accuracy. Even in diseases such as rheumatoid arthritis, where the appreciation of pain and discomfort is dependent on the central nervous system, accurate quantitation is difficult. Objective measures such as the measurement of digital joint size exist, but are not very sensitive to anti-inflammatory drugs. Appreciation of pain is revealed by such tests as the duration of morning stiffness, and the articular index of joint tenderness but undoubtedly the development of analogue pain scores has helped considerably in the quantitation of drug action in this area of therapeutics (Revill et al., 1976). In this test the patient is confronted with a line of fixed length and marks on it with a pen how severe he feels his pain has been using the two indicators — one at each end of the line to help him (fig. 24). No other helping marks should be used. The patient's pain is then quantitated by measurement (in cms) from the 'no pain' end of the line and the scale can be made as large as is needed. In practice the scale loses sensitivity if, over a length of 10cm, it is divided up into more than 20 parts. Thus maximum pain is, in this case, scored as 20. More usually, smaller scales are used. This test is remarkably sensitive to changes in pain and is also repeatable with little variation by the patient. Such scales can be extended to quantitate other subjective phenomena such as sedation, or severity of dry mouth with an anticholinergic drug.

In epilepsy, it is conventional to rely on the patient's own assessment of his fit frequency to determine the effectiveness of drug therapy. This is unreliable since most patients have no warning of a fit, and some have no knowledge that a fit has taken place, particularly if fits occur only at night. Epileptic fits can be monitored by closed circuit television and EEG records but this is only practicable in a few specialised units. The EEG can be recorded in the same way as the ECG, using a few leads only, and a portable transmitter. However, analysis of the spike and wave activity has to be done by hand. There is promise for computer based analysis and within a few years a readily usable method should be available for the monitoring of response to anticonvulsant drugs. Hypnotics, antipsychotic, antianxiety and antidepressant drugs are probably the most difficult group of drugs to assess clinically in patients. A variety of different methods has been evolved, some objective and some subjective. With sedative drugs, tests of mental concentration have been devised, particularly as related to driving automobiles, and performance in such tests can be related to the plasma concentration of the drug in question (Seppala et al., 1979). A variety of rating scales have been proposed for the quantitation of the degree of anxiety or depression, but most are complicated and require skilled persons to undertake them (Hamilton, 1976). Certainly, in these fields, reliable and accurate methods of assessing drug action are badly needed. Considerable sophistication now exists in using rating scales in psychiatry but most of these were not developed for measuring drug effects.

In phase I trials of antipsychotic and antidepressant drugs, biochemical assessment of drug effects is possible by measuring changes in monoamine metabolism in cerebrospinal fluid.

7.4 Side Effects

It is important to realise that not only the benefits of drug therapy, but also its adverse effects should be closely assessed, particularly in clinical trials. It is no longer acceptable to ask the patients if the tablets are upsetting them or if they have had any ill effects they attribute to the drug. Such nonspecific questions should be accompanied by a self administered questionnaire which can be completed by the patient. Such a questionnaire will list most of the side effects which have been linked with the particular drug under study and the patient will be asked to indicate their presence or absence (Bulpitt et al., 1976). Such an approach reveals a much higher incidence of ill effects than traditional methods, not all of which will be associated with the drug. However, by comparison with a placebo or other treatment group, it will be much easier when studying numbers of patients to see which side effects are, and which are not, associated with the use of a particular drug.

8. Principles of Controlled Clinical Trials

There is no doubt that in the best hands the controlled clinical trial is a most powerful tool for the investigation of both new and old drugs. When a drug is administered to a patient, the response to it is dependent on a number of variable factors (table XXI). The aims of a controlled clinical (therapeutic) trial are to standardise or minimise those factors as far as possible. Many considerations and much careful planning are necessary for the successful conduct of a clinical trial. This section is only intended as a very brief overview of some important general principles. For more detailed discussion a number of useful general reference works are available (e.g. Good, 1976; Harris and Fitzgerald, 1970; WHO, 1975).

8.1 Initial Clinical Trials

When a new drug is first tested in man, it is likely that the study will in fact be an open one, with little attempt to overcome bias. In some cases the drug will be given to a normal volunteer and the pharmacological response assessed by ap-

Fig. 24. Line of fixed length (no more than 10cm) for patient to mark severity of pain (see text).

Table XXI. Factors affecting drug response in patients (after Lawrence, 1973)

1. Pharmacodynamics of drug
2. Pharmacokinetics of drug
3. Potential drug interactions
4. Receptor sensitivity
5. Mood, personality and attitude of patient
6. Mood, personality and attitude of doctor
7. Doctor's explanation to patient
8. Patient's prior experience of doctors and drugs
9. Patient's estimate of what ought to happen
10. Social environment of patient

propriate tests. In other cases, the drug will be given first to patients with the disease for which the drug has been developed. This is especially the case with new cytotoxic drugs. The drug is likely to be given to a very few patients, perhaps 6 to 10, under closely supervised conditions. The main aim is to see if the pharmacodynamics and pharmacokinetics of the drug are similar to what has been predicted from studies in animals. To this end, it is very useful if a method is already available for measuring plasma concentrations of the drug.

It is not a main aim at this stage to look for toxic effects, although comprehensive side effect and biochemical screening will be undertaken. The clinician has to satisfy himself that the animal toxicity studies are adequate to justify the risk of administering the drug for the first time to man. However, there is no doubt that it is possible to waste too much time in testing a drug in animals before studying it in man. The correct balance of information is difficult to achieve (Dollery and Davies, 1970).

8.2 Design of Clinical Trials

Much has been written about the need for clinical trials to be randomised and double blind for reliable evaluation of the efficacy of treatments (e.g. Byar et al., 1976). It is probably in the field of cancer that the randomised trial has attained its most sophisticated and rigid form (see Peto et al., 1976, 1977). In some situations this design is unnecessary and unsuitable. Thus, in early drug studies in man the double blind technique is not appropriate and in specialised techniques, where perhaps the rate of onset of a drug's action is being studied, the open study may be more appropriate, provided the observations are made as bias free as possible. The requirements for adequate design of

a trial depend on the disease and drug effect being investigated.

The aims of a clinical trial may vary from trial to trial but must always be very carefully formulated before the start of the study. The aim should be to answer *one* precisely framed question — with perhaps one or two subsidiary questions. The more questions that are posed initially, the more complicated the trial becomes, and the more likely is it that the trial will break down in practice. Questions that may be asked include 'is this drug effective?'; 'how does it compare with other drugs?'; 'in what patients is it of value?'; 'what is the most appropriate dosage?'

The clinical trial should be carried out in like or equivalent (homogeneous) groups of patients, so that the patients in each treatment group are as closely matched as possible for all known variables — such as age, sex, race, duration and severity of disease, etc. The best way of achieving homogeneous groups of patients is by random allocation — it is not acceptable to allot patients alternatively to the two treatments under test as the clinician will almost certainly become biased in his allocation of patients to the regimens. Once the decision to enter the patient into the trial is taken, he is allotted treatment A or B depending on an agreed randomisation schedule — such as the use of random number tables. In some trials it is important to stratify patients at random into evenly divided subgroups according to defined criteria that may affect outcome — such as trials in acute myocardial infarction in which patients are stratified according to the factors known to influence prognosis. Such stratification produces more homogeneous subgroups in which significant results may be obtained, that would otherwise be less apparent if only the group as a whole was considered. Random allocation does not guarantee like groups and it is still necessary to show that the treatment groups are comparable. The larger the number of patients in each group or subgroup, the greater the chance that they will be reasonably well matched.

Treatments should ideally be carried out *concurrently* because diseases may vary in severity with time. However, consecutive or crossover studies are acceptable in some diseases where the severity of the disease is known to be relatively stable (e.g. hypertension). Any ancillary treatments should be the same for each study group and also be defined, since they may influence the outcome. This requires much co-ordination of treatments in multicentre (multiclinic) trials, in which it is also particularly important to achieve comparable groups both within and between centres.

The methods of assessment of response should obviously be relevant to the aim of the trial and the drug effect being studied. The persons who should make the assessments (patient, doctor, auxiliary), their nature (subjective and/or objective), type (particularly in relation to statistical considerations) and timing (daily, weekly, etc. or before and after) require much consideration prior to commencing the trial.

Before the start of the trial it is important to formulate as simple an aim as possible, to write out a detailed protocol and to adhere to the protocol throughout the study. This latter requirement may seem trite but it is surprising how often the design of a trial is altered half way through because of an observation in an early patient. This will destroy the results of the whole trial.

8.3 Use of Controls

Although in early clinical trials, controls may not be needed, it is vital to introduce control observations as soon as possible (Hill, 1960). Controls may consist of patients receiving no treatment, a different treatment (active or inactive pharmacologically), or patients receiving the same treatment but at a different dose or according to a different schedule.

Whichever control method is used, it must be both valid and suitable in relation to the aim of the trial. Historical controls in most cases are not satisfactory, since with the passage of time many variables may have changed the course of the disease or influenced outcome. Usually, the treatments are studied in comparable groups of patients studied over the same period of time. It is hoped that the groups will be large enough to minimise any interpatient variability. When the variability of disease between individuals is a cause for concern, it is sometimes useful to use a patient as his own control, provided the disease process is stable. Here each patient is exposed to every available treatment having first one and then the other. In such a crossover design it is then important to ensure that each treatment both precedes and follows each other treatment the same number of times to avoid the risk of systematic bias or 'carry over' effect. It is sometimes necessary to include a control 'washout' period of adequate duration between

active treatment periods. The most usual way to arrange this is the use of a 'latin square' design (fig. 25), where each treatment is as likely to precede as to follow each other.

Having decided to include a control — should a placebo or pharmacologically active medication be used? In some circumstances it is unethical to give a placebo medication (e.g. in epilepsy or tuberculosis) and thus comparison of the active drug is made not with a pharmacologically inert placebo preparation but with the best available therapy. The placebo, which should match the active drug as closely as possible in colour, texture, shape and *taste*, will help to distinguish between the pharmacological effects of the drug and the psychological effects associated with the trial (e.g. more doctor interest, more frequent visits etc). It will also help to avoid false positive and false negative conclusions. It is important to realise that in clinical trials an inert placebo will produce benefit in a certain proportion of patients and will produce side effects in some patients (see Blackwell et al., 1972; Lasagna et al., 1958). Placebos are not totally inactive; rather they are pharmacologically inactive.

8.4 Double Blind Technique

Since both doctors and patients are capable of bias due to previously held beliefs, the double blind technique is used as a control device to prevent this bias from influencing the results. However, the use of a double blind technique does not guarantee that the results of the trial will be either the whole truth or beyond reproach. Many factors other than the design of the trial influence the adequacy and interpretation of the results (see section 9.2). However, if a double blind technique is used properly, it is a most useful way of assessing the therapeutic efficacy of a drug, since neither the patient nor the doctor will know the true nature of the medication

	Treatment periods			
	1	2	3	4
Patient No. 1	A	B	D	C
Patient No. 2	B	C	A	D
Patient No. 3	C	D	B	A
Patient No. 4	D	A	C	B

Fig. 25. 'Latin square' design to assign patients to treatments (viz A, B, C, D) so that each is as likely to precede as to follow each other.

that is taken, until the *end* of the trial. The temptation to break open a code half way through a trial should be resisted, even with drop-outs, since it makes it more likely that the true nature of the other treatments will be discovered.

When two active drug treatments are compared it is often difficult to arrange a double blind study. It is tempting to arrange for drug A to be reformulated to make it appear to be identical to drug B. This, however, will mean that the bioavailability of drug A might be different from the original formulation and tests to ensure that this is not so, are necessary. It is easier to use a double dummy technique where active drug A plus placebo drug B is compared with placebo drug A plus active drug B.

8.5 Statistical Considerations

It is possible only to consider this, as with many other aspects of controlled trials, in brief in this section. Readers are referred elsewhere for more detailed discussions (Hill, 1971). In designing a clinical trial, the initial hypothesis is usually that of 'no difference'; i.e. that there is no difference between treatment A and treatment B. It then has to be decided if the results obtained could be due to chance or if there is a real probability of difference between the two treatments. In most cases it can be assumed that the data is normally distributed and relatively simple statistical tests can be used. However, in some cases the normal distribution does not apply and then more sophisticated statistics are necessary.

Before the start of a trial it is usual to assume that a given level of probability (p) will be accepted. Thus, if p is less than 0.05, a difference would be found by chance only 5 times in every 100 studies. Thus, by implication, the null hypothesis would be considered wrong and the conclusion be that a statistical difference existed between the treatments. In some cases, it may be preferred only to accept a result if p is less than 0.01. It is important to realise however, that even here, there is a 1 in 100 risk of the treatments being different by chance alone. Thus, it is not surprising that, with many similar trials being performed with a drug in different population groups and with a different design, results sometimes appear to be conflicting.

Sometimes too, results may be found that suggest that treatment A tends to be better than treatment B but in statistical terms there is no signifi-

cant difference between them. This may be seen with small patient numbers. It should be noted that failure to find a difference between two treatments does not necessarily mean that they are equal, but rather that any difference which might exist could not be detected with the number of patients studied. It may sometimes mean (e.g. where the response rate is high with both treatments) that any difference is not of much clinical importance. On the other hand, a statistically significant difference between two treatments may not be clinically important (i.e. is the magnitude of the difference worthwhile), such as on average an extra 15 minutes sleep between two hypnotics (Wade and Waterhouse, 1977). Similar considerations apply in bioavailability studies (see chapter VI).

It must be emphasised that statistical analysis, however good, will not salvage a trial that is poorly designed or poorly conducted.

8.6 Patient Numbers

It is often very difficult to know how many patients will be needed in a clinical trial in order that the result will be meaningful. In general, the mistake is to use too few patients. The smaller the expected difference between two treatments, the greater the number of patients required to achieve a significant result (fig. 26). The clinical investigator is best advised to consult with a statistician at the design stage of a trial. The statistician will need to know what magnitude of difference the clinician is interested in detecting (e.g. halving the death rate) and what risks he will tolerate of missing a difference that does genuinely exist. It is particularly difficult to obtain adequate numbers of patients in long term studies; for example, in the assessment of whether long term β-adrenoceptor blockade will reduce the death rate from myocardial infarction. The study of a few dozen patients can in most cases detect an ideal treatment which prevents more than 2 thirds of the deaths. However, in cases like the example quoted, where the death rate is small, and the interest is in detecting a small reduction in the death rate, then it will be necessary to follow several hundred patients over a number of years.

8.7 Sequential Analysis

This sophisticated technique has been widely used for trials on acute disease and allows a trial to

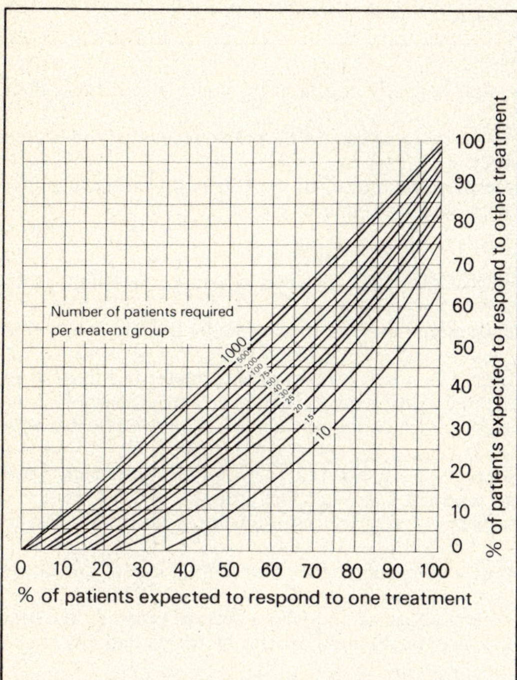

Fig. 26. Number of patients required for a clinical trial — assuming a minimum chance (50%) of successful conclusion at 5% level of significance ($p < 0.05$) [after Clark and Downie: Lancet 2: 1357, 1966; by permission of author and editor).

The treatment with the greater response is plotted on the horizontal scale. The graph can be used as a guide to:

a) Indicate the smallest number of patients likely to provide results from which significant conclusions can be drawn.

b) Determine from the actual number of patients studied, whether the observed difference in response is large enough to be significant at the 5% level.

be continually monitored and to be stopped when a significant result is achieved. In this way the numbers of patients involved can be kept to a minimum, and ethical objections can be best resolved. The most familiar of these procedures requires allocation of the subjects in pairs to two treatments (Armitage, 1960). Other designs have been developed which do not involve pairwise allocation (Day, 1969).

8.8 Ethical Considerations

In the conduct of a controlled clinical trial, whether in normal volunteers or patients, it is important to consider the ethical aspects of the study and nowadays all protocols should be vetted by an independent ethical review body. In addition, each participant in the study should give their informed consent to the study. Some of the important and vexed ethical aspects which can arise are considered in more detailed clinical trial publications (e.g. Smith, 1977; Vere, 1976) and in the original concepts outlined by Bradford Hill (Hill, 1963). Scientific medical ethics are founded on the moral principles and standards of reason that are a part of ethics generally, and on the cumulative wisdom and experience of scientific knowledge and practice (see Reiser et al., 1977).

Table XXII. Rational drug prescribing — decisions and considerations

---

A. Decision
1. Diagnosis
   a) Accurate, or
   b) At least probable
2. Disease understanding
   a) Pathophysiology
   b) Natural history
3. To treat or not
   a) Is a drug necessary at all?
     i) no need to treat?
     ii) other form of treatment more appropriate?
   b) If a drug is necessary
     i) what benefit is expected?
     ii) what harm may result from a drug?
     iii) what harm will result if a drug is not used?
4. Drug and regimen
   a) Choice of drug, preparation, route of administration
   b) Selection of an appropriate dosage and dose schedule (patient factors)
   c) Duration of treatment (nature of disease)

B. Consideration
1. Compatibility between drug and patient (adverse effects)
2. Compatibility between drugs (interactions)
3. Review decision in 4a, b above if necessary

C. Action
1. Write prescription (legibly)
2. Instruct the patient about:
   a) The therapeutic aim and that the potential benefit is expected to outweigh the risk of side effects
   b) Reporting and action to take on any important side effects
   c) How to take or use the medication (e.g. oral dose in relation to food, need to complete prescribed course, correct use of an aerosol asthma inhaler, etc)
3. Follow up
   a) Of symptoms. Titration of dose
   b) Check compliance with medication instructions

Table XXIII. Principles of assessing reports of therapeutic trials

1. *Basic principles*
   a) Any individual trial provides limited information — what happens in a selected group of patients under defined conditions
   b) One study cannot provide all evidence — the answers to the many questions that may need to be considered in evaluating a drug cannot be provided by any one study
   c) Statements made must be critically evaluated — statements made and conclusions drawn by authors cannot necessarily be accepted as read — critical faculties must be maintained at all times

2. *Important general requirements*
   a) Appropriate controls — were controls adequate or not necessary to avoid bias or reduce variation which might influence the results?
   b) Appropriate and adequate method of assessing therapeutic effects — were methods fully defined, relevant to aims and reproducible?
   c) Adequate number of subjects — the smaller the difference between two drugs the greater the number of patients required to achieve a significant result (failure to find a difference between two drugs does not necessarily mean that they are equal, but rather that any difference which might exist could not be detected with the number of patients used)
   d) Homogeneous population — when two or more treatments are compared, were groups sufficiently well matched (allocation of patients at random to treatment does not guarantee like groups)
   e) Appropriate duration of treatment — was therapy sufficiently long for optimum drug effect (adverse or favourable) and for the nature of the disease?
   f) Appropriate dosage — were dosages chosen adequate (if a dose-effect study) or comparable (if two drugs being compared)?
   g) Measurement of side effects — were methods of assessment adequate and with a defined protocol (the incidence of side effects depends on the care with which they are sought and how and by whom patients are interrogated)?
   h) Appropriate statistical validation — where necessary (most trials fall down before this point is reached)
      N.B. Elaborate statistics cannot validate a poorly designed or executed trial, make unlike treatment groups equal, or be used to extend the results obtained in a selected group of patients under defined conditions to individualised use of a drug in actual clinical practice

3. *Interpretation of results and conclusions*
   a) Is the result clinically significant (would the patient benefit) or acceptable (does it satisfy *current* desirable criteria)?
   b) Are comparisons with other drug trials (e.g. in discussion) valid? — was a comparison made with the *currently* accepted treatment of choice? If so, was the comparison valid. If not, was such a comparison unnecessary or was a comparison made against a superseded treatment of choice? Is the discussion a fair review of reliable results?
   c) Are the author's conclusions justified? — conclusions must be made on the basis of what has been established in the trial and not extended beyond these findings.

9. Clinical Pharmacological Principles in Drug Prescribing

9.1 The Drug Prescription

The decisions and considerations to be made in connection with the prescribing of modern drugs involve the same analytical principles as does sophisticated differential diagnosis (Binns, 1975; Smithells, 1975; see table XXII). Yet, the prescription is traditionally made in a hurry at the very last moment of the consultation or at the crowded time of discharge from hospital, with insufficient time left for informing the patient about the therapeutic aims or for providing appropriate instructions in use of the medication (Kellaway and McCrae, 1975, 1979). Worse than this, the illegibility of prescriptions is a well known joke, even within the medical profession. It is high time to change these poor habits.

The causes of unnecessary, unsuitable or ineffective therapy include inadequacy of time and facilities available for proper diagnosis, ignorance of the cause and natural history of disease, inadequacies of teaching in clinical pharmacology and drug evaluation, ineffectiveness of official advice about drug usage relative to that given by industry, and pressures exerted by patients and colleagues (see Hemminiki, 1975; Modell and Houde, 1958). Many patients expect a remedy for any symptom and it is the doctor's duty to explain to them that drugs are not needed for self limiting diseases or short lasting minor symptoms of unknown nature. It is a regrettable fact that many prescriptions in these situations come to resemble conditioned reflexes. It is even more regrettable that many drugs are used in a stereotyped manner, in fixed, often too low dosage schedules, and with little regard to basic principles of pharmacokinetics and drug response (Boethius and Sjoqvist, 1978).

9.2 Assessing Reports of Therapeutic Trials

New drugs are not necessarily better than the old; but they are almost always more expensive. Unexpected and important side effects can still occur after marketing of a new drug, even though it has complied with all the required tests. Familiarity with the use of a particular drug is a valid reason for continuing to use it until adequate and convincing reasons for change are apparent. Such evidence is generally based on the results of therapeutic trials, but they must be evaluated critically (table XXIII) because clinical trials vary greatly in quality and value (Lionel and Herxheimer, 1970). Statements made cannot neces-

sarily be accepted as read.

The fundamental problem with assessment of drug literature lies in the varying acceptability of published reports and in the subsequent interpretation and use of the data. Many factors, apart from study design (see section 8), may influence date in therapeutic trials. For example, even if randomisation was made were the treatment groups reasonably well matched, were doses of drugs under study equivalent, were patient numbers large enough to detect any differences, was the drug taken as intended, who made the observations and how were they made, etc (see Lionel and Herxheimer, 1970). The enthusiasm for a new drug generally changes with the passage of time and thus the nature and quality of evidence depends on the adequacy of study and extent of actual clinical experience at any given time of publication (fig. 27).

As discussed in section 8, in its most rigorous form, a therapeutic trial to establish the efficacy of a new drug demands homogeneous groups of patients, concurrently treated in different ways (i.e. other standard drug or treatment). The less the differences within the groups and between them (apart from the treatment) the better the design of the trial. What constitutes an adequately designed trial necessarily varies, depending on the disease and drug effect being evaluated. Each trial however, affords precise and limited information and can only show what on average is likely to happen

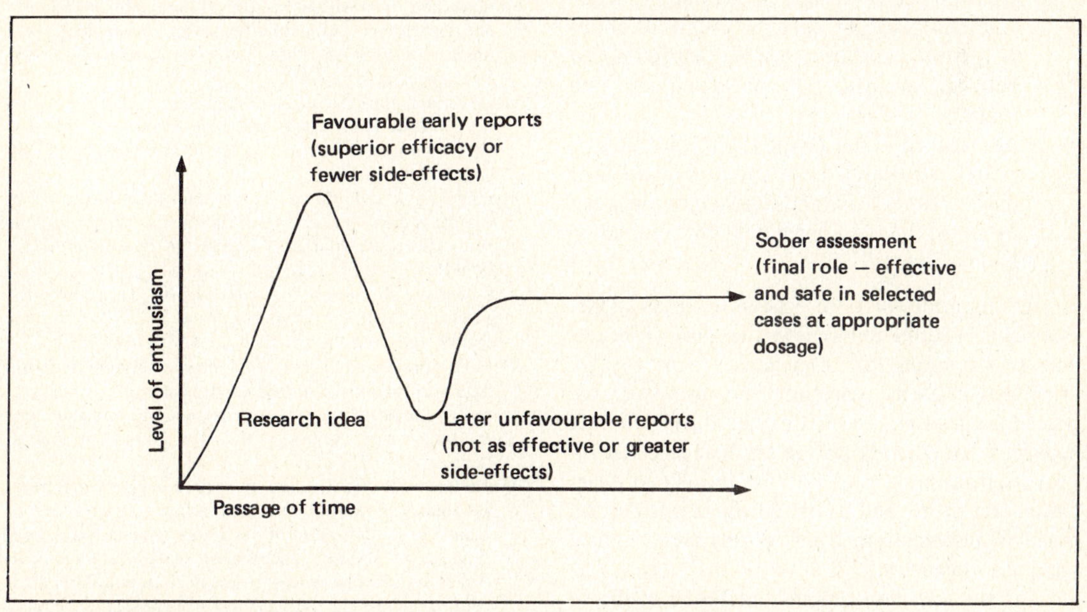

Fig. 27. Enthusiasm and therapeutic role for a new drug with the passage of time.

to a selected group of patients under defined conditions. Indeed, the more rigid the methodology of the trial the more artificial the conditions are likely to be and the narrower the general applicability of the results. These limitations must be borne in mind when extending the results (efficacy or adverse effects) of a particular therapeutic trial to clinical practice. Thus many trials are conducted under conditions that are far removed from those in which drugs are ultimately used, and it is a major objective for the future to evaluate drugs and monitor drug use under actual conditions of practice (Lasagna, 1974). There is an important balance between clinical sense and clinical science (Armstrong, 1977).

9.3 Utilisation of Existing Drugs and Individualisation of Therapy

Better utilisation of existing drugs and individualisation of drug therapy have increased in importance for three reasons:

1) The development of new, effective drugs is becoming more difficult, because the pharmaceutical industry is facing complex and far reaching demands from governmental health authorities regarding the documentation of drug safety and efficacy.
2) There is a tendency among patients and pressure groups to be sceptical about drugs and their usage by doctors. Decisions about drugs must not be made by self-interested political groups, but by scientists (see Melmon, 1976).
3) As outlined in this chapter, clinical pharmacological research has shown that much of the variability in drug response between patients can be explained by individual kinetic factors.

One important task for academic clinical pharmacology is active involvement in drug information programmes for clinicians, focussing on principles of drug selection and use (e.g. see Breckenridge et al., 1978; Levy et al., 1977) — a necessary complement to the product oriented information reaching doctors from individual pharmaceutical firms, and to the consumer protection oriented information from governmental drug regulatory agencies.

This and the other chapters in this book aim to make a start in this direction.

Further Reading

Bergman, U.; Grimsson, A. and Westerholm, B.: Drug Utilization Studies — Methods and Applications (World Health Organization, Regional Office of Europe, Copenhagen 1978).

Breckenridge, A.: Advanced Medicine Symposia: Topics in Therapeutics 1 (Pitman, London 1975).

Brodie, B.B. and Gillette, J.R.: Handbook of Experimental Pharmacology, Vol. XXVIII Concepts in Biochemical Pharmacology I and II (Springer-Verlag, Berlin 1971).

Gibaldi, M.: Biopharmaceutics and Clinical Pharmacokinetics 2nd ed (Lea and Febiger, Philadelphia 1977).

Gillette, J.R. and Mitchell, J.R.: Handbook of Experimental Pharmacology, Vol. XXVIII Concepts in Biochemical Pharmacology III (Springer-Verlag, Berlin 1975).

Goldstein, A.; Aronow, L. and Kalman, S.M.: Principles of Drug Action: The Basis of Pharmacology, 2nd ed (Wiley, New York 1974).

Goodman, L.S. and Gilman, A.: The Pharmacological Basis of Therapeutics, 5th ed (Macmillan, New York 1975).

Jouhar, A.J. and Grayson, M.F.: International Aspects of Drug Evaluation and Usage (Churchill Livingstone, Edinburgh 1973).

Laurence, D.R.: Clinical Pharmacology, 5th ed (Churchill Livingstone, London 1979).

Melmon, K.L. and Morelli, H.F.: Clinical Pharmacology: Basic Principles in Therapeutics, 2nd ed (Macmillan, New York 1978).

World Health Organisation: Technical Report Series No. 446, Clinical Pharmacology: Scope, Organization, Training (WHO, Geneva 1972).

References

Aarbakke, J.: Clinical pharmacokinetics of phenylbutazone. Clinical Pharmacokinetics 3: 369 (1978).

Alexanderson, B.: Pharmacokinetics of desmethylimipramine and nortriptyline in man after single and multiple oral doses — a crossover study. European Journal of Clinical Pharmacology 5: 1 (1972).

Alexanderson, B.: Prediction of steady-state plasma levels of nortriptyline from single oral dose kinetics: A study in twins. European Journal of Clinical Pharmacology 6: 44 (1973).

Alexanderson, B. and Borga, O.: Interindividual differences in plasma protein binding of nortriptyline in man — a twin study. European Journal of Clinical Pharmacology 4: 196 (1972).

Alexanderson, B.; Evans, D.A. and Sjoqvist, F.: Steady-state plasma levels of nortriptyline in twins: Influence of genetic factors and drug therapy. Brit. Med. J. 4: 764 (1969).

Alexanderson, B. and Sjoqvist, F.: Individual differences in the pharmacokinetics of monomethylated tricyclic antidepressants; role of genetic and environmental factors and clinical importance. Annals of the New York Academy of Sciences 179: 739 (1971).

Alexanderson, B. and Sjoqvist, F.: Pharmacokinetic and genetic studies of nortriptyline and desmethylimipramine in man. The predictability of therapeutic plasma levels from single-dose plasma concentration data; in Okita and Acheson (Eds) Pharmacology and the Future of Man, Proceedings of the 5th International Congress of Pharmacology, Vol. 3, p.150 (Karger, Basel 1973).

Alvan, G.: Individual differences in the disposition of drugs metabolised in the body. Clinical Pharmacokinetics 3: 155 (1978).

Alvan, G.; Lindgren, J.E.; Bogentoft, C. and Ericsson, O.: Plasma kinetics of methaqualone in man after single oral doses. European Journal of Clinical Pharmacology 6: 187 (1973).

Alvan, G.; Piafsky, K.; Lind, M.; von Bahr, C.: Effect of pentobarbital on the disposition of alprenolol. Clinical Pharmacology and Therapeutics 22: 316 (1977).

Alvares, A.P.: Interactions between environmental chemicals and drug biotransformation in man. Clinical Pharmacokinetics 3: 462 (1978).

Amdisen, A.: Serum level monitoring and clinical pharmacokinetics of lithium. Clinical Pharmacokinetics 2: 73 (1977).

Armitage, P.: Sequential Medical Trials (Blackwell, Oxford 1960).

Armstrong, D.: Clinical sense and clinical science. Social Science and Medicine 11: 599 (1977).

Arvidsson, A.; Borga, O. and Alvan, G.: Renal excretion of cefapyrin and cefaloridine: evidence for saturable reabsorption. Clinical Pharmacology and Therapeutics. In press (1979).

Asberg, M. and Sjoqvist, F.: On the role of plasma level monitoring of tricyclic antidepressants in clinical practice. Communications in Psychopharmacology 2: 381 (1978).

Azarnoff, D.L.: Proceedings of conference on implications of blood level assays of therapeutic agents. Clinical Pharmacology and Therapeutics 16 (pt 2): 129 (1975).

Balter, M.B.; Levine, J. and Manheimer, D.I.: Cross-national study of the extent of antianxiety/sedative drug use. New England Journal of Medicine 290: 769 (1974).

Benowitz, N.L. and Meister, W.: Clinical pharmacokinetics of lignocaine. Clinical Pharmacokinetics 3: 177 (1978).

Bertilsson, L.: Clinical pharmacokinetics of carbamazepine. Clinical Pharmacokinetics 3: 128 (1978).

Binns, T.B.: The absorption of drugs from the alimentary tract, lungs and skin. British Journal of Hospital Medicine 6: 133 (1971).

Binns, T.B.: Sensible prescribing. I — The context of prescribing. Practitioner 214: 118 (1975).

Blackwell, B.: The drug defaulter. Clinical Pharmacology and Therapeutics 13: 841 (1972).

Blackwell, B.: Patient compliance. New England Journal of Medicine 289: 249 (1973).

Blackwell, B.: Treatment adherence. British Journal of Psychiatry 129: 513 (1976).

Blackwell, B.; Bloomfield, S.S. and Buncher, C.R.: Demonstration to medical students of placebo-responses and non-drug factors. Lancet 1: 1279 (1972).

Blaschke, T.F.: Protein binding and kinetics of drugs in liver disease. Clinical Pharmacokinetics 2: 32 (1977).

Bloom, P.M. and Nelp, W.P.: Relationship of the excretion of tritiated digoxin to renal function. American Journal of the Medical Sciences 251: 133 (1966).

Bochner, F.; Hooper, W.D.; Tyrer, J.H. and Eadie, M.J.: Factors involved in an outbreak of phenytoin intoxication. Journal of Neurological Sciences 16: 481 (1972).

Boethius, G.: Recording of drug prescriptions in the county of Jamtland, Sweden. Pattern of drug usage in 16,600 individuals 1970-1975. Acta Medica Scandinavica 202: 241 (1977).

Boethius, G. and Sjoqvist, F.: Doses and dosage intervals of drugs — clinical practice versus pharmacokinetic principles. Clinical Pharmacology and Therapeutics 24: 255 (1978).

Bolme, P.; Eriksson, M. and Stintzing, G.: The gastrointestinal absorption of penicillin V in children with suspected coeliac disease. Acta Paediatrica Scandinavica 66: 573 (1977).

Boman, G.; Lundgren, P. and Stjernstrom, G.: Mechanism of the inhibitory effect of PAS granules, on the absorption of rifampicin: Adsorption of rifampicin by an excipient, bentonite, European Journal of Clinical Pharmacology 8: 293 (1975).

Borga, O.; Piafsky, K.M. and Nilsen, O.G.: Plasma protein binding of basic drugs. I. Selective displacement from α_1-acid glycoprotein by tris (2-butoxyethyl) phosphate. Clinical Pharmacology and Therapeutics 22: 539 (1977).

Breckenridge, A.; Orme, M.L'E.; Wesseling, H.; Bending, M. and Lewis, R.J.: Increased rates of drug oxidation in man; in Morselli, Garattini and Cohen (Eds) Drug Interactions, p.223 (Raven Press, New York 1974).

Breckenridge, A.; Orme, M.; Serlin, M.J.; Davidson, A.S. and Lowe, J.F.: Postgraduate education in therapeutics: experience in Merseyside. British Medical Journal 2: 671 (1978).

Breimer, D.D.: Clinical pharmacokinetics of hypnotics. Clinical Pharmacokinetics 2: 93 (1977).

Brodie, B.B.: in Binns (Ed) Absorption and Distribution of Drugs (Livingstone, London 1964).

Buchtal, F. and Lennox-Buchtal, M.A.: Phenobarbital. Relation of serum concentration to control of seizures; in Woodbury, Penry and Schmidt (Eds) Antiepileptic Drugs p.335 (Raven Press, New York 1972).

Bulpitt, C.J.; Shaw, K.M.; Hodes, C. and Bloom, A.: The symptom patterns of treated diabetic patients. Journal of Chronic Diseases 29: 571 (1976).

Byar, D.P.; Simon, R.M.; Friedewald, W.T.; Schlesselman, J.J.; DeMets, D.L.; Ellenberg, J.H.; Gail, M.H. and Ware, J.H.: Randomized clinical trials. New England Journal of Medicine 295: 74 (1976).

Caffruny, E.L.: Renal tubular handling of drugs. American Journal of Medicine 62: 491 (1977).

Clark, C.J. and Downie, C.C.: A method for the rapid determination of the number of patients to include in a controlled clinical trial. Lancet 2: 1357 (1966).

Clark, T.J.H. and Hetzel, M.R.: Diurnal variation of asthma. British Journal of Diseases of the Chest 71: 87 (1977).

Clarke, J.M.; Hamer, J.; Skeleton, J.R.; Taylor, S. and Venning, G.R.: The rhythm of the normal human heart. Lancet 2: 508 (1976).

Conney, A.H.; Pantuck, E.J.; Hsiao, K.C.; Garland, W.A.; Anderson, K.E.; Alvares, A.P. and Kappas, A.: Enhanced phenacetin metabolism in humans fed charcoal broiled beef. Clinical Pharmacology and Therapeutics 20: 633 (1976).

Conney, A.H.; Pantuck, E.J.; Pantuck, C.B.; Buening, M.; Jerina, D.M.; Fortner, J.G.; Alvares, A.P.; Anderson, K.E. and Kappas, A.: Role of environment and diet in the regulation of human drug metabolism; in Estabrook and Lindenlaub (Eds) The Induction of Drug Metabolism (Schattauer Verlag, Stuttgart 1979).

Crossland, J.: Modern views on pharmacology II — Drug metabolism. Practitioner 206: 293 (1971).

Danhof, M. and Breimer, D.D.: Therapeutic drug monitoring in saliva. Clinical Pharmacokinetics 3: 39 (1978).

Davies, D.S. and Prichard, B.N.C.: Biological Effects of Drugs in Relation to their Plasma Concentrations (Macmillan,

London 1973).

Day, N.E.: Two-stage designs for clinical trials. Biometrics 25: 111 (1969).

Dettli, L.: Drug dosage in renal disease. Clinical Pharmacokinetics 1: 126 (1976).

Dollery, C.T. and Davies, D.S.: The conduct of initial drug studies in man. British Medical Bulletin 26: 233 (1970).

Drayer, D.E.: Pathways of drug metabolism in man. Medical Clinics of North America 58: 927 (1974).

Drayer, D.E.: Pharmacologically active metabolites: Therapeutic and toxic activities, plasma and urine data in man, accumulation in renal failure. Clinical Pharmacokinetics 1: 426 (1976).

Drayer, D.E.: Active drug metabolites and renal failure. American Journal of Medicine 62: 486 (1977).

Drayer, D.E. and Reidenberg, M.M.: Clinical consequences of polymorphic acetylation of basic drugs. Clinical Pharmacology and Therapeutics 22: 251 (1977).

Duggan, D.E.: The accumulation of chlorothiazide and related saluretic agents by isolated renal tubules. Journal of Pharmacology and Experimental Therapeutics 152: 122 (1966).

du Souich, P.; McLean, A.L.; Lalka, D.; Erill, S. and Gibaldi, M.: Pulmonary disease and drug kinetics. Clinical Pharmacokinetics 3: 257 (1978).

Eichelbaum, M.: Drug metabolism in thyroid disease. Clinical Pharmacokinetics 1: 339 (1976).

Eichelbaum, M.; Spannbrucker, N. and Dengler, H.J.: A probably genetic defect of the metabolism of sparteine; in Gorrod (Ed) Biological Oxidation of Nitrogen p.113 (Elsevier/North Holland Biomedical Press, Amsterdam 1978).

Elfstrom, J.: Drug pharmacokinetics in the postoperative period. Clinical Pharmacokinetics 4: 16 (1979).

Ellard, G.A.: Variations between individuals and populations in the acetylation of isoniazid and its significance for the treatment of pulmonary tuberculosis. Clinical Pharmacology and Therapeutics 19: 610 (1976).

Ellard, G.A. and Gammon, P.T.: Pharmacokinetics of isoniazid metabolism in man. Journal of Pharmacokinetics and Biopharmaceutics 4: 83 (1976).

Ellard, G.A. and Gammon, P.T.: Acetylator phenotyping of tuberculosis patients using matrix isoniazid or sulphadimidine and its prognostic significance for treatment with several intermittent isoniazid-containing regimens. British Journal of Clinical Pharmacology 4: 5 (1977).

Ellard, G.A.; Mitchison, D.A.; Girling, D.J.; Nunn, A.J. and Fox, W.: The hepatic toxicity of isoniazid among rapid and slow acetylators of the drug. American Review of Respiratory Disease 118: 628 (1978).

Estabrook, R.W. and Lindenlaub, E. (Eds): The Induction of Drug Metabolism. Symposia Medica Hoechst 14 (Schattauer Verlag, Stuttgart 1979).

Estabrook, R.; Gillette, J. and Leibman, K.: Microsomes and Drug Oxidation (Williams and Wilkins, Baltimore 1972).

Fabre, J. and Balant, L.: Renal failure, drug pharmacokinetics and drug action. Clinical Pharmacokinetics 1: 99 (1976).

Fremstad, D.; Bergerud, K.; Haffner, J.F.W. and Lunde, P.K.M.: Increased protein binding of quinidine after surgery: A preliminary report. European Journal of Clinical Pharmacology 10: 441 (1976).

Garrett, E.R.: The physico-chemical and pharmacokinetic bases for the biopharmaceutical evaluation of drug biological availability in pharmaceutical formulations. Acta Pharmacologica et Toxicologica 29 (Suppl. 3): 1 (1971).

Gibaldi, M.: Biopharmaceutics and Clinical Pharmacokinetics, 2nd ed (Lea and Febiger, Philadelphia 1977).

Gibaldi, M.; Boyes, R.M. and Feldman, S.: Influence of first-pass effect on availability of drugs on oral administration. Journal of Pharmaceutical Sciences 60: 1338 (1971).

Gillette, J.R.: A perspective on the role of chemically reactive metabolites of foreign compounds in toxicity. Biochemical Pharmacology 23: 2785 (1974).

Glauser, S.C.: Drug metabolism: Conjugations and multiple pathways. Medical Clinics of North America 58: 945 (1974).

Goldman, P.; Peppercorn, M.A. and Goldin, B.R.: Drugs metabolized by intestinal microflora; in Morselli, Garattini and Cohen (Eds) Drug Interactions, p.91 (Raven Press, New York 1974).

Goldstein, A.; Aronow, L. and Kalman, S.M.: Principles of Drug Action: The Basis of Pharmacology, 2nd ed (Wiley, New York 1974).

Good, C.S.: The Principles and Practice of Clinical Trials (Churchill Livingstone, Edinburgh 1976).

Gram, L.: Plasma level monitoring of tricyclic antidepressant therapy. Clinical Pharmacokinetics 2: 237 (1977).

Greenblatt, D.J. and Koch-Weser, J.: Intramuscular injection of drugs. New England Journal of Medicine 295: 542 (1976).

Grundin, R.; Moldeus, P.; Orrenius, S.; Borg, K.O.; Skanberg, I. and Bahr, von C.: The possible role of cytochrome P-450 in the liver "first pass elimination" of a β-receptor blocking drug. Acta Pharmacologica et Toxicologica 35: 242 (1974).

Gugler, R. and Azarnoff, D.L.: The clinical use of plasma drug concentrations. Rational Drug Therapy 10: 1 (Nov. 1976).

Hamilton, M.: Comparative value of rating scales. British Journal of Clinical Pharmacology (Suppl. 1) 3: 58 (1976).

Hammer, W. and Sjoqvist, F.: Plasma levels of monomethylated tricyclic antidepressants during treatment with imipramine-like compounds. Life Sciences 6: 1895 (1967).

Hanngren, A.; Borga, O. and Sjoqvist, F.: Inactivation of isoniazid (INH) in Swedish tuberculous patients before and during treatment with para-aminosalicylic acid (PAS). Scandinavian Journal of Respiratory Diseases 51: 61 (1970).

Hansen, J.M. and Christensen, L.K.: Drug interactions with oral sulphonylurea hypoglycaemic drugs. Drugs 13: 24 (1977).

Harris, E.L. and Fitzgerald, J.D.: The Principles and Practice of Clinical Trials (Livingstone, Edinburgh 1970).

Hayes, A.H.: Intravenous infusion of lidocaine in the control of ventricular arrhythmias; in Scott and Julian (Eds) Lidocaine in the Treatment of Ventricular Arrhythmias, p.189 (Livingstone, Edinburgh 1971).

Heilman, K.: Therapeutic Systems. Pattern-Specific Drug Delivery: Concept and Development, p.52 (Thieme, Stuttgart 1978).

Hemminki, E.: Review of literature on the factors affecting drug prescribing. Social Science and Medicine 9: 111 (1975).

Hill, A.B.: Controlled Clinical Trials (Blackwell, Oxford 1960).

Hill, A.B.: Medical ethics and controlled trials. British Medical Journal 1: 1043 (1963).

Hill, A.B.: Principles of Medical Statistics, 9th ed (Lancet, London 1971).

Holman, R.R. and Turner, R.C.: Basal normoglycaemia attained with chlorpropamide in mild diabetes. Metabolism 27: 539 (1978).

Howe-Davies, S.; Holman, R.R.; Phillips, M. and Turner, R.C.: Home blood sampling for plasma glucose assay in control of diabetes. British Medical Journal 2: 596 (1978).

Hvidberg, E. and Dam, M.: Clinical pharmacokinetics of anticonvulsants. Clinical Pharmacokinetics 1: 161 (1976).

Iisalo, E.: Clinical pharmacokinetics of digoxin. Clinical Pharmacokinetics 2: 1 (1977).

Jeffery, W.H.; Ahlin, T.A.; Goren, C. and Hardy, W.R.: Loss of warfarin effect after occupational insecticide exposure. Journal of the American Medical Association 236: 2881 (1976).

Johnsson, G. and Regardh, C-G.: Clinical pharmacokinetics of β-adrenoreceptor blocking drugs. Clinical Pharmacokinetics 1: 233 (1976).

Jusko, W.J.: Role of tobacco smoking in pharmacokinetics. Journal of Pharmacokinetics and Biopharmaceutics 6: 7 (1978).

Jusko, W.J. and Gretch, M.: Plasma and tissue protein binding of drugs in pharmacokinetics. Drug Metabolism Reviews 5: 43 (1976).

Kalow, W.: Pharmacogenetics: Heredity and the Response to Drugs (Saunders, Philadelphia 1962).

Kalow, W.: Contributions of hereditary factors in the response to drugs. Federation Proceedings 24: 1259 (1965).

Kalow, W.; Kadar, D.; Inaba, T. and Tang, B.K.: A case of deficiency of N-hydroxylation of amobarbital. Clinical Pharmacology and Therapeutics 21: 530 (1977).

Kalow, W.; Tang, B.K.; Kadar, D. and Inaba, T.: Distinctive patterns of amobarbital metabolites. Clinical Pharmacology and Therapeutics 24: 576 (1978).

Karlsson, E.: Clinical pharmacokinetics of procainamide. Clinical Pharmacokinetics 3: 97 (1978).

Karlsson, E. and Molin, L.: Polymorphic acetylation of procaine amide in healthy subjects. Acta Medica Scandinavica 197: 299 (1975).

Kato, R.: Drug metabolism under pathological and abnormal physiological states in animals and man. Xenobiotica 7: 25 (1977).

Keberle, H.: Physico-chemical factors of drugs affecting absorption, distribution, and excretion. Acta Pharmacologica et Toxicologica 29 (Suppl. 3): 30 (1971).

Kellaway, G.S.M. and McCrae, E.: Non-compliance and errors of drug administration in patients discharged from acute general medical wards. New Zealand Medical Journal 81: 508 (1975).

Kellaway, G.S.M. and McCrae, E.: The effect of counselling on compliance-failure in patient drug therapy. New Zealand Medical Journal 89: 161 (1979).

Klotz, U.: Pathophysiological and disease-induced changes in drug distribution volume: Pharmacokinetic implications. Clinical Pharmacokinetics 1: 204 (1976).

Koch-Weser, J.: Correlation of serum concentrations and pharmacological effects of antiarrhythmic drugs. Proceedings of the 5th International Congress on Pharmacology, San Francisco 1972, vol. 3, p.69 (Karger, Basel 1973).

Koch-Weser, J.: Serum procainamide levels as therapeutic guides. Clinical Pharmacokinetics 2: 389 (1977).

Kragh-Sorenson, P.W.: Correlation between plasma levels of nortriptyline and clinical effects. Communications in Psychopharmacology 2: 451 (1978).

Krishnaswamy, K.: Drug metabolism and pharmacokinetics in malnutrition. Clinical Pharmacokinetics 3: 216 (1978).

Kristensen, M.B.: Drug interactions and clinical pharmacokinetics. Clinical Pharmacokinetics 1: 351 (1976).

Kutt, H.: Pharmacodynamic and pharmacokinetic measurements of antiepileptic drugs. Clinical Pharmacology and Therapeutics 16: 243 (1974).

Kutt, H.; Wolk, M.; Scherman, R. and McDowell, F.: Insufficient parahydroxylation as a cause of diphenylhydantoin toxicity. Neurology 14: 542 (1964).

Lasagna, L.: A plea for 'naturalistic' study of medicines. European Journal of Clinical Pharmacology 7: 1 (1974).

Lasagna, L.; Laties, V.G. and Dihan, J.L.: Further studies on the pharmacology of placebo administration. Journal of Clinical Investigation 37: 533 (1958).

Lawrence, D.: Clinical Pharmacology (Churchill Livingstone, London 1973).

Levy, M.; Kletter-Hemo, D.; Nir, I. and Eliakim, M.: Drug utilization and adverse drug reactions in medical patients. Comparison of two persons, 1969-72 and 1973-76. Israel Journal of Medical Sciences 13: 1065 (1977).

Lionel, N.D.W. and Herxheimer, A.: Assessing reports of therapeutic trials. British Medical Journal 3: 637 (1970).

Lund, L.: Bestamning av fenytoin i plasma — Kliniska erfarenheter. Lakartidningen 68: 73 (1971).

Lund, L.: Anticonvulsant effect of diphenylhydantoin relative to plasma levels. A prospective three-year study in ambulant patients with generalised epileptic seizures. Archives of Neurology 31: 289 (1974).

Lunde, P.K.M.; Frislid, K. and Hansteen, V.: Disease and acetylation polymorphism. Clinical Pharmacokinetics 2: 182 (1977).

Mahgoub, A.; Idel, J.R.; Dring, L.G.; Lancaster, K. and Smith, R.L.: Polymorphic hydroxylation of debrisoquine in man. Lancet 2: 584 (1977).

Mandelli, M.; Tognoni, G. and Garattini, S.: Clinical pharmacokinetics of diazepam. Clinical Pharmacokinetics 3: 72 (1978).

Martin, B.K.: Potential effect of the plasma proteins on drug distribution. Nature 207: 274 (1965).

Mattson, R.H.; Cramer, J.A.; Williamson, P.D. and Novelly, R.A.: Valproic acid in epilepsy: clinical and pharmacological effects. Annals of Neurology 3: 20 (1978).

Mazullo, J.M.: The non-pharmacologic basis of therapeutics. Clinical Pharmacology and Therapeutics 13: 157 (1972).

Meffin, P.J.; Birkett, D.J. and Wing, L.M.H.: Fundamentals of clinical pharmacology 2. How drugs act. Current Therapeutics 20: 87 (Apr 1979).

Melander, A.: Influence of food on the bioavailability of drugs. Clinical Pharmacokinetics 3: 337 (1978).

Melmon, K.L.: The clinical pharmacologist and scientifically unsound regulations for drug development. Clinical Pharmacology and Therapeutics 20: 125 (1976).

Meyer, M.B. and Zelechowski, K.: Intramuscular lidocaine in normal subjects; in Scott and Julian (Eds) Lidocaine in Treatment of Ventricular Arrhythmias, p.161 (Livingstone, Edinburgh 1971).

Milne, M.D.: Drug interactions and the kidney; in Cluff and Petrie (Eds) Clinical Effects of Interaction Between Drugs, p.193 (Excerpta Medica Amsterdam 1975).

Mitchell, J.R.; Jollow, D.J.; Gillette, J.R. and Brodie, B.B.: Drug metabolism as a cause of drug toxicity. Drug Metabolism and Disposition 1: 418 (1973).

Mitchell, J.R.; Thorgeirsson, U.P.; Black, M.; Timbrell, J.A.; Snodgrass, N.R.; Potter, W.Z.; Jollow, D.J. and Keiser, H.R.: Increased incidence of isoniazid hepatitis in rapid acetylators: possible relation to hydrazine metabolites. Clinical Pharmacology and Therapeutics 18: 70 (1975).

Modell, W. and Houde, R.W.: Factors influencing clinical evaluation of drugs. Journal of the American Medical Association 167: 2190 (1958).

Motulsky, A.G.: Pharmacogenetics. Progress in Medical Genetics 3: 49 (1964).

Mucklow, J.C. and Dollery, C.T.: Compliance with anticonvulsant therapy in a hospital clinic and in the community. British Journal of Clinical Pharmacology 6: 75 (1978).

Mucklow, J.C.; Bending, M.R.; Kahn, G.C. and Dollery, C.T.: Drug concentration in saliva. Clinical Pharmacology and Therapeutics 24: 563 (1978).

Neal, E.A.; Meffin, P.J.; Gregory, P.B. and Blaschke, T.F.: Enhanced bioavailability and decreased clearance of analgesics in patients with cirrhosis. Gastroenterology 77: 55 (1979).

Nebert, D.W. and Bausserman, L.L.: Genetic differences in the extent of aryl hydrocarbon hydroxylase induction in mouse fetal cell cultures. Journal of Biological Chemistry 245: 6373 (1970).

Neuvonen, P.J.: Interactions with the absorption of tetracyclines. Drugs 11: 45 (1976).

Neuvonen, P.J.: Bioavailability of phenytoin: Clinical pharmacokinetic and therapeutic implications. Clinical Pharmacokinetics 4: 91 (1979).

Nies, A.S.; Shand, D.G. and Wilkinson, G.R.: Altered hepatic blood flow and drug disposition. Clinical Pharmacokinetics 1: 135 (1976).

Nilsen, O.G.; Storstein, L. and Jacobsen, S.: Effect of heparin and fatty acids on the binding of quinidine and warfarin in plasma. Biochemical Pharmacology 26: 229 (1977).

Nimmo, W.S.: Drugs, diseases and altered gastric emptying. Clinical Pharmacokinetics 1: 189 (1976).

Odar-Cederlof, I.: Plasma protein binding of phenytoin and warfarin in patients undergoing renal transplantation. Clinical Pharmacokinetics 2: 147 (1977).

Odar-Cederlof, I. and Borga, O.: Kinetics of diphenylhydantoin in uraemic patients: Consequences of decreased plasma protein binding. European Journal of Clinical Pharmacology 7: 31 (1974).

Odar-Cederlof, I.; Vessman, J.; Alvan, G. and Sjoqvist, F.: Oxazepam disposition in uraemic subjects. Acta Pharmacologica et Toxicologica 40 (Suppl. I): 52 (1977).

Ogilvie, R.I.: Clinical pharmacokinetics of theophylline. Clinical Pharmacokinetics 3: 267 (1978).

O'Reilly, R.A.; Ageler, P.M. and Leong, L.S.: Studies on the coumarin anticoagulant drugs: a comparison of the pharmacodynamics of dicoumarol and warfarin in man. Thrombosis et Diathesis Haemorrhagica 11: 1 (1964).

Orme, M.L'E.; Borga, O.; Cook, C.E. and Sjoqvist, F.: Measurements of diphenylhydantoin in 0.1ml plasma samples: Gas chromatography and radioimmunoassay compared. Clinical Chemistry 22: 246 (1976).

Pantuck, E.J.; Pantuck, C.B.; Garland, W.A.; Min, B.H.; Wattenberg, L.W.; Anderson, K.E.; Kappas, A. and Conney, A.H.: Stimulatory effect of brussels sprouts and cabbage on human drug metabolism. Clinical Pharmacology and Therapeutics 25: 88 (1979).

Parsons, R.L.: Drug absorption in gastrointestinal disease with particular reference to malabsorption syndromes. Clinical Pharmacokinetics 2: 45 (1977).

Pelkonen, O.: Prenatal and neonatal development of drug and carcinogen metabolism; in Estabrook and Lindenlaub (Eds) The Induction of Drug Metabolism. Symposia Medica Hoechst 14, p.507 (Schattauer Verlag, Stuttgart 1979).

Penner, J.A. and Abbrecht, P.H.: Lack of interaction between ibuprofen and warfarin. Current Therapeutic Research 18: 862 (1975).

Penry, J.K.: Correlation of serum ethosuximide levels with clinical effect; in Schneider, Janz, Gardner-Thorpe, Meinardi and Sherwin (Eds) Clinical Pharmacology of Antiepileptic Drugs, p.217 (Springer-Verlag, Berlin 1975).

Perrel, J.M.; Stiller, R.L. and Glassman, A.H.: Studies on plasma level/effect relationships in imipramine therapy. Communications in Psychopharmacology 2: 429 (1978).

Perrier, D.; Moyersohn, M. and Marcus, F.I.: Clinical pharmacokinetics of digitoxin. Clinical Pharmacokinetics 2: 292 (1977).

Peto, R.; Pike, M.C.; Armitage, P.; Breslow, N.E.; Cox, D.R.; Howard, S.V.; Mantel, N.; McPherson, K.; Peto, J. and Smith, P.G.: Design and analysis of randomized clinical trials requiring prolonged observation of each patient. I. Introduction and design. British Journal of Cancer 34: 485 (1976).

Peto, R.; Pike, M.C.; Armitage, P.; Breslow, N.E.; Cox, D.R.; Howard, S.V.; Mantel, N.; McPherson, K.; Peto, J. and Smith, P.G.: Design and analysis of randomized clinical trials requiring prolonged observation of each patient II. Analysis and examples. British Journal of Cancer 35: 1 (1977).

Piafsky, K.M.; Borga, O.; Odar-Cederlof, I.; Johansson, C. and Sjoqvist, F.: Increased plasma protein binding of propranolol and chlorpromazine mediated by disease-induced elevations of plasma α_1-acid glycoprotein. New England Journal of Medicine 299: 1435 (1978).

Pippenger, C.; Penry, J.K.; White, B.G.; Daly, D.D. and Buddington, R.: Interlaboratory variability in determination of plasma antiepileptic drug concentrations. Archives of Neurology 33: 351 (1976).

Plaa, G.L.: The enterohepatic circulation; in Gillette and Mitchell (Eds) Handbook of Experimental Pharmacology, Vol. XXVIII Concepts in Biochemical Pharmacology III, p.130 (Springer-Verlag, Berlin 1975).

Prescott, L.F.: Variation in drug response due to disease; in Jouhar and Grayson (Eds) International Aspects of Drug Evaluation and Usage, p.231 (Churchill Livingstone, Edinburgh 1973).

Prescott, L.F.: Gastrointestinal absorption of drugs. Medical Clinics of North America 58: 907 (1974).

Prescott, L.F.: Pathological and physiological factors affecting drug absorption, distribution, elimination and response in man; in Gillette and Mitchell (Eds) Handbook of Experimental Pharmacology, Concepts in Biochemical Pharmacology Part 3, p234 (Springer-Verlag, Berlin 1975).

Rane, A.; Sjoqvist, F. and Orrenius, S.: Drugs and fetal metabolism. Clinical Pharmacology and Therapeutics 14: 666 (1973).

Reidenberg, M.M.: The binding of drugs to plasma proteins from patients with poor renal function. Clinical Pharmacokinetics 1: 121 (1976).

Reidenberg, M.: The binding of drugs to plasma proteins and the interpretation of measurements of plasma concentrations of drugs in patients with poor kidney function. American Journal of Medicine 62: 466 (1977a).

Reidenberg, M.M.: The biotransformation of drugs in renal failure. American Journal of Medicine 62: 482 (1977b).

Reiser, S.J.; Dyck, A.J. and Curran, W.J.: Ethics in Medicine (MIT Press, Cambridge, Mass. 1977).

Remmer, H.: The role of the liver in drug metabolism. American Journal of Medicine 49: 617 (1970).

Revill, S.; Robinson, J.O.; Rosen, M. and Hogg, M.I.J.: The reliability of a linear analogue for evaluating pain. Anaesthesia 31: 1191 (1976).

Richens, A.: Drug level monitoring — quality and quantity. British Journal of Clinical Pharmacology 5: 285 (1978).

Richens, A.: When should plasma drug levels be monitored? Drugs 17: 488 (1979).

Roberton, Y.R. and Johnson, E.S.: Interactions between oral contraceptives and other drugs: a review. Current Medical Research and Opinion 3: 647 (1976).

Rowland, M.: Drug administration and regimens; in Melmon and Morelli (Eds) Clinical Pharmacology, Basic Principles in Therapeutics, 1st ed, p.21 (Macmillan, New York 1972).

Rumack, B.H.: Aspirin and acetaminophen — a comparative view for the pediatric patient with particular regard to toxicity, both in therapeutic dose and in overdose. Pediatrics 62 (Suppl): 865 (1978).

Scott, J. and Poffenbarger, P.L.: Pharmacogenetics of tolbutamide metabolism in humans. Diabetes 28: 41 (1979).

Sellers, E.M. and Holloway, M.R.: Drug kinetics and alcohol ingestion. Clinical Pharmacokinetics 3: 440 (1978).

Seppala, T.; Linnoila, M. and Mattila, M.J.: Drugs, alcohol and driving. Drugs 17: 389 (1979).

Sjoholm, I.: Binding of drugs to human serum albumin. Proceedings of the XIth FEBS Meeting, Copenhagen 1977, 50: 71 (1978).

Sjoholm, I.; Ekman, B.; Kober, A.; Ljungstedt-Pahlman, I.; Seiving, B. and Sjodin, T.: The specificity of three binding sites as studied with albumin immobilized in microparticles. Molecular Pharmacology. In press (1979).

Sjoholm, I.; Kober, A.; Odar-Cederlof, I. and Borga, O.: Protein binding od drugs in uraemic and normal serum: The role of endogenous binding inhibitors. Biochemical Pharmacology 25: 1205 (1976).

Sjoqvist, F.: Clinical use of drug plasma level determinations; in Yearbook of Drug Therapy, p.13 (Yearbook, Chicago 1977).

Sjoqvist, F. and Alexanderson, B.: Drug interactions: A critical look at their documentation and clinical importance; in Baker and Neuhaus (Eds) Toxicological Problems of Drug Combinations, vol. 13, p.167 (Excerpta Medica, Amsterdam 1972).

Sjoqvist, F. and von Bahr, C.: Interindividual differences in drug oxidation: Clinical importance. Drug Metabolism and Disposition 1: 469 (1973).

Skovsted, L.; Hansen, J.M.; Kirstensen, M. and Christensen, L.K.: Inhibition of drug metabolism in man; in Morselli, Garattini and Cohen (Eds) Drug Interactions, p.81 (Raven Press, New York 1974).

Smith, R.N.: Ethical aspects of drug evaluation; in Johnson and Johnson (Eds) Clinical Trials (Blackwell, Oxford 1977).

Smith, T.W.; Butler, V.P. and Haber, E.: Determination of therapeutic and toxic serum digoxin concentrations by radioimmunoassay. New England Journal of Medicine 281: 1212 (1969).

Smithells, R.W.: Iatrogenic hazards and their effects. Postgraduate Medical Journal 51 (Suppl. 2): 39 (1975).

Snyder, S.: Receptors, neurotransmitters and drug responses. New England Journal of Medicine 300: 465 (1979).

Storstein, L.: The effect of heparin on serum protein binding of digitoxin and digoxin. Clinical Pharmacology and Therapeutics 20: 15 (1976).

Sudlow, G.: The specificity of binding sites on serum albumin. Proceedings of the 7th International Congress on Pharmacology, Paris, 1978 (Pergamon, Oxford 1979).

Sudlow, G.; Birkett, D.J. and Wade, D.N.: The characterization of two specific drug binding sites on human serum albumin. Molecular Pharmacology 11: 824 (1975).

Sudlow, G.; Birkett, D.J. and Wade, D.N.: Further characterization of specific drug binding sites on human serum albumin. Molecular Pharmacology 12: 1052 (1976).

Thorgeirsson, S.S. and Nebert, D.W.: The Ah Locus and the metabolism of chemical carcinogens and other foreign compounds. Advances in Cancer Research 25: 149 (1977).

Tikkanen, M.J.; Aldercreutz, H. and Pulkkinen, M.P.: Effects of antibiotics on oestrogen metabolism. British Medical Journal 2: 369 (1973).

Tillement, J.P.; Lhoste, F. and Giudicelli, J.F.: Diseases and drug protein binding. Clinical Pharmacokinetics 3: 144 (1978).

Vere, D.W.: Ethics of clinical trials; in Good (Ed) The Principles and Practice of Clinical Trials, p.3 (Churchill Livingstone, London 1976).

Vesell, E.S.: Pharmacogenetics. Biochemical Pharmacology 24: 445 (1975).

Vesell, E.S.: Genetic and environmental factors affecting drug disposition in man. Clinical Pharmacology and Therapeutics 22: 659 (1977).

Vesell, E.S.: Pharmacogenetics: Multiple interactions between genes and environment as determinants of drug response. American Journal of Medicine 66: 183 (1979).

von Bahr, C.: Metabolism of tricyclic antidepressants: Pharmacokinetic and molecular aspects. MD Thesis, Karolinska Institutet (1972).

von Bahr, C. and Collste, P.: Interindividual differences in plasma concentrations and effect of alprenolol and 4-hydroxyalprenolol in man; in Symposium on The Individual Factor in Drug Response. Proceedings of the 7th International Congress on Pharmacology, Paris, 1978 (Pergamon, Oxford 1979).

Wade, O.L. and Waterhouse, J.A.H.: Significant or important? British Journal of Clinical Pharmacology 4: 411 (1977).

Weintraub, M.: Interpretation of the serum digoxin concentration. Clinical Pharmacokinetics 2: 205 (1977).

Wilding, G.; Blumberg, B. and Vesell, G.: Reduced warfarin binding of albumin variants. Science 195: 991 (1977).

Wilkinson, G.R. and Shand, D.G.: A physiological approach to hepatic drug clearance. Clinical Pharmacology and Therapeutics 18: 377 (1975).

World Health Organisation: Guidelines for Evaluation of Drugs for Use in Man, Technical Report Series No. 563 (World Health Organisation, Geneva 1975).

Zilly, W.; Breimer, D.D. and Richter, E.: Pharmacokinetic interactions with rifampicin. Clinical Pharmacokinetics 2: 61 (1977).

Chapter II
Embryonic Clinical Pharmacology

H. Tuchmann-Duplessis

Synopsis of Important Principles

1) The embryo, which constitutes one of the most dynamic biological systems is characterised by continuous cellular changes.

2) During its intrauterine development, the embryo is more sensitive to harmful actions of the environment than at any other period of the life cycle. Such actions can result in congenital malformations, non-reversible morphological defects present at birth, or other adverse effects (behavioural, biochemical, etc) which may not appear until later postnatal life.

3) For its development, the embryo depends upon nutrients furnished by the mother through placental exchanges. All drugs can cross the placenta if given in sufficient quantity.

4) A drug will have an embryotoxic or dysmorphogenic potential if it accumulates in a genetically susceptible embryo. Accumulation appears to largely depend on the disposition inter-relationship of the drug or active metabolite between the mother, placenta and embryo.

5) To produce a congenital malformation, the dysmorphogenic drug not only has to be given at an appropriate dosage, but also it has to act at a very precise moment during the morphogenesis of the embryo. The morphological type(s) of anomaly depends on the developmental stage(s) at which the agent reaches the primordia.

6) The period in which a dysmorphogenic agent can affect the development of the human embryo is very short, and is over by the 8th week (postconception) of pregnancy — about the time that a woman knows that she is pregnant. Adverse effects can however, still occur during the fetal period of development.

7) Besides the developmental stage and the genetic constitution of the embryo, the action of a dysmorphogenic drug is also dependent on the physiological and pathological status of the mother.

8) Despite the many dysmorphogenic drugs discovered in animals, in only a few cases has it been possible to provide proof of their harmful effects in humans.

9) Very complex conditions have to be fulfilled in order to compete with the various mechanisms which control human prenatal development, and drugs are only one of a number of factors involved in the aetiology of a particular congenital abnormality.

10) Nevertheless, drugs should only be used in pregnancy if they are of specific and proven benefit to the mother or fetus.

The scientific achievements and therapeutic advances of the last 30 years have changed the priorities of paediatric problems and revealed the importance of impairment of prenatal development in the destiny of children. For centuries infection has been the main concern of the medical profession. Chances of survival were limited, a high percentage of children dying within their second year. The life expectancy of the subjects of Louis XIV (17th century) did not exceed 25 years. Now that the infant mortality rate has been reduced to less than 2% in developed countries, impairment of prenatal development which leads to congenital malformations, currently represents a major medicosocial problem. In more than half of spontaneous abortions, morphological abnormalities and chromosomal aberrations are found (Symposium, 1974).

Congenital malformations, whether due to heredity or not, can be defined as non-reversible morphological defects present at birth. They can be external, internal or only microscopically detectable. They are of an irreversible nature since the organism cannot repair them during its subsequent development by growth or regenerative processes. An exogenous factor which can be associated with a congenital abnormality is termed a dysmorphogen.[1] The majority of developmental defects involve deficiencies of tissue elements or of their biochemical products. Cell death in early phases plays an important part in the production of morphological abnormalities.

The study of developmental defects involves not only congenital malformations present at birth, but also any adverse effects (morphological, behavioural, biochemical etc) induced during embryonic or fetal life, detected at birth or later (World Health Organisation, 1967). It should be emphasised that the general considerations and principles discussed in this chapter have been derived from animal experimentation. However, reference to human conditions is made whenever such information exists.

---

1   An agent which produces major anatomical abnormalities such as cleft palate, phocomelia or anencephaly is a true teratogen (i.e. monster-producing), a word derived from the Greek term for monster. Less obvious congenital abnormalities can also occur, hence use of the *general* term dysmorphogen to describe functional abnormalities or structural abnormalities of either a minor or major degree. The term teratogen has therefore been reserved for major or gross abnormalities.

1. General Considerations

In no other field of medicine is the therapeutic risk higher than in the treatment of pregnant women. While in the adult most of the unexpected side effects of drugs are reversible, they are irreversible in the embryo and can lead to abnormalities in the newborn. Well before the practical implications of experimental dysmorphology were appreciated by practitioners, Corner (1944), in a brilliant series of lectures, 'Ourselves Unborn', stressed the importance of the prenatal life in the destiny of the adult:

> 'The months before birth are the most eventful part of life and we spend them at rapid pace. At the beginning the body consists of one cell: by the time of birth it has two hundred billion cells. Some time in the third week of life your heart began to beat, you had the beginning of a brain before you had hands, and of arms before legs, you developed muscles and nerves and began your struggle: in the darkness you faced strange perils and you came at last to the threshold of the world'.

From a few tragic experiences of recent years, it is known that during intrauterine development, the embryo is more sensitive to harmful actions of the environment than at any other period of the life cycle.

1.1 Prenatal Physiology

The embryo, which constitutes one of the most dynamic biological systems, is characterised by continuous changes of cell division, cell migration and cell differentiation (Tuchmann-Duplessis et al., 1972). The physiological activity of the conceptus can be divided into two main periods: the embryonic and the fetal periods. The fundamental cell components, nucleic acids, proteins and lipids are synthesised by the embryo. The cells of each individual have genetically controlled specific molecules or groups of molecules, which give them their specific character. Nutrients necessary for the various embryonic syntheses are furnished by the maternal organism through placental exchanges.

The initial stages of the growing conceptus are, in fact, governed by effects at the cellular level. Thereafter, morphogenetic movements determined by sequential protein induction processes mark the modelling of the early embryo. In this most critical period, the specific organ functions have not yet developed and thus drug elimination mechanisms such as possessed by the adult organism are not available to it. It is the phase of greatest sensitivity to dysmorphogens (Waddell and Marlowe, 1976). Specific enzyme functions characteristic of the future organs begin to form in the primordium. The general metabolic functions involve anaerobic glycolysis in the metabolism of carbohydrate. Later, when the embryo differentiates into a fetus, most metabolic functions are still taken care of by the maternal organism, the interrelating fetal functions being restricted to the circulation and hepatic and renal elimination.

Certain organ systems which differentiate at later stages like the external genitalia, or histogenetic processes which last for the entire prenatal period like the nervous system, remain vulnerable to factors which may interfere with their development. Some such adverse effects may not appear until later postnatal life (see section 4.1.3) or even in the next generation (see chapter III; sect. 5.3), although induced during the prenatal period.

1.2 Placental Function

The placenta mediates the attachment of the embryo to the uterine wall through an intimate apposition of maternal and fetal tissues. It is responsible for all nutrition of the embryo and develops secretory and regulatory functions essential for the maintenance of pregnancy (Tuchmann-Duplessis, 1974). All the supplies to the embryo must pass through the placenta. It can be a limiting factor for nutrition if it is not functioning properly. The placenta also has an important role in hormone synthesis and in various metabolic processes. Although a number of enzyme systems capable of being involved in drug biotransformation have been identified in the placenta, and the human placenta is capable of metabolising drugs, the clinical significance of these findings remains to be elucidated (see chapter III; sect. 1.2.7).

The placenta does not usually constitute a 'barrier' for various agents, since any substance administered to the mother in sufficient quantity will eventually reach the embryo or fetus (Ginsburg, 1971). The rate of placental drug transfer (as free or unbound drug) largely depends on the physicochemical properties of the compound: small molecular weight or highly lipid soluble (non-polar) drugs or metabolites pass rapidly across the membranes of the placenta, whereas large molecular weight or highly water soluble (polar) drugs or metabolites tend to pass such

membranes at slower rates (see chapter III; sect. 1.2). However, the placenta is only one factor in determining the time course of total drug concentration in the embryo or fetus. The amount of drug and rate at which it reaches the conceptus is dependent on the inter-relationship between the disposition of the drug in the mother (i.e. interaction of pathophysiological status of the mother and the pharmacokinetic properties of the drug) and the physiological activity of the placenta (see also fig. 3).

Although a large number of investigations have been devoted to the placenta structures and function, little is known of its role during the early stages of maximum dysmorphogenic susceptibility of the embryo. From the available data, it does not seem that placental transfer *per se* is a main determinant in the embryotoxic or dysmorphogenic action of exogenous factors, including drugs. The important determinant of toxicity is the physicochemical and pharmacological nature of the compound or of its metabolites, and the possibility of its accumulation in sufficient amounts in a genetically susceptible embryo (see section 2.4; 4).

1.3 Nutrition of the Embryo

The embryo requires building and energy producing materials simultaneously. Because the mammalian ovum is practically devoid of nutritional stores, the intrauterine development of the embryo is highly dependent on the food of the mother (Giroud, 1970; 1973). During development of the embryo, a lack or an excess of a specific nutrient (e.g. certain minerals and vitamins, low protein and deficiency of particular amino acids) can in experimental animals, result in severe impairment of the pregnancy, including embryonic death and congenital malformation. During the fetal stage, which is characterised by an intense general growth, a specific nutritional deficiency will result in growth inhibition. It has not been possible to demonstrate the same predictable effects in humans. The reasons for the disparity between experimental and clinical data are not clear, but it may be that in humans marked changes similar to those induced in experimental animals, never occur, except in cases of chronic malnutrition or severe deficiencies such as due to folate antagonism (see also section 4.3.1). In a susceptible individual, the combination of a drug, an induced nutritional deficiency and a disease which itself may be dysmorphogenic, can however, lead to an increased risk of congenital abnormalities — e.g. the triad of phenytoin (diphenylhydantoin), folate deficiency and epilepsy (see chapter III, sect. 3.10.2; chapter XXV, sect. 4.8).

1.4 Drugs and Other Agents as Dysmorphogens

Drug dysmorphogenicity has been demonstrated experimentally for more than 20 years. However, the clinical implications of the experimental results were only fully recognised with the discovery of the thalidomide induced embryopathies. However, at that time, and subsequently, the potential danger to the embryo and fetus of drugs taken by the mother was so overemphasised that it has inhibited research directed at therapeutic progress in obstetrics. At the present time, experimental and clinical data have led to a more realistic appreciation of the dysmorphogenic danger of drugs used in early pregnancy (see chapter XV; sect. 2.1).

Experimentally, hundreds of dysmorphogenic agents have been discovered. Among them are: (a) physical factors, like X-rays and anoxia; (b) viral infections such as rubella, varicella and cytomegalovirus; (c) endotoxins, and (d) a very large variety of chemicals, such as poisons, industrial and agricultural chemicals, and various therapeutic drugs. Some of these chemical compounds have a low or no general toxicity, like hormones; others are much more toxic, like the cytotoxic or antineoplastic drugs. Despite the numerous dysmorphogens discovered in animals, in only a few cases has it been possible to provide proof of their noxious effects in the human embryo (Tuchmann-Duplessis, 1975). It is now understood that very complex conditions have to be fulfilled in order to compete with the various mechanisms which control human prenatal development, and drugs are only one of a number of factors involved in the aetiology of a particular congenital abnormality (see sections 2.3; 4).

2. Epidemiology of Congenital Malformations

The epidemiological study of congenital abnormalities is fraught with problems and much evidence is required before an agent can be incriminated as an established dysmorphogen. Not only is the normal expected incidence of a particular abnormality difficult to establish, but also the results of methods to detect abnormalities are often difficult to interpret. Moreover, most congenital abnormalities are of a multifactorial aetiology and comprise an interaction between genetic and environmental factors and are due to complex and as yet inadequately understood mechanisms (Cohlan, 1969; Wilson, 1973).

2.1 Incidence of Congenital Malformations

Estimation of the incidence of congenital malformations varies according to the investigators and the sources used — hospital records of delivery, autopsy records, or death certificates. From an analysis of various reports, the incidence of obvious malformations in Western countries can be estimated at approximately 2 to 3 % at birth, which, in countries like France or Great Britain, means that approximately 20,000 to 25,000 abnormal children are born every year. The real frequency of congenital malformations is, in fact, nearly twice as high. Many anomalies of the cardiovascular system, kidneys and central nervous system are discovered only several months or even several years after birth; general statistics do not include them (Saxen and Rapola, 1969; Warkany, 1971). Moreover, differences in the frequency of some specific malformations have been found between various populations and races. For example, anencephalia is more frequent in Great Britain than in France. Significant differences exist even between different geographical areas of France (Tuchmann-Duplessis, 1975).

2.2 Detection of Congenital Abnormalities

The aetiology of congenital malformations (see section 2.3) can be explored by two methods — epidemiological and experimental. Epidemiological methods are difficult to conduct and results difficult to interpret, but they can provide valuable information. Epidemiological studies are of two types — retrospective and prospective (Bowes, 1970; Smithells, 1974; Yerushalmy, 1972).

A retrospective inquiry starts with the birth of a malformed child. A careful maternal history is retraced asking the mother about and recording any unusual events that occurred during the pregnancy and which may be possible aetiological factors in the malformation. Such inquiries done systematically on a large scale, may suggest a common factor, one of the intermingled agents, to be a dysmorphogen. Then, subsequent experimental studies may confirm this suspicion. Such methods established rubella virus (Gregg, 1941) and thalidomide (Lenz, 1961; McBride, 1961) as dysmorphogens in humans. The major problem with retrospective studies lies in the possible unreliability of the mother's replies.

Prospective inquiries exclude a number of sources of bias inherent in retrospective studies. They start at the beginning of the gestation: every drug prescription and possible infection is recorded throughout the pregnancy, so that the collected data are quite objective (Nelson and Forfar, 1971; Spira et al., 1972). But prospective studies are difficult to conduct; very large numbers of cases must be examined before it is possible to collect a reasonable number of malformations for statistical analysis. For instance, in order to obtain information about 100 spina bifida cases, the inquiry would need to investigate more than 100,000 pregnancies. Therefore, such prospective studies must be undertaken at a national or multiregional level in a number of countries (Shapiro et al., 1976; Heinonen et al., 1977). They aim to determine if the incidence of a particular abnormality is significantly higher than that observed in a control group, or that normally expected in a large population suitable for comparison (see further chapter XV; sect. 1.1.1; 2.1).

Experimental methods (see section 3) which give rapid results and can be established under strictly planned conditions also often result in difficulties in interpretation and for a number of reasons are of low predictive value to results in man.

2.3 Causes of Congenital Malformations

Development of the embryo is the resultant of two factors: the genetic information which contains the programming of the whole phenotype of

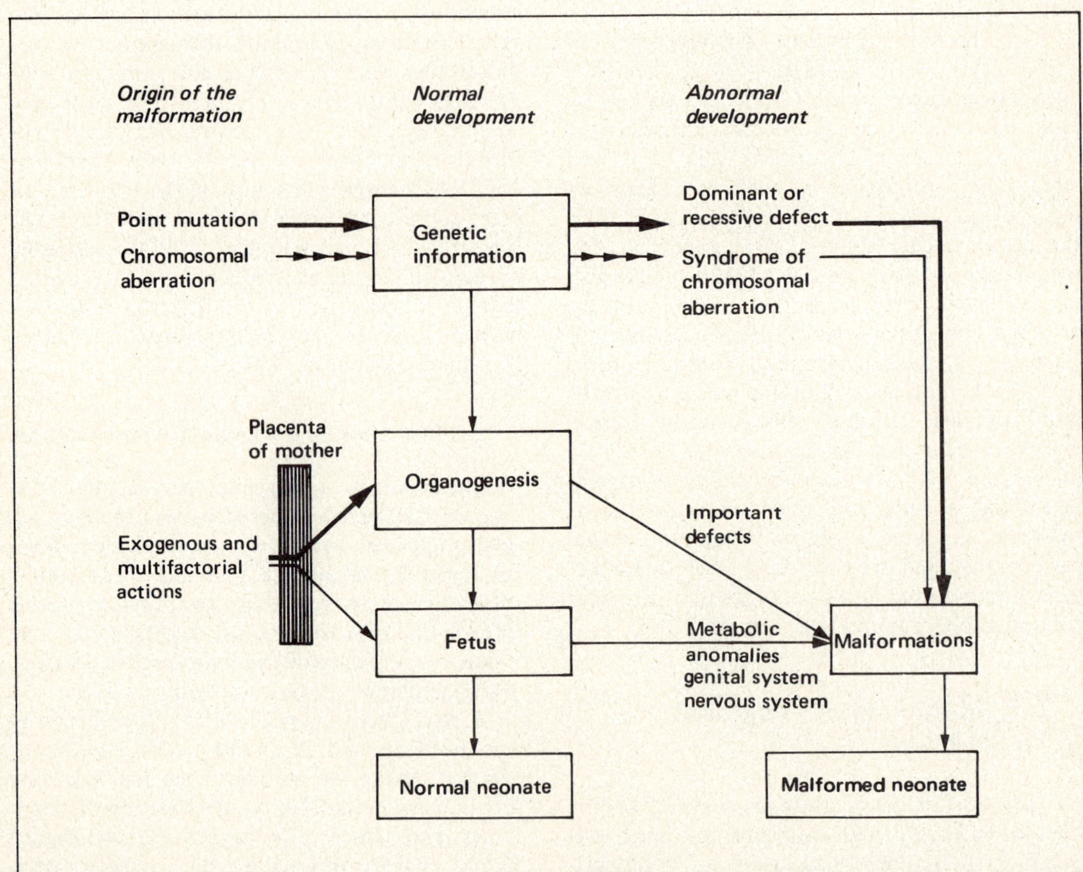

Fig. 1 Schematic representation of the aetiology of congenital malformations (after Tuchmann-Duplessis, 1975).

the future child and the environment which supplies the nutrients necessary for growth and differentiation of the embryo. The origin of developmental anomalies is complex. Schematically, four main causes can be defined: genetic, chromosomal, exogenous and, most frequently, multifactorial (fig. 1). The same type of congenital malformation can arise for example, from genetic or exogenous factors.

1) *Genetic malformations* — A defect in a genetic factor is produced at the origin by a mutation and is transmitted hereditarily.

2) *Chromosomal aberrations* — Chromosomal aberrations represent a gross imbalance in a genome and result in important and complex malformation syndromes, even though the individual genes are normal. These aberrations originate before, during or after conception.

3) *Exogenous malformations* — The genome is normal and well balanced, but its expression is impaired by exogenous factors present in the environment acting in the course of the embryonic development and having a dysmorphogenic effect.

4) *Multifactorial malformations* — in which exogenous factors including drugs contribute to an unknown extent. The particular liability of certain individuals (see section 2.4) is not necessarily due to the presence of a single gene, but frequently to several genes with an additive action. This polygenic trait is not transmitted in a Mendelian way, but represents an increased risk of dysmorphogenesis in some families which are likely to exhibit malformations when exposed to slight external causes that do not determine malformations in other individuals. When such a liability exists, an anomaly is both exogenous and genetic, since neither the genotype alone, nor the exogenous factor alone, is responsible for the malformation.

The problem is further complicated by the fact that all types of disturbed development may also occur through spontaneous mutation. In such a situation, the intervention of an exogenous agent can only be assumed if the incidence of a particular change is significantly higher than that observed in a control or other group suitable for comparison (see section 2.2). Most common malformations, both major and minor, have a multifactorial aetiology and drugs are therefore only one of the factors involved. Thus, where the polygenic background (fig. 2) provides susceptibility to malformation, the consumption of drugs in early pregnancy is sufficient to enhance the susceptibility and provoke an embryological anomaly.

2.4 Mechanisms of Congenital Abnormalities

Mechanisms involved in the adverse effects of exogenous factors on the embryo have only been partially explored, but can be conveniently classified as follows:

1) *General mechanisms involving the feto-maternal unit* — either a direct action on the embryo or fetus, an indirect action on the embryo or fetus (e.g. impaired nutrition) or a modification of maternal metabolism (e.g. impaired carbohydrate metabolism).

2) *Genetic mechanisms* — which are responsible for the different susceptibilities of the embryo to dysmorphogenic agents.

Hybridation experiments in inbred strains of mice show that the susceptibility to a drug may depend on one or several genes, the effects of which can be followed through successive generations (Fraser, 1965; Fraser et al., 1957). The susceptibility is not a general one: the gene action is organ-specific. The tendency to malformation of one organ may depend on several genes, each being affected by various dysmorphogens: a strain susceptible to one agent may be found to be resistant if a different dysmorphogen is used. These facts indicate that it is not possible to predict the susceptibility of one breed or strain to a compound, from known susceptibility to another compound, even if the compounds are structurally or pharmacologically related.

Polygenic heredity, which is widely represented for a number of characters in man, is certainly responsible for the susceptibility of a conceptus to different exogenous actions. It is perhaps the most important determinant in the multifactorial aetiology of congenital malformations. The results of extensive familial studies suggest that the usual type of malformation depends on a polygenic type of heredity (Symposium, 1974). This shows a transmission which as discussed above does not fit Mendelian laws.

Since dysmorphogenic substances may act by interfering with the expression of genes commanding the development of an organ or system, a threshold effect would explain the occurrence or non-occurrence of a congenital malformation, suggesting that normal development is possible only if the genetic activity is above the threshold. The closer this activity is to the threshold in normal conditions the greater will be the susceptibility to the dysmorphogen (see fig. 2).

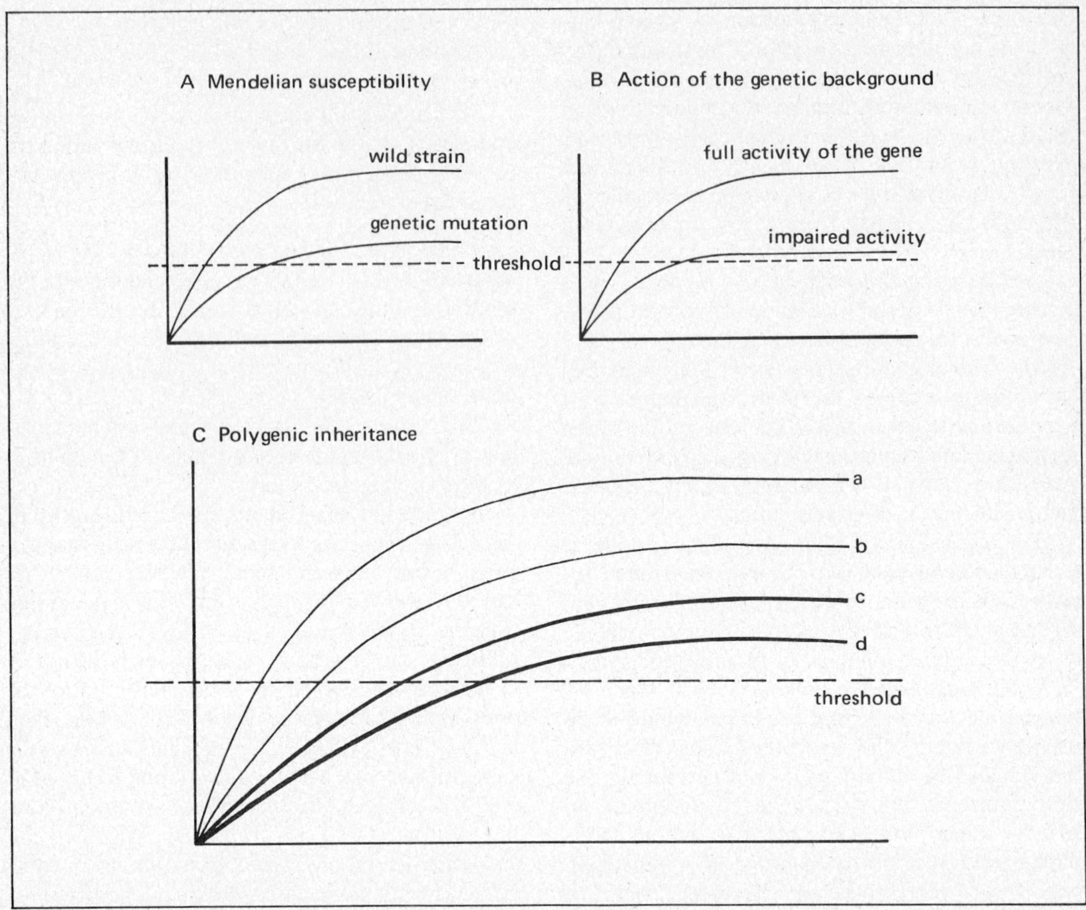

Fig. 2. Models for the different genetic mechanisms of susceptibility to dysmorphogenic factors.

Model A. Mendelian susceptibility: The new gene resulting from the mutation has a lower activity. It is close to the threshold. A slight dysmorphogenic agent can bring it below the threshold, resulting in a malformation.

Model B. Action of the genetic background. Activity of the gene is impaired by an unfavourable genetic background. Its susceptibility to dysmorphogenic agents is increased.

Model C. Polygenic inheritance. A great number of genes with an additive action are implicated in the normal development of an organ. The distribution of these genes in the population is a Gaussian one, so that the genetic activity is a continuous variable. Individuals having the lower number of genes at the extreme end of the variable (c,d) show the highest susceptibility to a dysmorphogenic agent, since the genetic activity is close to the threshold (after Tuchmann-Duplessis, 1975).

3) *Mechanisms acting on cell proliferation in the embryo* — a number of agents are able to impair division of the cell or to kill actively proliferating cells specifically (e.g. cytotoxic drugs, irradiation).

4) *Mechanisms acting on the basic physiological activities of the embryonic cells* — agents which interfere with the complex system of protein synthesis or in the enzymic activities of the embryonic cell, the basic aspects of cellular life (e.g. certain antibiotics and cytotoxic agents).

3. Prediction of Dysmorphogenic Effects

Analysis of experimental methods, which are designed to discover the harmful potential of an environmental agent including drugs, pesticides or environmental pollutants, reveals that the basic principles of testing for dysmorphogenicity are similar to those involved in the detection of drug toxicity in general (Tuchmann-Duplessis, 1971,

1972, 1974; Wilson and Warkany, 1965; Robson et al., 1965). In both cases, one has to consider the pharmacodynamic action, the dosage and its relationship to the pharmacokinetic properties of the drug. However, the action of an injurious agent on the embryo is more complex than its action on the adult. In dysmorphogenesis, in which one deals with two interdependent biological systems, the pregnant female and the embryo, the specific reactions of each may be entirely different. An agent harmless to the mother is capable of impairing the development of the embryo and causing congenital malformations, and is largely dependent on the disposition of the drug (or active metabolite) between the mother, placenta and embryo. This remains a virtually unexplored area in humans (Nishimura, 1973). However, in animals, recent approaches involving use of highly sensitive and specific assays, will allow measurement of drugs and metabolites and other substances in both the maternal organism and growing embryo, and may help to elucidate mechanisms of dysmorphogenic action of a drug as well as strain or species susceptibility differences (Nau, 1975).

3.1 Drug Class and Dysmorphogenic Effects

Experimental and clinical data show that there is no direct relationship between the chemical structure, the pharmacological activity, or the toxicity of a drug in the adult and its specific action on the embryo (Tuchmann-Duplessis, 1975). Among the various glutarimides, thalidomide is dysmorphogenic, while the others appear to be harmless to the embryo. A similar situation is observed with various sulphonylurea hypoglycaemic agents. Although their pharmacological action on carbohydrate metabolism is comparable, some of them (carbutamide) cause a high percentage of congenital malformations in experimental animals, while others have a low or no dysmorphogenic activity. Further examples are furnished by antiemetics and various cytotoxic drugs.

3.2 Species Specificity and Dysmorphogenic Effects

One of the greatest handicaps of experimental methods in the evaluation of the dysmorphogenic

potential of a drug lies in the different reactions to it of various animal species (Tuchmann-Duplessis, 1975). This difficulty has been partially overcome by using several animal species in dysmorphogenic screening procedures. Cortisone, a potent dysmorphogenic agent in the rabbit and in the mouse, does not produce malformations in the rat. Thalidomide, which produces obvious malformations in certain strains of rabbit (New Zealand white and Himalayan but not silver greys), is apparently safer or non-injurious in the rat. The immunosuppressive drug azathioprine, which is highly dysmorphogenic in the rabbit, does not produce anomalies in the rat. Furthermore, the type of malformations produced by a specific dysmorphogen can be different in each species. For example, carbutamide in the rat and in the mouse, essentially produces eye anomalies, while in the rabbit, facial and visceral malformations are observed.

Despite their limitations, experimental methods constitute the only approach available to evaluating the dysmorphogenic potential of drugs and other environmental agents to which pregnant women may be exposed.

3.3 Dosage and Dysmorphogenic Effects

In experimental dysmorphology, many malformations are significantly related to the dose of the suspected dysmorphogen and, as in most toxicological considerations, dysmorphogenicity follows a dose-effect relationship. In general, the dose range which causes dysmorphogenicity is narrow and the dose-effect curve has a steep slope; a notable exception is thalidomide, where a large increase in dose is associated with only a slight increase in morbidity of the conceptus. The duration of the total dosage is also of major potential importance (Yaffe and Stern, 1976).

In a human epidemiological survey it is probable that doses are almost all within the narrow therapeutic range. Therefore, for this reason alone, it is unlikely that epidemiological investigations would detect the variable effects observed in animals when large doses much closer to the toxic range are employed. This also means that when drugs suspected of dysmorphogenicity are specifically indicated for use in early pregnancy (see chapter XV; sect. 2.1), every effort should be made to use the lowest effective dose.

4. Dysmorphogenic Conditions

To produce a congenital malformation, the dysmorphogenic drug not only has to be given at an appropriate dosage, but it also has to act at a very precise moment during the morphogenesis of the embryo. In addition, the embryo must have a suitable genetic susceptibility to be capable of reacting to the dysmorphogenic agent (see section 2.4). All of these conditions, which can be easily attained in large numbers of experimental animals, occur only exceptionally in the development of the human fetus (fig. 3).

The action of a dysmorphogenic agent on the conceptus depends mainly on three conditions: the developmental stage of the embryo, the genetic susceptibility of the embryo and the physiological or pathological status of the mother (Tuchmann-Duplessis, 1975).

4.1 The Developmental Stage

The period in which environmental agents can affect the development of the human embryo is very short, and is over by the 8th week of pregnancy — about the time that a woman knows that she is pregnant.

4.1.1 Blastogenesis

Drugs can be transferred into the luminal secretions of the fallopian tube and uterine cavity (through which the ovum and blastocyst must

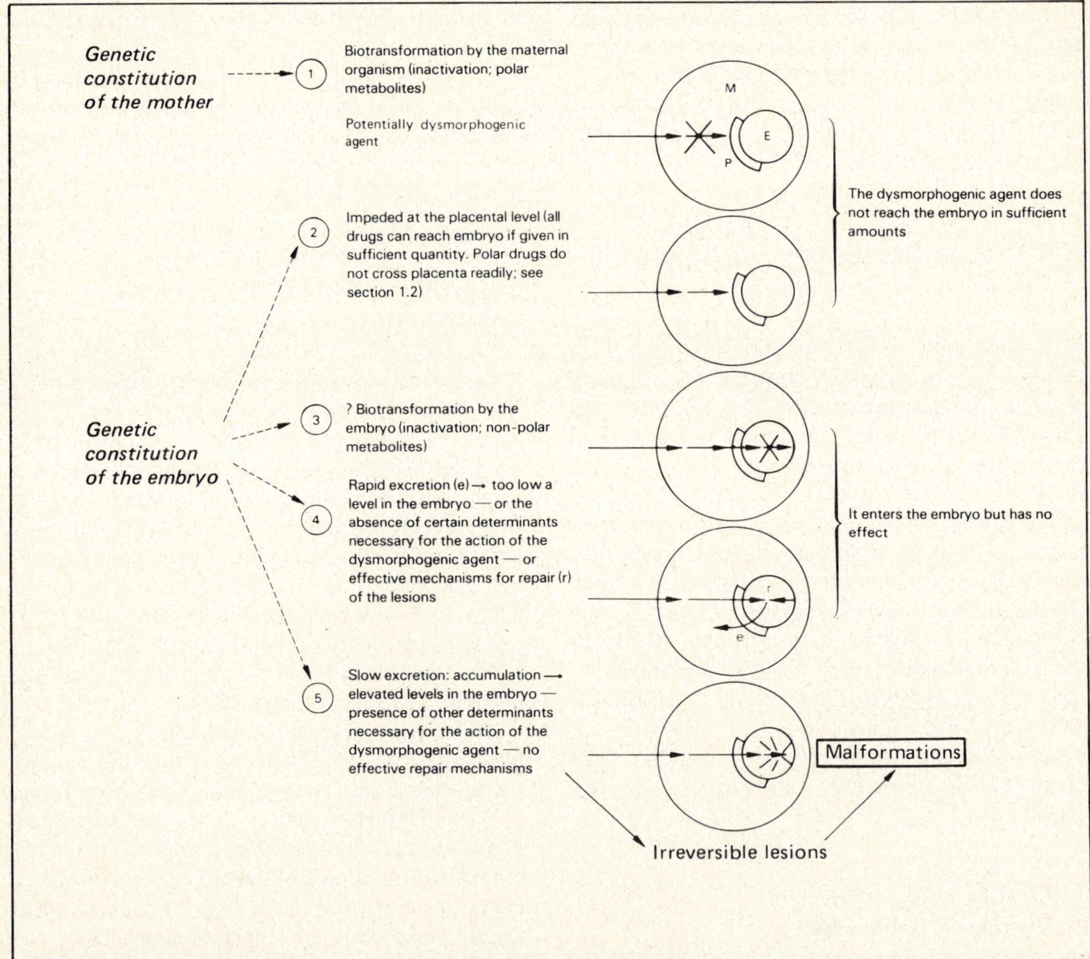

Fig. 3. Mechanisms which might explain the difference in susceptibility to potential dysmorphogenic agents between individuals, ethnic groups and animal species. M = mother; P = placenta; E = embryo (after Tuchmann-Duplessis, 1975).

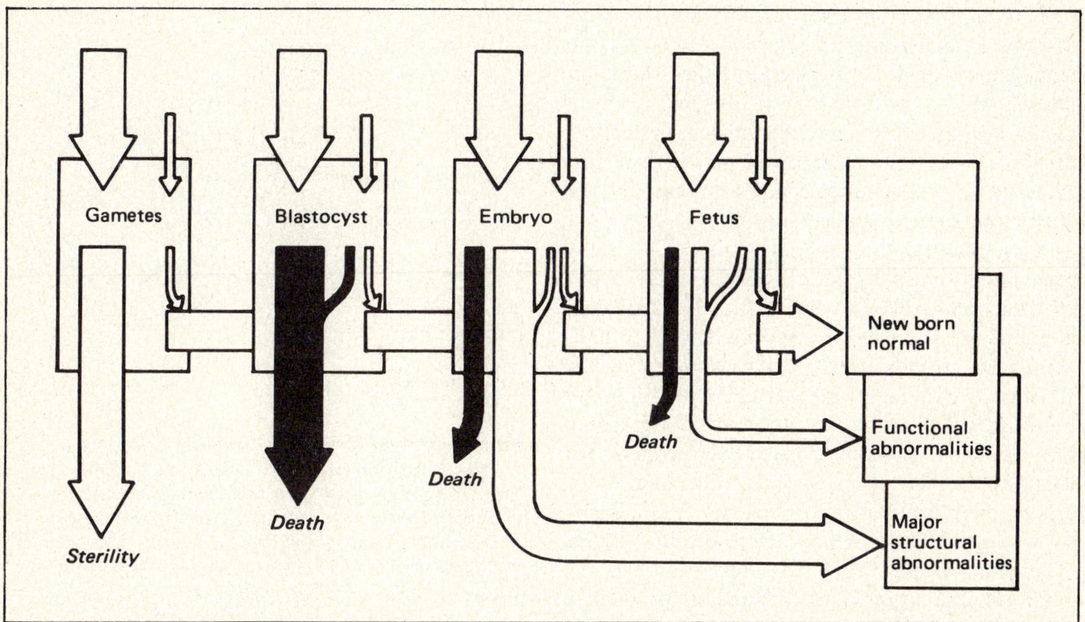

Fig. 4. Schematic representation of the influence of dysmorphogenic factors on gametogenesis and various stages of prenatal development. Strong dysmorphogenic agents: wide arrows; weak agents: narrow arrows (after Tuchmann-Duplessis, 1975).

pass during the early stages of embryogenesis) and also into the preimplantation blastocyst (Fabro, 1973; Lutwak-Mann, 1973). During the pre-implantation period (the period of maximum embryotoxicity) when the blastocyst lies free with-in the uterus and depends for its nutrition on the uterine secretions, exogenous agents can kill the embryo (fig. 4), but there is no evidence that they would produce congenital malformations. Slight injuries can be overcome without obvious harmful consequences on the growing embryo because dur-ing the segmentation stage, many blastomeres re-tain their totipotency[2], being able to replace damaged cells by newly formed cells.

4.1.2 Embryogenesis

Once implantation has occurred in the human, at 7 to 8 days after fertilisation, the embryo under-goes very rapid and important transformations, which will be briefly summarised.

At the end of the 2nd week, the primitive streak appears, converting the embryo into a trilaminar leaf-shaped structure. In the 3rd week,

the neural groove appears and the future heart is already visible. Thereafter, the neuropores close, and the optic vessels become discernible in the 4th week. Simultaneously, the digestive system differ-entiates, the foregut and hindgut appear, the buc-copharyngeal membrane ruptures and the primor-dia of the liver and pancreas become visible. At the end of the 4th week, at the 26th and 28th days, the arm and the leg buds are indicated as mesodermal thickenings. In the 5th week, the olfactory pits ap-pear, the superficial ectoderm of the optic vesicle forms the lens primordium, and in the heart the interatrial septum divides the atrial cavity into right and left portions.

From this moment, the growth of the embryo is accelerated: the heart structures and the limb buds differentiate and the Mullerian ducts appear in the 6th week. During the next 2 weeks, the atrial and interventricular septa of the heart are completed, the primary ossification centres ap-pear, the anal membrane ruptures and the sex of the embryo becomes well determined (fig. 5).

The sequence of the embryonic events shows that each organ and each system undergoes a criti-cal stage of differentiation at a precise moment of the prenatal development. It is during this critical period that the vulnerability of the developing

---

2   The potentiality inherent in the cell to produce the many and varied cells of the complete individual to come.

embryo is greatest and that specific *gross* malformations or fetal death can be produced. This is the teratogenic period. If the dosage of the drug is increased above the minimal teratogenic level, it would be possible to produce congenital malformations over a somewhat longer period than this, as noted in the schematic representation of the 'dysmorphogenic calendar' (fig. 6).

Since many organs are developing at the same time, the dysmorphogenic effect often represents a combination of different anomalies. Moreover, it is frequently possible for a specific cluster of malformations to indicate when the dysmorphogenic effect occurred (Yaffe and Stern, 1976). Although the morphological type of anomaly is dependent on the developmental stage(s) at which the dysmorphogenic agent reaches the primordia, among the various dysmorphogenic drugs, a few show a preferential action upon specific organs (Tuchmann-Duplessis, 1975). For example, the cytotoxic drug aminopterin will mainly produce in humans, general growth retardation and central nervous system anomalies; while thalidomide embryopathies are characterised by skeletal malformations, normal growth and well developed intelligence. Comparative experimental investigations in the rabbit with purine analogues (e.g. 6-mercaptopurine) and thalidomide, administered at the same embryonic stage, also show differences in the morphological type of malformations. While purine analogues determine characteristic skeletal malformations, thalidomide mainly induces (in the rabbit) nervous system anomalies.

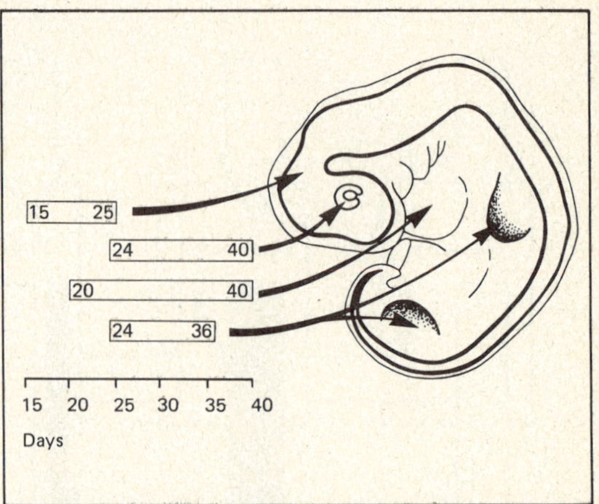

Fig. 6. Critical periods, i.e. days in pregnancy in the human embryo. [*Note* that the development ages given are *postconception* ages which for clinical purposes need to be translated into *postmenstrual* ages, ordinarily by adding 2 weeks]. After Tuchmann-Duplessis (1975).

4.1.3 Fetogenesis

The fetal period begins at the end of the 8th week, when little further differentiation of organs remains to be completed. The most important events of this stage are the complete closure of the palate, the reduction of the umbilical hernia at the end of the 9th week, the differentiation of the external genitalia, as well as the histogenesis of the central nervous system. The latter process lasts for the entire intrauterine development period and is completed only several months after birth. Consequently during the fetal period, dysmorphogenic agents do not determine major morphological malformations but can impair the differentiation of external genitalia, leading, in severe cases, to pseudohermaphrodism. Interference with the histogenesis of the central nervous system (fig. 7) can lead to various types of behavioural changes or impaired mental development in postnatal life (Brazelton, 1970; Thornburg and Moore, 1976). The great susceptibility of the nervous system to drugs administered during the period of myelinisation is related to the high metabolic stability of the constituents of myelin sheaths.

4.2 Genetic Susceptibility and Species Differences

The reaction of the embryo to exogenous agents depends upon its genetic constitution (see section 2.4). There is a constant interaction bet-

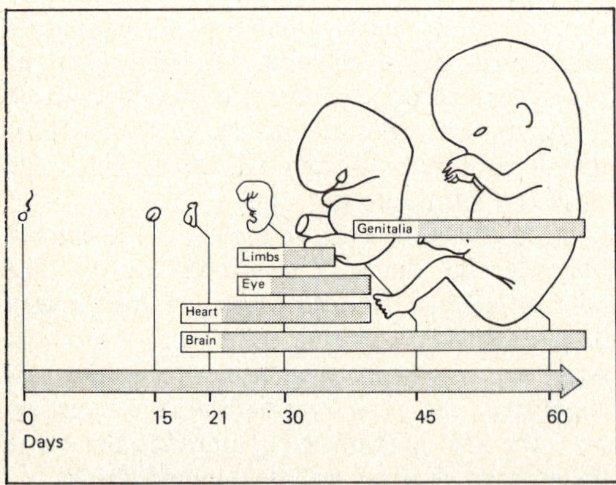

Fig. 5. The critical stages of development of the main structures of the human embryo. [*Note* that the development ages given are *postconception* ages which for clinical purposes need to be translated into *postmenstrual* ages, ordinarily by adding 2 weeks]. After Tuchmann-Duplessis (1975).

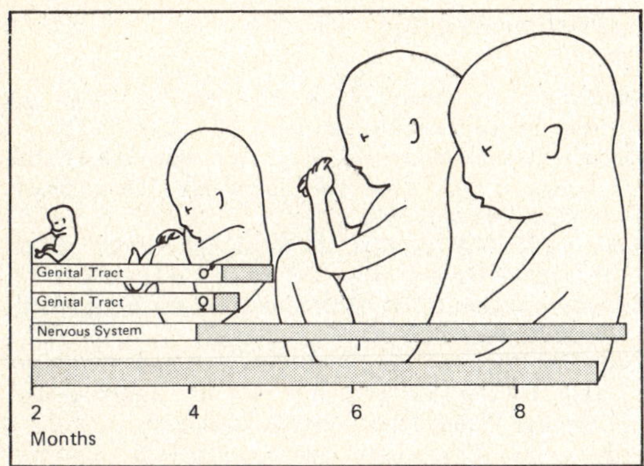

Fig. 7. The stages critical for the human fetus. [*Note* that the developmental ages given are *postconception* ages which for clinical purposes need to be translated into *postmenstrual* ages, ordinarily by adding 2 weeks]. After Tuchmann-Duplessis (1975).

ween the genes and exogenous agents. Differences in the reaction to a harmful agent between individuals, animal strains and species are ascribed to biochemical peculiarities related to genes (see also section 2.4). A striking example is the high susceptibility of the mouse embryo to induction of cleft palate by corticosteroids. The biochemical background of this action is still unknown but seems to be related to metabolic differences between the mouse and other species in the rate of absorption or of the rate of degradation of the hormone (Saxen and Saxen, 1975). Clinical observations have yielded comparable information on variations between individuals in susceptibility to dysmorphogens. Among women who took thalidomide in the critical period of pregnancy, less than 25 % had deformed babies, the remainder escaping the noxious effects of the drug (Lenz and Knapp, 1962). Similarly, congenital abnormality did not occur in all cases of infants born of mothers who were treated with warfarin during the first 3 months of pregnancy (Warkany, 1976). The incidence of rubella induced deafness is higher in children with a genetic susceptibility for impairment of hearing (Anderson et al., 1970).

4.3 Physiological or Pathological Status of the Mother

Besides the developmental stage and the genetic constitution of the embryo, the action of a drug is dependent on the physiological and pathological conditions of the mother.

Among the physiological factors, age, diet, local uterine condition, hormonal balance and environmental conditions are of great importance (fig. 8). Experimental and clinical data show that the risks of malformations and of perinatal mortality are higher in very young mothers and even more so in the older age groups (Tuchmann-Duplessis, 1974).

4.3.1 Nutritional Status

Particular emphasis must be placed on the nutritional condition. Among environmental factors, deficiencies or excess of nutrients can affect the expression of genes and may enhance the harmful effects of drugs with consequent irreversible results (Tuchmann-Duplessis, 1975). An excess of vitamin D is dysmorphogenic by itself, as it can lead to hypercalcaemia and the supravalvular aortic syndrome. Nutritional requirements are considerably increased during pregnancy for the requirements of energy and building material of the growing conceptus. This applies not only to organic substances and some vitamins, but also to certain inorganic elements. In humans, iron deficiency is frequent, and folate deficiency much less so. They must be detected in time and corrected

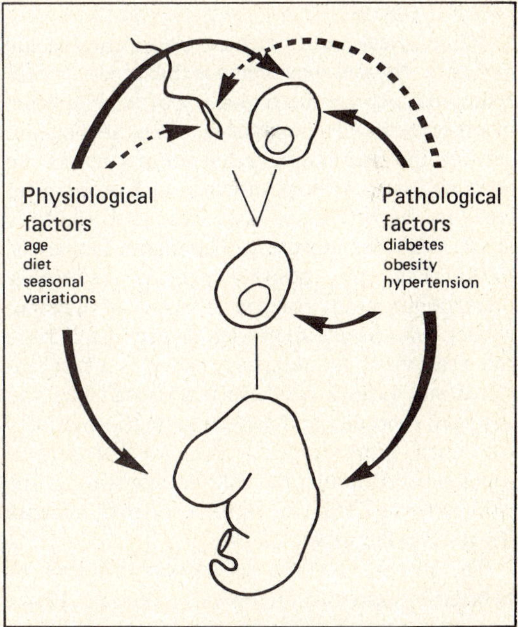

Fig. 8. The physiological and pathological status of the mother showing factors capable of modifying the action of dysmorphogenic agents (after Tuchmann-Duplessis, 1975).

(see chapter XV; sect. 3.1, 3.2). Calcium deficient women may give birth to infants with lesions of the skeleton and teeth. Milk and cheese are the best sources of dietary calcium.

Although the precise role of vitamins in human reproduction is not clearly established it seems necessary to ensure that pregnant women take sufficient dietary amounts of essential vitamins, since those compounds are involved in basic metabolic processes, including protein synthesis.

General feeding restrictions impair the maternal fertility and increase the frequency of prematurity, stunting, and fetal death. Specific deficiencies usually have worse consequences, as not only growth inhibition but also congenital malformations can be produced.

4.3.2 Socio-economic Status

In man, the physiological status of the mother depends not only upon her intake of food, but also on her socio-economic status, the climate and seasonal variations. The larger number of malformations in lower socio-economic groups is generally ascribed to malnutrition, alcoholism and chronic diseases.

4.3.3 Disease

Pathological factors such as certain chronic and metabolic diseases may enhance the toxic action of drugs and increase the frequency of fetal damage. In experimental dysmorphology, drug disposition between the fetal and maternal compartments can be modified by various diseases such as diabetes mellitus, hypertension, toxaemia and systemic lupus erythematosus (Tuchmann-Duplessis, 1974). This may possibly explain the higher susceptibility to environmental factors of pregnant women who have a metabolic disease. In diabetic and prediabetic women, pregnancy is often impaired and various accidents (abortions, fetal and postnatal mortality and congenital malformations) are much more frequent than in the general population. Although the data are conflicting, the estimates vary from a 5- to a 10-fold increase (Tuchmann-Duplessis, 1974).

The reasons for the deleterious influence of diabetes on reproduction are still unknown. However, it seems that besides impairment of carbohydrate metabolism, other disorders, particularly of fatty acid metabolism, may also be involved in these accidents.

Further Reading

Klingberg, M.A.; Abramovici, A. and Chemke, J.: Drugs and Fetal Development (Plenum Press, New York 1972).

Neubert, D. and Merker, H.J. (Eds): New Approaches to the Evaluation of Abnormal Embryonic Development (Thieme, Stuttgart 1975).

Robson, J.N.; Sullivan, F.M. and Smith, R.L.: Embryopathic Activity of Drugs (Churchill, London 1965).

Tuchmann-Duplessis, H.: Drug Effects on the Fetus (ADIS Press, Sydney 1975).

Tuchmann-Duplessis, H.; David, G. and Haegel, P.: Illustrated Human Embryology, vol. 1, Embryogenesis (Springer-Verlag, New York and Masson, Paris 1972).

Wilson, J.G.: Environment and Birth Defects (Academic Press, New York 1973).

Wilson, J.G. and Warkany, J.: Teratology, Principles and Techniques (University of Chicago Press, Chicago 1965).

World Health Organisation: Principles for the testing of drugs for teratogenicity. Report of a WHO scientific group. World Health Organisation Technical Report Series No. 364 (WHO, Geneva 1967).

References

Anderson, H.; Barr, B. and Wedenberg, E.: Genetic disposition — a prerequisite for maternal rubella deafness. Archives of Otolaryngology 91: 141 (1970).

Bowes, W.A.: Obstetrical medication and infant outcome: A review of the literature. Monographs of the Society for Research in Child Development 35: 3 (1970).

Brazelton, B.: Effect of prenatal drugs on the behaviour of the neonate. American Journal of Psychiatry 126: 1261 (1970).

Cohlan, S.Q.: The teratogenicity of drugs in man. Pharmacology for Physicians 3 (8): 1 (1969).

Corner, G.W.: Ourselves Unborn (Yale University Press, Yale 1944).

Fabro, S.: Passage of drugs and other chemicals into the uterine fluids and preimplantation blastocyst; in Boreus (Ed) Fetal Pharmacology, p.443 (Raven Press, New York 1973).

Fraser, F.C.: Some genetic aspects of teratology; in Wilson and Warkany (Eds) Teratology, Principles and Techniques, p.21 (University of Chicago Press, Chicago 1965).

Fraser, F.C.; Walker, B.E. and Trasler, D.G.: The experimental production of congenital cleft palate: genetic and environmental factors. Pediatrics 19: 782 (1957).

Ginsburg, J.: Placental drug transfer. Annual Review of Pharmacology 11: 387 (1971).

Giroud, A.: The Nutrition of the Embryo (Thomas, Springfield 1970).

Giroud, A.: Nutritional requirements of the embryo. World Review of Nutrition and Dietetics 18: 195 (1973).

Gregg, N.: Congenital cataract following German measles in the mother. Transactions of the Ophthalmological Society of Australia 3: 35 (1941).

Heinonen, O.P.; Slone, D. and Shapiro, S.: Birth Defects and Drugs in Pregnancy (Publishing Sciences Group, Littleton, Mass. 1977).

Lenz, W. Von: Die thalidomid-embryopathie. Deutsche Medizinische Wochenschrift 86: 2555 (1961).

Lenz, W. and Knapp, K.: Die thalidomid-embryopathie. Deutsche Medizinische Wochenschrift 87: 1232 (1962).

Lutwak-Mann, C.: Drugs and the blastocyst; in Boreus (Ed) Fetal Pharmacology, p.419 (Raven Press, New York 1973).

McBride, W.G.: Teratogenic action of thalidomide. Lancet 2: 1358 (1961).

Nau, H.: Determination of drugs and metabolites by CG MS computer system; in Neubert and Merker (Eds) New Approaches to the Evaluation of Abnormal Embryonic Development (Thieme, Stuttgart 1975).

Nelson, M.N. and Forfar, J.O.: Associations between drugs administered during pregnancy and congenital abnormalities of the fetus. British Medical Journal 1: 523 (1971).

Nishimura, H.: Comparative study on maternal-embryonic transfer of drugs in man and laboratory animals; in Boreus (Ed) Fetal Pharmacology, p.47 (Raven Press, New York 1973).

Robson, J.N.: Sullivan, F.M. and Smith, R.L.: Embryopathic Activity of Drugs (Churchill, London 1965).

Saxen, L. and Rapola, J.: Congenital Defects (Holt, Rinehart and Winston, New York 1969).

Saxen, I. and Saxen, L.: Organ culture in teratology: closure of the palatal shelves as a model system; in Neubert and Merker (Eds) New Approaches to the Evaluation of Abnormal Embryonic Development (Thieme, Stuttgart 1975).

Shapiro, S.; Hartz, S.C.; Siskind, V.; Mitchell, A.A.; Slone, D.; Rosenberg, Lynn; Monson, R.R.; Heinonen, O.P.; Idanpaan-Heikkila, J.: Haro, S. and Saxen, L.: Anticonvulsants and parental epilepsy in the development of birth defects. Lancet 1: 276 (1976).

Smithells, R.W.: Epidemiology of malformation: Inspiration and perspiration. Teratology 10: 217 (1974).

Spira, N.; Goujard, J.; Huel, G. and Rumeau-Rouquette, C.: Etude teratogene des hormones sexuelles. Premiers resultats d'une enquete epidemiologique portant sur 20,000 femmes. Rev. Med. Franc. 41: 2683 (1972).

Symposium: Evaluation of drugs and other chemical agents for teratogenicity. Bulletin der Schweizerischen Akademie der Medizinischen Wissenschaften 30: 1-62 (1974).

Thornburg, J.E. and Moore, K.E.: Pharmacologically induced modifications of behavioural and neurochemical development; in Mirkin (Ed) Perinatal Pharmacology and Therapeutics, p.270 (Academic Press, New York 1976).

Tuchmann-Duplessis, H.: Malformations Congenitales des Mammiferes (Masson, Paris 1971).

Tuchmann-Duplessis, H.: Teratogenic drug screening. Present procedures and requirements. Teratology 5: 221 (1972).

Tuchmann-Duplessis, H.: Methodes experimentales pour la detection des agents teratogenes. Biologie Medicale 3: 91 (1974).

Tuchmann-Duplessis, H.: Drug Effects on the Fetus (ADIS Press, Sydney 1975).

Tuchmann-Duplessis, H.; David, G. and Haegel, P.: Illustrated Human Embryology, vol. 1, Embryogenesis (Springer-Verlag, New York and Masson, Paris 1972).

Waddell, W.J. and Marlowe, G.C.: Disposition of drugs in the fetus; in Mirkin (Ed) Perinatal Pharmacology and Therapeutics, p.119 (Academic Press, New York 1976).

Warkany, J.: Congenital Malformations (Year Book, Chicago 1971).

Warkany, J.: Warfarin embryopathy. Teratology 14: 205 (1976).

Wilson, J.G.: Environment and Birth Defects (Academic Press, New York 1973).

Wilson, J.G. and Warkany, J.: Teratology, Principles and Techniques (University of Chicago Press, Chicago 1965).

World Health Organisation: Principles for the testing of drugs for teratogenicity. Report of a WHO scientific group. World Health Organisation Technical Report Series No. 364 (WHO, Geneva 1967).

Yaffe, S.J. and Stern, L.: Clinical implications of perinatal pharmacology; in Mirkin (Ed) Perinatal Pharmacology and Therapeutics, p.355 (Academic Press, New York 1976).

Yerushalmy, J.: Methodologic problems encountered in investigating the teratogenic effects of drugs; in Klingberg, Abramovici, Chemke (Eds) Drugs and Fetal Development (Plenum Press, New York 1972).

Chapter III
Fetal Clinical Pharmacology

R.M. Ward, S. Singh and B.L. Mirkin

Synopsis of Important Principles

1) All drugs entering the maternal circulation may be expected to cross the placenta in larger or smaller amounts, although the transfer of a few compounds is limited (e.g. ionised, relatively lipid insoluble compounds such as tubocurarine).

2) The many factors which regulate placental drug transfer and fetal drug localisation, inter-react concurrently and the mother and fetus can be regarded as an integrated system — the maternal-placento-fetal unit.

3) The disposition and effects of drugs on the fetus is governed by the physicochemical characteristics of the drug administered, and various physiological functions relating to the mother, placenta and fetus.

4) Many drugs which can be safely administered to an adult animal may cause unusual and unexpected effects on the fetus, but there is considerable uncertainty regarding extrapolation of data obtained in one animal species to another, let alone to man.

5) Under appropriate circumstances, administration of a drug during the initial trimester of pregnancy can lead to a variety of functional or structural abnormalities in the fetus. In contrast, drugs given to the mother at parturition tend to produce more immediate and generally transient effects in the fetus, which under some circumstances may persist into neonatal life.

6) Many of these effects are minor, uncommon or questionable, but apart from those mentioned below, the clinically more important effects include those of tetracyclines (tooth discolouration), narcotics and barbiturates in labour (neonatal depression: maternal narcotic addiction can also lead to neonatal withdrawal reactions), sulphonamides (increasing the risk of kernicterus by displacing bilirubin from albumin binding), iodides and antithyroid drugs (fetal goitre) and maternal use of oestrogen (vaginal adenocarcinoma in young girls).

7) The only drugs proven to cause congenital abnormalities are: anticonvulsants, warfarin, thalidomide, androgens and virilising progestagens, and cytotoxic drugs such as aminopterin.

Various therapeutic mishaps, such as the fetal malformation induced by the maternal administration of thalidomide, have pointed out the vulnerability of the fetus to drugs. Despite many clinical and laboratory observations there has not been a significant decrease in the utilisation of drugs during human gestation. In fact, if one considers the use of over-the-counter remedies to be in the realm of active therapeutic intervention, there probably has been an increase in maternal drug intake during pregnancy.

The discipline of fetal clinical pharmacology is primarily concerned with the multiple factors which regulate the disposition of drugs in the maternal-placento-fetal unit (for review, see Mirkin, 1976). This chapter will describe some of the effects of pharmacologically active molecules on the fetus and neonate, as well as the manner in which the feto-placental unit may influence their pharmacodynamic characteristics. Chapter II discusses the complex conditions which have to be met before an adverse drug effect on the embryo leads to congenital abnormality, and chapter XV (section 2.1) the principles governing the prescribing of drugs in pregnancy.

1. Transfer of Drugs From the Maternal to the Fetal Organism (fig. 1)

1.1 Maternal Factors

During pregnancy profound biochemical and physiological changes occur in the female organism which may influence the disposition of drugs (see chapter XV; sect. 1.1.4). Gastrointestinal motility may be decreased, the distribution of many drugs may be altered, glomerular filtration rate is greater and hepatic biotransformation capacity may be changed as pregnancy advances. In addition, altered drug distribution and disposition will be further anticipated as the fetus participates in these processes.

The amount of drug transferred from the mother to the fetus depends upon the concentration delivered to the fetus per unit time. In this regard, the route and duration of administration of the drug to the mother is of great significance. Maternal hypoproteinaemia may increase the quantity of free drug in the plasma, particularly of those compounds which are highly bound to plasma proteins, so that increased diffusion across

the placenta will occur. Maternal obesity is also an important consideration, as highly lipid soluble drugs will be sequestrated within body fat and less or lower concentrations of the drug will be available for transfer to the fetus per unit time.

The dynamics of blood flow to the uterus and placenta influences the transfer of drugs to the fetus. Changes in the uterine circulation, either due to maternal hypotension, hypoxia or direct local vasoconstrictive effects will alter the exchange of drugs, as will fetal hypotension resulting from blood loss (premature placental separation). As a consequence, the fetal effects of maternally administered analgesics and sedatives will be potentiated.

1.2 Placental Factors

The placenta is a highly complex organ through which the exchange of substrates between the fetus and the mother occurs. Most of the evidence points towards the placenta as the preferred route for the transport of drugs; however, substances may reach the fetus by other routes as well. *In vitro* preparations of the amniotic membranes have been demonstrated to be permeable to several ions and drugs, e.g. Na^+, Cl^-, I^-, Fe^{++}, guanine, creatinine and serum albumin. While it is conceivable that transfer of drugs via the yolk sac may have some importance in early gestation and in subprimate species, the significance of this route in humans remains unclear.

The placenta functions as a somewhat inefficient barrier for the partition of foreign molecules between the mother and the fetus. The permeability of the placenta to drugs is dependent upon the following factors.

1.2.1 Partition Coefficient and Lipid Solubility

Non-ionised, lipophilic compounds diffuse readily across the placenta, while polar compounds which are highly ionised at physiological pH tend to pass at a slower rate. Bases with extremely high pKa's and acids with extremely low pKa's diffuse poorly. Quaternary bases such as suxamethonium (succinylcholine), d-tubocurarine and THAM traverse the placenta slowly and achieve low concentrations in the fetus, whereas phenazone (antipyrine) and thiopentone (thiopental) cross the placenta very rapidly.

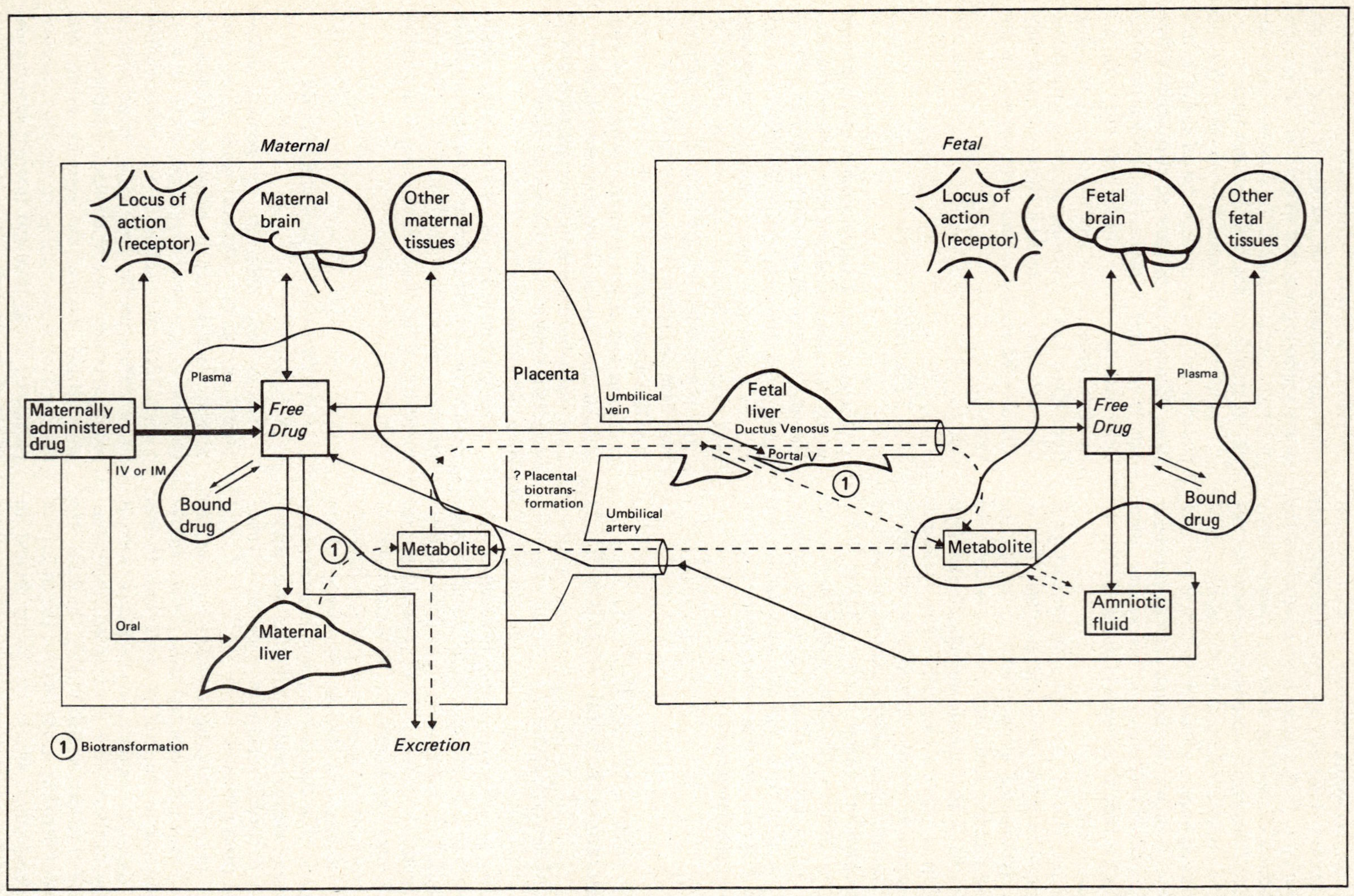

Fig. 1. Drug disposition in a model of the maternal-placento-fetal unit [after Mirkin: in Boreus (Ed) Fetal Pharmacology, Raven Press, New York 1973; by permission of author and publisher].

1.2.2 Molecular Weight

Compounds with low molecular weights diffuse most rapidly across the placenta; generally speaking, drugs with molecular weight less than 600 cross the placenta readily, while those with molecular weight greater than 1,000 do so poorly. (It should be noted that digoxin, mol. wt. 782, readily traverses the placenta). As the molecular weight increases, lipid solubility becomes a more important determinant of placental transfer.

1.2.3 Surface Area and Thickness

The thickness of tissue layers interposed between the capillaries and blood decreases from 25μ early in gestation to 2μ at birth. While few detailed studies have been performed throughout gestation, it has been demonstrated that the permeability of the fetal membranes to sodium and certain antibiotics increases greatly as pregnancy advances.

1.2.4 Protein Binding of Drugs

The free drug crosses the placenta to achieve equilibrium between the maternal and fetal circulation. A large quantity of drug has to be transferred to the fetus in order to establish maternal-fetal equilibrium, because fetal plasma and tissue proteins may act as a 'sink' for free drug molecules once they cross the placenta. Protein binding does not have any important influence on the placental passage of drugs which are highly lipophilic and non-polar, since the rate limiting step in the transfer of these drugs appears to be placental blood flow. In contrast, agents which move across the placenta at moderate or low rates are significantly affected by protein binding because diffusion is rate limiting.

1.2.5 Maternal and Fetal Blood pH

The influence of pH needs to be considered when dealing with drugs having pK_a's close to the pH of blood. The pH of umbilical vessel blood is normally 0.10 to 0.15 pH units lower than maternal blood pH. Consequently the concentration of dissociated basic drugs (pK_a above 7.0) will be higher in the maternal as compared with the fetal blood. This causes a net transfer of basic drug from mother to fetus, so that the total concentration of drug will be higher in the fetus than the mother at equilibrium.

1.2.6 Concentration Gradient and Rates of Equilibrium

The rate at which equilibrium is established between maternal and fetal blood depends upon the rate of delivery of the drug to the placenta, its rate of diffusion across the placenta and its removal from the fetal circulation.

Theoretical multiple compartment models used to calculate apparent rates of equilibration between maternal blood and fetal tissues demonstrate that the equilibrium is not established instantaneously. Using drugs with different characteristics (i.e. pK_a, mol. wt., lipid solubility), this model predicted that for some drugs, when constant maternal blood levels were established, half equilibration of fetal tissues takes place in about 13 minutes and 90 % equilibrium did not occur for almost an hour. On the other hand, when the maternal levels are falling the equilibration is faster, but occurs at lower concentrations and may be of no apparent clinical significance.

The rates of drug equilibration between the fetal and the maternal circuits may be affected by maternal diseases affecting placental function such as diabetes mellitus, systemic lupus erythematosus, hypertension and toxaemia of pregnancy (see chapter II; sect. 4.3).

1.2.7 Drug Metabolism in the Placenta and Fetal Liver

Metabolism may diminish the concentrations of drug passing the placenta and thus influence the availability of drugs to the fetus. It is also possible that drug metabolites may inhibit specific energy requiring transport functions of the placenta, leading to an impairment of active transport systems for substrates such as glucose.

The capacity of the fetus and the placenta to metabolise endogenous steroids has been well documented and the physiological relationship between the fetus and the placenta has led to the concept of the 'feto-placental' unit. The metabolism of drugs and foreign compounds by the fetus and placenta has been intensively investigated and the following is a brief summary of general considerations.

Drug Biotransformation Reactions in Placental Tissue

The placenta contains a considerable number of enzymes which are representative of those involved in drug biotransformation reactions. A number of studies have confirmed that human and animal placental tissue can catalyse the biotransformation of some drugs and foreign compounds by each of the four basic processes of drug metabolism: oxidation, reduction, hydrolysis and conjugation with endogenous molecules. Some studies have suggested that the capacity of human placental tissue for some biotransformation reactions may be lacking during the first trimester (Juchau, 1976).

The significance of these findings remains to be elucidated, particularly their relevance to drug disposition and responses in the fetus, neonate, or mother.

Drug Metabolism by the Fetal Liver
Morphological studies of human fetal liver obtained at legal abortion suggest that early in gestation an enzyme system is present which is capable of metabolising drugs. Indeed, drug metabolising enzyme studies have shown that the human fetal liver is capable of oxidising certain drugs, although in some cases the rate of metabolism is less than that which occurs in human adult liver microsomes. Conjugation reactions are also important for the excretion of drugs. However, studies of glucuronide synthesis by the human fetal liver and kidney show that conjugation capacity is very low, reflecting the low concentration of uridine diphosphate glucuronic acid (UDPGA) and glucuronyl transferase. Indeed, the induction of glucuronyl transferase by phenobarbitone administration has been used for the clinical management of hyperbilirubinaemia in the newborn. Possibly, because of deficiencies in experimental methodology, drug metabolising activity has been barely detectable or absent in tissues obtained from fetal animals of most phylogenetic groups.

While only limited data are available regarding the metabolism of drugs by human fetal liver it is clear that the fetus can extensively metabolise certain xenobiotics (foreign biologically active compounds) to form both inactive and potentially harmful dysmorphogenic and mutagenic metabolites (Mitchell and Corcoran, 1978).

2. Effects of Therapeutic Agents on the Fetus

Many drugs which can be safely administered to an adult may cause unusual and unexpected effects upon the fetus. Most of the experimental work reported in this area has been carried out in various subhuman animal models and considerable uncertainty prevails regarding the extrapolation of data obtained in one species to another. Consequently, extreme caution must be utilised, particularly when these observations are used to predict responses of the human fetus to pharmacological agents.

The ensuing discussion will summarise the effects of some commonly used drugs on the developing fetus (see also table I).

3. Drugs Acting on the Central Nervous System

3.1 Narcotic Analgesics

Drug abuse among teenagers and adults in the reproductive age range is widely prevalent in some countries and has created great concern regarding the effects of maternal drug abuse upon the fetus and neonate. The true magnitude of this problem is difficult to assess because of the illicit nature of drug abuse, the absence of reliable obstetric histories and the observation that narcotic addiction is associated with impaired menstrual function and increased fetal wastage.

All narcotics readily cross the placenta and studies in pregnant animals consistently show accumulation in fetal brain tissues. Methadone concentrations in cord blood and neonatal serum were half those obtained simultaneously in the mothers (Rosen and Pippenger, 1976). Stillborn human infant brain concentrations have not been reported. The dysmorphogenic effects of narcotics in lower animals have not been observed in humans.

Infants born to narcotic addicted mothers have an increased incidence of prematurity, intrauterine growth retardation, fetal distress, perinatal mortality and possibly materno-fetal infections (Fricker and Segal, 1978). Many of these findings may eventually be attributed to the socio-economic milieu which accompanies drug abuse. Connaughton et al. (1977) have shown that close comprehensive prenatal management with attention to nutrition improves the infant's outcome.

Withdrawal may be manifest by tremors, irritability, high pitched cry, hypertonicity, seizures, poor feeding in spite of vigorous sucking, vomiting, diarrhoea or tachypnoea. Although the symptoms of withdrawal are the same, infants of mothers addicted to methadone show symptoms of withdrawal with a later onset, greater frequency, and longer duration than infants whose mothers were addicted to heroin. The severity of an infant's withdrawal from methadone increases with a maternal maintenance dose above 20mg/day and with a more rapid clearance from the infant's serum. The onset of withdrawal is inversely related to the interval between last methadone dose and delivery. Late withdrawal from methadone has been observed beginning 10 to 32 days after birth (Rothstein and Gould, 1,974).

Long term follow-up studies have failed to confirm an early report of a high incidence of sudden infant death in children of narcotic addicted mothers. Although difficult to carry out in this elusive population, follow-up developmental studies have revealed an increased incidence of sleep disturbances, tremors, hypertonicity, and developmental problems (Rothstein and Gould, 1974).

Pethidine (meperidine) is considered to be one of the least depressing of the narcotics used for obstetric practice. The effect on the fetus, however, is related to maternal metabolism, placental transfer, fetal metabolism and fetal CNS penetration. Mean cord blood concentrations are reported at delivery to be 75% to 91% of maternal vein concentrations (Cooper et al., 1977; Caldwell et al., 1977). The fetus continues to acquire pethidine for at least 5 hours after maternal administration (Hogg et al., 1977) so that cord blood concentrations may exceed maternal levels by 2 1/2 to 3 hours after maternal administration. This reflects the slower fetal elimination half-life (22.7 hours) compared with that of the mother (2.8 hours) [Caldwell et al., 1977]. The fetus acquires high concentrations of pethidine within the first hour after maternal administration (Cooper et al., 1977; Caldwell et al., 1977), but low Apgar scores are usually *not* observed when delivery occurs within one hour of pethidine administration (Shnider and Moya, 1964; Morrison et al., 1976). This incongruity has led to speculation that neonatal depression is due to metabolites which do not reach significant CNS concentrations until 1 hour or more after maternal administration. One study correlated depression both with the interval after intravenous administration and the maternal pattern of elimination, but the assay did not separate pethidine from its metabolites (Morrison et al., 1976). Since fetal metabolism is slow and maternal metabolism makes pethidine more polar, the metabolites should cross the placenta less readily

than pethidine. The observations of the delay in neonatal depression may simply reflect the time course required for pethidine to enter the fetal central nervous system and produce depression. Beyond neonatal depression (low apgar scores, acidosis, delayed onset of sustained respiration), less obvious effects on feeding and ventilation up to 48 hours after delivery have been attributed to pethidine (Wiener et al., 1977).

Other synthetic narcotic analgesics such as alphaprodine and anileridine depress the newborn to about the same degree as morphine and pethidine. Pentazocine has not been thoroughly evaluated regarding its safety for the fetus and newborn even though it appears in the cord blood shortly after administration. Fetal blood concentrations do not however, appear to exceed those in the maternal blood at any time (Moore et al., 1973).

Nalorphine or naloxone (Wiener et al., 1977) can reverse the depressant effect of narcotic analgesics when administered to the mother prior to delivery or injected into the umbilical vein. It should also be noted that administration of these agents to narcotic addicts may be hazardous to the fetus.

3.2 Simple Analgesics and Non-Steroidal Anti-inflammatory Analgesics

Salicylates readily cross the placenta in the human (Palmisano and Cassady, 1969). Levy and Garrettson (1974) reported that plasma salicylate concentrations in infants ranged from 8.3 to 30.8µg/ml at birth, whereas the maternal salicylate concentrations 8 to 30 minutes after delivery varied between 2.0 and 26.0µg/ml. Approximately 2.3% of the dose of aspirin ingested by the mothers could be recovered in the urine of the neonates. The elimination half-life of salicylate in these infants ranged from 4.5 to 11.5 hours compared with an average value of 3 hours in the adult. Salicylate was eliminated by neonates mainly by conversion to glycine and glucuronic acid conjugates.

Regular salicylate ingestion during pregnancy has been reported to reduce birth weight and increase the risk of perinatal death (Turner and Collins, 1975). In contrast, Shapiro et al. (1975), based on data from the Collaborative Perinatal Project, found no evidence that aspirin ingested irregularly by pregnant women is related to

Table I. Possible adverse effects in the human fetus and neonate attributed to maternally administered drugs

Drug class	Agent	Possible fetal or neonatal effect (see also text)
Drugs acting on CNS	Strong analgesics (narcotics)	Neonatal depression; 'withdrawal symptoms'
	Simple analgesics (large doses salicylates)	Transient coagulation defects in newborn
	Barbiturates	Neonatal depression and 'withdrawal symptoms' Increased rate of neonatal drug metabolism Fetal asphyxia (if maternal hypotension induced by barbiturate)
	Ethanol	? Congenital abnormalities
	Local anaesthetics	Fetal bradycardia; neonatal depression Maternal hypotension (spinal anaesthesia) Methaemoglobinaemia (large doses prilocaine)
	Phenothiazines	Neonatal sedation Extrapyramidal reactions
	Anticonvulsants/antianxiety drugs benzodiazepines	Neonatal hypotonia, hypothermia, depression, altered fetal heart rate (large doses); ? congenital abnormalities (cleft lip, palate)
	phenytoin	Congenital abnormalities, coagulopathy
	trimethadione	Congenital abnormalities
	Lithium	Fetal goitre; ? congenital abnormalities
Drugs acting on hormonally regulated processes	Antithyroid agents iodides (NB cough mixtures)	Fetal euthyroid goitre
	radio-iodine	Severe hypothyroidism in fetus
	propylthiouracil, carbimazole	Fetal goitre, hypothyroidism
	Oral hypoglycaemic agents	? Prolonged hypoglycaemia
	Androgens and certain progestagens	Virilisation of female
	Oestrogens	Feminisation of male Adenocarcinoma of vagina in children
	Progestagen-oestrogens	Congenital abnormalities
	Corticosteroids	? Adrenal crisis on withdrawal (theoretically possible)
Anticoagulants	Coumarins	? Fetal and neonatal haemorrhage Congenital malformations (warfarin)
Antimicrobial agents	Aminoglycosides (streptomycin; kanamycin; gentamicin; amikacin; tobramycin)	Ototoxicity
	Tetracyclines	Abnormal dentition; impaired fetal bone growth Maternal hepatotoxicity (large doses)
	Chloramphenicol	Cardiovascular collapse, 'grey syndrome' (excessive doses to neonate)
	Sulphonamides	Neonatal kernicterus (highly protein bound compds) Haemolytic anaemia in those with G6PD deficiency
	Nitrofurantoin	Haemolytic anaemia in those with G6PD deficiency
	Antimalarials quinine	Thrombocytopenia
	chloroquine	Retinopathy Ototoxicity

Table I. (continued)

Drug class	Agent	Possible fetal or neonatal effect (see also text)
Drugs acting on cardiovascular system	β-Adrenoceptor blocking drugs (propranolol)	Fetal bradycardia (potential effects ?); hypoglycaemia
	β-Adrenoceptor stimulant drugs (agonists)	Fetal cardiac arrhythmias
	Antihypertensives	
	reserpine	Fetal bradycardia, nasal stuffiness, lethargy
	magnesium sulphate	Neuromuscular weakness, lethargy
	thiazides	Electrolyte imbalance, ? thrombocytopenia (very rare)
	diazoxide	Decreased uterine tone, hyperglycaemia
Antineoplastic agents	Cytotoxic drugs (aminopterin)	Congenital abnormalities

perinatal mortality or low birth weight. These contradictory findings are also related, at least in part, to the very different methods of selection of patients in the 2 studies. Aspirin may also prolong gestation and labour by inhibiting prostaglandin synthesis. Dysmorphogenic effects observed in experimental animals and suggested in retrospective surveys in humans have not been confirmed in large prospective studies in the human (Turner and Collins, 1975; Slone et al., 1976).

Bleyer and Breckenridge (1970) have demonstrated inhibition of collagen induced platelet aggregation and diminished coagulation factor XII activity in infants born to mothers exposed to aspirin during the last weeks of pregnancy. The clinical significance of aspirin induced abnormalities in platelet function and their role in bleeding disorders of the newborn remain to be clarified.

Phenacetin ingested by adults is rapidly and almost completely converted to paracetamol (acetaminophen). The placental transfer of paracetamol has been reported in humans. Placentally acquired paracetamol is however, excreted by the neonate mainly as paracetamol sulphate along with smaller quantities of glucuronide conjugate and the unchanged compound (see chapter IV; sect. 2.3.1; Levy et al., 1975). Although some reports indicate that phenacetin (acetophenetidin) can produce methaemoglobinaemia in the newborn, clinical experience shows that in conventional doses this does not constitute a hazard to the fetus.

Indomethacin has been used successfully to inhibit premature labour (Reiss et al., 1976), but it may have deleterious effects on the fetus and newborn. Indomethacin crosses the placenta in the rabbit, but the fetal levels are consistently less than those in the doe (Parks, 1977). Elimination of indomethacin in the newborn is significantly slower than that in adults (Traeger et al., 1973; Friedman et al., 1978; Evans et al., 1978).

Prostaglandin synthetase inhibitors have produced constriction of the ductus arteriosus and pulmonary arteries in the sheep fetus (Heymann and Rudolph, 1976). Following exposure to indomethacin during labour, several neonates have developed primary pulmonary artery hypertension (persistence of fetal vascularity), some fatally (Csaba et al., 1978; Manchester et al., 1976). Indomethacin administered to neonates has produced impaired platelet (Friedman et al., 1978) and renal function (Friedman et al., 1976; Heymann et al., 1976). Due to potentially severe fetal and neonatal complications, the risk of using indomethacin to inhibit premature labour may outweigh its benefits.

3.3 Barbiturates

All barbiturates are rapidly transferred across the placenta. Thiopentone can be detected in the fetal circulation within 45 seconds after maternal administration. Accumulation of thiopentone in the fetal liver has been reported with concentrations in this organ being 2 to 4 times greater than those detectable in other tissues. Barbitone, amylobarbitone (amobarbital) and phenobarbitone appear to concentrate in the human fetal brain and liver.

When barbiturates are administered to the mother during delivery, significant respiratory depression of the neonate may be observed. There is however, a poor correlation between the degree of respiratory depression and the neonatal blood barbiturate level. While depression of the perinate by barbiturates has been extensively studied, there is meagre information regarding their effects on the fetus. In conventional dosages, little more than mild sedation of the fetus will be anticipated. However, if maternal hypotension has been induced by barbiturate administration, more devastating effects may occur as a consequence of fetal asphyxia secondary to decreased placental blood flow.

Phenobarbitone has been demonstrated to induce hepatic microsomal drug metabolising enzyme activity (see section 1.2.7). Clinically, this is manifest by an increased capacity of the neonate to conjugate bilirubin. The magnitude and duration of physiological jaundice in the newborn is significantly decreased in infants delivered by mothers who have received phenobarbitone for 14 days before delivery (Maurer et al., 1968).

3.4 Ethanol

Although narcotics, 'street drugs' and marihuana use have attracted more attention in recent years, alcohol remains the most frequent worldwide drug of abuse. Ethanol readily crosses the placenta, resulting in equal maternal:fetal serum concentrations within 1 hour. The newborn, however, clears ethanol more slowly than the adult, and acute intoxication may further retard its elimination.

The direct toxicity of ethanol for the developing fetus is difficult to prove due to the pregnant alcoholic's altered nutritional and metabolic status. The intake of many other pharmacologically active agents in varying quantities further confounds the situation. The discovery of a consistent pattern of abnormalities in the offspring of 8 unrelated alcoholic mothers from 3 different ethnic backgrounds supported ethanol or one of its metabolites as the cause (Jones et al., 1973). The features attributed to the 'fetal alcohol syndrome' included prenatal and postnatal growth delay, developmental delay, microcephaly, narrow palpebral fissures, prominent mandible, limited joint mobility, abnormal palmar creases, cardiac anomalies and anomalous external genitalia. Subsequent reports have confirmed these associations and roughly correlated the degree of mental and growth retardation with

the degree to which these abnormalities are expressed (Streissguth et al., 1978).

3.5 Marihuana

As with other natural products, quantitative studies of *Cannabis* have been delayed by the need for isolation or synthesis of active compounds coupled with sensitive analytical techniques. The psychological effects from marihuana are primarily attributed to Δ^9-tetrahydrocannabinol (Δ^9-THC), although other cannabinoids are possibly involved. Δ^9-THC crosses the murine placenta to a limited degree with a fetal distribution similar to that in the mother. Numerous studies in pregnant animals of the effects of various dosages of Δ^9-THC have demonstrated reduction in litter size, increased fetal resorption and runting, but no dysmorphogenic changes (Harris et al., 1977).

3.6 General Anaesthetics

Gaseous and volatile liquid agents are used alone or in combination to provide anaesthesia or analgesia during labour. The halogenated hydrocarbons (halothane, chloroform, trichloroethylene) and cyclopropane are highly lipid soluble compounds which readily enter the fetal circulation. The effects of general anaesthetics on fetal function are difficult to assess since they are generally used in combination with sedatives, hypnotics or tranquillisers. In addition, the influence of changes in maternal ventilation, circulation and uterine perfusion are factors which must be taken into account.

Clinical experience with mothers undergoing surgery during pregnancy suggests that in the absence of maternal hypotension or respiratory depression no detrimental effects on the fetus are seen. It has been suggested that the fetus is more resistant to the pharmacodynamic actions of halogenated hydrocarbons than the adult and the fetal liver has been demonstrated to be resistant to damage by carbon tetrachloride and chloroform.

3.7 Phenothiazines

Phenothiazines have been shown to traverse the placenta readily. Chlorpromazine has been demonstrated in the fetal plasma and its metabolites in the amniotic fluid. Promazine has been identified in umbilical cord blood with peak levels achieved about 4 minutes after maternal administration, but only approximately 0.5 % of the maternal dose was estimated to have reached the fetus.

In contrast to the toxicity (cholestatic jaundice) observed in the adult liver, phenothiazines have not been demonstrated to produce such effects in the fetus, nor is neonatal jaundice accentuated. This is not unexpected as the phenothiazines are known to induce fetal liver enzymes.

In animals, antenatal phenothiazine exposure produces a number of abnormalities, possibly involving depletion of riboflavine. Two large multicentre studies have produced conflicting findings regarding an association between phenothiazine intake during the first trimester and the occurrence of congenital malformations. The larger study (50,000 women) found no increased incidence (Slone et al., 1977), whereas the smaller study (12,000 women) found an overall increase in malformations of various types associated with the intake of phenothiazines with a 3 carbon side chain (chlorpromazine) [Rumeau-Rouquette et al., 1977]. Neither study reported cases of retinopathy which is observed in adults treated with large dosage prolonged courses of phenothiazine drugs (see chapter XII; sect. 11.1.1).

Since phenothiazines can produce a significant degree of α-adrenoceptor blockade, non-shivering thermogenesis (which is dependent upon adrenergic stimulation) and temperature regulation may be impaired in neonates delivered from mothers receiving the drug.

3.8 Lithium

Lithium crosses the placenta producing similar maternal and cord blood concentrations at delivery (Weinstein and Goldfield, 1969; Fries, 1970; Rane et al., 1978). Neonatal hypotonia, poor suck and diminished reflexes have been reported, but this does not appear to be dose related (Wilbanks et al., 1970; Stothers et al., 1973). These symptoms may persist for several hours to days (Wilbanks et al., 1970) which likely reflects the delayed elimination rate observed in newborns (Rane et al., 1978).

From the late 1960's, a collaborative survey has sought case reports of congenital anomalies following exposure to lithium during the first trimester. Such retrospective case reporting does not

allow assessment of the prevalence of such anomalies or the risk for a given patient. In spite of these reservations, the reports of malformations following first trimester exposures to lithium do show a preponderance of serious cardiac malformations, particularly of the tricuspid valve (Weinstein and Goldfield, 1975). Prospective, appropriately controlled studies are needed to validate and analyse this association.

3.9 Antiemetics

Although the antiemetics meclozine and cyclizine readily cause fetal abnormalities in animals, allegations of similar effects in humans have not been substantiated. In fact, during pregnancies producing children with major congenital anomalies compared with normal children, antiemetic use and morning sickness are significantly less frequent (Kullander and Kallen, 1976). A careful prospective study from Sweden revealed an association between congenital hip dislocation and promethazine (a phenothiazine antihistamine) used during the first trimester. Since vomiting as well as congenital hip dislocation are associated with elevated human chorionic gonadotrophin during pregnancy, this association more likely reflects the cause of the vomiting. The most frequently used antiemetic in this study (promethazine, 79 %) would then have an apparent association with congenital hip dislocation (Kullander and Kallen, 1976). Most antiemetics commonly used in pregnancy have now been carefully studied. A small, questionably significant increase in congenital anomalies was noted only for trimethobenzamide (Milkovich and van den Berg, 1976; Shapiro et al., 1977).

3.10 Anticonvulsants and Antianxiety Drugs

3.10.1 Benzodiazepines

Diazepam and its metabolites are rapidly transferred across the placenta, with higher concentrations present in cord blood than in maternal blood shortly after administration. The fetus can N-demethylate diazepam but appears unable to hydroxylate this compound, so that diazepam and N-desmethyldiazepam can be recovered from cord blood (Mandelli et al., 1975). Concentrations above 3 to 400μg/ml of either of these compounds are associated with adverse effects in the fetus. Chlordiazepoxide also crosses the placenta and during labour cord levels of drug approximate maternal blood concentrations.

Chlordiazepoxide and diazepam are widely employed in toxaemia of pregnancy as muscle relaxants and anticonvulsants, but they must be used judiciously. Infants born to mothers treated with *high* doses of intravenous or intramuscular chlordiazepoxide or diazepam may have low Apgar scores, apnoeic spells and be reluctant to feed, unresponsive, hypotonic and hypothermic (Cree et al., 1973; Stirrat et al., 1974). Diazepam may alter fetal heart rate patterns but their clinical significance has not been determined. Elimination of diazepam by the neonate is slow and the drug and its active metabolites may persist in the neonate for a week after administration of high doses during labour (Cree et al., 1973). For a review see Mandelli et al. (1978).

Long term use of low doses of diazepam during pregnancy can also cause a hypotonic, unresponsive state in the neonate ('floppy infant syndrome'). Nitrazepam can produce similar effects (Speight, 1977). When used over long periods the benzodiazepines can produce physical dependence and withdrawal symptoms have occurred in neonates born of mothers who had taken chlordiazepoxide or diazepam during pregnancy (Athinarayanam et al., 1976; Rementeria and Bhatt, 1977).

3.10.2 Phenytoin (diphenylhydantoin)

Phenytoin is also transferred across the placenta; after a single intravenous maternal dose, the highest fetal concentrations are found in the liver, heart and adrenal gland. On repeat dose administration, umbilical artery and venous concentrations are similar to those of maternal plasma at parturition. The mean plasma half-life in the newborn is estimated to be 60 to 70 hours and the drug is present in the plasma of these neonates as late as the fifth postpartum day. A relatively large quantity of p-hydroxyphenyl-phenylhydantoin-glucuronide can also be identified in the urine. Cleft palate and lip was present in 3 of the 8 neonates studied in the investigation on which the above data are based (Mirkin, 1971a). Other reports have also suggested, but not conclusively proven, an increased incidence of congenital abnormalities in the offspring of mothers receiving anticonvulsant therapy during pregnancy.

A constellation of craniofacial malformations including broad, low nasal bridge and short upturned nose as well as cleft palate, pilonidal sinus,

hypoplasia of the distal phalanges and nails has been associated with the so-called 'fetal hydantoin syndrome' (Hill, 1978). The presence of epilepsy in either parent may contribute to an increased occurrence of congenital defects (Shapiro et al., 1976a). Despite these reports, the risk of congenital abnormalities (2 to 3-fold over normal) in patients receiving this agent may be regarded as acceptable when weighed against the hazards of uncontrolled epilepsy (see further chapter XXV; sect. 4.8). In addition, maternal phenytoin and phenobarbitone administration can induce depletion of the fetal vitamin K dependent clotting factors (II, VII, IX, X) [Solomon et al., 1972]. The resulting coagulopathy can produce serious neonatal haemorrhages unless treated adequately with vitamin K.

3.10.3 Other Anticonvulsants

In addition, carbamazepine and its metabolite carbamazepine-10-11-oxide have been identified in neonates delivered from mothers receiving this agent during gestation (Rane et al., 1975).

4. Drugs Acting on Peripheral Nervous System

4.1 Local Anaesthetics

Local anaesthetics can be classified into two general categories: (1) the ester derivatives such as procaine, 2-chloroprocaine, amethocaine (tetracaine), and (2) amide derivatives such as lignocaine (lidocaine), prilocaine, bupivacaine, etidocaine and mepivacaine. Except for amethocaine, the amides are more potent and longer lasting than the ester derivatives, but the longer acting agents have a slower onset of action.

Both types of local anaesthetics are employed for regional obstetric anaesthesia and readily cross the placenta after paracervical, caudal, spinal and epidural applications. They are not selectively concentrated in the fetus. The extent of placental passage from mother to fetus varies inversely with the degree of protein binding. Prilocaine, which is 55 % protein bound, results in equal maternal and umbilical venous concentrations. In contrast, bupivacaine, which is highly protein bound (94 %) produces umbilical venous concentrations which are only 1/7 that found in maternal serum (Finster, 1976). An hepatic amidase, often immature in the fetus, is responsible for the breakdown of the amides, whereas the esters are rapidly cleaved by plasma esterase which is present in the fetus in adequate concentrations. This results in a prolonged elevated fetal concentration of the amide anaesthetics such as lignocaine.

Fetal bradycardia and even death following paracervical and caudal anaesthesia has occurred with all the local anaesthetics and has been associated with high fetal concentrations of the drug. The frequency of fetal bradycardia or death following paracervical block, however, varies significantly among the available anaesthetics and may be influenced by dose. Bupivacaine was associated with a relatively large number of fetal deaths. Fetal bradycardia after prilocaine was half as frequent as after lignocaine and mepivacaine, but the clinical significance of methaemoglobinaemia seen after prilocaine is debated (Schnider and Gildea, 1973). Chlorprocaine, which is rapidly broken down in both fetal and maternal serum, caused fetal bradycardia in only 5% of cases (Freeman and Arnold, 1975).

Although the local anaesthetics are known to decrease myocardial conduction and contractility, detailed studies of fetal ECG during bradycardia following paracervical blocks have not revealed these changes except after direct fetal administration. The fetal ECG changes are more typical of fetal hypoperfusion and may be a result of anaesthetic induced changes in uterine tone or blood flow rather than a direct effect of the anaesthetic on the fetal heart (Freeman et al., 1972). Fetal acidosis and seizures produced by high concentrations of local anaesthetics in animal studies may also be involved in the fetal cardiovascular response after obstetric regional anaesthesia.

4.2 Neuromuscular Blocking Agents

Compounds employed for their neuromuscular blocking action are generally characterised by the presence of a quarternary nitrogen group. This radical imparts low lipid solubility and high polarity, consequently drugs like curare, suxamethonium (succinylcholine), gallamine and decamethonium cross the placenta poorly. Despite this, however, there are several clinical reports of flaccid infants with respiratory distress having been delivered to mothers receiving suxamethonium. If these neuromuscular blocking agents are inadvertently administered directly to the fetus, their effects are similar to those observed

in the adult and neuromuscular blockade of the fetus has been associated with skeletal deformities.

4.3 Anticholinergic Drugs

Atropine sulphate is readily transferred across the placenta, whereas more polar cholinergic blocking agents such as atropine methylbromide and glycopyrronium bromide (glycopyrrolate) cross the placenta less rapidly (Proakis and Harris, 1978). After the intravenous injection of atropine to pregnant women, fetal plasma levels are almost half of those attained in maternal plasma (Kivalo and Saarikoski, 1977). The maternal administration of atropine results in fetal tachycardia which may be preceded by a period of bradycardia (dePadua and Gravenstein, 1969). Atropine transferred across the placenta may also result in mydriasis and perhaps other cholinergic effects in newborn infants.

4.4 Anticholinesterases

A number of cases of transient neonatal myasthenia have been reported following administration of anticholinesterase agents to pregnant women afflicted with myasthenia gravis (Blackhall et al., 1969). Pyridostigmine is transferred across the placenta with a resultant significant decrease of fetal plasma cholinesterase activity. Pyridostigmine concentrations in the fetus are substantially lower than that in the mother, but clearance of the drug in the fetus is slower, consequently fetal accumulation of the drug can occur on repeated administration to the mother (Roberts et al., 1970).

5. Drugs Acting on Hormonally Regulated Processes

5.1 Antithyroid Agents

The fetal thyroid begins to function at about the fourth month of gestation and its activity is influenced by fetal rather than maternal thyroid stimulating hormone (TSH). Iodides are transferred across the placenta and ingestion of iodides by the mother can lead to fetal euthyroid goitre, sometimes large enough to cause severe obstruction or even death. The maternal administration of radioactive iodine can produce severe hypothyroidism in the fetus, whereas agents such as propylthiouracil and tapazole may lead to the development of a fetal goitre (see also chapter XVI; sect. 5.2.4).

5.2 Hypoglycaemic Agents

Studies with ^{131}I-labelled insulin in rhesus monkeys show that the isotope appears in the fetal blood within minutes of administration to the mother. However, the permeability must be limited since insulin in the usual doses produces no significant effects upon the fetus.

Oral hypoglycaemic agents freely cross the placenta and prolonged hypoglycaemia has been observed in an infant whose mother had been taking chlorpropamide. Dysmorphogenic effects have been reported in man and animals (Tuchmann-Duplessis, 1975), but those in man are difficult to evaluate because of the expected higher incidence of malformations in infants of diabetic mothers (Pedersen et al., 1964; see also chapter XV, sect. 21.2; XVI; sect. 3.4.4).

5.3 Hormonal Steroids

Masculinisation of the urogenital sinus of the female fetus can result from a variety of progestational compounds or other agents possessing androgenic potential. These compounds differ from naturally occurring steroids by having an hydroxyl group at carbon 17 in the β rather than the α position of the steroid nucleus. Methyltestosterone which possesses a similar chemical structure has also produced such effects on female fetuses.

Diethylstilboestrol, a synthetic oestrogen, has been noted to produce a similar effect, presumably by stimulating androgen production in the fetal adrenal gland. The report of vaginal changes in young women exposed to diethylstilboestrol *in utero,* including an extraordinary increase in incidence of clear cell adenocarcinoma in 1970, drew attention to the carcinogenic potential of diethylstilboestrol in the next generation. The risk for clear cell adenocarcinoma has been estimated at 0.14 to 1.4 per 1000 diethylstilboestrol exposed women, with a peak incidence between ages 14 and 22 (Herbst et al., 1977). These findings have been confirmed along with recent reports of an increased incidence of cervical carcinoma *in situ* in this population (Mattingly and Stafl, 1976). Although no increased incidence of cancer in males has been reported at this time, anatomical and functional genitourinary abnormalities have been reported in the analogous male population (Gill et al., 1977).

An association has been suggested, but not definitely shown, between first trimester exposure to female sex hormones and various congenital anomalies, especially cardiovascular and skeletal. Major problems of patient selection, inadequate control of compounding variables, and retrospective recall of information exist in some studies (Janerich et al., 1974, 1977; Greenberg et al., 1977). The resolution of this issue needs definitive study due to the frequency of such exposures via oral contraceptives, sex hormone pregnancy tests, and progestagen supplementation during pregnancy.

Both the Collaborative Perinatal Project (50,282 pregnancies) [Heinonen et al., 1977] and the Jerusalem Perinatal Study (11,468 babies) [Harlap et al., 1975] examined this association prospectively and found an overall increase in malformations associated with first trimester exposures to female sex hormones. In the Jerusalem study, cardiovascular malformations, including hemangiomata, telangiectasia and cardiac malformations, were increased but cardiac malformations alone were not. Progestagens were more frequently associated with anomalies than were oestrogens. No limb reduction anomalies were reported in Jerusalem during the study period, 1966-1968.

In contrast, the Perinatal Collaborative Study showed no difference in incidence between progestagens and oestrogens, but an overall increase in cardiac malformation, especially transpositions and truncoconal anomalies. Many compounding variables known to be associated with cardiovascular malformations were controlled in this study. The rate of cardiovascular malformations increased from 7.82 to 18.2 per 1,000 births ($p < 0.05$) with the ingestion of female sex hormones, particularly during the second and third months of gestation. No increased incidence occurred with later fetal exposures.

Although the risks may be small, this data would indicate the use of female sex hormones early in pregnancy should be avoided whenever possible. Specifically, with the availability of sensitive, inexpensive immunological tests, progestagens alone or combined with oestrogens should not be utilised for pregnancy testing in a potentially susceptible population during a critical period of embryogenesis.

5.4 Corticosteroids

Corticosteroids, frequently cortisone or prednisone, have been widely used in pregnant women and the evidence that they may cause harm in humans (in contrast to rats and mice) is minimal. Although adrenal corticosteroids have been shown to pass across the placenta of the mouse and rat and distribute widely, chemical assays and studies of human fetal adrenal suppression indicate differences in placental passage and biotransformation (inactivation) among individual corticosteroids (Jorgensen, 1969). While the more potent halogenated corticosteroids such as dexamethasone and betamethasone appear to cross the placenta with minimal inactivation, cortisol and prednisone undergo extensive placental dehydrogenation to their respective inactive products (Blanford and Murphy, 1977). This may account for the apparent lack of fetal toxicity with these two particular agents in usual clinical practice. A possible risk of cleft palate is slight, if it exists at all.

Since Liggins' finding that maternal betamethasone treatment reduced the incidence of hyaline membrane disease in 26 to 32 week gestation premature infants (Liggins and Howie, 1972), many more pregnant women and their offspring are being exposed to these potent corticosteroids. Evidence of adverse effects in these mothers and infants has been minimal, but central nervous system abnormalities have been suggested in humans (Fitzhardinge et al., 1974) and in primates (Epstein et al., 1977). Considering these findings, as well as the experience with diethylstilboesterol (see section 5.3), before using corticosteroids to prevent hyaline membrane disease, benefits must be carefully balanced against the risks with consideration of potential unforeseen toxicity. Maternal treatment with corticosteroids should be carefully documented in the infants' medical records to assist in follow-up (see further chapter XV; sect. 9; 21.1).

6. Anticoagulants

Heparin, because of its relatively large molecule and electronegative charge, does not cross the placenta in pharmacologically significant amounts; consequently, no untoward coagulation defects are encountered when heparin is given to the mother prior to delivery (Flessa et al., 1965). In view of the rather slow clearance of heparin from the fetus, fetal transfusion with heparinised blood may lead to prolonged anticoagulation. Citrate has been proposed as an alternative choice for this procedure.

Vitamin K antagonist anticoagulants (warfarin and dicoumarol), despite their high degree of protein binding which should limit placental passage, do get across to the fetus and interfere with prothrombin synthesis by the fetal liver (Saidi et al., 1965). The administration of oral anticoagulants during the latter part of pregnancy is known to cause fetal and placental haemorrhage (Bloomfield, 1970). Administration of warfarin (and possibly other oral anticoagulants) during the first 8 weeks of gestation may result in congenital malformations. The most consistent malformations include nasal hypoplasia, stippling of bones, ophthalmologic abnormalities, intrauterine growth retardation and developmental delay (Shaul and Hall, 1977). Whether these malformations result from microhaemorrhages in embryonic cartilage, fetal vitamin K deficiency or a more widespread dysmorphogenic defect remains to be clarified.

7. Antimicrobial Agents

While the untoward effects of antibiotics such as the 'grey syndrome' following chloramphenicol administration to the neonate are well known, there is little quantitative data describing the pharmacokinetics of antimicrobial agents during early gestation. Most studies have involved pulse injections to the mother during labour, followed by analysis of paired maternal and cord samples obtained at delivery. Despite the limitations of such data most of the information available suggests that all antibiotics are capable of being transferred across the placenta, at varying rates.

7.1 Penicillins and Cephalosporins

Penicillins rapidly pass across the placenta and therapeutic concentrations are present in fetal body fluids following administration of conventional doses to the mother. Both the penicillins and cephalosporins enter the amniotic fluid more extensively at term than during the first trimester (Wasz-Hockert et al., 1970; Bernard et al., 1977b). The penicillins have been used extensively in pregnancy without ill effects. After repeated dosage and constant infusion, neither the cephalosporins nor the penicillins accumulate in the fetus. In the newborn however, the renal clearance of the penicillins and cephalosporins is decreased, thus prolonging their half-life so that drug levels persist for a longer time in body fluids and tissues (see chapter IV; sect. 2.3.2).

The cephalosporins are also transferred rapidly across the placenta. As many new cephalosporins have become available for clinical use, some differences have appeared with respect to placental passage and fetal-neonatal clearance. For example, after comparable maternal dosages, cephaloridine and cephacetrile resulted in higher sustained fetal cord serum concentrations than after cephalothin (Stewart et al., 1973; Hirsch et al., 1974). Although the cephalosporins appear in the amniotic fluid as quickly as in the fetal serum, the cord serum reaches a maximal concentration faster (Stewart et al., 1973). Cephalosporins attain quite high concentrations in neonatal-fetal urine. No neonatal toxicity from maternal cephalosporins has been noted.

7.2 Aminoglycosides

Streptomycin and dihydrostreptomycin readily undergo transplacental passage and are detectable in fetal blood. After an intravenous injection to the mother, fetal blood and amniotic fluid concentrations are about 50% that of maternal blood, but still within the therapeutic range (Charles, 1954). Gentamicin administered by continuous infusion following a loading dose reaches equal serum concentration in the mother and fetus after 4 to 7 hours. Amniotic fluid concentrations rise later and subsequently exceed maternal serum concentrations by 20 to 30% (Daubenfeld et al., 1974). This likely reflects voiding and the capacity of the fetal kidney to concentrate and excrete gentamicin, which has been demonstrated as early as the first trimester (Kaufman et al., 1975). Higher than usual maternal dosages of gentamicin are required during pregnancy to achieve the desired serum concentrations (see chapter XV; sect. 1.4). Studies employing single intramuscular injections at intervals less than 4 hours before delivery may measure maternal-fetal distribution ratios prior to equilibrium.

Ototoxicity in the form of decreased eighth nerve function and abnormal audiograms have been described in young children whose mothers were given streptomycin during pregnancy (Robinson and Cambon, 1964). There are also poorly documented reports of ototoxicity in the offspring following kanamycin therapy of the pregnant mother. Definite neonatal toxicity from maternal gentamicin has not yet been observed.

Recently, amikacin, a semisynthetic aminoglycoside, was shown to cross the placenta and achieve significant levels in fetal tissues. It differed from other aminoglycosides in that high concentrations were established in fetal lungs ($8.0\mu g/g$) as well as kidneys ($22\mu g/kg$) [Bernard et al., 1977a].

7.3 Tetracyclines

Transmission of tetracyclines across the placenta results in cord blood levels which are 50 to 60% of simultaneously drawn maternal blood levels. Tetracyclines circulating in the fetal blood are selectively concentrated in both the dentine and enamel of teeth, which calcify towards the end of the fourth month of gestation. Tooth discolouration, enamel hypoplasia and a tendency to caries are side effects of tetracycline treatment in the third trimester of fetal life. Teeth discoloured by tetracyclines fluoresce and the fluorophor is a chelated complex of calcium and unaltered tetracycline. Tetracycline administration has also been reported to cause a significant depression of skeletal growth in premature infants (see also chapter XIII, sect.13.3; XXII, sect.14.5).

7.4 Chloramphenicol

Chloramphenicol achieves fetal plasma concentrations which range between one-third to four-fifths that of maternal blood levels. Biotransformation of chloramphenicol occurs primarily via glucuronidation and elimination by renal filtration of the unmetabolised drug and tubular secretion of its metabolites. The neonate, due to its renal and hepatic immaturity, is at a disadvantage when chloramphenicol is administered and large doses can produce cardiovascular collapse in the form of the 'grey syndrome' (see chapter IV; sect. 2.3.1). In contrast, the fetus has not been reported to be adversely affected by chloramphenicol, partly because the usual dosage in the adult is smaller on a weight basis when compared with that employed for the neonate.

7.5 Antimalarial Agents

Quinine has been falsely implicated as resulting in increased fetal wastage. This has not been borne out in carefully conducted studies and the passage of meconium *in utero* is more likely to be the result of a direct effect of the drug on fetal intestinal motility, rather than a sign of fetal disorder.

Primaquine, pentaquine, and other antimalarial agents could be expected to cause adverse effects only in the fetus with glucose-6-phosphate dehydrogenase (G6PD) deficiency (see chapter VII; sect. 4.2.2).

Chloroquine has been associated with abnormal retinal pigmentation and severe cochleovestibular paresis in the progeny of a mother taking chloroquine for chronic discoid lupus erythematosus during pregnancy (Hart and Nauton, 1964).

8. Drugs Acting on the Cardiovascular System

8.1 Catecholamines and β-Adrenoceptor Stimulant Drugs

The transfer of ^{3}H-noradrenaline (norepinephrine) from maternal to fetal circulation has been investigated in pregnant rats (Mirkin, 1972). Relatively large concentrations of ^{3}H-noradrenaline and metabolites were present in the placenta, whereas fetal heart, adrenals or spleen showed no uptake of ^{3}H-noradrenaline. Studies in pregnant dogs also failed to show any significant placental passage or fetal uptake of ^{3}H-noradrenaline (Mirkin, 1971b). The administration of ^{14}C-dl-noradrenaline to pregnant women resulted in cord levels which ranged from 2 to 18 % of the maternal concentration (Sandler et al., 1963). Despite the active metabolism of catecholamines to a variety of methylated and deaminated metabolites by the placenta, concentrations of noradrenaline reaching the fetal circulation may be sufficient to cause fetal bradycardia (Sandler et al., 1964), whereas adrenaline (epinephrine) causes fetal tachycardia or arrhythmias (Beard, 1962). Other investigators, however, suggest that catecholamines influence fetal heart rate indirectly by altering uterine blood flow (Dornhorst and Young, 1952).

Various β-adrenoceptor agonists (ritodrine, isoxsuprine, orciprenaline/metaproterenol, salbutamol/albuterol etc) have been employed recently to inhibit undesirable uterine activity and premature labour (see chapter XV; sect. 9). These agents are transferred across the placenta and in-

crease in fetal heart rate is usually observed during maternal infusion of β-adrenoceptor agonists (Eskes and Haan, 1972), although fetal cardiac arrhythmias have also been reported (Miller et al., 1976). The use of these agents is sometimes associated with a decrease in fetal pH, an increase in fetal glucose (Miller et al., 1976) and a fall in maternal blood pressure, all of which can be detrimental to the fetus.

8.2 β-Adrenoceptor Blocking Drugs

Relatively non-polar β-adrenoceptor antagonists (β-blockers) such as propranolol, oxprenolol, bunolol and butidrine are readily transferred across the ovine placenta and produce a measurable degree of β-blockade in the fetus, whereas, more polar β-blockers such as practolol and sotalol are impeded in their transfer across the placenta (Van Petten, 1975). The fetal plasma levels produced by single dose, intravenous administration of propranolol to the pregnant ewe are extremely low, yet the duration of β-blockade, as determined by chronotropic response to isoprenaline (isoproterenol), is 3 times longer in the fetus than in the pregnant ewe (Van Petten, 1975; Singh et al., 1977). Although transplacentally acquired propranolol decreases umbilical blood flow and fetal heart rate, fetal haemodynamics and acid-base status are not significantly affected at rest (Oakes et al., 1976). In contrast, the ability of the fetal lamb to respond to stress such as hypoxia or haemorrhage is seriously impaired (Singh et al., 1978b).

Propranolol is transferred across the human placenta and cord levels of propranolol in infants of mothers receiving the drug prenatally are usually in the therapeutic range (Habib and McCarthy, 1977). Numerous adverse effects have been attributed to the administration of propranolol during pregnancy and labour, included among which are intrauterine growth retardation, decreased placental size, prolonged labour, neonatal respiratory depression, hypoglycaemia and bradycardia (Gladstone et al., 1975; Habib and McCarthy, 1977). Despite these reported associations a clear cause and effect relationship between maternal administration of propranolol and impairment of the response of the human fetus and neonate to stress remains to be established. More recent clinical studies have not revealed any adverse effects in the neonate resulting from the administration of propranolol during gestation (Mirkin and Teramo, unpublished data 1978). See also chapter XV (sect. 5.1).

8.3 Antihypertensive Agents

8.3.1 Reserpine

Infants born to mothers who have received rauwolfia alkaloids during the third trimester of pregnancy are frequently lethargic during the first 24 hours and have nasal congestion which disappears in about a week. Despite this type of neonatal morbidity, fetal mortality is not increased (Budnick et al., 1955; Desmond et al., 1957).

8.3.2 Magnesium Sulphate

Magnesium ions produce neuromuscular weakness and lethargy in the neonate and these infants may have a delayed onset of respiration.

8.4 Cardiac Glycosides

The placental transfer of digoxin has been demonstrated to occur in the human (Saarikoski, 1976) and in a variety of animal species such as the rat, guinea pig, dog and sheep. The fetal digoxin concentrations ranged from 20 to 36 % of respective maternal levels 20 minutes after administering single intravenous doses of digoxin to pregnant rats and the value increased to 50 % after 40 minutes. The distribution pattern of digoxin differed in maternal and fetal tissue of the rat. Maternal digoxin levels were highest in the liver followed in descending order by the heart, kidney and skeletal muscle, whereas in fetal tissues the myocardial concentrations exceeded that of the kidney, which were higher than liver (Singh and Mirkin, 1978).

Investigations in pregnant ewes revealed major differences between the ovine and rodent maternal-placental-fetal unit with respect to the placental transfer of digoxin. Although digoxin was transferred rapidly across the ovine placenta, digoxin concentrations in umbilical and fetal circulations were very low. Digoxin could not be detected in fetal plasma 4 hours after intravenous administration to the ewe whereas maternal levels remained elevated for 12 to 24 hours (Singh et al., 1978a).

The ^{3}H-digoxin concentration of umbilical venous and arterial blood was reported to be similar to that of maternal blood 30 minutes after injection to women undergoing therapeutic abortion (Saarikoski, 1976). Long term administration of digoxin during pregnancy results in the establishment of a fetal-maternal equilibrium state and digoxin levels in cord blood and maternal venous blood samples obtained at parturition are similar (Rogers et al., 1972).

Long term digoxin therapy of pregnant women has not been associated with adverse effects in the fetus, although the pharmacodynamic consequences resulting from the placental transfer of digoxin have not been clearly elucidated.

8.5 Diuretics

Thiazide diuretics readily cross the placenta and have allegedly been associated with neonatal thrombocytopenia on very rare occasions (Rodriguez et al., 1964). Considering the low incidence of this complication, considerable doubt exists regarding the validity of this association.

9. Antineoplastic Drugs

Although the dysmorphogenic effects of cytotoxic drugs in rodents and the chick are well known, there are major discrepancies between such animal studies and clinical observations. During the first trimester, the risk of malformations from cytotoxic drugs appears to be increased, although the risk is low except for aminopterin (Nicholson, 1968). Besides a high incidence of spontaneous abortion and perinatal death (Lilleyman et al., 1977), chromosomal abnormalities, myelomeningocoele, skeletal anomalies, leucopenia and hypogammaglobulinaemia have occurred after cancer therapy and immunosuppression during pregnancy. More sophisticated follow-up and testing may reveal toxic effects on the developing brain or reproductive system as well as a predisposition to cancer in the offspring.

Further Reading

Boreus, L.O.: Fetal Pharmacology (Raven Press, New York 1973).

Cohen, S.N. and Olson, W.A.: Drugs that depress the newborn infant. Pediatric Clinics of North America 17: 835 (1970).

Mirkin, B.L.: Perinatal Pharmacology and Therapeutics (Academic Press, New York 1976).

Mirkin, B.L.: Clinical Pharmacology and Therapeutics: A Pediatric Perspective (Year Book, Chicago 1978).

Morselli, P.L.; Garattini, S. and Sereni, F.: Basic and Therapeutic Aspects of Perinatal Pharmacology (Raven Press, New York 1975).

Various Authors: Symposium on drugs and the unborn child. Clinical Pharmacology and Therapeutics 14(4, Part 2): 619 (1973).

References

Athinarayanan, P.; Pierog, Sophie, H.; Nigam, S.K. and Glass, L.: Chlordiazepoxide withdrawal in the neonate. American Journal of Obstetrics and Gynecology 124: 212 (1976).

Beard, R.W.: Response of human foetal heart and maternal circulation to adrenaline and noradrenaline, British Medical Journal 1: 443 (1962).

Bernard, B.; Abate, M.; Thielen, P.F.; Attar, H.; Ballard, C.A. and Wehrle, P.F.: Maternal-fetal pharmacological activity of amikacin. Journal of Infectious Diseases 135: 925 (1977a).

Bernard, B.; Barton, L.; Abate, M. and Ballard, C.A.: Maternal-fetal transfer of cephazolin in the first twenty weeks of pregnancy. Journal of Infectious Diseases 136: 377 (1977b).

Blackhall, M.I.; Buckley, G.A.; Roberts, D.V.; Roberts, J.B.; Thomas, B.H. and Wilson, A.: Drug induced myasthenia. Journal of Obstetrics and Gynaecology, British Commonwealth 76: 157 (1969).

Blanford, A.T. and Murphy, B.E.P.: *In vitro* metabolism of prednisolone, dexamethasone, betamethasone, and cortisol by the human placenta. American Journal of Obstetrics and Gynecology 127: 264 (1977).

Bleyer, W.A. and Breckenridge, R.T.: Studies on the detection of adverse drug reactions in the newborn II. The effects of prenatal aspirin on newborn hemostasis. Journal of the American Medical Association 213: 2049 (1970).

Bloomfield, D.K.: Fetal deaths and malformations associated with the use of coumarin derivatives in pregnancy. American Journal of Obstetrics and Gynecology 107: 883 (1970).

Budnick, I.S.; Leikin, S. and Hoeck, L.E.: Effect in the newborn infant of reserpine administered antepartum. American Journal of Diseases in Childhood 90: 286 (1955).

Caldwell, J.; Wakile, L.A.; Notarianni, L.J.; Smith, R.L.; Lieberman, B.A.; Jeffs, J.; Coy, Y. and Beard, R.W.: Transplacental passage and neonatal elimination of pethidine given to mothers in childbirth. British Journal of Clinical Pharmacology 4: 715P (1977).

Charles, D.: Placental transmission of antibiotics. Journal of Obstetrics and Gynaecology, British Empire 61: 750 (1954).

Connaughton, J.F.; Reeser, D.; Schut, J. and Finnegan, L.P.: Perinatal addiction: Outcome and management. American Journal of Obstetrics and Gynecology 129: 679 (1977).

Cooper, L.V.; Stephen, G.W. and Aggett, P.J.A.: Elimination of pethidine and bupivicaine in the newborn. Archives of Disease in Childhood 52: 638 (1977).

Cottrill, C.M.; McAllister, R.G.; Gettes, L. and Noonan, J.A.: Propranolol therapy during pregnancy, labor, and delivery: Evidence for transplacental drug transfer and impaired neonatal drug disposition. Journal of Pediatrics 91: 812 (1977).

Cree, Jean E.; Meyer, J. and Hailey, D.M.: Diazepam in labour: Its metabolism and effect on the clinical condition and thermogenesis of the newborn. British Medical Journal 4: 251 (1973).

Csaba, I.F.; Sulyak, E. and Ertl, T.: Relationship of maternal treatment with indomethacin to persistence of fetal circulation syndrome. Journal of Pediatrics 92: 484 (1978).

Daubenfeld, O.; Modde, H. and Hirsch, H.A.: Transfer of gentamicin to the foetus and the amniotic fluid during a steady-state in the mother. Archiv fur Gynakologie 217: 233 (1974).

dePadua, C.B. and Gravenstein, J.S.: Atropine sulfate vs atropine methyl bromide: Effect on maternal and fetal heart rate. Journal of the American Medical Association 208: 1022 (1969).

Desmond, M.M.; Rogers, S.F.; Lindley, J.E. and Moyer, J.H.: Management of toxemia of pregnancy with reserpine II. The newborn infant. Obstetrics and Gynecology 10: 140 (1957).

Dornhorst, A.C. and Young, I.M.: The action of adrenaline and noradrenaline on the placenta and foetal circulations in the rabbit and guinea pig. Journal of Physiology 118: 282 (1952).

Epstein, M.F.; Farrell, P.M.; Sparks, J.W.; Pepe, G.; Driscoll, S.G. and Chez, R.A.: Maternal betamethasone and fetal growth and development in the monkey. American Journal of Obstetrics and Gynecology 127: 261 (1977).

Eskes, T.K.A.B. and deHann, J.: The influence of beta-mimetic catecholamines upon the fetal circulation. Zeitschrift fur Geburtshilfe perinatologie 176: 97 (1972).

Evans, M.; Bhat, R.; Vadepalli, M.; Fisher, E.; Hastreiter, A. and Vidyasagar, D.: Disposition of indomethacin in premature infants. Pediatrics Research 12: 404 Abs. 245 (1978).

Finster, M.: Toxicity of local anesthetics in the fetus and the newborn. Bulletin of the New York Academy of Medicine 52: 222 (1976).

Fitzhardinge, P.M.; Eisen, A.; Lejtenyi, C.; Metrakos, K. and Ramsay, M.: Sequelae of early steroid administration to the newborn infant. Pediatrics 53: 877 (1974).

Flessa, H.C.; Kapstrom, A.B.; Glueck, H.I. and Will, J.J.: Placental transport of heparin. American Journal of Obstetrics and Gynecology 93: 570 (1965).

Freeman, D.W. and Arnold, N.I.: Paracervical block with low doses of chlorprocaine. Journal of the American Medical Association 231: 56 (1975).

Freeman, R.K.; Gutierrez, N.A.; Ray, M.L.; Stovall, D.; Paul, R.H. and Hon, E.H.: Fetal cardiac response to paracervical block anesthesia. American Journal of Obstetrics and Gynecology 113: 583 (1972).

Fricker, H.S. and Segal, S.: Narcotic addiction, pregnancy, and the newborn. American Journal of Diseases in Childhood 132: 360 (1978).

Friedman, W.F.; Hirshklaw, M.J.; Printz, M.P.; Pitlick, P.T. and Kirkpatrick, S.E.: Pharmacologic closure of patent ductus arteriosus in the premature infant. New England Journal of Medicine 295: 526 (1976).

Friedman, Z.; Whitman, V.; Maisels, M.J.; Berman, W.; Marks, K.H. and Vesell, E.S.: Indomethacin disposition in premature infants: Bleeding due to platelet dysfunction after single doses of indomethacin. Pediatrics Research 12: 405 Abs. 250 (1978).

Fries, H.: Lithium in pregnancy. Lancet 1: 1233 (1970).

Gill, W.B.; Schumacher, G.F.B. and Bibbo, M.: Pathological semen and antomical abnormalities of the genital tract in human male subjects exposed to diethylstilbesterol *in utero*. Journal of Urology 117: 477 (1977).

Gladstone, G.G.; Hordof, A. and Gersony, W.M.: Propranolol administration during pregnancy: Effects on the fetus. Journal of Pediatrics 86: 962 (1975).

Greenberg, G.; Inman, W.H.; Weatherall, J.A.C.; Adelstein, A.M. and Haskey, J.C.: Maternal drug histories and congenital abnormalities. British Medical Journal 2: 853 (1977).

Habib, A. and McCarthy, J.S.: Effects on the neonate of propranolol administered during pregnancy. Journal of Pediatrics 91: 808 (1977).

Harlap, S.; Prywes, R. and Davies, A.M.: Birth defects and oestrogens and progesterones in pregnancy. Lancet 1: 682 (1975).

Harris, L.S.; Dewey, W.L.; Razdan, R.K.: Cannabis, its chemistry, pharmacology and toxicology; in Martin (Ed) Handbook of Experimental Pharmacology, Vol. 45/II: Drug Addiction, p.371 (Springer, Berlin 1977).

Hart, C.W. and Nauton, R.F.: The ototoxicity of chloroquine phosphate. Archives of Otolaryngology 80: 407 (1964).

Heinonen, O.P.; Slone, D.; Monson, R.R.; Hook, E.B. and Shapiro, S.: Cardiovascular birth defects and antenatal exposure to female sex hormones. New England Journal of Medicine 296: 67 (1977).

Herbst, A.L.; Cole, P.; Colton, T.; Robboy, S.J. and Scully, R.C.: Age-incidence and risk of DES-related clear cell adenocarcinoma of the vagina and cervix. American Journal of Obstetrics and Gynecology 128: 43 (1977).

Heymann, M.A. and Rudolph, A.M.: Effects of acetylsalicylic acid on the ductus arteriosus and circulation in fetal lambs *in utero*. Circulation Research 38: 418 (1976).

Heymann, M.A.; Rudolph, A.M. and Silverman, N.H.: Closure of the ductus arteriosus in premature infants by inhibition of prostaglandin synthesis. New England Journal of Medicine 295: 530 (1976).

Hill, R.M.: Adverse effects of prenatal drug therapy; in Mirkin (Ed) Clinical Pharmacology and Therapeutics: A Pediatric Perspective (Year Book, Chicago 1978).

Hirsch, H.A.; Herbst, S.; Lang, R.; Dettli, L. and Gablinger, A.: Transfer of a new cephalosporin antibiotic to the foetus and amniotic fluid during a continuous infusion (steady state) and single repeated intravenous injections to the mother. Archiv fur Gynakologie 216: 1 (1974).

Hogg, M.I.J.; Wiener, P.C.; Rosen, M. and Mapleson, W.W.: Urinary excretion and metabolism of pethidine and norpethidine in the newborn. British Journal of Anaesthesiology 49: 891 (1977).

Jackson, A.V.: Toxic effects of salicylate on the fetus and mother. Journal of Pathology and Bacteriology 60: 587 (1948).

Janerich, D.T.; Piper, J.M. and Glebatis, D.M.: Oral contraceptives and congenital limb-reduction defects. New England Journal of Medicine 291: 697 (1974).

Janerich, D.T.; Dugan, J.M.; Standfast, S.J. and Strite, L.: Congenital heart disease and prenatal exposure to exogenous sex hormones. British Medical Journal 1: 1058 (1977).

Jones, K.L.; Smith, D.W.; Ulleland, C.N. and Streissguth, A.P.: Pattern of malformation in offspring of chronic alcoholic mothers. Lancet 1: 1267 (1973).

Jorgensen, P.I.: Influence of corticosteroids on the excretion of oestrogens in pregnancy. Journal of Steroids and Biochemistry 1: 33 (1969).

Juchau, M.R.: Drug biotransformation reactions in the placenta; in Mirkin (Ed) Perinatal Pharmacology and Therapeutics, p.71 (Academic Press, New York 1976).

Kauffman, R.E.; Azarnoff, D.L. and Morris, J.A.: Placental transfer and fetal urinary excretion of gentamicin — comparison between an animal model and the human fetus; in Morselli, Garattini and Sereni (Eds) Basic and Therapeutic Aspects of Perinatal Pharmacology, p.75 (Raven Press, New York 1975).

Kivalo, I. and Saarikoski, S.: Placental transmission of atropine at full-term pregnancy. British Journal of Anaesthesiology 49: 1017 (1977).

Kullander, S. and Kallen, B.: A prospective study of drugs and pregnancy. Archives of Obstetrics and Gynecology, Scandinavia 55: 105 (1976).

Levin, D.L.; Fixler, D.E.; Morriss, F.C. and Tyson, J.: Morphologic analysis of the pulmonary vascular bed in infants exposed *in utero* to prostaglandin synthetase inhibitors. Journal of Pediatrics 92: 478 (1978).

Levy, G. and Garrettson, L.K.: Kinetics of salicylate elimination by newborn infants of mothers who ingested aspirin before delivery. Pediatrics 53: 201 (1974).

Levy, G.; Garrettson, L.K. and Soda, D.M.: Evidence of placental transfer of acetaminophen. Pediatrics 55: 895 (1975).

Liggins, G.C. and Howie, R.N.: A controlled trial of antepartum glucocorticoid treatment for prevention of the respiratory distress syndrome in premature infants. Pediatrics 50: 515 (1972).

Lilleyman, J.S.; Hill, A.S. and Anderton, K.J.: Consequence of acute myelogenous leukemia in pregnancy. Cancer 40: 1300 (1977).

Manchester, D.; Margolis, H.S. and Sheldon, R.E.: Possible association between maternal indomethacin therapy and primary pulmonary hypertension of the newborn. American Journal of Obstetrics and Gynecology 126: 467 (1976).

Mandelli, M.; Morselli, P.L.; Nordio, S.; Pardi, G.; Principi, N.; Sereni, F. and Tognoni, G.: Placental transfer of diazepam and its disposition in the newborn. Clinical Pharmacology and Therapeutics 17: 564 (1975).

Mandelli, M.; Tognoni, G. and Garattini, S.: Clinical pharmacokinetics of diazepam. Clinical Pharmacokinetics 3: 72 (1978).

Mattingly, R.F. and Stafl, A.: Cancer risk in diethylstilbesterol-exposed offspring. American Journal of Obstetrics and Gynecology 126: 543 (1976).

Maurer, H.M.; Wolff, J.A.; Finster, M.; Poppers, P.J.; Pantuck, E.; Kuntzman, R. and Conney, A.H.: Reduction in concentration of total serum-bilirubin in offspring of women treated with phenobarbitone during pregnancy. Lancet 2: 122 (1968).

Milkovich, L. and van den Berg, B.J.: An evaluation of the teratogenicity of certain antinauseant drugs. American Journal of Obstetrics and Gynecology 125: 244 (1976).

Miller, F.C.; Nochimson, D.J.; Paul, R.H. and Hon, E.H.: Effects of ritodrine hydrochloride on uterine activity and the cardiovascular system in toxemic patients. Obstetrics and Gynecology 47: 50 (1976).

Mirkin, B.L.: Diphenylhydantoin: Placental transport, fetal localization, neonatal metabolism and possible teratogenic effects. Journal of Pediatrics 78: 329 (1971a).

Mirkin, B.L.: Unpublished data (1971b).

Mirkin, B.L.: Ontogenesis of the adrenergic nervous system: Functional and pharmacologic implications. Federation Proceedings 31: 65 (1972).

Mirkin, B.L.: Perinatal Pharmacology and Therapeutics (Academic Press, New York 1976).

Mirkin, B.L.: Clinical Pharmacology and Therapeutics: A Pediatric Perspective (Year Book, Chicago 1978).

Mitchell, J.R. and Corcoran, G.B.: Pharmacologic and toxic drug reactions in adult and pediatric medicine; in Mirkin (Ed) Clinical Pharmacology and Therapeutics: A Pediatric Perspective, p.49 (Year Book, Chicago 1978).

Moore, J.; McNabb, T.G. and Glynn, J.P.: The placental transfer of pentazocine and pethidine. British Journal of Anaesthesiology 45(Suppl.): 798 (1973).

Morrison, J.C.; Whybrew, W.D.; Rosser, S.I.; Bucovaz, E.T.; Wiser, W.L. and Fish, S.A.: Metabolites of meperidine in the fetal and maternal serum. American Journal of Obstetrics and Gynecology 126: 997 (1976).

Nicholson, H.O.: Cytotoxic drugs in pregnancy. Journal of Obstetrics and Gynaecology, British Commonwealth 75: 307 (1968).

Oakes, G.K.; Walker, A.M.; Ehrenkranz, R.A. and Chez, R.A.: Effect of propranolol infusion on the umbilical and uterine circulations of pregnant sheep. American Journal of Obstetrics and Gynecology 126: 1038 (1976).

Palmisano, P.A. and Cassady, G.: Salicylate exposure in the perinate. Journal of the American Medical Association 209: 556 (1969).

Parks, B.R.; Jordan, R.L.; Rawson, J.E. and Douglas, B.H.: Indomethacin: Studies of absorption and placental transfer. American Journal of Obstetrics and Gynecology 129: 464 (1977).

Pedersen, L.M.; Tygstrup, I. and Pedersen, J.: Congenital malformations in newborn infants of diabetic women. Correlation with maternal diabetic vascular complications. Lancet 1: 1124 (1964).

Proakis, A.G. and Harris, G.B.: Comparative penetration of glycopyrrolate and atropine across the blood-brain and placental barriers in anesthetized dogs. Anesthesiology 48: 339 (1978).

Rane, A.; Bertilsson, L. and Palmer, L.: Disposition of placentally transferred carbamazepine in the newborn. European Journal of Clinical Pharmacology 8: 283 (1975).

Rane, A.; Tomson, G. and Bjarke, B.: Effects of maternal lithium therapy in a newborn infant. Journal of Pediatrics 93: 296 (1978).

Reiss, U.; Atad, J.; Rubinstein, I. and Zuckerman, H.: The Effect of indomethacin in labour at term. International Journal of Gynecology and Obstetrics 14: 369 (1976).

Rementeria, J.L. and Bhatt, K.: Withdrawal symptoms in neonates due to diazepam. Journal of Pediatrics 90: 123 (1977).

Roberts, J.B.; Thomas, B.H. and Wilson, A.: Placental transfer of pyridostigmine in the rat. British Journal of Pharmacology 38: 202 (1970).

Robinson, G.C. and Cambon, K.G.: Hearing loss in infants of tuberculous mothers treated with streptomycin during pregnancy. New England Journal of Medicine 271: 949 (1964).

Rodriguez, S.U.; Leiken, S.L. and Hiller, M.C.: Neonatal thrombocytopenia associated with antepartum administration of thiazide drugs. New England Journal of Medicine 270: 887 (1964).

Rogers, M.C.; Willerson, J.T.; Goldblatt, A. and Smith, T.W.: Serum digoxin concentrations in the human fetus, neonate and infant. New England Journal of Medicine 287: 1010 (1972).

Rosen, T.S. and Pippenger, C.E.: Pharmacologic observations on the neonatal withdrawal syndrome. Journal of Pediatrics 88: 1044 (1976).

Rothstein, P. and Gould, J.B.: Born with a habit. Pediatric Clinics of North America 21: 307 (1974).

Rumeau-Rouquette, C.; Gaujard, J. and Huel, G.: Possible teratogenic effect of phenothiazines in human beings. Teratology 15: 57 (1977).

Saarikoski, S.: Placental transfer and fetal uptake of H^3-digoxin in infants. British Journal of Obstetrics and Gynecology 83: 879 (1976).

Saidi, P.; Hoag, M.S. and Aggeler, P.M.: Transplacental transfer of bishydroxycoumarin in the human. Journal of the American Medical Association 191: 157 (1965).

Sandler, M.; Ruthven, C.R.J.; Contractor, S.F.; Wood, C.; Booth, R.T. and Pinkerton, J.H.M.: Transmission of noradrenaline across the human placenta. Nature 197: 598 (1963).

Sandler, M.; Ruthven, C.R.J. and Wood, C.: Metabolism of C^{14}-norepinephrine and C^{14}-epinephrine and their transmission across the human placenta. International Journal of Neuropharmacology 3: 123 (1964).

Shapiro, S.; Hartz, S.C.; Siskind, V.; Mitchell, H.A.; Slone, D.; Rosenberg, L.; Monson, R.R.; Heinonen, O.P.; Indanpaan-Heikkila, J.; Haro, S. and Saxen, L.: Anticonvulsants and parental epilepsy in the development of birth defects. Lancet 1: 272 (1976a).

Shapiro, S.; Heinonen, O.P.; Siskind, V.; Kaufman, D.W.; Monson, R.R. and Slone, D.: Antenatal exposure to doxylamine succinate and dicyclomine hydrochloride (Bendectin) in relation to congenital malformations, perinatal mortality rate, birth weights, and intelligence quotient score. American Journal of Obstetrics and Gynecology 128: 480 (1977).

Shapiro, S.; Monson, R.R.; Kaufman, D.W.; Siskind, V.; Heinonen, O.P. and Slone, D.: Perinatal mortality and birth weight in relation to aspirin taken during pregnancy. Lancet 2: 1375 (1976b).

Shaul, W.L. and Hall, J.G.: Multiple congenital anomalies associated with oral anticoagulants. American Journal of Obstetrics and Gynecology 127: 191 (1977).

Shnider, S.M. and Gildea, J.: Paracervical block anesthesia in obstetrics. American Journal of Obstetrics and Gynecology 116: 320 (1973).

Shnider, S.M. and Moya, F.: Effects of meperidine on the newborn infant. American Journal of Obstetrics and Gynecology 89: 1009 (1964).

Singh, S.; Fehr, P.E. and Mirkin, B.L.: Elimination kinetics and placental transfer of digoxin in pregnant and nonpregnant ewes. Research Communications in Chemical Pathology and Pharmacology 20: 31 (1978a).

Singh, S.; Ward, R.M. and Mirkin, B.L.: Effect of β-adrenergic blockade on cardiovascular adaptation of pregnant ewes and fetal lambs to asphyxia. American Journal of Obstetrics and Gynecology. In review (1978b).

Singh, S.; Mirkin, B.L.; Cooper, M.J. and Anders, M.W.: Metabolism and placental transfer of propranolol (P) in the ovine maternal-placental-fetal unit (OMPFU). Federation Proceedings 36: 1033 (1977).

Singh, S. and Mirkin, B.L.: Placental transfer and tissue localization of digoxin in the pregnant rat. Toxicology and Applied Pharmacology 46: 395 (1978).

Slone, D.; Siskind, V.; Heinonen, O.P.; Monson, R.R.; Kaufman, D.W. and Shapiro, S.: Aspirin and congenital malformations. Lancet 1: 1373 (1976).

Slone, D.; Siskind, V.; Heinonen, O.P.; Monson, R.R.; Kaufman, D.W. and Shapiro, S.: Antenatal exposure to the phenothiazines in relation to congenital malformations, perinatal mortality rate, birth weight and intelligence quotient score. American Journal of Obstetrics and Gynecology 128: 486 (1977).

Solomon, G.E.; Hilgartner, M.W. and Kutt, H.: Coagulation defects caused by diphenylhydantoin. Neurology 22: 1165 (1972).

Speight, A.N.P.: Floppy-infant syndrome and maternal diazepam and/or nitrazepam. Lancet 2: 878 (1977).

Stewart, K.S.; Shafi, M.; Andrews, J. and Williams, J.D.: Distribution of parenteral ampicillin and cephalosporins in late pregnancy. Journal of Obstetrics and Gynecology, British Commonwealth 80: 902 (1973).

Stirrat, G.M.; Edington, P.T. and Berry, D.J.: Transplacental passage of chlordiazepoxide. British Medical Journal 2: 729 (1974).

Stothers, J.K.; Wilson, D.W. and Royston, N.: Lithium toxicity in the newborn. Brit. Med. J. 3: 233 (1973).

Streissguth, A.P.; Herman, C.S. and Smith, D.W.: Intelligence, behavior, and dysmorphogenesis in the fetal alcohol syndrome: A report on 20 patients. Journal of Pediatrics 92: 363 (1978).

Traeger, A.; Noschel, H. and Zaumseil, J.: Zur Pharmakokinetik von indomethazin bei schwangeren, kreissenden und deren neugeborenen. Zentralblatt fur Gynakologie 95: 635 (1973).

Tuchmann-Duplessis, H.: Disorders of metabolism; in Drug Effects on the Fetus, p.195 (ADIS Press, Sydney 1975).

Turner, G. and Collins, E.: Fetal effects of regular salicylate ingestion in pregnancy. Lancet 2: 338 (1975).

Van Petten, G.R.: Pharmacology and the fetus. British Medical Bulletin 31: 75 (1975).

Wasz-Hockert, O.; Nummi, S.; Vuopala, S. and Jarvinen, P.A.: Transplacental passage of Azidocillin, ampicillin and penicillin G during early and late pregnancy. Scandinavian Journal of Infectious Diseases 2: 125 (1970).

Weinstein, M.R. and Goldfield, M.: Lithium carbonate treatment during pregnancy. Diseases of the Nervous System 30: 828 (1969).

Weinstein, M.R. and Goldfield, M.D.: Cardiovascular malformations with lithium use during pregnancy. American Journal of Psychiatry 132: 529 (1975).

Wiener, P.C.; Hogg, M.I.J. and Rosen, M.: Effects of naloxone on pethidine-induced neonatal depression. British Medical Journal 2: 228 (1977).

Wilbanks, G.D.; Bressler, B.; Peete, C.H.; Cherney, W.B. and London, W.L.: Toxic effects of lithium carbonate in a mother and child. Journal of the American Medical Association 213: 865 (1970).

Chapter IV
Paediatric Clinical Pharmacology and Therapeutics

H.C. Shirkey

Synopsis of Important Principles

1) A number of factors other than age and size affect drug response and drug administration in infants and children. Unique problems exist during the neonatal period of life.

2) Responsiveness to drugs is altered in infants and young children because of progressive changes, with growth and development, in the processes of drug pharmacokinetics in the body, and with a few drugs, by altered tissue responsiveness.

3) Absorption of oral and parenterally administered drugs is not affected, but percutaneous absorption of topically applied drugs is significantly enhanced in infants and children, particularly in prematures and if the skin is burnt or excoriated.

4) Drug distribution is affected by changes in body composition and development of the blood-brain 'barrier' with increasing age, and by metabolic disturbances such as acidosis. The rate and efficiency of drug elimination processes is greatly diminished in neonates, especially premature infants, but for many drugs elimination processes may be 'supra normal' by late infancy and/or childhood.

5) Safe and effective drug therapy in the neonatal period is not only complicated by the functional immaturity of drug metabolising and renal excretory capacity, but also by the rapid increase in their activity as a function of postnatal age.

6) The early postnatal period also involves problems with drugs born with the baby, with a few drugs excreted in breast milk, and with difficulties in the administration of drugs.

7) Problems in drug administration, with special forms of medication and with drug handling, decrease with increasing age, but drug effects on growth must be considered at all ages.

8) When prescribing drugs, a decision on the particular drug prescribed, the route of administration, and the dosage form and dose used, should be made with the particular age group of the child in mind.

9) The average dose is not necessarily the correct dose. Dosage should be individualised for the drug, patient and disease. The dose-frequency schedule should be the most simple possible.

10) The parent and child should be taught to understand his disease and drugs and of the importance of taking medication regularly or completing the prescribed course of treatment. The clinician should further cooperate by providing adequate instruction in the correct administration of the drug.

Growth and development separate paediatrics from adult medicine and surgery. Nowhere have adult and paediatric differences been more clearly exemplified than in the use of drugs. The child is not a little man, and the need to understand the pharmacokinetics of his drugs vary inversely according to his age and size. Unique problems with drugs found in different paediatric age (growth and development) groups may likewise clearly separate the age groups from one another. Clinical pharmacological and therapeutic considerations therefore need to be adapted to each period of growth and development, which can be broadly divided into intrauterine and extrauterine periods. The periods of intrauterine growth and development relevant to drug action and response are:

a) Embryogenesis and organogenesis, which comprises most of the first trimester (see chapter II).
b) Fetal maturation, the second trimester to the beginning of labour (see chapter III, XV).
c) Period before birth or during labour — drugs born with the baby (see chapter III, XV).

This chapter concerns itself with the extrauterine period. It can be divided into five growth and development stages which can be related to problems in drug handling (pharmacokinetics), drug administration, drug acceptance, drug response and drug experimentation:

a) Early postnatal period — period of physiological immaturity and constant change and the period of most marked and important alteration in pharmacokinetics of drugs. Difficulties with administration of drugs.
b) Second through the twelfth month — period of improved pharmacokinetic handling and administration of drugs.
c) Ambulatory childhood (the toddler) — the dependent toddler tries the patience of many who administer drugs orally, yet he freely takes poison himself.
d) Kindergarten and early school age — these children are generally cooperative in many ways. Their ability to eliminate drugs can be superior to that in young adults.
e) Adolescence — the degree of cooperation varies and experimentation with non-medical drugs begins.

1. General Considerations

Much of drug action in children, particularly in infants, has been learned by scaling down the adult dose, and treating the paediatric patient as though he were in all ways a small adult. A second way of learning has been during paediatric growth periods by the occurrence of markedly different adverse drug reactions from those seen in adult life. A third and strongly advocated one is by planned paediatric drug studies (Shirkey, 1968a; 1972).

Most severe adverse reaction problems in children are discovered by catastrophe. Few prospective studies are available. That knowledge which is not gained by serendipity, is interpolated from adult data and either method overlooks much valuable information. Drug surveillance should be a responsibility of every hospital and many clinicians treating non-hospitalised children. Conscientious documentation of drug use experience (i.e. efficacy as well as toxicity), undertaken with the same zeal as infectious disease case reporting, would prove to be an invaluable source of current drug data for clinicians. Adult drug surveillance studies pointedly emphasise the need for closer supervision in paediatric practice. It is surprising indeed that although the greatest drug catastrophies have been paediatric ones, little effort is directed toward drug studies for infants and children by clinicians who profess to 'care' for them.

The history of paediatric pharmacology and therapy has been bitter. Greater concern for diagnostic prowess than for efficacious therapy, a paucity of hard data, interpolation from adult dosage and experience, lack of controlled paediatric studies, and 'trial by ordeal' have been the hallmarks of this branch of clinical pharmacology. Those who do not learn from history often must relive it. The history of paediatric pharmacology has been riddled with catastrophe and loss of life. To retread this same path is too costly. Yet, the legislative events in many countries following for example, the 'elixir' of sulphanilamide disaster in 1937 and that of thalidomide in 1961 turned out to be detrimental to children. Intended to protect infants and children, the legislation and regulations have resulted in allowing release of drugs for children without necessary studies.

In some countries, such as the United States, many of the newest drugs are considered not adequately evaluated for use in infants and children with studies which explore a drug's clinical potential. The result is that in the USA and some other countries children are denied the use of many potentially valuable drugs, and thus the drugs and children have been called 'therapeutic orphans' (Shirkey, 1968b; 1970). Certainly, most drugs need, but often do not receive, adequate study in infants and children, but to allow the use of a drug in infants and children with lack of controlled studies is most dangerous. Monitored drug use experience under the conditions of actual planned clinical studies can provide much useful information. Unless concerted efforts are made to take an interest in and responsibility for drug therapy and to change attitudes to clinical 'research' and to methods of gaining drug use experience, new drugs and infants and children will remain 'therapeutic orphans'. Eternal vigilance is required if childrens' therapy is not to fall far behind or require dependence on often unrelated adult data.

2. Determinants of Altered Drug Responsiveness in Infants and Children

A number of factors determine drug response and drug dosage in infants and children. From the time a drug enters the body until it is eliminated there may be developmental differences in drug pharmacokinetics in infants and young children (for reviews, see Morselli, 1976a, 1977; Rane and Wilson, 1976). Altered absorption, distribution and elimination is most marked in the newborn, especially in premature babies, but for many drugs elimination processes may be 'supra normal' by late infancy and/or childhood. Changes in drug effect can also be due to metabolic disturbances, altered tissue responsiveness and to the disease being treated. Other factors include problems of drug administration and acceptance of the drug by the infant or child (see section 3). All of these factors and others express themselves in children living in a tropical environment; in whom the potential for altered drug responsiveness is particularly marked (see chapter XXX; section 2; 11).

2.1 Drug Absorption and Bioavailability

The morphology and functions of the gastrointestinal tract are not constant; varying almost continuously from birth till senescence (Yaffe and Juchau, 1974). The most marked changes occur in the first month of life, after which there is a gradual maturation toward the condition in adults. Newborns, particularly prematures, have greatly reduced gastric acid secretion with a condition of more or less relative achlorhydria (except for hyperacidity shortly after birth). Adult values for gastric acidity are usually attained only after 3 years of age (Smith, 1951). Gastric emptying rate has an important influence on gastrointestinal absorption of many drugs (see chapter XIX; sect. 1.1). In the neonate, gastric emptying time is considerably prolonged and approaches adult values only after 6 to 8 months. Peristalsis is very irregular, completely unpredictable and only in part dependent on the feeding pattern (Smith, 1951).

2.1.1 Oral Absorption

Few studies have been conducted on the absorption of orally administered drugs in infants; many drugs are given parenterally. On the basis of the achlorhydria, the increased rate and extent of absorption of orally administered penicillins such as benzylpenicillin, ampicillin, amoxycillin, nafcillin and flucloxacillin, observed in newborns is understandable (Morselli, 1976a, 1977; Simon and Toeller, 1974). Phenobarbitone absorption is however, decreased in newborns up to 15 days of age (Boreus et al., 1975). There may be a delay in absorption of drugs such as phenytoin and rifampicin (rifampin) in newborns but absorption of cotrimoxazole (trimethoprim-sulphamethoxazole), digoxin and diazepam is normal (Morselli, 1976a; 1977). Although the peak concentration of cephalexin is less in neonates than in older infants, children and adults, the amount absorbed is similar (Marget, 1971). With some drugs such as riboflavine this is because absorption in newborns proceeds for longer than in the older infant or adult (Jusko et al., 1970); at least in part because of delayed gastric emptying.

Gastrointestinal absorption of many drugs is not altered in older infants and children compared with adults, although for some drugs such as diazepam, clonazepam, phenobarbitone, sodium valproate, ethosuximide and imipramine, the rate of absorption may be more rapid (Morselli, 1977). Bioavailability of orally administered drugs with a high hepatic clearance (see chapter I; sect. 3.3.3) such as propranolol and dextropropoxyphene, may however, be low and show great interindividual variability in children as in adults — consistent with their high hepatic first-pass elimination (Wilson et al., 1976).

Disorders of gastrointestinal function can have an important effect on absorption of orally administered drugs (see chapter XIX; sect. 1.1) and should also be considered in infants and children. Thus, absorption of cephalexin can be impaired in infants with coeliac disease (Marget, 1971), as can the absorption of ampicillin in children with diarrhoea (Elliott et al., 1964). Steatorrhoea impairs the absorption of fat soluble preparations of vitamin A and D.

2.1.2 Intramuscular Absorption

Absorption of some drugs following intramuscular administration is erratic in newborns; e.g. digoxin (Morselli, 1976b), gentamicin and kanamycin (Assael et al., 1977). Absorption of drugs after intramuscular administration depends mainly on the regional blood flow, which may be very different among specific muscles (Evans et al., 1975), and in certain pathophysiological states (e.g. oedema of nephrosis). In newborns, the rate and extent of intramuscular absorption may change considerably during the first 2 weeks of extrauterine life in relation to maturational changes of the relative blood flow of the various muscles and adaptation to the presence of any hypoxic conditions.

2.1.3 Percutaneous Absorption

Percutaneous absorption of drugs is significantly enhanced in infants and children, particularly if the skin area of application is burnt or excoriated. Significant percutaneous absorption of strong topical corticosteroids occurs following their continuous use in infants and children with severe or moderately severe eczema, and when repeatedly applied for napkin (diaper) rash, especially babies wearing disposable napkins or waterproof plastic pants (Feiwel, 1969). The weakest topical steroid which will achieve desirable control should be used in infantile eczema (Keipert, 1971). Topical steroids are generally unsuitable for napkin rash (see section 5.7). Boric acid, a useless and dangerous drug formerly used in babies' dusting powders and as a napkin rinse, is absorbed through broken skin. Systemic absorption leads to diarrhoea, further soreness of the napkin area and more liberal application of the powder. This vicious circle may end fatally (Valdes-Dapena and Arey, 1962; Skipworth, 1967). Aniline dyes used in marking inks can be absorbed through unbroken skin and give rise to methaemoglobinaemia. If such inks must be used

the dye should be fixed by boiling the napkins and baby clothes before use. The sulphonamide topical antiseptic mafenide acetate may also cause methaemoglobinaemia when applied to large areas of burned skin in infants (Ohlgisser et al., 1978). Excessive use of topical aminoglycoside-polymyxin sprays on burned skin of young children has led to permanent hearing loss (Bamford and Jones, 1978). Many other examples of percutaneous drug absorption and toxicity exist (Gadeke, 1972). Babies' clothes stored in mothballs (naphthalene) are a potential danger to the infant with glucose-6-phosphate dehydrogenase deficiency as percutaneous absorption of naphthalene can lead to haemolytic anaemia and jaundice (see chapter XIX; sect. 14.6.6).

In some neonatal nurseries, 3% hexachlorophane emulsion or an 0.33% or 0.5% powder is used routinely as an effective aid in the control of staphylococcal sepsis (Plueckhahn et al., 1978). Its use is not without risk of neurotoxicity from percutaneous absorption if used inappropriately. Premature or small birth-weight infants should not undergo routine antiseptic skin care with hexachlorophane preparations (Tyrala et al., 1977). Absorption across the skin of small newborn infants may be so rapid that even if hexachlorophane is apparently removed, absorption will have already occurred and this will be quantitatively related to the amount of hexachlorophane emulsion actually applied (Greaves et al., 1975). Certainly, the use of 3% hexachlorophane emulsion or an 0.33% or 0.5% powder on burnt or excoriated skin of any infant or young child is strongly contraindicated and may be fatal (Plueckhahn et al., 1978; Chilcote et al., 1977); as may accidental use of grossly excessive concentrations (6% powder) on normal skin (Goutieres and Aicardi, 1977).

2.2 Drug Distribution

Differences in distribution of drugs in the various paediatric age groups will depend on the relative sizes of body water compartments, plasma protein binding capacity, circulatory factors, the degree of development of the blood-brain barrier and drug specificity for tissue receptor sites.

2.2.1 Body Water

The body composition of the newborn infant is quite different from that in the older infant and adult. Newborn infants have a much higher extracellular fluid volume, particularly prematures (50% of body weight) than full term newborns (45%), older infants (30% at 4 to 6 months; 25% at 1 year; 20 to 25% over 1 year) or adults (20 to 25%). Total body water is also much greater in neonates and varies from about 85% of bodyweight in a small premature baby to about 75% in a full term infant, compared with 60% in the younger adult. Adult values for extracellular fluid volume are reached at around 13 to 15 years of age, whereas total body water increases slightly around puberty after which time a gradual decrease occurs throughout adult life (Friis-Hansen, 1961; 1971). Fat content, on the other hand, is decreased in the premature infant (3%) compared with the normal full term infant (12%), infant at 1 year (30%) and the young adult male (18%). Since drugs are distributed between extracellular water and depot fat according to their lipid:water partition coefficient, the relative variations of these two body compartments can alter drug distribution according to the physicochemical properties of the particular drug. Body composition is never constant, changes being greatest and most rapid in early life and becoming less rapid with advancing age. Because of the rapid changes in body composition in infants and children, changes in drug distribution with development are to be expected.

In terms of drug dosage, these changes are usually interpreted to mean that water soluble drugs without extensive tissue binding (e.g. sulphonamides, benzylpenicillin, amoxycillin) circulate freely through the extracellular fluid such that the dose required to achieve the same plasma concentration decreases during childhood in relation to weight. For such drugs dosage on the basis of extracellular water would be more accurate than on a body weight basis. Many drugs are in fact dosed indirectly in relation to extracellular water since this correlates closely with body surface area. In states of dehydration or shock, when the extracellular fluid falls, the 'usual' dose of a water soluble drug attains a higher concentration. On the other hand, the plasma concentration of a water soluble drug is reduced in an oedematous child with expanded extracellular fluid volume.

2.2.2 Protein Binding

Plasma protein binding of drugs is decreased in the newborn compared with adults (table I). The difference may be due not only to a lower concentration of plasma proteins (particularly albu-

min) but there may also be qualitative differences in the binding capacity of proteins (Krasner et al., 1973; Wallace, 1976, 1977). Reduced binding to globulins or interaction between albumin and globulin in the newborn may also be important for some drugs (Kurz et al., 1977). In addition, it is possible that high concentrations of free fatty acids or bilirubin (Ehrnebo et al., 1971; Fredholm et al., 1975) and endogenous substances during the first few days of life, especially hormones transferred across the placenta *in utero,* may occupy binding sites and thus reduce binding capacity (Windorfer et al., 1974). Furthermore, the sick newborn infant is often treated with multiple drug therapy and, also as a consequence of his disease, often has metabolic disturbances (e.g. acidosis). These factors may contribute to additional alterations in plasma protein binding leading to an increase in the fraction of unbound pharmacologically active drug in the plasma. The reduced plasma albumin levels of the newborn probably reach adult values by the end of the first year of life (Metcoff and Stare, 1947), but in premature infants plasma albumin is even lower and takes longer to reach mature levels (Brown, 1973). Total protein concentration and albumin binding capacity approach adult values by around 12 months (Ecobichon and Stephens, 1973; Metcoff and Stare, 1947; Windorfer et al., 1974).

The reduced albumin binding capacity for acidic drugs may explain, in part, why some drugs administered to the newborn are often associated with side effects, even though the dose used is proportionately smaller. For some drugs the fraction of unbound drug is related to the total concentration of bilirubin. In the case of phenobarbitone, the fraction of unbound drug which is already high (60 to 65%) in newborns with normal bilirubin levels, may reach values of around 70% or more in the presence of hyperbilirubinaemia (Ehrnebo et al., 1971; Ganshorn and Kurz, 1968). The fraction of unbound active phenytoin (diphenylhydantoin) in the plasma of neonates is increased about 2-fold compared with adults. When hyperbilirubinaemia is also present, the unbound fraction of phenytoin is up to 3 times greater than in adult plasma (Rane et al., 1971). At high doses in adults, phenytoin displays dose dependent elimination kinetics (see chapter I; sect. 2.1.1). Thus, when the plasma concentration of unbound phenytoin exceeds the capacity to eliminate the drug, phenytoin may accumulate with toxicity. At lower plasma phenytoin concentrations however,

Table I. Plasma protein binding and apparent volume of distribution of various drugs in newborn infants and adults (after Morselli, 1976a)

Drug	% Bound		Apparent V_d (L/kg)	
	newborns	adults	newborns	adults
Ampicillin	9-11	15-29	—	0.40-0.70
Benzylpenicillin	~60	~65	—	~0.3
Methicillin	~26	~37	—	~0.3
Nafcillin	68-69	87-90	—	0.60-0.70
Sulphafurazole (sulfisoxazole)	65-70	~84	0.35-0.43	~0.16
Sulphamethoxypyridazine	~57	65-70	0.36-0.47	0.18-0.20
Salicylate	63-84	80-85	0.15-0.35	0.13-0.20
Phenylbutazone	85-90	96-98	0.20-0.25	0.12-0.15
Digoxin	14-26	23-40	4.90-10.16	5.17-7.35
Diazepam	~84	94-98	1.40-1.82	2.20-2.60
Phenytoin	80-85	89-92	1.20-1.40	0.60-0.67
Phenobarbitone	28-36	46-48	0.59-1.54	0.50-0.60
Pentobarbitone	37-40	39-45	—	0.90-0.99
Imipramine	~74	85-92	—	20.0-40.0
Desipramine	64-71	80-94	—	22.0-59.0

an increase in the fraction of unbound drug may lead to an increased rate of elimination, since more drug is available for metabolism (see section 2.3.1).

As a consequence of the decreased protein binding in newborns, the apparent volume of distribution of many drugs increases (table I). This means that a given plasma concentration of a drug in the newborn may reflect a plasma/tissue ratio higher than in the adult and consequently a larger amount of drug in the body tissues than the same concentration would reflect in older children and adults. Thus, myocardial and skeletal concentrations of digoxin in newborns can be higher than those found in children and adults (Kim et al., 1974; see further section 2.3.2).

Altered protein binding of drugs in young children is most likely to arise as a consequence of disorders such as uraemia, the nephrotic syndrome and liver diseases (see chapter XXI, sect. 1.2; XIX, sect. 1.3) or in cases of poisoning with drugs which display concentration dependent binding (e.g. salicylate).

Malnutrition states characterised by hypoalbuminaemia can also influence protein binding of acidic drugs (see chapter XXX; sect. 2.2). Thus, binding of salicylate, warfarin and thiopentone is markedly decreased in children with kwashiorkor when drug concentrations exceed the binding capacity of available plasma proteins (Buchanan, 1977).

The concentration dependence of salicylate binding to plasma proteins has important implications to interpretation of plasma salicylate concentrations, particularly in cases of acute poisoning with salicylates in infants and young children. In salicylate poisoning, there is a poor correlation between plasma salicylate concentrations at a given time and the clinical severity of intoxication at that time. This can be explained by the increase in apparent volume of distribution of the drug with increasing doses and which seems to be due to decreased binding to plasma proteins at the higher doses (Levy and Yaffe, 1974). This means that a given plasma concentration in an individual who has taken a large dose of salicylate reflects a larger amount of drug in the body than the same plasma concentration in another individual who has taken a smaller dose of salicylate. Presumably the larger distribution at higher doses includes the central nervous system, the probable site of most of the very severe and potentially lethal manifestations of toxicity.

Drugs themselves may alter binding of endogenous substances in newborns. In newborn infants the hepatic conjugation of bilirubin is limited and increased plasma levels often occur. Acidic drugs such as salicylates and most sulphonamides (e.g. sulphafurazole/sulfisoxazole, sulphaphenazole, sulphadimethoxine, sulphapyridine including that formed from sulphasalazine), which are highly bound to plasma albumin, compete with and can displace bilirubin from albumin binding sites. This has serious consequences in newborns if hepatic metabolism of bilirubin is already compromised (Silverman et al., 1956; Schiff et al., 1973). The increased amount of unbound unconjugated (lipid soluble) bilirubin readily traverses the blood-brain 'barrier' and may lead to kernicterus, particularly in the presence of other factors such as acidosis, hypothermia, hypoglycaemia, haemolysis, and so on.

Aqueous preparations of synthetic vitamin K derivatives, when used in excessive doses to prevent or reverse hypoprothrombinaemia in the newborn, apart from causing instability of the immature erythrocyte, can also compete with and displace bilirubin from plasma albumin binding sites and may cause haemolytic anaemia and kernicterus (Done, 1964). As large doses of natural vitamin K_1 oxide generally do not lead to hyperbilirubinaemia, it is to be preferred.

2.2.3 Blood-Brain 'Barrier'

Development of the blood-brain 'barrier' in newborn animals is incomplete and as a consequence there is increased permeability of certain substances into the brain (Brown, 1973). Lipid soluble drugs (general anaesthetics, sedatives, narcotic analgesics, tetracyclines) and endogenous substances (unconjugated bilirubin) readily enter the brain. Due to increased brain uptake, morphine reaches higher concentrations in the brains of infant than adult rats, and human infants are considered to be relatively more 'sensitive' to the respiratory depressant effects of morphine than older children (Done, 1964). At equianalgesic doses (as fraction of adult dose), the respiratory depressant effects of pethidine (meperidine) are less than those of morphine since brain uptake in infants seems to be the same as in adults (Way et al., 1965).

There seems to be an increased uptake of barbiturates in young infants (Done, 1964). The more ready penetration of some lipid soluble drugs into the central nervous system in the newborn cannot only be due to immaturity of the blood-brain 'barrier'. Other factors such as acidosis, hypoxia, hypothermia, hypoglycaemia and the sparseness of myelination are also clearly involved. In anaesthetic practice, intravenous barbiturates are avoided as induction agents during the neonatal period, and morphine is not often used in infants under 6 months of age, and between 6 and 12 months it is used in reduced dosage (chapt. X; sect. 3.1).

2.2.4 Drug Receptor Sensitivity

The response to muscle relaxant drugs differs in infants and young children, particularly in newborns (see chapter X; sect. 3.1). Although neuromuscular transmission in the newborn is similar to that in the adult, the response to non-depolarising neuromuscular blocking drugs (e.g. curare-type) may be enhanced and resembles that seen in myasthenic patients, particularly in prematures during the first weeks of life (Churchill Davidson and Wise, 1963, 1964; Goudsouzian et al., 1975). The activity of plasma cholinesterase in newborns is about half of that of the older child and adult, and increases gradually to that of the adult by age 1 year (Ecobichon and Stephens, 1973; Zsigmond and Down, 1971). These low cholinesterase levels do not as expected prolong the duration of action of suxamethonium (succinylcholine). In fact, when dosed on a mg/kg basis, neonates and infants are relatively resistant to suxamethonium; whereas response is the same as in older children and adults when dosage is based on a body surface area basis. This discrepancy is probably largely due to the relatively greater surface area to body weight ratio in the newborn and to redistribution of the relaxant into a larger extracellular fluid volume (see chapter X; sect. 2.2.1).

Infants and small children appear to have increased responsiveness to vagal stimulation (Lipton et al., 1965); blockade of reflex bradycardia in anaesthetic practice necessitates doses of atropine much larger than those required to suppress salivation or prevent bradycardia (Brown, 1973). The neonatal dose of atropine for premedication is also larger than that used in older infants and children. Children tolerate relatively large doses of adrenaline and again the dose is greater in newborns than in the older infant and child (Brown, 1973). The physiological differences in the various paediatric age groups do not always necessitate reduced dosage (see also chapter X; sect. 3.1).

2.3 Drug Elimination

There are important differences in the rate of elimination of drugs in neonates, infants and children which can be related to the different developmental physiological states of the various age groups (see Morselli, 1976a; 1977; table II). This is reflected in a successive increase in the rate of elimination with increasing age. A decreased capacity to eliminate drugs is most marked and of greatest importance in the newborn, particularly premature infants. The postnatal adaptation to extrauterine life is characterised by very rapid physiological changes. Thus safe and effective drug therapy in the neonate is not only complicated by the functional immaturity of drug metabolising and renal excretory processes but also by the rapid increase in their activity as a function of postnatal age. As the age dependent rate of elimination varies with the particular drug and the individual patient, no general rule or guide can apply to the calculation of dosage for all drugs. In neonates in particular, proper clinical assessment, and where feasible, plasma monitoring of drug concentrations, must constitute the basis for proper adjustment of drug dosage.

2.3.1 Hepatic Metabolism

Diminished drug metabolising capacity in young animals has been well documented (Done, 1964). There is also evidence in man that the activity of many of the drug metabolising enzyme processes is low in neonates and that attainment of values approaching those of adults takes varying periods of time after birth (Morselli et al., 1974; Rane and Sjoqvist, 1972). In most cases a decreased drug metabolising capacity has been in-

Table II. Plasma half-lives (hours) of different drugs in newborn infants, children and adults[1] (after Morselli, 1976a, 1977; Morselli and Baruzzi, 1978)

Drug	Newborns (< 7 days)	Infants (> 1 month)	Children (1 to 15 years)	Adults[2]
Drugs mainly eliminated by hepatic metabolism				
Amylobarbitone	17-60			12-27
Carbamazepine	8-28		14; 19	16-27
Diazepam	22-46	10-12	15-21	24-48
	38-120 (prematures)			
Ethosuximide			24-41	30-60
Indomethacin	∼15			4-11
	13-24 (prematures)			
Lignocaine[4] (lidocaine)	∼3			1-2
Mepivacaine	∼9			∼2
Nalidixic acid	∼4	∼3	∼2	1.5-2.5
Nortriptyline	∼56			18-22
Paracetamol (acetaminophen)	2-5			∼2
	∼5[3].		∼4.5[3]	∼4[3]
Pethidine (meperidine)	∼23			∼3
Phenobarbitone[6]	70-500	20-70	20-80	60-180
Phenylbutazone[4]	∼27	∼18	∼18; 23[5]	∼70
Phenytoin[4,6]	30-60	2-7	2-20	20-30
Salicylate[4]	4.5-11[3]		2-3[3]	2-4[3]
Theophylline	14-58 (prematures)	∼5.6	1.4-8	3.5-8
Tolbutamide	10-40			4-10
Drugs mainly eliminated as unchanged drug by renal excretion				
Benzylpenicillin[7]	3.2	1.4	0.8	0.5
Digoxin	26-170	11-37	19-50	30-60
	90 (prematures)			
Gentamicin[7]	4-5	2-5	∼2-4	2-3

1   Mean values or ranges shown are only intended to show trend in elimination with postnatal development. Some values in children and adults are not from the same laboratory as those for newborns and infants.
2   Younger adults. Values can vary widely among individuals but those indicated are the usual mean values.
3   Based on urinary excretion, rather than plasma concentration.
4   Dose dependent elimination kinetics. Values given are for those at or around therapeutic concentrations.
5   Value of ∼18h in children aged 2 to 7 years; ∼23h for older children.
6   See also table III for values in the perinatal period.
7   See also table IV for values in the perinatal period and also for other antibacterial drugs.

ferred by a slow elimination rate from plasma, which for all the drugs studied shows a progressive increase with age (table II). As in adults (see chapter I; sect. 4.2), there is a marked variation in the rate of elimination among individual infants and children.

Changing Rate of Metabolism After Birth

The extent of decreased metabolising capacity and the age after birth at which the rate of elimination approaches that for adults varies with the drug and its biotransformation or metabolism pathways and is applicable only for those drugs mainly eliminated by hepatic metabolism. Liver function and hence drug metabolising capacity changes very rapidly after birth and in general, it would seem that for drugs extensively metabolised (e.g. diazepam, phenytoin, phenobarbitone), a decreased rate of elimination is likely to be of most clinical significance during the first few weeks of life for full term infants, but for longer periods in prematures (Morselli et al., 1974; Loughnan et al., 1977; Pitlick et al., 1978).

The rapid change in rate of elimination following birth is well illustrated in the case of phenobarbitone and phenytoin (Loughnan et al., 1977; Pitlick et al., 1978). In both cases, plasma concentrations and half-life decline rapidly after the first 1 to 2 weeks of life (table III). Plasma concentrations of phenytoin are very variable, particularly in prematures, and can readily reach the toxic range in the first week of life, necessitating individualised dosage and monitoring of therapy by plasma concentration estimation (Loughnan et al., 1977).

Diminished drug metabolism appears to have been the basis for many of the adverse effects which have been noted in infants born of mothers who received drugs prior to delivery (see chapter III) and when drugs have been prescribed to newborn infants on the basis of body size. There is some evidence which suggests that some drugs (e.g. phenytoin, carbamazepine) can be metabolised by newborn infants at adult rates, particularly following continuous exposure of the fetal liver to the drug during pregnancy (Rane et al., 1974, 1975).

Pathways of Metabolism in Infants and Young Children

As discussed in chapter I (sect. 3.3.4), drugs are usually metabolised through different conjugation processes such as glucuronidation, sulphation or glycine coupling, with or without prior oxidation, reduction (e.g. acetylation) or hydrolysis. Most of these reactions are catalysed by enzymes located in microsomes of the liver. Not all metabolic processes however, are impaired in the newborn infant. For example, the newborn seem to have a reasonably well developed capacity for conjugation reactions involving sulphation (Levy et al., 1975) and for oxidative reactions involving demethylation (Morselli et al., 1974; Meffin et al., 1973).

Conjugation processes in the neonate have received the most attention. Those involving glucuronidation are markedly deficient in some premature and newborn full term infants (Stern et al., 1970; Vest, 1965), reflecting the low concentration of the enzymes glucuronyl transferase and uridine disphosphate glucuronic dehydrogenase (chapter I; fig. 15b). Thus, chloramphenicol given in 'usual' doses based on weight to a newborn infant may cause serious toxicity (circulatory collapse or the 'grey baby' syndrome), because defective conjugation (and renal excretion of free drug) leads to high plasma concentrations of the unchanged drug. The same dose to the same infant at 2 to 3 weeks of life may not give concentrations high enough to be effective (see section 3.1.2). Nalidixic acid is also conjugated by glucuronidation (following prior hydroxylation) and is eliminated slowly in the newborn (Rohwedder et al., 1970). Elimination of salicylate is significantly delayed in the neonate compared with adults, because of immaturity of both metabolic transformation (glucuronidation) and renal excretory pathways (Levy and Garrettson, 1974; see also below). In adults, indomethacin is mainly eliminated in the urine, as glucuronidated metabolites and to a lesser extent (10 to 20 % of a dose) as unchanged drug. A decreased glucuronidation capacity may explain in large part the prolonged elimination and platelet dysfunction following use of indomethacin for closure of the patent ductus arteriosus in premature newborns (Friedman et al., 1978). Conjugation processes involving sulphation do not seem to be deficient. For example, the impaired phenolic glucuronidation of paracetamol (acetaminophen) in the newborn is offset, to a degree, by a well developed capacity for sulphate conjugation (Levy et al., 1975) and the rate of elimination is the same in newborns as in children and adults (Miller et al., 1976). Similarly, the low production of the conjugated metabolite of phenobarbitone (?glucuronide) in sick newborns, is well compensated by efficient output of the non-

Table III. Plasma half-lives and concentrations of phenytoin and phenobarbitone in the perinatal period after fixed dosage in each age group

	Phenytoin[1]		Phenobarbitone[2]	
	$t_{1/2}$ (h)	plasma conc (mg/L)	$t_{1/2}$ (h)	plasma conc (mg/L)
Prematures	16-160	> 40	—	—
Infants (< 7 days)	7-42	0.9-28.6	115	37
Infants (⩾ 14 days)	9-15	0.6-3.8	78	> 20
Infants (⩾ 1 month)	5-7	0.5-5.7	67	~ 15

1   After Loughnan et al. (1977): Loading dose of 12mg/kg intravenously, followed by 8mg/kg per 24h orally.
2   After Pitlick et al. (1978): Loading dose of 20mg/kg intravenously, followed by 5mg/kg in 2 divided doses per 24h. Mean values.

conjugated metabolite and unchanged drug, such that total renal elimination of the administered drug is almost as rapid in newborns as in adults (Boreus et al., 1978). The clinical significance of a decreased metabolic capacity can therefore depend on the existence of alternative metabolic pathways and routes of elimination.

Oxidative metabolism is the most important pathway for many drugs and hydroxylation of drugs has generally been shown to be deficient in the newborn, particularly prematures. Thus the rate of elimination from plasma of drugs such as amylobarbitone, phenobarbitone, mepivacaine, phenytoin and diazepam is decreased in newborn infants compared with older infants, children and adults (Morselli, 1976a, 1977; Meffin et al., 1973). The metabolism of diazepam has been studied in detail (Morselli et al., 1973, 1974; Mandelli et al., 1975). Premature infants have higher and more sustained plasma concentrations than children and the ability to hydroxylate the drug is significantly reduced in prematures and full term infants compared with children (4 to 8 years) and adults. The plasma half-lives show a progressive decrease with age; being 38 to 120 hours in prematures, 22 to 46 hours in full term newborn infants, and 15 to 21 hours in the children. Newborn infants born of mothers who received diazepam prior to delivery also show a reduced ability to hydroxylate the drug. Significant accumulation of diazepam and desmethyldiazepam (an active metabolite) occurs in the fetus after repeated administration of diazepam to the mother (Mandelli et al., 1975) and this may give a basis for the unwanted effects noted in newborns whose mothers received *excessive* dosage of diazepam in labour or for management of eclampsia and severe pre-eclampsia (see chapter III; sect. 3.10.1).

Ester hydrolysis is low in newborns and esterase activity in plasma appears to be significantly related to the developmental stage. The activity of various esterases and rate of hydrolysis of drugs such as procaine and aspirin is considerably slower in prematures than full term newborns, and in turn infants aged 1 year, when adult values are attained (Ecobichon and Stephens, 1973; Windorfer et al., 1974). The low activity of blood esterases in newborns may at least in part explain the cardiorespiratory depression observed in newborns when compounds containing ester bonds (e.g. some local anaesthetics) are used in obstetric procedures (see chapter X; sect. 2.5, 3.4). Some antibacterial drugs such as pivampicillin are esters of parent compounds. Pivampicillin, the pivaloyloxymethyl ester of ampicillin, is well absorbed after oral administration when it undergoes simultaneous hydrolysis by enzymes present in the blood and tissues with liberation of ampicillin. It is not as well absorbed in children under 1 year of age as in those over 1 year (Pedersen-Bjergaard and Petersen, 1977); possibly because of a developmental deficiency of blood and tissue esterases.

Factors Influencing the Rate of Metabolism in the Newborn

Apart from the capacity for drug metabolism and renal excretion (section 2.3), plasma protein binding may also influence the total elimination rate (see chapter I; sect. 3.2.3). Thus the decreased protein binding of phenytoin in the newborn (see sect. 2.2.2) may tend to increase the rate of metabolism as compared with adults, since more unbound drug is available for metabolism. For example, plasma concentrations of phenytoin in newborn infants treated with 10mg/kg daily for convulsive disorders have been noted to be half those of adults treated with 5mg/kg daily (Jalling et al., 1970). In adults, low steady-state plasma concentrations of phenytoin are compatible with rapid metabolism.

The rate of neonatal drug metabolism may also be altered by changes in the activity of the liver microsomal metabolising enzyme system. Thus continuous exposure to certain drugs may increase (induce) the activity of the hepatic microsomal enzyme system (see chapter I; sect. 3.3.5). Induction of enzyme activity by drugs such as phenobarbitone is nonspecific, but has been used therapeutically in neonatal hyperbilirubinaemia to enhance the activity of the enzyme glucuronyl transferase (Stern et al., 1970). Thus when phenobarbitone is given to the mother prenatally or to the infant at birth, there is a significant reduction in the degree of hyperbilirubinaemia in the late neonatal period (Thomas, 1976). Phototherapy (?photo-oxidation of bilirubin) or exchange transfusion has however, largely replaced phenobarbitone for this purpose. Enzyme induction can also influence the rate of metabolism of other drugs given to the neonate. Administration of phenobarbitone to the mother or newborn infant increases both the rate of elimination of diazepam as well as the concentration of hydroxylated metabolites excreted in the urine, presumably by inducing the hydroxylating activity of the liver microsomal enzymes (Morselli et al., 1974).

Continuous administration of drugs throughout pregnancy may possibly lead to induction of drug metabolising enzymes during fetal life. Some studies have shown that infants born of mothers who have been treated with drugs such as phenytoin or carbamazepine, seem to be capable of metabolising the transplacentally acquired drug at adult rates immediately after birth (Rane et al., 1974, 1975). Continuous fetal exposure to salicylate also seems to increase the rate of elimination by the neonate, apparently by causing a more rapid maturation of the major biotransformation pathway (salicyluric acid formation). Thus, the elimination of salicylate in an infant born of a mother who took 6.5g aspirin daily for arthritis throughout pregnancy, although relatively slower than in normal adults, was more rapid than in newborn infants of mothers who had taken only a single small dose of aspirin shortly before delivery (Garrettson et al., 1975). Reduced elimination compared with adults is due to immaturity of the renal excretory and other biotransformation (glucuronidation) pathways.

Drug Metabolism in Older Children

Drug metabolising capacity in older children has been studied less than in newborns and young infants, but for many drugs subject to hepatic metabolism (table II), children seem to have a more rapid rate of elimination; possibly due to increased hepatic drug metabolising activity (Rane and Wilson, 1976). The elimination of theophylline in particular is more rapid in young children than in adults (Ellis et al., 1976) and explains the need for an increase in the weight adjusted dose in young patients. Thus in one study, doses averaging 24mg/kg daily were required to maintain plasma concentrations of theophylline in the therapeutic range in children under 9 years, while there was a progressive decrease in the weight adjusted dose through adolescence until average dosage requirements of 13mg/kg daily were observed for adults (Wyatt et al., 1978). On the other hand, clearance of theophylline is decreased in newborns, particularly prematures, compared with children and adults (Ogilvie, 1978). Diazepam also seems to exhibit a similar developmental pattern in rate of elimination; being prolonged in newborns but more rapid in young children than in adults (Mandelli et al., 1978). The rate of elimination of other drugs such as phenobarbitone, phenytoin, carbamazepine, ethosuximide and dextropropoxyphene in young children is similar to or more rapid than in adults. In the case of phenobarbitone, phenytoin and ethosuximide, the plasma concentration/dose ratio is lower in children than in adults (Rane and Wilson, 1976). Children exhibit similar low bioavailability and significant hepatic first-pass metabolism of high clearance drugs such as propranolol and dextropropoxyphene, as do adults (Wilson et al., 1976).

For some drugs, although pathways of metabolism may differ in various age groups, the overall rate of elimination is similar. Thus, for paracetamol (acetaminophen), a higher rate of sulphate conjugation in newborns and young children (aged 3 to 9 years) compensates for a deficiency of phenolic glucuronidation and the rate of elimination is the same as in 12-year-old children and adults (Miller et al., 1976).

2.3.2 Renal Excretion

Renal excretory capacity is immature at birth and shows a successive maturation with postnatal age (West et al., 1948; Gladtke and Heimann, 1975). Adult values for glomerular filtration rate are gradually reached over several postnatal months and for tubular function some time later. Renal function in the neonate is about 30 to 40% (per unit of body surface area) less than that of an adult, as determined by usual measurements of glomerular filtration rate and renal blood flow.

Urinary excretion is the final route by which most drugs are eliminated from the body. Drugs are excreted either as more polar (water soluble) metabolites or mainly in unchanged form if they have not been metabolised to a significant extent. Many drugs in neonatal therapeutics are mainly eliminated unchanged by the kidneys (e.g. most antibacterial drugs, digoxin). In adults, tubular mechanisms are important for the excretion of some drugs (e.g. penicillins) whereas glomerular filtration is important for others (e.g. kanamycin, gentamicin, digoxin). However, in newborn and young infants, glomerular filtration becomes relatively more important for elimination of penicillins than tubular excretion, which is the primary mechanism in older infants and children (McCracken, 1974). Maturation of renal excretory mechanisms markedly alters elimination rates for the penicillins, such that urinary excretion increases and serum half-lives decrease with increasing postnatal age (Axline et al., 1967; Barnett et al., 1949). Patterns of elimination for gentamicin and kanamycin (Axline and Simon, 1964; McCracken, 1974) are very similar to those of the penicillins (table IV). For these drugs, rate of elimination is also inversely related to gestational age (Howard and McCracken, 1975; fig. 1).

Drugs Mainly Eliminated by Renal Excretion

In general, for antibacterial drugs mainly excreted unchanged by the kidneys, the plasma half-life is prolonged during the first 2 weeks of life (particularly week 1), but the rate of elimination increases rapidly during the remainder of the first month such that at 4 weeks the plasma half-life is similar to that for adults. For sulphonamides such as sulphafurazole/sulfisoxazole, a further but smaller increase in the rate of elimination occurs

during the first year. Consequently, in a 1-year-old child the plasma half-life of sulphafurazole is shorter than in adults (Krauer, 1974). After this age, a slow and constant increase in plasma half-life occurs until age 20 years when adult values are reached. Sulphafurazole is distributed primarily within the extracellular fluid compartment of the body. The observed changes in plasma half-life of sulphafurazole reflects both a change in the rate of renal elimination and a decrease in distribution consequent upon the decrease in extracellular fluid volume with growth and development (see also section 2.2.1).

In terms of serum concentrations, certain generalisations can be made for most antibacterial drugs. In the first days of life, peak serum concentrations are higher and sustained for considerably longer than those in older infants and children. With increasing postnatal age there is a gradual decline, but peak concentrations tend to be higher than those in older infants and children until the end of the first month. This pattern is exaggerated in the premature infant, in whom serum concentrations are higher and more sustained at any given age than the term infant. Knowledge of the plasma half-life and peak serum concentrations of antibacterial drugs therefore provides the basis for determination of appropriate dosage and dose in-

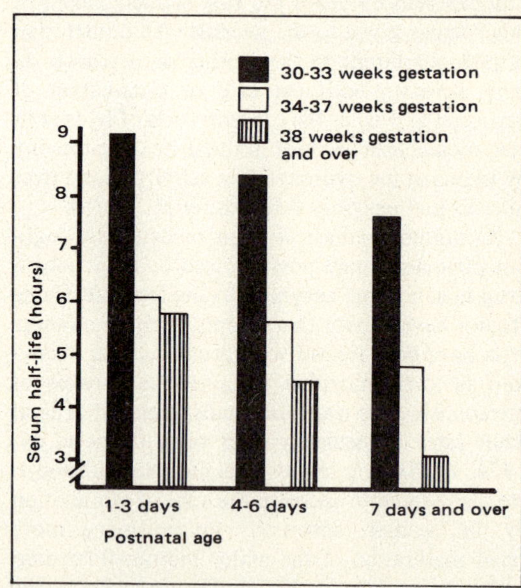

Fig. 1. Relationship between kanamycin plasma half-lives and gestational and postnatal ages (after Howard and McCracken: J. Ped. 86: 949, 1975; by permission of author and editor).

Table IV. Plasma half-lives (mean values or ranges in hours) of some antibacterial drugs in premature and term newborns and young infants (after McCracken, 1974; Tognoni, 1977)

Drug	Prematures (< 7 days)	Newborns (< 7 days)	Infants (7-14 days)	Infants (> 14 days)	Adults
Ampicillin	~4-6	4	2.8	1.7	1-1.5
Benzylpenicillin		3.2	1.7	1.4	0.5
Carbenicillin	~5-6	~5; ~3[1]	~2	~1.5	1-1.5
Chloramphenicol	15-22 24-28	~6			1.5-3
Gentamicin	~5-6	4-5.5	~3-3.5		2-3
Kanamycin[2]	~9	5-5.7[3]	3.8		3-5
Methicillin	2.4[4]	3.3; 1.3[5]	0.9	0.8	0.5
Tobramycin	8.0-8.7	4.6	3.9		2-3

1   At 3 days around 5h; at 4 to 7 days around 3h.
2   See also figure 1.
3   At 1 to 3 days around 5.7h; at 4 to 7 days around 5.0h.
4   At 4 to 7 days.
5   At 1 day 3.3h; at 4 to 5 days 1.3h.

terval for each individual agent (McCracken, 1974). Suggested dosages for some important antibacterial drugs which take these factors into account are given in table V. It must be remembered that the physiology of an infant is a dynamic process, changing rapidly from one week to the next. Thus for example, in a neonate with meningitis, the dose of an antibacterial drug such as gentamicin which is effective and safe when started in the first week of life may be inadequate during the second and third weeks of therapy. Serum assay of antibacterial concentrations is therefore highly desirable, particularly with potentially toxic drugs such as the aminoglycosides (e.g. gentamicin, kanamycin).

Digoxin disposition is also governed by the changing renal function in neonates and young infants (see Wettrell and Andersson, 1977; Nyberg and Wettrell, 1978). Renal clearance of digoxin is low during the first month of life but increases with increasing age, and in some studies, as in the elderly, shows a good correlation with creatinine clearance (Halkin et al., 1978a; Wettrell et al., 1974), but is greater than creatinine clearance in all paediatric age groups (Halkin et al., 1978a; Gorodischer et al., 1977). However, the plasma half-life of digoxin is shorter in infants aged 1 month to 2 years than in both adults and neonates (Morselli et al., 1975; Wettrell, 1977) and is

reflected in the higher dosage requirements (on a weight basis) for this age group than in older or younger subjects (table XI). The reason for the change in plasma half-life and increased dosage requirements in neonates and infants is not completely clear. Alteration in distribution and changed elimination capacities in the different developmental age groups are all probably involved (Gorodischer et al., 1976; Wettrell, 1977). With equivalent doses on a body weight basis, plasma concentrations are higher in infants (and also in neonates) than those considered to be optimum in adults for obtaining an adequate inotropic effect (table VI).

The higher plasma concentrations in the neonate appear most likely to be due to the low renal clearance of digoxin, which lessens rapidly after 3 months of age and does not increase further after age 12 months (Halkin et al., 1978a; Wettrell et al., 1974). The need for higher plasma concentrations of digoxin in neonates and infants has been questioned (Wettrell and Andersson, 1977; Nyberg and Wettrell, 1978), particularly since young patients can be intoxicated at plasma concentrations commonly regarded as safe for paediatric practice (Halkin et al., 1978b). Moreover, in one study no correlation existed between plasma concentration of digoxin and degree of control of heart failure (Neutze et al., 1977).

Premature newborns in particular may have a very low clearance of digoxin which often necessitates a large reduction of the maintenance dose but also a reduction of the loading dose (Nyberg and Wettrell, 1978). In one series, a reduction of the loading dose of digoxin from 30µg/kg to 20µg/kg in premature infants was associated with the same inotropic effects and a reduction in plasma concentrations from a potentially toxic to a non-toxic range (Pinsky et al., 1979).

Drugs Eliminated by Both Renal and Hepatic Mechanisms

Frusemide (furosemide) is eliminated about equally by hepatic and renal mechanisms and indomethacin by hepatic but also to a lesser extent by renal excretion of unchanged drug. Elimination of both is markedly prolonged in newborns. In the case of indomethacin, elimination is particularly prolonged in prematures (Friedman et al., 1978) and appears likely to be due primarily to impaired glucuronidation (see section 2.3.1), but immaturity of the glomerular filtration and tubular secretion mechanisms for elimination of the increased proportion of unchanged indomethacin could also possibly be involved (Traeger et al., 1973). The usual standard single daily dose range

of frusemide in the neonate should not lead to excessive accumulation, but any need for repeat dosing should take into account the markedly decreased clearance of the drug in the neonate (Aranda et al., 1978).

2.4 Metabolic Disturbances and Drug Response

Apart from immaturity of physiological processes or disease, the sensitivity to drugs in infants and young children may be influenced indirectly through complications such as dehydration, fever, and acid-base disturbances. Acidosis is common in sick children and the distribution of some drugs into cells can be altered by changes in acid-base balance. Thus the tissue uptake of acidic drugs is increased in acidosis whereas that of basic drugs is decreased. This phenomenon is due to the effect of pH on the ionisation of weak electrolytes (see chapter I; sect. 1.1) and is of major importance in acute poisoning with salicylates in young children and infants (Hill, 1973). Excessive dosage of aspirin in the young can cause serious toxicity, partly because infants and young children seem particularly susceptible to the consequences of metabolic acidosis and hypoglycaemia. Small

Table V. Daily dosage schedules (total dose per 24h) of some antibacterial drugs in infants (after Eichenwald and McCracken, 1978)

Drug	Route	Infants (< 1 week)	Infants (1 to 4 weeks)
Ampicillin sodium	IV, IM	50mg/kg (2)[1]	75 to 100mg/kg (3) 200mg/kg (3)[2]
Carbenicillin disodium	IV, IM	200mg/kg (2)	300mg/kg (3)[3] 400mg/kg (4)[4]
Chloramphenicol sodium succinate	IV	25mg/kg (1)	50mg/kg (1 or 2)
Gentamicin	IM	5mg/kg (2)	7.5mg/kg (3)
Kanamycin	IM	15mg/kg (2)[3] 20mg/kg (2)[4]	20mg/kg (2)[3] 30mg/kg (3)[4]
Methicillin	IV, IM	50mg/kg (2)	75 to 100mg/kg (3)
Penicillin G (soluble)	IV, IM	100,000u to 250,000u/kg (2)	100,000u to 250,000u/kg (2-3)

1   Number in parenthesis indicates the number of doses into which the daily dose should be divided.
2   Dosage for meningitis (see also text).
3   In infants < 2000g birth weight.
4   In infants > 2000g birth weight.

Table VI. Plasma concentrations of digoxin in neonates, infants, children and adults with heart disease (after Wettrell et al., 1974)

Age	Digoxin dosage (mg/kg/day)	Digoxin dosage (mg/m²/day)	Plasma digoxin (ng/ml)
Neonates and young infants (0-1 month)	0.013	0.20	2.1
Infants (1-12 months)	0.019 0.012	0.31 0.21	2.1 1.2
Children (1-10 years)	0.012	0.28	1.4
Adults	0.005	0.19	1.2 (0.7 to 1.9)

decreases in pH markedly affect the degree of ionisation of salicylate (pK_a3) and are associated with rather large increases in the non-ionised penetrating form of the drug. Thus acidosis accentuates salicylate penetration into brain and other tissues. Steady control of acidosis is therefore a primary therapeutic goal in cases of acute aspirin poisoning, particularly in the acidotic young child. Renal excretion of salicylate increases markedly as urine pH rises above 7 (Davidson, 1971; see chapter IX; sect. 5.5.1). Tubular secretion is an important mechanism of elimination of some drugs and acid-base disturbances such as metabolic acidosis may alter urine pH and hence the renal clearance of drugs (see chapter I; sect. 3.4).

The state of hydration can be of major importance and severe dehydration is common in infancy. In diabetic acidosis, a larger dose of insulin is required if the child is given insulin prior to rehydration. Fever readily occurs in older infants, especially in an underhydrated infant, and may modify the response to some drugs. Underhydration may tend to increase the effect of aspirin since most of the drug at usual doses is distributed in the body fluid (see section 2.2.1).

2.5 Genetically Determined Abnormal Drug Responses

Most studies of genetically determined abnormal responses to drugs have involved adults. However, in family studies, a number of children have been shown to have the same genetically determined propensity to suffer adverse reactions as the adults (Cohen and Weber, 1972). Moreover, some genetically determined abnormalities in drug response have been noted first in children

with the individual's first exposure to the drug (e.g. in glucose-6-phosphate dehydrogenase deficiency) and in others, children seem to react more frequently (e.g. general anaesthesia and malignant hyperpyrexia) or to a greater degree than adults (e.g. sulphonamides and nitrofurantoin in individuals with G6PD deficiency).

Patients with glucose-6-phosphate dehydrogenase deficiency (G6PD) are extremely sensitive to a number of drugs (see chapter XXIII; sect. 8.4). This is especially important in neonates as the resulting haemolysis can readily lead to jaundice (see chapter XIX; sect. 14.6.6). Because of erythrocyte immaturity in newborns, many of the drugs causing haemolysis in G6PD deficient individuals at older age also affect normal newborns. Malignant hyperpyrexia following general anaesthesia is rare in infants under 3 years of age. In one series, the condition was not reported in infants and children under 3 years of age, but almost 25% of all cases occurred in patients under 5 years of age and more than a third during the first 10 years of life (Kalow, 1970). The condition is often fatal and treatment is not well defined (see chapter X; sect. 5.6). The prolonged apnoea which can follow suxamethonium (succinylcholine) in individuals with variant forms of the enzyme which normally hydrolyses the drug (pseudocholinesterase), can be a disastrous drug effect. The pharmacological basis and other examples of genetically determined abnormal responses to drugs are discussed in chapter I (sect. 4.2) and VII (sect. 4.2).

The alert clinician therefore has the opportunity and the responsibility to recognise abnormal responses to drugs, to prevent them in known susceptible groups, or by early observation after treating a patient in a standard manner. A suspicion by ethnic or racial group (e.g. G6PD; see chapter VII, sect. 4.2.2; XXX, sect. 2.1.1), or a family history of abnormal response in other relatives should also call the clinician's attention to the possibility for adverse reactions with use of certain drugs. Children in families known to have G6PD deficiency should be educated along with their parents in the hazards of exposure to drugs which can precipitate episodes of haemolytic anaemia.

3. Problems with Drugs and Drug Therapy

Although arbitrarily chosen, the postnatal periods are distinctive and may be delineated from each other in many ways as growth and development progresses. Drugs serve as a tool for distinguishing these age groups, particularly at each end of the paediatric age spectrum beginning with prematurity and ending with adolescence. Adverse reactions to drugs depend on the particular developmental stage (Gadeke, 1972).

3.1 Early Postnatal Period

This period concerns problems with drugs born with the baby (see chapter III) and with drugs excreted in breast milk. It involves the use of drugs when there is a strong suspicion of disease (e.g. neonatal sepsis). Reactions largely relate to problems of administration and elimination of drugs (Done, 1964; Nyhan, 1961), particularly in premature infants (see section 2.3).

3.1.1 Problems with Administration of Drugs

Oral administration of drugs to newborns may result in aspiration, or much of the drug may be lost. However, less of an oral dose may be lost than in the older child or stronger toddler who refuses medication more vigorously. Infants requiring antibacterial drugs often have very little tissue into which intramuscular injections can be given and intravenous administration may be difficult or hazardous. Problems with intramuscular therapy include the all too frequent use of the buttocks for administration. Sciatic neuropathy with permanent stunting of leg growth and subsequent crippling is a hazard of this practice. Gangrene of the foot has followed injection into the lateral thigh, although this area is preferred over the gluteal area as an injection site. A number of difficulties can arise in small infants with handling of intravenous fluids containing dissolved drugs. Local necrosis and loss of drug activity are common after fluid extravasation. Certain drugs, particularly antibiotics, can deteriorate in the infusion bottle while it hangs above the baby and become inactive by the time of its delivery into the child. Chemical and physical interactions between drugs added to intravenous fluids compound the problems with this route of administration (see section 5.1.1).

3.1.2 Problems with Therapy

Problems with therapy generally result from higher or lower plasma concentrations than are desired. Careful monitoring of plasma concentrations, although often extremely difficult in sick small infants, is necessary to ensure effective and safe therapy. Without constant supervision, a dose which is toxic soon after birth may be ineffective 1 or 2 weeks later. Dosages, therefore, should be individualised. The chloramphenicol grey baby syndrome is an excellent example of the need for drug dose tailoring in the neonatal period.

Immaturity of hepatic glucuronyl transferase activity results in diminished conjugation of chloramphenicol to the inactive acid glucuronide. Non-conjugated chloramphenicol is excreted by glomerular filtration, while the conjugated drug is eliminated by tubular excretion. Diminished glucuronidation combined with decreased glomerular and tubular function in newborn infants, therefore results in elevated serum concentrations of both non-conjugated and conjugated chloramphenicol (Weiss et al., 1960). Accumulation of the non-conjugated drug rather than metabolites is believed to be responsible for the toxic effects. Within 3 to 4 days signs of toxicity appear (ashen grey cyanosis, poor feeding, abdominal distension) and death may result from circulatory collapse. At 2 to 3 weeks of age, however, the dose toxic to a newborn may not result in therapeutic serum levels for the older infant (Hodgman and Burns, 1961).

Special needs exist during the neonatal period of life. For example, the prophylactic or therapeutic need for vitamin K. This arises at the time that red blood cells are unstable and are readily haemolysed. Consequently, excessive dosage of aqueous preparations of synthetic vitamin K can lead to haemolytic anaemia during this period of life (see section 2.2.2). These circumstances very rarely occur later in life. The couplet of pulmonary atelectasis and oxygen therapy is another unique neonatal problem not found in later years. The as yet unexpanded lungs require oxygen to prevent anoxia at a critical time of brain development. On the other hand, retrolental fibroplasia may be produced by excessive oxygen therapy. Here again proper monitoring of dosage permits tailored therapy for each newborn's need.

Growth itself may be altered by drugs administered to the baby. Tetracyclines are avid bone seekers and may delay bone growth if given during this period of life (Cohlan et al., 1963). They may also cause staining of teeth and enamel hypoplasia when given during the time of tooth development (see chapter XIII; sect. 13.3).

3.1.3 Drug Excretion in Breast Milk

Many drugs taken by the nursing mother will be excreted in her milk. However, for most drugs the amounts are very small and will usually not be harmful (see Anderson, 1977). Nevertheless, for a few drugs, particularly those with a low therapeutic ratio, although the concentration in breast milk may appear small, the total amount of drug ingested by the infant may reach pharmacologically active levels if the infant consumes say 500 to 700ml of milk daily. Many factors determine the passage and concentration of a particular drug in breast milk and the likely consequences, if any, to the breast fed infant (Catz and Giacoia, 1972). A general statement which applies to all drugs cannot therefore be made. This is a poorly studied area.

There is a paucity of studies which provide information on maternal plasma drug concentration, amounts in breast milk and plasma concentrations in the infant (table VII). Such serial monitoring of drug concentrations is essential if meaningful information is to become available about any risks involved with individual drugs.

Factors Which Influence Excretion of Drugs in Breast Milk

The concentration of pharmacologically active drug in breast milk depends on the drug concentration in the maternal plasma at the time of breast feeding, and the physicochemical properties of the drug such as pK_a, lipid solubility and protein binding, which affect its ease of passage into breast milk. Drugs are transferred to breast milk in accordance with the pH partition theory (see further chapter I; sect. 1.1). Thus, lipid soluble drugs will diffuse readily into breast milk in their non-ionised form. Drugs with low lipid solubility in their non-ionised form will diffuse more slowly into breast milk. Breast milk generally being of a lower pH than plasma encourages concentration of weak bases, whereas the concentration of weak acids in milk is generally lower than in plasma (Rasmussen, 1971; fig.2). A high concentration or prolonged presence of the drug in the general circulation (e.g. delayed elimination) will enhance its passage into breast milk. 'Back diffusion' of some drugs may also possibly occur during periods of

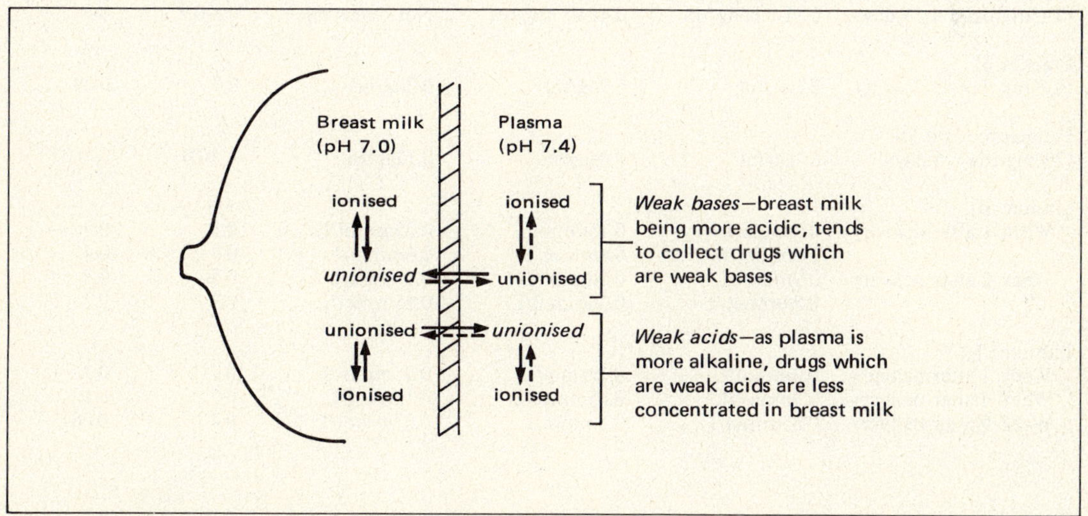

Fig. 2. Transfer of drugs to breast milk according to pH partition hypothesis. One of many factors determining drug concentration in milk.

Table VII. Concentration of drugs in maternal plasma and breast milk and infant's plasma (measured serially)

Drug[1] [and reference]	Maternal plasma	Breast milk	Infant's plasma	Milk: maternal plasma ratio	Infant's plasma: maternal plasma ratio
Carbamazepine [a] (6mg/kg daily)					
Day 2 after delivery	3.2µg/ml	1.8µg/ml	1.1µg/ml	0.6	0.3
Day 3 after delivery	2.0µg/ml	1.3µg/ml	1.3µg/ml	0.7	0.7
Day 28 after delivery	3.1µg/ml	1.8µg/ml	1.8µg/ml	0.6	0.6
Epoxycarbamazepine (active metabolite)					
Day 2 after delivery	0.7µg/ml	0.7µg/ml	0.3µg/ml	1.0	0.4
Day 3 after delivery	0.8µg/ml	0.5µg/ml	0µg/ml	0.6	0
Day 28 after delivery	1.1µg/ml	1.1µg/ml	0µg/ml	1.0	0
Carbamazepine [b] (8mg/kg daily)					
Day 2 after delivery	13.5µmol/L	7.5µmol/L	4.5µmol/L	0.6	0.3
Day 3 after delivery	8.5µmol/L	5.5µmol/L	5.5µmol/L	0.7	0.6
Day 30 after delivery	13.0µmol/L	7.5µmol/L	7.5µmol/L	0.6	0.6
Epoxycarbamazepine					
Day 2 after delivery	2.8µmol/L	3.0µmol/L	4.2µmol/L	1.1	1.5
Day 3 after delivery	3.0µmol/L	1.8µmol/L	0µmol/L	0.6	0
Day 30 after delivery	4.2µmol/L	4.4µmol/L	0µmol/L	1.1	0
Diazepam (10mg tds) [c]					
Day 4 after delivery	491ng/ml	51ng/ml	172ng/ml	0.1	0.4
Day 6 after delivery	601ng/ml	78ng/ml	74ng/ml	0.1	0.1
Desmethyldiazepam (active metabolite)					
Day 4 after delivery	340ng/ml	28ng/ml	243ng/ml	0.1	0.7
Day 6 after delivery	483ng/ml	52ng/ml	31ng/ml	0.1	0.1
Digoxin [d] (0.25mg daily x 14 days)	0.51-0.86ng/ml	0.41-0.78ng/ml	Not detectable[2]	0.8-0.9	—
Digoxin [l] (0.75mg daily x 7 days)	2.1ng/ml	1.9ng/ml	0.2ng/ml	0.9	0.09
Flufenamic acid [e] (200mg tds x 4 days)	6.4µg/ml[3]	0.05µg/ml[3]	0.12µg/ml[3]	< 0.01	~0.02
Lithium [f]					
Week 1 after delivery	0.34mmol/L	0.16mmol/L	0.22mmol/L	0.5	0.7
	1.5mmol/L	0.6mmol/L	0.6mmol/L	0.4	0.4
Week 2 after delivery	0.9mmol/L	0.3mmol/L	0.3mmol/L	0.3	0.3
	0.84mmol/L	0.56mmol/L	0.15mmol/L	0.7	0.2
Lithium[4] [g]					
Week 1 after delivery	0.3mmol/L	0.2mmol/L	0.05mmol/L	0.7	0.2
Week 4 after delivery	0.9mmol/L	0.65mmol/L	0.1mmol/L	0.7	0.1
Week 9 after delivery	0.85mmol/L	0.3mmol/L	0.07mmol/L	0.4	0.08

Table VII. (continued)

Metronidazole [h]					
(200mg PO, single dose)	2.6-3.9µg/ml	2.0-5.5µg/ml	0-0.4µg/ml	0.6-1.4	0-0.15
d-Norgestrel [i]					
(30µg)	0.4ng/ml	Not detectable[5]	Not detectable[5]		
(150µg)	3.1ng/ml	0.54ng/ml[6]		0.2	
(250µg)	3.9ng/ml	0.65ng/ml[6]	~0.1ng/ml	0.2	~0.03
Phenylbutazone [j]					
(750mg IM)	2-5mg/100ml	≤ 0.63mg/100ml	0.3-2mg/100ml	~0.1-0.3	~0.2-0.4
Tetracycline [k]					
(500mg PO q6h x 3 days)	0.8-3.2µg/ml	0.5-2.6µg/ml	Not detectable[7]	0.6-0.8	

1 References
    a = Pynnonen et al.: Acta Pharmacol. et Toxicol 41: 244 (1977)
    b = Erkkola and Kanto: Lancet 1: 1235 (1972)
    c = Pynnonen and Sillanpaa: Lancet 2: 563 (1975)
    d = Loughnan: J. Ped. 92: 1019 (1978)
    e = Buchanan et al.: Curr. Ther. Res. 11: 533 (1969)
    f = Schou and Amdisen: Brit. Med. J. 2: 138 (1973)
    g = Sykes et al.: Brit. Med. J. 2: 1299 (1976)
    h = Gray and Squires: Brit. J. Vener. Dis. 37: 278 (1961)
    i = Nilsson et al.: Am. J. Obstet. Gyn. 129: 178 (1977)
    j = Leuxner and Pulver: Munch. Med. Wschr. 98: 84 (1956)
    k = Posner et al.: Antibiot. Ann., p.594 (1954-1955)
    l = Finley et al.: J. Ped. 94: 339 (1979).
2 Detection limit 0.1ng/ml.
3 Figures are free drug in maternal plasma and breast milk and free plus conjugated drug in infant's plasma.
4 Figures shown are approximate values only, being extracted from a graph.
5 Detection limit approximately 100pg/ml.
6 Concentration in postnursing milk samples (slightly higher than prenursing concentrations).
7 Detection limit 0.05µg/ml.

rapidly decreasing maternal plasma levels (Catz and Giacoia, 1972). The degree of protein binding of a drug also influences the amount of unbound pharmacologically active drug in breast milk compared with plasma. Certain drugs such as sulphonamides are bound to milk proteins to a varying extent. Thus the milk to plasma ratio of unbound sulphanilamide is 1.03, whereas that for sulphadimidine is 0.31 and sulphathiazole is 0.25 (Rasmussen, 1971).

Factors Which Determine Adverse Effects in the Infant

Although the quantity of most drugs excreted in breast milk is small, it has been generally held that an important relationship for some drugs is the milk to plasma ratio (M:P ratio) of the unchanged drug or active metabolite, and for others the potential toxicity of the drug, particularly to the infant. For only a few drugs is the concentration in milk equal or greater than in maternal plasma (table VIII). Moreover, even if a drug has a relatively high milk to plasma ratio, it may not necessarily reach important concentrations in the plasma of the breast fed infant; for example, digoxin (Loughnan, 1978), tetracycline (Posner, 1955) and the active 10,11-epoxide metabolite of carbamazepine (Pynnonen et al., 1977). Although propranolol can attain concentrations in breast milk comparable with those in maternal plasma (Anderson and Salter, 1976), use at a dosage of up to 240mg daily was not associated with untoward effects in the breast fed infant (Bauer et al., 1979).

Some drugs may possibly appear in breast milk as pharmacologically inactive metabolites, others may not be absorbed at all by the infant. On the other hand, immaturity of the infant's renal or hepatic function (see section 2.3) might sufficiently delay elimination of some drugs, such that continuous passage from the mother's milk could lead to a clinically significant plasma concentration in the infant. Convulsions occurred in a breast fed newborn infant of a mother treated with large doses of indomethacin (Eeg-Olofsson et al., 1978); a drug known to be slowly eliminated in newborns (see section 2.3.2). Passage into breast milk of minute amounts of some drugs can cause toxicity in susceptible infants. For example, some sulphonamides are excreted in very small amounts in breast milk, but haemolytic anaemia has occurred in a breast fed G6PD-deficient infant following use of a sulphonamide (sulphamethoxy-pyridazine) by the mother (Harley and Robin, 1966). Some drugs which would otherwise be excreted in breast milk in small and clinically unharmful amounts for the breast fed infant, may accumulate if the nursing mother has impaired renal function. Haemolytic anaemia and jaundice has occurred in a breast fed infant of a mother with uraemia who was treated with nalidixic acid for pyelonephritis (Belton and Jones, 1965). The concentration of dihydrostreptomycin in breast milk increases 25-fold in the presence of renal failure (Fujimori and Imai, 1957).

The potential toxicity or contribution to toxicity of pharmacologically active metabolites of some drugs must also be considered (e.g. diazepam, carbamazepine; table VII). Adequate studies in this area do not appear to have been conducted. Toxicity seemed to be due to a pharmacologically active metabolite in one study with the oral anticoagulant ethylbiscoumacetate, which rapidly accumulated in breast milk as a metabolite with haemorrhagic activity unrelated to vitamin K-dependent clotting factor synthesis (Gostof et al., 1952). The concentration of ethylbiscoumacetate in the plasma of nursing mothers was much less than in those mothers not breast feeding, and that of the metabolite considerably less in maternal plasma than in breast milk. Addition of the unchanged drug to maternal milk collected from non-anticoagulated mothers did not result in any bleeding problems. Haemorrhages of the umbilical stump and cephalohaematoma in the infants of the anticoagulated mothers only seemed to occur when there had been previous vascular damage and this may be the reason why other studies with ethylbiscoumacetate have not revealed any bleeding problems in breast fed infants (Illingworth and Finch, 1959). The indane-

Table VIII. Some drugs which can reach concentrations in breast milk comparable or greater than in maternal plasma[1]

Carbamazepine[2]
(and its active metabolite)
Carisoprodol
Cycloserine
Digoxin[2]
Erythromycin
Isoniazid
Lincomycin
Lithium[2]
Meprobamate
Metoprolol
Metronidazole[2]
Propranolol
Radio-iodine
Streptomycin
Tetracyclines (most)[2]
Thiouracil
Trimethoprim

1   Such drugs may not necessarily attain high concentrations or cause adverse effects in the breast fed infant (see text).
2   See also table VII.

dione anticoagulant phenindione seems to accumulate in maternal plasma in breast feeding mothers. Five weeks after commencing breast feeding an infant developed a massive haematoma at the site of repair of an inguinal hernia. The prothrombin time of the mother fell from 50 to 23% of normal when breast feeding was stopped, indicating accumulation of phenindione in the maternal plasma when the mother stopped breast feeding (Eckstein and Jack, 1970).

Although severe bleeding has occurred in some nursing infants of mothers given ethylbiscoumacetate and phenindione, in extensive investigations involving large numbers of infants when prothrombin time of the mothers has been well controlled, no *spontaneous* bleeding problems have occurred with other oral anticoagulants such as dicoumarol, phenprocoumon or warfarin (see chapter XXIII; sect. 3.2.2, 3.2.6). Warfarin is not excreted in breast milk (Orme et al., 1977). However, in prophylaxis of puerperal thrombosis, initial laboratory control with oral anticoagulants is not easy to attain quickly and heparin or dextran 70 are preferred in mothers at risk who contemplate breast feeding (see chapter XV; sect.6). Some consider that oral anticoagulants can be used in other situations, provided that the mother's prothrombin time is well controlled. The prothrombin time of the infant should also be monitored. It would seem desirable however, that oral anticoagulants be temporarily discontinued if a surgical operation is performed on the child.

General Recommendations

In general, most drugs are excreted in breast milk in small and insignificant amounts, but there are rare occasions when it would seem desirable to avoid or temporarily stop breast feeding (Knowles, 1974):

1) When the drug is known to have harmful effects on the breast fed infant (table IX).
2) When the drug is so potent that even small amounts in breast milk could have profound effects on the infant (e.g. cytotoxic drugs, large doses of corticosteroids, radioactive agents).
3) If the mother has impaired renal function or severe liver disease such that a drug mainly eliminated by these routes might accumulate in the plasma or use the breast as an alternative means of excretion.

The value of breast feeding is well founded. Apart from the above exceptions, it is generally desirable to permit breast feeding in women who need treatment with drugs during lactation, but the infant should be continuously observed for possible adverse effects.

3.2 Second Through Twelfth Month

The infant in the first 2 to 3 months of life develops in a number of ways which are evidenced by his tolerance of drugs not handled successfully earlier. Thus, his red cells no longer act as though he had G6PD deficiency (if indeed he does not), and renal and hepatic development progresses giving him an increased drug elimination capacity (see section 2.3). At this age he begins to have more adequate muscle mass for intramuscular injections, and veins large enough for easier intravenous administration of drugs. Administration through all routes is more successful than in the newborn period.

3.3 Ambulatory Childhood (the toddler)

In this age group, behavioural development has its expression in relation to drugs. Oral drug administration is difficult at this age, yet the inquisitive toddler is the very one who by himself ingests drugs and other household chemicals, often bad tasting to adults, in large and often poisonous quantities. He is more frequently exposed to infectious and febrile diseases, and thus meets up with antibacterial drugs, which often may not be effective, and antipyretics and other drugs, which sometimes may not be necessary (see section 4). Diseases appear requiring decisions which pit proper drug therapy against continued growth, e.g. systemic corticosteroids for the nephrotic syndrome, or severe chronic asthma not responsive to other therapy. Weight gain slows normally at this age which may further complicate the issue. It does not require treatment with tonics, and certainly not anabolic steroids, with resultant precocious puberty and risk of premature closure of the epiphyses (Jackson et al., 1973; Zangeneh and Steiner, 1967), or with appetite stimulants such as cyproheptadine, with possible risk of reduced release of growth hormone (see chapter XVI; sect. 13.4).

3.4 Kindergarten and Early School Age

As the child becomes more civilised, he presents fewer anatomical and behavioural problems related to drug administration. As physiological maturity progresses, he eliminates drugs in a manner similar to or even more rapid than in adults (see section 2.3). His exposure to infectious diseases broadens as he enters school. Convulsive seizures may have appeared by this time requiring therapy replete with problems of side effects. This should not however, be a deterrent to use of effective doses (Borofsky et al., 1972; see chapter XXV, sect. 2.3).

3.5 Adolescence

During adolescence, the many problems of puberty carry over into drug use and therapy. Endocrine imbalance, behavioural upsets, increased opportunities for accidents to occur, and exposure to illicit drugs all necessitate reassessment of the adolescent's drug needs and drug taking habits. What was once an accidental ingestion of toxic drugs by the toddler now becomes an attempt at suicide by the teenager. Suicide is one of the top five causes of death in adolescents in the USA. Drug therapy at this paediatric age most closely resembles adult therapy. There are few problems related to administration, to special forms of

Table IX. Some drugs which have been known to cause adverse effects in breast fed infants (after Anderson, 1977; Catz and Giacoia, 1972; Knowles, 1974)

Drugs[1,2]	Effect	Notes[3]
Alcohol, narcotics, tobacco		
Alcohol	Intoxication	Mother ingested 750ml of port wine in 24 hours. Usual amounts have little or no effect on infant
Heroin	Withdrawal symptoms	Symptoms present in 13 of 22 infants in one study; heroin in breast milk may lessen withdrawal symptoms but is not the best way to care for addicted infants
Nicotine	Restlessness, insomnia, vomiting, diarrhoea, tachycardia, circulatory disturbances	Mother smoked 20 cigarettes per day
Anaesthetics		
Chloroform	Deep sleep for 8 hours	Mother given chloroform for 'afterpains'
Analgesics and anti-inflammatory agents		
Salicylates	Rash	High doses (5 g/day) have caused rash. Not a problem with lower doses
Indomethacin	Convulsions	Mother treated with large doses (up to 200mg daily)
Anticoagulants		
Ethylbiscoumacetate	Spontaneous bleeding	Bleeding occurred in those infants with evidence of previous vascular damage (see text, section 3.1.3)
Phenindione	Haematoma formation	Following surgery in the infant (see text, section 3.1.3)
Anticonvulsants and antianxiety drugs		
Diazepam	Lethargy (EEG evidence of sedative medication); weight loss	Mother received 10mg 3 times daily. Variable concentrations in breast milk (see table VII); 10mg daily not likely to cause untoward effects in breast fed infant
Phenobarbitone	Drowsiness, difficult to awaken	Mothers receiving phenobarbitone 100mg hs as hypnotic
Phenytoin	Methaemaglobinaemia	Mother receiving phenytoin and phenobarbitone
Antihypertensive drugs		
Reserpine	Nasal stuffiness and choanal atresia symptoms. Increased tracheobronchial secretions	Effects reported especially with combination of reserpine and diuretics
Antimicrobial agents		
Ampicillin	Diarrhoea and candidosis	
Benzylpenicillin	Apparent hypersensitivity reaction (fever, rash)	
Nalidixic acid	Haemolytic anaemia	Mother had azotaemia which would delay the elimination of the drug (given in a dose of 1g daily)
Sulphafurazole (sulfisoxazole)	May cause kernicterus in neonate	Concentration in breast milk comparable with that in maternal plasma
Sulphamethoxy-pyridazine	Haemolytic anaemia	In an infant with G6PD deficiency (see also chapter VIII, sect. 4.2.2; XXIII, sect. 8.4)
Sulphapyridine (metabolite of sulphasalazine)	Skin rash	Concentration in breast milk comparable with that in maternal plasma

Table IX. (continued)

Drug[1,2]	Effect	Notes[3]
Antipsychotic agents		
Chlorpromazine	Drowsiness, lethargy	Occurred at a chlorpromazine milk concentration of 92ng/ml
Environmental pollutants		
Hexachlorobenzene	Skin rash, diarrhoea, vomiting, death	Ingested by mother as a fungicide contaminated seed wheat
Mercury	Brain damage	Infants breast fed by mothers who ate mercury-contaminated fish
Hormonal steroids		
Oral contraceptives	Decreased weight gain. Gynaecomastia in male infant	Gynaecomastia occurred when dose of oral contraceptive was doubled. Probable that such adverse effects most likely with early high dose preparations (see also chapter XV; sect. 13.7)
Pregnane	Reversible hyperbilirubinaemia	This effect observed in those infants of mothers whose milk contains pregnane 3α-20β-diol instead of pregnane 3α-20α-diol
Laxatives		
Cascara	Diarrhoea	
Danthron	Diarrhoea	Regularly causes increased bowel activity
Senna	Diarrhoea	More likely with larger doses
Miscellaneous drugs		
Bromides	Drowsiness, rash	Non-prescription sedatives and hypnotics
Ergot	Ergotism (vomiting, diarrhoea, weak pulse, unstable blood pressure, convulsions)	In one study 90% of babies affected
Fava beans	Haemolytic anaemia	Occurred in presence of G6PD deficiency (see chapter VIII, sect. 4.2.2; XXIII, sect. 8.4)
Theophylline	Irritability, restlessness	Mother took drug sporadically; symptoms noted on days drug ingested

1   Other drugs which might cause adverse effects include in particular those which have a concentration in breast milk comparable or greater than that in maternal plasma (see table VIII).

2   Drugs which have a lower concentration in breast milk than maternal plasma but whose use in breast feeding mothers should be avoided or monitored closely include lithium; cytotoxic drugs, especially the lipid soluble drugs carmustine (BCNU) and lomustine (CCNU); large doses of corticosteroids; aminoglycoside antibacterial drugs; iodides; and drugs which can cause haemolytic anaemia in the presence of glucose-6-phosphate dehydrogenase deficiency (see chapter VIII, sect. 4.2.2; XXIII, sect. 8.4).

3   The likelihood of an adverse effect in general depends on the amount of drug ingested — i.e. quantity of milk taken and maternal drug concentration, particularly the presence of factors in mother or infant which can lead to abnormally high plasma drug concentrations (see also text section 3.1.3).

medication, or to drug elimination, but drug effects on growth must still be considered whenever a therapeutic measure is contemplated. Tetracyclines, avoided at all previous ages, may now be indicated. Attempts to control acne with self-administered excessive doses of vitamin A may present as pseudotumour cerebri.

4. Principles of Prescribing Drugs for Infants and Children

Because of the problems with drug administration in infants and young children and the many problems which can occur with therapy, as well as the need for parents to obtain an understanding of the nature of a number of common childhood illnesses and the reasons for medication, it is important to define certain basic principles of prescribing for this age group (see also table X).

1) *Is drug therapy required?*

Drug treatment is not always required, but parental pressure or expectation in paediatric practice is often hard to resist. Some examples serve to illustrate the therapeutic decisions required. Acute febrile illnesses in childhood are a concern of mothers, yet they do not necessarily require treatment, apart from removal of excessive clothing and tepid sponging. Although febrile convulsions are a concern, fever *per se* is not usually of any significant danger to the child. Antipyretic drugs are therefore not always necessary (Done, 1972). Antibacterial drugs also may not be needed at all, as in many respiratory illnesses of childhood (see section 5.1.4) and most cases of acute gastroenteritis (see section 5.1.6). An antibacterial drug should not, of course, be withheld when it is necessary, but if no benefit is possible, even minor risks should be avoided. Rational use of stimulant drugs is of benefit in hyperkinetic children (see chapter XXVI; sect. 10.1), but parental demands for something to 'quieten down' a typically energetic child should be resisted. The hyperkinetic child syndrome must not be diagnosed casually.

2) *If drug therapy is required, which drug is appropriate?*

Choice of an antibacterial drug should be largely guided by the causative organism and its demonstrated sensitivity to a drug appropriate for the patient and the disease (see chapter XXVII). Some antibacterial agents are unsuitable in children. The risk of toxicity from chloramphenicol is too great and it should generally only be considered in meningitis, in particular that due to *Haemophilus influenzae* (see chapter XXV; sect. 13), and typhoid fever (see chapter XXVII; sect. 5.4.1). Sulphonamides, including co-trimoxazole (trimethoprim-sulphamethoxazole), should always be avoided in the newborn because of the risk of kernicterus (see section 2.2.2). Tetracyclines should not be used in infancy and early childhood because of unacceptable problems of teeth damage and staining (see chapter XIII; sect. 13.3). There are very few, if any indications where tetracyclines are preferred choices in paediatric practice. Sometimes, side effects have to be accepted; for example, gingival hyperplasia in epileptic children treated with phenytoin. Because of the possibility of overenthusiastic use, some clinicians consider the risk of toxicity of aspirin to be too great in infants and young children (see section 5.2), and also it is not available in liquid form as is paracetamol (acetaminophen). Topical corticosteroids are unsuitable for routine use in napkin rash. Corticosteroids do not attack the cause of the eruption (see section 5.7) and repeated application of strong steroids can readily lead to systemic absorption with risk of growth retardation (Feiwel, 1969). There are few indications for topical antibiotics for use on the skin in children. Gentle thorough cleansing and protection of the area until healing occurs, is usually adequate for minor wounds and burns. In pyodermas such as impetigo, systemic antibiotics are preferable in all but localised cases in which removal of crusts and gentle washing of infected areas with mild soap or a mild saline solution is generally adequate. Antibiotics when used topically are those generally not used systemically; e.g. neomycin, bacitracin (see chapter XIV; sect. 2.1.1).

3) *Which route of administration and preparation?*

The oral route is preferable whenever possible, except in cases of proven or possible critical illness (e.g. meningitis, osteomyelitis). There is always the problem of whether the child takes the medication regularly or completes the course of therapy (see below). Preparations which can be given in single or twice-daily dose regimens should be used whenever possible as compliance is made easier, particularly for children at school. When com-

Table X. Summary of principles of drug prescribing in infants and children

1. *Is drug therapy required?*
   a) Acute febrile illnesses do not always require treatment with antipyretic drugs; other measures are safer (see section 5.2)
   b) Antibacterial drugs should not be withheld when necessary, but they are not indicated, for example, in every respiratory infection (see section 5.1.1, 5.1.4)

2. *Choice of preparation and dosage form*
   a) Should a particular drug be avoided in a particular age group? — e.g. increased risk of side effects (sulphonamides in neonates; aspirin in young children)
   b) Is a particular drug unsuitable for routine use in infants and children? — e.g. tetracyclines and tooth staining; chloramphenicol and blood dyscrasias
   c) Life saving drugs should not be withheld because of fear of side effects — e.g. penicillin in streptococcal disease
   d) Which preparation? — consider dosage form and route of administration (palatability, convenience and ease of administration, compliance) and cost

3. *Dose and dosage regimen*
   a) In neonates, use drugs and doses well studied in that age group; in general use smaller doses than estimates on body size alone — altered pharmacokinetic handling
   b) The average dose is not necessarily the correct dose — dosage should be individualised for the drug, patient and disease. Monitoring, clinical and by plasma levels, is ideal
   c) Prescribe the most convenient dose regimen — not a 4 times daily schedule if less frequent administration is feasible

4. *Medication instruction*
   a) Teach the parent and older child to understand his disease and drugs; especially the importance of regular administration (long term therapy) and of the need to complete the prescribed course (short term therapy)
   b) Instruct the parent and child in the administration of the drug or proper use of a drug delivery system

pliance cannot be guaranteed (e.g. prevention of rheumatic fever recurrence), parenteral administration is more appropriate. Parenteral therapy is mandatory in very sick children (e.g. meningitis) and is also indicated in those who are vomiting. To avoid injury to the sciatic nerve, intramuscular injections should not be given in the gluteal region in infants (see section 3.1.1). Few children enjoy receiving medication as a suppository; moreover, absorption is erratic, with consequent inadequate dosage or toxicity.

For oral administration, liquid preparations are most suitable for children under 5 years. Tablets can be hard to crush and may be difficult to divide except when scored. Capsules are often easier to use as the emptied contents can be more readily disguised in some jam or honey. The decision on choice of a particular oral preparation is based on factors such as palatability, convenience of administration (e.g. availability of liquid dosage form, feasibility of single or twice daily administration), cost, stability and toxicity. If tablets of drugs which are highly toxic on overdosage are prescribed (e.g. aspirin, paracetamol; imipramine, amitriptyline for enuresis; oral iron) they should be ordered and dispensed in strip foil packing or an appropriate safety closure container.

The inhaler is an important means of drug delivery in asthma, but for the drug to be effective, the device must be properly used. Very young children may find the inhaler difficult to manage, despite proper education of the parent. A nebuliser and face mask can be used for intensive drug therapy regimens involving inhaled drugs, as in cystic fibrosis or an acute attack of severe asthma, and can be adapted for use even in small infants.

The possibility of percutaneous absorption of topically applied drugs should always be considered, especially in premature infants and when the skin is burnt or excoriated or when medication is repeatedly applied to flexural areas (see section 2.1).

4) *Estimation of drug dosage*

Dosage is the heart of drug therapy. Many factors, including tissue responsiveness or pharmacokinetic handling of a drug contribute to correct dosage in an individual patient (see chapter I). Yet, children's dosages have been for the most part poorly derived as fractions of average adult doses.

Many formulae have been devised for calculating from the adult dose, the dose for a child (e.g. Young's, Clark's and Dilling's rules, percentage method, etc). However, the average adult dose can hardly be an accurate guide, since dosages given to adults should be individualised because of the variables involved, but as discussed in section 2 the variables become even more important in children, particularly in premature and newborn infants.

Doses based on age alone are not sufficiently accurate to compensate for the great variability of weights, particularly that related to fat in the paediatric age groups. Dosage based on weight is better but not ideal. With most drugs, adults and older children receive excessive dosage if satisfactory infant doses in mg/kg are given. Conversely, infants receive an underdosage if they are given mg/kg doses satisfactory for adults and large children. The surface area method of calculating drug doses gives a more consistent dose throughout all age groups, but is not suitable for the premature and the newly born full term infant. It requires measurement of height and weight and derivation from a nomogram or equivalent chart (Shirkey, 1965).

Whichever method is used depends on personal beliefs and experience. In any case, such dosage rules and guides as available (table XI) are only rough estimates of doses, i.e. average doses, and not necessarily correct for an individual child with a particular disease. For example, the dose of an antibacterial agent should be appropriate for the disease (see section 5.1). For urinary infections, the dose of penicillins and aminoglycosides should be reduced from those used in other infections (table XI), because these drugs are concentrated in the urine. An adequate dose of an anticonvulsant drug in epilepsy means good control of seizures with minimum side effects, but for patients with a severe seizure process, higher doses may have to be used at the expense of some adverse effects (see chapter XXV; sect. 2.3). In general, drug underdosage in children is much more common than overdosage, particularly in the treatment of epilepsy.

There are no rules that are adequate to guarantee safety or adequacy of dosage in the newborn infant, nor at any age does any method of calculating drug dosage anticipate all variables, particularly those due to individual differences in response to drugs. The correct dose for all ages of man, which is *enough but not too much,* must be determined and adjusted for each particular patient by the clinician.

5) *Duration of treatment*

The nature of the disease dictates the duration of treatment. This may be standardised in some instances; for example, a lifetime of thyroxine in the athyroid child, or 9 months or less of antituberculosis therapy for tuberculosis (see chapter XX; sect. 8.3). There may be a measurable end point, such as with iron therapy. In other situations, no fixed time can be set, as the course of the condition is subject to individual variation; as for example in asthma.

Some important childhood diseases require a certain minimum period of therapy — for example, acute otitis media, streptococcal pharyngitis and urinary tract infections. Medication is often discontinued when the child appears better and in many other cases, for a variety of reasons (see below), the full course of prescribed doses of treatment is not completed. Doctors must give easily remembered information and clear explanation about the illness and of the importance of completing treatment and taking medication exactly as prescribed. Provision of printed material is helpful.

6) *Compliance, medication instructions and education about the disease*

Non-compliance with medication instructions can result in inadequate therapy for necessary indications and is a particular problem in acute streptococcal tonsillitis or otitis media in children (Mohler et al., 1955; Mattar et al., 1975). It can occur at any point in the sequence of medication — from failure to have the prescription made up, parents forgetting to offer the drug, difficulty in getting the child to take the medication, omission of doses, incorrect dose or route, misunderstanding instructions, or discontinuing therapy or failing to complete the recommended course of therapy (because the child appeared better, occurrence of side effects, a broken or spilled bottle of liquid medication, insufficient quantity dispensed, and so on).

Sometimes errors result because parents feel that more medication will be more effective, or conversely less will be better because the medicine is 'too strong' or the dosage excessive (they may sometimes be right!). The parent's perception of the severity of the disease may have a significant influence on her cooperation in administering the

Table XI. Usual doses for older infants and children of some commonly used drugs (normal renal and hepatic function)

Drug	Dosage[1]	Notes[2]
Mild analgesics/antipyretics		
Aspirin	65mg/kg/24h divided into 4-6 doses (oral)	Avoid overdosage, particularly in infants and young children; avoid dehydration (see section 5.2)
Paracetamol (acetaminophen)	Under 1 yr: 60mg; 1 to 3 yr: 60-120mg; 3 to 6 yr: 120mg; 6 to 12 yr: 240mg. Single dose repeated every 4 to 6h (oral)	Accidental poisoning may cause hepatic damage (see section 5.2)
Narcotic analgesics		
Morphine	0.1-0.2mg/kg/dose SC (maximum 15mg)	Not usually given preoperatively to children under 1 yr of age
Pethidine (meperidine)	6mg/kg/24h (max. 100mg/dose) divided into 6 doses (oral, IM, SC)	
Anthelmintics (see also chapter XIX; table VII)		
Pyrantel pamoate	11mg/kg single dose (oral). Max. 1g	
Piperazine (as salts)	*Oxyuriasis:* < 7kg: 250mg; 7 to 14kg: 500mg; 14 to 27kg: 1g; > 27kg: 2g or 1g/m² — once daily for 7 consecutive days (oral) *Ascariasis:* < 14kg: 1g; 14 to 23kg: 2g; 23-45kg: 3g; > 45kg: 3.5g or 2g/m² — once daily for 2 consecutive days (oral)	Contraindicated in patients with predisposition to grand or petit mal epilepsy
Antibacterial agents (see also sect. 5.1; table V for doses in infants and neonates)		
Amikacin	15mg/kg daily divided into 2 or 3 doses (IM)	Monitor serum concentrations in renal impairment
Amoxycillin	20mg/kg daily divided into 3 doses (oral) *Severe infections and lower respiratory infections:* 40mg/kg daily divided into 3 doses (oral)	Oral absorption better than ampicillin
Ampicillin	*Moderately severe infections:* 50-100mg/kg daily divided into 3 or 4 doses (oral; IM; IV) *Severe infections:* 200mg/kg daily divided into 4 doses (IV, IM) *Very severe infections:* 400mg/kg daily (IV, IM)	Use parenteral solutions within 1h of reconstitution. Give orally 0.5h ac or 2h pc.
Carbenicillin	*Urinary tract infections — Pseudomonas, Proteus, Esch. coli,* 100-250mg/kg daily in divided doses every 4-6h (IM or IV) *Severe systemic infections, respiratory and soft tissue infections — Pseudomonas;* 400-600mg/kg daily IV in divided doses or by drip infusion; *Proteus and Esch. coli;* 250-400mg/kg daily IV continuous or in divided doses	Modify dose in impaired renal function (see appendix E)
Cephalexin	*Mild to moderate infections:* 25-50mg/kg daily divided into 4 doses (oral) *Severe infections:* 50-100mg/kg daily divided into 4 doses (oral)	
Cephaloridine	*Mild to moderately severe infections:* 30-50mg/kg/day (max. 4g daily) divided into 3 doses (IM, IV) *Severe infections:* 100mg/kg daily divided into 4 doses (IM, IV)	Contraindicated in azotaemia. Store freshly made solution not more than 96h

Table XI. (continued)

Drug	Dosage[1]	Notes[2]
Antibacterial agents (continued)		
Cephalothin	80-160mg/kg/day divided into 4 doses (IM or IV) in normal renal function	Store solution in refrigerator not more than 48h
Chloramphenicol	50mg/kg daily divided into 4 doses. Severe infections may require 100mg/kg (see table V for neonates). Oral or IV	To be used only for treatment of the following: Acute infections caused by *S. typhi*, serious infections caused by susceptible strains of *Salmonella* spp, initial use in infections suspected to be due to and use in those proven due to *H. influenzae* resistant to ampicillin; other susceptible organisms that have been shown to be resistant to all other appropriate antimicrobial agents
Co-trimoxazole (trimethoprim + sulphamethoxazole)	8mg/kg daily trimethoprim, 40mg/kg daily sulphamethoxazole. Divide into 2 doses (oral); 0.5 to 5y: Half above; 6w to 5m: Quarter above	Effective against *Pneumocystis carinii* (1.5 times dose). See sulphadiazine. Avoid use in severely impaired renal function and in megaloblastic anaemia
Dicloxacillin	*Mild to moderate infections:* 12.5mg/kg/day divided into 4 doses (oral) *Severe infections:* 25mg/kg/day divided into 4 doses	
Erythromycin	*Oral:* 30-50mg/kg daily divided into 4-6 doses *Parenteral:* 10-20mg/kg daily divided into 4 doses (continuous IV infusion). Double dose for very severe infections	Avoid intramuscular injection because of pain and necrosis. Care required in liver disease (especially estolate)
Gentamcin	6 to 7.5mg/kg daily divided into 3 doses (IM, IV)	Monitor serum concentrations in renal impairment
Kanamycin	15 to 30mg/kg daily divided into 3 doses (IM, very slow IV)	Monitor serum concentrations in renal impairment
Methicillin	100 to 200mg/kg daily divided into 4 doses (IM)	
Penicillin G (benzylpenicillin)	25,000-50,000 units/kg daily (IM or IV) *Severe infections:* 200,000-400,000u/kg/day (IV)	
Penicillin V	15-30mg/kg daily divided into 4 doses (oral)	Give 0.5h ac or 2h pc
Sulphadiazine (or combinations of sulphonamides)	*Oral* (over age 2 months): Initial — 75mg/kg single dose; maintenance — 150mg/kg daily divided into 4-6 doses (maximum 6g/24h) *Parenteral* (over age 2 months): Initial — 50mg/kg single dose; maintenance — 100mg/kg daily divided into 3 doses (SC) or 4 doses (IV)	Use cautiously in patients with impaired renal or hepatic function and in those with G6PD deficiency. Adequate fluid intake is required to prevent crystalluria. Avoid in infants under 2 months, breast feeding mothers
Sulphafurazole (sulfisoxazole)	*Initial:* 75mg/kg single dose (oral) *Maintenance:* 150mg/kg daily divided into 4 to 6 doses	As above
Sulphamethoxazole	*Initial:* 60mg/kg (max 2g) single oral dose *Maintenance:* 60mg/kg daily divided into 2 doses	As above

Table XI. (continued)

Drug	Dosage[1]	Notes[2]
Antibacterial agents (continued)		
Tetracycline (hydrochloride)	*Oral:* 25-50mg/kg daily divided into 4 doses 1h pc *Parenteral:* 10-25mg/kg daily divided into 2-3 doses IM (maximum 250mg per injection); 10-15mg/kg daily divided into 2 doses IV	Avoid tetracycline and its analogues during period of tooth development, unless alternative agents have been shown to be ineffective *in vitro.* Avoid in renal impairment and neonates
Ticarcillin	*Urinary tract infections:* Complicated, 150 to 200mg/kg daily IV divided into 4 to 6 doses. Uncomplicated, 50 to 100mg/kg daily IM or IV divided into 3 or 4 doses. *Severe infections, respiratory, skin and soft tissue infections:* 200 to 300mg/kg daily IV divided into 4 to 6 doses	Modify dose in impaired renal function (see appendix E)
Tobramycin	3 to 5mg/kg daily divided into 3 doses (IM)	Monitor serum concentrations in impaired renal function
Antidepressants/antipsychotics		
Imipramine	*Enuresis:* 6yr and older — initially, 25mg 1h before bedtime. If necessary increase to 50mg in children under 12yr and to 75mg in those over 12yr. In early night bedwetters divide into 2 doses, afternoon and bedtime (oral)	Avoid toxic dosage (disturbances of cardiac rhythm and conduction)
Chlorpromazine	2mg/kg daily divided into 4 to 6 doses (oral)	Extrapyramidal symptoms common on overdosage
Antidiarrhoeal drugs		
Diphenoxylate with atropine	2 to 5yr: 6mg/24h divided into 3 doses (oral); 5 to 8yr: 8mg/24h divided into 4 doses; 8 to 12yr: 10mg/24h divided into 5 doses	Contraindicated in children under 2yr
Loperamide	Over 8yr: 2mg, then adjusted as needed. Max. 8 to 12mg daily as single or divided doses. Under 8yr: 0.08mg/kg daily	
Sulphasalazine (salicylazosulpha-pyridine)	*Initial:* 75-150mg/kg daily divided into 4, 6 or 8 doses (oral). Severe colitis: 37.5-150mg/kg daily in 3, 4 or 6 doses *Maintenance:* 40mg/kg daily divided into 4 doses	An orange-yellow colour develops in alkaline urine; similar discolouration of skin has also been reported

Table XI. (continued)

Drug	Dosage[1]	Notes[2]
Antiemetics		
Cyclizine	3mg/kg daily divided into 3 doses (oral, IM). Rectal dose: double oral or IM dose	
Prochlorperazine	*Oral:* 1 to 5yr: 5mg daily in 2 equal doses; 6 to 12yr: 10-15mg daily in 2 or 3 equal doses *IM:* 0.2mg/kg daily in 2 or 3 doses *Rectal:* (suppository): 1 to 2yr: 7.5mg daily (maximum); 2 to 5yr: 10mg daily (maximum); 5 to 12yr: 15mg daily (maximum)	Not recommended in children weighing less than 10kg. Extrapyramidal symptoms common on overdosage
Promethazine	0.25-0.5mg/kg every 4-6h (oral, rectal, IM)	Extrapyramidal symptoms common on overdosage
Antifungal drugs		
Amphotericin B	Test dose: 0.1mg/kg/24h given intravenously over period of 6h. Increase to 0.25mg/kg initially, and as tolerance permits, to a maintenance dose of 1mg/kg daily	Use primarily for treatment of patients with progressive and life threatening fungal infections. Total daily dose must not exceed 1.5mg/kg
Griseofulvin (fine particle)	10mg/kg daily divided into 2-4 doses (oral)	
Nystatin	*Oral moniliasis:* 100,000u 4 times daily (oral drops)	
Antihistamines		
Chlorpheniramine	0.35mg/kg daily divided into 4 doses (oral, SC); 0.2mg/kg daily as single dose (prolonged action, oral)	
Dextrochlorpheniramine	0.15mg/kg daily divided into 4 doses (oral); 0.1mg/kg daily as single dose (prolonged action, oral)	
Promethazine	0.5mg/kg at night and 0.125mg/kg in the morning or as required (oral, rectal, IM)	Extrapyramidal symptoms on overdosage
Trimeprazine	Under 2yr: 3.75mg daily (maximum); 3 to 12yr: 7.5mg daily (maximum). Divided into 3 doses (oral)	
Antineoplastic drugs (see chapter XXIV; table VI)		
Antituberculosis drugs		
p-Aminosalicylic acid (PAS)	300mg/kg daily divided into 3 doses (oral) after meals	Do not use solutions older than 24h or if darker than when prepared
Ethambutol	15mg/kg (new cases); 25mg/kg for 2 months then 15mg/kg (retreatment) as single oral dose daily (children over 13yr)	Use with caution in patients with reduced visual acuity or impaired renal function
Isoniazid	*Active tuberculosis:* 10-30mg/kg daily divided into 2 or 3 doses (oral, IM). Max. 300-500mg in 24h *Prevention:* 10mg/kg daily, single or divided into 2 doses (oral, IM). Max. 300mg in 24h	Contraindication in patients who develop drug induced hepatitis
Rifampicin (rifampin)	10-20mg/kg (not exceeding 600mg in 24h) as a single daily dose (children over 5yr age)	Use with caution in the presence of liver disease. Colours urine, faeces, tears etc. red-orange
Streptomycin	20mg/kg daily as a single dose (IM)	Use with caution in impaired renal function

Table XI. (continued)

Drug	Dosage[1]	Notes[2]
Antitussives		
Pholcodine	2 to 6yr: 2mg; 6 to 9yr: 2-4mg; 9 to 12yr: 4mg per dose 3 or 4 times daily	
Dextromethorphan	1mg/kg daily divided into 3-4 doses (oral)	Do not mix in same bottle with penicillins, tetracyclines, salicylates, sodium phenobarbitone, iodides
Bronchodilators (see chapter XX; sect. 2.3.1)		
Cardiac glycosides (see also sect. 2.3.2)		
Digoxin	*Infants 2w — 2yr:* Digitalising dose — 0.06-0.08mg/kg (oral); 0.04-0.06mg/kg (IV) Maintenance dose — 1/5 to 1/3 of digitalising dose (oral) daily *Children over 2yr:* digitalising dose — 0.04-0.06mg/kg (oral); 0.02-0.04mg/kg (IV) Maintenance dose — 1/5 to 1/3 of digitalising dose (oral) daily *Premature and full term infants or reduced renal function or myocarditis:* Digitalising dose — 0.02-0.03mg/kg (oral, IV) Maintenance dose — 1/10 to 1/5 digitalising dose daily. Divide total digitalising dose into 3, 4 portions with 6h or more between doses	
Central stimulants (see also chapter XXVI; sect. 10.1)		
Dextroamphetamine	*Minimal brain dysfunction:* Age 3 to 5yr — initial, 2.5mg/24h (oral) increase daily dose in increments of 2.5mg weekly to obtain optimum response (2.5-40mg) Age 6yr and over: initial 5mg weekly (2.5-40mg) *Narcolepsy:* Age 6 to 12yr — initial 5mg/24 h (oral), increase daily dose by 5mg at weekly intervals to optimum response (5-60mg); 12yr and over: double above dose	Not recommended for use in children under 3yr
Methylphenidate	*Minimal brain dysfunction:* 6yr and older — 5mg before breakfast and lunch, increments 5-10mg weekly [max. 60mg/24h (oral)]	Contraindicated in marked anxiety, tension and agitation. Should not be used in children under 6yr
Corticosteroids		
Cortisone acetate	*Physiological replacement dose:* 0.7mg/kg daily divided into 3 doses (oral). Use 1/3-1/2 of oral dose intramuscularly once daily or a dose equal to the oral dose every third day. *Adrenocortical virilism:* 1.75mg/kg daily divided into 3 to 4 doses (oral). IM: give same as oral dose every third day or 1/3-1/2 the oral dose once daily *Pharmacological dose* varies according to the disease: 2.5 to 10mg/kg daily divided into 3 or 4 doses (oral). IM: 1/3-1/2 oral dose once or twice daily	

Table XI. (continued)

Drug	Dosage[1]	Notes[2]
Corticosteroids (continued)		
Hydrocortisone	4/5 cortisone dosage	
Prednisolone	*General:* 1/5 cortisone dosage (oral, IM, IV)	
Prednisone	*Nephrosis* (initial dose/24h): 18m to 4yr: 30-40mg; 4 to 10yr: 60mg; 11yr and over: 80mg *Rheumatic carditis, leukaemia, tumours:* 2mg/kg daily for 2-3 weeks, 1.5mg/kg daily for 4-6 weeks divided into 4 oral doses	
Haematinics		
Iron requirements (elemental iron)	*Prophylaxis:* 1-2mg/kg daily (single or divided oral doses) *Treatment:* 6mg/kg daily divided into 3 doses (oral)	
Laxatives		
Bisacodyl	0.3mg/kg (oral) swallowed whole	Tablets should be swallowed whole and not chewed or crushed and should not be taken within 1h of antacids or milk
Senna	Powder: 40mg/kg per dose (oral) Syrup: 0.15ml/kg per dose	
Sedatives and hypnotics (see also antihistamines)		
Amylobarbitone	*Sedation:* 2mg/kg daily divided into 4 doses (oral, rectal)	
Chloral hydrate	*Hypnotic dose:* 50mg/kg daily (maximum 1g per dose) (oral, rectal) *Sedative dose:* half hypnotic dose divided into 3 or 4 doses daily (oral)	
Diazepam	0.12-0.8mg/kg daily divided into 3 or 4 doses (oral)	
Vitamins		
Vitamin D_2 (calciferol)	*Prophylactic:* 400-1,000u daily (all ages) *Therapeutic:* 2,000-4,000u daily. Rarely 20,000u-1 mega u daily in resistant cases *Hypoparathyroidism:* 50,000-200,000 u/d	Avoid overdosage (hypercalcaemia)
Vitamin K Phytomenadione (vit K_1)	*Haemorrhagic disease of newborn* Prophylaxis — 1mg single dose (IV, IM, SC) Treatment — 5 to 10mg single dose (IV, IM, SC) *Other prothrombin deficiencies* Older infants and children: 5-10mg single dose (oral). Aqueous (IV, IM, SC); Infants: 2mg single dose (oral)	Overdose may cause kernicterus in premature infants. Avoid rapid intravenous injection ($\frac{1}{2}$ 3mg/m² or total 5mg)
Menaphthone (menadione)	*Haemorrhagic disease of newborn:* 1mg single dose (IM)	Overdose may cause kernicterus in premature infants

1   Dosage listed is not specifically intended for newborn premature and term infants unless so indicated. All doses are average doses and are approximate. Variability of response may require alteration of dosage (see section 2). Doses based on different criteria (body weight, surface area etc) frequently do not correspond. Specific dosage described in an individual chapter or section in this chapter should take precedence for the diseases discussed.

2   See also relevant discussion in this and other chapters.

complete course as prescribed (Charney et al., 1967). Sociocultural beliefs in particular can have a significant influence on how parents perceive disease, its aetiology and treatment.

Unfortunately there are no practical ways of determining or predicting who will be a non-complier. Clinicians and nurses may be the worst for their own children. The risk of non-compliance is a function of many variable factors, including the nature and severity of the disease and attitudes of mothers (Wilson, 1973). However, compliance can be improved and medication errors reduced by limiting the number of medications on a prescription, providing printed instructions with drugs such as corticosteroids (see section 5.5), and by encouraging parents to call when there is difficulty in administering the medication because of some side effect (e.g. diarrhoea or vomiting) or refusal by the child to take the medication. Education of the parents about the nature of the illness and reasons for the medication (Becker et al., 1972; Mattar et al., 1975), and advising them of the difficulty they may have in completing the course or getting the child to take the medication indefinitely, but of the importance of doing so, should be of major help. The character and quality of the doctor-patient relationship are clearly of prime importance in gaining compliance with medication instructions (Elling et al., 1960; Korsch et al., 1968). The child's sweet tooth and the parent's fear of a serious complication may need to be invoked. If compliance is likely to be unreliable or proper supervision cannot be guaranteed, parenteral therapy is preferable (e.g. prevention of rheumatic fever recurrence). Children may not necessarily be greater offenders than adults in not complying with medication requirements and in comparison with some adult situations (e.g. maintenance therapy of schizophrenia and tuberculosis) may be better than their elders (Haggerty and Roghmann, 1972; Wilson, 1973). However, for some common childhood diseases it is essential to complete the minimum short course of treatment as prescribed.

The clinician can also contribute to medication errors and non-compliance by prescribing an unmeasurable dose (e.g. fractions of a spoonful) and dose interval (4 times daily when less may be feasible), by failing to write a legible prescription or to give clear and adequate instructions to the parent about administration of the drug or instruction in the proper use of a drug delivery system (e.g. asthma inhaler). The absorption of many antibacterial drugs is affected by food and the parent should be instructed to give these drugs about 30 minutes to an hour before meals (see chapter VI; table IV). On the other hand, drugs such as iron are better tolerated if given with meals. Parents should be advised that forcing of oral medication can cause aspiration. Parents should also always be instructed on how to measure liquid doses and of the need to use standard metric measuring devices or spoons and not household teaspoons, which may vary from 2.5 to 9ml or more (Mattar et al., 1975). Toxicity can arise from the failure to shake the bottle of a suspension such as phenytoin — initial doses being dilute and inadequate and later doses too concentrated. The doctor must not necessarily expect the chemist to correctly label medication. Unreliability of drug administration, thought to be worst in outpatients, exists as well for hospitalised patients (Wilson and Wilkinson, 1974).

Effective drug treatment involves much more than the writing of a prescription. The clinician, parent and child must cooperate to comply with the intentions and aim of therapy. In many childhood diseases education of the parent and older child about the nature of the disease is just as important as the drug treatment — for example, epilepsy (see section 5.3).

5. Drug Treatment in Infants and Children

The principles which pertain to use of drugs in paediatric practice can be illustrated by a discussion of treatment of some common childhood conditions. Further discussion on some of these and other conditions is given in other chapters. Clinicians caring for children must be most familiar with the drugs they frequently use. (They will use fewer drugs and gain valuable experience undiluted by the spreading of experience to the use of many drugs). Special knowledge is required prior to using drugs infrequently prescribed.

5.1 Infections

Infectious diseases are the most common conditions encountered in the early years of life. Viral infection occurs frequently at all ages but accompanying illness is more common in young children than in older patients. However, the clinical course is generally self limited and of short duration.

Some viral diseases in childhood may however, be associated with fatal complications or sequelae. The prevention and symptomatic management of specific viral diseases is discussed in chapter XXVIII. This discussion concerns itself with general treatment of infections of childhood and the indications for use of antibacterial drugs (for reviews, see Eichenwald and McCracken, 1978; McCracken and Eichenwald, 1978; Spratt et al., 1978).

5.1.1 General Principles of Use of Antibacterial Drugs in Paediatric Practice

Precise diagnosis is the basis of rational therapy. Some viral diseases (e.g. herpetic stomatitis) and some bacterial diseases (e.g. scarlet fever) are diagnosed clinically — many require culture.

In prescribing antibacterial drugs for any patient, the clinician should always familiarise himself with factors peculiar to the causative organism and those unique to the host (see chapter XXVII). This is of especial importance in paediatric practice. In general, problems with antibacterial therapy are inversely related to the size and age of the child and the risk of infection is greatest in the newborn.

1) *Is antibacterial therapy required?* An antibacterial drug should always be given when it is necessary; not only for those conditions diagnosed but also for those suspected (e.g. septicaemia in the newborn), but should not be prescribed automatically for fever alone for there is no antibacterial agent which can be given without some risk. Moreover, in some conditions antibacterial drugs may not be of any benefit. Acute respiratory infections are the most common clinical problems facing the primary care practitioner in the paediatric age group. The overwhelming evidence is that most of these infections are due to viruses, not bacteria, and in the absence of effective antiviral agents or vaccines against the common respiratory viruses, treatment must be symptomatic rather than 'curative' (see chapter XXVIII; sect. 3.2). Parents are becoming more sophisticated medically and more readily convinced that antibacterial drugs are not always necessary for every respiratory infection or febrile illness. Antibacterial drugs are clearly indicated in acute otitis media and most pneumonias, but in common croup and acute bronchiolitis (both viral illnesses) and acute bronchitis, supportive treatment, clearing the airway, postural coughing, adequate hydration and oxygen rather than antibacterials are indicated initially and are more important. If a child has a sore throat it is wise to take a throat culture, but there is generally no need to immediately prescribe an antibacterial drug unless group A β-haemolytic streptococci are grown or strongly suspected (see chapter XI; sect. 2.7). On the other hand, antibacterial drugs can be commenced on clinical grounds in other situations and ceased with negative culture. The characteristic epiglottitis of *Haemophilus influenzae* 'croup' is diagnosed by the symptoms; airway control and then antibacterial drugs are necessary (see section 5.1.4).

The majority of cases of gastroenteritis in children are due to unknown causes or viral infection and treatment is directed at replacement of fluid loss and correction of acid-base and electrolyte balance. Antibacterial drugs are used when there is evidence of systemic spread and only indicated routinely in acute bacillary dysentery, in a minority of cases of *Salmonella* enteritis (young infants and in children in whom complications are likely) and although of no proven benefit are tradionally used in the few cases of bacterial diarrhoea due to *Escherichia coli* (see further in section 5.1.6).

2) *Factors relating to the causative organism:* Before prescribing an antibacterial drug, a diagnosis should be formed which is strongly suggestive of the presence of a given bacterial infection. To a large extent *initiation* of treatment is based on intelligent clinical or bacteriological guesswork (see chapter XXVII; sect. 3). In some acute infections, such as those of the upper respiratory tract, if good evidence is available on the most likely causative organism the appropriate agent for initial therapy can be selected with confidence (see chapter XI; sect. 1.1, 2). In life threatening infections such as meningitis, suspected septicaemia or severe penumonia, a bacteriological diagnosis is mandatory. But therapy must be started immediately with the most likely active agent(s). In neonatal infections in particular it is rare for the type and antibacterial sensitivities of the infecting organism to be known when treatment is started. The current patterns of bacterial infection, antibacterial sensitivities and the best agents for treatment can be found in the literature, but these patterns (see below; appendix D) can change and may vary from area to area. 'Antibiograms' in hospitals may be most helpful for the local situation.

Every major neonatal care centre has records of the current bacteriological flora of its nursery, and patterns of resistance and antibacterial sensitivities. It is therefore a simple matter for each centre to use these data to devise its own regimen for initial antibacterial therapy. Such data and regimens should also be made available for the benefit of practitioners in the surrounding areas who have to initiate treatment. The outcome of treatment usually depends on the first 24 hours of therapy, but when the organisms have been cultured and the sensitivities known, the antibacterial therapy can then be modified if necessary on the basis of this new information and patient response. Drugs which are not needed can be stopped and needed ones, if any, added to the regimen.

Multiple drug resistance is more commonly met in the treatment of acute bacterial gastrointestinal infections than elsewhere, but only a minority of instances of acute gastroenteritis are of primary bacterial aetiology (see section 5.1.6). Other resistance of significance is mentioned under the individual antibacterial agents in table XII.

3) *Factors relating to the patient:* Among the important host factors are an understanding of the pharmacology of the agents as related to the particular age of the child being treated. Factors such as absorption, distribution, metabolism, excretion, and overall effectiveness of a drug are of greatest importance (see section 2; table XII).

Also of fundamental significance is an understanding of how antibacterial drugs change the normal microbial flora and the importance of such change related to the particular infant or child. The normal flora of the infant's throat, gut and skin have a protective function that is often overlooked. When antibacterial drugs are used that inhibit the growth or kill *Streptococcus viridans, Neisseria* and other normal flora in his throat, and some of the *Escherichia coli* and anaerobes in his gut, the child is deprived of some of his natural protection. Such change in flora is greatest with broad spectrum agents and of most importance in the newborn. A sensible rule is to always use the antibacterial drug with the narrowest spectrum that is effective against the causative organism. Use a rifle, not a shotgun!

4) *Dosage of antibacterial drugs:* In general, the problems in determining an effective and safe dose are inversely related to the size and age of the child (section 2; table II, IV). This is well illustrated by chloramphenicol where the same dose to prematures within the first week of life which would produce toxic or fatal plasma concentrations, at 2 weeks of age would be ineffective (see section 3.1.2). Dosage also needs to be appropriate for the disease. For example the dosage of an antibacterial agent in an infant with meningitis is greater than that for other severe infections. Special considerations apply to tailoring of dosage to attain adequate CSF concentrations in meningitis (see section 5.1.2). For urinary infections, the dose of penicillins and aminoglycosides should be reduced from those used in other infections (table XI), because these drugs are concentrated in the urine.

Although reasonably well worked out for adults, the necessary dosage adjustments for antibacterial agents have not been studied sufficiently in variable degrees of renal failure in children. Dosage must be interpolated from these adult data and experience (see chapter XXI; sect. 14.1). Monitoring of plasma drug concentration is the only way to ensure adequate and safe levels of toxic agents which are eliminated by the kidneys, particularly in the neonatal period when renal function is changing rapidly. If this service is not available, serum inhibition tests which can be done by any routine laboratory, are helpful. In most situations the serum inhibition titre against the patient's infecting organism should be at least 1:4 or 1:8. If the titre exceeds 1:64 it represents an indication that dangerously high plasma concentrations are being approached and that dosage must be reduced appropriately (see chapter XXI; sect. 2.1, 14.1).

5) *Administration of antibacterial drugs:* The ease of administration of drugs also varies inversely with the age and size of the child (see section 3). The general considerations which relate to an appropriate systemic drug dosage form and route of administration (see section 4) are most applicable to antibacterial drugs. Clearly, parenteral administration is needed for severe infections and in cases of vomiting.

Stability and compatibility of antibacterial drugs in intravenous solutions can be a problem. Indeed, failure of intravenous antibacterial therapy has been ascribed to use of a degraded or inactivated drug. Ampicillin, for example, should be administered within 1 hour if diluted with sterile water. Some antibacterial drugs are inactivated by

Table XII. Principal properties and uses of antibacterial drugs in infants and children

Drug	Principal anti-bacterial activity	Indications (due to susceptible organisms shown opposite)[1]	Notes[2]
Cephalosporins	Staphylococcus aureus (pencillin resistant) *Str. pneumoniae* Some *Esch. coli, Klebsiella-Enterobacter* and *Proteus mirabilis*	1 Severe penicillin resistant staphylococcal infections in patients allergic to penicillin (great majority of patients tolerate without reaction) 2 Pneumonia due to *Str. pneumoniae* in patients allergic to penicillin 3 Alternative to gentamicin, kanamycin for severe infections due to Gram-negative bacilli (use only on basis of sensitivity tests)	Thrombophlebitis limits IV use of cephalothin. With the possible exception of cefamandole, cephalosporins show poor penetration into CSF and should not be used in meningitis. Cephalothin causes elevated SGOT levels in neonates and positive Coombs test. Large doses of cephalori-dine (and to lesser extent cephalothin) may cause nephrotoxicity
Chloramphenicol	*Salmonella* spp. *H. influenzae* *Bacteroides fragilis*	1 Brain abscess, peritonitis, septicaemia caused by *Bacteroides fragilis*[3] 2 Alternative to ampicillin in septic arthritis, meningitis, and lobar pneumonia caused by ampicillin resistant *H. influenzae* 3 Typhoid fever 4 Salmonellosis (invasive)	Readily penetrates into CSF. Causes 'grey syndrome' in neonates (see section 3.1.2). Irreversible bone marrow aplasia occurs in a few patients; risk increased when high dosage used
Co-trimoxazole (trimethoprim-sulphamethoxazole)	*H. influenzae* *Esch. coli* *Proteus mirabilis* *Shigella* spp. *Salmonella* spp. *Brucella* spp. *Pneumocystis carinii*	1 Urinary tract infection (chronic or recurrent; suppressive therapy) 2 Shigellosis (alternative to ampicillin) 3 Typhoid fever (alternative to chloramphenicol) 4 Salmonellosis, invasive (alternative to chloramphenicol or ampicillin) 5 Acute otitis media (alternative to ampicillin/ amoxycillin) 6 Brucellosis (alternative to tetracycline)	See sulphonamides
Erythromycin	Group A streptococci *Str. pneumoniae* *Mycoplasma pneumoniae* *B. pertussis*	1 Pertussis 2 Pneumonia *(M. pneumoniae)* 3 Acute otitis media (children over 6 years) 4 Impetigo, pharyngitis (alternative to penicillin) 5 Diphtheria 6 Legionnaire's disease	The oral route is preferred: erythromycin ethyl-succinate causes pain when given by intramuscular injection; erythromycin lactobionate must be given slowly intravenously (over 30 to 60 minutes) to avoid venous irritation. Erythromycin estolate can cause jaundice when used for longer than 10-14 days

Gentamicin.	*Esch. coli* *Klebsiella-Enterobacter-* *Serratia* spp. *Proteus* spp. *Pseudomonas* spp. *Mima-Moraxella-Herellea* spp.	1 Septicaemia 2 Meningitis 3 Lung abscess 4 Pneumonia *(Klebsiella pneumoniae)* 5 Urinary tract infection (chronic, recurrent or hospital acquired) 6 Proved *Pseudomonas* infection 7 Suspected *Pseudomonas* infection (combined with carbenicillin)	Absorption from intramuscular injection is erratic in newborn and serum concentrations should be monitored. Serum concentrations must also be monitored in the presence of renal impairment to avoid ototoxicity
Kanamycin	*Esch. coli* *Klebsiella-Enterobacter* spp. *Proteus* spp.	1 Septicaemia 2 Meningitis 3 Urinary tract infection (alternative to gentamicin) 4 Pneumonia *(Klebsiella pneumoniae)*	Drug of choice in preference to gentamicin when the causative organisms are susceptible (*Esch. coli* and *Klebsiella-Enterobacter* resistance occurs often). Monitor serum concentrations for same reasons as gentamicin
Neomycin, colistin, polymyxin B	*Esch. coli*	Bacterial diarrhoea in infants due to enteropathogenic *Esch. coli*. If neomycin resistant strains, use oral colistin or polymyxin B (see section 5.1.6).	Treatment limited to 3 to 5 days to avoid neomycin induced malabsorption
Nitrofurantoin	*Esch. coli* Some *Klebsiella-Enterobacter* and *Proteus* spp.	Prolonged therapy to prevent recurrence of chronic urinary tract infection after specific curative antibacterial treatment (see section 5.1.5)	Not suitable for use in infants < 3 months of age due to impaired elimination and risk of haemolysis of neonatal erythrocyte. Unsuitable for deep tissue infections because of poor serum concentrations. Preferred to nalidixic acid
Nalidixic acid	Gram-negative organisms, except *Pseudomonas* spp.	As above	Not suitable for use in neonates due to impaired elimination and risk of haemolysis of neonatal erythrocyte

Table XII. (continued)

Drug	Principal anti-bacterial activity	Indications (due to susceptible organisms shown opposite)[1]	Notes[2]
Penicillins Benzylpenicillin (penicillin G)	Streptococci (groups A, B) *Str. pneumoniae* *Staphylococcus aureus* (non-penicillinase-producing strains) *Clostridium* spp. *Neisseria* spp.	1 Septicaemia 2 Meningitis 3 Lung abscess 4 Pneumonia 5 Bacterial endocarditis — *Str. viridans* (alone or with streptomycin); *Str. faecalis* (plus streptomycin) 6 Suppurative pericarditis 7 Gonorrhoea (plus probenecid), gonococcal ophthalmia, meningitis, arthritis 8 Syphilis (procaine or benzathine salt) 9 Diphtheria 10 Tetanus (plus antitoxin) 11 Gas gangrene (plus antitoxin) 12 Prophylaxis of rheumatic fever (benzathine salt)	Avoid in patients allergic to penicillin (for most infections substitute erythromycin, or in severe infection, a cephalosporin)
Ampicillin Amoxycillin	*H. influenzae* (non β-lactamase producing) *Esch. coli* *Proteus mirabilis* (non β-lactamase producing) *Salmonella* spp. *Shigella* spp. *Listeria monocytogenes* *Str. faecalis*	1 Septicaemia 2 Meningitis 3 Lobar pneumonia (*H. influenzae*) 4 Acute otitis media 5 Acute sinusitis (*H. influenzae*) 6 Croup; acute epiglottitis (plus tracheostomy) 7 Urinary tract infection (*Proteus mirabilis;* *Esch. coli* as alternative to sulphonamides) 8 Shigellosis (not amoxycillin) 9 Typhoid fever (alternative to chloramphenicol) 10 Salmonellosis (invasive) 11 Septic arthritis (*H. influenzae*) 12 Osteomyelitis (*Salmonella* spp.) 13 Bacterial endocarditis (*Str. faecalis*), alone or preferably plus streptomycin; pericarditis (*H. influenzae*) 14 Cellulitis (*H. influenzae*) 15 Gonorrhoea (alternative to penicillin G)	Avoid in penicillin allergic patients and in patients with infectious mononucleosis (because of high incidence of skin rash). Intravenous solutions must be freshly prepared and not kept for the next dose. Laboratory confirmation of susceptibility is especially important if infection with Gram-negative enterobacteria is suspected, since sensitivity of such organisms shows considerable variability

Drug	Organism	Indication	Comment
Carbenicillin	*Pseudomonas* spp. *Proteus* spp. (indole positive)	1 Septicaemia 2 Meningitis 3 Urinary tract infection (chronic or recurrent)	Avoid in penicillin allergic patients. Serum levels can be enhanced by probenecid

Cloxacillin
Dicloxacillin
Flucloxacillin
Methicillin
Nafcillin
Oxacillin
	Penicillinase producing
	staphylococci
		1 Septicaemia
		2 Lobar pneumonia (suspected staphylococcal)
		3 Osteomyelitis[4] (initial therapy in infants)
		4 Septic arthritis of unknown aetiology
		  (plus gentamicin)
		5 Bacterial endocarditis
		6 Suppurative pericarditis in infants (plus
		  ampicillin)
		7 Abscesses, major wound infections
		8 Scalded skin syndrome, necrotising fasciitis
			Avoid in penicillin allergic patients. Inferior
			to penicillin G in treating penicillin sensitive
			staphylococci or other penicillin sensitive organisms

Phenoxymethyl penicillin (penicillin V; oral use)	Streptococci (groups A, B) *Staphylococcus aureus* (non-penicillinase- producing)	1 Acute sinusitis (*Str. pneumoniae*) 2 Streptococcal pharyngitis, scarlet fever 3 Impetigo, erysipelas 4 Acute otitis media (children over 6 years) 5 Prophylaxis of rheumatic fever (where compliance can be guaranteed)	Avoid in penicillin allergic patients
Sulphonamides	*Esch. coli* *Klebsiella-Enterobacter* spp. *Proteus mirabilis* *H. influenzae*	1 Urinary tract infections (initial therapy) 2 Otitis media (*H. influenzae*, in combination with full doses of ampicillin)	Avoid in patients with G6PD deficiency and in premature infants (risk of acute haemolysis and jaundice). See chapter XIX (sect. 14.6.6); XXIII (sect. 8.4)
Tetracyclines	*Borrelia* spp. *Brucella* spp. *Chlamydia* spp. *Leptospira* spp. *Listeria monocytogenes* *Mycoplasma pneumoniae* *Clostridia* spp.	1 Relapsing fever (*Borrelia* spp.) 2 Brucellosis 3 Psittacosis 4 Leptospirosis 5 Inclusion blennorrhoea (*Chlamydia* spp.; topical) 6 Syphilis (alternative to penicillin) 7 Mycoplasma pneumonia 8 Listeria septicaemia, meningitis (alternative to ampicillin) 9 Tetanus, gas gangrene (alternative to penicillin) 10 Acne vulgaris (see chapter XIV; sect. 4)	Avoid in infants and children (especially under 8y) because of tooth staining and damage to enamel (see chapter XIII; sect. 13.3)

1 See also text, particularly for choice and use of drugs in septicaemia, meningitis.
2 See also appendix D and other chapters.
3 Clindamycin can be used as an alternative.
4 Lincomycin can be used as an alternative.

particular solutions (e.g. benzylpenicillin and ampicillin with acidic infusion fluids such as dextrose and fructose) or incompatible with other antibacterial drugs (e.g. gentamicin and carbenicillin) or commonly used drugs with which they are mixed in parenteral therapy (e.g. kanamycin with heparin or hydrocortisone sodium succinate). These problems can be overcome by injecting drugs separately into drip tubing near the needle with due aseptic precautions and by giving each drug separately as a bolus over a period of about 5 minutes. It is not permissible to accept only visual incompatibility as an indication of which drugs do not mix in parenteral solutions. The hospital or clinical pharmacist should be asked for advice on relevant drug stability and compatibility information. Data and directions are published elsewhere (Kramer et al., 1971; Shirkey, 1975).

6) *Duration of antibacterial treatment:* In general, treatment of septicaemia in neonates must be continued for considerably longer than in older infants and adults (who are more easily monitored clinically), but the decision to stop must be made for each individual infant after review of the clinical and laboratory evidence. In the absence of deep tissue involvement or abscess formation, antibacterial therapy is usually continued for 5 to 7 days after clinical improvement. In some cases (e.g. involvement of multiple organs, slow clinical response), treatment may need to be continued for 2 to 3 or more weeks. Duration of treatment in meningitis is based upon the results of blood and CSF examination and cultures and the clinical condition of the patient. The duration of intraventricular or intrathecal administration is dependent upon the clinical condition of the patient, the causative organism and the time necessary to sterilise the cerebrospinal fluid.

Pulmonary infection in certain patients (e.g. cystic fibrosis) requires longer treatment. A number of important infections in childhood such as acute otitis media, acute urinary tract infection and streptococcal pharyngitis require a minimum of therapy which must be completed if complications or recurrence are to be avoided. Parents and children must be educated in the reasons why the full course of treatment must be taken as prescribed (see also section 4).

5.1.2 Septicaemia, Meningitis and Pneumonia in Newborn Infants

Clinically, the neonate has a poorly developed intrinsic defence mechanism and limited response to many pathogenic bacteria and viruses, so that when his outer defences are breached, infections are commonly generalised and severe. He may have acquired transient protection from his mother *in utero* for other infections (e.g. *H. influenzae*).

Septicaemia in the Neonate: Early suspicion and diagnosis and prompt treatment of neonatal septicaemia are essential. It is a disease which must be treated on suspicion and then confirmation attempted. The risk of unnecessarily giving antibacterials is weighed against the need for early treatment. Disease is suspected when there is abnormal behaviour such as hypo- or hyperthermia, unexpectedly poor feeding, vomiting, undue lethargy or irritability, or apnoea etc. The clinician must be ever alert to the possibility of bacterial infection in a vaguely unwell baby. Suspicion of illness by nurses or attendants identify problem babies. A history of complicated pregnancy or delivery is helpful in identifying high risk infants. Sick infants housed in intensive care units, particularly those requiring assisted ventilation and blood gas monitoring, are especially prone to bloodstream and tissue infection. In all infants suspected of sepsis, cultures of blood, urine, cerebrospinal fluid and other appropriate areas (skin, external auditory meatus) should be obtained prior to commencing antibacterial therapy. In addition, cultures and stained smear of material from a rectal swab (for *Listeria* spp., group B streptococci) or gastric aspirate may sometimes be helpful.

Since treatment usually must commence before the results of laboratory tests are available, a knowledge of the epidemiological experience in a particular neonatal nursery or intensive care unit is important in guiding initial therapy (Davies, 1978; McCracken and Eichenwald, 1978). *Escherichia coli* and group B β-haemolytic streptococci are the usual predominant pathogens, while *Staphylococcus aureus* phage group II, *Klebsiella-Enterobacter-Serratia* spp., *Pseudomonas aeruginosa, Proteus* spp. and *Listeria monocytogenes* cause disease less often but may be more common in particular units. Anaerobic organisms may occasionally be implicated. Resistance in organisms changes and may be related to local or widespread overusage or underdosage of antibacterial agents.

The aim of treatment is to maintain the wellbeing of the infant while giving him antibacterial therapy of sufficiently broad range to cover the pathogens most likely to be encountered during this period. Ampicillin with either kanamycin or gentamicin (choice based on susceptibility of coliform organisms in a particular nursery) give bactericidal activity against most potential pathogens. In units where group B β-haemolytic streptococci and *E. coli* are known to be the most prevalent, the combination of benzylpenicillin (most active of the penicillins against group B β-haemolytic streptococcus) and kanamycin or gentamicin will be suitable initially. Once the pathogen is identified and sensitivities known, the most appropriate drug or drugs are used (see table XIII). Supportive therapy will include intravenous fluids and may also involve treatment of shock and acidosis, and also in meningitis, treatment of convulsions.

Monitoring antibacterial therapy by serum concentrations should develop from the necessity which has existed unconsidered for too long. A number of neonatal units already have such support. It certainly seems as wise to ascertain the concentrations of an antibacterial agent in the serum of an infant as to know the BUN or creatinine in a patient followed for renal disease. Added expense is not as limiting as tradition and attitude in preventing the development of necessary monitoring. Monitoring of antibacterial drug concentrations requires attention as to time of blood sample, number of samples, especially as related to paediatric drug use (Shirkey, 1977). A simple test which can be done in any laboratory is to set up the infant's serum in various dilutions against the organism to ascertain the effective level of antibacterial drug in the serum (sect. 5.1.1).

Meningitis in the Neonate: Neonatal meningitis essentially follows neonatal septicaemia, of which it represents a complication. Making for difficulty in diagnosis are the facts that as many as 26 polymorphonuclear cells and 16 mononuclear cells/mm^3 may be present and a protein greater than 100mg/ml in the cerebrospinal fluid of normal babies, especially in prematures. Remembering that hypoglycaemia is common in neonates, a low CSF must be interpreted in relation to the blood sugar. Spinal fluid smears and Gram-stain offer an opportunity to identify organisms far in advance of culture. Hours are important in the treatment of meningitis in infants and children.

Initial antibacterial therapy is again based on the pathogens most likely to be encountered (usually group B β-haemolytic streptococci and *Esch. coli*), and dosage schedules are directed at maintaining a plasma concentration which will result in a CSF concentration of the drug well above the minimum inhibitory concentration for the causative organism. In suspected or proven purulent meningitis in neonates, ampicillin with gentamicin is an ideal initial combination when the organism is unknown. After the organism has been identified and appropriate antibacterial sensitivities known, therapy may need to be altered. Chloramphenicol, in suitably monitored dosage, is considered by some when organisms are susceptible to it. Duration of treatment is based upon results of blood and cerebrospinal fluid cultures and the clinical condition of the infant. Intraventricular administration of gentamicin may be necessary to sterilise the CSF (McCracken and Eichenwald, 1978). Further details of treatment of meningitis in both neonates and children are given in chapter XXV (sect. 13). Some suggested paediatric dosage schedules for initial therapy are given in table XIII.

In infants and children with immunological deficiency, prior neurosurgery, endocarditis, or malignant or other diseases treated with corticosteroids or immunosuppressive agents, the opportunistic pathogens are often different from those encountered in normal children. Therapy must be adjusted accordingly.

Pneumonia in the Neonate: Pneumonia may be but part of a generalised congenital infection caused by a virus (e.g. herpes virus, cytomegalovirus, rubella), toxoplasmosis, syphilis and *Listeria monocytogenes* or bacteria acquired in the pre- or postnatal period. Aspiration pneumonia is especially common in babies who are distressed *in utero,* or while passing through the birth canal or after feeding of milk. It is particularly common in infants with tracheoesophageal and gastrointestinal anomalies. Acquired pneumonias are generally from organisms present in the hospital personnel and the nursery. Staphylococcal and coliform organisms are especially common in the neonatal period and particularly before 1 year of age. Antistaphylococcal penicillins such as methicillin (50mg/kg daily in 2 doses in first 2 weeks life, then 75 to 100mg/kg/day in 3 doses) and gentamicin for coliform organisms (5mg/kg/day in 2 doses in the first week of life, then 7.5mg/kg/day in 3 doses) represent therapy of choice for these infections in neonates.

Table XIII. Antibacterial drugs for neonatal septicaemia and meningitis (after McCracken and Eichenwald, 1978)

Clinical condition	Initial therapy	Dosage[1]
1. *Septicaemia* Unknown aetiology[2]	Ampicillin + kanamycin[3] or gentamicin[3]	Ampicillin: 50mg/kg daily in 2 IV or IM doses (under 7 days old); 100mg/kg/day in 3 doses (prematures), 150mg/kg/day in 3 doses (over 7 days) Kanamycin: 20mg/kg daily in 2 IM doses for first 7 days (infants > 2kg at birth), then 30mg/kg daily in 3 doses; 15mg/kg daily in 2 IM doses for first 7 days (infants < 2kg at birth), then 20mg/kg daily in 2 doses Gentamicin: 5mg/kg daily IM in 2 doses (under 7 days); 7.5mg/kg/day IM in 3 doses (over 7 days). (Some clinicians use 6mg/kg daily; in 2 doses < 7 days, in 3 doses > 7 days.)
Group B streptococci	Soluble penicillin G	50,000 to 100,000u/kg daily IM or IV in 2 doses (under 7 days), 3 doses (over 7 days)
Listeria monocytogenes *Pr. mirabilis, Str. faecalis*	Ampicillin	As above
Pseudomonas Indole positive *Proteus*	Carbenicillin or ticarcillin (alone or combined with gentamicin)	Carbenicillin: 100mg/kg every 12 hours for first 7 days (infants > 2kg at birth), then 100mg/kg every 6 hours; 100mg/kg every 12 hours for first 7 days (infants < 2kg at birth), then 100mg/kg every 8 hours Gentamicin: As above Ticarcillin: Half of the dosage of carbenicillin
Esch. coli	Gentamicin (kanamycin if organism susceptible)	Gentamicin: As above Kanamycin: As above

2. *Meningitis*

Unknown aetiology[2]	Ampicillin + gentamicin	Ampicillin: 100mg/kg daily in 2 IV or IM doses (under 7 days); 200mg/kg daily in 3 doses (over 7 days) Gentamicin: As for septicaemia. If organisms are still present 24 to 36h after beginning therapy, gentamicin 1 to 2mg daily should be given intrathecally
Group B streptococci	Soluble penicillin G	100,000 to 250,000u/kg daily in 2 to 4 doses
Listeria monocytogenes *Str. faecalis*	Ampicillin	As above
Esch. coli	Ampicillin + gentamicin	As above under unknown aetiology
Pseudomonas spp.	Carbenicillin	400mg/kg daily IV in 4 doses (gentamicin may be added to this regimen)

1 See section 2.3 for dosage rationale.
2 Once the organism is identified and susceptibilities are known, the most appropriate drug or drugs are used. Drugs which are not needed may be stopped and needed ones added to the regimen.
3 It is advisable to monitor plasma concentrations of gentamicin and kanamycin since apart from variable rates of elimination, absorption from intramuscular injection may be erratic in some neonates, which may result in inadequate or excessive plasma concentrations.

5.1.3 Septicaemia and Meningitis Beyond the Neonatal Period

The pathogens which commonly cause sepsis differ after the neonatal period and most often include *Streptococcus (Diplococcus) pneumoniae, Neisseria meningitidis* and *Haemophilus influenzae* (McCracken and Eichenwald, 1978). Occasionally, coliform bacteria may be encountered in children with infections or abnormalities of the genitourinary tract. Septicaemia in older children is rare and usually associated with infections of the urinary tract or skeletal system. *Staphylococcus aureus* and group A streptococci can be cultured from the blood of about 50% of children older than 2 years with septic arthritis or osteomyelitis. *H. influenzae* is a ubiquitous pathogen of early childhood and may also be cultured. Children with malignancy or altered immunological responsiveness are especially at risk of developing septicaemia and deep tissue infections caused by the usual or uncommon bacterial pathogens, as well as fungi, protozoa and viruses (e.g. varicella).

When the bacteriological diagnosis is uncertain in older infants and children, ampicillin (150 to 200mg/kg daily in 4 divided doses) can be given together with either kanamycin (30mg/kg daily in 3 divided doses), or gentamicin (6 to 7.5mg/kg daily in 3 divided doses) if kanamycin resistant coliform bacteria or *Pseudomonas* spp are suspected. Monitoring of serum kanamycin or gentamicin concentrations is advised in those with proved Gram-negative sepsis, particularly if renal function is impaired. A change in therapy is indicated if the pathogen is subsequently identified as a penicillin sensitive Gram-positive coccus (benzylpenicillin 100,000 to 150,000u/kg daily in 4 divided doses) or penicillin resistant staphylococcus (methicillin 200mg/kg in 4 divided doses. Carbenicillin (400 to 600mg/kg in 4 divided doses) or ticarcillin (in half this dosage) can be given alone or in combination with gentamicin in *Pseudomonas* infections.

A combination of carbenicillin and gentamicin should also be given when septicaemia is suspected in patients with altered immunological responsiveness. A change in therapy is made on the basis of blood culture which, if negative for bacterial pathogens, necessitates special cultures for identification of fungal, protozoan or viral agents. Broad spectrum antibacterial therapy should not be continued in the absence of proven bacterial infection because of likely overgrowth of the gastrointestinal and respiratory tract with resistant organisms.

Bacterial meningitis beyond the neonatal period is treated initially with ampicillin alone — 100mg/kg by rapid intravenous infusion, followed by 50mg/kg intravenously in a 15 to 20 minute infusion every 6 hours (200mg/kg daily) or preferably in combination with chloramphenicol (100mg/kg daily in 4 divided doses intravenously). In some areas, the emergence of β-lactamase producing *H. influenzae* type b strains and resultant resistance to ampicillin, has necessitated the addition of chloramphenicol to the initial regimen (Jacobson et al., 1976). Continuation of either ampicillin or chloramphenicol depends on the sensitivity of the organism isolated (table XIII). If a type b strain *H. influenzae* is cultured, it must be tested for β-lactamase production and chloramphenicol continued for positive organisms.

5.1.4 Respiratory Infections

The majority of respiratory tract infections are due to viruses and are not affected by antibacterial agents. When antibacterial drugs are indicated, only a few agents are useful.

Acute Upper Respiratory Tract Infection (colds), Pharyngitis, Tonsillitis: Viruses cause most infections of the upper respiratory tract and routine antibacterial drugs are unlikely to be helpful. When group A β-haemolytic streptococci is suspected or proven by culture, penicillin is the drug of choice and should be given for at least 10 days. Symptomatic treatment of upper respiratory conditions is discussed in chapter XI (sect. 2).

Pseudomembranous pharyngitis may occur in diphtheria, infectious mononucleosis and sometimes in streptococcal and viral illnesses. In diphtheria, penicillin or erythromycin for 5 to 7 days can be used to eradicate the bacteria, but they have no effect on toxic manifestations. Antitoxin is indicated.

Otitis Media and Sinusitis: Antibacterial drugs are indicated in acute otitis media, mastoiditis and sinusitis. Chronic otitis media may not usually require systemic antibacterial agents. The treatment of these conditions is discussed in chapter XI (sect. 2.2, 3.2). Middle ear cultures (myringocentesis) are most valuable for diagnosis and monitoring therapy.

Croup, Acute Epiglottitis: These are the most common causes of acute upper airway obstruction in children. Croup has many aetiologies; most often it is a viral infection, usually due to parainfluenza 1, occasionally to parainfluenza 3, and less often to parainfluenza 2 and other viruses (Glezen and Denny, 1973). Antibacterials are not indicated initially. Immediate treatment is directed at relief of emotional stress and difficult breathing, with the head of the child over the mother's shoulder, in an humidified atmosphere (e.g. bathroom filled with steam). The child should be admitted to hospital if there is any doubt about hypoxia. Humidified oxygen is necessary in all but the mildest cases and is the foundation of therapy. Bronchodilators delivered in nebulised form with an intermittent positive pressure breathing apparatus can be used to terminate the relatively rare cases of obstruction from croup. The role of corticosteroids is controversial, but high dose short term use of steroids may be of value in severe cases of croup (Lockhart and Battaglia, 1977; Shaw and Marsmann, 1977). If all these measures fail to provide relief of airway obstruction, there should be no hesitation in providing an artificial airway before the child tires or hypercapnia or hypoxia occur. Sedatives are to be avoided.

Simple croup (acute infectious croup or laryngotracheobronchitis) must be differentiated from three other croup causing illnesses — diphtheria, acute epiglottitis due to *Haemophilus influenzae* type b strains and allergic croup. Acute epiglottitis is an emergency disease of children, usually under the age of 5; the age plagued by infections due to *H. influenzae*. The onset is more rapid than the usual case of croup and lacks the preceding coryza. The child is more toxic and can be proven by blood culture to have a bacteraemia if not a septicaemia. The first symptoms are fever, headache, and a very sore throat leading to difficulty in swallowing and even drooling of saliva. Stridor is severe and most children are either cyanosed or pale and shocked when first seen. Lower respiratory tract signs are usually absent (Holdaway, 1977). Immediate and orderly securing of relief of airway obstruction at the time of suspected diagnosis is essential. Preparation for laryngeal intubation or tracheostomy should precede any examination of the throat if the disease is suspected, since depression of the posterior portion of the tongue has been the terminal event in precipitating complete respiratory obstruction.

In many institutions laryngeal intubation or tracheostomy is done 'on the spot' without taking the child to the operating theatre. These patients are not watched for progress, because complete laryngeal obstruction due to spasm and oedema occurs precipitously. In some institutions laryngeal intubation is used in preference to tracheostomy; however, danger of pressure necrosis exists. The period of tracheostomy need only be very short because the condition rapidly responds to ampicillin and/or chloramphenicol; each given in a dose of 100mg/kg daily in 4 divided doses intravenously. In areas where ampicillin resistant strains of *H. influenzae* are prevalent, both agents or chloramphenicol are given. Therapy is continued with one or the other of these agents after the pathogen has been tested for β-lactamase production (chloramphenicol if positive) for 7 to 10 days. After the acute state, the antibiotics can be given orally.

Diphtheritic laryngitis, although less frequently seen in these days of nearly complete vaccination, represents an emergency situation but not quite that of acute epiglottitis.

Diphtheria: In the United States after a steady decline of diphtheria over the past 65 years it has, since 1965, become a major medical problem in several outbreaks, particularly in the Southern States where cutaneous diphtheria adds additional cases. In prevention, diphtheria toxoid remains the treatment of choice for exposed individuals previously actively immunised. In those not immunised actively and who are ill, antitoxin should be given as soon as the diagnosis is suspected. Infectious mononucleosis is more frequently encountered in association with a pseudomembrane than is diphtheria in the USA. Many cases of diphtheria are diagnosed quite late. The dangers of serum sickness (antitoxin) remain about the same as in former years. However, serum sickness responds to antihistamines or steroid therapy.

Exposed individuals are studied by throat cultures. All should be treated with a 5 to 7 day course of erythromycin or penicillin to eradicate the bacteria. Previously immunised (active) individuals should receive a dose of diphtheria toxoid.

Bronchitis: Antibacterial drugs are of little help in the early stages of acute bronchitis in children. Most success will be achieved by attention to hydration and teaching the mother to assist the child to get rid of retained secretions. Bronchodilators are of little demonstrated benefit in infants and children under 2 (oedema of the mucosa plus retained secretions causes the spasm in this age group) [Rutter et al., 1975], but may be helpful in older children. In hospital practice, the child can be placed in an humidified atmosphere to ease breathing. In the home, the child can be placed on the mother's lap in the bathroom with the hot shower running and this is less of a contamination hazard than unsterilised hospital equipment.

Persisting bronchitis lasting for more than 4 or 5 days is suggestive of secondary bacterial infection and an indication for culture and penicillin, since the most likely causative organism is *Streptococcus pneumoniae*. Persistent or recurrent wheezy bronchitis suggests a likelihood of underlying asthma, particularly if there is a strong family history or if the child had eczema in early infancy (see chapter XX; sect. 3.1.2 for details of treatment).

General antiallergic environmental prophylaxis is preferred to continuing drug therapy.

Pertussis: The reservoir of pertussis is now believed to be in adults and those with atypical mild disease. Consequently, adults with persistent bronchitis may be the source of infection to children (Nelson, 1978a). Paroxysms of coughing, the leucocytosis and lymphocytosis are variable and may occur late. Immunity from pertussis vaccination is of short duration and occurrence of disease in older children and adults indicates the inadequacy of the current vaccine. Without data to so indicate, boosters are not usually given after the age of 6 years.

There is no specific therapy for pertussis, but children with pertussis may be treated with erythromycin, given immediately following the first symptoms, for a period of 14 days (Bass et al., 1969). The basic treatment of pertussis is good supportive care. Susceptible family contacts should also probably be treated with erythromycin. Exposed susceptible infants are best treated with erythromycin (Altemeier and Ayoub, 1977; Linneman et al., 1974). Pertussis immune globulin (human) in daily doses for 3 to 5 days is modestly effective for prophylaxis but antibiotic treatment is preferred.

Fluorescent antibody examination may be helpful in reducing the period of isolation, which ordinarily is for 4 or more weeks. Without any solid data, clinical impression has caused immunisation for pertussis to be denied to older children and adults.

Acute Bronchiolitis: This dangerous condition is due to viral infection, usually respiratory syncytial virus. It is rare after the age of 2 years and has a peak incidence at about age 6 months. Deterioration in the infant's condition is likely to be rapid over the 24 to 48 hours after the onset of dyspnoea. The child should therefore preferably be hospitalised.

Treatment consists of humidified oxygen, which needs to be monitored, often by blood gas analysis, and adequate hydration, frequently intravenously. Corticosteroids have no place in routine management as they do not favourably influence the course of the condition (Leer et al., 1969), but are used by some paediatricians in the seriously ill infant. Most large institutions will withhold antibacterial drugs unless there are good indications of secondary bacterial invasion.

Pneumonia: When penumonia is suspected every effort should be made to identify the causative organism prior to commencing antibacterial therapy. Blood cultures should be obtained, and sputum or tracheal aspirates and pleural fluid, if present, examined by Gram stain and cultured. Culture from the throat and nasopharynx are valueless and often misleading.

The treatment of bacterial pneumonia in neonates is discussed in section 5.1.2. Bronchopneumonia in older infants and children is mainly due to viruses and to a lesser extent *Mycoplasma pneumoniae*. Supportive therapy is all that is necessary in viral pneumonia, while erythromycin (40mg/kg daily in 4 divided doses) is the preferred agent for *Mycoplasma* infections of childhood, since tetracyclines are undesirable because of the risk of teeth staining and enamel hypoplasia.

Empyema in early infancy can be due to viruses or to *Staphylococcus aureus* or *H. influenzae*. Initial treatment is based on clinical judgment and if the staphylococcus is suspected, a penicillinase resistant penicillin is given (e.g. methicillin 200mg/kg daily in 4 divided doses, or 50 to 100mg/kg daily in 2 or 3 divided doses in neonates, intramuscularly or intravenously). If *H. influenzae* infection is suspected, chloramphenicol (100mg/kg daily) and a penicillinase resistant penicillin such as methicillin is usually given. Ampicillin might be used initially in areas where resistance is known not to exist. Treatment is continued on the basis of the Gram stain of pleural fluid; methicillin being continued for *Staph. aureus* and ampicillin (100 to150mg/kg daily intravenously or intramuscularly in 4 divided doses) for non β-lactamase producing *H. influenzae* infection. Chloramphenicol is continued for ampicillin resistant strains of *H. influenzae*. Penicillin is used initially in empyema in childhood since *Str. pneumoniae* and *Staph. aureus* are the most likely aetiological agents. It is given intramuscularly or intravenously in a dosage of 50,000 to 100,000u/kg daily, divided into 4 or 6 doses. A penicillinase resistant penicillin can be used as an alternative.

Penicillin is the drug of choice for initial treatment of consolidating lobar pneumonia, since *Str. pneumoniae* is the most likely causative organism. It is given in a dosage of 25,000 to 50,000u/kg daily in 4 divided intravenous or intramuscular doses, followed by oral therapy (50,000u/kg daily) for a total of 7 to 10 days treatment in uncomplicated cases. Other agents are used as appropriate for specific infections — e.g. carbenicillin or ticarcillin for *Pseudomonas aeruginosa* and gentamicin or kanamycin for *Klebsiella pneumoniae*.

Supportive treatment for pneumonia is just as important as the choice of antibacterial agent. Regular postural coughing 3 to 4 times daily helps to clear the lungs of infected secretions. The state of hydration is important since a dehydrated child becomes more acidotic and has thick tenacious secretions. Bronchodilators are useful in children over 2 years if there is associated bronchospasm (see above). Hypoxia should always be looked for. Oxygen remains choice treatment for cyanosis. Contaminated respiratory apparatus, however, is common in hospitals and may represent greater hazard than value in milder cases.

5.1.5 Urinary Tract Infections

Urinary tract infections in children are both common and recurrent. The major problem in the prevention of chronic pyelonephritis is the detection of the patient at risk in early childhood (Heale, 1973). True urinary infections are difficult to diagnose on the basis of symptoms, and accurate bacteriological investigation is therefore essential. This also means the collection of an accurate urine sample (e.g. bladder puncture or carefully monitored clean-catch specimens). Acute infections are treated with a short course of a curative regimen of an appropriate drug (e.g. sulphafurazole/sulfisoxazole 100 to 150mg/kg daily orally in 4 doses for 7 to 10 days). Other agents can be given if needed on the basis of culture results (see

chapter XXI; sect. 3). It is important to impress upon parents that although relief of symptoms will probably be rapid, the full course of treatment must be completed. Subsequent management is determined on the basis of repeated cultures and the X-ray findings. Most infections are associated with little or no reflux and can be managed medically. Some infants and young children require admission to hospital for management of fluid and electrolyte disturbances, jaundice and septicaemia, and investigations to detect any severe underlying abnormalities.

Maintenance therapy is particularly useful in children who have recurrent symptomatic attacks; a 6 to 12 months course of antibacterial therapy usually breaks up the pattern of attacks. Infants with severe reflux and older children with moderate reflux are often placed on prolonged maintenance therapy until reflux is corrected surgically or ceases spontaneously. In young non-toilet trained children, a quarter of the full daily dose of antibacterial agent is given morning and night to maintain effective bladder levels over 24 hours. In older children a quarter of the full dose at night is given. Nitrofurantoin (4mg/kg in 4 doses) or co-trimoxazole (5mg trimethoprim/25mg sulphamethoxazole/kg daily in 2 doses) are the drugs commonly used at present in maintenance therapy; full doses given in parentheses (Smellie et al., 1976; White, 1977).

The most important group of patients are those with established chronic pyelonephritis, and life-long follow-up is mandatory in all these children to detect recurrent infections and hypertension. Detection in early childhood before severe renal damage occurs is the keystone to prevention of chronic renal failure in these children.

5.1.6 Gastrointestinal Infections

Diarrhoea, with or without vomiting, can be due to numerous causes. In children, that due to primary infection of the gut, or gastroenteritis, is an important cause of morbidity and mortality in many countries, and in developing countries is often the most common paediatric illness. Gastroenteritis is most often seen in children under 2 years of age, but rarely in breast fed infants.

Most cases of gastroenteritis in young children are due to viral infection; the rotavirus (orbivirus, duovirus, reo-like virus) having recently been implicated, particularly as the major cause of winter diarrhoea in infants in temperate climates in developed countries and a very common and predominant agent in developing countries (Kapikian et al., 1976; Ryder et al., 1976). Some cases are due to enteropathogenic bacteria, i.e. *Escherichia coli, Shigella* and *Salmonella* species (Nalin et al., 1978). Treatment depends on the severity of dehydration, as assessed clinically, and in all cases is guided by the following general principles (Ironside, 1973; Holdaway, 1977):

1) Arrest the diarrhoea — in most cases this can be achieved by gut rest. Antidiarrhoeal agents are of no value in controlling the diarrhoea.
2) Replacement of fluid loss, and correction of electrolyte and/or acid base imbalance.
3) Maintenance of hydration and electrolyte balance in the presence of continuing diarrhoea.

In children with mild dehydration the prime objective is rehydration and maintenance of adequate fluid intake by early treatment *in the home.* Gut rest is achieved by giving oral fluids in the form of glucose electrolyte or alternatively sucrose electrolyte solutions after stopping all milk and solid feeds (Nalin et al., 1978; Sack et al., 1978). After a period of 24 to 48 hours the diarrhoea in most instances will have lessened, following which graduated strengths of milk feeds can then be introduced, the strength being gradually increased as diarrhoea subsides.

Patients with moderate and severe dehydration require intravenous fluids and correction of acid-base and electrolyte imbalance. The diarrhoea in most cases also improves after 24 to 48 hours of complete gut rest when the child is on intravenous drip. Following this, the regimen as for patients with mild dehydration is then introduced.

Intractable diarrhoea requires intravenous hyperalimentation for days or even weeks until the child can tolerate oral feeds again. Therapy of the occasional case of hypernatraemic (hyperosmolar) dehydration is slightly modified, in that no replacement saline is given. Any child with severe dehydration and circulatory collapse should be regarded as an emergency, requiring immediate measures to prevent or minimise further brain damage.

Antibacterial drugs are not indicated in the routine case of bacterial diarrhoea, unless there is evidence of systemic spread (see chapter XIX; sect. 11.1), but they are of benefit in shigellosis and certain cases of salmonellosis.

Shigellosis: Antibacterial therapy is not indicated in simple self limited diarrhoea, but in true dysentery when used early it shortens the duration of symptoms and duration of faecal excretion of the organism (Haltalin et al., 1969). Ampicillin (100mg/kg daily in 4 doses) is given orally or parenterally for 5 days. Co-trimoxazole (8 to 12mg/kg trimethoprim + 40 to 60mg/kg daily sulphamethoxazole orally or parenterally in 2 doses) for 5 days can be used in cases of disease due to organisms resistant to ampicillin and other agents such as tetracyclines. Despite similar MIC's to ampicillin, for unexplained reasons amoxycillin does not appear to be effective in shigellosis (Nelson and Haltalin, 1974).

Salmonellosis: Because of the greater risk of bloodstream invasion, antibacterial therapy is indicated routinely if the illness occurs in young infants (especially prematures), in patients with immunodeficiency states, or in a child with a chronic or debilitating disease. In other cases, antibacterial therapy does not shorten the duration of symptoms and may prolong the carrier state (Aserkoff and Bennett, 1969; Joint Report, 1970). When therapy is indicated, ampicillin or chloramphenicol may be used; each given orally, 75 to 100mg/kg daily in 4 doses for 7 to 10 days. Amoxycillin or co-trimoxazole are suitable alternatives. Antibacterial agents are not indicated in the convalescent carrier state. Treatment of typhoid fever is discussed in chapter XXVII (sect. 5.4.1).

Pathogenic E. coli *enteritis in infants:* Therapy with neomycin is of benefit and is advisable in nosocomial outbreaks of diarrhoea or in specific patients with protracted watery diarrhoea associated with enteropathogenic *Esch. coli* on rectal culture (McCracken and Eichenwald, 1978). Neomycin (100mg/kg daily in 4 to 6 doses) is given orally for 5 days; longer periods are unnecessary and may be associated with drug induced malabsorption. Oral colistin (15 to 20mg/kg daily) may be used in cases of neomycin resistance.

Management of other gastrointestinal infections, including intestinal parasitic infestation, is discussed in chapter XIX (sect. 11).

5.1.7 Septic Arthritis and Osteomyelitis

Early management is based on needle aspiration or surgical drainage, culture of blood and specimens from the bone or joint lesions and on rational and adequate antibacterial therapy. Surgical treatment is of equal importance as antibacterial drugs.

In neonates, suspected staphylococcal or group B streptococcal arthritis is treated with parenteral methicillin (100 to 150mg/kg daily in 2 or 3 doses) or penicillin G (50,000 to 100,000 units in 2 or 3 doses) respectively and Gram-negative infection with gentamicin (5 to 7.5mg/kg daily in 2 or 3 divided doses). Therapy may need to be changed on the basis of culture data. A combination of methicillin and gentamicin is used if the causative organism cannot be identified. Beyond the neonatal period, *H. influenzae* type b is the major cause of suppurative arthritis but *Staph. aureus* may also be implicated. When the causative organism is not known, initial therapy is with a combination of a penicillinase resistant penicillin such as methicillin (150mg/kg daily in 4 doses) and chloramphenicol (100mg/kg daily in 4 doses). Treatment is continued with chloramphenicol if β-lactamase producing *H. influenzae* strains are isolated and with ampicillin (150mg/kg daily in 4 doses) if they are non-lactamase producing. Penicillin G (100,000u/kg daily in 4 doses) is substituted if the staphylococcus, or other Gram-positive organism, is susceptible. Beyond infancy, a penicillinase resistant penicillin such as methicillin (150 to 200mg/kg daily depending on age and to maximum of 6g daily in adolescents) provides adequate cover for the organisms usually encountered. Soluble penicillin G can be substituted (100,000u/kg daily in 4 doses) if the organism proves to be penicillin sensitive. Treatment of septic arthritis is continued for 2 to 3 weeks depending on the pathogen, the joints involved and the clinical condition of the patient. Gonococcal arthritis can be effectively treated with soluble penicillin G (100,000u daily in 4 doses) for about 7 days.

Staphylococcus aureus is the most common cause of osteomyelitis in infancy and childhood. Initial therapy consists of methicillin 200mg/kg daily in 4 or 6 doses intramuscularly or intravenously. Penicillin G (100,000u/kg daily) is substituted if the organism proves to be penicillin sensitive. Patients allergic to penicillin can be treated with lincomycin or fusidic acid. Parenteral treatment is continued for a minimum of 3 to 6 weeks. In some cases therapy must be given for months; it may be permissible to use oral antibacterial drugs in some patients after 5 to 10 days of effective parenteral therapy, provided the organisms are susceptible to the oral agents, complete patient compliance is guaranteed and serum concentrations are monitored, and the patient's condition followed closely (Nelson, 1978b; Nelson et al., 1978; Tetzlaff et al., 1978). Antibacterial therapy is not a substitute for adequate surgical drainage.

Ampicillin (150 to 200mg/kg daily) is the preferred drug for *Salmonella* osteomyelitis in patients with sickle cell anaemia or other haemoglobinopathies. Carbenicillin (400 to 600mg/kg daily in 4 doses) or ticarcillin in half this dosage can be used in *Pseudomonas* osteomyelitis, alone or with gentamicin.

5.1.8 Infections of the Heart

Streptococcus viridans is the most common cause of bacterial endocarditis and is treated by soluble penicillin G (100,000u/kg intravenously to maximum of 4 to 6 mega u daily) for a total of 4 weeks, preferably with streptomycin 30mg/kg daily in 2 doses intramuscularly for 2 weeks. Enterococcal endocarditis requires larger doses of penicillin (250,000u/kg daily to maximum 20 mega u) combined with streptomycin for 4 weeks. Staphylococci may also cause endocarditis and are the most common cause of suppurative pericarditis in children, for which intravenous methicillin (200mg/kg in 4 to 6 doses daily) is given. Penicillin G (20 mega u daily) is substituted if the organism is susceptible. Because *H. influenzae* pericarditis may occur during infancy, chloramphenicol (100mg/kg daily) should be added to methicillin as initial therapy in this age group, unless Gram-positive cocci have been definitely isolated. Soluble penicillin G (100,000u/kg in 4 to 6 doses daily intravenously or intramuscularly) is given for pericarditis caused by *Str. pneumoniae* or *N. meningitidis*. Treatment is continued in all cases for a minimum of 2 to 3 weeks.

5.1.9 Skin Infections and Infestations

Treatment of common bacterial skin infections such as impetigo and recurrent boils, fungal infections such as ringworm and parasitic infestations such as scabies and pediculosis are discussed in chapter XIV; sect. 2, 3.

The 'scalded skin syndrome' is a term used to denote a group of skin disorders due to *Staph. aureus* phage group II (Melish and Glasgow, 1971). The syndrome includes bullous impetigo, non-streptococcal scarlatina and toxic epidermal necrolysis of infancy and childhood (Lyell's disease). Methicillin, 150mg/kg daily intramuscularly in 4 doses, is used initially and substituted by soluble penicillin G if the organism is penicillin sensitive.

Life threatening necrotising fasciitis is usually caused by staphylococci or streptococci and occasionally by both. Extensive surgery involving resection of necrotic tissue is essential. Initial antibacterial therapy is with methicillin (dose as above) which is replaced by soluble penicillin G if the organism is susceptible.

5.1.10 Sexually Transmissible Diseases

With greater promiscuity and the 'pill', gonorrhoea has again returned to plague the clinician who treats children. In countries where the disease is pandemic, such as the United States, where during 1976 more than a million new cases occurred, nearly 25% of them were in the age group between 15 and 19, and about 1% of cases in children below puberty. In one series in prepubertal children, 55% of cases involved children 5 years of age or less (Nelson et al., 1976). Associated with the sexual mores of the times, pharyngitis and proctitis represent areas of infection and spread. Gonococcal arthritis and tenosynovitis occur with some frequency, especially in infants. Gonococcal conjunctivitis in the neonate has returned with its blinding potential. In infants and children parenteral therapy is mandatory. A single dose regimen of soluble or procaine penicillin G (75,000 to 100,000u/kg) intramuscularly in 1 or 2 sites, preceded by 25mg/kg probenecid 1 hour before the injection, can be used in children weighing less than 45kg. Amoxycillin 50mg/kg plus probenecid 25mg/kg as a single oral dose regimen may be used as an alternative. Spectinomycin 40mg/kg as a single intramuscular injection is used in patients with penicillinase producing strains of gonococci or who are allergic to penicillin. Those over 45kg and adolescents are treated as for adults. Whenever gonorrhoea is treated, concomitant syphilis must be diagnosed and treated, or ruled out.

Treatment of syphilis, neonatal gonococcal infection, and the principles of treatment of gonorrhoea and recommendations for therapy in adolescents and adults are discussed in chapter XXIX.

5.1.11 Tuberculosis

Treatment of pulmonary disease is discussed in chapter XX (sect. 8), meningitis in chapter XXV (sect. 13) and urinary infection in chapter XXI (sect. 3.3). Much larger doses of isoniazid are given to children (on a weight basis) than to adults. Toxicity is less frequently encountered.

5.1.12 Tetanus

Tetanus still constitutes a major treatment problem, especially in developing countries where neonatal tetanus in particular is associated with a high mortality.

Treatment has a number of objectives which can be summarised as follows (Saady and Torda, 1973):

1) Sedation of the patient prior to admission to hospital (e.g. phenobarbitone intramuscularly).
2) Establishment and maintenance of a safe airway and adequate ventilation.
3) Management of the source of infection and neutralisation of the circulating toxin (cleansing of wound, penicillin, tetanus immune globulin).
4) Control of muscle spasms (large doses of muscle relaxants).
5) Correction of acid-base imbalance, maintenance of adequate nutrition and hydration (intravenous and later, intragastric feeding).
6) Control of autonomic manifestations (e.g. hyperpyrexia, supraventricular or ventricular arrhythmias, episodic hypertension).
7) Prevention and control of complications (e.g. sputum retention, bronchopneumonia, gastrointestinal bleeding).

On admission, adequacy of the airway and ventilation is first assured. Tetanus immune human globulin or if not available tetanus antitoxin (animal), is given intramuscularly or slowly intravenously. After proper sedation and muscle relaxation, the wound, if present, is cleansed by surgical excision and foreign bodies and necrotic tissue removed. In neonatal tetanus, the umbilical cord must be cleansed. Soluble penicillin G is given in large doses 4 to 8-hourly intravenously for 10 days.

Initial control of spasms is achieved by large doses of diazepam, which can be given intravenously or later by nasogastric tube or intramuscularly. An intravenous regimen involves increments of 0.1mg/kg at 5 minute intervals until the desired result is achieved, with a variable maintenance dose ranging from 4 to 10mg/kg daily by continuous intravenous infusion. Small doses of narcotic analgesics such as pethidine (meperidine) can be given for significant pain.

If diazepam proves inadequate in non-coma producing dosage and vital functions threatened by spasms, the patient is paralysed with a neuromuscular blocking agent such as pancuronium and an endotracheal tube inserted. Tracheostomy should be performed early. Most patients require assisted ventilation. When the patient has been free of spasms for 24 hours, medication is gradually reduced. The effects of neuromuscular blockade should be allowed to wear off, not reversed.

Physiotherapy (e.g. prevention of chest complications) and skilled nursing care are major aids to survival. Upon recovery, a programme of special exercises is used to treat persistent hypertonus, rigidity and joint stiffness. Active immunisation of the recovered patient, the population at risk, proper wound care, and in developing countries, maternal immunisation, is the best means of preventing the disease (Rothstein and Baker, 1978; Schofield, 1973).

5.2 Fever

The best treatment for any problem is its prevention. Mothers should be taught the importance of avoiding overclothing, excessive blankets in bed and the need for ample fluid to allow normal frequency of voiding. Fever in an otherwise healthy child need not necessarily be treated. Indeed, it may actually be a valuable indicator of progress of the disease (Done, 1972). Low fever *per se* is usually of no significant danger to the child, provided that the increased insensible water loss is replaced.

Except in overclothed or overblanketed children, dangerously elevated body temperatures are extraordinarily rare and generally tend to occur as either a terminal event or in patients with serious central nervous system disease affecting temperature regulation. If skin is accessible to dissipate heat, even if temperature is left untreated, it seldom rises above 41°C. Except for febrile convulsions, temperatures as high as 40°C are unlikely to be harmful, as long as fluid intake is maintained. Many children are surprisingly well despite fairly high fever, while others can be miserable with little fever. Unless the fever is very high, the temperature of a febrile child who is reasonably well need not necessarily be reduced.

Febrile convulsions in children are a concern, but it is the rapidity of change of temperature in a febrile child, rather than the level, which determines whether febrile seizures are likely to occur. In most such cases in non-epileptic children, the seizure is frequently the presenting complaint and therefore occurs before a decision on antipyretic therapy can be made (see further section 5.3).

When reduction of fever is considered necessary, excessive clothing should be removed, perspiration be allowed to evaporate and tepid sponge baths (not cold water) given. An antipyretic drug can then be given if still needed. Some clinicians find tepid sponging combined with an antipyretic to be more effective than sponging alone (Steele et al., 1970; Hunter, 1973). Excessively rapid reduction of fever is to be avoided as it can lead to peripheral vascular collapse and death, especially in critically ill infants. Aspirin and paracetamol (acetaminophen) given in the doses in table XI are both highly effective (Koch-Weser, 1976), but because an initial dose of aspirin repeated too often can readily lead to respiratory alkalosis then metabolic acidosis and other evidence of toxicity in an underhydrated febrile infant or young child (Craig et al., 1966; see sect. 2.2.2; 2.4) paracetamol has been preferred by many clinicians.

Paracetamol is available as a liquid preparation (aspirin is insoluble) and may also therefore prove more convenient to administer. However, serious toxicity (acute hepatic necrosis and less commonly acute tubular necrosis) may arise in some cases of accidental poisoning with paracetamol in infants and children (Nogen and Bremner, 1978); as can CNS toxicity in the case of poisoning with aspirin (Craig et al., 1966). In one series, paracetamol poisoning was not severe in children under 5, most of whom ingested less than 5g; whereas liver damage occurred in some children aged 11 to 13, most of whom had ingested more than 5g (Meredith et al., 1978). The pathways of metabolism of paracetamol are different in neonates and infants than in older children and adults (see section 2.3.1), but whether this difference influences the formation of the toxic intermediate metabolite of paracetamol is not known. Certainly, severe paracetamol poisoning requires active treatment in those who have ingested large amounts of the drug (see chapter IX; sect. 6.3). Poisoning is especially difficult to manage in those who have ingested paracetamol in combination with dextropropoxyphene.

5.3 Convulsive Disorders

5.3.1 Febrile Seizures

Febrile seizures are the most common convulsive disorders of early childhood. They usually occur between the ages of 6 months and 5 years, but should be diagnosed only with circumspection after age 3 years. The seizure is major in type and although it is generally brief, it can be prolonged, sometimes leading to status epilepticus and rarely death.

Management of the initial febrile seizure involves prompt treatment with an adequate dose of an antiepileptic drug to control the convulsion, reduction of body temperature by tepid sponging (*not* cold water or alcohol) and administration of an antipyretic (see section 5.2), and recognition and treatment of any infection (e.g. acute bacterial meningitis). Correction of electrolyte imbalance may be required if seizures are resistant to treatment. Phenobarbitone (phenobarbital) sodium was the anticonvulsant most often used but diazepam (0.1 to 0.3mg/kg) slowly intravenously is now more widely used. Initial dosage of phenobarbitone should be of the order of 30 to 60mg per year of age up to a maximum of 250mg, given slowly intravenously. The subcutaneous or intramuscular routes give slower and less predictable results. Intravenous administration is given slowly and well diluted, closely monitoring respiration while the seizure abates. When the child regains consciousness, a relatively large dose of oral phenobarbitone 5mg/kg daily in 3 or 4 divided doses) is usually required to prevent recurrence of seizures until the fever has been reduced and any infection controlled.

Most children have one febrile seizure and no more. However, further febrile seizures must be avoided, particularly in those at risk of epilepsy or other possible neurological sequelae (Nelson and Ellenberg, 1976; Annegers et al., 1979). The approach to prevention after the first seizure is controversial (Fishman, 1979; Wolf, 1979). Some advocate preventive treatment with daily phenobarbitone only in those at most risk while others believe that all children with febrile seizures should be given daily anticonvulsant therapy. A middle course is to instruct parents of a child who has already had a febrile seizure of the importance of detecting and lowering fever, and treating infection. Children with increased risk (e.g. a very severe or atypical first seizure, evidence of prior neurological abnormality) should be treated with daily phenobarbitone (3 to 4mg/kg) after the first seizure and all children after a second seizure. An additional 30mg of phenobarbitone is given at the onset of any fever with an increase in daily dose to 5mg/kg during the fever (Wolf, 1977).

Daily phenobarbitone is continued until age 4, or for 1 seizure-free year (whichever occurs later), and then slowly tapered over at least a month. Compliance is frequently a problem in long term therapy of asymptomatic children. Serum level monitoring aids in evaluating the degree of compliance.

5.3.2 Epilepsy

The treatment of epilepsy in childhood can be divided into drug treatment and general management (see Livingston, 1978; chapter XXV, sect. 2 and 4).

The choice of drug treatment should be based on a precise diagnosis of the type of epilepsy; however, especially in mixed convulsions therapeutic trial is often reverted to. Antiepileptic drugs must be used in adequate dosage, which in the patient with severe seizures sometimes means effective control at the expense of some side effects. The child or parent should be informed of the possible occurrence of side effects and asked to report any unusual symptoms, particularly those (e.g. skin rash, fever and sore throat) related to the agent(s) being prescribed. The importance of omission of even one or two doses should be impressed upon the child and parent. Cooperation of the parent is important during the initiation of drug treatment in order to determine the most effective agent and dosage for an individual child. Monitoring of plasma concentrations is necessary for adequate control of therapy. Psychological testing can be used to monitor the response to therapy in children with epilepsy complicated by learning disabilities.

The duration of treatment cannot be decided in advance and is a difficult decision. It depends on the age of the child and onset of epilepsy, frequency of seizures, type of seizure pattern, aetiological or precipitating factors, results of neurological examination, and so on (Holowach et al., 1972). In general, continuation of antiepileptic drugs for 2 to 3 years after the last seizure is recommended. If the EEG still shows numerous discharges after this time, treatment should be continued with annual review (see below). Otherwise, treatment in the young child can be withdrawn gradually over a period of at least 2 or 3 months. The possibility of seizures recurring cannot be excluded and the child and parent should be informed of this so that they may not be unduly upset by a recurrence, particularly if the child is of school age. An early age of onset of epilepsy and prompt seizure control seem to be associated with the lowest recurrence rate (Holowach et al., 1972).

If the end of a 3 year period of freedom from seizures coincides with adolescence, antiepileptic drug therapy should be continued because the threshold to seizures is reduced and withdrawal of therapy particularly hazardous during adolescence. Drugs used to control absence (petit mal) seizures can be withdrawn (gradually, *not* abruptly) without danger, but small doses of phenobarbitone should be substituted and continued through adolescence to prevent the possible occurrence of major generalised (grand mal) seizures.

Focal seizures and the persistence of a focal abnormality in the EEG are indications to continue anticonvulsants for much longer periods. Similarly, children with psychomotor or temporal lobe seizures may require therapy into adult life. If there is any doubt, antiepileptic drugs should be continued. When therapy is discontinued some patients may be given a supply of phenobarbitone to take when factors known to increase susceptibility to seizures are experienced (e.g. excessive fatigue, immunisation, fever, emotional disturbance etc). Drugs known to precipitate seizures (see chapter XXV; sect. 15.3) should be avoided or used only when essential.

The management of the child with epilepsy is very much more than the prescribing of drugs and involves not merely the child, but his whole family, school and social environment. Education of parents and teachers about the nature of the disease leads to better acceptance of the child at home, at school and in social activities. The aim is to allow as full and normal a life as possible and to promote maximum development of the child's potential. In general, diet, exercise and life itself should proceed according to plans — the best life for all children.

5.4 Vomiting

Vomiting is a symptom, not a diagnosis. It is associated with a number of disorders in infancy and childhood. Vomiting is most commonly caused by overfeeding and/or air swallowing and thus gastric distension. Prevention is the best means of treatment. Symptomatic relief is not a substitute for seeking a diagnosis, particularly since persistent vomiting at all ages of childhood can be the earliest indication of serious underlying disease (e.g. bowel obstruction, septicaemia, gastroenteritis, head trauma).

Vomiting after feeds in early infancy is probably most often due to gastro-oesophageal reflux and not an incorrect milk formula or intolerance of cows' milk. Vomiting due to gastro-oesophageal reflux can be markedly alleviated by positioning. Congenital pyloric stenosis is best treated surgically.

Antiemetic drugs (see chapter XIX; sect. 5.2) must never be used before the cause of vomiting is established and seldom otherwise. Although they can be useful in cases of severe vomiting, even small dosage of metoclopramide and phenothiazines such as prochlorperazine can readily lead to acute dystonic reactions and trismus in young children which are easily confused with tetanus (see chapter XXV; sect. 15.5). The large number of antiemetic drugs speaks against any one being superior. Some examples of the drugs available are given in table XI.

5.5 Corticosteroids in Children

Corticosteroids are valuable agents in a number of diseases in children such as atopic eczema (see section 5.7), severe acute asthma (chapter XX; sect. 3), acute leukaemia (chapt. XXIV; sect. 5.1), the nephrotic syndrome (chapt. XXI; sect. 5), chronic inflammatory bowel disease (chapter XIX; sect. 8), rheumatic carditis (chapter XXII; sect. 2), idiopathic thrombocytopenic purpura (chapter XXIII; sect. 5.3.1) and the adrenogenital syndrome (chapter XVI; sect. 9.4). Systemic corticosteroids, particularly physiological doses, should not be withheld when indicated because of fear of side effects. The clinical pharmacology of corticosteroids, including aspects relating to their use in children is discussed in chapter XVI (sect. 9.1). The rational use and risks of topical corticosteroids in infants and young children are discussed in section 5.7 and chapter XIV (see section 7).

Dosage of systemic corticosteroids in children depends on the disease being treated, the degree of control desired and the extent to which side effects can be accepted (Pearn, 1975). In terms of prednisone, a dose of 10mg in adults is equivalent to a dose of 0.2mg/kg in children or 6mg/m^2 (adults and children) and this relationship can be used for approximate conversion purposes where only adult doses are given in specific disease discussions elsewhere in this book.

Maintenance dosage schedules in children should be divided according to normal diurnal rhythm. For twice daily administration, a common practice is to give two thirds of the dose in the morning and one third in the afternoon. A change to alternate day therapy (double daily dose given on alternate mornings) may be possible if relapse does not occur. If the child can be maintained on the alternate day regimen, it might be possible to minimise growth retardation and suppression of cortisol production rate. Dosage reduction after a short initial phase of high dose therapy must as in adults, be gradual; not more rapidly than halved decremental steps every 3 to 4 days, to the minimum effective level which is possible. Children who have received corticosteroids during the previous year should be given a supply of prednisone tablets to take in the event of stress from accident or illness (e.g. $6mg/m^2$ or $0.2mg/kg$ prednisone per 24h).

Children on corticosteroid therapy readily develop a cushingoid appearance with full red cheeks, striae and abnormal fat deposits. None of these effects are permanent, except the striae which fortunately occur mainly on parts of the body covered by clothes. Overeating may be troublesome in young children. Some children on long term therapy become euphoric, but corticosteroid induced depression and peptic ulcer are rare in children. Other side effects which occur in adults (e.g. osteoporosis) are also rare, but should be watched for in every child on prolonged therapy, especially older children. Specific corticosteroid induced pancreatitis has been described in children (see chapter XIX; sect. 14.5), as have cataracts (see chapter XII; table VI). Growth retardation is by far the most important effect of long term high dosage steroid therapy in children and emphasises the importance of always using the smallest maintenance dose possible to control the disease (see chapter XVI; sect. 14.3). Alternate day regimens (see above) are well worth trying in an attempt to decrease growth suppression. The advent of steroid inhalers such as beclomethasone dipropionate, has allowed many children with severe chronic asthma to avoid the use of systemic steroids and their consequent side effects, including growth retardation (see further chapter XX; section 3.1.2).

A major acute risk with corticosteroid therapy is that an underlying or superimposed infection may proceed unrecognised. Some virus diseases of childhood, particularly varicella, are dangerous in this context (see chapter XXVIII; sect. 3.8). Varicella may be no worse than usual, but occasionally a fulminating attack may occur which results in death. A logical step would be rapid modification of the dose to the equivalent of hydrocortisone 25 to $50mg/m^2$ per 24 hours (i.e. reduced to levels equivalent of endogenous cortisol production during the 'stress reaction'). If reduction cannot be reached within time for varicella to become manifest, then the previous dose should be maintained.

For a further discussion on corticosteroid side effects in both adults and children see chapter XVI (sect. 9.1, 14.3).

5.6 Iron Deficiency Anaemia

Iron deficiency is the most common cause of anaemia in paediatric practice. It is due to nutritional iron deficiency in children between the ages of 6 months and 3 years and may be related to deficiency of maternal stores of iron, blood loss, and especially to excessive ingestion of cow's milk. In those over 3 years of age blood loss is a common cause. Nutritional iron deficiency anaemia can be prevented by identification of children at risk (e.g. babies of anaemic mothers, prematures, small-for-dates, multiple births and those with perinatal blood loss) and through proper balanced nutrition (e.g. avoidance of excessive milk intake, i.e. > 1 litre daily, and/or diet rich in carbohydrate such as cereals, ice cream and tinned non-meat baby foods).

In infants at risk, oral iron therapy (2mg elemental iron/kg daily) should commence from the third month of age and continue for 3 months. In established iron deficiency anaemia, oral iron (6mg elemental iron/kg daily) should be given for at least 2 months. A suitable preparation is ferrous gluconate (1ml = 6mg elemental iron) or ferrous sulphate elixir given in 3 divided doses with fluids other than milk. Parents should be advised that the faeces will change to a black colour. Oral iron is well tolerated. Deciduous teeth may occasionally become temporarily discoloured, but this will not affect permanent teeth. Older children can avoid the staining by drinking a diluted iron solution through a straw. Instructions about proper nutrition are an integral part of iron therapy.

5.7 Skin Diseases

In *napkin (diaper) dermatitis,* the primary irritant is often ammonia released from the urine by the action of bacterial enzymes found in the faeces bacteria (Levin and Hayden-Smith, 1969). It is therefore important to change napkins as soon as they are wet or dirty to prevent urine and faeces soiling the skin for any length of time. Disposable paper napkins offer advantage over reusable cloth ones. Reusable cloth napkins should be boiled (there is no substitute) during washing and rinsed well; soap or detergents exacerbate the eruption. Liberal application of a zinc and castor oil or silicone cream to the napkin area after each change of napkins is often the only local measure required. A topical anticandidal preparation can be used if the eruption is complicated by secondary yeast infection (Montes et al., 1971). Leaving the napkin off with exposure to the air as much as possible is the best treatment.

Seborrhoeic dermatitis of infancy can usually be successfully managed with simple care such as sodium bicarbonate mother made pastes, finally resorting to a low potency topical corticosteroid/antibacterial preparation. Affected infants are remarkably free of deep irritation and rarely scratch. Strong steroid preparations (especially fluorinated ones) should not be used for long periods to treat extensive or resistant areas as there is a significant risk of systemic absorption and local atrophy (Feiwel, 1969). Moreover, large unsightly striae may be formed, especially in the groins and axillae. Hydrocortisone preparations are safer than strong steroids for long term use but less effective. Zinc and crude coal tar (0.5 %) ointment is a useful alternative in babies with widespread eruptions. Scaling of the scalp can be treated with 2 % sulphur and 2 % salicylic acid in white soft paraffin rubbed in well twice daily. The hair should be washed frequently with a good shampoo. A selenium sulphide or other antiseborrhoeic shampoo alone may control mild cases.

Atopic dermatitis or eczema is characterised by marked irritation with scratching and loss of sleep (Norins, 1971). A 1 % hydrocortisone cream or lotion or frequent (4-hourly) wet dressings of diluted (1:8) Burrow's solution are useful in the acute vesicular and weeping phase. When the dermatitis becomes dry and scaly, hydrocortisone ointment can be applied and covered with pieces of bandage coated with 1 to 10 % crude coal tar (strength depending on response and extent of lichenification) in zinc ointment. The covering prevents the child scratching and ensures that the ointment remains in contact with the affected area; however, arm restraints may be necessary to prevent loss of months of improvement in seconds of itching. Zinc paste and ichthamol bandage and zinc paste and coal tar bandage are suitable alternatives. Placing the child on a smooth surface (i.e. plastic) may also prevent the devastation of itching.

Care should be taken to avoid continuous or excessive use of topical corticosteroids. Low potency preparations are used for maintenance, but these may not always be adequate for reasonable control of the disease. Such patients can then be treated for short periods with a preparation of higher potency (see chapter XIV; table III). Trimeprazine can be used as an antipruritic and night time sedative. Infants and children tolerate antihistamines well, although photosensitivity with phenothiazines, such as is trimeprazine, is potentially important in sunny climates. A short course of systemic steroids may be needed in patients with severe atopic eczema and severe asthma to gain more rapid improvement and emotional support for parents (see further chapter XIV; sect. 7).

Some limitation should be placed on bathing; generally adolescents may shower daily but not with hot water or for long periods. Minimal or a neutral soap should be used and the use of emulsifying creams or equivalent can be useful. Sea water is usually tolerated but chlorinated pools may be irritant to some. Secondary impetiginisation is a problem in infants and the risk of viral complication is always present. Kaposi's varicelliform eruption especially associated with herpes simplex is not uncommon. Smallpox vaccination is not absolutely contraindicated (Kempe et al., 1968; Goldstein et al., 1975). Those at greatest risk of developing serious complications from vaccination are also at greatest risk of death from smallpox. Also, risk of a severe reaction decreases with increasing age. Those who must or wish to travel can be vaccinated (in an eczema free body area) in the usual way, provided vaccinia immune globulin is given at the same time. It is, of course, wise to warn the patient of the possible risks (see also chapter XXVIII; sect. 3.5). Patients should avoid other children (sibs or playmates) with fresh vaccination. Other immunisations can be given without risk.

Treatment of some other skin disorders which can affect children are discussed in section 5.1.9 above and in chapter XIV.

5.8 Other Diseases in Children

Treatment of many other diseases which can affect children are discussed in other chapters. Management of diabetes is discussed in chapter XVI (sect. 3.4) and asthma in chapter XX (sect. 3).

Further Reading

Burland, W.L. and Laurance, B.M.: The Therapeutic Choice in Paediatrics (Churchill Livingstone, Edinburgh 1972).

Mirkin, B.L. (Ed): Clinical Pharmacology and Therapeutics: A Pediatric Perspective (Year Book, Chicago 1978).

Morselli, P.L.: Drug Disposition During Development (Spectrum, New York 1977).

Morselli, P.L.; Garattini, S. and Sereni, F.: Basic and Therapeutic Aspects of Perinatal Pharmacology (Raven Press, New York; North-Holland, Amsterdam 1975).

Shirkey, H.C.: Pediatric Therapy, 6th Ed (Mosby, St. Louis 1980).

Yaffe, S.J. (Ed): Pediatric pharmacology. Pediatric Clinics of North America 19: 1 (1972).

References

Altemeier, W.A. and Ayoub, E.M.: Erythromycin prophylaxis for pertussis. Pediatrics 59: 623 (1977).

Anderson, P.O. and Salter, F.J.: Propranolol therapy during pregnancy and lactation. American Journal of Cardiology 37: 325 (1976).

Anderson, P.O.: Drugs and breast feeding — a review. Drug Intelligence and Clinical Pharmacy 11: 208 (1977).

Annegers, J.F.; Hauser, W.A.; Elveback, L.R. and Kurland, L.T.: The risk of epilepsy following febrile convulsions. Neurology 29: 297 (1979).

Aranda, J.V.; Perez, J.; Sitar, D.S.; Collinge, J.; Portuguez-Malavasi, A.; Duffey, B. and Dupont, C.: Pharmacokinetic disposition and protein binding of furosemide in newborn infants. Journal of Pediatrics 93: 507 (1978).

Aserkoff, B. and Bennett, J.V.: Effect of antibiotic therapy in acute salmonellosis on the fecal excretion of salmonellae. New England Journal of Medicine 281: 636 (1969).

Assael, B.M.; Gianni, V.; Marini, A.; Peneff, P. and Sereni, F.: Gentamicin dosage in preterm and term neonates. Archives of Disease in Childhood 52: 883 (1977).

Axline, S.G. and Simon, H.J.: Clinical pharmacology of antimicrobial agents in premature infants. I. Kanamycin, streptomycin and neomycin; in Antimicrobial Agents and Chemotherapy, p.135 (American Society for Microbiology, Ann Arbor 1964).

Axline, S.G.; Yaffe, S.J. and Simon, H.J.: Clinical pharmacology of antimicrobials in premature infants: II. Ampicillin, methicillin, oxacillin, neomycin and colistin. Pediatrics 39: 97 (1967).

Bamford, M.F.M. and Jones, L.F.: Deafness and biochemical imbalance after burns treatment with topical antibiotics in young children. Archives of Disease in Childhood 53: 326 (1978).

Barnett, H.L.; McNammara, H.; Schultz, S. and Tompsett, R.: Renal clearances of sodium penicillin G, procaine penicillin G, and inulin in infants and children. Pediatrics 3: 418 (1949).

Bass, J.W.; Klenk, E.L.; Kotheimer, J.B.; Linnemann, C.C. and Smith, M.H.D.: Antimicrobial treatment of pertussis. Journal of Pediatrics 75: 768 (1969).

Bauer, J.H.; Pape, B.; Zajicek, J. and Groshong, T.: Propranolol in human plasma and breast milk. American Journal of Cardiology 43: 860 (1979).

Becker, M.H.; Drachman, R.H. and Kirscht, J.P.: Predicting mothers' compliance with pediatric medical regimens. Journal of Pediatrics 81: 843 (1972).

Belton, E.M. and Jones, R.V.: Hemolytic anemia due to nalidixic acid. Lancet 2: 691 (1965).

Boreus, L.O.; Jalling, B. and Kallberg, N.: Clinical pharmacology of phenobarbital in the neonatal period; in Morselli, Garattini and Sereni (Eds) Basic and Therapeutic Aspects of Perinatal Pharmacology, p.331 (Raven Press, New York 1975).

Boreus, L.O.; Jalling, B. and Kallberg, N.: Phenobarbital metabolism in adults and in newborn infants. Acta Paediatrica Scandinavica 67: 193 (1978).

Borofsky, L.G.; Louis, S.; Kutt, H. and Roginsky, M.: Diphenylhydantoin: efficacy, toxicity, and dose-serum level relationships in children. Journal of Pediatrics 81: 995 (1972).

Brown, T.C.K.: Paediatric pharmacology. Anaesthesia and Intensive Care 1: 473 (1973).

Buchanan, N.: Drug-protein binding and protein-energy malnutrition. South African Medical Journal 52: 733 (1977).

Catz, C.S. and Giacoia, G.P.: Drugs and breast milk. Pediatric Clinics of North America 19: 151 (1972).

Charney, E.; Bynum, R.; Eldredge, D.; Frank, D.; MacWhinney, J.B.; McNab, M.; Scheiner, A.; Sumpter, E. and Iker, H.: How well do patients take oral penicillin? A collaborative study in private practice. Pediatrics 40: 188 (1967).

Chilcote, R.; Curley, A.; Loughlin, H.H. and Jupin, J.A.: Hexachlorophene storage in a burn patient associated with encephalopathy. Pediatrics 59: 457 (1977).

Churchill Davidson, H.C. and Wise, R.P.: Neuromuscular transmission in the newborn infant. Anesthesiology 24: 271 (1963).

Churchill Davidson, H.C. and Wise, R.P.: The response of the newborn infant to muscle relaxants. Canadian Anaesthetists Society Journal 11: 1 (1964).

Cohen, S.N. and Weber, W.W.: Pharmacogenetics. Pediatric Clinics of North America 19: 21 (1972).

Cohlan, S.Q.; Bevelander, G. and Tiamsic, T.: Growth inhibition of prematures receiving tetracycline. American Journal of Diseases of Children 105: 453 (1963).

Craig, J.O.; Ferguson, I.C. and Syme, J.: Infants, toddlers and aspirin. British Medical Journal 1: 757 (1966).

Davidson, C.: Salicylate metabolism in man. Annals of the New York Academy of Sciences 179: 249 (1971).

Davies, P.A.: Treatment of neonatal bacterial infection. British Medical Journal 2: 676 (1978).

Done, A.K.: Developmental pharmacology. Clinical Pharmacology and Therapeutics 5: 432 (1964).

Done, A.K.: Antipyretics. Pediatric Clinics of North America 19: 167 (1972).

Eckstein, H.B. and Jack, B.: Breast-feeding and anticoagulant therapy. Lancet 1: 672 (1970).

Ecobichon, D.J. and Stephens, D.S.: Perinatal development of blood esterases. Clinical Pharmacology and Therapeutics 14: 41 (1973).

Eeg-Olofsson, O.; Malmros, I.; Elwin, C-E. and Steen, B.: Convulsions in a breast-fed infant after maternal indomethacin. Lancet 2: 215 (1978).

Ehrnebo, M.; Agurell, S.; Jalling, B. and Boreus, L.O.: Age differences in drug binding by plasma proteins: studies on human foetuses, neonates and adults. European Journal of Clinical Pharmacology 3: 189 (1971).

Eichenwald, H.F. and McCracken, G.H.: Antimicrobial therapy in infants and children. Part I. Review of antimicrobial agents. Journal of Pediatrics 93: 337 (1978).

Elling, R.; Wittemore, R. and Green, M.: Patient participation in a pediatric program. Journal of Health and Human Behaviour 1: 183 (1960).

Elliott, R.B.; Stokes, E.J. and Maxwell, G.M.: Ampicillin paediatrics. Archives of Disease in Childhood 39: 1304 (1964).

Ellis, E.F.; Koysooko, R. and Levy, G.: Pharmacokinetics of theophylline in children with asthma. Pediatrics 58: 542 (1976).

Evans, E.F.; Proctor, J.D.; Fratkin, M.J.; Velandia, J. and Wasserman, A.J.: Blood flow in muscle groups and drug absorption. Clinical Pharmacology and Therapeutics 17: 44 (1975).

Feiwel, M.; Percutaneous absorption of topical steroids in children. British Journal of Dermatology 81 (Suppl. 4): 113 (1969).

Fishman, M.A.: Febrile seizures: The treatment controversy. Journal of Pediatrics 94: 177 (1979).

Fredholm, B.B.; Rane, A. and Persson, B.: Diphenylhydantoin binding to proteins in plasma and its dependence on free fatty acid and bilirubin concentration in dogs and newborn infants. Pediatric Research 9: 26 (1975).

Friedman, Z.; Whitman, V.; Maisels, M.J.; Berman, W.; Marks, K.H. and Vesell, E.S.: Indomethacin disposition and indomethacin-induced platelet dysfunction in premature infants. Journal of Clinical Pharmacology 18: 272 (1978).

Friis-Hansen, B.: Body water compartments in children: Changes during growth and related changes in body composition. Pediatrics 28: 169 (1961).

Friis-Hansen, B.: Body composition during growth. Pediatrics 47: 264 (1971).

Fujimori, H. and Imai, S.: Studies on dihydrostreptomycin administered to the pregnant and transmitted to their fetuses. Journal of the Japanese Obstetrics and Gynecological Society 4: 133 (1957).

Gadeke, R.: Unwanted effects of drugs in the neonate, premature and young child; in Meyler and Peck (Eds) Drug-Induced Diseases, vol. 4, p.585 (Excerpta Medica, Amsterdam 1972).

Ganshorn, A. and Kurz, H.: Unterschiede zwischen der Proteinbindung Neugeborener und Erwaschsener und ihre Bedeutung fur die pharmacologische Wirkung. Naunyn-Schmiedebergs Archiv fur Pharmakologie und Experimentelle Pathologie 260: 117 (1968).

Garrettson, L.K.; Procknal, J.A. and Levy, G.: Fetal acquisition and neonatal elimination of a large amount of salicylate. Clinical Pharmacology and Therapeutics 17: 98 (1975).

Gladtke, E. and Heimann, G.: The rate of development of elimination functions in kidney and liver of young infants; in Morselli, Garattini and Sereni (Eds) Basic and Therapeutic Aspects of Perinatal Pharmacology, p.393 (Raven Press, New York 1975).

Glezen, W.P. and Denny, F.W.: Epidemiology of acute lower respiratory disease in children. New England Journal of Medicine 288: 499 (1973).

Goldstein, J.A.; Neff, J.M.; Lane, J.M. and Koplan, J.P.: Smallpox vaccination reactions, prophylaxis, and therapy of complications. Pediatrics 55: 342 (1975).

Gorodischer, R.; Jusko, W.J. and Yaffe, S.J.: Tissue and erythrocyte distribution of digoxin in infants. Clinical Pharmacology and Therapeutics 19: 256 (1976).

Gorodischer, R.; Jusko, W.J. and Yaffe, S.J.: Renal clearance of digoxin in young infants. Research Communications in Chemical Pathology and Pharmacology 16: 363 (1977).

Gostof, P.; Homolka and Zelenka: Les substances derivees du tromexane dans le lait maternel et leurs actions paradoxales sur la prothrombine. Schweizerische Medizinische Wochenschrift 82: 764 (1952).

Goudsouzian, N.G.; Donlon, J.V.; Savarese, J.J. and Ryan, J.F.: Re-evaluation of dosage and duration of action of d-tubocurarine in the pediatric age group. Anesthesiology 43: 416 (1975).

Goutieres, F. and Aicardi, J.: Accidental percutaneous hexachlorophane intoxication in children. British Medical Journal 2: 663 (1977).

Greaves, S.J.; Ferry, D.G.; McQueen, E.G.; Malcolm, D.S. and Buckfield, P.M.: Serial hexachlorophane blood levels in premature infants. New Zealand Medical Journal 81: 334 (1975).

Haggerty, R.J. and Roghmann, K.J.: Noncompliance and self medication in paediatric practice. Pediatric Clinics of North America 19: 101 (1972).

Halkin, H.; Radomsky, M.; Millman, P.; Almog, S.; Blieden, L. and Boichis, H.: Steady state serum concentrations and renal clearance of digoxin in neonates, infants and children. European Journal of Clinical Pharmacology 13: 113 (1978a).

Halkin, H.; Radomsky, M.; Blieden, L.; Frand, M.; Millman, P. and Boichis, H.: Steady state serum digoxin concentration in relation to digitalis toxicity in neonates and infants. Pediatrics 61: 184 (1978b).

Haltalin, K.C.; Nelson, J.D.; Kusmiesz, H.T. and Hinton, L.V.: Optimal dosage of ampicillin for shigellosis. Journal of Pediatrics 74: 626 (1969).

Harley, J.D. and Robin, H.: Jaundice of late onset. Pediatrics 37: 856 (1966).

Heale, W.F.: Management of urinary infections in children. Drugs 6: 230 (1973).

Hill, J.B.: Current concepts: Salicylate intoxication. New England Journal of Medicine 288: 1110 (1973).

Hodgman, J.E. and Burns, L.E.: Safe and effective chloramphenicol dosages for premature infants. American Journal of Diseases of Children 101: 140 (1961).

Holdaway, M.D.: Management of gastroenteritis in early childhood. Drugs 14: 383 (1977).

Holdaway, M.D.: Croup and epiglottitis: Diagnosis and action. Drugs 13: 452 (1977).

Holowach, J.; Thurston, D.L. and O'Leary, J.: Prognosis in childhood epilepsy. New England Journal of Medicine 286: 169 (1972).

Howard, J.B. and McCracken, G.H.: Reappraisal of kanamycin usage in neonates. Journal of Pediatrics 86: 949 (1975).

Hunter, J.: Study of antipyretic therapy in current use. Archives of Disease in Childhood 48: 313 (1973).

Illingworth, R.S. and Finch, E.: Ethylbiscoumacetate (tromexan) in human milk. Journal of Obstetrics and Gynaecology of the British Commonwealth 66: 487 (1959).

Ironside, A.G.: Gastroenteritis of infancy. British Medical Journal 1: 284 (1973).

Jackson, S.T.; Rallison, M.L.; Buntin, W.H.; Johnson, S.B. and Flynn, R.R.: Use of oxandrolone for growth stimulation in children. American Journal of Diseases of Children 126: 481 (1973).

Jacobson, J.A.; McCormick, J.B.; Hayes, P.; Thornsberry, C. and Kirvin, L.: Epidemiologic characteristics of infections caused by ampicillin-resistant Hemophilus influenzae. Pediatrics 58: 388 (1976).

Jalling, B.; Boreus, L.O.; Rane, A. and Sjoqvist, F.: Plasma concentrations of diphenylhydantoin in young infants. Pharmacologia Clinica 2: 200 (1970).

Joint Report by Members of the Association for the Study of Infectious Disease: Effect of neomycin in non-invasive Salmonella infections of the gastrointestinal tract. Lancet 2: 1159 (1970).

Jusko, W.J.; Khanna, N.; Levy, G.; Stern, L. and Yaffe, S.J.: Riboflavin absorption and excretion in the neonate. Pediatrics 45: 945 (1970).

Kalow, W.: Malignant hyperthermia. Proceedings of the Royal Society of Medicine 63: 178 (1970).

Kapikian, A.Z.; Kim, H.W.; Wyatt, R.G.; Cline, W.L.; Arrobio, J.O.; Brandt, C.D.; Rodriguez, W.J.; Sack, D.A.; Chanock, R.M. and Parrott, R.H.: Human reovirus-like agent associated with 'winter' gastroenteritis. New England Journal of Medicine 294: 965 (1976).

Keipert, J.A.: Therapeutic implications of percutaneous absorption of topical corticosteroid in infancy and childhood. Medical Journal of Australia 2: 315 (1971).

Kempe, C.H.; Fulginiti, V.; Minamitani, M. and Shinefield, H.: Smallpox vaccination of eczema patients with a strain of attenuated live vaccinia (CVI-78). Pediatrics 42: 980 (1968).

Kim, P.W.; Yanagi, R.; Krasula, R.W.; Soyka, L.F.; Levitsky, S. and Hastreiter, A.R.: Post-mortem digoxin concentrations in infants; in Proceedings 47th Scientific Session, American Heart Association, Nov. 18-21, Dallas, Texas (1974).

Knowles, J.A.: Breast milk: A source of more than nutrition for the neonate. Clinical Toxicology 7: 69 (1974).

Koch-Weser, J.: Drug therapy: Acetaminophen. New England Journal of Medicine 295: 1297 (1976).

Korsch, B.M.; Gozzi, E.K. and Francis, V.: Gaps in doctor-patient communication. I. Doctor-patient interaction and patient satisfaction. Pediatrics 42: 855 (1968).

Kramer, W.; Inglott, A. and Cluxton, R.: Some physical and chemical incompatibilities of drugs for I.V. administration. Drug Intelligence and Clinical Pharmacy 5: 211 (1971).

Krasner, J.; Giacoia, P. and Yaffe, S.J.: Drug-protein binding in the newborn infant. Annals of the New York Academy of Sciences 226: 101 (1973).

Krauer, B.: Antibacterial therapy under special conditions: Paediatrics Antibiotics and Chemotherapy, vol. 18, p.89 (Karger, Basel 1974).

Kurz, H.; Michels, H. and Stickel, H.H.: Differences in the binding of drugs to plasma proteins from newborn and adult man. II. European Journal of Clinical Pharmacology 11: 469 (1977).

Leer, J.A.; Green, J.L.; Heimlich, E.M.; Hyde, J.S.; Moffet, H.L. and Barron, B.A.: Corticosteroid treatment in bronchiolitis: A controlled, collaborative study in 297 infants

and children. American Journal of Diseases of Children 117: 495 (1969).

Levin, S. and Hayden-Smith, S.: Ammonia dermatitis: 'Nappy rash'. South African Medical Journal 43: 61 (1969).

Levy, G. and Garrettson, L.K.: Kinetics of salicylate elimination by newborn infants of mothers who ingested aspirin before delivery. Pediatrics 53: 201 (1974).

Levy, G. and Yaffe, S.J.: Relationship between dose and apparent volume of distribution of salicylate in children. Pediatrics 54: 713 (1974).

Levy, G.; Khanna, N.N.; Soda, D.M.; Tsuzuki, O. and Stern, L.: Pharmacokinetics of acetaminophen in the human neonate: Formation of acetaminophen glucuronide and sulfate in relation to plasma bilirubin concentration and D-glucaric acid excretion. Pediatrics 55: 818 (1975).

Linnemann, C.C.; Partin, J.C.; Perlstein, P.H. and Englender, G.S.: Pertussis: Persistent problems. Journal of Pediatrics 85: 589 (1974).

Lipton, E.L.; Steinschneider, A. and Richmond, J.B.: The autonomic nervous system in early life. New England Journal of Medicine 273: 147, 201 (1965).

Livingston, S.: Medical treatment of epilepsy. Southern Medical Journal 71: 298, 432 (1978).

Lockhart, C.H. and Battaglia, J.D.: Croup (laryngotracheal bronchitis) and epiglottitis. Pediatric Annals 6: 262 (1977).

Loughnan, P.M.: Digoxin excretion in human breast milk. Journal of Pediatrics 92: 1019 (1978).

Loughnan, P.M.; Greenwald, A.; Purton, W.W.; Aranda, J.V.; Watters, G. and Neims, A.H.: Pharmacokinetic observations of phenytoin disposition in the newborn and young infant. Archives of Disease in Childhood 52: 302 (1977).

McCracken, G.H.: Pharmacological basis for antimicrobial therapy in newborn infants. American Journal of Diseases of Children 128: 407 (1974).

McCracken, G.H. and Eichenwald, H.F.: Antimicrobial therapy in infants and children. Part II. Therapy of infectious conditions. Journal of Pediatrics 93: 357 (1978).

Mandelli, M.; Morselli, P.L.; Nordio, S.; Pardi, G.; Principi, N.; Sereni, F. and Tognoni, G.: Placental transfer of diazepam and its disposition in the newborn. Clinical Pharmacology and Therapeutics 17: 564 (1975).

Mandelli, M.; Tognoni, G. and Garattini, S.: Clinical pharmacokinetics of diazepam. Clinical Pharmacokinetics 3: 72 (1978).

Marget, W.: Special aspects of cephalosporin therapy in infants and children. Postgraduate Medical Journal 47 (Suppl.): 54 (Feb. 1971).

Mattar, M.E.; Markello, J. and Yaffe, S.J.: Inadequacies in the pharmacologic management of ambulatory children. Journal of Pediatrics 87: 137 (1975).

Meffin, P.; Long, G.I. and Thomas, J.: Clearance and metabolism of mepivacaine in the human neonate. Clinical Pharmacology and Therapeutics 14: 218 (1973).

Melish, M.E. and Glasgow, L.A.: Staphylococcal scalded skin syndrome: The expanded clinical syndrome. Journal of Pediatrics 78: 958 (1971).

Meredith, T.J.; Newman, B. and Goulding, R.: Paracetamol poisoning in children. Brit. Med. J. 2: 478 (1978).

Metcoff, J. and Stare, F.: The physiologic and clinical significance of plasma proteins and protein metabolites. New England Journal of Medicine 236: 26 (1947).

Miller, R.P.; Roberts, R.J. and Fischer, L.J.: Acetaminophen elimination kinetics in neonates, children, and adults. Clinical Pharmacology and Therapeutics 19: 284 (1976).

Mohler, D.N.; Wallin, D.G. and Dreyfus, E.G.: Studies in the home treatment of streptococcal disease. New England Journal of Medicine 252: 1116 (1955).

Montes, L.F.; Pittillo, R.F.; Hunt, D.; Narkates, A.J. and Dillon, H.C.: Microbial flora of infant's skin. Comparison of types of microorganisms between normal skin and diaper dermatitis. Archives of Dermatology 103: 400 (1971).

Morselli, P.L.: Clinical pharmacokinetics in neonates. Clinical Pharmacokinetics 1: 81 (1976a).

Morselli, P.L.: Pediatric clinical pharmacology: routine monitoring or clinical trials; in Gouveia, Tognoni and van der Kleijn (Eds) Clinical Pharmacy and Clinical Pharmacology, p.277 (Elsevier/North-Holland, Amsterdam 1976b).

Morselli, P.L.: Drug Disposition During Development (Spectrum, New York 1977).

Morselli, P.L.; Principi, N.; Tognoni, G.; Reali, E.; Belvedere, G.; Standen, S.M. and Sereni, F.: Diazepam elimination in premature and full term infants and children. Journal of Perinatal Medicine 1: 133 (1973).

Morselli, P.L.; Mandelli, M.; Tognoni, G.; Principi, N.; Pardi, G. and Sereni, F.: Drug interactions in the human fetus and in the newborn infant; in Morselli, Cohen and Garattini (Eds) Drug Interactions, p.259 (Raven Press, New York 1974).

Morselli, P.L.; Assael, B.M.; Gomeni, R.; Mandelli, M.; Marini, A.; Reali, E.; Visconti, U. and Sereni, F.: Digoxin pharmacokinetics during human development; in Morselli, Garattini and Sereni (Eds) Basic and Therapeutic Aspects of Perinatal Pharmacology, p.377 (Raven Press, New York 1975).

Morselli, P.L. and Baruzzi, A.: Serum levels and pharmacokinetics of anticonvulsants in the management of seizure disorders; in Mirkin (Ed) Clinical Pharmacology and Therapeutics. A Pediatric Perspective, p.89 (Year Book, Chicago 1978).

Nalin, D.R.; Levine, M.M.; Mata, L.; De Cespedes, C.; Vargas, W.; Lizano, C.; Loria, A.R.; Simhon, A. and Mohs, E.: Comparison of sucrose with glucose in oral therapy of infant diarrhoea. Lancet 2: 277 (1978).

Nelson, J.D.: The changing epidemiology of pertussis in young infants. American Journal of Diseases of Children 132: 371 (1978).

Nelson, J.D.: Oral antibiotic therapy for serious infections in hospitalized patients. Journal of Pediatrics 92: 175 (1978b).

Nelson, J.D. and Haltalin, K.C.: Amoxicillin less effective than ampicillin against Shigella in vitro and in vivo: Relationship of efficacy to activity in serum. Journal of Infectious Diseases 129(Suppl.): 222 (June 1974).

Nelson, K. and Ellenberg, K.: Predictors of epilepsy in children who have experienced febrile seizures. New England Journal of Medicine 295: 1029 (1976).

Nelson, J.D.; Howard, J.B. and Shelton, S.: Oral antibiotic therapy for skeletal infections of children. I. Antibiotic concentrations in suppurative synovial fluid. Journal of Pediatrics 92: 131 (1978a).

Nelson, J.D.; Mohs, E.; Dajani, A.S. and Plotkin, S.A.: Gonorrhea in preschool- and school-aged children. Journal of the American Medical Association 236: 1359 (1976).

Neutze, J.M.; Rutherford, J.D. and Hurley, P.J.: Serum digoxin levels in neonates, infants and children with heart disease. New Zealand Medical Journal 86: 7 (1977).

Nogen, A.G. and Bremner, J.E.: Fatal acetaminophen overdosage in a young child. Journal of Pediatrics 92: 832 (1978).

Norins, A.L.: Atopic dermatitis. Pediatric Clinics of North America 18: 801 (1971).

Nyberg, L. and Wettrell, G.: Digoxin dosage schedules for neonates and infants based on pharmacokinetic considerations. Clinical Pharmacokinetics 3: 453 (1978).

Nyhan, W.L.: Toxicity of drugs in the neonatal period. Journal of Pediatrics 59: 1 (1961).

Ogilvie, R.I.: Clinical pharmacokinetics of theophylline Clinical Pharmacokinetics 3: 267 (1978).

Ohlgisser, M.; Adler, M.; Ben-Dov, D.; Toutelman, U.; Birkhan, H.J. and Bursztein, S.: Methaemoglobinaemia induced by mafenide acetate in children. A report of two cases. British Journal of Anaesthesia 50: 299 (1978).

Orme, M.L.'E.; Lewis, P.J.; de Swiet, M.; Serlin, M.J.; Sibeon, R.; Baty, J.D. and Breckenridge, A.M.: May mothers given warfarin breast-feed their infants? British Medical Journal 1: 1564 (1977).

Pearn, J.H.: Use of corticosteroids in childhood disease. Drugs 10: 426 (1975).

Pedersen-Bjergaard, L. and Petersen, K.E.: Oral absorption of pivampicillin and ampicillin in young children: Cross-over study using equimolar doses of a suspension. Clinical Pharmacokinetics 2: 451 (1977).

Pinsky, W.W.; Jacobsen, J.R.; Gillette, P.C.; Adams, J.; Monroe, L. and McNamara, D.G.: Dosage of digoxin in premature infants. Journal of Pediatrics 94: 639 (1979).

Pitlick, W.; Painter, M. and Pippenger, C.: Phenobarbital pharmacokinetics in neonates. Clinical Pharmacology and Therapeutics 23: 346 (1978).

Pleuckhahn, V.D.; Ballard, B.A.; Banks, J.M.; Collins, R.B. and Flett, P.T.: Hexachlorophane preparations in infant antiseptic skin care: Benefits, risks and the future. Medical Journal of Australia 2: 555 (1978).

Posner, A.C.: Further observations on the use of tetracycline hydrochloride in prophylaxis and treatment of obstetric infections. Antibiotics Annual 1954-1955, p.594 (Antibiotica Inc., New York 1955).

Pynnonen, S.; Kanto, J.; Sillanpaa, M. and Erkkola, R.: Carbamazepine: placental transport, tissue concentrations in foetus and newborn and level in milk. Acta Pharmacologica et Toxicologica 41: 244 (1977).

Rane, A. and Sjoqvist, F.: Drug metabolism in the human fetus and newborn infant. Pediatric Clinics of North America 19: 37 (1972).

Rane, A. and Wilson, J.T.: Clinical pharmacokinetics in infants and children. Clinical Pharmacokinetics 1:2 (1976).

Rane, A.; Lunde, P.K.M.; Jalling, B.; Yaffe, S.J. and Sjoqvist, F.: Plasma protein binding of diphenylhydantoin in normal and hyperbilirubinemic infants. Journal of Pediatrics 78: 877 (1971).

Rane, A.; Garle, M.; Borga, O. and Sjoqvist, F.: Plasma disappearance of transplacentally transferred diphenylhydantoin in the newborn studied by mass fragmentography. Clinical Pharmacology and Therapeutics 15: 39 (1974).

Rane, A.; Bertilsson, L. and Palmer, L.: Disposition of placentally transferred carbamazepine (Tegretol) in the newborn. European Journal of Clinical Pharmacology 8: 283 (1975).

Rasmussen, F.: Excretion of drugs by milk; in Brodie and Gillette (Eds) Handbook of Experimental Pharmacology, Vol. 28 Concepts in Biochemical Pharmacology, pt 1, p.390 (Springer, Berlin 1971).

Rohwedder, H-J.; Simon, C.; Kubler, W. and Hohfnauer, M.: Untersuchungen uber die Pharmacokinetik von Nalidixin-saure bei Kindern Verschiedenen Alters. Zeitschrift fur Kinderheilkunde 109: 124 (1970).

Rothstein, R.J. and Baker, F.J.: Tetanus: Prevention and treatment. J. Amer. Med. Ass. 240: 675 (1978).

Rutter, N.; Milner, A.D. and Hiller, E.J.: Effect of bronchodilators on respiratory resistance in infants and young children with bronchiolitis and wheezy bronchitis. Archives of Disease in Childhood 50: 719 (1975).

Ryder, R.W.; Sack, D.A.; Kapikian, A.Z.; McLaughlin, J.C.; Chakraborty, J.; Rahman, A.S.M.M.; Merson, M.H. and Wells, J.G.: Enterotoxigenic escherichia coli and reovirus-like agent in rural Bangladesh. Lancet 1: 659 (1976).

Saady, A. and Torda, T.A.: Tetanus: Principles of management and review of 37 cases. Anaesthesia and Intensive Care 1: 226 (1973).

Sack, D.A.; Chowdhury, A.M.A.K.; Eusof, A.; Ali, M.A.; Morson, M.H.; Islam, S.; Black, R.E. and Brown, K.H.: Oral hydration in rotavirus diarrhoea. A double blind comparison of sucrose with glucose electrolyte solution. Lancet 2: 280 (1978).

Schiff, D.; Chan, G. and Stern, L.: Clinical implications of bilirubin-albumin binding in the newborn. Revue Canadienne de Biologie 32: 135 (1973).

Schofield, F.D.: Prevention and management of tetanus. Tropical Doctor 3: 103 (1973).

Shaw, L.L. and Marsmann, H.C.: Decisions in the evaluation and treatment of acute viral croup. Pediatric Annals 6: 476 (1977).

Shirkey, H.C.; Drug dosage for infants and children. Journal of the American Medical Association 193: 105 (1965).

Shirkey, H.C.: Clinical pharmacology in ambulatory children. Clinical Pediatrics 7: 639 (1968a).

Shirkey, H.C.: Editorial comment: Therapeutic orphans. Journal of Pediatrics 72: 119 (1968b).

Shirkey, H.C.: Therapeutic orphans 1970. Journal of Infectious Diseases 121: 348 (1970).

Shirkey, H.C.: Clinical pharmacology in pediatrics. Clinical Pharmacology and Therapeutics 13: 827 (1972).

Shirkey, H.C.: Pediatric Therapy, 5th ed (Mosby, St. Louis 1975).

Shirkey, H.C.: Handbook of Paediatric Drugs (Saunders, Philadelphia 1977).

Silverman, W.A.; Anderson, D.H.; Blanc, W.A. and Crozier, D.N.: A difference in mortality rate and in incidence of kernicterus among premature infants allotted to two prophylactic antibacterial regimens. Pediatrics 18: 614 (1956).

Simon, C. and Toeller, W.: Amoxycillin, ein neues Amino-benzylpenicillin. Arzneimittel-Forschung 24: 181 (1974).

Skipworth, G.B.: Boric acid intoxication from 'medicated talcum powder.' Archives of Dermatology 95: 83 (1967).

Smellie, J.M.; Gruneberg, R.N.; Leakey, A. and Atkin, W.S.: Long-term low-dose co-trimoxazole in prophylaxis of childhood urinary tract infection: Clinical aspects. British Medical Journal 2: 203 (1976).

Smith, C.A.: The Physiology of the Newborn Infant, 2nd Ed, p.180 (Thomas, Springfield 1951).

Spratt, H.C.; Ahronheim, G.A. and Marks, M.I.: Common bacterial infections in infancy and childhood (7 parts). Drugs 16: 115, 136, 147, 202, 210, 219, 226 (1978).

Steele, R.W.; Tanaka, P.T.; Lara, R.P. and Bass, J.W.: Evaluation of sponging and of oral antipyretic therapy to reduce fever. Journal of Pediatrics 77: 824 (1970).

Stern, L.; Khanna, N.N.; Levy, G. and Yaffe, S.: Effect of phenobarbital on hyperbilirubinemia and glucuronide formation in newborns. American Journal of Diseases of Children 120: 26 (1970).

Tetzlaff, T.R.; McCracken, G.H. and Nelson, J.D.: Oral antibiotic therapy for skeletal infections of children. II. Therapy of osteomyelitis and suppurative arthritis. Journal of Pediatrics 92: 485 (1978).

Thomas, C.R.: Routine phenobarbital for prevention of neonatal hyperbilirubinemia. Obstetrics and Gynecology 47: 304 (1976).

Tognoni, G.: Antibiotics; in Morselli (Ed) Drug Disposition During Development, p.123 (Spectrum, New York 1977).

Traeger, A.; Noschel, H. and Zaumseil, J.: Zur pharmacokinetik von Indomethazin bei Schwangeren, Kreissenden und deren Neugeborenen. Zentralblatt Fur Gynaekologie 95: 635 (1973).

Tyrala, E.E.; Hillman, L.S.; Hillman, R.E. and Dodson, W.E.: Clinical pharmacology of hexachlorophene in newborn infants. Journal of Pediatrics 91: 481 (1977).

Valdes-Dapena, M.A. and Arey, J.B.: Boric acid poisoning. Three fatal cases with pancreatic inclusions and a review of the literature. Journal of Pediatrics 61: 531 (1962).

Vest, M.F.: The development of conjugation mechanisms and drug toxicity in the newborn. Biology of the Neonate 8: 258 (1965).

Wallace, S.: Factors affecting drug-protein binding in the plasma of newborn infants. British Journal of Clinical Pharmacology 3: 510 (1976).

Wallace, S.: Altered plasma albumin in the newborn infant. British Journal of Clinical Pharmacology 4: 82 (1977).

Way, W.L.; Costley, E.C. and Way, E.L.: Respiratory sensitivity of the newborn infant to meperidine and morphine. Clinical Pharmacology and Therapeutics 6: 454 (1965).

Weiss, C.F.; Glazko, A.J. and Weston, J.K.: Chloramphenicol in the newborn. A physiologic explanation of its toxicity when given in excessive doses. New England Journal of Medicine 262: 787 (1960).

West, J.R.; Smith, H.W. and Chasis, H.: Glomerular filtration rate, effective renal blood flow, and maximal tubular excretory capacity in infancy. Journal of Pediatrics 32: 10 (1948).

Wettrell, G.: Distribution and elimination of digoxin in infants. European Journal of Clinical Pharmacology 11: 329 (1977).

Wettrell, G. and Andersson, K-E.: Clinical pharmacokinetics of digoxin in infants. Clinical Pharmacokinetics 2: 17 (1977).

Wettrell, G.; Andersson, K.-E.; Bertler, A. and Lundstrom, N.R.: Concentrations of digoxin in plasma and urine in neonates, infants, and children with heart disease. Acta Pediatria Scandinavica 63: 705 (1974).

White, R.H.R.: Diseases of the urinary system. Urinary tract infections in children. British Medical Journal 1: 1650 (1977).

Wilson, J.T.: Compliance with instructions in the evaluation of therapeutic efficacy. A common but frequently unrecognised major variable. Clinical Pediatrics 12: 333 (1973).

Wilson, J.T. and Wilkinson, G.R.: Delivery of anticonvulsant drug therapy in epileptic patients assessed by plasma level analyses. Neurology 24: 614 (1974).

Wilson, J.T.; Atwood, G.F. and Shand, D.G.: Disposition of propoxyphene and propranolol in children. Clinical Pharmacology and Therapeutics 19: 264 (1976).

Windorfer, A.; Kuenzer, W. and Urbanek, R.: The influence of age on the activity of acetylsalicylic acid-esterase and protein salicylate binding. European Journal of Clinical Pharmacology 7: 227 (1974).

Wolf, S.M.: The effectiveness of phenobarbital in the prevention of recurrent febrile convulsions in children with and without a history of pre-, peri-, and postnatal abnormalities. Acta Paediatrica Scandinavica 66: 585 (1977).

Wolf, S.M.: Controversies in the treatment of febrile convulsions. Neurology 29: 287 (1979).

Wyatt, R.; Weinberger, M. and Hendeles, L.: Oral theophylline dosage for the management of chronic asthma. Journal of Pediatrics 92: 125 (1978).

Yaffe, S.J. and Juchau, M.R.: Perinatal pharmacology. Annual Review of Pharmacology 14: 219 (1974).

Zangeneh, F. and Steiner, M.M.: Oxandrolone therapy in growth retardation of children. American Journal of Diseases of Children 113: 234 (1967).

Zsigmond, E. and Down, J.R.: Plasma cholinesterase activity in newborns and infants. Canadian Anaesthetists Society Journal 18: 278 (1971).

Chapter V
Geriatric Clinical Pharmacology and Therapeutics

K. O'Malley, T.G. Judge and J. Crooks

Synopsis of Important Principles

1) Elderly patients are particularly susceptible to adverse drug reactions and bear the brunt of unwanted drug effects.

2) Responsiveness to drugs is altered in old age because of change in the processes of drug disposition in the body, altered tissue responsiveness and concurrent influence of associated disease states.

3) Absorption of drugs is probably unaltered. Drug distribution is likely to be affected by the changes in body composition and serum proteins which are known to occur. In particular, the rate and efficiency of drug elimination by the kidney is greatly diminished in old age. Diminished rate of elimination has been shown for some but not for other metabolised drugs.

4) Homeostasis in general becomes less responsive with advancing years so that the compensatory mechanisms which in younger patients help to buffer the body against troublesome side effects are not as effective.

5) Because of the added risks of prescribing for the elderly, particular care must be taken when drug therapy is being considered.

6) The clinician should be clear in his mind that drug treatment is needed at all — many diseases from which the elderly suffer do not require drug treatment.

7) A decision on the type of drug prescribed and on the preparation and dose used should be made with the patient's age and general condition in mind. In general, the elderly patient requires smaller doses of drugs than are customarily given to the young adult.

8) Only those drugs which the patient really needs should be prescribed — the likelihood of medication errors and adverse reactions or interactions increases as the number of drugs prescribed rises.

9) Dose regimens should be made as simple as possible. Special packaging and clear labelling will help to minimise non-compliance with medication instructions. Not infrequently it may be necessary to have a responsible neighbour or relative or community nurse manage drug therapy.

10) Drug regimens should be reviewed regularly so that unnecessary drugs are discontinued.

It has long been known that physiological and pathological changes occur with increasing age and thus the deterioration of organs and enzyme systems may be expected to lead to altered responsiveness to drugs in the elderly. However, because of the wide individual differences in the rates of development and the nature of these changes, and often the presence of multiple disease, in contrast to the fetus (see chapters II, III) and child (see chapter IV), it is not possible to establish a time table of changing drug responsiveness in the elderly. The effective and safe use of drugs in old people therefore becomes an individualised matter with a number of important prescribing and treatment considerations to be kept in mind.

1. General Considerations

The proportion of elderly people in a community varies with its degree of development. Figure 1 shows the percentage of persons 65 years of age and above from 1900 onwards in different countries. This percentage is rising for a number of reasons. In developed countries it is loaded artificially by a falling birth rate due to increasing use of efficient means of contraception, and more

recently by more liberal attitudes towards legalised abortion. At the other end of the scale, medical, economic and social factors operate to prolong life. Although in the United Kingdom for example, the elderly represent only 12 % of the population, they are responsible for approximately 30 % of National Health expenditure on drug prescriptions. With current trends, including increasing application of medical knowledge to the elderly, this figure is likely to increase. Similar patterns exist in the USA (Vestal, 1978), where it is estimated that about 11 % of the population are now aged over 65 years, rising to 17 % by the year 2030. In 1976 the elderly spent about 25 % of the national total expenditure for drugs and sundries.

In hospital practice the rate of adverse drug reactions increases with advancing years so that the incidence in the eighth and ninth decades is approximately 3 times that observed in adult patients under 50 years of age (Hurwitz, 1969). The pattern of adverse drug reactions outside of hospital is different because the factor of misuse of drugs by the elderly must also be considered (Learoyd, 1972). When the multiple disease states in the elderly and the large number of drugs prescribed for the elderly are considered in combination with the increased susceptibility to adverse drug reactions in this age group, it becomes apparent that a large proportion of all unwanted drug effects occur in geriatric patients. The necessity for a critical and conservative approach to drug therapy in the elderly is therefore obvious.

2. Determinants of Altered Drug Responsiveness in the Elderly

There are a number of variables in drug kinetics and tissue sensitivity which may alter the elderly patient's response to drugs. The intensity and duration of drug action is determined mainly by the concentration of free drug at the site of action (see chapter I; sect. 3). The principal factors which operate in determining the amount of free drug at its site of action are represented schematically in figure 2 and the probable changes in these inter-related pharmacokinetic processes which occur with aging indicated (see Crooks et al., 1976; Vestal, 1978). In addition, changes in drug effect may also be due to altered homeostasis, organ sensitivity and to disease. Consideration of adverse drug reactions in general practice reveals that domiciliary patients may be subject to a num-

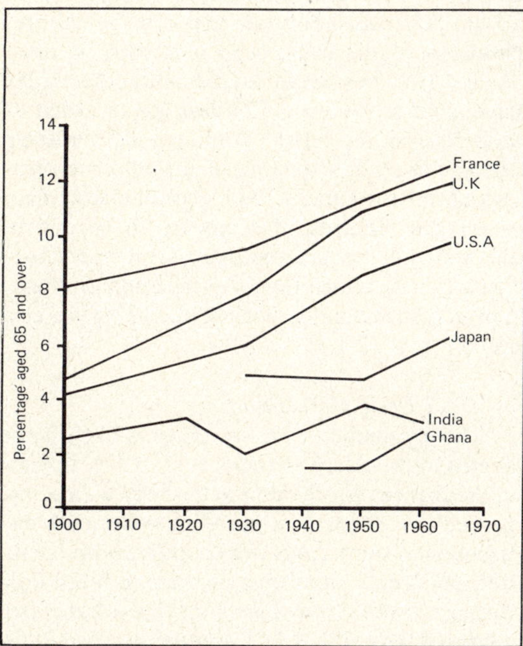

Fig. 1. Percentage of people aged 65 and above from 1900 onwards in 6 countries.

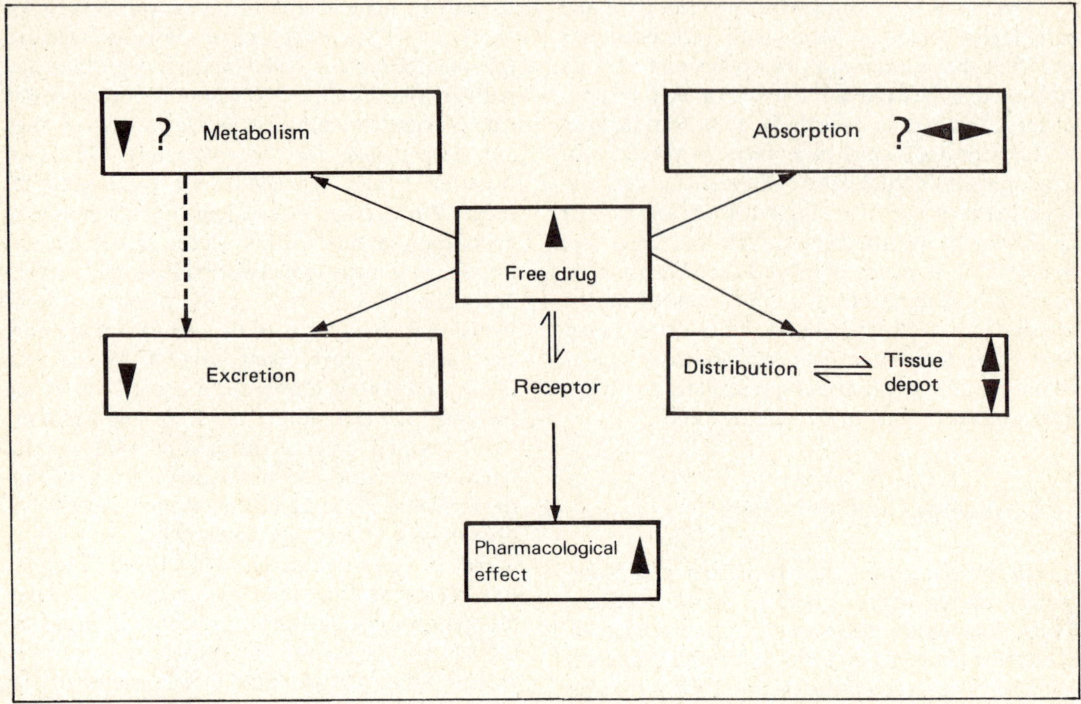

Fig. 2. Highly simplified schematic representation of pharmacokinetic changes (heavy arrows) in the elderly which may influence drug effect (see further chapter I). Absorption is probably unaltered.

ber of *additional* factors which do not apply to the hospitalised patient (see section 3).

2.1 Pharmacokinetic Factors

2.1.1 Drug Absorption

There are a number of changes in the gastrointestinal tract in the elderly which might be expected to alter drug absorption (Bender, 1968). For example, gastric pH rises with advancing years and intestinal blood flow diminishes, and possibly there is also a reduction in the number of absorbing cells, a delay in gastric emptying and a decrease in gastrointestinal motility. There is some evidence to suggest that absorption of some sugars, minerals and vitamins is diminished in the elderly, for example: 3-methylglucose, thiamine, galactose, calcium and organic iron. However, these compounds are absorbed by active transport whereas nearly all drugs are absorbed by passive diffusion (see chapter I; sect. 3.1). There is evidence from one study that the rate and extent of absorption of sulphamethizole, paracetamol (acetaminophen) and phenylbutazone is not affected by increasing age (Triggs et al., 1975). It should be stressed however that commercial preparations of the drugs were not used in these studies. However, recent studies with other drugs have failed to show a diminished rate or extent of absorption in the elderly. Although plasma levels of some drugs at some time after oral administration have been found to be higher in elderly than in younger patients, this appears to be due to alteration in other pharmacokinetic processes, particularly a decreased rate of elimination or alteration in distribution (Crooks et al., 1976; see also section 2.1.2; 2.1.3).

2.1.2 Drug Distribution

The distribution of many drugs is likely to be altered in the elderly (Crooks et al., 1976) in view of the changes which occur in the body with aging, particularly changes in apparent volume of distribution of some drugs (which differs with the individual drug). Although a decrease in blood flow through various vital organs may be a factor (see chapter I; sect. 3.2, 4.3.2), another possible factor may be that under nutrition becomes increasingly common over the age of 70 years. Total body water and lean body mass fall with advancing age. Initially, the loss in lean body mass may be made up on a weight basis by an increase in body fat but eventually even fat tends to be lost.

Probably the most important single factor changing drug distribution in the elderly is simply that these patients are, on average, smaller in body size than younger patients. For example, the smaller body size of the elderly contributes in part to the higher blood levels of digoxin in the elderly following the same intravenous dose to young and elderly patients (see also section 4.1).

Also, as plasma albumin levels are lower in the older age group (Woodford-Williams et al., 1968; Cammarata et al., 1967), important changes in pharmacokinetic behaviour (see chapter I; sect. 3.2) and possibly in response (see chapter VII; sect. 5.1) would be expected for drugs that are highly albumin bound. In fact, the extent of phenytoin (diphenylhydantoin) [Hayes et al., 1975b] and carbenoxolone (Hayes et al., 1977) binding to plasma protein is decreased in the elderly, and these differences correlate with serum albumin levels. However, as a consequence of the decrease in albumin binding, plasma clearance of phenytoin is increased whereas clearance of carbenoxolone is decreased in the elderly (see section 2.1.3). The position with regard to warfarin is not clear (Hayes et al., 1975a; Shepherd and Stevenson, 1978). In a systematic study of the effect of age on the disposition of diazepam (Klotz et al., 1975), a positive correlation was found between age and apparent volume of distribution at steady-state, but no alteration of plasma protein binding was observed and plasma clearance was unaltered (see section 2.1.3). It is reasonable to expect that changes in apparent volume of distribution and correspondingly prolonged plasma clearance of such drugs, may lead to altered pharmacological effect (see chapter I; sect. 3.2.3).

2.1.3 Drug Elimination

In general, drugs are either excreted unchanged by the kidney or are metabolised in the liver to less active or totally inactive compounds before excretion. Renal excretion, and for some drugs metabolism, becomes less efficient with advancing years (for review, see Crooks et al., 1976; Vestal, 1978). This decreased capacity to eliminate some drugs is probably one of the main reasons for the increased sensitivity of the elderly patient to therapeutic agents.

Metabolism

Diminished drug metabolising capacity in aged animals has been well documented. It has been felt for some time that the elderly have a diminished capacity to metabolise drugs (Crooks et al., 1976). The plasma half-lives of antipyrine[1], phenobarbitone and paracetamol (acetaminophen) — drugs which are totally or mainly metabolised by hepatic microsomal enzymes — are prolonged in the elderly. Similarly, the plasma half-lives of diazepam and lignocaine are lengthened in the elderly (Klotz et al., 1975; Nation et al., 1977). However, their volume of distribution is also increased and plasma clearance is, in fact, unaltered. Phenytoin (diphenylhydantoin) binding to albumin is decreased in the elderly; the increase in fraction of unbound drug leading to a shorter plasma half-life and more rapid plasma clearance than in young people (Hayes et al., 1975b). On the other hand, while binding of carbenoxolone to albumin is also decreased in the elderly, the plasma half-life is prolonged and, in the absence of a change in volume of distribution, plasma clearance of carbenoxolone is decreased (Hayes et al., 1977). It is apparent that plasma half-lives do not necessarily reflect the rate of drug metabolism as volume of distribution is an important determinant of rate of elimination, and that the consequences of a change in protein binding differ with individual drugs (see chapter I, sect. 2.1.3; 3.2.3). Interestingly, the rate of ethanol elimination is unaffected by age (Vestal et al., 1977). Similarly the rate of elimination of isoniazid is unaltered (Farah et al., 1977). Ethanol is mainly metabolised by alcohol dehydrogenase and isoniazid is acetylated. Neither of these occur in the microsomal fraction whereas the other examples discussed are all of drugs metabolised by hepatic microsomal enzymes.

Thus, while there is some evidence for a decreased rate of hepatic microsomal metabolism of particular drugs (table I), the importance of age-related changes in drug metabolising capacity is not yet clear. In the absence of a change in volume of distribution, diminished rate of drug metabol-

---

1   The rate of elimination of antipyrine is used as an index of hepatic microsomal (oxidation) drug metabolising ability as it is completely metabolised in the liver and is not bound to plasma protein to a significant extent. The rate of elimination therefore is considered to be dependent mainly on hepatic microsomal oxidation ability. Antipyrine elimination rate cannot be used to predict drug metabolising ability by other pathways (see also chapter I; sect. 4.1).

Table I. Pharmacokinetic parameters for some hepatically metabolised drugs showing altered disposition in the elderly (see also Crooks et al., 1976)

Drug	'Young' subjects (< 50 years)[1]				'Old' subjects (> 50 years)[1]				Reference[2]
	$t_{1/2}\beta$ (h)	Vd (L/kg)	plasma clearance	protein binding	$t_{1/2}\beta$ (h)	Vd (L/kg)	plasma clearance	protein binding	
High clearance drugs[3]									
Chlormethiazole	6.2		222ml/min/kg	69%	6.3		35ml/min/kg	60%	a
Desipramine[4]	34				76				b
Imipramine	19				24				b
Lignocaine	1.3	0.9	7.6ml/min/kg		2.3	1.6	8.1ml/min/kg		c
Morphine	3	3.2	14.7ml/min/kg		4.5[5]	4.7	12.4ml/min/kg		d
Propranolol (IV)	2.5	3.0	13.2ml/min/kg		4.3	2.7	7.8ml/min/kg		e
(oral)	3.5				3.5				
Low clearance drugs (binding sensitive)[3]									
Carbenoxolone	16.3	0.1	4.7ml/h/kg	798μmol/L	22.9	0.1	3.3ml/h/kg	640μmol/L	f
Chlordiazepoxide	10.1	0.4	36ml/h/kg	97%	18.2	0.5	24ml/h/kg	97%	g
Diazepam									
males	38.7	1.2	22.2ml/h/kg		93.8	1.7	14.4ml/h/kg		h
	24	1.0	34.5ml/min		35.8	1.6	32.8ml/min		i
females	44	1.7	28.2ml/h/kg		86.3	3	25.8ml/h/kg		h
	43.9	1.3	20.7ml/min		56.6	1.9	25.5ml/min		i
both sexes[6]	20	0.7	25ml/min	97%	90	1.7	25ml/min	97%	j
Desmethyldiazepam[7]	51	0.6	11.3ml/min		151	0.9	4.3ml/min		k
Lorazepam	14.3	1.1	59.4ml/h/kg		15.9	1.0	46.8ml/h/kg		h
Oxazepam	5.1	0.6	113.5ml/min	87%	5.6	0.8	136ml/min	89%	la
Nitrazepam	29	2.4	4.1L/h		40	4.8	4.7L/h		l
Phenylbutazone[8]	81	0.2	0.09L/h		105	0.1	0.07L/h		m
	110	0.2			87	0.2			n
				96%				94%	o
Phenytoin (oral)			26ml/h/kg	727μmol/L			42ml/h/kg	595μmol/L	p
(IV)			44.3ml/h/kg				67.3ml/h/kg		p
Quinidine	7.3	2.4	240ml/h/kg	75%	9.7	2.2	156ml/h/kg	72%	q
Sulphamethizole	1.75	0.4	167ml/min/1.73m²		3.0	0.4	90ml/min/1.73m²		n
Warfarin	37	0.2	3.8ml/h/kg		44	0.2	3.3ml/h/kg		r
				561μmol/L				451μmol/L	s
				98%				97%	t

Low clearance drugs (binding insensitive)[3]							
Antipyrine							
males	12.7	0.6	35ml/h/kg	14.8	0.5	28ml/h/kg	u
	12.2	0.6		17.5	0.6		v
females	12.7	0.6		16.1	0.5		v
both sexes[9]	12			17.4			m
Paracetamol	1.8	1.0	477ml/min/1.73m^2	2.2	1.0	379ml/min/1.73m^2	n
(acetaminophen)	1.8			2.3			w
Theophylline	5.8	0.5	57ml/h/kg	7.7	0.4	35.7ml/h/kg	x, y[10]

1   All data are expressed as mean values.

2   References:

a = Nation et al.: Euro. J. Clin. Pharm. 12: 137 (1977)

b = Robinson et al.: Clin. Pharm. Ther. 21: 116 (1977)

c = Nation et al.: Brit. J. Clin. Pharm. 4: 439 (1977)

d = Stanski et al.: Clin. Pharm. Ther. 24: 52 (1978)

e = Castleden and George: Brit. J. Clin. Pharm. 7: 49 (1979)

f = Hayes et al.: Gut 18: 1054 (1977)

g = Shader et al.: J. Clin. Pharm. 17: 709 (1977)

h = Greenblatt et al.: Clin. Pharm. Ther. 25: 227 (1979)

i = MacLeod et al.: J. Clin. Pharm. 19: 15 (1979)

j = Klotz et al.: J. Clin. Invest. 55: 347 (1975)

k = Klotz and Muller-Seydlitz: Brit. J. Clin. Pharm. 7: 119 (1979)

l = Ilsala et al.: Brit. J. Clin. Pharm. 4: 646P (1977)

la = Shull et al.: Ann. Int. Med. 84: 420 (1976)

m = O'Malley et al.: Brit. Med. J. 3: 607 (1971)

n = Triggs and Nation: J. Pharmacokin. Biopharm. 3: 387 (1975)

o = Wallace et al.: Brit. J. Clin. Pharm. 3: 327 (1976)

p = Hayes et al.: Brit. J. Clin. Pharm. 2: 73 (1975)

q = Ochs et al.: Amer. J. Card. 42: 481 (1978)

r = Hewick et al.: Brit. J. Clin. Pharm. 2: 189P (1975)

s = Hayes et al.: Brit. J. Clin. Pharm. 2: 69 (1975)

t = Shepherd and Stevenson: Clin. Pharm. Ther. 23: 129 (1978)

u = Vestal et al.: Clin. Pharm. Ther. 18: 425 (1975)

v = Liddell et al.: Clin. Exp. Pharm. Phys. 2: 481 (1975)

w = Briant et al.: N.Z. Med. J. 82: 136 (1975)

x = Ellis et al.: Pediatrics 58: 542 (1976)

y = Nielsen-Kudsk et al.: Acta Pharm. Toxicol. 42: 226 (1978)

3   See chapter I (sect. 4.3.3), chapter XIX (sect. 1.4).

4   Studied as a metabolite of imipramine.

5   'Old' subjects were surgical patients, 'young' subjects were healthy volunteers.

6   Mainly males (27 males, 6 females). Age was examined as a continuous variable; values quoted are approximate.

7   Desmethyldiazepam is the major active metabolite of diazepam (see chapter XXVI; sect. 1.4.3). Study was in male subjects only.

8   In reference m the geriatric group was mainly female (15 vs 6); in reference n only male subjects were studied. Differences in $t_{1/2\beta}$ were not statistically significant between age groups in either study.

9   In 'young' subjects sex ratio was about equal, but mainly females (15 vs 4) in 'old' group. In 'young' group $t_{1/2\beta}$ was 30% longer in males than in females.

10   Data for 'young' and 'old' subjects are from 2 separate studies in 'healthy' subjects.

ism would lead to a rise in plasma levels of active drug, and hence an increased intensity of pharmacological action for a given dosage (see chapter I; sect. 3.3.1).

The possible contribution and clinical importance of nutritional and environmental factors and enzyme induction response on rate of drug metabolism in the elderly also requires clarification (Vestal, 1978; see also chapter I, sect. 3.3.5).

Renal Excretion

Many drugs are eliminated either solely by the kidney or in large part by this route. In many cases the drugs are excreted by glomerular filtration and their rate of excretion correlates with glomerular filtration rate (and hence with creatinine clearance) — e.g. digoxin and the aminoglycoside antibiotics (see chapter XXI; sect. 14.1, 14.2). In old age renal function diminishes, even in the absence of apparent renal disease, so that at the age of 65 years there is a reduction of approximately 30% in glomerular filtration rate compared with normal young adults (Davies and Shock, 1950; Rowe et al., 1976). Similarly, tubular function deteriorates with age (Miller et al., 1952) so that drugs such as penicillin, which are secreted by the renal tubule, have diminished rates of elimination in the elderly (Hansen et al., 1970). In addition to the physiological decline in tubular and glomerular filtration, the geriatric patient is particularly liable to renal impairment due to dehydration, congestive heart failure, hypotension and urinary retention, or to intrinsic renal involvement, e.g. diabetic nephropathy or pyelonephritis (see also chapter XXI; sect. 1).

Where there is obvious renal disease, reference should be made to tables of recommended drug dosage for guidance (see also table III; chapter I, sect. 4.3.4; chapter XXI, sect. 14 and appendix E). It should also be remembered that even when blood urea or creatinine is normal, elderly patients have a smaller renal reserve than do younger people and therefore the dose of renally excreted drugs employed should always be chosen with this in mind. With some drugs this is particularly important because of the seriousness of the effects of overdosage; e.g. digoxin (Caird, 1974; Ewy et al., 1969), aminoglycoside antibiotics (Kristensen et al., 1974), lithium (Hewick et al., 1977) and chlorpropamide. In general, elderly patients are best treated with lower doses of renally excreted drugs than are younger patients (Crooks et al., 1976).

2.2 Pharmacodynamic Factors

Despite the presence of many differences in drug handling which help to account for the dissimilarities between the old and the young, there is still a residue of altered responsiveness which seems to be explicable only by differences in tissue 'sensitivity' to drugs. This age-dependent difference in responsiveness is so great with some drugs that the difference appears almost to be qualitative. The reaction of elderly patients to barbiturates provides a well known example (Bender, 1964); the response to this group of drugs may vary from mild restlessness to frank psychosis in a significant proportion of patients. While the increased susceptibility may in part be explained by a diminished capacity to metabolise these drugs, inappropriate responses may occur following a single dose, suggesting that there is an actual difference in the sensitivity of the elderly brain to these agents. Adverse reactions are so common with barbiturates in the elderly that they should be used very sparingly, indeed.

'Sensitivity' may also be altered by the presence of disease, either directly by the pathological process of aging or indirectly by associated complications such as peripheral circulatory failure, anaemia, malnutrition, or hepatic, cardiac and renal failure (see relevant sections in other chapters). The increased risk of haemorrhagic complications of anticoagulants in the elderly is, in part at least, due to degenerative vascular disease diminishing the haemostatic response. In the case of warfarin there appears to be an increased sensitivity at the level of clotting factor synthesis (Shepherd et al., 1977; see also section 4.6). Other homeostatic mechanisms are also considerably blunted in geriatric patients. Postural hypotension is particularly evident in this age group and many non-specific unwanted drug effects in the elderly such as dizziness, confusion, agitation, weakness, altered bowel habit etc. may reflect effects that in the younger patient would be prevented by more efficient homeostatic mechanisms.

While impaired homeostasis appears to be an integral part of the aging process it may be difficult on occasion to decide what degree of degenerative change is normal in aging. Advancing age brings about an interplay of the aging process and chronic degenerative disease and they frequently merge imperceptibly. However, from the point of view of those factors affecting response to drugs, the distinction between aging and associated pathology is often only an academic one.

Table II. Summary of principles of drug prescribing in the elderly

1. *Is drug therapy required?*
   a) Many diseases from which the elderly suffer do not require drug treatment.
   b) But, do not withhold drugs on account of old age, particularly when appropriate drug treatment can improve the quality of life.
   c) Only use those drugs which the patient really needs.
   d) Drug regimens should be reviewed regularly so that unnecessary drugs are discontinued.
   e) Remember that drugs may cause illness.

2. *Choice of appropriate drug and preparation*
   a) Is a particular drug which is satisfactory for the younger patient suitable for the elderly? — e.g. increased likelihood of side effects.
   b) Which preparation? — consider dosage form (syrup, effervescent tablet, suppository instead of capsule or tablet); its size, shape and colour.

3. *Dose and dosage regimen*
   a) In general, use smaller doses than are usually given to younger adults.
   b) Intermittent schedules should be avoided. Once daily dosage is ideal.

4. *Medication instructions*
   a) Teach the patient to understand his drugs, especially their relative importance to his well being, and their correct use and administration.
   b) Drugs prescribed should be clearly labelled in large print and packaged in readily opened containers.
   c) Supervision of therapy may sometimes be desirable or necessary — e.g. a responsible and interested neighbour, relative or friend, or a community nurse.

3. Principles of Prescribing Drugs for the Elderly

Because of multiple disease states and the wide use of drugs in the elderly, the potential for altered responsiveness to drugs and the higher incidence of adverse effects compared with the younger patient, it is important to define certain basic principles of prescribing for the older patient (Anderson, 1974; Vestal, 1978; table II).

1) Is drug therapy required?

It is important to realise that many of the diseases from which the elderly suffer are doing the patient no immediate harm and do not require treatment. Certainly there is no need to prescribe a different drug for each disease or symptom simply because of the multiple pathology present in the elderly. Indeed, it is surprising how often the elderly are better off without some drugs. Many old people admitted to hospital or reviewed during long term hospitalisation improve greatly when the regimen of drugs that they have been taking is stopped (Burr et al., 1977; Learoyd, 1972). This also means that a drug should not be used for longer than necessary: the need for repeat prescriptions should be reviewed at periodic intervals. These edicts do not mean, however, that drugs should be withheld on account of old age, particularly when appropriate drug treatment can improve the elderly person's quality of life.

2) If drug treatment is required, which drug is appropriate?

The margin between therapeutic effect and toxicity is so small in many cases that a drug which is indicated for a particular condition in younger patients (for example, carbenoxolone for gastric ulceration) may be unsuitable in the elderly with the same condition. Similarly the age related toxicity of barbiturates (section 2.2) makes the use of this group of drugs undesirable in the elderly. Other types of hypnotics will be more appropriate (see section 4.7.1).

3) Is the patient being asked to take more drugs than he can tolerate or manage?

The fewest drugs that the patient *needs* should always be used. The more drugs prescribed the greater the chance of adverse drug reactions (see also chapter VII; sect. 3) or drug interactions (see chapter VIII) — the likelihood of toxicity increases as the number of drugs prescribed rises. In addition, there is an increased likelihood of errors by the patient in taking the medication, leading to a possible lack of efficacy or an increase in toxicity. Medication errors, especially of omission, non-comprehension and non-compliance with medication instructions are common in the elderly (Schwartz et al., 1962; Parkin et al., 1976). Slowness of comprehension and lapses of memory, particularly short term memory which deteriorates with age, make it difficult for the elderly to manage complex drug regimens (see also below).

4) Which type of preparation to be used?

Apart from the total number of drugs prescribed, the dosage form, and the size, shape and colour of tablets and capsules and their similarity to one another, are all important con-

Table III. Examples of drugs usually given in reduced dosage in the elderly

Drug	Dosage	Comments (see also text)
Carbamazepine	100mg daily, increasing by 100mg every 4th or 5th day. Reduce dose if drowsiness or ataxia develop	See further, chapter XXV (sect. 3.4)
Chlormethiazole	250mg 3 times daily	See section 4.7.1
Chlorpropamide	50 to 500mg daily	Danger of cumulation See further, section 4.3
Digoxin	62.5 to 250µg daily	See further section 4.1.1; chapter XVII, section 8.1.3, 8.1.5
Flurazepam	5.0 to 15mg	Unwanted CNS depression more common with larger doses (see section 4.7.1)
Frusemide (furosemide)	20 to 80mg daily	May need to be given very early in the morning (see section 4.1.2)
Haloperidol	0.5 to 1mg 2 or 3 times daily	Danger of severe extrapyramidal signs (see section 4.7.2)
Levodopa	50mg daily at first, increasing by 50mg at weekly intervals	
Metoclopramide	5mg	Confusion common with larger doses
Nitrazepam	2.5 to 5mg	Cumulation common and unwanted CNS depression more common with larger doses (see section 4.7.1)
Pethidine (meperidine)	Orally: 50 to 100mg IM/IV: 25 to 100mg	50mg usual limit in those with respiratory failure (see further chapter X; sect. 8.4)
Sulthiame	100mg 3 times daily	Can be increased to 600mg daily if needed (see section 4.7.4)
Thioridazine	10mg 3 times daily	Confusion common in larger dose
Thyroxine	50µg daily, increasing by 50µg at weekly intervals	See further chapter XVI (sect. 5.1)
Vitamin D	1,000 units daily or 100,000 units by injection on every 3rd month	See further chapter XXII (sect. 11.2)
Warfarin	10mg as a loading dose, 3 to 8mg on the 3rd day and daily thereafter as per test of clotting time	Many factors can influence response to oral anticoagulants (see section 4.6; chapter XXIII; sect. 3.2.4)

siderations (Mazullo, 1972). Many older people have difficulty in swallowing, consequently large tablets and capsules should be avoided. There is a good case for the use of liquid preparations such as syrups for many patients, or of effervescent tablets. On occasion, the suppository may be the most suitable method of administration, for example, indomethacin at night for relief of nocturnal pain and morning stiffness of rheumatoid arthritis, or oxycodone as a substitute for morphine or pethidine (meperidine).

Many tablets and capsules of widely differing pharmacological actions are of similar size, shape and colour. This causes confusion for the patient; the loss of vision of the elderly in particular makes it difficult for them to determine which preparation they are taking. Touch and colour vision are however, well preserved in the elderly. Thus preparations to be used together should not be of the same colour or the same shape.

'The more distinctive the pill is, the easier and safer it is to use.'

5) Should the standard dosage or dosage schedule be modified?

As a rule the elderly patient requires smaller doses of drugs than are customarily given to the young adult, e.g. the starting dose of thyroxine and the maintenance dose of digoxin (see also section 2.1.3). Drugs usually given in reduced dosage in the elderly are listed in table III. Whenever possible, intermittent schedules, such as drugs given on alternate days or 5 days a week should be avoided, since they are rarely followed with accuracy. Once daily dosage is the ideal, whenever feasible (see also chapter I; sect. 3.3.1). Apart from convenience to the patient and thereby better patient compliance, once daily dosage at night, for example of psychotherapeutic drugs (Ayd, 1972, 1974), may well avoid troublesome adverse reactions since the patient would be asleep when these effects would be most annoying (see also section 4.7; chapter XXVI, sect. 2). Other drugs may be best given as a single dose in the morning, for example diuretics (see section 4.1.2).

6) Which side effects are likely to occur? Which drugs should be avoided if possible? (see tables IV and V).

The elderly differ from the young in that drugs more frequently lead to confusion and vague ill health. Drugs which act on various systems such as the gastrointestinal tract for example, are more apt to produce gastrointestinal upset in the aged.

Table IV. Drugs with potentially severe or unusual side effects in the elderly

Drug	Unwanted effect
Benzhexol (trihexphenidyl)	Visual and auditory hallucinations
Chlorpromazine	Postural hypotension, hypothermia
Emepronium bromide	Mouth ulceration (if tablet not swallowed), bromidism
Ethacrynic acid	Deafness
Mefenamic acid	Diarrhoea
Methyldopa	Drowsiness and depression
Oestrogens	Fluid retention and congestive cardiac failure
Disopyramide	Urinary retention
Isoniazid	Hepatotoxicity

Similarly, psychotherapeutic drugs may frequently induce markedly abnormal behavioural responses in older patients, while in younger patients these are much less common (see section 4.7; Davison, 1971, 1972).

7) Should the drug be specially packed and labelled?

Where possible, drugs prescribed for the elderly living at home should be packaged in readily opened containers so that disabled patients in particular are able to use them (Law and Chambers, 1976). Clear labelling in large print is also very important.

8) Can the patient living at home manage self medication?

The elderly patient should be taught to under stand his drugs, particularly their relative importance to his well being, and time should be spent to educate him in their use and administration (Gibson and O'Hare, 1968). Sometimes it may be necessary to provide clear instruction in writing about the manner in which a drug should be taken or to suggest the use of a diary or calendar to record daily drug administration (Wandles and Davie, 1977).

Collaboration with a responsible and interested relative, neighbour or friend can be helpful. Even with these and other considerations, discussed above, some drugs are best kept in the custody of others. Recent surveys have shown that many elderly patients living at home have potent drugs prescribed for them when they are mentally unfit to be responsible for their use (Shaw and Opit, 1976). It is imperative in such cases that a responsible relative should have charge of drug treatment. If there are no relatives it may be necessary to ask the community nurse to administer drug therapy. Sometimes these arrangements are necessary for physical reasons, for example, an elderly diabetic with impaired vision cannot be expected to measure out an injection of insulin with safety.

9) Is there a need for continued medication?

Because a drug such as digoxin has been prescribed in an acute episode, for example, atrial fibrillation complicating pneumonia, there is no reason for its continued use once the acute episode is satisfactorily treated. The same is true of many drugs commonly prescribed. It is useful to review treatment regularly and discontinue drugs no longer wanted (Burr et al., 1977; Learoyd, 1972).

Table V. Drugs to be avoided in the elderly if possible

Drug	Reason
All barbiturates	Confusion (see section 2.2)
Bethanidine	Severe postural hypotension (see chapter XVIII; sect. 5.4)
Carbenoxolone	Fluid retention and congestive cardiac failure (see chapter XIX; sect. 4.3.4)
Chlorthalidone	Prolonged diuresis, incontinence (see section 4.1.2)
Debrisoquine	Postural hypotension (see chapter XVIII; sect. 5.4)
Guanethidine	Postural hypotension (see chapter XVIII; sect. 5.4)
Pentazocine	Confusion. Variable efficacy (see chapter X; sect. 8.4)
Reserpine	Depression (see chapter XXVI; sect. 15.2)
Streptomycin	Ototoxicity (see chapter XI; sect. 7.1.1)
Tetracycline	Rising blood urea in the presence of impaired renal function (see chapter XXI; sect. 15.2.2)

Elderly patients tend to hoard drugs (Law and Chambers, 1976). Accumulation of medication will only serve to confuse the patient and encourage use of drugs from prior treatment programmes. To aid in the review of old, and current medication, patients should be encouraged to bring their containers to consultations in private practice and also in hospital outpatient departments. Any medication not required can then be destroyed.

4. Drug Treatment in the Elderly

The principles of treatment which pertain especially to older patients can be illustrated by a discussion of a variety of clinical syndromes and symptoms frequently found in the aged and in which the response to drugs commonly used for the conditions can be different from that occurring in younger patients. Further discussion on these and other conditions occurring in the elderly is given in other chapters (see also reviews by Crooks and Stevenson, 1979; Judge and Caird, 1978; Vestal, 1978).

4.1 Congestive Heart Failure

Causative and precipitating factors require careful attention and specific treatment, e.g. paroxysmal arrhythmias. The mainstays of treatment in congestive heart failure are the cardiac glycosides and diuretics. Many of the problems encountered in the treatment of cardiac failure are not peculiar to geriatric patients. However, older patients are particularly susceptible to certain hazards of the drugs which are used in the treatment of this condition.

4.1.1 Digitalis Glycosides

Side effects of this group of drugs are particularly common in the elderly (Evered and Chapman, 1971; Ogilvie and Ruedy, 1972). Digoxin is the glycoside most commonly used in clinical practice. It is excreted almost completely unchanged by the kidney (normal plasma half-life, 30 to 40 hours approximately), only about 10% being metabolised. Digitoxin (normal plasma half-life, 5 to 7 days) is occasionally used and is extensively metabolised in the liver and is excreted mostly in the urine as cardioinactive metabolites; a small proportion is however, excreted as digoxin and unchanged digitoxin. Other cardiac glycosides include lanatoside C and deslanoside. Lanatoside C is poorly absorbed following oral administration but deslanoside enjoys some popularity for parenteral administration (chapter XVII; sect. 8.1.3).

Determinants of Digitalis Toxicity in the Elderly: The following factors probably contribute to the very narrow gap between therapeutic and toxic doses of digoxin in the elderly:

1) Decreased body size.
2) Impaired renal function.
3) Presence of advanced cardiac vascular disease.
4) Frequency of electrolyte imbalance.

Manifestations of Digoxin Toxicity in the Elderly: In the elderly, the manifestations of digoxin toxicity may be quite different from those found in younger patients (Church and Marriott, 1959; Dall, 1965). The older patients frequently present with psychiatric disturbances such as confusion, depression and even psychosis. Inquiry should always be made about visual disturbances whenever digitalis intoxication is suspected. While digitalis glycosides may cause virtually any disturbance of cardiac rhythm known, some of the classical findings such as nausea, vomiting and bradycardia are frequently absent in this age group. Two pitfalls for the unwary should be mentioned:

1) A clinically detected change in rhythm from atrial fibrillation to a regular rhythm of say 100 per minute should always be checked electrocardiographically because regular nodal rhythm can be a manifestation of digoxin overdose.

2) In the absence of nausea and vomiting, digoxin toxicity may manifest itself by worsening of congestive heart failure accompanied frequently by a rise in pulse rate. Stopping digoxin for 48 to 60 hours may result in dramatic improvement.

Digoxin Dosage: While an accurate assessment of body mass is not practicable, a rough estimate should be consciously made, such as large, medium and small, and the digitalising dose tailored accordingly. Because of the increased risk of toxicity in the elderly and since even a small dose of digitalis produces a useful therapeutic effect in heart failure, many clinicians now avoid, or use a very much smaller than normal loading dose in the elderly. Thus, for digitalisation, unless there is great urgency, the proposed initial maintenance dose is adequate (Caird, 1974; see also chapter XVII; sect. 8.1.5).

Maintenance dose must be related to renal function (Ewy et al., 1969; Whiting et al., 1978), bearing in mind that a normal blood urea does not exclude renal impairment. Glomerular filtration must fall to approximately 25ml per minute before the blood urea rises. In other words, about 75% of glomeruli have to be non-functioning before the blood urea rises above the normal range.

While not always practicable, one way of deciding on the size of maintenance dose of digoxin is to measure creatinine clearance. In the complete absence of renal function (anephric) 14% of digoxin in the body is lost daily, mostly by compensatory faecal excretion. With normal renal function 30% appears in the urine daily and a total of about 33% of body stores (of a loading dose) of digoxin is lost in 24 hours. For degrees of renal impairment between these extremes, urinary excretion of digoxin is proportional to glomerular filtration rate and hence to creatinine clearance.

More usually, to take into account small body size and diminished glomerular filtration, a low loading dose — up to 0.5mg (500µg), or a maintenance dose of 0.25mg (250µg) per day is used initially. The dose for each patient is then titrated carefully. Often the dose may have to be reduced to 62.5µg/day.

One of the most important factors in the causation of digoxin toxicity is hypokalaemia. There are many possible reasons for hypokalaemia in elderly patients, including diuretic use (see section 4.1.2), so it is very important to check potassium status when undertaking digitalisation. These patients may also be dehydrated.

Digoxin Dose Regimen: As the digoxin plasma half-life is well over 30 hours in the elderly, there is little point in giving the daily requirement in divided doses. In fact, dividing the dose means the elderly mind has to remember two events rather than one in the day. Also, in the interests of simplifying dose regimens it is probably best that patients are not asked to take the digoxin for 5 days of the week only, and then to miss out their dose for 2 days. This may lead to confusion. With the availability of smaller dose tablets of digoxin this practice hardly seems justified.

Plasma Digoxin Estimation: The value of measuring plasma digoxin levels as a *sole* guide to the optimum therapeutic dose is very limited (see chapter XVII; sect. 8.1.5). The situation in which it is most likely to be of value in the clinical setting in management of the elderly, is in a patient suspected of having digitalis toxicity in whom very high plasma drug levels indicate toxicity. However, plasma values in the normal range do not exclude digitalis toxicity. It seems therefore that while plasma digoxin estimations may be useful, one must rely in many cases on clinical judgment (see also chapter I; sect. 5.2).

Is There a Need for Digitalis? Elderly patients without evidence of heart disease who are on digitalis glycosides may have these stopped without detrimental effect (Dall, 1970; chapter XVII, sect. 8.1.2). Other surveys have also shown that many elderly patients receive digitalis therapy without proper indications (Landahl et al., 1977). The clinician therefore has a very real responsibility to consider carefully the indications for digoxin in each case, and also must assess from time to time if the indication still exists. In some series, 20% of patients receiving digitalis have exhibited side effects, and the elderly were more likely to suffer digitalis intoxication (Ogilvie and Ruedy, 1972). It is important therefore to realise the limitations of this drug. There is little doubt that a diuretic alone will suffice in the majority of cases of congestive heart failure in the elderly.

4.1.2 Diuretics

The difficulties involved in the use of diuretics in the elderly are similar to those found in younger adults. The elderly are however, more susceptible to complications (see table VI). It is important to only use diuretics in the elderly for proper indications (only occasionally is ankle oedema associated with heart failure) and also to get an objective measure of the effectiveness of the diuretic used. However, with elderly patients it may not be practicable to make accurate urine collections. Because of urinary incontinence or inability of elderly patients to cooperate, regular weighings (daily or perhaps less frequently) will usually give a good indication of the effectiveness of the diuretic.

Choice of Drug: The combination of duration of action and of the various side effects that occur with each type of diuretic dictate in large measure the agent used in any individual case.

In the treatment of congestive heart failure in the elderly, one of the thiazides usually suffices (see chapter XVII; section 8.1.7). However, if a rapid diuretic response is required, one of the shorter acting drugs will be used. The action of the thiazide is spread over more than 10 hours so that the likelihood of acute retention and incontinence is less with this group than it is with potent short acting diuretics such as frusemide (furosemide), ethacrynic acid and bumetanide. On the other hand, a morning dose of a long acting diuretic such as chlorthalidone may cause nocturia and insomnia. The choice of diuretic may depend on balancing the risk of retention and incontinence on the one hand against nocturia and insomnia on the other.

While some patients may be resistant to one or other diuretic, in general, there is little difference between thiazides and frusemide or bumetanide as

Table VI. The main complications of use of diuretics in the elderly

Hypokalaemia, digitalis toxicity
Impaired glucose tolerance, diabetes
Hyperuricaemia, gout
Hypovolaemia, hypotension
Dehydration, uraemia
Acid-base imbalance
Urine incontinence, retention

regards sodium excretion over the full 24 hours after therapeutic doses. The use of frusemide, bumetanide and ethacrynic acid in emergencies is facilitated by their availability in a formulation suitable for intravenous administration. If these diuretics are used, and particularly if given intravenously, a small dose, e.g. 20mg of frusemide, should be used initially in case the patient is very sensitive. With larger doses a massive diuresis can ensue and hypotension and collapse may result.

Impaired Glucose Tolerance, Hyperuricaemia: Elderly patients are likely to be susceptible to the complication of carbohydrate intolerance and the diabetic state with the thiazide diuretics (Amery et al., 1978). Hyperuricaemia and gout may also develop. There is however, no evidence that gout and diabetes may be caused directly by these agents. Ethacrynic acid, frusemide and bumetanide may also occasionally cause decreased glucose tolerance and hyperuricaemia (see also chapter XVI; sect. 14.1; chapter XXII; sect. 14.4).

Hypokalaemia, Potassium Supplements: As all the above diuretics have their main site of action proximal to the distal tubular site for potassium-sodium exchange they may cause hypokalaemia when used on a long term basis, particularly in oedematous patients (see chapter XXI; sect. 7.1). The currently available slow release potassium chloride tablets (e.g. 'Slow-K') appear rather large for elderly patients to swallow, and if difficulty arises effervescent potassium chloride tablets should be used instead. A tablet of 'Slow-K' contains 8 mEq of potassium. About 32 to 48 mEq of potassium a day will suffice to supplement the average elderly patient's daily intake of potassium which is of the order of 30 to 60 mEq. Elderly patients with congestive heart failure may, however, have a decreased appetite and so potassium supplements are particularly important for this reason (Jellet, 1978).

While potassium deficiency causes lethargy, muscle weakness, bowel symptoms and mental confusion, the main complication of hypokalaemia if often the precipitation of digoxin toxicity. In the elderly therefore, it is very important to monitor patients who are on the combination of digoxin and potassium-losing diuretics for evidence of disturbed potassium balance and digoxin toxicity. The so-called potassium-sparing diuretics (e.g. amiloride, spironolactone, triamterene) do not seem to provide any special features in the elderly and in fact must be used with caution. Normally they are not used alone, but in conjunction with those diuretics which tend to cause increased potassium excretion. The two diuretics used in this way will potentiate each other and potassium supplementation will not then be required; indeed potassium supplements are contraindicated. Serum potassium should be monitored where possible, as there is a real risk of hyperkalaemia, particularly if renal function is significantly impaired or if the dietary intake of potassium suddenly increases (see chapter XXI; sect. 7.1.

4.2 Cardiac Arrhythmias

A number of cardiac arrhythmias merit special attention in the elderly by virtue of their high incidence.

4.2.1 Heart Block
Idiopathic chronic heart block occurs most commonly in patients over 65 years of age, the most consistent microscopic finding being fibrosis in the conducting system. Many of these patients do not require therapy and active intervention should be reserved for those patients with:

a) Significant decrease in effort tolerance. These usually occur as a result of a decrease in heart rate below 50/minute and reflect diminished cardiac output.

b) Stokes-Adams attacks. Often the history is vague and differentiation from a cerebrovascular problem may be difficult. Heart rate may be increased by use of atropine or isoprenaline (isoproterenol) but usually these should be temporary measures. The treatment of first choice is electrical pacing and the indications are as defined in chapter XVII (sect. 7).

4.2.2 Atrial Fibrillation
Atrial fibrillation is quite common in the elderly and most often there is no apparent cause.

The majority of patients manage quite well and the most common indication for intervention is heart failure. Therapy follows the conventional pattern (see chapter XVII; sect. 6.2.5). Digitalis increases cardiac output by decreasing ventricular rate. Usually a maintenance dose can be prescribed but in the presence of severe failure, more rapid digitalisation may be necessary (see section 4.1.1).

4.2.3 Premature Ventricular Contractions and Ventricular Tachycardia
Isolated premature ventricular contractions, often asymptomatic, do not necessitate therapy. However, in the case of ventricular tachycardia and if premature ventricular contractions are associated with symptoms, or recent myocardial infarction, therapy should be instituted. Orally effective antiarrhythmic agents such as disopyramide, mexiletine or phenytoin may be used. Disopyramide must be used with caution because urinary retention is not uncommon. There is a tendency to avoid β-adrenoceptor blocking agents in the elderly, presumably because of fear of their negative inotropic action. Procainamide is not suitable for long term therapy (see further chapter XVII; sect. 6.2.6, 6.2.7).

4.3 Diabetes Mellitus

The main difficulties which may arise in the management of diabetes in the elderly are:

1) Raised renal threshold for glucose which occurs as part of the aging process and which delays the onset of glycosuria.
2) Difficulties of obtaining specimens of urine.
3) Interaction of cerebrovascular accidents and glucose metabolism.
4) Problems of fluid replacement.
5) Practical and economic problems of dietary control.
6) Difficulty in the administration of insulin.

Control of therapy based on urinalysis alone is difficult and may be inadequate because of the change in renal threshold for glucose. Initially, blood sugar levels should be correlated with urinary sugar in each patient. This is most readily done by collecting blood and urine samples at various times on different days until a profile has been built up. It is important to avoid over vigorous treatment of the elderly diabetic. The aging brain often adapts itself to higher than normal blood sugar levels and in such circumstances the reduction of blood sugar level to 'normal' results in a relative hypoglycaemia and an acute confusional state.

When incontinence is a major problem and specimens of urine cannot be obtained, the diabetic state must be controlled on blood sugar measurements alone in the first instance. Once a stable state has been reached, however, such estimations need not be carried out with great frequency.

Glycosuria is quite common following a cerebrovascular accident. It is important to recognise that such glycosuria is usually trivial. Diabetes itself rarely results in coma in the elderly. Furthermore, glycosuria secondary to brain damage does not indicate serious disturbance of carbohydrate metabolism and therapy is not indicated.

Hypoglycaemia in the elderly may follow the classic pattern of hunger, sweating, tachycardia and dyspnoea, or may present as a confusional state, or occasionally as a hemiplegia. This hemiplegia is usually reversible, provided the blood sugar is raised to normal levels within a reasonable period of time. However, on occasion, despite rapid correction of blood sugar levels, permanent damage may still result. This is particularly likely to occur with repeated episodes of hypoglycaemia.

Hyperosmolor diabetic states occur in the elderly and their management is identical to that in younger patients. However, fluid overdose is more easily induced in the elderly. If massive fluid therapy is given it is wise to monitor central venous pressure. The elderly are particularly at risk of developing potassium depletion during the recovery period.

Many older people have great difficulty in following complicated diet sheets. These diet sheets are usually prepared for younger patients and they are not usually satisfactory for the elderly. Simplicity of the dietary regimen is essential for compliance. The help of a dietitian is invaluable.

The majority of elderly patients with diabetes can be controlled satisfactorily on diet alone. Where drug treatment is deemed necessary a sulphonylurea can be used in conjunction with diet (see chapter XVI; sect. 3.4). Some clinicians prefer conservative doses of chlorpropamide (table III) because it has the advantage of once daily dosage, but it is not without risk of symptomatic hypoglycaemia, particularly if renal function is impaired (60 % is excreted unchanged in the urine). To avoid this risk of dangerous hypoglycaemia

(see also above), others prefer tolbutamide in the elderly since it has a shorter half-life and is transformed in the liver to metabolites with no hypoglycaemic activity and hence is less likely to cause hypoglycaemia in the presence of decreased renal function (see also chapter XVI; sect. 3.3.3). If insulin is required at home, and should impairment of vision render the patient unable to measure or administer insulin with safety, then either a responsible relative must be trained in its administration or a community nurse called in. However, it must be realised that elderly patients rarely require insulin and careful consideration of the indications for insulin therapy must precede starting a patient on this drug (see chapter XVI; sect. 3.2). Usually when a patient is started on insulin he is condemned to its use for the rest of his life. Hence it is important when seeing an elderly diabetic patient who is already on insulin (or oral hypoglycaemic agents) for the first time, to ask the question: is drug treatment really required? Appropriate dietary control may be all that is necessary.

4.4 Hypertension

Hypertension in the elderly predisposes to strokes and heart failure: some rise in blood pressure occurs in most 'normal' older people with advancing years. Over the age of 80 systolic pressures of up to 200 mm Hg are frequently found in apparently healthy people. A diastolic pressure of 100 mm Hg in people aged 70 years or more as an isolated finding is not uncommon (Kaplan, 1973). It is important to remember that nonspecific symptoms such as headache and dizziness are frequently not due to hypertension and alone do not constitute an indication for antihypertensive treatment.

Probably more harm is done in the management of elderly patients by the *injudicious* use of antihypertensive agents than by failure to treat hypertension (Jackson et al., 1976). Postural hypotension is common in the elderly (Caird et al., 1973) and the main complications of incorrect lowering of the blood pressure in the elderly are syncopal episodes related to postural hypotension and coronary insufficiency. In some elderly patients an acute confusional state can be induced with loss of memory and intellectual impairment. These mental symptoms disappear on withdrawing drug treatment.

The investigation of hypertension is simpler in the elderly patient since it is unusual for patients with an untreated organic cause to survive to a great age. In the great majority of elderly people with hypertension no cause can be discovered and evidence can be adduced (family, pregnancy history; previous BP measurements) that the condition has been present, in a latent or manifest form, for many years. On the other hand, hypertension arising *de novo* may warrant a search for an underlying and possibly remedial cause such as renal artery stenosis. However, there is no point in subjecting an older patient to the rigors of an exhaustive and expensive workup for renal vascular hypertension unless surgery is planned in the event of positive results. Chronic renal disease is occasionally the cause and the rare case of aortic coarctation is not discovered until late in life.

4.4.1 Indications for Treating Hypertension in the Elderly

At present, the precise significance of elevated blood pressure in the elderly is not known. Indeed, it is not clear what constitutes high blood pressure in this population. Moreover, we do not really know the value of prescribing antihypertensive agents to those elderly patients who seem to have unduly high blood pressure, particularly in the absence of complications. Nevertheless, available data indicates that elevated diastolic and systolic blood pressures are both important risk factors for cardiovascular disease in those over 65 years of age as well as in those aged less than 65 (Dyer et al., 1977). Ongoing studies, notably the European working party study on hypertension in the elderly, will hopefully provide guidelines for optimum treatment in this difficult area in the near future. On the basis of current knowledge, a reasonable approach is to treat hypertension in the 'younger' elderly patients (less than 75 years) whose systolic blood pressure is more than 200mm Hg with a diastolic pressure exceeding 110mm Hg even in the absence of complications. The subject has recently been reviewed by Koch-Weser (1979) who advocates a more active approach to treatment of hypertension in the elderly than is currently practised by most clinicians.

The value of antihypertensive therapy in the elderly hypertensive patient who has suffered a stroke is controversial. Some suggest that the hypertensive patient suffering a severe stroke has a better prognosis than a similar patient with normal blood pressure, since reduction of cerebral perfusion pressure might result in further cerebral ischaemia and infarction, and hence antihypertensive therapy should be avoided in such a case. Others suggest that the hypertensive patient who suffers recurrent small strokes or transient cerebral ischaemic attacks is protected from further similar episodes by antihypertensive therapy. The available evidence indicates that therapy does have a beneficial effect on stroke recurrence in patients with hypertension who have had a stroke. Also antihypertensive therapy decreases the incidence of congestive heart failure complicating hypertension.

In many elderly hypertensive patients, systolic pressure is mainly raised while diastolic may be normal or only slightly raised. The potential of this form of hypertension to cause cardiovascular complications is not clear and it is therefore difficult to suggest guidelines for its management (Koch-Weser, 1973).

When treatment is decided upon, it is most important to avoid postural hypotension and excessive reductions of pressure. In patients over 65, a diastolic pressure of 100mm Hg whilst standing is the minimum which is desirable (see also chapter XVIII; sect. 9).

4.4.2 Drug Regimen

The decision to treat or not to treat hypertension in the elderly must therefore remain an individual one, especially since well supervised blood pressure control and patient cooperation over a long term is crucial to success. In patients who are not overweight, treatment should be initiated with an oral thiazide diuretic, such as bendrofluazide in a dose of 5mg once each day. Although potassium depletion is less common in patients who are given thiazide diuretics for essential hypertension compared with those treated for heart failure, it can occur, but with low doses of thiazides (e.g. 2.5 to 5mg bendrofluazide once daily) routine potassium supplements are probably not required (Kassirer and Harrington, 1977; Jellett, 1978).

If reduction in diastolic pressure to 100mm Hg is not achieved with bendrofluazide then methyldopa in a dose of 250mg twice per day or a β-adrenoceptor blocking drug should be added. In addition to the unwanted effects associated with antihypertensive agents in general (see chapter XVIII; sect. 6.2), methyldopa in the elderly is more liable to cause drowsiness and psychiatric disturbances such as depression and paranoid states (Dollery and Harington, 1962). The postural hypotension with methyldopa, though much less marked than with adrenergic neurone blocking drugs such as guanethidine or bethanidine, may be sufficiently severe to cause unconsciousness and it is imperative that the blood pressure be measured with the patient lying and standing in each case.

When effective, β-blockers have the advantage of lowering lying as well as standing blood pressure with minimal side effects. However, in common with all antihypertensive drugs they should be used cautiously with a close watch for potentially troublesome pharmacological side effects (see chapter XVIII; section 5.6.8). The broad acceptance of these drugs in younger patients has encouraged their more extensive use in the elderly and present trends indicate that the β-blockers may be preferrable to methyldopa.

4.5 Rheumatic Diseases

4.5.1 Rheumatoid Arthritis

Rheumatoid arthritis is part of a systemic disease the manifestations of which are embraced by the term rheumatoid disease. While the usual age of onset is in the thirties it not infrequently starts after the age of 60 or even 70. Most of the drugs employed in the treatment of rheumatoid arthritis have 3 main effects — anti-inflammatory, analgesic and antipyretic.

Acetylsalicylic Acid (aspirin): In a dose of 5g or more per day, salicylates have an anti-inflammatory effect. In lower doses this effect is not clinically detectable. However, some of the benefit derived in rheumatoid arthritis is from the analgesic effect which is evident at much lower doses.

Aspirin was formerly the drug of first choice in rheumatoid arthritis and is used to the limit of tolerance. However, because of better tolerance, the propionic acid derivatives are being increasingly preferred for initial therapy (see chapter XXII; sect. 3). The dose of aspirin tolerated is less in the elderly than in younger patients and is of the order of 3 to 4g per day. When given in high dosage many elderly patients experience tinnitus, nausea, anorexia and gastrointestinal irritation. The latter symptom may be controlled by reduction of dose or changing to soluble aspirin, glycinated aspirin or aloxiprin, which may be tolerated better.

Gastrointestinal haemorrhage may complicate salicylate use in two ways. Firstly, occult bleeding due to long term use occurs in most cases and in a small number of these may lead to iron deficiency anaemia (Davies, 1977). This is particularly likely to occur in those elderly patients whose dietary iron intake may already be marginal. Secondly, salicylates may rarely cause massive blood loss in peptic ulcer cases or indeed in the absence of any previously demonstrable lesion, gastric or duodenal. Alcohol and vitamin C deficiency may increase the risk of gastrointestinal bleeding. There does not appear to be a link between dyspeptic symptoms and the occurrence of occult bleeding. Therefore the absence of a history of dyspepsia does not help to exclude chronic gastrointestinal blood loss.

Despite having a long list of side effects in addition to those mentioned above, salicylates are relatively safe when the truly massive scale of their use is taken into account.

Propionic Acid Derivatives (e.g. ibuprofen, naproxen, fenoprofen): In full doses, these drugs have a useful analgesic and anti-inflammatory effect. The more active propionic acid derivatives such as naproxen and fenoprofen are as effective as full doses of aspirin, phenylbutazone or indomethacin but are better tolerated by most patients. They are increasingly being used as first choice drugs in rheumatoid arthritis (see chapter XXII; sect. 3.2.5).

Phenylbutazone: While aspirin often suffices it may not be suitable because of adverse effects or because of failure to respond. Phenylbutazone is a possible alternative to aspirin or one of the propionic acid derivatives, although like aspirin it has many side effects (see chapter XXII; sect. 3.2.2). The most serious of these include: blood dyscrasias, allergic reactions of varying severity, peptic ulceration with massive haemorrhage, sodium and fluid retention (which may precipitate heart failure in the elderly) and jaundice.

The elderly are particularly at risk from the bone marrow effects (Bottiger and Westerholm, 1973), the mortality associated with these effects being higher than in younger patients. Furthermore, aplastic anaemia occurs more frequently in older patients while agranulocytosis is more common in younger patients. Aplastic anaemia may not develop for up to a year after starting the drug. While many of the effects of phenylbutazone are dose dependent some cases of blood dyscrasia have occurred after relatively small doses of the drug.

Using doses less than 300mg per day will diminish the risk of serious side effects considerably. However, the benefits expected must be balanced against possible adverse effects. Some clinicians consider that the attendant risks with phenylbutazone are unacceptable and that it should not be used in the elderly. There are a number of other pyrazoles (e.g. oxyphenbutazone, nifenazone), the effectiveness and toxicity of which have not been shown to be more favourable than is found with phenylbutazone.

Indomethacin: The beneficial effects of this drug are comparable with those of phenylbutazone. While the frequency of side effects with the two drugs is roughly the same, the incidence of severe adverse effects associated with indomethacin is possibly less (Wade, 1970) and it is the preferred alternative to aspirin in the elderly. Indomethacin suppositories at night are useful to relieve early morning joint stiffness in particular. Headaches and unpleasant cerebral sensations and gastrointestinal disturbances may limit the tolerance of indomethacin in the elderly (see also chapter XXII; sect. 3.2.3).

Gold, D-Penicillamine and Corticosteroids: The use of these drugs should be considered only in that minority of patients whose disease is progressing rapidly despite adequate supportive treatment and therapy with non-steroid anti-inflammatory drugs, or where certain systemic manifestations are present. In younger patients some would advocate a trial of gold therapy, D-penicillamine or chloroquine before resorting to steroids, but there is less case for these toxic drugs in the elderly patient (see chapter XXII; sect. 3.3). The decision to prescribe steroids is a particularly difficult one, since many of the adverse effects of steroids are enhanced by old age, e.g. glucose intolerance, osteoporosis, susceptibility to infections, bruising, mental changes and oedema.

Most of the side effects of corticosteroids are related to dose and duration of treatment (see chapter XXII, sect. 3.4; chapter XVI, sect. 9.1.3). The dose tolerated is lower in old age and if possible the maintenance dose should be kept below 5mg of prednisolone (or its equivalent) per day.

Simple Analgesics: Many of these drugs are available without prescription and may have been tried by the patient, before being seen by his doctor. Frequently, inadequate doses will have been used. Paracetamol (acetaminophen) is probably the safest for long term use. However, overdose with as few as 20 tablets can cause death from hepatic necrosis (see further chapter IX; section 6.3). Phenacetin containing preparations should not be used. Phenacetin is metabolised mainly to paracetamol which is the active form. Because of the incrimination of phenacetin in analgesic nephropathy, paracetamol itself is to be preferred. Dextropropoxyphene, codeine and dihydrocodeine may be used on a short term basis but are not recommended for continued use. Constipation, dizziness and sleepiness which they cause may be particularly troublesome in the elderly. All have dependence producing potential and may cause respiratory depression. Pentazocine has a low abuse potential but causes confusion in the elderly and is mainly used for the short term relief of pain. In the inflammatory arthritides, pure analgesic agents have only a small part to play in management. Relief of pain in arthritis is usually secondary to the anti-inflammatory activity of the standard drugs (see chapter XXII; sect. 3).

4.5.2 Osteoarthrosis

There are two main types — primary nodal osteoarthrosis which typically presents in women in middle age, and secondary osteoarthrosis which may occur at any age and comprises degenerative change following damage to articular cartilage. Drugs have a secondary role. Initially, mild analgesics such as paracetamol or aspirin in low dose may suffice, but frequently it may be necessary to use indomethacin or phenylbutazone. Systemic corticosteroids are of course never indicated (see also chapter XXII; sect. 4).

4.5.3 Polymyalgia Rheumatica

This is a fairly common syndrome occurring almost exclusively in the elderly and of unknown origin. It involves the proximal muscle group and characteristically is associated with a very high erythrocyte sedimentation rate. It may also be associated with giant cell arteritis or temporal arteritis and therefore blindness. Response to drugs such as salicylates is poor, but corticosteroids (in high dose initially) produce dramatic relief and are specifically indicated in temporal arteritis to prevent the onset of blindness. The dose of steroid can usually be reduced rapidly, but it may be months or years before the steroids can be stopped (see also chapter XXII; sect. 6).

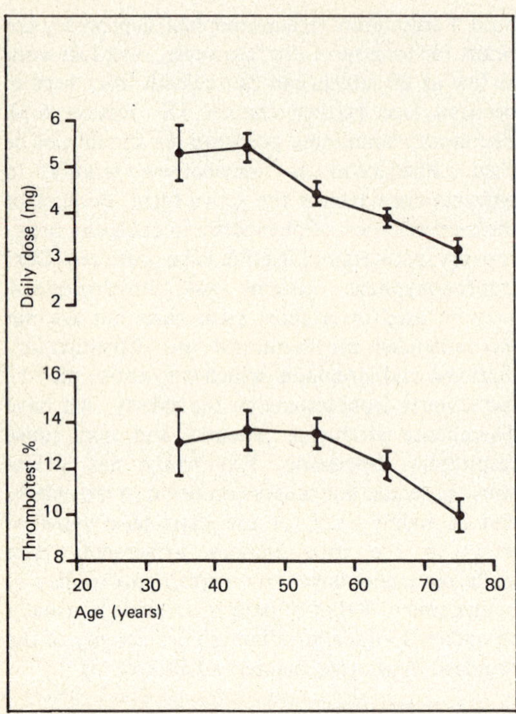

Fig. 3. The effect of age on warfarin dose and anti-coagulant effect in 177 patients. Dose decreased and anticoagulant effect increased with advancing age indicating a marked increase in responsiveness to this drug in the elderly. Values are means ± SEM. Age group size ranged from 10 to 56 patients (after O'Malley et al.: British Journal of Clinical Pharmacology 4: 30, 1977; by permission of author and editor).

4.6 Thromboembolic Disease

Many of the risk factors (heart disease, surgical operations, varicose veins, obesity, immobilisation, diuretic therapy, compression of calves in bed) involved in deep venous thrombosis and pulmonary embolism occur more commonly in the elderly so that this age group is particularly vulnerable. When it is realised that a higher proportion of hospital deaths are attributable to pulmonary embolism, the importance of early diagnosis and prompt treatment of deep venous thrombosis and pulmonary embolism becomes apparent.

While there is some uncertainty as to the value of anticoagulants in some situations, e.g. after acute myocardial infarction (see further chapter XXIII; sect. 4.1), there is little doubt that a definite diagnosis of deep venous thrombosis or pulmonary embolism is an indication for immediate anti-coagulant therapy. The patient should be heparinised rapidly (to avoid delay associated with oral anticoagulants in achieving anticoagulation) and oral anticoagulation with warfarin then instituted (table III).

It is generally held that the risks of anticoagulation are greater in the elderly. This applies particularly to heparinisation (Jick et al., 1968), but probably also applies to the oral anticoagulants (Husted and Andreasen, 1976) and is due presumably to the frequency of advanced vascular disease and poor renal and hepatic function. The data presented in figure 3 demonstrate an increased responsiveness to warfarin with advancing years. Even though the dose given is less in the elderly, the anticoagulant effect is greater (O'Malley et al., 1977). In addition, Husted and Andreasen (1977) have found increased responsiveness to other coumarin compounds. The likely explanation is that clotting factor synthesis inhibition by oral anticoagulants is more marked in elderly patients (Shepherd et al., 1977).

As the clinically used oral anticoagulants are metabolised to inactive compounds in the liver before elimination (see chapter XXIII; sect. 3.2.2), the increased incidence of haemorrhage associated with renal impairment is probably due to other haemostatic derangement secondary to the renal disease itself. Similarly, in the case of liver disease the dose requirement is independent of any effect of rate of metabolism of the drug. It is due mainly to altered rate of synthesis of clotting factors.

If adequate caution is exercised in using oral anticoagulants in the elderly and in particular if the relative contraindications such as renal failure are kept in mind, there is no doubt that the dangers of haemorrhage are far less than the sequelae of deep venous thrombosis and pulmonary embolism. However, the clinical situation is very often complicated. Frequently one is in doubt with regard to diagnosis of deep venous thrombosis and/or pulmonary embolism and an assessment of whether possible benefits outweigh risks becomes virtually impossible. With recent advances in the diagnosis of deep venous thrombosis and pulmonary embolism such as angiography and the ^{125}I-fibrinogen technique a definite diagnosis will be reached in a greater number of cases.

It is usually recommended that oral anticoagulant therapy should be continued for 6 months after a pulmonary embolism. When the acute phase is over in the elderly a second decision must therefore be made. Should oral anticoagulation be continued on an outpatient basis? The likelihood is that the geriatric patient will be unable to manage oral anticoagulants at home. Usually, therefore, anticoagulants will be stopped within a month or so of the clinical episode.

In summary, age in itself is not a contraindication to use of anticoagulants. However, extra caution should be used in the use of these agents in the elderly patient because of an increased risk of haemorrhagic complications. Satisfactory anticoagulation is unlikely to be achieved when organised on an outpatient basis.

4.7 Some Common Symptoms

The elderly commonly complain of symptoms as a result of the multiple diseases associated with the aging process. In addition, they have difficulties in adapting to their physical, psychological and social environments, which may be expressed as symptoms. It is important to recognise that the symptoms of elderly patients do not invariably require the use of drugs, and even when they are indicated they must be used carefully. This applies particularly to the psychotherapeutic drugs (Hollister, 1975; Learoyd, 1972).

4.7.1 Insomnia

Many relatively minor problems may give rise to insomnia such as a full bladder, a loaded or impacted rectum, hunger, a cold room or an uncomfortable bed, or by any disease process which results in hypoxia. Many old people do not realise that the consumption of tea or coffee before retiring leds to cerebral stimulation and diuresis. The latter problem may also arise due to the prescription of long acting diuretics (see section 4.1.2).

Depression is very common in older people and may be difficult to diagnose, especially in the early stages. Often the first manifestation is difficulty in getting off to sleep on retiring, or wakening in the early hours and being unable to get back to sleep again. This variety of insomnia is often helped by tricyclic antidepressant drugs after careful assessment of the various aetiological factors. These drugs should be used cautiously in the elderly as their anticholinergic activity may lead to troublesome side effects (e.g. severe confusional states, postural hypotension, urinary retention, dry mouth, constipation). Dosage should be conservative; very low doses initially and adjusted with great care (see chapter XXVI; sect. 7.5, 11).

Incipient cardiac failure in the elderly, due for example to myocardial insufficiency, may present not as nocturnal dyspnoea but as insomnia. Accurate diagnosis is obviously imperative as a basis for rational treatment.

Pain causes sleeplessness in old people as in the young, and must be treated appropriately before hypnotics are prescribed. The position is more complicated however, in the older patient with diminished pain sensitivity or pain awareness resulting from the aging process. Here restlessness and sleeplessness may appear as pain equivalents in association for example with myocardial infarction or peptic ulceration.

If treatment with hypnotics is required the choice of drug is restricted. The barbiturates should be rarely used in this age group (see section 2.2). A chloral derivative such as triclofos in a dose of 2.5g and the benzodiazepines, nitrazepam (2.5 to 5mg) or flurazepam (5 to 15mg), and chlormethiazole (250 to 500mg) are safe and effective hypnotics used judiciously as a short course of therapy to restore the patients 'normal' sleep pattern (see chapter XXVI; sect. 9.1). Triclofos and chlormethiazole have the advantage of being available as a syrup. Occasionally, confusion is seen following the use of hypnotics (this seems to be less with chlormethiazole; Magnus, 1978) and even more uncommonly, prolonged action leads to daytime drowsiness. Unwanted effects with nitrazepam and flurazepam in the elderly are more common if doses larger than those given above are used (fig. 4; Greenblatt et al., 1977; Greenblatt and Allen, 1978). The enhanced response to

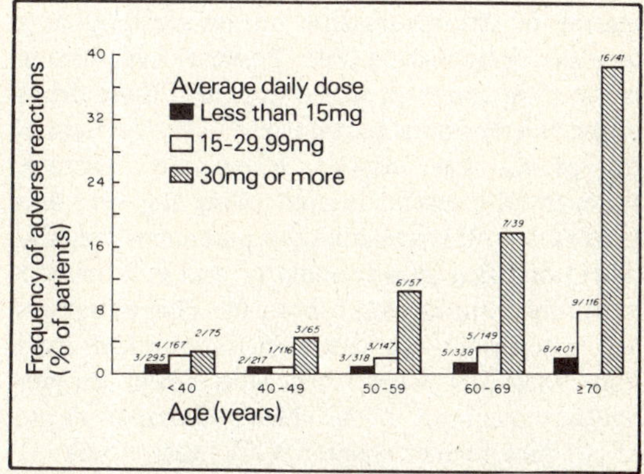

Fig. 4. Frequency of adverse reactions to flurazepam in relation to age and average daily dose (after Greenblatt et al.: Clinical Pharmacology and Therapeutics 21: 355-361, 1977; by permission of author and editor).

nitrazepam in the elderly seems to be related to increased 'sensitivity' of the aging brain (Castleden et al., 1977), and similarly also to diazepam (Reidenberg et al., 1978). Alcohol is often used as a hypnotic in this age group and is safe and effective.

4.7.2 Confusion

This is a symptom which has many causes and the following should be considered before symptomatic treatment is given.

1) Drug side effects, e.g. digitalis glycosides, reserpine, methyldopa, sedatives, tranquillisers, tricyclic antidepressants, etc (see chapter XXV; sect. 15.1).
2) Structural brain damage, e.g. due to a space occupying intracranial lesion.
3) Diminished cerebral blood flow, e.g. hypotension, carotid insufficiency, vertebro basilar disease, cerebral thrombosis.
4) Infection, e.g. pneumonia, urinary tract infection, meningitis, tuberculosis.
5 Metabolic and endocrine disease, e.g. thyroid disease, potassium deficiency.
6) Anaemia.

If no cause can be discovered, or if specific treatment is unsuccessful, then symptomatic treatment with one of the phenothiazine drugs should be tried. Thioridazine is probably the drug of choice for mild and moderate confusional states in an initial dose of 10 to 12.5mg 3 to 4 times a day. A total daily dose of 100mg should rarely be exceeded. A syrup is available which contains 25mg of thioridazine per 5ml. This is particularly suitable for patients who have difficulty in swallowing. If a parenteral preparation is required, then promazine or chlorpromazine intramuscularly in a dose of 25mg may be used. Postural hypotension is the most common side effect from these drugs in the elderly and is particularly likely to occur if the patient has organic neurological disease. Haloperidol is useful in controlling the very agitated patient. It is available as a parenteral preparation (5 or 10mg intramuscularly) and as drops (0.5 to 1.5mg 3 times daily). Both the phenothiazines and haloperidol can cause extrapyramidal reactions (table III). Choreiform side effects are particularly common in the elderly (Salzman et al., 1976). [See further chapter XXV; sect. 15.5].

On rare occasions paraldehyde is still required for the acutely confused patient. No more than 5ml should be given into one site intramuscularly, and it should be remembered that this drug rapidly dissolves most makes of plastic syringe. Its action can be potentiated by the simultaneous administration of a phenothiazine.

4.7.3 Anxiety

Anxiety in older people is commonly due to worry about finance, housing, health, etc. Drug treatment is not always indicated as it may be possible to alleviate the underlying cause. Anxiety as an isolated symptom responds well to chlordiazepoxide or diazepam. The phenothiazine drugs, in a dose similar to that suggested above for confusional states, are also effective in many cases. Meprobamate is also a useful drug but can cause confusion in older people. It is wise to start with a small dose, say 200mg once a day, and to increase slowly. All these drugs may produce postural hypotension or lead to unsteadiness or falls in the elderly. Anxiety may be a manifestation of a depressive illness and care should be taken to look for this, since treatment with conservative doses of a tricyclic antidepressant drug may be extremely effective (see further chapter XXVI; section 8.1).

4.7.4 Behaviour Disorders

The most common cause of behaviour disorder is confusion and its management is as outlined in section 4.7.2. Where the behaviour disorder contains a psychotic element, psychiatric help will be required (see chapter XXVI; sect. 11). Occasionally, however, disorders of behaviour are seen in hemiplegia. This should not be confused with the depression which often results from insight on the patient's part into their condition. The latter requires reassurance and possibly tricyclic antidepressant drugs.

A condition which can be difficult to manage is the apparent emotional incontinence sometimes seen in unilateral cerebrovascular disease and which resembles that of pseudobulbar palsy. Both these disturbances are motor in nature and are in fact disorders of expression of emotion, as can be demonstrated if the patient who is weeping uncontrollably is asked to put his thumb up if he is quite happy. It is important to recognise the condition since antidepressant therapy is inappropriate.

If therapy is deemed necessary, then a drug which depresses motor activity such as thioridazine or chlorpromazine should be used. A few hemiplegic patients develop a bizarre behaviour disorder which resembles epilepsy. There is some experimental evidence that an anticonvulsant drug such as sulthiame (100mg 3 times daily initially) may be of value.

4.7.5 Mental Deterioration

Many conditions, as well as problems of living, can contribute to the impaired recent memory and decreased mental alertness associated with old age. While careful use of drugs can be used to treat symptoms such as confusion and behaviour disturbances (see sections 4.7.2, 4.7.4), there is no good evidence that drugs which may modify the changes in cerebral function found in patients with senile dementia (Altzeiman's syndrome) or cerebral arteriosclerosis are of proven value in clinical practice (see further chapter XXVI; sect. 11).

4.7.6 Constipation

Constipation is probably the most common symptom in the elderly, particularly in women. It is important not only because of its increasing prevalence with age but also because of the variety of complications, notably those arising from faecal impaction, which may arise (Exton-Smith, 1972). Nevertheless, constipation may not be truly present in old people as their obsession with their bowels is such that they consider they have constipation if they do not have at least one bowel motion daily. Much of the laxative taking by the elderly is unnecessary. Thus in every case it is not only important to establish the cause of the constipation (functional or secondary) but also whether any laxative taking is really necessary.

A number of hazards can result from inappropriate choice and use of laxatives in the elderly (see appendix B). The most appropriate laxative for the elderly is standardised senna ('Senokot') in the minimum effective dose. After a few weeks, when bowel habit has become regular, the dose can be gradually reduced and often stopped altogether. Regular use of laxatives is however, often required to prevent faecal impaction in those who have had more than one episode not due to a temporary illness or confinement to bed. Small volume enemas such as the phosphate or citrate type are usually required in the initial treatment of severe constipation and in faecal impaction.

General measures such as instruction about what constitutes a regular bowel action, the desirability of physical activity, an adequate fluid intake, and the use of high residue diets and bran should not be forgotten. Naturally, any secondary causes (e.g. colonic, anorectal lesions) must be treated appropriately. Some drugs may also be a cause of constipation (see chapter XIX; sect. 14.4.1).

Further Reading

Crooks, J.; O'Malley, K. and Stevenson, I.H.: Pharmacokinetics in the elderly. Clinical Pharmacokinetics 1: 280 (1976).

Crooks, J. and Stevenson, I.H. (Eds): Drugs and the Elderly (Macmillan, London 1979).

Hall, M.R.P.(Ed): Symposium on evaluation of drug therapy in the elderly. Gerontologia Clinica 16: 1 (1974).

Judge, T. and Caird, F.: Drug Treatment of the Elderly Patient (Pitman, London 1978).

Lasagna, L.: Drug effects as modified by aging. Journal of Chronic Diseases 3: 567 (1956).

Vestal, R.E.: Drug use in the elderly: A review of problems and special considerations. Drugs 16: 358 (1978).

References

Amery, A. et al.: Glucose tolerance during diuretic therapy. Results of trial by the European Working Party on Hypertension in the Elderly. Lancet 1: 681 (1978).

Anderson, W.F.: Administration, labelling and general principles of drug prescription in the elderly. Gerontologia Clinica 16: 4 (1974).

Ayd, F.J.: Once-a-day neuroleptic and tricyclic antidepressant therapy. International Drug Therapy Newsletter 7: 33 (1972).

Ayd, F.J.: Single daily dose of antidepressants. Journal of the American Medical Association 230: 263 (1974).

Bender, A.D.: Pharmacologic aspects of aging. A survey of the effect of age on drug activity in adults. Journal of the American Geriatric Society 12: 114 (1964).

Bender, A.D.: Effect of age on intestinal absorption: Implications for drug absorption in the elderly. Journal of the American Geriatric Society 16: 1331 (1968).

Bottiger, L.E. and Westerholm, B.: Drug-induced blood dyscrasias in Sweden. British Medical Journal 2: 339 (1973).

Burr, M.L.; King, S.; Davies, H.E.F. and Pathy, M.S.: The effects of discontinuing long term diuretic therapy in the elderly. Age and Ageing 6: 38 (1977).

Caird, F.I.: Metabolism of digoxin in relation to therapy in the elderly. Gerontologia Clinica 16: 68 (1974).

Caird, F.I.; Andrews, G.R. and Kennedy, R.D.: Effect of posture on blood pressure in the elderly. British Heart Journal 35: 527 (1973).

Cammarata, R.J.; Rodnan, G.P. and Fennell, R.H.: Serum anti-gamma-globulin and anti-nuclear factors in the aged. Journal of the American Medical Association 199: 115 (1967).

Castleden, C.M.; George, C.F.; Marcer, D. and Hallett, C.: Increased sensitivity to nitrazepam in old age. British Medical Journal 1: 10 (1977).

Church, G. and Marriott, H.: Digitalis delirium. Circulation 20: 549 (1959).

Crooks, J.; O'Malley, K. and Stevenson, I.H. Pharmacokinetics in the elderly. Clinical Pharmacokinetics 1: 280 (1976).

Crooks, J. and Stevenson, I.H. (Eds): Drugs and the Elderly (Macmillan, London (1979).

Dall, J.L.C.: Digitalis intoxication in elderly patients. Lancet 1: 194 (1965).

Dall, J.L.C.: Maintenance digoxin in the elderly. British Medical Journal 2: 705 (1970).

Davies, D.M. (Ed): Textbook of Adverse Drug Reactions, p.137 (Oxford University Press, Oxford 1977).

Davies, D.F. and Shock, N.W.: Age changes in glomerular filtration rate, effective renal plasma flow, and tubular excretory capacity in adult males. Journal of Clinical Investigation 29: 496 (1950).

Davison, W.: Drug hazards in the elderly. British Journal of Hospital Medicine 6: 83 (1971).

Davison, W.: Unwanted drug effects in the elderly; in Meyler and Peck (Eds) Drug Induced Diseases, vol. 4. p.617 (Excerpta Medica, Amsterdam 1972).

Dollery, C.T. and Harington, J.: Methyldopa in hypertension. Clinical and pharmacological studies. Lancet 1: 759 (1962).

Dyer, A.R.; Stamler, J.; Shekelle, R.B.; Schoenberger, J.A. and Farinaro, E.: Hypertension in the elderly. Medical Clinics of North America 61: 513 (1977).

Evered, D.C. and Chapman, C.: Plasma digoxin concentrations and digoxin toxicity in hospital patients. British Heart Journal 33: 540 (1971).

Ewy, G.A.; Kapadia, G.G.; Yao, Linda; Lullin, Muriel and Marcus, F.I.: Digoxin metabolism in the elderly. Circulation 39: 449 (1969).

Exton-Smith, A.N.: Constipation in geriatrics; in Avery Jones and Godding (Eds) Management of Constipation, p.156 (Blackwell, Oxford 1972).

Farah, F.; Taylor, W.; Rawlins, M. and James, O.: Hepatic drug acetylation and oxidation: Effects of aging in man. British Medical Journal 11: 155 (1977).

Gibson, I.J. and O'Hare, M.O.: Prescription of drugs for old people at home. Gerontologia Clinica 10: 271 (1968).

Greenblatt, D.J.; Allen, Marcia D. and Shader, R.I.: Toxicity of high dose flurazepam in the elderly. Clinical Pharmacology and Therapeutics 21: 355 (1977).

Greenblatt, D.J. and Allen, Marcia D.: Toxicity of nitrazepam in the elderly: A report from the Boston Collaborative Drug Surveillance Program. British Journal of Clinical Pharmacology 5: 407 (1978).

Hansen, J.M.; Kampmann, J. and Laursen, H.: Renal excretion of drugs in the elderly. Lancet 1: 1170 (1970).

Hayes, M.J.; Sprackling, M. and Langman, M.J.S.: Changes in the plasma clearance and protein binding of carbenoxolone with age and their possible relationship with adverse drug effects. Gut 18: 1054 (1977).

Hayes, M.J.; Langman, M.J.S. and Short, A.H.: Changes in drug metabolism with increasing age. I. Warfarin binding and plasma proteins. British Journal of Clinical Pharmacology 2: 73 (1975a).

Hayes, M.J.; Langman, M.J.S. and Short, A.H.: Changes in drug metabolism with increasing age. II. Phenytoin clearance and protein binding. British Journal of Clinical Pharmacology 2: 69 (1975b).

Hewick, D.S.; Newbury, P.; Hopward, S.; Naylor, G.; Moody, J.: Age as a factor affecting lithium therapy. British Journal of Clinical Pharmacology 4: 201 (1977).

Hollister, L.E.: Drugs for mental disorders of old age. Journal of the American Medical Association 234: 195 (1975).

Hurwitz, N.: Predisposing factors in adverse reactions to drugs. British Medical Journal 1: 536 (1969).

Husted, S. and Andreasen, F.: Problems encountered in long term treatment with anticoagulants. Acta Medica Scandinavica 200: 379 (1976).

Husted, S. and Andreasen, F.: The influence of age on the response to anticoagulants. British Journal of Clinical Pharmacology 4: 559 (1977).

Jackson, G.; Mahon, W.; Pierscianowski, T.A. and Condon, J.: Inappropriate antihypertensive therapy in the elderly. Lancet 2: 1317 (1976).

Jellett, L.B.: Potassium therapy: When is it indicated? Drugs 16: 88 (1978).

Jick, H.; Slone, D.; Borda, I.T. and Shapiro, S.: Efficacy and toxicity of heparin in relation to age and sex. New England Journal of Medicine 279: 284 (1968).

Judge, T. and Caird, F.: Drug Treatment of the Elderly Patient (Pitman, London 1978).

Kaplan, N.: Clinical Hypertension (Medcom, New York 1973).

Kassirer, J.P. and Harrington, J.T.: Diuretics and potassium metabolism: A reassessment of the need, effectiveness and safety of potassium therapy. Kidney International 11: 505 (1977).

Klotz, U.; Avant, G.R.; Hoyumpa, A.; Schenker, S. and Wilkinson, G.R.: The effects of age and liver disease on the disposition and elimination of diazepam in adult man. Journal of Clinical Investigation 55: 347 (1975).

Koch-Weser, J.: The therapeutic challenge of systolic hypertension. New England Journal of Medicine 289: 481 (1973).

Koch-Weser, J.: Treatment of hypertension in the elderly; in Crooks and Stevenson (Ed) Drugs and the Elderly, p.247. (Macmillan, London 1979).

Kristensen, M.; Molholm Hansen, J.; Kampmann, J.; Lumholtz, B. and Siersback-Nielsen, K.: Drug elimination and renal function. Journal of Clinical Pharmacology 14: 307 (1974).

Landahl, S.; Lindblad, B.; Roupe, S.; Steen, B. and Svanborg, A.: Digitalis therapy in a 70-year-old population. Acta Medica Scandinavica 202: 437 (1977).

Law, R. and Chambers. C.: Medicines and elderly people: A general practice survey. British Medical Journal 1: 565 (1976).

Learoyd, B.M.: Psychotropic drugs and the elderly patient. Medical Journal of Australia 1: 1131 (1972).

Magnus, R.V.: A controlled trial of chlormethiazole in the management of symptoms of the organic dementias in the elderly. Clinical Therapeutics 1: 387 (1978).

Mazullo, J.M.: The nonpharmacologic basis of therapeutics. Clinical Pharmacology and Therapeutics 13: 157 (1972).

Miller, J.H.; McDonald, R.K. and Shock, N.W.: Age changes in the maximal rate of renal tubular reabsorption of glucose. Journal of Gerontology 7: 196 (1952).

Nation, R.L.; Triggs, E.J. and Selig, M.: Lignocaine kinetics in cardiac patients and aged subjects. British Journal of Clinical Pharmacology 4: 439 (1977).

Ogilvie, R.I. and Ruedy, J.: An educational program in digitalis therapy. Journal of the American Medical Association 222: 50 (1972).

O'Malley, K.; Stevenson, I.H.; Ward, C.A.; Wood, A.J. and Crooks, J.: Determinants of anticoagulant control in patients receiving warfarin. British Journal of Clinical Pharmacology 4: 309 (1977).

Parkin, D.M.; Henney, C.R.; Quirk, J. and Crooks, J.: Deviation from prescribed drug treatment after discharge from hospital. British Medical Journal 2: 686 (1976).

Reidenberg, M.M.; Levy, M.; Warner, H.; Coutinho, C.B.; Schwartz, M.A.; Yu, G. and Cheriplco, J.: The relationship between diazepam dose, plasma level, age and central nervous system depression in adults. Clinical Pharmacology and Therapeutics 23: 371 (1978).

Rowe, J.W.; Andres, R.; Tobin, J.D.; Noris, A.H. and Shock, N.W.: The effect of age on creatinine clearance in man: A cross-sectional and longitudinal study. Journal of Gerontology 31: 155 (1976).

Salzmann, C.; Shader, R.I. and Van der Kolk, B.A.: Clinical psychopharmacology and the elderly patient. New York State Journal of Medicine 76: 71 (1976).

Schwartz, D.; Wang, M.; Feitz, L. and Goss, M.E.W.: Medication errors made by elderly, chronically ill patients. American Journal of Public Health 52: 2018 (1962).

Shaw, S.M. and Opit, L.J.: Need for supervision in the elderly receiving long term prescribed medication. British Medical Journal 1: 505 (1976).

Shepherd, A.M.M. and Stevenson, I.H.: Warfarin protein binding in young and elderly subjects. Clinical Pharmacology and Therapeutics 23: 129 (1978).

Shepherd, A.M.M.; Hewick, D.S.; Moreland, T.A. and Stevenson, I.H.: Age as a determinant of sensitivity to warfarin. British Journal of Clinical Pharmacology 4: 315 (1977).

Triggs, E.J.; Nation, R.L.; Long, Ann and Ashley, J.J.: Pharmacokinetics in the elderly. European Journal of Clinical Pharmacology 8: 55 (1975).

Vestal, R.E.; McGuire, E.A.; Tobin, J.D.; Andres, R.; Norris, A.H. and Mezew, E.: Aging and ethanol metabolism. Clinical Pharmacology and Therapeutics 21: 343 (1977).

Wade, O.L.: Pattern of drug-induced disease in the community: an unsolved enigma. British Medical Bulletin 26: 240 (1970).

Wandless, I. and Davie, J.W.: Can drug compliance in the elderly be improved? British Medical Journal 1: 359 (1977).

Whiting, B.; Wandless, Irene; Sumner, D.J. and Goldberg, A.: Computer assisted review of digoxin therapy in the elderly. British Heart Journal 40: 8 (1978).

Woodford-Williams, E.; Alvares, A.S.; Webster, D.; Landless, B. and Dixon, M.P.: Serum protein patterns in 'normal' and pathological aging. Gerontologia Clinica 10: 86 (1968).

Chapter VI
The Therapeutic Performance of Drug Products

D.N. Wade

Synopsis of Important Principles

1) Administration of a known dose of an active drug substance alone is rarely practical and often impossible. The addition of other substances is usually necessary to make a manageable dosage form.

2) Differences in the pharmaceutical formulation of a drug can lead to marked variability in biological effect or availability (bioavailability) among different brands or generic equivalents of the same drug substance and is of major importance in the context of product substitution.

3) The bioavailability of a dosage form therefore refers to a particular drug product and reflects these formulation differences, as well as the many factors relating to the drug and individual patient which influence the processes of absorption, distribution and elimination.

4) The effects of formulation variables apply particularly to oral dosage forms and may be manifest at all stages of the absorption process — disintegration, dissolution or absorption, although most problems arise because of changes in the rate of dissolution. Parenteral dosage forms can also show incomplete bioavailability.

5) *In vitro* tests provide valuable information on the speed of disintegration of the tablet or capsule and the rate of solution of the particles of drug substance, but are not necessarily a reliable guide to the bioavailability or therapeutic performance of the product.

6) While differences in bioavailability between drug products can be shown to occur in man (bioinequivalence) they may not always be clinically significant.

7) The real frequency of significant differences in bioavailability during actual clinical use (therapeutic inequivalence) is unknown, but the therapeutic effectiveness or toxic potential of some drugs has been clearly shown to be altered by drug product formulation factors.

8) It is not possible to test all drugs or to specify optimum standards of bioavailability that apply equally to all formulations of all products. Standards for individual products can only be established in the context of the therapeutic ratio and the clinical situation for which the drug is intended.

9) Therapeutic equivalence between like formulations should not be assumed, unless therapeutic equivalence or bioequivalence have been demonstrated in man. Nor should therapeutic equivalence be assumed simply because therapeutic non-equivalence has not been reported.

10) Drugs should always be named as a specific drug product in a written prescription, and patients should not be changed from one formulation or dosage form to another without good reason and the knowledge of the clinician.

The therapeutic or toxic response to a drug is often influenced by factors other than the quantity of active drug substance administered in a particular dosage form. This is especially so with oral dosage forms, many of which are associated with incomplete and variable absorption such that different formulations of the same drug substance may be associated with marked variability in resultant biological effect or availability ('bioavailability'). Consequently, as discussed in chapter I, the relationship between the concentration of active drug substance in the circulation and a particular pharmacological effect is often much closer than the relationship between the dose administered and the drug induced effect.

1. Concept of Bioavailability and Non-equivalence of Drug Products

The bioavailability of a dosage form refers to the relationship between the administration of a particular formulation and the amount of drug substance that reaches the systemic circulation. As such, bioavailability reflects a number of variables including numerous aspects of formulation, the absorptive process itself, and the many factors governing drug distribution, metabolism and excretion (see Blanchard et al., 1979; Brodie and Heller, 1972; Koch-Weser, 1974). Thus, some drugs have poor bioavailability after oral administration because the rate of absorption is so slow that it is difficult to attain therapeutically useful or sustained plasma levels. Other drugs, although well absorbed, have a low oral bioavailability because of extensive metabolism of the drug during the first passage through the intestinal mucosa and/or liver (see chapter I; sect. 3.3.3). Some of these drugs cannot be given orally, because the 'first-pass' hepatic metabolism is so rapid and extensive (e.g. morphine; lignocaine/lidocaine), and for others (e.g. propranolol) the oral dose must be considerably larger than an intravenous dose to obtain the same pharmacological response. These drugs may also show differences in bioavailability among individuals due to differences in the extent of 'first-pass' metabolism. Changes in gastrointestinal function may also influence oral bioavailability, particularly with poorly absorbed drugs or with drugs which are metabolised in the gut wall (see section 5).

The concept of bioavailability has its major therapeutic importance in the context of product substitution due to differences in bioavailability from particular formulations, whether oral, parenteral or rectal dosage forms. Although the term is widely used, there is no internationally accepted definition or set of standards. The simple operational definition adopted by the United States Food and Drug Administration (FDA) serves to define the area of involvement; thus

> 'bioavailability simply means the degree and rate of absorption of a drug as determined by blood levels or urinary excretion rates, or by appropriate short term *in vivo* pharmacological studies. It is not meant to include therapeutic equivalence as determined by clinical trials' (Edwards, 1972)

It is important to emphasise that bioavailability measurements relate to particular formulations or dosage forms and that questions of efficacy and therapeutic equivalence are separate problems involving different experimental designs and methods. Furthermore, there may be specific features of the bioavailability of a formulation that are of special importance depending on the clinical use for which it is intended. It is therefore difficult to specify optimum standards for the bioavailability characteristics that apply to all drugs.

1.1 Factors Which Influence Bioavailability

The optimum bioavailability characteristics for a particular drug formulation depends on many factors, including the pharmacokinetics of the drug, the clinical situations in which it is used, its safety and efficacy, the known relationships between plasma concentration and drug related effects, and the proposed dosage regimen (Koch-Weser, 1974). Only some of these factors are under the control of the pharmaceutical chemist (table I). Factors such as the crystal form of the drug, the particle size, the salt form, the excipients in the tablet or capsule, and the speed with which the tablet or capsule liberates the drug substance, may all be related to significant variations in the availability of active drug within the body (see section 4).

1.2 Non-equivalence of Drug Products

Differences between various formulations of the same drug have, on occasions, been so large that certain preparations have been associated with

Table I. Factors which can influence bioavailability of oral drugs

1. Formulation and physicochemical characteristics of drug product
   a) Tablet disintegration time (e.g. degree of compaction)
   b) Dissolution time (e.g. particle size; salt and crystal form)
   c) Excipients and adjuvants

2. Patient characteristics
   a) Gastric emptying rate
   b) Intestinal transit time
   c) Gastrointestinal disease
   d) Individual ability to eliminate drug (biotransformation, excretion)
   e) Disease being treated (pathophysiological determinants affecting absorption, distribution or elimination)

3. Presence of other substances in the gastrointestinal tract
   a) Interaction with other drugs (e.g. antacids, anticholinergic compounds, cholestyramine, metoclopramide), ions
   b) Food (large meal)

4. Pharmacokinetic characteristics of drug
   a) Incomplete or erratic absorption
   b) First-pass drug metabolism by gut bacteria
   c) First-pass drug metabolism in gut wall and/or liver
   d) Dose (concentration) dependent hepatic metabolism.

toxicity whilst other preparations containing the same quantity of active drug have resulted in very low blood levels and therapeutic failure. Other drugs are readily absorbed and are less subject to variations in bioavailability associated with these factors. Variable availability may be less important if there is a wide margin of safety, but even in this case, it may be associated with an inability to 'titrate' a drug effect.

There have been remarkably few good studies in this field and the extent of the problem is far from clear. Strong opinions are often expressed because of the economic and political implications associated with the choice between the generic and brand name specification of drugs in prescriptions, but this is really a side issue. The basic problem is one of difference in bioavailability (bioinequivalence) between preparations (brand or generic) containing the same active drug substance, and the clinical significance of the variations in bioavailability (therapeutic inequivalence).

There is a need for much more work in this area, but significant clinical problems do arise, particularly when bioinequivalent drug products are substituted without the knowledge of the clinician.

Drug products that meet the statutory requirements in terms of quantity of active drug substance and dosage form are often deemed to be generically equivalent without bioequivalence having been demonstrated. Generically equivalent formulations may be interchangably dispensed if a prescription is written with the drug specified only by its approved generic name. This method of prescribing assumes that preparations listed as generically equivalent are equivalent therapeutically, but in some cases this is not so. Therapeutic non-equivalence of drug preparations arising because of differing bioavailability has clear implications for the prescribing doctor (see section 8).

2.The Problem of Therapeutic Inequivalence

Although there are well documented examples of significantly different bioavailability associated with formulations that are generically equivalent, the overall extent of the problem is far from clear. Thus, in the United Kingdom, the Sainsbury Committee recommended that drugs should be prescribed by their official generic name and other influential authors have made similar recommendations (Dollery, 1970). On the other hand, the mounting number of reports indicating that different preparations of the same drug may be associated with significant variability in biological effect or bioavailability, suggests that these recommendations should be reviewed. From a practical point of view, several basic questions arise.

1) Are demonstrable differences in bioavailability between different formulations clinically significant?
2) If so, how frequently are significant differences likely to be encountered?
3) Are problems of bioavailability likely to be restricted to a small finite number of drugs which should be subject to special standards of *in vivo* testing?
4) Are *in vitro* tests for formulations sufficient to ensure that generically equivalent drug products are equivalent therapeutically?

The answers to these questions are central to any meaningful discussion of therapeutic equivalence, but with the available information, all cannot be answered with certainty. Confusion about the extent of the problem is highlighted by events in the United States, including the Massachusetts 'generic drug law' which permits substitution of drug products, and the more recent regulations proposed by the FDA (Federal Register 42: 1618-1619, 1977) which indicates that new drug formulations should be studied with appropriate *in vivo* studies in man. Waiver of evidence of *in vivo* bioavailability may be granted in some limited circumstances, but there is a large number of drugs that must be tested in man (table II). The implication of these proposed regulations is that significant differences in bioavailability are not rare. On the other hand, the Massachusetts Drug Formulary Commission in 1971 concluded that therapeutic inequivalence was a 'rare bird' (Burack, 1971), a conclusion that did not at the time receive universal acceptance (Beck, 1971; Kurtz, 1971).

2.1 Evidence for Bioinequivalence

There have been remarkably few carefully controlled comparative studies in man of similar dosage forms of the same drug from different manufacturers. In a review published in 1971, data tabulated from all the published controlled bioavailability studies at the time, comprised 24 studies of only 12 drugs. Of the 12 drugs, 7 were associated with large differences in bioavailability between different preparations (Wagner, 1971). If this represents the entire extent of bioinequivalence, then it might be reasonable to dismiss the problem of therapeutic inequivalence as a 'rare bird'. The state of our knowledge in this field must be seen in perspective. The 12 drugs adequately studied come from a list of about 2000 preparations currently available. When 7 of the 12 drugs (58 %), are associated with significant bioinequivalence, then to assume this represents the entire extent of the potential problem is surely dangerous, even if most of the drugs adequately studied were those with solubility problems.

Apart from the carefully controlled clinical trials there are other laboratory studies in man and *in vitro* studies which indicate that significant differences in bioavailability between preparations may not be rare. Some of these reports will be discussed later. It is now well documented that significant differences in bioavailability have existed between different preparations of widely used

compounds amongst which may be listed phenytoin (diphenylhydantoin), prednisone, aspirin, phenylbutazone, dicoumarol (bishydroxycoumarin), penicillin V, chloramphenicol, oxytetracycline, tetracycline, tolbutamide, nitrofurantoin, digoxin and various thyroid preparations (see Brodie and Heller, 1972; Burkholder and Barr, 1969; Greenblatt et al., 1976; Wagner, 1971).

The importance of these considerations was very clearly demonstrated by the careful comparison of the bioavailability of four preparations of digoxin available in the USA. All the tablets met current USP standards of potency, disintegration time and dissolution rate. The relative bioavailability following one preparation was considerably higher than after another (Lindenbaum et al., 1971; fig. 1). This variation of blood level profile spans the range from potential therapeutic failure to dangerous toxicity. Significant differences in the quantity of active agent between different preparations of digoxin are also apparently frequent. In late 1970, the FDA instituted a voluntary certification programme based on systematic testing of dosage forms by the National Center for Drug Analysis (NCDA). There were 79 recalls of digoxin preparations during one 8 month period soon after the programme started. Problems with the bioavailability of digoxin formulations in the United Kingdom further demonstrate the widespread nature of difficulties with formula-

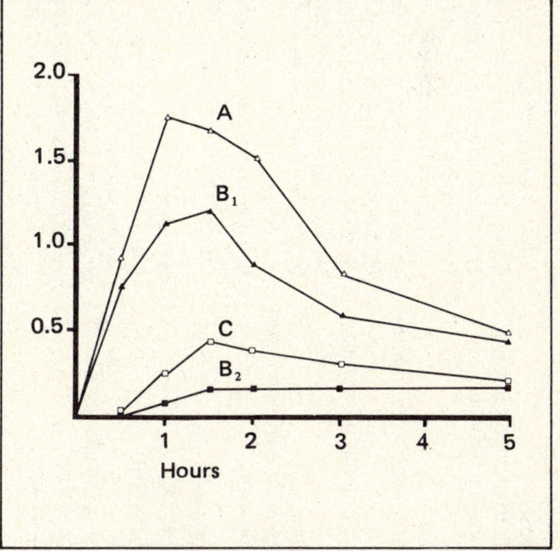

Fig. 1. Plasma level profile attained after oral administration of 0.5mg of each of four digoxin products to four subjects (after Lindenbaum et al.: New England Journal of Medicine 285: 1344, 1971; by permission).

Table II. A list of drugs for which waivers of *in vivo* bioavailability are not granted by the FDA[1,2]

Antiarrhythmics
Procainamide hydrochloride caps
Quinidine polygalacturonate
 	
Anticoagulants
Dicoumarol (bishydroxycoumarin)
  (and caps)
Warfarin, sodium and potassium
 	
Anticonvulsants
Phenytoin (diphenylhydantoin) susp
Ethosuximide caps
Ethotoin
Methoin (mephenytoin)
Methsuximide caps
Paramethadione caps
Phenacemide
Phensuximide caps and susp
Primidone (and susp)
Trimethadione caps
 	
Antihypertensive drugs/Diuretics
Alseroxylon
Bendroflumethiazide
Benzthiazide
Chlorothiazide
Deserpidine
Hydrochlorothiazide
Hydroflumethiazide
Methyclothiazide
Polythiazide
Quinethazone
Rauwolfia serpentina
Rescinnamine
Reserpine
Trichlormethiazide
	Antihypertensive/Diuretics in Combination
	Chlorothiazide and reserpine
	Hydrallazine and reserpine
	Hydrallazine hydrochloride and
	  hydrochlorothiazide
	Hydrochlorothiazide and deserpidine
	Hydrochlorothiazide and reserpine
	Hydroflumethiazide and reserpine
	Methyclothiazide and deserpidine
	Reserpine, hydrallazine hydrochloride and
	  hydrochlorothiazide
	Spironolactone and hydrochlorothiazide
	Trichloromethiazide and reserpine
	
	Anti-infectives
	Nitrofurantoin (and susp)
	Sulphasalazine (salicylazosulfapyridine)
	Sulphadiazine Na bicarbonate susp
	Sulphadiazine, sulphamethazine, and
	  sulphamerazine (triple sulpha) (and susp)
	Sulphadiazine
	Sulphadimethoxine (and drops and susp)
	Sulfamerazine
	Sulphamethoxypyridazine acetyl (and susp)
	Sulphaphenzole susp
	Sulphapyridine
	Sulphasomidine
	Sulphafurazole (sulfisoxazole) acetyl susp
	Sulphafurazole
	
	Antimalarials
	Pyrimethamine
	
	Antineoplastic drugs
	Chlorambucil
	Methotrexate
	Triethylene melamine
	Uracil mustard caps
		Antithyroid drugs
		Propylthiouracil
		
		Antituberculosis drugs
		Aminosalicylic acid and isoniazid
		Aminosalicylic acid (and powder and resin)
		Aminosalicylic Ca granules (and caps)
		Aminosalicylic K (and caps and powder)
		Aminosalicylic Na powder (and granules)
		Benzoylpas Ca (and Powder)
		Para-aminosalicylate Na and isoniazid
		Phenylaminosalicylate (and powder)
		
		Bronchodilators
		Aminophylline
		Dyphylline
		Oxtriphylline
		Theophylline Na glycinate
		
		Carbonic anhydrase inhibitors
		Acetazolamide
		Dichlorphenamide
		Ethoxzolamide
		Methazolamide
		
		Cardiac glycosides
		Acetyldigitoxin
		
		Corticosteroids
		Betamethasone
		Cortisone acetate
		Dexamethasone
		Fludrocortisone acetate
		Fluprednisolone
		Hydrocortisone acetate (and powder)
		Hydrocortisone
		Methylprednisolone
		Paramethasone acetate
		Prednisolone
		Prednisone
		Triamcinolone
			Oestrogens
			Dienoestrol
			Diethylstilboestrol diphosphate
			Diethylstilboestrol
			Ethinyl oestradiol
			
			Hypoglycaemics
			Tolbutamide
			
			Thyroid supplements
			Liothyronine sodium
			
			Tranquillisers
			Chlordiazepoxide hydrochloride caps
			Chlorpromazine
			Fluphenazine hydrochloride
			Perphenazine
			Prochlorperazine
			Promazine
			Promethazine
			Thioridazine
			Trifluoperazine
			Triflupromazine
			Trimeprazine
			
			Vitamin K
			Menaphthone (menadione)
			Phytomenadione (phytonadione)
			
			Miscellaneous drugs
			Imipramine hydrochloride
			Isoprenaline (isoproterenol) sublingual
			Methyltestosterone
			Probenecid
			Sodium sulfoxone

1   All dosage forms are tablets, unless otherwise noted. When tablets plus other dosage forms are involved, this is indicated by use of parens plus and (and caps).
2   Federal Register 42: 1619 (1977).

tions of this drug (Shaw, 1974; Shaw et al., 1973). There is clearly a potential hazard when patients are changed to an alternative digoxin formulation, although regulatory bodies in some countries have taken steps to ensure that all marketed digoxin preparations are of clinically satisfactory bioavailability (Greenblatt et al., 1976). The FDA now demands the demonstration of bioequivalence in man before licensing new formulations or products in the USA.

A more recent review of the published literature indicates that there are about 70 drugs for which there is good evidence of differences in bioavailability between like oral formulations (Chodos and DiSanto, 1973). There are very few studies that demonstrate no difference between like oral formulations, but it must be remembered that negative data of this type would be less likely to be published. While it can generally be assumed that bioequivalence usually guarantees therapeutic equivalence, the converse is not necessarily true. A 'statistically significant' difference in the bioavailability of a drug from different products does not mean that the products will differ to a therapeutically important extent. Bioinequivalence does not necessarily imply therapeutic inequivalence. The term 'clinically significant difference in bioavailability' must not be misunderstood. It not only describes bioinequivalence but also implies therapeutic inequivalence (Koch-Weser, 1974).

2.2 Evidence for Therapeutic Inequivalence

The frequency of therapeutically important differences in bioavailability of drugs from different products during actual clinical use is unknown. Nevertheless, the therapeutic effectiveness or toxic potential of some drugs has been clearly shown, by accidental detection or experimental demonstration to be altered by drug product formulation factors. The relatively small number of drugs so far implicated in therapeutic inequivalence does not mean that it does not occur.

Therapeutic inequivalence is very difficult to detect, because so many factors other than formulation differences can influence the response to drugs (see chapter I). Thus differences between patients are likely to be greater than differences in therapeutic performance between drug products. Although marked differences in bioavailability of drugs with a low therapeutic ratio like digoxin (see

section 2.1) are clearly of clinical significance, it is not possible to define arbitrary levels of bioinequivalence which would be universally applicable and likely to be associated with therapeutic inequivalence. This depends on many other factors such as the pharmacokinetic properties of the drug, its dosage and the clinical situation in which it is used (section 8.1).

Formulation related differences in bioavailability may be of little importance at the start of therapy for drugs like oral anticoagulants whose dosage must be individualised (see chapter XXIII; sect. 3.2.2), although bioavailability differences may make dose titration and anticoagulant control more difficult to attain. However, when the optimum dose of any such drug product has been established in an individual patient, substitution of another product with a marked difference in bioavailability could have serious consequences, particularly if it occurs without the clinician's knowledge. It is in the context of product substitution that differences in bioavailability are most important (see section 8.3). The implications are well illustrated by an epidemic of phenytoin intoxication which followed a change in formulation of a widely used brand (see section 4.4).

There is some truth in both opposing arguments about the therapeutic importance of bioinequivalence. Differences in bioavailability do occur and may be clinically important. On the other hand, they may not always be clinically significant (see section 8). Further, there are some drugs which are most unlikely to be associated with bioinequivalence problems given normal good manufacturing practices. It is clearly difficult to subject all existing drug formulations to *in vivo* tests of bioavailability. There is a need to identify those drugs with which bioinequivalence should be expected or suspected (Smith, 1975). Appropriate *in vivo* testing should be mandatory in these cases. Little reliance should be placed on *in vitro* tests unless these have been demonstrated to provide a reliable guide to bioavailability with the particular formulation, bearing in mind the various formulation variables and patient characteristics that determine the bioavailability of drug products.

3. Drug Substance and Drug Product — What is the Difference?

Central to this question is the clear distinction between the active drug substance and the final pharmaceutical formulation or drug product in which the drug is administered to the patient (see Burkholder and Barr, 1969). Administration of the active drug substance by itself is rarely practical and often impossible. Thus the active drug itself may be unstable at the pH of gastric juice — for example, erythromycin base and stearate must be protected from the stomach contents by formulation or coating that will release the base in the small intestine where it is absorbed. The simple matter of administering a known dose of the drug usually requires the addition of other substances to make up a manageable oral dosage form such as a tablet, capsule or pill. Parenteral administration obviously requires suitable solvents, buffers, antioxidants or emulsificants to produce a stable solution or suspension. Thus we rarely, if ever, administer only the pure drug substance.

The absorption of drug substance from orally administered dosage forms involves several separate steps. The formulation must first break up to release the particulate components of the formulation (disintegration). The drug substance must then dissolve in the fluid contents of the stomach or intestine (dissolution), and finally the drug substance in solution must be absorbed across the mucosal barrier into the circulation (fig. 2). Any one of these processes may represent the rate

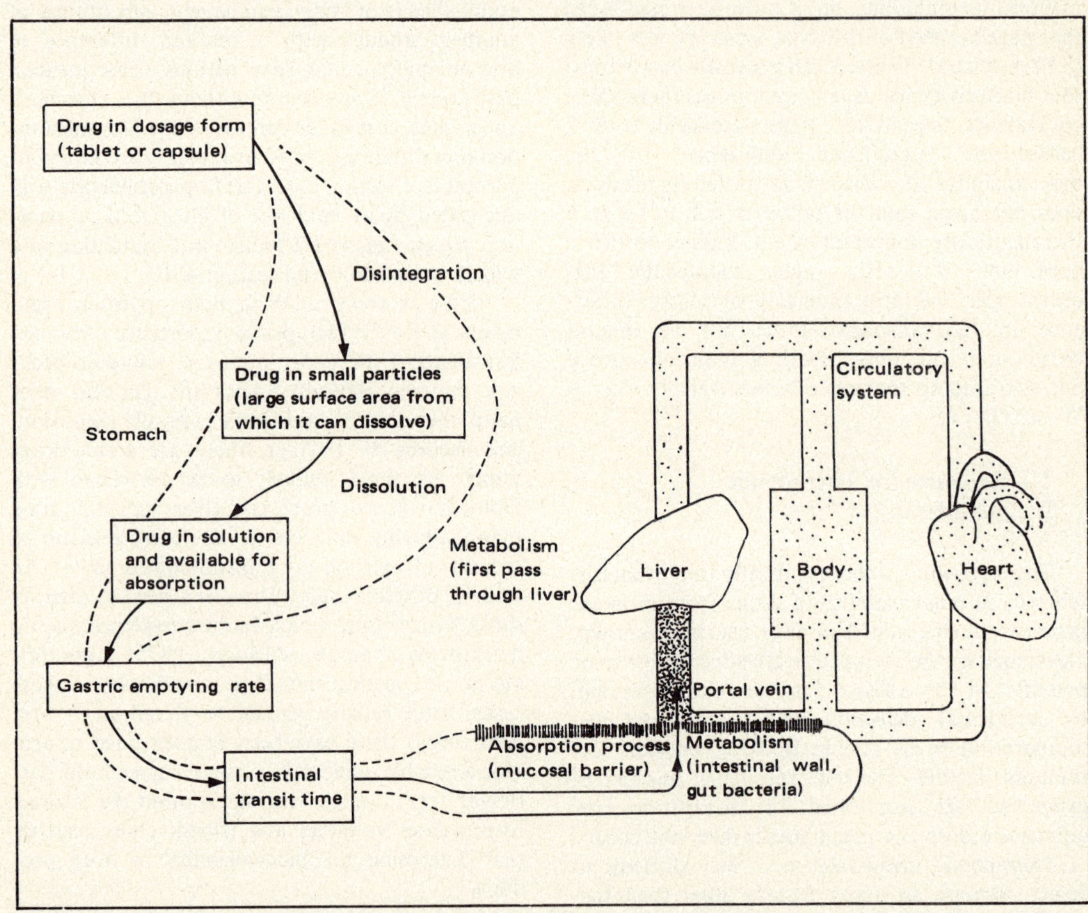

Fig. 2. Schematic representation of the processes of drug absorption and metabolism which influence bioavailability of oral dosage forms. The solid dosage form must disintegrate and the drug particles must dissolve before absorption occurs. The rate and extent of absorption can be influenced by gastrointestinal function and by metabolism in the gut or liver, prior to reaching the systemic circulation. The shaded area represents an orally administered drug which undergoes hepatic first-pass metabolism. The liver removes the drug from the portal venous blood during its transfer from the gut to the systemic circulation (adapted after Nies and Shand: Circulation 52: 6, 1975).

limiting step for the absorption of a particular drug (see chapter I; sect. 3.1). Poor or irregular absorption is not only confined to oral dosage forms. Intramuscularly administered formulations of diazepam, chlordiazepoxide and phenytoin, for instance, are usually associated with incomplete bioavailability (Editorial, 1975).

It is not surprising that different routes of administration and gross differences in formulation should be associated with different therapeutic responses. However, there are many pharmaceutical variables involved in the preparation of the final oral dosage form of any drug, and it is now appreciated that some of the more subtle aspects of formulation may exert a significant influence on the overall properties of the product. The effects of formulation variables may be manifest at all stages of the absorption process — disintegration, dissolution or absorption — although most problems arise because of changes in the rate of dissolution. Enteric coated tablets are a special case — some of these formulations may never disintegrate while absorption may be poor and erratic from others (Leonards and Levy, 1965). Sustained release tablet formulations are also associated with variation in bioavailability between products (Spangler et al., 1978).

4. Pharmaceutical Variables and Therapeutic Performance

4.1 Particle Size

The rate at which the drug goes into solution within the gastrointestinal tract is often the rate limiting step in the absorptive process. The particle size of the pure substance within the product very often influences significantly this dissolution rate. There is a direct relationship between the bioavailability of griseofulvin measured as the area under the blood concentration-time curve and the log of specific surface area of the particles. Small particles of about 2.5μm are absorbed at twice the rate of larger particles with a mean size of about 10μm (Atkinson et al., 1962; fig. 3).

Variation in particle size is known to affect the systemic availability of other drugs, particularly those with low intrinsic solubility (Barr, 1969). The production of small particles of drug substance (micronised particles) is a well recognised method used to improve the absorption of some poorly absorbed compounds. The particles of

spironolactone in preparations of 'Aldactone' currently available are much smaller than those in the product marketed some years ago. The absorption of drug from the presently available preparation is considerably enhanced due to a faster dissolution rate, with the result that the equivalent dose of the new preparation is smaller by several orders of magnitude (Karim et al., 1976).

4.2 Salt Form

Most drugs in common use are either weak acids or bases. The non-ionised form of both is more lipid soluble than the ionised form and thus more readily absorbed. The extent of dissociation depends on the dissociation constant (pK_a) and the pH of the intestinal lumen (see chapter I; sect. 1.1). The extent of dissociation, together with the intrinsic lipid solubility of the drug, are important determinants of the absorption rate. With an individual compound, these parameters are not easily modified, but the rate at which active substance is released from the preparation into solution

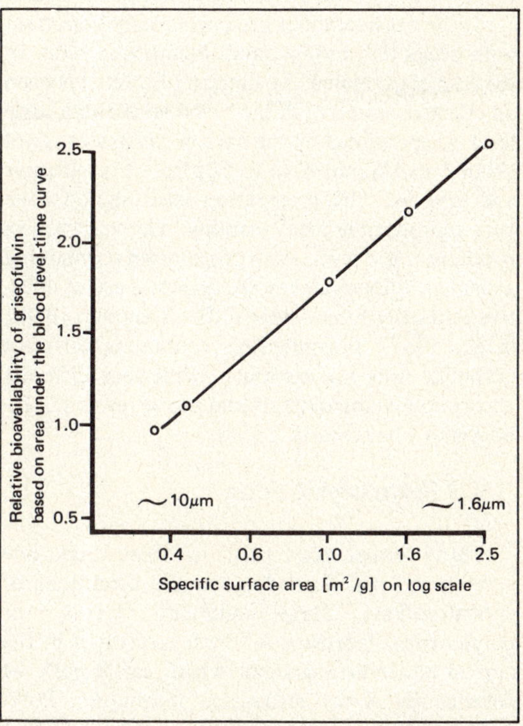

Fig. 3. Effect of particle size and surface area on plasma levels of griseofulvin (after Atkinson et al.: Antibiotics and Chemotherapy 12: 232, 1962; by permission of author and editor).

Table III. The effect of salt form on dissolution rate and the bioavailability of tolbutamide (Nelson et al., 1962)

Form of tolbutamide	Dissolution rate *in vitro* (mg/cm^2/h)		Drug in body[1]	Differences in blood sugars[2] (mg/100ml)
	pH = 1	pH = 7.2		
Acid	21	3.1	14	7.0
Sodium salt	1069	868	251	23.7

1 mg of tolbutamide (as free acid) 1 hour after oral load of 500mg (mean from 4 subjects).
2 In 23 normal subjects 2 hours after oral load of 1g.

can be influenced by the use of salts rather than the free acid or base. The more water soluble salts of weak acids are often associated with much faster dissolution rates. In the acid environment of the stomach, free acid may again be precipitated but usually in the form of very fine particles which facilitate solution and subsequent absorption (Munzel, 1971). This is clearly illustrated in table III which shows the greater bioavailability of the sodium salt of tolbutamide compared with the free acid (Nelson et al., 1962). The same principle underlies the differing availabilities of the various forms of aspirin (Morrison and Campbell, 1965).

These considerations are particularly important with drugs that have a small therapeutic ratio. In the case of quinidine, the margin of safety between an effective antiarrhythmic blood level and a toxic level is represented by the narrow plasma range of about 6 to 15µmol/L (2 to 5µg/ml). For effective and safe use, the preparation used should have very reproducible bioavailability. The variation in resultant blood levels with preparations containing a single salt form makes the maintenance of effective antiarrhythmic levels difficult enough (Bellet et al., 1957). Formulations containing different quinidine salts are associated with very different absorption characteristics and blood levels (Goldberg and Chakrabarti, 1964).

4.3 Polymorphic Form

Many drugs may exist in more than one crystalline form depending on the conditions of crystallisation. These alternate forms, or polymorphs, represent different structures in the crystal lattice arrangement which can usually be detected by X-ray diffraction techniques. Polymorphic forms usually have slightly differing physical properties. Differences in solubility are of particular importance. The less stable polymorphs are usually most soluble but their instability almost always precludes their use in pharmaceuticals. Polymorphs of intermediate stability — metastable forms — are sometimes appropriate in pharmaceuticals where the solubility of the drug is a problem, but the transformation of the metastable form to the stable polymorph results in decreasing availability of the drug as the preparation ages. This is one reason for the limited shelf life of some formulations.

The effect of polymorphic form on the bioavailability of drugs has been well illustrated with one or two drugs and is probably a much more important point than is generally appreciated. Differing bioavailability related to alternate polymorphic forms has been demonstrated in the case of subcutaneous methylprednisolone (Hamlin et al., 1962) and with oral chloramphenicol (Aguiar, 1969). Both chloramphenicol palmitate and chloramphenicol stearate exist in two polymorphic forms. In solution, the esters are hydrolysed by esterases to chloramphenicol which is then absorbed. The rate at which the esters dissolve is the rate limiting step in the absorptive process and is influenced by the polymorphic form of the crystals. The amorphous form of most compounds is more soluble than the crystalline form and in the case of chloramphenicol, this difference is so marked as to render preparations containing the crystalline forms of the stearate or palmitate of little therapeutic use. Blood concentrations of chloramphenicol from some preparations may be up to 10 times higher in the same patient than those from other preparations containing differing forms of chloramphenicol. Comparison of standard 'generically equivalent' forms of chloramphenicol on the USA market has shown mean peak plasma levels from a single 500mg dose ranging from 2 to 10µg/ml (Aguiar, 1969). These marked differences in the bioavailability of chloramphenicol preparations were not only due to varying proportions of different forms of chloramphenicol, but also to variations associated with the tablet or capsule formulation. As the drug must be in solution to be hydrolysed and absorbed, the rate at which the dosage form liberates particles of the drug substance is clearly an important determinant of the bioavailability.

4.4 Excipients and Adjuvants

Components in the dosage form other than the active drug substance may influence the absorption and thus the performance of the drug product. These additives or excipients may either facilitate or inhibit the absorptive process. Polyvalent cations such as calcium markedly reduce the absorption of various tetracyclines with which they complex (Neuvonen, 1976). In other cases, complexes such as ion-pairs may facilitate absorption. Complexes of inorganic iron with citrate, EDTA, or pyrophosphate are well established methods of increasing the absorption of this element, presumably by reducing the charge and increasing lipid solubility.

The importance of excipients in the determination of the final drug effect was clearly demonstrated by an outbreak of phenytoin (diphenylhydantoin) toxicity in Australasia (Bochner et al., 1972; McQueen, 1968). Patients previously maintained on a stable dose of 'Dilantin' capsules were noted to develop the clinical features associated with phenytoin overdosage. The toxicity was associated with higher than expected concentrations in the plasma, although the quantity of active substance in the capsules was unaltered. Subsequently, the high plasma concentrations were shown to be related to the substitution of lactose for calcium sulphate as an 'inert' excipient in the capsules. Presumably, the inorganic ion had complexed with the phenytoin reducing the absorption. Bentonite, a constituent in PAS granules, is responsible for a marked impairment of the absorption of rifampicin when given concurrently with PAS, due to adsorption of rifampicin on to bentonite (Boman et al., 1975).

The role of surface active agents is more complex and not always easy to predict. These substances are frequently used to increase solubility or act as emulsificants. The effect of a surface active agent (Tween 80) and of particle size on the absorption of phenacetin (acetophenetidin) was clearly shown by Prescott et al. (1970). However, surface active agents may either increase or decrease absorption depending on the agent used, the route of administration, the drug in question and the nature of the formulation. Furthermore, it is now clear that such agents may change the absorptive surface itself in the small intestine. In other cases, the surface active agent promotes micelle formation, thus enabling lipid soluble molecules to disperse in an aqueous medium.

4.5 Complex Formulations

A number of complex formulations are now being used to improve or control the drug delivery from oral formulations. Some of these employ novel approaches including the use of special excipients such as chelating agents to increase the absorption of polar drugs. Drugs may also be combined with ion exchange resins, contained in matrices of various types, or encapsulated in films or membranes.

The behaviour of these formulations *in vivo* is critically dependent on physiological variables and is difficult to predict from *in vitro* dissolution studies. Their performance can only be assessed by direct measurements in man.

4.6 Physical Properties of the Dosage Form

With many oral dosage forms, the rate at which the active drug can pass across the gut is not the rate limiting step in the absorptive process. It is often the rate at which the tablet or capsule disintegrates in the stomach or intestinal lumen and the rate at which the released drug dissolves that determines the speed and extent of absorption.

In general, a drug given in solution is absorbed faster than one in suspension which, in turn, is absorbed faster than the same substance administered in a tablet or capsule. Thus the physical properties of the tablet or capsule have an important influence on the ultimate performance and properties of the drug product. The modern compressed tablets present some special problems. Small changes in the composition of constituents or in the degree of compaction can lead to important changes in the performance of the tablet. These factors are now widely recognised, but a detailed discussion is beyond the scope of this chapter (see Kaplan, 1973). Drug manufacturers and regulatory bodies have set standards for the performance of tablets by the establishment of various *in vitro* 'disintegration' and 'dissolution rate' tests. Absolute values are of limited use, but relative rates between different preparations of the same drug often help to explain variation in the therapeutic performance of drug products which are 'generic equivalents'. Thus, in the case of the markedly different performance of chloramphenicol preparations (section 4.3), one brand was shown to release 92% of the drug in 10 minutes whilst in other brands, 20% of the drug was released in 30 minutes (Aguiar, 1969). Considered together with the plasma concentration data, it is clear that chloramphenicol preparations are not necessarily equivalent in terms of biological availability, even if they meet all the existing requirements to be listed as 'generic equivalents'.

It is important to remember that a disintegration test measures only the speed at which the tablet or capsule breaks up liberating particles of the drug substance. It does not indicate the rate of solution or absorption. Similarly, a 'dissolution test' provides valuable information on this aspect of the product's performance, but not necessarily a reliable guide to the bioavailability or therapeutic performance (WHO, 1974). The ultimate test is a study of the performance of the formulation in man. For a review of the influence of formulation on drug bioavailability and action, see Munzel (1971).

5. Gastrointestinal Function and Bioavailability

The physicochemical properties of the drug substance and the nature of the particular formulation are not the only variables that influence drug absorption and availability. Gastrointestinal function and first pass metabolism in the gut or liver (Gibaldi et al., 1972; Riegelman and Rowland, 1973) can play an important role, particularly when added to by drug product formulation defects. Some of the principles are well illustrated by the problems associated with the bioavailability of levodopa and digoxin.

Levodopa is a moderately water soluble amino acid absorbed by an active transport mechanism in the small intestine (Wade et al., 1973a). In addition to auto-oxidation and other loss within the lumen of the gut, there is a significant 'first-pass' decarboxylation of the drug during passage through the gut wall (Mearrick et al., 1974a). The availability of dopa is therefore very variable and critically dependent on the rate of gastric emptying (Wade et al., 1973b). Agents such as meto-

clopramide which accelerate gastric emptying increase the availability of the drug by delivering it more rapidly to the site of absorption and metabolism (Mearrick et al., 1974b). As the gut metabolism has a more limited capacity than the transport mechanism, there is an increase in the availability when gastric emptying is stimulated and a nonlinear relationship between dose and availability results. Furthermore, the time to obtain peak plasma concentrations is reduced and multiple peaks in the absorption profile are eliminated (Wade et al., 1973b; Mearrick et al., 1974b). Slowing gastric emptying has the opposite effect, decreasing the availability of dopa. Thus the rate and extent of 'first-pass' metabolism together with gastric and intestinal motility are the main factors responsible for the variable availability of levodopa. Formulation variables are of minor importance in this case.

Intestinal motility has the opposite effect on the absorption of sparingly soluble drugs such as digoxin. Drug induced acceleration of intestinal transit limits the time for dissolution and absorption of digoxin from tablets and thus decreases the bioavailability, whilst decreased gastrointestinal transit induced by propantheline bromide increases absorption; effects which are only likely to be clinically significant with formulations of digoxin which have slow dissolution characteristics (Manninen et al., 1973a,b). Phenolsulfonphthalein, another poorly absorbed drug, behaves similarly (Ashley and Levy, 1973). Slowing gastric emptying and increasing intestinal transit time may decrease the early rate of absorption although the total bioavailability is increased. This has been shown clearly with phenolsulfonphthalein (Ashley and Levy, 1973) and with riboflavine (Levy et al., 1972).

The rate of gastric emptying and small intestinal transit are very important determinants of bioavailability with many drug formulations. Drugs that alter the rate of gastric emptying have been shown to influence the *rate* of absorption of a number of drugs, including paracetamol (acetaminophen), lithium, digoxin, ampicillin, desipramine, PAS, phenylbutazone, tetracycline and pivampicillin (see Nimmo, 1976; Parsons, 1977). When defects in formulation with some of these drugs exist; for example, with slowly dissolving tablets of sparingly soluble drugs such as digoxin, sustained release preparations which release drug too slowly (e.g. lithium) or enteric coated preparations which normally give erratic release and require time to initiate release of drug substance, alteration of the *amount* of drug absorbed (i.e. bioavailability) can occur as a consequence of altered gastric emptying rate or intestinal transit time (Amdisen, 1977; Crammer et al., 1977; Manninen et al., 1973a,b). The importance of disease and drug induced changes in intestinal blood flow is unfortunately not clear. The absorption of some drugs is known to be dependent on intestinal blood flow; e.g. aspirin, salicylamide and antipyrine; and the absorption of salicylate and sulphamethoxypyridazine has been shown to decrease at the time of a simple faint (Rowland et al., 1972). The differences between blood sampling by intermittent venepuncture and an indwelling venous cannula may be important because of different levels of anxiety, autonomic tone and thus splanchnic blood flow. However, the magnitude of blood flow related changes in availability is unknown, as changes in intestinal blood flow rarely occur as isolated events. Thus, lying supine increases intestinal blood flow but also reduces intestinal motility and delays gastric emptying. This decrease in gastric emptying is most marked with the subject lying on the left side. Failure to control many of these physiological variables undoubtedly contributes to the confusion that abounds in the literature on drug absorption and bioavailability. These factors are of special relevance to the design and interpretation of bioavailability studies.

The effect of food in the gastrointestinal tract on gastric emptying rate and bioavailability has been inadequately studied and only recently have the complex and variable effects of food intake on bioavailability of drugs been demonstrated (see Melander, 1978). Food may interfere not only with tablet disintegration, drug dissolution and drug transit through the gastrointestinal tract, but it may also affect the first-pass metabolism of drugs in the gut wall and in the liver. Different food components can have different effects, and food may interact in opposite ways, even with drugs that are chemically related (table IV). Therefore, the net effect of food on drug bioavailability can be predicted only by direct clinical studies of the drug in question.

Gastrointestinal disease may modify the bioavailability of drugs, but the effects are variable and difficult to predict (see Parsons, 1977; chapter XIX, sect. 1.1). Extensive loss of the absorptive surface area such as that resulting from ileojejunal bypass for gross obesity is associated with malabsorption of sparingly soluble drugs such as pheny-

toin (Kennedy and Wade, 1979), although the absorption of digoxin from currently used formulations appears to be normal (Marcus et al., 1977). However, as drug absorption may be severely impaired in these patients, parenteral administration should be used when drugs are given for important indications. There is some evidence that oral contraceptives may have a higher failure rate in these patients (Johansson and Krai, 1976); presumably for the same reason.

Small bowel disease of mild to moderate severity may be associated with malabsorption of drugs but this problem correlates poorly with the extent of fat malabsorption. Patients with coeliac disease absorb most drugs normally and some a little better than normal, but there is evidence that thyroxine, dessicated thyroid, digoxin, amoxycillin and pivampicillin may be poorly absorbed. Drug malabsorption in patients with Crohn's disease may be a problem but the effects are also variable and unpredictable. Disproportionate changes in the absorption of trimethoprim and sulphamethoxazole may be important as the optimum ratio between the two agents in the plasma may not be achieved.

Plasma concentrations of propranolol after an oral dose are very much higher in patients with Crohn's disease and may also be higher in some patients with coeliac disease. The reason for the increased bioavailability is not clear, but the magnitude of the phenomenon may indicate a need for reduced dosage in these patients. Malabsorption due to pancreatic disease is usually associated with normal drug absorption, although cephalexin plasma concentrations have been reported to be lower in patients with cystic fibrosis.

This disparity between nutrient and drug malabsorption presumably reflects the factors that are rate limiting in the absorption of different solutes. Dissolution is the rate limiting process in the absorption of most drugs; it is therefore likely that gastric emptying, intestinal transit time and dispersion within the gut lumen are more important than a moderate loss of absorptive surface area.

Changes in drug absorption seen in acute gastroenteritis support this concept. Children with acute shigellosis may have impaired absorption of ampicillin and nalidixic acid, especially if the diarrhoea is severe. Similarly, there have been several reports of failure of oral contraceptives thought to be due to malabsorption in association with acute gastroenteritis.

Table IV. Effect of food intake on bioavailability of drugs (after Melander, 1978)

Drug	Possible mechanism/notes
1. *Increased bioavailability*[1]	
Propranolol Metoprolol	?Reduced hepatic first-pass metabolism
Hydrallazine (not slow release tablets)	Reduced first-pass metabolism in gut wall
Hydrochlorothiazide Nitrofurantoin	Reduced gastric emptying rate. Effect with nitrofurantoin most pronounced with slow dissolution formulations
Carbamazepine Spironolactone Dicoumarol Phenytoin	Improved drug dissolution due to food induced bile secretion
Griseofulvin	Fatty meal enhances absorption; presumably because of improved dissolution of griseofulvin which is very lipophilic
Erythromycin stearate	?
2. *Decreased bioavailability*	
Isoniazid	Reduced gastric emptying rate and increased gastrointestinal pH
Levodopa	Reduced gastric emptying rate and increased first-pass metabolism in gut wall
Phenacetin (acetophenetidin)	Charcoal broiled beef diet enhances first-pass metabolism
Tetracyclines (except doxycycline and minocycline)	Chelation with Ca in dairy foodstuffs; increased gastrointestinal pH
Penicillins Ampicillin Erythromycin base	Increased gastrointestinal pH
Rifampicin	?
3. *No or an inconsistent effect on bioavailability*	
Digoxin Diazepam Paracetamol (acetaminophen)	Food decreases rate of absorption but not amount absorbed
Theophylline	No effect on bioavailability but some diets can influence rate of hepatic elimination (see chapter I; sect. 3.3.5)
Aspirin	Some enteric coated preparations show decreased bioavailability; no effect with aspirin given as acid form
Amoxycillin Doxycycline Minocycline Erythromycin estolate Spiramycin Metronidazole Oxazepam Propylthiouracil Sulphonylureas	No significant effect

---

1   Increased bioavailability may only occur in some individuals and with particular formulations (i.e. with lesser bioavailability characteristics). Nevertheless, these drugs should always be taken in the same way in relation to meals.

Although the gastric contents and gastric motility are known to be important determinants of dissolution from solid dosage forms, there is surprisingly little good data on the effects of achlorhydria on bioavailability. Phenoxymethylpenicillin and cephalexin are not absorbed as well as normal, and there are conflicting reports suggesting that aspirin may be poorly absorbed (Parsons, 1977). There is an urgent need to obtain more data in this area because of the extensive use of cimetidine in the management of peptic ulcers.

The effects of gastrectomy on drug absorption are very similar to the actions of metoclopramide, suggesting that rapid dumping of the drug into the small bowel is the major functional effect. Again, the problem has been little studied but there is evidence that cephalexin, ethionamide and digoxin may be poorly absorbed (Parsons, 1977).

Antacids interfere with the absorption of several important drugs. The main mechanism involved is likely to be the induced change in gastric pH which alters dissolution characteristics and the rate of gastric emptying (see Hurwitz, 1977). Drug interactions involving changes in drug availability are not uncommon (see chapter VIII; sect. 2.3.1). Most result in decreased bioavailability and should be remembered as an unnecessary cause of therapeutic failure. Formulation variables in bioavailability become of greater importance when associated with disease or drug induced effects on the absorption process. Bioavailability therefore needs to be viewed in the clinical context in which the drug is used.

6. The Design and Interpretation of Bioavailability Studies

The bioavailability of oral formulations is commonly measured in healthy adult subjects. This is usually appropriate in studies of both relative and absolute bioavailability. However, it is more meaningful in some situations to study the formulation in the patient population for which the drug is intended (Brodie and Heller, 1972; Koch-Weser, 1974). Disease and age changes can alter significantly the physiological and pharmacokinetic parameters that influence bioavailability (see chapter I, sect. 4.3; IV, sect. 2; V, sect. 2). The effects of coincident drug therapy is another variable not estimated when bioavailability is measured in normal subjects.

The normal healthy volunteer, however, should never be assumed to be drug free, even when claiming no recent drug exposure. Experience has indicated the absolute necessity to examine pretest plasma and urine samples to confirm the drug free state. Similarly, every effort should be made to ensure compliance with the test drug and the programme of specimen collection.

There are two general types of experimental design appropriate to the study of bioavailability in man — single dose studies, and substitution studies during the 'steady-state' (Koch-Weser, 1974).

6.1 Single Dose Studies

Bioavailability may be measured after a single oral dose of the test formulation, the appearance of drug substance in the systemic circulation being followed by measurement in timed venous blood samples. Alternatively, when the drug is largely excreted unchanged by the kidney, the rate of appearance in the urine may be followed. Estimations based on the urinary excretion of drug are, in general, less satisfactory as they assume complete urine collection, near normal renal function and no other factors influencing renal elimination (see chapter XXI; sect. 1). If there is extensive first-pass hepatic metabolism of the drug, estimations based on urinary excretion are unsatisfactory as the bioavailability may be significantly overestimated.

The bioavailability of the test formulation can be tested against a standard reference drug product (relative bioavailability) or against the same quantity of pure drug substance given as an intravenous infusion (absolute bioavailability). Unless the variation between subjects is large, between 6 to 10 subjects should be included in the study, and the test and reference formulations should be administered using a randomised crossover experimental design. When measuring the absolute bioavailability, it is advisable that the reference intravenous preparation be administered at the same rate that the drug substance is absorbed from the oral formulation. This is to avoid errors due to very different plasma concentrations which may be associated with differing effects on drug distribution, biotransformation and renal excretion. It may be necessary to obtain preliminary estimates of the approximate absorption rate constants.

The concentration of drug in the timed plasma samples is plotted against time to graphically reproduce the absorption profile. When measuring relative bioavailability, there are three characteristics of the absorption profile of particular interest: (1) the peak concentration achieved in the plasma; (2) the time between dosage and the peak concentration; and (3) the area under the plasma level-time curve. These are illustrated in figure 4.

The time between dosage and the appearance of peak concentrations in the plasma reflects the overall speed of the absorptive process. Differences between like formulations in the time to attain peak concentrations may reflect differences in the characteristics of the formulation such as the speed of disintegration or dissolution, or alternatively, some effect on physiological determinants such as gastrointestinal motility. In general, formulations with more rapid absorption are usually associated with higher peak concentrations in the plasma and greater total bioavailability. These relationships do not always hold, especially with poorly soluble drugs. For example, the overall bioavailability of digoxin from slowly dissolving tablets is increased by slowing intestinal motility, allowing more time for dissolution see section 5). Peak concentrations in the plasma are, however, lower and delayed (Manninen et al., 1973a,b). The meaning of the peak concentration

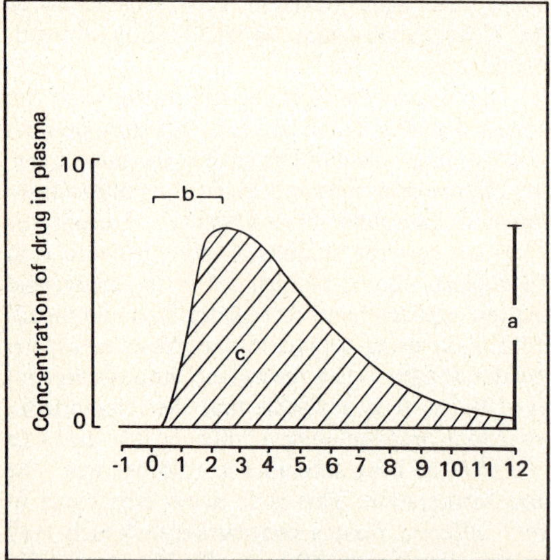

Fig. 4. Typical plasma concentration profile following the administration of an oral dosage form. (a) = peak plasma concentration; (b) = time between dosage and peak concentration in the plasma; (c) = area under the plasma concentration-time curve to 12 hours.

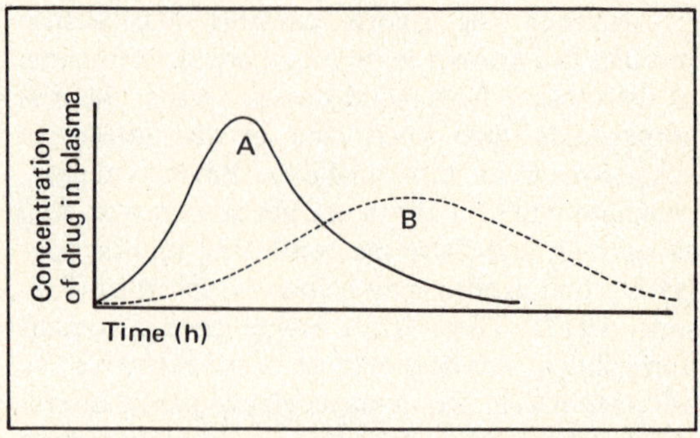

Fig. 5. Plasma level profile of two drug products given at zero time. Product A is more rapidly absorbed and gives higher peak concentration, but product B, although it is absorbed more slowly, has the same total bioavailability — i.e. the area under the plasma concentration-time curve is identical for both products.

should be understood. It does not signify that maximum absorption has been reached or that a higher peak necessarily implies better bioavailability (fig. 5). Absorption is far from complete when peak concentrations are seen. The peak simply represents the point at which the rate of drug addition to the plasma by absorption is balanced by the rate of removal by processes such as distribution, biotransformation and excretion.

The area under the plasma concentration-time curve is proportional to the quantity of total drug substance reaching the systemic circulation, and has the dimensions of mass and time. In most cases, the units used are $\mu g \cdot min \cdot ml^{-1}$. As drug elimination is usually a first order process (see chapter I; sect. 2.1.1), the drug is incompletely eliminated during the period of most bioavailability studies. It is usual therefore to measure the bioavailability (area under the plasma concentration-time curve) over a fixed period after dosage — say, 8 or 10 hours. Provided the absorptive phase is complete and the plasma concentration is measured until it has fallen to about 10% of the peak value, then little error results when comparing the relative bioavailability of like formulations. Under these circumstances, the area under the curve from completion of the study to infinite time can be calculated simply.

It must be stressed that the experimental design described is quite inappropriate to derive the pharmacokinetic properties of the drug. The determination of the terminal plasma half-life time and apparent volume of distribution requires that plasma concentrations be measured during the terminal exponential phase of the plasma decay, over at least 3 times the half-time (see chapter I; sect. 2.1.1).

Studies of the type described can be carried out in the fasting state or after meals or other drugs to test the influence of these factors on bio-availability.

6.2 Studies in the Steady-state

Alternatively, relative bioavailability may be assessed by substituting the test formulation with the reference formulation, once equilibrium or steady-state kinetics is achieved (see chapter I; sect. 2.2). This type of experimental design has particular relevance to studies in patient populations where complete drug withdrawal may not be possible, or where the disease state or other obligatory drug therapy may make alternate experimental designs impossible. The analytical procedures are likely to be simpler with this type of design, as plasma concentrations are invariably higher than those in the single dose studies.

The test formulation is substituted for the reference product only after the steady-state has been maintained and measured for at least a week. This delay is necessary to avoid errors due to gradually changing plasma concentrations associated with mechanisms such as enzyme induction or kinetic properties of the drug such as a long terminal elimination rate constant.

After substitution of the test formulation in the same dosage regimen, the relative bioavailability may be measured by following the plasma concentration over a period of 3 to 4 times the plasma half-time to allow the establishment of a new steady-state. If plasma concentrations should rise or fall near toxic or ineffective levels, the study can be terminated or dosage altered to restore the original steady-state. In some cases, it is possible to follow changes in the rate of urinary elimination following dosage substitution. The same limitations apply as in single dose studies, but if the drug is suitable to be studied in this way, measurement of the 24 hour urinary elimination of the drug gives a good estimate of overall bioavailability.

6.3 Number and Selection of Subjects

The number of subjects to be included in any bioavailability study depends on the variation bet-ween subjects and the differences in bioavailability that would be regarded as clinically significant. It is easy to demonstrate differences between formulations that are 'significant' in the mathematical sense, but they may have no therapeutic importance whatsoever. Further, it must be remembered that extreme care must be exercised in the selection of subjects and in the correct use of randomisation techniques. If there is any confusion on these points, a competent biostatistician should be involved at the early stages of experimental design.

7. Optimum Bioavailability

For reasons discussed, it is not possible to specify standards of bioavailability that apply equally to all formulations of all drugs, but some generalisations can be made. Formulations associated with the least variability are obviously to be preferred, and as a general rule, the least variable formulations also have the best total bioavailability. In some circumstances, it is important to distinguish clearly between different parameters of bioavailability. For example, the total drug absorbed may be more important than peak concentrations achieved when a drug is given over a long period of time. Bioavailability studies can only be interpreted meaningfully when considered in the context of the clinical situation for which the drug is intended.

8. Clinical Implications of Bioinequivalence

Differences in bioavailability between similar formulations of the same drug are common. In fact, bioinequivalence of this type is found much more frequently than bioequivalence (similar bioavailability). However, the important question is: what level of bioinequivalence is associated with significant therapeutic inequivalence?

8.1 Clinical Significance of Difference in Bioavailability

It is reasonable to assume that similar bioavailability characteristics will be associated with similar therapeutic performance, but the converse is not necessarily true. Further, the difference in bioavailability necessary to produce a significant clinical difference between two formulations depends on the particular drug and the clinical situation in which it is being used. Minor differences in bioavailability between formulations containing digoxin, quinidine, coumarins, anticonvulsants, cytotoxic agents and other drugs with low therapeutic ratios are likely to be clinically significant. On the other hand, much larger differences in availability are necessary to produce significant therapeutic inequivalence with many other drugs. Thus, it is not possible to specify universal standards of bioavailability equally applicable to all drugs. Standards must be established for like formulations of all drugs based on the known absorption characteristics of the drug, its therapeutic ratio, the dosage regimen employed and the pathophysiological features of the patient population in which it is to be used (see also section 5). Even if bioequivalence of all formulations of important drugs is ever attained, the major interindividual differences in response to drugs, and such problems as patient compliance will always remain. Differences in bioavailability are likely to be of most clinical significance when a patient is changed to another brand or formulation of a drug which has a low therapeutic ratio, and particularly if the elimination kinetics of the drug are concentration dependent (e.g. dicoumarol and phenytoin; Neuvonen, 1979) and the clinician is not aware of the substitution (section 8.3, 8.4).

8.2 Relationship of *In Vitro* Tests to *In Vivo* Studies in Man

It is clearly difficult to evaluate all available formulations by appropriate *in vivo* studies in man. At the present time, considerable reliance is placed on various *in vitro* test systems, including measures of the speed with which the formulation disintegrates and/or the drug substance dissolves.

Many drugs of limited solubility have absorption rates critically dependent on the speed of dissolution. The *in vitro* dissolution rate in these cases often correlates well with *in vivo* measurements of bioavailability. There are, however, a number of exceptions which make it clear that presently available *in vitro* tests are no substitute for well designed studies in man. Dissolution tests have been grossly misleading. One study with various formulations of oxytetracycline demonstrated the poorest oral bioavailability from a formulation with the fastest *in vitro* dissolution rate (Barber et al., 1974). Similarly, almost identical dissolution rates of formulations of dextropropoxyphene were associated with very different oral bioavailability (De Sante et al., 1977). Even in the case of digoxin, where there has been shown to be a reasonable correlation between the *in vitro* dissolution rate and the oral bioavailability of various formulations (Shaw et al., 1973), the FDA now demands well controlled *in vivo* tests to establish bioequivalence.

Dissolution tests do have an important place in the quality control of formulations, but their low predictive value indicates that they should not be used to compare formulations, and that they can not be relied on to predict the *in vivo* outcome if there is a change in formulation factors such as excipients or crystal form.

These limitations associated with *in vitro* dissolution tests reflect the complex physiological mechanisms involved in drug release and absorption. Furthermore, it is not generally appreciated that components in a formulation may themselves alter physiological mechanisms involved in determining bioavailability. Currently used dissolution tests do not predict the effects of these physiological changes. New types of oral dosage forms which involve the use of osmotic matrices, ion exchange resins, films, membranes and polymers are often designed to produce controlled sustained release of active drug substance. Dissolution tests may indicate the type of release, but the *in vivo* performance can only be determined by *in vivo* measurements in man. Some of the important factors not measured by *in vitro* tests are listed in table I (items 2, 3 and 4).

8.3 Implications for the Prescriber

The clinical implications for the prescriber are clear. Therapeutic equivalence between formulations of the same drug substance should not be assumed unless it has been demonstrated by appropriate studies in man. Therapeutic equivalence should never be assumed simply because therapeutic inequivalence has not been reported. This is usually the last considered cause of therapeutic failure or unexpected toxicity. Recent problems with the bioavailability of digoxin in the United States of America, Great Britain and Australia illustrate the importance of this point.

Drugs should therefore be specified as a particular drug product in every written prescription, and patients should not be changed from one formulation or dosage form to another without good reason. This is well illustrated with phenytoin, when bioavailability between products of the same or different salt forms can vary markedly; as can bioavailability of phenytoin in different dosage forms (see Neuvonen, 1979). If a change is necessary, then the patient should be closely observed, lest therapeutic failure or toxicity result. In such cases, if there is no clear clinical endpoint, but there is a known relationship between the plasma concentration of active drug and efficacy or toxicity, then the blood concentration should be monitored. Digoxin, phenytoin (diphenylhydantoin), quinidine, procainamide, and lithium are important examples in this category (see also chapter I; sect. 5.2).

Particular problems arise when formulations are changed without the knowledge of the prescriber or the patient. This arises in situations when hospitals or institutions change the supplies of 'generic' drugs, as is illustrated by an outbreak of digoxin intoxication following an unannounced change to an 'improved' formulation (Danon et al., 1977). This should never take place without the knowledge of all the clinicians involved and particular attention should be taken lest bioinequivalence results.

These considerations relate directly to the quality of patient care and it is difficult to see how any other conclusions can be drawn from the available data.

8.4 Implications of Drug Product Substitution

It is unfortunate that the clinical implications of bioinequivalence have become clouded by the acrimonious debate on 'generic' or 'trade name' drug prescribing (Lasagna, 1975; Strom et al., 1975). Similarly, it is sad that this issue has been chosen by professional bodies to pursue sectional interests. The position of the American Pharmaceutical Association is particularly hard to understand. This influential body advocates generic prescribing by the physician with the pharmacist free to select the formulation he thinks best (Editorial, 1973). Formulations would be changed from time to time without the knowledge of the prescriber, a situation that is bound to make therapeutic inequivalence more likely to occur and certainly more difficult to detect.

All prescribers should be aware of the real and potential problems associated with variable bioavailability. Improvement in the therapeutic performance of drugs is best achieved by the co-operative efforts of pharmaceutical manufacturers, prescribers, regulatory bodies and others involved in the design and evaluation of drug products.

Further Reading

Blanchard, J.; Sawchuk, R.J. and Brodie, B.B.: Principles and Perspectives in Drug Bioavailability (Karger, Basel 1979).

Brodie, B.B. and Heller, W.M.: Proceedings of conference on bioavailability of drugs. Pharmacology 8: 1 (1972).

Burkholder, D.F. and Barr, W.: Proceedings of the symposium on formulation factors affecting therapeutic performance of drug products. Drug Information Bulletin 3: 6 (1969).

Koch-Weser, J.: Drug Therapy: Bioavailability of drugs. New England Journal of Medicine 291: 233, 503 (1974).

World Health Organisation: Technical Report Series No. 536, Bioavailability of Drugs: Principles and Problems (WHO, Geneva 1974).

References

Aguiar, A.J.: Physical properties and pharmaceutical factors influencing absorption of chloramphenicol and chloramphenicol palmitate. Drug Information Bulletin 3: 17 (1969).

Amdisen, A.: Serum level monitoring and clinical pharmacokinetics of lithium. Clinical Pharmacokinetics 2: 73 (1977).

Ashley, J.J. and Levy, G.: Effect of vehicle viscosity and an anticholinergic agent on bioavailability of a poorly absorbed drug (phenosulfonphthalein) in man. Journal of Pharmaceutical Sciences 62: 688 (1973).

Atkinson, R.M; Bedford, C.; Child, K.J. and Tomich, E.G.: The effect of griseofulvin particle size on blood levels in man. Antibiotics and Chemotherapy 12: 232 (1962).

Barber, H.E.; Calvey, T.N. and Muir, K.: Biological availability and dissolution of oxytetracycline dihydrate tablets. British Journal of Clinical Pharmacology 1:405 (1974).

Barr, W.H.: Factors involved in the assessment of systemic or biologic availability of drug products. Drug Information Association Bulletin 3: 27 (1969).

Beck, J.R.: Massachusetts 'Generic Drug Law'. New England Journal of Medicine 285: 1328 (1971).

Bellet, S.; Finkelstein, D. and Gilmore, H.: Study of a long-acting quinidine preparation. Archives of Internal Medicine 100: 750 (1957).

Blanchard, J.; Sawchuk, R.J. and Brodie, B.B.: Principles and Perspectives in Drug Bioavailability (Karger, Basel 1979).

Bochner, F.; Hooper, W.D.; Tyrer, J.H. and Eadie, M.J.: The cause of an outbreak of phenytoin intoxication. Journal of Neurological Science 16: 481 (1972).

Boman, G.; Lundgren, P. and Stjernstrom, G.: Mechanism of the inhibitory effect of PAS granules on the absorption of rifampicin: Adsorption of rifampicin by an excipient, bentonite. European Journal of Clinical Pharmacology 8: 293 (1975).

Brodie, B.B. and Heller, W.M.: Proceedings of conference on bioavailability of drugs. Pharmacology 8: 1 (1972).

Burack, R.: Massachusetts 'Generic Drug Law'. New England Journal of Medicine 285: 1327 (1971).

Burkholder, D.F. and Barr, W.: Proceedings of the symposium on formulation factors affecting therapeutic performance of drug products. Drug Information Bulletin 3: 6 (1969).

Chodos, D.J. and Disanto, A.R.: Basis of Bioavailability (Upjohn, Kalamazoo 1973).

Crammer, J.L.; Rosser, R.M. and Crane, G.: Blood levels and management of lithium treatment. British Medical Journal 3: 650 (1974).

Danon, A.; Horowitz, J.; Ben-Zul, Z.; Kaplanski, J. and Glick, S.: An outbreak of digoxin intoxication. Clinical Pharmacology and Therapeutics 21: 643 (1977).

DeSante, K.A.; Stoll, R.G.; Kaiser, D.G. and Disanto, A.R.: Generic propoxyphene:Need for clinical bioavailability evaluation. Journal of Pharmaceutical Sciences 66: 1713 (1977).

Dollery, C.T.: Drug names. Prescribers' Journal 9: 97 (1970).

Editorial: APhA's bioavailability project. Journal of Pharmaceutical Sciences 62: 1 (1973).

Editorial: Bioavailability after intramuscular injection. Lancet 1: 261 (1975).

Edwards, C.C.: in Brodie and Heller (Eds) Bioavailability of drugs. Pharmacology 8: 11 (1972).

Gibaldi, M.; Boyes, R.N. and Feldman, S.: Influence of first-pass effect on availability of drugs on oral administration. Journal of Pharmaceutical Sciences 61: 70 (1972).

Goldberg, W.M. and Chakrabarti, S.G.: The relationship of dosage schedule to the blood level of quinidine using all available quinidine preparations. Canadian Medical Association Journal 91:991 (1964).

Greenblatt, D.J.; Smith, T.W. and Koch-Weser, J.: Bioavailability of drugs: The digoxin dilemma. Clinical Pharmacokinetics 1: 36 (1976).

Hamlin, W.E.; Nelson, E.; Ballard, B.E. and Wagner, J.G.: Loss of sensitivity in distinguishing real differences in dissolution rates due to increasing intensity of agitation. Journal of Pharmaceutical Sciences 51: 432 (1962).

Hurwitz, A.: Antacid therapy and drug kinetics. Clinical Pharmacokinetics 2: 269 (1977).

Johansson, E.D.B. and Krai, J.G.: Oral contraceptives after intestinal bypass operations. Journal of the American Medical Association 236: 2847 (1976).

Kaplan, S.A.: Biopharmaceutics in the preformulation stages of drug development; in Swarbrick (Ed) Dosage Form Design and Bioavailability, p.1-31 (Lea and Febiger, Philadelphia 1973).

Karim, A.; Zagarella, J.; Hutsell, T.C.; Chao, A. and Baltes, B.J.: Spironolactone. II. Bioavailability. Clinical Pharmacology and Therapeutics 19: 170 (1976).

Kennedy, M.C. and Wade, D.N.: Phenytoin absorption in patients with ileojejunal bypass. British Journal of Clinical Pharmacology 7: 515 (1979).

Kurtz, P.H.: Massachusetts 'Generic Drug Law'. New England Journal of Medicine 285: 1328 (1971).

Koch-Weser, J.: Drug therapy: Bioavailability of drugs. New England Journal of Medicine 291: 233, 503 (1974).

Lasagna, L.: Drug costs and drug quality. Annals of Internal Medicine 81: 261 (1975).

Leonards, J.R. and Levy, G.: Absorption and metabolism of aspirin administered in enteric-coated tablets. Journal of the American Medical Association 193: 99 (1965).

Levy, G.; Gibaldi, M. and Procknal, J.A.: Effect of an anticholinergic agent on riboflavin absorption in man. Journal of Pharmaceutical Sciences 61: 798 (1972).

Lindenbaum, J.; Mellow, M.H.; Blackstone, M.O. and Butler, V.P.: Variation in biologic availability of digoxin from four preparations. New England Journal of Medicine 285: 1344 (1971).

McQueen, E.G.: Phenytoin intoxication. New Zealand Medical Journal 68: 332 (1968).

Manninen, V.; Apajalahti, A.; Simonen, H. and Reissell, P.: Effect of propantheline and metoclopramide on absorption of digoxin. Lancet 1: 1118 (1973a).

Manninen, V.; Melin, J.; Apajalahti, A. and Karesoja, M.: Altered absorption of digoxin in patients given propantheline and metoclopramide. Lancet 1: 398 (1973b).

Marcus, F.I.; Quinn, E.J.; Horton, H.; Jacobs, S.; Pippin, S.; Stafford, M. and Zukoski, C.: The effect of jejunoileal bypass on the pharmacokinetics of digoxin in man. Circulation 55: 537 (1977).

Mearrick, P.T.; Graham, G.G. and Wade, D.N.: The role of the liver in the clearance of l-dopa from plasma. Journal of Pharmacokinetics and Biopharmaceutics 3: 13 (1974a).

Mearrick, P.T.; Wade, D.N.; Birkett, D.J. and Morris, J.: Metoclopramide, gastric emptying and l-dopa absorption. Australian and New Zealand Journal of Medicine 4: 144 (1974b).

Melander, A.: Influence of food on the bioavailability of drugs. Clinical Pharmacokinetics 3: 337 (1978).

Morrison, A.B. and Campbell, J.A.: Tablet disintegration and physiological availability of drugs. Journal of Pharmaceutical Sciences 54: 1 (1965).

Munzel, K.: The influence of formulation on drug action. Pharmaceutica Acta Helvetiae 46: 513 (1971).

Nelson, E.; Knoechel, E.L.; Hamlin, W.E. and Wagner, J.G.: Influence of the absorption rate of tolbutamide on the rate of decline of blood sugar levels in normal humans. Journal of Pharmaceutical Sciences 51: 509 (1962).

Neuvonen, P.J.: Interactions with the absorption of tetracyclines. Drugs 11: 45 (1976).

Neuvonen, P.J.: Bioavailability of phenytoin: Clinical pharmacokinetic and therapeutic implications. Clinical Pharmacokinetics 4: 91 (1979).

Nies, A.S. and Shand, D.G.: Clinical pharmacology of propranolol. Circulation 52: 6 (1975).

Nimmo, W.S.: Drugs, diseases and altered gastric emptying. Clinical Pharmacokinetics 1: 189 (1976).

Parsons, R.L.: Drug absorption in gastrointestinal disease with particular reference to malabsorption syndromes. Clinical Pharmacokinetics 2: 45 (1977).

Prescott, L.F.; Steel, R.F. and Ferrier, W.R.: The effect of particle size on the absorption of phenacetin in man. Clinical Pharmacology and Therapeutics 11: 496 (1970).

Riegelman, S. and Rowland, M.: Effect of route of administration on drug disposition. Journal of Pharmacokinetics and Biopharmaceutics 1: 419 (1973).

Rowland, M.; Riegelman, S.; Harris, P.A. and Sholkoff, S.D.: Absorption kinetics of aspirin in man following oral administration of an aqueous solution. Journal of Pharmaceutical Sciences 61: 379 (1972).

Shaw, T.R.D.: The digoxin affair. Postgraduate Medical Journal 50: 98 (1974).

Shaw, T.R.D.; Raymond, K.; Howard, M.R. and Hamer, J.: Therapeutic non-equivalence of digoxin tablets in the United Kingdom: Correlation with tablet dissolution rate. British Medical Journal 4: 763 (1973).

Smith, R.N.: Which drugs should we be testing for bioavailability. British Journal of Clinical Pharmacology 2: 5 (1975).

Spangler, D.L.; Kalof, D.D.; Bloom, F.L. and Wittig, H.J.: Theophylline bioavailability following oral administration of six sustained-release preparations. Annals of Allergy 40: 6 (1978).

Strom, B.L.; Stolley, P.D. and Brown, T.C.: Antisubstitution law controversy. Annals of Internal Medicine 81: 254 (1975).

Wade, D.N.; Mearrick, P.T. and Morris, J.L.: Active transport of l-dopa in the intestine. Nature 242: 463 (1973a).

Wade, D.N.; Mearrick, P.T.; Birkett, D.J. and Morris, J.: Variability of l-dopa absorption in man. Australian and New Zealand Journal of Medicine 4: 138 (1973b).

Wagner, J.G.: Generic equivalence and inequivalence of oral products. Drug Intell. Clin. Pharm. 5: 115 (1971).

World Health Organisation: Technical Report Series No. 536, Bioavailability of Drugs: Principles and Problems (WHO, Geneva 1974).

Chapter VII
Pharmacological Basis of Adverse Drug Reactions

E.G. McQueen

Synopsis of Important Principles

1) The risk of adverse drug reactions is an inevitable consequence of potent modern drugs. Few reactions are life threatening, but almost all effective drugs, no matter how skilfully used, can cause serious adverse effects in some patients.

2) Risk of a serious reaction is generally acceptable if the disease being treated is itself very serious. Use of a potentially toxic drug for a trivial illness is unacceptable.

3) The liability of a particular drug to cause adverse reactions, the profile of reactions and their seriousness dictate both the choice of drugs and the risks which are acceptable.

4) All drug effects are the result of complex interaction between the drug, the patient and his pathophysiological condition, and a number of extrinsic factors which can modify drug response.

5) With a knowledge of the pharmacological properties of a particular drug, the mechanisms of adverse reactions, and an awareness of the predisposing factors, particularly those determining special susceptibility of an individual patient, many drug reactions may be avoided.

6) Adverse drug reactions can result from inherent anomalies in patient response such as allergy, genetic factors and physiological variables, from acquired patient anomalies such as associated disease or intercurrent illness, from anomalies of drug presentation and administration, or from interaction of drugs.

7) Important general predisposing factors include an excessive amount of the drug due to non-individualised dosage, prolonged therapy, very young or old age, previous history of allergy or reaction to drugs and multiple drug therapy.

8) Disease and pathophysiological variables are the most important determinants for drug reactions, especially renal disease. Pregnancy and labour are also times of altered drug responsiveness.

9) The incidence of adverse reactions increases with the number of drugs prescribed. Only a few adverse effects of drugs can be attributed to drug interaction, but some important reactions are predictable and can be avoided.

10) The clinician has a responsibility to recognise the presence of an adverse drug reaction, to instruct and forewarn the patient about important reactions, and to report major adverse drug effects to the appropriate committee or registry.

Modern drugs are capable of modifying fundamental biological processes profoundly and their use is inevitably associated with the risk of adverse drug reactions. National and international agencies and a number of hospital-based programmes have been established for monitoring the occurrence of reactions, collating the data, and presenting it to the medical profession in various ways. The aim has been to promote awareness of possible adverse reactions in all therapeutic fields and to assist in early recognition of reactions. Complementary to the documentation and interpretation of reaction data is an adequate understanding of the processes underlying the production of adverse drug reactions. This chapter constitutes an endeavour to promote this better understanding through a systematised approach to the factors determining the development of adverse reactions in particular patients.

Although practising clinicians are seldom in serious doubt as to what constitutes an adverse drug reaction, both inclusive and exclusive criteria are required for deciding what may be designated appropriately as such. An adverse drug reaction may be defined as a reaction to one, or possibly a combination of therapeutic substances which is unsought, is of a potentially harmful character and occurs at a dosage level within the usual therapeutic range. Such reactions may be of an expected and appropriate character for that drug but of inordinate severity. Or they may be side effects; i.e. predictable but inappropriate responses. Many are allergic in origin. Some are the result of true cytotoxic effects of the drug or active metabolite. Lastly, but pre-eminently importantly, they take the form of congenital malformations.

However, a more clinically rewarding approach may be via the mechanisms whereby the above types of reactions are promoted and in the present chapter discussion will be orientated towards the aetiological or pathogenetic factors underlying the development of adverse reactions.

1. Aetiological Basis of Adverse Drug Reactions

1) *Inherent anomalies in patient response* — reactions resulting from allergy or idiosyncrasy, including those due to genetic factors; physiological variables such as age, sex, pregnancy.

2) *Acquired patient abnormalities* — reactions due to the presence of associated disease states or intercurrent illnesses which may modify the response to the drug.

3) *Anomalies of drug presentation and administration* — reactions as a consequence of excessive dosage; changed bioavailability characteristics such as a new dosage form or substitution of a drug product; inappropriate route or method of administration; medication errors.

4) *Interaction of drugs* — reactions resulting from the combined effects of more than one drug prescribed or taken at the same time.

In applying this approach to the problems of adverse reactions in general, its deficiencies become clear by virtue of the large areas of the field left outside the classification, e.g. where the adverse reaction involves a saprophyte such as the fetus, or the bacterial flora of the gut. The approach is however, based on the fundamental understanding that all drug effects are the result of complex interactions between the drug, the patient and his pathophysiological condition, and a number of known and/or unknown extrinsic factors which can modify drug response (Gysling and Heisler, 1975; see further table I). Throughout this book much emphasis has been placed on the individual patient and his disease as central to drug response. Thus, with a knowledge of the pharmacological characteristics of a particular drug (i.e. its actions, physicochemical and pharmacokinetic properties), and an appreciation of the possibility of special susceptibility of an individual patient under specific circumstances, many drug reactions may be averted or at least mitigated.

2. General Considerations

In general, most drugs are remarkably nontoxic but at times serious and even life threatening reactions can occur (Jenner et al., 1976; Jick, 1974). A few drugs have such a low therapeutic ratio that the margin between the effective and toxic dose is narrow. The indication for the use of such drugs must be very sound. Other drugs may cause severe or occasionally fatal reactions even when administered quite appropriately and for sound indications; with present knowledge the reactions are neither predictable nor avoidable. All potent drugs, no matter how skilfully used, can cause serious untoward effects in some patients. Nevertheless, adverse drug reactions due to inappropriate or inadequately supervised therapy do occur, and these can be avoided (Koch-Weser, 1974; Melmon, 1971).

Table I. Important determinants of adverse drug reactions.

___

1. *The administered drug*
   a) Physicochemical and pharmacokinetic characteristics
   b) Formulation characteristics
   c) Dose
   d) Rate and route of administration

2. *The patient and his condition*
   a) Physiological variables
      i) Age
      ii) Sex
      iii) Pregnancy
      iv) Malnutrition
   b) Pathological variables
      i) Associated disease
      ii) Intercurrent illness
   c) Allergic state
   d) Genetic predisposition

3. *Additional extrinsic factors*
   a) Other drugs given
   b) Alcohol consumption
   c) Environmental pollutants
      (heavy occupational exposure to insecticides)
   d) Cigarette smoking

___

2.1 Evaluating the Risk of Adverse Reactions

The risks of serious reactions are generally acceptable if the disease being treated is itself very serious. Sometimes, however, the illness is trivial and use of a drug which can cause a serious reaction, even if only rarely, then becomes completely unacceptable (Girdwood, 1974). Some of the worst drug reactions have occurred with use of potentially toxic drugs for trivial or inappropriate indications (e.g. aplastic anaemia with chloramphenicol for an upper respiratory illness, or with phenylbutazone for a sports injury).

The liability of a particular drug to cause adverse reactions, the profile of the reactions and their seriousness, influence both the choice of drugs and the risks which are acceptable (Wade, 1970). For example, ampicillin causes rashes in many patients, but they are seldom of serious consequence. Chloramphenicol causes relatively few reactions, but those it does, carry a high mortality. Cytotoxic drugs frequently cause serious unwanted side effects, but nobody would argue that they are too dangerous for use in leukaemia and solid tumours.

2.2 Awareness and Recognition of Adverse Reactions

The prescriber cannot be expected to memorise all the likely possibilities, but he should be aware of the most important risks involved with the drugs he employs (see appendix B), particularly those drugs used infrequently. He should be alert also to the possibility of a drug as the cause of or a causative factor in the occurrence of a particular disorder. Some adverse reactions to drugs are easily overlooked (Vere, 1976) because they so closely resemble naturally occurring conditions (e.g. digitalis induced diarrhoea), or because the disorder is so unusual that it does not seem possible that it should be associated with the use of a drug (e.g. sclerosing peritonitis associated with practolol). In some instances, however, it is especially difficult to incriminate a drug as a cause of a particular reaction — e.g. skin eruptions (see chapter XIII; sect. 12.1) and liver disease (see chapter XVIII; sect. 14.6.2). It is just as important for the clinician to recognise the presence of an adverse drug reaction as it is to recognise malignant disease, septicaemia, a metabolic abnormality, or any other of the previously known and well established disease processes. Although such recognition can be difficult, it is nevertheless important, since prompt withdrawal of the drug may be essential to recovery from the drug induced illness, and, with some types of reaction (e.g. hypersensitivity, genetic enzyme defects), to avoidance of a repeat illness from the drug in the future.

2.3 Instruction of the Patient and Reporting of Reactions

The clinician also has a responsibility to warn the patient about possible important reactions, particularly those which may cause the patient to discontinue or modify medication, and to instruct him to report any unusual symptoms or premonitory signs of major drug side effects (e.g. fever, sore mouth, rash as a warning of marrow dysplasia with gold or carbimazole). He also has a duty to report to the appropriate committee or registry any adverse reaction with a new drug, however trivial, for it may be the first of its kind. Unusual, unexpected or serious reactions to established drugs should also be reported, for even if they are known, it is still important to accumulate sufficient information to assess their true significance (McQueen, 1977; Finney, 1977).

Quantitative assessment of the frequency of adverse reactions requires formal monitoring studies such as the Boston Collaborative Drug Surveillance Program (Jick et al., 1970) which enables scrutiny of possible patient/drug interactions in large numbers of hospital patients in specialist units. *Ad hoc* studies have given information on overall frequency in general hospital populations (Smidt and McQueen, 1972; 1973) or in general practice (Jenner et al., 1976). Special characteristics of suspected reactions may require exercise of particular techniques from amongst a range of options for discerning drug related hazards, depending on the rarity or otherwise of the reaction as a drug sequel or as an unrelated event (Jick, 1977). Extrapolation from data gathered on specific patient groups is only justifiable when rigorously defined criteria are complied with (Karch and Lasagna, 1975). However, community health record linkage facilities may provide valuable quantitative data for investigations on suspect drugs within particular health districts (Skegg and Doll, 1977) or even whole nations (Idaanpaan-Heikkila, 1977). See further Lawson (1979).

3. Determinants of Adverse Reactions

With an understanding of the mechanisms and predisposing factors, a proportion of adverse drug reactions is predictable and can be avoided.

1) *Onset of reactions:* Abnormal responses to drugs can occur at any time during a course of treatment or after its completion (Hurwitz and Wade, 1969; Hurwitz, 1969b; Siedl et al., 1966). Many reactions occur early in the course of treatment, e.g. anaphylaxis or reactions due to genetic enzyme defects, even with the first dose. Alternatively, important reactions can develop insidiously over a prolonged period of treatment (e.g. corticosteroid induced posterior or subcapsular cataracts, retroperitoneal fibrosis from methysergide). Other reactions (e.g. sclerosing peritonitis due to practolol) may only become apparent long after the drug is discontinued.

Similar time scales may apply to adverse drug interactions. Some, such as those involving monoamine oxidase inhibitors (see chapter VIII; sect. 3) occur with the first dose of interactant, e.g. phenylpropanolamine. The effects of some drugs such as the monoamine oxidase inhibitors (MAOI) or anticholinesterases such as ecothiopate eye drops, persist when they are discontinued and may still interact with a drug started several days or weeks (MAOI) or months (ecothiopate) later (see chapter VIII, sect. 3; XI, table IIIb).

2) *Amount of drug administered:* Many, but not all drug effects are dose related. Because of individual differences in pharmacokinetic handling of the drug (see chapter I; sect. 3), a dose tolerated by one patient may cause side effects in another. Thus, an excessive amount of the drug resulting from non-individualised dosage and/or prolonged therapy, is likely to be a common predisposing factor for adverse drug reactions. Medication errors may also lead to an excessive amount of a drug being given, as may differences in bioavailability due to substitution of products of the same drug substance (see section 6; chapter VI).

3) *Age:* Reactions are much more likely to occur in the very young and the old (Hurwitz, 1969a; Smith et al., 1966). Response to drugs is significantly altered at the two extremes of life. Because of deficiencies in physiological function compared with young adults and older children, elimination of some drugs is markedly delayed in the elderly and newborn. A decreased capacity for protein binding of acidic drugs and other changes in distribution may also contribute to altered responsiveness. Tissue sensitivity and altered homeostasis are other contributory factors. In both these age groups, a lower dosage than that dictated by body size alone is generally indicated (see further chapters IV, V).

4) *Disease and pathophysiological variables:* The presence of associated disease or intercurrent illness, by altering pharmacokinetic handling or tissue sensitivity, can markedly influence drug response and the occurrence of adverse drug reactions. Pathophysiological variables are the most important determinants for drug reactions and many examples are discussed elsewhere in this book (see table II). Renal disease in particular, significantly increases the risk of adverse reactions of a predictable type, as well as occasionally contributing to unexpected abnormal responses such as neuropsychiatric reactions (see section 5.3).

Pregnancy and labour are also times of altered drug responsiveness (see chapter XV; sect. 1.1.4, 1.1.5). Drug dosage therefore needs to be individualised because of pathophysiological variables.

5) *Sex:* More adverse reactions are reported in women than in men. Average distribution bet-

Table II. Examples of adverse drug reactions due to influence of associated disease or intercurrent illness[1]

Condition	Drug	Possible effect or risk[2]	Mechanism[3]	Further information
Renal disease (see also appendix E)				
Renal failure	Aminoglycoside antibacterials	Ototoxicity	PKe	See chapter XI (sect. 7.1.1); XXI (sect. 14.1.2)
	Colistin	Neuropsychiatric reactions in chronic renal failure (better tolerated acute renal failure)	PKe PDt	
	Tetracyclines	Rise in blood urea, aggravation of renal insufficiency	PDd	See chapter XXI (sect. 14.1.5)
	Digoxin	Digitalis toxicity	PKe	See chapter XXI (sect. 14.2.1)
	Ethacrynic acid Frusemide	Risk of ototoxicity (more likely with large doses)	?PDd	See chapter XI (sect. 7.1.2)
	Aspirin	Enhances bleeding tendency of uraemia and itself may cause blood loss due to gastric mucosal irritation	PDd	See chapter XIX (sect. 14.2.2); XXI (sect. 14.4.6)
Nephrotic syndrome	Clofibrate	Myopathy	PKd	See chapter XXI (sect. 14.7)
	Prednisolone	Increased incidence side effects	PKd	See chapter XXI (sect. 1.2)
	Diuretics	Incautious use can precipitate acute renal failure	PDd	See chapter XXI (sect. 5.2)
Liver disease				
Hepatic pre-coma	Morphine Barbiturates	Precipitate encephalopathy	PDd ?PKm	See chapter XIX (sect. 13.4)
Cirrhotic oedema and ascites	Diuretics	Incautious use can precipitate encephaopathy	PDd	See chapter XIX (sect. 10.3.3)
Obstructive jaundice Hepatitis Cirrhosis	Oral anticoagulants	Enhanced response	PDt	See chapter XXIII (sect. 3.2.4)
Cirrhosis	Lignocaine (lidocaine)	Severe CNS toxicity	PKm	See chapter XIX (sect. 1.4, 13.4)
Hepatitis	Ergot drugs	Ergot poisoning	PKm	See chapter XIX (sect. 1.4, 13.4)

Gastroduodenal disease Peptic ulcer	Aspirin Corticosteroids Indomethacin Phenylbutazone	Risk of bleeding or perforation of a peptic ulcer	PDd	See chapter XIX (sect. 13.1.1, 14.2.2)
Acute gastroenteritis	Oral contraceptives	Pregnancy may result	PKa	See chapter XIX (sect. 13.1.2)
Cardiovascular disease Heart failure	β-Adrenoceptor blocking drugs Phenylbutazone Tricyclic antidepressants	Aggravate or precipitate heart failure	PDd	See chapter XVII (sect. 10.1)
	Lignocaine	CNS toxicity if dose not reduced in advanced heart failure	PKd,m	See chapter XVII (sect. 6.1.3)
Pulmonary heart disease	Digitalis	Digitalis toxicity	PDt	See chapter XVII (sect. 8.1.4); XX (sect. 10.2)
Myocardial ischaemia	Tricyclic antidepressants	Disturbances of cardiac rate, rhythm and conduction	PDd	See chapter XVII (sect. 10.2)
	Digitalis	Arrhythmias	PDt	See chapter XVII (sect. 8.1.4)
	Procainamide	Reduced cardiac output	PDd	See chapter XVII (sect. 10.2)
Bradycardia Conduction abnormality	Quinidine Procainamide Lignocaine Propranolol	Cardiac standstill	PDd	See chapter XVII (sect. 10.2)
Hypertension	Carbenoxolone Oral contraceptives Vasoconstrictors	Rise in blood pressure	PDd	See chapter XVIII (sect. 12)
	Phenothiazines Glyceryl trinitrate	Fall in blood pressure	PDd	See chapter XVIII (sect. 10)
	Tricyclic antidepressants Amphetamines Vasoconstrictors	Antagonise guanethidine-type antihypertensive agents with rise in blood pressure	PDd	See chapter XVIII (sect. 10)

Table II. (continued)

Condition	Drug	Possible effect or risk[2]	Mechanism[3]	Further information
Haematological disease Bleeding disorders	Aspirin	Increased risk haemorrhage	PDd	See chapter XXIII (sect. 7.3)
Thromboembolic disorders	Oral anticoagulants	Many drugs can modify response of oral anticoagulant	PD PK	See chapter XXIII (sect. 3.2.5)
Inherited abnormalities of erythrocyte	Many drugs	Haemolytic anaemia in those with G6PD deficiency	PDd	See chapter XXIII (sect. 8.4)
Megaloblastic anaemia	Co-trimoxazole	Haemopoietic depression	PDd	See chapter XXIII (sect. 7.2)
Psychological disorders	Corticosteroids	May aggravate schizophrenia	PDd	See chapter XXVI (sect. 14)
Neurological disorders Myasthenia gravis	Aminoglycoside antibacterials Polymyxins	Aggravate muscle weakness	PDd	See chapter XXV (sect. 14.1)
Epilepsy	Nalidixic acid Phenothiazines Tricyclic antidepressants	May aggravate seizures	PDd	See chapter XXV (sect. 14.3)
Cerebrovascular disease	Ergotamine	Ischaemic episodes	PDd	See chapter XXV (sect. 11.4)
Rheumatic diseases Systemic lupus	Drugs	Increased incidence drug reactions in general	PDd	See chapter XXII (sect. 13)
Hyperuricaemia	Thiazides	Attack of gout	PDd	See chapter XXII (sect. 13)
Respiratory diseases Asthma	β-Adrenoceptor blocking drugs Prostaglandin $F_{2\alpha}$	Acute bronchospasm	PDd	See chapter XX (sect. 10.1)
Pulmonary heart disease	Digitalis	Digitalis toxicity	PDt	See chapter XVII (sect. 8.1.4); XX (sect. 10.2)

Endocrine disorders				
Diabetes mellitus	Thiazides Ethacrynic acid Frusemide (furosemide) Corticosteroids Oral contraceptives	May aggravate diabetes or make control more difficult	PDd	See chapter XVI (sect. 13.1)
Hypothyroidism	Digoxin Oral anticoagulants	Enhanced response Decreased response	PK/PD PDt	See chapter XVI (sect. 13.2) See chapter XVI (sect. 13.2)
Hyperthyroidism	Digoxin Oral anticoagulants	Decreased response Enhanced response		
Hypopituitarism	Morphine and analogues	Precipitate coma		
Ocular disease				
Glaucoma (narrow angle)	Anticholinergics	Risk precipitation angle closure glaucoma	PDd	See chapter XII (sect. 10.1)
Glaucoma (open angle)	Corticosteroids (systemic)	Sudden rise in intraocular pressure	PDd	
Infections	Corticosteroids (topical)	Exacerbate infection	PDd	See chapter XII (sect. 10.2)
Hypoalbuminaemia	Prednis(ol)one Phenytoin	Increased incidence of side effects	PKd	See this chapter (sect. 5.1)

1 Examples relating to drugs used in anaesthetic practice are given in chapter X (sect. 6). For drug interactions see chapter VIII, appendix C.
2 Some adverse reactions are predictable, others may not necessarily occur or occur in all patients. Many can be avoided by appropriate adjustment of dosage.
3 PK = Due to altered pharmacokinetic handling
   a = inhibition of absorption
   d = altered distribution
   m = inhibition of hepatic metabolism
   e = inhibition of renal excretion
   PD = Due to pharmacodynamic mode of action of the drug
   d = direct effect of drug
   t = altered tissue sensitivity

ween the sexes amongst cases reported to the New Zealand Committee on Adverse Drug Reactions over a 12 year period was 64% female (annual range 61 to 69) and 36% male. Sex distribution amongst the 231 deaths attributed to adverse drug reactions was very similar, 62% female, 38% male. Some of the reactions amongst women have been related to therapy for obstetric or gynaecological conditions. Oral contraceptives accounted for 15 deaths. However, the disparity was less obvious in a general hospital population (Smidt and McQueen, 1972, 1973), 56% of reactions only being in females in two successive 6 month periods. In another general hospital population, 64% of reactions occurred in women (Klein et al., 1976).

There may be a greater tendency on the part of women to seek medical attention and hence to receive drugs. In some contexts however, there is possibly a sex hormone determined predisposition to drug reactions in humans comparable to the regularly observable differences in dose responses seen in experimental animals.

Kellerman et al. (1976) showed that the half-life of antipyrine varied significantly with the phase of the menstrual cycle. Giudicelli and Tillement (1977) have reviewed a number of contexts in which drug kinetics appeared to be significantly modified by the sex of the recipient. Sex linked genetic factors are obvious causes of disparity; e.g. oxidant drug haemolysis with glucose-6-phosphate dehydrogenase deficiency, which affects males preponderantly (see section 4.2.2).

Table III. Incidence of adverse drug reactions in hospitalised patients in relation to previous history of reactions or drug allergy

	USA study[1] (rate %)	UK study[2] (rate %)
History of prior reaction	14.1	27.9
No history of prior reaction	9.0	8.6
History of allergic disease	12.5	28.4
No history of allergic disease	10.5	9.0

1 USA study = Smith et al. (1966).
2 UK study = Hurwitz (1969a).

Table IV. Incidence of adverse drug reactions in hospitalised patients in relation to number of drugs given

USA study[1]		UK study[2]	
drugs given	reaction rate (%)	drugs given	reaction rate (%)
0-5	4.2	1-5	3.3
6-10	7.4	6+	19.8
11-15	24.2		
16-20	40.0		
21+	45.0		

1 Smith et al. (1966).
2 Hurwitz (1969a).

6) *Previous history of allergy or reaction to drugs:* Adverse reactions are much more likely to occur in patients with a history of previous reaction to drugs (table III). In a New Zealand hospital study, 28% of those having an adverse reaction had experienced one before (Smidt and McQueen, 1972). A history of allergic disease is also associated with an increased risk of adverse reactions (table III), based primarily on a genetically determined liability to anaphylactic type reactions, in turn the sequel of a propensity to form inordinately large amounts of IgE.

7) *Multiple drug therapy:* The incidence of adverse reactions increases with the number of drugs given (table IV). The average inpatient in an American hospital receives 9 drugs during hospitalisation compared with 6 for the average Israeli inpatient (Levy et al., 1973), and around 5 for the average British one (Hurwitz and Wade, 1969; Crooks et al., 1977; Lawson and Jick, 1976). In studies in the USA, hospitalised patients who had experienced adverse drug reactions had received an average of 14 (Siedl et al., 1966) or 15 (May et al., 1977) drugs. Outpatients are also prescribed a number of drugs at the same time (Kellaway and McCrae, 1973; Petrie et al., 1975). In some cases, reactions resulting from use of a larger number of drugs is partly due to severe or multiple disease processes for which multiple therapy is unavoidable.

8) *Ethnic and genetic factors:* Heritable characteristics can lead to an abnormal drug response or an increased risk of adverse reactions, by either altering pharmacokinetic handling of the drug, or

altering tissue responsiveness to it (see section 4.2). Genetically determined differences exist in the rate of metabolism of many drugs and the same dose in mg/kg may be associated with wide variations in plasma levels — from subtherapeutic to toxic (see chapter I; sect. 4.2). The importance of monitoring therapy by blood level estimation is being increasingly recognised.

Genetic factors additionally can lead to unique and unexpected responses, some of which may be fatal (e.g. malignant hyperpyrexia with general anaesthesia). Recognition of genetically determined reactions can lead to their prevention. For example, patients with genetic enzyme defects such as glucose-6-phosphate dehydrogenase deficiency should avoid certain drugs (see section 4.2.2; chapter XXIII; sect. 8.4).

4. Reactions Due to Inherent Anomalies in Patient Response

4.1 Drug Allergy

In categorising reactions under this heading it is important to establish clearly what is intended by the term 'allergy'. Originally introduced by von Pirquet in 1906 to describe a state of *'changed reactivity'* resulting from exposure to a foreign substance acting as an 'allergen', the allergic state is one of specifically altered potential reactivity to a particular chemically definable substance — in this case a drug or breakdown product of a drug. However, the term 'drug allergy' is used more often than not to refer to the *'allergic reaction'* to the drug concerned in a patient who already had the specifically altered or allergic state established as a result of prior exposure.

Recognition of a drug reaction as an allergic one classically follows its conformity to the pattern characteristically associated with allergy (for review, see Samter and Parker, 1972):

a) There is a delay in the establishment of the allergic state following the initial exposure.
b) Once an allergic state has been established the allergic reaction can be precipitated by minute amounts of the drug.
c) There is recurrence of the reaction on repeated exposure.
d) The reaction does not resemble the pharmacological activity of the drug.

e) The symptoms are suggestive of some form of allergic response, e.g. urticaria, serum sickness, anaphylaxis etc, and may be accompanied by other stigmata such as eosinophilia.

However, none of these criteria may be apparent and differentiation from genetically determined anomalies of drug response may be difficult; reactions now believed to be due to an immune mechanism may, in the future, prove to be due to enzymatic or other abnormalities in the patient.

4.1.1 Mechanisms of Drug Allergy

All allergic mechanisms depend upon interaction between a foreign antigen and host antibodies or sensitised lymphocytes (for review, see Parker, 1975; Whittingham and Mackay, 1976).

Before a drug can act as an allergen it must have two properties:

a) It must be able to form a macromolecular, covalently bonded, complex in the body — in other words, it must be able to form an antigen.
b) This antigen must be able to produce an allergic response.

Most drugs are small molecules and therefore cannot themselves act as antigens and stimulate immunological responses, but they may do so if they are of sufficient chemical reactivity to combine with endogenous carrier macromolecules, usually proteins. When small molecules react in this way they are known as haptens. Binding to a carrier macromolecule need not necessarily involve the drug itself. In fact, the drugs themselves may be chemically incapable of covalent linkage in this way. Under these circumstances it must be presumed that a metabolite of the drug is responsible. In the case of penicillin, the unmodified molecule circulates bound to serum albumin, but in a loose readily dissociable combination not capable of acting as an antigen. A number of its breakdown products however, do readily couple with larger peptide or protein molecules by amide, carbonyl, or disulphide linkages to form a series of potent 'antigenic determinants' (Parker, 1975). Thus, antibodies which can be detected in the serum of patients receiving penicillin are not directed towards penicillin itself, but to its breakdown products, especially the penicilloyl group, which are capable of existing in covalent linkage to protein (Batchelor et al., 1967).

The immunogenicity of the carrier itself seems to be important, since haptens combined with foreign proteins are more effective in promoting an immune response than haptens on native proteins. Interaction with thymus derived (T) lymphocytes initiates the immune response. Once T cells have been activated hapten specific activation is produced in bone marrow derived (B) lymphocytes and antihapten (antidrug) antibodies are formed (fig. 1).

To elicit a reaction, the antigen must be capable of forming a bridge between antibody molecules. A bridge between antibody molecules permits them to react with complement to release cytoactive peptides. A bridge between cell bound antibody molecules or antigen receptors on lymphocytes produces the conformational change in the cell membrane required for activation of mediator release or lymphocyte transformation.

Precipitation of a reaction in the already sen-

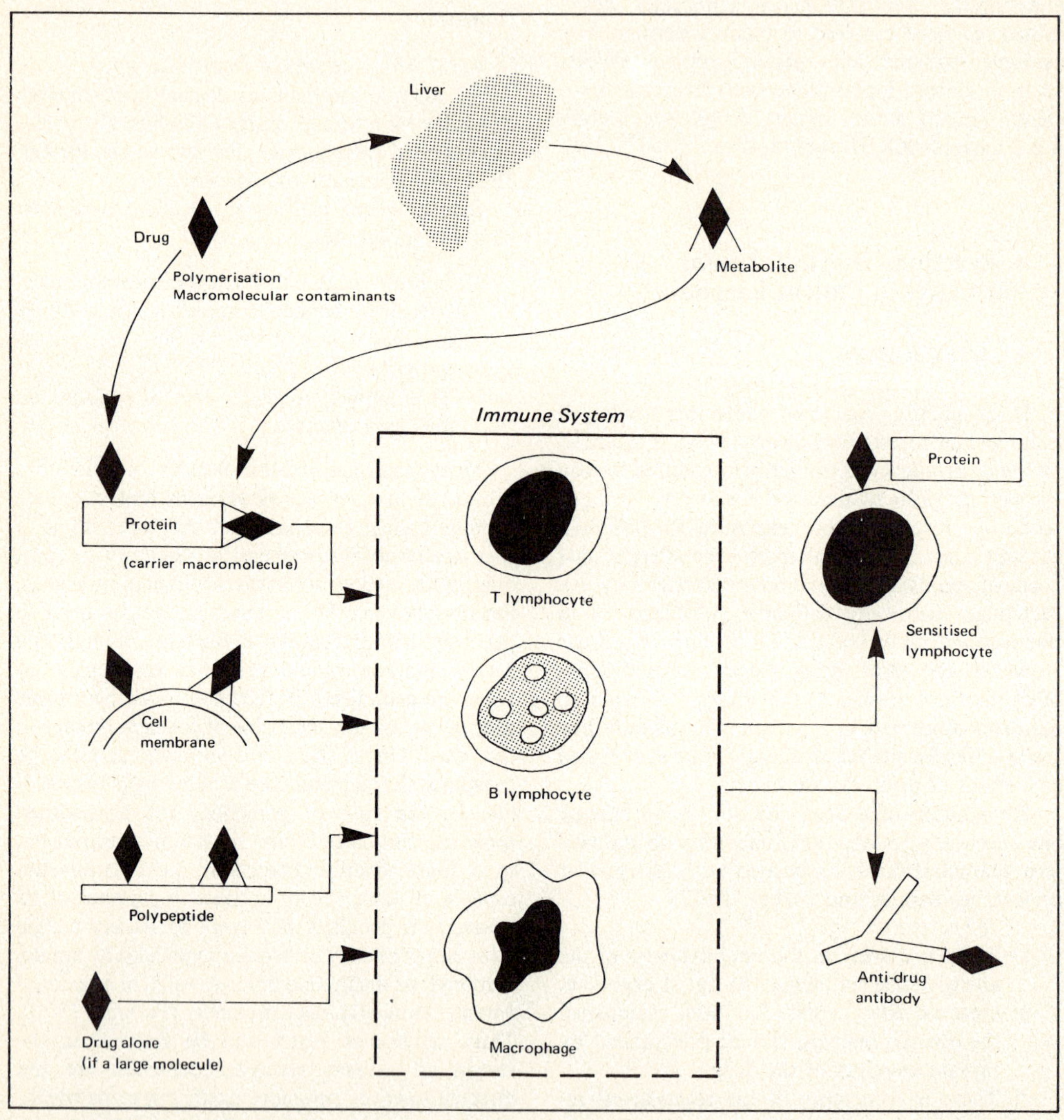

Fig. 1. Schematic representation of general process of drug allergy. The drug, metabolite or other breakdown product combines with host protein or cell membrane. This is regarded as 'foreign' and an immune response results (after Wilson: Patient Management 4: 32, Nov. 1975; by permission of author and editor).

Table V. Examples of allergic drug reactions and drug reactions suspected of being allergic (after Parker, 1975)

Type	Example (see also text and other chapters)
Anaphylaxis	Penicillins[1], Dextrans, Foreign antisera, Iodinated radiographic contrast media, Intravenous anaesthetics and relaxants
Serum sickness	Penicillins (notably long acting forms), Sulphonamides[2], Thiouracils
Immune haemolytic anaemia	Penicillins, Cephalothin, Quinidine, Rifampicin (more likely intermittent regimen, especially large dose), PAS, Sulphonamides, Phenacetin
Autoimmune haemolytic anaemia	Methyldopa
Immune thrombocytopenia	Quinidine, Quinine, Thiouracils, Sulphonamides, Rifampicin (more likely intermittent regimen, especially large dose), Thiazides
Immune granulocytopenia	Phenylbutazone, Thiouracils, Sulphonamides, Penicillins, Chlorpropamide, Aminopyrine

Cutaneous eruptions
  Urticaria
  Contact dermatitis
  Maculopapular
	
	Aspirin, Penicillin
	Topical neomycin[2], Paraben vehicle preservatives
	Barbiturates, Sulphonamides

Fever (as isolated manifestation)	Penicillins, PAS, Amphotericin B, Phenytoin (diphenylhydantoin), Quinidine
Hepatitis	PAS, Sulphonamides, Phenothiazines, ?Halothane
Pulmonary eosinophilia	Nitrofurantoin[2], PAS, Sulphonamides
Interstitial nephritis	Penicillins (high dose, especially methicillin)
Vasculitis	Penicillins, Sulphonamides, Thiouracils
Systemic lupus syndrome	Hydrallazine, Procainamide, Isoniazid, Phenytoin

1   Anaphylaxis most common with parenteral benzylpenicillin (penicillin G).
2   Examples of chemically related drugs: Sulphonamides — thiazides, sulphonylureas; Neomycin — framycetin, gentamicin topical preparations; Nitrofurantoin — furazolidone.

sitised patient however, need not necessarily involve the complete macromolecular antigen necessary for creation of the allergic state. Thus, penicillin may precipitate anaphylactic shock by virtue of polymeric complexes of the drug itself, already formed in the preparation prior to administration (Stewart, 1967). The pharmacological (humoral) mediators of the sequelae of the antigen-antibody response include histamine, kinins, 'slow reacting substance of anaphylaxis' (SRS-A), serotonin and prostaglandins (see chapter XX, fig. 1).

Antibodies formed against drug-protein complexes may be of the IgG or IgM types, i.e. circulating antibodies, or of the 'reaginic' IgE type, with its propensity for cell coating and sequestration in tissues. In the latter case, rechallenge with the antigen may lead to typical anaphylactic-type reactions. IgG and IgM may however, act as 'blocking antibodies', combining with antigen before it can reach fixed IgE antibodies. Blocking antibodies may prevent anaphylaxis. They only rarely cause a clinical syndrome themselves. They are very widespread, and can be found in non-allergic subjects as often as in allergic subjects. Competition between the blocking antibodies and the reaginic antibody IgE may explain the apparent discrepancies between skin testing and the development of acute anaphylactic reactions. Additionally, free drug or non-conjugated metabolite may pre-empt binding sites on antibodies, denying access to complete antigens.

4.1.2 Clinical Manifestations of Drug Allergy

The symptoms of drug allergy will depend upon which mechanism is involved (for review, see Parker, 1975). Sometimes more than one mechanism appears to contribute to the allergic response. The symptoms produced are those of an allergic reaction and will not be specific for any particular drug. Some drugs such as penicillin can produce a number of types of allergic symptoms. Table V lists examples of drug reactions known or suspected to be due to allergic mechanisms. Some of these reactions to particular drugs are used to illustrate the clinical presentation of allergy in the sections which follow.

1) *Anaphylactic Reactions* (Coombs-Gell type I hypersensitivity; Coombs and Gell, 1968): Reactions of this, the 'immediate' type, are largely IgE mediated (fig. 2a). They may be generalised, when they take the form of acute systemic anaphylactic shock, or localised. Reactions of the latter type are presumably determined by the preponderant site of interaction of the allergen with IgE. This may be in the skin with production of acute urticaria or angio-oedema, in the respiratory tract causing bronchial asthma, or in the gastrointestinal tract giving rise to vomiting, abdominal pain and diarrhoea.

Generalised systemic anaphylaxis is an acute, life threatening allergic reaction with hypotension, plus bronchospasm, urticaria, laryngeal oedema etc, either in combination or as isolated features. Anaphylaxis is most common with drugs given intramuscularly or intravenously, although oral, percutaneous or even respiratory exposure may produce the response. The reaction typically develops rapidly (reaching a maximum within 5 to 30 minutes) and usually occurs at the start of treatment with a drug to which the patient has been exposed previously. Allergic symptoms may not necessarily have occurred during previous courses of treatment. Indeed, anaphylactic shock to penicillin has been known to occur with the 17th course of treatment, the previous 16 courses having been given without incident (Parker, 1975). Contrariwise, there may be no history of prior therapeutic exposure. Penicillin is the most frequent cause of such acute immunologically

mediated reactions, although even it causes anaphylaxis very infrequently. The risk of anaphylactic reactions to penicillin is 2 to 3 times greater in atopic subjects than in the general population (De Warte, 1972), but individuals who experience anaphylactic reactions to drugs need not have a personal or family history of allergy. Some other drugs which can cause anaphylaxis by allergic mechanisms are given in table V. Acute anaphylaxis may be related to any of the intravenous anaesthetics or relaxants (Fisher, 1977; see chapter X, section 2.1.2, 2.2).

'Anaphylactoid' reactions may present with features resembling those of genuine allergic reactions (bronchospasm, urticaria, etc) following administration of certain drugs which act directly as histamine releasers (i.e. by a pharmacological mechanism). Intravenous opiates (e.g. heroin, codeine, morphine) may produce this effect, as may intravenous dextran, which however, is a potent allergen as well.

2) *Serum Sickness* (Coombs-Gell type III hypersensitivity; Coombs and Gell, 1968): Serum sickness is a less acute systemic allergic reaction which results from damage produced by circulating immune complexes. It results when antigens remain in the circulation for a prolonged period of time, so that when antibody is first formed, intravascular antigen is still present and permits the formation of circulating antigen-antibody (i.e. drug-hapten-antibody) complexes. Such immune complexes may, with or without complement, produce a serum sickness syndrome.

The serum sickness-type reaction to drugs associated with circulating antibodies and antigen excess in serum or tissue fluid, corresponds to type III hypersensitivity of the Coombs-Gell classification. The antibodies are largely of the IgG class and possibly IgM (fig. 2b). IgE antibodies may also contribute to the response (see below).

In the presence of a relative excess of antigen, the immune complexes are small and not readily removed, and lodge in small blood vessels leading to inflammation. Such reactions may take the form of fever only, or involve generalised lymphadenopathy and joint swellings, and be accompanied by anaphylactic (IgE) features as well, such as bronchospasm, urticaria, and angio-oedema. Neutropenia is likely to be evident early on; eosinophilia is not a feature of this condition, but thrombocytopenia may occur. Skin rashes are particularly common and may occur locally at a previous injection site. Glomerulonephritis, pericar-

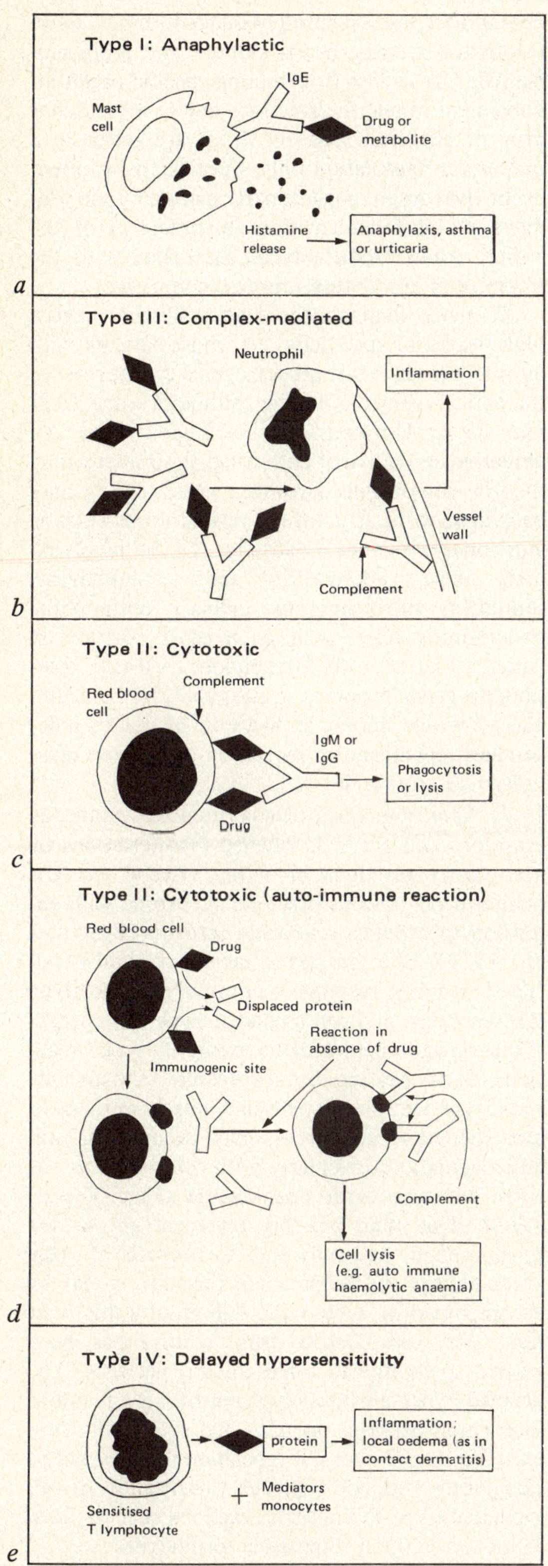

ditis, myocarditis, meningitis, meningoencephalitis, peripheral neuritis, myelitis may also occur.

Serum sickness, seldom now seen as the result of the classical foreign serum injection (e.g. ATS), may also result from the injection of contaminant foreign proteins, e.g. egg protein in influenza vaccine. Penicillin is again a frequent cause, the long acting procaine penicillin perhaps particularly so. Streptomycin, para aminosalicylic acid (PAS), sulphonamides and a few other drugs (table V) have also been implicated reasonably often. In the initial exposure to a drug, symptoms of the serum sickness syndrome generally develop after a latent period of 6 days or more, reflecting the time taken to synthesise appreciable amounts of antibody. However, symptoms may first appear as long as 3 weeks after the last dose. Generally, symptoms last for from a few days to a week, but may persist for as long as 6 weeks.

3) *Immunologically Mediated Reactions Against Specific Tissues:* IgE antibody mediated drug allergy may result in consistent involvement of specific organs, particularly the skin and bronchial tree, by reason of preponderant localisation of IgE antibody, high frequency of mediator-containing mast cells, or hyper-reactivity of target tissue. However, drug allergy may also develop as a result of interaction between drug (or a metabolite) acting as a hapten, and tissue constituents, with the conferral of antigenicity and production of antibodies (IgG type), specifically directed against those tissues.

By reason of their accessibility, reactions of this kind involving the formed elements of the blood have been most extensively studied. Immune haemolytic anaemias have been described with numerous drugs (table V), the mechanism in most cases apparently being combination of hapten with a serum protein macromolecule, production of anti-drug antibody, and, on further administration of the drug, adsorption of the drug-antibody complex onto red cells. Activation of the complement mechanism produces haemolysis (Beutler, 1969). Similarly drug/anti-drug antibody complex may localise on platelets with aggregation and platelet sequestration. The apparently vicarious involve-

Fig. 2. Mechanisms of cell damage by allergic response, representing: (a) anaphylaxis; (b) serum sickness; (c) cytotoxic reaction directed against individual organ; (d) cytotoxic reaction of auto-immune type; (e) contact dermatitis due to delayed hypersensitivity (after Wilson: Patient Management 4: 32, Nov. 1975; by permission of author and editor).

ment of red cells or platelets has led to the description of these reactions as of the 'innocent bystander' type (Damashek, 1965). However, although a number of drugs such as quinine or quinidine are common to the lists of agents responsible for either haemolysis or thrombocytopenia, there is a consistent reproduction of the same reaction in a given patient, e.g. thrombocytopenia with quinidine. This suggests specific involvement of the platelet as a component of the antigen, as originally postulated by Ackroyd, 1954). However, rifampicin can apparently produce either or both, generally in association with intermittent regimens (Kronig et al., 1972; Lakshminarayan, 1973; Pujet et al., 1974).

At excessively high blood levels of penicillin (e.g. dose of 15 mega units per day with tubular blockade and/or renal disease), circulating red cells become modified by hapten and bind anti-hapten antibody resulting in a positive Coombs test (fig. 2c). Under these circumstances they are primed to undergo phagocytosis and lysis (Parker, 1975). Penicillin induced haemolytic anaemia has been described with quite low dosage (Dove et al., 1975, McPherson et al., 1976), and cephalothin induced haemolysis with a positive Coombs test occurs at regular dose levels in the absence of renal disease (Gralnick et al., 1971; Rubin and Burka, 1977).

Some drugs can induce an autoimmune state. Methyldopa induced haemolytic anaemia appears to arise in this way. Antibodies develop which are directed towards native antigens on the red cell surface and often have Rh specificity (fig. 2d). Existence of the process is manifest by a positive Coombs test, but only a minority of such patients develop overt haemolysis (see further chapter XXIII; sect. 8.4). The autoimmune disturbance is evidenced also in a few patients by the presence of LE cells, antibodies and hepatitis.

High titres of antinuclear autoantibody can be demonstrated in drug triggered chronic active hepatitis (Lindberg et al., 1975). Drugs involved have included particularly oxyphenisatin but also methyldopa, isoniazid, sulphonamides, phenylbutazone and nitrofurantoin (Maddrey and Boitnott, 1977; Zimmerman, 1978). Antineutrophil antibody activity of various types may be demonstrable in patients with neutropenia associated with various drugs (Weitzman and Stossel, 1978).

Other drug reactions, either involving entrapment of circulating immune complexes or the interaction of circulating antibodies with tissue bound drug, may result in damage to lungs, liver, locomotor system, heart, kidneys and peripheral nerves. The factors determining specific organ involvement in allergic reactions due to a particular drug or chemical series of drugs are generally a matter for speculation only. Specific involvement of the liver might suggest participation by the products of biotransformation. Involvement of the kidney could predictably be associated with the trapping of circulating immune complexes.

In many contexts, the drug antibodies have a high degree of specificity, e.g. most patients with quinine-sensitive thrombocytopenia do not react to the optical isomer quinidine, although some 20 % may do so (Horowitz and Nachman, 1965). An oxidative derivative of both drugs (quininone) may then be responsible. However, cross allergy may be evident with structurally related drugs such as sulphonamides (see Goldstein, 1974) involving drug fever, dermatitis and conjunctivitis. Similarly, nitrofurantoin induced eosinophilic pneumonitis may occur as a cross reaction in patients treated with furazolidone. Allergic reactions to cephalosporins in persons with penicillin allergy would appear as likely to be due to independent cephalosporin sensitivity as to cross reactivity (see section 4.1.3).

4) *Skin Reactions:* Drug induced cutaneous eruptions can occur as isolated manifestations or accompany reactions involving viscera, e.g. the oculomucocutaneous practolol syndrome with extension to produce sclerosing serositis (Brown et al., 1974). Skin reactions include Coombs-Gell type I (reaginic reactions), immune complex (type III) reactions, and cell mediated (type IV) allergy. Urticaria and angio-oedema exemplify type I reactions. A devastating, but fortunately very uncommon, type III reaction of blood vessels in the skin and subcutaneous tissues, may occur with oral anticoagulants particularly with coumarin derivatives but also with phenindione (Koch-Weser, 1968). This may possibly represent an Arthus phenomenon, and may lead to necrosis of large areas of skin and subcutaneous tissues. It may be accompanied by acute renal failure, and this in at least one case (Dixon, pers. comm) has been shown to be due to renal cortical necrosis. The delayed hypersensitivity type reaction is a result of interaction between the drug and specifically sensitised cells and does not depend on the presence of circulating antibody (fig. 2e). Localisation of cell mediated (type IV) allergic reactions such as fixed eruptions is often impossible to interpret.

5) *Fever:* Fever may occur as an isolated manifestation of drug allergy, for example with sulphonamides and aminosalicylic acid (PAS). Marked and sustained fever is usually associated with definite inflammation of small vessels, and if the drug is continued, serious visceral or cutaneous complications can result. Thus, aminosalicylate may produce some or all of the components of a generalised hypersensitivity syndrome including general malaise, fever, headache, rash, encephalopathy, splenomegaly, sometimes hepatomegaly and atypical lymphocytes in the blood, possibly with eosinophilia (NZ Committee on Adverse Drug Reactions, unpublished data). An acute systemic hypersensitivity reaction accompanied by nephropathy, hepatitis and variable haematological abnormalities may complicate the use of phenindione (NZ Committee on Adverse Drug Reactions, 1970).

4.1.3 Penicillin Allergy

Penicillin can cause many types of allergic reaction (table V; for review, see Isbister, 1971; Stewart and McGovern, 1970; Girard and Cueras, 1975). Its peculiarly high capacity to generate allergens is possibly because a proteinaceous fermentation residue may be present in commercial penicillin, certified as pure by ordinary standards, with which penicilloyl groups and minor determinants conjugate readily. This may explain why life threatening anaphylactic responses are characteristically observed with the natural penicillin G. The deacylation and replacement of side-chains which are involved in manufacture of the semi-synthetic penicillins presumably remove the proteinaceous residue. However, acute anaphylaxis may occur with ampicillin, even when given orally (NZ Committee Adverse Drug Reactions, 1972; Hoffmann, 1968). Acute anaphylaxis is possibly less common when drugs are given orally, because alimentary digestion may also remove proteinaceous allergens. Precipitation of an allergic reaction in a sensitised subject does not necessarily require complete antigen and may be elicited by polymeric complexes forming spontaneously in solutions of penicillins (see section 4.1.1).

The incidence of allergic reactions to all cephalosporins in patients not hypersensitive to penicillin is about 1.7% while the incidence in patients who are hypersensitive to penicillin is about 8.2% (Petz, 1971). This does not necessarily mean that there is cross allergenicity, but it does mean that allergic reactions to cephalosporins are about 5 times more common in patients with a history of penicillin allergy. This is not far from the 6-fold increase in reactions noted among patients with bacterial endocarditis who were treated with penicillin itself, despite a history of allergy to penicillin (Green et al., 1966, 1967). It may be that the incidence of cephalosporin reactions in penicillin sensitive subjects merely reflects that to be expected in an atopic population.

4.1.4 Occurrence of Allergic Drug Reactions

The factors which determine the likelihood of an allergic reaction to a drug can be classified as follows (Parker, 1975):

1) *Duration and number of courses of treatment:* In general, the likelihood of a reaction increases with the number of courses of treatment; e.g. a patient may have been given penicillin on a number of occasions without incident, but suffer anaphylactic shock with the next course. The incidence of anaphylaxis itself increases with repeat courses (Girard and Cueras, 1975). With drugs given in a single course over a prolonged period of time, the likelihood of a reaction is much greater in the first 2 or 3 weeks, although reactions may occur later, even after years of treatment. Anaphylaxis should not be a problem once treatment is under way, provided different batches of the drug are of comparable purity.

2) *Route of drug administration:* Any route of administration can result in allergic symptoms. With topical application, the site of entry can be the main target area for the reaction. Anaphylaxis is much less common with oral than with parenteral administration (Simmonds et al., 1978).

3) *Atopic subjects:* The risk of anaphylaxis is substantially increased in atopic individuals, as is that of other reaginic (type I) allergic reactions, but other types of allergic reaction seem to occur with about the same frequency as in the general population.

4) *Previous history of allergic reactions:* The likelihood of another reaction is increased in those who have suffered a previous allergic reaction, but the allergy may not necessarily persist indefinitely. Cross allergy can occur between chemically related drugs (see table V).

5) *Age:* Allergic reactions to drugs seem to be less common in children. The reasons for the lower prevalence are not clear.

6) *Disease:* Impaired renal function increases the risk of haemolytic anaemia with high dose penicillin therapy (see section 4.1.2). There does not seem to be an increased prevalence of drug allergy in patients with systemic lupus erythematosus (Becker, 1973). Patients with infectious mononucleosis, lymphoid leukaemia, or hyperuricaemia (with or without allopurinol therapy), have a very much greater likelihood of maculopapular rash with ampicillin (Pullen et al., 1967; Boston Collaborative Drug Surveillance Program, 1972a; Cameron and Richmond, 1971). This may result from a reaction involving polymeric adducts of penicillin, which have the capacity to induce lymphocyte proliferation and abnormal lymphocytes (Parker and Richmond, 1976). The incidence of the rash appears to be able to be reduced by use of polymer free ampicillin.

4.2 Genetically Determined Drug Reactions

Individual patients vary widely in their response and reaction to drugs. Even if allowance has been made for the patient's age, sex, weight, disease state and other drugs he is taking, there is still variation between individuals. The patient's unique genetic constitution is one contribution to this variability. Depending on the drug, some patients do not obtain the desired therapeutic effect, while others experience severe adverse reactions when given what is considered to be the average and safe dose. The discipline of pharmacogenetics deals with those variations in drug response which are under hereditary control (for reviews, see Kalow, 1962; La Du, 1972; Motulsky, 1964; World Health Organisation, 1973). Its rapid development has permitted a high degree of discrimination within major genetically determined adverse drug reactions (Vesell, 1972, 1975). These can be divided into two types:

a) Those which are due to altered pharmacokinetic handling of the drug in the body — i.e. the effect of the body on drugs.
b) Those which are due to altered tissue responsiveness and hence are pharmacodynamic in origin — i.e. the effect of drugs on the body.

Variability in the response to a drug in the general population may take the form of a continuous unimodal (or Gaussian) distribution curve or a discontinuous polymodal (or discrete) curve

(fig. 3). Multiple genetic influences presumably determine the continuous type of variability. The discontinuous type gives bimodal or even trimodal distribution and suggests a simpler genetic system, but it can also indicate extraneous influences or even artefacts. Other genetic terms of relevance to a basic understanding of pharmacogenetics include the phenotype and genetic polymorphism (see Evans, 1969b). The phenotype is the manifestation of the genetic constitution of an individual which, in the case of a 'gene of large effect' can produce manifest characteristics, or characteristics which can be discovered by examination (e.g. acetylation phenotype of isoniazid). Genetic polymorphism is a type of variation in which individuals with sharply distinct qualities (i.e. discontinuous variability) coexist as normal members of a population. Polymorphism is a property of the population which has in it different kinds of person (i.e. genotypes). A genetic polymorphism is maintained from one generation to the next by inheritance of the appropriate allelic genes. Allelic genes are alternative genes which can occupy the same location (locus) on a chromosome. Anomalous drug responses of this type which achieve recognition as adverse drug reactions derive from the extremes of continuous distribution curves or from sharply discontinuous variation in genetically determined frequency distributions. It is in the latter area that the most dramatic manifestations, which may still merit the term 'idiosyncrasy', occur.

4.2.1 Genetically Determined Pharmacokinetic Reactions

As discussed in chapter I (sect. 4) and elsewhere in this book, differences between individuals in drug absorption, distribution, metabolism and excretion can have profound effects on the response to drugs. Genetic factors have not been shown to be important in influencing drug absorption and distribution. For some drugs (e.g. nortriptyline), there are small interindividual differences in drug distribution and plasma protein binding which appear to be partially under genetic control (Rawlins, 1975). Genetic factors do not seem to be directly related to altered rates of renal excretion, although genetic disorders associated with abnormal renal function (e.g. renal tubular acidosis) may influence drug excretion indirectly.

Drug metabolism however, is markedly influenced by genetic factors, such that wide interindividual differences exist in the rate of drug elimination. Individual differences also exist in the pattern of drug metabolites. For a variety of drugs, wide differences in steady-state plasma concentrations exist between individuals given the same dose of the drug (see chapter I; sect. 4.2; see also review by Alvan, 1978). Such differences help to explain why some patients have a poor therapeutic response and others severe side effects to a standard dose of the drug. Moreover, drug metabolites may have pharmacological or toxic potential themselves (Drayer, 1976; Mitchell and Jollows, 1975; Orme, 1977). Genetically determined differences in metabolism have been shown to be of particular importance for a number of drugs initially metabolised by hydrolysis, acetylation or oxidation pathways.

The classical example of altered drug response due to individual differences in drug metabolism is suxamethonium (succinylcholine) apnoea, which led to the recognition of plasma pseudocholinesterase polymorphism. Suxamethonium usually exerts its neuromuscular blocking effect for only a few minutes as it is rapidly hydrolysed by a cholinesterase (pseudocholinesterase) present in the plasma and liver. In about 1 in 2,500 individuals of the population, the neuromuscular blockade of suxamethonium lasts for as long as 3 hours, because of low plasma pseudocholinesterase activity due to an 'atypical' plasma

pseudocholinesterase which has a markedly reduced affinity for suxamethonium. One-sixtieth the dose of suxamethonium in these subjects produces the same effect as a full dose in a subject with normal enzyme activity (Kalow and Genest, 1957; Kalow and Gunn, 1957). Only about two-thirds of patients with prolonged apnoea after suxamethonium have recognisable genetic abnormalities (Simpson and Kalow, 1966). Liver disease, malnutrition, other drugs and occupational exposure to organophosphorus insecticides can also influence the activity of plasma pseudocholinesterase (see chapter X; sect. 2.2, table VII). Atypical resistance to suxamethonium has also been described in members of one family (Neitlich, 1966). The decreased response is due to the presence of a form of pseudocholinesterase with an activity 3 times that of the normal enzyme.

A number of drugs are metabolised by acetylation. The rate at which some drugs are acetylated (e.g. isoniazid) varies widely between individuals and shows a bimodal distribution in the population, permitting categorisation of individuals as either slow or rapid inactivators (acetylators) [for review, see Lunde et al., 1977]. The variability is predominantly genetic in origin and is due to differences in the activity of the liver enzyme N-acetyltransferase. Slow acetylators are homo-

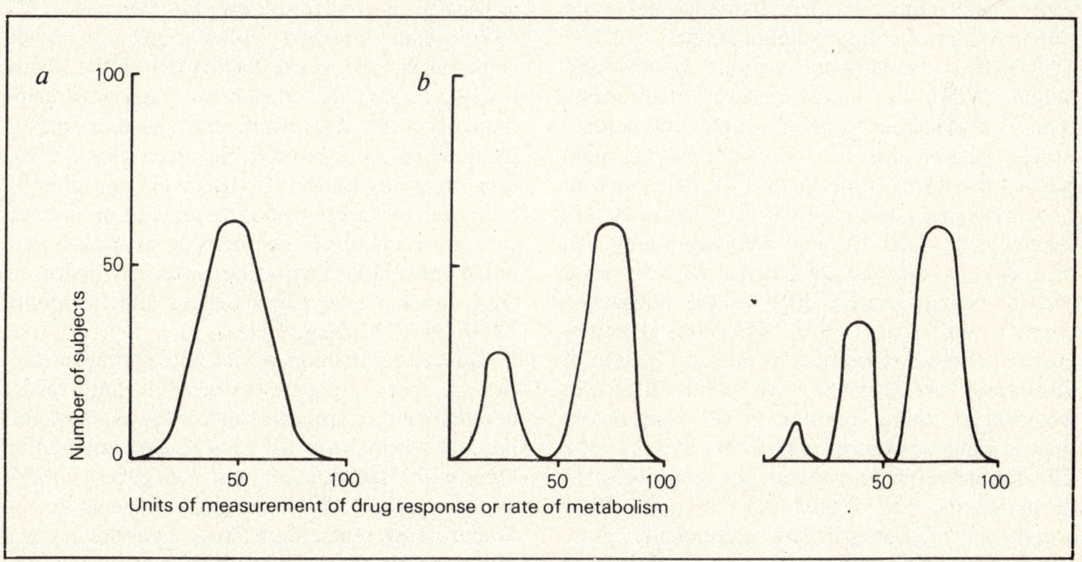

Fig. 3. Two types of variability or frequency distributions which may be observed when a large number of subjects are given a standard dose of a drug under identical circumstances.

(a) Continuous unimodal or Gaussian distribution; (b) Discontinuous polymodal or discrete variation. Left: bimodal; Right: trimodal.

Table VI. Adverse reactions according to acetylation (metabolism) phenotype (after Lunde et al., 1977; Drayer and Reidenberg, 1977)

Drug	Phenotype	Adverse effects[1]
Isoniazid	Slow	Increased incidence of peripheral neuropathy (overcome by pyridoxine) Systemic lupus syndrome more likely Increased risk interaction with phenytoin Increased risk hepatitis when combined with rifampicin
Hydrallazine	Slow	Systemic lupus syndrome more likely, particularly with higher doses Other unwanted effects more common than in rapid acetylators
Procainamide	Slow	Systemic lupus syndrome more likely and of earlier development
Phenelzine	Slow	?Severe reactions more likely
Sulphasalazine[2]	Slow	Severe reactions more likely when large doses used
Dapsone	Slow	? Haematological effects more likely

1　See also text.
2　Salicylazosulphapyridine. Metabolised by colonic bacteria to 5-amino salicylic acid and sulphapyridine, which are both metabolised in the liver by enzyme acetyl transferase. Sulphapyridine also undergoes metabolism by hydroxylation followed by glucuronide conjugation (Cowan et al., 1977; Das and Dubin, 1976).

zygous for an autosomal recessive gene. Fast acetylators are either heterozygous or homozygous for a dominant gene.

Other drugs subjected to polymorphic acetylation by the liver enzyme N-acetyltransferase include hydrallazine, procainamide, phenelzine, dapsone, sulphadimidine (sulphamethazine) and sulphapyridine. Other sulphonamides are N-acetylated by a different enzyme (Evans and White, 1964). The amine metabolite of nitrazepam is also subject to polymorphic acetylation.

The plasma half-life of isoniazid in rapid acetylators ranges from 45 to 80 minutes and in slow acetylators from 140 to 200 minutes (see chapter I; fig. 18a). In rapid acetylators only 3% of a dose is excreted unchanged whereas slow acetylators may excrete 30% as the unchanged drug (Evans et al., 1960). The clinical consequences of these differences in rate and pattern of metabolism are that the neuropathic effects of isoniazid are more common in slow acetylators than in rapid acetylators (Devadatta et al., 1960). This can however, be overcome by administration of pyridoxine (see chapter XX; sect. 8). Slow acetylators of isoniazid are additionally more susceptible to certain drug interactions involving drug metabolism. Thus phenytoin (diphenylhydantoin) toxicity associated with concurrent isoniazid treatment is confined to slow acetylators

(Kutt et al., 1970; see chapter XXV; sect. 3.1) and the risk of liver toxicity with antituberculosis regimens containing isoniazid and rifampicin appears to be increased in those who are slow acetylators of isoniazid (see chapter XIX, sect. 14.6.4). There is some dubiety as to whether or not susceptibility to hepatitis is greater amongst fast (Mitchell et al., 1975) than amongst slow acetylators when isoniazid is used alone. Formation of the highly reactive acetylated metabolite acetylhydrazine thought to be responsible for hepatotoxicity is likely to be more rapid in fast acetylators. However, acetylhydrazine is itself polymorphically acetylated to diacetylhydrazine and this process occurs more rapidly in fast acetylators who excrete much more acetylhydrazine as diacetylhydrazine than do slow acetylators (Ellard and Gammon, 1976, 1977; Girling, 1978).

Concensus opinion would now appear to indicate a more frequent association and earlier development of procainamide induced systemic lupus erythematosus (SLE) with slow acetylation than with fast (Drayer and Reidenberg, 1977; Woosley et al., 1978). Similarly, patients on hydrallazine are much more likely to develop lupus if they are slow than if they are fast acetylators and Drayer and Reidenberg (1977) suggest that the body content of procainamide and hydrallazine, especially the aromatic amino or hydrazine moiety, is likely to contribute to the development of procainamide and hydrallazine induced SLE. The drug induced syndrome is likely to be relatively mild but this may be due to inhibition of its full development by prompt withdrawal of the offending agent; but where withdrawal is impractical the full pathological picture including the typical renal changes may be seen (Levo et al., 1976; Whittle and Ainsworth, 1976).

The proportion of rapid and slow acetylators in a given population varies according to the ethnic group; rapid acetylation is most common among Eskimos, Polynesians and Asians and lowest among some Mediterranean Jews and Egyptians (table VII). Acetylation status can be most conveniently determined by giving the patient a single dose of sulphadimidine (sulphamethazine) and measuring the proportions of free and acetylated drug which appear in the plasma and urine (Evans, 1969a; Eze and Evans, 1972). The possibility that other factors such as pathophysiological states may also affect the acetylator phenotype must always be considered; patients with renal failure often appear to be slow acetylators (see Lunde et al., 1977).

Oxidation is the major pathway of metabolism of many commonly used drugs (e.g. phenytoin, phenylbutazone, dicoumarol, nortriptyline). Rates of drug oxidation can vary widely between individuals, but unlike acetylation, the frequency distribution curve is unimodal (see fig. 3). Studies in twins and in families have shown that drug oxidation is under genetic control, and individuals who so metabolise one drug slowly are likely also to metabolise other drugs slowly which similarly undergo oxidative metabolism (Alexanderson et al., 1969; Asberg et al., 1971; Vesell et al., 1971). A decreased rate of metabolism may lead to toxicity with continuous therapy, particularly if the drug also has dose dependent elimination kinetics; for example, the rates of metabolism of drugs such as phenylbutazone, dicoumarol and phenytoin decrease as their dosage increases (see further chapter I; sect. 2.1.1, 3.3). The liver enzymes involved in drug oxidation can be induced by other drugs and environmental pollutants; the degree of induction also being under genetic control (Vesell and Page, 1969).

Examples of rare phenotypes determining aberrant responses to drugs via metabolic anomalies in drug oxidation include a peculiar inability to metabolise phenytoin by hydroxylation, with resultant accumulation and toxicity (Kutt et al., 1964; see

Table VII. Distribution of rapid acetylation phenotype according to ethnic origin (after Ellard, 1976; Lunde et al., 1977; Motulsky, 1964; Vivien et al., 1973)

Ethnic group	Rapid acetylators (%)
Asiatic origin	
Canadian Eskimo	95-100
New Zealand Polynesians	93
Korean	89
Japanese	88-90
Ainu	87
Ryukyuan	85
Saame Lapps	80
Alaskan Eskimo	79
American Indians	79
Chinese	78-85
Thais	72
Filipino	72
Canadian Indians	63
Burmese	62
Skolt Lapps	50
Hindu Indians	40
African origin	
South African Negro	59
American Negro	49-58
Africans	43-51
Sudanese Negro	35
Ethiopian Negro	20-50
European origin	
Latin Americans	67
Italian	51
USA Whites	43-48
Norwegians	44
German	43
French	41
USA Greek	40
Czechoslovakians	40
Swiss	39
British	38-40
Finns	36-39
USA Italian	36
USA Scandinavian	33
Swedes	32-49
Canadians	30-41
Mediterranean origin	
USA Askenazi	45
Israeli Askenazi	33
Israeli Non-Askenazi	31
Israeli Baghdad Jews	25
Egyptians	18

chapter XXV; sect. 3.1); a decreased capacity to hydroxylate phenytoin in an individual who showed an increased response to warfarin, which is also hydroxylated in the liver (Bochner et al., 1975); and an inability to perform a de-ethylation step (a form of oxidation) in the metabolism of

Table VIII. Examples of genetically determined adverse reactions of pharmacodynamic origin (after La Du, 1972; World Health Organisation, 1973)

Condition	Drug	Effects (see also text)
1. *Quantitatively abnormal reactions*		
Angle closure glaucoma	Atropine	Intraocular pressure increased
Mongolism	Atropine	Response increased
Muscular subaortic stenosis	Digitalis	Decreased cardiac output
2. *Qualitatively abnormal reactions*		
Erythrocyte enzymatic deficiencies		
Glucose-6-phosphate dehydrogenase	Oxidant drugs[1]	Haemolytic anaemia
Methaemoglobin reductase	Oxidant drugs[1] Nitrites	Methaemoglobinaemia
Haemoglobin variants		
Haemoglobin H	Oxidant drugs[1]	Haemolytic anaemia
Haemoglobin Zurich	Sulphonamides	Haemolytic anaemia
Malignant hyperpyrexia	General anaesthetics (halothane) Muscle relaxants (suxamethonium)	Hyperthermia with prolonged muscle rigidity, acidosis
Genetic predisposition to open angle glaucoma, diabetes, pre-diabetes, certain myopes	Topical corticosteroids	Increased intraocular pressure. This may also make underlying open angle glaucoma more difficult to treat
Porphyria (hepatic)	Barbiturates[2] Griseofulvin	Precipitate attack of porphyria

1 See text and chapter XXIII (sect. 8.4).
2 See text for other drugs.

phenacetin (acetophenetidin), with resultant methaemoglobinaemia (Shahidi, 1968). On the other hand, a genetically determined inability to hydroxylate the antihypertensive drug debrisoquine, which is active as unchanged drug, explains why such patients have a greater response to the drug (Mahgoub et al., 1977). Extensive metabolism of debrisoquine to 4-hydroxydebrisoquine is associated with a poor response (Silas et al., 1977).

4.2.2 Genetically Determined Pharmacodynamic Reactions

Such adverse reactions may be either normal responses which occur to an exaggerated extent, i.e. quantitatively abnormal, or novel pharmacodynamic effects, i.e. qualitatively abnormal (table VIII). The latter are well illustrated by acute haemolytic anaemia precipitated by oxidant drugs.

Drug induced haemolytic anaemia may depend upon several genetically determined peculiarities of red cell metabolism (for review, see Beutler, 1971; World Health Organisation, 1973; Marks and Banks, 1965). The best known of these depends upon an autonomous sex linked deficiency of glucose-6-phosphate dehydrogenase (G6PD) activity (table IX). G6PD in sufficient amounts is required for the stability of red blood cells, particularly to protect them against the oxidative stresses of substances such as the 8-aminoquinoline, primaquine. Other haemolytic oxidant drugs include many sulphonamides, nitrofurans (e.g. nitrofurantoin), sulphones (e.g. dapsone), quinine, quinidine, and a variety of other drugs and chemicals, including naphthalene (see chapter XXIII; sect. 8.4). Affected males carry the defect on their one X chromosome. Heterozygous females show intermediate sensitivity as both the defective gene on one of the X chromosomes and the normal allele on the other receive expression, the latter mitigating the effects of the former.

There is a great degree of genetic heterogeneity of G6PD, more than 80 different and fairly well characterised variants being recognised. The severity and duration of haemolytic anaemia varies, according to the variant enzymatic defect (see Motulsky et al., 1971; World Health Organisation, 1973). The African (A – type) variant which includes Negroes, and the Mediterranean (B – type) variant have been studied in most detail. The Mediterranean type which is found in Greeks, Sardinians, Sephardic Jews, Asian and North West Indian peoples is the more severe deficiency. It is affected by the widest range of drugs and haemolytic episodes are not necessarily self limiting. The variants of G6PD that are common in East and Southeast Asia (i.e. Canton and Union variants) differ from the Mediterranean and A – types. It is likely that at least some of these may be as severe as the Mediterranean types of G6PD deficiency (Chan et al., 1976). In patients with the (A – type) variant, haemolytic episodes may be arrested at intermediate levels of haemoglobin, even with continuation of the drug. The G6PD deficiency induced defect renders only the older red cells vulnerable and the initial haemolysis, destroying older cells, has the effect of replacing old cells with young ones. In the Mediterranean type, red cells of all ages are destroyed. The offending drug should be discontinued in both types. Individuals with haemolytic anaemia due to the Mediterranean type deficiency may require transfusion. Acute infection (Chan et al., 1971), diabetic acidosis, liver failure and uraemia may also promote haemolysis. In some variants the G6PD defect is associated with spontaneous haemolysis.

A deficiency of G6PD can lead to marked neonatal jaundice (see chapter XIX; sect. 14.6.6). In some cases this may appear spontaneously, but other factors, particularly drugs, are usually involved. Any patient with haemolytic episodes (e.g. shivers, fever, often with back pain and dark urine due to free haemoglobin), particularly after administration of an oxidant drug, should come under suspicion of G6PD deficiency. Family studies should be made in proven cases and affected individuals given appropriate advice about medication to avoid, and also genetic counselling (World Health Organisation, 1973). A number of

Table IX. Populations with more than 1% frequency of glucose-6-phosphate dehydrogenase deficiency in males (after World Health Organisation, 1973)

Africans
All populations with African ancestry
  (i.e. American Negroes, Puerto Ricans)
Arabs (Egyptians, Kuwaiti, Lebanese)
Filipinos
Greeks
Indians from the Indian subcontinent
Indonesians
Jews (primarily Oriental and Sephardic)
Kurds
Malaysians
New Guineans
Pakistanis
Persians
Romanians
Sardinians
Sicilians
Southern Chinese
Thais

---

tests are available for detecting G6PD deficiency; of these, the fluorescent spot test on blood collected on filter paper is the most specific and simple to perform (Beutler, 1973; Dow et al., 1974).

Other genetically determined red cell abnormalities, including unstable haemoglobin mutants, may result in the production of haemolysis by drugs (see chapter XXIII; sect. 8.4); e.g. haemolysis induced by oxidant drugs in haemoglobin H and by sulphonamides and primaquine in patients with haemoglobin Zurich. Several inherited biochemical lesions of the red blood cell are associated with the development of methaemoglobinaemia following administration of oxidant drugs. Patients with for example, a deficiency of the enzyme methaemoglobin reductase, are more likely than normal to develop methaemoglobinaemia and cyanosis when given drugs such as primaquine, chloroquine and dapsone (Cohen et al., 1968). Virtually anyone may develop methaemoglobinaemia and a degree of haemolysis when challenged with a sufficient dose of a strongly oxidant drug such as phenacetin (acetophenetidin). Such modifications are evident if sought in many patients with analgesic nephropathy at presentation.

Malignant hyperpyrexia is a rare complication of general anaesthesia which presents as a desperate emergency demanding immediate and expert management (see chapter X; sect. 5.6). The basic defect is unknown, but is probably related to an abnormality of calcium regulation within the voluntary muscle cell. The condition is inherited in all or at least a substantial number of cases. Affected members of a family usually have high resting serum creatine phosphokinase activity. The possibility cannot be excluded that some cases might occur without genetic predisposition (Britt, 1975).

Continuous use of *topical corticosteroid eye drops* may produce a marked rise in intraocular pressure in some individuals (see chapter XII; sect. 11.1.2). The extent of increase in intraocular pressure depends on the age of the subject, being greater in those over 40 years, and his genetic constitution. Caucasian population studies show a trimodal distribution — 66 % with low, 29 % intermediate and 5 % with high pressure changes (Armaly, 1968).

4.2.3 Possible Genetically Determined Reactions of Undetermined Origin

Jaundice on oral contraceptives is rare, except in Sweden (Sotaniemi et al., 1964) and in Chile (Popper, 1968). A genetically determined propensity to develop hormonal steroid induced cholestasis appears to be likely (chapter XIX; sect. 13.4).

Impairment of erythropoiesis can regularly be seen in patients receiving chloramphenicol. In the great majority, normal haemopoiesis is rapidly restored following cessation of the drug. An additional factor would seem to be implicated in those cases which go on to develop aplastic anaemia which is irreversible or reversible only after a prolonged period (Yunis, 1973). An indication that the development of aplastic anaemia after chloramphenicol may involve a genetically determined factor has been suggested by its occurrence in identical twins exposed to it (Nagao and Mauer, 1969).

Phenothiazine induced agranulocytosis may involve a mechanism of a different character from that operative in the case of chloramphenicol (Pisciotta, 1978). If the patient negotiates 3 months without adverse effect, agranulocytosis is not likely to develop. Low dose phenothiazines, such as prochlorperazine produce agranulocytosis less often than those with which higher dosage is required, such as chlorpromazine. Chlorpromazine sensitive patients may have a cellular defect, involving the final step of DNA synthesis, which limits incorporation of thymidine triphosphate into DNA. This type of reaction is

associated with production of bone marrow insufficiency in a patient who is believed to have a limited proliferative potential of bone marrow cells, which limit compensatory bone marrow response during treatment with a drug which ordinarily has limited bone marrow toxicity. Introduction of the antipsychotic drug clozapine into Finland was shortly followed by a disconcerting incidence of agranulocytosis following quite extensive prior safe use elsewhere in Europe. A trait determining particular susceptibility within the Finnish population seems possible (Anderman and Griffith, 1977; Idanpaan-Heikkila et al., 1977).

Extreme inherent susceptibility may also be encountered from time to time, e.g. to anticoagulants (Bochner et al., 1975). Although such reactions are of the same character as the anticipated therapeutic effect, the potentially highly dangerous and even fatal effects that may result from extreme susceptibility must lead them to be regarded as adverse reactions.

4.2.4 Genetic Diseases Associated with Abnormal Responses to Drugs

An important example of genetic disorders with altered drug sensitivity is precipitation of acute intermittent porphyria by drugs (de Matteis, 1967; Eales, 1971). The hepatic porphyrias constitute several genetically distinct disorders which involve the metabolic pathway of porphyrins and haem biosynthesis in the liver. One feature of the disorders is overproduction of the rate limiting enzyme δ-aminolevulinic acid (ALA) synthetase in the liver. Variation in an operator gene which is poorly responsive to the normal repressor (haem) may underly the disorder. A number of drugs which induce hepatic ALA synthetase may precipitate exacerbations when given in usual therapeutic doses to patients in remission or with latent disease. In particular barbiturates, but also non-barbiturate hypnotics (glutethimide, dichloralphenazone), aminopyrine, the antifungal agent griseofulvin, oral sulphonylurea hypoglycaemics (tolbutamide, chlorpropamide), antianxiety drugs (chlordiazepoxide), anticonvulsants (phenytoin), and oral contraceptives. The clinical features include a combination of abdominal colic, vomiting and severe constipation, peripheral neuritis, and severe psychological disturbances. An attack may be precipitated by a single dose of one of these drugs but may not necessarily occur each time it is taken or may require a number of relatively large doses in another patient. Porphyria cutanea tarda which is associated with photodermatoses may also be precipitated by drugs (see chapter XIV; sect. 21, 22.3.11).

4.3 Other Reactions Due to Inherent Patient Susceptibility

Side effects, i.e. effects which, although unwanted, are regular effects of the drug in use, may also be modified by inherent differences in patient susceptibility; for example dystonic reactions to the phenothiazines, with which there appears to be linked a genetically determined sensitivity to the taste of quinine (Knopp et al., 1966). The quite remarkable severity these may assume after small doses, particularly of the piperazine substituted phenothiazines (e.g. fluphenazine, perphenazine), in healthy young people is a matter for continued astonishment. The dystonic side effects of phenothiazines appear to affect females more often than males, and children under 15 years show the severest and most bizarre neuromuscular symptoms (Ayd, 1961). Metoclopramide can also cause acute dystonic reactions in young children (see further chapter XXV; sect. 15.5).

Abnormal drug responses due to inherent physiological factors are particularly likely to occur in the elderly (see chapter V) and the newborn (see chapter IV). Altered responsiveness to drugs can also occur in pregnancy (see chapter XV; sect. 1.1.5).

5. Reactions Due to Acquired Patient Anomalies

The pathophysiological condition of the patient, by altering the pharmacokinetic handling or tissue response to a drug can increase the susceptibility to adverse reactions. Thus, an associated disease (i.e. a disease for which treatment is not primarily intended) or intercurrent illness is a most important determinant of adverse drug effects.

5.1 Hypoalbuminaemia and Plasma Protein Binding

With highly protein bound acidic drugs having ordinarily a low volume of distribution, in the presence of hypoproteinaemia there will be a relative increase in the fraction of free, unbound drug. However, this does not necessarily increase the pharmacological effects as the consequent increase

Table X. Incidence of adverse drug reactions of highly protein bound drugs in relation to serum albumin levels

Serum albumin (g/100ml)	Incidence (%)	Effects noted (for groups as a whole)[1]
Prednisone (Lewis et al., 1971)		
< 2.5	37.1	Facial plethora, haemorrhage,
⩾ 2.6	14.6	psychoses, hyperglycaemia, myopathy
Phenytoin (BCDSP, 1973)		
< 2.5	13.3	Neurological (ataxia, confusion,
2.5-2.9	10.3	drowsiness, convulsions); haema-
3.0-3.4	6.7	tological (anaemia, leucopenia,
3.5-3.9	5.0	pancytopenia); rashes; other
⩾ 4.0	1.0[2]	(fever, gum hyperplasia, gastrointestinal)
Diazepam (Greenblatt and Koch-Weser, 1974)		
< 3-3.9	8.5	Unwanted CNS depression
⩾ 4	2.9	
Chlordiazepoxide (Greenblatt and Koch-Weser, 1974)		
< 3-3.9	12.2	Unwanted CNS depression
⩾ 4	9.5	

1 See text for correlation of phenytoin effects with serum albumin levels.
2 Patient also taking isoniazid.

in the apparent volume of distribution and increased rate of elimination will lead to a lower total plasma drug level but unchanged unbound concentration. If however, the elimination of the drug is also reduced, as in some cases of the nephrotic syndrome when the hypoproteinaemia is accompanied by markedly reduced renal function (see chapter XXI; sect. 1.2), or when, in the case of drugs eliminated by hepatic metabolism, clearance is prejudiced (see chapter XIX; sect. 1.3), the total plasma concentration may remain in the usual range or increase, and the unbound drug concentration will rise. In this situation pharmacological effects may be increased (fig. 4). Hypoalbuminaemic patients receiving phenytoin have been shown to have an increased risk of side effects (table X). However, possibly the most serious sequelae may arise from misinterpretation of the significance of blood levels where treatment is being monitored. Plasma total drug levels will be substantially lower for a given unbound concentration in hypoproteinaemic patients than in normals (see further chapter I; sect. 4.3.2, 5.1.2).

Serum albumin depletion, with consequent diminution in storage capacity for corticosteroids can also, with high dose therapy, lead to unusually high levels of free unbound drug and an enhanced susceptibility to steroid side effects (table X; also Uribe et al., 1976, 1977). At physiological concentrations cortisol is bound to a specific α-glycoprotein, corticosteroid binding globulin (CBG or transcortin), which has high affinity but low capacity for certain corticosteroids. When the capacity of this protein is exceeded, binding takes place increasingly to albumin, which has low affinity but high capacity for cortisol. Corticosteroids other than cortisol which bind to transcortin, include prednisolone. With high doses, the percentage of bound prednisolone decreases about 50% when serum albumin falls from 4g/100ml to 2.5g/100ml (Lewis et al., 1971).

An increased incidence of CNS depressant effects of diazepam and chlordiazepoxide has been described in the presence of hypoalbuminaemia (Greenblatt and Koch-Weser, 1974). The contribution of the disorders (e.g. liver disease) underlying the hypoalbuminaemia to other pharmacokinetic processes such as clearance of the drug must always be considered (see above and Tillement et al., 1978; Blaschke, 1977).

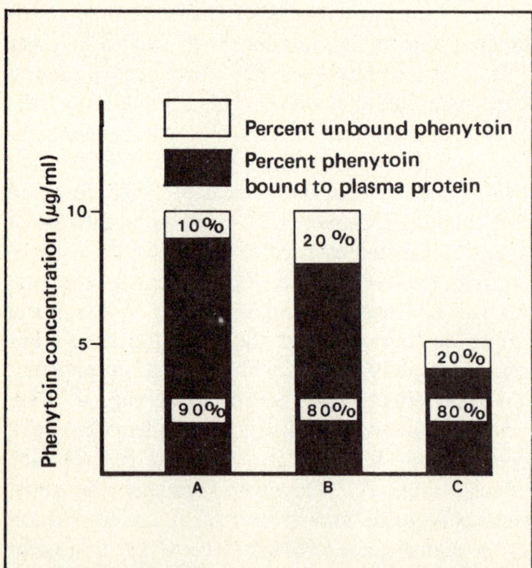

Fig. 4. Effect of reduction in plasma protein binding of phenytoin from 90% (A) to 80% (B). Unbound phenytoin concentration would remain unchanged if increase in unbound fraction from 10% to 20% were associated with decrease in total concentration to one half (C) [after Gugler and Azarnoff, 1976].

5.2 Liver Disease

An increased susceptibility to drug reactions in liver disease can occur as a result of altered pharmacokinetic handling (particularly reduced protein binding or a decreased rate of metabolism) and also possibly of altered sensitivity. The processing of drugs by the liver to permit their elimination from the body gives the liver a central role in drug disposal. Consequently, liver disease would seem likely to be of special importance as a potential source of untoward reactions resulting from excessively high plasma levels of drugs mainly eliminated by this route. It has, however, been quite difficult to demonstrate impairment of drug metabolism in patients with hepatic disease directly, and indeed many such patients may react normally to drugs (Blaschke, 1977). Nevertheless, in some studies when care was taken to exclude pretreatment with drugs of any kind, enzyme induction by which may have confused the issue, it was possible to demonstrate a prolonged half-life of phenylbutazone in patients with liver disease compared with normals (Levi et al., 1968). Although some mechanisms such as bilirubin secretion may be impaired, liver enzymes may continue to metabolise drugs normally. It appears that the efficiency with which a drug is metabolised by the liver, the extent of binding to blood constituents, and the aetiology and stage of hepatic disorder are each important in determining whether significant alterations in drug disposition will occur. If liver disease is severe (as in hepatic cirrhosis), the rate of metabolism of drugs such as lignocaine can be markedly impaired and there are other occasional examples of excessive clinical susceptibility to adverse reactions (Naranjo et al., 1978; see table II).

Abnormal responses to drugs in liver disease may also occur as a result of inordinate susceptibility to the pharmacological action of the drug. It is a common clinical experience that morphine may precipitate coma and hypnotics cause profound sleep in patients with severe hepatic disease (Laidlaw et al., 1961; Sherlock, 1968). Patients with cirrhosis are also extremely sensitive to chlorpromazine and to monoamine oxidase inhibitors (Read et al., 1969). Incautious diuretic therapy can precipitate hepatic coma in susceptible patients with cirrhotic oedema and ascites (Sherlock et al., 1966; Naranjo et al., 1978). The pharmacological basis for adverse drug effects in liver disease is discussed in more detail in chapter

XIX (sect. 1.3, 1.4, 13.4). This chapter also gives a number of examples of untoward effects and provides guidelines for safe prescribing in liver disease (sect. 13.4).

5.3 Renal Disease

Diseases of the kidney may profoundly alter drug pharmacokinetics and occasionally alter sensitivity to drugs. Some drugs may themselves exacerbate renal disease (see chapter XXI; sect. 1, 14, 15). It is not surprising therefore that renal disease frequently leads to adverse reactions especially when renal excretion contributes importantly to elimination of the particular drug or pharmacologically active metabolite. Digoxin clearance is approximately equivalent to creatinine clearance and when this is reduced, dosage appropriate for patients with normal renal function will inevitably lead to establishment of an inordinately high plasma level with serious risk of digitalis toxicity (Iisalo, 1977; Whiting et al., 1978). Aminoglycoside antibiotic ototoxicity is inevitable in patients with renal insufficiency, unless appropriate adjustment of dosage is made (Jackson and Arcieri, 1971).

Some adverse drug reactions are virtually confined to patients with impaired renal function. Peripheral neuritis, due to nitrofurantoin, occurs almost (although not quite) exclusively in patients with impaired renal function (Toole and Parrish, 1973). Transient or permanent deafness may follow the use of ethacrynic acid in patients with renal failure (Pillay et al., 1969).

Patients with chronic renal failure are especially prone to neuropsychiatric reactions (Richet et al., 1970; see chapter XXV; sect. 15). Such drug intoxication is thought to be due partly to an accumulation of drugs normally excreted by the kidney, and partly to susceptibility of the CNS in uraemic patients (e.g. synergism between uraemic somnolence and the CNS depressant effects of barbiturates and narcotics). Synergism between pathological substrates in uraemia and drugs which increase myocardial irritability may promote arrhythmias. It is possible that uraemic patients may suffer alteration of the body membranes in general so that drugs may enter anatomical areas from which they are normally excluded (Schreiner and Maher, 1965; Richet et al., 1970).

Cephaloridine and cephalothin can cause reversible renal damage when given with aminoglycoside antibiotics or potent diuretics such as frusemide or ethacrynic acid. The dose of the cephalosporin required to produce nephrotoxicity is decreased in the presence of impaired renal function (Appel and Neu, 1977). Tetracyclines cause a marked increase in blood urea concentration in patients with impaired renal function and often lead to further acute deterioration in renal function (Ribush and Morgan, 1972; Phillips et al., 1974; see chapter XXI, sect. 14.1.5). Polar drug derivatives ordinarily eliminated promptly by the kidney may accumulate in the presence of renal disease, e.g. the glucuronide conjugates of clofibrate (Gugler, 1978; Faed and McQueen, 1979). Additional examples of enhanced susceptibility to drug toxicity in renal disease are discussed in chapter XXI (sect. 14, 15).

Guidelines for modification of usual drug dosage and the principles of safe prescribing of drugs in renal disease are also given in chapter XXI (sect. 1, 14) and in appendix E.

5.4 Acquired Drug Receptor Anomalies

Occasionally, acquired drug receptor anomalies may determine excessively intense primary or secondary pharmacological responses in the absence of excessive levels of drug at the receptor sites. The basis of enhanced susceptibility may be in some metabolic alteration of the target organ, e.g. enhanced susceptibility to the toxic effects of digitalis in the presence of potassium depletion, or the excessive depressant effects which may result from hypnotics in patients with respiratory depression or hypopituitarism. Other examples are given elsewhere in this book (see also table II).

6. Reactions Due to Anomalies of Drug Presentation

Substitution of drug products with different bioavailability characteristics is an important potential cause of toxicity with certain drugs (see chapter VI). This is illustrated by the epidemic of phenytoin intoxication which occurred in Australia (Tyrer et al., 1970) and New Zealand (McQueen, 1968) due to increased absorption following removal of calcium sulphate from the capsule excipient. Outdated and poorly stored products may also cause toxicity (Fulop and Drapkin, 1965). Poorly formulated liquid preparations permitting unduly rapid sedimentation of the active ingredient may lead to dangerous inequality of dosage.

Occasional instances of toxicity have resulted from accidental introduction of toxic substances via an inappropriate route, e.g. entry of barium sulphate into the blood stream during urethrography as a result of breach of the urethral mucous membrane (NZ Committee on Adverse Drug Reactions, unpublished data). Unduly rapid infusion is a potential cause of reactions, some of which may be of an unexpected character, e.g. hypocalcaemic tetany from rapid intravenous infusion of tetracyclines (Azarnoff and Hurwitz, 1970) and cardiac arrhythmias from rapid intravenous infusion of lincomycin (Paturaud and Gut, 1975). With some drugs, frequency of dosage may be of more importance in determining adverse reactions than total dosage. For example, in patients receiving methotrexate for treatment of recalcitrant psoriasis the prevalence of cirrhosis and fibrosis is significantly greater in those treated by frequent small dosage than in those treated by intermittent large dosage, though the dose level (mg/month) is similar in both groups (Bahl et al., 1972).

7. Reactions Due to Interaction of Drugs

This is an area where responsible authority is at a premium. With the rather belated appreciation of drug interaction as a potentially hazardous consequence of multiple drug therapy there was a pronounced over-reaction. Reports of interactions based on isolated anecdotal events were collected like postage stamps and elaborately categorised, particularly if there appeared to be some academic mileage in their theoretical implication. As a result, a backlash of scepticism towards the subject set in when it was found that predicted interactions frequently failed to manifest themselves in clinical practice (Crooks et al., 1977; Puckett and Visconti, 1971; Starr and Petrie, 1972; see also chapter VIII, sect. 1.1).

Nevertheless, the area is one of real practical importance, as is illustrated by occasional examples of remarkable therapeutic ingenuousness on the subject, e.g. use together of β-adrenoceptor agonists and antagonists, an event probably only possible when drug trade names are used. The reality of the risk of interaction must always be borne in mind when more than one drug is being prescribed.

The incidence of adverse reactions increases with the number of drugs in use. Thus in one survey, in patients given 1 to 5 drugs, the incidence of reactions was 3.3% while in those who received 6 or more drugs the incidence rose to 19.8% (table IV). Drug interactions however appear to make up only a small proportion of all adverse reactions. In reports to the New Zealand Committee on Adverse Drug Reactions, interactions account for only some 2%. In a published report of interaction frequency (Boston Collaborative Drug Surveillance Program, 1972b), of 3,600 reactions involving 83,200 drugs administered, 6.9% were considered to be due to drug interactions.

7.1 Mechanisms of Drug Interactions

Chapter VIII discusses the mechanisms of drug interactions in detail and provides many examples of clinically significant effects. Interactions involving commonly used drugs or potentially interacting drugs which are often likely to be given together are of more importance than those involving drugs that are infrequently used. Many of these interactions can be avoided by an awareness of the risks involved and by a knowledge of the ways in which drugs can interact. Interactions can occur when a drug is added to, or withdrawn from, a previously stable therapeutic regimen, and by many different mechanisms. These occur at many different sites and can be broadly classified as follows:

1) *Pharmacokinetic interactions* — due to modification of the action of the body on drugs. Such interactions occur when one agent changes the plasma concentration of another drug as a consequence of alteration of its absorption, distribution, metabolism or excretion (see chapter VIII; sect. 2.3). Sometimes, more than one of these mechanisms is involved (e.g. some oral coumarin anticoagulant interactions).

2) *Pharmacodynamic interactions* — due to modification of the action of drugs on the body, as reflected in a change caused by one drug in the sensitivity or responsiveness of the tissues to another, when drugs which act at the same site or on the same physiological system are used concurrently (see chapter VIII; sect. 2.2).

Interaction at the level of the pharmacodynamic response may be in the direction of enhancement or inhibition, or it may create circumstances in which the combined effect could

Table XI. Examples of clinically important drug interactions[1]

Primary drug	Interacts with	Mechanism[2]	Potential result
1. *Interactions leading to harmful effects*			
Warfarin	Phenylbutazone	AD+IM	Haemorrhage
	Clofibrate	PD	
	Aspirin	PD	
	Barbiturates	AM	Haemorrhage on withdrawal interacting
	Rifampicin		drug if dose warfarin not decreased
Tolbutamide	Phenylbutazone	AD+IM	Hypoglycaemia
Chlorpropamide	Phenylbutazone	AD+IE/IM	
Phenytoin	Phenylbutazone	IM	Nystagmus, ataxia, lethargy
	Isoniazid (slow acetylators)	IM	
	Sulthiame	IM	
Azathioprine	Allopurinol	IM	Bone marrow suppression
6-Mercaptopurine	Allopurinol		
Methotrexate	Salicylate	IE	
Digitalis	Diuretics	EB	Digitalis intoxication in presence of hypokalaemia
Antidepressants	Alcohol	PD	Excessive sedation
Antipsychotics	Other CNS		
Antianxiety drugs	depressants		
Monoamine oxidase inhibitors	Amphetamine	PD	Hypertensive crisis
	Pseudoephedrine etc		
	Tyramine- and dopamine-rich foodstuffs		
	Pethidine	?IM	Excitation, hyper- or hypotension, coma
Aminoglycoside antibiotics (gentamicin etc)	Frusemide	PD	Acute renal failure (especially with high doses of the aminoglycoside and in presence renal insufficiency)
	Ethacrynic acid		
2. *Interactions leading to ineffective therapy*			
Guanethidine	Amitriptyline	PD	Loss of blood pressure control
	Imipramine		
	Phenylbutazone		
Warfarin	Barbiturates	AM	Loss of anticoagulant control (see also above)
	Rifampicin		
Prednisone	Barbiturates	AM	Reduced steroid effect
Oral contraceptives	Rifampicin	AM	Loss of contraceptive effect
Tetracycline	Oral iron	IA	Mutual loss of effect if given simultaneously
Tolbutamide	Thiazides	PD	Control of blood sugar may be more difficult
Chlorpropamide	Corticosteroids		

1　Excluding interactions in anaesthetic practice (see chapter X; sect. 6). For a complete list of potentially important interactions see appendix C and specific chapter discussions.
2　AD　=　Albumin binding displacement.
　　AM　=　Accelerated drug metabolism.
　　EB　=　Altered electrolyte balance.
　　IA　=　Inhibition drug absorption.
　　IE　=　Inhibition renal excretion.
　　IM　=　Inhibition drug metabolism.
　　PD　=　Pharmacodynamic effect (see relevant chapter discussion).

promote entirely unexpected adverse reactions. The action of oral anticoagulants may be potentiated by the antiplatelet aggregating action of salicylates, but further, the anticoagulant state may render gastric haemorrhage induced by salicylates especially hazardous. Phenylbutazone, in addition to the enhancing effect produced by displacement of warfarin from plasma proteins and inhibition of its metabolism, may promote peptic ulceration with serious gastric haemorrhage in the anticoagulated state. Additionally, an antiplatelet effect may produce inhibition of primary haemostatis (O'Reilly and Aggeler, 1970).

The potential vasospastic effects of ergotamine have been elicited when the addition of triacetyloleandomycin, presumably as a consequence of induced liver dysfunction, retarded the rate of ergotamine biotransformation (Hayton, 1969).

3) *Pharmaceutical interactions* — due to the action of drugs outside the body. Such interactions occur prior to administration of the drug as a result of incompatibilities between drugs or between drug and vehicle. They usually lead to inactivation rather than overt untoward effect and are most important with intravenous antibacterial therapy. For example, kanamycin and methicillin, and gentamicin and carbenicillin inactivate each other, while dextrose solutions of inappropriately low pH inactivate benzylpenicillin. Heparin is incompatible with erythromycin, hydrocortisone, kanamycin, benzylpenicillin, polymyxin and tetracycline, as well as with a number of more improbable combinations. If in doubt the hospital or clinical pharmacist should always be consulted for relevant incompatibility information (Kramer et al., 1971).

7.2 Determinants of Interactions

In theory at least and depending on the pharmacological properties of the individual drugs, clinically significant interactions would in general appear more likely to occur if large doses of the potentially interacting drugs are used, if they are ingested simultaneously or close together, or if they are given in the presence of associated renal or severe liver disease, and when therapy is continued for several days or more. Genetic differences affecting drug metabolism and other acquired differences between patients may also influence the occurrence or intensity of interactions (see section 4.2).

Although a few studies have followed up patients taking potentially interacting drugs and suggest that adverse or undesirable effects are not very common (see chapter VIII; sect. 1.1), a few drugs can predictably cause an unwanted interaction. Phenylbutazone can affect protein binding and inhibit drug metabolism as well as renal excretion mechanisms (table XI; Aarbakke, 1978) and is best avoided in regimens involving oral coumarin anticoagulants (see chapter XXIII; sect. 3.2.5) or oral sulphonylurea hypoglycaemic drugs (see chapter XVI; sect. 3.3.5). When an interaction predictably affects dosage requirements and one of the interacting drugs is withdrawn, modification of dosage may be necessary, as with oral coumarin anticoagulant dosage when barbiturates or other potent hepatic microsomal enzyme inducing agents are withdrawn or reduced in dosage. Interactions between monoamine oxidase inhibitors and indirect acting sympathomimetic amines (e.g. appetite suppressants, common cold remedies) or foodstuffs rich in tyramine (e.g. matured cheeses such as cheddar, wines such as chianti, protein extracts) or dopamine (e.g. broad beans) are important because of their alarming nature (see chapter VIII; sect. 3).

An awareness of the more important interactions (see appendix C) and the ways in which interactions occur can help to avoid, or at least minimise, adverse drug effects or ineffective treatment as a result of drug interactions.

Further Reading

Cluff, L.E.; Caranasos, G.J. and Stewart, R.B.: Clinical Problems with Drugs (Saunders, Philadelphia 1975).

Davies, D.M.: Textbook of Adverse Drug Reactions (Oxford University Press, Oxford 1977).

Gross, F.H. and Inman, W.H.W.: Drug Monitoring (Academic Press, London 1977).

Miller, R.R. and Greenblatt, D.J.: Drug Effects in Hospitalized Patients (Wiley, New York 1976).

Smith, S.E. and Rawlins, M.D.: Variability in Human Drug Response (Butterworths, London 1973).

Wade, O.L.: Adverse Reactions to Drugs (Heinemann, London 1970).

Wolstenholme, G. and Porter, Ruth: Drug Responses in Man (Churchill, London 1967).

Reference Texts

Cluff, L.E.; Caranasos, G.J. and Stewart, R.B.: Clinical Problems with Drugs (Saunders, Philadelphia 1975).

Davies, D.M.: Textbook of Adverse Drug Reactions (Oxford University Press, Oxford 1977).

Dukes, M.N.G.: Meylers Side Effects of Drugs, vol. 8 and Annual supplements (Excerpta Medica, Amsterdam 1976).

Meyler, L. and Peck, H.M.: Drug-Induced Diseases, vol. 4 (Excerpta Medica, Amsterdam 1972)

References

Aarbakke, J.: Clinical Pharmacokinetics of phenylbutazone. Clinical Pharmacokinetics 3: 369 (1978).

Ackroyd, J.F.: The role of sedormid in the immunological reaction that results in plateletlysis in sedormid purpura. Clinical Science 13: 409 (1954).

Alexanderson, B.; Evans, D.A.P. and Sjoqvist, R.: Steady-state plasma levels of nortriptyline in twins: Influence of genetic factors and drug therapy. British Medical Journal 4: 764 (1969).

Alvan, G.: Individual differences in the disposition of drugs metabolised in the body. Clinical Pharmacokinetics 3: 155 (1978).

Anderman, B. and Griffith, R.W.: Clozapine-induced agranulocytosis: A situation report up to August 1976. European Journal of Clinical Pharmacology 11: 199 (1977).

Appel, G.B. and Neu, H.C.: The nephrotoxicity of anti-microbial agents. New England Journal of Medicine 296: 663 (1977).

Armaly, M.F.: Genetic factors related to glaucoma. Annals of the New York Academy of Sciences 151: 861 (1968).

Asberg, M.; Evans, D.A.P. and Sjoqvist, F.: Genetic control of nortriptyline kinetics in man: A study of relatives of propositi with high plasma concentrations. Journal of Medical Genetics 8: 129 (1971).

Ayd, F.J.: Toxic somatic and psychopathologic reactions to antidepressant drugs. Journal of Neuropsychiatry 2 (Suppl. 1): 119 (1961).

Azarnoff, D.L. and Hurwitz, A.: Drug Interactions. Pharmacology for Physicians 4 (2): 1 (1970).

Bahl, M.G.C.; Gregory, M.M. and Scheuer, P.J.: Methotrexate hepatotoxicity in psoriasis - comparison of different dose regimens. British Medical Journal 1: 654 (1972).

Batchelor, F.R.; Dewdney, Janet; Feinberg, J.G. and Weston, R.D.: A penicilloylated protein impurity as a source of allergy to benzylpenicillin and 6-aminopenicillanic acid. Lancet 1: 1175 (1967).

Becker, L.C.: Allergy in systemic lupus erythematosus. John Hopkins Medical Journal 133: 38 (1973).

Beutler, E.: Drug-induced haemolytic anaemia. Pharmacological Reviews 21: 73 (1969).

Beutler, E.: Abnormalities of the hexose monophosphate shunt. Seminars in Haematology 8: 311 (1971).

Beutler, E.: Screening for glucose-6-phosphate dehydrogenase deficiency. Israel Journal of Medical Sciences 9: 1350 (1973).

Blaschke, T.F.: Protein binding and kinetics of drugs in liver disease. Clinical Pharmacokinetics 2: 32 (1977).

Bochner, F.; Hooper, W.D.; Eadie, M.J. and Tyrer, J.H.: Decreased capacity to metabolize diphenylhydantoin in a patient with hypersensitivity to warfarin. Australia and New Zealand Journal of Medicine 5: 462 (1975).

Boston Collaborative Drug Surveillance Program: Excess of ampicillin rashes associated with allopurinol or hyperuricaemia. New England Journal of Medicine 286: 505 (1972a).

Boston Collaborative Drug Surveillance Program: Adverse drug reactions. Journal of the American Medical Association 220: 1238 (1972b).

Boston Collaborative Drug Surveillance Program: Diphenylhydantoin side effects and serum albumin levels. Clinical Pharmacology and Therapeutics 14: 529 (1973).

Britt, B.A.: Malignant hyperthermia. Clinical Anesthesia 11: 61 (1975).

Brown, P.; Baddeley, H.; Read, A.E.; Davies, J.D. and McGarry, J.: Sclerosing peritonitis, an unusual reaction to a β-adrenergic-blocking drug (practolol). Lancet 2: 1477 (1974).

Cameron, S.J. and Richmond, J.: Ampicillin hypersensitivity in lymphatic leukaemia. Scottish Medical Journal 16: 425 (1971).

Chan, T.K.; Chesterman, C.N.; McFadzean, A.J.S. and Todd, D.: The survival of glucose-6-phosphate dehydrogenase-deficient erythrocytes in patients with typhoid fever on chloramphenicol therapy. Journal of Laboratory and Clinical Medicine 77: 177 (1971).

Chan, T.K.; Todd, D. and Tso, S.C.: Drug-induced haemolysis in glucose-6-phosphate dehydrogenase deficiency. British Medical Journal 2: 1227 (1976).

Cohen, R.J.; Sachs, J.R.; Wicker, D.J. and Conrad, M.E.: Methemoglobinemia provoked by malarial chemoprophylaxis in Vietnam. New England Journal of Medicine 279: 1127 (1968).

Coombs, R.R.A. and Gell, P.G.H.: Classification of allergic reactions responsible for clinical hypersensitivity and disease; in Gell and Coombs (Eds) Clinical Aspects of Immunology, p. 575, 2nd ed (Blackwell, Oxford 1968).

Cowan, G.O.; Das, K.M. and Eastwood, M.A.: Further studies of sulphasalazine metabolism in the treatment of ulcerative colitis. British Medical Journal 2: 1057 (1977).

Crooks, J.; Stevenson, I.H.; Shepherd, A.M.M. and Moir, D.C.: The clinical significance and importance of drug interactions; in Grahame-Smith (Ed) Drug Interactions, p. 3 (Macmillan, London 1977).

Damashek, W.: Concepts of autoimmunity and their applications in haematology; in Bjorkman (Ed) Series Haematologica 19: 317 (1965).

Das, K.M. and Dubin, R.: Clinical pharmacokinetics of sulphasalazine. Clinical Pharmacokinetics 1: 406 (1976).

de Matteis, F.: Disturbances of liver porphyrin metabolism caused by drugs. Pharmacological Reviews 19: 523 (1967).

Devadatta, S.; Gangadharam, P.R.J.; Andrews, R.H.; Fox, W.; Ramakrishnan, C.V.; Selhon, J.B. and Veru, S.: Peripheral neuritis due to isoniazid. Bulletin of the World Health Organisation 23: 587 (1960).

DeWarte, R.D.: Drug allergy; in Patterson (Ed) Allergic Diseases: Diagnosis and Management, p. 393 (Lippincott, Philadelphia 1972).

Dove, A.F.; Thomas, D.J.B.; Aronstam, A. and Chant, R.D.: Haemolytic anaemia due to penicillin. British Medical Journal 3: 684 (1975).

Dow, Patricia A.; Mozellar, B.; Petteway, B.A. and Alperin, J.B.: Simplified method for G6PD screening using blood collected on filter paper. American Journal of Clinical Pathology 61: 333 (1974).

Drayer, D.E.: Pharmacologically active drug metabolites: Therapeutic and toxic activities, plasma and urine data in man, accumulation in renal failure. Clinical Pharmacokinetics 1: 426 (1976).

Drayer, D.E. and Reidenberg, M.M.: Clinical consequences of polymorphic acetylation of basic drugs. Clinical Pharmacology and Therapeutics 22: 251 (1977).

Eales, L.: Acute porphyria: The precipitating and aggravating factors. South African Journal of Laboratory and Clinical Medicine 17: 120 (1971).

Ellard, G.A.: Variations between individuals and populations in the acetylation of isoniazid and its significance for the treatment of pulmonary tuberculosis. Clinical Pharmacology and Therapeutics 19: 610 (1976).

Ellard, G.A. and Gammon, P.T.: Pharmacokinetics of isoniazid metabolism in man. Journal of Pharmacokinetics and Biopharmaceutics 4: 83 (1976).

Ellard, G.A. and Gammon, P.T.: Acetylator phenotyping of tuberculosis patients using matrix isoniazid on sulphadimidine and its prognostic significance for treatment with several intermittent isoniazid-containing regimens. British Journal of Clinical Pharmacology 4: 5 (1977).

Evans, D.A.P.: An improved and simplified method of detecting the acetylator phenotype. Journal of Medical Genetics 6: 405 (1969a).

Evans, D.A.P.: Recent advances in knowledge of genetically controlled idiosyncratic reaction to drugs. Sensitisation to Drugs; in Baker and Tripod (Eds) Proceedings of the European Society of the Study of Drug Toxicity, vol. 10, p. 11 (Excerpta Medica Foundation, Amsterdam 1969b).

Evans, D.A.P. and White, T.A.: Human acetylation polymorphism. Journal of Laboratory and Clinical Medicine 63: 394 (1964).

Evans, D.A.P.; Manley, K.A. and McKusick, V.A.: Genetic control of isoniazid metabolism in man. British Medical Journal 2: 485 (1960).

Eze, L.C. and Evans, D.A.P.: The use of the autoanalyser to determine the acetylator phenotype. Journal of Medical Genetics 9: 57 (1972).

Faed, E.M. and McQueen, E.G.: Measurement of clofibric acid (CPIB) metabolites in plasma of patients on clofibrate therapy. Clinical and Experimental Pharmacology and Physiology. In press (1979).

Finney, D.J.: Theoretical objectives of international collaboration; in Gross and Inman (Eds) Drug Monitoring, p.207 (Academic Press, London 1977).

Fisher, M.: Blood volume replacement in acute anaphylactic cardiac collapse related to anaesthesia. British Journal of Anaesthesia 49: 1023 (1977).

Fulop, M. and Drapkin, A.: Potassium-depletion syndrome secondary to nephropathy caused by 'outdated tetracycline'. New England Journal of Medicine 272: 986 (1965).

Girard, J.P. and Cuevas, M.: Clinical and immunologic analysis of 1047 allergic reactions to penicillin. Schweizerische Medizinische Wochenschrift 105: 953 (1975).

Girdwood, R.H.: Death after taking medicaments. British Medical Journal 1: 501 (1974).

Girling, D.J.: The hepatic toxicity of antituberculosis regimens containing isoniazid, rifampicin and pyrazinamide. Tubercle 59: 13 (1978).

Giudicelli, J.F. and Tillement, J.P.: Influence of sex on drug kinetics in man. Clinical Pharmacokinetics 2: 157 (1977).

Goldstein, A.; Aronow, L. and Kalman, S.M.: Principles of Drug Action, 2nd ed, p. 504 (Wiley, New York 1974).

Gralnick, H.R.; McGuiness, M.; Elton, W. and McCurdy, P.: Haemolytic anaemia associated with cephalothin. Journal of the American Medical Association 217: 1102 (1971).

Green, G.R.; Peters, G.A. and Geraci, J.E.: Treatment of bacterial endocarditis in patients with penicillin hypersensitivity. Annals of Internal Medicine 64: 1170 (1966); 67: 235 (1967).

Greenblatt, D.J. and Koch-Weser, J.: Clinical toxicity of chlordiazepoxide and diazepam in relation to serum albumin concentration: A report from the Boston Collaborative Drug Surveillance Program. European Journal of Clinical Pharmacology 7: 259 (1974).

Gugler, R. and Azarnoff, D.L.: Drug protein binding and the nephrotic syndrome. Clinical Pharmacokinetics 1: 25 (1976).

Gugler, R.: Clinical pharmacokinetics of hypolipidaemic drugs. Clinical Pharmacokinetics 3: 425 (1978).

Gysling, E. and Heisler, S.: A practical classification of untoward drug effects. Canadian Medical Association Journal 113: 32 (1975).

Hayton, A.C.: Precipitation of acute ergotism by triacetyloleandomycin. N.Z. Medical Journal 69: 42 (1969).

Hoffmann, K.F.: Anaphylactic shock after oral ampicillin. Proceedings of the Rudolf Virchow Medical Society New York 27: 93 (1968).

Horowitz, H.I. and Nachman, R.L.: Drug Purpura. Seminars in Haematology 2: 287 (1965).

Hurwitz, Natalie: Predisposing factors in adverse reactions to drugs. British Medical Journal 1: 536 (1969a).

Hurwitz, Natalie: Admissions to hospital due to drugs. British Medical Journal 1: 539 (1969b).

Hurwitz, Natalie, and Wade, O.L.: Intensive hospital monitoring of adverse reactions to drugs. British Medical Journal 1: 531 (1969).

Idanpaan-Heikkila, J.: Population monitoring: medical record linkage for drug safety surveillance; in Gross and Inman (Eds) Drug Monitoring, p.17 (Academic Press, London 1977).

Idanpaan-Heikkila, J.: Alhava, E.; Olkinuora, M. and Palva, I.P.: Agranulocytosis during treatment with clozapine. European Journal of Clinical Pharmacology 11: 193 (1977).

Iisalo, E.: Clinical pharmacokinetics of digoxin. Clinical Pharmacokinetics 2: 1 (1977).

Isbister, J.P.: Penicillin allergy: A review of the immunological and clinical aspects. Medical Journal of Australia 1: 1067 (1971).

Jackson, G.G. and Arcieri, G.: Ototoxicity of gentamicin in man: A survey and controlled analysis of clinical experience in the United States. Journal of Infectious Diseases 124 (Suppl.): S130 (1971).

Jenner, G.G.; Macintosh, D.; West, S.R. and McQueen, E.G.: Intensive monitoring of adverse reactions in general practice. New Zealand Medical Journal 83: 378 (1976).

Jick, H.: Drugs - Remarkably nontoxic. New England Journal of Medicine 291: 824 (1974).

Jick, H.: The discovery of drug-induced illness. New England Journal of Medicine 296: 481-485 (1977).

Jick, H.; Miettinen, O.S.; Shapiro, S.; Lewis, G.P.; Suokind, V. and Slone, D.: Comprehensive drug surveillance. Journal of the American Medical Association 213: 1455-1460 (1970).

Kalow, W.: Pharmacogenetics: Heredity and the Response to Drugs (Saunders, Philadelphia 1962).

Kalow, W. and Genest, K.: A method for the detection of atypical forms of human serum cholinesterase: Determination of dibucaine numbers. Canadian Journal of Biochemistry 35: 339 (1957).

Kalow, W. and Gunn, D.R.: The relation between dose of succinylcholine and duration of apnoea in man. Journal of Pharmacology and Experimental Therapeutics 120: 203 (1957).

Karch, F.E. and Lasagna, L.: Adverse drug reactions. Journal of the American Medical Association 234: 1236 (1975).

Kellaway, G.S. and McCrae, Ellen: Intensive monitoring for adverse drug effects in patients discharged from acute medical wards. New Zealand Medical Journal 78:525 (1973).

Kellermann, G.; Luyten-Kellermann, M.; Homing, M.G. and Stafford, M.: Elimination of antipyrine and benzo:a:pyrene metabolism in cultured human lymphocytes. Clinical Pharmacology and Therapeutics 20: 72 (1976).

Klein, U.; Klein, M.; Sturm, H.; Rothenbuhler, M.; Huber, R.; Stucki, P.; Gikalov, I.; Keller, M. and Hoigne, R.: The frequency of adverse drug reactions as dependent upon age, sex and duration of hospitalization. International Journal of Clinical Pharmacology and Biopharmacy 13: 187 (1976).

Knopp, W.; Fischer, R.; Beck, J. and Teitelbaum, A.: Clinical implications of the relation between taste sensitivity and the appearance of extrapyramidal side effects. Diseases of the Nervous System 27: 729 (1966).

Koch-Weser, J.: Coumarin necrosis. Annals of Internal Medicine 68: 1365 (1968).

Koch-Weser, J.: Fatal reactions to drug therapy. New England Journal of Medicine 291: 302 (1974).

Kramer, W.; Inglott, A. and Cluxton, R.: Some physical and chemical incompatibilities of drugs for I.V. administration. Drug Intelligence and Clinical Pharmacy 5: 211 (1971).

Kronig, B.; Fiegel, P.; Weihrauch, Th.; Hoffler, D.; Jahnecke, J. and Arndt-Hanser, A.: A case of severe repeated immunological reactions to intermittent rifampicin treatment. European Journal of Clinical Pharmacology 5: 53 (1972).

Kutt, H.; Wolk, M.; Scherman, R. and McDowell, F.: Insufficient parahydroxylation as a cause of diphenylhydantoin toxicity. Neurology 14: 542 (1964).

Kutt, H.; Brennan, R.; Dehejia, H. and Verebely, K.: Diphenylhydantoin intoxication. A complication of isoniazid therapy. American Review of Respiratory Disease 101: 377 (1970).

La Du, B.N.: Pharmacogenetics: Defective enzymes in relation to reactions to drugs. Annual Review of Medicine 23: 453 (1972).

Laidlaw, J.; Read, A.E. and Sherlock, S.: Morphine tolerance in hepatic cirrhosis. Gastroenterology 40: 389 (1961).

Lakshminarayan, S.; Sahn, S.A. and Hudson, L.D.: Massive haemolysis caused by rifampicin. British Medical Journal 2: 282 (1973).

Lawson, D.H.: Detection of drug-induced disease. British Journal of Clinical Pharmacology 7: 13 (1979).

Lawson, D.H. and Jick, H.: Drug prescribing in hospitals: an international comparison. American Journal of Public Health 66: 644 (1976).

Levi, A.J.; Sherlock, S. and Walker, D.: Phenylbutazone and isoniazid metabolism in patients with liver disease in relation to previous drug therapy. Lancet 1: 1275 (1968).

Levo, Y.; Pick, A.I.; Avidor, I. and Ben-Bassat, M.: Clinicopathological study of a patient with procainamide-induced systemic lupus erythematosus. Annals of the Rheumatic Diseases 35: 181 (1976).

Levy, M.; Nir, I.; Birnbaum, D.; Superstine, E. and Eliakim, M.: Adverse reactions to drugs in hospitalised medical patients. Israel Journal of Medical Sciences 9: 617 (1973).

Lewis, G.P.; Jusko, W.J.; Burke, C.W.; Graves, Linda: Prednisone side-effects and serum-protein levels. Lancet 2: 778 (1971).

Lindberg, J.; Lindholdm A.; Lundin, P. and Iwarson, S.: Trigger factors and HL-A antigens in chronic active hepatitis. British Medical Journal 4: 77 (1975).

Lunde, P.K.M.; Frislid, K. and Hansteen, V.: Disease and acetylation polymorphism. Clinical Pharmacokinetics 2: 182 (1977).

McPherson, A.J.; Parkin, J.D. and Hope, R.: Penicillin-induced haemolytic anaemia associated with microangiopathy. Australian and New Zealand Journal of Medicine 6: 152 (1976).

McQueen, E.G.: Voluntary reporting systems; in Gross and Inman (Eds) Drug Monitoring, p.11 (Academic Press, London 1977).

McQueen, E.G.: Phenytoin intoxication. New Zealand Medical Journal 68: 332 (1968).

Maddrey, W.C. and Boitnott, J.K.: Drug-induced chronic liver disease. Gastroenterology 72: 1348 (1977).

Mahgoub, A.; Idle, J.R.; Dring, L.C.; Lancaster, R. and Smith, R.L.: Polymorphic hydroxylation of debrisoquine in man. Lancet 2: 584 (1977).

Marks, P.A. and Banks, J.: Drug-induced hemolytic anemias associated with glucose-6-phosphate dehydrogenase deficiency: A genetically heterogeneous trait. Annals of the New York Academy of Sciences 123: 198 (1965).

May, F.E.; Stewart, R.B. and Cluff, L.E.: Drug interactions and multiple drug administration. Clinical Pharmacology and Therapeutics 22: 322 (1977).

Melmon, K.L.: Preventable drug reactions - Causes and cures. New England Journal of Medicine 284: 1361 (1971).

Mitchell, J.R. and Jollows, D.J.: Metabolic activation of drugs to toxic substances. Gastroenterology 68: 392 (1975).

Mitchell, J.R.; Thorgeirsson, U.P.; Black, M.; Timbrell, J.A.; Snodgrass, W.R.; Potter, W.Z.; Jollow, D.J. and Keiser, H.R.: Increased incidence of isoniazid hepatitis in rapid acetylators: possible relation to hydrazine metabolites. Clinical Pharmacology and Therapeutics 18: 70 (1975).

Motulsky, A.G.: Pharmacogenetics. Progress in Medical Genetics 3: 49 (1964).

Motulsky, A.G.; Yoshida, A. and Stamatoyannopoulos, G.:Variants of glucose-6-phosphate dehydrogenase. Annals of the New York Academy of Sciences 179: 636 (1971).

Nagao, T. and Mauer, A.M.: Concordance for drug-induced aplastic anaemia in identical twins. New England Journal of Medicine 281: 7 (1969).

Naranjo, C.A.; Busto, U. and Mardones, R.: Adverse drug reactions in liver cirrhosis. European Journal of Clinical Pharmacology 13: 429 (1978).

Neitlich, H.W.: Increased plasma cholinesterase activity and succinylcholine resistant: A genetic variant. Journal of Clinical Investigation 45: 380 (1966).

New Zealand Committee on Adverse Drug Reactions, 5th Annual Report (1970).

New Zealand Committee on Adverse Drug Reactions. Seventh annual report. New Zealand Medical Journal 76: 357 (1972).

O'Reilly, R.A. and Aggeler, P.M.: Determinants of response to oral anticoagulant drugs in man. Pharmacological Reviews 22: 35 (1970).

Orme, M.: Adverse reactions caused by drug metabolites. Adverse Drug Reaction Bulletin 64: 224 (June 1977).

Parker, C.W.: Drug allergy. New England Journal of Medicine 292: 511, 732, 957 (1975).

Parker, A.C. and Richmond, J.: Reduction in incidence of rash using polymer-free ampicillin. British Medical Journal 1: 998 (1976).

Paturaud, J-P. and Gut, J-P.: Cardiac arrest following the rapid intravenous injection of lincomycin. Nouvelle Presse Medicale 4: 1593 (1975).

Petrie, J.C.; Durno, D. and Howie, J.G.R.: Drug interaction in general practice; in Cluff and Petrie (Eds) Clinical Effects of Interaction Between Drugs, p. 237 (Excerpta Medica,

Amsterdam 1975).

Petz, L.D.: Immunologic reactions of humans to cephalosporins. Postgraduate Medical Journal 47 (Suppl.): 64 (Feb. 1971).

Phillips, M.E.; Eastwood, J.B.; Curtis, J.R.; Gower, P.E. and de Wardener, H.E.: Tetracycline poisoning in renal failure. British Medical Journal 2: 149 (1974).

Pillay, V.K.G.; Schwerta, F.D.; Aimi, K. and Kark, R.M.: Transient and permanent deafness following treatment with ethacrynic acid in renal failure. Lancet 1: 77 (1969).

Pisciotta, V.: Drug-induced agranulocytosis. Drugs 15: 132 (1978).

Popper, H.: Cholestasis. Annual Review of Medicine 19: 39 (1968).

Puckett, W.H. and Visconti, J.A.: An epidemiological study of the clinical significance of drug-drug interactions in a private community hospital. American Journal of Hospital Pharmacy 28: 247 (1971).

Pujet, J-C.; Homberg, J-C. and Decroix, G.: Sensitivity to rifampicin: Incidence, mechanism and prevention. British Medical Journal 2: 415 (1974).

Pullen, H.: Wright, N. and Murdoch, J.McC.: Hypersensitivity reactions to antibacterial drugs in infectious mononucleosis. Lancet 2: 1176 (1967).

Rawlins, M.D.: Inheritance and adverse drug reactions. Adverse Drug Reaction Bulletin No. 53: 180 (1975).

Read, A.E.; Laidlaw, J. and McCarthy, C.F.: Effects of chlorpromazine in patients with hepatic disease. British Medical Journal 3: 497 (1969).

Ribush, N. and Morgan, T.: Tetracyclines and renal failure. Medical Journal of Australia 1: 53 (1972).

Richet, G.; Lopex de Novales, E. and Verroust, P.: Drug intoxication and neurological episodes in chronic renal failure. British Medical Journal 2: 394 (1970).

Rubin, R.N. and Burka, E.R.: Anti-cephalothin antibody and Coombs-positive hemolytic anemia. Annals of Internal Medicine 86: 64 (1977).

Samter, M. and Parker, C.W.: International Encyclopaedia of Pharmacology and Therapeutics, Section 75, Hypersensitivity to Drugs, vol. 1 (Pergamon, Oxford 1972).

Schreiner, G. and Maher, J.F.: Drugs and the kidney. Annals of the New York Academy of Sciences 123: 326 (1965).

Seidl, L.G.; Thornton, G.F.; Smith, Jay W. and Cluff, L.E.: Studies on the epidemiology of adverse drug reactions. Bulletin of the Johns Hopkins Hospital 119: 299 (1966).

Shahidi, N.T.: Acetophenetidin-induced methaemoglobinemia. Annals of the New York Academy of Sciences 151: 822 (1968).

Sherlock, S.: Drugs and the liver. British Medical Journal 1: 227 (1968).

Sherlock, S.; Senewirante, B.; Scott, A. and Walker, J.G.: Complications of diuretic therapy in hepatic cirrhosis. Lancet 1: 1049 (1966).

Silas, J.H.; Lennard, M.S.; Tucker, G.T.; Smith, A.J.; Malcolm, S.L. and Marten, T.R.: Why hypertensive patients vary in their response to oral debrisoquine. British Medical Journal 1: 422 (1977).

Simmonds, J.; Hodges, S.; Nicol, F. and Barnett, D.: Anaphylaxis after oral penicillin. British Medical Journal 2: 1404 (1978).

Simpson, N.E. and Kalow, W.: Pharmacology and biological variation. Annals of New York Academy of Science 134: 864 (1966).

Skegg, D.C.G. and Doll, R.: Frequency of eye complaints and rashes among patients receiving practolol and propranolol.

Lancet 2: 475 (1977).

Smidt, Ngaire A. and McQueen, E.G.: Adverse reactions to drugs: A comprehensive hospital inpatient survey. New Zealand Medical Journal 76: 397 (1972).

Smidt, Ngaire A. and McQueen, E.G.: Adverse drug reactions in a general hospital. New Zealand Medical Journal 78: 39 (1973).

Smith, J.W.; Seidl, L.G. and Cluff, L.E.: Studies on the epidemiology of adverse drug reactions. Annals of Internal Medicine 65: 629 (1966).

Sotaniemi, E.; Krens, K.E. and Schinin, T.M.: Oral contraception and liver damage. British Medical Journal 2: 1264 (1964).

Starr, K.J. and Petrie, J.C.: Drug interactions in patients on long-term oral anticoagulant and antihypertensive adrenergic neurone-blocking drugs. British Medical Journal 4: 133 (1972).

Stewart, G.T.: Allergenic residues in penicillins. Lancet 1: 1177 (1967).

Stewart, G.T. and McGovern, J.P.: Penicillin Allergy (Thomas, Springfield 1970).

Tillement, J.P.; Lhoste, F. and Giudicelli, J..: Diseases and drug protein binding. Clinical Pharmacokinetics 3: 144 (1978).

Toole, J.F. and Parrish, M.L.: Nitrofurantoin polyneuropathy. Neurology 23: 554 (1973).

Tyrer, J.H.; Eadie, M.J.; Sutherland, J.M. and Hooper, W.D.: Outbreak of anticonvulsant intoxication in an Australian city. British Medical Journal 4: 271 (1970).

Uribe, M.; Wolf, A.M. and Summerskill, W.H.J.: Steroid side effects during therapy of chronic active liver disease: What to expect. Gastroenterology 71: 932 (1976).

Uribe, M.; Summerskill, W.H.J. and Go, V.L.W.: Why hyperbilirubinemia and hypoalbuminaemia predispose to steroid side effects during treatment of chronic active liver disease. Gastroenterology 72: 1143 (1977).

Vere, D.W.: Drug adverse reactions as masqueraders. Adverse Drug Reaction Bulletin 60: 208 (Oct. 1976).

Vesell, E.S.: Individual variations in drug response; in Orlandi and Jezequel (Eds) Liver and Drugs, p. 1 (Academic Press, London 1972).

Vesell, E.S.: Pharmacogenetics: Biochemical Pharmacology 24: 445 (1975).

Vesell, E.S. and Page, J.G.: Genetic control of the phenobarbital-induced shortening of plasma antipyrine half-lives in man. Journal of Clinical Investigation 48: 2202 (1969).

Vesell, E.S.; Page, J.G. and Passananti, G.T.: Genetic and environmental factors affecting ethanol metabolism in man. Clinical Pharmacology and Therapeutics 12: 192 (1971).

Vivien, J.N.; Thiebier, R. and Lepeuple, A.: La pharmacocinetique de L'isoniazide dans la race blanche. Revue Francaise des Maladies Respiratoires 1: 753 (1973).

Wade, O.L.: Pattern of drug induced disease in the community. British Medical Bulletin 26: 240 (1970).

Weitzman, S.A. and Stossel, T.P.: Drug-induced immunological neutropenia. Lancet 1: 1068 (1978).

Whiting, B.; Wandless, Irene; Sumner, D.G. and Goldberg, A.: Computer-assisted review of digoxin therapy in the elderly. British Heart Hournal 40: 8 (1978).

Whittingham, Senga and Mackay, I.R.: Adverse reactions to drugs: Relationship to immunopathic disease. Medical Journal of Australia 1: 486 (1976).

Whittle, T.S. and Ainsworth, S.K.: Procainamide-induced systemic lupus erythematosus. Renal involvement with deposition of immune complexes. Archives of Pathology and Laboratory Medicine 100: 469 (1976).

Woosley, R.L.; Drayer, D.E.; Reidenberg, M.M.; Nies, A.S.; Carr, K. and Oates, J.A.: Effect of acetylator phenotype on the rate at which procainamide induces antinuclear antibodies and the lupus syndrome. New England Journal of Medicine 298: 1157 (1978).

World Health Organisation: Technical Report Series No. 524, Pharmacogenetics (WHO, Geneva 1973).

Yunis, A.A.: Chloramphenicol-induced bone marrow suppression. Seminars in Haematology 10: 225 (1973).

Zimmerman, H.J.: Drug-induced liver disease. Drugs 16: 25 (1978).

Chapter VIII
Clinically Important Drug Interactions

L.F. Prescott

Synopsis of Important Principles

1) The effects of one drug can be increased or decreased by the previous or concurrent administration of another drug.

2) Many drug interactions can be predicted if the pharmacodynamic effects, pharmacokinetic properties and mechanisms of action are known. Most could be avoided by the application of this knowledge and the simple use of common sense.

3) Drug interactions occur through several different mechanisms, including actions on the same receptors or physiological systems and alteration in pharmacokinetic handling of the drug. Drug induced disease or changes in fluid and electrolyte balance may modify response or enhance toxicity of another drug.

4) It can never be assumed that interactions observed *in vitro* or in animals will necessarily occur in man.

5) Interactions will not necessarily occur in all patients receiving a given combination of drugs known to have a potential for interaction in man.

6) Many clinically important interactions, especially those of a pharmacokinetic nature, depend on a variety of factors additional to the drugs given.

7) Pharmacokinetic interactions demonstrated with one drug combination should not be extrapolated to other combinations involving closely related drugs.

8) Because of the practice of multiple drug therapy, the potential for interactions is large, but at present it is difficult to assess the overall clinical importance of drug interactions, and their dangers have probably been exaggerated.

9) By far the most common interactions are those involving mutual potentiation of central nervous system depression by hypnotics, tranquillisers, antidepressants, ethanol, analgesics, antihistamines, anticonvulsants and miscellaneous centrally acting drugs.

10) The most obvious interactions are those involving oral anticoagulants, hypoglycaemic agents, cardiac glycosides and cytotoxic drugs. These drugs have a low therapeutic ratio and an exaggerated response is potentially lethal. Interactions involving certain antihypertensive drugs and anticonvulsants can also be important.

When two or more drugs are given in combination the response may be greater or smaller than the sum of the effects of the two drugs given separately. Thus one drug may antagonise or potentiate the effects of another and in some cases there may be qualitative differences in response. Drugs are of course often given in combination to obtain enhanced therapeutic effects with reduced toxicity. Familiar examples include combinations of antihypertensive drugs, antibiotics and cytotoxic drugs. Advantage is also taken of specific interactions in the treatment of drug overdosage and the actions of narcotic analgesics, levodopa and cholinesterase inhibitors can be reversed by naloxone, pyridoxine and atropine respectively. Only the undesirable consequences of drug interaction will be considered here.

The problems of drug interaction have attracted much attention in recent years. Doctors have always practised polypharmacy, and until fairly recently this mattered little because the great majority of drugs had little or no pharmacological activity. At the present time, however, scores of potent drugs are prescribed on an enormous scale to a public with an insatiable appetite for medication. The average hospital inpatient is at times treated with 5 or more drugs simultaneously; some with as many as 15 drugs concurrently. In one London hospital one patient in 10 received 10 drugs at once, and one was apparently assaulted with no less than 21 drugs in a period of 24 hours. In another hospital a patient was given more than 50 different drugs during a single admission (Koch-Weser, 1975; also chapter VII, sect. 3). The elderly are particularly susceptible to drugs (see chapter V; sect. 1, 2) yet 87 % of individuals aged more than 75 years in a London general practice were taking drugs regularly and a third were taking 3 or 4 different drugs each day (Law and Chalmers, 1976). The incidence of adverse reactions increases disproportionately as the number of drugs prescribed rises (table I; see also chapter VII, sect. 3), and this is probably due in part, to drug interaction (May et al., 1977).

1. General Considerations

Although drug interactions are probably an important cause of drug toxicity, there has been an almost hysterical over-reaction on the part of pharmacists and pharmacologists. Enormous lists of real or imaginary interactions have been

Table I. Incidence of adverse drug reactions in medical hospital patients in relation to the number of drugs prescribed concurrently (after May et al., 1977)

	Number of drugs prescribed			
	0-5	6-10	11-15	16-20
No. of patients	4009	3861	1713	641
No. of reactions	142	397	478	347
Adverse reaction rate	4%	10%	28%	54%

published with warnings of dire consequences if virtually any two drugs are given at the same time. For all that has been written on the subject, the clinical importance of drug interactions is largely unknown. The action of many drugs cannot be measured readily under clinical conditions and interactions are unlikely to be recognised unless they cause grossly exaggerated responses or serious toxicity. Considerable difficulties arise through inadequate clinical documentation of drug effects and drug administration, failure of communication between doctors so that one may be totally unaware of drugs prescribed for his patients by other doctors, and inability to differentiate between drug effects and manifestations of disease. Not only is the awareness and recognition of adverse drug interactions by prescribers low (Howie et al., 1977; Petrie et al., 1974), but also there are serious gaps in their knowledge of the contents of the preparations which they order for their patients (Biron, 1973).

Many drug interactions can be predicted if the pharmacokinetic characteristics and mechanisms of drug action are known. Quantitative changes in response can be anticipated with combinations of drugs acting at the same site or on the same physiological systems. Unfortunately, animal studies are of limited predictive value because of species differences and it can never be assumed that interactions observed in animals will necessarily occur in man (Brodie, 1962; Conney et al., 1972). A number of factors must be taken into account in the assessment of the clinical importance of drug interactions.

1.1 Incidence of Important Drug Interactions

The overall incidence of clinically important drug interactions is difficult to assess. There have been a few surveys with selected drugs, but these cannot be compared directly because methods and criteria vary greatly. In 4 recent surveys, of a total of 716 patients taking oral anticoagulants, 34 to 63% were also given potentially interacting drugs (Kleinman and Griner, 1970; Starr and Petrie, 1972; Husted and Andreasen, 1976; Williams et al., 1976). The incidence of observed interaction (which varied from poor control to a few cases of overt life threatening haemorrhage) ranged from 1.4 to 56%. In other studies, 34% of 64 hypertensive patients treated with guanethidine, bethanidine or debrisoquine and 75% of 709 diabetics were taking potentially interfering drugs. Only 3 probable interactions were noted in the hypertensive group, but diabetic control was significantly impaired in patients receiving sulphonylureas (Starr and Petrie, 1972; Logie et al., 1976). The incidence of prescription of potentially interacting drugs seems to be 4 to 5% in teaching hospitals (Simborg, 1976). Some well documented interactions do not seem to be important in clinical practice (e.g. tetracycline and iron salts — probably because they are not taken simultaneously), while others can cause lethal toxicity (spironolactone plus potassium chloride and phenylbutazone plus warfarin).

1.2 The Consequences

Drug interactions are only important for the clinician when they influence the efficacy or safety of treatment (Koch-Weser and Greenblatt, 1977).

Potentially lethal interactions involving anticoagulants, hypoglycaemic agents and cytotoxic drugs are obviously important, but therapeutic failure — not so easily recognised as an interaction — is also of clinical significance. Similarly, doctors may not be directly involved in the immediate consequences of serious interaction, as in the case of a patient who drives his car into a tree after the prescription of inappropriate combinations of CNS depressants such as benzodiazepines, tricyclic antidepressants, methyldopa and analgesic combinations containing dextropropoxyphene. Drug interactions are likely to be more serious in vulnerable patients such as the elderly, the very ill, and the poisoned. Particular care is needed with drugs which have dose dependent metabolism, a steep dose-response curve or a low therapeutic ratio.

The time sequence and order in which interacting drugs are started and stopped may greatly influence the response. For example, addition of a tricyclic antidepressant such as imipramine or amitriptyline in a hypertensive patient already stabilised on bethanidine might cause a rapid loss of control of blood pressure. On the other hand, withdrawal of long term tricyclic antidepressant therapy in a patient adequately controlled with large doses of bethanidine could result in a calamitous fall in blood pressure due to the unopposed action of an excessive dose of bethanidine.

The minority of clinically important interactions must be distinguished from the majority which are only of chance occurrence or academic interest.

1.3 Drug Usage

Interactions between commonly used drugs, or drugs often given together in the treatment of specific conditions, are clearly more important than those occurring with rarely used drugs. This is a particular problem with some drugs available without prescription. For instance, ethanol and salicylate can interact with many drugs, yet both compounds are consumed on an enormous scale and are rarely thought of as drugs either by the public or by doctors (Seixas, 1975).

1.4 Documentation and Reliability of Clinical Data

This is often hopelessly inadequate. Many reports are based on anecdote or single case reports without studies to elucidate the mechanisms of interactions or the conditions under which they occur (Sjoqvist and Alexanderson, 1972). In 1967, hypoglycaemia was reported in a patient receiving chlorpromazine and orphenadrine. Although these drugs are frequently prescribed together, no further studies seem to have been carried out and it can only be presumed that this interaction is very rare. Some authors have described interactions with far reaching clinical implications which have not been confirmed by others in subsequent studies. Some examples include impairment of indomethacin absorption by aspirin, and inhibition of drug metabolism by nortriptyline and allopurinol. Such discrepancies are not readily explicable and add greatly to the confusion. Even worse, many of the 'interactions' included in the exhaustive lists compiled by some authors exist only in their minds since they have never been shown to occur in man.

1.5 Individual Variation

Interactions may occur in some individuals but not in others (Vesell et al., 1975). Although the anticoagulant action of warfarin is invariably potentiated by phenylbutazone (Bull and Mackinnon, 1975; Aggeler et al., 1967), there is usually considerable variation between patients in the extent to which one drug modifies the response of another. Indeed, some interactions involving monoamine oxidase inhibitors seem only to occur in a very small proportion of patients at risk (see section 3). The effects of interactions involving drug metabolism may vary greatly in different patients because of individual differences in the initial rates of drug metabolism and in susceptibility to hepatic microsomal enzyme induction (see chapter I; sect. 4.2). Interactions may also be controlled on a genetic basis. For instance, the inhibitory effect of isoniazid on phenytoin (diphenylhydantoin) metabolism is usually only of clinical importance in slow acetylators of isoniazid (see chapter XXV; sect. 3.1).

1.6 Effects of Disease

Some interactions are likely to be modified by disease states, but there is very little reliable information on this point. The effects of plasma protein binding displacement interactions are likely to be more marked in patients with hypoalbuminaemia and renal failure or severe liver disease (see section 2.3.2), while muscle weakness caused by the combination of aminoglycoside antibiotics (e.g. kanamycin) and non-depolarising muscle relaxants (e.g. d-tubocurarine) is aggravated by myopathy, hypokalaemia or uraemia (Davie, 1977).

2. Mechanisms of Drug Interaction

Drugs may interact on a pharmaceutical, pharmacodynamic or pharmacokinetic basis (Ariens, 1972; Birkett and Pond, 1975; Kramer et al., 1971; Kristensen, 1976). Pharmaceutical interactions may occur when drugs are mixed inappropriately in syringes and infusion fluids prior to administration, while pharmacodynamic interactions arise with drugs acting on the same receptors, sites of action or physiological systems. In pharmacokinetic interactions one drug interferes with the absorption, transport, distribution or elimination of another. Some mechanisms of in-

Table II. Mechanisms of drug interactions

1. Pharmaceutical incompatibility

2. Mutual antagonism or potentiation of drugs acting at the same site or influencing the same physiological system

3. Competition at receptor sites

4. Changes in fluid or electrolyte balance

5. Intracellular transport (interference with amine uptake by sympathetic neurones)

6. Interference with absorption
   a) Change in pH of gastrointestinal fluids
   b) Effects on gastric emptying and gastrointestinal motility
   c) Binding and chelation of drugs
   d) Toxic effect on gastrointestinal tract
   e) Unknown

7. Drug distribution (plasma protein binding displacement)

8. Modification of drug metabolism
   a) Stimulation
   b) Inhibition
   c) Changes in hepatic blood flow

9. Interference with biliary excretion and enterohepatic circulation

10. Modification of renal excretion
    a) Competition for active renal tubular secretion
    b) Changes in urine pH

11. Miscellaneous
    a) Monoamine oxidase inhibition
    b) Antagonism of antibacterial drugs

teraction are listed in table II, while some examples likely to be of potential clinical significance are given in table III. Since the first edition of this book, there have been scores of further drug interaction reports. Although many have been isolated anecdotal accounts, some would be of great importance if confirmed. It is becoming increasingly difficult to assess these reports and a few unconfirmed but potentially important interactions with a reasonably sound theoretical basis have been included. Those unlikely to influence the result of drug therapy have generally been omitted, even if adequately documented in man, and none have been included solely on the basis of animal or 'in vitro' studies.

A number of drugs may interact simultaneously at several different sites so that it may be difficult to attribute interaction to a single mechanism. For instance, aspirin could interfere with the absorption, plasma protein binding and active renal tubular secretion of other acidic drugs, and in addition might increase the toxicity of oral anticoagulants through effects on the bleeding time, capillary fragility, platelet adhesiveness, intrinsic inhibition of clotting factor synthesis and production of gastrointestinal erosions and ulcers which may bleed. Alcohol can also alter both the pharmacodynamics and pharmacokinetics of other drugs (Sellers and Holloway, 1978). Phenylbutazone can enhance or inhibit drug metabolism, as well as being capable of inhibiting renal excretion and displacing other highly albumin bound drugs. It is a predictable cause of important interactions with warfarin and oral sulphonylurea hypoglycaemic drugs (Aarbakke, 1978; see chapter XVI, sect. 3.3.5; XXIII, sect. 3.2.5).

Many lists of interactions extrapolate reactions demonstrated with one compound to other combinations involving closely related drugs. Such extrapolations might be relevant when an interaction involves a pharmacodynamic mechanism, but should not be made with pharmacokinetic interactions (Pond et al., 1975). Indeed, pharmacodynamic interactions involving one drug should generally be anticipated with other related drugs, even though confirmation in man is lacking. For example, cardiovascular effects attributed to propranolol may well be observed with other β-adrenoceptor blocking agents. The situation is different with interactions involving pharmacokinetic mechanisms. As discussed in chapter I, drugs have characteristic physicochemical and pharmacokinetic properties. For example, all the various pharmacokinetic interactions which can occur with dicoumarol do not necessarily occur with other coumarin anticoagulants (see chapter XXIII; table V). Similarly, an interaction with tolbutamide and sulphaphenazole cannot be extrapolated to apply to all sulphonamides (see chapter XVI; table V). It must also be emphasised that interactions will not necessarily occur in all patients receiving a given combination of potentially interacting drugs — not only because of individual variation (sect. 1.5), but also because the occurrence of a clinically important interaction often depends on a variety of factors additional to the combination of drugs given (Sellers and Koch-Weser, 1971; Koch-Weser and Greenblatt, 1977).

Most pharmacodynamic interactions are entirely predictable and could be avoided with knowledge of the actions of drugs and the use of commonsense. Many reports of such 'interactions' only confirm what is already known of the effects of the drugs and underline the lack of awareness of the prescriber on this point. It should come as no surprise to find the combined use of full doses of potent vasodilators such as diazoxide and hydrallazine can cause catastrophic hypotension, that combinations of hypnotics, tranquillisers, antidepressants and narcotic analgesics cause depression, ataxia, confusion and dementia in the elderly and that dopamine and ergotamine combined may cause gangrene of the extremities.

2.1 Pharmaceutical Incompatibility

Drugs may be inactivated or precipitated from solution if mixed in syringes or added to blood or infusion fluids prior to administration. Numerous incompatibilities have been demonstrated and drugs should never be mixed in this fashion unless the absence of reaction has been clearly established (Kramer et al., 1971; Davie, 1977).

2.2 Pharmacodynamic Interactions

Pharmacodynamic interactions involving additive, synergistic or antagonistic effects of drugs acting on the same receptors or physiological systems probably account for most clinically important drug interactions, although they have not received the attention they deserve. The greatest problems appear to be caused by multiple prescription of drugs acting on the CNS (Boston Collaborative Drug Surveillance Program, 1972). The toll in respect of physical and mental depression, particularly in the elderly, is frightening (see further chapter V; sect. 4.7). Many fashionable psychotherapeutic drugs and their active metabolites have very long elimination half-lives, and since the full effects do not become apparent for several weeks, neither the patient nor her doctor may associate slow deterioration with drug therapy. The inappropriate prescription of depressants with antidepressants, convulsants with anticonvulsants, and even β-adrenoceptor blockers wth β-adrenoceptor stimulants is not uncommon. Interaction between psychotherapeutic drugs and ethanol is a major problem, and in some countries, contributes significantly to death and injury in road traffic accidents (Seppala et al., 1979). An

Table III. Mechanisms and examples of potential drug interaction (see also text and appendix C)

Mechanism	Effect	Examples[1]
Pharmaceutical incompatibility	Inactivation of drug *in vitro*	Inactivation of carbenicillin by gentamicin, reaction between hydrocortisone and heparin, penicillins and phenytoin (diphenylhydantoin) etc, when drugs mixed in syringes and infusion bottles *Many other examples known*
Mutual potentiation or antagonism by drugs acting at the same site or influencing the same physiological system	Exaggerated or reduced effects	Potentiation of central nervous system depression caused by ethanol, hypnotics, sedatives, tranquillisers, antidepressants, narcotic analgesics, anticonvulsants, antihistamines, methyldopa, clonidine, reserpine and miscellaneous drugs
		Non-depolarising muscle relaxants potentiated by aminoglycoside antibiotics, colistin, local anaesthetics, and quinidine
		Risk of catastrophic hypotension if diazoxide given with other potent antihypertensive agents, especially hydrallazine
		Potentiation of antihypertensive agents by central nervous system depressants, anaesthetic drugs, diuretics, antidepressants and tranquillisers
		Antagonism of some antihypertensive agents by sympathomimetics
		Inhibition of blood pressure lowering effect of pindolol and propranolol by indomethacin
		Potentiation of hypoglycaemic agents by salicylates, β-adrenoceptor blockers and monoamine oxidase inhibitors
		Antagonism of hypoglycaemic agents by thiazide diuretics, diazoxide, corticosteroids and oral contraceptives
		Potentiation of cephaloridine and cephalothin nephrotoxicity by frusemide (all produce nephrotoxic metabolites)
		Increased risk of aminoglycoside antibiotic ototoxicity with frusemide and ethacrynic acid
		Clofibrate and thyroxine potentiate effects of coumarins
		Potentiation of anticoagulants (increased risk of bleeding) by aspirin and other acidic non-steroidal anti-inflammatory drugs
		Reduced cardiac output caused by β-adrenoceptor blockers in patients premedicated with atropine under anaesthesia with cardiac depressants (e.g. ether)
		Mutual potentiation of parasympathetic block by atropine, propantheline, antihistamines, tricyclic antidepressants, pethidine, orphenadrine, benzhexol trihexphenidyl), procyclidine, amantidine, disopyramide etc
		Irreversible dementia, tremor, confusion and extrapyramidal reactions when lithium combined with haloperidol or methyldopa and haloperidol combined with methyldopa
		Extrapyramidal reaction to phenothiazines precipitated by ethanol
		Antagonism of amphetamine stimulation by lithium
		Hypothermia with combined use of lithium and diazepam
		Long term use of 'long acting' nitrates (e.g. isosorbide dinitrate) results in tolerance and greatly reduced therapeutic response to sublingual glyceryl trinitrate

Table III. (continued)

Mechanism	Effect	Examples[1]
Competition at receptor sites	Usually antagonism	Antihistamines, atropine, d-tubocurarine, β-adrenoceptor blockers, phentolamine etc, combine reversibly with receptors and compete with and antagonise physiological transmitters
		Naloxone is a specific narcotic antagonist
		Neostigmine antagonises non-depolarising muscle relaxants (e.g. d-tubocurarine) and potentiates polarisation block caused by suxamethonium (succinylcholine)
		Physostigmine antagonises central effects of anticholinergics such as atropine and tricyclic antidepressants
		Mutual antagonism of β-adrenoceptor stimulants (e.g. salbutamol) and β-adrenoceptor blockers (e.g. propranolol)
		Vitamin K antagonises coumarin anticoagulants
		Anabolic steroids thought to potentiate oral anticoagulants by altering receptor affinity for vitamin K (other mechanisms suggested include increased rate of decay or impaired synthesis of clotting factors). Thyroxine may act similarly
		Broad spectrum antibiotics are said to potentiate oral anticoagulants by reducing vitamin K synthesis by gut flora
Changes in electrolyte or fluid balance	Antagonism or potentiation	Potentiation of effects of digitalis and non-depolarising muscle relaxants by hypokalaemia induced by diuretics, carbenoxolone and amphotericin B
		Prolonged paralysis after suxamethonium (succinylcholine) in patients given lithium
		Precipitation of lithium toxicity by diuretic induced natriuresis
		Therapeutic failure of lithium if renal excretion enhanced by high sodium intake (e.g. sodium bicarbonate)
		Acetazolamide renders urine alkaline, increases calcium excretion and predisposes to osteomalacia in patients taking anticonvulsants
		Ventricular arrhythmias in patients receiving digitalis caused by release of K^+ following injection of suxamethonium, especially in patients with trauma, burns or muscle disorders
		Antagonism of antiarrhythmic action of lignocaine (lidocaine), quinidine, phenytoin (diphenylhydantoin) and procainamide by drugs which cause hypokalaemia
		Antagonism of effects of antihypertensive agents (e.g. guanethidine, β-adrenoceptor blockers, and diuretics) by phenylbutazone and related pyrazolones, indomethacin and carbenoxolone
Interference with amine uptake by sympathetic neurones	Antagonism of hypotensive action of adrenergic neurone blocking drugs	Antagonism of blood pressure lowering action of guanethidine, bethanidine and debrisoquine by tricyclic antidepressants, maprotiline, antihistamines, chlorpromazine, sympathomimetic agents (e.g. amphetamines, phenyl-propanolamine, phenylephrine, pseudoephedrine, ephedrine), pizotifen and mazindol
		? Antagonism of antihypertensive effects of clonidine by tricyclic antidepressants

Table III. (continued)

Mechanism	Effect	Examples[1]
Interference with drug absorption	Increased or decreased rate of absorption or amount of drug absorbed	
Change in pH of gastrointestinal fluids		Sodium bicarbonate reduces absorption of tetracycline, increases absorption of levodopa and increases the rate of absorption of acetylsalicylic acid
		Some antacids increase levodopa absorption
Effects on gastric emptying and gastrointestinal motility		Anticholinergics such as propantheline and tricyclic antidepressants, slow absorption of ethanol, paracetamol, diazepam, propranolol, phenylbutazone and lithium (slow release tablets) and decrease absorption of levodopa
		Narcotic analgesics such as heroin (diamorphine), morphine, pethidine (meperidine) and pentazocine strongly inhibit gastric emptying and greatly reduce the rate of absorption of paracetamol (and probably many other drugs). Morphine and heroin slow down and reduce the absorption of mexiletine in patients with myocardial infarction. Similar effects are likely with other oral antiarrhythmic drugs
		Lithium decreases chlorpromazine absorption
		Aluminium hydroxide gel decreases isoniazid absorption
		Metoclopramide accelerates absorption of paracetamol, ethanol, diazepam, propranolol and lithium (slow release tablets), and increases absorption of levodopa
		Tricyclic antidepressants increase bioavailability of dicoumarol
Binding or chelation of drugs		Kaolin-pectin reduces digoxin absorption and prevents lincomycin absorption. Some antacids reduce digoxin absorption
		Cholestyramine interferes with absorption of warfarin, thyroxine, digoxin and digitoxin absorption; colestipol reduces absorption of digitoxin
		Tetracycline absorption reduced by Ca^{++}, Mg^{++}, Al^{+++}, Fe^{++}
Toxic effect on gastrointestinal tract		Mefenamic acid, phenformin, p-aminosalicylate, neomycin, and colchicine may cause malabsorption syndromes
		Neomycin interferes with penicillin absorption
Unknown		Aluminium hydroxide reduces absorption of propranolol and indomethacin; phenytoin (diphenylhydantoin) and chlorpromazine absorption reduced by antacids
		Phenytoin absorption reduced by frusemide; digoxin by neomycin and sulphasalazine (salicylazosulphapyridine); propranolol by halofenate; phenobarbitone interferes with griseofulvin absorption; and warfarin absorption reduced by heptabarbitone

Table III. (continued)

Mechanism	Effect	Examples[1]
Plasma protein binding displacement	Potentiation due to temporary increase in concentration of active unbound drug; drug elimination can be accelerated	Potentiation of anticoagulant action of warfarin by phenylbutazone, oxyphenbutazone, sulphaphenazole, co-trimoxazole, ? sulphafurazole (sulphisoxazole), clofibrate, feprazone and azapropazone
		Potentiation of tolbutamide and chlorpropamide by phenylbutazone, oxyphenbutazone, salicylate, sulphaphenazole and halofenate. Methotrexate potentiated by salicylate and sulphonamides
		Phenytoin (diphenylhydantoin) potentiated by phenylbutazone, oxyphenbutazone, salicylate and valproate
		Sulphafurazole (sulphisoxazole) potentiates thiopentone
		Diazoxide decreases plasma concentrations of phenytoin (diphenylhydantoin) and greatly increases elimination
Stimulation of hepatic drug metabolism	Increased rate of drug metabolism. Drug effects usually reduced, but enhanced if metabolites more active than parent drug. Similarly, increased or decreased toxicity	Accelerated metabolism and reduced effects of oral anticoagulants, phenytoin (diphenylhydantoin) barbiturates, methadone, desipramine, digitoxin, alprenolol, phenylbutazone, corticosteroids, oral contraceptives and many other drugs possible with administration of enzyme inducing agents — barbiturates (especially phenobarbitone), phenytoin, primidone, carbamazepine, glutethimide, antipyrine, rifampicin and ethanol (chronic use)
		N.B. If drug dose increased to regain initial response, overdosage will occur 1 to 3 weeks after the inducing drug is discontinued. This effect is particularly hazardous with oral anticoagulants
		Pregnancy in women on oral contraceptives and renal transplant rejection in patients receiving corticosteroids may occur if rifampicin taken as well
		? Rifampicin may enhance hepatotoxicity of isoniazid
		Paracetamol hepatotoxicity and nephrotoxicity increased in chronic alcoholics and patients taking barbiturates and anticonvulsants
		Stimulation of salicylate metabolism by corticosteroids

Table III. (continued)

Mechanism	Effect	Examples[1]
Inhibition of drug metabolism	Reduced rate of drug metabolism. Usually prolonged action, cumulation and toxicity	Inhibition of tolbutamide metabolism by dicoumarol, sulphaphenazole, phenylbutazone, oxyphenbutazone and chloramphenicol
		Potentiation of warfarin by phenylbutazone, oxyphenbutazone, sulphaphenazole, co-trimoxazole, disulfiram, metronidazole and dextropropoxyphene
		Potentiation of dicoumarol by allopurinol and chloramphenicol
		Serious potentiation of azathioprine and 6-mercaptopurine by allopurinol
		Phenytoin intoxication caused by administration of isoniazid (slow acetylators), sulthiame, dicoumarol, disulfiram, chloramphenicol, phenylbutazone, sulphaphenazole, sulphamethizole, chlordiazepoxide, diazepam, chlorpromazine, prochlorperazine, imipramine, dextropropoxyphene
		Perphenazine may inhibit nortriptyline metabolism; chlorpromazine and haloperidol slow down metabolism of imipramine
		Warfarin, meprobamate and pentobarbitone metabolism slowed by acute ethanol intoxication
		Suxamethonium (succinylcholine) paralysis prolonged by propanidid, hexafluorenium, ecothiopate and procaine
		'Antabuse'-like syndrome following ethanol in some patients taking chlorpropamide, metronidazole and procarbazine
Interference with biliary excretion	Prolonged drug action	Inhibition of hepatic uptake and delayed plasma clearance of rifampicin by probenecid in some subjects
		Probenecid reduces non-renal clearance of indomethacin, possibly by reducing biliary clearance
		Paracetamol reduces bromsulphthalein (BSP) clearance
Competition for active renal tubular secretion	Reduced renal clearance, prolonged effects, cumulation and toxicity	Phenylbutazone and dicoumarol cause accumulation of chlorpropamide with hypoglycaemia
		Salicylate, probenecid and sulphonamides inhibit excretion of methotrexate
		Probenecid reduces the renal clearance of penicillins, dapsone, frusemide, sulphinpyrazone and p-aminosalicylate
		Frusemide reduces the renal excretion of gentamicin and cephaloridine
		Salicylate (low doses) inhibits the actions of uricosuric drugs
		Diuretic effect of thiazides and frusemide antagonised by phenylbutazone and indomethacin
Changes in urine pH	Renal clearance of basic drugs (pK_a 7-10 increased in acid urine, clearance of acidic drugs (pK_a 3 to 7.5) enhanced in alkaline urine, decreased in acid urine	Renal excretion of amphetamine, ephedrine, fenfluramine and quinidine increased in acid urine (e.g. following ammonium chloride), decreased in alkaline urine (e.g. following administration of sodium bicarbonate or acetazolamide)
		Renal clearance of salicylate enhanced in alkaline urine (e.g. following antacid therapy)

Table III. (continued)

Mechanism	Effect	Examples[1]
Monoamine oxidase inhibition	Hypertensive reactions, coma and hyperpyrexia. Potentiation of hypoglycaemic agents and antihypertensive drugs	Acute hypertensive crisis or exaggerated and prolonged rise in blood pressure following foods containing tyramine or dopamine (matured cheese, chianti-type wine, yeast extracts, pickled herrings, broad beans), pressor agents (amphetamine, mephentermine), nasal decongestants (ephedrine, phenylephrine), proprietary cold 'cures' (phenylpropanolamine, pseudoephedrine) and levodopa
		Central excitation with α-methyldopa
		Hypotension, agitation, tremor, convulsions, hyperpyrexia and coma in minority of patients given pethidine, tricyclic antidepressants and anaesthetics
		Potentiation of hypoglycaemic and antihypertensive agents
Antagonism of antibacterial agents	Reduced antibacterial activity	Mutual antagonism between bactericidal and bacteriostatic drugs when both drugs used at minimum effective levels, e.g. penicillins and tetracycline
Mechanisms unknown	Antagonism or potentiation	Antagonism of effects of levodopa by pyridoxine
		Paradoxical rise in blood pressure in some patients when clonidine combined with sotalol
		Increased nephrotoxicity of methoxyflurane in patients receiving tetracycline
		Potentiation of aminoglycoside antibiotic (streptomycin, kanamycin, gentamicin) ototoxicity by frusemide and ethacrynic acid
		Potentiation of cephaloridine and cephalothin nephrotoxicity by aminoglycoside antibiotics
		Antagonism of the diuretic action of spironolactone by aspirin

---

1   Examples given which refer only to the mechanism involved (e.g. reduced rate of absorption, inhibition of metabolism), may not necessarily be of clinical significance.

It is important to realise that a particular interaction may not occur in all patients (see text).

---

enormous number of interactions could be included in table III, but only examples of the most important are listed.

2.2.1 Interactions at Receptors

One drug may have a greater affinity than another for a receptor. If it has little or no intrinsic activity, the actions of the second drug are antagonised (see chapter I; sect. 1.2.1). This is a common mechanism of drug action, and compounds such as atropine and d-tubocurarine act by combining reversibly with receptors and thus prevent access of the normal physiological transmitter (acetylcholine). Since the drug-receptor combination is reversible, it is possible to overcome the antagonism by increasing the amount of agonist at the receptor. Thus muscle paralysis induced by non-depolarising relaxants such as d-tubocurarine can be reversed by neostigmine which inhibits cholinesterase and increases the concentration of acetylcholine at receptors (Davie, 1977). Many other interactions occur at receptors and familiar examples include the antagonism of narcotic analgesics by naloxone and the competition between isoprenaline and propranolol for adrenergic β-receptors. Drugs may also modify receptor sensitivity. Thus the pressor response to noradrenaline is markedly increased by chronic administration of guanethidine. This effect is analogous to denervation hypersensitivity caused in this instance by 'pharmacological sympathectomy' (Stafford and Fann, 1977).

Serious interactions characterised by extrapyramidal syndromes and irreversible dementia have been reported with lithium combined with methyldopa or haloperidol and methyldopa combined with haloperidol (Thornton, 1976). The mechanisms are unknown but all 3 drugs act on central dopaminergic receptors.

2.2.2 Drugs Acting at the Same Site or on the Same Physiological System

Combinations of drugs acting at the same site or influencing the same physiological system may cause reduced or exaggerated responses. For example, the effects of hypnotics on the central nervous system are potentiated by ethanol, narcotic analgesics, antihistamines, tranquillisers, antidepressants, anticonvulsants, etc. Similarly, diuretics, propranolol, monoamine oxidase inhibitors, anaesthetics and central nervous system depressants may potentiate the blood pressure lowering effects of antihypertensive agents (Crook and Nies, 1978). The autonomic reflex control of cardiac function is abolished by the combination of atropine and propranolol, and in these circumstances anaesthetic agents such as ether may cause a marked reduction in cardiac output.

2.2.3 Changes in Fluid and Electrolyte Balance

Changes in electrolyte balance may alter the effects of drugs, particularly those acting on the myocardium, neuromuscular transmission and on the kidney. One of the most important interactions is the potentiation of the action of cardiac glycosides by diuretic induced hypokalaemia (Koch-Weser, 1975), although some question the importance of this effect (Binnion, 1978). The antiarrhythmic actions of phenytoin (diphenylhydantoin), procainamide, lignocaine (lidocaine) and quinidine are antagonised by hypokalaemia, and the sudden release of potassium from muscle following the injection of suxamethonium (succinylcholine) could cause ventricular arrhythmias in patients receiving digitalis (Dreifus et al., 1974; Evers et al., 1969). Non-depolarising muscle

relaxants may produce prolonged paralysis in the presence of hypokalaemia in patients taking thiazide diuretics or carbenoxolone; hypokalaemia causes hyperpolarisation of the motor end plate and thereby antagonises the action of acetylcholine (see chapter X; fig. 1).

Potassium chloride is obviously contraindicated in patients also taking potassium-retaining diuretics and this combination can cause fatal hyperkalaemia in patients with impaired renal function (Greenblatt and Koch-Weser, 1973). Nevertheless, in one study no less than 42 % of 245 patients on spironolactone were also prescribed potassium chloride and of these, 52 % developed hyperkalaemia (Simborg, 1976). There is a direct relationship between lithium excretion and sodium balance, and lithium intoxication can be precipitated by the unwise use of diuretics (Himmelhoch et al., 1977).

Interactions may also occur as a result of drug induced water and electrolyte retention. Phenylbutazone and related pyrazolone drugs regularly cause water and salt retention, and thus can inhibit the actions of diuretics and antihyper-

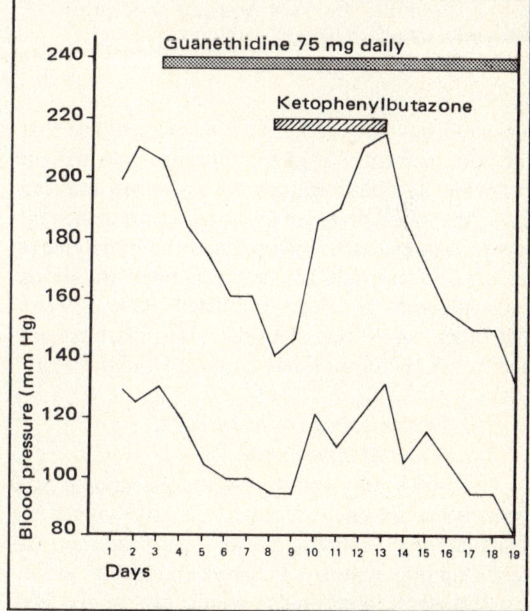

Fig. 1. Change in fluid and electrolyte balance: Inhibitory effect of ketophenylbutazone (750mg daily) on the blood pressure lowering effect of guanethidine. The upper and lower lines represent systolic and diastolic pressures respectively (after Polak: Zeitschrift fur die Gesamte Innere Medizin und Ihre Grenzgebiete 22: 375, 1967; by permission of author and editor).

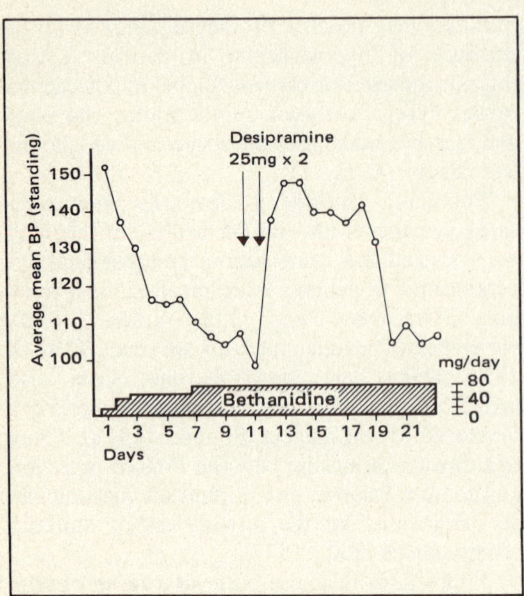

Fig. 2. Interference with amine uptake by sympathetic neurones: Antagonism of hypotensive action of bethanidine by desipramine. Bethanidine was given in increasing doses until the blood pressure was controlled on 80mg daily. This dose was maintained during the experimental period. Two doses of desipramine were administered as indicated by the arrows (after Oates et al.: Annals of the New York Academy of Sciences 179: 302, 1971; by permission of author and editor).

tensive drugs (see fig. 1). Few doctors realise that the administration of phenylbutazone to a patient receiving adequate therapy for hypertension can cause the blood pressure to return to pretreatment levels. Indomethacin also reduces the hypotensive action of frusemide and a mechanism involving prostaglandins has been postulated (Patak, 1975). All other acidic non-steroidal anti-inflammatory agents are therefore likely to have similar effects.

2.2.4 Interference with Intracellular Transport Mechanisms

One drug may interfere with the uptake and transport of another to intracellular sites of action. Guanethidine, bethanidine and debrisoquine are taken up into sympathetic nerve endings by an active transport mechanism which can be blocked competitively by sympathomimetic amines (e.g. some appetite suppressants, common cold remedies), chlorpromazine, some antihistamines and tricyclic antidepressants. Therapeutic doses of ephedrine, amphetamines, phenylpropanolamine, pseudoephedrine, phenylephrine, chlorpromazine,

amitriptyline, imipramine and desipramine can inhibit the blood pressure lowering action of guanethidine, bethanidine and debrisoquine (see fig. 2). Tricyclic antidepressants such as imipramine may potentiate the pressor effects of adrenaline and noradrenaline (see also chapter X, sect. 6.2.1, 6.2.2; XVIII, sect. 10.1) [Koch-Weser, 1975; Stafford and Fann, 1977; Crook and Nies, 1978].

2.3 Pharmacokinetic Interactions

2.3.1 Drug Absorption Interactions

One drug may alter the rate of absorption or the completeness of absorption of other drugs from the gastrointestinal tract. Several different mechanisms may be involved, many of which are poorly understood. Moreover, because of the complex processes involved in drug absorption from the gastrointestinal tract and the different physicochemical and pharmacokinetic properties of individual drugs, these mechanisms may vary from one drug to another. This makes prediction of drug absorption interactions very difficult (Prescott, 1977).

It is important to differentiate between interactions which alter the *rate* of drug absorption and those which increase or decrease the *total amount* of drug absorbed (i.e. alter bioavailability), since the consequences may be quite different. A change in the rate of absorption of a drug with a long plasma half-life such as warfarin would probably have little or no effect if all the drug were eventually absorbed, whereas a change in the total amount absorbed may be disastrous. On the other hand, if the rate of absorption of a drug with a short plasma half-life, such as procainamide is reduced, therapeutic plasma concentrations may never be reached. Delayed absorption is also important when a rapid effect is required, e.g. with analgesics and hypnotics.

Change in pH of Gastrointestinal Fluids

The rate of absorption of many drugs may be limited by the rate at which the drug passes into solution from tablets or capsules. Basic drugs are more soluble in acid gastrointestinal contents and acidic drugs are more soluble in alkaline fluids. On the other hand, basic drugs will tend to be ionised and less lipid soluble in acid solution and hence absorbed less rapidly, but these theoretical concepts do not always hold in practice in man. For example, weak acids such as aspirin are absorbed more rapidly from buffered alkaline solutions than from unbuffered solutions at pH 2.8. Drugs which alter pH such as antacids may therefore have complex and unpredictable effects on the absorption of other drugs (Prescott, 1974a; Hurwitz, 1977). Sodium bicarbonate may however, decrease the absorption of some basic drugs through effects on solubility (e.g. decreased absorption of some tetracycline products). Other antacids decrease the absorption of tetracycline by chelation mechanisms (see below). Antacids may also alter gastrointestinal motility (Hurwitz, 1977).

Effects on Gastric Emptying and Gastrointestinal Motility

Drugs are absorbed much more rapidly from the small intestine than from the stomach. It follows that agents which increase or decrease the rate of gastric emptying may influence the rate of absorption of other drugs given at the same time (Prescott, 1974b; Nimmo, 1976). Drugs such as levodopa are metabolised by gastric mucosa, and if gastric emptying is delayed, less unchanged drug would be available for absorption (see chapter VI; sect. 5). Very rapid gastrointestinal transit may decrease the absorption of poorly soluble drugs (e.g. digoxin and corticosteroids) or drugs which are actively absorbed from a limited area of the intestine (e.g. riboflavine).

Drugs which alter gastrointestinal motility or the rate of gastric emptying can have significant effects on the rate, and in some cases, the extent of absorption of other drugs. Anticholinergic drugs such as propantheline decrease gastrointestinal motility (Hurwitz et al., 1977) and slow down the rate of absorption of paracetamol (acetaminophen)[1], but not the total amount of drug absorbed (fig. 3; Nimmo et al., 1973). On the other hand, the bioavailability of poorly absorbed drugs such as dicoumarol is increased by tricyclic antidepressants (Pond et al., 1975). The tricyclic antidepressants have marked anticholinergic effects which probably slow gastrointestinal motility. This may increase the time available for dissolution and absorption of dicoumarol. A similar effect has been suggested with slowly dissolving tablets of digoxin after administration of pro-

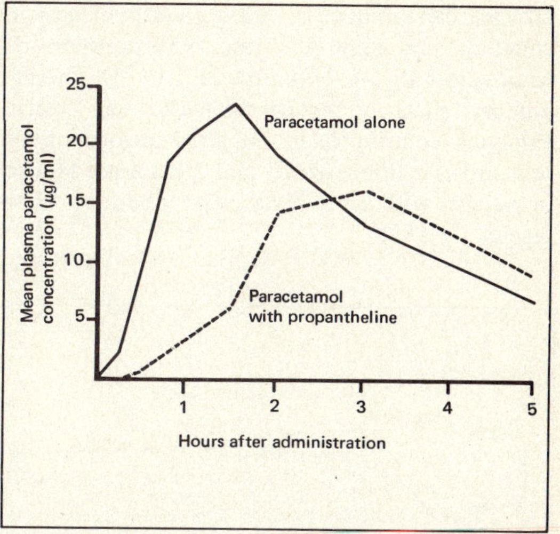

Fig. 3. Change in the rate of drug absorption: Reduced rate of absorption of oral paracetamol (1.5g) by propantheline (30mg IV). After Nimmo et al.: British Medical Journal 1: 587 (1973); by permission of author and editor.

pantheline (Manninen et al., 1973a,b; see chapter VI, sect. 5). Other drugs with anticholinergic activity which might influence intestinal motility include antipsychotic drugs (e.g. phenothiazines), anti-Parkinsonian drugs and certain antihistamines (e.g. diphenhydramine, phenindamine, promethazine). Antacids such as aluminium hydroxide gel delay gastric emptying and can decrease the rate of absorption of highly soluble and rapidly absorbed drugs; for example, pentobarbitone, isoniazid (Hurwitz, 1977). In the case of isoniazid, which has a rapid rate of elimination and undergoes significant hepatic metabolism, the delay in absorption following aluminium hydroxide gel leads to lower peak plasma concentrations of isoniazid, as well as the total amount absorbed unchanged. This could be of therapeutic importance with intermittent dosage regimens. By contrast, aluminium hydroxide gel does not decrease the rate or amount absorbed of ampicillin trihydrate, a drug which is slowly and incompletely absorbed, and further illustrates the unpredictable nature of drug absorption interactions. Lithium reduces the bioavailability of chlorpromazine, possibly by decreasing gastrointestinal motility, slowing absorption and increasing the gastrointestinal metabolism of chlorpromazine (Rivera-Calimlim et al., 1978).

Narcotic analgesics such as pethidine (meperidine), heroin (diamorphine) and pen-

---

1　Paracetamol is used as a model for drug absorption studies because it is a weak acid (pKa 9.5) that is largely unionised in both gastric and intestinal fluids and its rate of absorption in man is directly related to the gastric emptying rate.

tazocine can produce a marked delay in gastric emptying and slow the rate of absorption of paracetamol (fig. 4; Nimmo et al., 1975). The inhibitory effect of strong analgesics on gastric emptying contributes to impaired absorption of oral antiarrhythmic agents and therapeutic failure in patients with acute myocardial infarction (Pottage et al., 1978).

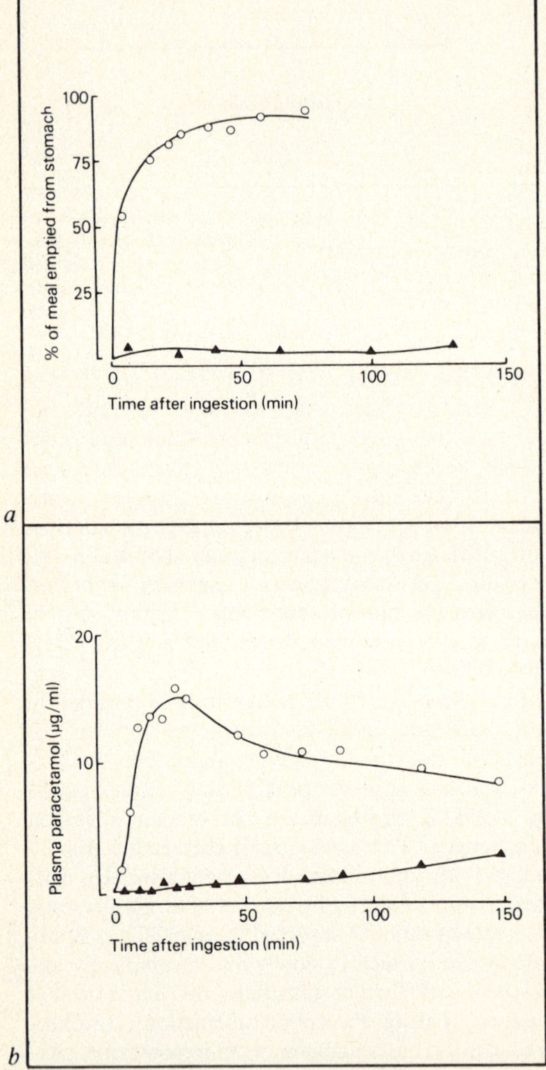

Fig. 4. Change in rate of gastric emptying (a) and rate of drug absorption (b). The effect of heroin (10mg intramuscularly ▲) on rate of gastric emptying (a) and on paracetamol absorption (b) compared with saline injection (o) in one volunteer (after Nimmo et al.: British Journal of Clinical Pharmacology 2: 509, 1975; by permission of author and editor).

Metoclopramide accelerates the rate of gastric emptying and increases the rate of absorption of paracetamol (fig. 5). Metoclopramide has also been shown to increase the rate of absorption and peak plasma levels of diazepam, propranolol, ethanol, and lithium from slow release tablets (Nimmo, 1976). On the other hand, plasma concentrations of digoxin from slowly dissolving tablets are decreased, possibly as a result of the decreased time available for dissolution and absorption of digoxin, a poorly soluble drug (Manninen et al., 1973a,b). The results of interactions involving changes in gastrointestinal motility may depend critically on dissolution characteristics and completely opposite effects may be seen depending on whether the drug or formulation is readily soluble or poorly soluble (see chapter VI; sect. 5).

Binding or Chelation of Drugs

Drugs may react directly within the gastrointestinal tract to form insoluble chelates which cannot be absorbed, for example iron and tetracycline (see fig. 6), or aluminium, calcium or magnesium containing antacids and tetracycline (Neuvonen, 1976). In some cases more rapidly absorbed soluble complexes are formed (e.g. caffeine and ergotamine). The absorption of dicoumarol is increased by the formation of a more soluble complex with magnesium hydroxide (Ambre and Fischer, 1973). Many other examples are known. Absorption of drugs may also be reduced if they are given with adsorbents such as kaolin or charcoal, or ionic binding agents such as cholestyramine. Thus, digoxin absorption is seriously impaired by some antacids and kaolin-pectin (Brown and Juhl, 1976).

Competition for Active Absorption Mechanisms

Drugs which are analogues of naturally occurring purines, pyrimidines, sugars and amino acids (e.g. 6-mercaptopurine, levodopa, methyldopa) may be absorbed by specialised active transport systems which occur primarily in the small intestine, and absorption could be inhibited on a competitive basis. For example, there may be competition between levodopa and phenylalanine derived from dietary sources. Consequently, a high protein diet (2g/kg/day) may decrease the therapeutic effect of levodopa, while a low protein diet (0.5g/kg/day) may increase the therapeutic effect (Mena and Cotzias, 1975). It is also possible for one drug to inhibit enzymes involved in the active

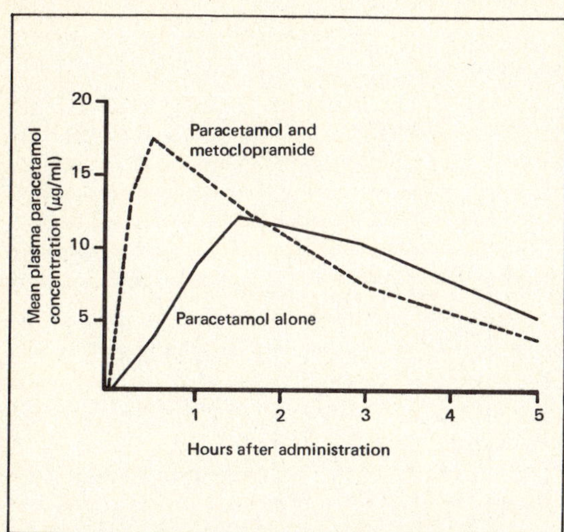

Fig. 5. Change in the rate of drug absorption: Increased rate of absorption of paracetamol (1.5g) by metoclopramide (10mg IV). After Nimmo et al.: British Medical Journal 1: 587 (1973); by permission of author and editor.

transport of another drug, as has been postulated between chlorpromazine and levodopa (Rivera-Calimlim, 1972).

Toxic Effects on the Gastrointestinal Tract

Patients receiving chronic therapy with p-aminosalicylic acid, neomycin, mefenamic acid, phenformin and colchicine may develop a malabsorption syndrome (see chapter XIX; sect. 14.3.1). In such circumstances the absorption of other drugs might be impaired. Thus colchicine may cause megaloblastic anaemia through interference with vitamin B_{12} absorption.

Other Possible Mechanisms

Some drugs are metabolised extensively (sulphasalazine) or in part (levodopa) by the gut bacterial flora. This process might be altered by concurrent administration of antibacterial drugs. Suppression of the gut bacterial flora by antibiotics might limit the metabolic conversion of sulphasalazine to its active component (Das and Dubin, 1976; see also chapter XIX, sect. 8.1.2). The intestinal metabolism and absorption of levodopa is abnormal in germ free animals and in patients after treatment with neomycin (Goldman et al., 1974).

Drugs can also influence the volume and composition of gastrointestinal secretions, including bile, and changes in viscosity may modify drug ab-

sorption. Interference with micelle formation may limit the solubility of lipids — e.g. inhibition of absorption of cholesterol, bile acids and vitamin A by long term neomycin therapy (see chapter XIX; sect. 14.3.1). Other possible mechanisms include changes in portal blood flow and permeability of the gastrointestinal epithelium. The mechanisms of many drug absorption interactions are unknown.

2.3.2 Drug Distribution

One drug may change the distribution of another and thereby alter the concentration of unbound active drug at sites of action. The most important interactions in this category are those in which drugs are displaced from plasma protein binding sites.

Plasma Protein Binding

Many acidic drugs *(vide infra)* and drug metabolites are highly bound to plasma albumin and one may displace another depending on their relative plasma concentrations and particular binding characteristics (Koch-Weser and Sellers, 1976). Depending on the circumstances (see chapter I; sect. 3.2.3), the plasma concentration of unbound active drug can be increased and drug effects correspondingly enhanced. This potentiation of action only occurs with those highly bound drugs which

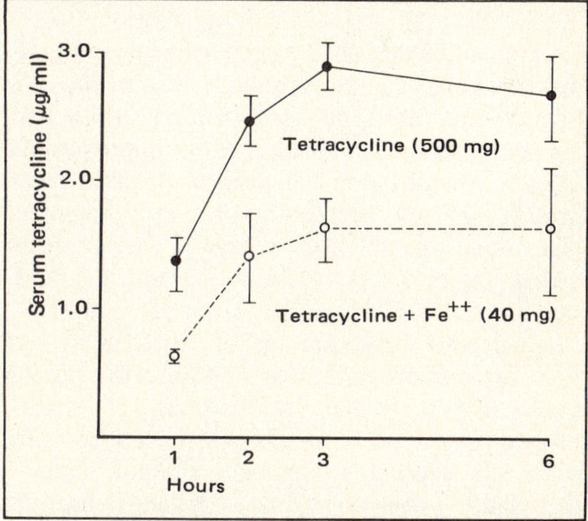

Fig. 6. Interference with drug absorption: Reduced absorption of tetracycline caused by simultaneous ingestion of ferrous sulphate. Serum concentrations of tetracyclines (µg/ml) are given on the y axis. ●———● = tetracycline alone, ○-----○ = tetracycline with ferrous sulphate (after Neuvonen et al.: British Medical Journal 4: 532, 1970; by permission of author and editor).

have a small apparent volume of distribution and bind to the same site on plasma albumin (see chapter I; sect. 3.2.3). Unless clearance of the drug is decreased (see below), it is a temporary phenomenon, since the decreased protein binding makes more unbound drug available for metabolism or glomerular filtration, and the concentration of total and free (unbound) drug in the plasma decreases progressively until a new steady-state is reached. If drug dosage has not been changed, the new steady-state is characterised by a lower total plasma concentration of the drug, but the same free drug concentration, and consequently intensity of effect, as before the addition of the displacing drug to therapy. This sequence proceeds in reverse when a displacing drug is withdrawn from therapy. Thus, an increased intensity of drug action as a consequence of albumin binding displacement eventually corrects itself, but may cause serious effects before it can do so; for example, with oral anticoagulants (see further chapter XXIII; sect. 3.2.5). With some drugs, clearance is decreased and progressive accumulation might occur as a consequence of protein binding displacement if dosage is not reduced. Thus a decreased rate of elimination due to albumin binding displacement may occur at high plasma concentrations of drugs with concentration (dose) dependent elimination kinetics such as phenytoin, salicylate and dicoumarol when hepatic metabolising capacity is 'saturated' (see further chapter I; sect. 3.2.3).

A small change in the proportion bound is of much greater significance with drugs that are highly bound (90 % or more) than with those that are poorly bound, and drugs present in the plasma in high concentration will tend to displace those present in low concentration. For example, phenylbutazone (therapeutic plasma concentration 100μg/ml) displaces warfarin (2μg/ml), the binding of which may be reduced from 98 % to 96 %. The effective concentration of warfarin would then increase from 2 to 4 % with resultant increase in prothrombin time (see fig. 7). Highly protein bound acidic drugs which can compete with one another for plasma albumin include salicylates, phenylbutazone, oxyphenbutazone, mefenamic and flufenamic acids, indomethacin, other acidic non-steroidal anti-inflammatory drugs, sulphinpyrazone, probenecid, coumarin anticoagulants, thiopentone, other barbiturates, phenytoin, valproic acid (sodium valproate) tolbutamide, chlorpropamide, diazoxide, ethacrynic acid, frusemide (furosemide), thiazide diuretics,

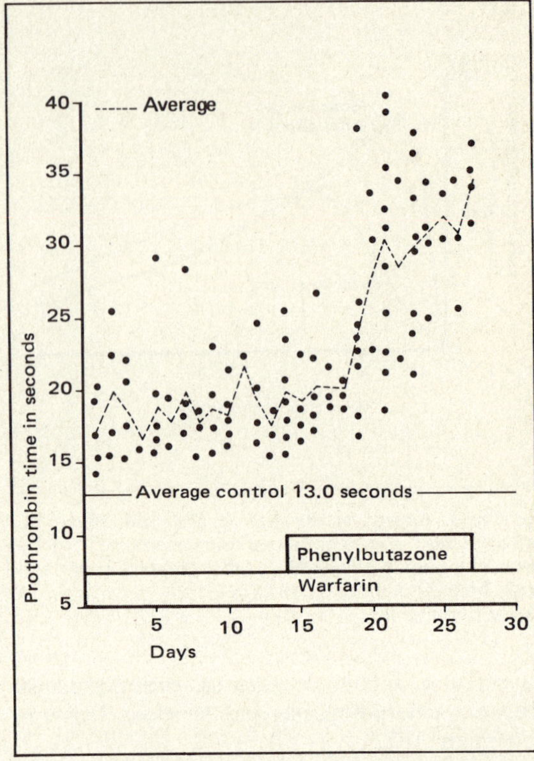

Fig. 7. Plasma protein binding displacement: Effect of phenylbutazone (300mg daily) on prothrombin time in 10 patients receiving long term warfarin therapy (after Udall: Clinical Medicine 77: 20, 1970; by permission of author and editor).

penicillins, many sulphonamides, nalidixic acid, clofibric acid (metabolite of clofibrate), halofenate, trichloracetic acid (a persistent metabolite of chloral), methotrexate and radiographic contrast media. However, clinically important interactions have only been documented with a few of these drugs (e.g. Sellers and Koch-Weser, 1971; Udall, 1974). Although many basic drugs are highly bound to plasma proteins, corresponding displacement interactions have not been described — basic drugs such as tricyclic antidepressants are more avidly bound to a different protein (α_1-acid glycoprotein) and also, most basic drugs have a very large volume of distribution and plasma contains only a very small proportion of the total amount of drug in the body (see chapter I; sect. 3.2.1, 3.2.3).

As discussed above, the net consequence of a protein binding displacement interaction depends on whether clearance of the drug changes. Thus, depending on the pharmacokinetic properties of the particular drugs, plasma protein binding interactions are likely to be exaggerated or only occur in patients with hypoalbuminaemia and renal failure (in which the binding of acidic drugs is reduced) or certain types of severe liver disease (in which the binding and clearance of acidic drugs can be altered) [Reidenberg, 1976; Blaschke, 1977; Tillement et al., 1978]. Many of the drugs mentioned above also compete for active renal tubular and biliary excretion, and some inhibit drug metabolism. Although interactions involving these drugs are often attributed to displacement from plasma proteins, these other mechanisms may be more important. The interaction between diazoxide and phenytoin is remarkable in that elimination of the latter is enhanced to such a degree that it is virtually impossible to maintain therapeutic plasma concentations (Roe et al., 1975).

Tissue Binding

It is conceivable that drugs might compete for binding sites (other than receptors) in the tissues. The considerable elevation of plasma digoxin concentrations in patients also given quinidine could be explained on this basis (Ejvinsson, 1978).

2.3.3 Stimulation of Drug Metabolism

Many lipid soluble drugs cause nonspecific stimulation of drug metabolism in animals through induction of hepatic microsomal enzyme activity (Conney, 1967). A similar effect has been demonstrated in man with barbiturates, glutethimide, phenytoin (diphenylhydantoin), primidone, carbamazepine, ethanol, antipyrine (phenazone), the combination of methaqualone and diphenhydramine ('Mandrax'), rifampicin, griseofulvin and insecticides such as DDT (dicophane) and gamma benzene hexachloride (lindane). The list is undoubtedly very much longer. The administration of an inducing drug causes stimulation of not only its own metabolism, but also the metabolism of many other unrelated drugs and physiological compounds which are substrates for microsomal enzymes. Depending on the dose and drug, induction usually develops over a period of several days or weeks, and persists for a similar period following withdrawal of the inducing agent (Breckenridge and Orme, 1971; Kristensen, 1976). The effects of chlorinated hydrocarbon insecticides such as dicophane and gamma benzene hexachloride are more persistent since they are stored in body fat and have very long biological half-lives. Other environmental chemicals such as polychlorinated biphenyls and charcoal broiling of food, which introduces polycyclic hydrocarbons, can also stimulate drug metabolism (Alvares, 1978).

Induction of drug metabolism is a complex, dose related phenomenon. Initially, there may be transient inhibition, and one inducing agent may accelerate the metabolism of some drugs but have no effect on that of others. There have been conflicting reports on the stimulatory effects of some compounds (e.g. hydrocortisone) on drug metabolism. Complex interactions may occur between anticonvulsants with stimulation or inhibition of metabolism and displacement from plasma proteins (Kutt, 1975; Richens, 1977).

Drug metabolites often have little or no pharmacological activity (see chapter I; sect. 3.3), and in such circumstances drug effects are reduced by inducing drugs. This may partly explain the development of tolerance to some drugs. On the other hand, drug effects may be enhanced if metabolites are more active than the parent compound. Sometimes toxicity is caused by drug metabolites and toxicity is then enhanced by previous exposure to inducing agents. For example, hepatic necrosis following paracetamol overdosage is more severe in chronic alcoholics and patients who have previously taken inducing drugs, (Wright and Prescott, 1973), while methaemoglobinaemia and haemolysis produced by phenacetin is increased by prior consumption of phenobarbitone (Shahidi, 1968). Acute hepatic necrosis has been reported in patients previously taking inducing drugs following anaesthesia with halogenated hydrocarbons. Similarly, prior use of inducing drugs increases the risk of nephrotoxicity after methoxyflurane anaesthesia (Churchill et al., 1976).

Enzyme induction interactions have other subtle but potentially important clinical implications. Tobacco smoking for example, can stimulate metabolism of some drugs such as theophylline, pentazocine, phenacetin and dextropropoxyphene and should as a consequence be considered as an important contributory factor in drug interactions (Alvares, 1978; Jusko, 1978).

Stimulation of the metabolism of oral anticoagulants by barbiturates, other hypnotics and rifampicin is one of the most important induction interactions (Koch-Weser and Sellers, 1971; MacLeod and Sellers, 1976; Zilly et al., 1977). If barbiturates are given to a patient on long term warfarin therapy, the anticoagulant effect is reduced over a period of several weeks and the dose of warfarin may have to be doubled or quadrupled to regain the original effect on the prothrombin time. Satisfactory control can of course be maintained with the higher dose but the patient's life is endangered if the inducing drug is suddenly withdrawn. Drug metabolising enzyme activity returns to normal in 1 to 4 weeks, and unless the dose of warfarin is correspondingly reduced the patient is at risk from haemorrhage (see fig. 8). Patients are particularly vulnerable at the time of discharge from hospital since sedatives and hypnotics are often discontinued then. Induction interactions are particularly difficult to recognise since the enhanced effect of one drug occurs gradually days or weeks after stopping another unrelated drug. Figure 8 illustrates how dosage requirements may be greatly increased when inducing drugs are also taken — more than 200mg of warfarin was required to maintain anticoagulation and therapeutic plasma concentrations while the patient was taking barbiturates. When these were discontinued, the warfarin dose was progressively reduced over several months to a small fraction of the original dose. Therapeutic doses of chlordiazepoxide, diazepam and nitrazepam do not seem to stimulate drug metabolism in man and can probably be given safely to patients receiving warfarin (see also chapter XXIII; sect. 3.2.5). Other important induction interactions include

failure of oral contraceptive therapy (Roberton and Johnson, 1976; Hempel and Klinger, 1976; Gelbke et al., 1977), renal transplant rejection in patients receiving corticosteroids for immunosuppression (Buffington et al., 1976) and methadone withdrawal reactions in patients on methadone maintenance (Kreek et al., 1976).

Stimulation of drug metabolism can have significant effects on the amount of unchanged drug reaching the systemic circulation after an oral dose. This effect is particularly marked with drugs which are extensively metabolised in the liver during absorption ('hepatic first-pass metabolism') [see chapter I; sect. 3.3.3]. Thus, administration of 100mg of pentobarbitone daily for 10 to 14 days had no significant effect on the elimination rate of alprenolol, but the amount of an oral dose reaching the circulation unchanged was reduced almost 5-fold (Alvan et al., 1977).

2.3.4 Inhibition of Drug Metabolism

Inhibition of drug metabolism may result in exaggerated and prolonged responses with an increased risk of toxicity (see fig. 9). Many interactions of this type involve liver microsomal enzymes and mechanisms include substrate com-

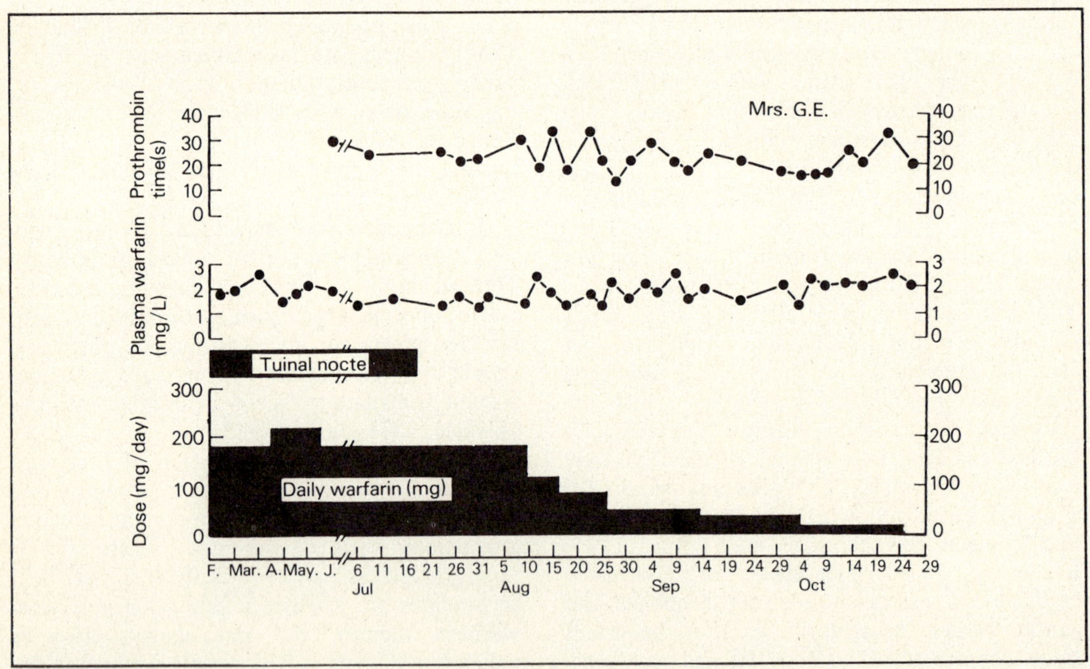

Fig. 8. *Stimulation of hepatic drug metabolism:* Warfarin resistance in a patient taking 'Tuinal' (amylobarbitone plus quinalbarbitone). Progressive reduction in warfarin dose was needed when the barbiturates were discontinued [after Breckenridge and Orme: in Davies and Prichard (Eds) Biological Effects of Drugs in Relation to their Plasma Concentrations, p.150, Macmillan, London 1973; by permission of author and publisher].

petition, interference with drug transport, depletion of hepatic glycogen and functional impairment of enzyme activity due to hepatotoxicity (Kristensen, 1976). Inhibition of drug metabolism may be stereospecific. For example, metronidazole and phenylbutazone inhibit the metabolism of the S (−) enantiomer of warfarin but have little or no effect on the R (+) form (Lewis et al., 1974; O'Reilly, 1976). Some interactions arise through inhibition of other enzymes. For example, hexafluorenium and propranidid prolong muscle paralysis produced by suxamethonium (succinylcholine) by competing with it for plasma pseudocholinesterase. This enzyme is also irreversibly inhibited by organophosphorus cholinesterase inhibitors such as ecothiopate (Davie, 1977).

6-Mercaptopurine is metabolised by xanthine oxidase, and its toxicity is enhanced if xanthine oxidase is inhibited by allopurinol. Azathioprine is converted in the body to 6-mercaptopurine, and like the latter drug must be given in reduced dosage (to about 33 %) to patients receiving allopurinol (Rundles et al., 1963). The failure of doctors to recognise this relatively well publicised interaction is illustrated by a report in a well known medical journal of a clinicopathological conference in which the patient died of azathioprine toxicity soon after being given allopurinol (Anon, 1970). It is quite clear from the description that the patient died because the dose of azathioprine was not reduced when allopurinol was given, yet this fatal interaction was not recognised by the clinicians, pathologists or the journal editor.

The efficacy of certain popular drug combinations could be due in part to the inhibitory effect of one drug on the metabolism of the other and the same therapeutic result could conceivably be obtained with a higher dose of just one drug. For example, anticonvulsants such as sulthiame and pheneturide (ethylphenacemide) inhibit the metabolism of phenytoin; p-aminosalicylic acid inhibits the metabolism of isoniazid; and perphenazine may inhibit the metabolism of nortriptyline (Richens, 1977; Gram and Fredricson Overo, 1972).

The clinical significance of interactions due to inhibition of drug metabolism depends on the therapeutic ratio of the drug involved and on the initial plasma concentration before the inhibiting drug is given. Suppose that the steady-state plasma concentration of phenytoin in a patient on chronic therapy is 5μg/ml and that this increases to

15μg/ml when chloramphenicol is added. In this case the increase in plasma concentration would probably result in better control of fits rather than toxicity. But if the initial concentration of phenytoin had been 15μg/ml, an increase beyond the desirable therapeutic range (upper limit 20μg/ml) to 45μg/ml would have caused severe toxicity (see chapter XXV; sect. 2.2). Particular care is needed with known inhibitors of drug metabolism such as phenylbutazone, oxyphenbutazone, sulphonamides, dextropropoxyphene, dicoumarol, disulfiram, chloramphenicol and possibly metronidazole and isoniazid (Kristensen, 1976; Pond et al., 1977; Hansen and Christensen, 1977). The result of inhibition may be exaggerated with drugs which have dose dependent metabolism (see chapter I; sect. 2.1.1).

2.3.5 Changes in Hepatic Blood Flow

Hepatic blood flow is an important determinant of the elimination of drugs which are extensively and rapidly removed from the plasma by the liver (e.g. propranolol and lignocaine/lidocaine), such that their disposition can be affected by drug induced changes in blood flow to the liver (Nies et al., 1974; 1976). As a consequence of the reduced cardiac output which it causes, propranolol not only decreases hepatic blood flow and affects its own clearance, but also decreases the plasma clearance of other drugs with a high hepatic extraction ratio given simultaneously (e.g. lignocaine). Some vasoactive drugs such as glucagon and isoprenaline (isoproterenol) increase hepatic blood flow and can increase the rate of elimination of propranolol and lignocaine. Phenobarbitone also increases hepatic blood flow and with drugs such as propranolol given intravenously, the change in blood flow may have a greater role than enzyme induction in enhancing drug clearance. Thus with some drugs, interactions, with phenobarbitone can be understood and predicted only by taking into account possible effects on hepatic blood flow as well as enzyme induction. The full clinical significance of these experimental findings has yet to be assessed, but the clinician should be aware of the potential of haemodynamic drug interactions, especially in patients requiring acute intensive care with cardiovascular drugs given intravenously (Nies et al., 1974; Koch-Weser, 1975).

2.3.6 Interference with Biliary Excretion and Enterohepatic Circulation

Many polar compounds with molecular weights above about 400 are actively secreted into bile either unchanged or conjugated (e.g. with glucuronide or glutathione). Drugs and their metabolites may compete for biliary excretion or for the essential preliminary conjugation step. Thus, probenecid reduces the biliary excretion of rifampicin and possibly indomethacin (Kenwright and Levi, 1973; Baber et al., 1978) while paracetamol metabolites compete with bromsulphthalein (BSP) for glutathione conjugation, and reduce the biliary clearance of BSP (Davis et al., 1975). Some drug conjugates are hydrolysed (sometimes by bacteria) in the intestine and the parent drug is then reabsorbed and so enters an enterohepatic circulation which may greatly prolong the half-life. Such enterohepatic circulation can be interrupted by suppression of intestinal bacteria with neomycin (Brewster et al., 1977) and reabsorption of the original drug prevented by administration of a binding agent such as cholestyramine. The latter may significantly reduce the half-lives of digitoxin and phenprocoumon by this mechanism (Meinertz et al., 1977).

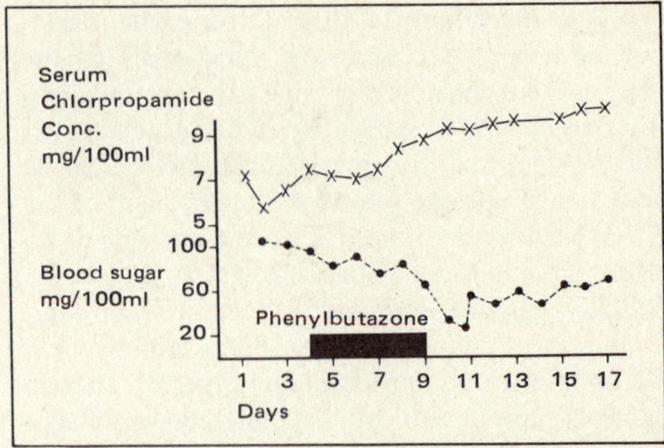

Fig. 10. Competition for active renal tubular secretion: Effect of phenylbutazone (600mg daily) on serum chlorpropamide and blood sugar concentrations. This interaction was thought to be due to inhibition of renal excretion and displacement of chlorpropamide from plasma proteins (after Thomsen et al.: Ugeskrift for Laeger 137: 1722, 1970; by permission of author and editor).

2.3.7 Competition for Active Renal Tubular Secretion

Many acidic drugs and drug metabolites share the same proximal tubular active transport system and can compete with each other for secretion (Kristensen, 1976). One drug may therefore interfere with the renal excretion of another and cause accumulation and toxicity (see fig. 10). Drugs which may interact by this mechanism include p-aminohippurate, phenolsulphonphthalein (PSP), sulphonamides, acetazolamide, thiazide diuretics, diazoxide, chlorpropamide, indomethacin, salicylate, phenylbutazone, oxyphenbutazone, sulphinpyrazone, probenecid, penicillins, dicoumarol and methotrexate. Many of these drugs can also displace one another from plasma protein binding sites (see section 2.3.2), and their interactions may have a dual basis. Such competition between drugs can be used to therapeutic advantage when for example, probenecid is given to increase the serum concentration of penicillins by altering their distribution and delaying their renal excretion (Kabins, 1972). The serum half-life of penicillin is also significantly prolonged by phenylbutazone, sulphinpyrazone, aspirin, indomethacin and sulphaphenazole. Salicylate antagonises the actions of uricosuric drugs and complex interactions may occur between this group of therapeutic agents (Yu et al., 1977).

2.3.8 Change in Urine pH

The renal clearance of weak organic bases with pK_a values of 7.5 to 10 is increased if the urine is

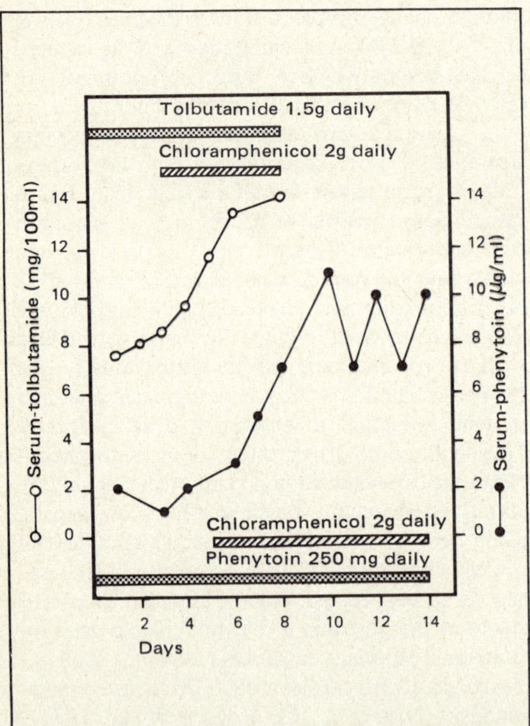

Fig. 9. Inhibition of drug metabolism: Chloramphenicol-induced increase in serum tolbutamide and serum phenytoin (diphenylhydantoin) concentrations (single cases) [after Christensen and Skovsted: Lancet 2: 1397, 1969; by permission of author and editor].

made acid and decreased in alkaline urine. Conversely, the clearance of weak organic acids (pK_a 3.0 to 7.5) is higher in alkaline than acid urine (Milne et al., 1958). Strong acids and bases are virtually completely ionised over the physiological range of urine pH and their clearance is unaffected by changes in pH. With a few exceptions (see fig. 11), interference with pH dependent renal excretion is of no clinical significance because most weak organic acids and bases are inactivated by hepatic metabolism rather than renal excretion. Even if the amount of drug excreted in the urine is increased from 2 to 20%, the effect on the plasma half-life would be of no practical importance. Furthermore, it is rarely necessary to give drugs which produce large changes in urine pH.

A few basic drugs (e.g. quinidine and amphetamine) are normally excreted unchanged in the urine to a significant extent (more than 30%), and their effects may be prolonged if the urine is made strongly alkaline. Overdosage of amphetamine or fenfluramine can be treated by forced acid diuresis, and forced alkaline diuresis is normally carried out in patients with severe salicylate or phenobar-

bitone intoxication (Levy, 1965; see also chapter IX; sect. 5.5.1). Therapeutic doses of antacids such as aluminium and magnesium hydroxide, and sodium bicarbonate also markedly decrease serum levels of salicylate, as a consequence of increased renal clearance caused by the rise in urinary pH (Gibaldi et al., 1974; Levy et al., 1975). Acetazolamide and other carbonic anhydrase inhibitors render the urine alkaline by interfering with bicarbonate reabsorption. The urinary excretion of calcium is thereby increased and this may lead to renal calculi and aggravation of osteomalacia induced by long term anticonvulsant therapy (Mallette, 1977). Antibiotics such as streptomycin are very much more effective in the treatment of urinary tract infections if the urine is made alkaline (Kabins, 1972).

3. Monoamine Oxidase Inhibitors

These drugs can cause serious interactions through a number of different mechanisms (Sjoqvist, 1965), although the extent of their interac-

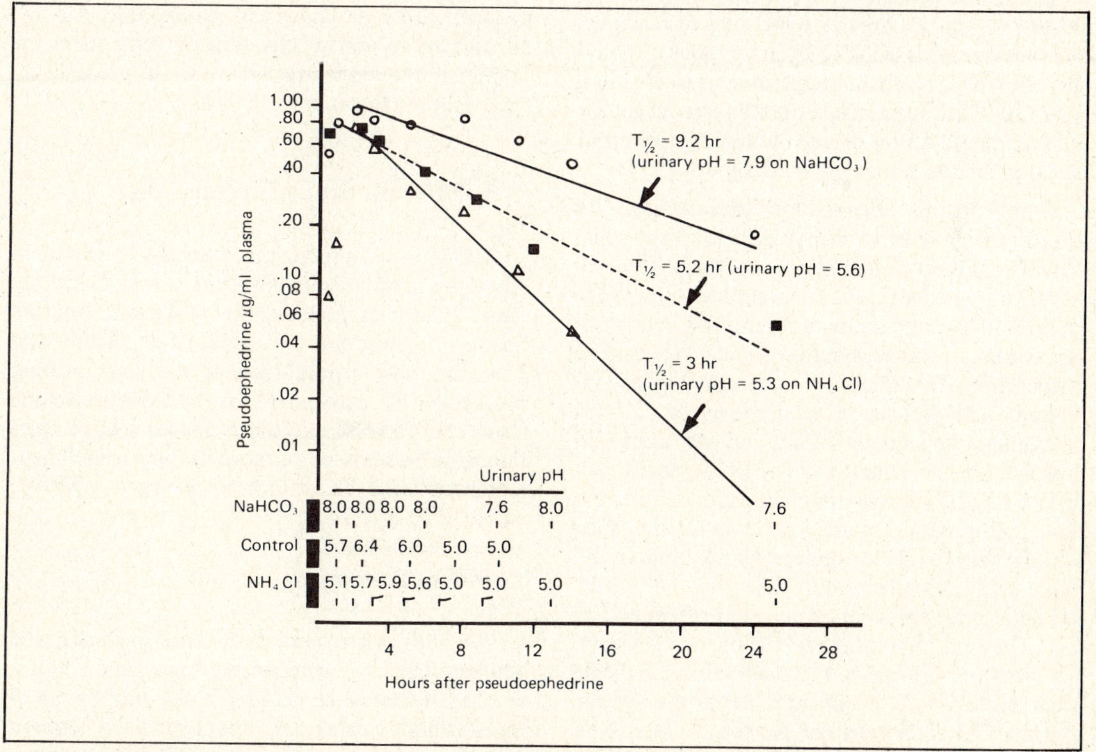

Fig. 11. Change in urine pH: Effect of changes in urine pH on the plasma half-life of pseudoephedrine in man (after Kuntzman et al.: Clinical Pharmacology and Therapeutics 12: 62, 1971; by permission).

tion potential has probably been overestimated. Inhibition of monoamine oxidase results in the accumulation of large amounts of noradrenaline in sympathetic nerve endings, and a decrease in the rate of intracellular metabolism of biogenic amines such as catecholamines, dopamine and 5-hydroxytryptamine (serotonin). If a patient receiving a monoamine oxidase inhibitor is given indirectly acting sympathomimetic agents such as amphetamine, phenylpropanolamine, pseudoephedrine, phenylephrine or tyramine, large amounts of noradrenaline are released causing an alarming reaction with severe headache, marked hypertension, and in some cases acute left ventricular failure or fatal intracerebral haemorrhage. This is the basis of the notorious 'cheese reaction' (Blackwell et al., 1967). Foods such as matured cheese, Chianti and Alicante type wine, yeast extracts and pickled herrings can contain large amounts of tyramine (Marley, 1977). Dietary tyramine is normally metabolised by monoamine oxidase in the intestinal mucosa and the liver before it can reach the systemic circulation, but in patients receiving monoamine oxidase inhibitors it is absorbed intact and releases the large amounts of stored noradrenaline causing a hypertensive crisis (see chapter X; fig. 2). Similar hypertensive reactions have occurred following ingestion of pods of broad beans, which contain dopamine rather than tyramine. Such reactions should be treated by the intravenous injection of an α-adrenergic receptor blocking agent such as phentolamine.

Other serious interactions characterised by agitation, hypotension, tachycardia, hyperpyrexia, convulsions, and coma have occasionally been observed in patients taking monoamine oxidase inhibitors following administration of tricyclic antidepressants, anaesthetics and pethidine (meperidine). In addition, monoamine oxidase inhibitors may potentiate antihypertensive drugs, insulin and the sulphonylureas and are said to inhibit drug metabolism (Sjoqvist, 1965; see also appendix C). Interactions involving monoamine oxidase inhibitors are unpredictable and some, such as those with tricyclic antidepressants (Spiker and Pugh, 1976; Goldberg and Thornton, 1978), occur only in a very small proportion of patients at risk. They are important because of their severity, and since the enzyme is irreversibly inhibited, can occur up to 2 to 3 weeks after the drugs are discontinued (see also chapter X; sect. 6.2.1). Notwithstanding the above comments, serious interactions with monoamine oxidase inhibitors are rare and the risks with sensible prescribing have probably been overestimated (McGilchrist, 1975; Sargent, 1975; Stewart, 1976).

4. Antibiotics and Chemotherapeutic Agents

Antibacterial agents are often given in combination, but there may be mutual antagonism if bactericidal and bacteriostatic drugs are given together (see also chapter XXVII; sect. 3.4). Penicillins act on dividing bacteria by interfering with cell wall synthesis and may be less effective if cell division is prevented by bacteriostatic drugs such as tetracycline or chloramphenicol. Although the activity of antibacterial combinations can be studied readily *in vitro,* it is very difficult to assess their effects under clinical conditions (Kabins, 1972). Indeed, apparently antagonistic combinations of antibacterial drugs are sometimes employed to good therapeutic purpose (e.g. ampicillin and chloramphenicol in typhoid fever). In general, antagonism is likely to be serious only when both agents are near their minimum effective level. Other examples include antagonism of miconazole by amphotericin B, oxolinic acid by nitrofurantoin and inactivation of gentamicin by carbenicillin *in vitro,* and *in vivo* in the presence of renal failure (Ervin et al., 1976).

5. Miscellaneous Interactions

Many drug interactions cannot be classified since the mechanisms involved are not entirely clear. Examples include, the antagonism of the action of levodopa by pyridoxine (Yahr and Duvoisin, 1972), inhibition of the ulcer healing properties of carbenoxolone by spironolactone (Doll et al., 1968), and the increased risk of renal failure in patients on tetracycline when methoxyflurane is used for anaesthesia (Kuzucu, 1970).

6. Conclusions

It is difficult to assess the true incidence and ultimate clinical significance of drug interactions. Published clinical reports represent only the tip of an enormous iceberg, and it is particularly difficult to know how often drug interactions are responsible for therapeutic failure. Not all drug interactions are predictable, and the results of studies in experimental animals cannot be extrapolated directly to man because of species differences. The dangers of multiple drug therapy may have been exaggerated and clinicians are confused rather than helped by exhaustive tabulations of largely theoretical and unconfirmed interactions.

It is unrealistic to expect doctors to be familiar with all known interactions.[2] But it is not unreasonable to expect them to know that the lives of their patients receiving anticoagulants, hypoglycaemic agents, cardiac glycosides and cytotoxic drugs can be at risk if other drugs are thoughtlessly added or discontinued. Clinical pharmacology has had little influence so far on the teaching of therapeutics. But if doctors had a sound knowledge of basic pharmacological principles and were aware of the mechanisms of action and elimination of the drugs they use, the present period of uncontrolled pharmacomania would surely give way to a more enlightened and successful therapeutic era.

Further Reading

Baker, S.B. de C. and Neuhaus, G.A.: Toxicological Problems of Drug Combinations: Proceedings of the European Society for the Study of Drug Toxicity, vol. 13 (Excerpta Medica, Amsterdam 1972).

Cluff, L.E. and Petrie, J.C.: Clinical Effects of Interaction Between Drugs (Excerpta Medica, Amsterdam 1975).

Grahame-Smith, D.G.: Drug Interactions (Macmillan, London 1977).

Morselli, P.L.; Cohen, S.N. and Garattini, S.: Drug Interactions (Raven Press, New York 1974).

Reference Texts

American Pharmaceutical Association: Evaluations of Drug Interactions, 2nd ed (American Pharmaceutical Association, Washington 1976).

Cohen, S.T. and Armstrong, Marsha, F.: Drug Interactions: A Handbook for Clinical Use (Williams and Wilkins, Baltimore 1974).

Hansten, P.D.: Drug Interactions, 3rd ed (Lea and Febiger, Philadelphia 1975).

Interactions Involving Specific Drug Groups

Bender, R.A.; Zwelling, L.A.; Doroshow, J.H.; Gershon, Y.L.; Hande, K.R.; Murinson, D.S.; Cohen, M.; Myers, C.E. and Chabner, B.A.: Antineoplastic drugs: Clinical Pharmacology and Therapeutic Use. Drugs 16: 46 (1978).

Binnion, P.F.: Drug interactions with digitalis glycosides. Drugs 15: 369 (1978).

Crook, J.E. and Nies, A.S.: Drug interactions with antihypertensive drugs. Drugs 15: 72 (1978).

Davie, I.T.: Specific drug interactions in anaesthesia. Anaesthesia 32: 1000 (1977).

Hansen, J.M. and Christensen, L.K.: Drug interactions with oral sulphonylurea hypoglycaemic drugs. Drugs 13: 24 (1977).

Hempel, E. and Klinger, W.: Drug stimulated biotransformation of hormonal steroid contraceptives. Clinical implications. Practical Therapeutics. Drugs 12: 442 (1976).

Hurwitz, A.: Antacid therapy and drug kinetics. Clinical Pharmacokinetics 2: 269 (1977).

Kabins, S.A.: Interactions among antibiotics and other drugs. Journal of the American Medical Association 219: 206 (1972).

Koch-Weser, J.: Drug interactions in cardiovascular therapy. American Heart Journal 90: 93 (1975).

Koch-Weser, J. and Sellers, E.M.: Drug interactions with coumarin anticoagulants. New England Journal of Medicine 285: 487, 547 (1971).

Kutt, H.: Interactions of antiepileptic drugs. Epilepsia 16: 393 (1975).

MacLeod, S.M. and Sellers, E.M.: Pharmacodynamic and pharmacokinetic drug interactions with coumarin anticoagulants. Drugs 11: 461 (1976).

Neuvonen, P.J.: Interactions with the absorption of tetracyclines. Drugs 11: 45 (1976).

Nies, A.A.: Adverse reactions and interactions limiting the use of antihypertensive drugs. American Journal of Medicine 58: 495 (1975).

Richens, A.: Interactions with antiepileptic drugs. Drugs 13: 266 (1977).

Roberton, Y.R. and Johnson, E.S.: Interactions between oral contraceptives and other drugs: A review. Current Medical Research and Opinion 3: 647 (1976).

Seixas, F.A.: Alcohol and its drug interactions. Annals of Internal Medicine 83: 86 (1975).

Sellers, E.M. and Holloway, M.R.: Drug kinetics and alcohol ingestion. Clinical Pharmacokinetics 3: 440 (1978).

Sjoqvist, F.: Interaction between monoamine oxidase (MAO) inhibitors and other drugs. Proceedings of the Royal Society of Medicine 58 (2): 967 (1965).

Stafford, J.R. and Fann, W.E.: Drug interactions with guanidinium antihypertensives. Drugs 13: 57 (1977).

Udall, J.A.: Clinical implications of warfarin interactions with five sedatives. American Journal of Cardiology 35: 67 (1975).

References

Aarbakke, J.: Clinical pharmacokinetics of phenylbutazone. Clinical Pharmacokinetics 3: 369 (1978).

Aggeler, P.M.; O'Reilly, R.A.; Leong, L. and Kowitz, P.E.: Potentiation of anticoagulant effect of warfarin by phenylbutazone. New England Journal of Medicine 276: 496 (1967).

Alvan, G.; Piafsky, K.; Lind, M. and Bahr, C.: Effect of pentobarbitone on the disposition of alprenolol. Clinical Pharmacology and Therapeutics 22: 316 (1977).

Alvares, A.P.: Interactions between environmental chemicals and drug biotransformation in man. Clinical Pharmacokinetics 3: 462 (1978).

---

2   For a guide to clinically important interactions see table III this chapter and drug interactions check list, appendix C.

Ambre, J.J. and Fischer, L.J.: Effect of coadministration of aluminium and magnesium hydroxides on absorption of anticoagulants in man. Clinical Pharmacology and Therapeutics 14: 231 (1973).

Anon: Clinicopathologic conference: Hypertension and the lupus syndrome. American Journal of Medicine 49: 519 (1970).

Ariens, E.J.: Adverse drug interactions. Interactions of drugs on the pharmacodynamic level; in Baker and Neuhaus (Eds) Toxicological Problems of Drug Combinations: Proceedings of the European Society for the Study of Drug Toxicity, vol. 13, p.137 (Excerpta Medica, Amsterdam 1972).

Baber, N.; Halliday, L.; Sibeon, R.; Littler, T. and Orme, M.L'E.: The interaction between indomethacin and probenecid. A clinical and pharmacokinetic study. Clinical Pharmacology and Therapeutics 24: 298 (1978).

Binnion, P.F.: Drug interactions with digitalis glycosides. Drugs 15: 369 (1978).

Birkett, D.J. and Pond, S.M.: Metabolic drug interactions. A critical review. Medical Journal of Australia 1: 687 (1975).

Biron, P.: A hopefully biased pilot survey of physicians' knowledge of the content of drug combinations. Canadian Medical Association Journal 109: 35 (1973).

Blackwell, B.; Marley, E.; Price, J. and Taylor, D.: Hypertensive interactions between monoamine oxidase inhibitors and foodstuffs. British Journal of Psychiatry 113: 349 (1967).

Blaschke, T.F.: Protein binding and kinetics of drugs in liver diseases. Clinical Pharmacokinetics 2: 32 (1977).

Boston Collaborative Drug Surveillance Program: Adverse drug reactions. Journal of the American Medical Association 220: 1238 (1972).

Breckenridge, A. and Orme, M.: Clinical implications of enzyme induction. Annals of the New York Academy of Science 179: 421 (1971).

Breckenridge, A. and Orme, M.L'E.: Measurement of plasma warfarin concentrations in clinical practice; in Davies and Prichard (Eds) Biological Effects of Drugs in Relation to their Plasma Concentrations, p.150 (Macmillan, London 1973).

Brewster, D.; Jones, R.S. and Symons, A.M.: Effects of neomycin on the biliary excretion and enterohepatic circulation of mestranol and 17 β-oestradiol. Biochemical Pharmacology 26: 943 (1977).

Brodie, B.B.: Difficulties in extrapolating data on metabolism of drugs from animals to man. Clinical Pharmacology and Therapeutics 3: 374 (1962).

Brown, D.D. and Juhl, R.P.: Decreased bioavailability of digoxin due to antacids and kaolin-pectin. New England Journal of Medicine 295: 1034 (1976).

Buffington, G.A.; Dominguez, J.H.; Piering, W.F.; Hebert, L.A.; Kauffman, M.H. and Lemann, J.: Interaction of rifampicin and glucocorticoids. Adverse effect on renal allograft function. Journal of the American Medical Association 236: 1958 (1976).

Bull, J. and Mackinnon, J.: Phenylbutazone and anticoagulant control. Practitioner 215: 767 (1975).

Christensen, L.K. and Skovsted, L.: Inhibition of drug metabolism by chloramphenicol. Lancet 2: 1397 (1969).

Churchill, D.; Yacomb, J.M.; Siu, K.P.; Symes, A. and Gault, M.H.: Toxic nephropathy after low-dose methoxyflurane anesthesia: drug interaction with secobarbital? Canadian Medical Association Journal 114: 326 (1976).

Conney, A.H.: Pharmacological implications of microsomal enzyme induction. Pharmacological Reviews 19: 317 (1967).

Conney, A.H.; Chang, R.; Levin, W.M.; Garbut, A.; Munro-Faure, A.D.; Peck, A.W. and Bye, A.: Effects of piperonyl butoxide on drug metabolism in rodents and man. Archives of Environmental Health 24: 97 (1972).

Crook, J.E. and Nies, A.S.: Drug interactions with antihypertensive drugs. Drugs 15: 72 (1978).

Das, K.M. and Dubin, R.: Clinical pharmacokinetics of sulphasalazine. Clinical Pharmacokinetics 1: 406 (1976).

Davie, I.T.: Specific drug interactions in anaesthesia. Anaesthesia 32: 1000 (1977).

Davis, M.; Ideo, G.; Harrison, N.G. and Williams, R.: Hepatic glutathione depletion and impaired bromosulphthalein clearance early after paracetamol overdosage in man and the rat. Clinical Science and Molecular Medicine 49: 495 (1975).

Doll, R.; Langman, M.J.S. and Shawdon, H.H.: Treatment of gastric ulcer with carbenoxolone: Antagonistic effect of spironolactone. Gut 9: 42 (1968).

Dreifus, L.S.; de Azevedo, I.M. and Watanabe, Y.: Electrolyte and antiarrhythmic drug interaction. American Heart Journal 88: 95 (1974).

Ejvinsson, G.: Effect of quinidine on plasma concentrations of digoxin. British Medical Journal 1: 279 (1978).

Ervin, F.R.; Bullock, W.E. and Nuttall, C.E.: Inactivation of gentamicin by penicillins in patients with renal failure. Antimicrobial Agents and Chemotherapy 9: 1004 (1976).

Evers, W.; Racz, G.B. and Dobkin, A.B.: A study of plasma potassium and electrocardiographic changes after single dose of succinylcholine. Canadian Anaesthetists Society Journal 16: 273 (1969).

Gelbke, H.P.; Gethmann, U. and Knuppen, R.: Influence of rifampicin treatment on the metabolic fate of $4^{14}C$ mestranol in women. Hormone and Metabolic Research 9: 415 (1977).

Gibaldi, M.; Grundhofer, B. and Levy, G.: Effect of antacids on pH of urine. Clinical Pharmacology and Therapeutics 16: 520 (1974).

Goldberg, R.S. and Thornton, W.E.: Combined tricyclic-MAOI therapy for refractory depression: A review with guidelines for appropriate usage. Journal of Clinical Pharmacology 18: 143 (1978).

Goldman, P.; Peppercorn, M.A. and Goldin, B.R.: Drugs metabolized by intestinal microflora; in Morselli, Cohen and Garattini (Eds) Drug Interactions, p.91 (Raven Press, New York 1974).

Gram, L.F. and Fredricson Overø, K.: Inhibitory effect of neuroleptics on metabolism of tricyclic antidepressants in man. British Medical Journal 1: 463 (1972).

Greenblatt, D.J. and Koch-Weser, J.: Adverse reactions to spironolactone: A report from the Boston Collaborative Drug Surveillance Program. Journal of the American Medical Association 225: 40 (1973).

Hansen, J.M. and Christensen, L.K.: Drug interactions with oral sulphonylurea hypoglycaemic drugs. Drugs 13: 24 (1977).

Hempel, E. and Klinger, W.: Drug stimulated biotransformation of hormonal steroid contraceptives: Clinical implications. Practical Therapeutics. Drugs 12: 442 (1976).

Himmelhoch, J.M.; Poust, R.I.; Mallinger, A.G.; Hanin, I. and Neil, J.F.: Adjustment of lithium dose during lithium-chlorothiazide therapy. Clinical Pharmacology and Therapeutics 22: 225 (1977).

Howie, J.G.R.; Jeffers, T.A.; Millar, H.R. and Petrie, J.C.: Prevention of adverse drug interactions. British Journal of Clinical Pharmacology 4: 611 (1977).

Hurwitz, A.: Antacid therapy and drug kinetics. Clinical Pharmacokinetics 2: 269 (1977).

Hurwitz, A.; Robinson, R.G.; Herrin, W.F.: Prolongation of gastric emptying by oral propantheline. Clinical Pharmacology and Therapeutics 22: 206 (1977).

Husted, S. and Andreasen, F.: Problems encountered in long-term treatment with anticoagulants. Acta Medica Scandinavica 200: 379 (1976).

Jusko, W.J.: Role of tobacco smoking in pharmacokinetics. Journal of Pharmacokinetics and Biopharmaceutics 6: 7 (1978).

Kabins, S.A.: Interactions among antibiotics and other drugs. Journal of the American Medical Association 219: 206 (1972).

Kenwright, S. and Levi, A.J.: Impairment of hepatic uptake of rifamycin antibiotics by probenecid and its therapeutic implications. Lancet 2: 1401 (1973).

Kleinman, P.D. and Griner, P.F.: Studies of the epidemiology of anticoagulant-drug interactions. Archives of Internal Medicine 126: 522 (1970).

Koch-Weser, J.: Drug interactions in cardiovascular therapy. American Heart Journal 90: 93 (1975).

Koch-Weser, J. and Sellers, E.M.: Drug interactions with coumarin anticoagulants. New England Journal of Medicine 285: 487, 547 (1971).

Koch-Weser, J. and Sellers, E.M.: Binding of drugs to serum albumin. New England Journal of Medicine 294: 311, 526 (1976).

Koch-Weser, J. and Greenblatt, D.J.: Drug interactions in clinical perspective. European Journal of Clinical Pharmacology 11: 405 (1977).

Kramer, W.; Inglott, A. and Cluxton, R.: I.V. Additive review: Some physical and chemical incompatibilities of drugs for I.V. administration. Drug Intelligence and Clinical Pharmacy 5: 211 (1971).

Kreek, M.J.; Garfield, J.W.; Gutjahr, C.L. and Giusti, L.M.: Rifampicin-induced methadone withdrawal. New England Journal of Medicine 294: 1104 (1976).

Kristensen, M.B.: Drug interactions and clinical pharmacokinetics. Clinical Pharmacokinetics 1: 351 (1976).

Kuntzman, R.G.; Tsai, Irene; Brand, L. and Mark, L.C.: The influence of urinary pH on the plasma half-life of pseudoephedrine in man and dog and a sensitive assay for its determination in human plasma. Clinical Pharmacology and Therapeutics 12: 62 (1971).

Kutt, H.: Interactions of antiepileptic drugs. Epilepsia 16: 393 (1975).

Kuzucu, E.Y.: Methoxyflurane, tetracycline, and renal failure. Journal of the American Medical Association 211: 1162 (1970).

Law, R. and Chalmers, C.: Medicines and elderly people: a general practice survey. British Medical Journal 1: 565 (1976).

Levy, G.: Pharmacokinetics of salicylate elimination in man. Journal of Pharmaceutical Sciences 54: 959 (1965).

Levy, G.; Lampman, T.; Kamath, B.L. and Garrettson, L.K.: Decreased serum salicylate concentrations in children with rheumatic fever treated with antacid. New England Journal of Medicine 293: 323 (1975).

Lewis, R.J.; Trager, W.F.; Chan, K.K.; Breckenridge, A.; Orme, M.; Roland, M. and Schary, W.: Warfarin: Stereochemical aspects of its metabolism and the inter-action with phenylbutazone. Journal of Clinical Investigation 53: 1607 (1974).

Logie, A.W.; Galloway, D.B. and Petrie, J.C.: Drug interactions and long-term antidiabetic therapy. British Journal of Clinical Pharmacology 3: 1027 (1976).

MacLeod, S.M. and Sellers, E.M.: Pharmacodynamic and pharmacokinetic drug interactions with coumarin anticoagulants. Drugs 11: 461 (1976).

McGilchrist, J.M.: Interactions with monoamine oxidase inhibitors. British Medical Journal 3: 591 (1975).

Mallette, L.E.: Acetazolamide-accelerated anticonvulsant osteomalacia. Archives of Internal Medicine 137: 1013 (1977).

Manninen, V.; Apajalahti, A.; Simonen, H. and Reissell, P.: Effect of propantheline and metoclopramide on absorption of digoxin. Lancet 1: 1118 (1973a).

Manninen, V.; Melin, J.; Apajalahti, A. and Karesoja, M.: Altered absorption of digoxin in patients given propantheline and metoclopramide. Lancet 1: 398 (1973b).

Marley, E.: Monoamine oxidase inhibitors and drug interactions; in Grahame-Smith (Ed) Drug Interactions, p.171 (Macmillan, London 1977).

May, F.E.; Stewart, R.B. and Cluff, L.E.: Drug interactions and multiple drug administration. Clinical Pharmacology and Therapeutics 22: 322 (1977).

Meinertz, T.; Gilfrich, H.-J.; Groth, U.; Jonen, H.G. and Jahnchen, E.: Interruption of the enterohepatic circulation of phenprocoumon by cholestyramine. Clinical Pharmacology and Therapeutics 21: 731 (1977).

Mena, I. and Cotzias, G.C.: Protein intake and treatment of Parkinson's disease with levodopa. New England Journal of Medicine 292: 181 (1975).

Milne, M.D.; Scribner, B.H. and Crawford, M.A.: Non-ionic diffusion and the excretion of weak acids and bases. American Journal of Medicine 24: 709 (1958).

Neuvonen, P.J.: Interactions with the absorption of tetracyclines. Drugs 11: 45 (1976).

Neuvonen, P.J.; Gothoni, G.; Hackman, R. and Bjorksten, K.: Interference of iron with the absorption of tetracyclines in man. British Medical Journal 4: 532 (1970).

Nies, A.A.; Adverse reactions and interactions limiting the use of antihypertensive drugs. American Journal of Medicine 58: 495 (1975).

Nies, A.S.; Shand, D.G. and Branch, R.A.: Hemodynamic drug interactions: The effects of altering hepatic blood flow on drug disposition; in Morselli, Cohen and Garattini (Eds) Drug Interactions, p.231 (Raven Press, New York 1974).

Nies, A.S.; Shand, D.G. and Wilkinson, G.R.: Altered hepatic blood flow and drug disposition. Clinical Pharmacokinetics 1: 135 (1976).

Nimmo, W.S.: Drugs, diseases and gastric emptying. Clinical Pharmacokinetics 1: 189 (1976).

Nimmo, J.; Heading, R.C.; Tothill, P. and Prescott, L.F.: Pharmacological modification of gastric emptying: Effects of propantheline and metoclopromide on paracetamol absorption. British Medical Journal 1: 587 (1973).

Nimmo, W.S.; Heading, R.C.; Wilson, J.; Tothill, P. and Prescott, L.F.: Inhibition of gastric emptying and drug absorption by narcotic analgesics. British Journal of Clinical Pharmacology 2: 509 (1975).

O'Reilly, R.A.: The stereoselective interaction of warfarin and metronidazole in man. New England Journal of Medicine 295: 354 (1976).

Patak, R.V.; Mookerjee, B.K.; Bentzel, C.J.; Hysert, P.E.;

Babej, M. and Lee, J.B.: Antagonism of the effects of furosemide by indomethacin in normal and hypertensive man. Prostaglandins 10: 649 (1975).

Petrie, J.C.; Howie, J.G.R. and Dumo, D.: Awareness and experience of general practitioners of selected drug interactions. British Medical Journal 2: 262 (1974).

Polak, F.: Die hemmende Wirkung von Phenylbutazon auf die durch einige Antihypertonika hervorgerufene Blutdrucksenkung bei Hypertonikern. Zeitschrift fur die Gesamte Innere Medizin und Ihre Grenzgebiete 22: 375 (1967).

Pond, S.M.; Graham, G.G.; Birkett, D.J. and Wade, D.N.: Effect of tricyclic antidepressants on drug metabolism. Clinical Pharmacology and Therapeutics 18: 191 (1975).

Pond, S.M.; Birkett, D.J. and Wade, D.N.: Mechanisms of inhibition of tolbutamide metabolism: Phenylbutazone oxyphenbutazone, sulphaphenazole. Clinical Pharmacology and Therapeutics 22: 573 (1977).

Pottage, A.; Campbell, R.W.F.; Achuff, S.C.; Murray, A.; Julian, D.G. and Prescott, L.F.: The absorption of oral mexiletine in coronary care patients. European Journal of Clinical Pharmacology 13: 393 (1978).

Prescott, L.F.: Gastro-intestinal absorption of drugs. Medical Clinics of North America 58: 907 (1974a).

Prescott, L.F.: Gastric emptying and drug absorption. British Journal of Clinical Pharmacology 1: 189 (1974b).

Prescott, L.F.; Nimmo, W.S. and Heading, R.C.: Drug absorption interactions; Grahame-Smith (Ed) Drug Interactions, p.45 (Macmillan, London 1977).

Reidenberg, M.M.: The binding of drugs to plasma proteins from patients with poor renal function. Clinical Pharmacokinetics 1: 121 (1976).

Richens, A.: Interactions with antiepileptic drugs. Drugs 13: 266 (1977).

Rivera-Calimlim, L.: Effect of chronic drug treatment on intestinal membrane transport of ^{14}C-L-Dopa. British Journal of Pharmacology 46: 708 (1972).

Rivera-Calimlim, L.; Kerzner, B. and Karch, F.E.: Effect of lithium on plasma chlorpromazine levels. Clinical Pharmacology and Therapeutics 23: 451 (1978).

Roberton, Y.R. and Johnson, E.S.: Interactions between oral contraceptives and other drugs: a review. Current Medical Research and Opinion 3: 647 (1976).

Roe, T.F.; Podosin, R.L.; Blaskovics, M.E.: Drug interaction: Diazoxide and diphenylhydantoin. Journal of Pediatrics 87: 480 (1975).

Rundles, R.W. et al.: Effects of a xanthine oxidase inhibitor on thiopurine metabolism, hyperuricaemia and gout. Transactions of the Association of American Physicians 76: 126 (1963).

Sargent, W.: Interactions with monoamine oxidase inhibitors. British Medical Journal 4: 101 (1975).

Seixas, F.A.: Alcohol and its drug interactions. Annals of Internal Medicine 83: 86 (1975).

Sellers, E.M. and Holloway, M.R.: Drug kinetics and alcohol ingestion. Clinical Pharmacokinetics 3: 440 (1978).

Sellers, E.M. and Koch-Weser, J.: Kinetics and clinical importance of displacement of warfarin from albumin by acidic drugs. Annals of the New York Academy of Sciences 179: 213 (1971).

Seppala, T.; Linnoila, M. and Mattila, M.J.: Drugs, alcohol and driving. Drugs 17: 389 (1979).

Shahidi, N.T.: Acetophenetidin induced methaemoglobinemia. Annals of the New York Academy of Science 151: 822 (1968).

Simborg, D.W.: Medication prescribing on a university medical service — the incidence of drug combinations with potential adverse interactions. Johns Hopkins Medical Journal 139: 23 (1976).

Sjoqvist, F.: Interaction between monoamine oxidase (MAO) inhibitors and other drugs. Proceedings of the Royal Society of Medicine 58 (2): 967 (1965).

Sjoqvist, F. and Alexanderson, B.: Drug interactions. A critical look at their documentation and clinical importance; in Baker and Neuhaus (Eds) Proceedings of the European Society for the Study of Drug Toxicity, vol. 13, Toxicological Problems of Drug Combinations, p.167 (Excerpta Medica, Amsterdam 1972).

Spiker, D.G. and Pugh, D.D.: Combining tricyclic and monoamine oxidase inhibitor antidepressants. Archives of General Psychiatry 33: 828 (1976).

Stafford, J.R. and Fann, W.E.: Drug interactions with guanidinium antihypertensives. Drugs 13: 57 (1977).

Starr, K.J. and Petrie, J.C.: Drug interactions in patients on long-term oral anticoagulant and antihypertensive adrenergic neurone-blocking drugs. British Medical Journal 4: 133 (1972).

Stewart, M.M.: MAOIs and Food: Fact and fiction. Adverse Drug Reaction Bulletin No. 58: 200 (June 1976).

Thornton, W.E.: Dementia induced by methyldopa with haloperidol. New England Journal of Medicine 294: 1222 (1976).

Tillement, J.P.; Lhoste, F. and Giudicelli, J.F.: Diseases and drug protein binding. Clinical Pharmacokinetics 3: 144 (1978).

Thomsen, P.E.B.; Ostenfeld, H.O.L. and Kristensen, M.: Chlorpropamide-phenylbutazone as the cause of hypoglycaemia. A case of an unfortunate drug combination. Ugeskrift for Laeger 137: 1722 (1970).

Udall, J.A.: Drug interference with warfarin therapy. Clinical Medicine 77: 20 (1970).

Udall, J.A.: Warfarin-chloral hydrate interaction. Annals of Internal Medicine 81: 341 (1974).

Vessell, E.S.; Passananti, G.T. and Glenwright, P.: Anomalous results of studies of drug interaction in man. Pharmacology 13: 481 (1975).

Williams, J.R.B.; Griffin, J.P. and Parkins, A.: Effect of concomitantly administered drugs on the control of long term anticoagulant therapy. Quarterly Journal of Medicine 45: 63 (1976).

Wright, N. and Prescott, L.F.: Potentiation by previous drug therapy of hepatotoxicity following paracetamol overdosage. Scottish Medical Journal 18: 56 (1973).

Yahr, M.D. and Duvoisin, R.C.: Pyridoxine and levodopa in the treatment of Parkinsonism. Journal of the American Medical Association 220: 861 (1972).

Yu, T.F.; Perel, J.; Berger, L.; Roboz, J.; Israili, Z.H. and Dayton, P.G.: The effect of the interaction of pyrazinamide and probenicid on urinary uric acid excretion in man. American Journal of Medicine 63: 723 (1977).

Zilly, W.; Breimer, D.D. and Richter, E.: Pharmacokinetic interactions with rifampicin. Clinical Pharmacokinetics 2: 61 (1977).

Chapter IX
Drug Overdosage and Poisoning

L.F. Prescott

Synopsis of Important Principles

1) Specific antidotal therapy is available for very few poisons. The mainstay of treatment of poisoning is intensive supportive therapy, good nursing care and a minimum of meddlesome medical interference.

2) The great majority of poisoned patients recover with intensive supportive therapy alone, and enthusiastic claims for the success of other treatment often cannot be justified.

3) With some important exceptions, the management of poisoning is not altered by knowledge of plasma drug concentrations. There are many pitfalls in the interpretation of drug concentrations in poisoned patients, and the use of nonspecific analytical methods causes great confusion.

4) Gastric lavage and induction of emesis soon after ingestion may be effective in removing unabsorbed drug, but are unreliable. Adsorbents such as activated charcoal are ineffective when given more than 1 hour after ingestion.

5) Poisoned patients are often subjected to unnecessary and potentially harmful haemodialysis, peritoneal dialysis and diuresis. The efficacy of these measures has rarely been established in terms of reduction in morbidity and mortality or removal of toxicologically significant amounts of active drug or poison.

6) The efficacy of haemodialysis for the removal of drugs from the body depends on molecular size, plasma protein binding, volume of drug distribution and clearance relative to the endogenous total body clearance.

7) Haemoperfusion with activated charcoal or exchange resins is more effective than haemodialysis in removing drugs from the blood. Peritoneal dialysis is less effective than haemodialysis. Drugs with large volumes of distribution cannot be removed rapidly by any of these techniques, and indications for their use are limited.

8) Forced diuresis increases the renal clearance of reabsorbed compounds, and clearance may be further increased by appropriate manipulation of urine pH. However, the renal excretion of most drugs is insignificant in relation to the metabolic clearance. Forced alkaline diuresis is largely restricted to salicylate and phenobarbitone poisoning.

9) The toxicity of a few drugs and poisons can be reversed by specific antidotal therapy. Mechanisms include pharmacological antagonism, inhibition of conversion to toxic metabolites, inactivation of highly reactive alkylating intermediates and chelation.

The incidence of self poisoning with drugs and toxic substances is increasing in many countries. Although intensive supportive therapy is the mainstay of treatment, proper management also depends on an understanding of the pharmacodynamic, toxicological and pharmacokinetic principles involved. Unfortunately, recent advances in knowledge of the mechanisms of toxicity, drug disposition and drug analysis have not always been matched by corresponding progress in clinical toxicology.

There are many practical difficulties. The number of toxic substances likely to be taken is enormous and includes not only drugs, but the whole range of household, agricultural and industrial chemicals, and animal and plant toxins. No single individual could possibly have the necessary knowledge and experience to deal with even a tiny fraction of these and Poisons Information Centres have been established in many countries to provide emergency information. With many of the less common poisons, clinical and toxicological data are very limited. Household products are most often taken by young children but contrary to popular belief, rarely cause serious trouble (Goulding et al., 1978). It must also be remembered that the pattern of drugs used for self poisoning changes with time (Proudfoot and Park, 1978).

1. General Principles

The folklore of poisoning is riddled with myths and misconceptions (Matthew, 1971), and the efficacy or otherwise of much fashionable 'treatment' has never been established. Therapeutic measures should be assessed by the same strict scientific criteria as for other medical treatment (Prescott, 1978a). Unfortunately, this is rarely practicable because of ethical constraints on the proper use of controls and difficulty in obtaining adequate numbers of patients for clinical trials in any one centre. The literature is full of glowing accounts of recovery from poisoning after various treatments. The fact that a seriously ill patient has survived is no proof of efficacy of treatment since the great majority of poisoned patients recover with intensive supportive therapy alone (Matthew, 1971; Matthew and Lawson, 1975).

The basis of drug toxicity in poisoning often differs from that encountered with adverse reactions from the therapeutic use of drugs. The so-called 'hypersensitivity' and immunological reactions beloved of so many clinicians are rarely seen, and most forms of acute toxicity represent exaggerated therapeutic responses, secondary pharmacological actions, drug-specific organ toxicity and interference with vital enzyme systems. Some examples are shown in table I.

In practice, the issue is more complex. In Edinburgh, about 40 % of patients take more than 1 drug in overdosage and in addition alcohol is taken beforehand by 70 % of men and 40 % of women. There is great potential for toxic drug interaction in such circumstances. Some popular drug combinations cause particular problems. In the UK for example, there is an epidemic of poisoning with the highly dangerous combination of paracetamol (acetaminophen) and dextropropoxyphene ('Distalgesic') [Carson and Carson, 1977; Whittington, 1977]. Many patients die rapidly from respiratory depression caused by the dextropropoxyphene, and those who survive this initial phase then run the risk of severe liver damage, sometimes fatal, from the paracetamol. There is obviously considerable individual variation in susceptibility to toxicity depending on such factors as rate of absorption (which is influenced by food and alcohol), age, genetic factors, underlying disease, drug metabolising enzyme activity, tolerance, and previous drug therapy not to mention other drugs and alcohol taken at the same time (see chapters I; VIII).

Many drugs and poisons produce reversible effects related to the concentrations of active compound at the sites of action. Effects may be non-specific or caused by stimulation or blockade of receptors. Within limits, the severity of intoxication is related to the concentration at the sites of action, and the duration of intoxication depends on the rate of elimination from the body. Other compounds however, behave as 'hit and run' poisons and manifestations of toxicity may not become apparent until most of the poison has disappeared (e.g. carbon tetrachloride).

The basic treatment of poisoning is intensive supportive therapy since specific antidotal therapy is available for relatively few drugs and poisons. Additional measures include removal of unabsorbed drug from the gastrointestinal tract and enhancement of elimination of drug from the body by dialysis, haemoperfusion and diuresis.

2. Drug Identification and Measurement

Identification of a drug and measurement of its plasma concentration is often thought to be of

Table I. Examples of different types of toxicity in drug overdosage and poisoning

Mechanism	Drug or poison	Principal use	Manifestations of poisoning
Exaggerated therapeutic effect	Amylobarbitone (amobarbital)	Sedative/hypnotic	Deep coma
	Propranolol	β-Adrenoceptor blockade	Bradycardia, hypotension
Secondary pharmacological actions	Morphine Dextropropoxyphene	Analgesic	Coma, severe respiratory depression
	Amitriptyline	Antidepressant	Anticholinergic syndrome
Drug specific organ toxicity	Paracetamol (acetaminophen)	Antipyretic analgesic	Acute hepatic necrosis
	Paraquat	Herbicide	Progressive pulmonary fibrosis
Enzyme inhibition	Cyanide	Industrial	Inactivation of cytochrome oxidase
	Organophosphorus compounds	Insecticide	Inhibition of cholinesterase

value in the management of poisoning. However, there are relatively few situations where treatment will actually be influenced by this knowledge, since the management of most patients depends solely on intensive supportive therapy (Newton, 1974; Matthew and Lawson, 1975).

2.1 Identification of the Drug

The nature of the drug taken can usually be established from the clinical signs and circumstantial evidence. It must be remembered that poisoned patients are notoriously unreliable historians and frequently overestimate the amounts taken. Emergency and supportive treatment must never be delayed pending laboratory confirmation of poisoning. In most cases, the toxicology laboratory provides reassurance for the doctor rather than benefit for the patient. However, drug identification and measurement of plasma concentrations is necessary for the proper treatment of certain intoxications and before undertaking such measures as dialysis, haemoperfusion and diuresis. Serial estimations are helpful in the assessment of prognosis and the efficacy of treatment. Comprehensive screening for the identification of drugs and their metabolites in urine may occasionally be

useful to determine what has been taken, but otherwise is of little or no value. Measurement of plasma concentrations may sometimes be helpful in poisoning with the compounds listed in table II.

2.2 Plasma Drug Concentrations

There are many pitfalls in the interpretation of plasma drug concentrations in poisoned patients, and the relationship between concentrations and toxicity is complex (Prescott et al., 1973). Previous consumption of some drugs may result in marked tolerance, and there is often cross tolerance between central nervous system depressants including ethanol. Several drugs may be contributing to toxicity and it is pointless to measure one but not the others. There may also be doubt concerning continuing absorption. The specificity of analytical methods must also be considered. Many polar drug metabolites have little or no pharmacological activity. Since they usually have a much smaller volume of distribution than the parent drug, their concentrations in plasma may be much higher. The use of nonspecific methods which also measure metabolites may give highly misleading results (Prescott, 1974). Conversely, active metabolites may contribute to toxicity. For example, it has been suggested that deepening coma with delayed apnoea in glutethimide poisoning is due to the combined effects of the unchanged drug and cumulation of an active metabolite, 4-hydroxy-glutethimide (Hansen et al., 1975). Similarly, delayed prolonged deep coma in methsuximide overdosage has been attributed to increasing concentrations of the metabolite methylphenyl-succinimide rather than the parent drug (Karch, 1973).

With poisons which produce delayed toxicity and are rapidly eliminated (e.g. paracetamol/acetaminophen) or rapidly taken up into tissues (e.g. paraquat), plasma concentrations can only be interpreted in relation to the time of ingestion, and serial estimations are desirable. Prediction of the duration of coma on the basis of a single estimation of drug concentration is unreliable as there is great individual variation in the rate of drug elimination, and acute tolerance to central nervous system depressants may occur. In overdosage, barbiturates cause induction of hepatic microsomal enzymes with a progressive shortening of their plasma half-life (Forrest et al., 1974). The metabolism of drugs such as salicylate and phenytoin (diphenylhydantoin) is dose dependent because of early saturation of drug metabolising enzymes and the rate of elimination, initially slow, increases rapidly with the transition from zero order to first order kinetics (see chapter I; sect. 2.1.1).

Finally, attention must be drawn to the inappropriate and misleading tabulation of 'toxic' and 'lethal' plasma or blood concentrations of drugs and poisons. Because of individual variation in susceptibility, frequent ingestion of more than 1 drug and common use of nonspecific analytical methods, such data are often meaningless in practical clinical terms. Unfortunately, information in some publications is also grossly inaccurate such as the statements that 'lethal concentrations' of phenobarbitone and salicylate are 80 to 150 and 500µg/ml respectively (Winek, 1976).

3. General Management of Drug Overdosage and Poisoning

3.1 Emergency Treatment

Most deaths from poisoning with central nervous system depressants are caused by respiratory obstruction or depression. The first priority is the

Table II. Some compounds for which measurement of plasma concentrations may be helpful in the management of poisoning

Drug or poison	Indication
Paracetamol	Specific antidotal therapy
Iron salts	Specific antidotal therapy
Salicylates	Active removal
Phenobarbitone	Active removal
Paraquat	? Active removal
Lithium	Active removal
Methanol	Active removal
Bromide	Clinical diagnosis difficult, active removal
Medium duration of action barbiturates (e.g. amylobarbitone, butobarbitone)	In very severe poisoning if active removal being considered
Glutethimide	
Meprobamate	
Ethchlorvynol	
Chloral hydrate	
Quinine, quinidine	

establishment and maintenance of an adequate airway with endotracheal intubation, administration of oxygen and assisted ventilation if necessary. The adequacy of ventilation should be checked by blood gas analysis if there is doubt. In severe poisoning with depressant drugs cardiac output falls, normal cardiovascular reflexes are impaired and the venous return to the heart is reduced because loss of venous tone results in a disproportion between vascular capacity and blood volume (Shubin and Weil, 1971). The resultant hypotension often causes alarm, but is rarely, if ever, of consequence in the presence of warm extremities. Our practice is never to use vasopressors. The blood pressure and circulation can usually be improved simply by elevation of the foot of the bed, and if necessary, infusion of plasma or albumin. Many poisons cause severe disturbances of acid-base and electrolyte balance. Metabolic acidosis and hypo- and hyperkalaemia are potentially dangerous and may require appropriate treatment. The condition of a severely poisoned patient may be transformed by the simple measures outlined above.

3.2 Intensive Supportive Therapy

Intensive supportive therapy is based on the general principles of intensive care. The object is to support and maintain vital functions to allow spontaneous elimination of the poison and recovery (Matthew and Lawson, 1975). Continued close attention is given to ventilation, the circulation and acid-base, electrolyte and fluid balance. Complications must be anticipated, and dealt with if necessary and expert nursing care is essential. The latter includes frequent turning, attention to pressure areas, prompt removal of bronchial secretions, passive limb movements, physiotherapy and care of the mouth and eyes. Routine bladder catheterisation is unnecessary since the bladder can usually be emptied satisfactorily by fundal pressure.

A close watch is kept for signs of infection but there is no case for the prophylactic use of antibiotics, except perhaps in aspiration pneumonia. It must be remembered that some drugs and poisons cause pyrexia (e.g. central nervous system stimulants and salicylates) and fever often occurs during recovery from prolonged deep coma with hypothermia. Administration of unnecessary drugs to an already seriously poisoned patient can turn a critical situation into a disaster and meddlesome medical interference must be kept to an absolute minimum.

3.3 Treatment of Complications

Hypothermia is a common complication of poisoning with central nervous system depressants, particularly if alcohol has also been taken. It almost always responds to a warm environment and simple commonsense measures to minimise further heat loss. Active rewarming is rarely, if ever, necessary.

Cardiac arrhythmias are always alarming, but again are usually transient and self limiting. Correction of hypoxia and abnormalities of acid-base and electrolyte balance may be all that is required. Treatment with antiarrhythmic drugs (chapter XVII; sect. 6.1) is usually only indicated for ventricular fibrillation or when the arrhythmia is seriously reducing cardiac output. Unnecessary administration of such drugs may cause further myocardial depression and can convert a benign arrhythmia into a dangerous one. The cardiac effects of tricyclic antidepressants may be cited as an example. These drugs have sympathomimetic, anticholinergic and quinidine-like actions, and increasing toxic doses produce progressively, sinus tachycardia, disappearance of 'P' waves and widening of the QRS complexes (fig. 1a). These

changes are easily mistaken for ventricular tachycardia, but almost always regress spontaneously without antiarrhythmic therapy (fig. 1b). In one report, electrocardiographic changes similar to those shown in figure 1a were diagnosed as ventricular tachycardia and lignocaine (lidocaine) and physostigmine (22mg) were given. This was hailed as 'successful treatment', despite the fact that the patient would almost certainly have recovered without it (Tobis and Das, 1976). Administration of unnecessary cardiotoxic antiarrhythmic agents may end in disaster (Greenblatt et al., 1974).

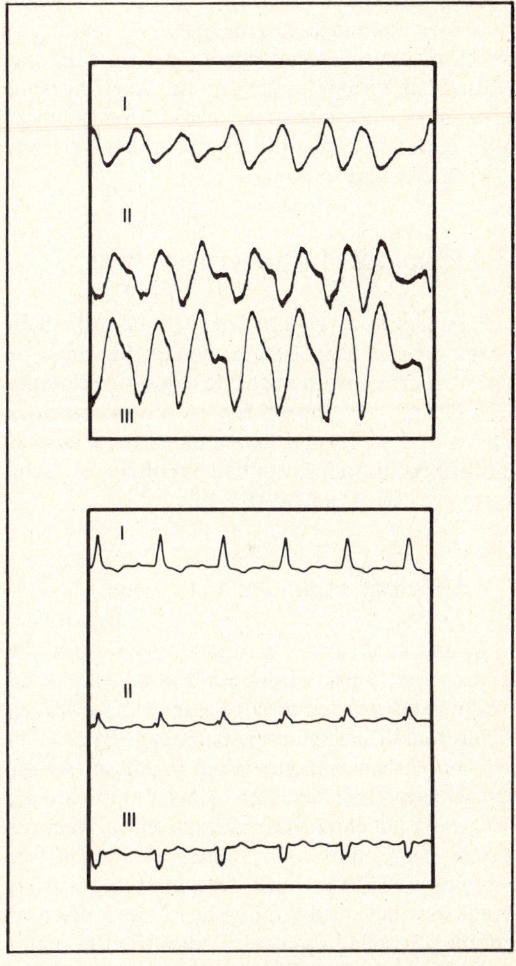

Fig. 1. a (top panel): Electrocardiogram (standard leads I to III) in a patient with tricyclic antidepressant poisoning showing supraventricular tachycardia, disappearance of 'P' waves and gross widening of the QRS complexes.

b (lower panel): Repeat electrocardiogram 12 hours later showing spontaneous improvement without drug therapy.

Serious impairment of A-V conduction (e.g. complete heart block) may require insertion of a cardiac pacemaker (see chapter XVII; sect. 7).

Convulsions may occur in a variety of intoxications, but treatment of isolated events is unnecessary. Repeated convulsions should be controlled with intravenous diazepam. Uncontrolled status epilepticus is better treated by curarisation and assisted ventilation than by large doses of diazepam, barbiturates or chlormethiazole. Other complications such as cerebral and pulmonary oedema, and renal and hepatic failure are treated conventionally.

These aspects of intensive supportive therapy have been discussed to emphasise the basic approach of physiological support, anticipation and treatment of serious complications, expert nursing care, and the least possible medical interference. With such measures, the overall mortality from poisoning is very low.

4. Removal of Unabsorbed Drug

It is logical to assume that removal of unabsorbed drug is beneficial. Although this must be true with gross overdosage and ingestion of highly toxic compounds, the efficacy of current methods for removal of poisons leaves much to be desired and efforts to remove small amounts of 'safe' drugs are clearly not worthwhile.

4.1 Gastric Aspiration and Lavage

Unabsorbed drug in the stomach may be removed by gastric aspiration and lavage. However, most drugs and poisons seem to be absorbed rapidly and this technique is unlikely to be productive more than 4 hours after ingestion, unless gastric emptying has been delayed by narcotic analgesics, anticholinergic agents, central nervous system depressants and possibly salicylates (see Nimmo, 1976). In such circumstances gastric lavage may be worthwhile up to 12 hours after ingestion. It is said to be contraindicated after ingestion of corrosives and hydrocarbons such as paraffin because of the risks of perforation and lipoid pneumonia respectively.

The patient must be correctly positioned head down in the left lateral position and a cuffed endotracheal tube inserted beforehand if the protective pharyngeal reflexes are depressed. It is essential to use a large bore tube (e.g. Jacques 30 gauge) and in adults lavage should be carried out with 300ml portions of warm tap water until the return is clear (Matthew and Lawson, 1975). Complications include pulmonary aspiration of stomach contents, and rarely, oesophageal rupture.

Although gastric lavage is often unrewarding, large amounts of drug are occasionally recovered. A common cause of failure is the use of too small a tube — an ordinary nasogastric tube is virtually useless (Matthew, 1971). Large amounts of residual drug have been found in the stomach postmortem after attempts at lavage with a nasogastric tube (Jenis et al., 1969), and in 1 case a large drug mass containing 25g of meprobamate was removed by gastrotomy 40 hours after ingestion despite gastric lavage (Schwartz, 1977).

4.2 Emetics

The comparative efficacy of induced emesis and gastric lavage is still debated. Neither guarantees emptying of the stomach. Lavage is not always practicable in children because of the physical difficulty in passing a tube large enough to allow the passage of tablets, and emesis is probably preferable in young children. In 1 study in children poisoned with salicylates, emesis was claimed to be more effective than lavage (Boxer et al., 1969), but in another, only 10 to 15 % of the amount of salicylate taken was recovered, even when emesis occurred within 1 hour of ingestion (Yaffe et al., 1970).

The major disadvantages are failure of emesis, particularly if central nervous system depressants have been taken, and toxicity, sometimes fatal, from the retained emetic. Syrup of ipecac given with water is probably the best emetic, and is often effective within 20 to 30 minutes (Cashman and Shirkey, 1970). Other agents which have been used include sodium chloride, copper sulphate, zinc sulphate, tartar emetic (antimony potassium tartrate) apomorphine and mustard. The overenthusiastic use of sodium chloride and heavy metals can be extremely dangerous and fatal poisoning with salt and copper sulphate has been reported (Roberts and Noakes, 1974; Stein et al., 1976). Two patients with trivial overdosage seen personally died with severe hypernatraemia after being given grossly excessive amounts of salt in water as an emetic, prepared in one case by a doctor.

4.3 Cathartics and Enemas

Although the use of cathartics and enemas is traditional, these measures are most unlikely to reduce absorption since this usually occurs rapidly in the upper small intestine. They can only add to the misery and discomfort of the patient. Efficacy in removal of drug has never been established, but regrettably such 'treatment' is still practised and continues to be recommended.

4.4 Whole Gut Lavage

One situation where attempts to empty the bowel may be helpful is in poisoning with 'slow' or 'timed release' formulations. The number of such preparations on the market is increasing and since they usually contain a much larger dose of drug than ordinary tablets, intoxication may be severe and prolonged. In such circumstances, rapid emptying of the bowel might limit absorption. The preferred technique is 'whole gut lavage' in which normal saline is given by nasogastric tube at a rate of 2 litres an hour (Woo et al., 1976). Although this technique is readily controlled and rapidly effective in emptying the bowel in conscious patients being prepared for abdominal surgery, its efficacy in removing unabsorbed drug has yet to be established. It may not be effective and could possibly be dangerous in poisoned patients with grossly depressed gastrointestinal motility.

4.5 Activated Charcoal

Activated charcoal has great adsorptive capacity and can reduce the absorption of many compounds if taken orally at the same time (Picchioni, 1970; Dordoni et al., 1973; Neuvonen et al., 1978). The charcoal must be given in great excess (at least 10 times the weight of the drug) and efficacy falls off rapidly as the time interval between ingestion of the poison and administration of the charcoal increases. After 1 hour, there is little inhibitory effect on the absorption of most drugs, although a significant reduction has been reported with phenytoin (Neuvonen et al., 1978). Repeated administration of charcoal after 1 hour confers no additional benefit. There is no clear evidence of extensive subsequent dissociation of the drug-charcoal complex. Unfortunately, the delay between ingestion of the poison and arrival at hospital is usually such that little will be achieved by the use of activated charcoal. On the other hand, there are no known adverse effects, and it may be of value for the home treatment of childhood poisoning.

4.6 Other Binding Agents

Other agents have been used in attempts to bind unabsorbed drug in the gastrointestinal tract. Paraquat, a lethal weedkiller for which there is no known antidote, binds very strongly to Fuller's earth and bentonite, and these adsorbents are used routinely in the treatment of paraquat poisoning. Although bentonite may reduce the normally slow absorption of paraquat in pure aqueous solution in rats (Smith et al., 1974), all the evidence points to extremely rapid absorption of paraquat from commercial weedkillers in man. Our experience of paraquat poisoning has been disastrous, with no apparent benefit from the early use of bentonite. Cholestyramine binds acidic drugs and can reduce the absorption of paracetamol (acetaminophen) taken at the same time. Like activated charcoal, however, it is virtually useless when the delay between ingestion and administration exceeds 1 hour (Dordoni et al., 1973). The use of desferrioxamine for iron poisoning is described below (see section 6.4).

4.7 Interruption of Enterohepatic Circulation

Polar compounds with molecular weight exceeding 400 to 500 may be actively secreted into the bile, and drugs and compounds of lower molecular weight may be secreted as conjugates. The latter may be hydrolysed by intestinal enzymes to liberate the parent compound. Administration of activated charcoal and ion exchange resins such as cholestyramine and colestipol may prevent intestinal reabsorption of drugs which undergo enterohepatic cycling and enhance their rate of elimination from the body. In 1 study, colestipol shortened the plasma half-life of digitoxin from 9.3 to 2.75 days (Bazzano and Bazzano, 1972) and in another, the half-life of phenprocoumon was halved by administration of cholestyramine (Meinertz et al., 1977). This approach has received little attention, but is likely to be of value in the management of poisoning with many other compounds.

5. Methods for Enhancement of Drug Elimination

5.1 General Principles

Haemodialysis, peritoneal dialysis, haemoperfusion, exchange transfusion and forced diuresis have all been used in attempts to increase the rate of removal of drugs and poisons. However, the amount of active drug removed is often disappointingly small, and the indications for the use of such measures is very limited. Nevertheless, poisoned patients are often subjected to unnecessary and potentially harmful dialysis, haemoperfusion and diuresis (Matthew, 1971; Prescott, 1974), and the literature is full of enthusiastic but anecdotal accounts of miraculous recovery attributed to such treatment (Winchester et al., 1977). Properly controlled clinical trials are difficult to carry out, and very few have been published. With the possible exception of forced alkaline diuresis for poisoning with salicylate and long acting barbiturates such as phenobarbitone, none of the methods used for enhancement of drug removal has ever been shown to reduce morbidity or mortality in poisoned patients. Indeed, some studies suggest the opposite result (Chazan and Cohen, 1969; Gazzard et al., 1974). This is not to say that such measures are never necessary, or indeed sometimes life saving, but a more critical appraisal of their role is required.

In some cases, the drug presumed to have been taken has never been chemically identified, while in others, haemodialysis has been carried out in patients with less than therapeutic plasma concentrations of the drug in question (Prescott, 1974). Other studies have shown removal of only a very small and insignificant fraction of the ingested dose, sometimes amounting to the equivalent of less than 1 tablet or capsule (Woie and Oyri, 1974; Mauer et al., 1975). A misleading impression of efficacy may be gained by the use of nonspecific analytical methods for drug assay (Prescott, 1974).

The efficacy of these techniques for drug removal in poisoned patients can be predicted from well established toxicological and pharmacokinetic principles. They obviously have no place following overdosage with 'safe' drugs such as benzodiazepines or drugs such as paracetamol or narcotic analgesics for which specific antidotal therapy is available. They are unlikely to be helpful with rapidly acting metabolic poisons (e.g.

cyanide) and 'hit and run' or irreversibly acting poisons (e.g. organophosphorus pesticides). Whatever the mechanisms and time course of toxicity, the ultimate pharmacokinetic criteria for the effectiveness of assisted removal is that drug clearance by the technique used should be similar to or greater than the endogenous total body clearance. From a clinical point of view, the use of such measures can only be justified by the results of controlled clinical trials or biochemical evidence of removal of toxicologically significant amounts of active drug.

5.2 Haemodialysis

The rate of transfer of drugs across a dialysis membrane depends on many factors including molecular size and weight, concentration gradient, permeability and surface area of the membrane, blood and dialysate flow rates, pH differences between blood and dialysate and plasma protein binding. Within limits, which depend on molecular size, the clearance by dialysis increases with the flow rate. Drugs with molecular weights exceeding about 350 permeate most membranes poorly and the clearance is not increased with flow rates above 200 to 300ml/minute (Winchester et al., 1977). Attempts have been made to trap highly protein bound drugs in the dialysate by the addition of albumin, and to increase the removal of highly lipid soluble compounds by dialysis against soybean oil (Welch et al., 1972). In practice, the clearance of drugs by dialysis rarely exceeds 100ml/minute. There is considerable variation, depending on the actual drug and the haemodialysis system used (Gibson et al., 1976; Gibson and Nelson, 1977). The most reliable measure of drug removal is estimation of the amount recovered in the dialysis bath.

5.2.1 Effectiveness and Role of Haemodialysis

The amount of drug actually removed by haemodialysis is the product of the clearance, plasma concentration and duration of dialysis. An impressive value for clearance therefore means little if the plasma concentration is very low in relation to the total amount of drug in the body. Thus, the effectiveness of haemodialysis depends on the apparent volume of drug distribution (see chapter I; sect. 2.1.2). It is virtually useless for compounds such as digoxin, tricyclic antidepressants and paraquat which are extensively taken up by tissues since at steady-state only a tiny fraction of the dose is in the circulation. Removal by haemodialysis is further impeded by slow redistribution from peripheral tissues to blood. A further disadvantage is that haemodialysis is of necessity an intermittent procedure.

An example of the lack of effect of intensive haemodialysis on the overall plasma concentration-time curve in paraquat poisoning is shown in figure 2. Although plasma concentrations always fell substantially during dialysis, there was a prompt return to previous levels when it was stopped. Calculations showed that paraquat was only removed from a volume corresponding to the plasma volume, and only a tiny fraction of 1% of the ingested dose was removed by 24 hours of dialysis. Despite impairment of renal function, much more paraquat was excreted in the urine in this period than was removed by dialysis.

On the other hand, drugs which have a small volume of distribution (e.g. salicylate, about 0.15L/kg) are accessible for removal by dialysis. Plasma concentrations are high in relation to the total amount of drug in the body and there is a high concentration gradient between blood and dialysate. Some drugs in this category are extensively bound to plasma proteins and have a low endogenous total body clearance. Plasma protein binding may limit the clearance by dialysis,

Table III. Limited use of haemodialysis for removal of drugs at the Edinburgh Regional Poisoning Treatment Centre, January 1975 to June 1978

	No. of patients
Total admissions	7756
Haemodialysis for drug removal	3[a]
Haemodialysis for removal of paraquat	20
Deaths from poisoning	32 (0.4%)
Unavoidable deaths	14[b]
Terminal illness	6
Death within 3 hours of admission	7
Death possibly preventable by haemodialysis	2

a   Includes 1 haemoperfusion.
b   Paraquat 8; late paracetamol 3; 1; colchicine brain death on admission 2.

although binding is usually less at higher plasma concentrations.

Claims for efficacy are sometimes based on a shortening of the plasma half-life during haemodialysis (Prescott, 1974). As can be seen from figure 2, unless concentrations are followed during the period after dialysis is discontinued, the rebound rise will be missed, giving a false impression of efficacy. A similar phenomenon has been observed with other compounds (Welch et al., 1972) and there may be clinical improvement during dialysis followed by relapse after it is stopped.

Large lists of drugs and poisons said to be actively removed by dialysis have been published with the implication that haemodialysis would be effective treatment for poisoning. Included are drugs for which dialysis would never be indicated (e.g. paracetamol, benzodiazepines and heroin), and many others for which it would be ineffective (e.g. digoxin, chloroquine, 5-fluorouracil and antidepressants) [Winchester et al., 1977]. The limited role of haemodialysis in the modern treatment of poisoning is shown in table III. It was used for the removal of drugs in only 2 of 7756 consecutive admissions to the Edinburgh Regional Poisoning Treatment Centre 1975-1978. 32 patients died from poisoning (0.4%), but the outcome in the majority would not have been influenced by haemodialysis. Death was unavoidable in 14 patients, 6 had terminal illness and a further 7 died within 3 hours of admission. In retrospect, it is conceivable (but impossible to prove) that haemodialysis might have prevented death in 2 patients, one of whom took aspirin and the other a

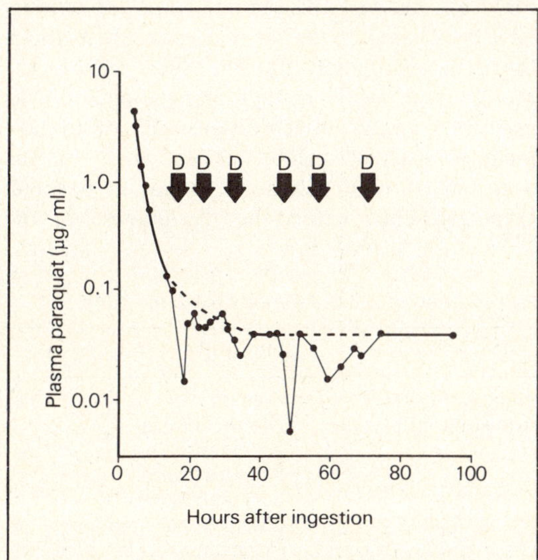

Fig. 2. Lack of effect of repeated haemodialysis (D) on the overall plasma concentration-time curve in a patient with paraquat poisoning. Note the logarithmic scale and the very low steady-state paraquat level.

Table IV. Properties required for rapid removal of a drug or poison from the body by haemodialysis

1. Low molecular size and weight
2. Rapid diffusion across dialysis membrane
3. Rapid transfer from tissues to blood
4. Small volume of distribution
5. Minimal binding to plasma proteins
6. Haemodialysis clearance similar to or greater than endogenous total body clearance
7. Toxicity directly related to amount of drug in body

combination of aminophylline, ephedrine and barbiturate.

5.2.2 Indications for Haemodialysis

Clearcut indications for haemodialysis are difficult to define. The decision must rest primarily on the clinical state of the patient, the anticipated prognosis and the effectiveness of dialysis in the removal of the particular drug or poison. Failure of spontaneous improvement with adequate intensive supportive therapy within a reasonable time, old age, serious complications such as severe pneumonia and impairment of normal mechanisms of elimination caused by underlying cardiac, hepatic and renal disease, are also factors which must be taken into account. The properties required of a drug for rapid removal from the body by haemodialysis are summarised in table IV, and the relative efficacy of removal of a number of compounds is shown in table V. The drug should be identified if possible and its plasma concentration measured before, during and after dialysis. A decision to undertake haemodialysis should not be based solely on the plasma concentration. It has been stated repeatedly that concentrations of short-medium duration and long

duration of action barbiturates of more than 35 and 80µg/ml respectively are potentially fatal and an indication for haemodialysis (Winchester et al., 1977). This is certainly not the case and some patients may be conscious at these levels (Prescott et al., 1973).

Although haemodialysis is a safe elective procedure, there are well recognised hazards which include air embolism, haemolysis, haemorrhage and disturbance of electrolyte and fluid balance. The risks are probably greater with emergency dialysis of a seriously ill patient and suicidal intent must not be forgotten. One of our patients disconnected her shunt during the night and almost bled to death.

5.3 Peritoneal Dialysis

The clearance of drugs by peritoneal dialysis is much less than by haemodialysis and rarely exceeds 20ml/minute. However, unlike haemodialysis, it is a continual process which can be kept going for days. The same general principles regarding drug removal apply as for haemodialysis. The clearance of drugs which are highly protein bound can be increased somewhat by the addition of albumin to the dialysate and the removal of weakly acidic drugs is enhanced if the dialysate is made alkaline with THAM buffer (Winchester et al., 1977). As with other methods for drug removal, misleading claims for efficacy have been based on the use of nonspecific methods for drug estimation. In one such report, the grossly nonspecific methyl orange method was used for tricyclic antidepressants and would have included inactive metabolites and many of the drugs given with therapeutic intent in hospital. Hyperglycaemia caused by the glucose in the

Table V. Relative efficacy of haemodialysis for the removal of some drugs and poisons from the body

Effective	Relatively ineffective	Ineffective
Alcohols	Medium duration of action barbiturates	Digoxin
Chloral hydrate	(e.g. amylobarbitone, butobarbitone)	Amphetamines
Salicylate	Meprobamate	Antidepressants
Phenobarbitone	Ethchlorvynol	Phenothiazines
Barbitone	Phenytoin	Butyrophenones
Theophylline	Lithium	Chloroquine
Many antibiotics	Glutethimide	Colchicine
Inorganic salts	Methaqualone	Dextropropoxyphene
? Sulphonylureas	Procainamide	(propoxyphene)
		Paraquat, etc

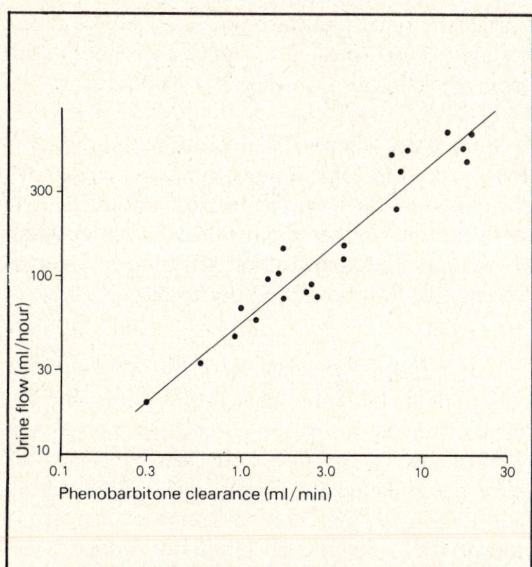

Fig. 3. The relationship between urine flow rate and renal clearance of drug in 3 patients with phenobarbitone intoxication.

peritoneal fluid was even suggested as a useful clinical sign of tricyclic antidepressant poisoning (Royds and Knight, 1970). Peritoneal dialysis is only indicated in severe poisoning with readily removable drugs when haemodialysis or haemoperfusion is not available. Complications of peritoneal dialysis include perforation, peritonitis, adhesions, and disturbances of acid-base electrolyte and fluid balance.

5.4 Haemoperfusion

Drugs can also be removed by passing heparinised blood through a column packed with adsorbents such as activated charcoal or exchange resins. The procedure is technically simpler than haemodialysis and charcoal columns are commercially available. The charcoal is coated (e.g. with acrylic hydrogel) to reduce the risk of embolism, damage to blood cells and pyrexial reactions (Vale et al., 1975). The clearance of many drugs, including barbiturates, glutethimide and salicylate is considerably greater than can be achieved by haemodialysis and barbiturate clearances of 100 to 125ml/min have been obtained with flow rates of about 200ml/minute (Vale et al., 1975; Winchester et al., 1977).

Even more efficient removal of drugs has been reported with haemoperfusion through ion ex-

change resins such as Amberlite XAD-2 and XAD-4 (Rosenbaum et al., 1976). Unlike charcoal haemoperfusion, saturation of the column is not usually encountered and the clearances of barbiturates and glutethimide may approach the blood flow rate (Gibson et al., 1976; Trafford et al., 1977; Winchester et al., 1977). Drugs which can be effectively removed by charcoal or resin perfusion include barbiturates, glutethimide, meprobamate, ethchlorvynol, salicylate and theophylline. However, the same limitations concerning removal of drugs from the body apply as for haemodialysis, and the clinical indications are essentially the same. Contrary to claims made by some investigators, haemoperfusion cannot be effective with drugs which have a large volume of distribution such as tricyclic antidepressants (Crome et al., 1978). In their enthusiasm for this technique, some workers have compared the amounts of extensively metabolised drugs such as barbiturates, glutethimide and meprobamate removed by haemoperfusion with the amounts recovered in the urine (Vale et al., 1975; Crome et al., 1977). This is misleading since very small amounts of these drugs would be excreted unchanged in the urine. The complications of haemoperfusion include embolism, loss of white cells, platelets and fibrinogen and haemorrhage.

5.5 Forced Diuresis

The renal clearance of lipid soluble compounds which undergo passive reabsorption is related to the urine flow rate. Reabsorption depends on the concentration gradient between the tubular lumen and peritubular capillaries, and this is reduced by dilution as urine flow increases. If reabsorption is complete, the concentrations of drug in the plasma and final urine are the same and the renal clearance then equals the urine flow rate (Prescott, 1972). In such circumstances, diuresis increases the rate of urinary excretion of the drug. The effect of urine flow on the renal clearance of phenobarbitone is shown in figure 3. It follows that diuresis cannot increase the renal clearance of compounds which are not reabsorbed.

The renal clearance of weak organic acids and bases with pK_a values between 3.0 to 7.5 and 7.5 to 10.5 respectively can be further influenced by manipulation of the urine pH (Milne, 1965). If the urine is made alkaline, the ionisation of weakly acidic drugs is increased and lipid solubility and tubular reabsorption decreased. As less drug is reabsorbed, the renal clearance is increased. The converse applies to weakly basic drugs (see chapter I; sect. 2.1).

The effectiveness of forced alkaline or acid diuresis depends on the relative contribution of renal clearance to the total body clearance of active drug. Many drugs are extensively metabolised and renal excretion is a minor route of elimination. If only 1 % of a dose is normally excreted unchanged in the urine, even a 20-fold increase in renal clearance will have no clinically significant effect on the overall rate of removal.

5.5.1 Indications for Forced Diuresis

In practice, forced alkaline diuresis is virtually restricted to salicylate and phenobarbitone poisoning. Fluids may be infused at rates of 2 litres an hour for 3 hours for salicylate (Lawson et al., 1969) and 12 to 24 litres in 24 hours for phenobarbitone intoxication (Matthew and Lawson, 1975). Sodium bicarbonate is given to keep the urine pH in the range 7.5 to 8.0. Acetazolamide may cause metabolic acidosis and increases mortality in experimental salicylate poisoning. It is not recommended.

Salicylate poisoning represents a rather special case. Its elimination is highly dose dependent because of early saturation of the mechanisms for conjugation with glycine to form salicyluric acid (Levy and Tsuchiya, 1972). In adults, a single therapeutic dose is eliminated with a half-life of about 3 hours, irrespective of urine flow and pH, since about 80 to 90 % is metabolised to salicyluric acid which is actively secreted by the renal tubules. With high therapeutic and toxic doses, salicylurate conjugation is saturated, plasma concentrations of this metabolite are no higher than with therapeutic doses, and the salicylate half-life is 20 to 30 hours. However, elimination of the unmetabolised salicylate can be greatly enhanced by forced alkaline diuresis (Lawson et al., 1969).

The removal of other less commonly encountered organic acids may also be greatly enhanced by forced alkaline diuresis. Poisoning with the commonly used weedkiller 2,4-dichlorophenoxyacetic acid (2,4-D) carries a high mortality. It is excreted largely unchanged in the urine and its renal clearance is directly related to the urine pH (figure 4). In one seriously ill patient there was no significant spontaneous fall in plasma 2,4-D levels over 2 days (fig. 5), but when alkaline diuresis was

started the renal clearance increased 100-fold and the plasma half-life fell to less than 4 hours with dramatic clinical improvement (Prescott et al., 1979).

Forced acid diuresis is probably a more hazardous procedure and although recommended for poisoning with amphetamines, quinine and fenfluramine, its benefit in terms of clinical improvement and removal of active drug in such patients has not been well documented.

5.5.2 Inappropriate Use of Forced Diuresis

Unjustified claims have been made for the value of forced diuresis in a variety of poisonings. With a few exceptions, there have been no properly controlled clinical trials, and a false impression of efficacy has been obtained by the use of nonspecific analytical methods which also measure inactive metabolites present in urine in high concentrations (Prescott, 1974). Linton et al. (1967) advocated forced alkaline diuresis for poisoning with short-medium duration of action barbiturates on the basis of urinary recovery using a nonspecific method of assay. However, with a specific assay it was subsequently shown to be of no therapeutic value in poisoning with pentobar-

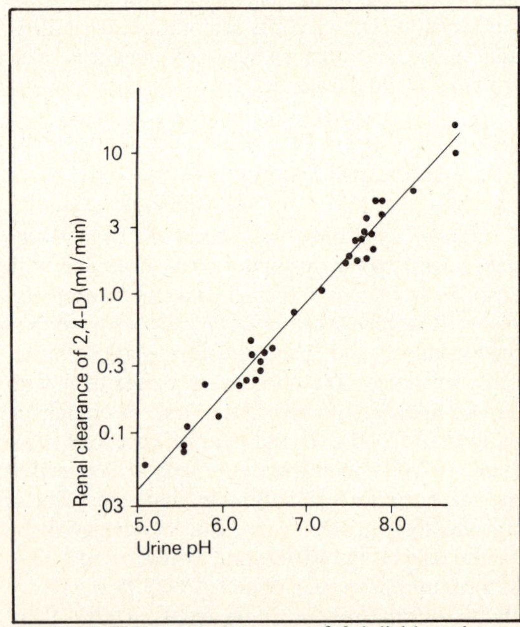

Fig. 4. The renal clearance of 2,4-dichlorophenoxyacetic acid in relation to urine pH in a poisoned patient. The renal clearance was corrected to a urine flow of 1ml/minute.

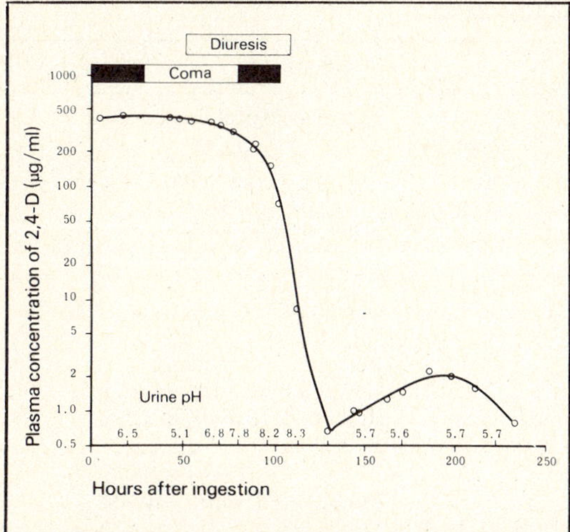

Fig. 5. The effects of alkaline diuresis on plasma concentrations and clinical state in a patient with severe intoxication with 2,4-dichlorophenoxyacetic acid. Note changes in urine pH and the minor rebound after the alkaline diuresis was discontinued.

bitone, amylobarbitone and quinalbarbitone. Only a small fraction of the 'barbiturate' in the urine was unchanged drug (Mawer and Lee, 1968). Similar misleading claims have been made for the efficacy of forced diuresis for intoxication with tricyclic antidepressants (Royds and Knight, 1970), and in 1 patient who had taken a 'massive' overdose of these drugs a diuresis amounting to 23,370ml yielded the equivalent of only 1.5 tablets of imipramine including metabolites (Bailey et al., 1974). Acidification of the urine increases the renal clearance of tricyclic antidepressants, but even so, renal excretion is insignificant in relation to the metabolic clearance (Sjoqvist et al., 1969). The inappropriate use of forced *alkaline* diuresis for amitriptyline intoxication has been reported (Beighton and Hardingham, 1966), and regrettably, this is still recommended by some manufacturers (Prescott, 1978).

Forced diuresis is potentially hazardous, particularly in poisoning with cardiotoxic drugs such as tricyclic antidepressants and in the elderly. Extreme caution is required in patients with impaired cardiac and renal function. Complications include fluid overload, pulmonary oedema, cerebral oedema, disturbances of acid-base and electrolyte balance, and urinary retention. On the other hand, diuresis may protect against renal damage, and administration of alkali and acidifying agents may

have a beneficial effect on redistribution of drug from the tissues to the blood (Waddell and Butler, 1957).

6. Specific Antidotal Therapy

Unfortunately, specific antidotes or antagonists are available for very few commonly taken drugs and poisons. Furthermore, their usefulness is sometimes limited because they must be given very soon after ingestion to be effective. Toxicity may be reversed by several different mechanisms and some examples are shown in table VI.

6.1 Drug-Receptor Interactions

The effects of compounds which produce toxicity by stimulation or blockade of specific receptors can sometimes be reversed by the appropriate pharmacological antagonists or agonists respectively. Thus narcotic induced coma and respiratory depression can be reversed with naloxone (Evans et al., 1973) and physostigmine antagonises many of the effects of anticholinergic agents such as tricyclic antidepressants (Newton, 1975). However, physostigmine causes convulsions and it is not known whether it can safely reverse A-V conduction block and the serious quinidine-like cardiotoxicity of the tricyclic antidepressants. Its use is not recommended (see section 3.3).

Bradycardia and myocardial depression in poisoning with β-adrenoceptor blockers can often be reversed with atropine and isoprenaline (isoproterenol), but they may have little or no effect in gross overdosage. In such circumstances myocardial function can be restored with glucagon, which probably activates adenylcyclase by a mechanism different from that of isoprenaline (Kosinski and Malindzak, 1973). The result of the combined action of an agonist and antagonist depends on their relative concentrations, affinities for the receptor and intrinsic activities. The correct dose to reverse toxicity thus depends on the actual drugs involved and the severity of intoxication. In the example shown in figure 6, severe central nervous system and respiratory depression caused by dipipanone was not reversed by 'therapeutic' doses of naloxone and a larger dose was eventually required. The relative duration of action of the drugs involved must also be considered. Naloxone has a short half-life and may

Table VI. Specific antidotal therapy for drug overdosage and poisoning

Drug or poison	Specific therapy	Mechanism
Narcotic analgesics, including pentazocine and dextropropoxyphene	Naloxone	Pharmacological antagonist
Paracetamol (acetaminophen)	N-Acetylcysteine, cysteamine, methionine	Sulphydryl donors, inactivation of toxic metabolite
Iron salts	Desferrioxamine	Chelation
Metoclopramide, phenothiazines, butyrophenones (extrapyramidal reactions)	Anticholinergics (e.g. benztropine, procyclidine, orphenadrine)	Restoration of balance between dopaminergic and cholinergic activity in CNS
β-Adrenoceptor blockers	Atropine	Inhibition of vagal activity
	Isoprenaline (isoproterenol)	Pharmacological antagonist
	Glucagon	Direct stimulation of myocardial adenylcyclase
Sympathomimetics	β-Adrenoceptor blockers	Pharmacological antagonist
Methanol, ethylene glycol	Ethanol	Inhibition of conversion to toxic metabolites
Heavy metals	Edetate, penicillamine dimercaprol	Chelation
Anticholinergic agents	Physostigmine	Cholinesterase inhibition and pharmacological antagonism
Cholinesterase inhibitors	Atropine	Pharmacological antagonism
	Pralidoxime	Regeneration of cholinesterase
Cyanide	Cobalt edetate	Chelation
	Nitrite	Methaemoglobinaemia
	Thiosulphate	Provision of sulphur for metabolism to thiocyanate
Oxidising agents causing methaemoglobinaemia	Methylene blue	Reduction of Fe^{+++} to Fe^{++}, conversion to haemoglobin
Coumarin anticoagulants	Clotting factors	Replacement of clotting factors
	Vitamin K_1	Pharmacological antagonist
Methotrexate	Tetrahydrofolic acid	Bypass of inhibited enzyme reaction

have to be given repeatedly for as long as 48 to 72 hours in poisoning with long acting narcotics such as dipipanone and methadone.

6.2 Enzyme Inhibition

Toxicity may be caused by inhibition of vital enzymes. Thus cyanide inactivates cytochrome oxidases, organophosphorus compounds combine irreversibly with cholinesterase and salicylate uncouples oxidative phosphorylation and thereby interferes with the function of enzymes dependent on adenosine triphosphate. If a single enzyme is inhibited it may be possible to restore function by increasing the concentration of the substrate or administration of the product of the inhibited reaction. Thus, the toxicity of the antifolate drug methotrexate can be reduced by tetrahydrofolic acid. The toxicity of organophosphorus compounds is related to excessive action of acetylcholine, and muscarinic effects can be partially reversed by atropine. However, eventual recovery depends on resynthesis or regeneration of cholinesterase, and the enzyme-phosphate bond can be hydrolysed with pralidoxime to regenerate the enzyme if treatment is not delayed (Sidell, 1974).

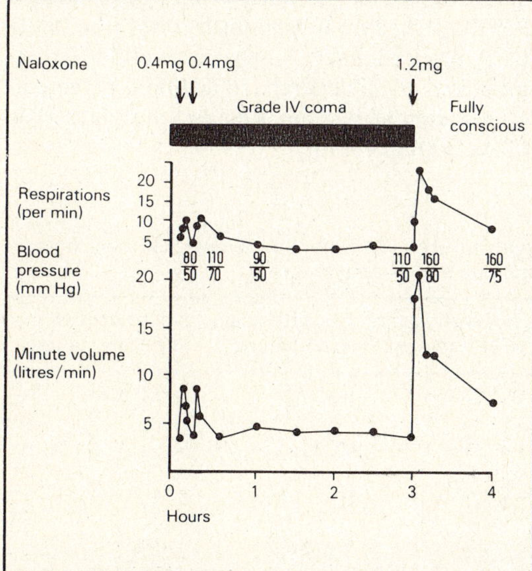

Fig. 6. The effect of naloxone on coma, respiratory depression and blood pressure in a patient with severe dipipanone intoxication. Note the slight transient response to inadequate doses of 0.4mg and subsequent complete reversal of toxicity with 1.2mg.

6.3 Toxic Metabolites

Many compounds are converted to toxic metabolites. In some cases, toxicity can be reduced by inhibiting the biotransformation or by administration of agents which inactivate the toxic metabolite.

Methanol is converted by alcohol and aldehyde dehydrogenases to formaldehyde and formic acid and these metabolites are thought to be responsible for the blindness and metabolic acidosis associated with severe methanol poisoning. The oxidation of methanol can be slowed and toxicity reduced by administration of ethanol which competitively inhibits the dehydrogenases (Lancet, 1978). Similarly, ethanol reduces the toxicity of ethylene glycol which is caused by the formation of intermediate aldehydes and acids including oxalic acid.

Minor highly reactive metabolites are responsible for methaemoglobinaemia and haemolysis induced by phenacetin (acetophenetidin) and the hepatotoxicity or nephrotoxicity produced by a variety of compounds including paracetamol, phenacetin, salicylates, cephaloridine, methyldopa, isoniazid and frusemide (Mitchell et al., 1973; Mitchell et al., 1974; Mitchell et al., 1977). Paracetamol in overdosage causes acute hepatic necrosis which may be fatal, and acute tubular necrosis is a less common complication (Prescott, 1978b). About 5 to 10 % of a therapeutic dose of paracetamol is converted by cytochrome P-450 dependent mixed function oxidase to a toxic alkylating intermediate metabolite. With therapeutic doses, this is normally inactivated by preferential conjugation with hepatic reduced glutathione. With hepatotoxic doses, however, glutathione is rapidly depleted and the excess metabolite binds covalently to liver macromolecules causing cell damage and necrosis (Mitchell et al., 1973; Mitchell et al., 1974). Susceptibility to paracetamol hepatotoxicity is increased if microsomal enzymes are induced by prior heavy consumption of ethanol or drugs such as barbiturates and anticonvulsants.

Paracetamol hepatotoxicity and nephrotoxicity can be prevented by the intravenous administration of sulphydryl donors such as cysteamine, L-methionine and N-acetylcysteine given within 10 hours of ingestion (Prescott et al., 1976; Prescott et al., 1977, 1978b). Treatment after 12 hours is not effective. The results of treatment of severe paracetamol poisoning with these agents compared with supportive therapy only are shown in table VII. Only a minority of patients are at risk of severe liver damage, and treatment is indicated in those with potentially toxic plasma paracetamol concentrations above a danger line joining plots of 200µg/ml at 4 hours and 50µg/ml at 12 hours after ingestion, on a semilogarithmic graph (fig. 7). On the basis of efficacy, safety and availability, N-acetylcysteine is the current treatment of choice.

These sulphydryl compounds also protect against ionising radiation and the toxicity of alkylating agents, carbon tetrachloride, bromobenzene and heavy metals such as mercury. They probably act by the common mechanism of trapping reactive metabolites and radicals which would otherwise bind irreversibly to sulphydryl or other functional groups of essential proteins and enzymes. Reduced glutathione probably plays a vital role in protecting vulnerable functional groups from attack by reactive metabolites and alkylating agents (Mitchell et al., 1974).

6.4 Chelation

Heavy metals can form highly stable soluble complexes with chelating agents such as desferrioxamine (iron), calcium disodium edetate (lead), dimercaprol and penicillamine (mercury, gold, copper, arsenic) and dithiocarb (thallium) [Westein, 1966; Chenoweth, 1968; Beattie et al., 1975; Peterson and Rumack, 1977]. The toxicity of these metals can be reduced by early administration of chelating agents but their efficacy is reduced once the metals have become firmly bound in the tissues. Iron poisoning is relatively common,

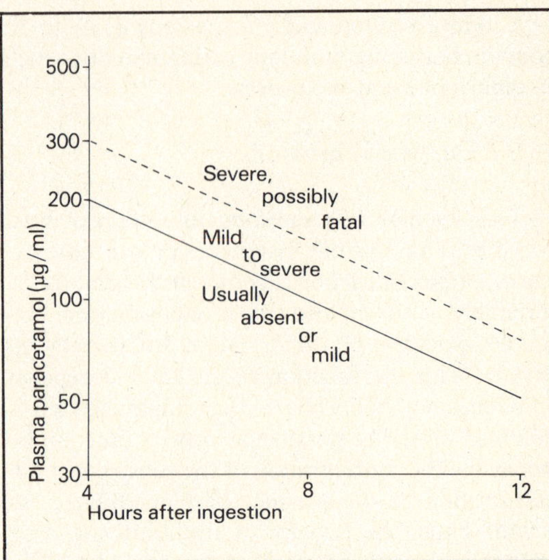

Fig. 7. Relationship of plasma paracetamol concentration and time after ingestion to liver damage following overdosage. Treatment with sulphydryl compounds such as N-acetylcysteine is indicated with values above the solid line. Severe, possibly fatal liver damage is likely above the upper interrupted line. Values obtained before 4 hours are unreliable.

especially in young children (Greengard, 1975). Gastric lavage is usually carried out with a solution containing 2g/litre of desferrioxamine, and in adults 10g in 50ml of water is left in the stomach after the procedure to bind unabsorbed iron in the gut. A proportionately smaller dose of desferrioxamine is used in children. In addition, parenteral desferrioxamine is given if the serum iron exceeds 700 to 800µg/100ml.

Table VII. Incidence of serious complications in patients with severe paracetamol poisoning[1] receiving supportive therapy only and specific therapy with cysteamine, methionine and N-acetylcysteine

Treatment	No. patients	No. with severe liver damage[2]	No. with acute renal failure	No. of deaths in hepatic failure
Supportive therapy only	52	31 (60%)	6 (12%)	3 (6%)
Specific therapy within 10h of ingestion	96	4 (4%)	0	0
Specific therapy 10 to 12h after ingestion	20	5 (25%)	0	0
Specific therapy 12 to 24h after ingestion	29	21 (72%)	5 (17%)	2 (7%)

1   Admission plasma paracetamol above 'treatment' line joining semilogarithmic plots of 200µg/ml at 4 hours and 50µg/ml at 12 hours after ingestion.

2   Aminotransferases > 1000 U/litre. 40 patients received cysteamine, 20 methionine and 85 N-acetylcysteine in specific therapy groups.

Cyanide is a very rapidly acting poison which inhibits cell respiration by combining with cytochrome oxidase. It is avidly bound by many compounds containing cobalt, and the current treatment of choice for cyanide poisoning is cobalt edetate ('Kelocyanor'). Previously, treatment consisted of intravenous sodium nitrite and thiosulphate. The nitrite converts haemoglobin to methaemoglobin which has a high affinity for cyanide. Inactivation and elimination of cyanide is further enhanced by the sodium thiosulphate which provides sulphur for its conversion to thiocyanate in the presence of the enzyme rhodanese (Chen and Rose, 1952). The value of this traditional therapy has been questioned, and hydroxocobalamin proposed as alternative therapy (Graham et al., 1977). Although hydroxocobalamin reduces blood cyanide and prevents acidosis when given in large doses during infusions of sodium nitroprusside (Cottrell et al., 1978), it has been calculated that 10 litres of the standard solution would be required to neutralise a fatal dose of cyanide.

6.5 Immunotherapy

The use of anti-drug antibodies to bind and inactivate drugs is an interesting new approach which unfortunately is limited by the availability of antibody. Severe digoxin poisoning in a 39 year old man was successfully treated with Fab fragments of sheep digoxin specific antibodies. Before treatment there was extreme bradycardia with intractable hyperkalaemia and the serum digoxin concentration was 18ng/ml. Toxicity was dramatically reversed and the serum digoxin concentration fell precipitously to less than 1ng/ml after infusion of 1.1g of digoxin specific Fab fragments (Smith et al., 1976).

6.6 Methaemoglobinaemia

Oxidising agents such as chlorate and drugs such as phenacetin may cause methaemoglobinaemia in which the iron is converted into the ferric form. Minor degrees are of little consequence, but the oxygen carrying capacity of blood is significantly impaired when more than about 30% of the haemoglobin is converted to methaemoglobin. The usual treatment is administration of methylene blue which reduces the methaemoglobin back to haemoglobin by a cyclic reaction involving conversion of the dye to its colourless form, leucomethylene blue.

Further Reading

Cashman, T.M. and Shirkey, H.C.: Emergency management of poisoning. Pediatric Clinics of North America 17: 525 (1970).

Goulding, R.; Ashforth, G.K. and Jenkins, H.: Household products and poisoning. British Medical Journal 1: 286 (1978).

Matthew, H. and Lawson, A.A.H.: Treatment of Common Acute Poisonings, 3rd Ed. (Churchill Livingstone, Edinburgh 1975).

Proudfoot, A.T. and Park, J.: Changing pattern of drugs used for self-poisoning. British Medical Journal 1: 90 (1978).

Symposium: The Poisoned Patient: The Role of the Laboratory. CIBA Foundation Symposium 26 (new series) [Associated Scientific Publishers, Oxford 1974].

Yaffe, S.J.; Sjoqvist, F. and Alvan, G.: Pharmacological principles in the management of accidental poisoning. Pediatric Clinics of North America 17: 495 (1970).

References

Bailey, R.R.; Sharman, J.R.; O'Rourke, J. and Buttimore, A.L.: Haemodialysis and forced diuresis for tricyclic antidepressant poisoning. British Medical Journal 4: 230 (1974).

Bazzano, G. and Bazzano, G.S.: Digitalis Intoxication — Treatment with a new steroid-binding resin. Journal of the American Medical Association 220: 828 (1972).

Beattie, A.D.; Briggs, J.D.; Canavan, J.S.F.; Doyle, D.; Mullin, P.J. and Watson, A.A.: Acute lead poisoning — Five cases resulting from self-injection of lead and opium. Quarterly Journal of Medicine, New Series 44: 275 (1975).

Beighton, P. and Hardingham, M.: Amitriptyline poisoning treated by forced diuresis. Practitioner 197: 354 (1966).

Boxer, L.; Anderson, F.P. and Rowe, D.S.: Comparison of ipecac-induced emesis with gastric lavage in the treatment of acute salicylate ingestion. Journal of Pediatrics 74: 800 (1969).

Carson, D.J.L. and Carson, E.D.: Fatal dextropropoxyphene poisoning in Northern Ireland. Lancet 1: 894 (1977).

Cashman, T.M. and Shirkey, H.C.: Emergency management of poisoning. Pediatric Clinics of North America 17: 525 (1970).

Chazan, J.A. and Cohen, J.J.: Clinical spectrum of glutethimide intoxication. Journal of the American Medical Association 208: 837 (1969).

Chen, K.K. and Rose, C.L.: Nitrite and thiosulphate therapy in cyanide poisoning. Journal of the American Medical Association 149: 113 (1952).

Chenoweth, M.B.: Clinical use of metal-binding drugs. Clinical Pharmacology and Therapeutics 9: 365 (1968).

Cottrell, J.E.; Casthely, P.; Brodie, J.D.; Patel, K.; Klein, A. and Turndorf, H.: Prevention of nitroprusside-induced cyanide toxicity with hydroxocobalamin. New England Journal of Medicine 298: 809 (1978).

Crome, P.; Higgenbottom, T. and Elliott, J.A.: Severe meprobamate poisoning: successful treatment with haemoperfusion. Postgraduate Medical Journal 53: 698 (1977).

Crome, P.; Volans, G.N.; Hampel, G.; Widdop, B.; Vale, J.A. and Goulding, R.: Haemoperfusion in treatment of drug intoxication. British Medical Journal 1: 174 (1978).

Dordoni, B.; Willson, R.A.; Thompson, R.P.H. and Williams, R.: Reduction of absorption of paracetamol by activated charcoal and cholestyramine: a possible therapeutic measure. British Medical Journal 3: 86 (1973).

Evans, L.E.; Roscoe, P.; Swainson, C.P. and Prescott, L.F.: Treatment of drug overdosage with naloxone, a specific narcotic antagonist. Lancet 1: 452 (1973).

Forrest, J.A.H.; Roscoe, P.; Stevenson, I.H. and Prescott, L.F.: Abnormal drug metabolism following barbiturate and paracetamol overdose. British Medical Journal 4: 499 (1974).

Gazzard, B.G.; Willson, R.A.; Weston, M.J.; Thompson, R.P.H. and Williams, R.: Charcoal haemoperfusion for paracetamol overdose. British Journal of Clinical Pharmacology 1: 271 (1974).

Gibson, T.P. and Nelson, H.A.: Drug kinetics and artificial kidneys. Clinical Pharmacokinetics 2: 403 (1977).

Gibson, T.P.; Matusik, E.; Nelson, L.D. and Briggs, W.A.: Artificial kidneys and clearance calculations. Clinical Pharmacology and Therapeutics 20: 720 (1976).

Goulding, R.; Ashforth, G.K. and Jenkins, H.: Household products and poisoning. British Medical Journal 1: 286 (1978).

Graham, D.L.; Laman, D.; Theodore, J. and Robin, E.D.: Acute cyanide poisoning complicated by lactic acidosis and pulmonary edema. Archives of Internal Medicine 137: 1051 (1977).

Greenblatt, D.J.; Koch-Weser, J. and Shader, R.I.: Multiple complications and death following protriptyline overdosage. Journal of the American Medical Association 229: 556 (1974).

Greengard, J.: Iron poisoning in children. Clinical Toxicology 8: 575 (1975).

Hansen, A.R.; Kennedy, K.A.; Ambre, J.J. and Fischer, L.J.: Glutethimide poisoning — A metabolite contributes to morbidity and mortality. New England Journal of Medicine 292: 250 (1975).

Jenis, E.H.; Payne, R.J. and Goldbaum, L.R.: Acute meprobamate poisonong — A fatal case following a lucid interval. Journal of the American Medical Association 207: 361 (1969).

Karch, S.B.: Methsuximide overdose — Delayed onset of profound coma. Journal of the American Medical Association 223: 1463 (1973).

Kosinski, E.J. and Malindzak, G.S.: Glucagon and isoproterenol in reversing propranolol toxicity. Archives of Internal Medicine 132: 840 (1973).

Lancet: Methanol poisoning. 2: 510 (1978).

Lawson, A.A.H.; Proudfoot, A.T.; Brown, S.S.; Macdonald, R.H.; Fraser, A.G.; Cameron, J.C. and Matthew, H.: Forced diuresis in the treatment of acute salicylate poisoning in adults. Quarterly Journal of Medicine, New Series 38: 31 (1969).

Levy, G. and Tsuchiya, T.: Salicylate accumulation kinetics in man. New England Journal of Medicine 287: 430 (1972).

Linton, A.L.; Luke, R.G. and Briggs, J.D.: Methods of forced diuresis and its application in barbiturate poisoning. Lancet 2: 377 (1967).

Matthew, H.: Acute poisoning: Some myths and misconceptions. British Medical Journal 1: 519 (1971).

Matthew, H. and Lawson, A.A.H.: Treatment of common acute poisonings, 3rd Ed. (Churchill Livingstone, Edinburgh 1975).

Mauer, S.M.; Paxson, C.L.; Hartizch, B.; Buselmeier, T.J. and Kjellstrand, C.M.: Hemodialysis in an infant with propoxyphene intoxication. Clinical Pharmacology and Therapeutics 17: 88 (1975).

Mawer, G.E. and Lee, H.A.: Value of forced diuresis in acute barbiturate poisoning. British Medical Journal 2: 790 (1968).

Meinertz, T.; Gilfrich, H.-J.; Bork, R. and Jahnchen, E.: Treatment of phenprocoumon intoxication with cholestyramine. British Medical Journal 2: 439 (1977).

Milne, M.D.: Influence of acid-base balance on efficacy and toxicity of drugs. Proceedings of the Royal Society of Medicine 58: 961 (1965).

Mitchell, J.R.; Jollow, D.J.; Gillette, J.R. and Brodie, B.B.: Drug metabolism as a cause of drug toxicity. Drug Metabolism and Disposition 1: 418 (1973).

Mitchell, J.R.; McMurtry, R.J.; Statham, C.N. and Nelson, S.D. Molecular basis for several drug-induced nephropathies. American Journal of Medicine 62: 518 (1977).

Mitchell, J.R.; Thorgeirsson, S.S.; Potter, W.Z.; Jollow, D.J. and Keiser, H.: Acetaminophen-induced hepatic injury: Protective role of glutathione in man and rationale for therapy. Clinical Pharmacology and Therapeutics 16: 676 (1974).

Neuvonen, P.J.; Elfving, S.M. and Elonen, E.: Reduction of absorption of digoxin, phenytoin and aspirin by activated charcoal in man. European Journal of Clinical Pharmacology 13: 213 (1978).

Newton, R.W.: The clinician's requirements from the laboratory in the treatment of the acutely poisoned patient; in The Poisoned Patient: The Role of the Laboratory. Ciba Foundation Symposium 26 (New Series), p. 5 (Associated Scientific Publishers, Oxford 1974).

Newton, R.W.: Physostigmine salicylate in the treatment of tricyclic antidepressant poisoning. Journal of American Medical Association 231: 941 (1975).

Nimmo, W.S.: Drugs, diseases and altered gastric emptying. Clinical Pharmacokinetics 1: 189 (1976).

Peterson, R.G. and Rumack, B.H.: D-Penicillamine therapy of acute arsenic poisoning. Journal of Pediatrics 91: 661 (1977).

Picchioni, A.L.: Activated charcoal — A neglected antidote. Pediatric Clinics of North America 17: 535 (1970).

Prescott, L.F.: Mechanisms of renal excretion of drugs (with special reference to drugs used by anaesthetists). British Journal of Anaesthesia 44: 246 (1972).

Prescott, L.F.: Limitations of haemodialysis and forced diuresis; in The Poisoned Patient : The Role of the Laboratory. Ciba Foundation Symposium 26 (New Series), p. 269 (Associated Scientific Publishers, Oxford 1974).

Prescott, L.F.: Clinical toxicology. British Journal of Clinical Pharmacology. In press (1978a).

Prescott, L.F.: Prevention of hepatic necrosis following paracetamol overdosage. Health Bulletin 36: 204 (1978b).

Prescott, L.F.; Park, J.; Ballantyne, A.; Adriaenssens, P. and Proudfoot, A.T.: Treatment of paracetamol (acetaminophen) poisoning with N-acetylcysteine. Lancet 2: 432 (1977).

Prescott, L.F.; Park, J. and Darrien, I.: Treatment of severe 2, 4-D and mecoprop intoxication with alkaline diuresis. British Journal of Clinical Pharmacology 7: 111 (1979).

Prescott, L.F.; Park, J.; Sutherland, G.R.; Smith, I.J. and Proudfoot, A.T.: Cysteamine, methionine and penicillamine in the treatment of paracetamol poisoning. Lancet 2: 109 (1976).

Prescott, L.F.; Roscoe, P. and Forrest, J.A.H.: Plasma concentrations and drug toxicity in man; in Davies and Prichard (Eds) Biological Effects of Drugs in Relation to Their Plasma Concentration, p. 51 (Macmillan, London 1973).

Proudfoot, A.T. and Park, J.: Changing pattern of drugs used for self-poisoning. British Medical Journal 1: 90 (1978).

Roberts, C.J.C. and Noakes, M.J.: Fatal outcome from administration of a salt emetic. Postgraduate Medical Journal 50: 513 (1974).

Rosenbaum, J.L.; Kramer, M.S. and Raja, R.: Resin haemoperfusion for acute drug intoxication, Archives of Internal Medicine 136: 263 (1976).

Royds, R.B. and Knight, A.H.: Tricyclic antidepressant poisoning. Practitioner 204: 282 (1970).

Schwartz, H.S.: Acute meprobamate poisoning with gastrotomy and removal of a drug-containing mass. New England Journal of Medicine 295: 1177 (1977).

Shubin, H. and Weil, M.H.: Shock associated with barbiturate intoxication; in Matthew (Ed) Acute Barbiturate Poisoning, p. 135 (Excerpta Medica, Amsterdam 1971).

Sidell, F.R.: Soman and Sarin: clinical manifestations and treatment of accidental poisoning by organophosphates Clinical Toxicology 7: 1 (1974).

Sjoqvist, F.; Berglund, F.; Borga, O.; Hammer, W.; Andersson, S. and Thorstrand, C.: The pH-dependent excretion of monomethylated tricyclic antidepressants in dog and man. Clinical Pharmacology and Therapeutics 10: 826 (1969).

Smith, T.W.; Haber, E.; Yeatman, L. and Butler, V.P.: Reversal of advanced digoxin intoxication with Fab fragments of digoxin-specific antibodies. New England Journal of Medicine 294: 797 (1976).

Smith, L.L.; Wright, A.; Wyatt, I. and Rose, M.S.: Effective treatment for paraquat poisoning in rats and its relevance to treatment of paraquat poisoning in man. British Medical Journal 4: 569 (1974).

Stein, R.S.; Jenkins, D. and Korns, M.E.: Death after use of cupric sulfate as emetic. Journal of the American Medical Association 235: 801 (1976).

Tobis, J. and Das, .B.N.: Cardiac complications in amitriptyline poisoning — Successful treatment with physostigmine. Journal of the American Medical Association 235: 1474 (1976).

Trafford, J.A.P.; Jones, R.H.; Evans, R.; Sharp, P.; Sharpstone, P. and Cook, J.: Haemoperfusion with R-004 amberlite resin for treating acute poisoning. British Medical Journal 2: 1453 (1977).

Vale, J.A.; Rees, A.J.; Widdop, B. and Goulding, R.: Use of charcoal haemoperfusion in the management of severely poisoned patients. British Medical Journal 1: 5 (1975).

Waddell, W.J. and Butler, T.C.: The distribution and excretion of phenobarbital. Journal of Clinical Investigation 36: 1217 (1957).

Welch, L.T.; Bower, J.D.; Ott, C.E. and Hume, A.S.: Oil dialysis for ethchlorvynol intoxication. Clinical Pharmacology and Therapeutics 13: 745 (1972).

Westein, W.F.: Deferoxamine in the treatment of acute iron poisoning. Clinical Paediatrics 5: 531 (1966).

Whittington, R.M.: Dextropropoxyphene (Distalgesic) overdosage in the West Midlands. British Medical Journal 2: 172 (1977).

Winchester, J.F.; Gelfand, M.C.; Knepshield, J.H. and Schreiner, G.E.: Dialysis and hemoperfusion of poisons and drugs. Transactions of the American Society for Artificial Internal Organs 23: 762 (1977).

Winek, C.L.: Tabulation of therapeutic, toxic, and lethal concentrations of drugs and chemicals in blood. Clinical Chemistry 22: 832 (1976).

Woie, L. and Oyri, A.: Quinidine intoxication treated with hemodialysis. Acta medica scandinavica 195: 237 (1974).

Woo, P.; Hatfield, A.; Green, J.R. and Hamilton, S.M.: Whole-gut perfusion for therapeutic purgation. British Medical Journal 1: 433 (1976).

Yaffe, S.J.; Sjoqvist, F. and Alvan, G.: Pharmacological principles in the management of accidental poisoning. Pediatric Clinics of North America 17: 495 (1970).

Chapter X
Drugs in Anaesthetic Practice

J.W. Dundee and W. McCaughey

Synopsis of Important Principles

1) The main aim of anaesthesia is the prevention of pain during surgery and at other times.

2) Anaesthesia involves a balanced approach, in which the individual patient's psyche and pathophysiology are taken into account and drugs are used to modify and control any aspect as required.

3) The decision to use a particular drug or technique must be made after careful consideration of the pathophysiological features of the individual case and how these may affect the pharmacokinetic handling and tissue response to the drugs available.

4) Any associated disease or pathophysiological abnormality should wherever possible be treated or corrected before operation, and potentially dangerous physiological disturbances avoided during and after anaesthesia.

5) Anaesthetic drugs are relatively non-toxic but there are some important effects. Halothane is occasionally associated with hepatitis and methoxyflurane with kidney damage. Malignant hyperpyrexia, the aetiology of which is uncertain, is a rare but often fatal condition which can be triggered off by several anaesthetic drugs in genetically susceptible individuals.

6) Drugs used in anaesthesia can be involved in significant unwanted interactions with other drugs.

7) The treatment of respiratory failure is usually the responsibility of the anaesthetist. Although ventilatory assistance, physiotherapy etc are often the mainstay of treatment, drugs of different pharmacological classes are used.

8) Pain perception is an individual sensation. Symptomatic treatment of acute pain should not therefore be based on a concept of the painfulness of certain conditions, although some analgesics may be more appropriate for pain of certain conditions.

9) Strong analgesics for severe chronic pain preferably should be given orally, in adequate dosage and on a regular individualised dosage schedule.

Although achieving insensibility to pain and to unpleasant surroundings has been the goal of much human activity since prehistoric times, it is only since 1846 with the introduction of ether by Morton that this could be done with any reliable chance of success. Anaesthesia has developed and been refined considerably since that time, and several important milestones are recognised and worthy of recall. These include the discovery of the local anaesthetic action of cocaine by Koller in 1884 and its use to produce spinal anaesthesia by Bier in 1898, the perfection of endotracheal anaesthesia by Magill and Rowbotham about 1920, the introduction of the first barbiturate for induction of anaesthesia in 1932, and the introduction of curare in 1942.

1. General Considerations

Of recent years the specialty of anaesthesia has been broadened, and its scope is well described in a recent definition for the US Department of Labor (Dripps, 1966).

'Anesthesiology is a practice of medicine dealing with:

1) The management of procedures for rendering a patient insensible to pain during surgical procedures.
2) The support of life functions under the stress of anesthetic and surgical manipulations.
3) The clinical management of the patient unconscious from whatever cause.
4) The management of problems in pain relief.
5) The management of problems in cardiac and respiratory resuscitation.
6) The application of specific methods of inhalational therapy.
7) The clinical management of various fluid electrolyte and metabolic disturbances.'

The modern concept is one of 'balanced anaesthesia', in which the whole of the patient's psyche and pathophysiology are taken into account and drugs are used to modify and control any aspect as required. Thus, as well as general anaesthetic agents, drugs of many classes — tranquillisers, analgesics, muscle relaxants, drugs affecting the autonomic system etc — all fall within the sphere of interest of the anaesthetist. Some of the more important of these will be discussed in the following sections.

2. Drugs Used in Anaesthesia

2.1 General Anaesthetic Agents

The mechanism by which anaesthetic drugs produce unconsciousness is still unknown. Meyer in 1899 and Overton in 1901 noted that within any group of drugs, anaesthetic potency correlates well with lipid solubility, and most modern theories agree that the site of action is probably the lipid bilayer of nerve-cell membranes, or possibly a protein receptor in this situation, but further knowledge is limited.

2.1.1 Inhalational Agents

Anaesthetic practice is unique in that a high proportion of the drugs are administered by the inhalational route. Such agents must either be gaseous, or the vapour of volatile liquids (Various Authors, 1965).

Of the original three inhalational agents — nitrous oxide, ether and chloroform — the first two are still used widely. The greatest disadvantage of many of the volatile liquids and gases has been their flammable nature; the main reason for the decline of cyclopropane, which enjoyed wide popularity until the advent of halothane in 1956. Halothane, now firmly established as the basis of many general anaesthetic techniques, is not without its drawbacks, and investigation of new compounds continues. However methoxyflurane, which does avoid some of the problems associated with halothane, is overall no more safe, and the more recently discovered isoflurane and enflurane do not at present seem likely to replace halothane.

Disposition and Pharmacological Properties: The uptake and distribution of inhalational anaesthetics is complex (Eger, 1974). One must distinguish between an effective gas tension (partial pressure) and the total amount of drug dissolved in blood; it is the tension which determines the depth of anaesthesia. When a constant concentration of the anaesthetic is inhaled, the concentration in the alveoli rises gradually toward the inhaled level. How quickly it rises will depend on the ventilation of the alveoli (which may be reduced if the drug is irritant or depresses respiration) and on the rate at which the drug is taken up into the blood from the alveoli. If the solubility (blood/gas solubility coefficient) of the drug is high, then it will take longer for equilibrium to be attained, because (a) more of the drug needs to be dissolved in the blood

Table I. A summary of the major pharmacological properties of inhalational anaesthetics

Agent	Physical charac-teristics	Onset of action	Cardio-vascular effect[1]	Respiratory effect	Elimination	Notes[2]
Nitrous oxide	Non-volatile, non-flam-mable gas	Rapid	? Stable	Mild respiratory depression	Lungs	Weak anaesthetic unless supple-mented Good analgesic
Trichloro-ethylene	Non-volatile, flammable liquid	Slow	Bradycardia Sensitises myocardium to adrenaline	Tachypnoea	Lungs; hepatic metabolism and renal excretion	Good analgesic with limited clinical use
Diethyl ether	Volatile, flammable liquid	Slow	BP stable CO↑	Respiratory stimulation Tracheo-bronchial irritation	Lungs; hepatic metabolism and renal excretion (minor)	Analgesic in subanaesthetic concentrations
Halothane	Volatile, non-flam-mable liquid	Rapid	BP↓ Bradycardia CO↓ (minor) Sensitises myocardium to adrenaline	Respiratory depression	Lungs; hepatic metabolism (wide interindividual variation) and renal excretion of potentially toxic metabolites	? Hepatitis Increases intra-cranial pressure Inhibits uterine contractility
Methoxy-flurane	Volatile, non-flam-mable liquid	Slow	BP↓ CO↓ (minor)	Respiratory depression	Lungs; hepatic metabolism and renal excretion of nephrotoxic metabolite (fluoride ion)	High output renal failure Analgesic in low concentrations
Enflurane	Volatile, non-flam-mable liquid	Rapid	BP↓ Sensitises myocardium to adrenaline	Respiratory depression	Lungs, hepatic metabolism (biotrans-formation to fluoride ion much less than methoxyflurane)	Convulsions and other muscle movements
Isoflurane	Volatile, non-flam-mable liquid	Rapid	BP↓	Marked respiratory depression	Lungs; minimal biotrans-formation	

---

1   BP = blood pressure; CO = cardiac output.
2   See also table VII.

for a given tension to be reached, and (b) the more rapid removal of the drug from the alveoli reduces the concentration here, and therefore reduces the gradient driving it from alveolus to capillary blood. A less soluble drug will likewise reach equilibrium more rapidly. The rate of removal of drug into the blood will also depend on the cardiac output, which may be influenced by the drug itself; and finally the rate at which the tension of the drug in the blood rises toward that in alveoli will also depend on the rate at which it is distributed to other tissues, not only the target organ, brain; but also muscle, fat depots etc. Such differences between infants and adults helps to explain the more rapid alveolar uptake of inhalational anaesthetics in the neonate (Cook, 1976; Eger et al., 1971).

The ability of the drug in the blood to produce anaesthesia will depend on the anaesthetic potency of the drug. The minimal alveolar concentration (MAC) of the drug which will cause anaesthesia in 50% of patients is a measure often used to compare the potencies of different inhalational agents. Therefore, to produce most rapid induction and emergence from anaesthesia, an inhalational agent will have as many as possible of the following attributes: high potency, low solubility in blood, low solubility in fat depots, lack of irritant and respiratory depressant effects, lack of cardiac depressant effects, and in the case of a volatile liquid, a relatively low boiling point, so that adequate vapour pressure can be attained. Due to the time taken to reach equilibrium, anaesthesia is induced using a relatively high concentration of inhaled drug, and this is gradually reduced, at a rate depending on the above factors.

Inhalational anaesthetics which by definition enter the body through the lungs, were thought to leave unchanged by the same route, however, it is now known that appreciable proportions of all inhaled anaesthetics are metabolised in the body (Cohen, 1971; Cascorbi, 1973) — varying from a small amount in the case of nitrous oxide to over 40% of the amount inhaled of methoxyflurane (Mazze and Hitt, 1976), and that there is an association between the biotransformation of inhalational anaesthetics and the development of toxicity (see section 5; for review, see Cohen, 1978). The rate of metabolism of an inhaled anaesthetic may be influenced by the concentration being inhaled. Thus, high concentrations of halothane inhibit its own biotransformation, while in trace concentrations halothane is extensively metabolised (Sawyer et al., 1971; see also

section 5.2). Inhaled anaesthetics can inhibit the rate of metabolism of other drugs in a dose dependent manner (Cohen, 1971).

Nitrous oxide: All inhalational anaesthetic methods involve the use of a gas containing oxygen and an anaesthetic agent. It is common practice for this carrier gas to contain 50 to 75% nitrous oxide which may be the main anaesthetic, but more often it is supplemented by a more powerful volatile or intravenous agent. Nitrous oxide itself is a weak anaesthetic and in the absence of hypoxia, it will not produce anaesthesia in all persons. It is analgesic in subanaesthetic concentrations and this is useful in obstetric practice, where a 50% mixture with oxygen is commonly used (see section 8.3.2). As it is relatively insoluble in blood and tissues, its action is rapid and recovery time short; the rapidity of action is helped by its being non-irritant and almost without smell.

Ether: Diethyl ether is still used, especially in developing countries where its low cost is an important factor. It is a volatile liquid, flammable in air but explosive in oxygen. It is a potent anaesthetic, but is irritant to the tracheobronchial tree and is relatively unpleasant to inhale. As it is quite soluble in blood and in tissues, the concentration in the blood builds up only slowly, and induction of anaesthesia is slow, as is recovery. Diethyl ether is a comparatively safe drug to use, as it is less depressant to the heart and cardiovascular system than halothane, and in overdosage respiratory depression will become apparent before there is dangerous depression of the circulation. Clinically, it is used in concentrations of 10 to 20 volumes per cent. Despite its good features, its properties of flammability and slowness of action have led to a lessening in popularity.

Halothane, introduced in 1956, was the first important member of the new generation of halogenated anaesthetic compounds arising from the new chemical technology of fluorine which was developed during World War II for the purification of uranium. Halothane is a volatile liquid with the fairly low boiling point of 50.2°C and has a sweet and not unpleasant smell. It is also a powerful anaesthetic agent. Because of this and its non-flammability, it rapidly became the most popular general anaesthetic agent in use. It is pleasant to use, rapid in action, its side effects are few, and recovery is rapid and not accompanied by much nausea.

Its effects on the cardiovascular system are important and because of these it must be given in carefully controlled concentrations. It depresses smooth muscle and causes dilatation of blood vessels, with a consequent fall in peripheral vascular resistance and fall in blood pressure, which is also augmented by some depression of cardiac output. Halothane (and many other halogenated anaesthetics) sensitises the myocardium to the effects of catecholamines, so that if adrenaline (epinephrine) is injected, or if the body secretes excess adrenaline in response to a raised carbon dioxide level, there is an increased likelihood of cardiac arrhythmias, which can occasionally be dangerous (Katz and Epstein, 1968).

'Halothane hepatitis' is a diagnosis which has been widely misapplied in recent years. Jaundice, hepatitis or occasionally fulminant liver failure may follow surgery and anaesthesia with halothane — or with another anaesthetic technique. Halothane does not consistently or commonly cause clinically apparent liver damage. However, liver damage detectable by electron microscopy can be demonstrated following prolonged exposure in animals (Stevens et al., 1975). Some feel that halothane hepatitis should be regarded as a clinical entity (Sherlock, 1978), while others are not yet satisfied that there is clear cut evidence of a direct relationship between halothane and postoperative hepatitis (Simpson et al., 1975; Strunin, 1976; Johnstone, 1978). There is no way at present in which hepatitis following halothane anaesthesia can be positively identified as being due to halothane, and suspicion (the clinical features resemble severe viral hepatitis), must rest on the inability to find an alternative explanation for the occurrence of jaundice. The results of most early studies are invalid because they were based on intrinsically biased reporting of cases, while the National Halothane Study in the USA showed halothane to have a record of safety as compared with other techniques (Committee, 1966).

If halothane is not directly hepatotoxic, there are two main theories as to why halothane might cause liver damage; its biotransformation being central to each: (a) a hypersensitivity phenomenon, possibly manifesting itself on a second exposure, due to formation of metabolites, which when complexed to proteins, act as haptens; or (b) formation of reactive intermediates or an accumulation of toxic metabolites (see Cohen, 1978).

There is an increased incidence of jaundice following multiple exposure to halothane anaesthesia, especially within 28 days (Inman and Mushin, 1974; 1978) and a controlled prospective study of repeat halothane anaesthesia (Dundee et al., 1978) has shown that abnormal postoperative liver function tests occurred in a proportion of patients and that the incidence of abnormal liver function tests increased with each subsequent halothane anaesthetic, but not in the control enflurane series. However, the incidence of clinical jaundice is increased after repeated exposure to other anaesthetic methods (McEwan, 1976; McPeek and Gilbert, 1974), a fact which is widely ignored. The Medical Research Council (1976), in Britain, considers that 'there is insufficient evidence to indicate whether repeated exposure to halothane carries a greater overall risk than the substitution of other general anaesthesia after the first use of halothane; nor is there sufficient comparable information on the risks associated with repeated exposure to anaesthetics other than halothane. When the need arises for repeated anaesthesia within a short time, it clearly remains a matter for the clinical judgment of the anaesthetist to decide whether a further halothane or non-halothane anaesthetic is in the best overall interests of the patient.'

Certainly, halothane should not be used if unexplained jaundice or delayed fever has occurred following a previous exposure, although there is no contraindication to its use in patients with other forms of liver disease or those undergoing biliary tract surgery (Moult and Sherlock, 1975). Obesity may be a risk factor since halothane is stored in adipose tissue (see Sherlock, 1978). The incidence of jaundice following halothane is low — probably only occurring in about 1 in 6,000 to 20,000 exposures (Inman and Mushin, 1974). While it is a real risk, it should not be over dramatised.

Methoxyflurane was introduced a few years after halothane. It also is non-flammable, relatively easy to administer and pleasant to inhale. However, although quite potent, it has a high boiling point (104.6°C) and a high solubility in blood and fat — which makes induction of anaesthesia slow. Unlike halothane, it does not, to any significant extent, sensitise the heart to catecholamines, but it does depress blood pressure. There are some differences in the response of the peripheral blood vessels to methoxyflurane and halothane (Black, 1965), and there is generally slightly less blood loss during surgery under methoxyflurane anaesthesia, which has proved to be of some advantage in plastic surgery.

Methoxyflurane is analgesic when inhaled in low concentrations and this has led to its use in obstetrics and as an analgesic for burns dressings and similar procedures. For this purpose a special inhaler has been developed and a simple disposable inhaler (e.g. Analgizer) is also available.

A serious disadvantage of methoxyflurane is its ability to cause a high output renal failure in some patients. This is due to the nephrotoxic effect of inorganic fluoride ion to which a large proportion of absorbed methoxyflurane is metabolised (Mazze and Hitt, 1976), and may occur when the serum level of this metabolite reaches $50\mu M$. Peak levels are reached 48 hours after anaesthesia, and the level depends mainly on the dosage and duration of administration (Cousins and Mazze, 1973), and is lower in infants and children than adults (Stoelting and Peterson, 1975). Toxicity is more likely following prolonged anaesthesia with high concentrations of methoxyflurane, especially in obese patients (Young et al., 1975). Induction of metabolism, for example by barbiturate pretreatment, may also increase toxicity by increasing the production of inorganic fluoride (Cousins et al., 1974). Methoxyflurane should not be administered concurrently with other drugs with nephrotoxic potential (see table VII; chapter XXI; sect. 15) and it should be avoided in patients with renal disease, or in patients undergoing surgery with an added risk of renal complications, such as surgery of the abdominal aorta or renal vessels. With appreciation of the risks associated with excessive dosage, methoxyflurane anaesthesia can be safe, and authoritative opinion does not consider that it should be withdrawn on the present evidence (Committee on Anesthesia, 1971).

Enflurane and Isoflurane: These drugs are isomers. Like methoxyflurane, they are halogenated ethers. Both are potent inhalational anaesthetics, and in many ways similar in use to halothane (Various Authors, 1971a; Prys-Roberts, 1977). They were developed in the search for safer alternatives to halothane and other older drugs. Initially, they were thought to be minimally metabolised in the body, but this has proved not to be so, and enflurane, although much less metabolised to inorganic fluoride than methoxyflurane (Cousins et al., 1976), can cause renal damage if

kidney function is already depressed (Cohen, 1978). However, there is some evidence that it may be preferable to halothane for repeated anaesthesia (Dundee et al., 1978). Although isoflurane is metabolised only slightly and is overall the more promising drug, it is still undergoing investigation, while enflurane has been available for clinical use for some years. Despite this, there is still some cause for concern about enflurane (Prys-Roberts, 1977). Isoflurane is compatible with use of adrenaline (epinephrine) infiltration, but enflurane is not, although causing less dysrhythmias than halothane. Both drugs produce good muscle relaxation, so that reduced doses of muscle relaxants are required. Respiratory depression caused by isoflurane means that controlled ventilation is essential, while the main disadvantage of enflurane is the occasional occurrence of convulsive movements due to increased CNS excitability. Enflurane also causes some cardiovascular depression, and, in contrast to halothane, this depression is markedly enhanced by β-adrenoceptor blockade. At present, neither drug has been proved to represent a significant advance over halothane.

Inhalational Anaesthesia plus Narcotics: Light general anaesthesia with nitrous oxide supplemented by narcotic analgesics is becoming increasingly used, particularly since the advent of the short acting narcotics such as fentanyl and phenoperidine (see also section 2.3.1) and the availability of a more effective and safer narcotic antagonist, naloxone, to control ventilatory depression and postoperative sedation (see section 8.4.4).

2.1.2 Intravenous Anaesthetic Agents

The intravenous route is simple and pleasant for the patient. As the drugs enter the circulation directly, the effects are rapid in onset and can be readily controlled. Unlike inhalational agents, drugs given by this route depend mainly on hepatic mechanisms for their elimination, so inadvertent overdosage is less easily remedied and dosage may therefore need to be modified in the elderly, and in shocked and poor risk patients. Intravenous anaesthetic agents are widely used for the induction of anaesthesia, and as sole agents for short procedures, but for operations longer than a few minutes maintenance of anaesthesia is commonly continued by inhalational agents.

The barbiturates were introduced as intravenous anaesthetic agents in 1932, and remained

Table IIa. A summary of the major pharmacological properties of intravenous anaesthetics

Agent	Onset of action	Duration (single dose)	Recovery	Cardio-vascular effects[1]	Respiratory or other effects	Inactivation and elimination
Thiopentone	Rapid	Short	Short	BP↓ CO↓	Marked respiratory depression Laryngospasm Bronchospasm Increases intracranial pressure	Redistribution and slow hepatic metabolism
Metho-hexitone	Rapid	Short	Moderately rapid	BP↓ CO↓ Tachycardia	Respiratory depression Abnormal muscle movements Cough, hiccough	Redistribution and fairly rapid hepatic metabolism
Propanidid	Rapid	Brief	Very rapid	BP↓ (can be marked) CO↓ Tachycardia ?Quinidine-like effect (ECG)	Initial respiratory stimulation followed by respiratory depression	Redistribution (minor) and rapid metabolism by plasma pseudocholinesterase and hepatic microsomal cholinesterases (aliesterases)
Althesin (alfathesin)	Rapid	Short	Rapid	BP↓ CO↔ Tachycardia	Respiratory depression	Redistribution and hepatic metabolism (elimination may be prolonged in severe liver disease and in renal failure)
Etomidate	Rapid	Short	Moderately rapid	Minimal	Marked muscle movements. Pain on injection	Redistribution and hepatic metabolism
Diazepam	Slow	Long	Very slow		Mild respiratory depression Marked amnesia	Very slow hepatic metabolism; prolonged in the elderly and in liver disease (metabolites are active). Enterohepatic recirculation may occur (evidence contradictory). Halothane reduces plasma clearance of diazepam
Ketamine[2]	Slow	Short (longer than others)	Slow	BP↑ CO↑ Tachycardia	Transient respiratory depression Increases intra-cranial pressure Hallucinations, dreams on recovery (except children and elderly)	Redistribution and slow hepatic metabolism (some metabolites are active). Induces own metabolism. Diazepam inhibits metabolism of ketamine

1   See also table VII.
2   Can also be given intramuscularly to induce anaesthesia. See also section 2.3.2.

virtually unchallenged until within the past decade. Thiopentone remains the standard intravenous induction agent and methohexitone is also widely used, but several newer non-barbiturate drugs are now used (table IIa,b; see Dundee and Wyant, 1974; Dundee, 1979).

Pharmacokinetic Properties and Action: Intravenous anaesthetics comprise a variety of drugs that differ in chemical structure but share a suitable combination of physical properties that confer ready penetration of the blood-brain barrier. Lipid solubility is particularly important in this respect. Rapid entry into the brain is associated with rapid distribution and redistribution in the body for most of these drugs. They all readily cross the placenta to the fetus. Rate of elimination varies between the rapidly biotransformed drugs like propanidid and the slowly metabolised ones like thiopentone and diazepam and its major active metabolite desmethyldiazepam. The liver is the main site of biotransformation, with the exception of propanidid which is hydrolysed by plasma pseudocholinesterase and etomidate which is hydrolysed by esterases in the plasma and liver. Protein binding may also influence the elimination of some agents. Diazepam is highly protein bound and decreased binding in liver diseases is associated with delayed plasma clearance. Thiopentone is also relatively highly protein bound and decreased protein binding may in part explain the 'sensitivity' to thiopentone of patients with renal or liver disease. Biotransformation leads to the formation of active metabolites in the case of diazepam, ketamine and possibly with alfathesin (alphaxalone plus alphadione). Recovery of mental and psychomotor functions depends on redistribution and hepatic metabolism and takes longer than with the inhalation anaesthetics, except after propanidid, which is due to its rapid hydrolysis in plasma. Use of intravenous anaesthetics therefore needs to take into account the individual pharmacokinetic properties of the various agents (for review, see Ghoneim and Korttila, 1977; see also table IIa and appendix A).

Adverse Reactions: These may relate to induction complications; tissue irritation and damage (drug and solvent used for insoluble drugs), with for example pain on injection and venous complications; recovery complications; and hypersensitivity or idiosyncratic reactions, which can be caused by most of the drugs administered intra-venously during anaesthesia. Hypersensitivity reactions are being increasingly reported (see section 5.7). The precise mechanism of the hypersensitivity response with the individual agents remains to be clarified but may be due to direct pharmacological effects causing histamine release (thiopentone, methohexitone, althesin and propanidid cause an increase in plasma histamine concentration; etomidate does not appear to stimulate histamine release); immune-mediated type I anaphylactic reactions; or chemical activation of complement C3 leading to histamine release. Other amines and peptides may also be involved in many of these reactions. The principal adverse reactions of the individual intravenous anaesthetics are discussed below and summarised in table IIa,b (for review, see Whitwam, 1978; Watkins and Ward, 1978). Drug interactions are discussed in section 6.

Thiopentone and Methohexitone: These are rapid acting barbiturates. They cross the blood-brain barrier very rapidly, and induce sleep in one arm-to-brain circulation time. This time will vary between 8 to 10 seconds in patients with a hyperdynamic circulation, but can be up to 2 minutes in patients with cardiac disease or in shock. Acidosis favours penetration of the drug through the blood-brain barrier while alkalosis has the opposite effect. Acidosis will thus deepen a barbiturate anaesthetic, while alkalosis will lighten it; a metabolic alteration of pH having a greater effect on distribution of the drug than a respiratory change.

With average doses (around 4mg/kg thiopentone or 1.6mg/kg methohexitone) sleep will last for a few minutes, and the patient will re-awaken as the drug concentration falls due to redistribution to other parts of the body, particularly muscle and later fat depots in the case of thiopentone. In hypovolaemia, blood flow to muscle is reduced and the rate of loss of thiopentone to muscle will be decreased, leading to sustained high concentrations in the brain and heart and therefore marked cerebral and cardiac depression. Hepatic metabolism is not important in the immediate recovery from thiopentone, but contributes significantly to the more rapid initial recovery from methohexitone (Breimer, 1976). If sleep is maintained by giving incremental small doses of the drug, these will become progressively smaller as the sites of redistribution become saturated. As this method leads to slow recovery, it is more common to maintain anaesthesia by an inhalational agent.

Table IIb. Comparison of the principal characteristics of common induction agents

---

1. Barbiturates
   All water soluble, rapidly acting induction agents; delay in time to full recovery, which depends mainly on redistribution; isolated cases of hypersensitivity reactions.
   a) Thiobarbiturates (yellow solution)
      Thiopentone, thiamylal: Approximately equally potent (1.0); smooth induction; few complications; isolated cases of hypersensitivity reactions.
      Thiobutobarbitone: Potency approximately 0.7 to 0.8; smooth induction; few complications.
   b) Methylated barbiturates (clear solution)
      Hexobarbitone: Potency approximately 0.5; high incidence of muscle movement.
      Methohexitone: Potency 2 to 3; dose related incidence of muscle movement and respiratory upset; tachycardia; more rapid recovery than after thiopentone (due partly to rapid metabolism), minimal risk of damage after intravenous injection; occasional pain on injection.
      Enibomal: Potency approximately 1.0; long shelf life in commercially available solution; high incidence of muscle movement (dose related).

2. Eugenols
   Non-water soluble, rapidly acting induction agents, with quick recovery due to biotransformation.
   Propanidid: Potency approximately 1.0; usually smooth induction with normal doses; hypotension with high doses; hypersensitivity occurs.

3. Steroids
   Non-water soluble, rapidly acting induction agents, with moderately rapid recovery.
   Alfathesin (althesin): Mixture of two steroids (alphaxalone, alphadolone; also known as alphadione); small volume required; smooth induction, muscle movements with large doses; hypersensitivity occurs.

4. Imidazoles
   Etomidate: Water soluble, rapidly acting induction agent. High incidence of injection pain, muscle movement and venous thrombosis.

5. *Neurolept analgesia*
   State of analgesia and detachment produced by a mixture of an opiate and a neuroleptic (antipsychotic) drug, but can be used for full induction of anaesthesia; slow onset of effect; prolonged action; respiratory depression is main side effect; best used for basal narcosis.

6. *Diazepam*
   Slowly acting antianxiety agent which produces a high incidence of amnesia; can be used for full induction of anaesthesia; prolonged action; best employed as a basal sedative.

7. *Ketamine*
   Slowly acting agent with a quite different effect from that of conventional anaesthetics or 'tranquillisers'; stimulation of cardiovascular system; can be routinely given by both the intravenous and intramuscular routes; undesirable sequelae when used for minor procedures in the absence of depressant premedication; very useful when specifically indicated.

The barbiturates produce depression of the heart, cardiovascular reflexes and respiration. As they enter the body rapidly, these effects will often be more marked than with inhalational agents, particularly if the intravenous injection is rapid or if the circulatory state is already precarious.

Thiopentone should not be given extravenously, as it may cause local tissue death. Also, should it be given intra-arterially, thrombosis of the artery with distal gangrene often occurs. This is less likely with weaker solutions (2.5%) and with methohexitone. Should it occur immediate treatment is necessary.

Propanidid belongs to the eugenol group of drugs. It is not water soluble and is made up with a solubilising agent, 'Cremophor EL'. Like the barbiturates, it produces sleep in one arm-to-brain circulation time, but unlike the barbiturates, propanidid is very rapidly metabolised; initially, as a result of hydrolysis by plasma pseudocholinesterase and subsequently by hepatic microsomal cholinesterates (aliesterases). This has considerable advantages in situations such as dental and outpatient work, where the 'hangover' from barbiturates can be dangerous should the patient drive or drink alcohol soon after anaesthesia. The usual dosage is 5 to 10mg/kg. Duration of sleep is age dependent; indicating the need to reduce dosage of propanidid in older patients (Ghonheim and Kortilla, 1977).

As with the barbiturates, there is a depression of myocardial function and hypotension occurs. This is dose related and can be more profound than with the barbiturates, and although it is generally of short duration, the drug should be used with caution in poor risk subjects. Initially, it stimulates respiration which is followed by a short period of respiratory depression. Eugenols prolong the action of suxamethonium, another ester hydrolysed by plasma pseudocholinesterase, by about 50% (Clarke et al., 1964). Propanidid causes a slightly higher incidence of venous thrombosis at the injection site than barbiturates.

Steroids: It has been known for a long time that many steroids have some central effect, but until recently no acceptable anaesthetic drug has been developed from this nucleus, though hydroxydione did have a small use. Althesin (Alfathesin; CT 1341) is a mixture of two pregnanedione steroids, alphaxalone and alphadolone acetate, which virtually have no hormonal activity (Brogden et al., 1974). It is also made up with 'Cremophor EL' and shares with propanidid the advantage of rapid metabolism in the body, so that there is little 'hangover', but on the other hand, its action is not so brief as propanidid and thus a smoother course of anaesthesia can be achieved. There is some evidence which suggests the possibility of active metabolites and prolonged recovery time in patients with severe liver disease or renal failure (Ghonheim and Korttila, 1977). Depression of the respiratory and cardiovascular systems is rather less than after thiopentone. The usual dosage is 50 to 75μL/kg. Involuntary muscle movements are the most common unwanted effects, especially after higher doses or when hyoscine is used for premedication. Cardiovascular collapse may rarely occur, as after propanidid, probably as a hypersensitivity response (see above; section 5.7).

Etomidate: This rapidly acting non-barbiturate agent is approximately 12 times more potent (w/w) than thiopentone, the usual induction dose being 0.3mg/kg. It is rapidly broken down in the body, being mainly hydrolysed by esterases both in the liver and plasma (Heykants et al., 1975). Although soluble in water, the aqueous solution causes too high an incidence of pain on injection, and propylene glycol is used as solvent (Zacharias et al., 1978). All preparations are followed by an unacceptably high incidence of venous thrombosis. Induction is accompanied by spontaneous involuntary muscle movements, although opinions differ as to the frequency and significance of this (Dundee and Zacharias, 1979; Doenicke, 1974). It is claimed that etomidate causes a negligible incidence of cardiovascular depression; but its induction characteristics will have to be studied in detail before recommending its introduction into clinical practice.

Benzodiazepines: Diazepam can be used for induction of anaesthesia in doses of 0.2 to 0.8mg/kg. It does not cause anaesthesia in one arm-to-brain circulation time, taking 30 to 60 seconds. Recovery is also slow, with dizziness persisting for up to 24 hours. It also has a powerful amnesic effect even in patients who have not lost consciousness, so that when used in poor risk patients, as for example for cardioversion, dosage sufficient to cause sleep need not be given. This makes it a valuable adjuvant to local anaesthesia. The elderly are more sensitive to the CNS depressant effects of diazepam than the young; plasma concentrations and dosage being lower in the elderly than in younger patients to achieve the same degree of CNS depression (Reidenberg et al., 1978).

The pharmacokinetic properties of diazepam have been well studied and have important implications for its clinical use in anaesthetic practice (see Ghonheim and Korttila, 1977; Mandelli et al., 1978). Diazepam is highly bound to plasma albumin; the degree of binding varying between 96 to 98%. Binding is significantly decreased in patients with liver disease and plasma clearance is delayed, indicating a need to modify dosage. The elimination half-life in younger adults following intravenous administration ranges from about 24 to 48 hours, but is prolonged up to 90 hours in the elderly due to a larger initial distribution space and volume of distribution (but plasma clearance is not altered [Klotz et al., 1975]; for explanation see chapter I, sect. 2.1.3). N-Desmethyldiazepam, the major metabolite, accumulates in the plasma after repeated doses of diazepam because of its long plasma half-life of 51 to 120 hours, and can reach concentrations of up to 2 to 3 times those of the parent drug (Gamble et al., 1976). There is a consistent rise in plasma diazepam concentration 6 to

8 hours after administration, and this is accompanied by the subjective recurrence of drowsiness (Gamble et al., 1975). The mechanism of this 'second peak' effect is not clear; it may be due to enterohepatic recirculation of diazepam. Placental transfer of diazepam and its clinical implications is discussed in chapter III (sect. 3.10.1). It appears to preferentially accumulate in the fetus, with fetal:maternal concentrations of 1.3:1 (Gamble et al., 1977). Elimination of diazepam is slower in the premature infant and the mature infant at term than in older infants, children and adults and the nature of diazepam metabolites formed varies according to age (see chapter IV; sect. 2.3.1).

Flunitrazepam is about 10 to 20 times as potent as diazepam, with a slightly longer duration of action. It is variable in action but the clinical effects are similar to those of diazepam (Dundee et al., 1976). Otherwise the effect of the two drugs is very similar. Lorazepam is a much longer acting drug, with amnesia lasting up to 4 hours after a 4mg dose. It also has a much slower onset of action. The incidence of painless thrombosis is much less after flunitrazepam and lorazepam than after diazepam (Hegarty and Dundee, 1977).

2.2 Muscle Relaxants

2.2.1 Neuromuscular Blocking Agents

Muscle relaxation or paralysis results from an interruption in the pathways for nervous impulses between the nervous system and the muscle (fig. 1). Those drugs in use in anaesthetic practice act at the neuromuscular junction and are of two types — non-depolarising (competitive blocking) and depolarising relaxants (table III). Competitive blocking drugs like curare prevent acetylcholine from reaching the receptors on the end plate, and thus prevent depolarisation occurring. These can be antagonised by anticholinesterase drugs such as neostigmine which prevent breakdown of acetylcholine so that more of it is present to compete with the relaxant drug. The second type comprises the depolarising muscle relaxants, of which suxamethonium (succinylcholine) is the common example. These act by causing a prolonged depolarisation of the muscle end plate and are not antagonised by neostigmine (except in the complicated circumstance of a 'dual' block, where the type of myoneural block changes to a competitive type after large doses, over a long period of time,

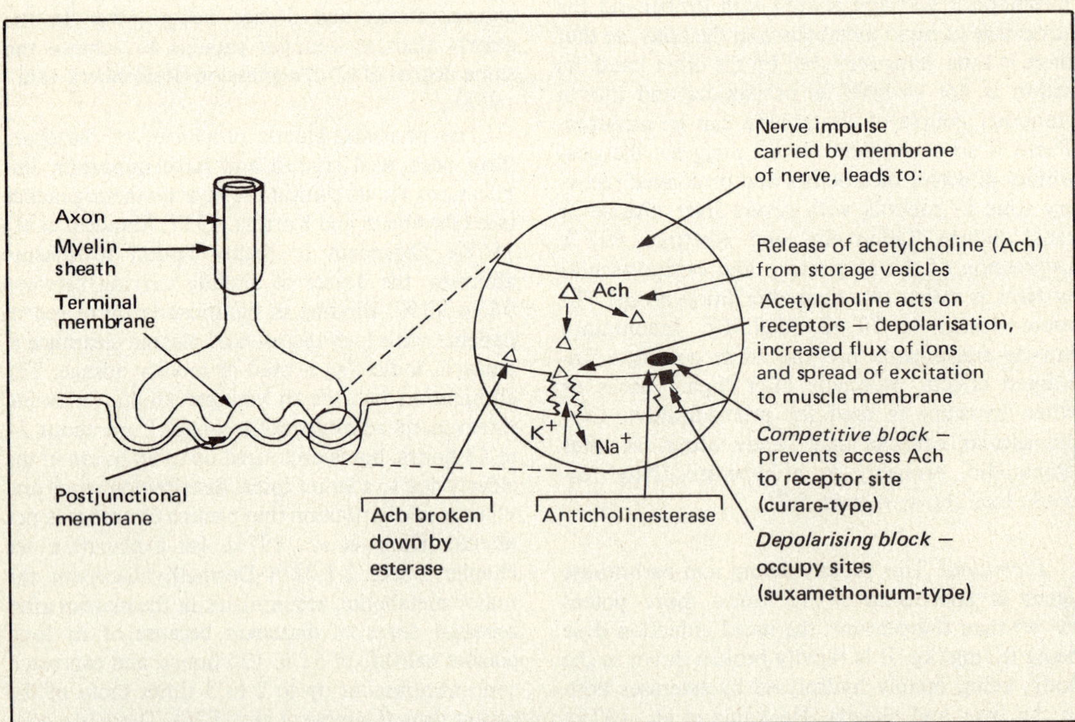

Fig. 1. Simplified anatomy and physiology of motor end-plate and action of neuromuscular blocking agents.

Table III. A summary of the major properties of muscle relaxants

Agent	Dose[1] (mg/60kg)	Duration of action	Cardio-vascular effects	Respiratory and other effects[2]	Hista-mine re-lease	Inactivation and elimination
Depolarising Suxa-methonium	60 to 100	Short	Bradycardia Arrhythmias	Increases serum K^+ Increases bronchial secretions Bronchospasm (rare) Increases intraocular pressure	Yes	Rapid hydrolysis and virtually complete metabolism by plasma cholinesterase (NB genetically deter-mined)
Non-depolarising Tubocurarine	15 to 30	Long	BP↓	Bronchospasm (rare)	Yes	Redistribution, hepatic metabolism and renal excretion of unchanged drug[3]
Gallamine	100 to 150	Medium	Tachycardia		Yes	Redistribution; renal excretion of unchanged drug (major importance)
Alcuronium	8 to 15	Long	BP↓	Bronchospasm (rare)	Yes	? Redistribution, hepatic metabolism and renal excretion of unchanged drug
Pancuronium	3 to 6	Long	BP↑ Chronotropic effect		Min-imal	Redistribution, hepatic metabolism and renal excretion of unchanged drug[3] (important with usual dosage)
Fazadinium	30 to 45	Long	BP↓ Tachycardia		Min-imal	Redistribution, renal excretion, some hepatic metabolism

1   Some workers using volatile agents which potentiate muscle relaxants may recommend lower doses of these.
2   See also table VII.
3   In renal failure, usual standard doses are possibly eliminated by biliary excretion, but large or repeated doses may lead to prolonged neuromuscular blockade.

or in an abnormal patient). For a review of the clinical types and pharmacology of neuromuscular blockade and factors which may alter neuromuscular function or normal responses to muscle relaxant drugs, see Ali and Savarese (1976).

Pharmacokinetic Properties: All these neuro-muscular blocking agents have 1 to 3 quaternary ammonium groups and are thus ionised and positively charged, irrespective of the pH, and are poorly lipid soluble. The muscle relaxants are usually administered intravenously. They are rapidly distributed by blood flow and diffusion into the extracellular fluids throughout the body. Because of the abundant blood supply of the neuromuscular junction, transfer of neuromuscular blockers from the plasma to the motor endplate is rapid and may take place in 7 to 12 seconds. Because of their physicochemical properties, they do not readily cross the lipoid intestinal wall, blood-brain barrier, cell membranes, or placenta. Changes in cardiac output or muscle blood flow can change the speed of onset of neuromuscular blockade. None of the muscle relaxants are metabolised at their site of action. The neuromuscular block with non-depolarising agents wears off because of biotransformation and excretion following redistribution into inactive sites with relatively less abundant blood supply than that of the neuromuscular junction. Only when the inactive sites of uptake have been saturated (e.g. after an excessive single dose or repeated fractional doses) will elimination processes become the rate determining factors for clearance of the drug and termination of the neuromuscular block (Foldes, 1972). This has important implications in the dosage and use of these agents in patients with poor renal function (see below). The neuromuscular block with suxamethonium is terminated by rediffusion into the plasma, where the drug is relatively rapidly hydrolysed by plasma cholinesterase. The clinically important pharmacokinetic properties of the individual agents are summarised in table III and discussed below (for review, see Wingard and Cook, 1977).

Adverse Reactions: As with intravenous anaesthetics (see section 2.1.2), hypersensitivity reactions to neuromuscular blocking agents are being increasingly reported; these reactions may be due to direct pharmacological effects causing histamine release or immune-mediated type I anaphylactic reactions (Clarke et al., 1977; Fisher, 1978; Fisher et al., 1978). Other important reactions are summarised in table III. A variety of drugs may modify, usually by enhancement, the neuromuscular blocking effects of the muscle relaxants (see section 6).

Clinical Application: Neuromuscular blocking drugs are used mainly as part of balanced anaesthesia, to produce profound muscular paralysis and so facilitate surgical procedures (see Foldes, 1966). Their use to block the reflex arc at the neuromuscular level will mean that less general anaesthesia is required, although ventilation of the lungs and endotracheal intubation will be nececessary. The depolarising drug, suxamethonium, is used to provide paralysis of short duration for intubation of the trachea, or for electroconvulsive therapy. Although it can be given intermittently or by infusion for longer procedures, it is usual to employ non-depolarising relaxants in these situations. Muscle relaxants are also used in intensive care treatment of tetanus (to control the convulsions) and in other situations such as crushed chest injuries and so on, which are being treated by artificial ventilation.

Tubocurarine, introduced in 1942, remains the standard by which others are assessed. It is the active principle of 'tube' curare, while from 'calabash' or 'gourd' curare, toxiferine is isolated. After a dose of 0.3 to 0.6mg/kg it causes a competitive neuromuscular block lasting for about 40 minutes. It also causes a fall in blood pressure, mainly due to a ganglion blocking action, although histamine release is also a contributory factor.

Tubocurarine is eliminated by hepatic metabolism and renal excretion of unchanged drug; about 40% of a dose being eliminated unchanged in the urine in 24 hours after injection in patients with normal renal function. In patients with impaired renal function, the duration of neuromuscular blockade is near normal following standard doses of tubocurarine, but can be markedly prolonged after large or repeated doses. Dosage should be halved for anephric patients (Ali and Savarese, 1976; Wingard and Cook, 1977). A newly transplanted kidney can eliminate tubocurarine effectively, but the rate of excretion is prolonged; an effect augmented by frusemide (Miller et al., 1976; 1977). Although it does cross the placenta in small amounts, tubocurarine can be used in obstetrics. Newborns are more sensitive than children and adults to tubocurarine (see section 3.1). A dose of 0.25mg/kg can be used in neonates at birth increasing to 0.5mg/kg at age 28 days, with reduction of dosage in the event of prematurity, acidosis or hypothermia (Bennett et al., 1976).

Gallamine, which is a synthetic drug, has the advantage of a shorter duration of action than tubocurarine, but because of an atropine-like action it causes tachycardia. Indirect evidence suggests that an appreciable fraction of a dose is excreted unchanged by the kidneys and prolongation of blockade follows use of gallamine in patients with renal failure. It is therefore contraindicated in renal disease of any severity.

Alcuronium (diallylnortoxiferine), was claimed to have a shorter duration of action than tubocurarine, to be more readily reversed by neostigmine, and to cause less fall in blood pressure. More extensive use has shown that any differences between alcuronium and tubocurarine are in fact very small.

Pancuronium (Speight and Avery, 1972) is unusual in that its structure includes a steroid nucleus. It is free from hormonal activity. The duration of action is similar to that of tubocurarine, although its onset is slightly more rapid and intubation with its aid is more easily accomplished. Pancuronium causes little histamine release (Bodman, 1978), and unlike tubocurarine its use is not followed by a fall in blood pressure — in fact it usually causes a slight rise. This is an advantage in many situations, such as in cardiac surgery, or in patients who are shocked or hypovolaemic. It does, however, consistently cause a variable degree of tachycardia.

As with tubocurarine, a large fraction of an injected dose is eliminated unchanged in the urine in patients with normal renal function; about 40% as unchanged drug and 10% as metabolites, the major mono-hydroxy metabolite possessing some muscle relaxant activity. A further 10% of the dose is eliminated through the bile. Prolongation of pancuronium blockade and delayed elimination has been reported in patients with renal failure following usual dosage (Miller et al., 1972; Somogyi et al., 1977). Accumulation is particularly likely after repeated doses in renal failure (Buzello and Agoston, 1978). Pancuronium is thought to be over 87% protein bound and reduction in binding in patients with poor renal function may contribute to its altered disposition in renal failure (Somogyi et al., 1977). Dosage should be reduced about 50% in anephric patients (Ali and Savarese, 1976). Patients with liver disease require a high initial dose for adequate muscle relaxation, but repeated doses should be conservative because of delayed elimination and risk of prolongation of pancuronium blockade (Duvaldestin et al., 1978a). Pancuronium does not appear to cross the placenta in appreciable amounts (Booth et al., 1977; Duvaldestin et al., 1978b). It appears that corticosteroids may cause a rapid termination of the action of pancuronium (Laflin, 1977).

Fazadinium, which has recently been introduced, has the advantage of a more rapid onset of action than other non-depolarising drugs, but with full doses, it may be more difficult to antagonise its action than that of tubocurarine (Hughes et al., 1976).

Suxamethonium (succinylcholine) is the most commonly used depolarising relaxant, producing paralysis lasting 2 to 4 minutes after a dose of 1 to 2mg/kg. As well as acting at the neuromuscular junction it also has an action on autonomic transmission, particularly a parasympathomimetic effect, so that salivation and slowing of the heart are seen if a drug such as atropine has not been given. The bradycardia is usually seen with a second dose of suxamethonium given within a few minutes of the first.

Suxamethonium is normally hydrolysed relatively rapidly by the enzyme plasma (pseudo) cholinesterase, but the action may be prolonged if the level of this enzyme is low — as occasionally occurs in malnutrition, uraemia and liver disease, following occupational exposure to anticholinesterase drugs such as the organophosphorus insecticides, other drugs (table VII), or if the cholinesterase is an abnormal genetic variant, which occurs as an hereditary condition (Kalow and Gunn, 1959; see also chapter VIII; sect. 4.2.1) and in such cases the dose of suxamethonium must be reduced by as much as a factor of 10 or more (Lee-Son et al., 1975).

On a mg/kg basis, less suxamethonium is required to obtain a desired degree of neuromuscular blockade as the age of the patient increases; with infants requiring more than children or adults. This may be due to changes in the relative volumes of extracellular fluid in the different age groups (see also section 3.1; chapter IV; sect. 2.2.1, 2.2.4). Although plasma cholinesterase levels of the neonate are about a half of those of the older child, recovery rates are comparable in infants and older children; this suggests that redistribution of suxamethonium from the neuromuscular junction in a limited muscle mass into a large extracellular fluid volume compensates well for the low plasma cholinesterase levels (Cook and Fischer, 1975). Little data are available on the placental transfer of suxamethonium in humans, but a dose of 1mg/kg during obstetric anaesthesia should not endanger the fetus, provided repeated doses are not needed or atypical plasma cholinesterase is not encountered.

When given to a patient there is transient muscle contraction, seen as fasciculations, before paralysis occurs. Some patients have muscular aches postoperatively, which may possibly be related to this. This is thought to be due to direct damage to the muscle during the period of fasciculation and it can be reduced by pretreatment with small doses of non-depolarising drugs, which will also minimise fasciculations (Bali et al., 1975). A rise in serum potassium levels may occur when suxamethonium is given (Gronert and Theye, 1975), but this is only important in burned and traumatised patients, in those with muscular disorders and in some with central nervous system lesions, where the rise in serum potassium can be quite large and lead to cardiac arrest (Mazze et al., 1969; Cooperman et al., 1970).

Because of its short duration of action, suxamethonium is often used for short procedures such as intubation of the trachea, but intermittent doses or administration by continuous infusion may be used for longer relaxation. In these situations, or in prolonged paralysis due to abnormal cholinesterase, the block produced by the suxamethonium may begin to change to a competitive type, becoming a 'dual block'.

2.2.2 Antagonists to Muscle Relaxants

Neostigmine is the most commonly used drug. It is an anticholinesterase which allows an accumulation of acetylcholine at the end plate to compete with the muscle relaxants. Atropine is given with neostigmine to prevent its parasympathomimetic effects (Rosner et al., 1971; Wilkins et al., 1970); the dose of neostigmine being 2.5 to 5mg. Neostigmine and its relative pyridostigmine are used in the treatment of myasthenia gravis (see chapter XXV; sect. 9).

Physostigmine, which crosses the blood-brain barrier, has been used to improve the level of consciousness and treat some tachydysrhythmias occurring after tricyclic antidepressant drug overdose (but see chapter IX; sect. 3.3, 6.1). It has also been claimed to be of use in arousing patients from postanaesthetic drowsiness following tranquillisers and antihistamines, but not anaesthetic drugs (Brebner and Hadley, 1976).

Germine Diacetate (GDA) is a new antagonist to muscle relaxants (Flacke et al., 1968). It is not an anticholinesterase, and although it increases the amount of acetylcholine produced at motor nerve terminals, its main action is postjunctional on the muscle fibres. It will antagonise not only non-depolarising relaxants but also the depolarising type, and even reverses the neuromuscular block caused by certain antibiotics (see section 6.2.5). GDA has also been used in treating myasthenia gravis.

2.3 Dissociative Anaesthesia

The 'triad of anaesthesia', hypnosis, analgesia and muscular relaxation, is generally achieved by a combination of drugs as outlined above. Recently some potent agents have been developed which dissociate' the patient from his surroundings, rather than produce sleep, and these form the basis of new techniques which are interesting, if somewhat limited in their application (Pender, 1971).

2.3.1 Neuroleptanalgesia

Neuroleptanalgesia, a term introduced in 1959 by de Castro and Mundeleer, describes a technique based on the use of the narcotic analgesics fentanyl and phenoperidine and the 'neuroleptic' drug droperidol (dehydrobenzperidol). With this technique the patient can be awake and cooperative and yet in a state of analgesia (see Morrison, 1974).

The technique is also claimed to provide an exceptionally stable cardiovascular system, a mild α-adrenoceptor blockade (to protect against shock) and good recovery. Droperidol, a butyrophenone derivative, causes a catatonia-like state where the patient is sedated and motionless. However, although at rest, frequently the patient is extremely agitated although unable to show this. Whereas a procedure such as bronchoscopy can be performed without apparent distress, the patient will often later state that it was extremely unpleasant. Droperidol can also produce extrapyramidal symptoms which are reduced by concomitant use of an opiate. It is a potent antiemetic.

Fentanyl is exceptionally potent; having about 100 times the analgesic activity of morphine, with a rapid onset of action and short peak effect (20 to 30 minutes). It has an elimination half-life of 1 to 4 hours, depending on dosage and may therefore accumulate in the body after large or multiple doses. Redistribution appears to be responsible for the short duration of action after standard dosage. Despite its brevity of action, there has been a report that the respiratory depressant effect may occasionally outlast the analgesia (Adams and Pybus, 1978). Droperidol has an elimination half-life of about 2 hours and accumulates in certain areas of the brain. Both fentanyl and droperidol are extensively metabolised in the liver (Ghonheim and Korttila, 1977).

More recently the combination of diazepam and pentazocine has become extremely popular (Aldrete et al., 1971). Diazepam when given intravenously causes a short period of anterograde amnesia, as well as drowsiness and tranquillisation. When combined with the analgesic effects of pentazocine many minor procedures such as reduction of simple fractures, or wound dressings can be carried out satisfactorily. Diazepam is used in a dose of approximately 0.1 to 0.3mg/kg, and pentazocine 0.5mg/kg. Pentazocine should be given sufficiently slowly that the dosage can be titrated so as not to cause significant respiratory depression. It must be realised by casualty department staff, however, that such a combination does depress the protective laryngeal reflexes, and that it should not be considered safer than general anaesthesia where the patient has a potentially full stomach, or in similar situations.

Often neuroleptanalgesia is converted to neuroleptanaesthesia by the addition of a nitrous oxide-oxygen inhalation.

2.3.2 Ketamine

Ketamine is a member of the cyclohexylamine group of drugs and is a successor to the earlier drug phencyclidine. Its actions are definitely different from other general anaesthetic agents and from tranquillisers such as diazepam or droperidol (Dundee and Wyant, 1974).

The site of action is claimed to be the midbrain, whereas barbiturates, for example, act on the reticular formation. Characteristically, it produces a state of complete analgesia with only superficial sleep, and with a tendency to keep the eyes open, some degree of nystagmus and often hypertonus of skeletal musculature. It can be given intravenously or intramuscularly.

Metabolism is important in the elimination of ketamine (Ghonheim and Korttila, 1977). Biotransformation to its active N-dealkyl metabolite is inhibited by diazepam, with a prolongation of half-life of ketamine and increased sleeping time. In rats halothane slows the uptake, distribution and redistribution (probably responsible for termination of action) of ketamine and the active dealkyl metabolite. The plasma clearance of ketamine is reduced in pregnant patients during delivery, which since ketamine readily crosses the placenta, may account for depression of the newborn after relatively large doses of ketamine to the mother. Also, there is little metabolism of ketamine in the newborn (Chang and Glazko, 1974). The relationship between plasma concentrations of ketamine and its metabolites and incidence of perceptual disturbances during recovery (see below) requires study.

Unlike other anaesthetic agents, ketamine has a cardiovascular stimulating effect (table II). This is associated with some degree of tachycardia and an increased cardiac output. It can be explained by a cocaine-like action of ketamine resulting in increased blood noradrenaline levels and sensitisation of the baroreceptors. Whether this makes it a good choice of induction agent in shocked patients is not known. It also increases cerebral blood flow with a resulting rise in intracranial pressure.

Recovery from ketamine is often complicated by delirium or excitement which can be minimised by intravenous diazepam shortly before the conclusion of anaesthesia. Alternatively, premedication with 3.5 to 4mg lorazepam, given 60 to 90 minutes preoperatively will reduce sequelae (Lilburn et al., 1978a). More troublesome are perceptual disturbances during recovery. Patients may have hallucinations and dreams, which may be pleasant or unpleasant, sometimes terrifying. These however, appear much less often in children and in the aged. Reflex activities, including maintenance of a good airway, are generally only slightly depressed by ketamine in comparison with other general anaesthetic drugs but this cannot be relied on, and both airway obstruction and aspiration of vomit can occur.

The place of ketamine in anaesthesia is being slowly defined. Certainly its side effects are too marked for it to become widely used as a routine anaesthetic. It is very useful for surgical procedures requiring multiple frequent anaesthetics, such as dressing of burns, especially in children. It would appear to be very suitable for mass casualties. Also it is a good choice in some procedures such as cardiac catheterisation, where it is an advantage for the patient to breathe air. Its use in obstetrics has been increasing, but the uncertainty of the competence of the laryngeal reflex is a danger in this context. It may be the drug of choice in the asthmatic patient. Ketamine infusions are being investigated as one possible answer to theatre pollution from volatile anaesthetics, and while they are very effective when given with neuromuscular blocking drugs, the possibility of the hepatotoxic effect of large doses of ketamine must be considered (Lilburn et al., 1978b).

2.4 Drugs Used in Premedication

Premedication was introduced in the 1860s to make easier the induction of anaesthesia by the methods then in use. Traditionally, a combination of morphine or another opiate with an atropine-like drug has been used, and until recently this combination undoubtedly did give the best results. The use of tranquillising and sedative drugs has become more common in the past 20 years. Since induction of anaesthesia is now simple and not unpleasant, the chief aim of premedication is to allay anxiety in the patient awaiting surgery (Mushin, 1960; Forrest et al., 1977), and the opiate drugs with their side effects of emesis and sometimes dysphoria are not ideal in this context. It is also worth noting that a preoperative visit from the anaesthetist has been shown to be as effective as an opiate or barbiturate! (Egbert et al., 1963).

2.4.1 Drugs Used as Preoperative Sedation

The opiates, pethidine (meperidine), morphine, diamorphine (heroin) and methadone, and other strong analgesics are still the most commonly used premedicants.

Barbiturates may be given by a variety of routes. They give sedation comparable with that from opiates, but postoperative restlessness is common, probably because they lack analgesic action or may be antianalgesic. Oral and intramuscular routes are used, and in infants, rectal thiopentone in a dose of 30 to 40mg/kg body weight is a useful basal sedative. Thiopentone has the disadvantage of occasionally causing excessive depression, so that a child must never be left alone after receiving this drug.

Tranquillisers: Phenothiazine drugs, which are widely used in psychiatry (see chapter XXVI; sect. 3), are disappointing as preoperative sedatives, as although quite good tranquillisation may be achieved, restlessness is common, and side effects such as Parkinsonian tremors, and hypotension may occur. Promethazine is the most frequently used phenothiazine and is usually given with pethidine, while trimeprazine syrup is popular for children.

Droperidol is also used and, like the phenothiazines, is generally disappointing as although patients are actually calm, they often inwardly feel extremely apprehensive (Morrison, 1970). However, this may not be so if it is given with pethidine (Tornetta, 1977), or with other opiates, when its antiemetic effect is useful.

Benzodiazepines: These include chlordiazepoxide, diazepam, nitrazepam, flurazepam, flunitrazepam and lorazepam. Diazepam is effective as a premedicant by oral, intramuscular and intravenous routes, but intramuscular injection is painful and reliable absorption depends on the site of intramuscular injection and injection technique (Assaf et al., 1975; Gamble et al., 1975). Orally it is effective at least as rapidly as when given intramuscularly; 10 to 20mg is commonly used in adults. When given intravenously the dose can be titrated, and for premedication will be in the range 2.5 to 10mg (0.04 to 0.16mg/kg). Dosage of diazepam is dependent on age (see sect. 2.1.2) and previous use of the drug (Giles et al., 1978). Side effects are few and it causes little respiratory depression (although depression by an opiate may be potentiated), nor is there nausea after its use. When given intravenously, diazepam has an intense but short lived amnesic action, which makes it useful, for example, as a sedation for cardioversion or conservative dentistry (Dundee et al., 1972).

Lorazepam is 4 to 5 times more potent than diazepam and is an effective tranquilliser with a slow onset and prolonged duration of action. It is particularly useful for night sedation prior to operation and in circumstances where accurate timing of preanaesthetic medication is difficult. Amnesia may persist for 6 hours after administration by any route (Dundee et al., 1979).

Flunitrazepam is very similar to diazepam in its actions as a premedicant, in its cardiovascular effects and in its ability to cause amnesia. Like diazepam it has been used as an induction agent, but it shows the variation in response and slight delay in onset which characterises the older drug (Dundee et al., 1976). Flunitrazepam is 10 to 20 times more potent than diazepam. One important difference between these three injectable benzodiazepines is the incidence and severity of venous thrombosis. This is greatest with diazepam, particularly in the elderly. Thromboses extending into the axilla have been found on the 7th to 10th day after injection. The incidence is much less with lorazepam and flunitrazepam is virtually free from this complication (Hegarty and Dundee 1977).

Miscellaneous Drugs: Many other sedative drugs have been used, such as hydroxyzine, methaqualone + diphenhydramine, meprobamate, chloral, methylpentynol and so on. Some of these are effective in some patients; in other cases the benefit may be marginal.

2.4.2 Antiparasympathetic Drugs

It is also common practice to give a drug to dry secretions and prevent overactivity of the parasympathetic nervous system which could lead to excessive bradycardia. Some feel that the former objective is seldom necessary with modern drugs (ketamine excepted), and that the latter objective is better achieved by administration of the drug as part of the anaesthetic technique than as a premedicant (see Mirakhur et al., 1978a).

Atropine blocks the action of acetylcholine at parasympathetic nerve endings. The main effects are drying of secretions and tachycardia. It is a mild cerebral stimulant. The adult dose is 0.6mg for most purposes, but at least 2mg are required for nearly complete vagal blockade. It is also used locally in the eye to produce cycloplegia (see chapter XII; sect. 9.6, 9.7).

Hyoscine differs from atropine chiefly in having a cerebral depressant effect, and it may cause confusion in the elderly. It is antiemetic to a greater extent than atropine. It has little effect on heart rate.

Glycopyrrolate (glycopyrronium) methobromide, a synthetic quaternary ammonium compound, shows promise as an anticholinergic agent (Oduro, 1975). It is twice as potent, on a mg per mg basis, as atropine, and has the advantage of being effective when given orally. Preliminary results suggest that it may be particularly effective in antagonising the muscarinic effects of neostigmine (Mirakhur et al., 1977; 1978b).

2.5 Local Anaesthetic Drugs

Sensory information, including pain, travels to the brain along nerves, the action potential being propagated by a local flow of sodium ions into, and potassium out of, the axon. Local anaesthetic drugs can cause a localised and reversible block to conduction by reducing the permeability of the membrane to sodium. The smaller the nerve fibre the more sensitive it will be, so that a differential block may occur, where for example autonomic and pain fibres may be blocked, leaving coarse touch and movement spared (see Covino, 1972; Various Authors, 1975). The clinical use of local anaesthetics depends upon knowledge of their clinical pharmacological properties and the physiological basis of neural blockade (Mather and Cousins, 1979).

Pharmacokinetic Properties: Unlike most drugs, local anaesthetics do not rely on the circulation to transport them to their sites of action on the nerve membrane or in the neural fluids, but uptake into the systemic circulation is important in terminating their action. The pharmacokinetic properties of local anaesthetics are therefore important determinants of their local and systemic effects. Other factors such as vascularity at the injection site, concentration to volume relationship of the dose used and rate of injection are also important determinants of the pattern of systemic absorption. Following most regional anaesthesia procedures, maximum arterial blood concentrations of anaesthetic develop within about 10 to 25 minutes, as typified by epidural administration (Tucker and Mather, 1975), and thus the most intensive surveillance of the patient should be during the first half hour after injection.

Local anaesthetics are weak bases, with pK_a's between 7.5 (mepivacaine) and 8.9 (procaine) so that significant changes in the ratio of ionised to unionised lipid soluble drug may occur with changes of acid-base balance; acidosis favouring ionisation and trapping of unbound drug (see chapter I; sect. 1.1). Local anaesthetics are bound to plasma and tissue proteins, the amide type more firmly than the ester type; plasma binding varying from 95% (bupivacaine) to 55% (prilocaine) and being lower at higher plasma concentrations (Tucker et al., 1970). Most of this binding is to α_1-acid glycoproteins. Differences in plasma protein binding contribute to the extent of placental transfer and concentration of unbound drug in the fetal blood; highly protein bound agents attaining a lower total drug concentration in fetal blood but a higher fraction being in the unbound (active) form (Scott, 1977; see also chapter III, sect. 4.1). Protein binding also influences the intensity and duration of effect; binding being more extensive for agents with greater anaesthetic potency and duration of effect (Tucker and Mather, 1975). Hepatic metabolism is important for elimination of local anaesthetics. Although the ester type agents are at least partially metabolised by plasma esterases (pseudocholinesterase), the amide type local anaesthetics are extensively metabolised in the liver (Boyes, 1975). Clearance of amide-type agents is critically dependent on hepatic blood flow

Table IV. A summary of the major properties of local anaesthetics (after Mather and Cousins, 1979)

Agent	Lipid solubility (at pH 7.4)	Plasma protein binding (%)	Equi-anaesthetic concentration (cocaine = 1)	Onset of action	Duration (single dose)	Principal uses	Primary site of metabolism
Amide type							
Bupivacaine	High	95	0.25	Slow	Long	Obstetric analgesia Postoperative pain	Liver
Cinchocaine	High	?	0.25	Rapid	Long	Spinal	Liver
Etidocaine	High	94	0.5	Rapid	Long	Surgical blocks requiring muscle relaxation	Liver
Lignocaine	Medium	64	1	Rapid	Medium	All block techniques Topical	Liver
Mepivacaine	Medium	78	1	Slower	Medium	All block techniques except topical	Liver
Prilocaine	Medium	55	1	Slower	Medium	IV regional Single dose nerve block	Liver
Ester type							
Amethocaine (tetracaine)	High	?	0.25	Slow	Long	Topical	Plasma
Cocaine	Medium	?	1	Slow	Medium	Topical	Liver
Procaine	Low	?	2	Slow	Short	Infiltration	Plasma

(Tucker and Mather, 1975), but because at any one time the liver has access to only a small fraction of drug in the body, the rate of plasma clearance is relatively slow. Thus, accumulation of amide anaesthetics and their active metabolites can occur when large doses are used frequently over a prolonged period (Moore et al., 1970) or when hepatic blood flow is reduced (e.g. cardiac failure; see chapter XVII, sect. 1.4). The physicochemical and pharmacokinetic properties of individual local anaesthetics are summarised in table IV and appendix A (for review, see Ralston and Shnider, 1978; Tucker and Mather, 1975, 1979).

Adverse Reactions: Hypersensitivity reactions are very rare and virtually limited to the ester type agents. Otherwise, the most important risk of local anaesthetics is a dose (plasma concentration) related CNS toxicity which progresses from drowsiness through to convulsions (de Jong, 1978). CNS toxicity can be minimised by careful attention to dosage and injection technique (Moore et al., 1977). Cardiac depression may occur with very high concentrations, and is more likely to be

a problem in obstetric use in the presence of fetal distress or likely acidosis (Ralston and Shnider, 1978; see section 8.3.3). Families susceptible to malignant hyperpyrexia (see section 5.6) should only receive ester type local anaesthetics since amide-type agents have been implicated in this serious reaction.

2.5.1 Cocaine

Cocaine was the first drug to be used as a local anaesthetic. As well as its local anaesthetic action, it is a vasoconstrictor. Its effects on the central nervous system are stimulatory, accounting for its abuse, and convulsions may occur. It is too toxic for general use but is still used as a topical anaesthetic in nose and throat surgery and ophthalmology (see chapter XII; sect 4).

2.5.2 Lignocaine (lidocaine)

Lignocaine is presently the most widely used local anaesthetic drug. It can be used in all the various sites for conduction block. Thus, an 0.5 % solution may be used for infiltration, with or without adrenaline (never with adrenaline in digits); 1

to 2% for nerve blocks, either individual nerves or plexus blocks; 15 to 50ml of a 1.5% solution is usual for epidural and caudal block; 0.5 to 2ml of a 5% solution for spinal blocks. For topical analgesia of the pharynx and larynx, 2% or 4% are used.

Lignocaine may also be given intravenously beyond a tourniquet to give anaesthesia of an arm, and also by infusion (up to 800mg/6 hours) to give pain relief in patients with crushed chests. As an antiarrhythmic drug for ventricular tachyarrhythmias it is used in 'coronary care' units (see chapter XVII; sect. 6.1.3).

As a local anaesthetic it has a rapid onset of action which lasts for 60 to 90 minutes. The toxic dose will vary with the route of administration and use of adrenaline, but in most situations the appropriate figure is 200mg. Like most local anaesthetic drugs, its action on the central nervous system is biphasic, causing stimulation followed by depression. Should convulsions occur, the essential part of treatment is to maintain oxygenation of the patient, control of convulsions being by use of thiopentone, or preferably suxamethonium. Its action on the cardiovascular system is depressant.

2.5.3 Procaine

Procaine, although dissimilar chemically, is similar to but shorter in its actions than lignocaine, which has largely displaced it. Use of procaine in large doses in the management of the malignant hyperpyrexia syndrome is controversial, while lignocaine is definitely contraindicated (see section 5.6).

2.5.4 Prilocaine

Prilocaine is similar in its properties to lignocaine, but slightly less toxic. Methaemoglobinaemia may however, occur after large doses (800mg).

2.5.5 Bupivacaine

This drug is both more toxic and more potent than lignocaine. Its advantage is a longer duration of action which may be from 4 to 5 hours after epidural block, up to 10 hours after specific nerve block. This longer duration of action combined with its minimal motor block and relative lack of effect on the fetus, makes bupivacaine particularly suitable for single dose epidural injection, where the duration of action of other local anaesthetic drugs is likely to be inadequate.

2.5.6 Etidocaine

Etidocaine, an acetanilide derivative, is a newer drug, which has a duration of action similar to that of bupivacaine. The time of onset is shorter with etidocaine, and the motor blockade produced may be more intense. A concentration of 0.5% is, like bupivacaine 0.25 to 0.5%, suitable for peripheral nerve blocks, while 1.0% etidocaine or 0.5% bupivacaine is suitable for epidural block (Lofstrom, 1975). The systemic toxicity of etidocaine is similar to, or slightly less than that of bupivacaine, and in particular it has been reported to give significantly lower fetal blood levels when used for epidural block in labour (Lund et al., 1977), although the analgesia which it produces is accompanied by marked motor blockade (Mather and Cousins, 1979).

2.5.7 Mepivacaine

Mepivacaine is similar in physiochemical and general properties to lignocaine. It has a slightly greater duration of action, but as it is more cumulative it may be less safe than lignocaine.

2.5.8 Adjuvants in Local Anaesthetics

The penetration of a local anaesthetic can be enhanced by increasing the concentration of the solution injected or by maintaining a high concentration around the nerve by means of a vasoconstrictor. Adrenaline, noradrenaline and felypressin are the vasoconstrictors which are chiefly used. They have the effect of: (a) reducing the toxic effects of the agent by retarding absorption of the drug; (b) confining the anaesthetic to a local area, hence increasing the depth and duration of anaesthesia, and (c) producing a relatively bloodless field for surgery. The effects of adrenaline vary with the agent used; for example, the action of lignocaine is markedly prolonged whereas that of prilocaine is less affected since its intrinsic vasodilator activity is not marked (Scott et al., 1972). Solutions containing vasoconstrictors must never be used in digits. Adrenaline containing solutions must not be used in conjunction with halothane or cyclopropane (these agents sensitise the myocardium to catecholamines), and except in skilled hands, are not normally recommended for use in patients with cardiovascular disease, poorly controlled diabetes, thyrotoxicosis or peripheral vascular disorders.

The onset of action of local anaesthetics can be hastened by use of carbonated solutions. Spread is also enhanced but toxicity is not increased (Bromage, 1965). Such solutions are not readily available.

2.6 Drugs Acting on the Sympathetic Nervous System

The autonomic nervous system, consisting of two divisions — sympathetic and parasympathetic — serves to control the automatic functions of the body. Most important is control of the cardiovascular system, but most other systems are also affected.

From controlling centres in the mid brain, autonomic nerve fibres leave the central nervous system, and synapse once before reaching their ultimate destination. In the case of the parasympathetic, the outflow is in cranial nerves and sacral nerve roots and synapses are near to or in the organs served, while sympathetic nerves leave the spinal cord in the thoracolumbar region and synapse mainly in the ganglia of the sympathetic chain. The transmitter substance in the intermediate synapses, at parasympathetic endings and a few sympathetic endings is acetylcholine, while at most sympathetic endings it is noradrenaline (norepinephrine).

From the point of view of cardiovascular function, the important action of the parasympathetic nervous system is vagal activity on the heart, causing slowing, an action which may be antagonised by atropine.

The sympathetic nervous system is the body's main mechanism for controlling cardiac output, blood pressure and distribution of blood flow. Drugs may act at the sympathetic ganglion or at nerve endings. At the most important site, noradrenaline (norepinephrine) released from the nerve ending acts on a receptor. There are variants of these, which react differently to particular drugs. α-Adrenoceptors include those causing vasoconstriction; β-adrenoceptors include those causing stimulation of heart rate and contractility (β_1) and bronchodilation (β_2) [see also chapter I; sect. 1.2.2 and chapter XVIII; sect. 5.6.2].

At ganglia, many drugs act to block conduction and thus cause vasodilatation and hypotension. In anaesthesia, agents which are used most commonly in hypotensive techniques to reduce surgical blood loss, include hexamethonium (10 to 40mg iv) and trimetaphan (0.1 % solution given by infusion) The newer agent sodium nitroprusside (0.002 to 0.01 % solution given by infusion) acts directly on blood vessels (see below).

At nerve endings and receptor sites drugs may stimulate or block sympathetic activity. Several which interfere with noradrenaline synthesis, storage or release (e.g. guanethidine, methyldopa) are used in general medicine to control hypertension (see chapter XVIII). 'Vasopressors' are drugs which raise blood pressure by causing vasoconstriction (α-adrenoceptor stimulation) and in some cases also stimulate the heart (β-adrenoceptor stimulation). As vasoconstriction raises blood pressure at the expense of tissue perfusion, their use in states of shock other than cardiogenic shock (see chapter XVII; section 5.4) has fallen into disfavour, although the more recent introduction of drugs such as dopamine, which spares the renal circulation has led to some renewal of their use (Goldberg, 1972). Other drugs in this class include adrenaline and noradrenaline, metaraminol, methoxamine and many others.

Isoprenaline, which stimulates β-adrenoceptors, may be used for its chronotropic and inotropic action on the heart, where the intravenous dose is around 10 to 20µg; and as a bronchodilator where administration by inhalation is common. Newer drugs such as salbutamol and terbutaline which are more commonly used for the latter purpose, have a more selective action on the β_2-adrenoreceptors of the bronchi (see chapter XX; sect. 2.3.1).

β-Adrenoceptor blocking drugs such as propranolol (1 to 5mg IV dose) have many applications, particularly in controlling tachycardia and extrasystoles. Propranolol may cause hypotension (and is indeed used to treat hypertension; see chapter XVIII) or bronchospasm. These are less common with practolol which is more specific for β_1-receptors. Practolol is still available for parenteral use in some of those countries where it had been introduced. Because of a number of immunological and other side effects in long term treatment, its oral use has been abandoned.

Blockade of α-adrenoceptors causes vasodilatation and hypotension. Such blocking drugs may be used in the treatment of established shock states, to improve blood flow to the tissues (after adequate transfusion). They are also used in the diagnosis and treatment of phaeochromocytoma.

Labetalol, is a new drug with α and β-adrenoceptor blocking properties. While its main use is in treatment of hypertension, it has a use in inducing controlled hypotension during anaesthesia. Doses in the region of 25mg will augment the hypotensive action of halothane.

Table V. Alteration in drug response in paediatric anaesthetic practice (after Brown, 1973; Cook, 1976; Wingard and Cook, 1977)

Class	Drug	Dose response compared with adults[1]
General anaesthetics	Halothane	Neonates and children require 30 to 50% higher concentration for a given surgical stimulus (increased alveolar uptake and requirement of halothane)
	Thiopentone	Avoid as induction agent in neonates (?increased brain uptake; ?change in distribution due to decrease in serum albumin in neonates)
	Ketamine	Larger dose/kg in infants to prevent gross movements, but increased risk of respiratory depression
Muscle relaxants	Suxamethonium	Larger dose/kg in neonates (?change in distribution due to larger volume of ECF); dose on surface area basis unchanged
	Tubocurarine	Reduced dose/kg (where response is depression of respiratory function) and reduced dose on surface area but not per kg basis (where response measured directly) in neonates and infants under 3 months Larger dose however, in children with severe burns or cyanotic congenital heart disease
Adjuvants	Adrenaline Atropine Neostigmine	Relatively larger doses in neonate
Narcotic analgesics	Morphine	Generally avoid in neonate. Reduced dose in infants 6 to 12 months (increased brain penetration; ?decreased rate of metabolism)

1   In general, a smaller dose than that estimated on body size alone is required with most drugs used in neonates (see chapter IV; sect. 2).

Sodium nitroprusside acts directly on blood vessels to dilate them, and thus causes hypotension, and is a useful drug in hypotensive anaesthesia and in treatment of hypertensive crises (Tinker and Michenfelder, 1976; Cole, 1978). It is given by infusion, and its dose titrated according to the effects achieved, usually starting with 0.5 to 5µg/kg/minute. Close monitoring of arterial pressure is mandatory. Toxic effects (metabolic acidosis) may occur due to an excessive rate of infusion or accumulation of cyanide if large amounts are given; a maximum total dose of 3mg/kg (some recommend 1.5mg/kg maximum) should not be exceeded or 0.5mg/kg during short term infusions. Concomitant use of hydroxocobalamin may prevent toxicity due to cyanide release (Cottrell et al., 1978b). Sodium nitroprusside has a more rapid onset and more controllable action than other means of deliberately lowering blood pressure. In contrast to trimetaphan, tachyphylaxis is not a major problem with it (Cottrell et al., 1978a).

2.7 Antiemetic Drugs

Vomiting in anaesthesia is usually due to pre- or postoperative use of narcotic analgesics. Nausea and vomiting can occur before induction of anaesthesia with rapidly acting drugs such as pethidine, but are reduced by atropine or hyoscine premedication. Routine preoperative use of antiemetics is not justified. Occasionally antiemetics are used postoperatively if vomiting occurs after narcotic analgesics or anaesthetic agents, but mechanical or surgical causes must first be excluded. Cyclizine (50mg), a phenothiazine such as prochlorperazine (10mg) or perphenazine (5mg) can be used (see chapter XIX; sect. 5.2); they inhibit vomiting without aggravating the ileus which may accompany abdominal operations. Repeated administration of antiemetics is necessary after surgery on the middle ear due to the very high incidence of vomiting and dizziness.

3. Anaesthesia in Clinical Practice

The practice of anaesthesia is an exercise in applied physiology, clinical pharmacology and medicine. The decision to use a regional or general anaesthetic technique, to induce sleep by inhalational or intravenous drugs, to use or not to use muscle relaxants, to intubate the trachea or not — all must be decided not only after consideration of the pathophysiological features of the individual case, but also how these features may affect the pharmacokinetic handling (uptake/absorption, distribution, metabolism, excretion) and dosage of the individual drugs available (e.g. see tables V, VI, VII). Alteration of the pharmacokinetics of drugs may also occur following surgery, particularly in the early postoperative period (Elfstrom, 1979). Some specific points in particular situations are mentioned below.

3.1 Paediatric Anaesthesia

In anaesthesia, children over the age of 2 may be regarded almost as small adults. The main specialist problems lie with younger children, and in particular with neonates (for review, see Cook, 1976; Overton, 1976). Paediatric anaesthesia presents problems due mainly to the small size of the patient, whose anatomy is slightly different, whose small airways are easily obstructed and may be excessively narrowed by intubation, and whose large surface area to volume ratio and inefficient temperature control lead easily to the development of hypothermia. Assisted ventilation is required in any long procedure in small infants, as they tire easily; the inspired gases must be humified. Blood and fluid balance therapy are more critical than in the adult.

The young infant also differs from the adult in his quantitative responses to many anaesthetic drugs and adjuncts. In the neonate, the larger extracellular fluid volume and blood volume, the smaller muscle mass and fat stores, and presumable greater blood flow to the central organs, not only influence the distribution of drugs to their ac-

Table VI. Alteration in drug response in anaesthetic practice in the elderly (after Evans, 1973)

Class	Drug	Response compared with younger patient[1]
General anaesthetics	Inhalational agents	Reduced dose (more profound effects due to aging process in CNS tissue; increased risk of hypotension)
	Intravenous agents	Reduced dose of thiopentone (changed distribution due to decrease in serum albumin and total body water in elderly) and slower rate of injection (slower circulation time) recommended
Muscle relaxants	Gallamine Suxamethonium Tubocurarine Pancuronium	Reduced dose (decreased renal excretion — gallamine; ?pancuronium; degenerative changes in neuromuscular function)
	Suxamethonium	Onset of maximum block for endotracheal intubation delayed (slower circulation time)
Adjuvants	Atropine	Premedication for salivary effects may be unnecessary (atrophy of salivary gland)
	Phenothiazines	Reduced dose (increased risk of hypotension)
	Diazepam	Reduced dose (altered distribution and apparent increased sensitivity)
Narcotic analgesics	Morphine etc Pentazocine	Reduced dose (? decreased rate of metabolism; elderly report greater pain relief from standard dose)

1   In general, a reduced dose is required with drugs used in the elderly (see chapter V; sect. 2). In anaesthetic practice, dosage reductions will usually be considerable.

tive site but also secondary redistribution away from their site of action. There may also be differences in uptake and penetration of the blood-brain barrier in infants for some anaesthetics. Some, but not all, mechanisms for the elimination of drugs are immature in the neonate, but this has led to the generalised belief that most, if not all, therapeutic agents are more toxic to the newborn than the adult. However, this is not uniformly true (Mirkin, 1975). Some biotransformation pathways can be reasonably well developed in the neonate but glomerular filtration, important for excretion of some drugs, is inefficient compared with older children and adults (see chapter IV; sect. 2).

Thiopentone and other barbiturate induction agents are usually avoided, because (based on animal studies) there is an increased 'sensitivity' and prolonged sleeping time. However, redistribution of thiopentone is as important as metabolism in reducing brain concentration and plasma levels of thiopentone decrease about as rapidly in newborns as in their mothers, allowing safe use of doses in the order of 4 to 7mg/kg (Kosaka et al., 1969). The respiratory depressant effect of morphine is increased markedly and it should be avoided; this increase in toxicity may be largely due to increased penetration into the brain, or to increased sensitivity of opiate receptors in the brain. The sensitivity to pethidine (meperidine) may not be increased to the same extent (Way et al., 1965), possibly because brain uptake in infants seems to be about the same as in adults. The response to muscle relaxant drugs differs in the neonate (Walts and Dillon, 1969). There is a relative insensitivity of the neonate to depolarising agents such as suxamethonium when dosage is based on weight (which decreases as the age of the subject increases; Cook and Fischer, 1975), but because of the relatively larger surface area in relation to body weight of the infant, the response is the same in infants as in adults when dosage is based on body surface area (Walts and Dillon, 1969). The differences in dosage on a weight basis may be due in large part to altered distribution (section 2.2.1). When the response of muscle to non-depolarising agents like tubocurarine is measured directly, infants are not more sensitive than adults when dosage is based on body weight (Goudsouzian et al., 1975; Walts and Dillon, 1969), but if surface area is used in calculating dose, the neonate is more sensitive to non-depolarising agents. Where the criterion is the clinical one of depression of respiratory function however, there is a marked increase in the sensitivity of the neonate and very young infant, even when doses are calculated on a weight basis. This is probably due to the fact that the respiratory system of the newborn has little reserve. In practice, therefore, muscle relaxants should be used with caution.

Anaesthesia of the newborn and young infant is thus generally induced by inhalation. Relatively high concentrations of inhalational agent are likely to be required, due to more rapid alveolar uptake and increased anaesthetic requirement in infants and children. Analgesic drugs are used only with extreme caution, or not at all, and muscle relaxant drugs as noted above (see Cook, 1976; Wingard and Cook, 1977).

3.2 Anaesthesia in the Elderly

Anaesthesia in the elderly presents few problems specifically due to age (see Evans, 1973). Those which do arise are due to the increased incidence of associated disease in old age. Patients are also likely to be receiving a number of drugs for this disease, and side effects may be associated with these, particularly with digoxin, tranquillisers and antihypertensive agents. The respiratory and cardiovascular systems have less reserve, so that hypoxia will occur more easily, and be more important to avoid. Depression of respiratory function will be a danger, although elderly patients without respiratory disease tolerate opiate drugs well. Depression of cardiovascular function is an important danger, as many patients are already in incipient heart failure, and frank failure may be precipitated by drugs, or by the stress of operation, anaesthesia and the illness with which these are associated, or by incorrect fluid therapy. The cardiovascular depressant effects of anaesthetic drugs such as thiopentone and some of the inhalational agents will be exaggerated, and doses must be markedly reduced. Hypertensive elderly patients will show even more instability, and care must be taken not only to prevent hypotension, but also episodes of extreme hypertension.

Drug handling in the elderly in general is not consistently different from other age groups, but can be altered for some drugs, depending on their particular pharmacokinetic characteristics. Absorption or uptake of drugs is not significantly changed, but distribution may be altered, for example reduced binding to proteins or changes in total body water may be responsible for an increased effect of some highly protein bound drugs (e.g. thiopentone). Renal function deteriorates with age, so that there is inevitably some prolongation of elimination of renally excreted drugs (e.g. gallamine), and renal function may be further compromised by cardiac failure, or by stresses incurred at the time of operation. Drug induced confusion is easily caused in the elderly, and certain drugs known to cause this (e.g. hyoscine) should be avoided, and other psychotherapeutic drugs (in premedication for example) used cautiously. In particular, dosage of diazepam is very much age dependent; due to both altered distribution (see section 2.1.2) and an apparent increased sensitivity (Giles et al., 1978; Reidenberg et al., 1978).

In general therefore, there are few specific recommendations, but choice of drug dose is more critical, and often should be considerably reduced in the elderly patient (see table VI; also chapter V, sect. 2).

3.3 Neurosurgery

Anaesthesia for neurosurgery presents two specific problems: (1) positioning of the patient, which is mainly a mechanical problem, and (2) maintenance of perfusion of the brain with blood. This means that techniques must be used which avoid any rise in intracranial pressure, and also blood pressure must be maintained. A rise in mean arterial blood pressure above 125 to 140mm Hg causes a breakdown of autoregulation and the blood-brain barrier is breached, leading to forced vasodilatation and focal plasma leakage. With excessive hypotension, the pressure gradient between arterial and intracranial pressures may be insufficient for adequate blood flow (see McDowall and Norman, 1976; Michenfelder et al., 1969).

Intravenous induction agents such as thiopentone and althesin are suitable, as their use is followed by a fall in intracranial pressure, though care should be taken not to cause also a decrease in arterial pressure. The use of suxamethonium for intubation provides good conditions, while the hypertensive response to intubation and the concomitant increase in intracranial pressure may be attenuated by prior administration of a β-adrenoceptor blocking drug and by spraying of the larynx and trachea with lignocaine. All the volatile inhalational anaesthetic agents cause cerebral vasodilatation, and therefore are avoided in any patient at risk from increased intracranial pressure. Following induction, anaesthesia is maintained by use of a muscle relaxant with controlled ventilation, and a nitrous oxide analgesic, or neuroleptic technique (see section 2.3.1). Controlled hyperventilation, to give a P_{aCO_2} of 25 to 30mm Hg will further reduce intracranial pressure.

Intracranial pressure may be actively reduced by use of mannitol infusion; e.g. 0.5 to 1.0g/kg body weight over 10 minutes. Other pharmacological measures directed toward reduction of intracranial pressure in patients with head injury and others, includes use of corticosteroids — whose effectiveness is uncertain, and of thiopentone to reduce metabolic requirements — which is as yet experimental.

3.4 Obstetric Anaesthesia

In obstetric anaesthesia the requirements of both mother and fetus must be considered, as well as the altered disposition of drugs during labour (see chapter XV; sect. 1.1.6). Most drugs, including intravenous and inhalational anaesthetics and narcotic analgesics cross the placenta readily, so that their use is kept to a minimum to reduce the degree of depression of the neonate (see further chapter III). Muscle relaxants (except possibly gallamine) cross the placenta in insignificant amounts. The main problem presented by the mother is the occurrence of delayed emptying of the stomach, and decreased pH of the contents, with the potential danger of pulmonary aspiration of stomach contents during anaesthesia. Although practices vary in other parts of the world, in Britain the general principles of obstetric general anaesthesia are relatively standard (Moir, 1976).

Antacids are administered to combat gastric acidity (use of metoclopramide to increase emptying of the stomach or of cimetidine to reduce acidity are not yet accepted practice). Following preoxygenation and an intravenous induction, the trachea is intubated rapidly, usually under suxamethonium relaxation and using cricoid pressure. Anaesthesia is maintained with nitrous oxide/oxygen (50 to 66% O_2) which may be supplemented by low concentrations of a volatile agent. Halothane 0.5% is acceptable, although higher concentrations may interfere with uterine contraction. Muscle relaxation may be maintained using further suxamethonium, or a non-depolarising drug. Hyperventilation should be avoided as hypocapnia reduces uterine blood flow and fetal oxygenation, so ventilation should aim to maintain a normal P_aco_2. Following delivery, anaesthesia may be deepened and narcotic analgesics given. Also an oxytocic drug is normally given. Ergometrine causes generalised vasoconstriction and raised venous pressure may be a hazard in patients with cardiac disease or severe pre-eclampsia; oxytocin may be used instead.

Regional anaesthesia is widely used, particularly epidural blockade. This may be used for conduct of normal labour, but is also gaining popularity as an alternative method of anaesthesia for caesarian section. At present bupivacaine is the drug of choice, but etidocaine may give lower fetal and neonatal blood levels (see section 2.5.6). Pain relief in obstetric practice is discussed in section 8.3 (see also Various Authors, 1971b).

4. Anaesthesia in the Presence of Associated Disease

The general principle is wherever possible to treat the disease or correct any pathophysiological abnormality prior to operation, and to avoid potentially dangerous physiological disturbances during and after anaesthesia. In certain situations, some drugs are best avoided while in others modification of dosage will be necessary (see also table VII).

4.1 Cardiovascular Disease

Cardiovascular disease is often encountered in the preoperative patient. Correct diagnosis is important, and the patient's cardiovascular condition should be treated as effectively as time allows. This may include rest, and control of heart failure, hypertension etc, along usual medical lines, with particular care to avoid hyperkalaemia from diuretic therapy. Antihypertensive drugs should not be withdrawn prior to surgery (see Foex and Prys-Roberts, 1974; Prys-Roberts, 1976; section 6.2.3). Indeed, rebound hypertension which may follow sudden cessation of antihypertensive therapy is a very real hazard (Katz et al., 1976; Spotnitz, 1978). High doses of propranolol do not necessarily complicate anaesthesia and open heart surgery in patients with serious cardiac disease when continued throughout or just prior to the operative procedure (Kopriva et al., 1978a,b; Slogoff et al., 1978; see also chapter XVII, sect. 4.2.2).

With poor cardiac performance, there is usually a slow circulation time (making it easy to give an overdose of induction agent), a reduced tolerance of drugs which depress the cardiovascular system (see table I, II, III) and reduced tolerance of disturbances of circulating volume. While situations involving hypoxia and marked hypotension should obviously be avoided, the attitude to cardiac depressant drugs is changing (Hamilton, 1976). One of the main aims both in medical and anaesthetic management of patients with cardiac disease is to avoid myocardial ischaemia. Therefore, use of drugs which have some cardiac depressant effect (and so reduce myocardial oxygen demand) and drugs which have some vascular depressant effect (and so reduce the workload of the left ventricle), is not contraindicated. The aim during anaesthesia should be to maintain reasonable normality of the circulation, without hypertension and with only moderate hypotension. As in geriatric anaesthesia, the precise choice of drugs is of less importance than the skill with which they are used, but the principle stated above would indicate a definite place for the use of halothane, and warrant caution in the use of agents such as ketamine. The ischaemia seen following stresses such as tracheal intubation may be modified by β-adrenoceptor blockade.

Following myocardial infarction, elective surgery should be postponed for at least 3, and preferably 6 months, as operative mortality is very markedly increased in the immediate postinfarction period (Tarhan et al., 1972).

4.2 Respiratory Disease

Respiratory disease may be the reason for an operation, such as resection of carcinoma, or it may be encountered as an incidental problem in a patient with other pathology. The most common problem is chronic obstructive airways disease. Respiratory function should be fully assessed preoperatively, using both clinical and laboratory tests as indicated (Anderson, 1974). Commonly used criteria are vital capacity, forced expiratory volume in 1 second (FEV_1), and blood gases. Milledge and Nunn (1975) have defined criteria of fitness for surgery in chronic obstructive airways disease: the FEV_1 should be used as a screening test, and arterial blood gases measured in any patient whose FEV_1 is under 1 litre or 50% of predicted value. Patients with only a reduced FEV_1 can be treated normally. When there is also arterial hypoxaemia, oxygen therapy is needed; while a raised P_aco_2 is the most important aspect of pre-operative assessment — patients with this are likely to need postoperative respiratory support, often including ventilation of the lungs. Where lung resection is contemplated, measurement of vital capacity etc, and possibly separate assessment of each lung function, may be required to attempt forecast of postoperative function.

Details of anaesthetic management depend on the pathophysiology of the condition. Pre-operative physiotherapy, and drug therapy to reduce bronchoconstriction may help (see chapter XX; sect. 3, 4), while during anaesthesia drug administration will be modified mainly in that great care needs to be exercised in the use of drugs with respiratory depressant effects, or which cause laryngospasm or bronchospasm (see table I, II, III).

4.3 Allergy

Problems may develop in allergic patients during or after anaesthesia (Adriani, 1970). These may be in the form of adverse drug responses or technical difficulties in maintaining an adequate airway due to secretions, oedema and thickening of the nasal passages for example. It is therefore essential that the history of the allergic patient, particularly with respect to drug intake, be known before operation. Patients with a history of multiple allergies, particularly to drugs, should be given careful consideration, but repeated exposures are usually necessary to sensitise patients to drugs ordinarily used by the anaesthetist. In the light of recent experience althesin and propanidid are best avoided in such patients (see section 2.1.2).

4.4 Endocrine Disease

Diabetes Mellitus: The aim is to maintain control of diabetes in the operative and postoperative period, avoiding hyper- or hypoglycaemic episodes. Many anaesthetic agents cause some rise in blood sugar, although halothane does not.

Patients satisfactorily controlled on diet or oral hypoglycaemic drugs will often require no change in regimen for minor operations, but may be better stabilised on insulin for longer procedures. Patients on insulin are generally stabilised pre-operatively on soluble insulin. A minor procedure may be carried out early in the day, simply delaying the first dose of insulin, and breakfast, until afterwards. For larger procedures, requirements will be estimated as usual by tests on blood sugar and urine, and carbohydrate requirements given intravenously. The stress of operation and the postoperative period will often mean a greater need for insulin.

Corticosteroid Therapy: All patients who have had or are still taking systemic corticosteroids should be assessed and observed carefully. Routine prophylactic cover however, is only necessary for those who have ceased steroids recently (see section 6.2.4).

4.5 Renal Disease

Many of the problems encountered in this situation are due to hypertension, and to the water and electrolyte imbalance and acid-base disturbance (the patient tends to become acidotic) which may accompany renal failure (Slawson, 1972; Various Authors, 1972a). These should, so far as possible, be corrected before operation. Even so, however, it is common for patients in renal failure to have haemoglobin levels of 4 to 6g/100ml which cannot be raised. Compensatory changes to anaemia occur such that tissue perfusion increases and oxyhaemoglobin dissociates more readily. During operation these anaemic patients will obviously require great care to avoid hypoxic situations, and blood loss must be carefully replaced, preferably by whole blood.

Choice of anaesthetic technique will be to avoid agents which depend to an important extent on the kidneys for their elimination (see tables I, II, III), particularly methoxyflurane and the muscle relaxant gallamine, and to avoid techniques which might cause renal damage by hypotension. Normal (1mg/kg) or repeated doses of suxamethonium do not usually raise the serum potassium to dangerous levels (Powell and Miller, 1975) but large or repeated doses of tubocurarine or pancuronium may lead to prolonged curarisation in patients with renal failure (see section 2.2.1). Patients who are maintained by haemodialysis will be more sensitive to hypotension immediately after dialysis, when their circulating volume is lower. For small procedures, such as the establishment of an arteriovenous shunt, local nerve block techniques are often applicable. There is an increased sensitivity to barbiturates in uraemia (Dundee, 1956) — thus thiopentone should be given slowly and in suitably small doses in renal failure.

4.6 Hepatic Disease

Full assessment and careful management are as important for patients with liver disease as for those with respiratory or cardiovascular disease (Strunin, 1978). The most important factor in preventing further damage to the liver is the avoidance of hypotension, hypoxia or hypercarbia (Editorial, 1978; Various Authors, 1972b). Light general anaesthesia with inhalational agents and relaxants is preferred. Halothane can be used once except in those in whom unexplained jaundice occurred following a previous exposure (Moult and Sherlock, 1975; see section 2.1.1). Attention to renal function is an integral part of management Large doses of drugs, such as local anaesthetics or opiates, which depend on the liver for their elimination, should be avoided. The action of suxamethonium may be prolonged when liver disease is associated with low plasma cholinesterase levels, but this is not usually a problem. Larger than normal doses of tubocurarine and pancuronium may be required initially in some patients with liver disease but repeated doses may need to be reduced due to delayed elimination. In the early stages of alcoholic cirrhosis, there is resistance to barbiturates and anaesthesia, but in the later stages of the cirrhosis marked sensitivity to barbiturates develops (Shideman et al., 1949; see further chapter XIX; sect. 13.4).

4.7 Epilepsy

Epileptic patients usually tolerate anaesthesia without incident, but occasionally they present problems (Evans, 1975). There is not only a risk of convulsions in susceptible patients given certain anaesthetics (methohexitone, diethylether, enflurane, ketamine, ?althesin), but also a possibility of anticonvulsant drug neurotoxicity, particularly with phenytoin (diphenylhydantoin), as a result of the depressant effects of general anaesthesia on hepatic drug elimination processes. It is probably wise therefore to monitor serum phenytoin levels prior to elective surgery and to adjust dosage to attain the minimum desirable concentration (see section 6.1; also chapter XXV; sect. 3.1). As in patients with liver disease it is important to avoid hypoxia, hypercarbia or hypotension.

4.8 Thyroid Disease

Except in an emergency it is unlikely that operations will be carried out in patients whose thyroid disease is not controlled (Stehling, 1974). Many patients with hyperthyroidism will have been prepared for surgery with β-adrenoceptor blocking drugs. These may make patients sensitive to blood loss by blocking compensatory tachycardia and on occasion they may induce bronchospasm. In hypothyroidism the main problems will be increased sensitivity to depressant drugs, and diminished cardiovascular reserve. Treatment with triiodothyronine may help, but must be used very cautiously. In hyperthyroid states, there is a hyperdynamic circulation, and also the increased metabolic rate will make the patient more likely to become anoxic. 'Thyroid crisis', often seen in the past after thyroidectomy, is rare now as patients are controlled medically before operation. Should it occur, the main lines of treatment are sedation, cooling if required, and use of antithyroid drugs, and propranolol to control the effects of circulating thyroid hormones (chapt. XVI; sect. 5.2.3).

5. Toxicity of Anaesthetic Drugs

5.1 General Considerations

Virtually all drugs produce undesired effects as well as the effect for which they are prescribed, and anaesthetic drugs are no exception. The most common side effects of the drugs which induce sleep are depression of the cardiovascular system with reduced cardiac output, reduced peripheral resistance and lowering of blood pressure (ketamine being an exception). This is due both to direct effects on the heart and blood vessels, and to an effect on central autonomic control. Depression of respiration due to an action on the brain is also common.

To minimise these effects it is necessary to carefully choose the dose and monitor the action of the drugs. Dose is related not only to the size of the patient but also to his physical and pathophysiological condition, the clinical situation in question, and the response to the initial exposure (see also sections 3,4).

5.2 Effects on Cell Division and Occupational Exposure

Bone marrow depression has been reported after prolonged administration of nitrous oxide (for periods in excess of 24 hours) and in animals similar effects have been seen with other anaesthetic agents. Dysmorphogenicity of any anaesthetic agent has not been shown in man (although an effect on cell division in human cell cultures has been demonstrated), but many substances including nitrous oxide, ether, cyclopropane and methoxyflurane have produced congenital abnormalities in chick embryos. Nitrous oxide and halothane are also capable of producing abnormalities in the rat (Tuchmann-Duplessis, 1975). The only inference which can at present be drawn is that anaesthetic drugs, like all other drugs, are relatively contraindicated in the first trimester of pregnancy.

Long term exposure to trace amounts of anaesthetic agents is a different situation (Fink and Cullen, 1976). Operating theatre personnel have been shown in several surveys to have a higher incidence of disease than control groups (Spence et al., 1977; Pharoah et al., 1977). Among women there has been said to be an increased risk of infertility, spontaneous abortion and congenital abnormalities in their children; and of cancer, and hepatic and renal disease in both sexes. An increased risk of congenital abnormalities has also been noted in the unexposed wives of male operating room personnel. However, other studies have not supported all of these findings, and in particular, comparisons with other hospital groups suggest that the environmental factor to blame for spontaneous abortion may be the stressful way of life of operating theatre, intensive care or casualty departments, rather than pollution of the atmosphere (Rosenberg and Kirves, 1973). A prospective study found death rates in anaesthetists, including those from cancer, to be no higher than for the general population (Bruce et al., 1974). However, while it has not been unequivocally established that waste anaesthetics are responsible for the increased disease rate (Vessey, 1978), it seems highly desirable to scavenge all exhaust gases from anaesthetic circuits and the theatre atmosphere and vent them to the outside air.

Metabolism of anaesthetic gases may be an important factor in long term exposure to low concentrations, since a higher proportion of the small dose which is absorbed appears to be metabolised to non-volatile and possibly more harmful metabolites (Sawyer et al., 1971). Anaesthetists metabolise volatile agents such as halothane and methoxyflurane more readily than non-anaesthetists, probably as a consequence of hepatic enzyme induction (Cascorbi et al., 1970; Wood et al., 1974). See further section 2.1.1.

Study of the effect of trace quantities of anaesthetics on mental performance have been inconsistent, but some have indeed suggested a measurable decrease in performance of psychological tests by volunteers exposed to as little as 50ppm (parts per million) of nitrous oxide or 1ppm halothane. Halothane is metabolised to various substances including bromide, and after exposure to a typical anaesthetic dose, bromide levels rise to the psychoactive range by the second day and are still high by 9 days (Tinker et al., 1976).

5.3 Oxygen Toxicity

Oxygen in high concentrations is commonly used in anaesthesia and associated techniques. Breathing 80 to 100% oxygen produces signs of pulmonary oxygen toxicity within 24 hours, with substernal pain, fall in vital capacity and lung compliance. With hyperbaric therapy, these changes will occur more rapidly, and at over 2.5 atmospheres (1600mm Hg) central nervous system toxicity with convulsions occurs. The effects in the premature infant, where retrolental fibroplasia may occur, are well known (Clark and Lambertsen, 1971; Editorial, 1974). These factors mean that care must be taken with oxygen therapy, and in some cases monitoring of arterial blood oxygen tension and of inspired oxygen concentration is indicated. In long term intensive care therapy, the inspired oxygen concentrations should be kept to 40% or below when this is possible.

5.4 Renal Function

Few drugs used in anaesthesia have any direct damaging effect on the function of the kidneys, and by far the most common cause of damage during anaesthesia is inadequate renal blood flow (Rosen, 1972). It is well known that the body reacts to hypovolaemia by constricting the splanchnic, including the renal, blood vessels and that this may lead to tubular necrosis. However, the response to haemorrhage is different in conscious and anaesthetised animals, and renal vasoconstriction may be relatively more marked during anaesthesia (Vatner and Braunwald, 1975). Adrenaline and noradrenaline also reduce renal blood flow, so treatment of hypotension with these agents is likely to increase kidney damage. Dopamine may, however, be used in some conditions (e.g. some states of cardiogenic shock) as it causes a peripheral vasoconstriction while sparing the renal circulation (McDonald et al., 1964). It is given by infusion at a rate of 2 to $50\mu g/kg/min$. In susceptible patients, mannitol may be given intravenously during operation to maintain renal blood flow by producing an osmotic diuresis.

Methoxyflurane and its relationship to renal damage have been discussed in section 2.1.1 above.

5.5 Hepatic Function

The liver is the site of many of the important metabolic processes of the body, including synthesis of proteins and other substances, and the metabolism of most drugs (see chapter I; sect. 3.3). These include anaesthetic drugs administered parenterally and it is becoming apparent that most of the inhalational agents are also metabolised to a greater or lesser extent (see table I; for review, see Cohen, 1971; Cascorbi, 1973) and that toxicity can result as a consequence of metabolism of inhalational anaesthetics (Cohen, 1978; see section 2.1.1).

Damage to the liver caused during anaesthesia may occur by several mechanisms (Clarke et al., 1976; Strunin, 1977):

1. Due indirectly to drugs, anaesthetic technique or surgery:
   a) Hypoxia
   b) Hypercarbia
   c) Underperfusion due to splanchnic vasoconstriction in states of shock, or to hypotension after sympathetic blockade in hypotensive techniques or spinal anaesthesia, or prolonged hypotension from any cause.
2. Due to drugs:
   a) A direct toxic effect from the parent drug or a metabolite. Chloroform is generally acknowledged to be toxic to the liver, and severe damage has often occurred, so that the drug is now little used. Clinical doses of intravenous agents are not toxic, but liver dysfunction has been reported after large doses of thiopentone (Dundee, 1956).

b) A sensitisation process involving hapten formation. The relationship of halothane to liver damage and possible mechanisms including sensitisation (Vergani et al., 1978), have been discussed in section 2.1.1, but it must also be appreciated that liver damage has occurred after methoxyflurane, and cross sensitisation between these two drugs has also been suggested (Joshi and Conn, 1974).

5.6 Malignant Hyperpyrexia

Some susceptible patients, who suffer from an inherited subclinical myopathy, develop a fulminating and often fatal hyperpyrexia when given certain anaesthetic drugs or non-depolarising muscle relaxants (Britt, 1975; Britt and Kalow, 1970). Most patients develop muscle contracture, acidosis and hyperkalaemia. Unexplained tachypnoea, tachycardia, sweating, cyanosis or overheating of soda lime may be nonspecific early warnings. A working definition of malignant hyperpyrexia is an unexplained fever during anaesthesia in which the body temperature rises at a rate of at least $2°$ an hour, but sometimes the rise in body temperature may be a late sign.

The condition is inherited as a Mendelian autosomal dominant trait with variable expression and incomplete penetrance (Kelstrup et al., 1974), and may be due to a disorder of calcium binding by the sarcoplasmic reticulum and sarcolemma, but the full aetiology is unknown. Halothane and suxamethonium (succinylcholine) are the drugs which have most often been incriminated, but all the volatile anaesthetic drugs, and nitrous oxide, and several other drugs have been shown to cause hyperpyrexia or are under suspicion. Some patients at risk may have a family history of the condition, or of unexplained deaths under anaesthesia. However, positive identification of the susceptible patient is difficult. Some, but not all patients at risk may be recognised by a raised serum creatine phosphokinase level. *In vitro* testing of a muscle biopsy specimen from the patient is more reliable, but can only be carried out at a few centres in the world. Mortality from the established condition is over 60%, so that a high index of suspicion, and early recognition of the development of hyperthermia is essential.

Treatment is not well defined at present, and consists mainly in early withdrawal of the initiating drug, followed by symptomatic treatment including vigorous cooling, artificial ventilation, correction of acidosis using sodium bicarbonate, and in particular recognition and treatment of hyperkalaemia which often occurs. Specific remedies are still lacking. Use of procaine in high doses (Clarke and Ellis, 1975) is at present controversial (it may help in some cases but at doses at which it is a serious cardiac depressant), and the use of large doses of dexamethasone has been reported as successful (Ellis et al., 1974), but lacks confirmation. The antispasticity drug dantrolene sodium, a hydantoin, which appears to act by interference with the release of calcium from the sarcoplasmic reticulum of muscle fibrils, has been successful in both prevention and treatment of the syndrome in susceptible pigs. Recent reports (Austin and Denborough, 1977), of *in vitro* tests suggest that it should be specific and effective in treatment of the human condition and at doses which should be safe.

5.7 Hypersensitivity

Apart from halothane related hepatitis possibly being due to a sensitisation process (see section 2.1.1), intravenous anaesthetics are being increasingly incriminated in hypersensitivity reactions. In a recent review, Clarke (1979) gave details of 202 reports with althesin, 63 with thiopentone, 58 with propanidid, 11 with methohexitone and one with thiamylal. Considering the overall use of these drugs, and the almost complete abandonment of propanidid, it would appear that hypersensitivity reactions are more likely to occur with non-barbiturates. An alternative explanation for this frequency distribution may be the use of the solubilising agent, cremophor, with both althesin and propanidid. It has been estimated that abnormal reactions to althesin occur in about 1:10,000 administrations (Clarke, 1978), although some place it as high as 1:1000 (Evans and Keogh, 1977).

The acute reactions have been mainly characterised by hypotension and bronchospasm. The latter can be very severe and difficult to treat. The cardiovascular effects respond to rapid intravenous infusion of balanced salt solutions, but vasopressors and hydrocortisone may be required. Reactions usually occur within 2 minutes of injection and in a few instances they have immediately followed the administration of minute doses. Reactions seem more likely to occur in patients with a personal or family history of asthma or eczema and in those known to be sensitive to other drugs (Clarke et al., 1977; Dundee, 1976). Similar abnormal responses, which are presumably due to histamine release (see section 2.1.2), may occur with muscle relaxants. Contact dermatitis to propanidid has also occurred.

6. Drug Interactions and the Anaesthetist

The effects of one drug may modify the action of another given concurrently or subsequently, in a predictable and therapeutically desirable manner. This forms the basis of many drug combinations used before or during anaesthesia. There are, however, many other drugs, often not related to anaesthesia, which may profoundly alter the patient's response to drugs given during or following surgery (Davie, 1977). It is important to note that many of these effects bear no relation to the normal therapeutic action of the drugs, so that the patient may have no symptoms referable to the drugs he has been receiving and only show an abnormal reaction when another drug is given.

6.1 Mechanism of Drug Interactions

Where possible, interactions between drugs should be described in terms of mechanism and site of action (Dundee and McCaughey, 1972; Rawlins, 1978). In simple terms, the effects of one drug can be increased (potentiated) or decreased (antagonised) by the previous or concurrent administration of another drug (see chapters VII, VIII).

The site of interaction may be outside the body, when two chemically incompatible substances are mixed in the same syringe (e.g. thiopentone and pancuronium). Absorption of the drug may be modified — for example adrenaline slows the uptake of subcutaneous local anaesthetics. Distribution of the drug may be modified — for example, thiopentone can be displaced from plasma protein binding sites by sulphafurazole (Csogor and Kerek, 1970) and presumably by other drugs such as warfarin and phenylbutazone (Ghoneim and Korttila, 1977; see further chapter I; sect. 3.2.3). At the active receptor, there may be competition for the same receptor site — for example the competition between neostigmine and atropine. The hepatic metabolism of the drug may be modified, as for example by the process of enzyme induction,

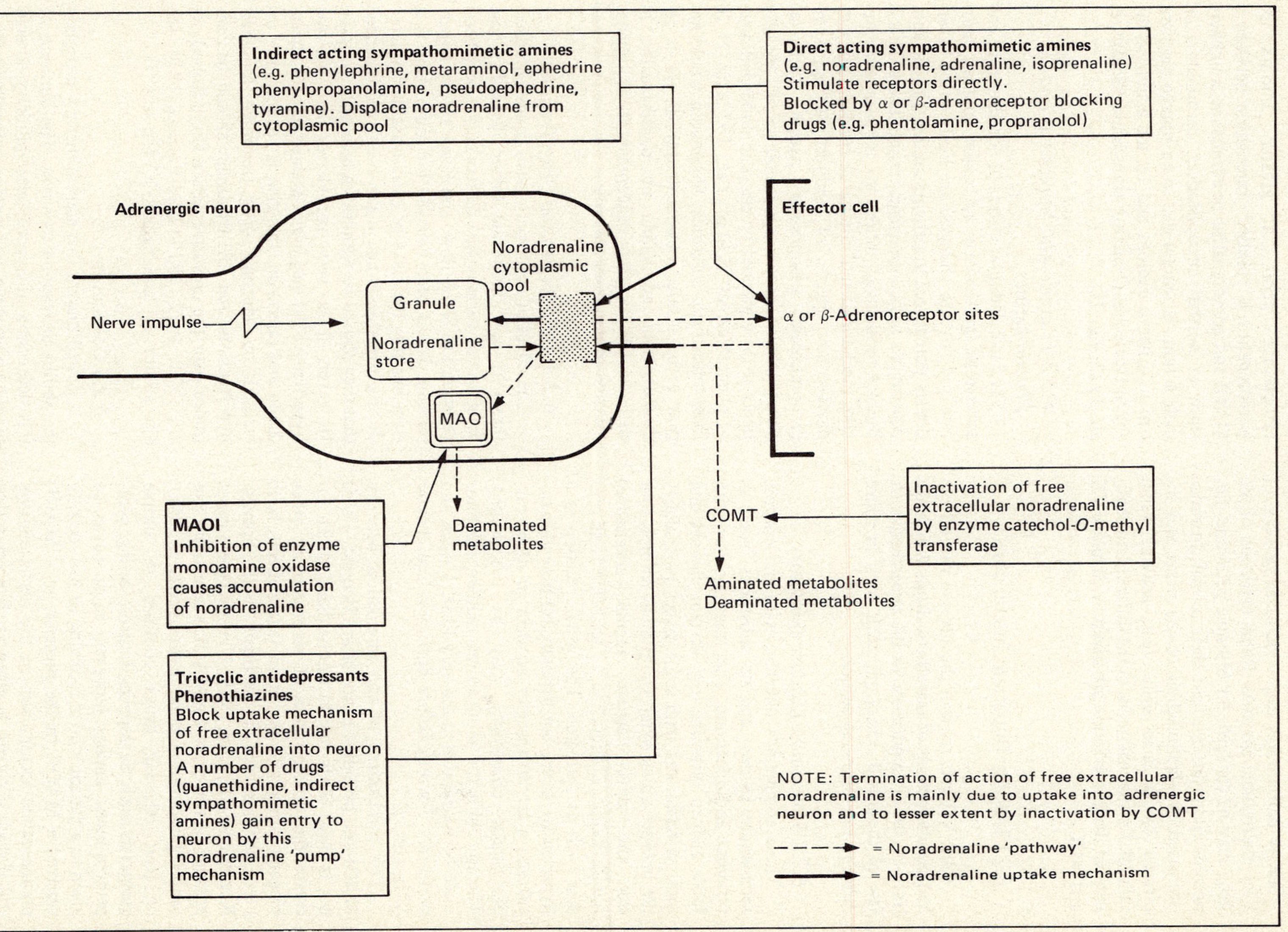

Fig. 2. Simplified schematic diagram of drugs that modify the uptake, release and actions of noradrenaline at adrenergic neurons.

whereby barbiturates cause increased activity of liver microsomal enzymes. Renal excretion of the drug may be changed, for example pethidine, lignocaine and prilocaine have their rate of clearance decreased by alkalinisation of the urine and increased by an acid urine (e.g. acidotic renal failure). Further examples of the different mechanisms of drug interaction are given in chapters VII and VIII.

6.2 Clinically Important Interactions

Table VII lists most of the adverse side effects and the interactions of anaesthetic drugs which are likely to be of importance to the anaesthetist. A few of these and others are dealt with in more detail in the following sections.

6.2.1 Monoamine Oxidase Inhibitors

These compounds interfere with the enzyme monoamine oxidase and its substrates, such as tyramine and dopamine. They may interact with foods rich in tyramine (e.g. certain cheeses and meat extracts), and with some drugs, particularly the indirect acting sympathomimetic amines (but not the direct acting agents adrenaline, noradrenaline, isoprenaline — see below) and opiates such as pethidine. The usual reaction is a hypertensive crisis, but hypotension may also occur and a cerebrovascular accident or other cardiovascular catastrophe may be precipitated. Therapy with the monoamine oxidase inhibitor must be withdrawn at the very least, 1 week and preferably 3 weeks before operation (see chapter VIII; sect. 3).

The mechanism of the interaction between MAOI and pethidine is not clear (Sjoqvist, 1965) but is most likely due to mechanisms which increase the concentration of serotonin or other biogenic amines in the brain (such effects have been demonstrated in animals with opiates; Rogers and Thornton, 1969). Thus, where it is not possible to withdraw the MAOI, a sensitivity test to the opiates can be done (Evans-Prosser, 1968), or pain relieving drugs confined to simple analgesics such as aspirin. Indirect acting sympathomimetic amines however, must never be given to a patient who is receiving or has recently received a MAOI. In the presence of a MAOI, noradrenaline accumulates in the nerve endings and if such a patient is given an indirect acting amine (which displaces noradrenaline from the

cytoplasmic pool), a greater amount of noradrenaline is released. Interaction between a MAOI and noradrenaline or adrenaline is unlikely since in normal circumstances, termination of their actions is mainly due to an uptake mechanism into nerve endings and by the action of the enzyme catechol-*O*-methyl transferase (Boakes et al., 1973; fig. 2).

6.2.2 Tricyclic Antidepressants and Phenothiazines

The cardiovascular effects of noradrenaline and adrenaline (particularly adrenaline induced heart rate and rhythm changes) are likely to be hazardously potentiated in patients taking tricyclic antidepressants or phenothiazine tranquillisers. This is because these drugs inhibit the noradrenaline uptake mechanism into the nerve endings. The cardiovascular effects of indirect acting sympathomimetic vasopressor agents such as phenylephrine, metaraminol and so on, are also likely to be enhanced by tricyclic antidepressants or phenothiazines (Boakes et al., 1973; fig. 2). In local anaesthetic solutions, felypressin would appear to be a safer vasoconstrictor (if one is required) than adrenaline or noradrenaline in patients on tricyclic antidepressant or phenothiazine tranquilliser therapy.

6.2.3 Antihypertensive Drug Treatment

The effect of antihypertensive drugs on anaesthesia is now becoming better defined. These drugs act at various sites to reduce the peripheral resistance to blood flow, and hence relieve hypertension. It has been believed for some years that they increase the risks of cardiovascular collapse during anaesthesia and it has been recommended that they should be withdrawn before anaesthesia. However, it is now considered that whereas hypertensive patients are at greater risk for anaesthesia and operation, this risk is reduced, not increased, by adequate drug treatment for their hypertension, and this treatment should be continued over the operative period (Prys-Roberts et al., 1971, 1972, 1973; Prys-Roberts, 1976; see also section 4.1 and chapter XVIII; sect. 11).

6.2.4 Corticosteroids

It is well known that steroid therapy depresses the ability to respond to stress. The duration of this depression of hypothalamic-pituitary-adrenal function is variable, and may occasionally be for a very long time. However, in general, it is very

Table VII. Drug reactions and interactions and some special risk situations with anaesthetic drugs[1]

Agent	Drug or clinical situation	Potential interaction or risk[2]
Inhalational anaesthetics		
Halothane	Liver disease	Can be used once except in those in whom unexplained jaundice occurred following a previous exposure
	Muscular disorders	May trigger malignant hyperpyrexia (see section 5.6)
	Adrenaline	Myocardium sensitised to adrenaline
	Phenytoin	Depressed liver blood flow or function may cause phenytoin toxicity in those with previously 'high' serum levels
Methoxyflurane	Renal disease Tetracycline	Increased risk of polyuric renal failure
Enflurane	Epilepsy	Risk of convulsions
	Adrenaline	Myocardium sensitised to adrenaline
Diethyl ether	β-Adrenoceptor blockers	Risk of heart failure, hypotension
	Epilepsy	Risk of convulsions
Cyclopropane Trichloroethylene	Adrenaline	Myocardium sensitised to adrenaline
Intravenous anaesthetics		
Thiopentone	Renal failure Cirrhosis	Decreased protein binding of thiopentone may enhance its activity
	Metabolic acidosis	Enhanced activity
	Pancuronium Suxamethonium	Chemically incompatible
Thiopentone Methohexitone	Porphyria	Precipitate attacks
Methohexitone	Epilepsy	Risk of convulsions
Propanidid	Suxamethonium	Activity of suxamethonium prolonged 50%
	Low serum cholinesterase activity	Prolonged activity
Thiopentone Methohexitone Propanidid Althesin	Allergy Asthma Eczema	Increased risk of anaphylactic response and bronchospasm
Ketamine	Quinalbarbitone Diazepam Hydroxyzine	Prolonged recovery time (by around 30 to 40%) with use of these drugs as premedicants
	Thyroid drugs	Severe hypertension and tachycardia
	Pancuronium	Excessive tachycardia
Althesin	Severe liver disease Renal failure	Prolonged activity
	Epilepsy	Risk of convulsions
Diazepam	Hypoalbuminaemia	Enhanced response (chapt. VII, sect. 5.1; XXVI, sect. 1.5.3)
	Liver disease	Delayed clearance from plasma

Table VII. (continued)

Agent	Drug or clinical situation	Potentiation interaction or risk[2]
Muscle relaxants Suxamethonium Gallamine Tubocurarine Alcuronium Pancuronium	Aminoglycosides (neomycin, gentamicin, etc) Polymyxins (colistin) Tetracycline Clindamycin ? Lincomycin Bronchial carcinoma	Prolonged apnoea; most likely if antibiotics given intraperitoneally and in presence of liver (clinda-mycin, lincomycin) or renal impairment or muscle weakness (see section 6.2.5)
	Quinidine Procainamide	Increased neuromuscular blocking activity (doubtful clinical significance)
Suxamethonium	Propanidid	Prolonged neuromuscular blocking activity
	Severe liver disease Uraemia Malnutrition Anticholinesterases (ecothiopate eye drops; exposure to pesticides) Cyclophosphamide Thiotepa Monoamine oxidase inhibitors (phenelzine)	Serum pseudocholinesterase levels decreased and prolonged neuromuscular blocking activity (see also section 2.2.1)
	Procaine (infusion or injection)	Prolonged action. Competes with pseudocholinesterase
	Trauma, burns, wounds Muscular disorders Renal failure (large doses) with peripheral neuropathy	Hyperkalaemia and risk of serious cardiac arrhythmias. Also risk of triggering malignant hyperpyrexia in those with muscular disorders. Avoid use
	Digitalis	Risk of digitalis toxicity due to sudden release of potassium, especially in presence of trauma, burns, wounds, muscular disorders
Gallamine	Renal failure	Prolonged apnoea due to delayed elimination. Avoid use
Tubocurarine Alcuronium Pancuronium	Renal failure	Safe, but large or repeated doses may lead to prolonged activity. Augmented by frusemide (furosemide). See section 2.2.1
Gallamine Tubocurarine Alcuronium Pancuronium	Severe liver disease Anticholinesterases	Serum pseudocholinesterase levels decreased and neuro-muscular blocking activity decreased in some patients. Increased binding to gamma globulin. Larger than normal initial doses required but repeated doses tubocurarine and pancuronium may need to be reduced due to delayed elimination
	Immunosuppressive therapy	Decreased neuromuscular blocking activity
	Hypokalaemia Metabolic acidosis	Prolonged neuromuscular blocking activity
Suxamethonium Pancuronium	Lithium	Prolonged neuromuscular blocking activity (? due to inhibition of acetylcholine release and/or synthesis)
Pancuronium	Corticosteroids	Rapid termination of action by large doses of corticosteroids

Table VII. (continued)

Agent	Drug or clinical situation	Potential interaction or risk[2]
Muscle relaxant antagonists		
Neostigmine	Bowel surgery	Increases peristalsis and may cause leakage from intestinal anastomosis (blocked by halothane but not by atropine)
Local anaesthetics		
All compounds	Metabolic acidosis	Increased risk of toxicity
Amethocaine (tetracaine) Procaine	Low serum cholinesterase activity	Prolonged activity
Prilocaine	Labour	Risk of methaemoglobinaemia in mother and newborn
Adrenaline Noradrenaline	Tricyclic antidepressants	Risk of marked increase in pressor response (NB not with MAOI)

1　For reactions with other drugs used in anaesthetic practice see chapter VIII and appendices B, C.

2　It does not necessarily follow that the effect described will automatically occur as its likelihood depends on a number of factors such as dose, severity of disease and so on. See also sections 3, 4, 5 and 6 for further information. In some situations certain drugs are best avoided; in others, modification of dose of the primary drug is needed.

unlikely that collapse from this cause will occur if surgery is undertaken more than 2 months after cessation of treatment, and whereas all patients who are or who have been on steroids must be carefully assessed, only those having had treatment recently need have routine cover. A fairly satisfactory method of cover is to give intramuscular hydrocortisone hemisuccinate, 100mg 6-hourly, starting with premedication and lasting from 24 hours to 3 days (Kehlet and Binder, 1973; Plumpton et al., 1969).

6.2.5 Antibacterial Agents

A large number of antibiotics has been found to possess some neuromuscular blocking activity or to be capable of enhancing the action of neuromuscular blocking agents. These fall chemically into different groups: (a) streptomycin and related aminoglycoside compounds; (b) the polymyxins; (c) the tetracyclines, and (d) in addition lincomycin and clindamycin. Some antibiotics, including the penicillins, have not been implicated. The mechanism of action is not certain (Pittinger et al., 1970; Pittinger and Adamson, 1972), but it appears that the aminoglycosides, like magnesium ions, primarily inhibit the prejunctional release of acetylcholine and also depress postjunctional sensitivity to the humoral agent. The mechanisms of action of the tetracycline and polymyxins, and of lincomycin and clindamycin are not known. The block produced by the aminoglycosides may sometimes be antagonised by calcium and also by neostigmine if incomplete, but neostigmine may prolong the blockade produced by other antibiotics. There is an enhanced effect of these antibiotics with the neuromuscular block produced by the non-depolarising muscle relaxants, which has led to difficulty in many cases in which antibiotics had been given parenterally by various routes during anaesthesia; especially in the presence of renal disease. On occasions, this effect was augmented by the curariform activity of diethyl ether and in some instances a combination of relaxant, antibiotic and ether resulted in prolonged apnoea. An enhanced effect can also occur with both non-depolarising and depolarising relaxants when the antibiotics are given immediately after surgery (Foldes et al., 1963). Weakness or paralysis have also occurred with parenteral antibiotics alone (especially aminoglycosides in those with renal disease and hypocalcaemia), and on rare occasions after oral neomycin, and after polymyxin applied topically to burns. The aminoglycoside and polymyxin antibiotics may also cause muscle weakness in patients with myasthenia gravis (see chapter XXV; sect. 14.1).

6.2.6 Anticoagulants

The anticoagulant drugs demonstrate interactions by many different mechanisms, from the direct physical antagonism between heparin and protamine, to a multiplicity of pharmacological interactions involving the coumarin type drugs (see chapter XXIII, sect. 3.2.5). While clinically significant interactions involving coumarin anticoagulants can occur with a number of different drugs these are not likely to be a particular problem in anaesthetic practice since most of the drugs involved are not likely to be directly encountered by the anaesthetist. Nevertheless, it should always be borne in mind that any factor which depresses liver function may enhance the action of the coumarin anticoagulants (e.g. postoperative jaundice). Paracetamol (acetaminophen) is preferable to aspirin as a postoperative simple analgesic in coumarin anticoagulated patients. Barbiturate hypnotics or sedatives should be avoided.

7. Respiratory Failure

This implies an inability of the respiratory system to achieve adequate oxygenation and removal of carbon dioxide. In most situations a Pco_2 over 55mm Hg (normal 40) or a Po_2 under 60 (normal 95 to 100) indicates a degree of failure. As shown in table VIII it may result from a defect in any one of the components of the respiratory system, from the central control in the brainstem, to the mechanical structures of the thoracic cage, to the various parts of the lungs.

7.1 Acute Respiratory Failure

The causes of acute respiratory failure are many, and often interrelated, so the treatment is complex. Simple procedures of pain relief or suction of airways etc, in patients with potential respiratory failure may halt deterioration in time to avoid the need for more radical treatment. Narcotic drug induced respiratory depression may be antagonised by a specific antagonist such as naloxone (0.4 to 0.8mg) or if this is ineffective (as with buprenorphine), by a nonspecific respiratory stimulant such as doxapram. Use of a nerve stimulator may be needed to differentiate respiratory depression from residual curarisation. Where hypoxia is present despite 'adequate' alveolar ventilation, oxygen therapy may relieve it.

More often, however, mechanical methods are the main line of treatment — endotracheal intubation to clear obstruction, suction of secretions from the bronchial tree (with the help of intensive

Table VIII. Classification of causes of respiratory insufficiency

1. Central depression
   a) Poisoning
   b) Increased intracranial pressure
   c) Head injury
   d) Cerebrovascular accident
   e) Miscellaneous — post hypoxia, hypoglycaemia
2. Impairment of respiratory mechanism
   a) Nervous tissue — poliomyelitis, polyneuritis, porphyria
   b) Myoneural junction — myasthenia gravis, carcinomatous neuropathy
   c) Muscle — polymyositis, progressive muscular atrophy, trauma to chest wall
   d) Obstruction to airway — including asthma
3. Lung damage
   a) Bronchitis and emphysema
   b) Pneumonia — including effects of aspiration of stomach content; — including postoperative pain; — crushed chest
   c) Post-traumatic pulmonary insufficiency (adult respiratory distress syndrome) is a complex of syndromes following non-thoracic insults
4. Mixed causes
5. Induced insufficiency
   a) Inadvertent — following muscle relaxants
   b) Therapeutic — control of convulsions

physiotherapy), and artificial ventilation to assist or replace inadequate spontaneous ventilation from many causes. The details and language of this are beyond the scope of this text — variations include spontaneous ventilation with continuous raised airway pressure (CRAP); intermittent positive pressure ventilation (IPPV), with or without patient triggering of the ventilator; IPPV with positive end-expiratory pressure (PEEP); intermittent mandatory ventilation (IMV) and other variations on these themes. Muscle relaxant drugs may be needed to induce apnoea in conditions where excessive muscle tone interferes with normal respiration, such as convulsions, or tetanus. In other conditions, the patient must not be allowed to breathe out of phase with the ventilator (except in IMV), and this may be achieved by patient triggering of the ventilator, or by use of muscle relaxants to paralyse the patient, or by depression of his respiratory drive by opiate drugs (Pontoppidan et al., 1972; 1977).

It is becoming apparent that respiratory failure in some degree is a feature of many conditions such as head injury, severe trauma not involving the chest, shock, and in postoperative cardiac surgery patients. In such situations artificial ventilation will help by removing the extra work of breathing, whereas drugs to stimulate respiration will to some extent be whipping an already exhausted horse.

7.2 Thoracic Injury

Thoracic injury may include danger to the chest wall and lung tissue and, if severe, is currently treated by artificial ventilation. Patients with minor degrees of injury, with only a few broken ribs, may be prevented from developing respiratory failure by providing adequate analgesia, so that deep respiration and good coughing are possible. General analgesia by intravenous infusion of lignocaine can give good results. Thoracic extradural block will produce complete analgesia, and in some cases block of intercostal nerves helps. In both situations the longer action of bupivacaine is useful.

7.3 Lung Disease

Diseases of the lungs which may lead to respiratory failure include bronchitis and emphysema, asthma and the various pneumoconioses. Treatment of these falls largely within the sphere of general medicine but acute respiratory failure may occur in exacerbations of the diseases. Exacerbations of bronchitis are usually due to infection, and appropriate antibacterial therapy is needed; supported by carefully controlled oxygen therapy, humidification, intensive physiotherapy and sometimes endotracheal intubation and suction of secretions. Some centres use artificial ventilation for some of these patients, whereas others may treat the most severe cases of respiratory failure by infusion of nikethamide, amiphenazole, doxapram or ethamivan (vanillic acid diethylamide). See chapter XX (section 5) for further information on treatment.

Status asthmaticus is the end state of asthma which has failed to respond to usual treatment. It requires intensive drug treatment in hospital (see chapter XX; sect. 3.2). Maintenance of the patient's hydration, humidification of the breathed gases and correction of acid-base disturbances are also of vital importance. Artificial ventilation (using a volume-limited ventilator) with clearance of blocked airways by suction may sometimes be necessary.

8. Pain Relief

Pain is a mode of sensation essential for the protection of the body from damaging influences. However, it may persist after it has played its part in this, and treatment of the pain is then desirable (Bonica, 1974; Katz, 1970).

Pain impulses are carried from their receptors by small unmyelinated C fibres, and by the delta group of A fibres in afferent neurones. They ascend in the spinal cord in the opposite lateral spinothalamic tract to the thalamus and to the cortex, where they are appreciated. This pathway may be modified at several points (fig. 3).

Local anaesthetic drugs (see section 2.5) will block conduction of nervous impulses past the area in which they are placed, and they may be used to block conduction at any point up to spinal cord level. However, they will to a lesser extent

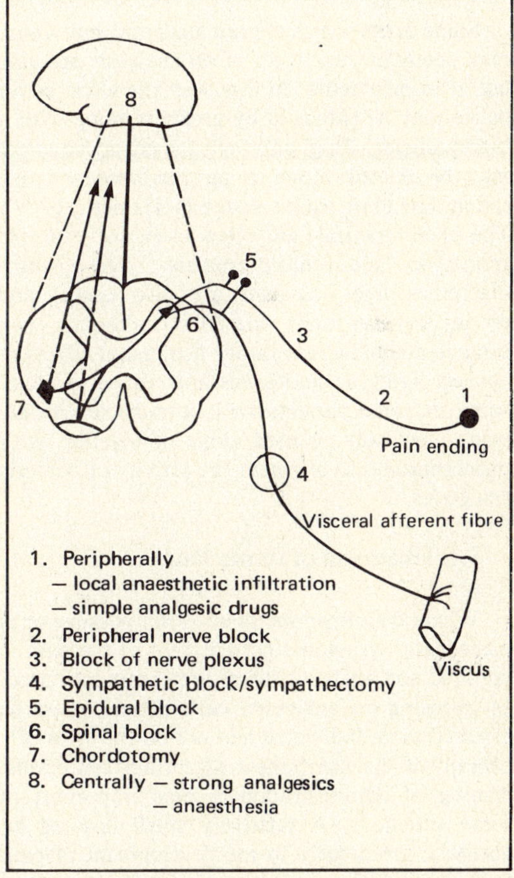

Fig. 3. Simplified concept of pain pathway: Points where it may be interrupted.

also block other modalities of sensation and motor impulses.

Drugs given systemically act by differing mechanisms. These might be taken as being in three groups:

1) Drugs which are not analgesic, but reduce pain by treating its cause — for example glyceryl trinitrate in angina (see chapter XVII; sect. 4.2).
2) Drugs which are analgesics, and act partly peripherally — these include the simple analgesics such as aspirin or paracetamol (acetaminophen).
3) Drugs which act mainly centrally on the perception of pain by the brain — these include morphine and its narcotic analgesic relatives, although there is some evidence that these may have some action at a spinal cord level (Jaffe and Martin, 1975).

Some drugs which are not analgesic, but which may potentiate the effect of an analgesic are also useful in pain relief. In this way the effect of an opiate may be enhanced by giving it along with a 'tranquillising' drug, although the enhanced effect may be related more to an increased sedative action than to increased analgesia (Halpern, 1977). The phenothiazines are often used, for example morphine and chlorpromazine. The benzodiazepines like diazepam are also useful and do not have so many side effects, although they can potentiate the respiratory depressant effects of opiates. Tricyclic antidepressants can also be of value in some patients with intractable chronic pain. They may be used alone or together with phenothiazines to augment the activity of narcotic analgesics.

8.1 Treatment of Acute Pain

Where definitive treatment is not possible or is inadequate, symptomatic treatment of the pain is required and analgesic drugs are commonly used. In choosing an analgesic, each patient must be assessed as an individual and not on the basis of a concept of the painfulness of certain conditions. Timing of administration is also important in some situations. A relatively small dose of an analgesic given early in the development of pain (e.g. postoperative period or after tooth extraction) is usually more effective than a larger dose given when the pain has become severe (Parkhouse, 1975).

In general, where the intensity of pain is not great, simple analgesics (section 8.5; table XI) are indicated, whereas with more intense pain the narcotic analgesics (section 8.4, table IX) will be required (Halpern, 1977). In treating severe acute pain, the intravenous route is often the best initially, as the dose of the drug can be adjusted to the need and side effects seen. When the opiate drugs are given, care must be taken not to cause respiratory depression of a significant degree. The elderly are both more sensitive to the depressant effects of narcotic analgesics and experience more analgesia for a given dose than younger patients (Belville et al., 1971).

Postoperative pain relief is often best achieved by extradural injection of local anaesthetics (Knight and Mehta, 1978), but too extensive or too prolonged a block may lead to hypotension. This method may also be useful after thoracotomy and for chest injuries, as may intravenous lignocaine. Extradural use of morphine has been described by Behar et al. (1979). This preliminary report suggests that pain relief may be obtained without side effects.

Analgesia by inhalational agents is of use in some situations in hospital practice (Baskett and Bennett, 1971). Nitrous oxide/oxygen mixtures are easily self administered from premixed cylinders while methoxyflurane may be given from specially designed vaporisers. These are used in obstetrics and are also used for burns dressings and other painful minor ward procedures.

8.2 Management of Chronic Pain

A number of situations exist where cure of pathology causing pain is not possible and measures to control the pain are required. Cancer patients are the most common group. Management will be by general measures, by systemic drugs, and by local nerve section or block.

8.2.1 General Measures

These are chiefly attention to comfort, explanations, good nursing, and drug treatment of distressing accompaniments such as vomiting etc. For the latter cyclizine (50mg) is reasonably satisfactory, and is less toxic though less effective than phenothiazines such as perphenazine (2 to 5mg), prochlorperazine (10mg) or thiethylperazine (6.5mg).

8.2.2 Administration of Analgesic Drugs

Preferably these should be given orally in adequate dosage, and on a regular dosage schedule. The next dose of an analgesic should be given before the effects of the previous dose have worn off. Analgesics will not remove the pain, but will make it more bearable. Success depends on finding an analgesic which is effective and well tolerated by the patient. The simple analgesics, except perhaps dihydrocodeine, are unlikely to be of use for any length of time and use is made mainly of the narcotics with their attendant problems of tolerance (Twycross, 1975; Halpern, 1977).

The choice of narcotic is largely a matter of personal experience, but best are the longer acting drugs, particularly those with good absorption and activity by the oral route (table IX). Morphine itself is the most widely used narcotic, but others such as levorphanol, methadone and dipipanone may be more suitable because they are effective orally. Oral pentazocine is of lesser effectiveness in severe pain but is suitable for use in pain of moderate severity, provided it is given in adequate dosage (75 to 100mg) — see section 8.4.3. Diamorphine (heroin) is a controversial drug which is claimed by some to be particularly indicated in terminal malignancy. In such cases, potentiation of opiates by other drugs such as alcohol or phenothiazines is useful, and several regimens have been employed.[1] As these are potent preparations they will be used only in the terminal stages (Editorial, 1975).

Specific drug therapy for facial pain is discussed in chapter XXV (sect. 6) and therapy for relief of pain in rheumatic disorders in chapter XXII (sect. 3).

8.2.3 Nerve Blocking

Whereas drug therapy does not completely remove pain an effective nerve block can do so (Mehta, 1973). However, it is not always possible to block the appropriate pain pathway, nor is it possible to block only pain without involving other modes of sensation, and in some cases the loss of sensation may be as distressing as the original pain.

Local anaesthetic drugs (section 2.5) act only for a short time, but surprisingly often the patient experiences pain relief even after the drugs have worn off, so they are worth trying. More permanent blocks are achieved using substances which destroy nerves, such as phenol and alcohol. These are most successful when used intrathecally to block carefully chosen dorsal nerve roots. Any such procedure must only be undertaken after careful consideration of the anatomy of the pain, and of the probable side effects of the block.

8.3 Obstetric Analgesia

Pain associated with childbirth differs from other types of discomfort in that it is intermittent in type and increases in severity as labour progresses. The patient's background, emotional status and her pain threshold are important factors in the response it evokes and this varies markedly. Consequently, set routines of analgesia may satisfy the majority but will leave a small proportion who find labour a very upsetting experience (see Moir, 1976; Scott, 1977).

8.3.1 Narcotic Analgesics

Conventional pain relief is provided by injected drugs given early in labour and, as the time of delivery approaches, inhalation analgesia. Intravenous administration of narcotic analgesics may cause transient high maternal plasma levels of the drug with resultant placental transmission of larger amounts to the baby (see chapter III; sect. 3.1). This effect may be minimised by dilution and very slow injection, or by intramuscular administration.

Pethidine (meperidine) is the most widely used systemic treatment and the average dose of 100mg intramuscularly may be repeated at 2-hourly intervals. However, if given late in labour, or in excessive amounts, depression of the newborn infant may occur (see chapter III; sect. 3.1). Sickness and dizziness are the two most frequent side effects. Almost all of the other potent narcotic analgesic drugs have been used for obstetric pain relief, but none have been shown to possess clear cut advantages over pethidine.

Pentazocine, a newer analgesic with a low abuse liability, offers little better pain relief than pethidine when used intramuscularly. However, if pain is increasing rapidly in severity, it can be given slowly intravenously with minimal side effects in the mother and with less risk to the infant.

---

1   An example is: diamorphine 5 to 10mg; cocaine 10mg; syrup of prochlorperazine 5mg; gin 3.6ml; syrup 7.2ml; aqua chloroform 0.75ml; water to 30ml.

Naloxone is the agent of choice for reversal of respiratory depression in the newborn induced by pethidine or pentazocine (Evans et al., 1976).

8.3.2 Inhalation Analgesia

Inhalational analgesia can be provided by nitrous oxide, trichloroethylene or methoxyflurane and these are usually administered by a non-rebreathing technique from apparatus delivering a fixed concentration. Premixed cylinders containing 50 % nitrous oxide in oxygen are available in some countries. It is difficult to ascertain which particular inhaler provides the best analgesia but all those commonly used have been shown to make the second stage of labour a less painful process.

8.3.3 Extradural Analgesia

For the patient with a low pain threshold, emotional instability, or who may find the process of labour exhausting, extradural analgesia, using the lumbar or sacral approach, will completely remove the pain of labour and the effort of the 2nd stage (Scott, 1977). Bupivacaine (0.5 %) has a duration of effect of 3 hours and has superseded the use of other local anaesthetics (section 2.5.5). Tachyphylaxis (i.e. tolerance to repeat doses) is not a problem when this drug is used and the interval between top up injections can be greatly increased. Hypotension is infrequent if the patient is in the lateral position and intravenous fluids are given to prevent dehydration. Local anaesthetics readily cross the placenta with potential risk of toxicity in the fetus and neonate (Ralston and Shnider, 1978; see also chapter III; sect. 4.1). Although bupivacaine has relatively little effect on the fetus, it should be given in the smallest effective volume and lowest concentration (0.25 to 0.5 %); doses being adjusted according to the patient's weight. Fetal acidosis favours increased drug ionisation, and thus, since it is the unionised form which crosses the placenta and is in equilibrium, this leads to accumulation of local anaesthetics in acidic compartments and increases the risk of CNS and cardiac toxicity (Dodson, 1976). Extradural techniques require the services of a skilled anaesthetist and the institution of a 24-hour service can be both demanding and expensive.

While the obstetrician can do much to relieve labour discomfort by the use of drugs, it should be remembered that antenatal training, sympathetic understanding and constant reassurance can do much to help the patient. The benefit of cheerful and understanding company for the patient during labour cannot be over emphasised. The effect of labour and delivery on the disposition of drugs is discussed in chapter XV (sect. 1.1.6).

8.4 The Narcotic Analgesics

Actions: Receptor sites exist in the brain and elsewhere, at which opiates such as morphine act to produce analgesia and their other effects. There also exist within the body naturally occurring 'opiate-like' substances, endorphins or more specifically enkephalins, which normally use these receptor sites (Hughes and Kosterlitz, 1977). All the details of the actions of the opiates, and their antagonists cannot be explained on the basis of actions and interactions at one receptor site, so there is probably more than one type of receptor (or the receptor may exist in more than one state), and one hypothesis uses three receptors to explain these complex relationships (see section 8.4.3). The various actions of morphine and related drugs are discussed in section 8.4.1.

Pharmacokinetic Properties: The narcotic analgesics are extensively metabolised in the liver and are sensitive to changes in hepatic blood flow for their elimination (Blaschke, 1977). Morphine, pethidine and pentazocine undergo significant hepatic first-pass metabolism (see chapter I; sect. 3.3.3) following oral administration, such that bioavailability is low and variable: indeed, hepatic first-pass metabolism is so marked with morphine that it cannot be effectively given orally. These and other analgesics such as methadone also display wide interindividual variability in plasma concentrations and rates of elimination following parenteral administration (Berkowitz, 1976; Ehrnebo et al., 1977; Mather and Meffin, 1978). Such individual differences in systemic availability and elimination rate, combined with wide variation in pain perception, emphasises the need to use individualised dosage schedules of narcotic analgesics.

Although elimination of pethidine is delayed and bioavailability is increased in patients with cirrhosis, oral dosage may not need to be reduced because common oral dosage regimens probably produce subanalgesic plasma concentrations (Mather and Meffin, 1978). Certain cirrhotic patients are however, susceptible to the depressant effects of opiates such as morphine (see chapter XIX; sect. 13.4). All the narcotic analgesics are

Table IX. Properties and principal uses of the narcotic analgesics

Drug	Usual intra-muscular dosage[1] (mg)	Duration of single i.m. dose (hours)	Oral efficacy for severe pain	Usual oral dosage[1] (mg)	Principal indication(s)[2]	Main adverse effects and interactions[3]
Natural opiates						
Morphine	8-16	4-6	Poor	—	Chronic pain, myocardial infarction	Dependence; nausea, vomiting; MAOI (see sect. 6.2.1)
Papaveretum	20	3-4	Poor	—		
Semi-synthetic						
Diamorphine (heroin)	4-8	2	Poor	5-10	Chronic pain, terminal malignancy	
Dihydro-morphinone	1-2	2-4				
Oxymorphone	1-3	4-6	—	—		
Oxycodone	10	4-6	Good	5-20		
Synthetic						
Anileridine	30-60	2-3	Good	25		
Buprenorphine	0.3-0.6	6-8	Good (sub-lingual)	0.4-0.8		Low dependence liability
Butorphanol	1-4	3-4	Good	4-8		Low dependence liability
Dextromoramide	5-8	2-3	Good	5-10		
Dipipanone	10-25	5-6	Good	10-25	Terminal pain	
Levorphanol	2-4	4-6	Good	1.5-4.5	Postoperative pain	
Methadone	5-15	6-8	Good	5-10	Postoperative pain, chronic pain	
Pentazocine	20-40	2-4	Fair	75-100	Labour, postoperative pain, moderately severe chronic pain	Low dependence liability; but inappropiate use has led to abuse; hallucinations; MAOI
Pethidine (meperidine)	75-125	2-3	Poor	50-100	Labour, premedication, renal and biliary colic, acute pancreatitis	MAOI (avoid; see section 6.2.1); phenobarbitone increases formation of toxic metabolite, norpethidine
Phenazocine	2-4	4-6	Good (sub-lingual)	10-20		
Piritramide	15-20	6-8	—	—		More soporific than morphine; fewer emetic complications

1   Dosage should be reduced:
    a)   if any respiratory depressant has been given
    b)   in patients with reduced respiratory reserve
    c)   in the elderly (see section 8.1)
    d)   in neonates and infants under 12m (older infants and children tolerate opiates well) — see table V
    e)   in patients with impaired renal function, especially methadone. Some patients with uraemia are extremely sensitive to depressant effects of strong analgesics (see appendix E)
    f)   in patients with severe liver disease (see also chapter XIX; sect. 1.4, 13.4)
  In the presence of hypovolaemia (e.g. after surgery, burns victim, trauma), give analgesic by cautious intravenous administration. Intramuscularly administered medication may be poorly absorbed.

2   Indications given are those where drugs are generally first choices. Other agents can be used as alternatives for specified indications. See also section 8.1 and 8.2.

3   Side effects of morphine apply to all other narcotic analgesics. See also section 8.3, 8.4 and appendices B, C.

eliminated by hepatic metabolism, but methadone (a variable proportion, up to 20% or more, of which is excreted unchanged in the urine) and a toxic (convulsive) metabolite of pethidine, (norpethidine), may accumulate in renal failure (see chapter XXI; sect. 14.4.6). Phenobarbitone, and presumably other enzyme inducing agents, by increasing the formation of norpethidine may lead to enhanced toxicity (Stambaugh et al., 1977; 1978). Narcotic analgesics such as pethidine, diamorphine (heroin) and pentazocine can produce a marked delay in gastric emptying and have the potential to alter absorption of other orally administered drugs (see chapter VIII; sect. 2.3.1). Dosage of narcotic analgesics should be reduced in the elderly not only because of increased 'sensitivity' (see section 8.1), but also because of increased plasma concentrations, as shown with morphine and pethidine (Berkowitz, 1976; Mather and Meffin, 1978). Neonates are also 'sensitive' to the effects of narcotic analgesics, probably only in small part due to impaired elimination (see section 3.1). The pharmacokinetic properties of individual narcotic analgesics are summarised in appendix A.

8.4.1 Morphine and Other Opiates

Morphine is the standard with which other narcotic analgesics are compared (Loan and Morrison, 1973; table IX). It causes analgesia due to a central action on pain perception, rather than a peripheral action, and it also causes drowsiness and euphoria (though sometimes dysphoria, particularly in those who are free of pain — such as preoperative patients). It depresses respiration, mainly by reducing the response to carbon dioxide, and overdose is characterised by extremely low respiratory rates. Stimulation of the vomiting centre leads to prolonged nausea or vomiting in a proportion of patients.

Morphine and related drugs strongly inhibit gastric emptying and decrease intestinal motility. Gastric, pancreatic and biliary secretions are decreased. The effects on intestinal motility can result in marked constipation or may impair the absorption of orally administered drugs (see chapter VIII; sect. 2.3.1). The tone in the anal and ileocolic sphincters and in the sphincter of Oddi is increased and marked rises in biliary pressure may occur, even to the extent of causing biliary colic. Ureteric tone and contractions are increased, as is the tone of the detrusor muscle which in association with increased tone of the vesicular sphincter

occasionally causes difficulty in micturition. Bronchoconstriction may follow large doses of morphine but this effect is rarely seen after therapeutic doses. All these effects on smooth muscle tone are quantitatively less with pethidine.

Ordinary doses of narcotic analgesics have no major effects on heart rate or blood pressure in normal subjects, although postural hypotension may occur with morphine as a result of venous pooling due to peripheral vasodilatation. This may in part be due to histamine release. Dilatation of the skin and blood vessels of the face may cause itching and sweating. Morphine and diamorphine (heroin) have little effect on the haemodynamic status of patients with acute myocardial infarction, whereas pethidine may cause a decrease in arterial blood pressure and pentazocine an increase in arterial and pulmonary artery pressure and in left ventricular minute work (see chapter XVII; sect. 5.1.1).

As is well known, morphine and its relatives are drugs of dependence, and although this is not a problem in short term treatment, such as in relief of postoperative pain, dependence, with the consequent requirement for increasing doses of the drug becomes a serious difficulty in treating chronic pain (section 8.2).

Heroin (diamorphine) is more potent than morphine (5mg equivalent to morphine 10mg), has an earlier onset of action, but a shorter duration of action and greater dependence potential. It is unstable in solution and should be freshly prepared before use.

Levorphanol (2mg = morphine 10mg) causes slightly less nausea than morphine. It and *methadone* (10mg) are probably the best of this group of drugs for postoperative pain relief.

Pethidine or meperidine (75 to 100mg = morphine 10mg) is very popular in premedication, but it is relatively toxic, causing more nausea and vomiting and more hypotension than most opiate drugs. It is also more soporific and has a very short, but intense action with a rapid onset. Bioavailability after oral and intramuscular administration is variable. As it has some antispasmodic activity it may be the analgesic of choice in renal colic, biliary colic and acute pancreatitis. Important pharmacokinetic properties of pethidine and situations in which dosage should be modified are summarised above (for review, see Mather and Meffin, 1978) and interactions with other drugs in table IX and appendix C.

Table X. Characteristics of the pharmacological actions of the μ, κ and σ receptors and their postulated relative role in the actions of mixed agonists and antagonists (modified from Martin et al., 1976)

Drug	Receptor type and some characteristics		
	μ (Morphine)	κ	σ
	analgesia morphine dependence	analgesia	delirium
Agonist Morphine	High affinity High activity	Moderate affinity High activity	No activity
Partial agonist Buprenorphine Butorphanol	High affinity Low activity		No activity
Agonist-antagonist Pentazocine	Low affinity No activity	Low affinity High activity	Low affinity High activity
Nalorphine	High affinity No activity	High affinity Low activity	Low affinity Low activity

8.4.2 Fentanyl and Phenoperidine

These drugs were developed primarily for the technique of neuroleptanalgesia (see section 2.3.1). They differ from other opiates chiefly in having a short duration of action — 20 to 30 minutes for fentanyl compared with 3 to 4 hours for pethidine or 4 to 6 hours for morphine. Doses of 0.2mg fentanyl or 2mg phenoperidine are roughly equivalent to morphine 10mg. Although they produce marked respiratory depression, because of their short action they can be given in relatively high dosage during anaesthesia, thus achieving intense analgesia with minimal postoperative respiratory effects. Excessive respiratory depression during anaesthesia can be antagonised by naloxone, and this may be necessary postoperatively, as the respiratory depressant action may outlast analgesia (see section 2.1.1).

8.4.3 Narcotic Agonist-Antagonist Drugs

Because of the dependence potential of all the opiate drugs, much research has been carried out to discover powerful analgesics without this drawback (Isbell, 1977). Studies of the actions of the endogenous 'opiate-like' substances or enkephalins (Hughes and Kosterlitz, 1977) and of the actions and interactions of opiate and related drugs, indicate that there may be multiple types of opioid receptors, and therefore that it may prove possible to separate wanted and unwanted effects. An apparently simple view of opiate actions is to regard them as having a spectrum of activity ranging from pure agonist activity (morphine) through partial agonists (buprenorphine, butorphanol) or agonist-antagonists such as pentazocine, with nalorphine and levallorphan more specific as antagonists, and at the end of the scale, pure antagonist drugs like naloxone, with affinity for the receptor but no agonist activity. However, this does not explain all the complex relationships between the drugs, and one theory (Martin et al., 1976) postulates three types of receptors, μ, κ and σ (table X). Morphine acts at the μ receptor to cause analgesia, respiratory depression, dependence, etc, and also has a slight action at the κ receptor to cause analgesia and sedation. A partial agonist such as buprenorphine acts likewise, but can cause some antagonism to morphine by displacing it at the receptor (because its intrinsic activity is less — i.e. more molecules of buprenorphine than of morphine are needed for the same effect). Nalorphine is a powerful antagonist, having a high affinity for the μ receptor, but no agonist activity, but it does have agonist activity at the κ receptor, causing analgesia and respiratory depression but without dependence. It is not clinically useful as an analgesic drug because of hallucinations and other psychological effects, which may be due to activity at a third, σ receptor.

Pentazocine was the first clinically useful result of research into the chemical relatives of the opioid antagonists, being a powerful analgesic (Brogden et al., 1973). It shares the hallucinatory side effect potential of nalorphine and levallorphan, and many of the side effects of the opiates, though it causes less nausea than most. However, pentazocine is for practical purposes non-dependence producing, and so is free of the restrictions and limitations applied to the opiates (Kelly, 1977), although inappropriate use has led to its reclassification as a drug of high abuse potential in some states in the USA (Annexton, 1978). Consequently it is useful in the treatment of chronic pain of moderate severity, particularly as it can be administered orally in large doses (75 to 100mg) with fairly reliable results. Its use in acute myocardial infarction is controversial as its effects on the cardiovascular system, in contrast to morphine, lead to an increased work load on the heart. For this reason, morphine or heroin is still preferred by some, but the theoretically adverse haemodynamic effects of pentazocine should not prevent its use by paramedical personnel in coronary care ambulances (see chapter XVII; sect. 5.1.1).

Buprenorphine is a new drug related to morphine, but with some antagonist activity (Heel et al., 1979). It is a powerful analgesic, 0.3 to 0.6mg being equivalent to morphine 10 to 15mg. It has a longer duration of action than morphine, and the incidence of side effects such as nausea is relatively low. Like pentazocine, dependence liability is likely to be low, but unlike pentazocine, hallucinatory effects are not a feature. Respiratory depression occurs as with other narcotic analgesics, and is not antagonised by nalorphine and levallorphan, and only partly by naloxone. It can be treated with the nonspecific respiratory stimulant, doxapram; in view of the prolonged action of buprenorphine, a doxapram infusion is preferred to a single administration.

Butorphanol is another new analgesic with agonist-antagonist activity (Heel et al., 1978). Butorphanol 1 to 4mg would seem to give similar analgesia to the normal clinically used doses of pentazocine, pethidine or morphine. It may produce fewer psychotomimetic side effects than pentazocine, and shares with it the advantage of a flatter dose-response curve for respiratory depression than morphine (i.e. at higher doses the degree of respiratory depression does not appear to increase as it would with morphine). As with buprenorphine, dependence liability is likely to be low.

Meptazinol, another analgesic which also has opiate antagonist properties, appears to be about equipotent with pethidine on a weight-for-weight basis and produces a similar profile of side effects (Paymaster, 1977).

8.4.4 Narcotic Antagonists

The *N*-allyl derivatives of the opiates, nalorphine and levallorphan, have been used for some time to antagonise overdosage of the opiates (Martin, 1967). Naloxone, the *N*-allyl derivative of oxymorphone, is more potent than nalorphine or levallorphan, and longer lasting than the latter. Unlike them it is a pure antagonist with little or no intrinsic narcotic activity. It is capable of reversing the actions (including analgesia) of relatively large doses of any narcotic and is the only specific antagonist to pentazocine, although it will only partially antagonise buprenorphine. It is able also to antagonise the emetic effect of pethidine (meperidine). Since the action of naloxone is short, repeated doses may be necessary with most narcotics. Naltrexone, an investigational drug, has a longer duration of action. Because a large dose may arouse the patient, it is probably best given in small intravenous increments in order to obtain a suitable balance between reversal of ventilatory depression and maintenance of analgesia (Martin, 1976). Alternatively, the respiratory stimulant drug doxapram, which will not antagonise analgesia, may be used.

These drugs probably act mainly by competing for drug receptor sites, but this is not a complete explanation of their mechanism of action. Since nalorphine and levallorphan do have some analgesic effects of their own, combinations such as pethidine + levallorphan have been quite widely used, but are less potent than pethidine alone, and have never been convincingly shown to have an advantage over the opiate alone. Mixtures with naloxone have also been used in labour in an attempt to avoid respiratory depression of the newborn, but these also reverse much of the analgesic effect of the opiate.

8.5 Simple Analgesics

Some of the less potent compounds related to morphine (codeine, dihydrocodeine, dextropropox-

Table XI. Properties and principal uses of the simple analgesics

Drug	Usual oral dosage[1] (mg)	Principal indications[2]	Main adverse effects and interactions[3]	Dependence liability
Peripherally acting				
Aspirin	300-600	Continuous, aching pain; acute pain of bone, joint trauma, tissue inflammation	Gastric irritation, haemorrhage; ? nephropathy (long term abuse); inhibits platelet aggregation (see chapter XXII; sect. 3.2.1)	Nil
Paracetamol (acetaminophen)	500-1,000	Pain, fever in children; alternative to aspirin	Hepatic necrosis (overdosage)	Nil
Phenacetin	—		Nephropathy (long term abuse); methaemoglobinaemia	Nil
Centrally acting				
Codeine	30-60	Visceral pain; cough with pain; synergistic with aspirin	Nausea, vomiting, dizziness, constipation	Low (morphine-like)
Dihydrocodeine	30-60	Moderately severe chronic pain	As for codeine (? better tolerated)	Low (morphine-like)
Dextropro-poxyphene	65-100	Visceral pain	Nausea, vomiting, dizziness, skin rash; coma, convulsions, respiratory depression (overdosage)	Low (morphine-like)

1   See chapter IV (table XI) for dosage in infants and children.
2   Indications given are those where drugs are generally first choices. See also section 8.5.
3   Refer also section 8.5 and appendices B, C.

yphene, ethoheptazine etc) may be used in the treatment of less severe pain. However, drugs mostly used for this purpose (e.g. aspirin, paracetamol) are unrelated to these, and act at peripheral sites to reduce pain (table XI). They are sometimes termed 'mild' analgesics, but this does not imply that they have no role in more severe pain. Indeed, some acute conditions, particularly those involving tissue inflammation or bone and joint trauma, may produce extremely severe pain which responds well to simple analgesics. Their use in postoperative pain is limited by the fear of inducing gastrointestinal irritation, or of interference with blood coagulation which may occur with aspirin and other non-steroidal anti-inflammatory analgesics. All analgesics, and particularly the simple analgesics, tend to be more effective against continuous, aching pain than against sudden, sharp pain or acute exacerbation. Aspirin and paracetamol tend to be much less effective against viscerally engendered pain than centrally acting drugs such as codeine and dextropropoxyphene (Parkhouse, 1975). Comparative evaluation of mild analgesics is difficult, and well designed and controlled trials have been conspicuously rare, particularly in view of the widespread use of these drugs. Moertel et al. (1972) could detect no difference between several popular drugs and placebo, while none was superior to aspirin; illustrating the difficulty of assessment of pain relief (Lasagna, 1977).

8.5.1 Aspirin

Aspirin has analgesic, antipyretic and anti-inflammatory properties, all of which can be explained as due to inhibition of prostaglandin synthesis (Ferreira and Vane, 1974). The analgesic action occurs peripherally, while the antipyretic activity is central. Its anti-inflammatory action and pharmacokinetic properties are discussed in chapter XXII (sect. 3.2). In usual therapeutic doses aspirin has no significant effects on the circulation or respiration. Overdose, however, is characterised by hyperventilation and respiratory alkalosis, and later by a metabolic acidosis, which is seen particularly in children with fever and dehydration (see chapter IV; sect. 2.4). In a small minority of patients, aspirin may cause serious gastric irritation and occasionally profuse gastric bleeding (see chapt. XIX; sect. 14.2.2). Because of its effect on platelet aggregation, a history of abnormal bleeding should demand caution in use of aspirin (see chapter XXIII; sect. 7.3). A few patients are allergic to aspirin, particularly asthmatics (see chapter XX; sect. 11.3) and those with allergic rhinitis. Despite these uncommon reactions, aspirin remains a very valuable and generally safe analgesic (Koch-Weser, 1976).

8.5.2 Paracetamol (acetaminophen)

Paracetamol also exerts its analgesic effect by a peripheral action. It is comparable to, and is used as an alternative to aspirin, particularly in children (Committee on Drugs, 1978). Gastrointestinal tolerance is better than aspirin, and paracetamol is preferable to aspirin in patients with a bleeding tendency and in those on coumarin anticoagulants (see chapter XXIII; sect. 3.2.5, 7.3). Prolonged use may lead to renal dysfunction. Overdose of paracetamol often leads to severe hepatic damage due to formation of a toxic metabolite (see chapter IX; sect. 6.3), but can also occur with prolonged use of normal doses (Johnson and Tolman, 1977). For a review of the properties and use of paracetamol, see Koch-Weser (1976).

8.5.3 Codeine

Codeine, a naturally occurring constituent of opium, shares the characteristic pharmacological properties of morphine. Indeed, metabolically produced morphine may influence or be responsible for the analgesic efficacy of codeine (Findlay et al., 1978). It is much less potent than morphine but can be given orally (32mg approx. equivalent to 600mg aspirin) and has a considerably lower dependence liability. Combination of codeine and aspirin has a synergistic analgesic effect. Codeine is particularly valuable for pain associated with coughing. Its main side effects are nausea, dizziness and drowsiness and sometimes vomiting.

8.5.4 Dextropropoxyphene

Dextropropoxyphene (propoxyphene), which is structurally related to the methadone group of compounds, has rather less analgesic activity than codeine. Side effects are similar to but more marked than with codeine, and skin rashes are more common. Dosage of dextropropoxyphene should probably be reduced in patients with renal failure due to accumulation of a potentially toxic metabolite, norpropoxyphene (Gibson et al., 1977). Recent reports of respiratory failure and convulsions as a result of dextropropoxyphene overdosage have been disturbing in view of its wide use as a mild analgesic, although the respiratory depression can be antagonised by naloxone. Complications following overdosage of combinations of dextropropoxyphene and paracetamol are particularly difficult to manage; the clinical features of overdose due to dextropropoxyphene occurring very early or before late liver damage caused by paracetamol overdosage (Whittington, 1977). Dependence of the morphine type can occur, the incidence probably being less or about the same as with codeine. For reviews on the properties and efficacy of dextropropoxyphene, see Miller (1977) and Lasagna (1977).

8.5.5 Dihydrocodeine

Dihydrocodeine also has many features in common with codeine, but can sometimes be very useful in moderately severe chronic pain, including that of malignancy, without producing side effects other than obstinate constipation. It has a similar dependence liability to codeine (Eddy et al., 1970).

8.5.6 New Analgesics

Several new analgesics have been synthesised and reports on floctafenine, nefopam and diflunisal are encouraging.

Floctafenine, a hydroxyquinoline derivative, 200mg gives comparable analgesia to other mild analgesics, and has been reported to cause fewer side effects (Lomas et al., 1976).

Nefopam, a benzoxazocine derivative, is effective orally (60mg = aspirin 600mg) or intramuscularly (15 to 30mg), when it may give analgesia comparable to some of the narcotic analgesics. It does not have respiratory depressant effects and does not cause gastrointestinal blood loss. Its site of action is uncertain (Beaver and Feise, 1977; Baltes, 1977).

Diflunisal, a salicylic acid derivative, 250 to 500mg has analgesic activity comparable with aspirin 500 to 750mg, but causes fewer gastrointestinal and other side effects. It also has anti-inflammatory activity but does not affect bleeding time or platelet function at normal analgesic blood levels, although it can enhance the action of coumarin anticoagulants such as acenocoumarol (nicoumalone). It is highly protein bound (98 to

99%) and is eliminated almost completely in the urine as unchanged drug or mainly as the glucuronide metabolite and has a long elimination half-life (8 to 12 hours), permitting twice daily dosage in conditions such as osteoarthritis (Symposium, 1977, 1978). Elimination of unchanged drug is prolonged in patients with impaired renal function, necessitating reduction of usual dosage (Verbeeck et al., 1979).

Further Reading

Covino, B.G. and Vassalo, H.G.: Local Anesthetics: Mechanisms of Action and Clinical Use (Grune and Stratton, New York 1976).

Dundee, J.W. and Wyant, G.M.: Intravenous Anaesthesia (Churchill Livingstone, Edinburgh 1974).

Various Authors: Symposium on anesthesia and clinical pharmacology. Anesthesiology 35: 111 (1971).

Vickers, M.D.; Wood-Smith, F.G. and Stewart, H.C.: Drugs in Anaesthetic Practice, 5th ed (Butterworths, London 1978).

Wylie, W.D. and Churchill-Davidson, H.C.: A Practice of Anaesthesia, 3rd ed (Lloyd-Luke, London 1972).

Zorab, J. and Baskett, P.: Immediate Care (Saunders, Philadelphia 1977).

References

Adams, A.P. and Pybus, D.A.: Delayed respiratory depression after use of fentanyl during anaesthesia. British Medical Journal 1; 278 (1978).

Adriani, J.: Adverse responses due to allergy and drug interactions during otorhinolaryngologic procedures. Southern Medical Journal 63: 537 (1970).

Aldrete, J.A.; Clapp, H.W.; Fishman, J. and O'Higgins, J.W.: 'Pentazepam': A supplementary agent. Anaesthesia and Analgesia: Current Researches 50: 498 (1971).

Ali, H.H. and Savarese, J.J.: Monitoring of neuromuscular function. Anesthesiology 45: 216 (1976).

Anderson, W.G.: Respiratory aspects of the preoperative examination. British Journal of Anaesthesia 46: 549 (1974).

Annexton, M.: Pentazocine reclassified in Illinois. Journal of the American Medical Association 240: 2234 (1978).

Assaf, R.A.E.; Dundee, J.W. and Gamble, J.A.S.: Influence of the route of administration of the clinical action of diazepam. Anaesthesia 30: 152 (1975).

Austin, K.L. and Denborough, M.A.: Drug treatment of malignant hyperpyrexia. Anaesthesia and Intensive Care 5: 207 (1977).

Bali, I.M.; Dundee, J.W. and Doggart, J.R.: The source of increased plasma potassium following succinylcholine. Anaesthesia and Analgesia: Current Researches 54: 680 (1975).

Baltes, B.J.: Gastrointestinal blood loss study with a new analgesic compound: nefopam hydrochloride. Journal of Clinical Pharmacology 17: 120 (1977).

Baskett, P.J.F. and Bennett, J.A.: Pain relief in hospital: The more widespread use of nitrous oxide. British Medical Journal 2: 509 (1971).

Beaver, W.T. and Feise, G.A.: A comparison of the analgesic effect of intramuscular nefopam and morphine in patients with postoperative pain. Journal of Clinical Pharmacology 17(pt.1): 579 (1977).

Behar, M.; Magora, F.; Olshwang, D. and Davidson, J.T.: Epidural morphine in treatment of pain. Lancet 1: 527 (1979).

Belville, J.W.; Forrest, W.H.; Miller, E. and Brown, B.W.: Influence of age on pain relief from analgesics. Journal of the American Medical Association 217: 1835 (1971).

Bennett, E.J.; Ignancio, A.; Patel, K.; Grundy, E.M. and Salem, M.R.: Tubocurarine and the neonate. British Journal of Anaesthesia 48: 687 (1976).

Berkowitz, B.A.: The relationship of pharmacokinetics to pharmacological activity: Morphine, methadone and naloxone. Clinical Pharmacokinetics 1: 219 (1976).

Black, G.W.: Effects of cyclopropane, halothane and methoxyflurane on the peripheral circulation; in Eckenhoff (Ed) Science and Practice in Anesthesia, p.53 (Lippincott, Philadelphia 1965).

Blaschke, T.F.: Protein binding and kinetics of drugs in liver diseases. Clinical Pharmacokinetics 2: 32 (1977).

Boakes, A.J.; Laurence, D.R.; Teoh, P.C.; Barar, F.S.K.; Benedikter, L.T. and Prichard, B.N.C.: Interactions between sympathomimetic amines and antidepressant agents in man. British Medical Journal 1: 311 (1973).

Bodman, R.I.: Pancuronium and histamine release. Canadian Anaesthetists Society Journal 25: 40 (1978).

Bonica, J.J.: International Symposium on pain. Advances in Neurology, vol. 4 (Raven Press, New York 1974).

Booth, P.N.; Watson, M.J. and McLeod, K.: Pancuronium and the placental barrier. Anaesthesia 32: 320 (1977).

Boyes, R.N.: A review of the metabolism of amide local anaesthetic agents. British Journal of Anaesthesia 47: 225 (1975).

Brebner, J. and Hadley, L.: Experiences with physostigmine in the reversal of adverse post-anaesthetic effects. Canadian Anaesthetists Society Journal 23: 574 (1976).

Breimer, D.D.: Pharmacokinetics of methohexitone following intravenous infusion in humans. British Journal of Anaesthesia 48: 643 (1976).

Britt, B.A.: Malignant hyperthermia. Clinical Anesthesia 11: 61 (1975).

Britt. B.A. and Kalow, W.: Malignant hyperthermia: A statistical review. Canadian Anaesthetists' Society Journal 17: 293 (1970).

Brogden, R.N.; Speight, T.M. and Avery, G.S.: Pentazocine: A review of its pharmacological properties, therapeutic efficacy and dependence liability. Drugs 5: 6 (1973).

Brogden, R.N.; Speight, T.M. and Avery, G.S.: Alfathesin: A Review. Drugs 8: 87 (1974).

Bromage, P.R.: A comparison of the hydrochloride and carbon dioxide salts of lidocaine and prilocaine. Acta Anaesthesiologica Scandinavica Suppl. 16: 55 (1965).

Brown, T.C.K.: Paediatric pharmacology. Anaesthesia and Intensive Care 1: 473 (1973).

Bruce, D.L.; Eide, K.A.; Smith, N.J.; Seltzer, F. and Dykes, M.H.M.: A prospective survey of anesthesiologist mortality, 1967-1971. Anesthesiology 41: 71 (1974).

Buzello, W. and Agoston, S.: Pharmacokinetics of pancuronium in patients with normal and impaired renal function. Anaesthesist 27: 291 (1978).

Cascorbi, H.F.; Blake, D.A. and Helrich, M.: Differences in biotransformation of halothane in man. Anesthesiology 32: 119 (1970).

Cascorbi, H.F.: Biotransformation of drugs used in anaesthesia. Anesthesiology 39: 115 (1973).

Change, T. and Glazko, T.: Biotransformation and distribution of ketamine. International Anesthesia Clinics 12: 157 (1974).

Clark, J.M. and Lambertsen, C.J.: Pulmonary oxygen toxicity: A review. Pharmacological Reviews 23: 37 (1971).

Clark, R.S.J.; Doggart, J.R. and Lavery, T.: Changes in liver function after different types of surgery. British Journal of Anaesthesia 48: 119 (1976).

Clarke, R.S.J.: Newer intravenous anesthetics. International Anesthesiology Clinics 7: No. 1 (1969).

Clarke, R.S.J.: Hypersensitivity reactions to intravenous anaesthetics; in Dundee (Ed) Current Concepts in Intravenous Anaesthesia (Saunders, London 1979).

Clarke, I.M.C. and Ellis, F.R.: An evaluation of procaine in the treatment of malignant hyperpyrexia. British Journal of Anaesthesia 47: 17 (1975).

Clarke, R.S.J.; Dundee, J.W. and Daw, R.H.: Clinical studies of induction agents XI: The influence of some intravenous anaesthetics on the respiratory effects and sequelae of suxamethonium. Br. J. Anaesth. 36: 307 (1964).

Clarke, R.S.J.; Fee, J.P.H.; and Dundee, J.W.: Factors predisposing to hypersensitivity reactions to intravenous anaesthetics. Proceedings of the Royal Society of Medicine 70: 782 (1977).

Cohen, E.N.: Metabolism of volatile anesthetics. Anesthesiology 35: 193 (1971).

Cohen, E.N.: Toxicity of inhalational anesthetic agents. British Journal of Anaesthesia 50: 665 (1978).

Cole, P.: The safe use of sodium nitroprusside. Anaesthesia 33: 473 (1978).

Committee on Anesthesia, National Academy of Sciences National Research Council: Summary of the national halothane study. Possible association between halothane, anesthesia and postoperative hepatic necrosis. Journal of the American Medical Association 197: 775 (1966).

Committee on Anesthesia, National Academy of Sciences-National Research Council: Statement regarding the role of methoxyflurane in the production of renal dysfunction. Anesthesiology 34: 505 (1971).

Committee on Drugs American Academy of Pediatrics: Commentary on acetaminophen. Pediatrics 61: 108 (1978).

Cook, D.R.: Paediatric anaesthesia: Pharmacological considerations. Drugs 12: 212 (1976).

Cook, D.R. and Fischer, C.G.: Neuromuscular blocking effects of succinylcholine in infants and children. Anesthesiology 42: 662 (1975).

Cooperman, L.H.: Succinylcholine-induced hyperkalaemia in neuromuscular disease. Journal of the American Medical Association 213: 1867 (1970).

Cottrell, J.E.; Patel, K.; Casthely, P.; Klein, A. and Turndorf, H.: Nitroprusside tachyphylaxis without acidosis. Anesthesiology 49: 141 (1978).

Cottrell, J.E.; Casthely, P.; Brodie, J.D.; Klein, A. and Turndorf, H.: Prevention of nitroprusside-induced cyanide toxicity with hydroxocobalamin. New England Journal of Medicine 298: 809 (1978).

Cousins, M.J. and Mazze, R.I.: Methoxyflurane nephrotoxicity: A study of dose response in man. Journal of the American Medical Association 225: 1611 (1973).

Cousins, M.J.; Mazze, R.I. and Kosek, J.C.: The etiology of methoxyflurane nephrotoxicity. Journal of Pharmacology and Experimental Therapeutics 190: 530 (1974).

Cousins, M.J.; Greenstein, L.R.; Hitt, B.A. and Mazze, R.I.: Metabolism and renal effects of enflurane in man. Anesthesiology 44: 44 (1976).

Covino, B.G.: Local anesthesia. New England Journal of Medicine 286: 975, 1035 (1972).

Csogor, S.I. and Kerek, S.F.: Enhancement of thiopentone anaesthesia by sulphafurazole. British Journal of Anaesthesia 42: 988 (1970).

Davie, I.T.: Specific drug interactions in anaesthesia. Anaesthesia 32: 1000 (1977).

de Jong, R.H.: Toxic effects of local anesthetics. Journal of the American Medical Association 239: 1166 (1978).

Dodson, W.E.: Neonatal drug intoxication: Local anesthetics. Pedicatric Clinics of North America 23: 399 (1976).

Doenicke, A.: Etomidate, a new intravenous hypnotic. Acta Anaesthesia Belgica 25: 307 (1974).

Dripps, R.D.: Objective analysis of a medical specialty: The anaesthesia survey; in White (Ed) Medical Education and Anaesthesia, p. 1 (Blackwell, Oxford 1966).

Dundee, J.W.: Thiopentone and Other Thiobarbiturates (Livingstone, Edinburgh 1956).

Dundee, J.W.: Editorial: Hypersensitivity to intravenous anaesthetic agents. Br. J. Anaesth. 48: 57 (1976).

Dundee, J.W. and McCaughey, W.: Interaction of drugs associated with anaesthesia; in Hewer (Ed) Recent Advances in Anaesthesia, 11th ed (Churchill, London 1972).

Dundee, J.W.; McGowan, W.A.W.; Lilburn, J.K.; McKay, A.C. and Hegarty, J.E.: Comparison of the actions of diazepam and lorazepam. Brit. J. Anaesth. 51: 439 (1979).

Dundee, J.W. and Pandit, S.K.: Anterograde amnesic effects of pethidine, hyoscine and diazepam in adults. British Journal of Pharmacology 44: 140 (1972).

Dundee, J.W. and Wyant, G.M.: Intravenous Anaesthesia (Churchill Livingstone, Edinburgh 1974).

Dundee, J.W. and Zacharias, M.: Etomidate: in Dundee (Ed) Current Topics in Anaesthesia: Intravenous Anaesthetic Agents (Arnold, London 1979).

Dundee, J.W.; Varadarajan, C.R.; Gaston, J.H. and Clarke, R.S.J.: Clinical studies of induction agents XLIII: Flunitrazepam. British Journal of Anaesthesia 48: 551 (1976).

Dundee, J.W.; Black, G.W.; Johnston, S.B. and Fee, J.P.H.: Liver function following repeat anaesthesia. Paper read at 5th European Congress of Anaesthesiology, Paris (1978).

Duvaldestin, P.; Agoston, S.; Henzel, D.; Kersten, U.W. and Desmonts, J.M.: Pancuronium pharmacokinetics in patients with liver cirrhosis. British Journal of Anaesthesia 50: 1131 (1978a).

Duvaldestin, P.; Demetriou, M.; Henzel, D. and Desmonts, J.M.: The placental transfer of pancuronium and its pharmacokinetics during caesarian section. Acta Anaesthesiologica Scandinavica 22: 327 (1978b).

Eddy, N.B.; Friebel, H.; Hahn, K-J, and Halbach, H.: Codeine and its alternatives for pain and cough relief (World Health Organisation, Geneva 1970).

Editorial: The pulmonary toxicity of oxygen. British Journal of Anaesthesia 46: 325 (1974).

Editorial: Narcotic analgesics in terminal cancer. Lancet 2: 694 (1975).

Editorial: Liver disease and anaesthesia. British Medical Journal 1: 1375 (1978).

Egbert, L.D.; Battit, G.E.; Turndoff, H. and Beecher, H.K.: The value of the preoperative visit by an anaesthetist. Journal of the American Medical Association 185: 553 (1963).

Eger, E.I.: Anesthetic Uptake and Action (Williams & Wilkins Company, Baltimore 1974).

Eger, E.I.; Bahlman, S.H. and Munson, E.S.: The effect of age on the rate of increase of alveolar anesthetic concentration. Anesthesiology 35: 365 (1971).

Ehrnebo, M.; Boreus, L.O. and Lonroth, U.: Bioavailability and first-pass metabolism of oral pentazocine in man. Clinical Pharmacology and Therapeutics 22: 888 (1977).

Elfstrom, J.: Drug pharmacokinetics in the postoperative period. Clinical Pharmacokinetics 4: 16 (1979).

Ellis, F.R.; Clarke, I.M.C.; Appleyard, T.N. and Dinsdale, R.C.W.: Malignant hyperpyrexia induced by nitrous oxide and treated with dexamethasone. British Medical Journal 4: 270 (1974).

Evans, T.I.: The physiological basis of geriatric general anaesthesia. Anaesthesia and Intensive Care 1: 319 (1973).

Evans, D.E.: Anaesthesia and the epileptic patient. Anaesthesia 30: 34 (1975).

Evans, J.M. and Keogh, J.A.M.: Adverse reactions to intravenous induction agents. British Medical Journal 2: 735 (1977).

Evans, J.M.; Hogg, M.I.J. and Rosen, M.: Reversal of narcotic depression in the neonate by naloxone. British Medical Journal 2: 1098 (1976).

Evans-Prosser, C.D.G.: The use of pethidine and morphine in the presence of monoamine oxidase inhibitors. British Journal of Anaesthesia 40: 279 (1968).

Ferreira, S.H. and Vane, J.R.: New aspects of the mode of action of nonsteroid anti-inflammatory drugs. Annual Review of Pharmacology 14: 57 (1974).

Findlay, J.W.A.; Jones, E.C; Butz, R.F. and Welch, R.M.: Plasma codeine and morphine concentrations after therapeutic oral doses of codeine-containing analgesics. Clinical Pharmacology and Therapeutics 24: 60 (1978).

Fink, R. and Cullen, B.F.: Anesthetic pollution: What is happening to us? Anesthesiology 45: 79 (1976).

Fisher, M.McD.: Anaphylactic reactions to gallamine triethiodide. Anaesthesia and Intensive Care 6: 62 (1978).

Fisher, M.McD.; Hallowes, R-C. and Wilson, R.M.: Anaphylaxis to alcuronium. Anaesthesia and Intensive Care 6: 125 (1978).

Flacke, W.; Katz, R.L.; Flacke, J.W. and Alper, M.: Germine diacetate as an antagonist of depolarising and nondepolarising neuromuscular blocking agents in man. Anesthesiology 29: 850 (1968).

Foex, P. and Prys Roberts, C.: Anaesthesia and the hypertensive patient. British Journal of Anaesthesia 46: 575 (1974).

Foldes, F.F.: Muscle Relaxants (Davis, Philadelphia 1966).

Foldes, F.F.: The rational use of neuromuscular blocking agents: The role of pancuronium. Drugs 4: 153 (1972).

Foldes, F.J.; Lunn, J.N. and Benz, H.G.: Prolonged respiratory depression caused by drug combinations. Muscle relaxants and intraperitoneal antibiotics as etiologic agents. Journal of the American Medical Association 183: 672 (1963).

Forrest, W.H.; Brown, C.R. and Brown, B.W.: Subjective responses to six common preoperative medications. Anesthesiology 47: 241 (1977).

Gamble, J.A.S.; Dundee, J.W. and Assaf, R.A.E.: Plasma diazepam levels after single dose oral and intramuscular administration. Anaesthesia 30: 164 (1975).

Gamble, J.A.S.; Dundee, J.W. and Gray, R.C.: Plasma diazepam concentrations following prolonged administration. British Journal of Anaesthesia 48: 1087 (1976).

Gamble, J.A.S.; Moore, J.; Lamki, H. and Howard, P.J.: A study of plasma diazepam levels in mother and infant. British Journal of Obstetrics and Gynaecology 84: 588 (1977).

Ghonheim, M.M. and Korttila, K.: Pharmacokinetics of intravenous anaesthetics: Implications for clinical use. Clinical Pharmacokinetics 2: 344 (1977).

Gibson, T.P.; Giacomini, K.M.; Briggs, W.A.; Whitman, W. and Levy, G.: Pharmacokinetics of d-propoxyphene in anephric patients. Clinical Pharmacology and Therapeutics 21: 103 (1977).

Giles, H.G.; MacLeod, S.M.; Wright, J.R. and Sellers, E.M.: Influence of age and previous use on diazepam dosage required for endoscopy. Canadian Medical Association Journal 118: 513 (1978).

Goldberg, L.I.: Cardiovascular and renal actions of dopamine: potential clinical applications. Pharmacological Reviews 24: 1 (1972).

Goudsouzian, N.G.; Donlon, J.V.; Savarese, J.J. and Ryan, J.F.: Re-evaluation of dosage and duration of action of d-tubocurarine in the pediatric age group. Anesthesiology 43: 416 (1975).

Gronert, G.A. and Theye, R.A.: Pathophysiology of hyperkalemia induced by succinylcholine. Anesthesiology 43: 89 (1975).

Halpern, L.M.: Analgesic drugs in the management of pain. Archives of Surgery 112: 861 (1977).

Hamilton, W.K.: Editorial Views: Do let the blood pressure drop and do use myocardial depressants. Anesthesiology 45: 273 (1976).

Heel, R.C.; Brogden, R.M.; Speight, T.M. and Avery, G.S.: Butorphanol: A review of its pharmacological properties and therapeutic efficacy. Drugs 16: 473 (1978).

Heel, R.C.; Brogden, R.N.; Speight, T.M. and Avery, G.S.: Buprenorphine: A review of its pharmacological properties and therapeutic efficacy. Drugs 17: 81 (1979).

Hegarty, J.E. and Dundee, J.W.: Sequelae after the intravenous injection of three benzodiazepines — diazepam, lorazepam and flunitrazepam. British Medical Journal 2: 1384 (1977).

Heykants, J.J.P.; Meuldermans, W.E.S.; Michiels, L.J.M.; Lewi, P.J. and Janssen, P.A.J.: Distribution, metabolism and excretion of etomidate, a short-acting hypnotic drug, in the rat. Archives internationale de Pharmacodynamie et de Therapie 216: 113 (1975).

Hughes, J. and Kosterlitz, H.W.: Opioid peptides. British Medical Bulletin 33: 157 (1977).

Hughes, R.; Payne, J.P. and Sugai, N.: Studies on fazadinium bromide (AH 8165); A new non-depolarizing neuromuscular blocking agent. Canadian Anaesthetists' Society Journal 23: 36 (1976)

Inman, W.H.W. and Mushin, W.W.: Jaundice after repeated exposure to halothane: An analysis of reports to the Committee on Safety of Medicines. British Medical Journal 1: 5 (1974).

Inman, W.H.W. and Mushin, W.W.: Jaundice after repeated exposure to halothane: a further analysis of reports to the Committee on Safety of Medicines. British Medical Journal 2: 1455 (1978).

Isbell, H.: Commentary: The search for a nonaddicting analgesic: Has it been worth it? Clinical Pharmacology and Therapeutics 22: 377 (1977).

Jaffe, J.H. and Martin, W.R.: Narcotic analgesics and antagonists: in Goodman and Gilman (Ed) The Pharmacological Basis of Therapeutics, p.249 (MacMillan, New York 1975).

Johnson, G.K. and Tolman, K.G.: Chronic liver disease and

acetaminophen. Annals of Internal Medicine 87: 302 (1977).

Johnstone, M.: Halothane hepatitis. Lancet 2: 526 (1978).

Joshi, P.H. and Conn, H.V. The syndrome of methoxyflurane associated hepatitis. Annals of Internal Medicine 80: 395 (1974).

Kalow, W. and Gunn, D.R.: Some statistical data on atypical cholinesterase of human serum. Annals of Human Genetics 23: 239 (1959).

Katz, J.: Pain: Theory and management; in Scurr and Feldman (Eds) Scientific Foundations of Anaesthetics, p. 266 (Heinemann, London 1970).

Katz, R.L. and Epstein, R.A.: The interaction of anaesthetic agents and adrenergic drugs to produce cardiac arrhythmias. Anesthesiology 29: 763 (1968).

Katz, J.D.; Croneau, L.H. and Barash, P.G.: Postoperative hypertension: A hazard of abrupt cessation of antihypertensive medication in the preoperative period. American Heart Journal 92: 79 (1976).

Kehlet, K. and Binder, C.: Adrenocortical function and clinical course during and after surgery in unsupplemented glucocorticoid-treated patients. British Journal of Anaesthesia 45: 1043 (1973).

Kelly, M.G.: Pentazocine — Strong analgesic with low abuse potential. British Journal of Addiction 72: 250 (1977).

Kelstrup, J.; Reske-Nielsen, E.; Haase, J. and Jorm, J.: Malignant hyperthermia in a family: a clinical and serological investigation of 139 members. Acta Anaesthesiologica Scandinavica 18: 58 (1974).

Klotz, U.; Avant, G.R.; Hoyumpa, A.; Schenker, S. and Wilkinson, G.R.: The effects of age and liver disease on the disposition and elimination of diazepam in adult man. Journal of Clinical Investigation 55: 347 (1975).

Knight, C.L. and Mehta, M.: Postoperative pain relief. British Journal of Hospital Medicine 19: 462 (1978).

Koch-Weser, J.: Drug Therapy: Acetaminophen. New England Journal of Medicine 295: 1297 (1976).

Kopriva, C.J.; Brown, A.C.D. and Pappas, G.: Hemodynamics during general anesthesia in patients receiving propranolol. Anesthesiology 48: 28 (1978a).

Kopriva, C.J.; Guinazu, A. and Barash, P.G.: Massive propranolol therapy and uncomplicated cardiac surgery. J. Amer. Med. Ass. 239: 1157 (1978b).

Kosaka, Y.; Takahashi, T. and Mark, L.C.: Intravenous thiobarbiturate anesthesia for cesarean section. Anesthesiology 31: 489 (1969).

Laflin, M.J.: Interaction of pancuronium and corticosteroids. Anesthesiology 47: 471 (1977).

Lasagna, L.: Propoxyphene and placebo: in comment. Annals of Internal Medicine 86: 506 (1977).

Lee-Son, S.; Pilon, R.N.; Nahor, A. and Waud, B.E.: Use of succinylcholine in the presence of atypical cholinesterase. Anesthesiology 43: 239 (1975).

Lilburn, J.K.; Dundee, J.W.; Nair, S.G.; Fee, J.P.H. and Johnston, H.M.L.: Ketamine sequelae. Evaluation of the ability of various premedicants to attenuate its psychic actions. Anaesthesia 33: 307 (1978a).

Lilburn, J.K.; Dundee, J.W. and Moore, J.: Ketamine infusions: Observations on technique, dosage and cardiovascular effects. Anaesthesia 33: 315 (1978b).

Loan, W.B. and Morrison, J.D.: Strong analgesics. Drugs 5: 108 (1973).

Lofstrom, B.: Clinical experience with long-acting local anaesthetics. Symposium, Madrid Sept 5, 1974. Acta Anaesthesiologica Scandinavica Suppl. 60 (1975).

Lomas, D.M.; Gay, J.; Midha, R.N.. and Postlethwaite, D.L.: A double-blind comparative clinical trial of floctafenine and four other analgesics conducted in general practice. Journal of International Medical Research 4: 179 (1976).

Lund, P.C.; Cwik, J.C.; Gannon, R.T. and Vassallo, H.G.: Etidocaine for caesarean section — effects on mother and baby. British Journal of Anaesthesia 49: 457 (1977).

McDonald, R.H. Jr.; Goldberg, L.I.; McNay, J.L. and Tuttle, E.P. Jr.: Effect of dopamine in man: Augmentation of sodium excretion, glomerular filtration rate and renal plasma flow. Journal of Clinical Investigation 43: 1116 (1964).

McDowall, D.G. and Norman, J.B.: Symposium on neurosurgical anaesthesia. British Journal of Anaesthesia 48: 717 (1976).

McEwan, J.: Liver function tests following anaesthesia. British Journal of Anaesthesia 48: 1065 (1976).

McPeek, B. and Gilbert, J.P.: Onset of postoperative jaundice related to anaesthetic history. British Medical Journal 3: 615 (1974).

Mandelli, M.; Tognoni, G. and Garattini, S.: Clinical pharmacokinetics of diazepam. Clinical Pharmacokinetics 3: 72 (1978).

Martin, W.R.: Opioid antagonists. Pharmacology Review 19: 463 (1967).

Martin, W.R.: Naloxone. Annals of Internal Medicine 85: 765 (1976).

Martin, W.R.; Eades, C.G.; Thompson, J.A.; Huppler, R.E. and Gilbert, P.E.: The effects of morphine and nalorphine-like drugs in the nondependent and morphine-dependent chronic spinal dog. Journal of Pharmacology and Experimental Therapeutics 197: 517 (1976).

Mather, L.E. and Meffin, P.J.: Clinical pharmacokinetics of pethidine. Clinical Pharmacokinetics 3: 352 (1978).

Mather, L.E. and Cousins, M.J.: Local anaesthetics and their use in general practice. Drugs. In press (1979).

Mazze, R.I. and Hitt, B.A.: Methoxyflurane metabolism. Anesthesiology 44: 369 (1976).

Mazze, R.I.; Escue, H.M. and Houston, J.B.: Hyperkalaemia and cardiovascular collapse following administration of succinylcholine to the traumatised patient. Anesthesiology 31: 540 (1969).

Medical Research Council: Conclusions of working party on the effect of repeated exposure to anaesthetics. British Journal of Anaesthesia 48: 1037 (1976).

Mehta, M.: Intractable Pain (Saunders, London 1973).

Meyer, H.H.: Welche eigenschaft der anaesthetica bedingt ihre narkitische wirkung. Archives of Experimental Pathology and Pharmacology 42: 109 (1899).

Michenfelder, J.D.; Gronert, G.A. and Rehder, K.: Neuroanaesthesia. Anesthesiology 30: 65 (1969).

Milledge, J.S. and Nunn, J.F.: Criteria of fitness for anaesthesia in patients with chronic obstructive lung disease. British Medical Journal 3: 670 (1975).

Miller, R.R.: Propoxyphene: a review. Journal of the Maine Medical Association 68: 86 (1977).

Miller, R.D.; Sohn, Y.J. and Matteo, R.S.: Enhancement of d-tubocurarine neuromuscular blockade by diuretics in man. Anesthesiology 45: 442 (1976).

Miller, R.D.; Stevens, W.C. and Way, W.L.: The effect of renal failure and hyperkalaemia on the duration of pancuronium neuromuscular blockade in man. Anesthesia and Analgesia 52: 661 (1972).

Miller, R.D.; Matteo, R.S.; Benet, L.Z. and Sohn, Y.J.: The pharmacokinetics of d-tubocurarine in man with and without renal failure. Journal of Pharmacology and Experimental Therapeutics 202: 1 (1977).

Mirakhur, R.K.; Clarke, R.S.J.; Dundee, J.W. and McDonald, J.R.: Anticholinergic drugs in anaesthesia. A survey of their present position. Anaesthesia 33: 133 (1978a).

Mirakhur, R.K.; Dundee, J.W. and Clark, R.S.J.: Glycopyrrolate — neostigmine mixture for the antagonism of neuromuscular block: comparison with atropine-neostigmine mixture. British Journal of Anaesthesia 49: 825 (1977).

Mirakhur, R.K.; Dundee, J.W. and Jones, C.J.: Evaluation of the anticholinergic actions of glycopyrronium bromide. British Journal of Clinical Pharmacology 5: 77 (1978b).

Mirkin, B.: Perinatal pharmacology. Anesthesiology 43: 156 (1975).

Moertel, C.G.; Ahmann, D.L.; Taylor, W.F. and Schwartau, N.: A comparative evaluation of marketed analgesic drugs. New England Journal of Medicine 286: 813 (1972).

Moir, D.D.: Obstetric Anaesthesia and Analgesia (Bailliere Tindall, London 1976).

Moore, D.C.; Bridenbaugh, L.D.; Bridenbaugh, P.O. and Tucker, G.T.: Bupivacaine: A review of 2,077 cases. Journal of the American Medical Association 214: 713 (1970).

Moore, D.C.; Bridenbaugh, L.D.; Thompson, G.E.; Balfour, R.I. and Horton, W.G.: Factors determining dosages of amide-type local anaesthetic drugs. Anesthesiology 47: 263 (1977).

Morrison, J.D.: Studies of drugs given before anaesthesia, XXII. Phenoperidine and fentanyl, alone and in combination with droperidol. British Journal of Anaesthesia 42: 1119 (1970).

Morrison, J.D.; Neurolept techniques; in Dundee and Wyant (Eds) Intravenous Anaesthesia (Churchill Livingstone, Edinburgh 1974).

Moult, P.J.A. and Sherlock, S.: Halothane-related hepatitis. Quarterly Journal of Medicine 44 (NS): 99 (1975).

Mushin, W.W.: Administration of drugs before anaesthesia. British Medical Journal 1: 1558 (1960).

Oduro, K.A.: Glycopyrrolate methobromide. II. Comparison with atropine sulphate in anaesthesia. Canadian Anaesthetists' Society Journal 22: 466 (1975).

Overton, E.: Studien uber die narkose (Fisher, Jena 1901).

Overton, J.H.: Common problems in paediatric anaesthesia. Medical Journal of Australia 2: 873 (1976).

Parkhouse, J.: Simple analgesics. Drugs 10: 366 (1975).

Paymaster, N.J.: Analgesia after operation. British Journal of Anaesthesia 49: 1139 (1977).

Pender, J.W.: Dissociative anesthesia. Journal of the American Medical Association 215: 1126 (1971).

Pharoah, P.O.D.; Alberman, E. and Doyle, P.: Outcome of pregnancy among women in anaesthetic practice. Lancet 1: 34 (1977).

Pittinger, C. and Adamson, R.: Antibiotic blockade of neuromuscular function. Annual Review of Pharmacology 12: 169 (1972).

Pittinger, C.B.; Eryasa, Y. and Adamson, R.: Antibiotic-induced paralysis. Anesthesia and Analgesia 49: 487 (1970).

Plumpton, F.S.; Besser, G.M. and Cole, P.V.: Corticosteroid treatment and surgery. Anaesthesia 24: 3, 12 (1969).

Pontoppidan, H.; Geffin, B. and Lowenstein, E.: Acute respiratory failure in the adult. New England Journal of Medicine 287: 690, 743, 799 (1972).

Pontoppidan, H.; Wilson, R.S.; Rie, M.A. and Schneider, R.C.: Respiratory intensive care. Anesthesiology 47: 96 (1977).

Powell, D.R. and Miller, R.: The effect of repeated doses of succinylcholine on serum potassium in patients with renal failure. Anesthesia and Analgesia 54: 746 (1975).

Prys-Roberts, C.: Medical problems of surgical patients: Hypertension and ischaemic heart disease. Annals of the Royal College of Surgeons of England 58: 465 (1976).

Prys-Roberts, C.: New wine in old bottles. British Journal of Anaesthesia 49: 845 (1977).

Prys-Roberts, C. et al.: Studies of anaesthesia in relation to hypertension. British Journal of Anaesthesia 43: 122, 531, 644 (1971); 44: 335 (1972); 45: 671 (1973).

Ralston, D.H. and Shnider, S.M.: The fetal and neonatal effects of regional anesthesia in obstetrics. Anesthesiology 48: 34 (1978).

Rawlings, M.D.: Drug interaction and anaesthesia. British Journal of Anaesthesia 50: 689 (1978).

Reidenberg, M.M.; Levy, M.; Warner, H.; Coutinho, C.B.; Schwartz, M.A.; Yu, G. and Cheripko, Joyce: Relationship between diazepam dose, plasma level, age and central nervous system depression. Clinical Pharmacology and Therapeutics 23: 371 (1978).

Rogers, K.J. and Thornton, J.A.: The interaction between monoamine oxidase inhibitors and narcotic analgesics in mice. British Journal of Pharmacology 36: 470 (1969).

Rosen, S.M.: Effects of anaesthesia and surgery on renal haemodynamics. British Journal of Anaesthesia 44: 252 (1972).

Rosenberg, P. and Kirves, A.: Miscarriages among operating theatre staff. Acta Anaesthesiologica Scandinavica 53 (Suppl.): 37 (1973).

Rosner, V.; Kepes, E.R. and Foldes, F.F.: The effects of atropine and neostigmine on heart rate and rhythm. British Journal of Anaesthesia 43: 1066 (1971).

Sawyer, D.C.; Eger, E.I.; Bahlman, S.H.; Cullen, B.F. and Impelman, D.: Concentration dependence of hepatic halothane metabolism. Anesthesiology 34: 230 (1971).

Scott, D.B.: Analgesia in labour. British Journal of Anaesthesia 49: 11 (1977).

Scott, D.B.; Jebson, P.J.R.: Braid, D.P.; Ortengren, B. and Frisch, P.: Factors affecting plasma levels of lignocaine and prilocaine. British Journal of Anaesthesia 44: 1040 (1972).

Sherlock, S.: Halothane hepatitis. Lancet 2: 364 (1978).

Shideman, F.E.; Kelly, A.R.; Lee, L.E. et al.: The role of the liver in the detoxification of thiopental (Pentothal) by man. Anesthesiology 10: 421 (1949).

Simpson, B.R.; Strunin, L. and Walton, B.: Halothane and jaundice. British Journal of Hospital Medicine 13: 433 (1975).

Sjoqvist, F.: Psychotropic drugs (2). Interaction between monoamine oxidase (MAO) inhibitors and other substances. Proceedings of the Royal Society of Medicine 58 (Pt 2): 967 (1965).

Slawson, K.B.: Anaesthesia for the patient in renal failure. British Journal of Anaesthesia 44: 277 (1972).

Slogoff, S.; Keats, A.S. and Ott, E.: Preoperative propranolol therapy and aortocoronary bypass operation. Journal of the American Medical Association 240: 1487 (1978).

Somogyi, A.A.; Shanks, C.A. and Triggs, E.J.: The effect of renal failure on the disposition and neuromuscular blocking action of pancuronium bromide. European Journal of Clinical Pharmacology 12: 23 (1977).

Speight, T.M. and Avery, G.S.: Pancuronium bromide: A review of its pharmacological properties and clinical application. Drugs 4: 163 (1972).

Spence, A.A.; Cohen, E.N.; Brown, B.W.; Knill-Jones, R.P. and Himmelberger, D.U.: Occupational hazards for operating room-based physicians. Analysis of data from the United States and the United Kingdom. Journal of the American Medical Association 238: 955 (1977).

Spotnitz, H.M.: Clonidine withdrawal. Annals of Thoracic Surgery 25: 179 (1978).

Stambaugh, J.E.; Wainer, I.W.; Hemphill, D.M. and Schwartz, I.: A potentially toxic drug interaction between pethidine (meperidine) and phenobarbitone. Lancet 1: 398 (1977).

Stambaugh, J.E.; Wainer, I.W. and Schwartz, I.: The effect of phenobarbital on the metabolism of meperidine in normal volunteers. Journal of Clinical Pharmacology 18: 482 (1978).

Stehling, L.C.: Anesthetic management of the patient with hyperthyroidism. Anesthesiology 41: 585 (1974).

Stevens, W.C; Eger, E.I.; White, A.; Halsey, M.J.; Munger, W.; Gibbons, R.D.; Dolan, W. and Shargel, R.: Comparative toxicities of halothane, isoflurane and diethyl ether at subanesthetic concentrations in laboratory animals. Anesthesiology 42: 408 (1975).

Stoelting, R.K. and Peterson, C.: Methoxyflurane anesthesia in pediatric patients: evaluation of anesthetic metabolism and renal function. Anesthesiology 42: 26 (1975).

Strunin, L.: Hepatitis and halothane. British Journal of Anaesthesia 48: 1035 (1976).

Strunin, L.: The Liver and Anaesthesia (Saunders, London 1977).

Strunin, L.: Preoperative assessment of the patient with liver dysfunction. British Journal of Anaesthesia 50: 25 (1978).

Symposium: Proceedings of a symposium on diflunisal held in London, 18th February 1977. British Journal of Clinical Pharmacology 4 (Suppl. 1): 5S (1977).

Symposium: held in conjunction with the 30th Anniversary Symposium of the European League Against Rheumatism (EULAR) Zurich, Switzerland, April 28-30 1977. Clinical Therapeutics 1(Suppl. A): 1 (1978).

Tarhan, S.; Moffitt, E.A.; Taylor, W.F. and Giuliani, E.R.: Myocardial infarction after general anaesthesia. Journal of the American Medical Association 220: 1451 (1972).

Tinker, J.H. and Michenfelder, J.D.: Sodium nitroprusside. Anesthesiology 45: 340 (1976).

Tinker, J.H.; Gandolfi, J. and Van Dyke, R.A.: Elevation of plasma bromide levels in patients following halothane anesthesia. Anesthesiology 44: 194 (1976).

Tornetta, F.J.: A comparison of droperidol, diazepam and hydroxyzine hydrochloride as premedication. Anaesthesia and Analgesia: Current Researches 56: 496 (1977).

Tuchmann-Duplessis, H.: Drug Effects on the Fetus, p. 162 (ADIS Press, Sydney 1975).

Tucker, G.T. and Mather, L.E.: Pharmacokinetics of local anaesthetic agents. British Journal of Anaesthesia 47: 213 (1975).

Tucker, G.T. and Mather, L.E.: Clinical pharmacokinetics of local anaesthetics. Clinical Pharmacokinetics. In press (1979).

Tucker, G.T.; Boyes, R.N.; Bridenbaugh, P.O. and Moore, D.C.: Binding of anilide-type local anaesthetics in human plasma. I. Relationship between binding, physicochemical properties, and anaesthetic activity. Anesthesiology 33: 287 (1970).

Twycross, R.G.: Diseases of the central nervous system. Relief of terminal pain. British Medical Journal 4: 212 (1975).

Various Authors: Symposium on inhalational anaesthetics. British Journal of Anaesthesia 37: 643 (1965).

Various Authors: Symposium on Forane. Anesthesiology 35: 4 (1971a).

Various Authors: Symposium on obstetric anaesthesia and analgesia. British Journal of Anaesthesia 43: 824 (1971b).

Various Authors: The kidney and the anaesthetist. British Journal of Anaesthesia 44: 235 (1972a).

Various Authors: Symposium on anaesthesia and the liver. British Journal of Anaesthesia 44: 909 (1972b).

Various Authors: Proceedings of a symposium on local anaesthesia. British Journal of Anaesthesia 47: 163 (1975).

Vatner, S.F. and Braunwald, E.: Cardiovascular control mechanisms in the conscious state. New England Journal of Medicine 293: 970 (1975).

Verbeek, R.; Tjandramaga, T.B.; Mullie, A.; Verbesselt, R.; Verberckmoes, R. and De Schepper, P.J.: Biotransformation of diflunisal and renal excretion of its glucuronides in renal insufficiency. British Journal of Clinical Pharmacology 7: 273 (1979).

Vergani, D.; Tsantoulas, D.; Eddleston, A.L.W.F.; Davis, M. and Williams, R.: Sensitisation to halothane-altered liver components in sever hepatic necrosis after halothane anaesthesia. Lancet 2: 801 (1978).

Vessey, M.P.: Epidemiological studies of the occupational hazards of anaesthesia — a review. Anaesthesia 33: 430 (1978).

Walts, L.F. and Dillon, J.B.: The response of newborns to succinylcholine and d-tubocurarine. Anesthesiology 31: 35 (1969).

Watkins, J. and Ward, A.M. (Ed): Adverse Responses to Intravenous Drugs (Academic Press, London; Grune and Stratton, New York 1978).

Way, W.L; Costley, E.C. and Way, E.L.: Respiratory sensitivity of the newborn infant to meperidine and morphine. Clinical Pharmacology and Therapeutics 6: 454 (1965).

Whittington, R.M.: Dextropropoxyphene (Distalgesic) overdosage in the West Midlands. British Medical Journal 2: 172 (1977).

Whitwam, J.G.: Adverse reactions to I.V. induction agents. British Journal of Anaesthesia 50: 677 (1978).

Wilkins, J.L.; Hardcastle, J.D.; Mann, C.V. and Kaufman, L.: Effects of neostigmine and atropine on motor activity of ileum, colon and rectum of anaesthetised subjects. British Medical Journal 1: 793 (1970).

Wingard, L.B. and Cook, D.R.: Clinical pharmacokinetics of muscle relaxants. Clinical Pharmacokinetics 2: 330 (1977).

Wood, M.; O'Malley, K. and Stevenson, I.H.: Drug metabolizing ability in operating theatre personnel. British Journal of Anaesthesia 46: 726 (1974).

Young, S.R.; Stoelting, R.K.; Peterson, C. and Madura, J.A.: Anesthetic biotransformation and renal function in obese patients during and after methoxyflurane or halothane anesthesia. Anesthesiology 42: 451 (1975).

Zacharias, M.; Clarke, R.S.J.; Dundee, J.W. and Johnston, S.B.: An evaluation of three preparations of etomidate. British Journal of Anaesthesia 50: 925 (1978).

Chapter XI
Ear, Nose and Throat Diseases

R.T. Jackson, J.H. Per-Lee, J.H. Burson and J.S. Turner, Jr

Synopsis of Important Principles

1) Drug therapy in ear, nose and throat disease is at present a balance between the practical and scientific bases for drug selection and use.

2) Apart from infections, in only a few situations is there a clear pharmacological basis for drug action and use (e.g. sympathetic control of nasal and eustachian tube function), but there are still good theoretical bases for rational selection and use of drugs in other situations.

3) In bacterial infections of the ear, nose or throat good evidence is available on the most likely causative organism in various situations. With this knowledge, the appropriate agent for initial therapy can be selected with confidence.

4) Penicillin, erythromycin or ampicillin/amoxycillin (when *Haemophilus influenzae* is likely to be involved) and gentamicin for topical use, cover the common causative organisms.

5) Measures directed at attaining a clear ear canal or nasal airway, and restoration of eustachian tube function, are also important in a number of disorders involving the ear or nose.

6) Allergy can be implicated in some nasal disorders and is often associated with secretory otitis media.

7) Treatment of vertigo is based upon a careful history and investigation such that the most likely cause can be identified and an appropriate antivertigo drug (or other treatment) selected.

8) Some drugs can cause ototoxicity, the aminoglycoside antibacterial drugs and potent diuretics when used in the patient with impaired renal function being the most important.

In recent years, government agencies and individuals have demanded objective evidence of the efficacy of a drug. Rigorous experimental design has largely supplanted the subjective responses of office 'clinical trials'. However, in otolaryngology in particular, objective evidence is scarce or conflicting in many instances (e.g. the treatment of sudden hearing loss, Meniere's disease and even otitis media) and the clinician must often rely on clinical experience. Occasionally, this may conflict with pharmacological rationale for treatment of a particular disease. Drug treatment in ear, nose and throat disease is therefore at present, a balance between the practical and scientific bases for drug selection and use.

1. Clinical Pharmacological Considerations and General Principles of Treatment

The drugs most often prescribed for ear, nose and throat diseases fall into the following classes: antimicrobial agents, antihistamines, antivertigo drugs, sympathomimetics and vasodilators.

1.1 Antibacterial Agents

A knowledgeable clinician can make intelligent predictions as to the likely organism or class of organisms he will be treating in many given situations in otolaryngology and need not await cultures to initiate therapy (see section 2.1; table I). However, it is a good rule that cultures should be made when treating severe infections, chronic infections not responsive to treatment and those in debilitated patients, or infections which produce life threatening complications (e.g. suppurative labyrinthitis). The selection of a suitable agent, its dose and route of administration, are functions of the aforementioned considerations. These considerations, as well as the pharmacological properties and activity of antibacterial drugs, are discussed further in chapter XXVII.

Use of antibacterial agents for routine uncomplicated cases of colds and upper respiratory symptoms of other viral diseases is to be condemned (see section 2.1). Once started, an antibacterial agent should be used in an adequate dose for sufficient time to completely control infection, and the patient (or parent of a young child) should be educated in the need to comply with medication instructions and to complete the prescribed course.

1.2 Antihistamines

The antihistamines used by otolaryngologists are histamine$_1$ (H$_1$)-receptor inhibitors. Although H$_2$-receptor inhibitors such as cimetidine (see chapter XIX; sect. 4.1.3) can interfere with histamine induced vascular responses in animals, their effects have not been tested in animals or patients on ear, nose or throat tissues. The H$_1$ antihistamines competitively inhibit the actions of histamine released from mast cells. They are more effective in preventing histamine induced leakage through capillaries than histamine induced vasodilation (Pearlman, 1976; Jackson and Burson, 1977). Antihistamines should not be expected to reverse the effects of any histamine already attached to receptors. They are only useful in competing for receptors with newly released histamine. Thus, they should be most effective if given *prior* to histamine release and onset of histamine induced symptoms (e.g. before exposure in allergic rhinitis). Also, histamine is not the only mediator of inflammation released in infected or allergic tissue (Kaliner et al., 1973). Other mediators like kinins, prostaglandins, complement fractions (e.g. C3A), slow reacting substance of anaphylaxis, lysosomal enzymes and the toxins elaborated by micro-organisms are also partially responsible for symptoms of the inflammatory response. It is unrealistic to expect that antihistamines could suppress the actions of all these mediators of inflammation.

Besides being inhibitors of histamine, antihistamines also have a number of other actions, including a weak anticholinergic effect, local anaesthetic effects, and they can act as a vasoconstrictor, prevent or control motion sickness and can be used as sedatives. The extent and nature of these multiple actions depends on the particular compound and the dose (Pearlman, 1976).

Antihistamines are useful in otolaryngology primarily in the relief of symptoms of certain allergic disorders such as mild, seasonal acute allergic rhinitis (section 2.4). Given alone, they are of little use for the relief of perennial vasomotor rhinitis (section 2.3). Some antihistamines, because of their weak anticholinergic and vasoconstrictor activity, occasionally have a palliative effect on the common cold by helping to counteract rhinorrhoea or nasal congestion, but this effect is probably slight and unpredictable (West et al., 1975).

1.3 Antivertigo Drugs

While several methods are available for judging the effectiveness of drugs used to treat vertigo and motion sickness, the pharmacological basis for drug selection, is not as yet well defined. Drugs used in vertigo are of many different types and actions. Selection depends upon the suspected diagnosis (see section 4).

1.4 Sympathomimetic Drugs

Normal nasal patency depends on a constant flow of sympathetic nerve impulses to nasal blood vessels. Augmentation of this flow by sympathomimetic drugs will decrease blood flow and increase the nasal airway (see Jackson, 1971). Interruption of this flow by sympathectomy or drugs that inhibit sympathetic transmission will increase vessel diameter and decrease the nasal airway. This on-going sympathetic activity has not been described in the vasculature of the sinus and eustachian tube mucosa. Sympathomimetic drugs are used in otolaryngology mainly for their effects on inflamed nasal, sinus and eustachian tube mucosa. These drugs act at the neuroeffector junction of the postganglionic adrenergic nerves and their effects mimic or resemble the response to stimulation of adrenergic nerves. The action can be at the axon terminal or at the receptor site on the structure innervated by the terminal (e.g. vascular smooth muscle of the nasal mucosa).

Sympathomimetic drugs used in otolaryngology practice thus include the topical and oral decongestants and also certain of the peripheral vasodilators (e.g. nylidrin). Sympathomimetic drugs stimulate adrenergic receptors (classed as α or β), by either a direct or indirect action (see fig. 1a). Some sympathomimetic drugs can interact with both α- and β-adrenoceptors (e.g. adrenaline or epinephrine) while others exert their effect by both a direct or indirect action (e.g. ephedrine), but usually one effect or action predominates. Direct acting drugs interact directly with the α- or β-receptors located on the structure innervated, whereas the indirect acting drugs increase the amount of free noradrenaline (norepinephrine) at the synaptic junction between the sympathetic nerve and the blood vessel (fig. 1a). The indirect acting sympathomimetic drugs, because of their mode of action, have important unwanted interactions with certain antihypertensive drugs and

monoamine oxidase inhibitors (see chapter X, fig. 2; XVIII, fig. 3).

Just as some drugs can stimulate sympathetic function, others, such as certain antihypertensives, can inhibit the function of sympathetic nerve activity by decreasing the amount of noradrenaline available for neurotransmitter functions (fig. 1b). This has the effect of inhibiting synaptic transmission (i.e. nerve terminal blockade). Thus, if the sympathetic fibres are innervating blood vessels, stimulation of these fibres will not produce the usual degree of vasoconstriction. If a particular group of blood vessels is usually partially constricted (e.g. in the nasal mucosa) because of a resting sympathetic activity or tone, nerve terminal blockade will produce a vasodilatation (e.g. nasal congestion).

1.5 Vasodilator Drugs

These drugs are used to treat sudden hearing loss (see section 6) and certain types of vertigo (see section 4). They dilate blood vessels and thereby increase blood flow. The use of these drugs raises two questions. Firstly, do they actually increase blood flow to the inner ear? Secondly, if the blood flow did increase, could one reasonably expect a therapeutic effect? There is a great deal of controversy concerning the effectiveness of these drugs, especially on intracranial vessels (Kuvayama et al., 1972). Many pharmacologists feel that only a few vascular beds (e.g., skin) are readily affected by vasodilators. They feel that autoregulatory mechanisms (local changes in pH, Po_2 and Pco_2) have already adjusted blood flow as much as possible in ischaemic areas. Besides local regulation, it is quite difficult to significantly change blood flow to intracranial vessels because of baroreceptor reflexes originating in the carotids and elsewhere. However, animal experiments have shown that several drugs (e.g. carbon dioxide, histamine, papaverine) induce an increased otic blood flow if given in adequate dosage (Suga and Snow, 1969; Clairmont et al., 1973; Pollock et al., 1974). This data forms the experimental basis for treating ischaemic inner ear disease with such drugs. If such medication is effective in the patient, and clinical experience suggests that at times it is, it may be that blood flow is restricted by functional (nervous or humoral) rather than structural (sclerotic) changes. The pharmacologist's cynicism is usually engendered by claims of relieving ischaemia during long term treatment of degenerative vascular diseases.

The vasodilators are of two types: (1) those that appear to react with a specific receptor on the blood vessel (e.g. nylidrin, histamine), and (2) those drugs that are smooth muscle relaxants (e.g. papaverine, nicotinic acid) whose mechanism of action appears to involve increasing the concentration of cyclic AMP (Andersson et al., 1975). Cyclic AMP inhibits smooth muscle contraction in blood vessels. The enzyme phosphodiesterase degrades cyclic AMP to an inactive product.

Drugs like papaverine and theophylline inhibit this degradation, raise the concentration of cyclic AMP and thus induce vasodilatation.

2. Upper Respiratory Conditions

2.1 Principles of Therapy

Upper respiratory tract dysfunction often reflects an alteration in the ciliated secretory epithelium which lines the tract from nose to

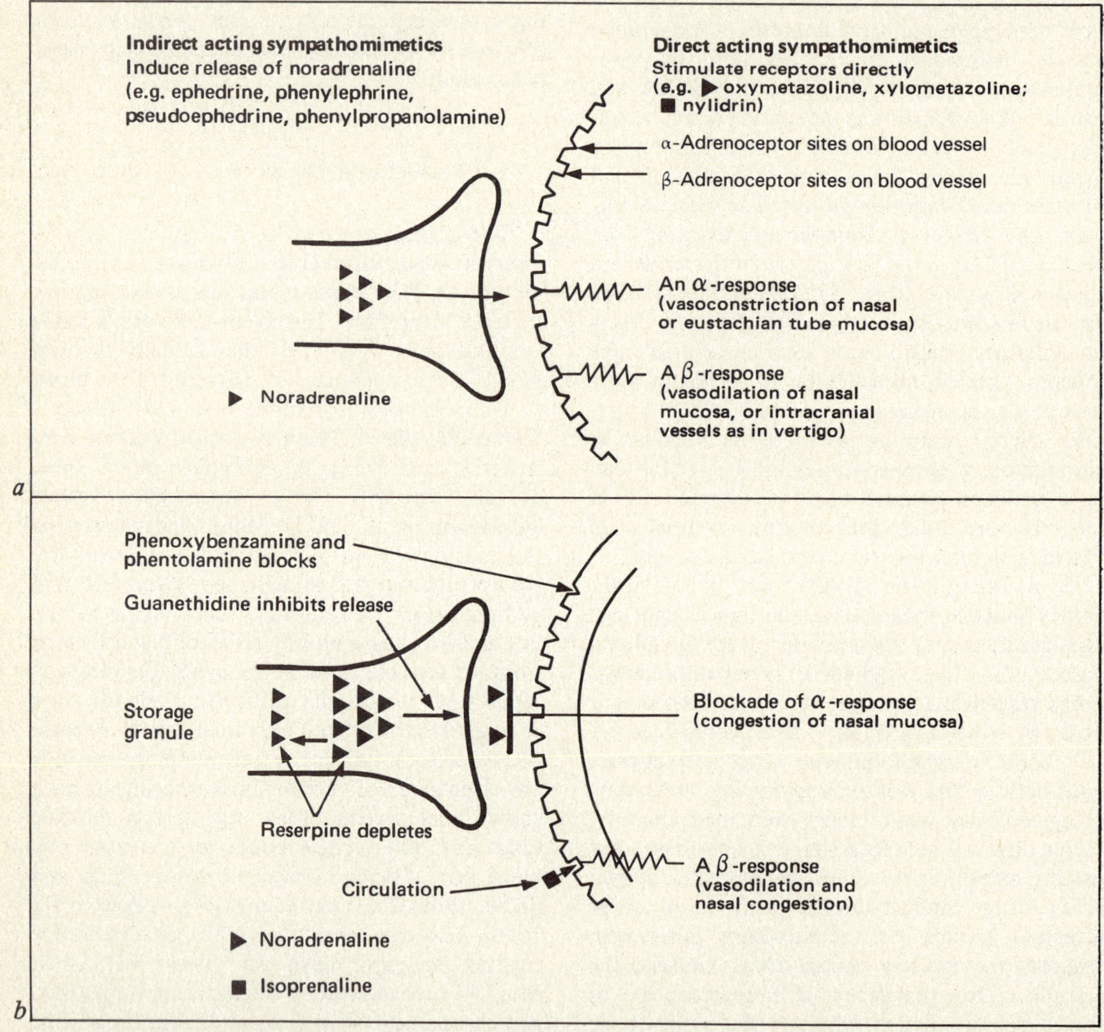

Fig. 1. Highly schematic and simplified representation of adrenergic mechanisms with particular reference to control of nasal patency and eustachian tube function. (a) Predominant action of direct and indirect acting sympathomimetics; (b) Blockade of adrenergic function by certain antihypertensive drugs, illustrating mechanism of nasal stuffiness (see also section 6.3). [After Jackson: Annals of Otology, Rhinology and Laryngology 80: 313, 1971; by permission of author and editor].

Table I. Systemic antibacterial drugs for initial treatment of common ear, nose and throat infections

Indication	Causative organisms[1] (those most likely to predominate)	Drug[2]	Usual dosage and duration[3]
Acute rhinosinusitis	Pneumococci *Str. pyogenes*	Penicillin V	250mg (6.25mg/kg) 4 times daily for 10 days minimum (parenteral penicillin in severe cases)
Pharyngitis	β-Haemolytic streptococcus	Penicillin V	250mg (6.25mg/kg) 4 times daily for 10 days minimum
Acute furunculosis	Staphylococci *Str. pyogenes*	Dicloxacillin	125mg (3.125mg/kg) 4 times daily for 10 days minimum
		Cloxacillin	500mg (12.5mg/kg) 4 times daily for 10 days minimum
		Flucloxacillin	250mg (6.25mg/kg) 4 times daily for 10 days minimum (a parenteral cloxacillin in severe cases)
Acute otitis media	Pneumococci *Str. pyogenes* *H. influenzae*	Amoxycillin	250mg (6.25mg/kg) 3 times daily for 10 days minimum
		Ampicillin[4]	500mg (12.5mg/kg) 4 times daily for 10 days minimum

1   See text for situations when culture necessary. See also appendix D.

2   In cases of penicillin allergy, erythromycin (250mg or 10mg/kg 4 times daily) or when *H. influenzae* is involved co-trimoxazole (2 tablets twice daily), can be used.

3   Oral unless stated otherwise. Children's dosage in parentheses — see also chapter IV, table XI. Penicillin, cloxacillins and ampicillin should be taken 1 hour before meals.

4   There is a 15 to 20% incidence of resistance to ampicillin in some areas (Schwartz et al., 1978).

lungs. This dysfunction may be the result of infection, allergy, anatomical factors, trauma, tumour, drug related processes or any combinations thereof. Despite the continuity of the upper respiratory epithelium, studies have demonstrated, within respiratory regions, a wide range of response to infectious organisms. There is also a variation in response to drugs (Jackson, 1970).

Given the appropriate conditions, pathogenic organisms breach the normal protective mucosal blanket and have a toxic effect upon mucosal cells. The results are hypertrophy, vacuolisation and necrosis. The products of tissue damage evoke an acute inflammatory response, the signs and symptoms of which are: fever, redness, swelling and pain. Cellular function is altered further and a secondary bacterial invasion of the damaged mucosal layer often follows. Drug treatment is generally 2-fold in nature. The initial goal is to resolve the inflammatory symptoms. This is accomplished by shrinking the swollen mucous membranes and reducing the profuse secretions associated with the process. Concomitantly, treatment may be directed at eliminating the offending aetiological agent with appropriate systemic therapy.

An organism responsible for the infection should be identified, at least presumptively, prior to choosing an antimicrobial drug. Identification may be by intelligent guesswork based on clinical evidence (table I), or by definitive culture isolation. Gram stained smears and cultures must be interpreted with caution from head and neck sites because the normal pharyngeal flora can include such usual pathogens as *Haemophilus influenzae, Streptococcus pneumoniae* and potentially pathogenic anaerobic species. The nose may also be inhabited by a commensal flora but the mastoid cells, middle ear and paranasal sinuses are thought to be normally sterile. Also, a very large number of viruses have been isolated from the upper respiratory tract and shown to have pathogenic potential. The routine use of viral cultures or acute and convalescent antibody titres is however, not generally performed and at present is of limited value in daily practice. Specific antiviral treatment is wanting, but research in this area is very active. Effective prevention and treatment of a few viral respiratory infections such as influenza is nevertheless possible (see chapter XXVIII; sect. 3.2).

The majority of all acute infections causing morbidity are of the upper respiratory tract and most of these are viral in aetiology (e.g. the common cold) and do not benefit from *routine* use of antibacterial drugs (Soyka et al., 1975; Taylor et al., 1977). The common cold may result from any of a large number of potential viral pathogens, most commonly from the rhinoviruses. The common cold generally is a self limiting illness requiring only symptomatic treatment. However, a great many patients present with a progression of symptoms that is highly suggestive of secondary bacterial involvement. Consequently, the use of antibacterial agents in these *more complicated* cases is gaining favour among many clinicians. This is not to suggest routine use of antibacterial agents for the uncomplicated common cold (see further chapter XXVIII; sect. 3.2). The choice of antimicrobial drugs recommended in the following sections is based on susceptibility studies, clinical trials and generally accepted alternative drugs for pathogenic organisms found in diseases of the upper respiratory tract.

It should be emphasised that functional anatomy is of paramount importance in all disorders of the middle ear, nose and paranasal sinuses. Complete resolution of infectious disorders of these areas is generally precluded unless adequate ventilation and drainage pathways are established. This may involve only pharmacological shrinkage of oedematous tissues with re-establishment of physiological drainage, or may require creation of surgical drainage pathways.

2.2 Acute Rhinosinusitis

Most nasal inflammatory disorders also involve, to a greater or lesser degree, the paranasal sinuses. The sinuses are formed as embryological and developmental outgrowths of nasal structures and thus have the same general histological and pharmacological properties as the nasal mucosa (for review, see Chapnick and Bach, 1976; Kutnick and Keith, 1976).

Acute rhinosinusitis presents as a mucoid or purulent discharge. The nature of the discharge forms the basis for an initial differential diagnosis.

A thin mucoid discharge is typical of vasomotor, allergic or viral infectious states. Purulent discharge is virtually pathognomonic of bacterial infection.

2.2.1 Initial Symptomatic Treatment

Acute allergic, vasomotor or viral disorders are generally treated initially with topical nasal sprays or oral decongestants (see section 1.4). Supplemental moisture at night is helpful in rehydrating dry air and is conveniently supplied by spinning disk atomisers, ultrasonic or pneumatic nebulisers or steam vaporisers. Topical sprays of decongestants such as oxymetazoline or xylometazoline are recommended for a period of not more than 5 to 7 days. Oral decongestants commonly available may contain only vasoconstrictors (sympathomimetic amines such as phenylpropanolamine, pseudoephedrine, phenylephrine) or may be combined with antihistamines. Well designed clinical studies have demonstrated the efficacy and synergism of oral sympathomimetic amines combined with antihistamines in the treatment of nasal mucosal congestion due to infection or allergy (Aschan, 1974). A large variety of decongestants, antihistamines and combinations thereof, with the addition of analgesics, stimulants, antitussives, expectorants, vitamins and laxatives, is available for both prescription and over the counter preparations. Possibilities for abuse and irrational use are plentiful. A single over the counter product may contain as many as 8 different drugs.

Topical decongestants have the advantage of selective site of action and more rapid action than do oral agents. However, there are significant problems associated with topical agents. All topical vasoconstrictor and mucolytic agents damage the mucociliary flow apparatus, but, the most serious objection to their use is the rebound or reactive hyperaemic state known as rhinitis medicamentosa that develops with repeated use (e.g. Walker, 1952). The longer acting imidazoline derivatives such as oxymetazoline and xylometazoline are apparently metabolised at a slower rate than the catecholamines such as ephedrine or phenylephrine and result in a longer duration of action and decreased rebound effect. However, they too can cause rebound phenomena after 5 to 7 days usage (Feinberg and Feinberg, 1971). Particular attention should be directed to the medically unsupervised use of nose drops in infants and children. Systemic effects such as tachycardia, somnolence and shock-like states have been reported in infants and children after administration of a large number of drops (Geimer and Geimer, 1966; Wick, 1966). Thus, caution should be used in prescribing topical decongestants and mucolytic agents. Ciliotoxicity with disruption of mucus flow and rebound congestion may be an unacceptable price for the short term symptomatic benefit associated with vasoconstriction from topical agents.

2.2.2 Secondary Bacterial Infection

Persistence of congestion for over 7 to 10 days and the appearance of purulent discharge are indicative of progression of disease to secondary bacterial involvement. Once bacterial infection has supervened, systemic antibacterial drugs should be administered for 10 to 14 days. Radiological evidence of maxillary air fluid levels after 3 to 7 days of therapy with nasal sprays or oral decongestants and antibacterial agents is an indication for irrigation, either via the natural ostia or inferior meatal puncture. Drainage of the sinuses is a procedure for a specialist, and the clinician should be willing to trephine the frontal sinuses if there is no symptomatic or radiological evidence of improvement. Culture and sensitivity tests of contained secretions should be performed. Oral decongestants should be continued (although they may thicken the secretions) but topical medications are normally stopped after 5 to 7 days. Local application of moist heat to the overlying facial tissues often provides symptomatic relief.

Penicillin remains the drug of choice for the initial treatment of acute upper respiratory conditions due to bacterial infection. The simple penicillins (benzylpenicillin, phenoxymethylpenicillin) are highly effective against pneumococci and streptococci, the most common organisms in acute rhinosinusitis (table I). They are also effective against practically all anaerobic species found in head and neck sites; the most notable exception being *Bacteroides fragilis,* which however, is uncommon in our area. Aminopenicillins (ampicillin and amoxycillin) are more effective than simple penicillins against *Escherichia coli* and *H. influenzae,* which can be implicated in some cases of acute rhinosinusitis. All aminopenicillins have the propensity to cause a maculopapular rash, which is not related to the IgE mediated penicillin urticarial rash. Unfortunately, the presence of such a rash often labels a patient as allergic to penicillin (Benn, 1977). Isoxazolyl penicillins (cloxacillin, oxacillin etc) extend the spectrum of the simple

penicillins to include the penicillinase producing *Staphylococcus aureus*. Penicillinase resistant penicillins, which are bactericidal for penicillinase producing staphylococci, are considerably less active than simple penicillins against penicillin sensitive staphylococci. Some authorities therefore recommend that initial therapy of serious suspected staphylococcal infections should involve use of both benzylpenicillin with an isoxazolyl penicillin, with cessation of one when sensitivities are known.

2.2.3 Recurrent Bouts of Acute Rhinosinusitis

Incompletely resolved bacterial infections or recurrent bouts of acute rhinosinusitis may give rise to mucosal ulcerations, inflammatory metaplasia and progressive fibrosis with resultant obstruction of the drainage orifices of the sinuses. Unless adequate drainage is re-established, the mucosa ultimately becomes irreversibly damaged and surgical intervention is required. Early drug treatment during this progression can sometimes halt the process. Saline lavage of the maxillary antrum is helpful, both in mechanically removing inspissated secretions and for identification of the predominant bacterial species.

Presumptive drug treatment for this condition should include antibacterial cover for *H. influenzae* which, along with anaerobic streptococci, are the predominant organisms in chronic rhinosinusitis. Full course therapy with ampicillin or amoxycillin (table I) and oral decongestants is indicated. Antihistamines are also indicated in allergic patients. Development of tolerance to a particular class of antihistamine or undesirable side effects such as somnolence can be a problem in drug treatment of chronic rhinosinusitis. Periodic changes among chemical classes of antihistamines (table II) may achieve the desired physiological effect while minimising undue side effects. According to some clinicians, such changes should be made from one class to another but not to other compounds within the same class since each congener within a class generally will have similar properties. However, others have questioned the need to change classes of antihistamines (Pearlman, 1976).

Patients with recurrent sinusitis should be carefully checked for chronic dental infections since these have been found responsible for between 10 and 25% of recurrent sinus infections (Dayal et al., 1976).

Table II. Chemical classes of antihistamines

Class	Drug
Ethanolamines	Bromodiphenhydramine
	Carbinoxamine
	d-Carbinoxamine
	Diphenhydramine
	Diphenylpyraline
	Doxylamine
Ethylenediamines	Antazoline
	Clemizole
	Mepyramine
	Methapyrilene
	Tripelenamine
Alkylamines	Brompheniramine
	d-Brompheniramine
	Chlorpheniramine
	d-Chlorpheniramine
	Dimethindene
	Pheniramine
	Triprolidine
Piperazines	Chlorcyclizine
	Meclozine
Phenothiazines	Dimethothiazine
	Isothipendyl
	Methdilazine
	Promethazine
	Trimeprazine
Miscellaneous	Azatadine
	Bamipine
	Cyproheptadine
	Mebhydrolin
	Meclastine
	Phenindamine

2.2.4 Complications

Intracranial and orbital extension are the most serious and life threatening complications of suppurative diseases of the nose and paranasal sinuses (Chandler et al., 1970). Meningitis, extradural, subdural and multifocal brain abscesses may complicate paranasal infections. Mild headache, malaise and low grade fever may be the only symptoms of cryptogenic intracranial infection. Neurosurgical consultation should be sought in all suspected cases.

2.3 Vasomotor Rhinitis

Vasomotor rhinitis is a poorly understood disease that is characterised by chronic nasal congestion; usually with an accompanying thin viscid rhinorrhoea associated with a hypertrophic red to red-blue mucosa. The most commonly evoked aetiology is an imbalance between the secretory-vasodilatory effect of the parasympathetic nerve supply and the drying-vasoconstrictive effect of the sympathetic nerve supply. Drug treatment is with oral decongestants (see section 1.4; Benson, 1971). Tachyphylaxis often develops and frequent changes of drugs are usually required. Many patients with this disorder are abusers of topical decongestant sprays and rhinitis medicamentosa is typically a feature of this syndrome. Complete cessation of topical decongestants and frequent nasal spray with normal saline containing 0.125% glycerine may be helpful in restoring the nasal mucosa to a more physiological state. Perhaps more effective is the use of an intranasal corticosteroid such as beclomethasone dipropionate as an aerosol — 1 jet to each nostril 4 times daily (Lofkvist and Svensson, 1976). Dexamethasone phosphate or flunisolide aerosol can be used as an alternative. The anti-inflammatory action is useful in restoring physiological function to the atrophic, denuded nasal mucosa seen as an end stage with vasomotor and allergic rhinitis.

2.4 Allergic Rhinitis

Nasal stuffiness, nasal discharge, sneezing, eye irritation with swelling and itching of the eyes, nose and throat are the common symptoms of allergic rhinitis. Offending allergens in a genetically predisposed patient have the capacity to alter the immune system with a resulting state of hypersensitivity to these agents. The rhinitis produced results from the release of chemical mediators of inflammation triggered by the antigen-antibody reaction. Symptoms of allergic rhinitis may begin at any age and may be categorised as seasonal, perennial, intermittent or continuous. The severity of the symptoms depends upon the amount of allergen exposure and the sensitivity of the nasal mucous membrane (for review, see Alberti, 1976; Mygind, 1978). Aspirin usage has been found in certain allergic individuals to cause rhinitis, asthma and polyposis (see chapter XX; sect. 11.3). Therefore, in allergic patients, particular attention should be given to a history of chronic analgesic use.

Early treatment is most effectively directed at control of allergen exposure. This requires exclusion of known or suspected food allergens from the diet, and where airborne antigens are concerned, is enhanced by air filtration and allergen avoidance. Subsequent treatment may involve hyposensitisation. Pharmacological treatment becomes necessary when avoidance of the offending allergen is impractical and hyposensitisation inconvenient or unsuccessful (Pearlman, 1975). Hyposensitisation can also be dangerous and in view of the efficacy of drugs in allergic rhinitis it should not be embarked upon lightly. Only one drug, sodium cromoglycate (cromolyn sodium), is available for prophylactic intranasal use in an attempt to prevent the allergic response (see chapter XX; sect. 2.3.2). While it can prevent the effects of experimental nasal challenge with pollen in sensitive subjects, and be used successfully in anticipation of exposure (e.g. house dust; anticipated exposure to an animal at a friend's house), it is not always practical to judge administration in this way. Intranasal cromoglycate (drops, spray or powder) used regularly during the pollen season has however, controlled nasal symptoms in less patients with seasonal allergic rhinitis, but results are convincing in those with perennial allergy (Brogden et al., 1974; Craig et al., 1977; Topilsky et al., 1976). The most convenient and successful treatments at present are symptomatic and thus directed at events occurring after antigen-antibody reaction — antihistamines to antagonise histamine liberated from sensitised mast cells, aerosol topical corticosteroids to suppress the inflammatory response elicited by released mediators, and nasal decongestants.

Topical nasal decongestants have a place in both seasonal and perennial allergies but, as in vasomotor rhinitis, can be over used. The large frequent doses required for relief in the acute stage of allergy lead to rapid sensitisation. Conversely, the unrelenting and drawn out clinical course of perennial allergies leads to a more insidious development of nose spray addiction. Therefore relief of nasal congestion should be obtained by other approaches and nasal sprays only used for brief periods during acute exacerbations. With the perennial form of rhinitis, use of a spray in one nasal chamber shortly before bed may give the patient adequate relief. Nasal congestion may be particularly bothersome at night due to passive venous congestion from the supine position and the low nocturnal circulating steroid level.

Antihistamines offer much relief from mild bouts of allergic rhinitis but they are unable to control severe episodes and are less effective in perennial than in seasonal allergic rhinitis (Fein-

berg, 1950). Since allergic rhinitis is often more troublesome at night and on rising, a long acting antihistamine is useful and avoids the drowsiness associated with daytime doses. Combined use of an antihistamine and an oral decongestant is helpful and offers an enhanced effect in the nose and also helps to combat drowsiness of daytime doses of the antihistamine (Empey et al., 1975). All oral decongestants have potential hypertensive and cardiac circulatory side effects and must be used cautiously in older patients. They may also interact with adrenergic neurone blocking antihypertensive drugs (see chapter XVIII; sect. 10.1.1) and with monoamine oxidase inhibitors (chapter VIII; sect. 3).

Numerous antihistaminic-decongestant drug combinations are available and undesirable side effects may occasionally be eliminated by switching drugs (see section 2.2.3). Patients may also rapidly develop tolerance to one particular combination but still respond to another preparation.

Nasal aerosols containing corticosteroids are effective in both seasonal and perennial allergic rhinitis and have largely replaced injections of long acting steroids into the nasal tissue although some clinicians still prefer long acting steroids such as methylprednisolone acetate in seasonal allergies, when 1, 2 or 3 injections only may suffice. In perennial allergies, the duration and efficacy gradually diminishes with each repeat injection.

Intrapolyp and intraturbinal injection of depot corticosteroids can be effective in inducing shrinkage of polyps, but unfortunately, there have been a very small but disturbing number of cases of blindness complicating this treatment (McGrew et al., 1978). Consequently, it is recommended that this treatment be used only by those skilled in the technique. Dexamethasone phosphate aerosol allows a high concentration in nasal tissues but low systemic levels and therefore minimal risk of adrenal suppression with usual doses. Beclomethasone dipropionate or flunisolide aerosol provides an even greater margin of safety and is to be preferred (Brogden et al., 1975; Mygind, 1977; Turkeltaub et al., 1976). Intranasal topical steroids allow a marked reduction in antihistamine requirements for rhinorrhoea but have little effect on eye symptoms. For maximum effectiveness, the intranasal aerosol must reach all or most of the nasal mucosa, and for this reason, polyps may need to be removed surgically prior to such therapy. A topical decongestant can also be used during the initial week of therapy to help distribute the subsequent steroid spray. A few patients may not tolerate topical steroid administration, but the only real disadvantage is the delayed onset of symptomatic relief. It usually takes 3 to 7 days to decongest a swollen nose since shrinkage begins anteriorly and progresses posteriorly. A 3 or 4 day course of oral steroids may be of use until the topical application becomes effective. The usual adult dosage of beclomethasone is 2 jets (100µg) into each nostril 4 times daily for 1 week, with subsequent reduction to 200 to 300µg daily. Patients should be instructed in the correct use of the nasal aerosol. Long term, high dose topical steroid use produces increased capillary fragility and mucosal atrophy, but there have been no important local or systemic side effects with clinical use of intranasal beclomethasone at recommended dosage (Poynter, 1977).

Surgical management may be required in advanced cases with hyperplastic sinusitis, anatomic obstruction, or massive polyposis. When irreversibly damaged tissues have been removed and adequate drainage re-established, medical management is usually successful.

2.5 Fungal Infections of the Nasal Cavity

Mucormycosis of the nasal and paranasal tissues is almost always found only in poorly controlled diabetics or renal transplant patients, who are susceptible to fungal infections from commensal or saprophytic organisms. Clinically, such mycotic infections differ little from bacterial infections. Treatment includes control of underlying systemic disease states, local surgical removal of infected tissues and a systemic antifungal agent (see chapter XXVII; sect. 5.8).

Aspergillosis is most commonly seen as an external ear infection but can also occur in the nose, sinuses and orbit. The pathogenicity of this organism is much less than other typical mycoses and is usually best treated by local removal and topical antifungal agents such as nystatin, miconazole or clotrimazole (see chapter XXVII; sect. 5.8).

2.6 Nasal Furuncles

Furuncles are often found in the nasal vestibular area and may occur as chronically recurring infections. Effective treatment consists of warm soaks and local incision and drainage after maturation has occurred. Topical antibacterial agents such as povidone iodine or bacitracin are helpful prophylactic measures. Neomycin containing preparations should be used with caution because of sensitisation that may occur. Persistent or progressive furunculosis demands systemic antibacterials. Since penicillinase producing *Staph. aureus* and streptococci are the usual organisms, a penicillinase resistant penicillin such as a cloxacillin (table I) is required.

2.7 Pharyngitis

The acute sore throat is a common illness with numerous aetiologies, including not only many infectious agents, but also nonspecific irritants and chemical pollutants. In most cases of acute pharyngitis, the clinician must decide between viral or streptococcal infection. Except in epidemics or in cases of scarlet fever, clinical findings alone do not distinguish viral from streptococcal sore throat with sufficient precision. For this reason, a culture of the posterior pharyngeal wall and both tonsils should be obtained to rule out streptococcal pharyngitis (Wannamaker, 1972, 1976).

Individual clinicians differ in their approach to treatment (and their enthusiasm for throat culture) depending on their attitude to the likelihood of streptococcal infection and the use and value of antibacterial dugs. Some administer antibacterial drugs empirically to all patients complaining of sore throat, but this is not the generally recommended authoritative practice. Sore throats are most often non-streptococcal (Glezen et al., 1967; Feery et al., 1976); many are viral and most of these require only supportive therapy and do not benefit from antibacterial drugs (Taylor et al., 1977). Antibacterial drugs are effective only in preventing the rheumatic sequelae of streptococcal pharyngitis. They do not alter the symptomatic course of streptococcal pharyngitis (Brink et al., 1951) and evidence that they prevent glomerulonephritis is not convincing (Weinstein and Le Frock, 1971). A delay in treatment of 24 to 48 hours for culture results does not appreciably prolong the patient's discomfort or increase the risk of developing rheumatic fever (Denny et al., 1971). For these reasons, apart from an epidemic of rheumatic fever, when all patients with pharyngitis should be treated, antibacterial drugs generally need only be administered after throat culture results are known (Pantell, 1977). Certain patients however, have a high likelihood of streptococcal infection and in practice should be given penicillin (or erythromycin in known cases of penicillin allergy) immediately. Such patients include those with a clinical diagnosis of scarlet fever, febrile patients with pus in the tonsillar crypts and tender enlarged anterior cervical glands, those with bacterial complications such as quinsy, those with rheumatic heart disease, and patients with any kind of sore throat if streptococcal infection is known to be prevalent in the family.

When used, antibacterials must be given in full dosage for 10 to 14 days. It must be impressed upon parents of young children in particular, that antibacterial treatment must be taken regularly as prescribed for the full course and not stop after 3 or 4 days when symptoms subside. A positive culture for group A β-haemolytic streptococcus, apart from indicating treatment with penicillin, may indicate the need to swab contacts in special risk situations, such as those in rheumatic families or groups where the risk of rheumatic fever may be greater (Wannamaker, 1976). While a negative culture is considered by some clinicians to be an indication to discontinue antibacterial therapy given before culture results are known, we feel that once treatment is started, it should be continued until the course is completed.

Effective symptomatic treatment consists of warm saline gargles or throat irrigations and antipyretic analgesics such as aspirin or paracetamol (acetaminophen).

Any of the viral infectious diseases, infectious mononucleosis in particular, may present as a pharyngitis. Treatment of the pharyngeal inflammation of infectious mononucleosis is usually symptomatic, with careful attention directed to development of hepatosplenomegaly and other protean manifestations of this disease. If there is airway obstruction however, high doses of corticosteroids (e.g. 40 to 80mg daily prednisone or equivalent) are indicated for 2 to 4 days and then rapidly tapered.

The role of adenoidectomy and tonsillectomy in the treatment of recurrent infections of the tonsils and adenoids remains one of the most controversial subjects in contemporary medicine (Sprinkle and Sorenson, 1977). At present, the most effective medical management consists of repeated courses of appropriate antibacterial drugs with supportive symptomatic care. While cultures are helpful, surface organisms do not always reflect what is found in the parenchyma. The dangers of repeated antibiotic therapy may range from dermatitis to death (Sprinkle and Sorenson, 1977). Recent studies have shown that the concentration of bacteria in tonsillar tissue may have a critical level above which one has symptomatic bacterial tonsillitis (Snow, 1978). Predictive assays from tonsillar biopsies may thus be helpful in assessing the likelihood of recurrent disease.

Peritonsillar abscesses are the most common parapharyngeal suppurative infections of the neck. They are rarely seen in children but are commonly seen after puberty and in young adults. The patient usually gives a history of a sore throat of several days duration and progressive difficulty with swallowing and talking. Treatment consists of surgical drainage and penicillin. Occasionally, the patient will be seen prior to development of a frank abscess and will have only peritonsillar cellulitis. Some clinicians prefer to treat peritonsillar abscesses with immediate tonsillectomy. Regardless of the surgical procedure chosen, and certainly with pre-abscess cellulitis, systemic antibacterial cover with penicillin or erythromycin is indicated for a full 10 to 14 days. Gargles or throat irrigations with warm saline provide symptomatic relief after incision and drainage.

Treatment of diphtheria and pertussis is discussed in chapter IV (section 5.1.4).

3. Ear Infections

3.1 Otitis Externa

Drugs for the control of disease in the external auditory canal are basically medications for various forms of dermatitis (Cassisi et al., 1977; Tonkin, 1973). The skin of the ear canal should have an acidic surface pH and variations of this lead to disease states. Therapy involves a thorough cleansing of the skin and is directed toward the restoration of pH; reduction of swelling; elimination of infection; and removal or control of predisposing causes, especially prevention of scratching or rubbing in and around the ear.

Five classifications of external ear disease requiring drug therapy are: (1) acute oedematous otitis externa (swimmer's ear); (2) eczematoid dermatitis with secondary infection; (3) true otomycosis; (4) acute furunculosis, and (5) malignant otitis externa.

3.1.1 Acute Oedematous Otitis Externa (swimmer's ear)

Following gentle and meticulous ear cleansing with a suction apparatus or with extremely small wire (e.g. dental broaches) cotton tipped applicators, a 70 to 95 % alcohol solution (may be painful), or a 1 % acetic solution is used to carefully wipe the ear canal. (The usual wooden applicator stick is far too large and must never be used). Following this, and removal of any excess alcohol with suction, a cotton wick saturated with an anti-bacterial-corticosteroid or acetic acid-corticosteroid solution is gently inserted and the patient instructed to use the same solution as a topical drop 3 times daily for a week (Special Report, 1978). The cotton wick is usually removed in 48 to 72 hours and the drops continued. Since the infection is often due to Gram-negative bacilli, preparations based on neomycin or framycetin, preferably with polymyxin, or on gentamicin, are the most appropriate.

Severe swelling may require injectable or oral corticosteroids for a few days in order to reduce the oedema to the point that the topical medication will be effective. An antipruritic, such as oral promethazine at night, is an essential part of management and should be continued for many days after apparent resolution of the infection. Patients must not scratch, poke or rub in and around the ear. Prevention of otitis externa, for example in competitive swimmers or professional scuba divers, is by avoiding this precipitating factor and by use of 5 % acetic acid in 50 % ethyl alcohol after immersion — to dry the skin, kill any bacteria or fungi and maintain the normal acidity of the skin (Wright et al., 1974).

3.1.2 Infected Eczematoid Dermatitis

This condition involves secondary infection of an existing neurodermatitis and is commonly induced by scratching skin with infected nails. Following careful ear cleaning by suction and wiping of the ear canal with 70 to 95 % alcohol, a cotton gauze wick is gently inserted into the external canal with a small wire applicator and is saturated with aluminium acetate (Burrow's solution) or aluminium acetate with acetic acid solution. The patient should be treated with these drops 3 times daily for 48 to 72 hours; the Burrow's solution should then be stopped, the wick removed and an antibacterial corticosteroid solution should be used for 1 week, together with an oral antipruritic at night (see section 3.1.1).

Recurrent crusting or itching of the meatus after the drops are stopped may necessitate the application of a steroid or steroid and antibacterial/antifungal ointment for a prolonged period of time as a prophylactic measure.

3.1.3 Otomycosis

Otomycosis is a relatively uncommon occurrence, but should be considered in cases of recurrent otitis externa. True fungus infection of the ear canal is not seen often (although it may be frequently mentioned by the patient as the primary complaint) and actual growth of fungus from the canal is rarely accomplished.

If inspection indicates probable mycelia, or a blackish accumulation, then the ear canal should be cleansed carefully with applicators and a suction (see section 3.1.1) and should be wiped several times with an antifungal solution such as diamthazole or tolnaftate. The ear canal may then be painted with a solution of gentian violet (10 %) or an antifungal powder such as nystatin or clioquinol (iodochlorhydroxyquinoline) may be insufflated into the canal. Usually, the application of this powder (once) weekly will keep the fungal inflammation under control. An occasional resistant case may require the tolnaftate solution to be applied daily (1 drop bid). The patient should be repeatedly instructed to keep the ears exquisitely dry and to avoid any picking, scratching or rubbing in and around the ear.

3.1.4 Acute Furunculosis

Acute infection around hair follicles in the ear canal may develop with subsequent boil formation and sudden onset of severe burning pain in one ear, which increases rapidly in severity. Unlike acute mastoiditis (see section 3.2.4), acute furunculosis is not related to a history of upper respiratory infection and acute otitis media. Narcotic analgesics such as morphine are necessary in the beginning, but after the first 24 hours aspirin with codeine is often adequate. Very careful cleansing of the ear canal should be carried out with suction and 70 % alcohol. A cotton wick saturated with gentamicin ointment is inserted.

Since most of these infections are due to staphylococcal or sometimes streptococcal infection, the patient should be started on oral antibiotics such as a cloxacillin (table I). In severe cases with signs of systemic spread (e.g. lymphadenitis, fever), parenteral administration of a cloxacillin is necessary. Surgical incision and drainage of obvious abscess is necessary. All patients should be treated for 7 days.

3.1.5 Malignant Otitis Externa

The proper management of this rapidly progressive disorder (Cohn, 1974) involves the rigid control of diabetes mellitus with which it is usually associated. The disease can also occur in children with malnutrition and anaemia (Joachims, 1976). In most cases, parenteral gentamicin in maximum dosage short of toxicity is required. This therapy should be given for a minimum of 2 weeks and then lower preventive dosage levels should be maintained for longer periods. Recent studies (Joachims, 1976) have shown *Pseudomonas* strains resistant to gentamicin and alternate therapy with intravenous carbenicillin may be indicated by sensitivity studies. Metronidazole has also been used in cases involving anaerobes (see further chapter XXVII; sect. 5.7).

Local cleansing and debridement is mandatory and very often extensive resection of infected cartilage and devitalised skin and soft tissue is required. Following this resection, the infected area should be packed with gentamicin ointment. Repeated daily local irrigation or douche with gentamicin solution is also helpful. After the immediate severe local infection is controlled, the patient should be placed on long term prophylaxis with topical application of gentamicin drops. This infection usually involves *Pseudomonas* or *Proteus* saprophytes and careful attention to recurrent infection must be maintained. After all infection has subsided, 95% alcohol drops in the ear canal once a day should be continued indefinitely.

3.2 Otitis Media

Drug treatment in otitis media is directed towards the control of infection, the ventilation of the middle ear, and the restoration of normal eustachian tube function. Very often there are associated systemic or generalised ear, nose and throat disorders which may also need therapy (Roydhouse, 1972, 1978; Symposium, 1976).

3.2.1 Acute Otitis Media

The patient usually complains of earache, so that initial treatment is directed toward immediate relief of pain. Topical solutions containing local analgesics (e.g. antipyrine/benzocaine; lignocaine/lidocaine) have been long used, warmed under running water, to fill the ear canal. Although they do appear to provide local pain relief in most cases (solutions containing antibacterials have no therapeutic benefit), supplemental systemic analgesics are still usually required. Codeine combined with aspirin is generally effective, but some patients may require an injection of pethidine (meperidine) for immediate relief of a severe throbbing pain.

Systemic antibacterial agents should be started immediately. The most common pathogens are pneumococci, *Streptococcus pyogenes,* and in children *Haemophilus influenzae* also. In under 6 year old children, *H. influenzae* occurs frequently but can also be common in older children (Bass et al., 1967; Howie et al., 1970; Schwartz et al., 1977). Ampicillin or amoxycillin is the agent of choice because of its spectrum of activity, in particular for its effectiveness against *H. influenzae* in children (Howard et al., 1976). However, strains of *H. influenzae* resistant to ampicillin are now being reported (Schwartz et al., 1978). Erythromycin combined with a sulphonamide, or co-trimoxazole (trimethoprim + sulphamethoxazole) is preferred in cases not responding to amoxycillin or ampicillin. Erythromycin in full doses or co-trimoxazole can be used in the penicillin allergic patient (for dosages table I). Cephalexin is not recommended in childhood otitis media because of inadequate activity against *H. influenzae* (Stechenberg et al., 1976).

Antibacterial therapy should be continued for a minimum of 10 days to prevent the development of serous (secretory) otitis media and if the ear has not cleared completely, for a period of 14 days or more. In order to prevent prolonged complications, the ear may have to be opened with myringotomy if pus is obviously present, if the appearance of the middle ear has not returned to normal after antibacterial therapy, or if there is persistent conductive hearing loss.

Topical nasal decongestants such as xylometazoline or oxymetazoline and oral eustachian tube decongestants such as phenylpropanolamine or pseudoephedrine (section 1.4) may be helpful, but should be used for limited periods only. Since the infection in most cases spreads from the nose, clearance of nasal and sinus secretions is logical.

3.2.2 Purulent Otitis Media

In simple practical terms, purulent or chronic suppurative otitis media indicates a middle ear infection which has persisted continuously for over

6 weeks, but it also includes recurrent ear infection which did not begin as an acute otitis media, for example, a non-painful discharge from the ear through a pre-existing perforation.

Initial treatment is directed at measures aimed at producing a healthy nose and paranasal sinuses — investigation for sinusitis, appropriate anti-allergy treatment, removal of adenoids and nasal septal operations if indicated. As soon as a clear nasal airway has been provided, the patient must be educated in how to breathe through it. At the same time, careful and adequate cleansing of the external ear canal and middle ear must be accomplished with use of a suction, and often with the pneumatic otoscope. Once the purulent exudate and debris is removed, an antibacterial solution may be displaced into the middle ear and mastoid, often with the assistance of the pneumatic otoscope. Solutions containing gentamicin, polymyxin with acetic acid, or 70% alcohol (may be painful) are appropriate.

This aural toilet should be repeated once weekly (or more frequently), together with topical application of antibacterial drops or powder[1] once daily for several weeks. Usually a saprophyte such as a *Pseudomonas* or *Proteus* spp. is involved and prolonged treatment is necessary to eradicate the organism. Systemic therapy with appropriate antibiotics such as gentamicin, colistin or kanamycin would be too toxic and because of the presence of a cavity and purulent exudate, these drugs usually do not reach the bacteria in sufficient concentration. Systemic antibiotics may however, be indicated if the culture is positive for a bacteria other than *Pseudomonas* or *Proteus* since such organisms can be more virulent and may have invaded tissue beyond the mastoid cavities. Occasionally, culture will indicate an overwhelming yeast infection, appropriate topical use of nystatin powder is then required. Otitis media from anaerobic infections occurs in some patients (Fulghum et al., 1977; Jokipii et al., 1977) and drugs appropriate

---

1   Medications recommended for topical application include: gentamicin solution (3mg/ml); polymyxin with acetic acid solution; 70% alcohol; 70% alcohol plus 2.5% boric acid solution; chloramphenicol powder; chloramphenicol solution 0.25%; 1 to 5% acetic acid solution. Our experience indicates no effect on sensorineural hearing from using topical gentamicin solution in the human middle ear. At least one report of toxicity from topical use of neomycin and colistin in guinea pigs has been published (Brummett et al., 1976). See further section 7.1.1.

for these bacteria (see chapter XXVII; sect. 5.7) need to be used in patients unresponsive to the usual antibiotics listed above.

Prolonged local antibacterial therapy with frequent cleansing will usually dry up most chronic infections where there is a large perforation. If drainage persists after 6 weeks of intensive therapy, or if cholesteatoma is present, tympano-mastoid surgery is necessary. Very often intense local therapy pre-operatively may convert an extremely infected ear into a quiescent one which will permit the surgeon to perform less radical mastoid surgery and permit more effective reconstruction of the sound-transformer mechanism.

3.2.3 Serous (secretory) Otitis Media and Mucoid Otitis Media

Serous or secretory otitis media is the most common form of deafness in children (Liu et al., 1975; Juhn et al., 1977). The condition is characterised by accumulation of thin serous fluid, or more often, thick tenacious mucus ('glue ear' or mucoid otitis media). It affects adults much less commonly than children. Some children with obvious evidence of middle ear fluid may have little or no earache and only very mild or very short lived hearing loss. Other children complain of frequent earache, often followed by discharge from the ear, with hearing loss which may be prolonged for months. Very occasionally, permanent hearing loss results.

Medical treatment should be tried first but may not always be satisfactory (Fraser et al., 1977): milk free diet, antihistamines and other appropriate antiallergy treatment, topical nasal decongestants, oral eustachian tube decongestants and eustachian autoinflation manoeuvres are often used (see below). Remission can occur spontaneously in many children (Fraser, 1971).

Persistent fluid behind the eardrum should be treated by myringotomy, followed by aspiration of exudate, with or without the insertion of ventilation tubes (grommets) [Oppenheimer, 1975]. When adequate drainage has been established topical clearing agents to the tube or middle ear may be necessary. 70% alcohol, 1 or 2 drops at a time, can be used to hold down the crusting. Glycerite of peroxide may be used also. These substances may burn slightly and if the burning persists, should be terminated. Antibacterial-corticosteroid solutions are often helpful in holding down the crusting and the recurrent exudate. Topical infection can also be contained with these agents (see section 3.2.2). There is no good case for systemic antibacterial agents (Riding et al., 1978).

Although they have not been proven to be of benefit (Fraser et al., 1977; Olsen et al., 1978), eustachian tube decongestants are often used as adjunctive treatment to the elimination of fluid from the middle ear. Persistent oedema and obstruction of the eustachian tube with failure of aeration of the middle ear, is the underlying cause of most serous otitis. Drugs used in decongestion (alone or with an antihistamine) are oral pseudoephedrine or phenylpropanolamine and oral plus intranasal phenylephrine. Alternate use of different classes of antihistamines (table II) may provide an improved clinical effect since some patients respond much better, with fewer side effects, to one class of agent than another. Azatadine, a recently introduced antihistamine, appears to have few side effects when used for these problems. Meclastine and mebhydrolin are also effective antihistamines with a low incidence of sedative side effects (see further section 1.2).

Corticosteroids are also helpful for their antiinflammatory action, either given intramuscularly or orally for a few days.

Allergy of the nose or respiratory tract is often associated with serous otitis media and suitable antiallergy treatent (e.g. milk free diet, avoidance of dust and animals, hyposensitisation to airborne allergens), including antihistamines or intranasal beclomethasone dipropionate or sodium cromoglycate, and treatment of obvious cases of allergic rhinitis (see section 2.4), may be required as indicated by appropriate testing measures (Dees and Lefkowitz, 1972; Phillips et al., 1974).

Replacement therapy for any metabolic deficiency should be considered. Hyperimmune gamma globulin in particular may be necessary as well as daily thyroid extract or synthetic thyroid preparations.

3.2.4 Mastoiditis

In acute mastoiditis, unlike acute furunculosis (see section 3.1.4), there is definite progression from upper respiratory infection to acute otitis media to acute mastoiditis, and the deafness which occurs with the stage of otitis media is frequently severe. Once the diagnosis of acute mastoiditis has been made, initial intravenous antibiotics followed by several weeks of maintenance oral antibacterials should be used. If no culture information is available, ampicillin (8g daily) or amoxycillin (4g

daily) should be started. Appropriate surgical procedures should be applied. Certain cases of acute mastoiditis may respond without surgery if adequate middle ear drainage is established. Chronic mastoiditis in association with any persistent purulent ear exudate will require surgical management as outlined under purulent otitis media (see section 3.2.2).

3.2.5 Perichondritis

Immediate incision and drainage of the infected pinna is necessary in order to separate the infected skin and cartilage and permit infusion of appropriate antibacterial agents into the relatively avascular cartilage. Perforated plastic or rubber drains should be inserted between the skin and cartilage and irrigation of topical antibiotic solution should be made through these drains at least twice a day.

Most infections associated with perichondritis are due to *Pseudomonas* or *Proteus* spp. Systemic antibacterials are generally not effective. Occasionally, a topical solution of 0.25% acetic acid will be effective in eliminating the infection. More rapid resolution can usually be obtained by irrigating with a gentamicin, colistin or polymyxin solution. Supplemental parenteral dosages of these drugs, in maximum amounts below the level of toxicity, for a period of 2 to 4 weeks may also be useful.

Debridement agents such as topical trypsin may be helpful. Resection of infected cartilage may become necessary if the measures described above do not yield results after a 2 week period.

4. Vertigo

Vertigo is a symptom, not a disease, and essentially denotes an hallucinatory sensation of movement (Dix, 1973; Roydhouse, 1973). Episodes of vertigo, whether fleeting or lasting, are generally referred to as dizziness by the patient. Vertiginous dizziness must be differentiated from syncopal dizziness. This is done by describing each of the two types. The patient then can identify with one or the other. There are a large number of conditions in which vertigo is a symptom. The disease process can involve the peripheral labyrinth, the 8th cranial nerve, or the central connections of the 8th nerve in the brain stem, cerebrum and cerebellum. Vertigo is classified in more than one way, but a scheme based on a symptomatic investigation which progresses logically to the most likely cause (fig. 2), is the most practical for treatment purposes (Turner, 1975). Vertigo is usually not life threatening but it sometimes heralds serious disease such as multiple sclerosis, intracranial tumours or focal epilepsy.

A variety of drugs have been used for vertigo and those types considered most useful are given in table III. Selection hopefully depends upon an aetiological diagnosis.

Since with vertigo, the aetiology often evades one's diagnostic capability, a conception of possible pathological mechanisms leads to intelligent trial and error treatment.

4.1 Vertigo of Sudden Onset

A sudden, severe, primary attack of vertigo in a patient less than 50 years old is usually due to a labyrinthitis or vestibular neuronitis as a sequel of bacterial or viral infection or metabolic disturbance. Most viral labyrinthine infections follow upper respiratory infection. Bacterial labyrinthitis is serious, destroys the end organ, can lead to meningitis but is fortunately rare. Most labyrinthine infections are viral. Viral end organ or neuronal disease is self limited and treatment consists of bed rest and oral labyrinthine suppres-

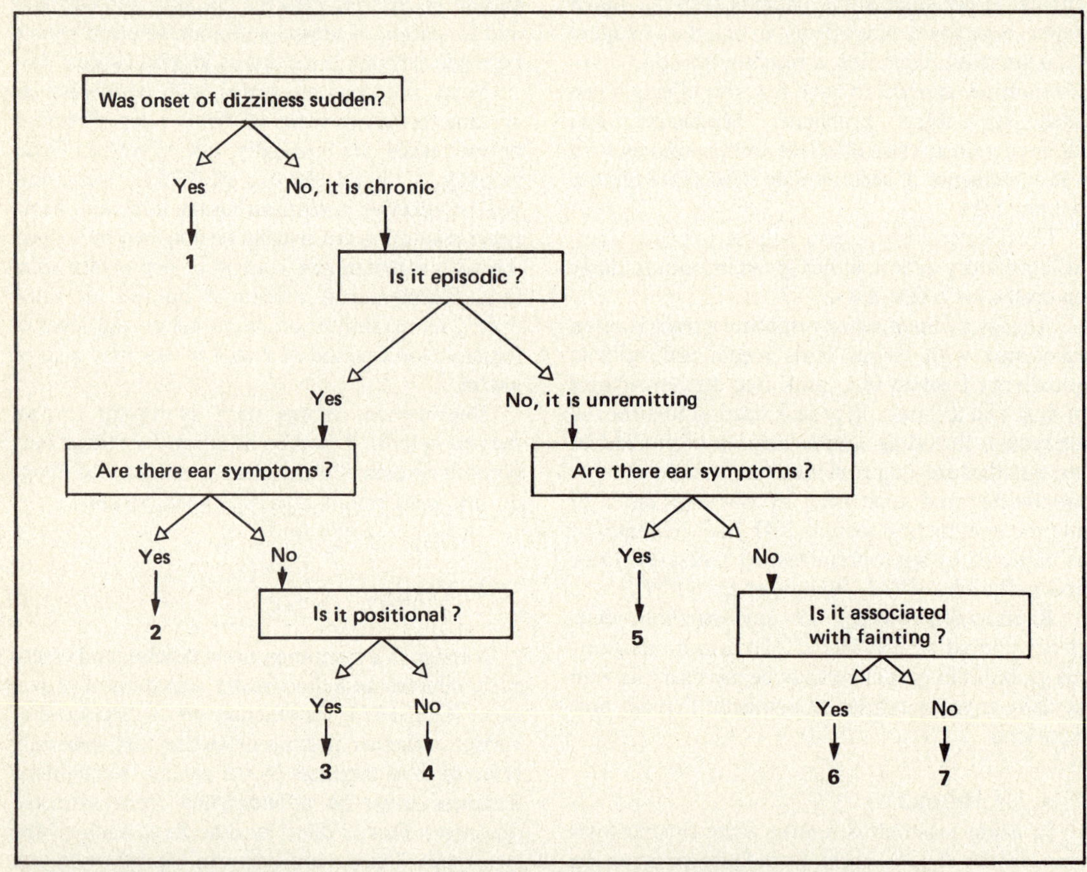

Fig. 2. Diagnostic approach to patient with vertigo and key to possible diagnoses which influence treatment (after Turner: Southern Medical Journal 68: 241, 1975; by permission of author and editor).
  (1) Exertional vertigo, vestibular neuronitis, labyrinthitis, vascular disorder of inner ear
  (2) Chronic suppurative otitis media or mastoiditis, Meniere's disease, acoustic neurinoma
  (3) Benign positional vertigo (e.g. head injury), cervical spine lesions
  (4) Drugs, hyperventilation, trauma to cervical spine, menopause, migraine
  (5) Acoustic neurinoma or other cerebello-pontine angle tumor
  (6) Vertebrobasilar artery insufficiency, or orthostatic hypotension, paroxysmal cardiac arrhythmias, carotid arteriosclerosis, carotid sinus sensitivity
  (7) Psychoneurosis, diabetes mellitus, thyroid disease, anaemia, hypertension, leukaemia

sants such as prochlorperazine or dimenhyrinate (table III) for a few weeks. Corticosteroids (table III) when given at the onset of symptoms may reduce the damage done by the virus. The patient may be left with a sensitive labyrinth which requires mild sedatives such as 2mg diazepam when travelling. If a patient with sudden vertigo has an associated severe and persistent headache, meningitis should be ruled out.

In a patient more than 50 years old, sudden vertigo is more likely due to a vascular disorder involving the labyrinthine blood supply. This includes a plexus of small arteries branching from the vertebral-basilar system. A previous history of peripheral arteriosclerotic or hypertensive vascular disease suggests such a mechanism. Treatment includes hospitalisation and vasodilatation by an intravenous infusion of histamine ($1\mu g/kg/min$) or papaverine ($0.5mg/kg/min$). Inhalation of 5% carbon dioxide and 95% oxygen, from a tight fitting anaesthesia mask with a large reservoir and one way valve, is also effective.

A sudden, unprecedented attack of vertigo with hearing loss, may follow physical activity (extreme exertion, intercourse), middle ear pressure changes (flying, scuba diving) or emotional stress. Otological examination for round window rupture and complete bed rest are required. Diazepam (10mg orally every 6 hours) is helpful in relieving symptoms.

4.2 Chronic, Episodic Vertigo with Ear Symptoms

4.2.1 Recurrent Vertigo due to Otological Causes

If the patient admits to associated ear symptoms (e.g. fullness in one ear, tinnitus or hearing loss), the cause of vertigo is probably otological. Obvious chronic suppurative otitis media, with or without mastoiditis, is treated with local secretion aspiration, mechanical cleaning, antibacterial drugs and often surgery. Bacterial flora varies, so cultures are wise in these chronic disorders (see also section 3.2.2).

4.2.2 Meniere's Disease (endolymphatic hydrops)

Only a few patients with recurrent vertigo have endolymphatic hydrops. However, it is possible to have labyrinthine hydrops without hearing loss and *vice versa*. Other symptoms in various combinations include fluctuating pressure, loudness intolerance, diplacusis and tinnitus. If there is hearing loss it should be intermittently fluctuant. Skilled audiometry is necessary to confirm the diagnosis when hearing loss is present and it will also help differentiate the unilateral hearing loss from that due to acoustic neuroma (Johnson, 1968).

Medical treatment does reduce the morbidity of endolymphatic hydrops but it is not clear whether treatment at an early stage can prevent advance of the condition. Surgical treatment is reserved for certain cases refractory to medical treatment. Endolymphatic hydrops has more than one cause or precipitating factor, although the pathological finding (distention of the endolymphatic space) is the same in all patients. Cigarettes, coffee and other CNS stimulants should be prohibited. Abnormalities of glucose metabolism (e.g. hyperglycaemia and hypoglycaemia) are corrected with the appropriate diet (see chapter XVI; sect. 3). Fat metabolism variations, as reflected in high triglyceride levels, are similarly corrected by appropriate diet (see chapter XVII; sect. 3.2.3). A suspected allergic diathesis is confirmed with appropriate testing and corrected insofar as possible with hyposensitisation and allergen withdrawal.

Theory rather than fact is the basis of our understanding of the pathophysiological events leading to hydrops. Drug therapy is empirical (Roydhouse, 1973; Arenberg and Bayer, 1977). It presently centres around vasodilation to increase cochlear and labyrinthine blood flow, diuretics or a salt restriction-diuretic regimen to remove water from the body in the aim of decreasing the supposed elevated intralabyrinthine fluid pressure, symptomatic antivertiginous antihistamines, and psychotherapeutic drugs to offset attacks precipitated by autonomic influences (table III). Correction of the metabolic aberrations mentioned above, where relevant, rounds out these choices. While several drugs are often used simultaneously, it is not known whether such combinations are more efficacious than each by itself.

Cochlear and labyrinthine blood flow studies in guinea pigs and dogs have been published with data to commend papaverine, intravenous histamine, betahistine and inhalations of 5% carbon dioxide and oxygen. Cyclandelate as a smooth muscle relaxant is possibly as good as papaverine. Nicotinic acid does not increase blood flow in these animals. Also, a flow increase from vasodilation can be offset by a reduced blood pressure (see further section 1.5).

Table III. Drugs used in treatment of vertigo (see also Leonard and Lawrence, 1971; Rubin, 1973)

Class[1]	Action	Drug	Initial dosage[2]	Notes[3]
Labyrinthine suppressants Antihistamines [1] (also have an anti- cholinergic and sedative effect)	Act by suppressing vestibular end organ receptors and inhibiting activation of central cholinergic pathways	Cinnarizine Cyclizine Dimenhydrinate Diphenidol (not antihistamine) Meclozine Promethazine	15mg 4 to 6-hourly 50mg 4 to 6-hourly 50mg 4 to 6 hourly 50mg 4 to 6-hourly 25-50mg 24-hourly 25mg 12-hourly	Hallucinations may occur: use initially only in hospital
Antiemetic phenothiazines [2]	Suppress central vestibular pathways	Prochlorperazine Thiethylperazine	10mg 4-hourly 10mg 8 to 24-hourly	Useful when nausea or vomiting prominent
Anticholinergics [3]	Inhibit activation of central cholinergic pathways	Atropine sulphate Hyoscine hydrobromide	0.4mg IM 0.6mg 3-hourly	Useful to abort an attack of vertigo resulting from endolymphatic hydrops
Vasodilators [4]	Improve blood flow to labyrinth and brain stem			Useful when vascular ischaemia suspected (e.g. Meniere's disease, sudden hearing loss and vertigo, positional vertigo). Probably not useful when atherosclerosis is the factor which limits blood flow.
		Histamine (diphosphate)	2.5mg in 250ml saline IV	Given after a meal, at rate (16-60 drops/min) to produce flushing. BP must not fall $>$ 10-15mm Hg.
		5% CO_2 + 95% O_2	Breathe over 20 min, 2-4 times daily	Use tight fitting mask (see section 4.1)
		Betahistine	32-48mg daily in 3 or 4 divided doses	
		Cyclandelate	200mg 6 to 8-hourly; up to 1,200mg daily if necessary	
		Nylidrin Papaverine	6mg 8-hourly 0.5mg/kg/min IV or 150mg 12-hourly (long acting capsule)	

Diuretics[5]	?Decrease intra-labyrinthine fluid pressure			Useful in women with premenstrual fluid retention (salt restriction alone may suffice)
		Acetazolamide	250mg daily for 2 days in every 3 days	To avoid acidosis, give 250mg a day for 2 days, discontinue on 3rd
		Hydrochlorothiazide (or equivalent)	25mg 12-hourly	Potassium supplements may be necessary if given long term
Psychotherapeutic drugs [6]	Modify subjective response to the vertigo			Useful in some cases of Meniere's disease, vasomotor labyrinthitis, psycho-genic dizziness
Antianxiety agents		Chlordiazepoxide	10mg 8-hourly	When anxiety is the predominant response to vertigo
		Diazepam	2-5mg 8-hourly	
		Phenobarbitone	15-45mg 8-hourly	
Antidepressants		Amitriptyline	25mg 8-hourly	When depression is the predominant response to vertigo
		Nortriptyline	10mg 8-hourly	
Corticosteroids [7]	Suppress labyrinthine oedema and swelling due to virus infection	Methylprednisolone	40-80mg daily for 4-5 days, then 20mg daily for next 4 days	May lessen damage of acute viral labyrinthitis if given within 1 or 2 days
Antibacterial drugs	Combat direct bacterial infection of labyrinth	Penicillin	High doses (10-20 mega u daily) by IV infusion	Used in suppurative labyrinthitis (NB life threatening illness) and in vertigo associated with chronic suppurative otitis media and mastoiditis

1   Numbers in brackets beside class name refer to putative site of action in figure 3.
2   The usual adult oral (unless specified) dosage for initial treatment. Some of the dosages (e.g. labyrinthine suppressants, vasodilators) may need to be reduced for maintenance treatment (i.e. decreased dose or less frequent dosage interval).
3   See also text.

Some clinicians have used diuretics (Hinchcliffe, 1973), while others favour a combination regimen of salt restriction diet (500mg of sodium) with a diuretic (Boles et al., 1975). Potassium supplements (50mEq or mmol daily) are required if diuretics are used long term. With increasing attention to the psychosomatic aspects of the disease, tricyclic antidepressants such as amitriptyline have proved useful, particularly in influencing the emotional response to the vertigo.

If an attack occurs, the maintenance dosage of vestibulosuppressive drugs should be increased, but not that of the diuretic. Vasodilatation is improved with daily intravenous histamine and 5% carbon dioxide inhalations 3 or 4 times daily. Bed rest and corticosteroid therapy help (oral betamethasone 48mg followed by 24mg every 12 hours for 4 doses, then rapidly tapered; or an equivalent dose of another steroid). After 2 weeks freedom from vertigo, the usual maintenance dosage of vestibulosuppressive drugs should be resumed.

Drug therapy has been of little or no benefit in conservation or improvement of hearing. Surgical approaches to treatment directed at the hearing as well as the vertiginous component of Meniere's disease have yielded promising results and are receiving increasing emphasis (Arenberg and Bayer, 1977).

4.3 Chronic, Episodic Vertigo without Ear Symptoms but Related to Position

Vertigo which occurs within seconds of assuming certain head positions and is reproducible by positional testing usually confirms the diagnosis of benign positional vertigo. A detailed neurological and medical examination may however, be necessary to rule out vertigo due to cervical spine lesions, a multiple sensory deficit, or a malignant posterior fossa lesion.

Benign positional vertigo, which includes post-traumatic vertigo following head injury, may improve spontaneously — usually within a matter of weeks. A mild sedative and reassurance that compensation to the head position will occur in time is generally sufficient, but in some cases labyrinthine suppressants (table III) may be more effective. If benign positional vertigo persists, exercises to habituate the vertiginous mechanism (McCabe, 1969), or even a singular neurectomy, add to available options.

4.4 Chronic, Episodic Vertigo without Ear Symptoms and not Related to Position

Overdosage of anticonvulsant drugs can cause severe imbalance and nystagmus (see chapter XXV; sect. 3) indistinguishable from a posterior fossa syndrome, and overdosage of streptomycin or gentamicin may lead to severe imbalance and vertigo with sudden movements (see section 7.1.1). A careful history may show other drugs such as antihypertensives, diuretics, the antibiotic minocycline or nasal decongestant sprays to be the cause of the dizziness. Relief in these cases can be obtained by discontinuing the drug or reducing the dosage. Oral contraceptives may also cause dizziness in some women; a change to a low dose preparation may help.

Other causes include trauma to the cervical spine when orthopaedic or neurosurgical examination is necessary, or the periodic dizziness associated with the menopause when diuretic and oestrogen replacement therapy may be of benefit. The dizziness associated with migraine headaches often responds to ergotamine and phenobarbitone.

4.5 Chronic, Unremitting Vertigo without Ear Symptoms or Fainting

The psychoneurotic patient may complain of lightheadedness or vertigo, sometimes over a period of years, and may be shown to be anxious or depressed on clinical examination. More serious disorders must however, be ruled out before a diagnosis of psychogenic dizziness is made. Such conditions include central nervous system disease, uncontrolled or poorly controlled diabetes mellitus, and untreated thyroid disease, anaemia or hypertension.

Treatment of psychogenic dizziness consists of an explanation of the relationship of the patient's dizziness to his environmental stress, together with diazepam for anxiety or a tricyclic antidepressant such as amitriptyline for depression

5. Motion Sickness

The subjective sensation in motion sickness is one of malaise rather than of vertigo. Evaluation of motion sickness drugs has greatly benefited by the sustained, practical interest of the armed services of many countries. Efficacy has been tested both subjectively and objectively, and the effectiveness of any one drug shown to have no relationship to its efficacy in other types of nausea and vomiting (Wood and Graybiel, 1970, 1972). The most effective single drug is 0.6mg of hyoscine hydrobromide (scopolamine), which is about a third more effective than 50mg of dimenhydrinate in inhibiting experimentally induced motion sickness. Surprisingly, 10 to 20mg of amphetamine is equal to hyoscine or better than antihistamines such as dimenhydrinate, promethazine or diphenidol. The

most effective and best tolerated regimen is a combination of 25mg promethazine with 10mg d-amphetamine, or 0.6mg hyoscine with 10mg d-amphetamine. Thus, drugs with central anticholinergic actions (e.g. hyoscine, promethazine) and drugs with central sympathomimetic activity (e.g. d-amphetamine) are effective against motion sickness and a combination of these actions produces a synergistic effect (fig. 3).

Hyoscine is also effective when given after symptoms of motion sickness have begun. An intramuscular injection of 0.2mg of hyoscine hy-

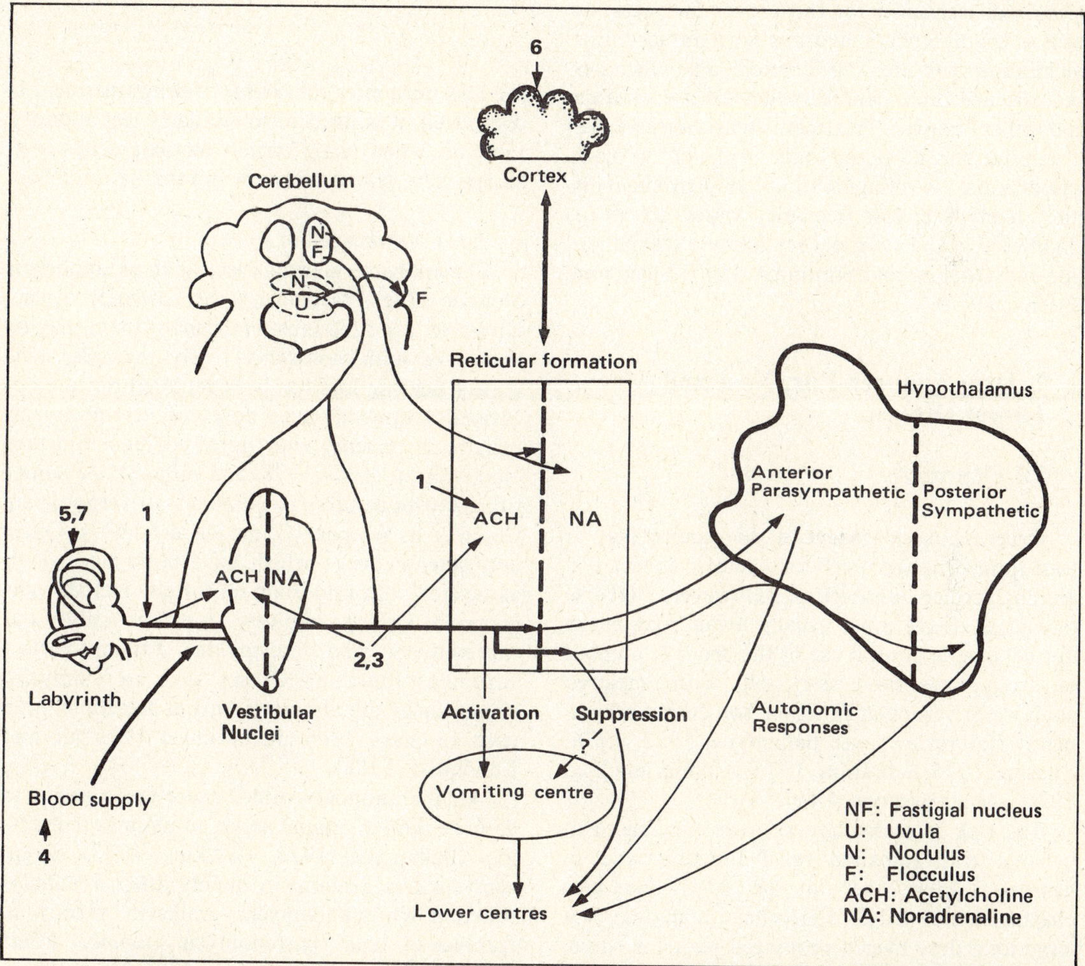

Fig. 3. Highly schematic and simplified representation of suggested site of action of antivertigo and antimotion sickness drugs. Based on the studies of the action of antimotion sickness drugs by Wood and Graybiel (Clinical Pharmacology and Therapeutics 11: 621, 1970; adapted by permission of author and editor).

The numbers refer to the antivertigo drug classes in table III.

1 = Antihistamines
2 = Antiemetic phenothiazines
3 = Anticholinergics
4 = Vasodilators
5 = Diuretics
6 = Psychotherapeutic drugs
7 = Corticosteroids.

drobromide is effective in 15 to 30 minutes and lasts for about 4 hours.

6. Sudden, Sensorineural Hearing Loss

This symptom can occur at any age but is fairly evenly distributed beyond age 30 years. Sudden unilateral hearing loss leads to complete or good recovery in 65% of cases, whether treated or not (Mattox and Simmons, 1977). Speculation on the cause favours viral infection for those under 50 years old, ischaemia for those over 50 years, as well as endolymphatic hydrops with intracochlear membrane rupture. Speculation also includes acoustic neuroma, demyelinating disease, trauma and other causes. Treatment with intravenous histamine, or corticosteroids with or without vasodilators, is disappointing. Improvement is more likely with low frequency losses, absent or slight vertigo and a normal erythrocyte sedimentation rate (Mattox and Simmons, 1977; Shaia and Sheehy, 1976).

7. Drug Induced Ear, Nose and Throat Disease

7.1 Ototoxicity

Drug regulatory agencies do require that at least some drugs be tested for ototoxic effects, e.g. aminoglycoside antibiotics. However, adverse otological effects must usually await recognition during general clinical use of the drug. A number of drugs have been associated with impaired auditory or vestibular function, sometimes permanently (for reviews, see Ballantyne, 1973, 1976; Lucente, 1975; Schramm, 1976; Ajodhia and Dix, 1976; see also section 4.4).

The risk of ototoxicity is greatly increased in patients with impaired renal function, and in general is more likely in the elderly (see also chapter V; sect. 2.1.3), following a high dose or a large total dose over a prolonged period of time, and if there has been a previous course or concurrent administration of another ototoxic drug. Some of the most important ototoxic drugs are also potentially nephrotoxic, thus it is highly desirable to adjust the dose of an ototoxic drug on the basis of renal function tests. Because the patient may sometimes not become aware of hear-

Table IV. Differential ototoxicity of aminoglycoside antibacterial drugs (relative effects)

Drug	Vestibular toxicity	Auditory toxicity	Early symptoms	
			tinnitus	vertigo
Streptomycin	+++	+	+	+
Gentamicin	++	+	+	+
Tobramycin	+	+	?+	?+
Amikacin	+	++	?+	?
Kanamycin	+	+++	++	?
Neomycin (framycetin, paromomycin)	++	++++	?	0

ing loss until after the course of drug treatment is completed, it is prudent to regularly test auditory function when using certain ototoxic drugs (e.g. kanamycin, potent diuretics in renal failure).

7.1.1 Antibacterial Agents

The antibacterial drugs are the most important ototoxic drugs, particularly the aminoglycosides. However, even the most innocent of them may be associated with ototoxicity — for example, temporary hearing loss has been reported on rare occasions following large doses of erythromycin, usually in patients with impaired renal function (van Marion et al., 1978) and minocycline sometimes causes troublesome dizziness or vertigo, particularly in women (Gump et al., 1977). Other antibacterial drugs which have been more often associated with important ototoxicity include vancomycin (affects auditory function only) and capreomycin and polymyxins (mainly affect vestibular function). Others such as viomycin, ristocetin or dihydrostreptomycin are either little used or have been discontinued (Wersall and Lundquist, 1968).

All the aminoglycosides share the capacity to damage the 8th cranial nerve, sometimes irreversibly (Ballantyne, 1973; Hawkins, 1973). Streptomycin and gentamicin mainly affect vestibular function while kanamycin, amikacin, neomycin, framycetin and paromomycin mainly affect auditory function. However, decreased auditory capacity can occur with gentamicin and hearing loss in young children has been attributed to use of streptomycin in infancy or in their mothers during pregnancy. Tobramycin, like gentamicin, can affect both auditory and vestibular function (table IV).

The early clinical features of ototoxicity differ with the individual aminoglycosides (table IV). In the case of streptomycin there is often a high pitched tinnitus and vertigo. In time, there is generally compensation for the vestibular disturbance, which is replaced by a chronic condition of uncertainty of balance in which only sudden movements cause vertigo. Loss of hearing (mainly high frequencies) with the aminoglycosides, particularly kanamycin, tends to appear after a latent period and usually becomes worse if treatment is continued. In some cases, onset of hearing loss may not occur until some time after treatment is discontinued, or may continue to progress even when treatment is stopped.

Risk of ototoxicity is greatly increased in the presence of impaired renal function. It is also more likely in the elderly, with excessive dosage or a large total dose, or following a previous course or concurrent administration of another ototoxic drug (Ballantyne, 1973; Jackson and Arcieri, 1971). The aminoglycosides are excreted unchanged in the urine and their ototoxicity is related to a prolonged high concentration in the inner ear. Thus, the rate of excretion by the kidney and the fact that the aminoglycosides are slowly reabsorbed from the endolymph once they have been secreted into it (Stupp et al., 1973), are the most important factors in determining ototoxicity. High dosage and use of ordinary doses in patients with renal failure will predictably cause ototoxic effects (see also chapter XXI; sect. 14.1.2).

Ototoxicity is not necessarily limited only to parenteral administration. Hearing loss has occurred with neomycin following irrigation of surgical wounds, superficial dressing of severe burns, aerosol inhalation, rectal and colonic irrigation, or even after oral administration (Ballantyne, 1973; Kalbian, 1972). Systemic absorption of neomycin is high following its use as an irrigating solution and probably only low strength solutions should be used (Anderson, 1978; Weinstein et al., 1977). Absorption of neomycin from the gastrointestinal tract is minimal. However, when there are gastric mucosal abnormalities (e.g. ulcerative colitis, gastroenteritis) or when large doses are used for prolonged periods (e.g. prophylaxis in chronic portal systemic encephalopathy) particularly if the patient also has impaired renal function, the amount absorbed and thus retained in the endolymph is sufficient to cause ototoxic effects.

Use of ototoxic antibiotics topically in the ear appears to be safe if administered properly and for correct indications (McKelvie et al., 1975; Turner et al., 1966). Severe ototoxicity has been associated with *direct* application (transtympanic) of streptomycin to the inner ear (Schuknecht, 1957); as can also be readily demonstrated with direct application to the inner ear of aminoglycosides, polymyxins, chloramphenicol and erythromycin in experimental animals (Mittleman, 1972; Stupp et al., 1973). Ototoxic antibiotics therefore should not be used locally during, or as preoperative prophylaxis before, inner ear surgery.

7.1.2 Diuretics

Transient and occasionally permanent hearing loss has been observed in some patients after ethacrynic acid and frusemide (furosemide). Deafness from ethacrynic acid may follow an intravenous dose or large oral doses in patients with impaired renal function, especially if given along with an aminoglycoside antibacterial drug (Matz, 1976; Mathog, 1976). Hearing loss from frusemide has also only occurred in patients with impaired renal function, generally after rapid intravenous administration of a high dose (Rupp, 1974), but gradually progressive and permanent deafness has developed up to 6 months after treatment with relatively small repeated doses of frusemide (Quick and Hoppe, 1975) and transient deafness has followed use of large oral doses in the nephrotic syndrome (Rifkin et al., 1978).

Since the uraemic patient is at special risk, it would seem prudent to monitor hearing during such treatment with ethacrynic acid or frusemide. This is especially true if the patient is also receiving or has recently received an ototoxic antibacterial drug (see section 7.1.1).

7.1.3 Salicylates

Symptoms of hearing loss, tinnitus and vertigo are observed with high doses of salicylates, particularly in patients with rheumatoid arthritis. Deafness is almost always reversible within a few days after cessation of the drug (Ballantyne, 1973; Porter and Jick, 1977).

7.1.4 Chloroquine, Quinine and Quinidine

Chloroquine can cause tinnitus and perceptive deafness. Hearing loss may become apparent after the drug has been discontinued; it tends to occur after long term high dosage and is usually irreversible (Toone et al., 1965). Vertigo, tinnitus and hearing loss can also occur with large doses or prolonged treatment with quinine. The ototoxic symptoms are however, usually reversible. Congenital deafness has been noted in infants born of mothers who attempted to induce abortion with high doses of quinine (McKinna, 1966). Vertigo and tinnitus, and rarely, reversible mild hearing loss, can occur with usual doses of quinidine (Rosketh and Storstein, 1963).

7.1.5 Miscellaneous Agents

Vertigo has been attributed to use of oral contraceptives and other commonly used drugs (see section 4.4). Regional perfusion of nitrogen mustard may cause vestibular symptoms and sometimes hearing loss (Ballantyne, 1973). Bleomycin may cause ototoxicity when used in high dosage (Dal et al., 1973), as may cis-platinum (see chapter XXIV; sect. 6.7). General poisons such as arsenic, lead, mercury, cadmium disulphide, phosphorus and carbon monoxide can cause deafness, tinnitus and vertigo. Chlorhexidine is unsuitable as a skin antiseptic prior to surgery on or in the region around the ear; especially for repair of a perforated eardrum when total and permanent deafness has been reported (Bicknell, 1971). Tinnitus and dizziness have also occurred. Gradual development of reversible deafness has been observed with the β-adrenoceptor blocking drug practolol, in association with, but months to years after the appearance of, the oculomucocutaneous syndrome seen with this drug (McNab Jones et al., 1977).

7.2 Nasal Congestion

It is well recognised that drugs can cause nasal congestion (Capel, 1976). Nasal blood vessels are kept in a state of partial constriction by a tonic sympathetic discharge (fig. 1a). Any drug that interferes with sympathetic transmission will induce a degree of nasal congestion, for example reserpine and drugs like guanethidine and methyldopa (fig. 1b). β-Adrenoceptor stimulant drugs such as isoprenaline (isoproterenol) are often used in the treatment of asthma. Although these drugs dilate the lower airway, they are capable of inducing both vasodilatation and congestion of the nasal passage and the eustachian tube (fig. 1b).

High circulating levels of female sex hormones, e.g. as with some oral contraceptives, can produce nasal congestion. The mechanism is unknown but is thought to be associated with fluid retention and increased blood volume. Conversely, 'the pill' can produce a patulous eustachian tube (Schiff, 1968). Allergic rhinitis has also been reported, usually in women with a history of perennial rhinitis or pollinosis (Pelikan, 1978).

As discussed in section 2.2.1, vasoconstrictors used in topical nasal sprays or drops will inevitably induce a rebound nasal congestion if used for prolonged periods. Some investigators feel that the rebound is due to reactive hyperaemia. Part of the rebound congestion may be due to the toxic effect of some drugs on the nasal mucosa. Several common topical nasal decongestants (but not 0.1% and 0.25% phenylephrine) have been shown to be ciliotoxic when tested in tracheal organ culture (Dudley and Cherry, 1978).

Further Reading

Ballenger, J.J. et al.: Diseases of the Nose, Throat and Ear, 12th Ed (Lea and Febiger, Philadelphia 1978).
De Weese, D.D. and Saunders, W.H.: Textbook of Otolaryngology, 5th Ed (Mosby, St Louis 1977).
Saunders, W.H. and Gardier, R.W.: Pharmacotherapy in Otolaryngology (Mosby, St Louis 1976).

References

Ajodhia, J.M. and Dix, M.R.: Drug-induced deafness and its treatment. Practitioner 216: 561 (1976).
Alberti, P.W.: Inflammatory disease of the maxillary sinus and its complications. Otolaryngologic Clinics of North America 9: 153 (1976).
Anderson, M.G.: Neomycin ototoxicity associated with wound irrigation in the local treatment of osteomyelitis. Journal of the Florida Medical Association 65: 20 (1978).
Andersson, R.; Nilsson, K.; Wikberg, J.; Johasson, S. and Lundholm, L.: Cyclic nucleotides and contraction of smooth muscle; in Drummond, Greengard and Robison (Eds) Advances in Cyclic Nucleotide Research, Vol. 5, p.491 (Raven Press, New York 1975).
Arenberg, I.K. and Bayer, R.F.: Therapeutic options in Meniere's disease. Archives of Otolaryngology 103: 589 (1977).
Ballantyne, J.: Ototoxicity: A clinical review. Audiology 12: 325 (1973).
Ballantyne, J.: Ototoxic drugs; in Hinchcliffe and Harrison (Eds) Scientific Foundations of Otolaryngology, p.849 (Year Book Medical Publishers, Chicago 1976).
Bass, J.W.; Cohen, S.H.; Corless, J.D. and Mamunes, P.: Ampicillin compared to other antimicrobials in acute otitis media. Journal of the American Medical Association 202: 697 (1967).
Benn, R.A.V.: Antibiotics: Use and abuse in office practice. Drugs 13: 297 (1977).
Benson, M.K.: Maximal nasal inspiratory flow rate: Its use in assessing the effect of pseudoephedrine in vasomotor

rhinitis. European Journal of Clinical Pharmacology 3: 182 (1971).

Bicknell, P.G.: Sensorineural deafness following myringoplasty operations. Journal of Laryngology and Otology 85: 957 (1971).

Boles, R.; Rice, D.H. and Hybels, R.: Conservative management of Meniere's disease: Furstenberg regimen revisited. Annals of Otology, Rhinology and Laryngology 84: 513 (1975).

Brink, W.R.; Rammelkamp, C.H.; Denny, F.W. et al.: Effect of penicillin and aureomycin on the natural course of streptococcal tonsillitis and pharyngitis. American Journal of Medicine 10: 300 (1951).

Brogden, R.N.; Speight, T.M. and Avery, G.S.: Sodium cromoglycate (cromolyn sodium): A review of its mode of action, pharmacology, therapeutic efficacy and use. Part II: Allergic rhinitis and other conditions. Drugs 7: 283 (1974).

Brogden, R.N.; Pinder, R.M.; Sawyer, P.R.; Speight, T.M. and Avery, G.S.: Beclomethasone dipropionate II: Allergic rhinitis and other conditions. Drugs 10: 211 (1975).

Brummett, R.E.; Harris, R.F.; Lindgren, J.A.: Detection of ototoxicity from drugs applied topically to the middle ear space. Laryngoscope 86: 1177 (1976).

Capel, L.H.: Rhinotoxic drugs; in Hinchcliffe and Harrison (Eds) Scientific Foundations of Otolaryngology, p.862 (Year Book Medical Publishers, Chicago 1976).

Cassisi, N.; Cohn, A.; Davidson, T. and Witten, B.R.: Diffuse otitis externa. Annals of Otology, Rhinology and Laryngology 86(Suppl. 39): 1 (1977).

Chandler, J.R.; Langenbrunner, D.J. and Stevens, E.R.: The pathogenesis of orbital complications in acute sinusitis. Laryngoscope 80: 1414 (1970).

Chapnick, J.S. and Bach, M.C.: Bacterial and fungal infections of the maxillary sinus. Otolaryngologic Clinics of North America 9: 43 (1976).

Clairmont, A.A.; Wright, R.; Dempsey, E.; Sheffield, P.A. and Jackson, R.T.: Blood flow in otorhinologic tissue after histamine and papaverine. Annals of Otology, Rhinology and Laryngology 82: 69 (1973).

Cohn, A.M.: Progressive necrotizing otitis. Archives of Otolaryngology 99: 136 (1974).

Craig, S.; Rubinstein, E.; Reisman, R.E.; Arbesman, C.E.: Treatment of ragweed hay fever with intranasally administered disodium cromoglycate. Clinical Allergy 7: 569 (1977).

Dal, I.; Edsmyr, R. and Stahle, J.: Bleomycin therapy and ototoxicity. Acta Oto-Laryngologica 75: 323 (1973).

Dayal, V.S.; Jones, J. and Noyek, A.M.: Management of odontogenic maxillary sinus disease. Otolaryngologic Clinics of North America 9: 213 (1976).

Dees, Susan C. and Lefkowitz, D.: Secretory otitis media in allergic children. American Journal of Diseases of Children 124: 364 (1972).

Denny, F.W.; Ayoub, E.M.; Dillon, H.C. et al.: Prevention of rheumatic fever. A statement prepared by the Rheumatic Fever Committee of the Council on Rheumatic Fever and Congenital Heart Disease of the American Heart Association. Circulation 43: 983 (1971).

Dix, M.R.: Vertigo. Practitioner 211: 295 (1973).

Dudley, J.P. and Cherry, J.D.: Effects of topical nasal decongestants on the cilia of a chicken embryo tracheal organ culture system. Laryngoscope 88: 110 (1978).

Empey, D.W.; Bye, C.; Hodder, M. and Hughes, D.T.D.: A double-blind crossover trial of pseudoephedrine and triprolidine, alone and in combination, for the treatment of allergenic rhinitis. Annals of Allergy 34: 41 (1975).

Feery, B.J.; Forsell, P. and Gulasekharam, J.: Streptococcal sore throat in general practice — a controlled study. Medical Journal of Australia 1: 989 (1976).

Feinberg, S.M.: Antihistamine therapy. Experimental and clinical correlation. Annals of the New York Academy of Sciences 123: 1186 (1950).

Feinberg, A.R. and Feinberg, S.M.: The 'nose drop nose' due to oxymetazoline (Afrin) and other topical vasoconstrictors. Illinois Medical Journal 140: 50 (1971).

Fraser, J.G.: Secretory otitis media in childhood. A survey of current understanding and management. Clinical Pediatrics 10: 261 (1971).

Fraser, J.G.; Mehta, M. and Fraser, P.M.: The medical treatment of secretory otitis media. Journal of Laryngology and Otology 91: 757 (1977).

Fulghum, R.S.; Daniel, H.J. and Yarborough, J.G.: Anaerobic bacteria in otitis media. Annals of Otology, Rhinology and Laryngology 86: 196 (1977).

Geimer, M. and Geimer, R.: Zur Wirksamkeit, Vertraglichkeit und therapeutischen Anwendung moderner Nasentropfen unter besonderer Berucksichtigung von Adrianol. Nasentropfen fur Sauglinge und Kleinkinder. Monatsschrift fur Kinderheilkunde 114: 553 (1966).

Glezen, W.P.; Clyde, W.A.; Senior, R.J.; Sheaffer, C.I. and Denny, F.W.: Group A Streptococci, mycoplasmas and viruses associated with acute pharyngitis. Journal of the American Medical Association 202: 455 (1967).

Gump, D.W.; Ashikaga, T.; Fink, T.J. and Radin, A.M.: Side effects of minocycline: different dosage regimens. Antimicrobial Agents and Chemotherapy 12: 642 (1977).

Hawkins, E.: Ototoxic mechanisms. Audiology 12: 383 (1973).

Hinchcliffe, R.: Review of treatment of Meniere's syndrome. Acta Oto-Laryngologica Suppl. 305: 10 (1973).

Howard, J.E.; Nelson, J.D.; Clahsen, J. and Jackson, L.H.: Otitis media of infancy and early childhood: A double-blind study of four treatment regimens. American Journal of Diseases of Children 130: 965 (1976).

Howie, V.M.; Ploussard, J.H. and Lester, R.L.: Otitis media: A clinical and bacteriological correlation. Pediatrics 45: 29 (1970).

Jackson, R.T.: Pharmacological responsiveness of the nasal mucosa. Annals of Otology, Rhinology and Laryngology 79: 461 (1970).

Jackson, R.T.: Pharmacological mechanisms in the eustachian tube. Annals of Otology, Rhinology and Laryngology 80: 313 (1971).

Jackson, G.G. and Arcieri, G.: Ototoxicity of gentamicin in man. A survey and controlled analysis of clinical experience in the United States. Journal of Infectious Diseases 124: S130 (Dec 1971).

Jackson, R.T. and Burson, J.H.: Effect of inflammatory mediators on nasal mucosa. Archives of Otolaryngology 103: 441 (1977).

Joachims, H.Z.: Malignant external otitis in children. Archives of Otolaryngology 102: 236 (1976).

Johnson, E.: Auditory findings in 200 cases of acoustic neuroma. Archives of Otolaryngology 88: 598 (1968).

Jokipii, A.M.M.; Karma, P.; Ojala, K. and Jokipii, L.: Anaerobic bacteria in chronic otitis media. Archives of Otolaryngology 103: 278 (1977).

Juhn, S.K.; Paparella, M.M.; Kim, C.S.; Goycollea, M.V. and Giebink, S.: Pathogenesis of otitis media. Annals of

Otology, Rhinology and Laryngology 86: 481 (1977).

Kalbian, V.V.: Deafness following oral use of neomycin. Southern Medical Journal 65: 499 (1972).

Kaliner, M.; Wasserman, S.I. and Austen, K.F.: Immunologic release of chemical mediators from human nasal polyps. New England Journal of Medicine 289: 277 (1973).

Kutnick, S.L. and Keith, J.D.: Acute sinusitis and otitis: their complications and surgical treatment. Otolaryngologic Clinics of North America 9: 689 (1976).

Kuvayama, A.; Zervas, N.T.; Shintani, A. and Pickren, K.S.: Papaverine hydrochloride and experimental hemorrhagic cerebral arterial spasm. Stroke 3: 27 (1972).

Leonard, J.R. and Lawrence, R.A.: Pharmacologic properties of antivertiginous drugs. Eye, Ear, Nose and Throat Monthly 50: 391, 417 (1971).

Liu, Y.S.; Lim, D.J.; Loang, R.W. and Birck, H.G.: Chronic middle ear effusions. Archives of Otolaryngology 101: 278 (1975).

Lofkvist, T. and Svensson, G.: Treatment of vasomotor rhinitis with intranasal beclomethasone dipropionate (Becotide). Results from a double-blind crossover study. Acta Allergologica 31: 227 (1976).

Lucente, F.E.: Drugs and the otolaryngologist. Laryngoscope 85: 2026 (1975).

McCabe, B.F.: Labyrinthine exercises in the treatment of diseases characterised by vertigo: Their physiological basis and methodology. Laryngoscope 79: 714 (1969).

McGrew, R.N.; Wilson, R.S. and Havenor, W.H.: Sudden blindness secondary to injections of common drugs in the head and neck. Otolaryngology 86: 147 (1978).

McKelvie, P.; Johnstone, I.; Jamieson, I.; Brooks, C.: The effect of gentamycin ear drops on the cochlea. British Journal of Audiology 9: 45 (1975).

McKinna, A.J.: Quinine induced hypoplasia and the optic nerve. Canadian Journal of Ophthalmology 1: 261 (1966).

McNab Jones, R.F.; Hammond, V.T.; Wright, D. and Ballantyne, J.C.: Practolol and deafness. Journal of Laryngology and Otology 91: 963 (1977).

Mathog, R.H.: Vestibulotoxicity of ethacrynic acid. Laryngoscope 87: 1791 (1977).

Mattox, D.E. and Simmons, F.B.: Natural history of sudden sensorineural hearing loss. Annals of Otology, Rhinology and Laryngology 86: 463 (1977).

Matz, G.L.: The ototoxic effects of ethacrynic acid in man and animals. Laryngoscope 86: 1065 (1976).

Mittelman, H.: Ototoxicity of 'ototopical' antibiotics: Past, present, and future. Transactions of the American Academy of Ophthalmology and Otolaryngology 76: 1432 (1972).

Mygind, N.: Intranasal beclomethasone dipropionate. ORL Digest 39: 19 (1977).

Mygind, N.: Immunohistopathology of allergic rhinitis and conditions allied. Clinical Otolaryngology 3: 325 (1978).

Olsen, A.L.; Klein, S.W.; Charney, E.; MacWhinney, J.B.; McInerny, T.K.; Miller, R.L.; Nazarian, L.F. and Cunningham, D.: Prevention and therapy of serous otitis media by oral decongestant: A double-blind study in pediatric practice. Pediatrics 61: 679 (1978).

Oppenheimer, R.P.: Serous otitis: Review of 922 cases. Eye, Ear, Nose and Throat Monthly 54: 316 (1975).

Pantell, R.H.: Cost-effectiveness of pharyngitis management and prevention of rheumatic fever. Annals of Internal Medicine 86: 497 (1977).

Pearlman, D.S.: Rationale for therapy of allergic disorders. Pediatric Clinics of North America 22: 101 (1975).

Pearlman, D.S.: Antihistamines: Pharmacology and clinical use. Drugs 12: 258 (1976).

Pelikan, Z.: Possible immediate hypersensitivity reaction of the nasal mucosa to oral contraceptives. Annals of Allergy 40: 211 (1978).

Phillips, M.J.; Knight, N.J.; Manning, Helen; Abott, A.L. and Tripp, W.G.: IgE and secretory otitis media. Lancet 2: 1176 (1974).

Pollock, R.A.; Jackson, R.T.; Clairmont, A.A. and Nicholson, W.L.: Carbon dioxide as an otic vasodilator. Archives of Otolaryngology 100: 309 (1974).

Porter, J. and Jick, H.: Drug-induced anaphylaxis, convulsions, deafness, and extrapyramidal symptoms. Lancet 1: 587 (1977).

Poynter, D.: Beclomethasone dipropionate aerosol and nasal mucosa. British Journal of Clinical Pharmacology 4: 295 (1977).

Quick, C. and Hoppe, W.: Permanent deafness associated with furosemide. Annals of Otology, Rhinology and Laryngology 84: 94 (1975).

Riding, K.H.; Bluestone, C.D.; Michaels, R.H.; Cantekin, E.I.; Doyle, W.J. and Poziviak, C.S.: Microbiology of recurrent and chronic otitis media with effusion. Journal of Pediatrics 93: 739 (1978).

Rifkin, S.I.; de Quesada, A.M.; Pickering, M.J. and Shires, D.L.: Deafness associated with oral furosemide. Southern Medical Journal 71: 86 (1978).

Rosketh, R. and Storstein, O.: Quinidine therapy of chronic auricular fibrillation. Archives of Internal Medicine 111: 184 (1963).

Roydhouse, N.: Management of otitis media in general practice. Drugs 3: 418 (1972).

Roydhouse, N.: Vertigo and its treatment. Drugs 7: 297 (1973).

Roydhouse, N.: Middle ear problems in children: Rational treatment. Drugs 15: 393 (1978).

Rubin, W.: Vestibular suppressant drugs. Archives of Otolaryngology 97: 135 (1973).

Rupp, W.: Pharmacokinetics and pharmacodynamics of lasix. Scottish Medical Journal 19: 5 (1974).

Schiff, M.: The 'pill' in otolaryngology. Transactions of the American Academy of Ophthalmology and Otolaryngology 72: 76 (1968).

Schramm, V.L.: Physician and patient-induced diseases in otolaryngology office practice. Laryngoscope 86: 1524 (1976).

Schuknecht, H.F.: Ablation therapy in the management of Meniere's disease. Acta Oto-Laryngologica Suppl. 132: 1 (1957).

Schwartz, R.; Rodriguez, W.J.; Khan, W.N. and Ross, S.: Acute purulent otitis media in children older than 5 years. Journal of the American Medical Association 238: 1032 (1977).

Schwartz, R.; Rodriguez, W.; Khan, W. and Ross, S.: The increasing incidence of ampicillin-resistant *Haemophilus influenzae*. A cause of otitis media. Journal of the American Medical Association 239: 320 (1978).

Shaia, F.T. and Sheehy, J.L.: Sudden sensorineural hearing impairment: a report of 1220 cases. Laryngoscope 86: 389 (1976).

Snow, J.B.: What's new in otolaryngology? Bulletin of the American College of Surgeons 63: 12 (1978).

Soyka, L.F.; Robinson, D.S.; Lachant, N. and Monaco, J.: The misuse of antibiotics for treatment of upper respiratory tract infections in children. Pediatrics 55: 552 (1975).

Special Report: Report of investigations on acute, diffuse otitis externa: Therapy with non-antibiotic and antibiotic topical otic medications. Current Therapeutic Research 23: SS1 (May 1978).

Sprinkle, P.M. and Sorenson, H.: Panel discussion on tonsillectomies and adenoidectomies. Otolaryngologic Clinics of North America 10: 245 (1977).

Stechenberg, B.W.; Anderson, D.; Change, M.J.; Dunkle, L.; Wong, M.; Van Reken, D.; Pickering, L.K. and Feigin, R.D.: Cephalexin compared to ampicillin treatment in otitis media. Pediatrics 58: 532 (1976).

Stupp, H.; Kupper, K.; Lagler, F.; Sous, H. and Quante, M.: Inner ear concentrations and ototoxicity of different antibiotics in local and systemic application. Audiology 12: 350 (1973).

Suga, F. and Snow, J.B.: Cochlear blood flow in response to vasodilating drugs and some related agents. Laryngoscope 79: 1956 (1969).

Symposium: Recent advances in middle ear effusions. Annals Oto. Rhino. Laryngol. 85 (Suppl. 25): 7 (1976).

Taylor, B.; Abbott, G.D.; Kerr, M.McK. and Fergusson, D.M.: Amoxycillin and co-trimoxazole in presumed viral respiratory infections of childhood: placebo-controlled trial. British Medical Journal 2: 552 (1977).

Tonkin, J.: Treatment of otitis externa. Drugs 6: 261 (1973).

Toone, E.C.; Hayden, G.D. and Ellman, H.M.: Ototoxicity of chloroquine. Arthritis and Rheumatism 8: 475 (1965).

Topilsky, M.; Greif, J.; Kurlat, D. and Spitzer, S.: Disodium cromoglycate in the treatment of seasonal and perennial rhinitis. Annals of Allergy 36: 246 (1976).

Turkeltaub, P.C.; Norman, P.S. and Crepea, S.: Treatment of ragweed hay fever with an intra nasal spray containing flunisolide, a new synthetic corticosteroid. Journal of Allergy and Clinical Immunology 58: 597 (1976).

Turner, J.S.: A practical guide to the patient with vertigo: An outline of diagnosis and management for the nonspecialist. Southern Medical Journal 68: 241 (1975).

Turner, J.S.; Staats, E.; Store, H. and Logon, R.: Preparation of the chronically infected ear for tympanoplastic surgery. Southern Medical Journal 59: 94 (1966).

Van Marion, W.F.; van der Meer, J.W.M.; Kalff, M.W. and Schicht, S.M.: Ototoxicity of erythromycin. Lancet 2: 214 (1978).

Walker, J.S.: Rhinitis medicamentosa. Journal of Allergy 23: 183 (1952).

Wannamaker, L.W.: Perplexity and precision in the diagnosis of streptococcal pharyngitis. American Journal of Diseases of Children 124: 352 (1972).

Wannamaker, L.W.: A penicillin shot without culturing the child's throat. Journal of the American Medical Association 235: 913 (1976).

Weinstein, L. and Le Frock, J.: Does antimicrobial therapy of streptococcal pharyngitis or pyoderma alter the risk of glomerulonephritis? Journal of Infectious Diseases 124: 229 (1971).

Weinstein, A.J.; McHenry, M.C. and Gavan, T.L.: Systemic absorption of neomycin irrigating solution. Journal of the American Medical Association 238: 152 (1977).

Wersall, J. and Lundquist, P.-G.: Ototoxic drugs; in Herxheimer (Ed) Drugs and Sensory Functions, p.142 (Churchill, London 1968).

West, S.; Brandon, B.; Stolley, P. and Rumrill, R.: A review of antihistamines and the common cold. Pediatrics 56: 100 (1975).

Wick, H.: Ueber Tyzine-Vergiftung. Praxis 55: 791 (1966).

Wood, C.D. and Graybiel, A.: A theory of motion sickness based on pharmacologic reactions. Clinical Pharmacology and Therapeutics 11: 621 (1970).

Wood, C.D. and Graybiel, A.: Theory of antimotion sickness drug mechanisms. Aerospace Medicine 43: 249 (1972).

Wright, D.N. and Alexander, J.M.: Effect of water on the bacterial flora of swimmer's ear. Archives of Otolaryngology 99: 15 (1974).

Chapter XII
Ocular Diseases

R. Abel and I.H. Leopold

Synopsis of Important Principles

1) Ocular diseases frequently pose a threat to vision and rapid diagnosis and appropriate treatment are imperative.

2) Therapy is largely directed at the eradication of infection, elimination of inflammation, the reduction of elevated intraocular pressure, and the use of artificial tears in dry eyes.

3) Applications of pharmacological agents in ophthalmology may be for diagnostic, therapeutic or investigatory purposes.

4) A number of physicochemical properties of the drug and its vehicle, and the physiological state of the eye, affect penetration of a topically applied drug into ocular structures.

5) Therapeutic drug levels in the cornea and aqueous humour can be maintained or increased by prolonging contact with the eye by means of ointments, iontophoresis, continuous irrigation or slow release inserts.

6) Intraocular drug levels which are adequate for treatment of anterior segment disease usually can be achieved by topical administration. Higher concentrations in the eye can be achieved with subconjunctival or subtenon injections.

7) The therapy of posterior ocular disorders requires retrobulbar or systemic drug administration.

8) Drug induced ocular disease may be produced by a wide variety of drugs used systemically and locally to treat diseases in all systems of the body, as well as in the eye. Locally and systemically administered corticosteroids and systemic phenothiazines are the most important.

9) In general, the unwanted effects of topically applied agents are reversible (except for angle closure glaucoma caused by mydriatic and cycloplegic agents and corticosteroid induced cataract formation) and do not usually affect visual function, whereas those effects caused by long term systemic administration are more likely to be irreversible as they may go unnoticed until the patient complains of decreased vision.

10) Topical eye medications, particularly mydriatic agents and those used in glaucoma therapy, can be responsible for adverse systemic effects.

The eye is an organ which is readily available for examination by virtue of the fact of its transparency and that many parameters of ophthalmic function can be quantitated. A therapeutic effect can be achieved by numerous drugs which can be applied topically, by local injection, or systemically. In addition to the desired therapeutic effect, many agents may have adverse reactions on the eye or on other organ systems. A wide variety of pharmaceutical agents may be employed in the therapy of ophthalmic conditions. Their effective use by clinicians depends on the awareness of specific considerations unique to ocular structures and disease.

1. Clinical Pharmacological Considerations

1.1 Ability of Drug to Penetrate Eye

Many factors determine the ability of a drug to penetrate into the eye (table I). These include the type of agent; its physicochemical properties such as differential solubility in water and lipids (partition coefficient) and dissociation constant; its concentration and pH of the vehicle; and the nature of the ocular structure (see Benson, 1974).

When administered topically, drugs can be absorbed through the cornea or through the conjunctiva and sclera. Subconjunctival or subtenon deposits of medication can penetrate through the sclera and ciliary body. Retrobulbar injections pass through the sclera while systemically administered drugs have to pass through the blood-eye barrier, which is similar to the blood-brain barrier in many ways.

The corneal nervous supply determines the degree of discomfort of topically applied medications. The corneal epithelium and endothelium are readily penetrated by lipid soluble substances and the stroma by water soluble agents. Therefore, substances combining polar (water soluble) and non-polar groups will penetrate the cornea more freely than totally polar or non-polar compounds. Weak acids and bases will have different lipid and water solubilities in their two different ionic states, which depends on the pH of the vehicle (see also chapter I; sect. 1.1).

The physicochemical properties of the drug, its concentration, and the osmolarity and the pH of the vehicle will therefore largely influence absorption. Hypotonic solutions tend to be more permeable. Wetting agents such as benzalkonium chloride, a commonly used preservative in ophthalmic medications, lower surface tension and can improve corneal permeability.

Table I. Factors which influence penetration of drugs into ocular structures

1. Nature of the drug.
   a) Chemical structure
   b) Molecular weight (occasionally)
   c) Physicochemical properties (lipid: water solubility ratio or partition coefficient; polarity; ionisation)

2. Nature of the pharmaceutical preparation.
   a) Drug concentration
   b) Vehicle characteristics (pH; osmolarity; inclusion of agents to lower surface tension; viscosity)

3. Method of administration
   a) Systemic
   b) Topical — increased duration of contact with eye (vehicle viscosity — ointment vs drops; continuous irrigation; diminution of tear production; prolonged drug release system — 'Ocusert'; cotton pledgets soaked in solution of drug; soft contact lenses)
   c) Subconjunctival subtenon or retrobulbar injection
   d) Carotid perfusion (only experimentally in the case of certain ocular tumours)

4. Nature of the ocular structure.
   a) Integrity of corneal epithelium (particularly polar compounds — abrasion; ulceration
   b) Inflammation (dilated vasculature). Increases the permeability of ciliary and iris vessels and increases drug concentration into the eye
   c) Status of lacrimal outflow passages and conjunctival vasculature (which carry drug away from the eye)
   d) Status of the gonio angle (ability to be enlarged or closed)
   e) Presence of the lens (influences drug penetration into the vitreous body)

1.2 Vehicle and Drug Delivery System

The topical route is effective for all alkaloids, corticosteroids (Cox et al., 1972b), local anaesthetics and various antibiotics. Therapeutic drug levels in contact with the cornea, aqueous humour and cul-de-sac can be maintained or increased by prolonging contact with the eye via ointments (Robin and Ellis, 1978), continuous irrigation, and rarely by iontophoresis.

Petrolatum, lanolin, and peanut oil are viscous vehicles commonly used as bases in ophthalmic ointments. These bases are toxic to the corneal endothelium and should not be used during or prior to intraocular surgery. Also, there is conflicting evidence as to whether ointments may delay healing of corneal abrasions. However, they protect the eye from exposure, soften discharges and are diluted less by tears than are suspensions, powders and solutions.

Continuous irrigation will provide constantly high antibiotic concentrations in the cul-de-sac and will remove necrotic debris. This method is used in treating acute chemical burns to be certain of ablution of all acid or alkali. However, continuous irrigation has been generally abandoned for the treatment of corneal ulcers because the irrigation washes away the polymorphonuclear leukocytes carried in the precorneal tear film which constitute the cornea's main line of immunological defence.

Cotton pledgets, soaked with ophthalmic solutions, inserted into the inferior cul-de-sac will prolong drug contact. This technique is used to facilitate mydriasis when posterior synechiae (iris adhesions) are present. Damage to the epithelium will enhance drug penetration.

The hydrophilic (soft) contact lenses and the Ocusert pilocarpine system (see section 5.2; table III) serve as drug reservoirs and maintain continuous intraocular drug levels in contrast to the transient drug levels produced by the standard topically applied medications (Dohlman et al., 1972; Maurice, 1972). Topically applied pilocarpine, phenylephrine and idoxuridine have more profound and prolonged effects when used in conjunction with a soft contact lens than without such a lens (Abel, 1975).

Sterility of all commercially available ophthalmic products is of the utmost importance since certain barriers to infection are frequently compromised at the time of their utilisation.

1.3 Physiological State of the Eye

The intraocular concentration of drugs is also determined by the rate of removal by the conjunctival and episcleral circulations and by the physiological egress of aqueous through the trabecular meshwork. The dilated vasculature in the inflamed eye facilitates penetration (Cox et al., 1972a) but also hastens the removal of medication. Thus drugs for ocular inflammation require more frequent topical application. Gentle lid closure to eliminate rapid blinking and occlusion of the lower punctum will partially negate rapid tear dilution and elimination of the drug. (This also will decrease the systemic absorption of certain drugs via the nasal epithelium).

1.4 Route and Mode of Administration

Topical medications do not penetrate well to the posterior portions of the globe. Therefore, their use is restricted to external and anterior segment disease. Intraocular drug levels can be increased by subconjunctival or subtenon injections, thus bypassing conjunctival and corneal barriers, allowing the drugs to penetrate the sclera and ciliary body by simple diffusion. This route is reserved for drugs which penetrate the cornea poorly, to minimise the number of topical applications to achieve equivalent drug levels, in the management of acute anterior segment inflammations, and to avoid the complications of systemic corticosteroids (O'Connor, 1976). Subtenon injections may however, have to be repeated.

Retrobulbar injections will provide a depot of medication adjacent to the globe for enhancement of drug levels in the posterior segment. This is mainly employed for steroid therapy in order to avoid systemic administration and may have to be repeated.

Systemic administration of drugs, notably antibiotics and carbonic anhydrase inhibitors, will provide adequate intraocular concentration for lipid soluble agents, which penetrate the blood-aqueous barrier freely. However, the studies on aqueous concentrations of medication have been performed on normal eyes prior to intraocular surgery and do not reflect the actual drug levels in the inflamed eye. It is known that penicillin, tetracycline and chlortetracycline, when given in large dosage systemically, do not penetrate the normal blood-aqueous barrier but will penetrate the inflamed eye in sufficient concentrations. Gentamicin shows increased penetration into the postoperative rabbit eye after subconjunctival administration (Abel et al., 1976). On the other hand, repository drug is more quickly carried away in the severely inflamed rabbit eye (Baum, 1978). Newer antimicrobial agents such as tobramycin (Furgiuele et al., 1978) penetrate the eye well after subconjunctival administration (Purnell and McPherson, 1974) and may become the agents of choice in cases due to gentamicin resistant strains. Probenecid inhibits renal excretion of penicillin (see chapter VIII; sect. 2.3.7) as well as a carrier mechanism in the ciliary body pigment epithelium, thereby increasing blood, aqueous and vitreous levels and helping to make this drug effective for intravitreal infections (Boger and Flippin, 1949; Martin and Wellman, 1967).

Carotid perfusion has been used in the treatment of malignant orbital and ocular tumours, especially in the presence of local and distant metastases. This route can cause severe side effects and is employed only when other modes of therapy seem likely to be ineffective.

2. General Principles of Treatment

Drug treatment in ophthalmology is largely directed to one of the following approaches:

1) Relief of inflammation by prompt and intensive treatment of microbial infection, or by identification and removal of the predisposing factor.
2) Reduction of raised intraocular pressure and corneal oedema.
3) Removal of an opacified corneal epithelium by pharmacological agents.
4) Physiological replacement of tears in dry eyes.
5) Use of dye solutions, mydriatic and cycloplegic drugs for diagnosis and investigative procedures.

2.1 Inflammation and Infection

The sequelae of an infective process can have a marked effect on vision. Even minimal scarring in the central pupillary zone of the cornea can markedly decrease visual acuity. Therefore, the treatment of acute ophthalmological inflammatory disorders such as blepharitis, conjunctivitis, corneal ulcer and endophthalmitis, consists of prompt and intensive antimicrobial therapy. In bacterial infections of the conjunctiva (which are less common than seborrhoeic or viral) this means frequent topical application (at least hourly during daytime for the first 2 to 3 days). Topical and sometimes systemic therapy should be used for corneal infections, depending on the extent of the infection (Jones, 1973). Subconjunctival injection should be considered if a higher antibacterial concentration is required. The dosages of antibiotics

for intraocular infections are generally much greater than those normally used, in order to guarantee adequate drug levels in the relatively sequestered intraocular tissues. It is often necessary to start broad spectrum antibacterial coverage on initial suspicion of bacterial infection and subsequently to alter therapy on clinical grounds. Ideally, the pathogen should be identified by conjunctival cultures and its sensitivity determined, but this is not always practicable. Most cases of bacterial conjunctivitis will respond rapidly to topical antibiotics. If after 2 days there is no improvement, the patient should be referred to an ophthalmologist for expert examination (see Sabiston, 1977).

Combined topical corticosteroid and antibacterial preparations should be used cautiously in superficial infections of the eye as suppression of inflammation by the corticosteroid may falsely suggest that the infection is being controlled. In blepharitis, a steroid-antibacterial combination often gives a dramatic response when an antibacterial agent alone does not.

The treatment of chronic conjunctivitis, which is frequently a problem, is aimed at eliminating predisposing factors (insufficient sleep, keratitis sicca, seborrhoea, trichiasis, abnormalities of the lid margins, heavy alcohol intake, and exophthalmic eyes) wherever possible, as well as treating any microbial pathogen. The treatment of seborrhoea is discussed in section 3.5. Staphylococcal hypersensitivity, caused by the organism's exotoxin, is treated by appropriate antibacterial therapy in conjunction with topical steroids (Leibowitz et al., 1976).

The treatment of uveitis and optic neuritis is based on careful diagnostic evaluation and specific therapy is employed whenever possible. However, nonspecific therapy (corticosteroids, mydriatics) is usually employed, even when the aetiology is determined (see section 6). Corticosteroid therapy is initiated and various criteria are followed for improvement, deterioration, or side effects, so that treatment can be altered as necessary.

Corticosteroids inhibit or minimise the signs of inflammation and have had dramatic effects in the treatment of a wide variety of ophthalmic inflammatory and allergic conditions — for example, allergic blepharitis and conjunctivitis, vernal catarrh, sarcoid conjunctivitis, temporal and cranial arteritis, and so on (Levine and Leopold, 1973; Dinning, 1976). Topical application is often sufficient for anterior segment disease, but occasionally, subtenon's injections or systemic administration is necessary. Many preparations and dosage forms are available. Acute processes may require high oral doses and necessitate full dosage for up to 2 weeks or more. The dosage of systemic steroids should be reduced as soon as possible. Retrobulbar injections can be utilised to avoid systemic administration of steroids.

Because of their potentially serious side effects, the route of administration of steroids must be carefully selected and the patient followed closely (see section 11.1.2).

2.2 Raised Intraocular Pressure

A number of pharmacological approaches are used to control intraocular pressure in chronic glaucoma, with miotics the basis of therapy. Topical β-adrenoceptor blocking drugs such as timolol, which act by decreasing aqueous humour production, may however, replace miotics as initial therapy in the future (see section 5). In general, it can be said that miosis changes the configuration of the angle structures thereby allowing a greater outflow of aqueous humour into the canal of Schlemm. This is useful in the therapy of both 'narrow' and 'open angle' types of glaucoma.

In the eye with anatomically narrow angles, dilatation (spontaneous or drug induced) may allow the peripheral iris to close off the drainage system from the anterior chamber and be followed by an acute rise in intraocular pressure. Thus, in the case of narrow angles, miosis would presumably be useful in keeping the peripheral iris away from the outflow system. In an acute angle closure attack, therapy is aimed at pulling the peripheral iris away from the drainage system by causing miosis (see Pollack, 1973).

It is important to note that the aqueous humour is secreted by the epithelium of the ciliary body in the posterior chamber of the eye, and must percolate around the lens and through the pupillary aperture to reach the drainage system. If miosis is marked, as occurs with the anticholinesterase drugs, the flow of aqueous humour from the posterior to the anterior chamber might be inhibited, not only by the smaller pupillary size but also by the valve-like action of the pupillary sphincter against the lens capsule. Under these circumstances there is a relative pupillary 'block', and the accumulation of aqueous humour in the posterior chamber could easily push the entire iris diaphragm forward. If the angles are anatomically narrow, an acute angle closure attack is possible. Therefore, anticholinesterase type miotics should be used with great caution in patients with anatomically narrow angles (see also table III).

2.3 Corneal Oedema

Corneal oedema resulting from intractable glaucoma and corneal degenerations and dystrophies can be reduced with various hypertonic agents (see table III). Glycerol is used for acute conditions in order to better evaluate the chamber angle and intraocular functions. For long term use, sodium chloride 2 to 8 % solutions or ointments, albumin solutions and cellulose gums are preferred. The soft contact lens appears to facilitate the use of these agents and serves as a therapeutic ocular bandage in a variety of refractory corneal conditions.

2.4 Removal of Opacified Corneal Epithelium

Epitheliolytic iodine, trichloracetic acid and ether solutions can be used to remove the corneal epithelium in the treatment of refractory herpes simplex keratitis and prior to decalcification treatment for band keratopathy, although manual removal is easier.

Chelating agents, primarily ethylenediamine tetra-acetate sodium (EDTA, sodium versenate), are used to decalcify Bowman's membrane in band keratopathy. After the epithelium is pharmacologically or mechanically removed, a cup containing the EDTA solution is applied to the cornea for several minutes, then washed off. The calcium ions become bonded into the inner ring of the molecule.

Tattooing has been used to conceal a corneal leukoma. After removal of the epithelium, palladium and platinum salts are introduced into the anterior stroma with a fine needle and blackened with oxidation to simulate a pupil. Lamellar and penetrating keratoplasty are the treatments of choice in an eye capable of useful vision.

2.5 Dry Eyes

Tear replacement for keratitis sicca or neuroparalytic keratitis (which often necessitates a therapeutic soft contact lens or tarsorrhaphy) consists of physiological replacement of a moist solution with various electrolytes. Methylcellulose, 0.25 to 1% in Ringer's solution or ointment, hypromellose or polyvinyl chloride solutions are currently employed. They are generally applied every hour or less frequently, but in warmer climates drops may have to be applied more often. It is often necessary to try several agents until the patient's discomfort has been alleviated (see Holly and Lemp, 1977). Flowbase, a new tear substitute, is currently under investigation. Lubricants are also necessary for lubrication of the sockets of prosthesis wearers. Mucolytic agents such as acetylcysteine can be usefully employed in order to break up the ropy mucoid secretions which are often a feature of this disease. Acetylcysteine and EDTA may have a role in binding the destructive collagenase enzymes which are produced by *Pseudomonas* species and after severe chemical burns when the cornea fails to re-epithelialise.

2.6 Diagnostic Dyes

Fluorescein and mercurochrome solutions are dyes which reveal corneal epithelial defects. Rose bengal solution will stain devitalised cornea and conjunctiva; it is used as part of the evaluation of keratitis sicca.

3. Ocular Inflammation and Ocular Infections

3.1 Acute Catarrhal Conjunctivitis

This may be bacterial, viral, or Bedsonial in origin. It must be treated early, because of occasional epidemics it can cause, and adequately, especially infections due to *Staphylococcus aureus* which can chronically involve the lid margins and peripheral cornea. Samples of exudate for bacteriological examination should be obtained and empirical therapy started before the results are available. Often, serological and fluorescent immunological studies are important in making the diagnosis of a viral disease.

Staphylococcus species, *Streptococcus (Diplococcus) pneumoniae* and *pyogenes* and occasionally *Haemophilus aegypitius* (Koch-Weeks bacillus) are among the more common bacterial causes of conjunctivitis. Topical sulphonamides (sulphacetamide, sulphafurazole or sulfisoxazole), neomycin-

polymyxin or bacitracin/gramicidin-neomycin-polymyxin combinations, or chlortetracycline are usually adequate. Chloramphenicol 0.5% and gentamicin 0.3% solutions are reserved for more refractory cases. Drops should be instilled frequently during the day (at least hourly for first 2 to 3 days) and an ointment at night for about a week. Discharges should be irrigated from the eye prior to instillation of drugs (see Furgiuele, 1978).

3.2 Corneal Ulcers and Dacryocystitis

Corneal ulcers and dacryocystitis often require oral and parenteral antibiotics to attain therapeutic drug levels. For dacryocystitis, nose drops and lacrimal sac massage are useful adjuncts. Dacryocystitis can be caused by any of the common external ocular pathogens; the most frequently implicated organism is *Streptococcus (Diplococcus) pneumoniae*. Bacterial organisms responsible for corneal ulcers (Jones, 1973) include the Gram-positive and Gram-negative cocci, and less frequently the Gram-negative bacilli. However, viruses (herpes simplex, vaccinia) and fungi (*Aspergillus, Fusarium, Nocardia, Actinomycoses, Cephalosporium*, and *Candida* spp.) may also be implicated (see section 3.3, 3.6). Herpes simplex virus is now the most common cause of corneal ulcers in North America.

Appropriate antimicrobial agents must be started immediately for corneal ulcers, after examining the corneal scrapings and while specimens are being cultured. An initial subconjunctival injection and full dosage parenteral therapy may be necessary to avoid such complications as diffuse scarring, perforation and endophthalmitis. Topical solutions should also be instilled every 10 to 60 minutes. Ointments are to be avoided. Occasionally a conjunctival flap or superficial keratectomy are performed to quiet a refractory ulceration (see Furgiuele, 1978).

3.3 Fungal Keratitis

In the treatment of keratitis due to *Candida* and other yeast-like fungi, amphotericin B (2.5 to 10mg/ml) or nystatin (100,000u/ml) can be used topically every two hours. Natamycin and clotrimazole are active against both dermatophytes and yeast-like fungi and have also been used successfully in ocular infections. Griseofulvin, 1 to 2g daily orally, can also be used for lid infections due to dermatophytes. Tincture of iodine, conjunctival flaps, and lamellar keratoplasty may be of some value.

Intravenous administration of amphotericin B (0.15 to 0.25mg/kg/day) remains the treatment of choice for intraocular fungal infections. *Candida* species are becoming increasingly prevalent as a cause of haematogenous endophthalmitis because of the increased use of immunosuppressive drugs and widespread use of systemic corticosteroid and antibiotic therapy and drug addiction (Fishman et al., 1972; Stone et al., 1975). 5-Fluorocytosine (6g/d) is orally administered and metabolised by the liver. It does not have a wide antifungal spectrum and has been disappointing in the treatment of *Candida* endocarditis and chronic mucocutaneous *Candida,* even when the isolate had been shown to be sensitive. There are some indications, that 5-fluorocytosine may have a synergistic activity with amphotericin B; therefore, the present recommendation for fungal endophthalmitis therapy is to use both agents if the organism is sensitive (see Jones, 1978). See further chapter XXVII (sect. 5.8).

3.4 Ophthalmia Neonatorum

Ophthalmia neonatorum refers to acute conjunctivitis in the newborn. It can be caused by *Chlamydiae* (inclusion blenorrhoea — an oculogenitally transmitted virus), *Staph. aureus* or other bacteria such as *N. gonorrhoea, Str. pneumoniae* and *pyogenes,* and *H. influenzae.* As the Crede prophylaxis regimen of mild silver nitrate often results in a prolific chemical conjunctivitis, it has been replaced with intramuscular penicillin in some centres. However, routine penicillin prophylaxis may only suppress rather than cure a gonococcal conjunctivitis, and, like silver nitrate, does not prevent conjunctivitis due to *Chlamydiae* which may be the most common cause of this disease in most countries, although fortunately not causing any serious permanent damage (Harris, 1973). Since penicillin administration may lead to adverse reactions, such as sensitisation, it is currently recommended that 1% silver nitrate drops should be used prophylactically (Armstrong et al., 1976).

Gonococcal conjunctivitis presents as a progressive purulent discharge, usually unilateral, which may produce corneal ulceration and even perforate quite rapidly. Thus, when it does occur (diagnosis proven by culture) it should be treated promptly with systemic penicillin augmented with a topical broad spectrum antibiotic. A suitable regimen is 50,000u/kg aqueous benzylpenicillin intramuscularly daily for 7 days. Penicillin, tetracycline or chloramphenicol eye drops, preceded by saline irrigation, are instilled every 15 minutes, initially, decreasing in frequency as response occurs. When there is corneal involvement penicillin may be given subconjunctivally or intravenously (Thatcher and Pettit, 1971; (see further chapter XXIX; sect. 3.2).

Dacryostenosis, with the accumulation of debris in the lacrimal sac, is a frequent cause of recurrent unilateral conjunctivitis in the neonate.

3.5 Blepharitis and Other Lid Lesions

Blepharitis is usually caused by the staphylococcus, and uncommonly by parasites such as lice and *Demodex folliculorum.* It may also present as an angular form. Rare causes such as anthrax, glanders, chancroid or tetanus may be seen in endemic areas. Since eye drops do not penetrate the upper lid, ointments are the major form of therapy for blepharitis, but even then penetration is still relatively poor.

Staphylococcal blepharitis is generally treated with a sulphonamide (15% sodium sulphacetamide drops qds) or erythromycin ointment and by removal of crusts, and manual expression of the meibomian glands. Recurrences are treated by the addition of topical steroids, desensitisation of the patient to staphylococcal toxoid, or applications of 1% silver nitrate.

Allergic blepharitis usually responds to topical antihistamine and dilute corticosteroid preparations. Watch out for steroid induced glaucoma with the more potent topical agents (see also section 11.1.2).

Angular blepharitis, which is often due to the Morax-Axenfeld Gram-negative rod, responds to sodium sulphacetamide, zinc sulphate, or gentamicin, topically applied several times daily.

Chronic blepharitis is frequently a mixture of seborrhoeic, staphylococcal and sicca forms; appropriately coined the term 'triples' syndrome. Some clinicians consider that the fungus *Pityrosporum ovale* may be of aetiological significance and should be carefully searched for in the smear, but this organism is very difficult to culture. Treatment is by removal of crusts and scales, shampooing the hair (selenium sulphide suspension) and even the eyelids (e.g. Johnson's baby shampoo or in more severe cases 0.5%

selenium sulphide and hydrocortisone), and often responds to a combination of sodium sulphacetamide, prednisolone and phenylephrine in polyvinyl alcohol. Expression of the meibomian glands can be tried by the capable patient.

A hordeolum (stye) is a staphylococcal infection of the sebaceous glands of the eyelids. It is usually self limited. Hot, moist compresses, sometimes removal of lashes to expedite drainage, and antibacterial ointments if needed are the basis of therapy.

Granulomatous lid lesions are usually seen as a chalazion (a sterile inflammation of the meibomian glands due to obstruction of the duct) or meibomianitis in the acute diffuse form. Warm moist compresses are usually adequate therapy, but systemic tetracycline does reduce the inflammation in the meibomian glands (see Furgiuele, 1978). Parasitic lid infestation is discussed in section 3.7.

3.6 Viral Infection

Viral lesions of the lids, conjunctiva and cornea can be caused by a number of different virus types (Kaufman, 1973), such as herpes zoster, which is treated with steroids (1 % hydrocortisone ointment), either alone or with an antibiotic, or Burrow's solution (boric acid and aluminium acetate 1:40) which may provide some relief; vaccinia, which may respond to vaccinia immune globulin (0.6ml/kg intramuscularly, 2 doses given 2 to 3 days apart) or to idoxuridine or vidarabine (adenine arabinoside) ointment; molluscum contagiosum, which responds best to excision or cautery of the lid lesions; and herpes simplex on the lid can be treated with vidarabine or idoxuridine ointment.

In acute herpes simplex keratitis, idoxuridine is helpful if application is frequent. This can be achieved by use of 0.1 % drops instilled 5 times during the day and an 0.5 % ointment at night for 5 to 14 days. Some clinicians occasionally use idoxuridine in conjunction with steroids, but corticosteroids should never be used alone in the treatment of this disease (Maloney and Kaufman, 1965; Gasset et al., 1969).

Topical vidarabine (3 % ointment 5 times daily initially) and trifluorothymidine (1 % solution 5 or more times daily) are newer agents which are effective against herpes simplex keratitis and are generally employed when resistance to or toxicity with idoxuridine develops. Vidarabine may how-

ever, prove to be superior to idoxuridine (McGill et al., 1974; Pavan-Langston, 1977). A controlled animal trial of acycloguanosine, an acyclic derivative of a purine nucleoside, as a 3 % ointment in a petrolatum base, has demonstrated significantly better results than idoxuridine and vidarabine (Pavan-Langston, 1978). This drug appears to be specifically activated by viral induced thymidine kinase and does not affect normal uninfected cells. Mechanical debridement and cryotherapy of the epithelium have been superseded by the growing number of effective antiviral agents, and are less frequently employed.

The topical application of human leukocyte interferon has been shown to prevent the emergence of herpetic keratitis in the primate (Kaufman and Goorha, 1970) but has not demonstrated significant effectiveness (perhaps because of potency of the preparations used) in a large controlled trial in the United States.

Epidemic keratoconjunctivitis (adenovirus type 8 among others) and the agent of superficial punctate keratitis can be suppressed (but not cured) by topical steroids. When EKC agent causes an iritis or corneal opacities in the visual axis, a definite indication for suppressive steroid therapy does exist. In cat scratch conjunctivitis, topical steroids and chlortetracycline 250mg 4 times a day may hasten recovery.

Trachoma and inclusion conjunctivitis *(Bedsonia* or *Chlamydia)* are large viruses which can invade the conjunctiva and cornea. Trachoma responds to treatment with systemic or topical sulphonamides and tetracycline, given for 3 to 6 weeks. Tetracycline ointment 1 % 3 to 4 times daily, sodium sulphacetamide ointment 10 % 3 to 4 times daily, and sulphafurazole (sulfisoxazole) drops 4 times daily, are topical agents useful for mass prophylaxis programmes in endemic areas. Systemically administered sulphonamides and tetracyclines provide more constant tissue levels of antibiotic, but are also more costly and have a greater incidence of adverse reactions. Systemic agents should be used for recurrences and progressive disease. A regimen of intramuscular benzathine penicillin and erythromycin once per week for 3 weeks has provided excellent results in limited studies (Havener, 1970a). It should be realised that communicable ophthalmia of the Middle East is caused by the combination of chronic trachoma and bacterial superinfection. Treatment must be directed against both infectious entities, as well as fly control (Jones et al., 1976).

3.7 Parasitic Infestations

Infections caused by *Phthirus palpebrum* (crab louse) or *P. pubis* (pubic louse) and the *Sarcoptes scabiei* mite are effectively treated by shampooing the cilia with gamma benzene hexachloride or Selsun Blue and repeating application in 5 to 7 days. Gamma benzene hexachloride cream may be used as an alternative, applied to the lid margins and repeated in 5 to 7 days. Lid infestation is associated with infection of abdominal skin and pubic areas, which should also be treated with gamma benzene hexachloride shampoo. Sex partners should also be treated. Physostigmine (eserine) and dyflos (DFP) solution have also been used but produce uncomfortable side effects due to ciliary spasm and miosis. *Demodex folliculorum,* a tenacious mite that resides in eyelid hair shafts, may contribute to chronic blepharitis, but responds to the same treatment as for louse infection; or if this fails to the organophosphate cholinesterase inhibitor (ecothiopate) eye drops and sulphur ointment.

3.8 Allergic External Ocular Diseases

All allergic external ocular diseases, after staphylococcal or tubercule phlyctenular conjunctivitis) hypersensitivity has been eliminated, are treated similarly (Allansmith, 1973). All possible contact allergens should be removed. Antihistamines can be given orally or topically as 0.5 % antazoline phosphate or 0.3 % chlorpheniramine maleate drops. Topically applied corticosteroid solutions, however, are often more effective. The topical administration of sodium cromoglycate (cromolyn sodium) as 2 % eye drops 4 times daily may be of some value. It has been particularly effective in vernal keratoconjunctivitis; reducing the need for and strength of steroid eye drops (Hyams et al., 1975; Kazdan et al., 1976).

Topical sympathomimetic agents are no longer used in the treatment of allergic eye disease. However, intramuscular adrenaline (epinephrine) 0.5 to 1ml of a 1:1,000 solution is given for angioneurotic oedema. Desensitisation to dust, grasses, foods, or moulds may be of benefit where there is an atopic history.

3.9 Keratitis Sicca

Keratitis sicca can be caused by deficiency of tear production (with or without Sjogren's syndrome — which is an autoimmune disease most frequently seen in postmenopausal women and in patients with rheumatoid arthritis — or due to the β-adrenoceptor blocking drug practolol) [Rahi et al., 1976], or to mucin deficiency caused by scarring of the conjunctiva [cicatricial trachoma, Stevens-Johnson syndrome, ocular pemphigoid, postirradiation, postdrug (DFP, fermethide) therapy and chemical burns]. Treatment consists of tear substitutes or sometimes mucolytic agents as outlined in section 2.5, replacement oestrogen therapy where applicable, and bland ointments such as 4 % boric acid, bacitracin, or methylcellulose. Occlusion of the inferior punctum may be very helpful. However, parotid duct transplants have given equivocal results at best. The soft contact lens may prove very beneficial in conjunction with tear substitutes in selected cases (Abel, 1975).

4. Ocular Anaesthesia

The pharmacological agents in most common use in ocular surgery are listed in table II.

Any of the topical anaesthetics is useful in removing a foreign body, in tonometry and in minor surgical procedures such as pterygium excision and conjunctival biopsy. The patient should be informed about the anaesthetic state and instructed not to rub or wipe his eyes for at least 30 minutes after the procedure. Most of the drugs have an onset of action within a minute or less, with a duration of effect up to 20 minutes. All can cause sensitivity and have a potential for epithelial toxicity (Henrotte and Weekers, 1972) and may produce punctate epithelial staining, with cocaine the major offender.

In intraocular surgery to be performed under local anaesthesia, the objective is to have the patient arrive in the operating room relaxed and cooperative. Barbiturates, opiates, and phenothiazines may be usefully combined and are given 30 to 90 minutes preoperatively.

Acetazolamide intramuscularly or mannitol intravenously, is administered routinely prior to cataract surgery to reduce the possible complications of operating on a hard eye. When planning cataract extractions in patients with smouldering uveitis, corticosteroids or ACTH should be given. If the patient has previously had dacryocystitis, prophylactic antibiotics should be given and all evidence of infection should be eradicated prior to surgery (see Leopold, 1974; Newell, 1975).

Table II. Drugs in common use in ocular surgery

1. *Pre-operative medication*
   a) Sedatives
      Barbiturates are excellent sedatives but they may occasionally cause idiosyncratic reactions such as agitation and delirium, especially in the elderly (see also chapter V; sect. 2.2).

Quinalbarbitone	50 to 100mg IM	If the only premedication
	100 to 200mg IM	
Pentobarbitone	50 to 100mg IM	
Chloral hydrate	0.75 to 1g orally	As substitute for barbiturates

   b) Opiates
      Since these agents possess little sedative effect they are usually employed in combination with other pre-medication.

Pethidine	
(meperidine)	50 to 100mg IM
Morphine	5 to 10mg IM
Methadone	5 to 10mg IM
Anileridine	25 to 100mg IM
Codeine	30 to 60mg orally

   c) Phenothiazines
      Phenothiazines act as tranquillisers, antiemetics and potentiate the action of barbiturates and opiates.

Chlorpromazine	— rarely used as it frequently causes hypotension
Promethazine	25 to 50mg IM
Triflupromazine	10 to 25mg IM
Hydroxyzine	
pamoate	25 to 50mg IM, orally

2. *Topical anaesthetics*
   Used for tonometry, foreign body removal, pterygium excision and conjunctival biopsy.

Amethocaine (tetracaine) 0.5%	
Benoxinate 0.4%	May cause less corneal epithelial staining
Butacaine 2%	May be the most sensitising
Cinchocaine (dibucaine) 0.1%	
Proxymetacaine (proparacaine) 0.5%	Less cross sensitivity with the others
Cocaine 4 to 10%	Potent topical anaesthetic but causes most corneal epithelial staining. Also used for pupillary testing and to achieve maximum mydriasis.

3. *Local anaesthetics*
   Used for intraocular and rarely strabismus surgery. Adverse reactions such as allergy, irritation, CNS stimulation and cardiovascular stimulation followed by collapse, must be remembered when using these agents.

Lignocaine (lidocaine) 1 to 4%	Some ophthalmologists add adrenaline (epinephrine) 1:50,000 or 1:100,000 to lower systemic absorption, or hyaluronidase to assist in distributing the drug retrobulbarly
Mepivacaine 1 to 4%	Only anaesthetic with vasoconstrictor efffect
Bupivacaine 0.25 to 0.75%	Longer duration of action

4. *General anaesthetics*
   In strabismus surgery, general anaesthesia is usually employed and many ophthalmologists prefer to use intramuscular atropine as an adjunct — this serves to block the oculocardiac reflexes which may be stimulated by traction on the eye muscles.

---

5. Glaucoma

Glaucoma can be conveniently discussed in terms of angle closure (or narrow angle), primary open angle, and other types. The diagnosis of acute angle closure glaucoma can be made almost immediately when a patient presents with blurred vision, coloured haloes, a painful eye, intense ciliary injection, and variably elevated intraocular pressure (IOP).

In contrast, the diagnosis of open angle glaucoma may be difficult to make. The diurnal variation in IOP, tonography, visual fields, the gonioangle, and optic cupping must be carefully evaluated and followed for diagnostic and treatment purposes. Ophthalmologists use varying criteria for initiating treatment, such as enlarging optic cup, progressive visual field changes, or a rising base line diurnal curve. Ingestion of 1 litre of water or 5% intravenous glucose (based on weight, sex and age) may be employed as tension or tonography provocative tests (see Kolker and Hetherington, 1970).

5.1 Narrow Angle Glaucoma

An attack of narrow angle glaucoma is treated medically until the pressure is normalised and the patient can be carefully evaluated, and then surgical treatment (iridectomy or filtering procedure) is standard. Pilocarpine 2 to 4% is administered every few minutes until the pressure is controlled, then less frequently. Concomitantly, the hyperosmotic agents such as glycerol orally or 20% mannitol intravenously (if glycerol cannot be taken because of nausea), and acetazolamide 500mg intravenously plus 500mg orally are employed until normal or subnormal pressures are attained. In certain cases, vigorous mydriasis will help break the attack. However, the pupils of elderly patients do not dilate well and peripheral anterior synechiae are minimised on miotic therapy (although posterior synechiae are maximised). Topical or intravenous corticosteroids may be required to reduce inflammation.

In terms of definitive therapy for narrow angle glaucoma, the risks of surgery (on the affected eye to cure glaucoma and on the fellow eye to prevent such an acute attack) are less than those which occur with long term medical maintenance (Imre and Bogi, 1976).

5.2 Primary Open Angle Glaucoma

Chronic simple glaucoma is a bilateral, asymmetric disease with variable degrees of severity and courses. Although topically applied β-adrenoceptor blocking drugs such as timolol, may become therapy of first choice (see section 5.4), miotics have been the basis of therapy. Pilocarpine 1 to 2%, 2 to 4 times daily is generally used for the initial treatment of open angle glaucoma when the intraocular pressure is not inordinately high. When resistance to pilocarpine develops, increasing the dosage may regain effectiveness.

The use of a pilocarpine ocusert will often lower intraocular pressure (IOP) as much as a daily instillation of pilocarpine drops, and it need be inserted only once weekly. A definite percentage of patients will not be able to keep the thin semipermeable diaphragm in the eye; the loss of the ocusert may be unnoticed. Others may not tolerate the foreign body sensation. The ocusert system would seem to be most useful for some patients who have marked side effects with pilocarpine eye drops and for unreliable users of eye drops (Bloch et al., 1977). Encouragement and instruction in use of the insert are very important during initial weeks of therapy (Armaly and Rao, 1973; Pollack et al., 1976). Glaucoma patients wearing a therapeutic soft contact lens may be able to maintain lower intraocular pressures with their daily pilocarpine therapy with the lens than without the lens. The soft contact lens, like the ocusert, acts as a drug reservoir (Podos et al., 1972).

Adrenaline (epinephrine) compounds in a strength of 1 to 2% 1 to 3 times daily, may be employed in addition. These may rarely increase intraocular pressure, and are contraindicated in patients with hypertension and narrow chamber angles. In special circumstances, e.g. young adults, or patients with axial lens opacities, adrenaline may be used initially to control the pressure. Because of risk of macular oedema (although reversible), adrenaline should be avoided in aphakic glaucomatous eyes if other therapy controls intraocular pressure; when used, fluorescein angiography should be conducted periodically, or with any change in visual acuity or symptoms that may suggest macular oedema (Mackool et al., 1977; Thomas et al., 1978).

If the intraocular pressure is not controlled, an anticholinesterase agent miotic (or aceclidine) can be substituted for pilocarpine, or the carbonic anhydrase inhibitors can be added to the previous regimen. Ecothiopate iodide or demecarium bromide are the most commonly used anticholinesterases; their use with other miotics or with each other is generally not to be recommended. Acetazolamide 62.5 to 250mg 2 to 4 times daily (or its equivalent such as dichlorphenamide) can be added to the miotic and adrenaline therapy. Slow release acetazolamide tablets may be better tolerated by some patients. The management of systemic hypertension often benefits glaucoma control; oral β-adrenoceptor blocking drugs being especially suitable since they decrease systemic and ocular hypertension (Borthne, 1976).

The properties and side effects of the various agents employed in glaucoma therapy are listed in

Table III. Drugs for medical management of glaucoma (Leopold and Keates, 1965; Grant, 1973)

1. *Miotics* (table IIIa)
   In open angle glaucoma these agents improve outflow facility which may be related to contraction of the ciliary musculature. In angle closure glaucoma, the miotics constrict the pupil, extracting the peripheral iris from the trabecular meshwork. This action can create an iris bombe and pupillary 'block' situation and must be kept in mind (see also section 2.2).

2. *Anticholinesterase agents* (table IIIb)
   These drugs potentiate the actions of locally produced acetylcholine on parasympathetically innervated structures. In general, they are more potent and require a longer time to develop tolerance, but frequently cause adverse effects which may or may not necessitate cessation of therapy. Their vascular congestive effect and pupillary blocking propensities make them unsuitable for narrow chamber angle patients.

3. *Sympathomimetic agents* (table IIIc)
   Adrenaline (epinephrine) primarily decreases the rate of aqueous production but also may increase the outflow facility somewhat. The other agents listed are generally less effective and not often employed.

4. *β-Adrenoceptor blocking drugs*
   This is the most exciting and promising new area in ocular hypotensive therapy, although the site of action of β-blockers has not been confirmed. Topical timolol is as effective as pilocarpine in moderate to weaker concentrations (up to 4%), is well tolerated and is given in less frequent applications. Other agents are also under investigation (see section 5.4).

5. *Hyperosmotic agents* (table IIId)
   These agents lower intraocular pressure by producing a rapid increase in blood osmolarity, creating an osmotic gradient between the plasma and the ocular fluids. They are used preoperatively in acute glaucoma and in self limited glaucoma states.

6. *Carbonic anhydrase inhibitors* (table IIIe)
   Carbonic anhydrase in the ciliary body epithelium contributes to the formation of aqueous humour. The blood acidifying action of these agents is important in causing ocular hypotension.

---

table III. Only after maximum medical therapy fails to control intraocular pressure can the medical management of open angle glaucoma be said to have failed and surgical intervention then undertaken.

5.3 Other Types of Glaucoma

Children with glaucoma may present with eye rubbing, photophobia, excess tearing, corneal enlargement and opacification and with abnormal anatomy of the trabeculum, iris or cornea. After infancy, headache, coloured haloes around lights are prominent symptoms and optic cupping and visual field changes may be observed. Goniotomy or trabeculectomy is usually preferable to medical management in this age group.

Low tension glaucoma (when normal IOP is associated with progressive disc and visual field changes because of vascular insufficiency) must be considered in certain cases of open angle glaucoma.

Trauma, inflammation, rubeosis (neovascularisation of the iris and trabeculum), extraocular venous congestion, pseudoexfoliation, Fuch's heterochromic cyclitis, essential iris atrophy and phakomatoses may cause unilateral open angle glaucoma. Early chronic simple glaucoma must also be ruled out. Secondary glaucoma is managed by controlling the primary ocular condition and by following the general treatment rules for open angle glaucoma. Pupillary dilation is preferable in cases where intraocular inflammation is present.

Malignant glaucoma following intraocular surgery, is treated by vigorous dilatation (with care not to create significant mydriasis in a susceptible fellow eye) and with acetazolamide. A flat anterior chamber must be reformed. Occasionally, rupture of the hyaloid face must be employed to break pupillary block. Transient pressure elevations following intraocular surgery frequently occur and may be caused by the α-chymotrypsin injected to break the zonular attachments of the cataractous lens.

When cells can be seen in the anterior chamber, haemorrhagic glaucoma, glaucoma cyclitic crisis, and uveitis must be suspected. However, an anterior chamber can be seen with angle closure attacks and after cycloplegic instillation.

5.4 New Approaches to Management

New ideas in glaucoma diagnoses and treatment are being explored. Prolonged reading and prone position testing of intraocular pressure have been used to elucidate 'position glaucoma', a more recently recognised narrow chamber angle variant. Acteroid, a fibrinolytic agent prepared from duodenal mucosa, is being tested for use in open angle glaucoma.

The use of β-adrenoceptor blocking drugs to lower intraocular pressure is an exciting new area in ocular hypotensive therapy. Systemic propranolol (Borthne, 1976) and labetalol are being studied in chronic open angle glaucoma. Topical application of β-blockers has also been investigated. Although atenolol drops produce a profound decrease in intraocular pressure, in some patients who show a good initial response the effect gradually decreases after several months use (Brenkman, 1978). Topical timolol (Heel et al., 1979), also produces a marked decrease in intraocular pressure and is as effective as weak to moderate concentrations of pilocarpine (up to 4 %), appears to be well tolerated and needs only to be applied twice daily; although pulse rate, blood pressure

Table IIIa. Therapeutic dosage and pharmacological properties of miotics used in glaucoma

Agent	Dosage	Onset and duration of effect	Notes and side effects
Pilocarpine hydrochloride or nitrate	0.5 to 4% every 5 to 15 min acutely 2 to 4 times/d regularly	Miosis begins in 15 min lasts 4 to 8 hours	Greater than 4% solutions generally provide no increase in effectiveness. Initial browache and accommodative spasm. Tolerance develops after a while . . . increase strength or switch miotics or add adrenaline (epinephrine). 0.5 to 1.0% methylcellulose base promotes better absorption and delays removal
Pilocarpine 'Ocusert'	20 to 80μg/h every day or week	Begins 10 to 15 min	Reduced incidence pilocarpine side effects and improved efficacy because of greater convenience to patient (i.e. better patient compliance through less frequent administration). The Ocusert unit is designed to fit in the conjunctival cul-de-sac and to release pilocarpine at a predictable rate on contact with an aqueous medium such as tears. See also text
Methacholine chloride	10 to 20%	Begins 5 to 10 min lasts 1 to 2 hours	Unstable, must be freshly prepared. Only short term use, sometimes in angle closure glaucoma. Main use in pupillomotor testing
Carbachol chloride	0.75 to 3%	Begins 10 to 20 min lasts 4 to 8 hours	Stronger than pilocarpine because of some anticholinesterase effect, but does not penetrate well. Irregular effectiveness and more rapid development of resistance. An alternative or replacement for pilocarpine
Aceclidine hydrochloride	2%	Begins 10 to 15 min lasts 4 to 8 hours	Penetrates well and is stable. Alternative or replacement for pilocarpine
Acetylcholine	1%	Immediate onset 15 min duration	For intraocular use during routine cataract surgery and intraocular lens implantation

Table IIIb. Therapeutic dosage, pharmacological properties and side effects of anticholinesterase agents used in glaucoma

Agent	Dosage	Onset and duration of effect	Notes and side effects
Physostigmine salicylate (eserine)	0.25 to 1.0% 4 to 8 hours	Miosis within 10 to 30 minutes lasts 24 to 48 hours	Follicular hypertrophy, browache, intense photophobia usually makes for short term use, especially as there are better agents
Neostigmine bromide	3 to 5% every 4 to 6 hours	Begins 15 to 30 min lasts 4 to 8 hours	More stable and better tolerated, but seldom used. Employed in the past with methacholine for narrow angle glaucoma
Dyflos (DFP)	0.01 to 0.1% usually 0.05 to 0.1% 1 to 2 times per day	Begins 15 to 30 min lasts 1 to 2 wks	Stable in peanut oil base. Do not contaminate with tears. Less follicular hypertrophy of the conjunctiva, rarely retinal detachment. Systemic adverse effects reversed by pralidoxime and atropine
Ecothiopate iodide	0.03 to 0.25% usually 0.12 to 0.25% bid	Begins 15 to 30 min lasts 1 to 2 weeks	Stable in water, less deterioration with refrigeration. Very effective and the standard drug of this type. Ocular adverse effects may limit usefulness (see section 11.1.4). Systemic absorption may lead to toxic effects including abdominal cramps, bradycardia, sweating and bronchospasm in asthmatics (stop drug and if severe give atropine). Long term use can lead to marked depression of serum pseudocholinesterase levels which persist long after the drug is discontinued. This is of relevance to use of neuromuscular blocking agents (see chapter X; sect. 2.2.1). Anticholinesterase drugs such as ecothiopate should be discontinued 4 to 6 weeks prior to elective surgery
Demecarium bromide	0.12 to 1% usually 0.25% bid	Begins 15 to 30 min lasts 12 to 48 hours	Stable. Alternative to ecothiopate

Table IIIc. Therapeutic dosage and pharmacological properties of sympathomimetic agents used in glaucoma

Agent	Dosage	Pharmacological properties
Adrenaline (epinephrine) hydrochloride, bitartrate, borate	1 to 2% every 12 to 24 hours	Decrease the rate of aqueous formation approximately 30 to 35%. Oxidises over 6 to 8 weeks. The borate compounds are more stable and have demonstrated fewer side effects (irritation, vasodilatation, conjunctival pigmentation). Reasonably effective when combined with miotics
Phenylephrine hydrochloride Naphazoline nitrate	10%	Decrease intraocular pressure when applied topically (see also section 10). Thymoxamine 5%, an α-adrenoreceptor blocking agent, prevents mydriasis of phenylephrine. Use with extreme caution in patients with hypertension or cardiovascular disease (risk of acute myocardial infarction, severe rise in blood pressure, arrhythmias). Elderly patients especially susceptible (Fraunfelder and Scafidi, 1978)
Dipivefrin (dipivalyl epinephrine; DPE)	0.1%	Addition of 2 pivalyl side-chains make dipivefrin a prodrug, more lipophilic than adrenaline (epinephrine) and is better absorbed and better tolerated (Mandel and Podos, 1977)

Table IIId. Therapeutic dosage, pharmacological properties and side effects of hyperosmotic agents used in glaucoma

Agent	Dosage	Therapeutic properties
Intravenous agents		
Mannitol	2.5 to 10ml/kg of a 20% solution given over 30 to 60 minutes	Confined to extracellular water, poor ocular penetration, rapidly excreted in urine. Drug of choice for IV use
Urea	2 to 7ml/kg (approx 30% solution) in 10% fructose	Rapid decrease in intraocular pressure, rapid excretion, good ocular penetration. Major disadvantage blood osmolarity falls below vitreous, creating a rebound phenomenon
Sodium ascorbate	0.2 to 5ml/kg of a 20% solution	Must be freshly prepared
Oral agents		
Glycerol	0.7 to 1.5ml/kg of 50% solution in fruit juice	Most widely used of this type for breaking acute glaucoma. Major disadvantage: GI side effects and high caloric intake for those with diabetes mellitus
Propylene glycol		Theoretically safer for those with diabetes mellitus
Isosorbide	2 to 4ml/kg of a 50% solution	Theoretically safer for those with diabetes mellitus
Ethyl alcohol	2 to 3ml/kg of a 50% solution	Alcohol inhibits antidiuretic hormone causing a hypotonic diuresis. Used in emergency situations
Sodium ascorbate	0.5g/kg per day in 4 doses	

and tear formation may be slightly reduced. It has retained effectiveness when used for periods of a year or more. If further studies confirm the continued efficacy and safety of topical agents such as timolol when used over long periods, they may well become the most appropriate drugs to use initially in primary open angle glaucoma.

6. Uveitis

The term uveitis signifies any inflammation of the uveal (vascular) coat of the eye and includes a variety of terms, such as iritis, cyclitis, iridocyclitis, peripheral retinitis, choroiditis, and chorioretinitis. Various classifications of uveitis are useful for descriptive and diagnostic purposes. However, they do not always indicate specific therapeutic regimens.

An anatomical classification dividing uveitis into anterior, posterior and mixed, does correlate with the knowledge that topical and subconjunctival administration of steroids produce high drug levels in the anterior segment of the eye and that retrobulbar and systemic routes will provide adequate drug levels in the posterior segment.

The histopathological classification (Hogan and Zimmerman, 1962) divides uveitis into exogenous and endogenous, suppurative and non-suppurative, and the latter into granulomatous. Exogenous uveitis is usually due to the introduction of foreign material or pathogens into the eye and is generally suppurative. Endogenous uveitis may be related to idiopathic ocular conditions, known ocular disease, or systemic disorders, and is generally non-suppurative.

6.1 Diagnosis

The diagnosis and treatment of uveitis conditions is frequently perplexing and frustrating. Table IV lists the more common specific causes of uveitis and specific treatment wherever this is possible. The basis of treatment is a thorough diagnostic work-up, details of which can be found in any current ophthalmology textbook (Duane,

1976). A nonspecific therapeutic approach to uveitis is discussed below. It cannot be over emphasised, that a thorough and continuing evaluation of a given patient's medical history, physical and general health, and a discerning approach to therapy is basic to successful management.

6.2 Nonspecific Treatment

Topical cycloplegics and corticosteroids are the mainstay of nonspecific therapy and are frequently sufficient to abate the uveal reaction (Havener, 1970b; Leopold, 1963). Solutions of 0.2 to 0.5% hyoscine (scopolamine), 1% atropine or 5% homatropine, are used to achieve pupillary dilatation and relaxation of the ciliary body; atropine also decreases vascular permeability. Dexamethasone or prednisolone (0.1 and 1.0% strengths respectively) should be instilled frequently during the day and their ointment forms applied at night.

The use of subconjunctival, subtenon, and retrobulbar steroid injections may provide higher intraocular levels for several days to several weeks. These routes are employed for acute exacerbations, focal chorioretinal lesions, to decrease the frequency of application of topical agents, and to avoid dependence upon systemic steroids.

Systemic corticosteroids are necessary for chronic refractory uveitis (Godfrey et al., 1977). The dose should be kept to a minimum and gradually reduced whenever possible. Guidelines for duration or cessation of therapy cannot be rigidly established. Relapses and rebound phenomena are common. Failure to respond to one steroid preparation may be overcome by changing to another. Non-steroid anti-inflammatory analgesics of antimalarials may be effective for the accompanying arthritis in certain selected cases.

Immunosuppressive agents have been used in selected cases of refractory ocular inflammatory conditions, including uveitis (Pirofsky et al., 1976). Methotrexate and cyclophosphamide have been usefully employed in the treatment of sympathetic ophthalmia, cystoid macular oedema due to chronic pars planitis, scleromalacia perforans and Wegener's granulomatosis. Also chlorambucil is of some value in cases of Behcet's disease (Dinning and Perkins, 1975). However, corticosteroids have remained the mainstay of therapy for chronic inflammatory conditions.

Table IIIe. Therapeutic dosage and pharmacological properties of carbonic anhydrase inhibitors used in glaucoma

Agent	Dosage	Onset and duration of effect	Pharmacological properties
Acetazolamide	Oral 62.5mg every 12h to 250mg (or more) every 4h, average 250mg qid IV or IM 500mg in 5 to 10ml of distilled water	Orally starts in 60 to 90 minutes, maximal 3 to 5 hours, lasting 4 to 8 hours IV and IM faster effect	Topically ineffective. Side effects include paraesthesias, GI distress, anorexia, weight loss, metabolic acidosis, renal and ureteric colic, rashes, and rarely blood dyscrasias; these drugs are sulphonamide derivatives. They can also precipitate urate stones in patients with gout, but this is rarely a clinical problem. A high fluid intake should be maintained during their use
Dichlor- phenamide	Oral 50 to 200mg every 6 to 8 hours average 50 to 100mg every 6 to 8 hours		Less metabolic acidosis. More renal potassium loss, but not likely to be clinically significant
Ethoxzolamide	Oral 50 to 250mg every 4 to 8 hours, average 125mg every 6 to 8 hours		
Methazolamide	Oral 25 to 100mg every 8 hours, average 50mg every 6 to 8 hours		Penetrates the CSF and aqueous humour 3 to 5 times more rapidly than acetazolamide. Renal calculi seem much less frequent than with acetazolamide

Table IV. Causes and treatment of uveitis

Cause	Notes and guide to treatment
1. Infection (gonococci, toxoplasmosis, herpes etc)	Appropriate systemic antimicrobial agent in full dosage. Desensitisation (e.g. staphylococcal) where relevant in bacterial infection since pathogen may act via a hypersensitivity mechanism
2. Associated systemic disease (rheumatoid arthritis, ankylosing spondylitis, SLE; sarcoidosis etc)	Therapy for underlying condition. Topical steroids, cycloplegia
3. Trauma	Uveitis usually acute, anterior and responsive to topical steroids and cycloplegia
4. Allergy (drug, foreign protein or bacterial hypersensitivity)	Treat as nonspecific uveitis (section 6.2), antihistamines usually not very effective
5. Toxic (external, intraocular foreign body)	Remove any foreign substances (esp. iron and copper) whenever possible
6. Sympathetic ophthalmia	Prophylaxis (surgery) may be only means of cure. For active sympathetic uveitis, cycloplegia, analgesics and intensive systemic and topical steroids as well as cytotoxic agents
7. Primary intraocular disease	Often refractory to treatment but spontaneous remissions and exacerbations occur (pars planitis or peripheral uveitis, cyclitis) or generally benign (heterochromic iridocyclitis). Some conditions may require maximum therapy as for sympathetic ophthalmia. The majority of cases are idiopathic in origin

7. Diseases of the Retina

7.1 Tapetoretinal Degeneration

Many pharmacological agents have been employed for the tapetoretinal degenerations, but with less than favourable results. Perhaps defining the specific cause of a patient's macular degeneration, such as diabetes mellitus, hypertension, carotid insufficiency, or sunstaring, would allow therapy to be directed more appropriately. Vitamin E (tocopherol) and B complex and clofibrate have not met with much success in preventing progression of this central degeneration. Therapy in this area remains nonspecific.

7.2 Retinal Dystrophies

Retinal dystrophies remain a therapeutic enigma. Hopefully, a specific enzyme deficiency can be isolated for the amaurotic familial idiocies, macular dystrophies, the mucolipidoses, and the mucopolysaccharidoses such as Apo-LP-serine which seems to be deficient in the small intestinal mucosa in a-β lipoproteinaemia (Bassen-Kornzweig syndrome). Phytanic acid is deficient in Refsum's disease.

7.3 Central Serous Maculopathy

Central serous maculopathy can be associated with hypersensitivity conditions, peripheral retinal disease, macular disorders, the presence of a congenital pit in the optic nerve, or may be idiopathic. It is characterised by a chronic course with spontaneous remissions and exacerbations. Sometimes, acute exacerbations, especially when the fovea is threatened, respond to high dose corticosteroids or to photocoagulation of a focal chorioretinal vessel leak, as demonstrated by fluorescein angiography. Otherwise, treatment is confined to an underlying cause, e.g. peripheral chorioretinal lesions, if discovered.

7.4 Retinal Vascular Disease

The patient with retinal vascular disease should be carefully evaluated for underlying conditions before therapy is initiated. Retinal vasculitis can be treated with corticosteroids, or anticoagulants when vascular occlusion is imminent, and by discontinuing drugs such as oral contraceptives. Retinal vein occlusions can be treated with short term intravenous heparin if the macular area is not completely involved, if there is only a branch vein occlusion, if this is the better eye, and to prevent the frequent (25 %) complication of haemorrhagic glaucoma. Many clinicians do not use anticoagulants in patients with retinal vein occlusions because the fellow eye does not become involved for an average of 6 to 7 years and because these patients generally have contraindications to such treatment. Currently a multicentre study is being conducted to evaluate photocoagulation on branch vein occlusions.

Thrombolytic agents such as streptokinase have a limited role in retinal vein occlusion, but may be useful in recent thromboses such as venous occlusion during oral contraceptive use (Kohner et al., 1976).

7.5 Retinal Arterial Occlusions

Retinal arterial occlusions, when diagnosed immediately, are treated with retrobulbar administration of the α-adrenoceptor blocking drug tolazoline, anterior chamber paracentesis, carbon dioxide rebreathing, or possibly with decompression of the retinal artery at the usual location of the occlusion by cutting the sclera adjacent to the entrance of the optic nerve. However, the visual loss is generally irreversible because therapy is ineffective after 15 minutes (Ffytche, 1974).

7.6 Diabetic Retinopathy

Diabetic retinopathy, a leading cause of severe visual impairment throughout the world, remains unpredictable and difficult to contain. Nonproliferative retinopathy and senile diabetic maculopathy should be carefully followed by fluorescein angiography. Vascular leaks in the macular region associated with sudden fluctuation in visual acuity might be amenable to photo-

coagulation with the ruby or argon laser. These lasers can occlude small blood vessels with less tissue necrosis. The xenon arc photocoagulator can be used to destroy deeper areas in the retina, hopefully eliminating the anoxic tissue which may stimulate the neovascular response.

Proliferative diabetic retinopathy constitutes a greater threat to vision because of the possibilities of recurrent vitreous haemorrhages, traction retinal detachments, and haemorrhagic (neovascular) glaucoma. Hypophysectomy, careful blood sugar control, calcium dobesilate (Larsen et al., 1977) and various vitamin therapies rarely alter the course of the retinopathy. Hard retinal exudates are not often influenced by lipid lowering agents such as clofibrate, as had been once hoped. The argon laser, which may coagulate tiny vascular tufts adjacent to the optic nerve, macula, and growing into the vitreous, offers the most promise at neutralising the neovascular proliferation. The use of xenon arc photocoagulation to destroy large areas of peripheral retina (by eliminating retinal anoxia) has demonstrated some surprising successes in eliminating proliferative retinopathy and should be considered in progressive cases (Diabetic Retinopathy Group, 1978). Diabetic patients should not be denied the hope of improvement as spontaneous decrudescences can sometimes occur.

7.7 Other Retinal Disorders

As a result of the dissemination of knowledge of peripheral retina examination and the continuing refinement and modification of the surgical approaches, retinal holes, tears, and detachments have become reversible entities. Retinal holes and tears can be effectively sealed off with cryotherapy, diathermy or photocoagulation. Scleral buckling procedures and release of the accumulated subretinal fluid are highly successful in repairing retinal detachment.

Trauma can lead to a number of retinal disorders. Berliner's macular oedema seems to be reversible, whereas macular hole formation, choroidal and scleral rupture lead to permanent visual impairment. Vitreous haemorrhage secondary to ocular trauma usually resolves completely and traumatic retinal detachments are quite amenable to therapy after the retinal break has been identified.

Systemic administration of urea compounds and cyanate may prove efficacious in the treatment of sickle cell disease.

8. Diseases of the Optic Nerve

8.1 Papilloedema

Papilloedema may be caused by increased intracranial pressure (Hedges, 1975) and less frequently by increased intraorbital pressure or sudden decreased intraocular pressure. Thorough radiological (which may include carotid angiography and pneumoencephalography) and laboratory evaluation are imperative. Causes of benign intracranial hypertension (e.g. tetracycline, triamcinolone, vitamin A excess) should be eliminated. Infectious causes should be immediately identified and treated, wherever possible. The intracranial pressure can be rapidly lowered with intravenous mannitol (or other hyperosmotic agents) and fluorescein angiography may demonstrate the reversal of some of the optic nerve inflammatory response.

The sudden appearance of papilloedema and papillitis due to leptomeningeal infiltration (e.g. leukaemias and lymphomas) has been dramatically reversed with localised radiotherapy, systemic corticosteroids, and specific intrathecal chemotherapy.

The presence of congenital drusen of the optic nerve head may simulate the appearance of papilloedema (Friedman, 1977).

8.2 Optic Neuritis

Optic neuritis should be carefully studied and treated before nerve fibre oedema is replaced by gliosis, leading to optic atrophy. Cranial or temporal arteritis may respond to corticosteroid therapy and vascular insufficiency in suitable cases may benefit by carotid endarterectomy. Drug induced optic neuritis is discussed in section 11.1.3. Intravenous 5% sodium bicarbonate is employed to counter the acidosis encountered in methanol toxicity. Calcium disodium versenate, 1g/kg over 24 hours for 10 days, may be used to reverse the signs of lead poisoning.

Optic nerve disorders due to thyroid disease, syphilis, and polycythaemia rubra vera are amenable to therapy if the diagnosis is made in time. When virus, demyelinating disease, tobacco, alcohol, diabetes, ischaemia or idiopathic causes are responsible for the papillitis, the results of therapy remain variable.

When optic atrophy is present, rapid diagnosis and therapy may be life saving. Hereditary optic atrophy, the cerebral scleroses, optic nerve tumours (glioma), intraorbital disease, syphilis, vascular insufficiency, anterior fossa meningioma, pituitary tumours, intoxicants and trauma, should be considered and appropriately treated whenever possible.

9. Miscellaneous Ophthalmological Conditions

9.1 Thyrotoxic Exophthalmos

The pathogenesis of thyrotoxic or thyrotropic exophthalmopathy remains unexplained and may be more frequently encountered after medical rather than surgical management of Graves' disease. When the exophthalmos becomes 'malignant', causing optic nerve compromise, multiple extraocular muscle pareses or exposure keratitis, several procedures have been employed. These include high dose systemic corticosteroids, low dosage radiation, orbital decompression, and short term cyclophosphamide.

Often the exophthalmos accompanying acute thyrotoxicosis disappears with appropriate treatment of the thyrotoxicosis.

9.2 Orbital Pseudotumour

Orbital pseudotumour, a cause of proptosis diagnosed by exclusion and biopsy, is also treated with corticosteroids and orbital decompression.

9.3 Cataracts

Cataracts are apparently formed as a result of single or multiple insults to the lens metabolism. Trauma, gamma irradiation, drugs (see table VII), retinopathies, diabetes, and galactosaemia may result in lens changes. Changing blood sugar levels cause alteration in the lens volume. Diabetics often develop changing refractive errors, retinopathy, chronic simple glaucoma and cataracts. A galactose free diet, when prescribed early, can lead to reversal of the cataractous changes which are due to dulcitol accumulation in the lens.

9.4 Accommodative Esotropia

Accommodative esotropia, occurring after the age of 1 year and manifest when focusing at near, is neutralised with the appropriate hyperopic correction or by anticholinesterase agents which eliminate much of the accommodative response.

Ecothiopate iodide 0.06 % drops at bedtime are employed for diagnosis or short term therapy, but are not without their adverse effects (see table III).

9.5 Intraocular Tumours

Drug therapy is usually the last choice in treatment of intraocular tumours. For retinoblastoma, the involved eye or worse eye (when binocular) is often enucleated and supravoltage radiation given for involvement of the second eye and for metastases. Genetic investigation and counselling are essential. Once convinced of the diagnosis of a choroidal melanoma, enucleation is often the treatment of choice (Shields, 1977). Ocular wall resection of localized choroidal melanomas is being performed at several centres. Vincristine, carmustine, and dacarbazine (imidazole carboxamide) are combined for treating a melanoma in an only eye or for metastatic disease (see also chapter XXIV; sect. 6.5). At least one case of sudden tumour necrosis and disruption of the globe has resulted after chemotherapy (Ferry, 1972). Photocoagulation to the adjacent retina has been employed to contain an overlying retinal detachment. Immunotherapy by use of BCG vaccine has not been successful.

Ocular complications may be associated with autoimmune disorders, leukaemia and lymphomas. The haematogenous neoplasms can infiltrate the conjunctiva, retina (leukaemia), the orbit, and rarely the cornea (leukaemia) and choroid (lymphoma). Treatment is usually directed at the systemic disease (see chapter XXIV). Orbital involvement usually responds to radiation.

9.6 Fundus Examination

The mydriatic drugs phenylephrine (2.5 to 10 %) and tropicamide (0.5 %) are routinely used to examine the fundus oculi. Cycloplegic agents such as cyclopentolate (1 %), homatropine (5 %) and atropine (1 %) may be employed during refraction, especially in younger children (Havener, 1970c). In susceptible individuals, a narrow angle glaucoma attack may be provoked in the ensuing 24 hours. Therefore, it is important to gonioscopy patients with shallow anterior chambers and to make them aware of the symptoms of increased intraocular pressure. Pupillary size may

return to normal in as little as 2 hours (tropicamide) or as long as several days (cyclopentolate). Patients should be informed about the possibility of large pupils for several days as many people become concerned about them. Patients with darkly pigmented irides usually respond poorly to any of the mydriatic drugs used. This seems to be due to an excess of parasympathetic over sympathetic tone which is genetically influenced (Smith and Rawlins, 1973).

Phenylephrine and cyclopentolate may cause the shedding of iris pigment cells leading to the erroneous diagnosis of iritis. Caution should be used when administering these agents to children because of their rapid absorption and relatively large dosages. Cyclopentolate, particularly with repeated instillation at short intervals or use of solutions greater than 1 %, can cause fever and convulsions and disorientation (see Binkhorst et al., 1963; Kennerdell and Wucher, 1972). Phenylephrine 10 % has been associated with subarachnoid bleeding in infants and in adults cardiac arrest and myocardial infarction (Fraunfelder and Scafidi, 1978), and atropine 1 % can cause fever, rash, disorientation and dehydration, particularly when several drops are applied.

Systemic absorption is most likely to occur in hot weather, especially in those living in the tropics (Shah, 1966).

9.7 Cycloplegia

The sympathomimetic agents (e.g. phenylephrine) are weaker mydriatic drugs and dilate the pupil without affecting accommodation (section 9.6), whereas the parasympatholytic agents (e.g. cyclopentolate, atropine, tropicamide) are longer acting and produce cycloplegia as well as mydriasis. These drug actions are essential for performing retinoscopy in paediatric ophthalmology, are helpful in determining the refractive error in young people, and may allow a better ophthalmoscopic examination (Havener, 1970c). Cyclopentolate exerts its maximum effect in less than 1 hour and usually has an effect for 4 to 24 hours. However, strict attention to dosage is necessary to avoid potentially serious side effects. Children under 2 years of age should have only one drop of a 1 % solution instilled in each eye while one drop of a 2 % solution is used in older children. Tropicamide is a weaker cycloplegic agent, acting within 15 to 20 minutes and lasting for 2 to 4 hours, and may be sufficient for dilated examination of the fundus or retinoscopy in older patients. Atropine ointment (0.5 %) can be applied to the conjunctival sac several days before the examination, but parents must be informed of the possible side effects (see section 9.6).

10. Use of Drugs in the Presence of Associated Ocular Disease

10.1 Glaucoma

The systemic administration of such agents as corticosteroids, anticholinergics (e.g. doses as used for peptic ulceration, anti-Parkinsonian drugs, tricyclic antidepressants, the antiarrhythmic drug disopyramide) and the topical use of corticosteroids and sympathomimetics (e.g. adrenaline and phenylephrine) may sometimes have adverse effects in patients with associated ocular diseases which are often unsuspected. The susceptibility to narrow angle and open angle glaucoma should always be anticipated when these agents are being used (see Grant, 1969; Lazenby et al., 1970).

The risk of aggravating glaucoma with systemic anticholinergic drugs is largely confined to patients with abnormally shallow anterior chambers and narrow angles, since if the systemic medication is given in doses large enough to cause the pupil to dilate, angle closure glaucoma could be precipitated. This is most likely to occur in the elderly patient who has hyperopia (far sightedness) and is developing early cataractous changes (see further section 2.2). Adrenaline and phenylephrine can also dilate the pupil when applied topically, and may also induce angle closure glaucoma in predisposed patients. The effect of systemically administered sympathomimetic drugs (e.g. anorexiants, common cold remedies) is unclear, but is probably only significant in those with very shallow anterior chambers and probably only rarely so. The narrow anterior chamber angle however, is difficult to diagnose unless by gonioscopy and is often only revealed after dilating the pupil to perform ophthalmoscopy. Mydriasis with one drop of 1 % tropicamide has been used as a provocative test for narrow angle glaucoma, the detection of which is valuable. Since the acute attack may occur several hours later when the patient is home, it is important to advise all patients to be mindful of any unusual symptoms.

The use of systemic anticholinergic drugs is much less of a problem in patients with chronic open angle glaucoma since their anterior chambers are much deeper, allowing pupillary dilatation without the danger of precipitating angle closure glaucoma. In only a minority of patients with chronic open angle glaucoma have systemic anticholinergic drugs caused a significant rise in intraocular pressure and this has usually been readily controlled by adjustment of the glaucoma treatment (Lazenby et al., 1970; Hiatt et al., 1970). Thus, systemic anticholinergic drugs may be safely given to most patients with open angle glaucoma, if the management is shared between the clinician and ophthalmologist. Gonioscopy helps to identify those patients who should be closely observed. If the patient is already on miotic drug therapy for glaucoma then the risks of pupillary dilatation with these drugs is infinitesimally small.

Systemic corticosteroids may sometimes make glaucoma more difficult to control in patients with chronic open angle disease. Topical corticosteroids certainly carry a risk of inducing a sudden rise in intraocular pressure in patients with open angle glaucoma and their use must be closely supervised (Becker and Hahn, 1964). Alternatively, agents such as medrysone, tetrahydrotriamcinolone and fluorometholone can be safely used for treatment of external inflammatory and allergic conditions (see also section 11.1.2).

10.2 Infections

Topical corticosteroids can exacerbate bacterial, herpes simplex, or vaccinia keratitis as well as tuberculosis of the eye and are therefore contraindicated in the presence of these infections until antimicrobial control has been achieved (David and Berkowitz, 1969). Some ophthalmologists do nevertheless use topical steroids in herpes simplex keratitis, especially with stromal involvement and iritis, but only under the cover of an antiviral agent (see section 3.6). Topical steroids however, will temporarily fade the subepithelial opacities of epidemic keratoconjunctivitis, quell the iritis of herpes zoster ophthalmicus and ameliorate the symptoms of Thygeson's punctate keratopathy (Hyndiuk, 1973).

If a hypersensitivity induced blepharitis, conjunctivitis, or keratitis is suspected, it is prudent not to treat the condition with any of the more sensitising topical antibiotic preparations (e.g. neomycin, bacitracin, sulphonamides).

Table V. Ocular complications with phenothiazines

Drug	Side effect	Notes
Thioridazine	Pigmentary retinopathy Optic atrophy Transient myopia and loss of accommodation Oculogyric crises Anterior cortical lens opacities	Night blindness occurs early but central vision becomes involved later. High dosage over prolonged period needed; can occur with doses in excess of 200mg daily for many months — but generally doses greater than 600 to 800mg daily are necessary
Chlorpromazine	Pigmentary retinopathy[1] Anterior cortical lens opacities[1] Oculomotor palsies Optic atrophy Stellate and polar lens changes Posterior corneal opacities	High dosage over prolonged period (in excess of 300mg for many months) Rare
Prochlorperazine	Pigmentary retinopathy	High dosage over prolonged period
Perphenazine	Optic atrophy	
Trifluoperazine	Posterior corneal opacities Anterior cortical lens opacities	In exposed areas yellow granular pigment deposits, partially reversible

1   Ocular changes appear to be positively correlated with severe photosensitivity responses to chlorpromazine; thus patients who develop photosensitivity reactions on light exposed areas (see also chapter XIV; sect. 22.3.11) should have an eye examination (Prien et al., 1970).

11. Drug Induced Ocular Disease

The eye may manifest side effects from a wide variety of drugs used in the treatment of diseases of all systems of the body. Some of these side effects, though undesirable, have to be accepted as unavoidable. The toxic effects of drugs such as the chloroquine antimalarials, corticosteroids and phenothiazines used in high dosage over long periods have caused serious irreversible visual defects. These effects and others indicate the need for safer agents and for all clinicians to be aware of the risks involved.

Many factors are concerned in the production of ocular side effects by a drug (see Willetts, 1969).

1) *The nature of the drug* determines its pharmacodynamic effects and ease of absorption and rate of metabolism and excretion (see chapter I). The ease with which a drug passes into the general circulation and thence into the eye determines the ability of systemically administered drugs to affect the eye directly. Some drugs cause ocular side effects indirectly by their effects on the general circulation — e.g. blindness from a precipitous fall of blood pressure due to antihypertensive agents and intraocular haemorrhage with anticoagulants.

2) *Amount of the drug.* Toxic levels of drugs may be reached in some instances by high daily dosage and in others by prolonged use.

3) *Route of administration.* Drugs may affect the eye when administered not only orally or parenterally but also topically, such as in the absorption of toxic substances applied to burns.

4) *Patient's general health and condition under treatment.* Severe liver and renal disease may affect the metabolism and excretion of drugs, allowing them to cumulate to toxic levels (see chapter I; sect. 4.3.3, 4.3.4). In some cases, it may be difficult to determine whether an ocular defect has arisen as a result of involvement with the general disease or as a toxic manifestation of a drug used in therapy.

5) *Individual idiosyncrasy.* Many cases of ocular side effects may be the result of individual idiosyncrasy and some of these abnormal responses may be genetically determined — e.g. increased intraocular pressure with topical corticosteroids (see table VI; chapter VII, sect. 4.2.2).

6) *Previous exposure to the drug* leading to drug hypersensitivity, particularly with topical applica-

tion over long periods of time — e.g. hypersensitivity to topical atropine or antibiotic preparations.

The evaluation of reports concerning possible or actual ocular side effects is very difficult and it is important not to condemn a drug of proven usefulness unless the evidence of drug induced toxicity is unequivocal, or the severity of the reaction warrants more careful investigation (see also chapter XIV; sect. 22).

11.1 Drugs which may Cause Numerous Reactions

11.1.1 Phenothiazines

The phenothiazine derivatives have been known to cause corneal and lens deposits and pigmentary retinopathy and myopia with large doses (e.g. in excess of 300mg daily chlorpromazine) given over a prolonged period. Total dosage also seems to be important, since about 1 in 3 patients receiving large doses of a phenothiazine for several years are at risk of developing an ocular side effect, while nearly all patients have some detectable ocular manifestations if therapy is used for over 10 years (De Long, 1968; Mathalone, 1967; Fraunfelder, 1976). The pigmentary deposits with chlorpromazine are first observed on the anterior lens capsule near the pupil; the ocular melanosis later appearing in Descemet's membrane, and rarely in the cornea. Cutaneous pigmentation, including melanosis of the lids and conjunctiva, is also sometimes seen (Greiner and Berry, 1964). No association seems to exist between extrapyramidal symptoms and ocular pigmentation (Wheeler et al., 1969). Thioridazine has been most frequently implicated in a dose related retinitis pigmentosa type deposition, with associated night blindness and decreased central vision among other complications (Hagopian et al., 1966; table V). Impairment of visual acuity may recover but the pigmentation remains (May et al., 1960; Davidorf, 1973). Transient myopia, oculomotor palsies and optic atrophy have also been reported (see table V).

11.1.2 Corticosteroids

Corticosteroid preparations have been both a blessing and a distress at times (David and Berkowitz, 1969; Dinning, 1976). The anti-inflammatory properties of the glucocorticoids are heavily relied upon in ophthalmology (see section 2.1). The side effects of long term administration of systemic steroids are primarily not related to the eyes, but the reverse holds true for topical steroid usage. Ocular complications of steroids are related to dosage and duration of treatment (see table VI). Topical steroids used indiscriminately in the eye are especially liable to cause a rise in intraocular pressure; a response which appears to be genetically determined (see chapter VII, sect. 4.2.2; Armaly, 1966; Becker, 1965) and may precipitate glaucoma in susceptible individuals and diabetics (Becker and Mills, 1963; Becker and Le Blanc, 1970). Some topical steroids developed for ocular use do not have this propensity (table VI), but hydrocortisone and other steroids can increase intraocular pressure in susceptible individuals if used in the eye frequently over several weeks and occasionally sooner. Prolonged or excessive application of topical steroids to the skin of the eyelids can also increase intraocular pressure and precipitate glaucoma (Cubey, 1976; Howell, 1976). Most ocular complications of steroids are reversible, but some such as posterior subcapsular cataracts following prolonged systemic use are generally irreversible.

11.1.3 Chloroquine Derivatives

The synthetic 4-amino quinolines are well known for their production of maculopathy with a bull's eye appearance. This occurs early in those susceptible to chloroquine, but can appear some time after cessation of therapy. The condition is usually irreversible and may progress despite withdrawal of the drug. It usually occurs when chloroquine (250 to 750mg daily), or hydroxychloroquine (200 to 400mg daily) are used for their anti-inflammatory properties in severe rheumatoid arthritis (see chapt. XXII; sect. 3.3.2) and does not seem to occur with the low doses used for prophylaxis and treatment of malaria. In severe cases there is a mottling of the fundus due to increased retinal pigmentation, and optic atrophy may later supervene with complete blindness. Reversible corneal deposits and posterior subcapsular lens opacities have also been described. Optic neuritis is a rare complication with chloroquine. Primaquine (an 8-aminoquinoline derivative) seems to have no ocular side effects (see Leopold, 1963; Nylander, 1966, 1967).

11.1.4 Miotics

Long term use of miotic therapy for the maintenance of normal intraocular pressure in chronic glaucoma can occasionally lead to anterior cortical

Table VI. Ocular complications of topical and systemic corticosteroids

	Complication	Description	Notes and action
1.	Increased intraocular pressure (IOP)	Loss of normal diurnal variation in IOP. Increased IOP in 1/3 population, probably as autosomal dominant genetic trait. Includes those destined for open angle glaucoma, diabetes, pre-diabetics, certain myopes. This increased IOP may make underlying open angle glaucoma more refractory to treatment	Topical — requires several weeks, 4 times daily of topical treatment (prednisone, hydrocortisone, triamcinolone, dexamethasone, betamethasone, etc). Medrysone 1% and tetrahydrotriamcinolone 0.15%, and fluorometholone do not cause the elevation of IOP and should be used for external allergy in susceptible patients and in those with glaucoma. Systemic — requires months to years with systemic administration; almost always reversible
2.	Posterior subcapsular cataracts	Bilateral posterior polar, well demarcated. Vision not affected immediately	Usually requires 15mg or more of prednisone or equivalent daily for 2 years or more (Kristensen, 1968; Williamson et al., 1969). Has also occurred with long term topical steroids in diabetics (Yablonski and Burde, 1978) Irreversible usually. May occur in children
3.	Exophthalmos		Dose related. Evidence indicates reversibility. Steroids also used to treat exophthalmos in certain conditions
4.	Mydriasis	1mm average enlargement of pupil	Topical Reversible
5.	Ptosis	Lid oedema	Topical
6.	Benign intracranial hypertension		Systemic steroids triamcinolone (most often implicated) on administration or shortly after withdrawal. Treat by increasing dosage and very gradual reduction (Ivey and Den Besten, 1969)
7.	Delayed wound healing	Fibroblast inhibition	Not clinically impressive in most cases, but must be remembered after intraocular surgery
8.	Enhancement of infection	Bacterial, fungal, viral	Watch out for vaccinia and herpes simplex. Treat PPD converter

vacuoles in the lens, cataracts (Levene, 1975), and changing refractive errors. These changes are dose related and are more common in the young and middle aged. Although the cholinesterase inhibitors (ecothiopate iodide, demecarium bromide, dyflos) will cause cataractous changes much more frequently than will pilocarpine, the incidence still remains tolerable. It must be remembered that glaucoma surgery will also induce lens opacities. Ecothiopate and dyflos can however, cause iris pigment epithelial cysts, especially in younger individuals. These are usually reversible on withdrawal of the drug. Use of 10% phenylephrine may reduce the chance of cyst formation. Rarely, ecothiopate has been associated with retinal detachments in aphakic patients and it should therefore be used cautiously in susceptible individuals (Pape and Forbes, 1978).

The side effects of increased absorption of topical cholinesterase inhibitors are similar to cholinergic crises in myasthenia gravis. These can be rapidly counteracted with pralidoxime and systemic atropine. These agents should be discontinued several weeks prior to general anaesthesia if the use of suxamethonium (succinylcholine) is anticipated (see chapter X; sect. 2.2.1, table VI).

Table VII. Ocular complications caused by specific drugs (after Willetts, 1969; Crombie, 1977)

Side effect	Examples	Notes
Conjunctiva and cornea		
Conjunctivitis	Cocaine	Keratitis, mydriasis
	Phenytoin, penicillin, sulphonamides	Allergic (Stevens-Johnson syndrome)
	Phenylbutazone, oxyphenbutazone	Allergic (Stevens-Johnson syndrome)
Contact dermatitis or follicular conjunctivitis	Idoxuridine, atropine, hyoscine, penicillin, neomycin, bacitracin	Rare with atropine
	Miotics	Pilocarpine infrequently; dyflos (DFP) and echothiopate iodide can cause significant follicular hypertrophy
Corneal reactions	Topical corneal anaesthetics	Keratitis; when applied frequently for days or weeks
	Carbimazole	Keratitis
	Adrenaline (local) 1%	Pigmentation
	Vitamin D (plus calcium)	Band shaped degeneration; with calcium deposits
	Chlorpropamide, thioridazine	Corneal opacities
	Chloroquine, hydroxychloroquine, mepacrine	Corneal oedema, deposits (usually reversible)
	Phenothiazines, copper, gold	Posterior corneal opacities (see table V)
	Oral contraceptives	Corneal oedema (rare); contact lens difficulties
	Practolol	Keratoconjunctivitis, decreased tear flow, corneal ulceration (Rahi et al., 1976)
	Clofazimine	Fine, linear brownish subepithelial opacifications (Ohman and Wahlberg, 1975)
	?Tamoxifen	Corneal opacities (?high dose; Kaiser-Kupfer and Lippman, 1978)
	?Indomethacin	Corneal deposits
Pupillary and accommodative changes	Adrenaline compounds	Slight mydriasis when used parenterally
	Morphine	Miosis
	Vasoconstrictors, ephedrine, amphetamines	May cause slight mydriasis, no effect on accommodation, rare to never causing narrow angle attack in susceptible patients
	Isoxsuprine	Can induce transient rise in intraocular pressure
	Anticholinergics	High doses used in Parkinsonism or peptic ulcer disease may cause cycloplegia and significant mydriasis (see also section 10)
	Antihistamines	Minimal mydriasis
	Amitriptyline etc	Rarely significant mydriasis, but disturbance of accommodation
Myopia	Organo-arsenicals	Transient reversible
	Diuretics (acetazolamide, thiazides)	Rare (more likely late pregnancy); transient
	Sulphonamides	Transient
	Phenothiazines	Especially with prochlorperazine
	Tetracyclines	Transient, rare
	Miotics	
Lens abnormalities	Gold salts	Chryseosis. Prolonged use
	Carbonic anhydrase inhibitors	Refractive changes
	Corticosteroids	Posterior subcapsular opacities (high doses)
	Chlorpropamide	Changes in refractive error
	Chlorpromazine, trifluoperazine, thioridazine	Anterior cortical lens opacities. High dosage over prolonged period (see table V)
Retrolental fibroplasia	Oxygen	Premature infants, early stages reversible
Cataracts	Miotics	See section 11.1.4
	Corticosteroids	Long term use (see table VI)

Table VII. (continued)

Side effect	Examples	Notes
Retina	Oral contraceptives	Retinal oedema, venous occlusions (rare) [Chizek and Franceshetti, 1968]
	Phenylbutazone	Haemorrhages
	Methysergide	Retinal vasospasm
	?Tamoxifen	Retinal opacities (? high dose; Kaiser-Kupfer and Lippman, 1978)
Pigmentary retinopathy	Chloroquine, hydroxychloroquine, mepacrine	See section 11.1.3
	Thioridazine, chlorpromazine, prochlorperazine	See table V
Optic nerve		
Optic neuritis	Phenothiazines	Optic atrophy (see table V)
	Chloramphenicol	Partially reversible; rare, usually with high dose
	Streptomycin	Usually reversible
	Isoniazid	Rare, usually in malnutrition
	Ethambutol	Retrobulbar neuritis dose dependent (Citron, 1969)
	Quinine	Rare at recommended doses
	Digitalis	Overdosage
	Sulphonamides	Rare, usually reversible
	Disulfiram	Occasional, usually reversible
	Para aminosalicylate	Probably rare
	Ethionamide	Rare at recommended doses
	Cycloserine	
	?Rifampicin, ?capreomycin, ?kanamycin	
	D-Penicillamine	
	Clioquinol (Selby, 1973)	
Papilloedema	Triamcinolone	See table VI
	Tetracyclines	Rare
	Vitamin A	Excess dosage; greater than 25,000 units daily
Vision effects		
Central vision effect	Allopurinol	Macular oedema
	Adrenaline	In aphakia; macular oedema
	Indomethacin	Central serous
	Phenylbutazone, oxyphenbutazone	Decreased vision
	Clomiphene	Blurred vision, photopsia
	Chlorpropamide	Central scotomata
	Nalidixic acid	Occasional, transient
	Reserpine	Blurred vision
Scotomata	Quinine, quinidine	Rare at recommended doses
	Ethambutol	Dose dependent
	Digitalis	Overdosage
	Mepacrine	
Colour vision (Lyle, 1974)	Anticonvulsants	Oxazolidines, e.g. trimethadione
	Ethambutol	Loss of green vision, red colour, bull's eye maculopathy (dose dependent)
	Digitalis	Green or yellow vision, photopsia (overdosage)
	Chlorothiazide	Xanthepsia
	Frusemide (furosemide)	Rare
Hallucinations	Propranolol	May occur with modest doses (Fleminger, 1978)
	Pentazocine	Tend to occur more frequently with larger doses
	Ketamine	May persist for months after use
	Anticholinergics	See section 9.6
	Cimetidine	High doses, elderly, renal impairment

Table VII. (continued)

Side effect	Examples	Notes
Raised intraocular pressure	Corticosteroids	Principally topical (see table VI)
	Anticholinergics	See section 10
	Tricyclic antidepressants	Occasional in narrow angle glaucoma, otherwise rare (see section 10)
Muscle palsies	Vincristine	
	Sulphonamides	
	Digitalis	
	Phenothiazines	Oculogyric crisis. Caused by thioridazine and prochlorperazine
	Gold salts	Secondary to encephalitis
Toxic amblyopia	Quinine	Rare with recommended doses
	Chloramphenicol	Long term or high dose systemic use (especially children)
	Heavy metals	Arsenicals, antimony compounds, lead compounds
	Many other drugs	
	?Tobacco, alcohol	
Infection	Fluorescein solutions	Contamination with *Pseudomonas* spp.
	Topical anaesthetics	Chronic use
	Topical corticosteroids	Increase susceptibility to infection

11.2 Ocular Disease Caused by Specific Drugs

Local and systemic administration of a wide variety of drugs has resulted in many forms of complications to the eye and vision (e.g. see Leopold, 1968; Willetts, 1969; Davidson, 1973). These include blurred vision, disturbances in colour vision, scotomata, pigmentary degeneration of the retina, and other adverse effects on the cornea, sclera, lens, retina, optic nerve and extraocular muscles. The factors which lead to these adverse effects by a drug are discussed above. The drugs responsible are summarised in table VII, and include those that are retinotoxic: the cardiac glycosides, the 4-amino quinolines (see also section 11.1.3); and the phenothiazines (see also section 11.1.1); and those that produce toxic optic neuropathies: chlorpropamide, the corticosteroids, and chloramphenicol.

Systemically administered drugs can have significant adverse effects on ocular structures. The untoward effects of some drugs can be predicted and occur shortly after drug administration. Other drugs produce adverse ocular effects which cannot be predicted and that occur only after long term administration. Most of the adverse ocular effects of drugs are transient but some may cause severe visual damage which is permanent. Careful ophthalmological screening is therefore desirable whenever possible for patients who are to receive long term systemically administered drugs, especially new drugs.

Further Reading

Duane, T.D.: Clinical Ophthalmology, vol. VI (Harper and Row, New York 1976).

Ellis, P.: Ocular Pharmacology and Therapeutics, 5th ed (Mosby, St. Louis 1977).

Fraunfelder, F.T.: Drug Induced Ocular Side Effects and Drug Interactions (Lea & Febiger, Philadelphia 1976).

Havener, W.H.: Ocular Pharmacology, 4th ed (Mosby, St. Louis 1978).

Levine, S. and Leopold, I.H.: Disorders of the eye. Medical Clinics of North America 57: 1167 (1973).

References

Abel, R. Jr.: Therapeutic indications for soft contact lenses. Delaware Medical Journal 47: 515 (1975).

Abel, R. Jr.; Masciulli, L. and Boyle, G.L.: Subconjunctival gentamicin prophylaxis against post-operative endophthalmitis in the rabbit. Ocular Surgery 7: 59 (1976).

Allansmith, M.R.: Treatment of external diseases with immunological properties; in Laibson and Troub (Eds) External ocular diseases: Diagnosis and therapy. International Ophthalmology Clinics 13: 193 (1973).

Armaly, M.F.: The heritable nature of dexamethasone induced ocular hypertension. Archives of Ophthalmology 75: 32 (1966).

Armaly, M.F. and Rao, K.R.: The effect of pilocarpine ocusert with different release rates on ocular pressure. Investigative Ophthalmology 12: 491 (1973).

Armstrong, J.H.; Zacarias, F. and Rein, M.F.: Ophthalmia neonatorum: A chart review. Pediatrics 57: 884 (1976).

Baum, J.L.: The treatment of bacterial endophthalmitis. Ophthalmologica 85: 350 (1978).

Becker, B.: Intraocular pressure response to topical corticosteroids. Investigative Ophthalmology 4: 198 (1965).

Becker, B. and Mills, D.: Corticosteroids and intraocular pressure. Archives of Ophthalmology 70: 106 (1963).

Becker, B. and Hahn, K.A.: Topical corticosteroids and heredity in primary open-angle glaucoma. American Journal of Ophthalmology 57: 543 (1964).

Becker, B. and Le Blanc, R.P.: The glucose tolerance test and the response of intraocular pressure to topical corticosteroids. Diabetes 19: 715 (1970).

Benson, Harriet: Permeability of the cornea to topically applied drugs. Archives of Ophthalmology 91: 313 (1974).

Binkhorst, R.D.; Weinstein, G.W.; Baretz, R.M. and Clahane, A.C.: Psychotic reaction induced by cyclopentolate (Cyclogyl). Results of a pilot study and a double-blind study. American Journal of Ophthalmology 55: 1243 (1963).

Bloch, S.; Rosenthal, A.R.; Friedman, L. and Caldarolla, P.: Patient compliance in glaucoma. British Journal of Ophthalmology 61: 531 (1977).

Boger, W.P. and Flippin, H.F.: Penicillin plasma concentrations. Journal of the American Medical Association 139: 1131 (1949).

Borthne, A.: The treatment of glaucoma with propranolol (Inderal). A clinical trial. Acta Ophthalmologica 54: 291 (1976).

Brenkman, R.F.: Long-term hypotensive effect of atenolol 4% eyedrops. British Journal of Ophthalmology 62: 287 (1978).

Chapman-Smith, J.S. and Crock, G.W.: Urokinase in the management of vitreous haemorrhage. British Journal of Ophthalmology 61: 500 (1977).

Chizek, D.J. and Franceshetti, A.T.: Oral contraceptives: Their side effects and ophthalmological manifestations. Survey of Ophthalmology 14: 90 (1968).

Citron, K.M.: Ethambutol: A review with special reference to ocular toxicity. Tubercle 50 (Suppl.): 32 (1969).

Cox, W.V.; Kupferman, A. and Leibowitz, H.M.: Topically applied steroids in corneal disease: I. The role of inflammation in stromal absorption of dexamethasone. Archives of Ophthalmology 88: 308 (1972a).

Cox, W.V.; Kupferman, A. and Leibowitz, H.M.: Topically applied steroids in corneal disease: II. The role of drug vehicle in stromal absorption of dexamethasone. Archives of Ophthalmology 88: 549 (1972b).

Crombie, A.L.: Eye disorders; in Davies (Ed) Textbook of Adverse Drug Reactions, p.313 (Oxford University Press, Oxford 1977).

Cubey, R.B.: Glaucoma following the application of corticosteroid to the skin of the eyelids. British Journal of Ophthalmology 95: 207 (1976).

David, D.S. and Berkowitz, J.S.: Ocular effects of topical and systemic corticosteroids. Lancet 2: 149 (1969).

Davidorf, F.H.: Thioridazine pigmentary retinopathy. Archives of Ophthalmology 90: 251 (1973).

Davidson, S.J.: Reports of ocular adverse reactions. Transactions of the Ophthalmological Societies of the United Kingdom 93: 495 (1973).

De Long, S.L.: Incidence and significance of chlorpromazine-induced eye changes. Diseases of the Nervous System 29 (Suppl.): 19 (1968).

Diabetic Retinopathy Study Research Group: Photocoagulation therapy of proliferative diabetic retinopathy. Ophthalmologica 85: 82 (1978).

Dinning, W.J.: Steroids and the eye — indications and complications. Postgraduate Medical Journal 52: 634 (1976).

Dinning, W.J. and Perkins, E.S.: Immunosuppressives in uveitis. A preliminary report of experience with chlorambucil. British Journal of Ophthalmology 59: 397 (1975).

Dohlman, C.H.; Pavan-Langston, D. and Rose, J.: A new ocular insert device for continuous constant-rate delivery of medication to the eye. Annals of Ophthalmology 4: 823 (1972).

Duane, T.D.: Clinical Ophthalmology, vol. VI (Harper and Row, New York 1976).

Ferry, A.P.: Primary malignant melanoma of the skin metastatic to the eye. American Journal of Ophthalmology 74: 12 (1972).

Ffytche, T.J.: A rationalization of treatment of central retinal artery occlusion. Transactions of the Ophthalmological Societies of the United Kingdom 94: 468-479 (1974).

Fishman, L.S.; Griffin, J.R.; Sapico, F.L. and Height, R.: Hematogenous Candida endophthalmitis. New England Journal of Medicine 286: 675 (1972).

Fleminger, R.: Visual hallucinations and illusions with propranolol. British Medical Journal 1: 1182 (1978).

Fraunfelder, F.T.: Drug Induced Ocular Side Effects and Drug Interactions, p.68 (Lea & Febiger, Philadelphia 1976).

Fraunfelder, F.T. and Scafidi, A.F.: Possible adverse effects from topical ocular 10% phenylephrine. American Journal of Ophthalmology 85: 447 (1978).

Friedman, A.H.; Beckerman, B.; Gold, D.H.; Walsh, J.B. and Gartner, S.: Drusen of the Optic Disc. 21(5): 375 (1977).

Furgiuele, F.P.: Eye and eyelid infections. Treatment and prevention. Drugs 15: 310 (1978).

Gasset, A.R.; Lorenzetti, D.W.C.; Ellison, E.M. and Kaufman, H.E.: Quantitative corticosteroid effect on corneal wound healing. Archives of Ophthalmology 81: 589 (1969).

Godfrey, W.A.; Smith, R.E. and Kimura, S.J.: Chronic cyclitis: Corticosteroid therapy. Transactions of the American Ophthalmological Society 74: 178 (1977).

Grant, W.M.: Ocular complications of drugs: Glaucoma. Journal of the American Medical Association 207: 2089 (1969).

Grant, W.M.: Antiglaucoma drugs: problems with carbonic anhydrase inhibitors; in Leopold (Ed) Symposium on Ocular Therapy, vol. 6, p.19 (Mosby, St. Louis 1973).

Greiner, A.C. and Berry, K.: Skin pigmentation and corneal and lens opacities with prolonged chlorpromazine therapy. Canadian Medical Association Journal 90: 663 (1964).

Hagopian, V.; Stratton, D.B. and Busiek, R.D.: Five cases of pigmentary retinopathy associated with thioridazine administration. American Journal of Psychiatry 123: 97 (1966).

Harris, J.E.: Prophylaxis of ophthalmia neonatorum; in

Leopold (Ed) Symposium on Ocular Therapy, vol. 6, p.39 (Mosby, St. Louis 1973).

Havener, W.H.: Ocular Pharmacology, 2nd ed, pp.103, 118 (Mosby, St. Louis 1970a).

Havener, W.H.: Ocular Pharmacology, 2nd ed, pp.190, 289, 528 (Mosby, St. Louis 1970b).

Havener, W.H.: Ocular Pharmacology, 2nd ed, p.188 (Mosby, St. Louis 1970c).

Hedges, T.R.: Papilledema: Its recognition and relation to increased intracranial pressure. Survey of Ophthalmology 19: 201 (1975).

Heel, R.C.; Brogden, R.N.; Speight, T.M. and Avery, G.S.: Timolol: A review of its therapeutic efficacy in the topical treatment of glaucoma. Drugs 17: 38 (1979).

Henrotte, J. and Weekers, J.: Corneal lesions from prolonged anesthetics. Archives of Ophthalmology 32: 449 (1972) abstract cited in American Journal of Ophthalmology 76: 408 (1973).

Hiatt, R.L.; Fuller, I.B.; Smith, L.; Swartz, J. and Risser, C.: Systemically administered anticholinergic drugs and intraocular pressure. Archives of Ophthalmology 84: 735 (1970).

Hogan, M.J. and Zimmerman, L.E.: Ophthalmic Pathology, 2nd ed, p.373 (Saunders, Philadelphia 1962).

Holly, F.J. and Lemp, M.A.: Tear physiology and dry eyes. Survey of Ophthalmology 22: 69 (1977).

Howell, J.B.: Eye diseases induced by topically applied steroids. The thin edge of the wedge. Archives of Dermatology 112: 1529 (1976).

Hyams, S.W.; Bialik, M. and Neumann, E.: Clinical trial of topical disodium cromoglycate in vernal kerato-conjunctivitis. Journal of Pediatric Ophthalmology 12: 116 (1975).

Hyndiuk, R.A. and Chin, G.N.: Corticosteroid therapy in corneal disease, I. International Ophthalmology Clinics 13: 112 (1973).

Imre, G. and Bogi, J.: The fellow eye in acute angle-closure glaucoma. Klinische Monatsblaetter fur Augenheilkunde 169: 264 (1976) abstract cited in American Journal of Ophthalmology 83: 437 (1977).

Ivey, K.J. and Den Besten, L.: Pseudotumor cerebri associated with corticosteroid therapy in an adult. Journal of the American Medical Association 208: 1698 (1969).

Jones, D.B.: Early diagnosis and therapy of bacterial corneal ulcers; in Laibson and Troub (Eds) External ocular diseases: Diagnosis and current therapy. International Ophthalmology Clinics 13: 1 (1973).

Jones, D.B.: Therapy of post-surgical fungal endophthalmitis. Ophthalmologica 85: 357 (1978).

Jones, B.R.; Darougar, S.; Mohsenine, H. and Poirier, R.H.: Communicable ophthalmia: The blinding scourge of the Middle East. British Journal of Ophthalmology 60: 492 (1976).

Kaiser-Kupfer, M.I. and Lippman, M.E.: Tamoxifen retinopathy. Cancer Treatment Reports 62: 315 (1978).

Kaufman, H.E.: Ocular virus disease. Annals of Clinical Research 5: 189 (1973).

Kaufman, H.E. and Goorha, R.: Interferon and ocular virus disease. Survey of Ophthalmology 15: 169 (1970).

Kazdan, J.J.; Crawford, J.S.; Langer, H. and MacDonald, A.L.: Sodium cromoglycate in the treatment of vernal kerato-conjunctivitis and allergic conjunctivitis. Canadian Journal of Ophthalmology 11(4): 300 (1976).

Kennerdell, J.S. and Wucher, F.P.: Cyclopentolate associated with two cases of grand mal seizure. Archives of Ophthalmology 87: 634 (1972).

Kohner, E.M.; Pettit, J.E.; Hamilton, A.M.; Bulpitt, C.J. and Dollery, C.T.: Streptokinase in central retinal vein occlusion: A controlled clinical trial. British Medical Journal 1: 550 (1976).

Kolker, A.E. and Hetherington, J. Jr.: Becker-Schaffer's Diagnosis and Therapy of the Glaucomas, 3rd ed (Mosby, St. Louis 1970).

Kristensen, P.: Posterior subcapsular cataract and systemic steroid therapy. Acta Ophthalmologica 46: 1025 (1968).

Larsen, H.W.; Sander, E. and Hoppe, R.: The value of calcium dobesilate in the treatment of diabetic retinopathy. A controlled clinical trial. Diabetologia 13: 105 (1977).

Lazenby, G.W.; Reed, J.W. and Grant, W.M.: Anticholinergic medication in open-angle glaucoma. Long-term tests. Archives of Ophthalmology 84: 719 (1970).

Leibowitz, H.M.; Pratt, Mary J.; Flagstad, I.J.; Berrospi, A.R. and Kundsin, Ruth: Human conjunctivitis. II treatment. Archives of Ophthalmology 94: 1752 (1976).

Leopold, I.H.: Drug therapy in uveitis. XVII Annual Francis I. Proctor Lecture. American Journal of Ophthalmology 56: 709 (1963).

Leopold, I.H.: Ocular complications of drugs: Visual changes. Journal of the American Medical Association 205: 631 (1968).

Leopold, I.H.: Advances in anaesthesia in ophthalmic surgery. Ophthalmic Surgery 5: 13 (1974).

Leopold, I.H. and Keates, E.: Drugs used in treatment of glaucoma. Clinical Pharmacology and Therapeutics 6: 130 (1965).

Levene, R.Z.: Uniocular miotic therapy. American Academy of Ophthalmology and Otolaryngology 79: OP376 (1975).

Levine, S.B. and Leopold, I.H.: Advances in ocular corticosteroid therapy. Medical Clinics of North America 57: 1167 (1973).

Lyle, W.M.: Drugs and conditions which may affect color vision. Part 1 — Drugs and Chemicals. Journal of the American Optometric Association 45: 47 (1974).

McGill, J.; Holt-Wilson, A.; McKinnon, J.; Williams, H. and Jones, B.: Some aspects of the clinical use of trifluorothymidine in the treatment of herpetic ulceration of the cornea. Transactions of the Ophthalmological Societies of the United Kingdom 94: 342 (1974).

Mackool, R.J.; Muldoon, T.; Fortier, A. and Nelson, D.: Epinephrine-induced cystoid macular edema in aphakic eyes. Archives of Ophthalmology 95: 791 (1977).

Maloney, E.D. and Kaufman, H.E.: Dissemination of corneal herpes simplex. Investigative Ophthalmology 4: 872 (1965).

Mandel, A.I. and Podos, S.M.: Dipivalyl epinephrine (DPE): A new product in the treatment of glaucoma; in Leopold and Burns (Eds) Symposium on Ocular Therapy, vol. 10 (Mosby, St. Louis 1977).

Martin, J.W. and Wellman, W.E.: Clinically useful antimicrobial agents. Postgraduate Medicine 42: 350 (1967).

Mathalone, M.R.B.: Eye and skin changes in psychiatric patients treated with chlorpromazine. British Journal of Ophthalmology 51: 86 (1967).

Maurice, D.M.: Prolonged release systems and topically applied drugs. Sight-Saving Review 42: 42 (1972).

May, R.H.; Selymes, P.; Weekley, R.D. and Potts, A.M.: Thioridazine therapy; results and complications. Journal of Nervous and Mental Disease 130: 230 (1960).

Newell, F.W.: Current trends in ophthalmic anaesthesia. Ophthalmic Surgery 6: 15 (1975).

Nylander, U.: Ocular damage in chloroquine therapy. Acta Ophthalmologica 44: 335 (1966); ibid 92 (Suppl.): 5 (1967).

O'Connor, G.R.: Periocular corticosteroid injections: Uses and abuses. Eye, Ear, Nose and Throat Monthly 55: 83 (1976).

Ohman, L. and Wahlberg, I.: Ocular side-effects of clofazimine. Lancet 2: 933 (1975).

Pape, L.G. and Forbes, M.: Retinal detachment and miotic therapy. American Journal of Ophthalmology 85: 558 (1978).

Pavan-Langston, D.: Use of vidarabine in ophthalmology: A review. Annals of Ophthalmology 9: 835 (1977).

Pavan-Langston, D.; Campbell, R. and Lass, J.: Acyclic antimetabolite treatment of experimental herpes simplex keratitis. American Journal of Ophthalmology 86: 618 (1978).

Pirofsky, B.: Immunosuppressive therapy of severe chronic uveitis. Transactions of the Pacific Coast Oto-ophthalmological Society 57: 291 (1976).

Podos, S.M.; Becker, B.; Asseff, C. and Hartstein, J.: Pilocarpine therapy with soft contact lenses. American Journal of Ophthalmology 73: 336 (1972).

Pollack, I.P.: Mechanisms of glaucoma. Sight Saving Review 45: 157 (Winter, 1973).

Pollack, I.P.; Quigley, H.A. and Harbin, T.S.: The ocusert pilocarpine system: Advantages and disadvantages. Southern Medical Journal 69: 1296 (1976).

Prien, R.F.; DeLong, S.; Cole, J.O. and Levine, J.: Ocular change occurring with prolonged high dose chlorpromazine therapy. Archives of General Psychiatry 23: 464 (1970).

Purnell, W.D. and McPherson, S.D. Jr.: The effect of tobramycin on rabbit eyes. American Journal of Ophthalmology 77: 578 (1974).

Rahi, A.H.S.; Chapman, C.M.; Garner, A. and Wright, P.: Pathology of practolol-induced ocular toxicity. British Journal of Ophthalmology 60: 312 (1976).

Robin, J.S. and Ellis, P.P.: Ophthalmic ointments. Survey of Ophthalmology 22: 335 (1978).

Sabiston, D.W.: The use of antibiotics in ophthalmology. Drugs 14: 207 (1977).

Selby, G.: Subacute myelo-optico-neuropathy (SMON) — neurotoxicity of clioquinol. Proceedings of the Australian Association of Neurologists 9: 23 (1973).

Shah, P.M.: Toxic effects of atropine eye drops. Indian Journal of Pediatrics 33: 13 (1966).

Shields, J.A.: Current approaches to the diagnosis and management of choroidal melanomas. Survey of Ophthalmology 21: 443 (1977).

Smith, S.E. and Rawlins, M.D.: Mydriatic drugs; in Variability in Human Drug Response, p.124 (Butterworth, London 1973).

Stone, R.D.; Irvine, A.R. and O'Connor, G.R.: Candida endophthalmitis: Report of an unusual case with isolation of the etiologic agent by vitreous biopsy. Annals of Ophthalmology 7: 757 (1975).

Thatcher, R.W. and Pettit, T.H.: Gonorrhoeal conjunctivitis. Journal of the American Medical Association 215: 1494 (1971).

Thomas, J.V.; Gragoudas, E.S.; Blair, N.P. and Lapus, J.V.: Correlation of epinephrine use and macular edema. Archives of Ophthalmology 96: 625 (1978).

Wheeler, R.H.; Bhalerao, V.R. and Gilkes, M.J.: Ocular pigmentation, extrapyramidal symptoms and phenothiazine dosage. British Journal of Psychiatry 115: 687 (1969).

Willetts, G.S.: Ocular side-effects of drugs. British Journal of Ophthalmology 53: 252 (1969).

Williamson, J.; Paterson, R.W.W.; McGavin, D.D.M.; Jasani, M.K.; Boyl, J.A. and Doig, W.M.: Posterior subcapsular cataracts and glaucoma associated with long-term oral corticosteroid therapy. British Journal of Ophthalmology 53: 361 (1969).

Yablonski, M.E. and Burde, R.M.: Cataracts induced by topical dexamethasone in diabetes. Archives of Ophthalmology 96: 474 (1978).

Chapter XIII
Diseases of the Oral Cavity

E. Zegarelli

Synopsis of Important Principles

1) Diseases of the oral cavity result from infection, local irritation or trauma, or they may be an oral manifestation of various systemic diseases.

2) As much of the treatment of disorders of the oral cavity is largely ameliorative, or directed at removal or elimination of causative factors or an underlying systemic disease, accurate diagnosis is an important prerequisite to effective therapy.

3) Most tissues and structures of the oral cavity are available for direct or topical administration of medications, and the majority of diseases of the oral cavity can be controlled satisfactorily by local therapeutic measures. Occasionally, a severe or resistant oral disease may require systemic therapy or the use of combined local and systemic drugs.

4) Consultation between medical and dental practitioners may be necessary, particularly when the patient's medical or dental treatment has to be modified because of systemic disease or concomitant drug therapy.

5) Drugs may induce oral ulceration, thus careful enquiry about concomitant or recent medication is important. The appearance of a sore mouth or stomatitis with gold or phenylbutazone is an indication of bone marrow depression and the drug must be stopped immediately.

6) Some drug induced diseases of the oral cavity are acceptable (e.g. phenytoin gingival hyperplasia) while others are not (e.g. tetracycline induced tooth staining and enamel hypoplasia).

There are at least 400, and quite possibly as many as 600 different diseases which may affect the tissues and structures of the mouth, teeth and jaws. This wide variety of disorders ranges from those resulting from local irritation or trauma, or allergic reactions; to infections (local and systemic) and inflammatory gingival diseases; to oral manifestations of systemic diseases such as malnutritional states, metabolic disease, bone disease, tumours including neoplasms and cysts, blood diseases, and numerous others.

1. Clinical Pharmacological Considerations

Many of these conditions are related to systemic disease, and the clinical pharmacological considerations and general principles of therapy which are used in the treatment of those illnesses are applicable in the treatment of associated disorders of the oral cavity (see chapter XVI; sect. 1.2).

A large number of diseases are however, more or less 'local' in nature, or at least 'localised' to the mouth in a geographic sense. As most of the tissues and structures of the oral cavity are readily available for direct or topical administration of medications, much greater utilisation of topical therapy is possible in oral medicine than perhaps any other area of therapeutics, with the possible exception of skin diseases. Furthermore, just as the mucosa of the nose, vagina or rectum is employed for the administration and absorption of drugs, so too is the mucosa of the mouth. Indeed, the sublingual and buccal route of administration have been found quite useful, not only for obtaining a 'local therapeutic response', but also for obtaining systemic action. Numerous drugs are therefore easily and effectively administered and absorbed via the oral mucosal route. These include antimicrobial agents, corticosteroids, sedatives, analgesics and others.

The topical application of drugs to the oral mucosa for local therapeutic purposes should be encouraged, provided that the drug employed is not a frequent sensitising agent. Although locally active agents are applied in a variety of vehicles, such as mouthwashes, suspensions, ointments and adhesive formulations, long lasting lozenges or pellets have proven remarkably effective and should become an increasingly popular and effective method of drug delivery to the oral mucosa (Kutscher et al., 1968, 1969).

2. General Principles of Treatment

Drug treatment in oral diseases is largely based on the following general principles (see Kutscher et al., 1964; Zegarelli et al., 1978):

1) In a number of clinical conditions of the oral cavity treatment is only ameliorative and not directed at the condition itself.

2) Diseases of the oral cavity may be a result of local factors or a manifestation of an underlying systemic disease, and management depends on accurate diagnosis and appropriate treatment or removal of the causative condition or factor(s).

3) Many oral diseases are relatively innocuous and can best be managed by removal and protection against local irritants, and improvement in nutrition and oral hygiene.

4) Local therapy is the most logical and practical approach to treatment of many diseases of the oral cavity. The various forms used include local protectants, local anaesthetics, medicated mouthwashes, lozenges or pellets, local drainage, and specific topical remedies for a particular symptom.

3. Oral Ulceration

A number of patients suffer from frequent or continuous oral ulceration which causes severe pain with associated difficulties in speaking and eating and sometimes loss of weight. In many cases oral ulcerations are accepted by doctor and patient as trivial. In general, they do not carry the threat of serious complications as do other ulcerations of the gastrointestinal tract, but some patients suffer much misery. There is no curative treatment, but ameliorative therapy can be provided following accurate differential diagnosis of the many types of oral ulcerations. In some cases, systemic diseases predispose to or cause oral ulcerations, and these should always be investigated and treated if recurrences are to be avoided (see Macalister, 1973; Zegarelli, 1970; Zegarelli et al., 1978).

3.1 Traumatic Ulcers

The traumatic ulcer of the mouth is undoubtedly the most frequently encountered ulcerative lesion of the many different diseases which may cause ulcerations in the oral cavity. It accounts for more than 50 % of all oral ulcerations. It may be single or multiple, small or large sized, flat or deep, and regular or irregular in shape. It may occur anywhere in the mouth, but usually in areas which are most predisposed to injury such as the lateral tongue, buccal mucosa (plane of occlusion), lips and vault of palate.

All traumatic ulcers result from the application of an externally applied injurious and destructive force or action, which acts directly on the surface of the oral mucosa. This may be due to physical, thermal or chemical and, much less commonly, electrical or irradiation insults. Thus, a careful mouth examination and thorough history aimed at identifying the causative factor, is essential.

3.1.1 Physically Induced Ulcers

In most cases of mild or even moderate sized ulcers, elimination of the cause (e.g. cheek biting, ill fitting dentures, etc) is followed by prompt healing (within 3 to 5 days) and this may be the only treatment necessary.

Where the lesions are more extensive and the symptoms quite severe, topically applied antibacterial formulations such as those containing bacitracin, benzalkonium chloride, or 2% gentian violet are recommended. Systemically administered antibacterial drugs are only advised for the control of traumatic ulcers which are affected with severe degrees of secondary bacterial infection. Topically applied corticosteroid preparations in an ointment or Orabase vehicle (triamcinolone acetonide 0.1% or prednisolone) may be useful in suppressing or shortening the healing time of mild ulcerations without a significant infectious component.

Where alleviation of the attendant pain is the prime concern, topically applied protectants such as denture adhesive powders or pastes, or tincture of benzoin compound (applied and dried) may be quite effective. Topically applied local anaesthetics (lignocaine/lidocaine viscous or benzocaine ointment) may be necessary to control unusually painful ulcerations.

3.1.2 Chemically Induced Ulcers

Chemically induced oral ulcerations are managed in essentially the same manner as those induced by physical trauma, with the exception that appropriate antidotes are immediately administered where the specific cause (an acid or alkali) has been established. In emergency situations, immediate and copious washing of the mouth with plain water or mild saline solution

may be effective as an initial approach. Where the aetiological agent is identified as an acid, neutralisation with dilute solution of sodium bicarbonate is indicated. Where an alkali has been identified as the causative factor, dilute lemon juice, vinegar or dilute solutions of other mild organic acids are recommended for use as a mouthwash.

Topical protectants such as emollient mixtures (Orabase), compound benzoin tincture or denture adhesives are often beneficial in alleviating attendant pain.

Aspirin may also induce a chemical burn lesion if allowed to remain in contact with the oral mucosa (Claman, 1967). Mild and asymptomatic lesions generally require no therapy. Healing proceeds uneventfully and is usually complete in 5 to 10 days. When tissue necrosis is severe, or when sloughing results in ulceration with accompanying pain, topical applications of antiseptic or antibacterial preparations may be used to combat or prevent infection. Coating the lesions with protective emollient mixture (Orabase) or with a denture adhesive will provide considerable comfort during the healing stages. Topically applied local anaesthetics may be employed if pain is intense.

Other drugs which have been implicated in oral ulceration type lesions, either directly or as an associated reaction to a systemic disease, are discussed in section 13.1.

3.2 Recurrent Aphthous (Ulcerative) Stomatitis (recurrent canker sores)

Recurrent aphthous stomatitis is another very common ulcerative disease, perhaps second in frequency only to the traumatic ulcers.

In most cases, the sole clinical manifestations are restricted entirely to the oral cavity — multiple (generally 3 to 10 in number), small sized (one to several millimetres in diameter), flat, round or oval shaped, discrete bordered ulcerations in scattered regions of the oral mucosa. There are no accompanying skin (see section 4), eye or genital lesions, and fever, malaise and regional lymphadenitis is absent. This presentation is true in the vast majority of cases, but there are occasional exceptions when numerous, large sized and deeply situated ulcers, accompanied by extreme pain, distress and occasionally lymphadenitis, are encountered (see section 3.3). Extraoral sites may also be involved. Thus, the patient should always be questioned as to whether or not ocular or genital conditions are present, since oral ulcers of the mucocutaneous neuro-ocular syndrome (e.g. Behcet's syndrome) are nonspecific.

Although the specific aetiology in most cases is difficult or impossible to establish with the present investigatory methods available, numerous theories have been offered. Occasional cases are indeed of herpetic aetiology and where the relationship is positive, the disease should be called recurrent herpetic ulcerative stomatitis. Others, similarly, are found to be allergic (fruits, chocolates, nuts, shellfish and others), while still others appear to be of hormonal origin, associated with deficiency or excess of sex hormone(s). Some cases are thought to be related to states of malnutrition or gastrointestinal diseases, or due to emotional factors.

With the exception of those comparatively few cases where the aetiology can be clearly established (allergy, malnutrition, gastrointestinal disease) and where treatment of these is successful, no therapeutic regimen has yet been developed which has proven to be consistently successful in curing and preventing recurrences of a significant number of cases of recurrent aphthous ulceration. And yet, numerous agents and approaches have been advocated and used, but not found to be completely effective when studied under the rigorous conditions of a controlled clinical trial. These remedies range from topically applied caustic agents (phenol, silver nitrate, trichloracetic acid), through topical protectants (Orabase, denture adhesives, tincture benzoin compound), to topically applied antibacterial solutions, ointments and lozenges, and administration of corticosteroids, or immunostimulants such as levamisole (Lehner, 1968; Lehner et al., 1976). In many cases 'successful' treatment has resulted from trying a host of medications empirically. Cauterisation of ulcers with a caustic such as phenol or silver nitrate is to be avoided, since while these agents will ameliorate a small ulcer, they will also cause a much wider area of necrosis and subsequent retardation of healing.

Most clinicians obtain best results from a regimen of a tetracycline mouthwash plus topical application of a corticosteroid-containing ointment or long acting pellet or lozenge. This treatment approach is not curative, but is highly successful in shortening the duration of episodes, in providing palliation of symptoms and in a considerable number of cases can reduce the number of episodes or even abort anticipated episodes (Graykowski and Barile, 1966).

A tetracycline suspension is used as a mouthwash, 125mg/5ml 4 times daily, rinsed for at least 1 to 2 minutes on each occasion, and continued for at least 2 days. There is little or no absorption and the rationale is directed at reduction of any secondary bacterial infection and hence relief of pain.

Of the many corticosteroid pellets and lozenges tried, those such as hydrocortisone succinate or betamethasone valerate have proved the most helpful (Lehner and Lyne, 1969, 1970). These pellets may be useful when the lesion is in the floor of the mouth or in the cheek sulcus — areas which lend themselves to having a pellet placed in contact for several hours. Pellets are of less value when the lesion is on a more mobile part of the mouth (tongue or cheek). In such cases 0.1% triamcinolone acetonide in an emollient ointment base or an adhesive paste (Orabase) is of some value. In either case, topical steroids are probably most helpful if they are applied during the prodromal phase of the ulceration. This means application when the first symptoms develop a day or two before the epithelium breaks down.

On occasion, where the episodes are of unusually high degree of severity, short courses of systemically administered corticosteroids are effective in reducing the healing time of the ulcers (see Graykowski and Holroyd, 1970; Zegarelli and Kutscher, 1970; Editorial, 1974).

3.3 Recurrent Ulcerative Scarifying Stomatitis (periadenitis mucosa necrotica recurrens, Sutton's disease)

This disease must be distinguished from recurrent aphthous stomatitis since treatment involves use of systemic rather than topical corticosteroids. The mouth lesions can be quite similar in appearance and behaviour. Recurrent scarifying stomatitis is however, generally identified easily by the presence of deeper ulcerations with greater degrees of tissue necrosis and oral mucosal scars at sites of previous ulcerations. Also, the lesions of recurrent scarifying stomatitis are often accompanied by regional lymphadenopathy and sometimes a low grade fever. The clinical presentation more closely resembles that of erythema multiforme (section 4.3).

Treatment is essentially the same as for recurrent aphthous ulceration, except that systemic corticosteroids are generally necessary to control the disease. Topical therapy is more often only adjunctive. Prednisone 30 to 60mg orally daily (or equivalent) can be used initially, with a gradual reduction to 5 or 10mg daily as soon as possible.

Antibacterial agents, such as phenoxymethyl-penicillin 1 to 2g daily, are often very effective in reducing the healing time when given in conjunction with orally administered corticosteroids.

3.4 Acute Ulcerative Necrotising Gingivitis (Vincent's infection, trench mouth etc)

The usual presenting complaint of the patient with Vincent's infection is 'painful gums, bleeding gums, bad taste or foul mouth odour'. The clinical features are striking. The condition occurs in a young adult, who is ambulatory and appears fairly well but has no fever. Gingivitis is invariably present, but most important from a diagnostic standpoint, is the presence of one or more blunted interproximal papilla, partially or totally covered with a greyish, loosely adherent, necrotic slough. Removal of the slough reveals the presence of a painful ulceration at the base of the papilla.

Occasionally, the infection is unusually severe and widespread, sometimes even affecting the buccal mucosa, retromolar regions and soft palate with large sized, irregular shaped greyish sloughs. In these cases especially, signs of systemic illness such as fever, pallor, fatigue and regional lymphadenitis, are apparent.

Immediate treatment is limited to local debridement. Supportive therapy is important and includes the recommendation of as much rest as possible, a bland and soft diet and a multivitamin preparation in therapeutic dosage. Home care should also include improved oral hygiene measures and mechanical lavages with warm saline, mild hydrogen peroxide or mild alkaline solutions.

Antimicrobial agents are rarely indicated, except when the condition is severe and widespread and accompanied by fever. In such instances, systemic antimicrobial agents may be prescribed. The causative organisms have been named as *Treponema (Borrelia) vincenti* (a spirochaete) and *Fusiformis fusiformis* (a Gram-negative bacillus). The acute phase of the infection may be reduced by a course of standard doses of phenoxymethyl-penicillin for 1 week, or by the use of metronidazole (200mg tablets tds for 1 week). Considerable improvement, both orally and systemically, should occur within 48 hours. If improvement is not noted within this time, investigation for blood dyscrasias and other systemic diseases should be initiated.

It is most important to realise that the initial resolution is not permanent, and until all primary foci (gum flaps, irregular gaps between teeth or overhanging fillings etc) have been eliminated, the disease is liable to flare up again with fluctuations in general and local resistance. Thus following initial treatment, the patient should be sent to his dental practitioner for more thorough periodontal therapy, including removal of local contributory factors.

Recommendations for overcoming systemic predisposing factors are also advisable if recurrences are to be avoided (see Graykowski and Holroyd, 1970).

3.5 Acute Herpetic Gingivo-Stomatitis (primary herpes, acute herpes)

Acute herpetic gingivo-stomatitis, caused by the herpes simplex virus, is a common childhood disease (85% of cases occur between 18 months and 11 years) with the most severe and clinically distinguishable lesions located in the mouth.

In the more acute and severe cases the patient shows signs of a generalised infection (pallor, fatigue and fever), has difficulty eating or talking, has tender bilateral submandibular lymphadenopathy and occasionally herpetic lesions on the lips. More important diagnostically, are the mouth lesions. These include multiple, small sized 'herpetic' ulcerations of the oral mucosa, an acute and severe gingivitis which is often accompanied by pharyngitis. The disease, fortunately, is self limiting, generally disappearing in from 7 to 14 days, but occasionally lasting longer.

At present, there is no topical chemotherapeutic agent which is consistently able to halt, alter or abort the course of acute herpes (see chapter XXVIII; sect. 4) and since the oral infection is self limiting treatment is symptomatic, palliative and supportive. Bed rest, maintenance of adequate fluid intake (particularly in young children) and a soft diet supplemented by proteins are recommended. Where the disease is unusually severe and accompanied by debility or prostration, hospital supportive care may be necessary.

Systemic therapy for symptoms may include, when indicated, an antipyretic such as paracetamol (acetaminophen) for fever; an antihistamine such as diphenhydramine or promethazine for sedation; and an appropriate systemic antibacterial agent for any secondary bacterial infection.

Local therapy to ameliorate symptoms may include dilute solutions of hydrogen peroxide, mild alkaline or saline mouthwashes; painting of lesions with 2% gentian violet, topical applications of antibacterial formulations containing bacitracin, neomycin, or both; and topical protectants, such as emollient mixtures (Orabase), compound benzoin tincture, or denture adhesives. Because of the very widespread nature of the ulceration, which makes application of antibiotic ointments and topical protectants difficult, some clinicians prefer to use tetracycline mouthwashes and have obtained good results (Cooke, 1960; see also section 3.2).

For the management of lip lesions, a water soluble emollient containing adequate quantities of bacitracin, neomycin, or both or idoxuridine ointment (see chapter XXVIII; sect. 4.3.1), may be beneficial (see further Graykowski and Holroyd, 1970).

3.6 Herpangina (summer grippe, three day fever, Coxsackie pharyngitis)

Herpangina is an acute, contagious, pyretic, seasonal, self limiting disease caused by group A or B Coxsackie virus. It is a childhood disease with clinical manifestations often simulating acute herpes (see section 3.5) but generally much shorter in duration, lasting from 2 to 6 days. In addition, the oral ulcerations are usually restricted to the posterior regions of the mouth and the gingivitis is mild rather than severe. However, in contradistinction to acute herpes, patients with herpangina often complain of anorexia, dysphagia, and sore throat. Headache, colic, diarrhoea and convulsions are less frequently encountered.

Since herpangina is a self limited disease, in most cases expending itself in less than a week, treatment is generally symptomatic and supportive (see acute herpes in section 3.5).

3.7 Benign Mucosal Pemphigoid

The oral mucosa is frequently affected in cases of chronic benign mucosal pemphigoid, formerly termed 'ocular pemphigus'. It is generally agreed that in a few cases, the oral tissues are the only ones involved throughout the course of the disease.

The oral lesions begin as vesicles, rapidly burst and form shallow ulcerations, their appearances often simulating pemphigus. However, histological examination of pemphigoid lesions reveal subepithelial bullae and absence of acantholysis. The gingiva are frequently affected, presenting an appearance similar to that of desquamative gingivitis.

There is no specific or curative treatment for pemphigoid. It is generally a persistent disease, but is usually reasonably satisfactorily controlled by systemic corticosteroids. An effective regimen is 30 to 50mg prednisone (or its equivalent) orally per day with gradual reductions to maintenance doses of 5 to 15mg daily.

Local treatment of the mouth lesions includes:

1) Topical corticosteroid ointment formulations, applied several times daily as adjunctive therapy;
2) Tetracycline suspension as a mouth rinse (5ml/125mg) 4 times daily for several days to reduce any secondary bacterial infection (see section 3.2);
3) Careful but thorough gingival therapy (curettage, mild water irrigations and improved oral hygiene at home) where the gingival tissues are involved.

Improvement of the patient's nutrition and supplemental multivitamins in therapeutic dosage are generally indicated and usually exert a beneficial effect.

4. Diseases Involving the Mouth and Skin

Severe inflammatory skin conditions such as lichen planus, pemphigus and erythema multiforme, can often involve the oral cavity as well. Sometimes, only oral lesions are present (Zegarelli et al., 1978).

4.1 Lichen Planus

Lichen planus is a relatively common chronic mucocutaneous disease which often affects the oral mucosa, with or without skin lesions (see chapter XIV; section 11). Although its aetiology has not been definitely established, numerous factors have been implicated. These include microbial pathogens, malnutrition, allergy, drug toxicity, chronic irritations and in particular, emotional disturbances. Unfortunately, lichen planus of the oral mucosa may present in any one or combination of several different clinical patterns, the nature of which influences treatment:

1) Reticular pattern — composed of narrow, slightly elevated, greyish lines or striae which form mesh or network arrangements. Undoubtedly the most common and easiest to recognise.
2) Annular pattern — circular rings of keratin.
3) Papular pattern — small pinhead sized, hemispherical, glistening white spots.
4) Plaque pattern — greyish coloured, raised, discrete patches; frequently resembling and misdiagnosed as hyperkeratosis or leucoplakia.
5) Bullous form — and its consequent, erosive or ulcerative lesions, generally in the midst of or surrounded by keratotic striae, is the most painful and troublesome.

Where the oral lesions are minimal and asymptomatic (reticular, papular and annular patterns), reassurance of the patient is the best and soundest approach, but the condition should be kept under observation. Obviously, local irritations, which may tend to intensify the mucosal lesions, should be removed or avoided.

Treatment of widespread, erosive or ulcerative lesions is ameliorative or suppressant, and not curative. The more successful approaches include administration of therapeutic doses of vitamin B complex (3 capsules per day) with additional nicotinamide (200mg daily), which may be beneficial in some instances of widespread lesions, and topical corticosteroids (ointment or pellets 4 or more times daily) to reduce the duration time of erosions or ulcerations. Local anaesthetics in lozenge or ointment form can be used as temporary palliative measures where the lesions are severely painful. Systemic (e.g. prednisone 30 to 60mg orally daily initially) or intralesional steroids (e.g. triamcinolone acetonide) are used when erosive or ulcerative lesions prove resistant to local therapy. Antianxiety agents such as diazepam, either alone or in combination with the above treatments, can be used in those patients where emotional factors definitely appear to have a precipitating role.

Surgical excision, electrocoagulation and radiation are indicated in those rare cases of ulcerative lichen planus, where histological findings suggest the presence of dyskeratosis or malignant neoplasia.

4.2 Pemphigus

Although pemphigus is a severe skin disease (see chapter XIV; sect. 12.1), well over half the patients have oral mucosal lesions. In some, the mouth and skin lesions appear simultaneously. In others, the mouth lesions just precede or just follow the onset of the skin lesions, but, in a significantly large number of cases the mouth lesions precede those of the skin by weeks or months and, in a few cases, skin lesions may not appear for as long as 3 or more years after the onset of the oral lesions.

Systemic corticosteroids are the most effective method of controlling the oral lesions of pemphigus (generally as much as 100mg of prednisone, or its equivalent, each day followed by reductions of 5mg in the daily dosage every 2 to 3 weeks). However, the more resistant oral lesions may respond more rapidly when topical corticosteroids (ointments, pellets or lozenges) are applied as adjunctive therapy. Topical corticosteroids alone are generally ineffective. A tetracycline mouth rinse (see section 3.2) is used to control any secondary bacterial infection. Occasionally, topical anaesthetics may be required for the control of severe pain or tenderness.

As in other severe skin diseases, nutrition of the patient becomes an important treatment problem and hence, general supportive measures are essential.

4.3 Erythema Multiforme

As with pemphigus, erythema multiforme is considered a severe inflammatory dermatological disease and exhibits a variety of skin, eye and genital lesions. Not infrequently, oral lesions accompany those on the skin, and not uncommonly, the mouth may be the only site of involvement. Oral lesions are basically the same as the skin lesions — they too, may begin as macules, papules, vesicles or bullae — but owing to the peculiar environment of the mouth (its moisture, heat, irritations and organisms) they invariably break down, usually leading to the formation of large sized, flat, irregularly shaped erosions and ulcerations.

Treatment is generally directed toward aborting the current painful episode, providing general supportive measures where necessary, and preventing recurrences whenever possible by eliminating or treating the causative factors (allergic, toxic, debilitating systemic diseases, etc).

Systemic therapy is often necessary and usually consists of moderately high doses of systemic corticosteroids (e.g. 30 to 60mg prednisone orally per day, decreasing the dosage over several weeks). Where secondary bacterial infection is considerable, as it is in most cases, an appropriate systemic antibacterial agent should be prescribed.

Local treatment may include any of the following, depending on the severity and extent of the mouth lesions: (1) a tetracycline mouth rinse (see section 3.2) several times per day; (2) anaesthetic lozenges, ointment or solutions where pain is severe; or (3) topical corticosteroid ointments or lozenges.

General supportive measures include a highly nutritious liquid or semisolid diet, and therapeutic dosages of vitamin B complex and vitamin C.

Where the disease is acute, generalised, severe and accompanied by fever, hospitalisation is often necessary in order to adequately control the problems of hydration, nutrition and secondary bacterial infection. In less severe cases bed rest at home is appropriate (see also chapter XIV; sect. 12.4).

5. Allergic Reactions in the Mouth

A variety of soft tissue reactions associated with allergic phenomena may occur in the oral cavity. The more common are inflammatory (stomatitis, glossitis or even merely gingivitis), oedematous (angioneurotic oedema of lips, tongue or elsewhere in mouth) and vesiculo-bullous-ulcerative lesions.

5.1 Allergic Stomatitis

Allergic stomatitis is usually the result of contact hypersensitivity. Identification and prompt removal of the allergen (dental material, toothpaste, mouthwash, cosmetic agent, medicated lozenge) may be the only measure necessary.

Occasionally, palliation or suppression of the lesion is facilitated by topical application of corticosteroid ointments. Topical anaesthetics (lignocaine/lidocaine viscous) in the form of a mouthwash are often effective. Systemic antihistamines may also be indicated, especially with the more persistent lesions.

5.2 Oedematous Reactions

The location and severity of the oedematous reaction invariably determines the selection of antiallergic therapy. Oedema of the lips, eyelids or even the face may require nothing more than identification and elimination of the allergen.

Oedema of the tongue, pharyngeal tissues, and especially oedema of the glottis, on the other hand, demand immediate emergency therapy if death through respiratory difficulty is to be avoided. Administration of oxygen is necessary and may be lifesaving. Intramuscular administration of 0.5 to 1ml of 1:1,000 adrenaline (epinephrine) usually provides rapid relief in such instances. Intravenously administered antihistamines (e.g. 50mg promethazine) may also be employed. Severe oedema requires parenteral administration of corticosteroids (e.g. 100mg hydrocortisone succinate) as an adjunct to the other emergency procedures.

If the oedematous reaction is moderate and not life threatening, systemic administration of antihistamines is indicated. Corticosteroids may be given orally to combat moderate to severe allergic oedema which is not life threatening.

5.3 Vesiculo-Bullous-Ulcerative Stomatitis

Although allergic ulcers of the mouth are often accompanied by severe discomfort, they generally are not emergency situations. Elimination of the allergen and palliative therapy are indicated. Systemic corticosteroids or antihistamines are indicated if the condition is severe. When the mouth pain is unusually severe, the lesions may be coated with topical anaesthetic ointments.

6. Oral Candidiasis (thrush, moniliasis)

Candidiasis is undoubtedly the most common fungal infection of the mouth. *Candida albicans* is considered a normal inhabitant of the oral cavity, but under certain conditions a state of overgrowth is induced with consequent oral infection, sometimes accompanied by gastrointestinal and vaginal infection. Overgrowth is most likely in the very young, in the aged or in states of malnutrition and/or general debilitation, particularly when several factors capable of promoting candidiasis are present (Lehner, 1964). Other precipitating factors include inhaled (Willey et al., 1976) or prolonged systemic use of corticosteroids, immunosuppressive therapy and poor oral hygiene (e.g. 'denture sore mouth'). A reduction in salivary flow, as a result of drug therapy (e.g. tricyclic antidepressants, phenothiazine antipsychotics) or as a sequel of radiotherapy, will also increase the likelihood of oral candidiasis (Bahn, 1972). Prolonged use of broad spectrum antibiotics may produce drug induced stomatitis in which *Candida* infection is usually implicated (see also chapter XIV; sect. 2.3.1).

The oral lesions of candidiasis respond readily to topical application of antifungal suspensions or lozenges. When using a suspension (e.g. nystatin, amphotericin B), about 3ml or more is swished around the mouth for 1 to 2 minutes and then either expectorated or swallowed. This should be repeated after each meal and prior to bedtime, although more numerous rinses may be desirable in the particularly severe or resistant case. Alternatively, 3 or 4 amphotericin B lozenges can be sucked each day, or amphotericin B incorporated in an adhesive vehicle such as Orabase (de Vries-Hospers and vander Waaij, 1978). At least 10 to 14 days of therapy is advisable to avoid relapse. Amphotericin B is much more palatable than nystatin. Lozenges of miconazole or clotrimazole are also effective (Kirkpatrick and Alling, 1978), as is a gel of miconazole. Nystatin or natamycin drops placed on the lesion are convenient for infants and young children. Otherwise, a topical cream or suspension may be tried.

When indicated (e.g. angular cheilitis), improvement of the patient's general nutrition contributes greatly to the overall management. Therapeutic doses of vitamin B complex are often effective as adjunctive therapy.

Chronic forms of candidiasis involving the mouth and sometimes also the skin are difficult to treat, but fortunately not common. Individuals with diabetes mellitus, some other endocrine disorders, immunodeficiency or genetic predisposition are susceptible (Wells et al., 1972). Treatment involves use of topical, and in diffuse forms, systemic, anticandidal agents. Latent iron deficiency must be looked for and treated. Administration of vitamin A and B complex may also be helpful.

7. Oral Herpes Labialis

No medication has consistently proved to be curative for the lip lesions of secondary or recurrent herpes simplex infections (Graykowski and Holroyd, 1970). The efficacy of idoxuridine remains controversial and, for the time being at least, it is not recommended for herpetic labialis, despite its apparent success in ophthalmic and cutaneous herpes simplex infections (see chapters XII, sect. 3.6, XIV, sect. 2.2.2). Smallpox vaccination has not proved successful and therefore, is also not recommended. Applications of caustic and escharotic agents such as phenol and silver nitrate are contraindicated.

Where lesions of herpetic labialis are known to be associated with or result from exposure to the sunlight or chronic irritation, avoidance of such irritants or protecting the lips with sun screening agents are advisable. Symptomatic treatment may include applications of bland emollient creams or ointments and protectants such as tincture of benzoin compound. Where secondary bacterial infection is apparent, applications of antibacterial creams or ointments (bacitracin, neomycin) is appropriate and effective.

8. Diseases of the Tongue

8.1 Hairy Tongue

Hairy tongue refers to the hypertrophy and elongation of the filiform papilla on the dorsum of the tongue, generally the region immediately anterior to the circumvallate papilla.

Successful treatment is usually dependent on the clinician's ability to identify and remove the causative factor(s). Thus, all agents which tend to stimulate hypertrophy of filiform papillae, such as irritating dentifrices, lozenges, mouthwashes and especially those containing oxygen liberating drugs, antibiotics and excessive smoking, should be eliminated or at least curtailed. Improved hygiene for the tongue, to remove food and other debris trapped by the elongated taste buds, should also be emphasised. Brushing the tongue with a toothbrush and rubbing it vigorously with a moistened washcloth wrapped around the index finger may be beneficial. Detergent foods such as apples and fresh vegetables may also be helpful.

Patients with severe and resistant hairy tongue should be referred to a dental practitioner. Very careful topical application of minute quantities of escharotic or caustic agents (phenol or trichloracetic acid) may be tried. Repeat treatment sessions at weekly intervals and spread over weeks and months may be necessary before complete disappearance of the condition is obtained.

8.2 Glossodynia (burning tongue)

Glossodynia refers to instances of burning tongue when all organic causes (anaemia, diabetes mellitus, allergy, malnutrition, etc.) have been eliminated and where a psychogenic factor has been established or strongly suspected. The condition is more often observed in postmenopausal women and is frequently a manifestation of depression precipitated by a sense of loss.

Although clinically detectable lesions associated with the burning are absent, a clear explanation of the condition and its cause should be given to the patient. This in itself may provide a measure of relief since a considerable number of patients are disturbed by a fear of cancer. Patience and repeated reassurance is therefore required in the management of such patients. The placebo effect of vitamin B complex, or antianxiety agents such as diazepam, may be tried if explanation and reassurance proves ineffective. If the condition persists or is severe, referral to a psychiatrist is indicated.

8.3 Geographic Tongue (wandering rash, benign migratory glossitis)

In most cases, geographic tongue is asymptomatic, of unknown aetiology and usually considered an anomaly of no pathological significance. Therefore, aside from reassuring the patient, treatment is unnecessary. In occasional instances, the areas of redness (atrophy of epithelium) or denudation of the epithelium are accompanied by burning, pain, tenderness or hypersensitivity during ingestion of fruit juices, spices, alcohol, etc. In such cases, applications of a protectant, non-medicated material may be palliative, such as sprinkling of a denture adhesive powder over the areas of redness. Therapeutic doses of vitamin B complex or improvement of nutrition may also be beneficial in some patients (e.g. in pregnancy). Palliative therapy leading to suppression of symptoms may be obtained through topical application of corticosteroid ointments or lozenges.

8.4 Fissured Tongue

The fissured tongue is a congenital or developmental condition of little or no pathological significance. It generally requires no treatment, except explanation and reassurance of its benign nature if there is concern or a fear of cancer. Improved hygiene of the tongue, and particularly cleansing of the fissures with mildly antiseptic mouthwashes, is occasionally needed when there is tenderness or pain due to trapping of food and bacteria in the deeper fissures.

9. Odontogenic Infections

Infectious processes in the mouth and jaws of odontogenic origin require accurate diagnosis and precise therapy for successful management. The stage and severity of the infection, the responsible organism and the extensions of the disease process should dictate the appropriate approach.

9.1 Cellulitis

Cellulitis is a diffuse inflammation of soft tissues which tends to spread through the tissue spaces. It generally occurs as a spreading infection resulting from a periapical abscess, osteomyelitis or periodontal disease. Streptococci are usually the chief offenders, although staphylococci may also give rise to cellulitis. Parenteral penicillin followed by oral maintenance doses is usually the best initial choice for common infections. Erythromycin can be used in patients with a history of penicillin allergy. Adequate doses should be maintained for at least 72 hours after acute symptoms have subsided. An antipyretic analgesic such as aspirin can be given if necessary. Hot saline oral lavage may aid in localising the process. Dental procedures such as opening into the pulp chamber, incision of a soft tissue abscess or tooth extraction, are indicated where drainage is required.

9.2 Lateral, Pericemental or Periodontal Abscess

This sequel of chronic periodontitis is more apt to be of limited involvement and amenable to local management, but where there are systemic signs of infection, such as fever and malaise, systemic antibacterial agents, analgesics and antiseptics as described above are indicated.

9.3 Pericoronal Abscess

Infections around partially erupted third molars are hazardous for several reasons, but particularly because they tend to spread readily into musculofascial planes and spaces. Simple drainage procedures, irrigation beneath flaps with antiseptic solutions and hot saline lavages are recommended for localisation of the process. Trauma to the site should be avoided. Antibacterial agents are indicated if symptoms of fever and malaise are present.

9.4 Severe Acute Infections

The potentially life threatening infection in the fascial spaces of the face and neck, as in Ludwig's angina, demands total hospital supportive care. Procedures should be available to assure a patent airway. The responsible organism(s) should be identified to determine the most appropriate antibacterial agent.

9.5 Chronic Soft Tissue Abscess, Chronic Osteomyelitis

The chronic persistent or resistant infection, such as a soft tissue abscess and osteomyelitis, also calls for intensive investigations aimed at identifying the causative organisms. The efficacy of blood borne antimicrobial agents may however, be inhibited by chronic infectious processes with their zones of necrosis and foreign material.

10. Teething

Teething is usually uneventful. At times, however, there may be tenderness at the site of eruption, oedema or inflammation causing a slight bulging of the overlapping gingival tissues, and fretfulness.

When the child's regular sleeping pattern is disturbed by symptomatic teething, simple palliative measures may be undertaken. The mucous membranes overlying the erupting tooth may be rubbed gently with a topical anaesthetic such as ethyl alcohol or paregoric, using a cotton tipped applicator. This is usually sufficient to relieve the local symptoms and permit the baby to fall asleep. It may be necessary to repeat this treatment for several nights if the symptoms persist. Proprietary teething aids which contain mercurial compounds should not be used.

In some cases, symptomatic teething may persist for long periods, at times until the primary dentition has erupted completely. If teething extends into seasons when other illnesses are common, such as upper respiratory and ear infections, the clinical presentation of these infections may include one or more symptoms which are also suggestive of teething. It is essential, therefore, that the infant with persistent fever, malaise, and crankiness during the teething period be examined for possible upper respiratory and ear infections (see Seward, 1972).

11. Miscellaneous Conditions

11.1 Angular Stomatitis (cheilitis, perleche and pseudocheilitis)

Angular stomatitis refers to any chronic inflammatory lesion at the corner of the mouth, usually beginning at the mucocutaneous junction and extending onto the skin. Most are of varying shades of red, fissured, eroded or ulcerated but others are encrusted and generally accompanied by soreness, tenderness or frank pain.

Since angular stomatitis may be associated with one or a combination of causes, every effort should be made to identify the cause(s) and remove or correct them.

When loss of intermaxillary distance due to lack of teeth is the sole or the principal contributing cause, as in pseudocheilosis, appropriate restorative procedures should be undertaken. Where new dentures are not expected to adequately remove the wrinkling or folds of skin, or when bite opening is contraindicated because of the age of the patient, instructions in local hygiene care will be helpful — avoidance of drooling of saliva, cleansing of folds of skin with bland emollients and their protection with non-medicated creams and ointments.

Where a nutritional and/or vitamin deficiency is suspected as the cause, i.e. cheilosis, a corrective and supportive diet and appropriate vitamin supplements (particularly vitamin B complex in therapeutic doses) is recommended.

Where secondary infection appears to be playing more than a minimal role, i.e. perleche, topical antimicrobial agents may be prescribed. If *Candida albicans* has been cultured or candidiasis is suspected clinically, antifungal agents such as nystatin or amphotericin B ointment may be prescribed (see also section 6; chapter XIV, sect. 2.3.1). Where infection is found to be nonspecific, ointment or cream preparations containing adequate concentrations of bacitracin or neomycin are recommended.

Angular stomatitis is often associated with multiple rather than single aetiological factors, thus necessitating combinations of the therapeutic approaches described above. Where the lesions remain persistent or prove to be recurrent, other causative factors should be suspected, such as allergy, repetitive trauma, drug toxicity and herpes simplex infection.

11.2 Xerostomia (dry mouth)

Dryness of the mouth often distresses patients, particularly those with advanced neoplastic disease. It can vary in degree from slight dryness involving only minor inconvenience to the patient, with a constant desire to drink, to marked dryness with difficulties in speech, stinging of the palate, glossitis and desquamation of the lips.

Since salivary gland secretion depends to some degree upon the status of body fluids, and because the salivary flow rate may be considerably or severely reduced by high fever, diarrhoea, severe renal disease, alcoholism and other systemic disorders, dry mouth is best managed by correcting, where possible, the associated systemic disease. Similarly, the underlying condition should be treated where the dry mouth is believed to be associated with mechanical obstruction of the duct (sialolithiasis) or infection of a salivary gland. Where the xerostomia is associated with radiation to the salivary glands (in the course of treating malignant neoplasms of the head, mouth and jaws), is part of Sjogren's syndrome, or where it is associated with senility, or drugs (e.g. tricyclic antidepressants, antipsychotics, clonidine, narcotic analgesics, antineoplastic drugs; see section 13.5), treatment directed at enhancing salivary flow is generally successful.

A high fluid intake should be encouraged where fluids are not contraindicated. For stimulating salivary flow, candy lozenges (particularly sugar free lemon drops) or sugar free chewing gum may be prescribed. Topical application of 2 % citric acid in glycerol also serves to stimulate salivary flow, and at the same time lubricates the dry mucosa. If these approaches are unsuccessful, cholinergic drugs such as pilocarpine and neostigmine, which increase salivary flow, may be tried. While they may be beneficial, their undesirable side effects generally limit their prolonged use and they are probably not suitable for use with drugs with anticholinergic activity (e.g. tricyclic antidepressants). Nicotinic acid, 300 to 400mg per day

in 6 to 8 divided doses, and choleretic drugs such as anetholtrithionine (Falkson, 1975), have also been recommended.

In those cases where the xerostomia is severe and resistant to treatment, substances which provide some degree of relief through their lubricating action or their tendency to increase the slippage of tissues, might provide temporary alleviation of symptoms. These include applications of cocoa butter, vaseline, mineral oil, olive oil, slippery elm, glycerol (as in glycerine cough drops) and solutions of wetting agents (surfactants).

11.3 Temporomandibular Joint Pain-Dysfunction Syndrome

The temporomandibular joint pain-dysfunction syndrome is a functional jaw abnormality. It usually presents as facial pain which arises in the mandibular joint and radiates to the face and temporal area. There are abnormal joint sounds, muscle spasms and limitation of mandibular movement. Any attempt to open the mouth fully produces additional facial pain. Most of the pain is due to reflex muscle spasm and palpation of the masseter muscle will often confirm this. Since there are many varieties of arthritic pathology which may affect the temporomandibular joint (traumatic, degenerative, infectious, rheumatoid) an accurate diagnosis is essential.

Treatment requires total patient appraisal and an immediate regimen of pain control, muscle relaxation, and rest to the articulation and jaw muscles. Malocclusal difficulties, habit patterns (clenching, grinding, etc) and emotional tensions and stresses (often the trigger of an acute episode) must receive attention.

Rest to the joint is accompanied by restricted movement, a soft diet and, in extreme cases, intermaxillary fixation. Heat applied to the masseteric and temporal regions may bring some relief. Aspirin and diazepam (for its anxiolytic and muscle relaxant properties) are useful when given in generous doses over several days. Persistent arthritic pain which is localised to the joint region and is without evidence of infection, may be treated by local steroid injection to reduce the inflammatory symptoms. The injection is made aseptically in the periarticular and intra-articular regions.

When pain and muscle spasms have subsided sufficiently to permit a more accurate evaluation of mandibular movement, adjustment of an unsatisfactory occlusion of the natural dentition (one of the major aetiological factors) can be started. In certain individuals, minor degrees of premature contact, unsatisfactory removable dentures, interferences and shifts in occlusion act as profound stimuli to the syndrome and require corrective equilibration procedures (see Lerman, 1973; Roydhouse and Horan, 1971; Griffin and Harris, 1975).

11.4 Denture Stomatitis

Denture stomatitis is an inflammatory reaction of those oral tissues which are in immediate contact and associated with the wearing of removable dentures. The symptoms vary greatly — from asymptomatic, to mild tenderness, dryness, or burning to outright pain. Denture stomatitis is not a treatment diagnosis, since any one or a combination of factors may be responsible. These may be due to mechanical, inadequate denture hygiene, nutritional, infectious and allergic causes.

Appropriate corrective procedures, such as relining or a new denture, are indicated with unstable or loose dentures or the very rare true allergic denture stomatitis. Instructions on the care and cleansing of the denture and its nightly immersion in a weak solution of sodium hypochlorite is often effective where inadequate denture hygiene is apparent. An antifungal mouthwash can be used in addition in cases of candidiasis (see section 6) and bacitracin or neomycin ointment or solution in cases of nonspecific infection. A corrective diet with therapeutic dosages of vitamin B complex is recommended when a nutritional or vitamin deficiency is suspected.

11.5 Halitosis

In most cases, halitosis is a sign of an underlying systemic illness of an abnormal or unhygienic local state. Obviously, whenever the aetiological factor is identified, every effort should be made to remove or correct it and to improve oral hygiene. Maxillary sinusitis, a postnasal drip, tonsillar infections, pharyngitis, bronchitis, pulmonary disease, diabetes mellitus and gastrointestinal diseases frequently induce or contribute to halitosis.

Diseases of the oral mucosa, teeth and gingiva may also be aetiological or contributory. Restriction or elimination of odour producing foods, tobacco and alcohol (which frequently contribute to halitosis) is advisable. The antianginal agent isosorbide dinitrate has been reported to cause halitosis (Bauman, 1975).

The use of mouthwashes containing antibacterial, oxygen liberating and/or antiodoriferous components are basically 'masking' agents and therefore are only of temporary benefit.

11.6 Hyperkeratosis and Leucoplakia

The terms 'hyperkeratosis' and 'leucoplakia' refer to somewhat similar appearing greyish or whitish coloured, adherent keratotic patches on the oral mucosa. However, they are different keratotic diseases from an histological standpoint. Hyperkeratosis is usually a greyish coloured, flat or slightly elevated, fairly soft keratotic patch, which histologically shows no signs of precancerous changes, epithelial dysplasia and/or dyskeratosis. Leucoplakia, on the other hand, is generally a raised, discrete, roughened surface, elevated and firm keratotic patch which is precancerous because it does contain histological signs of epithelial dysplasia and/or dyskeratosis. Initial treatment is aimed at identifying and removing *all* sources of local chronic irritations. These may be physical (trauma due to dental problems), chemical (tobacco habits and chronic use of lozenges), or thermal (habitual hot fluids or foods). If the lesion does not disappear or markedly improve in 2 to 3 weeks after correction of all local irritations, the patient should be referred to an oral surgeon for further investigation and treatment. A few cases of oral hyperkeratoses are associated with systemic illnesses (nutritional deficiencies, particularly of iron and vitamins A and/or B). Prolonged administration of oestrogens and hypercholesterolaemia may be rare causes. Where a greyish or whitish patch has been biopsied and the histological findings are those of leucoplakia, complete and thorough removal of the lesion is mandatory.

12. Inter-reactions of Medical and Dental Therapy

Interdisciplinary consultation between medical and dental practitioner may be required when a patient's medical or dental treatment has to be modified because of existing systemic disease or concomitant drug therapy. Due to the possibility of inter-reactions between medical and dental therapy, it is necessary that a thorough history be obtained before commencing dental treatment.

Table I. Penicillin dosage for prophylactic cover prior to oral surgery in patients with a history of rheumatic fever, rheumatic heart disease, congenital heart defect or bacterial endocarditis

Penicillin	
Day of procedure	600,000 units procaine penicillin supplemented with 1,000,000 units of benzylpenicillin intramuscularly, 30 min to 1h before procedure. Streptomycin 1g intramuscularly should also be given in high risk patients (e.g. prosthetic heart valves) *or* (when co-operation of patient assured) 2g phenoxymethylpenicillin orally 30 min to 1h before procedure
For 2 days after procedure	600,000 units of procaine penicillin intramuscularly each day *or* (when co-operation of patient assured) 500mg phenoxymethylpenicillin 4 times daily orally each day
Penicillin allergic patients	
Erythromycin	1g erythromycin orally 30 min to 1h before procedure, then 500mg 4 times daily for 2 days after procedure, *or*
Vancomycin	1g vancomycin intravenously 1h before procedure, then 500mg erythromycin orally 4 times daily for 2 days after procedure

12.1 Patients with Certain Cardiovascular Diseases

Patients with a history of rheumatic fever, rheumatic heart disease, congenital heart defect, or bacterial endocarditis who require dental or any other oral surgical procedure where organisms may be forced into the bloodstream, should receive prophylactic cover with an appropriate antibacterial agent. Some investigators advocate initiating prophylactic antibacterials 48 hours preoperatively, others recommend 24 hours and still others recommend only 1 or 2 hours prior to the surgical procedure.

The usual standard practice is to start penicillin 30 minutes to 1 hour before the procedure and continue for 2 successive days (American Heart Association, 1977; ADA, 1975-76). High doses of erythromycin may be substituted in patients with a history of hypersensitivity to penicillin. Optimum penicillin dosage has not been definitely established (see Durack, 1975; Petersdorf, 1978) but the doses given in table I may be regarded as

adequate precautionary measures against the hazards of postoperative bacteraemia. Intramuscular penicillin is the more reliable route of administration. However, because of practical considerations, some dentists and clinicians rely on oral penicillin when the full cooperation of the patient is assured. Children with a history of rheumatic fever who receive long term low dose penicillin as a prophylaxis against a recurrent attack, require special consideration. This antibacterial regimen does not provide adequate cover for potentially hazardous dental treatment. Serum levels of the drug are insufficient to protect against bacterial endocarditis, and sensitive strains of *Streptococcus viridans* in the mouth are replaced by resistant ones. These patients should also receive intramuscular penicillin, as outlined in table I. In those patients receiving continuous oral penicillin for secondary prevention of rheumatic fever, α-haemolytic streptococci which are relatively resistant to penicillin are occasionally found in the mouth. While it is likely that the doses of penicillin recommended above will be sufficient to control these organisms, the clinician or dentist may choose to supplement penicillin with streptomycin (1g intramuscularly).

12.2 Patients Receiving Anticoagulants or Antiplatelet Drugs

Patients receiving anticoagulants or drugs such as aspirin which inhibit platelet aggregation, should be given special consideration by the dentist, particularly where a surgical procedure is planned. Anticoagulants and antiplatelet aggregation drug therapy (Hepso et al., 1976) may predispose toward haemorrhage after surgery and in some cases, spontaneous bleeding from the gingiva may occur. However, with anticoagulants where the prothrombin time is not more than 2 to 2 1/4 the control time, and where the patient is thoroughly evaluated and closely managed by the clinician, the usual and uncomplicated oral surgical procedures may be successfully done without interrupting the anticoagulant therapy. If the prothrombin time is higher, or where extensive oral surgical procedures are anticipated, close cooperation of the dentist and clinician are essential. Any interruption or adjustment of the dosage of anticoagulant therapy should be authorised and supervised only by the clinician. Patients on anticoagulants are often concerned that postoperative haemorrhage will be excessive and in such cases pre- and postoperative sedation may be indicated, but with agents such as diazepam which do not interact with the anticoagulant (see chapter XXIII; sect. 3.2.5).

Where prolonged bleeding following a surgical procedure is encountered, careful local haemostatic procedures (pressure, topical haemostatic agents) will usually prove to be successful. If postoperative pain is a problem, analgesics containing aspirin should not be given (and the patient also instructed accordingly) since they adversely influence the precariously balanced coagulation mechanism (see chapter XXIII; sect. 3.2.5). Paracetamol (acetaminophen) is a suitable mild analgesic for these patients (Skjelbred et al., 1977).

12.3 Patients Receiving Antianginal or Antihypertensive Agents

Patients with a history of angina pectoris, recent myocardial infarction or hypertension and who are under treatment with 'vasodilators' such as glyceryl trinitrate or antihypertensive drugs also require consideration. It may be advisable for the dentist to consult the patient's clinician prior to instituting dental procedures.

Anginal attacks may be precipitated by pain, apprehension or excitement associated with dental procedures. Apprehension and long, fatiguing operative appointments should be minimised or avoided since they may serve as a stimulus to discharge of adrenaline (epinephrine) into the circulation and give rise to increases in cardiac rate and blood pressure. Patients taking β-adrenoceptor blocking drugs such as propranolol for angina may however, be protected from this potential problem.

Some antihypertensive drugs have a sedative effect (see chapter XVIII; sect. 4.2) and hence reduction of dosage of sedative drugs may be necessary. Antihypertensive drugs should not be stopped prior to general anaesthesia, but it is important that the anaesthetist is aware of the patient's therapy and considers this in management (see chapter XVIII; sect. 11).

12.4 Patients on Antidepressant Drugs

Clinically significant interactions between drugs used in anaesthetic practice and antidepressants of the monoamine oxidase inhibitor or tricyclic type are discussed in chapter VIII (sect. 3) and chapter X (sect. 6.2.1, 6.2.2). For the patient who is taking MAO inhibitors, there is little or no risk of interaction with adrenaline or noradrenaline (norepinephrine) employed as vasoconstrictors in local anaesthetic solutions (Boakes et al., 1972). However, it is possible that injection of adrenaline or noradrenaline, particularly if inadvertently intravascular, could be hazardous for the patient taking tricyclic antidepressants for depression or bedwetting (see chapter X; sect. 6.2.2).

12.5 Patients on Corticosteroids

General anaesthesia or multiple extractions are usually regarded as stressful situations, but corticosteroid cover is only considered necessary if patients have ceased steroids within the previous 2 months (see chapter X; sect. 6.2.4). Patients requiring general anaesthesia are probably best managed in hospital. Dental extractions under local anaesthesia may however, be conducted in the dental surgery and will usually require the cooperation of clinician and dentist.

13. Drug Induced Diseases of the Oral Cavity

13.1 Oral Ulceration

A number of drugs have been incriminated as a possible cause of oral ulcerations (Cawson, 1972). It is difficult however, to be certain what the role of particular drugs may be. For example, the presence of aphthous ulceration at the time of therapy may be purely coincidental and also with multiple drug therapy, identification of the responsible agent is difficult (see also chapter XIV; sect. 22). Moreover, cessation of the drug therapy may not slow up the pathological process which is already established. Some of the drugs alleged to have caused oral ulceration type reactions are given in table II. Ulceration as a consequence of a chemical burn is discussed in section 3.1.2.

The best known drug induced oral ulceration is associated with use of various cytotoxic drugs, which may act as toxic agents to oral mucosal tissues (e.g. Bonadonna et al., 1972; Jaffe, 1974). In the earlier stages of toxicity the oral lesions resemble the small sized ulcers of recurrent ulcerative stomatitis, but, with continued administration of the drug, large sized ulcerations resembling

Table II. Examples of drugs which may cause ulceration type reactions (Cawson, 1972; Walton, 1977)

Nature	Drug	Action
1. *Local reactions*		
Chemical burns	Aspirin	Prevent bad habits (see also section 3.1.2)
Local irritation	Isoprenaline (sublingual) Potassium chloride Pancreatin Emepronium	Replace drug (isoprenaline) or encourage to swallow drug (slow release potassium chloride and emepronium)
2. *Systemic or associated cause*		
Direct toxicity	Indomethacin Methotrexate	Reduce dose or replace drug (may be more likely with indomethacin in those with artificial dentures)
	Penicillamine	Discontinue drug
Bone marrow damage	Cytotoxic drugs Phenothiazines	Discontinue drug or if possible reduce dose
	Gold Phenylbutazone Oxyphenbutazone Carbimazole	Discontinue drug immediately
Immunodeficiency	Corticosteroids Immunosuppressives	Reduce dose if possible
Lichenoid reaction	Chloroquine	Discontinue drug
Erythema multiforme Stevens-Johnson syndrome	Sulphonamides Barbiturates	Discontinue drug
Collagen diseases (polyarteritis, SLE)	Hydrallazine Procainamide	Discontinue drug
Exfoliative dermatitis	Gold Heavy metals	Discontinue drug

those of erythema multiforme may occur. Indeed, the onset and progression of the oral lesions have been used as a measure of maximum drug tolerance, for reducing dosage or stopping the medication (Malaviya et al., 1968). Although the oral mucosal lesions may sometimes be the result of direct mucosal toxicity (methotrexate), in other cases they are secondary to bone marrow depression. Those associated with severe leucopenia (agranulocytosis) or pancytopenia consist of ulcerations of varying sizes, which are often covered with dirty grey necrotic sloughs.

The appearance of a sore mouth or stomatitis with drugs such as gold (Adams and Dippy, 1976), phenylbutazone or oxyphenbutazone or carbimazole is an indication to immediately stop the drug. Penicillamine has been associated with skin and oral mucosal ulceration resembling that of pemphigus. The lesions responded to withdrawal of the drug and oral corticosteroids (Hay et al., 1978).

13.2 Gingival Hyperplasia and Hypertrophy

The anticonvulsant phenytoin (diphenylhydantoin) has the peculiar effect of stimulating fibrous connective tissue of the attached gingiva in 25 to 50 % or more of patients who are on regular daily treatment (Livingston and Livingston, 1969; Keith, 1978). The degree or intensity of enlarged gums varies widely — from a minimal and barely detectable overgrowth covering a small or even insignificant portion of the crowns of teeth, to massive, firm, nodular masses of gum growth which practically bury major portions of the tooth crowns. Some studies suggest that the condition is related to dose and is more common in younger (adolescent) patients, and in those with poor oral hygiene (Angelopoulos, 1975; Klar, 1973; Little et al., 1975).

Treatment of phenytoin induced gingival hyperplasia varies, depending on the degree of gum overgrowth, but generally includes improvement of oral hygiene, elimination of local contributing factors (calculus, malocclusion, dental caries), and surgical gingivectomy. Despite the intensity of the gingival hyperplasia phenytoin should *not* be replaced by some other anticonvulsant when it has been found to be the most effective.

Oral contraceptives, especially when taken in excessive dosage, have been associated with hypertrophic gingivitis (Lynn, 1967; El-Ashiry et al., 1971).

13.3 Discoloration of Teeth

The tetracyclines, when administered during tooth formative periods, may be deposited not only in bone but also in developing teeth. Hence, following eruption, clinically observable discolorations of the teeth are noted. The deciduous and/or the permanent dentition may be affected, depending on the time and length of administration (see Storey, 1973).

The discoloration will vary, depending on the colour of the tetracycline used, from a light grey, yellow, or tan to darker shades of grey (almost bordering on black), yellow or brown (Antalovska et al., 1971; Weyman, 1965). It may be generalised throughout the crowns or, on the other hand, may affect varying portions of the crowns, depending upon the time of administration of the drugs and the duration of therapy during the formative period of the affected teeth. Occasionally, it may be so intense as to be cosmetically disfiguring. Histological investigations of teeth (under tungsten illumination or by fluorescent microscopy techniques) have demonstrated deposition of tetracycline in the dentine of the formative tooth, usually along the incremental lines of growth. Some investigators have also reported that tetracycline may be deposited in the enamel portion of the tooth as well and that such teeth are softer and more liable to attrition than normal.

In as much as teeth do not manifest the same mineral interchange as bone, tetracycline deposits are more or less permanent. Furthermore, since deposited tetracyclines may, apparently, be affected by exposure to light or other factors (becoming darker in intensity), teeth with such deposits may darken over a period of time.

The minimum dosage of tetracycline necessary to cause discoloration is unknown, although usual therapeutic dosages are known to be capable of producing this effect. The minimum duration of tetracycline therapy that may lead to discoloration of the teeth is also unknown, but discoloration has been noted in the offspring of women who received tetracycline during pregnancy in the usual therapeutic dosage for only 3 days (Kutscher et al., 1966).

Dental maturity is probably the single most important factor in determining whether a tetracycline will cause discoloration. This is usually closely related to chronological age — the younger the child the greater the risk. Tetracycline therapy in the later half of pregnancy, in premature children and in the first month of life induces more frequent and severe tooth changes than when therapy is given later in life (Antalovska et al., 1971; Zegarelli et al., 1963a,b). The total dose of tetracycline is therefore probably less important than the age at which the drug is administered, but the more courses of tetracycline given, the greater the chance that the compound will deposit near the tooth surface where it appears most aesthetically objectionable (Grossman et al, 1971). Thus, even a single course given at the wrong time is probably sufficient to cause discoloration.

Caution should therefore apply to the use of tetracyclines throughout pregnancy (see also chapter XV; sect. 1.1.5) and infancy and up to about 10 years of life. Other equally effective antibacterial agents for childhood infections are available (see Storey, 1973).

Occasionally, deciduous teeth may be temporarily discolored by oral liquid iron therapy. This is unlikely to contribute to caries and will not affect permanent teeth. Staining can be prevented in older children by drinking a diluted solution of iron through a straw.

13.4 Oral Candidiasis

A number of commonly used drugs, such as prolonged use of antibacterial agents, corticosteroids (inhaled or systemic), immunosuppressive drugs, tricyclic antidepressants and antipsychotics may lead or predispose to oral candidiasis. The condition is readily managed and need not interfere with treatment (see section 6).

13.5 Xerostomia and Salivary Gland Enlargement

Many drugs with anticholinergic activity such as tricyclic antidepressants and antipsychotics, or other drugs like clonidine, narcotic analgesics and antineoplastic drugs, can lead to dry mouth (see section 11.2; Bahn, 1972; Colon, 1972). For some patients the problem can be corrected, but for others it persists. The reduced salivary flow may result in an increased rate of dental decay, so that regular care and oral hygiene are of particular importance. If the mouth is dry, dentures may also be inadequately retained and may be sources of physical irritation, thus leading to complaints of tenderness.

Phenylbutazone and oxyphenbutazone have rarely been noted to produce enlargement of the salivary gland with fever and marked dryness of the mouth (Chen et al., 1977; Mirsky, 1970). The symptoms gradually subside on withdrawal of the drug and recur to a more severe degree when it is given again (Gross, 1969). Guanethidine and particularly bretylium have also caused parotid swelling and tenderness. 'Parotid pain' has sometimes been associated with dry mouth following clonidine (Onesti et al., 1971). Intoxication or excessive doses of iodides, including radiographic contrast media, can cause parotid swelling (Harden, 1968). Parotid swelling has also been reported after commencement of insulin or an increase in dose of insulin (Shaper, 1966; Lawrence, 1965).

13.6 Disturbances of Taste

Partial or total loss of taste can occur with penicillamine; the sensation being much less common in patients with Wilson's disease than in those receiving the drug for other conditions such as severe rheumatoid arthritis (Henkin et al., 1967). A metallic taste can occur with biguanide oral hypoglycaemic drugs such as phenformin and also with metronidazole (Powell, 1968) and iron sorbitol injection (McCurdy, 1964). Disturbances of taste have also been noted with griseofulvin (Fogan and Henlein, 1971), lithium (Duffield, 1973) and the antituberculosis drugs ethionamide and prothionamide (Fox et al., 1969).

Disturbances in taste may occur in pernicious anaemia and xerostomia, and these are probably related to atrophy of the nerve fibres and a decreased response of the taste buds.

Complaints of 'salty', 'bitter' or 'metallic' taste may not be related to organic disease or drug administration but to a functional disturbance or senescence. Emotional problems should also be investigated, and antianxiety drugs may be helpful.

Further Reading

ADA: Accepted Dental Therapeutics (American Dental Association, Chicago 1977-78).

Gayford, J.J. and Haskell, R.: Clinical Oral Medicine (Staples Press, London 1971).

Kutscher, A.H.; Zegarelli, E.V. and Hyman, G.A.: Pharmacotherapeutics of Oral Disease (McGraw-Hill, New York 1964).

Zegarelli, E.V.: Therapeutic management of certain acute and chronic soft tissue diseases of the mouth. Dental Clinics of North America 14: 733 (1970).

Zegarelli, E.V.; Kutscher, A.H. and Hyman, G.A.: Diagnosis of Diseases of the Mouth and Jaws, 2nd ed (Lea and Febiger, Philadelphia 1978).

References

ADA: Accepted Dental Therapeutics (American Dental Association, Chicago 1975-76).

Adams, D. and Dippy, J.: Oral ulceration and lymphocyte reactions in rheumatoid-arthritis patients on gold therapy. Rheumatology and Rehabilitation 15: 248 (1976).

American Heart Association, Committee on Prevention of Rheumatic Fever: Prevention of rheumatic fever. Circulation 55: 1 (1977).

Angelopoulos, A.P.: Diphenylhydantoin gingival hyperplasia: a clinicopathological review. 1. Incidence, clinical features, and histopathology. Journal of the Canadian Dental Association 41: 103 (1975).

Antalovska, Z.; Skalicka, H. and Sucha-Hodrova, J.: Changes in teeth after tetracycline therapy: Statistical evaluation of findings in 424 children. Sbornik vedeckych praci Lekarske fakulty KU v Hradci Kralove 14: 379 (1971).

Bahn, S.L.: Drug-related dental destruction. Oral Surgery, Oral Medicine and Oral Pathology 3: 49 (1972).

Bauman, D.: Halitosis from isosorbide dinitrate. Journal of the American Medical Association 234: 482 (1975).

Boakes, A.J.; Laurence, D.R.; Lovell, K.W.; O'Neil, R. and Verill, P.J.: Adverse reactions to local anaesthetic-vasoconstrictor preparations. A study of the cardiovascular responses to Xylestesin and Hostacain with Noradrenaline. British Dental Journal 133: 137 (1972).

Bonadonna, G.; De Lena, M.; Monfardini, S.; Bartoli, C.; Bajetta, E.; Beretta, G. and Fossati-Bellani, F.: Clinical trials with bleomycin in lymphomas and in solid tumours. European Journal of Cancer 8: 205 (1972).

Cawson, R.A.: Oral ulceration — clinical aspects. Oral Surgery, Oral Medicine and Oral Pathology 33: 912 (1972).

Chen, J.H.; Otolenghi, P. and Distenfeld, A.: Oxyphenbutazone-induced sialadenitis. Journal of the American Medical Association 238: 1399 (1977).

Claman, H.N.: Mouth ulcers associated with prolonged chewing of gum containing aspirin. Journal of the American Medical Association 202: 199 (1967).

Colon, P.G.: Dental disease in the narcotic addict. Journal of Oral Surgery, Oral Medicine and Oral Pathology 33: 905 (1972).

Cooke, B.E.D.: The diagnosis of bullous lesions affecting the oral mucosa. British Dental Journal 109: 83 (1960).

de Vries-Hospers, H.G. and van der Waaij, D.: Amphotericin B concentrations in saliva after application of 2% amphotericin B in Orabase. Infection 6: 16 (1978).

Duffield, J.E.: Side effects of lithium carbonate. British Medical Journal 1: 491 (1973).

Durack, D.T.: Current practice in prevention of bacterial endocarditis. British Heart Journal 37: 478 (1975).

Editorial: Recurrent oral ulceration. British Medical Journal 3: 757 (1974).

El-Ashiry, G.M.; El-Kafrawy, A.H.; Nasr, M.F. and Younis, N.: Effects of oral contraceptives on the gingiva. Journal of Periodontology 42: 273 (1971).

Falkson, H.C.: Relief of dry mouth. South African Medical Journal 49: 690 (1975).

Fogan, L. and Henlein, R.I.: Griseofulvin and dysgeusia: implications? Annals of Internal Medicine 74: 795 (1971).

Fox, W.; Robinson, D.K.; Tall, R.; Mitchison, D.A.; Kent, P.W. and Macfadyen, D.M.: A study of acute intolerance to ethionamide, including a comparison with prothionamide, and of the influence of vitamin B complex additive in prophylaxis. Tubercule 50: 125 (1969).

Graykowski, E.A. and Barile, M.F.: Clinical therapeutic, histopathologic and hypersensitivity aspect of recurrent aphthous stomatitis. Journal of the American Medical Association 196: 637 (1966).

Graykowski, E.A. and Holroyd, S.V.: Therapeutic management of primary herpes, recurrent labial herpes, aphthous stomatitis and Vincents infection. Dental Clinics of North America 14: 721 (1970).

Griffin, C.J. and Harris, R.: The Temporomandibular Joint Syndrome: the masticatory apparatus of man in normal and abnormal function. Monographs in Oral Science, vol. IV, p.205 (Karger, Basel 1975).

Gross, L.: Oxyphenbutazone-induced parotitis. Annals of Internal Medicine 70: 1229 (1969).

Grossman, E.R.; Walchek, A. and Freedman, H.: Tetracyclines and permanent teeth: The relation between dose and tooth color. Pediatrics 47: 567 (1971).

Harden, R. McG.: Submandibular adenitis due to iodide administration. British Medical Journal 1: 160 (1968).

Hay, K.D.; Muller, H.K. and Reade, P.C.: D-penicillamine-induced mycocutaneous lesions with features of pemphigus. Oral Surgery, Oral Medicine, Oral Pathology 45: 385 (1978).

Henkin, R.I.; Keiser, H.R.; Jaffe, I.A.; Sternlieb, I. and Scheinberg, I.H.: Decreased taste sensitivity after D-penicillamine reversed by copper administration. Lancet 2: 1268 (1967).

Hepso, H.U.; Lokken, P.; Bjornson, J. and Godal, H.C.: Double-blind crossover study of the effect of acetylsalicylic acid on bleeding and post-operative course after bilateral oral surgery. European Journal of Clinical Pharmacology 10: 217 (1976).

Jaffe, N.: Progress report on high dose methotrexate (NSC-740) with citrovorum rescue in the treatment of metastatic bone tumors. Cancer Chemotherapy Reports 58: 275 (1974).

Keith, D.A.: Side effects of diphenylhydantoin. Journal of Oral Surgery 36: 206 (1978).

Kirkpatrick, C.H. and Alling, D.W.: Treatment of chronic oral candidiasis with clotrimazole troches. A controlled clinical trial. New England Journal of Medicine 299: 1201 (1978).

Klar, L.A.: Gingival hyperplasia during dilantin-therapy: A survey of 312 patients. Journal of Public Health Dentistry 33: 180 (1973).

Kutscher, A.H. and Zegarelli, E.V.: A new long-lasting lozenge: properties and uses. Journal of Oral Therapy 4: 464 (1968).

Kutscher, A.H.; Zegarelli, E.V. and Hyman, G.A.: Pharmacotherapeutics of Oral Disease (McGraw-Hill, New York 1964).

Kutscher, A.H.; Zegarelli, E.V.; Tovell, H.M.; Hochberg, B. and Hauptman, J.: Discolouration of deciduous teeth induced by administration of tetracycline ante partum. American Journal of Obstetrics and Gynaecology 96: 291 (1966).

Kutscher, A.H.; Zegarelli, E.V. and Ruiz, L. et al.: New long-lasting lozenge protectant vehicle for oral mucosal disease. New York State Journal of Medicine 69: 687 (1969).

Lawrence, R.D.: Evanescent parotitis in diabetes. British Medical Journal 2: 1432 (1965).

Lehner, T.: Oral thrush, or acute pseudomembranous candidiasis. A clinicopathologic study of forty-four cases. Oral Surgery 18: 27 (1964).

Lehner, T.: Autoimmunity in oral diseases, with special reference to recurrent oral ulceration. Proceedings of the Royal Society of Medicine 61: 515 (1968).

Lehner, T. and Lyne, C.: Adrenal function during topical oral corticosteroid treatment. British Medical Journal 4: 138 (1969).

Lehner, T. and Lyne, C.: Adrenal function during topical oral treatment with triamcinolone acetonide. British Dental Journal 129: 164 (1970).

Lehner, T.; Wilton, J.M.A. and Ivanyi, L.: A double blind crossover trial of levamisole in recurrent aphthous ulceration. Lancet 2: 926 (1976).

Lerman, M.D.: A unifying concept of the TMJ pain-dysfunction syndrome. Journal of the American Dental Association 86: 833 (1973).

Little, T.M.; Girgis, S.S. and Masotti, R.E.: Diphenylhydantoin-induced gingival hyperplasia: its response to changes in drug dosage. Developmental Medicine and Child Neurology 17: 421 (1975).

Livingston, S. and Livingston, H.L.: Diphenylhydantoin gingival hyperplasia. American Journal of Diseases of Children 117: 265 (1969).

Lynn, B.D.: 'The Pill' as an etiologic agent in hypertrophic gingivitis. Oral Surgery 24: 333 (1967).

McCurdy, P.R.: Parenteral iron therapy. II. A new iron-sorbitol citric acid complex for intra-muscular injection. Annals of Internal Medicine 61: 1053 (1964).

Macalister, A.D.: The management of oral ulceration. Drugs 5: 453 (1973).

Malaviya, A.N.; Many, A. and Schwartz, R.S.: Treatment of dermatomyositis with methotrexate. Lancet 2: 485 (1968).

Mirsky, S.: Salivary gland reaction to phenylbutazone. Canadian Medical Association Journal 102: 91 (1970).

Onesti, G.; Bock, K.D.; Heimsoth, V.; Kim, K.E. and Merguet, P.: Clonidine: A new antihypertensive agent. American Journal of Cardiology 28: 74 (1971).

Petersdorf, R.G.: Antimicrobial prophylaxis of bacterial endocarditis. Prudent caution or bacterial overkill. American Journal of Medicine 65: 220 (1978).

Powell, S.J.: Metronidazole. An anti-infective agent of growing importance. Medicine Today 2: 44 (1968).

Roydhouse, N.H. and Horan, J.D.: Temporomandibular and mandibular dysfunction. Canadian Medical Association Journal 105: 1320 (1971).

Seward, M.H.: The treatment of teething in infants. British Dental Journal 132: 33 (1972).

Shaper, A.G.: Parotid gland enlargement and the insulin-oedema syndrome. British Medical Journal 1: 803 (1966).

Skjelbred, P.; Album, B. and Lokken, P.: Acetylsalicylic acid vs paracetamol: Effects on post-operative course. European Journal of Clinical Pharmacology 12: 257 (1977).

Storey, E.: Tetracyclines and children's teeth. Drugs 6: 321 (1973).

Walton, J.G.: Dental disorders; in Davies (Ed) Textbook of Adverse Drug Reactions, p.128 (Oxford University Press, Oxford 1977).

Wells, R.S.; Higgs, J.M.; Macdonald, A.; Valdimarsson, H. and Holt, P.J.L.: Familial chronic muco-cutaneous candidiasis. Journal of Medical Genetics 9: 302 (1972).

Weyman, J.: The clinical appearances of tetracycline staining of the teeth. British Dental Journal 118: 289 (1965).

Willey, R.F.; Milne, L.J.R.; Crompton, G.K. and Grant, I.W.B.: Beclomethasone dipropionate aerosol and oropharyngeal candidiasis. British Journal of Diseases of the Chest 70: 32 (1976).

Zegarelli, E.V.: Therapeutic management of certain acute and chronic soft tissue diseases of the mouth. Dental Clinics of North America 14: 733 (1970).

Zegarelli, E.V. and Kutscher, A.H.: Recurrent ulcerative stomatitis: current concepts of therapy. New York Dental Journal 36: 20 (1970).

Zegarelli, E.V.; Kutscher, A.H. and Fahn, B.: Discolouration of the teeth associated with intensive tetracycline therapy in infancy. New York State J. Med. 63: 2703 (1963a).

Zegarelli, E.V.; Rosenstein, S.N.; Kutscher, A.H.; Fahn, B.; Botwick, J. and Silverman, W.: Discolouration of teeth associated with oxytetracycline administration to premature birth children. Journal of Dentistry for Children 30: 69 (1963b).

Zegarelli, E.V.; Kutscher, A.H. and Hyman, G.A.: Diagnosis of Diseases of the Mouth and Jaws, 2nd ed (Lea and Febiger, Philadelphia 1978).

Chapter XIV
Skin Diseases

Janet Marks

Synopsis of Important Principles

1) There should be no great mystery about treatment of skin diseases for the same rules apply to the management of inflammation, infection, allergy and neoplasia here as elsewhere in the body.

2) In other disease processes which are special to the skin, some equally logical treatments exist; e.g. in psoriasis, effective control can be achieved by drugs directed towards reducing the abnormally high epidermal cell turnover.

3) In planning rational treatment, it is important to know whether the disease is confined to the skin, and when other organs are involved, to know whether the primary fault is internal or in the skin.

4) Especially when the disease is confined to the skin, topical as well as systemic treatment can often be used.

5) There is usually some good reason if topical treatment is unsatisfactory; e.g. the drug is irritant or sensitising, or does not adequately penetrate the skin.

6) The base in which a drug is applied to the skin is important — in general lotions and pastes are best for weeping lesions and greases for dry lesions, while creams are suitable for either.

7) In some skin diseases, considerable reliance is placed on the nonspecific effects of drugs and, as in disease of other organs, on symptomatic treatment.

8) The placebo effect is large in a number of skin diseases but if a placebo is to be used it should be a harmless one.

9) Drug induced skin disease is common and there are few drugs which have never caused a skin eruption. Drug rashes are of many different types. Only a few are produced by a known immunological mechanism.

10) Proof that a given drug is responsible for a rash is often very difficult to obtain. Nevertheless, in general, it is important to stop the drug or drugs thought most likely to be responsible, especially when the drug is known to have severe effects on the skin or adverse systemic effects.

Dermatology has not, over the last few years, made the progress in the clinical pharmacological basis of treatment that it has made in other aspects of skin disease. Its standards for the assessment of the efficacy of a new treatment also still fall far below those which would be considered acceptable in certain other specialities, and if dermatologists restricted themselves to treatments which had been unequivocally *proved* to be effective, they would be without much of their standard therapy. This is particularly true of the old remedies like tar, ultraviolet light and calamine lotion, but is also, and with less excuse, true of the more recently introduced drugs such as corticosteroids and antibiotics in some of the conditions for which they are used. Most of the modern drugs used in dermatological practice have been developed primarily for treatment of non-dermatological disease and have only indirectly been found to be useful in skin diseases. Even in cases where drugs have a known pharmacological effect on the skin, there is often little concrete evidence on the best way to use them or which drug of a particular group to choose.

'Placebos' are still an essential part of dermatological treatment and it is reasonable to use them provided they are recognised for what they are and are used only when there is nothing better to offer the patient. Placebos should preferably be harmless and inexpensive and, in these respects, many of the older treatments are still the best.

1. Clinical Pharmacological Considerations and General Principles of Treatment

It is, no doubt, mostly because of the paucity of evidence as to whether a particular dermatological treatment is effective or not, whether it is better than another treatment, and how the treatment is best administered, that management of a given dermatological situation is determined almost as much by local practice and personal choice as by scientific principles. Nevertheless, there are certain general rules to be followed, and before treatment is started the following aspects should be considered:

1.1 Fundamental Cause of Skin Eruption

Although much time has been spent in attempting to identify the precise biochemical defect responsible for the production of certain rashes, at present there are few skin diseases about which this information is available. In its absence treatment cannot be directed to the fundamental cause of the skin eruption. In some instances however, it is possible to get very close to this aim. In allergic urticaria for instance, specific pharmacological 'antagonists', antihistamines are available. In psoriasis, the rash can be resolved by agents which decrease the rate of epidermal cell 'turnover', even though the mechanism whereby the increased epidermal cell 'turnover' is brought about is not known.

When the cause of a rash is an extrinsic one, treatment by removal of the external agent responsible (e.g. avoiding contact with a primula which has produced contact dermatitis) might appear to be attacking the disease at a basic level, even though the equally important question of why that individual rather than another has developed an allergy to that particular plant, remains unanswered. It has been suggested that genetic factors play a small part in the development of contact dermatitis (Walker et al., 1967), although these are more obvious in certain other dermatoses such as atopic eczema. As yet, little can be done to alter such genetic influences. Nevertheless, in a number of skin diseases with a major genetic component, the disease can be approached at the level of the 'trigger' factors which precipitate the condition in those so genetically predisposed. For example, attacks of guttate psoriasis in certain individuals can be prevented by preventing recurrent streptococcal infections which in these individuals act as the 'trigger' (Whyte and Baughman, 1964).

For skin infections, more often than not, effective specific therapy is available, although it is important to remember that intact skin of normal individuals does not easily become infected and the real culprit may be not the infecting agent but some abnormality in the host's response to it: this, more often than not, remains untreatable or untreated. The altered host response resulting from the current use of immunosuppressive drugs in a whole host of diseases has led to an increase in extensive skin infections, sometimes of a bizarre nature (Savin and Noble, 1975).

Much treatment of the common dermatoses is still symptomatic, whether drugs like corticosteroids are used whose action is understood at least in part, or drugs like tar whose action is hardly understood at all. Often in the course of symptomatic treatment use is made of the nonspecific effects of drugs. The antihistamines for example, are less often used for their specific antihistamine effect than for their nonspecific sedative or antipruritic effect in diseases such as eczema, in which histamine plays little part.

In some skin diseases, especially chronic dermatoses, there may be nothing more to offer patients than a placebo. This may be good treatment even if it is bad science. There are even those who would argue that, in a disease like psoriasis, those who prescribe a harmless placebo such as vitamin B_{12}, which has been shown to be ineffective in the disease, are doing, if no more good, certainly less harm to their patients than those who prescribe effective cytotoxic drugs with their potentially serious side effects. But progress in putting skin therapeutics on a more rational basis will never be made this way.

1.2 Relationship of Skin Disease and Systemic Disease

In a patient with a rash the skin may be the only organ involved, but quite often the rash is associated with a systemic disease. When other organs are involved it is essential to know the relationship between the skin disease and the disease of the other organs, for only in this way can treatment be planned intelligently. Skin disease and systemic disease can be related in four different ways (Shuster and Marks, 1970):

a) Where the skin disease is due to an internal disease
b) Where the skin disease causes disease of other organs
c) Where the skin disease and internal disease have a common cause or common pathology
d) Where the skin disease and internal disease are related indirectly

Where the skin disease is due to an internal disease, e.g. when dermatomyositis arises in consequence of an internal carcinoma, when dry skin results from malabsorption or other wasting diseases, or when a purpuric rash is caused by thrombocytopenia. Here it is essential to treat the primary cause and, if this can be done effectively, the rash will disappear. Any topical treatment of the skin is only symptomatic.

Where the skin disease causes disease of other organs, e.g. when shunting of blood through the vessels of inflamed skin results in high output 'heart failure'. In this situation prompt treatment of the rash is essential and any treatment of the heart failure will not be fully effective until the skin is dealt with. The systemic effects of skin disease are many and varied and, while not all are serious, some are of practical importance in management of patients. For example, the hypoferraemia caused by eczema and psoriasis, like the hypoferraemia of infection, is not due to deficiency of iron but to inability to release it from the body stores where it is present in abundance. The hypoferraemia should be recognised for what it is, since it is not necessary or desirable to treat it by administration of iron, and indeed oral iron is not effective in increasing the serum iron level.

Where the skin disease and internal disease have a common cause or a common pathology, e.g. in the so called 'collagen vascular' diseases the skin is often affected along with a number of internal organs. If an effective treatment is available to deal with the basic cause, skin and internal organs will both respond. Often, however, e.g. in the majority of cases of systemic sclerosis, all that can be done is to treat the symptoms.

Where the skin disease and the internal disease are related indirectly, i.e. when they occur together more commonly than would be expected by chance, and yet relationships a, b and c do not apply. For example, the epilepsy which arises from glial proliferation, in 80 % of cases of epiloia needs treatment in its own right, quite independent of anything that is done to the hyperplastic vascular lesions of the skin (tuberous sclerosis).

1.3 Appropriate Route of Administration

The skin is ideally suited for topical therapy and at least when it is primarily implicated in the disease, this would seem the logical route of administration. But topical treatment is not always satisfactory. Several other factors need to be considered, of which the following are important:

1.3.1 Ability of the Applied Drug to Penetrate the Skin Adequately

A number of factors pertaining to the pharmaceutical preparation and also to the patient and his environment determine whether a medicament applied topically will penetrate to the required level in the skin and will act when it gets there. Many of

Table I. Factors which influence penetration of a drug into and through the skin

1. Physicochemical properties of the drug
   a) Esterification
   b) Solubility in base
   c) Solubility in lipids
   d) Stability

2. Nature of the pharmaceutical preparation
   a) Drug concentration
   b) Composition and physicochemical properties of the base
   c) Incompatible mixtures

3. Method of application (occlusion)

4. Nature of the skin
   a) Condition of horny cell layer of epidermis
   b) Flexural surfaces
   c) Age (penetration greater in infants, elderly)

5. External factors
   a) Temperature
   b) Ambient water vapour pressure

these (see table I) are poorly understood or their practical clinical importance ill defined (for review, see Scheuplein, 1976).

Penetration through the intact stratum corneum is the rate limiting step in percutaneous absorption of a drug, as once this barrier is passed it usually disperses freely through the rest of the epidermis and the dermis and thence into its blood vessels. There is a 'reservoir' in the stratum corneum (Vickers, 1963) where some drugs are held for a variable time to be absorbed later when conditions of keratin hydration or temperature change. Drugs can also pass into the body through pilosebaceous follicles and sweat glands, and although this movement can be rapid it is usually relatively little in amount, compared with absorption through intact stratum corneum (Scheuplein, 1976).

As a rule, lipid soluble compounds are more easily absorbed than water soluble ones, though this depends to some extent on the base in which the compound is applied and the partition coefficient between the base and the epidermis. Esterification of some drugs, e.g. methotrexate (McCullough et al., 1976), by conversion to a form which is more lipid soluble enhances their absorption.

Concentration of a drug in its base influences the total amount absorbed but although this increases with increased concentration in the base, the proportion absorbed may actually be less with increased concentration so that the more dilute some drugs are the more efficiently they are absorbed (Wester and Maibach, 1976).

In clinical practice there are various ways of increasing percutaneous absorption of a drug including:

a) Applying it under polythene occlusion, as for example in the case of corticosteroids.

b) Applying it with dimethylsulphoxide which enhances absorption without damaging the skin, as for example in the case of idoxuridine in cutaneous herpes simplex infection (section 2.2.2; MacCallum and Juel-Jensen, 1966).

c) Mixing it with substances which damage the stratum corneum and remove its barrier action, e.g. salicylic acid, sodium lauryl sulphate.

Other substances may reduce absorption of a drug with which they are mixed, e.g. corticosteroids, which probably do so by their vasoconstrictor effect.

Quite apart from adding 'active' substances to enhance absorption from a base, the composition of the base itself can alter absorption; e.g. propylene glycol in bases as a solvent for corticosteroids increases their release and therapeutic efficacy, but a base with an optimum amount of propylene glycol for one corticosteroid is not necessarily suitable for another (Poulsen et al., 1968). The type of base may also affect absorption; e.g. betamethasone benzoate is more active in a gel than in a cream or lotion (Stoughton, 1972) and fluocinolone acetonide is more active in an ointment than in a gel or cream (Coldman et al., 1971). In general, 'Betnovate' (betamethasone valerate) ointment is better than the cream (Munro et al., 1977; Stoughton, 1972). Usually it is not possible to forecast the best vehicle for penetration and each new steroid preparation has to be tried in a number of vehicles (Stoughton, 1971).

Just as there are 'incompatible' mixtures in internal medication (see chapter VIII), so there are substances which should not be mixed in topical preparations; e.g. salicylic acid combines with zinc to form zinc salicylate which no longer has the effect on the skin of salicylic acid: when dithranol is used in zinc paste the zinc oxide of the paste combines with the dithranol to form an inert compound, though in this case the presence of salicylic acid is helpful in preventing the unwanted interaction between dithranol and zinc (Comaish et al., 1971). Another undesirable effect of mixing is seen with dimethylsulphoxide, for although it enhances absorption of a number of substances, including corticosteroids, it may reduce the therapeutic effectiveness of certain steroids when it is mixed with them; presumably there is chemical alteration in the steroid.

There are regional differences in percutaneous absorption and some are related to differences in regional anatomy. Thickness of the stratum corneum of the palms and soles makes them relatively resistant to topical applications and for example topical corticosteroids, effective without occlusion on other parts of the body, may have to be applied with occlusion to be equally effective on these parts. This is true regardless of the large numbers of sweat glands opening onto palms and soles, which suggests that this latter anatomical peculiarity is relatively unimportant. Regional difference in construction of stratum corneum probably explains the increased permeability of facial skin compared with that of forearm skin (Craig et al., 1977). The flexures are well known sites for enhanced absorption partly because flexural skin is relatively thin and partly because of the occlusive effect of the apposing surfaces. Non-cornifying mucous membranes are other sites of increased absorption.

Age of skin affects percutaneous absorption too, and in general skins of the very young and very old are more permeable.

Damaged skin, whether as a result of experimental cellulose tape stripping, burns, disease, or the application of substances that break down the stratum corneum, is more permeable than normal skin. This can be clinically important; as in the case of boric acid, which in quantities which do not have toxic effects when applied to intact skin, produces systemic toxicity when applied to excoriated skin of the napkin area. Burnt skin also readily leads to enhanced percutaneous absorption, as in a case of fatal encephalopathy following use of hexachlorophane emulsion in an uncomplicated burn (Chilcote et al., 1977).

The ability of drugs to penetrate skin is probably reduced by the presence of scale and crust. It seems logical to try and remove 'heaped-up' scale; e.g. in the scalp in psoriasis with a preparation such as salicylic acid ointment before starting more specific treatment. In impetigo there is no evidence that removing the crust increases the effectiveness of topical antibiotics.

1.3.2 Undesirable Local Effects of Drug When Used Topically

Antihistamines, local anaesthetics (except amides such as lignocaine) and certain antibiotics, including penicillin and streptomycin, are so liable to produce contact dermatitis that they should never be applied to the skin. Consequently, their use in dermatology is restricted to oral or parenteral administration, or in the case of local anaesthetics, to local injections.

Some drugs have an adverse effect on the skin whether given systemically or topically. The deleterious effects of corticosteroids on the skin is a good example, whether they are produced as part of a Cushing's syndrome following systemic administration, or purely as the result of a local effect when applied to the skin directly (Sneddon, 1976).

In certain diseases (e.g. severe eczema) in which the choice may lie between treatment with a topical or a systemic corticosteroid, it may be that the adverse effects on the skin will prove to be greater with the topical preparation than with the systemic preparation given in the dose required to produce the same therapeutic effect. Thus, in certain special situations where adverse effects on the skin are particularly undesirable, the systemic route of administration might then be the one of choice.

1.3.3 Lack of Effect When Drug Used Topically

In some cases, local treatment is relatively unsatisfactory for reasons which are not understood. In severe eczema and certain bullous dermatoses of the pemphigus group, a systemic corticosteroid is often effective in cases where a topical corticosteroid was not, even though it can be calculated that the amount of corticosteroid reaching the skin is much less in the case of the systemically administered drug. It is not known why this should be so but there are several possible explanations. The most likely is that a central, as well as a peripheral, action of the systemic corticosteroid is necessary for maximum effect. The effectiveness of methotrexate in psoriasis (see section 6.2.2) also depends on it being given systemically, although *in vitro* it has a direct effect on epidermal cells, reducing their rate of turnover. The fact that it has been found to be ineffective when used topically is partly due to lack of penetration of the epidermis (McCullough et al., 1976), but the additional possibility that its action in psoriasis is due in part to the production of folic acid deficiency in the body as a whole has not been entirely ruled out.

1.4 Which Drug?

No league table is available to advise, for instance, which of the many presently available antihistamines is the most effective in reducing itch in urticaria. Even if it were, the most effective drug should not necessarily be chosen, for side effects per unit of effectiveness, and convenience of administration have also to be taken into consideration. Sedative side effects are especially important in the clinical choice of an antihistamine, for such a side effect may for instance be an advantage in helping with sleep at night time, but will be a distinct disadvantage if the patient has to continue an active working life during the day. It is a good general rule in therapeutics, that when there are many drugs available and little to choose between them, to confine prescribing to one or two and so get to know them well. Thus for example with the antihistamines, the more sedating trimeprazine might be used at night and the less sedating chlorpheniramine in the day. Only when these prove unsuccessful would another compound be tried (see also chapter XI; sect. 2.2.3; 2.4).

The choice of a topical corticosteroid can be equally difficult. In Britain for example there are at present over 30 proprietary corticosteroid preparations available for prescription in general practice. A number of them are available in a variety of different bases as well as in combination preparations with antibiotics, antiseptics, etc. To add to the complexities, the commercial preparations can be used diluted to any degree in the appropriate base. How can a clinician possibly choose between these preparations, especially when many of the published clinical trials comparing them are poorly documented and misleading? Therapeutic trials of topical preparations need planning to take into account a number of factors, of which choosing the right 'endpoint', the right base, the right disease and inclusion of an adequate number of patients are particularly important (Wilson, 1976). Selection of the right 'endpoint' is often not faced at all and vague terms like 'patient acceptability' and 'doctor preference' are quoted in the literature. The vasoconstrictor assay, much used in comparing topical corticosteroids is not necessarily a measure of their therapeutic efficacy in a given disease; in one such study the assay was shown to underestimate the clinical effect of

flurandrenolone and over rate that of triamcinolone acetonide (Wilson, 1976). While fluocinonide in its synthetic base causes more vasoconstriction than either betamethasone valerate cream or ointment, it is inferior therapeutically to the ointment of betamethasone although superior to betamethasone cream (Munro et al., 1977). Use of a small number of patients or patients with only mild disease, may mean that any difference between preparations does not become apparent. Thus on very slender evidence, clinicians may be urged to change their prescribing habits as each new topical corticosteroid to appear on the market is heralded as 'better' or 'equipotent but better accepted' than the last. Claims for the majority of new preparations do not stand the test of time and this is likely to be because the new product really was not 'better' or 'equipotent' at all. Choice of a suitable corticosteroid is discussed below (see section 6.1.3, 7.1; table III).

1.5 Which Base?

Many factors have to be taken into account and some of these have already been mentioned (see section 1.3.1; table II). In general, it is best to prescribe a lotion or a paste for application to a weeping skin surface and a greasy ointment for application to a dry, cracked surface. Creams are convenient since to some extent they can be used for either dry or wet surfaces, and have the advantage over ointments of being clean to use. Many ointments contain lanolin or wool alcohols and patients not uncommonly develop contact sensitivity to these substances. Creams less often contain lanolin, and in addition usually contain a preservative or stabiliser: the ones in general use (e.g. parabens or ethylenediamine hydrochloride) are known to be occasional sensitisers (Bandman et al., 1972; White et al., 1978). Thus choice of a base will be limited if the patient develops a contact dermatitis to one of its constituents. Manufacturers change the constituents of their bases from time to time, so it is always wise to check the current formulation before advising those with known contact sensitivity. Some bases contain propylene glycol (e.g. fluocinonide) or part of the base is propylene glycol and the remainder is the steroid in a microcrystalline phase (e.g. halcinonide) and avoid the need for a preservative.

The boundary line between creams and ointments has to some extent become blurred by the introduction of certain synthetic bases (e.g. fatty

Table II. Properties and uses of common dermatological bases (adapted after Hunter, 1973)

Surface, disease	Base	Effect	Examples/Notes
Dry and scaly (e.g. psoriasis, dry eczema, ichthyosis)	Ointment	Occlusive emollient	Soft white or soft yellow paraffin Emulsifying ointment Synthetic bases Lanoline (may sensitise)
Moist or dry (e.g. eczema in various stages)	Cream	Cooling, emollient and moisturising	Oily cream Aqueous cream Cetomacrogol cream Synthetic bases (preservatives may sensitise)
Acutely inflamed; wet and oozing (e.g. weeping eczema and other bullous diseases)	Lotions	Drying, soothing and cooling	Saline solution Calamine lotion Aluminium acetate solution Potassium permanganate solution
Lichenified (e.g. eczema); oozing (e.g. eczema)	Pastes	Protective, prevents spreading of active ingredient Dries wet areas	Zinc compound paste Lassar's paste Coal tar paste-impregnated bandages protect eczema from scratching Paste used as vehicle for dithranol in psoriasis
Flexures, especially if sore and moist (e.g. intertrigo, flexural eczema and psoriasis, candidiasis)	Dusting powders	Lessen friction and are drying	Talc dusting powder; zinc starch and talc can be used as a vehicle for other antifungal drugs
Flexures (e.g. intertrigo, candidiasis, ulcers)	Paints	Drying	Castellani's magenta paint Better than powders for very moist areas

alcohol propylene glycol or FAPG) which is said to have 'the properties of a cream and an ointment'. Early impressions that they are not very satisfactory when a truly greasy preparation is required have not altered with time.

Lotions are preferable to greasy applications for flexural sites, e.g. groin and toe clefts. Sprays are expensive and on the whole not to be recommended.

The choice of a base will to some extent be influenced by the drug in question, for as already mentioned in section 1.3.1 corticosteroids for example perform better in one base than in another.

2. Skin Infections

2.1 Bacterial Infections

2.1.1 Impetigo

This is a superficial infection of the skin caused by staphylococci, a mixture of staphylococci and streptococci or, less often, streptococci alone (Esterly and Markowitz, 1970). Because the lesion is so superficial it would be reasonable to expect it to respond to topical antibiotics and, indeed it usually does so, but systemic antibiotics are preferable in many cases, particularly in young children (see below). Ideally, the choice of antibiotic should be based on knowledge of the sensitivity of the organism but in practice this information is not always available and the choice of the topical antibiotic is then often a personal one.

All antibiotics which are used topically carry the risk of producing contact dermatitis, but in impetigo where the period of time over which application is required is short, this is not often a problem. Nevertheless, topical penicillin, chloramphenicol and streptomycin as well as sulphonamides, with their very great ability to produce contact dermatitis should always be avoided. Valuable antibiotics which may later be needed for treatment of a systemic illness should be avoided for topical use in order to minimise development of resistant organisms, particularly as the skin is a site likely to predispose to development of such resistance (Noble and Naidoo, 1978; see also chapter XXVII, sect. 2.3). Thus, fusidic acid and gentamicin are best not used topically but reserved for systemic use in serious infections. Antibiotics are usually preferable to antibacterials and vital dyes. Preparations such as 1 % neomycin, 1.5 % framycetin, 0.025 % gramicidin, or 3 % chlortetracycline are effective and cosmetically acceptable. They should not be used in preparations in combination with corticosteroids in impetigo; it is neither necessary nor desirable to use a corticosteroid in impetigo, which is an *infection*.

Patients with impetigo who present to hospital clinics often do so because they have failed to respond to topical antibiotics for one reason or another. It is first important to make sure that there is no underlying skin condition such as scabies, pediculosis, or herpes simplex. If not, information about the identity and sensitivity of the bacterial organism is especially desirable, but again it cannot always be obtained. In any case, the choice of antibacterial agent must be influenced by the fact that cases of nephritis following streptococcal infections of the skin have been described (Anthony et al., 1967; Bassett, 1971). Consequently, the antibacterial agent should be effective against streptococci as well as against staphylococci. The incidence of nephritis seems to be particularly great in certain geographical areas and in children aged 1 to 11 years, particularly if the rash is extensive (Anthony et al., 1967).

When there is a case for treating impetigo with systemic antibiotics one of the penicillinase resistant penicillins such as cloxacillin or flucloxacillin is the drug of choice, with erythromycin or co-trimoxazole (trimethoprim + sulphamethoxazole) as an alternative for patients known to have penicillin allergy. The full oral dosage, correspondingly reduced for small children, should be given and treatment should be continued for 10 days. The potential problem of resistant strains of bacteria readily emerging does not arise with penicillins or co-trimoxazole, and bacteriologists do not seem concerned about it arising with erythromycin, provided it is used only occasionally.

As a working rule, topical antibiotics should be used except in the following groups of patients who should have systemic treatment:

a) Children up to 11 years of age except those with a very small area of skin involved.

b) Anyone who has not responded to topical treatment.

c) Those with coexisting eczema.

d) Those immunosuppressed by drugs or disease and those receiving systemic or topical corticosteroids.

e) Those who develop systemic symptoms (e.g. pyrexia).

f) Those with existing renal and heart disease and those who have previously had guttate psoriasis.

g) Those who develop proteinuria, haematuria, oedema, hypertension or have a low third component of complement (C_3) level in the serum.

h) In 'epidemics' of dermatogenic nephritis.

2.1.2 Erysipelas

This is an infection of the skin and the superficial parts of the subcutaneous tissues by *Streptococcus pyogenes*. It differs from streptococcal cellulitis since in this condition the deeper tissues are also involved. The infecting bacteria usually enter through a small crack in the skin surface. Systemic symptoms are frequent and treatment should be with a systemic antibiotic. Oral penicillin V (phenoxymethylpenicillin) is the drug of choice and should be given in full dosage for 7 days, with a sulphonamide substituted for individuals with penicillin allergy. Recurrent attacks of erysipelas may occur in those patients, who for one reason or another, have inadequate lymphatic drainage of the part concerned. Whether this is due to congenital hypoplasia of the lymphatics or to damage to the lymphatics from the infection itself is usually impossible to determine, but in any case the situation will be made worse by recurrent attacks of infection, and in such patients long term maintenance therapy with low doses of penicillin should be given.

2.1.3 Recurrent Boils

A furuncle or boil is an acute infection of a hair follicle in which staphylococci are usually involved. While diabetes mellitus, an underlying immunological abnormality or uraemia are well known causes, boils most often occur in otherwise healthy individuals. Staphylococci of the same phage type may be isolated from the boil as from other parts of the skin and from the nose, throat and perineum. The role of these 'carrier' sites in the production of skin infection can be overstressed and in some cases there is evidence that the appearance of a given bacterium in the skin predates its appearance in the nose and throat. Nevertheless, if infection, clinical or subclinical, persists at any site after clearing of skin lesions, it is reasonable to deal with it.

In the acute stage, boils should be treated with full dosage of the appropriate antibacterial agent as indicated by sensitivity studies. Patients who develop boils at very frequent intervals may need long term treatment. Creams containing neomycin can be used if it is decided to treat the 'carrier' state.

The role of antiseptics such as chlorhexidine applied to the skin as a cream or added to a bath is not proven, but they may help to reduce skin carriage of bacteria, and spread of infection.

2.1.4 Tuberculosis of the Skin

Lupus vulgaris is the only tuberculous infection seen in dermatological clinics with any frequency nowadays, and even this is relatively rare. It is a low grade infection in an individual who has previously acquired some immunity and some hypersensitivity to the organism. In affected patients, tuberculosis may be present at sites other than the skin but this is by no means usual. The course of the skin lesion is often chronic and very slowly progressive with a tendency to self healing, and when some cases are referred for treatment the disease has already been present for many years and has all along run an entirely benign course. The few cases in which the infection is more aggressive leave little doubt, however, that all patients who present should be treated. The risks of leaving the disease untreated are mainly those of local extension. Spread to other organs is rare and, although cases of carcinoma arising at the site of

previous lupus vulgaris in the absence of treatment with irradiation or ultraviolet light are documented, there is no proof that carcinoma can be caused by lupus vulgaris itself.

Before starting treatment an attempt should be made to culture the organism and to establish its sensitivity. This is best done by culturing from a skin biopsy and although it is true that only in relatively few cases is it possible to culture the organism, there is no doubt that the harder one tries the better are the chances of doing so. The practice in most dermatological clinics is to treat lupus vulgaris with isoniazid alone. While this departure from normal combination drug therapy in tuberculosis (see chapter XX; sect. 8.1) is considered very undesirable by some, early worries about the emergence of resistant strains of *Mycobacteria* seem to have been unfounded. The dose of isoniazid should be 300 to 600mg daily, with pyridoxine 50mg daily given in addition to prevent isoniazid induced peripheral neuropathy. The use of streptomycin is probably never justifiable in tuberculosis confined to the skin and when PAS is prescribed a high proportion of patients with lupus vulgaris refuse to take it. Now that rifampicin and ethambutol are much used in tuberculosis and are relatively non-toxic and well tolerated, it is preferable to use one of these in combination with isoniazid, although there is no evidence yet that such a regimen is more effective. Rifampicin and ethambutol should be given in the usual dosage and all treatment should be continued for at least 18 months (see also chapter XX; sect. 8).

Some cases of lupus vulgaris respond dramatically to treatment but others, including some in whom the bacterial sensitivities are known and the appropriate antituberculosis drugs have been given in full doses, continue unabated. In some of these, intralesional injection of a corticosteroid such as triamcinolone acetonide is helpful, antituberculosis drugs being given at the same time.

2.2 Viral Infections

2.2.1 Warts

No specific antiviral agent is as yet available for dealing with this very common infection by the DNA containing wart virus (Bunney, 1977). Fortunately, the majority of warts do not need treatment as they undergo spontaneous regression in time. In one hospital for example, in 50% of patients with warts placed on a waiting list for 6 months, treatment was no longer necessary at the end of this time because of spontaneous regression (Marks, unpublished data). Warts are infectious, especially in children who presumably have little or no immunity to the virus which is almost ubiquitous. Present Public Health measures such as banning from swimming baths those with plantar warts are not very effective in stopping spread and are probably best abandoned.

The main indications for treatment are pain, uncertainty of diagnosis and serious cosmetic disability. Genital and perianal warts also usually need treatment. Once a decision to treat a wart has been made, therapy can be by destroying it by heat, cold, acid, alkali, etc., or by surgical removal. The chosen procedure will depend to some extent on the number of warts to be dealt with and upon the local facilities available for treatment. Warts should never be excised but should be removed by curettage. If this is done properly no scarring will result. Any treatment which requires general anaesthesia is rarely justifiable and, similarly, radiotherapy is not an acceptable treatment for this benign condition.

Common methods of destroying a wart include carbon dioxide snow, liquid nitrogen, trichloracetic acid or phenol — more than one application may be required. All can produce scarring if used injudiciously. Salicylic acid is the basis of most general purpose wart paints that patients buy themselves, a typical formula being salicylic acid 1 part, lactic acid 1 part, flexible collodion 4 parts. Formaldehyde and podophyllin are helpful in the management of plantar warts, although 5% formaldehyde soaks can lead to overdrying of the skin or to contact dermatitis, and podophyllin paint can lead to painful blistering and sloughing. Gluteraldehyde 10% is a possible alternative (Allenby, 1977). A 15 to 25% solution of podophyllin in spirit or compound benzoin tincture is the treatment of choice in genital and perianal warts. If weekly painting with this fails, curettage under general anaesthesia is usually required. General purpose wart paints should not be used on the face or anogenital regions and podophyllin should be used only in a limited area of skin in pregnancy because of its toxic action and possible dysmorphogenic effects (Chamberlain et al., 1972). A topical solution of the immunopotentiating agent dinitrochlorobenzene is being investigated in recalcitrant warts (Goihman-Yahr et al., 1978).

2.2.2 Herpes Simplex
(including herpetic whitlow)

Idoxuridine, which is known in its phosphorylated form to prevent the formation of DNA by competing with thymidic acid, is a logical treatment for infections caused by this DNA containing virus. It is effective in practice if enough is absorbed through the skin. This can be achieved by using a solution of 5% idoxuridine in dimethylsulphoxide applied 3 or 4 times a day (MacCallum and Juel-Jensen, 1966). An alternative treatment is by photoinactivation of the herpes virus by painting the lesion with a vital dye like proflavine and irradiating it with white fluorescent light (Felber et al., 1973). This is successful in getting rid of existing lesions and preventing recurrence in a number of cases, but has not proved a very popular treatment, partly because of one report of malignant change in animal cells after exposure to photoinactivated virus (Melnick and Wallis, 1977).

Treatment directed at 'drying up' the lesion may help the patient symptomatically and surgical spirit or calamine lotion are suitable applications for this purpose. Topical corticosteroids should not be used as these may facilitate dissemination of the infection. Treatment of herpes simplex of the eye should be left to the experts (see chapter XII; sect. 3.6).

2.2.3 Herpes Zoster and Varicella

These infections are also caused by a DNA containing virus. An appropriate formulation and dose regimen of idoxuridine can be effective in cutaneous herpes zoster (Juel-Jensen et al., 1970). Idoxuridine can be used intermittently as a 5% solution in dimethylsulphoxide (applied 3 or 4 times daily) or continuously as a 40% solution in dimethylsulphoxide, applied as a compress and renewed as it dries. There is no evidence that systemic corticosteroids given to patients with herpes zoster who are otherwise fit lead to an increased liability of the infection to disseminate and corticosteroids can be used in treatment, especially in an attempt to prevent postherpetic neuralgia (Eaglstein et al., 1976). Their use in zoster and other aspects of management of zoster and varicella is discussed in chapter XXVIII (sect. 3.8) and chapter XXV (sect. 6.2).

2.2.4 Kaposi's Varicelliform Eruption

This term is used to describe a widely disseminated infection of the skin with the herpes simplex or the vaccinia virus. Such infections are most common in patients with atopic eczema, and it is on this evidence that the advice not to vaccinate atopic individuals without good reason, such as the presence of an epidemic of smallpox, is based. Three main lines of treatment are available — idoxuridine, methisazone and vaccinia immune human globulin. When the herpes simplex virus is responsible, topical idoxuridine should be used as for localised infections (section 2.2.2). When the vaccinia virus is involved, vaccinia immune globulin (0.6ml/kg) should be given together with the oral antiviral agent methisazone — 200mg/kg initially followed by 8 doses of 50mg/kg 6-hourly. A compress of idoxuridine may also be effective in severe vaccinia lesions (see further chapter XXVIII; sect. 4.2, 4.3.2).

2.3 Fungal Infections

2.3.1 Candidiasis

Candida albicans rarely, if ever, invades intact skin of normal individuals, but patients with intertrigo and chronic paronychia as well as patients who have recently been treated with immunosuppressive drugs, certain antibiotics and oral contraceptives, or who are suffering from systemic diseases such as diabetes mellitus, hypoparathyroidism and various immunological abnormalities, are notoriously prone to *Candida* infection. In some patients who have an underlying systemic disease, the infection is particularly chronic and extensive, and sometimes *Candida* granulomata develop in these patients.

Management should include attention to the underlying condition if that is at all possible. It is unnecessary to give an anticandidal agent routinely with broad spectrum antibiotics but one should certainly be given with the antibiotic if clinical candidiasis develops in special risk patients. Drugs effective in mucocutaneous candidiasis include nystatin and amphotericin B. Griseofulvin is not effective against *Candida* spp. Nystatin and amphotericin B can be used topically as a cream, ointment, lotion, powder, oral suspension or lozenges, or be given systemically by mouth. Oral administration, except in massive dosage, is only of use in clearing the intestinal tract of the yeast, for both drugs are very poorly absorbed. Removal of 'reservoirs' of infection in the mouth (see chapter XIII; sect. 6), vagina or intestine is a rational adjunct to direct attack on the skin. A dose of nystatin of 1,500,000 units daily for 3 weeks is usually sufficient: both vaginal (pessary or cream) and oral treatment should be given for the same length of time. Of the more recently introduced but now well established anticandidal drugs, both clotrimazole and miconazole have proved very effective topical preparations for dermatological use.

2.3.2 Ringworm

Nystatin and amphotericin B are not effective in infections by filamentous fungi (i.e. dermatophytes). Griseofulvin is effective against dermatophytes, and with rare exceptions, treatment of scalp ringworm presents no difficulty. Griseofulvin is less dramatic though in its effect on fungal infections of the nails and toe webs, and on kerions or inflammatory ringworm at any site. It is not normally necessary to use griseofulvin in non-inflammatory ringworm of glabrous skin, although it is very effective and can be used if the rash is extensive.

The mechanism of action of griseofulvin is not fully understood but it is active only where new keratin is being formed. Consequently, it deals with the fungal hyphae present at this site only and treatment has to be continued until all affected keratin has been shed: this may be for as long as a year in the case of the toe nails. In the case of those scalp fungi which fluoresce under Wood's light, treatment should be continued until all fluorescent hairs have been shed or otherwise removed. Absorption of griseofulvin from the gastrointestinal tract is markedly affected by the particle size of the drug, micronised forms producing higher plasma concentrations (see Lin and Symchowicz, 1975). Absorption is increased if the drug is taken with fat. The concentration of griseofulvin in the stratum corneum exceeds by several-fold the concentration in plasma sampled at the same time (Epstein et al., 1972). Most of the drug is eliminated in the urine as metabolites, but about 18 to 36% of a dose is excreted in the faeces.

The standard dose of griseofulvin is 500mg once daily or as 2 divided doses, taken with a fatty meal for maximum absorption. It is on the whole a very safe drug but some patients may complain of headache or gastrointestinal disturbances. It can cause photosensitivity reactions and may, by reducing absorption, decrease the effect of coumarin anticoagulants such as warfarin in some cases (Cullen and Catalano, 1967; Koch-Weser and Sellers, 1971).

Effective topical fungicides include Castellani's magenta paint, which is particularly useful for flexural sites like toe webs and groins, and Whitfield's ointment (ung. benzoic acid co) which is a convenient preparation for other sites. There are many cosmetically more acceptable proprietary topical fungicides, of which the best are tolnaftate and miconazole. Clotrimazole is effective but is not as clinically impressive in dermatophyte infections as it is in cutaneous candidiasis (Sawyer et al., 1975). In a kerion or inflammatory ringworm usually transmitted from cattle or horses, fungal elements are relatively sparse and though it is usual to give griseofulvin it is not always very effective. Similarly, topical fungicides are not very effective. Fortunately, the natural history is such that spontaneous healing occurs, but often there is considerable scarring in the process. The usefulness of systemic or intralesional corticosteroids in treatment of a kerion is not established but there are theoretical reasons why they might be expected to be efficacious.

2.3.3 Tinea Versicolor

This is an infection of the skin, usually of the upper trunk, with *Malassezia furfur (Pityrosporon orbiculare)*. It is particularly common in patients with Cushing's syndrome, but occurs in healthy individuals as well. The usual topical fungicide preparations are used in its treatment and are reasonably effective, but the treatment of choice is a 10% sodium thiosulphate solution. This should be applied to the whole upper trunk and upper arms every day for 3 weeks. Alternatively a 2.5% selenium sulphide lotion may be used.

3. Skin Infestations

3.1 Scabies

The *Sarcoptes scabiei* var. *hominis* is a mite, the female of which lays her eggs in burrows in the skin. These are especially common in the finger webs and on the wrist flexures but are also found in palms, soles, breasts and penis. Lesions of other parts of the body are mostly due to 'sensitivity' reactions to the mite, or to secondary infection. Human scabies is spread from person to person by close contact only. An exception is the extremely infectious Norwegian or crusted scabies where all skin lesions are teeming with mites, and minimal contact with patient, clothing, bedding or furniture

can lead to infestation, for example, of medical and nursing personnel (Carslaw et al., 1975).

Benzyl benzoate remains a very effective treatment as long as attention is paid to details of application. For this reason, precise instructions should always be given to the patient. A 25% emulsion of benzyl benzoate should be painted on all areas of the skin except that of the face, head and neck where the sarcoptes are very rarely found. The application should be painted on the dried skin after a hot bath and left on for 24 hours, after which time another application should be made but without a further bath. At the end of the total of 48 hours all the emulsion should be washed off. All sarcoptes will have been killed. As benzyl benzoate is a highly irritant substance it is imperative that application of it should not be continued. Thus, it is important to explain to the patient that the itch may persist sometimes for as long as 3 weeks, but even so benzyl benzoate should not be reapplied. It is important too that all members of the affected family or bedmates should be treated at the same time, or reinfestation will occur — 'ping pong scabies'.

It is customary to tell patients to change their clothes and sheets after treatment, but, as the scabies mite can not survive for long outside the human skin, this is probably not very important except in crusted scabies (see above). It may be necessary to treat secondary infection, e.g. impetigo, as well (see section 2.1.1), but this will not usually respond until the antiscabetic treatment has been given. Several antiscabetic preparations have been advocated in an attempt to avoid the inconvenience and irritant effect of benzyl benzoate. Crotamiton is a weak antiscabetic and not to be recommended for use on its own: monosulfiram is effective but absorption can lead to severe symptoms in those who have taken alcohol (Antabuse is disulfiram). There is no doubt that the best alternative to benzyl benzoate is gamma benzene hexachloride.

Gamma benzene hexachloride is used as a 1% preparation and has to be applied as meticulously as benzyl benzoate though it is slightly less messy and less irritant. Because of enhanced percutaneous absorption (Ginsburg et al., 1977) and risk of toxicity (CNS disturbances, convulsions, respiratory failure) in infants, some do not use gamma benzene hexachloride in infants or young children. It should also be used with caution in pregnant women and in patients with massively excoriated skin. Gamma benzene hexachloride is used following a bath or shower, but to avoid excessive percutaneous absorption, it should be applied after the skin has been allowed to dry and cool. A cool bath or shower 24 hours later to remove the insecticide is also recommended lest too much be absorbed (Solomon et al., 1977). Personal experience is that it is not successful in quite as high a percentage of cases as benzyl benzoate but both are excellent treatments and individual preference and experience are usually the ultimate factors in choosing between them.

3.2 Pediculosis

Emulsions or creams containing 5% dicophane (DDT) have been the insecticide preparations most commonly used to kill head, body and pubic lice, but reports from Europe of 'superlice' resistant to dicophane have led to the more frequent use of 1% gamma benzene hexachloride cream or lotion. The hair or body is washed and the preparation applied daily for 4 or 5 days. Any secondary infection or exudative lesions should be treated before using insecticides. Lice resistant to gamma benzene hexachloride have also emerged in Europe. Resistance has not been reported with malathion: it is less irritant to the skin and also kills ova so repeated applications are not required (Maunder, 1971). For these reasons, it is considered by some to be the treatment of choice. It has been used mainly for infestations with head lice as a 1% shampoo but an 0.5% lotion can be used to deal with body and pubic lice as well. Thorough personal hygiene is essential and clothing and bedding must be disinfested — by steam autoclaving or liberal application of malathion or other insecticide powders, especially to garment seams. The chlorinated hydrocarbon insecticides have powerful metabolic effects and it goes without saying that they should be used only according to instructions in the concentration prescribed: they should never be taken by mouth. Treatment of pubic lice is discussed in chapter XXIX (sect. 8.1).

4. Acne

Acne is a very common skin disorder and indeed most teenagers have it in some degree. As a rule, it regresses with time but while it lasts it can, in its severe forms, be extremely disfiguring and it can result in scarring. Thus, patients often ask for treatment of their acne and although to some extent this is still symptomatic and empirical, it is, with increasing knowledge, becoming more and more directed to specific aspects of its pathogenesis (Kligman, 1974; Leyden and Kligman, 1976; Rasmussen, 1978). The following are believed to be factors in its production:

1) *Grease:* A very important abnormality is that the skin is more greasy than normal. In addition, the composition of the grease differs from normal although the significance of this is not known.

2) *Bacteria:* The anaerobic bacterium *Corynebacterium acnes (Propionibacterium acnes)* and other bacteria, usually not regarded as pathogens, are found on the surface of the skin and in the lesions of acne.

3) *Lipolysis: C. acnes* and other bacteria are able to split fats in sebum to form irritant fatty acids which probably contribute to pus formation.

4) *Blocking of ducts of sebaceous glands:* This is manifest clinically by the blackhead or comedone and may be important in the production of other lesions like pustules and cysts.

5) *Increased sensitivity of skin end organs to androgens.*

4.1 Primary Measures

Most patients who ask for treatment do need it and the majority of patients seen in hospitals need systemic treatment, usually with tetracycline.

Tetracycline is the most useful single measure in acne. It should be given orally in a dosage of 250mg daily half an hour before breakfast for maximal absorption. In this low dosage, toxic effects are almost unknown (Gould and Cunliffe, 1978) but vaginal candidiasis may occur in a small number of cases (Hall and Lupton, 1977). The treatment should be continued for at least 3 months and longer if new lesions are still appearing or if they do so on stopping the drug. Tetracycline should not be given in pregnancy (see chapter XV; sect. 1.1.5) or in young children because of staining of the teeth (see chapter XIII; sect. 13.3) and it should not be used in those with impaired renal function (see chapter XXI; sect. 14.1.5). The mechanism of action is not known, but it probably involves reduction of bacterial lipolysis. Tetracycline does not reduce sebum secretion.

Cleansers: Removal of grease by proprietary products such as 'pHisomed' or 'Brasivol' or frequent gentle washing with soapy water is helpful.

Peeling agents: These presumably help by unblocking follicles. Sulphur, benzoyl peroxide and sunlight produce peeling and probably work this way; benzoyl peroxide may also act by an antibacterial action, so suppressing *C. acnes* (Anderson et al., 1975). Retinoic acid (vitamin A acid; tretinoin), which is available as a gel and a lotion, produces redness and soreness more than the other agents, as well as peeling, and patients must be warned to reduce the frequency of application; e.g. to twice a week if this occurs, since a marked peeling effect is not needed for therapeutic benefit (Heel et al., 1977). Used correctly it is one of the best topical agents for acne. It can be applied in conjunction with systemic tetracycline.

4.2 Other Measures

The above three methods of treatment are satisfactory in the majority of cases and only rarely is it necessary to resort to other measures.

Other systemic antibacterial agents: If tetracycline is contraindicated or ineffective other antibacterial drugs active against *C. acnes* can be given systemically in an equivalent dose; e.g. co-trimoxazole two tablets, erythromycin 250mg or metronidazole 400mg once daily. Alternatively, in resistant cases tetracycline can be given in full dosage; i.e. 500 to 2000mg daily (Baer et al., 1976), although often this is no more effective than the smaller dose and patients cannot tolerate it for long. Such a regimen may however, serve as a useful temporary measure. Intracranial hypertension has occurred in adolescents on higher dose tetracycline regimens (Monaco et al., 1978; Stuart and Litt, 1978).

Topical antibiotics (except neomycin to which *C. acnes* is not sensitive) would be expected to be effective in acne and erythromycin base 250mg in 100ml methylated spirit has enjoyed some success; as has a tetracycline lotion (Frank, 1976).

Oestrogens have long been used in acne and can conveniently be given as the contraceptive pill, although the high oestrogen (and therefore less desirable) pills are generally best for acne and the androgenic effect of some progestagen containing pills (e.g. norgestrel) can make it worse (Pye et al., 1977; Woodward, 1974). In men, oestrogens to be effective, have to be given in doses which as a rule are unacceptably high.

Antiandrogens, especially cyproterone, can be used in severe acne and are effective. They should

Table III. Potency of topical corticosteroids

1. *Very Strong*
   Beclomethasone dipropionate 0.5%
   Clobetasol propionate 0.05%
   Diflucortolone valerate 0.3%
   Fluocinolone acetonide 0.2%

2. *Strong*
   Beclomethasone dipropionate 0.025%
   Betamethasone benzoate 0.025%
   Betamethasone dipropionate 0.05%
   Betamethasone valerate 0.1%
   Desonide 0.05%
   Desoxymethasone 0.25%
   Diflorasone diacetate 0.05%
   Diflucortolone valerate 0.1%
   Fluclorolone acetonide 0.025%
   Fluocinolone acetonide 0.025%
   Fluocinonide 0.05%
   Fluocortolone 0.5%
   Fluprednidene (fluprednylidene) acetate 0.1%
   Flurandrenolone 0.05%
   Halcinonide 0.1%
   Triamcinolone acetonide 0.1%, 0.2%

3. *Intermediate*
   Beclomethasone dipropionate 0.0125%
   Betamethasone valerate 0.05%
   Clobetasone butyrate 0.05%
   Flumethasone pivalate 0.02%
   Fluocinolone acetonide 0.01%
   Fluocortin butylester 0.75%
   Fluocortolone 0.2%
   Flurandrenolone 0.025%
   Halcinonide 0.05%
   Hydrocortisone 2.5%
   Hydrocortisone butyrate 0.1%
   Triamcinolone acetonide 0.05%

   Betamethasone valerate 0.02%
   Fluocortolone 0.08%
   Flurandrenolone 0.0125%
   Halcinonide 0.02%
   Triamcinolone acetonide 0.02%

4. *Weak*
   Betamethasone valerate 0.01%
   Hydrocortisone 0.1%, 0.5%, 1%
   Methylprednisolone 0.25%

Note: This is a rough guide as no direct comparison has been made between all these preparations. The borderline between groups 2 and 3 and between group 3 (the lower strengths) and 4 is not well defined and the decision to allocate a preparation to one or the other group will vary; e.g. with base and clinical situation.

never be given in pregnancy because they may cause feminisation of the male fetus. In men, their general antiandrogen effects make them unacceptable in all but the severest acne.

Zinc by mouth after meals has been reported to be as effective in acne as tetracycline (Michaelsson et al., 1977) but the experience of most is that it is not so (Orris et al., 1978).

Corticosteroids can be used for local injection into acne cysts but otherwise should not be used in acne.

Plastic surgery: Dermabrasion for severe scarring may be satisfactory in some cases of 'burnt out' acne.

4.3 General Measures

There is no evidence that diet influences acne significantly, but if patients are convinced that a particular food (e.g. chocolate) makes their acne worse they should be advised not to eat it. Local conditions (e.g. industrial oil, greasy make up, hot damp conditions), which often make acne worse, should obviously be avoided. Some drugs can also aggravate acne (table VIII; section 22.3.3).

5. Rosacea

Rosacea is a disease which affects an older age group than acne. It is characterised by a marked tendency of the skin to flush and by the formation of papules and pustules. The majority of cases at the present time are iatrogenic and have resulted from long term application of strong corticosteroids to the face (Sneddon, 1969). The mechanism of the production of the disorder is not known. The histological appearances of a papule resemble those seen in a tuberculoid granuloma, although there is no evidence that the disease is a manifestation of tuberculosis. *Corynebacterium acnes* is often found in the skin and may be important there. The presence of *Demodex folliculorum* is not thought to be important in pathogenesis. The skin is not always greasy.

The most effective treatment for rosacea is tetracycline 250mg daily (before food), and as with acne, may have to be continued for months or years (Knight and Vickers, 1975). Corticosteroids, if they are being used should be stopped immediately and the patient should be warned that this may well be followed by temporary worsening of the condition (Sneddon, 1969). It is quite illogical to use any topical corticosteroids in rosacea for any temporary improvement will be followed by worsening. Apart from systemic tetracycline, treatment can include the use of emulsifying ointment instead of soap for washing. Extremes of temperature and excess of sunlight as well as peeling agents (see section 4.1) often aggravate the condition and should be avoided. Topical sunscreens may help.

Other measures which can be used, especially in cases where tetracycline is contraindicated or ineffective, are systemic co-trimoxazole or metronidazole (Pye and Burton, 1976; see section 4.2). There is no need to put patients on a diet, although if foods and drinks which produce extreme flushing make the condition worse they are best omitted. Eye complications like keratitis and corneal ulcers will need specialist advice and rhinophyma can be dealt with by plastic surgery.

6. Psoriasis

Psoriasis is one of the most common dermatoses for which patients ask for specialist treatment, but a large number of cases, albeit usually the milder ones, put up with their affliction without seeking any advice. This attitude might well change now that psoralen and ultraviolet light wavelength A therapy (PUVA) is becoming more generally available, for it appears to be relatively safe and is certainly a clean treatment. The large hereditary element and the idea of 'trigger' factors producing overt disease in those with a predisposed hereditary background have been mentioned in section 1.1 (see also Watson et al., 1972). The only 'triggers' which are known at the moment to have any relevance to prevention and treatment are streptococcal infections and trauma. Streptococcal infections, especially in children, can produce attacks of guttate psoriasis and if such infections can be prevented then further attacks of psoriasis may be prevented too (Whyte and Baughman, 1964). Localised trauma to the skin, e.g. sunburn, vaccination, or an operation incision will often produce psoriasis at its site, but the practical application of this Koebner phenomenon to prevention and treatment of psoriasis is obviously very limited.

A great deal of information is now available about the many abnormalities which can be found in the skin and elsewhere in psoriasis (Shuster and Marks, 1970; Tickner, 1961). The majority, however, are the result and not the cause of the disease. A near fundamental fault is that epidermal cell 'turnover' (mitosis) is increased to about 10 times the rate found in normal skin. Drugs like the cytotoxic agent methotrexate, which reduce epidermal turnover certainly help psoriasis, and psoralens in combination with long wave length ultraviolet light (UVA) possibly act by a similar mechanism (Walter et al., 1973). All currently available effective treatments are capable of inhibiting epidermal mitosis, although in many cases (e.g. corticosteroids) there is no evidence that this is their mechanism of action.

It is important to remember that all measures available to treat psoriasis will suppress the disease while they are being used, but when they are stopped there is a good chance that the rash will recur, although the time taken for this recurrence is very variable. There is no evidence that permanent 'cure' is effected by any form of treatment, so that when the rash remains absent after treatment it is probably because of a coincidental natural remission. There are two separate problems in the treatment of psoriasis. The first is to clear the rash — which can usually be achieved. The second is to prevent recurrence of the rash — which with few exceptions, is an impossible task.

6.1 Topical Treatment in Psoriasis

Dithranol (anthralin), tar and to a lesser extent the stronger topical fluorinated corticosteroids (table III) are the three forms of treatment available. For the most part it is not known why they work. The anti-inflammatory action of the corticosteroids may not be the only mechanism or indeed the main mechanism by which they exert their effect in psoriasis. Dithranol was used empirically long before its effects on DNA synthesis, and thus lowering of cell proliferation, were known, although the precise mechanism of its action in psoriasis is still unknown. Even less is known about the mechanism of the action of tar in psoriasis.

The choice of dithranol, tar or topical corticosteroid in a given case of psoriasis will depend on many factors. For example, dithranol which stains the skin brown is not normally acceptable for treatment of the face. If topical corticosteroids are to be used over long periods of time the undesirable side effect of skin atrophy must be weighed against the good effect upon the rash. If treatment is to be carried out by the patient at home, he may find messy applications like dithranol and tar so impracticable as to be useless. Different treatment centres tend to concentrate on either the dithranol or the tar regimen as the mainstay of treatment for chronic psoriasis, and, as both forms of treatment depend for their success upon attention to detail, it is usually better to prescribe a treatment which is familiar to the local doctors and nurses who are administering it.

6.1.1 Dithranol Regimen

Dithranol is an irritant substance, but it is less irritant to psoriatic skin than to normal skin. Consequently, the best effect will only be obtained if the dithranol application remains confined to the psoriatic plaques: an important characteristic of dithranol preparations for glabrous skin therefore is their stiffness and 'non-spreadability'. This is achieved by using dithranol in Lassar's paste of which starch, zinc oxide, salicylic acid and hard paraffin are all essential ingredients; powdering the paste after it is applied also helps to stop it spreading (Seville, 1966). The concentration of dithranol which can be tolerated varies from individual to individual. It tends to be greater as treatment continues, and it varies from site to site, but strengths from 0.05 to 0.4 % are usually satisfactory.

The paste is applied accurately to psoriatic plaques after the patient has had a bath to which 120ml liquor picis carb and 30ml of liquid detergent (or proprietary tar-detergent preparation) have been added. After the bath and before the application of the dithranol the patient is exposed to intermediate wavelength ultraviolet light (UVB); either as sunlight or in a light box. In cases of psoriasis where the pattern of the rash is such that the paste cannot be applied to the individual lesions accurately, the dithranol is used in 'half strength' Lassar's paste; that is Lassar's paste diluted with equal quantities of soft paraffin. In either case the patient wears dressings until the next day when the whole procedure is repeated. A number of patients treat themselves at home overnight with the commercially available dithranol ointment (Seville, 1975), but its relatively high concentration of dithranol (0.5 %) is liable to burn a number of them, and though it is easier to apply it is not as effective as the stiff dithranol paste used by skilled personnel in hospital.

The scalp can be treated with dithranol too, though in fair haired people it may produce discolouration of the hair: stiff pastes are unsuitable for the scalp and a 'pomade' containing emulsifying ointment and a wetting agent such as polysorbate 20 ('Tween 20') is a better vehicle for the dithranol which is used at an 0.2 or 0.4 % concentration. The choice of shampoo is probably not important and cetrimide 3 % or a liquid detergent such as Teepol are as effective as most in removing scale and old pomade.

6.1.2 Tar Regimens

Here coal tar, usually as a 2 to 5% paste, is employed in conjunction with UVB radiation (Grupper, 1971; Perry et al., 1968). The variation between different treatment centres in the preparations of tar used as well as the methods of applying them and the number of times they and the ultraviolet light are applied during the day all mean that there is no standard regimen. There is no evidence that in good hands, tar is inferior to dithranol but few centres use the two regimens with equal enthusiasm, so no real comparisons are available.

6.1.3 Corticosteroid Regimens

The stronger topical corticosteroids (e.g. betamethasone valerate, fluocinolone acetonide, clobetasol propionate) are usually effective in psoriasis and are even more so if they are applied under polythene occlusion (Vickers, 1963; 1973). This can be effected in localised areas like hands and feet, by polythene gloves or polythene bags, and in the case of large areas, by a polythene suit. Occlusion encourages infection of the underlying skin, and whole body occlusion is perhaps the form of dressing most likely to lead to dangerous over-heating of the patient in cases of widespread skin disease, in which temperature control is already abnormal. The other great disadvantage of occlusion is that in addition to their desirable effects, the adverse local effects of corticosteroids on the skin (see table IV) are potentiated, so that some degree of atrophy commonly results. Systemic absorption, although it undoubtedly occurs, is not often of serious consequence unless large amounts of topical steroid are applied over a large body surface area (Scoggins and Kliman, 1965). The risk of clinically important absorption is greatest in infants (Feiwel, 1969; Keipert, 1971; see also chapter IV; sect. 2.1).

The main indications for using topical corticosteroids in psoriasis are:

a) In cases where the skin is particularly 'sore' or likely to be irritated by other applications. In some instances, a topical corticosteroid can be used together with dithranol or tar to decrease their irritant effect and to enable stronger concentrations of these to be used than would otherwise be possible.

Table IV. Principal side effects of topical corticosteroids applied to the skin (Burry, 1973; Sneddon, 1976)

Side effect	Influencing factors/notes
Epidermal and dermal atrophy manifest by clinical thinning of the skin, telangiectasia, corticosteroid purpura and striae	Prolonged use of potent corticosteroids More likely when occlusive dressings used, or waterproof plastic pants in babies treated for napkin eruptions and in deeper skin folds Combined dermal and epidermal atrophy is the most common form
Rosacea-like 'corticosteroid face' and 'perioral dermatitis'	Here the signs of atrophy with telangiectasia and corticosteroid purpura are accompanied by pustulation Corticosteroids, especially the strong ones, applied to the face can produce this picture whatever the primary facial condition
Impede healing	Particularly ulcers
Local hypertrichosis	Usually only after prolonged use Most noticeable on the face
Masking or spread of infection	When used in presence of fungal, viral or bacterial infection
Systemic absorption	Application in large quantities to large areas, particularly under occlusion. Risk of adrenal suppression greatest in infants

b) As a possible adjunct to systemic corticosteroid treatment in cases of erythrodermic psoriasis. Here, diminution of the inflammation of the skin is an urgent matter because if allowed to continue it can be expected to have adverse systemic consequences, such as hypothermia and heart failure.

c) For a limited period of use in particular areas of the body or in particular patients where other applications are cosmetically unacceptable. Note, however, that application, usually over long periods of time, of strong corticosteroids to the face produces a clinical picture indistinguishable from that of rosacea (Sneddon, 1969).

There is no doubt that a strong topical corticosteroid can be very effective and can produce a rapid and dramatic improvement in appearance in some cases of psoriasis. There is, however, an impression, although this has not been proved, that this rapid clearing is followed when treatment is stopped, by a more rapid return of the rash than after the standard treatment with dithranol or tar (Knudsen, 1965).

6.2 Systemic Treatment in Psoriasis

Treatment with systemic drugs is necessary in certain severe or recalcitrant cases of psoriasis, but is not advised outside hospital or without specialist dermatological supervision. It is to be hoped that treatment with PUVA will reduce the need for systemic corticosteroid and cytotoxic drugs in psoriasis in the future.

6.2.1 Corticosteroids

These are not effective and should not be given in chronic psoriasis, but have some part to play in erythrodermic, generalised pustular and severe arthropathic psoriasis. There is no good evidence on the relative effectiveness, dose for dose, of the different corticosteroids in psoriasis in spite of claims, based mainly on clinical impressions, that triamcinolone is the drug of choice. In the absence of this evidence there is no reason to use cortico-steroids other than prednisone or prednisolone. Doses of the order of 80 to 100mg daily may be required initially, but every effort should be made to reduce the dose gradually and to stop the drug as soon as possible. Rapid dose reduction is liable to result in a flare up of the psoriasis. Patients should be told about potential hazards of systemic steroids and should always carry a 'corticosteroid card' (see chapter XVI; sect. 9.1).

6.2.2 Cytotoxic Drugs

Cytotoxic drugs have a place in the treatment of the following types of psoriasis: (1) erythroder-mic psoriasis; (2) generalised pustular psoriasis; and (3) extensive chronic or recurrent plaque psoriasis which cannot be controlled by other means — but the decision to use them should never be taken without full consideration of their undesirable effects. The drugs which have been used systemically are listed in table V and it will be seen that they differ considerably in the mechanism whereby they reduce epidermal cell turnover rate.

At present, few comparative trials of the differ-ent drugs have been done and so the choice in a particular case depends mostly on personal im-pression and experience. Methotrexate is most commonly used in the UK, but in the USA a con-siderable amount of information on the use of azaribine has also accumulated. With all drugs there is a risk of marrow suppression, increased susceptibility to infection, interaction with other drugs, dysmorphogenicity, alopecia and possibly increased incidence of malignancy if used long term (see chapter XXIV). The drugs should never be given when pregnancy is a possibility and they should be given with care and in lower dosage in the presence of impaired renal function for they are mainly excreted as unchanged drug or active metabolites in the urine (see appendix E). In the dosage in which they are used in psoriasis there are other risks which will influence their exclusion in certain cases (table V). These drugs will not be discussed in detail here but a few remarks about methotrexate and azaribine are appropriate.

Methotrexate can be given orally or by in-tramuscular injection and a dose of 12.5 to 25mg every 2 weeks is a reasonable one to start with in patients with good renal function. This should be reduced as much and as soon as possible. Intermit-tent therapy is less toxic to the liver dose for dose than continuous therapy (Dahl et al., 1972). Pro-vided only severe psoriasis is treated with methotrexate the risk of liver toxicity is acceptable, although it may be greater in those with a high alcohol intake. Biopsy to assess liver architecture before treatment is wise and so is regular follow up in those who are on the drug for more than a few months. Acute toxicity, e.g. bone marrow suppression and mucosal ulceration, is reversible and folinic acid should be given if this occurs.

Azaribine: Unlike the other cytotoxic drugs used in psoriasis which are also used in malignant disease, the use of azaribine has been almost con-fined to psoriasis. In the dosage in which it has been used (125mg/kg/day) it is not universally successful in controlling psoriasis (Cornell et al., 1976) and further trials, possibly with different dose regimens, are necessary before its role in treatment is known. At present, it is obviously less effective than methotrexate without being signifi-cantly less toxic.

6.2.3 Oral Psoralen and Longwave Ultraviolet Light (PUVA)

This new photochemotherapy treatment (Par-rish et al., 1974; Wolff et al., 1976) is becoming more readily available in most major dermatologi-cal centres and there is little doubt that it has come to stay. It's therapeutic effect depends upon the binding with DNA in the skin of the photosen-

Table V. Cytotoxic drugs used in severe psoriasis: Action and major adverse effects

Drug	Action	Adverse effects
Methotrexate	Folic acid antagonist	Liver toxicity; gastrointestinal irritation
Azaribine	Pyrimidine antagonist	CNS toxicity; gastrointestinal irritation; megaloblastic anaemia; ? thromboembolism
Hydroxyurea	Blocks conversion of ribonucleotides to desoxyribonucleotides	Renal toxicity; macrocytic anaemia; hyperpigmentation
Azathioprine	Purine antagonist	Leucopenia
Cyclophosphamide	Alkylating agent	Bladder irritation
Razoxane	Blocks cell cycle in post DNA synthesis phase	Leucopenia

sitising drugs 8-methoxy-psoralen (8-MOP; methoxsalen) or trimethylpsoralen (trioxsalen) in the presence of long wave ultraviolet light (UVA) at 365nm. This suppresses skin cell division and it is a suggested mechanism of action.

Methoxypsoralen is generally given orally in a dosage of about 0.6mg/kg with food 2 hours before irradiation, although general rules about timing are not entirely satisfactory in view of interindividual (Steiner et al., 1978; Thune, 1978) and interproduct (Polano and Schothorst, 1977) variation in absorption and peak levels in blood and skin. Methoxypsoralen is metabolised in the liver and excreted in the urine as glucuronide and hydroxylated metabolites (Schalla et al., 1976). Special lamps are needed to deliver the UVA and are relatively expensive. Trimethylpsoralen is less well absorbed and produces a lesser photosensitivity response than methoxypsoralen. The dose of UVA is adjusted to the patient's history of burning and/or tanning on exposure to natural sunlight (Wolff et al., 1977) and a number of different regimens are in use. Generally, patients are treated 2, 3 or 4 times a week to clearing and in most this takes longer than with a dithranol regimen (Morrison et al., 1978; Rogers et al., 1979). Patients relapse without maintenance treatment and even if treated as often as once a week after clearing there is a high rate of relapse (Melski et al., 1977). Patients intolerant of or resistant to dithranol and patients who have previously needed cytotoxic drugs are amongst those who do well on PUVA therapy (Rogers et al., 1979), but with the usual regimens psoriasis of scalp, nails, flexures, palms and soles do not as a rule respond well and joints do not respond at all. Great care has to be taken with erythrodermic and generalised pustular psoriasis (Honigsmann et al., 1977), although some patients eventually improve in skilled hands.

Undesirable effects on liver, kidneys and blood have not been significant (Wolff et al., 1976) and although pruritus and nausea occur they have not often interfered with treatment. Accidental burns are serious but should not occur with skilled operators. Hyperpigmentation, although attractive and unavoidable, is undesirable as it interferes with subsequent response to treatment. Cataracts, a feature of high dose psoralen and UVA in animals, have not been seen in man. It is likely that there will be an increase in skin cancer in treated individuals (Hakim et al., 1960), but internal cancer and significant effect on germ cells seem unlikely.

Patients likely to become pregnant should not receive PUVA therapy and those with significant disease of the liver (where psoralen is metabolised) should be treated with caution, if at all. Great care should be taken to protect the eyes and prevent burning of the skin. The patient should wear goggles which protect from UVA; e.g. Hazemaster (American Optical), Cool-Ray (Polaroid) [Wennersten, 1978] during treatment and for at least 8 hours afterwards (the duration of significant psoralen levels in blood and skin), and skin should be protected by clothes for 8 hours after treatment from extraneous UVA in natural sunlight. Long term follow-up of eyes for cataract and skin for cancer is essential. Whole body radiation with

UVA should not at present be given to anyone with less than 10% skin surface involved with psoriasis. Lamps are available for treating smaller areas of skin.

The precise role of PUVA therapy in the management of psoriasis is still not clear but at present it can be regarded as an acceptable, effective adjunct to other therapies which is reasonably safe, at least in the short term, as long as it is used by those conversant with its potential hazards.

7. Eczema

Eczema or dermatitis is an inflammation of the skin which has special clinical and histological features. It may be caused by an external irritant or allergen, or it may be of unknown aetiology, when some call it 'constitutional'. Atopic eczema is a form of 'constitutional' eczema: it is associated with circulating IgE antibodies to one or more of a wide variety of antigens, although these antigens bear no obvious relationship to production of clinical disease. Recent work in certain aspects of the atopic state, including the role of early antigen exposure and the use of cromoglycates in treatment, has suggested possible new ways of managing atopic eczema. The effect of avoidance of antigen, especially cow's milk protein, on its development (Matthew et al., 1977) has not yet been fully assessed: the great practical inconvenience involved makes it unjustifiable to recommend this method of management until more is known. Disodium cromoglycate (cromolyn sodium), which is effective in the treatment of allergic asthma (see chapter XX; sect. 2.3.2), has not proved useful in atopic eczema in the hands of most clinical dermatologists (e.g. Thirumoorthy and Greaves, 1978), although one report suggests that it can be effective in some children (Haider, 1977). Further studies are needed. Thus, at the present time the treatment of this common form of eczema is still mainly symptomatic.

Different types of eczema need treatments which differ in some respects (table VI), but the basic drug treatment is common to all types. Nearly always an anti-inflammatory agent is required. At present, corticosteroids are the most appropriate and although topical non-steroid anti-inflammatory agents such as bufexamac are being tried as they become available they have not proved satisfactory so far (Christiansen et al., 1977).

Table VI. Therapeutic measures to be used in addition to general ones (see text) in different types of eczema

1. *Atopic*
It is particularly helpful to deal with dryness of skin, with itch and with secondary infection when it occurs. Paste bandages helpful in children.

2. *Seborrhoeic*
Antibacterial and less often anticandida drugs may be necessary.

3. *Discoid*
Antibacterial measures may be necessary.

4. *Varicose*
Bandages which reduce oedema and support varicose veins may be needed. Paste bandages sometimes aid healing of eczema. Contact dermatitis to applied medicaments should be watched for.

5. *Contact*
Patch testing for delayed hypersensitivity in cases of allergic contact dermatitis is extremely helpful in diagnosis and thus in management. Offending allergens should be removed. Patch testing is not helpful in diagnosis of non-allergic irritant dermatitis, but removal of irritants is equally important in management of these eczemas of external origin.

7.1 Topical Treatment of Eczema

In all but exceptional cases, if corticosteroids are to be used, they are used topically. The particular proprietary preparation chosen is largely a matter of personal preference. Nevertheless, some preparations 'suit' one patient better than another, and this depends on a number of factors, including the character of the base (see section 1.3.1, 1.5), as well as the potency of the corticosteroid (Sneddon, 1976). Many cases of eczema respond readily to 1% hydrocortisone or diluted fluorinated steroid preparations and it is obviously desirable to use these if they work. Nevertheless, it is quite useless to continue with weak preparations when they are having no effect and, especially in hospital practice stronger corticosteroids may be required temporarily to bring severe eczema under control. Their adverse effects on the skin (see section 6.1.3 and table IV), make it imperative that once the eczema is under control attempts should be made to stop the corticosteroid, or to reduce its concentration to the weakest which is effective, especially when used on the face (Sneddon, 1972;

1976). In severe chronic eczemas, one may have to choose between progressive skin atrophy and continuing eczema. This choice may not be easy, although most patients if they are asked seem to prefer the atrophy.

Because of the side effects of continued use of corticosteroids, a critical reappraisal is warranted of some of the treatments for eczema that were used in precorticosteroid days. Of these, tar preparations may prove the most rewarding. There is no doubt that they are effective in some hands, but it is not known which of their many constituents are the active ones, or how tar is best used. Its colour and smell make it unacceptable to most patients but it may be that in the future both can be removed from the crude tar preparations without reducing effectiveness.

Other topical preparations which are effective in eczema include potassium permanganate solution or aluminium acetate solution, which are useful for 'drying' acute weeping lesions, certain occlusive bandages which are useful both as a mechanical barrier to scratching and for the healing properties of the active ingredient they contain, and certain preparations which counteract the dryness of the skin which accompanies some types of eczema. In the latter group of preparations, simple greases like emulsifying ointment, and creams containing urea, which act by increasing hydration, are most used at the present time.

Some eczemas are particularly prone to secondary infection (Leyden and Kligman, 1977). Topical, or occasionally systemic, antibacterial or antiyeast agents (see below and section 2.3.1) are then prescribed as required. Some topical steroid preparations include an antibacterial and/or antiyeast agent. These agents should be used with discretion as they add little, if anything, to the efficacy of routine treatment and some increase the risk of contact dermatitis, especially in cases of stasis eczema and ulcers (Wereide, 1970). The contact sensitivity to the antibacterial agent is to some extent masked by the corticosteroid, and often the only evidence of sensitisation will be the persistence of the eczema. Patch testing to the antibacterial agent alone, i.e. without the corticosteroid, is necessary for diagnosis, and cross sensitivity (e.g. between neomycin and framycetin) is common.

7.2 Systemic Treatment of Eczema

Systemic corticosteroids have no place in the routine treatment of eczema, but are certainly very effective in acute disease. Situations in which they can be reasonably used are:

a) *In acute contact eczema* — where, if the offending substances can be identified and removed, the condition will not recur. Systemic corticosteroids will rapidly reduce the discomfort of the acute stage and the question of continuing the corticosteroid for more than a few days will not arise. A dose of 30mg prednisone daily is a reasonable one to start with and it is usually possible to stop the drug within 10 to 14 days.

b) *In very widespread or erythrodermic eczema* — in which, regardless of the cause of the eczema, the patient is at risk from the systemic consequences of the inflammation; e.g. hypothermia and heart failure. Here, an initial large dose of up to 100mg prednisone may be required in an emergency. The dose must be reduced gradually and only when the rash is under control, or otherwise the condition will recur. A small 'maintenance' dose of 10 to 15mg daily usually has to be given for several months or even longer.

c) *In certain cases of severe atopic eczema* — in which additional factors, e.g. the presence of severe asthma, influence the decision to give systemic corticosteroids.

The part played by other systemic treatment in eczema is unproven. Obviously, if sleep is a problem some form of sedation should be given. Trimeprazine or other antihistamines with a strong sedative action are usually satisfactory for this purpose, and in addition they reduce itch, possibly by virtue of their local anaesthetic action. Specific antihistamine action is not important in eczema for in this disease the inflammation is not in the main mediated by histamine. Antihistamines should never be used topically. Because of the frequency with which they produce contact dermatitis, the systemic route is the only one available. Children tolerate antihistamines well. A small baby with atopic eczema may for instance need and tolerate 30 to 50mg trimeprazine at night, while an adult will need only 10 to 20mg.

Systemic antibacterials e.g. cloxacillin/flucloxacillin or co-trimoxazole are useful alternatives to topical antibiotics in infected eczema, especially when it is severe or extensive or when there is evidence of contact sensitivity to topical preparations.

Psoriasiform napkin dermatitis of babies is rarely true psoriasis. It is usually a severe form of seborrhoeic eczema with secondary candidal infection; as such it responds to a weak corticosteroid cream, topical antibacterials such as clioquinol (iodochlorhydroxyquinoline), and measures directed towards eliminating *Candida albicans* from the gut.

8. Pruritus Vulvae and Pruritus Ani

The irritation in these regions that concerns the dermatologist is that due to skin disease which happens to be in these areas. In some instances, other areas of skin will also be involved and examination of the skin as a whole may well lead to the finding of typical lesions elsewhere which help in diagnosis.

8.1 Local and Systemic Conditions

Local conditions, such as tumours, warts and herpes simplex virus infections occasionally cause itch and examination including proctoscopy and culposcopy should always be done. In children especially, threadworms should be looked for. Care should be taken to exclude systemic disease, such as diabetes mellitus (especially in the case of pruritus vulvae), and altered gut flora from broad spectrum antibiotics (especially in the case of pruritus ani).

Pediculosis of pubic hair is unlikely to give rise to true vulval or perianal itch.

8.2 Skin Conditions

Eczema: This is not an uncommon site for atopic eczema and lichenification often occurs from persistent itch and scratching. Contact dermatitis; e.g. to proprietary creams (especially those containing local anaesthetics), suppositories and contraceptives, is another common cause of eczema here. Management is as for eczema elsewhere (section 7).

Topical corticosteroids are best used as lotions or creams and clioquinol is a useful mild anticandidal agent in these eczemas.

Psoriasis: Treatment is as for flexural psoriasis elsewhere; i.e. usually, dithranol is not well tolerated and topical corticosteroids have to be used (section 6.1.3).

Candidiasis may produce pruritus from genital tract or alimentary candidiasis and these conditions should be treated when appropriate, in addition to treatment of the skin. Topical preparations, such as nystatin and miconazole creams are suitable (see section 2.3.1).

Lichen sclerosus is a relatively rare but important disease of the vulva which can extend to involve perianal skin and very occasionally can be complicated by carcinoma. Topical corticosteroids are usually effective in relieving the itch.

9. Ichthyosis

Ichthyosis occurs in inherited and acquired forms. The common form is inherited as an autosomal dominant and is common in atopic individuals. The rarer sex linked recessive form is confined to males. Acquired ichthyosis can be secondary to changes in climatic conditions but should also give rise to suspicion about underlying wasting diseases such as a malabsorption or malignant disease. Some cases of acquired ichthyosis, e.g. those after small bowel resection, respond to topical linoleic acid (as sunflower seed oil), of which there is presumed to be a deficiency (Prottey et al., 1975). Otherwise, the treatment of ichthyosis is symptomatic with the application of grease (e.g. ung emulsificans or vaseline), or hygroscopic agents (e.g. glycerine; or urea, as Calmurid).

10. Urticaria

Urticaria is a common condition which may be acute or chronic. Certain different clinical patterns of rash are seen, e.g. papular urticaria, giant urticaria, but there is always some degree of whealing and some erythematous flare, so that the basic lesion mimics that produced by experimental intradermal injection of histamine.

The causes of urticaria include pressure on the skin (dermographism), heat, cold, ingestion of food allergens and systemic administration of drugs and antisera (see section 22.3.1). The mechanisms whereby they produce histamine release in the skin are many and varied; only a few urticarias being the end result of a 'type I' hypersensitivity reaction. Urticaria can be a manifestation of the atopic state; i.e. it can occur in families with eczema, hay fever and asthma. In such patients, circulating antibodies of the IgE class (reagins) are found, although the relationship of a specific reagin, or the antigen that produces it, to the urticaria is not a simple one of cause and effect.

10.1 Acute Urticaria

Usually, the cause is obvious to the patient who knows for instance that he has eaten shell fish or had a penicillin injection to which he is allergic. Future trouble is prevented by avoiding the offending substance. Intradermal testing is unnecessary and unlikely to elicit any more useful information than a good history: in addition of course it can be dangerous.

Treatment of the attacks is with oral antihistamines, e.g. chlorpheniramine up to 8mg 4 times during the day and trimeprazine 20mg at night. Occasionally, it is necessary to give the antihistamine intramuscularly.

Treatment of angioedema which may accompany acute urticaria or occur without the rash requires urgent treatment. When this involves or threatens to involve the mouth or upper respiratory passages it is a life threatening condition and if the patient is already showing signs of respiratory distress a tracheotomy should be done. In any case, attempts should be made to reduce the swelling and to deal with accompanying effects of histamine release such as hypotension. The following treatments should be given in this order: (1) adrenaline (epinephrine) by subcutaneous injection in a dosage of 0.5ml 1:1000 solution; (2) hydrocortisone sodium succinate 100mg intravenously, preferably in a saline 'drip' so that fluid and more hydrocortisone can be given if necessary; (3) antihistamine; e.g. chlorpheniramine 10mg intramuscularly.

10.2 Chronic Urticaria

In chronic urticaria, it is usually much more difficult to find a cause and indeed it is rare for the cause to be proven. Intradermal testing with suspected allergens is in general a waste of time: some positive reactions are to be expected in atopic individuals and give no clue to the cause of the urticaria.

Infections such as candidiasis, and food additives such as azo dyes are sometimes blamed, but response of the patient to elimination of the infection or withdrawal of the food is virtually impossible to assess in this disease whose natural history is one of eventual spontaneous remission.

Treatment is with adequate doses of oral antihistamines (H_1-receptor antagonists), taken regularly for a sufficiently long period of time. It is usually possible to find an antihistamine which is effective without producing oversedation. Patients tolerate up to 8mg chlorpheniramine 4 times daily and trimeprazine 20mg each night long term. The usual mistake is to give inadequate dosage and to stop treatment too soon. Systemic corticosteroids are rarely effective in chronic urticaria and are not a recommended form of treatment. Topical applications like calamine lotion serve only to 'cool' the skin. Nonspecific worsening of urticaria (of whatever cause) by aspirin is a common phenomenon and patients with urticaria should not take aspirin (see also section 22.3.1).

Histamine-H_2-receptor antagonists such as cimetidine, may prove to be of clinical use in urticaria, especially in combination with the H_1 antagonists already mentioned (Greaves et al., 1977): H_2 as well as H_1 histamine receptors are present in skin blood vessels and cimetidine reduces the vascular response to histamine.

10.3 Cholinergic Urticaria

This is a clinically recognisable variant of chronic urticaria which is seen particularly in fit young men after exercising or bathing, often in association with sweating. Although the lesions resemble those produced by injection of cholinergic drugs, the mechanism of their production is not known. The attacks can usually be prevented by regular or periodic oral antihistamines. Anticholinergic drugs such as propantheline bromide can be used in addition, although given alone they usually produce too many side effects if given in a dose large enough to suppress the skin lesions.

10.4 Familial Angioedema

This is a rare condition inherited as an autosomal dominant trait. It is not related to allergic or other urticarias or angioedemas and a useful diagnostic point is that the submucosal and subcutaneous swellings that occur are *not* accompanied by urticaria. There is a deficiency of the inhibitor of the enzyme C1 esterase, one of the components of complement. One of the consequences of the defect is that kinins are released and oedema results, though why this occurs in attacks is not fully understood. Local trauma is often a provoking factor and this is of course particularly dangerous if the mouth, neck or throat are traumatised. Death from respiratory obstruction often occurs in early adult life so that life expectancy is considerably reduced in affected individuals.

Treatment is by prompt relief of respiratory obstruction and by correcting the enzyme deficiency with a transfusion of fresh frozen or freeze dried plasma (Frank et al., 1976). Adrenaline and other measures used for allergic angioedema are not effective and should not be given. Few people have enough experience of treating these patients to enable any alternatives to plasma infusions to be assessed properly, but epsilon aminocaproic acid or tranexamic acid, inhibitors of C1 esterase (see chapter XXIII; section 5.4), are reported to control spontaneous attacks and can be used as an (expensive) long term maintenance treatment when this is required (Sheffer et al., 1972). More recently, there are reports that danazol, an antigonadotrophin with weak androgenic activity, can be effective in preventing attacks by increasing C1 esterase and C4 serum levels (Agostoni et al., 1978; Gelfand et al., 1976).

11. Lichen Planus

Lichen planus is a disease of unknown aetiology, except that rashes very similar to it have been seen in those who have survived bone marrow transplant as part of a graft-versus-host reaction. Rashes indistinguishable from it can be caused by drugs such as antimalarials and gold. Contact with chemicals used in colour photography processing occasionally produce a similar rash. There is no evidence that infection or emotional upsets produce the disease. Mouth lesions are common (see chapter XIII; section 4.1), and of other mucosal surfaces known to be involved, the glans penis is the most common. An attack of lichen planus usually lasts several months or more, and some patients have recurrent attacks.

The necessity to treat the condition depends on the extent of the rash and the amount of irritation present. Often only reassurance or symptomatic treatment is required. Both systemic antihistamines and topical corticosteroids will help to relieve the itch, and a strong corticosteroid, if necessary applied under polythene occlusion, will improve the appearance of the rash. Occasionally, a systemic corticosteroid is required if the rash is extensive: prednisone in an oral dose of about 40mg daily initially should suppress the rash but does not appear to alter the natural history of the disease.

12. Bullous Diseases

12.1 Pemphigus and Pemphigoid

In these diseases, the extensive blistering of the skin means that patients may lose heat, water, electrolytes and protein through the skin and consequently are in danger of death from their disease, especially if they are elderly. Corticosteroids in large doses, usually about 100mg prednisone daily, are generally needed to control the blistering and the maintenance dose required, though lower, may well be of an order likely to produce serious side effects.

It is known that autoantibodies are produced by the patient. In pemphigus, these are directed towards the intercellular cement substance between the epidermal cells, and in pemphigoid, to the basement membrane at the dermoepidermal junction. It is not known for certain that these antibodies are the cause rather than the result of the disease, but evidence is accumulating that immunosuppressive drugs, especially azathioprine, are useful in the treatment of the diseases when used in a dosage of about 150mg daily (2.5mg/kg body weight), assuming renal function to be normal (Greaves et al., 1971). Azathioprine is relatively safe, although leucopenia and deterioration in liver function are occasional complications. At this dosage a 'corticosteroid sparing' effect is usual (Burton et al., 1978), and in some cases it is even possible to take the patient off corticosteroid and maintain him on azathioprine alone.

General measures directed towards replacing lost fluid, electrolytes and protein and maintaining a normal temperature are obviously required in severe cases. An extensively blistered skin is extremely uncomfortable and the application of 'spread dressings' of a corticosteroid such as betamethasone valerate is soothing. Potassium permanganate baths to dry up the blisters and oozing surfaces also help.

12.2 Benign Mucous Membrane Pemphigoid ('ocular pemphigus')

Blisters occur in the mouth in the majority of patients with pemphigus and in some patients with pemphigoid: occasionally mouth lesions predate skin lesions by months or even longer (see chapter XIII; section 4.2). Benign mucous membrane pemphigoid has clinical and immunological differences from the other bullous diseases although it is most closely related to pemphigoid. In some cases the skin is not involved at all and in most patients the skin lesions are the least important feature of the disease. A topical corticosteroid may be all that is required to control the rash: otherwise systemic corticosteroids and immunosuppressive agents can be used as in pemphigoid and pemphigus. Treatment of the eye and mouth lesions is best left to the specialist in those fields.

12.3 Dermatitis Herpetiformis

This is a blistering disease with some resemblance to pemphigoid but usually without the very extensive large blisters. It does not as a rule respond to corticosteroids or to immunosuppressive drugs. Autoantibodies to particular components of skin have not been demonstrated, although deposits of IgA are found in the dermis. The rash is completely and promptly suppressed by sulphonamides and sulphones. Dapsone is the drug most used in England, the minimal effective dose ranging from 50mg weekly to 500mg daily in different individuals and also varying considerably from time to time in a given individual. Other sulphones act after conversion to dapsone and are as a rule less well absorbed and more rapidly excreted. Diasone is much used in the USA, 900mg being equivalent to 100mg dapsone.

Dapsone, an antileprotic drug, has been used in a number of dermatoses but it is most effective in dermatitis herpetiformis. It should be used in the smallest dose required to produce a clinical effect. It is most toxic in slow acetylators and those with glucose 6-phosphate dehydrogenase deficiency (see below). Laboratory evidence of haemolysis can be found in most people who take the drug, but in the absence of clinically important anaemia this is not an indication that the drug must be stopped.

It is well absorbed and peak plasma levels occur within a few hours of an oral dose, but it is still detectable in the blood 4 days later partly because of its secretion in the bile and enterohepatic circulation. It is distributed into all body tissues and secretions including breast milk and is concentrated in red cells, one of its main targets for toxicity, but not apparently in skin apart from the granulomatous lesions of leprosy. It circulates protein bound and is excreted as metabolites by the kidneys some of the drug appearing in the urine quickly but some is still present there several days after a single dose.

There is still relatively little known about the various metabolites of dapsone and it is not known in which form it is active in dermatitis herpetiformis. In the blood, in addition to dapsone itself, there are acetylated derivatives and small amounts of compounds formed by hydroxylation, oxidation, sulphation and conjugation with glucuronic acid. It is also assumed that hydroxylamino compounds are present, for these unlike other derivatives of dapsone that have been tested *in vitro*, are toxic to red cells. Acetylation of dapsone is by the same enzyme as that responsible for acetylation of isoniazid, and fast and slow acetylators are likewise genetically determined (see chapter VII; sect. 4.2.1). Slow acetylators of dapsone have higher peak levels in the blood and, although clinical effectiveness is no greater, toxic effects are more marked (Ellard et al., 1974). The main metabolite in the urine is the glucuronide, although it is not known in what tissue conjugation occurs. Urinary excretion is inhibited by probenecid.

Dapsone has been shown to have many effects but its mechanism of action in dermatitis herpetiformis is not known. It is a bacteriostatic by virtue of its inhibition of para aminobenzoic acid. Dermatitis herpetiformis is not an infection and this inhibition is not the mechanism of its action. It is an enzyme inhibitor. It is an oxidising agent and its toxic effects on red cells, but not apparently its therapeutic action, depend on this. Dapsone has a number of immunological effects and its effect in dermatitis herpetiformis is most likely due to one of these — perhaps its inhibition of complement activation by the 'alternative' pathway.

Although depression, rashes, leucopenia and neuropathy occur, the main effects are on red cells. These are detectable in nearly all patients taking dapsone but are only clinically important in a few cases (Cream and Scott, 1970). Oxidation of haemoglobin results in the formation of methaemoglobin and this is the main cause of the blue colour and in more extreme cases shortness of breath. Oxidation of globin results in the formation of Heinz bodies which are frequently found in patients' blood films. Oxidation of the red cell membrane results in haemolysis. This is dose related but in addition is worse in those with glucose 6-phosphate dehydrogenase deficiency (see chapter VII; sect. 4.2.2; chapter XXIII; sect. 8.4). Severe haemolytic anaemia and severe methaemoglobinaemia will mean that dapsone must be stopped but care should be taken to see that anaemia in patients with dermatitis herpetiformis, which is dapsone induced, is not confused with that due to coeliac disease (see below).

Dermatitis herpetiformis and coeliac disease: The discovery that at least two thirds of patients with dermatitis herpetiformis have structural changes in the small intestinal mucosa indistinguishable from those of coeliac disease (Marks et al., 1966), raised hopes that the rash, like the bowel, might respond to a gluten free diet. This has not universally been the case, even in those whose bowel has returned to normal on the diet. There is little doubt that some patients are able to reduce the dose of dapsone or do without it altogether, although some patients are reported who have developed dermatitis herpetiformis for the first time while on a gluten free diet for coeliac disease. The assessment of the effect of gluten on the rash is made especially difficult by the spontaneous improvement that can occur in people with dermatitis herpetiformis regardless of diet, and the fact that putting patients on a 'gluten free diet' has effects other than simple withdrawal of gluten.

Patients with dermatitis herpetiformis who also have coeliac disease should of course be put on a gluten free diet. Those without gut symptoms should be similarly treated if the structural changes in the bowel are severe or there is biochemical evidence of malabsorption. It is not known whether putting those with minor changes on a gluten free diet will decrease the risk of small bowel lymphoma which is a complication of coeliac disease. A gluten free diet is certainly worth trying for its effect on the rash, especially in patients in whom dapsone is ineffective or is producing adverse effects, but most dermatologists find that the majority of patients need some dapsone even after a long time on a strict gluten free diet.

12.4 Erythema Multiforme

This disease and its severe variant, the Stevens-Johnson syndrome, is almost certainly an immunological reaction to one of a number of insults. Some of the more common ones are infections such as herpes simplex virus; drugs, including antibiotics (see sect. 22.3.8); and malignant disease, especially after treatment which results in tissue destruction.

In the Stevens-Johnson syndrome there is fever, soreness or ulceration of the mouth (see also chapter XIII; sect. 4.3), eyes and genitalia, as well as a rash: the classical rash consists of 'target' or 'iris' lesions especially of the hands and feet, but erythematous, urticated, purpuric and bullous rashes also occur. Associated nephritis can result in death.

Treatment of the severe form, whatever its cause, is with oral prednisone 40mg daily. If an infection is thought to be the cause, the appropriate antibacterial or antiviral agent must also be given and any drug thought to be responsible must of course be stopped. Symptomatic treatment, including mouthwashes, soothing baths for the genital lesions and bathing the eyes, is also important in the severe forms.

13. Collagen Vascular Diseases

The skin is one of the organs most commonly involved in these diseases and consequently the dermatologist may be called upon to supervise treatment, especially in the less acute forms. All have in common the ability to produce skin abnormalities as a result of blockage of blood vessels of various sizes: the conditions include Raynaud's phenomenon, vasculitic purpura and gangrene. Some are amenable to treatment by vasodilators, anticoagulants and lowering of blood viscosity by such measures as infusion of low molecular weight dextran. Other skin manifestations which are not particularly associated with vascular disease need different treatment, depending upon the particular collagen vascular disease involved (see also chapter XXII; sect. 10.1).

13.1 Systemic Lupus Erythematosus

A variety of nonspecific rashes occur in this disease, often in light exposed areas (e.g. the butterfly area of the face) and some patients are helped by the application, especially in the summer, of sunscreen creams (section 21). The rash is usually helped by hydroxychloroquine in a dose of 200 to 400mg daily and this may also improve other aspects of the systemic disease. This drug and the related antimalarials have toxic effects of which those on the retina, which can lead to blindness, are most important. They should never be given without good reason, or for too long, or without frequent expert ophthalmological supervision (see chapter XII; section 11.1.3). The skin lesions of systemic lupus erythematosus rarely warrant other systemic treatment such as corticosteroids and immunosuppressive drugs, although they will respond if the drugs are used for other reasons. When skin lesions of discoid lupus erythematosus occur in the course of systemic lupus erythematosus they should be treated like all other lesions of discoid lupus (see section 13.4).

13.2 Systemic Sclerosis

The scleroderma usually most obvious in the fingers and the face in this condition is not treated in the absence of other abnormalities, and measures directed towards treating the vascular and internal aspects of systemic sclerosis rarely help the scleroderma. Antimalarials are not effective and systemic corticosteroids are less useful than in other collagen vascular diseases. Immunosuppressives are used with some apparent success in severe cases.

13.3 Dermatomyositis

In adults, this collagen vascular disease is more often than not a skin manifestation of underlying malignancy: removal of the tumour, if this is practicable, will result in improvement of the rash and the myopathy. In other cases, it is rarely necessary to treat the rash but the myopathy will need treatment when there is clinically important weakness of the proximal limb and trunk muscles, or dysphagia from weakness of the muscles of swallowing. In such cases, the rash will improve with the systemic corticosteroid or antimetabolite drug given. Large doses of corticosteroids (e.g. prednisone 100mg daily) may be required initially. As maintenance therapy a smaller dose with or without an antimetabolite such as methotrexate is usually effective (Malaviya et al., 1968).

13.4 Discoid Lupus Erythematosus and Morphoea

These are diseases related to the collagen vascular diseases but usually they are confined to the skin and so only rarely are they of more than cosmetic importance.

13.4.1 Discoid Lupus Erythematosus
This does occur as one of the skin manifestations of systemic lupus, and a minority of cases of discoid lupus do go on to develop systemic lupus. Nevertheless, discoid lupus erythematosus usually occurs in patients who are otherwise fit. The rash like that of systemic lupus is often on light exposed areas, especially the face. Unlike the nonspecific and often transient rashes of systemic lupus it goes on to scarring and when this occurs in the scalp it results in permanent baldness. In severe and widespread discoid lupus it may be necessary to give hydroxychloroquine or systemic corticosteroids as for systemic lupus but usually topical treatment with corticosteroids is sufficient. Hydrocortisone does not work and stronger preparations like betamethasone valerate or clobetasol propionate, or their equivalents (see table III), will have to be used. Their use, even on the face, is completely justifiable in this potentially scarring condition. An alternative route of administration is by intradermal injection and triamcinolone is a convenient preparation for this. Sunscreen creams may also help.

13.4.2 Morphoea
This form of scleroderma usually occurs in otherwise fit people, although it is occasionally seen in systemic sclerosis. Its only effects on internal structures are mechanical ones; e.g. if the chest wall is involved with large plaques they will interfere with respiration. Lathyrogenic agents like D-penicillamine (Nimni, 1977) have been used to 'dissolve' the collagen, but are only to be recommended in very severe cases for they are likely to cause collagen breakdown in vital organs as well as in the skin. Application of strong topical corticosteroid or intralesional triamcinolone injection may help, but the effects are difficult to assess in this disease whose natural history is one of slow regression.

Intralesional injection of triamcinolone acetonide can be done through a needle or with a 'Dermojet' painless injector. The quantity injected will vary according to the size and nature of the lesion but it is reasonable to start with 0.5ml of 10mg/ml suspension and to repeat it in 2 or 3 weeks if necessary. Atrophy of subcutaneous tissue can occur and if there is any sign of it, the injections should be stopped.

14. Leg Ulcers

Leg ulcers have many causes, but most result from arterial or arteriolar disease or venous 'stasis'. Often arterial and venous disease occur in the same patient.

14.1 Surgery and Systemic Treatment

Only rarely is it possible to improve the mechanical state of the blood vessels to any degree and operations (e.g. stripping of varicose veins) should only be undertaken by experts after due consideration of the pros and cons. The help most patients with leg ulcers get from vascular surgery is negligible. In the case of venous ulcers, venous drainage can be improved by raising the legs at night and when sitting down, by wearing elastic stockings or tights and by various external 'pumps'. Normal walking should usually be encouraged. Occasionally, in arterial and arteriolar disease the patients are helped by vasodilators, sympathectomy and lowering of blood viscosity (e.g. by infusion of low molecular weight dextran). Obviously, coexisting diabetes mellitus and other contributory disease should be treated and drugs such as corticosteroids which impede healing should not be given (except in some cases of arteritis when they may be necessary).

Zinc is essential for wound healing, but this does not mean it will heal leg ulcers and trials designed to test its efficacy have differed in their results. Zinc deficiency is difficult to assess (Hawkins et al., 1976), but on the present evidence it is reasonable to give oral zinc sulphate 220mg twice daily with or after meals for a few weeks in those with a low serum zinc concentration (Phillips et al., 1977). Systemic antibiotics should not be given routinely for colonisation of leg ulcers with such organisms as *Pseudomonas aeruginosa,* but when clinical erysipelas or cellulitis occur around the ulcer, systemic antistreptococcal drugs such as penicillin should be given. Pain should be treated with analgesics.

14.2 Topical Treatment

Possibilities for topical treatment are extremely numerous and only a few can be discussed.

Cleaning the ulcer: This can be done with normal saline solution, hydrogen peroxide or a solution of potassium permanganate. Occasionally slough has to be removed surgically or by proteolytic enzymes (e.g. trypsin, collagenase; Nierman, 1978), urea cream, or substances which act by adsorbing exudate, etc on a large surface (dextranomer; Floden and Wikstrom, 1978).

Topical antibacterials: Silver nitrate solution, vital dyes (e.g. gentian violet) and clioquinol (iodochlorhydroxyquinoline) are amongst the preparations used, but antibiotics are probably preferable as long as the general rules for use of topical antibiotics are observed (see section 2.1.1). In chronic leg ulcers, contact sensitivity to antibiotics and ointment bases is a considerable risk and may delay ulcer healing and should always be watched for (Perera, 1970; Wereide, 1970).

Dressings: Constant changing of dressings is detrimental to healing and unless discharge and/or pain dictate otherwise, the ulcer can be occluded for days or weeks at a time, either with traditional non-stick polyester film dressings such as 'Melolin' or hydrocortisone and silicone cream impregnated bandages such as 'Cortacream'. Firm crepe or elastic bandages should be applied on top to help reduce oedema, to support varicose veins and to protect the legs from further trauma.

Covering the ulcer with various preparations of porcine skin, which acts as a framework for epithelisation, does not seem as satisfactory as skin grafting and this is done with success in some cases (Millard et al., 1977).

Oxygen therapy: A variety of techniques have been used to provide supplemental oxygen to cutaneous ulcers on the basis that oxygen stimulates phagocytosis, granulation tissue growth and bacteriostasis. Success has been claimed in leg ulcers with hyperbaric oxygen (Olejniczak and Zielinski, 1977) and with application of dressings saturated in a 20% benzoyl peroxide emulsion (Pace, 1976).

15. Pressure Sores

Many of the principles of treatment of leg ulcers apply to management. Pressure sores are best prevented by frequent turning and where possible ambulation of incontinent, paralysed and immobile patients: if in spite of this, sores do develop, maximum activity is more than ever necessary. Special 'hammocks' and water beds are available for easier nursing.

16. Burns

Burns are only the concern of the dermatologist if they are superficial or of limited extent. Topical corticosteroids such as fluocinolone acetonide cream applied *early on* may be very helpful, especially in sunburn (see section 21.1). Exceptionally, a course of systemic corticosteroids may be required, and these should be given as soon as possible after the appearance of the burn. Then non-stick polyester film dressings such as 'Melolin' should be applied. Systemic analgesics can be used as required in more severe cases. Infection should be treated as it arises and lost fluid, electrolytes and protein should be replaced. Many of the principles of treating leg ulcers apply to management (section 14). Surgical intervention may be necessary for grafting, prevention of contractures and dealing with keloid formation.

17. Zinc Deficiency and the Skin

Acrodermatitis enteropathica is a rare disease, but an interesting and an important one to recognise and treat. Affected children 'fail to thrive', have diarrhoea, alopecia and recurrent blistering with secondary *Candida albicans* infections of the nail folds, mouth and perineum ('acrodermatitis'). Previously, treatment with di-iodohydroxyquinoline produced dramatic improvement, although the mechanism of action of the drug was not known and the children were at risk of developing optic atrophy from absorbed drug. It is now known that patients with acrodermatitis enteropathica have a low serum zinc concentration and the condition is completely controlled by zinc sulphate (Moynahan, 1974); the dosage depending on age, but being approximately 220mg daily.

Elemental feeding: Patients who are treated solely with elemental feeds develop rashes very similar to those of acrodermatitis enteropathica (Wexler and Pace, 1977). The skin lesions respond to zinc and correct management now consists of addition of zinc to elemental oral or intravenous feeds, for this will prevent the condition.

Wound healing: Zinc is necessary for healing and its possible role in healing stasis ulcers is discussed in section 14.1.

18. Vitiligo

This abnormality of pigmentation is probably of autoimmune aetiology. It is most unusual for spontaneous recovery to occur and treatment is unsatisfactory.

18.1 Symptomatic Treatment

Symptomatic treatment consists of: (1) sunscreen creams (see section 21.1.1) which pre-vent burning of the depigmented skin, and (2) cosmetic disguise with commercially available paints (e.g. artificial tanning preparations) or with dihydroxyacetone in 50:50 water and acetone. The concentration of dihydroxyacetone used determines the resultant skin colour and so it should be adjusted to suit the patient. 1% or 2% are reasonable concentrations to start with.

18.2 Attempts to Produce Repigmentation

These are usually not satisfactory but with increasing experience with psoralens in psoriasis, methods of using these drugs in vitiligo may improve and better results may follow. Trimethylpsoralen (trioxsalen) is the synthetic psoralen most used for photosensitising the skin in vitiligo. In sunny parts of the world, e.g. Egypt, it can be used with natural sunlight but in Western Europe and many parts of the USA this is unsatisfactory and the oral dose of psoralen must be followed in 2 hours by exposure to long wave ultraviolet light (UVA) from an artificial source. Management of the patient and precautions to be taken are similar to those of patients with psoriasis treated with PUVA therapy (see section 6.2.3). Trimethylpsoralen is used in a dosage of 40mg orally and the treatment given 2 or 3 times a week for about a year (Parrish et al., 1976). The minority show significant repigmentation in this time. Alternatively, trimethylpsoralen can be used as a paint; the application being followed 2 hours later by exposure to UVA.

18.3 Attempts to Counteract Autoimmune Reaction

This is a possible mechanism for the action of topical corticosteroids especially 0.05% clobetasol propionate which has been used in vitiligo and has been claimed to produce partial repigmentation, but only when used in amounts that also produced dermal atrophy (Clayton, 1977).

18.4 Attempts to Produce Depigmentation of Remaining Normal Skin

Permanent depigmentation can be produced by monobenzylether of hydroquinone (Mosher et al., 1977). It is only to be recommended in extensive vitiligo, or that which because of its site is particularly cosmetically disabling. A 20% paint is used twice daily and depigmentation usually takes from 3 to 12 months. Contact dermatitis is a possible complication.

19. Alopecia

There are many causes of hair loss, diffuse and patchy, scarring and non-scarring. The treatment of drug induced alopecia, scalp ringworm, and the scarring alopecia of discoid lupus erythematosus are discussed elsewhere (sections 22.2.3; 2.3.2; 13.4.1). A few other aspects are worth discussing here:

19.1 Alopecia Areata

This condition is related to the autoimmune group of diseases and as might be expected corticosteroids influence regrowth of hair. Except in very large doses however, systemic corticosteroid therapy does not alter the natural history of the disease so that the hair falls out again when the corticosteroid is stopped and this continues until spontaneous remission occurs (Winter et al., 1976). Systemic corticosteroids can rarely be justified in this disease. Intralesional triamcinolone injection can be used (see section 13.4.2) and corticosteroid creams can be tried. The immunopotentiating agent dinitrochlorobenzene, as a topical solution or ointment, is being investigated in persistent refractory cases (Happle and Echternacht, 1977; Daman et al., 1978).).

19.2 Male Pattern Alopecia

This requires the presence of circulating androgens as well as genetic factors for its production. The distribution of the hair loss with frontal recession and balding on the vertex is well known and these areas of scalp are most androgen sensitive. The success of hair transplants in this condition depends upon the fact that hair transplanted from the back (androgen insensitive) area to the bald area retains its properties at its new site and thus survives. The use of antiandrogens such as cyproterone in male pattern alopecia is still experimental.

19.3 Chronic Diffuse Alopecia

This type of alopecia is most troublesome in women and often has a hereditary basis so that results of treatment are extremely poor. It is important not to miss the relatively rare treatable causes of the condition, namely hypothyroidism and hypoferraemia. These should be treated by appropriate replacements.

19.4 Telogen Effluvium

The synchronous precipitation of hair into the resting (telogen) phase and its subsequent shedding is a not uncommon occurrence following serious illness or parturition. The prognosis is excellent and no treatment is required.

20. Skin Tumours and Naevi

Tumours both benign and malignant can arise from all anatomical components of skin including blood vessels, nerves, connective tissue, pigment cells and epidermis. Often, histological examination is necessary for diagnosis. Thus excision biopsy is the treatment of choice for the majority of solitary small tumours. Multiple benign tumours like skin tags and seborrhoeic warts (basal cell papillomata) can be removed by currettage or destroyed by heat, cold, acid or alkali.

20.1 Malignant and Premalignant Tumours

Malignant tumours of skin are often multiple and exposure to actinic radiation over the years is a common predisposing cause as in 'sailor's skin' and 'farmer's skin'. Those occupationally exposed to the sun should be encouraged to wear protective clothing or to use an effective sunscreen such as 5% para aminobenzoic acid in 55 to 75% ethyl alcohol on light exposed areas. Exposure to x-rays, contact with mineral oils, inorganic arsenic ingestion and hereditary factors are important in other cases. It is not uncommon for malignant epidermal tumours to be multiple and for premalignant tumours such as solar or senile keratoses to coexist.

Excision, radiotherapy and local destruction, e.g. by deep currettage and cautery, all have a role in treatment of malignant and premalignant tumours, but where they are multiple, chemotherapy is especially useful. 5-Fluorouracil cream (5%) is a commonly used preparation and is worth a trial in solar and senile keratoses, intraepidermal carcinomata and superficial basal cell carcinomata (Belisario, 1969; Klein, 1968). It should *not* be used for squamous cell carcinomata as these metastasise rapidly and require urgent treatment of a more radical nature: most basal cell carcinomata will not respond to chemotherapy either. Fluorouracil cream is irritant and patients should be told that inflammation may follow its use, although this is rarely severe enough to warrant stopping treatment.

Malignant melanomas are commonly treated by excision, sometimes together with removal of lymph nodes in the affected area. Chemotherapy with compounds with a special affinity for melanin is being investigated experimentally in animals and is not yet suitable for treatment in man.

20.2 Vascular Naevi

These constitute a considerable cosmetic problem whether they are of the 'strawberry' cavernous type or the 'port wine' capillary type.

The 'strawberry' naevus, although unsightly in infants, is likely to disappear within the first decade of life. The end result is best when the lesion is left to regress spontaneously but in certain situations (e.g. near the eye), active treatment with systemic corticosteroids, x-rays or plastic surgery may be necessary. The 'port wine' naevus does not as a rule regress and may increase in size with time. Usually, surgical removal is not practical and radiotherapy is ineffective. Fortunately, the lesion is as a rule flat and special opaquing cosmetics like 'Covermark' give satisfactory disguise, although they are time consuming to apply properly. Over tattooing with flesh coloured pigments is a possible alternative.

20.3 Mycosis Fungoides

Reticuloses such as Hodgkin's disease may involve the skin as well as other organs, but mycosis fungoides is by definition confined to the skin alone. It is a disease of abnormal T-cell proliferation and in extensive skin involvement systemic treatment with antimitotic drugs may be required as with other reticuloses, but generally topical treatment of the skin is preferable. Nitrogen mustard paint 0.5% or electron beam therapy are usually effective, at least for a time. Success has been claimed after deliberately sensitising the affected areas of the skin, for example with dinitrochlorbenzone: the consequent immunological reaction in the skin apparently results in disap-

Table VII. Rashes precipitated or aggravated by exposure to sunlight

---

1. *Rashes precipitated by sunlight*
   a) Lupus erythematosus (see section 13.1)
   b) Porphyria cutanea tarda (PCT) and erythropoetic protoporphyria (EPP)
   c) Solar urticaria
   d) Photosensitive drug eruptions (see section 22.3.11)
   e) Pellagra
   f) Polymorphic light eruption
   g) Some herpes simplex virus infections

2. *Rashes aggravated by sunlight*
   a) Eczema — especially atopic and seborrhoeic; 'actinic reticuloid'
   b) Rosacea
   c) Dermatomyositis
   d) Psoriasis (occasionally)

---

pearance of the tumour. Mycosis fungoides is one of the conditions in which PUVA therapy (see section 6.2.3) works for a time, although it is not yet known which of the many forms of the disease respond best or whether the treatment has any effect on the ultimate outcome of the disease.

21. Adverse Effects of Sunlight on the Skin

Sunlight has both acute and chronic effects on the skin. The acute ones are burning, the development of new rashes and the exacerbation of existing rashes: the chronic ones are hyperpigmentation, collagen degeneration and neoplasia. The precise wavelength involved is not always known but, except in industrial processes involving UVC (germicidal light 200 to 290nm), UVB (290 to 320nm) and/or UVA (320 to 400nm) are to blame. The wavelength responsible for some diseases is quite specific and can have important diagnostic and therapeutic consequences; e.g. radiation of wavelength 400nm produces the rash of porphyria and is transmitted through window glass, while light of shorter wavelength responsible for some other rashes is filtered off by this glass.

21.1 Acute Effects of Sunlight

21.1.1 Sunburn
When sunburn results from natural sunlight it is due to UVB, but high intensity UVA light as

part of PUVA treatment (see section 6.2.3) can produce a clinically similar (but pharmacologically different) response. Those with a relative or complete lack of protective melanin are particularly liable to sunburn and this includes fair skinned races, albinos and those with vitiligo. Those taking photosensitising drugs (table VIII) are also susceptible to sunburn.

Sunburn is most unpleasant and quite unnecessary. Prevention is far preferable to treatment and susceptible individuals should be particularly careful. It is most unwise to expose the skin to bright sunlight for long periods of time until a protective tan has developed, and some people never do tan. A number of sunscreen creams (see section 21.1.2) are available which do give some protection and aid tanning but they do not prevent burning completely in the susceptible. Vitamin A tablets are sold for prophylaxis of sunburn and are safe if the recommended dose is not exceeded, but the evidence that they work is not convincing (Furman, 1972). It is not safe for normal people to take antimalarials such as chloroquine, or psoralens (to produce a tan) merely to prevent sunburn. Principles of treatment of sunburn are discussed in section 16.

21.1.2 Photodermatoses

Rashes precipitated or made worse by the sun (photodermatoses) are summarised in table VII (Ramsay, 1975). Management involves protection of the skin from radiation, identification and treatment of specific photodermatoses and in some conditions use of systemic agents.

1) *Treat the specific disease* — e.g. porphyria cutanea tarda with venesection; vitiligo with psoralens and UVA; photosensitive drug eruptions by stopping the drug.

2) *Protect skin from radiation* with clothing and sunscreen creams (Lane-Brown, 1977; Poh-Fitzpatrick, 1977). Sunscreens can be divided into those that protect by physical and those that protect by chemical means. Physical sunscreens like zinc oxide, titanium dioxide and red veterinary petroleum are effective but are cosmetically unacceptable. Para aminobenzoic acid (PABA) 5% in alcohol, benzophenone 3% in alcohol and various preparations containing cinnamates are amongst the most commonly used chemical sunscreens. PABA is only effective in the ultraviolet light wavelength range 280 to 320nm, whereas the benzophenones absorb light up to about 360nm. Some mixtures containing cinnamates absorb light

up to the visible part of the spectrum and therefore are the most helpful preparations in 'actinic reticuloid' where the longer wavelength as well as the short often produces trouble. Should sunburn occur in spite of protection, principles of its treatment are discussed in section 16.

3) *Use of systemic drugs:* β-Carotene has been used in a number of photodermatoses but it is most worthwhile in erythropoetic protoporphyria (Pollitt, 1975). To be effective, it has to be used in doses which produce yellow discoloration of the skin. In an adult a reasonable starting dose would be 100mg daily.

Antimalarials are occasionally used. Hydroxychloroquine is probably less toxic that chloroquine and both are preferable to mepacrine because of the discoloration of the skin it produces. Hydroxychloroquine is most used in lupus erythematosus (section 13.1; 13.4.1) but is contraindicated in porphyria.

Indomethacin is an inhibitor of prostaglandin synthetase and in certain experimental situations is effective against UVB in preventing erythema. Its clinical use has not been proven. Antihistamines are effective in some cases of solar urticaria. Psoralens should *not* be used for tanning or for the prevention of sunburn, but only for serious dermatological disease.

21.2 Chronic Effects of Sunlight

Chronic effects of sunlight include hyperpigmentation, especially chloasma and poikiloderma of Civatte; collagen degeneration (e.g. 'solar elastosis') and importantly, malignant and premalignant changes. Solar keratoses, squamous cell carcinomas, basal cell carcinomas and possibly malignant melanomas are most common in light exposed skin. Patients with xeroderma pigmentosum who have a genetic defect of DNA repair after ultraviolet light damage are particularly liable to develop these skin cancers.

It is not known precisely what wavelengths are responsible for these skin effects of chronic ultraviolet light exposure in man, but susceptible individuals should be advised to use sunscreens which absorb over a wide range of the spectrum.

22. Drug Induced Skin Disease

The effects of drugs on the skin are legion (see Bruinsma, 1973) and the changes they produce are

Table VIII. Some dermatological reactions to drugs used systemically and topically

Skin reaction	Examples of implicated drugs (N.B. see also text. Not a comprehensive list)
Urticaria (possibly with accompanying angioneurotic oedema)	Penicillin; Aspirin; Sulphonamides; Barbiturates, Morphine
Erythematous rash	Barbiturates; Aspirin; Antibacterial agents
Acne or aggravation of existing acne	Corticosteroids; Androgenic and anabolic steroids; Phenobarbitone; Phenytoin (diphenylhydantoin); Oral contraceptives (some); Bromides; Iodides; Cytotoxic drugs; Isoniazid; PUVA therapy; Lithium; Danazol
Eczema from systemic drug (exfoliative dermatitis)	Gold; Organic arsenic
Eczema from contact with drug (contact dermatitis)	Topical antimicrobials (Penicillin; Streptomycin; Chloramphenicol; Neomycin; Sulphonamides); Topical local anaesthetics (except amide types); Topical antihistamines; Cream and lotion preservatives; Lanoline
Purpura (non-thrombocytopenic) (thrombocytopenic)	Corticosteroids; Anticoagulants; Aspirin; Carbromal, Meprobamate; Barbiturates; Thiazides; Sulphonamides; Sulphonylureas Cytotoxic drugs and other drugs which cause bone marrow suppression
Bullous reactions	Barbiturates (coma); Phenylbutazone (toxic epidermal necrolysis); Penicillamine (pemphigus); Nalidixic acid (photosensitivity); Frusemide/furosemide (photosensitivity; high doses in chronic renal failure)
Erythema multiforme (Stevens-Johnson syndrome; may be bullous)	Penicillin; Sulphonamides; Barbiturates; Phenylbutazone
Lichenoid eruptions	Gold; Antimalarials; Amiphenazole; PAS; Quinine; Quinidine
Fixed drug eruption	Phenolphthalein; Barbiturates; Phenylbutazone; Aspirin; Sulphonamides; Quinine; Tetracyclines
Photosensitivity from systemic and/or topical administration	Tetracyclines (e.g. demethylchlortetracycline); Phenothiazines (including some antihistamines); Griseofulvin; Nalidixic acid; Sulphonamides; Thiazides; Sulphonylureas; Frusemide/furosemide (high doses in chronic renal failure); Psoralens; Oral contraceptives (rarely). Topically applied Antihistamines, Sulphonamides, Halogenated salicylanilide antiseptics (e.g. soaps)
Systemic lupus erythematosus-like reaction	Hydrallazine; Procainamide; Phenytoin (diphenylhydantoin); Isoniazid; Practolol (psoriasiform rash but positive antinuclear factor)
Discolouration[1] (except due to drug induced jaundice, methaemoglobinaemia, etc.)	Brown — ACTH; Oral contraceptives (chloasma); Hydroxyurea; Iron; Silver; Arsenic Purple — Chlorpromazine Blue — Chloroquine; Hydroxychloroquine; Amodiaquine; Amantadine (elderly parkinsonian patients) Yellow — β-Carotene; Mepacrine (quinacrine) (greenish-bluish-grey discolouration of ears, nose, nail beds on prolonged use)
Alopecia	Anticoagulants, Cytotoxic drugs; Carbimazole; Trimethadione; Ethionamide; Oral contraceptives; Vitamin A (overdosage); Thallium; (not now used in therapeutics)

1   May be due to increased melanin deposition or to presence of drug or its metabolites in the skin. Sometimes drug and melanin are deposited together (e.g. haemosiderosis).

not always explicable on the basis of known pathological mechanisms: certainly, only the minority are strictly immunological reactions. Proof that a given drug is responsible is often extremely difficult, although in the majority of cases with careful history and examination, and where indicated rechallenge, it is possible to make a clinical diagnosis with some degree of confidence. Some of the more common dermatological reactions to drugs and those agents most often implicated are summarised in table VIII.

22.1 Diagnosis

Some of the difficulties which arise in the diagnosis of drug induced rashes and particularly in allocating the blame to a given drug are as follows:

1) *They are rarely specific,* so that a given drug is capable of producing different skin effects in different patients, and even in the same patient in different situations. The reverse is also true, since drugs of very different chemical structures and pharmacological actions are capable of producing the same rash.

2) *Direct proof that a given drug is responsible for a given rash is often difficult to obtain.* Few patients are given one drug at a time (see chapter VIII). Thus, even when it is fairly certain on morphological grounds that the rash is drug induced, it may be impossible to identify the culprit. Sometimes, the relationship in time of the appearance of the rash to the administration of the drug helps, but often it does not. Some rashes, e.g. those due to penicillin, have even been known to develop after the drug has been stopped. Diagnosis by stopping all drugs and then reintroducing them one by one is usually possible, but it is not entirely without its problems and dangers.

Some drugs such as ampicillin, may produce a rash in a given individual on one occasion but not necessarily on another; e.g. patients with infectious mononucleosis are prone to ampicillin rashes at that time (Almeyda and Levantine, 1972; McKenzie et al., 1976). In the case of serious drug reactions, systemic rechallenge may well be dangerous and this also applies to *in vivo* skin testing. For example, in true penicillin allergy death has been known to follow intradermal injection of as little as a few molecules of penicillin. *In vivo* skin testing in other situations may be unreliable, and unfortunately, of the many *in vitro* tests that

have been tried, none has proved infallible as a simple method of identifying the drug which has produced the rash.

Certainly, even after taking all the known facts into consideration it may still be impossible to say that the rash was *not* due to a given drug.

3) *Many of the diseases for which drugs are given can themselves produce rashes.* For instance, erythema multiforme and erythema nodosum, which are relatively common types of drug reactions, can be produced both by infections and by the antibiotic and other drugs used to combat them.

22.2 General Effects of Drugs on the Skin

22.2.1 Change in Skin Colour
When drugs do affect the skin they may do so by producing a diffuse or patchy change in skin colour. This may be due to deposition of the drug or its metabolites in the skin, as for instance in the case of silver and mepacrine, or to production of excessive melanin pigmentation as in the 'raindrop' pigmentation of arsenical poisoning. Often, the colour change is due to both accumulation of the drug and to increased melanin pigmentation, and this is known to be the case with iron and chlorpromazine.

Other colour changes in the skin are not due to alteration in the skin itself but reflect an alteration in the colour of the blood flowing through it. Such is the case in the various drug induced jaundices as well as in methaemoglobinaemia and sulphaemoglobinaemia caused by drugs such as the sulphonamides and sulphones (e.g. dapsone).

22.2.2 Skin Cancer: Infections
Drugs like arsenic and tar may predispose to skin cancer and produce precancerous lesions. Other drugs make the skin less resistant to infection with viruses, bacteria or fungi, such as can follow use of immunosuppressive and corticosteroid drugs (see section 2.3.1).

22.2.3 Effects on the Hair
Heparin, the coumarins, cytotoxic drugs, carbimazole, trimethadione, oral contraceptives, thallium and overdosage with vitamin A can all produce diffuse alopecia. With vitamin A intoxication, alopecia is accompanied by excessive dryness of the scalp and hair. In the case of the coumarin anticoagulants, there is shedding of large numbers

of club, resting or telogen hairs, while with cytotoxic drugs the hair is arrested in the growing or anagen phase, and then breaks off (Van Scott et al., 1957). Thallium is no longer used in therapeutics but cases of poisoning occasionally occur and the resulting alopecia seems to be the result of hairs being shed both in anagen and telogen phases.

Two types of alopecia have been described with oral contraceptives, a 'male pattern' alopecia with those containing the more androgenic progestagens and an excessive shedding of telogen hairs after stopping the more oestrogenic-containing preparations (Cormia, 1967; Editorial, 1973). Considering the numbers of contraceptive pills consumed at the present time, these side effects are found in a very small proportion of the population at risk.

The prognosis in the drug induced alopecias is excellent if the drug can be stopped and patients should be persuaded not to patronise expensive 'hair clinics' which have nothing to offer, that time will not also provide. A wig may be necessary during the acute episode.

Drugs which can cause hypertrichosis include minoxidil, a new antihypertensive agent (Earhart et al., 1977), oral diazoxide (Burton et al., 1976) and occasionally topical corticosteroids, usually after prolonged use (table IV).

22.2.4 Rashes

The greatest diagnostic difficulties arise with actual rashes induced by drugs. Here, an opinion from a dermatologist is worthwhile. As discussed in section 22.1, his task may well be impossible and he can often do no more than make an intelligent guess at the offending drug. This 'informed guess' may be no better than that of his non-dermatological colleagues. A dermatologist can however, describe the reaction in precise dermatological terms and allocate it to one of the clinical types, which may be useful for future reference. He is also usually the best person to advise on the management of the reaction which in severe cases, e.g. of erythroderma, toxic epidermal necrolysis, may be so serious that the correct treatment for the skin can make all the difference between life and death.

22.3 Clinical Types of Skin Reactions

Individual lesions may be urticarial, erythematous, acneform, eczematous, purpuric, bullous and lichenoid. Clinically recognisable patterns include erythema multiforme, erythema nodosum, the 'fixed' eruption and rashes which involve predominantly the light exposed areas of the skin. Rarely, drugs 'induce' lupus erythematosus (see chapter XXII; sect. 14.1) or porphyria and then the rashes characteristic of these diseases may appear. In psoriatic individuals, any rash, including one produced by a drug, may take on psoriatic features. The β-adrenoceptor blocking drug practolol has also caused a psoriasiform reaction (Felix et al., 1974), but its psoriatic appearance is not confined to those with a genetic predisposition to psoriasis and it is not a general property of other β-blockers (Brigden and Almeyda, 1976).

22.3.1 Urticaria

Many drugs can produce urticaria and this is one of the most common skin reactions produced by drugs. Such reactions are potentially dangerous since there may be accompanying swelling of the mouth and larynx from angioedema, as well as bronchospasm and hypotension. Some urticarias are produced by an allergic mechanism. Apart from the various antisera which may be responsible, penicillin and aspirin are two of the most common drug causes. In such patients, death may follow injection of as little as a few molecules in the course of skin testing, so these tests should never be carried out unless full resuscitative measures, including intravenous hydrocortisone succinate, are available. Urticaria can also be produced by drugs which act as histamine liberators; for example aspirin and morphine. Thus aspirin is one of the drugs which can cause urticaria by allergic or non-allergic mechanisms.

22.3.2 Erythema

Erythematous rashes of various patterns are another common form of drug rash. Barbiturates, aspirin and antibiotics are common culprits. In general, the rashes, although uncomfortable, are not dangerous and some disappear even with continued use of the responsible drug.

22.3.3 Acne

Corticosteroids, cytotoxic drugs and androgens produce acne, as do isoniazid, iodides and bromides when given over relatively long periods of time. Phenobarbitone and phenytoin (diphenylhydantoin) appear to aggravate existing acne. Some progestagens (e.g. certain oral contraceptive formulations) may also make acne worse (section 4.2).

22.3.4 Eczema (dermatitis)

Eczematous reactions to drugs are most often produced by contact with the drug — by topical application of the drug, or by the handling of the drug. Medicaments most likely to produce contact sensitivity are topical antibiotics, especially penicillin, streptomycin, chloramphenicol and neomycin (see also section 7.1); sulphonamides; and local anaesthetics (except amide types such as lignocaine) and antihistamines. Preservatives in creams and lotions (e.g. parabens, chlorocresol; Shorr, 1968) or their stabilisers (e.g. ethylene diamine hydrochloride; White et al., 1978) may occasionally cause contact sensitivity. Of the drugs handled by nurses, streptomycin and chlorpromazine have produced much trouble from contact sensitivity in the past, but now that the problem is recognised and efforts are made to prevent contact with the nurse's skin, such undesirable effects of these drugs should be almost completely preventable.

Contact dermatitis is one of the few adverse reactions of the skin to drugs in which it is relatively easy to make a firm diagnosis as a result of challenge with the suspected drug — in this case by patch testing with a small amount of the suspected substance (the exact amount and concentration suitable for patch testing and the form and base in which it should be applied is known for most substances as a result of previous trial and error, and this information is available in standard text books dealing with the subject). An eczematous reaction present at 48 to 96 hours after applying the substance under an occlusive dressing indicates a 'delayed' type of hypersensitivity reaction to that substance. Eczematous reactions to drugs are not all due to 'delayed' hypersensitivity, for some are due to nonspecific irritation by the substance. Formalin, for example, can produce a nonspecific eczema as well as a contact sensitivity. Patch testing is not designed to diagnose these nonspecific reactions.

Eczema is less often produced by drugs given systemically. Occasionally, there is 'lighting up' of a patch of contact dermatitis when the allergen or a related substance is given systemically. This may occur, for instance, in a suspender dermatitis due to contact with nickel when at a later date a blood transfusion is given through a needle which contains nickel. Other eczematous reactions to systemic medication do occur and extreme examples of this are the exfoliative dermatitis which sometimes follows injections of gold or organic arsenic. These reactions can be extremely serious and can result in death.

22.3.5 Vasculitis and Purpura

Drug induced purpura can arise by a number of different mechanisms. For example, by depression of platelet formation in the bone marrow as with the cytotoxic drugs or chloramphenicol, or by destruction of formed platelets by an allergic mechanism as in apronal (Sedormid) purpura. In either case there will be thrombocytopenia. In cases where the platelet count is normal, the drug may interfere with other aspects of the clotting mechanism, or there may be damage to the blood vessel walls or their supporting ground substance. Aspirin is an example of a drug which causes purpura partly by interfering with prothrombin formation.

A number of drugs can produce vasculitis, and purpura resembling that of Henoch Schonlein disease will result if small arteries are affected. The capillaries of the skin are often affected in drug reactions and the purpuras which then result are associated with a decreased capillary resistance, as shown by a positive Hess' test. One of the most easily recognisable drug eruptions is that produced by carbromal. The rash consists of fine purpura ('cayenne pepper') and scaling and is usually most marked on the lower legs. Histologically, there is eczema and capillaritis. Meprobamate and barbiturates occasionally produce an identical rash. Corticosteroids, by virtue of a deleterious action on the collagen of the ground substance which supports the capillaries, can produce purpura, which clinically resembles senile purpura (Shuster and Scarborough, 1961). Corticosteroids have this effect whether they are used topically or systemically.

22.3.6 Bullous Reactions

Blisters are not uncommonly seen in unconscious patients. The impression that such blisters are particularly common when the unconsciousness is due to a barbiturate is probably false, as blisters are seen in patients unconscious from other causes. The 'scalded skin' syndrome or toxic epidermal necrolysis (Lyell's disease) is characterised by extensive superficial blistering of the skin (Lyell, 1967). The disease is extremely serious, as a number of affected patients, especially adults, die. In adults, most of the cases are due to drugs and phenylbutazone is one of the most common responsible. A similar clinical picture can occur in children in whom it is more likely to be due to a staphylococcal infection eminently treatable by large doses of an appropriate antibiotic such as cloxacillin or flucloxacillin. Blisters also occur in the course of eczematous and urticarial drug reactions and of erythema multiforme, in 'fixed' drug reactions and in rashes induced by sunlight. Some drugs, e.g. griseofulvin, can produce blisters by precipitating porphyria in those with latent disease (Felsher and Redeker, 1967). Pemphigus has been associated with use of D-penicillamine in rheumatoid arthritis (Marsden et al., 1976) and can present with both oral and cutaneous lesions (Hay et al., 1978). Large doses of frusemide (furosemide) in patients with chronic renal failure can produce blisters in areas exposed to sunlight (Burry and Lawrence, 1976; Heydenreich et al., 1977).

22.3.7 Lichenoid Eruptions

Rashes indistinguishable from lichen planus may be induced by drugs, e.g. gold, antimalarials and amiphenazole.

22.3.8 Erythema Multiforme

The characteristic lesions consist of concentric circles of erythema and are 'target' or 'iris' like. They are usually most numerous on the hands and feet. Occasionally, blisters and purpura are seen. In the severe variant, the Stevens-Johnson syndrome, there is in addition pyrexia and lesions of the eyes, mouth and genitalia. The disease may be precipitated by an infection or by drugs and it may be difficult to decide whether to blame the infection or the drug given for the infection. The disease may be extremely serious and patients may die from renal involvement. Treatment is discussed in sections 12.4 and 22.4.2.

22.3.9 Erythema Nodosum

This may be drug induced, but streptococcal infection, sarcoidosis and tuberculosis, as well as less common causes like ulcerative colitis, have to be excluded.

22.3.10 'Fixed' Drug Eruption

This is a localised skin lesion in which there are plaques, usually of a dusky colour, which each time a drug is given systemically reappear in exactly the same site, i.e. the site is fixed. The plaques occasionally blister and afterwards leave areas of hyperpigmentation. The drug most often involved is probably phenolphthalein which the patient has taken as a constituent of one of a number of proprietary purgatives. Many other drugs have been implicated (e.g. barbiturates, phenylbutazone, salicylates, sulphonamides and derivatives; Sehgal et al., 1978).

22.3.11 Rashes on Light Exposed Areas

Photosensitivity may be induced by a drug applied to the skin or by a drug given systemically (Pathak and Fitzpatrick, 1972). The drug induced photosensitivities are usually eczematous. In some, there is evidence of an immunological reaction but in others there is not. Many of the drug induced photosensitivities are caused by ultraviolet light of longer wave length; i.e. about 350nm. In some cases, the wave length which does the damage corresponds to the maximum absorption spectrum of the drug. Drugs which induce lupus erythematosus (e.g. hydrallazine, procainamide) or porphyria (e.g. griseofulvin) will also lead to photosensitivity in those so predisposed. Topically applied drugs which produce UV light sensitivity reactions include antihistamines, sulphonamides and the halogenated salicylanilide antiseptics. Systemically administered drugs which produce photosensitivity include the tetracyclines, especially demethylchlortetracycline (demeclocycline) and doxycycline but probably not minocycline, the phenothiazines, some antihistamines, and psoralens, nalidixic acid, frusemide (high doses in chronic renal failure) and sulphonamides and their derivatives (e.g. oral sulphonylureas, thiazides). Oral contraceptives may occasionally cause photosensitivity (Erickson and Peterka, 1968).

22.3.12 Topical Corticosteroids

The adverse effects on the skin of topically applied corticosteroids are summarised in table IV (for review, see Burry, 1973).

22.4 Management of Rashes Induced by Drugs

22.4.1 Diagnosis by Challenge

The difficulty of precise diagnosis in a large number of cases has been discussed above. In general, it is not only the bedside diagnosis that is difficult, for laboratory tests as well as intradermal and patch tests (except in cases of contact dermatitis) on the patient at a later date, rarely help. The decision whether or not to challenge the patient with a drug that is suspected of causing the reaction is sometimes difficult, and must in the end depend upon the individual case.

If the initial drug reaction has been a serious one, e.g. a severe exfoliative dermatitis or a toxic epidermal necrolysis, it would be extremely unwise to give even a small dose of the suspected drug again. The usual advice is not to give the patient the implicated drug on any future occasion. Occasionally, however, it might be vital to know which of several possible drugs has caused a reaction so that it becomes necessary to challenge the patient; for example in a patient who had reacted to a combination of drugs he was taking for tuberculosis.

With less serious reactions, e.g. a possible carbromal induced purpura, challenge would almost certainly be a completely safe procedure. In all cases in which challenge is done, its limitations must of course be borne in mind. If a patient does not respond to the challenge, it does not rule out the possibility that the initial reaction was caused by the drug.

22.4.2 Treatment

The most important part of treatment is usually to stop the drug suspected of causing the rash. In the case of severe reactions, however, other measures may be required. Urgent treatment will of course be needed in severe urticarial reactions accompanied by collapse or difficulty in breathing. Intravenous hydrocortisone succinate should be given together with adrenaline (epinephrine), and measures should be taken to ensure that an airway is maintained, if necessary by tracheotomy (see section 10.1). Simple urticarial drug reactions, whether they are allergic or not, will nearly always be suppressed by adequate doses of a systemic antihistamine. Cases of toxic epidermal necrolysis as well as severe cases of exfoliative dermatitis, Stevens-Johnson syndrome and 'allergic vasculitis' due to drugs will usually need systemic corticosteroids. Other treatment will be symptomatic. If the rash is inflammatory and itches, a corticosteroid cream can be applied and an antihistamine given by mouth.

When it is essential for a drug to be continued, even though it is known to be responsible for a rash, it may be possible to suppress the reaction by giving systemic corticosteroids at the same time. It should be remembered though, that the skin is not necessarily the only organ which is reacting adversely and it is important not to assume that because the rash has disappeared, more important organs such as the kidneys, eyes, liver or bone marrow, are necessarily free from the adverse effects of the drug. If these are left unheeded the patient may die from toxic effects of the drug. On the other hand, in some cases, the appearance of a rash in a patient on a drug may be important in drawing attention to impaired renal function and the need to modify the dosage of the drug.

Further Reading

Rook, A.; Wilkinson, D.S. and Ebling, F.J.G.: Textbook of Dermatology, 3rd ed (Blackwell Scientific, Oxford 1978).

Soter, N.A.; Wilkinson, D.S. and Fitzpatrick, M.D.: Clinical dermatology. New England Journal of Medicine 289: 189, 242, 296 (1973).

References

Agostoni, A.; Marasoni, B.; Licardi, M. and Martignoni, G.C.: Intermittent therapy with danazol in hereditary angiodema. Lancet 1: 453 (1978).

Allenby, C.F.: The treatment of viral warts with glutaraldehyde. British Journal of Clinical Practice 31: 12 (1977).

Almeyda, J. and Levantine, A.: Adverse cutaneous reactions to the penicillins-ampicillin rashes. British Journal of Dermatology 87: 294 (1972).

Anderson, A.S.; Galdys, G.J.; Green, R.C.; Hohisel, D.W. and Brown, E.P.: Improved reduction of cutaneous bacteria and free fatty acids with new benzoyl peroxide gel. Cutis 16: 307 (1975).

Anthony, B.F.; Perlman, L.V. and Wannamaker, L.W.: Skin infection and acute glomerulonephritis in American Indian children. Pediatrics 39: 263 (1967).

Baer, R.L.; Leshaw, S.M. and Shalita, A.R.: High dose tetracycline therapy in severe acne. Archives of Dermatology 112: 479 (1976).

Bandman, N.H.; Calnan, C.D.; Cronin, E.; Fregert, S.; Hjorth, N.; Magnusson, B.; Maibach, H.; Malten, K.E.; Meneghini, C.J.; Pirila, V. and Wilkinson, D.S.: Dermatitis from applied medicaments. Archives of Dermatology 106: 335 (1972).

Bassett, D.C.J.: Streptococcal pyoderma and acute nephritis in Trinidad. British Journal of Dermatology 86(Suppl. 8): 55 (1971).

Belisario, J.C.: Topical cytotoxic therapy of solar keratoses with 5-fluorouracil. Medical Journal of Australia 2: 1136 (1969).

Brigden, W.D. and Almeyda, J.: Adverse reaction to the β-adrenergic blocking drugs. British Journal of Dermatology 95: 335 (1976).

Bruinsma, W.: A Guide to Drug Eruptions (Excerpta Medica, Amsterdam 1973).

Bunney, M.H.: The treatment of viral warts. Drugs 13: 445 (1977).

Burry, J.N.: Adverse effects of fluorinated corticosteroid creams and ointments. Medical Journal of Australia 1: 393 (1973).

Burry, J.N. and Lawrence, J.R.: Phototoxic blisters from high frusemide dosage. British Journal of Dermatology 94: 495 (1976).

Burton, J.L.; Schutt, W.H. and Caldwell, I.: Hypertrichosis due to diazoxide. British Journal of Dermatology 93: 707 (1976).

Burton, J.L.; Harman, R.R.M.; Peachey, R.D.G. and Warin, R.P.: Azathioprine plus prednisone in treatment of pemphigoid. British Medical Journal 2: 1190 (1978).

Carslaw, R.W.; Dobson, R.M.; Hood, A.J.K. and Taylor, R.N.: Mites in the environment of cases of Norwegian scabies. British Journal of Dermatology 92: 333 (1975).

Chamberlain, M.J.; Reynolds, A.L. and Yeoman, W.B.: Toxic effect of podophyllin application in pregnancy. British Medical Journal 3: 391 (1972).

Chilcote, R.; Curley, A.; Loughlin, H.H. and Jupin, J.A.: Hexachlorophene storage in a burn patient associated with encephalopathy. Pediatrics 59: 457 (1977).

Christiansen, J.V.; Gadborg, E.; Kleiter, I.; Ludvigsen, K.; Meier, C.H.K.; Norholm, A.; Reiter, H.; Reymann, F.; Raaschou-Nielsen, W.; Sondergaard, M.; Unna, P. and Wehnert, R.: Efficacy of bufexamac (NFN) cream in skin diseases. A double-blind multicentre trial. Dermatologica 154: 177 (1977).

Clayton, R.: Treatment of vitiligo with clobetasol propionate. British Journal of Dermatology 96: 71 (1977).

Coldman, M.F.; Lockerbie, L. and Laws, E.A.: The evaluation of several topical corticosteroid preparations in the blanching test. British Journal of Dermatology 85: 381 (1971).

Comaish, J.S.; Smith, J. and Seville, R.H.: Factors affecting the clearance of psoriasis with dithranol (anthralin). British Journal of Dermatology 84: 282 (1971).

Cormia, F.E.: Alopecia from oral contraceptives. Journal of the American Medical Association 201: 635 (1967).

Cornell, R.C.; Milstein, H.G.; Fox, R.M. and Stoughton, R.B.: Anaemia of azaribine in the treatment of psoriasis. Archives of Dermatology 112: 1717 (1976).

Craig, F.N.; Cummings, E.G. and Sim, V.M.: Environmental temperature and the absorption of a cholinesterase inhibitor, XV. Journal of Investigative Dermatology 68: 357 (1977).

Cream, J.J. and Scott, G.L.: Anaemia in dermatitis herpetiformis. The role of dapsone induced haemolysis and malabsorption. British Journal of Dermatology 82: 333 (1970).

Cullen, S.I. and Catalano, P.M.: Griseofulvin-warfarin antagonism. Journal of the American Medical Association 199: 582 (1967).

Dahl, M.G.C.; Gregory, M.M. and Scheuer, P.J.: Methotrexate hepatotoxicity in psoriasis — Comparison of different dose regimens. British Medical Journal 1: 654 (1972).

Daman, L.A.; Rosenberg, E.W. and Drake, L.: Treatment of alopecia areata with dinitrochlorobenzene. Archives of Dermatology 114: 1036 (1978).

Eaglstein, W.H.; Katz, R. and Brown, J.A.: Use of steroids in herpes zoster. Journal of the American Medical Association 211: 1681 (1970).

Earhart, R.N.; Ball, J.; Nuss, D.D. and Aeling, J.L.: Minoxidil-induced hypertrichosis: Treatment with calcium thioglycolate depilatory. Southern Medical Journal 70: 442 (1977).

Editorial: Hair loss and contraceptives. British Medical Journal 2: 499 (1973).

Ellard, G.A.; Gammon, P.T.; Savin, J.A. and Tan, R.S.H.: Dapsone acetylation in dermatitis herpetiformis. British Journal of Dermatology 90: 441 (1974).

Epstein, W.L.; Shah, V.P. and Riegelman, S.: Griseofulvin levels in stratum corneum. Study after oral administration in man. Archives of Dermatology 106: 344 (1972).

Erickson, I.R. and Peterka, E.S.: Sunlight sensitivity from oral contraceptives. Journal of the American Medical Association 201: 980 (1968).

Esterly, N.B. and Markowitz, M.: The treatment of pyoderma in children. Journal of the American Medical Association 212: 1667 (1970).

Feiwel, M.: Percutaneous absorption of topical steroids in children. British Journal of Dermatology 81(Suppl. 4): 113 (1969).

Felber, T.D.; Smith, E.B.; Knox, J.M.; Wallis, C. and Melnick, J.L.: Photodynamic inactivation of herpes simplex. Report of a clinical trial. Journal of the American Medical Association 223: 289 (1973).

Felix, R.H.; Ive, F.A. and Dahl, M.G.C.: Cutaneous and ocular reactions to practolol. British Medical Journal 4: 321 (1974).

Felsher, B.F. and Redeker, A.G.: Acute intermittent porphyria: effect of diet and griseofulvin. Medicine (Baltimore) 46: 217 (1967).

Floden, C.H. and Wikstrom, K.: Controlled clinical trial with dextranomer (Debrisan) on venous leg ulcers. Current Therapeutic Research 24: 753 (1978).

Frank, S.B.: Topical treatment of acne with a tetracycline preparation: Results of a multi-group study. Cutis 17: 539 (1976).

Frank, M.M.; Gelfand, J.A. and Atkinson, J.P.: Hereditary angioedema: the clinical syndrome and its management. Annals of Internal Medicine 84: 580 (1976).

Furman, K.I.: Sylvasun and prevention of sun-trauma. South African Medical Journal 46: 1670 (1972).

Gelfand, J.A.; Sherins, R.J.; Alling, D.W. and Frank, M.M.: Treatment of hereditary angioedema with danazol: Reversal of clinical and biochemical abnormalities. New England Journal of Medicine 295: 1444 (1976).

Ginsburg, C.M.; Lowry, W. and Reisch, J.S.: Absorption of lindane (gamma benzene hexachloride) in infants and children. Journal of Pediatrics 91: 998 (1977).

Goihman-Yahr, M.; Fernandez, J.; Boatswain, A. and Convit, J.: Unilateral dinitrochlorobenzene immunopathy of recalcitrant warts. Lancet 1: 447 (1978).

Gould, D.J. and Cunliffe, W.J.: The long-term treatment of acne vulgaris. Clinical and Experimental Dermatology 3: 249 (1978).

Greaves, M.W.; Burton, J.L.; Marks, Janet and Dawber, R.P.R.: Azathioprine in treatment of bullous pemphigoid. British Medical Journal 1: 144 (1971).

Greaves, M.; Marks, R. and Robertson, I.: Receptors for histamine in human skin blood vessels: a review. British Journal of Dermatology 97: 225 (1977).

Grupper, C.: The chemistry, pharmacology and use of tar in the treatment of psoriasis; in Farber and Cox (Eds) Psoriasis, Proceedings of the International Symposium, Stanford University 1971 (Stanford University Press, Stanford 1971).

Haider, S.A.: Treatment of atopic eczema in children: clinical trial of 10% sodium cromoglycate ointment. British Medical Journal 1: 1570 (1977).

Hakim, R.E.; Griffin, A.C. and Knox, J.M.: Erythema and tumour formation in methoxsalen treated mice exposed to fluorescent light. Archives of Dermatology 82: 572 (1960).

Hall, J.H. and Lupton, E.S.: Tetracycline therapy for acne: Incidence of vaginitis. Cutis 20: 97 (1977).

Happle, R. and Echternacht, K.: Induction of hair growth in alopecia areata with D.N.C.B. Lancet 2: 1002 (1977).

Hawkins, T.; Marks, J.M.; Plummer, V.M. and Greaves, M.W.: Whole body monitoring of zinc 65 retention in patients with leg ulceration and minimal dermatoses. Clinical and Experimental Dermatology 1: 243 (1976).

Hay, K.D.; Muller, H.K. and Reade, P.C.: D-penicillamine-induced mucocutaneous lesions with features of pemphigus. Oral Surgery, Oral Medicine, Oral Pathology 45: 385 (1978).

Heel, R.C.; Brogden, R.N.; Speight, T.M. and Avery, G.S.: Vitamin A acid: A review of its pharmacological properties and therapeutic use in the topical treatment of acne vulgaris. Drugs 14: 401 (1977).

Heydenreich, G.; Pindborg, T. and Schmidt, H.: Bullous dermatitis among patients with chronic renal failure on high dose frusemide. Acta Medica Scandinavica 202: 61 (1977).

Honigsmann, H.; Gschnait, F.; Konrad, K. and Wolff, K.: Photochemotherapy for psoriasis (Von Zumbusch). British Journal of Dermatology 97: 119 (1977).

Hunter, J.A.A.: The structure and function of skin in relation to therapy. British Medical Journal 4: 340 (1973). The basis of skin therapy. British Medical Journal 4: 411 (1973).

Juel-Jensen, B.E.; MacCallum, F.O.; Mackenzie, A.M.R. and Pike, M.C.: Treatment of zoster with idoxuridine in dimethyl sulphoxide. British Medical Journal 4: 776 (1970).

Keipert, J.A.: Therapeutic implications of percutaneous absorption of topical corticosteroid in infancy and childhood. Medical Journal of Australia 2: 315 (1971).

Klein, E.: Tumours of the skin. IX. Local cytotoxic therapy of cutaneous and mucosal premalignant and malignant lesions. New York State Journal of Medicine 68: 886 (1968).

Kligman, A.M.: An overview of acne. Journal of Investigative Dermatology 62: 268 (1974).

Knight, A.G. and Vickers, C.F.H.: A follow-up of tetracycline-treated rosacea with special reference to rosacea keratitis. British Journal of Dermatology 93: 577 (1975).

Knudsen, E.A.: Fluocinolone-plastic treatment in severe psoriasis: a comparative study. Acta Dermatovenereologica 45: 50 (1965).

Koch-Weser, J. and Sellers, E.M.: Drug interactions with coumarin anticoagulants. New England Journal of Medicine 285: 487, 547 (1971).

Lane-Brown, M.: New concepts in prevention and treatment of sunburn. Drugs 13: 366 (1977).

Leyden, J.J. and Kligman, A.M.: Acne vulgaris: New concepts in pathogenesis and treatment. Drugs 12: 292 (1976).

Leyden, J.J. and Kligman, A.H.: The case for steroid-antibiotic combinations. British Journal of Dermatology 96: 179 (1977).

Lin, C. and Symchowicz, S.: Absorption, distribution, metabolism and excretion of griseofulvin in man and animals. Drug Metabolism Reviews 4: 75 (1975).

Lyell, A.: A review of toxic epidermal necrolysis in Britain. British Journal of Dermatology 79: 662 (1967).

MacCallum, F.O. and Juel-Jensen, B.E.: Herpes simplex virus skin infections in man treated with idoxuridine in dimethyl sulphoxide. British Medical Journal 2: 805 (1966).

McCullough, J.L.; Snyder, D.S.; Weinstein, G.D.; Friedland, A. and Stein, B.: Factors affecting human percutaneous penetration of methotrexate and its analogues in vitro. Journal of Investigative Dermatology 66: 103 (1976).

McKenzie, H.; Parratt, D. and White, R.G.: IgM and IgG antibody levels to ampicillin in patients with infectious mononucleosis. Clinical and Experimental Immunology 26: 214 (1976).

Malaviya, A.N.; Many, A. and Schwartz, R.S.: Treatment of dermatomyositis with methotrexate. Lancet 2: 485 (1968).

Marks, J.; Shuster, S. and Watson, A.J.: Small bowel changes in dermatitis herpetiformis. Lancet 2: 1280 (1966).

Marsden, R.A.; Ryan, T.J.; Vanhegan, R.I.; Walshe, M.; Hill, H. and Mowat, A.G.: Pemphigus foliaceus induced by penicillamine. British Medical Journal 2: 1423 (1976).

Matthew, D.J.; Norman, A.P.; Taylor, B.; Turner, M.W. and Soothill, J.F.: Prevention of eczema. Lancet 1: 321 (1977).

Maunder, J.W.: Community Medicine 126: 145 (1971).

Melnick, J.L. and Wallis, C.: Photodynamic inactivation of herpes simplex virus: A status report. Annals of the New York Academy of Sciences 284: 171 (1977).

Melski, J.W.; Tanenbaum, L.; Parrish, J.A.; Fitzpatrick, T.B.; Bleich, H.L. et al.: Oral methoxsalen photochemotherapy for the treatment of psoriasis: a co-operative clinical trial. Journal of Investigative Dermatology 68: 328 (1977).

Michaelsson, G.; Juhlin, L. and Ljunghall, K.: A double-blind study of the effect of zinc and oxytetracycline in acne vulgaris. British Journal of Dermatology 97: 561 (1977).

Millard, L.G.; Roberts, M.M. and Gatecliffe, M.: Chronic leg ulcers treated by the pinch graft method. British Journal of Dermatology 97: 289 (1977).

Monaco, F.; Agnetti, V. and Mutani, R.: Benign intercranial hypertension after minocycline therapy. European Neurology 17: 48 (1978).

Morrison, W.I.; Parrish, J.A. and Fitzpatrick, T.B.: Controlled study of PUVA and adjunctive therapy in management of psoriasis. British Journal of Dermatology 98: 125 (1978).

Mosher, D.B.; Parrish, J.A. and Fitzpatrick, T.B.: Monobenzylether of hydroquinone. A retrospective study of 18 vitiligo patients and a review of the literature. British Journal of Dermatology 97: 669 (1977).

Moynahan, E.J.: Acrodermatitis enteropathica. A lethal inherited human zinc deficiency disorder. Lancet 2: 399 (1974).

Munro, D.D.; Robinson, T.W.E.; duVivier, A.W.P.; France, D.M.; Clayton, R. and Sparkes, C.G.: Betamethasone valerate ointment compared with fluocinonide FAPG. Use in the treatment of psoriasis and eczema. Archives of Dermatology 113: 599 (1977).

Nierman, M.M.: Treatment of dermal and decubitus ulcers. Drugs 15: 226 (1978).

Nimni, M.E.: Mechanism of inhibition of collagen cross-linking by penicillamine. Proceedings of the Royal Society of Medicine 70(Suppl. 3): 65 (1977).

Noble, W.C. and Naidoo, J.: Evolution of antibiotic resistance in Staphylococcus aureus: the role of the skin. British Journal of Dermatology 98: 481 (1978).

Olejniczak, S. and Zielinski, A.: Topical oxygen promotes healing of leg ulcers. Resident and Staff Physician 23(8): 16S (1977).

Orris, L.; Shalita, A.R.; Sibulkin, D. and Gans, E.H.: Oral zinc therapy of acne: Absorption and clinical effect. Archives of Dermatology 114: 1018 (1978).

Pace, W.E.: Treatment of cutaneous ulcers with benzoyl peroxide. Canadian Medical Association Journal 115: 1101 (1976).

Parrish, J.A.; Fitzpatrick, T.B.; Tanenbaum, L. and Pathak, M.A.: Photochemotherapy of psoriasis with oral methoxsalen and long wave ultraviolet light. New England Journal of Medicine 291: 1207 (1974).

Parrish, J.A.; Fitzpatrick, T.B.; Shea, C. and Pathak, M.A.: Photochemotherapy of vitiligo. Archives of Dermatology 112: 1531 (1976).

Pathak, M. and Fitzpatrick, T.B.: Photosensitivity caused by drugs. Rational Drug Therapy 6: 1 (June 1972).

Perera, P.: An investigation of varicose ulcers. Transactions of the St. Johns Hospital Dermatological Society 56: 175 (1970).

Perry, H.O.; Soderstrom, C.W. and Schulze, R.W.: The Goeckerman treatment of psoriasis. Archives of Dermatology 98: 178 (1968).

Phillips, A.; Davidson, M. and Greaves, M.W.: Venous leg ulceration: evaluation of zinc treatment, serum zinc and rate of healing. Clinical and Experimental Dermatology 2: 395 (1977).

Poh-Fitzpatrick, M.B.: The biologic actions of solar radiation on skin with a note on sunscreens. Journal of Dermatological Surgery and Oncology 3: 199 (1977).

Polano, M.K. and Schothorst, A.A.: Difference in the efficiency of two delivery forms of 8-methoxypsoralen. Dermatologica 154: 216 (1977).

Pollitt, N.: β-Carotene and the photodermatoses. British Journal of Dermatology 93: 721 (1975).

Poulson, B.J.; Young, E.; Coquilla, V. and Katz, M.: Effect of topical vehicle composition on the *in vitro* release of fluocinolone acetonide and its acetate ester. Journal of Pharmaceutical Sciences 57: 928 (1968).

Prottey, C.; Hartop, P.J. and Pross, M.: Correction of the cutaneous manifestations of fatty acid deficiency in man by application of sunflower-seed oil. Journal of Investigative Dermatology 64: 223 (1975).

Pye, R.J. and Burton, J.L.: Treatment of rosacea by metronidazole. Lancet 1: 1211 (1976).

Pye, R.J.; Meyrick, G.; Pye, M.J. and Burton, J.L.: Effect of oral contraceptives on sebum excretion rate. British Medical Journal 2: 1581 (1977).

Ramsay, C.A. Photosensitivity and the skin. British Journal of Hospital Medicine 13: 536 (1975).

Rasmussen, J.E.: A new look at old acne. Pediatric Clinics of North America 25: 285 (1978).

Rogers, S.; Marks, J.; Briffa, D.V.; Warin, A. and Greaves, M.: Comparison of photochemotherapy and dithranol in the treatment of chronic plaque psoriasis. Lancet 1: 455 (1979).

Savin, J.A. and Noble, W.C.: Immunosuppression and skin infection. British Journal of Dermatology 93: 115 (1975).

Sawyer, P.R.; Brogden, R.N.; Pinder, R.M.; Speight, T.M. and Avery, G.S.: Clotrimazole: A review of its antifungal activity and therapeutic efficacy. Drugs 9: 424 (1975).

Schalla, W.; Schaefer, H.; Kammerau, B. and Zesch, A.: Pharmacokinetics of 8-methoxypsoralen (8-MOP) after oral and local application. Journal of Investigative Dermatology 66: 258 (1976).

Scheuplein, R.J.: Percutaneous absorption after twenty-five years: or "old wine in new wineskins". Journal of Investigative Dermatology 69: 31 (1976).

Scoggins, R.B. and Kliman, B.: Percutaneous absorption of corticosteroids: Systemic effects. New England Journal of Medicine 273: 831 (1965).

Sehgal, V.N.; Rege, V.L. and Kharangate, V.N.: Fixed drug eruptions caused by medications: A report from India. International Journal of Dermatology 17: 78 (1978).

Seville, R.H.: Dithranol paste for psoriasis. British Journal of Dermatology 78: 269 (1966).

Seville, R.H.: Simplified dithranol treatment for psoriasis. British Journal of Dermatology 93: 205 (1975).

Sheffer, A.L.; Austen, K.F. and Rosen, F.S.: Tranexamic acid therapy in hereditary angioneurotic edema. New England Journal of Medicine 287: 452 (1972).

Shorr, W.F.: Paraben allergy. Journal of the American Medical Association 204: 859 (1968).

Shuster, S. and Marks, Janet: Systemic Effects of Skin Disease (Heinemann, London 1970).

Shuster, S. and Scarborough, H.: Corticosteroid purpura. Quarterly Journal of Medicine 30: 33 (1961).

Sneddon, I.: Adverse effect of topical fluorinated corticosteroids in rosacea. British Medical Journal 1: 671 (1969).

Sneddon, I.B.: Perioral dermatitis. British Journal of Dermatology 87: 430 (1972).

Sneddon, I.B.: Clinical use of topical corticosteroids. Drugs 11: 193 (1976).

Solomon, L.M.; Fahrner, L. and West, D.P.: Gamma benzene hexachloride toxicity. Archives of Dermatology 113: 353 (1977).

Steiner, I.; Prey, T.; Gschnait, F.; Washuttl, J. and Greiter, F.: Serum levels of 8-methoxypsoralen 2 hours after oral administration. Acta Dermatovenereologica 58: 185 (1978).

Stoughton, R.B.: Corticosteroids in psoriasis; in Farber and Cox (Eds) Psoriasis, Proceedings of the International Symposium, Stanford University, 1971 (Stanford University Press, Stanford 1971).

Stoughton, R.B.: Bioassay system for formulations of topically applied glucocorticosteroids. Archives of Dermatology 106: 825 (1972).

Stuart, B.H. and Litt, I.F.: Tetracycline-associated intercranial hypertension in an adolescent: A complication of systemic acne therapy. Journal of Pediatrics 92: 679 (1978).

Thirumoorthy, T. and Greaves, M.W.: Disodium cromoglycate ointment in atopic eczema. British Medical Journal 2: 500 (1978).

Thune, P.: Plasma levels of 8-methoxypsoralen and phototoxicity studies during PUVA treatment of psoriasis with meladinin tablets. Acta Dermatovenereologica 58: 149 (1978).

Tickner, A.: The biochemistry of psoriasis. British Journal of Dermatology 73: 87 (1961).

Van Scott, E.J.; Reinertson, R.P. and Steinmuller, R.: The growing hair roots of the human scalp and morphologic changes therein following amethopterin therapy. Journal of Investigative Dermatology 29: 197 (1957).

Vickers, C.F.H.: Existence of reservoirs in the stratum corneum. Archives of Dermatology 59: 10 (1963).

Vickers, C.F.H.: Dam, reservoir or filter. Transactions of the St. John's Hospital Dermatological Society 59: 10 (1973).

Walker, F.B.; Smith, P.D. and Maibach, H.I.: Genetic factors in human allergic contact dermatitis. International Archives of Allergy 32: 453 (1967).

Walter, J.F.; Voorhees, J.J.; Kelsey, W.H.; Duell, E.A. and Arbor, A.: Psoralen plus black light inhibits DNA synthesis. Archives of Dermatology 107: 861 (1973).

Watson, W.; Cann, H.M.; Farber, E.M. and Nall, M.L.: The genetics of psoriasis. Archives of Dermatology 105: 197 (1972).

Wennersten, G.: Photoprotection of the eye in PUVA therapy. British Journal of Dermatology 98: 137 (1978).

Wereide, K.: Neomycin sensitivity in atopic dermatitis and other eczematous conditions. Acta Dermatovenereologica 50: 114 (1970).

Wester, R.C. and Maibach, H.I.: Relationship of topical dose and percutaneous absorption in Rhesus monkey and man.

Journal of Investigative Dermatology 67: 518 (1976).

Wexler, D. and Pace, W.: Acquired zinc deficiency disease of skin. British Journal of Dermatology 96: 669 (1977).

White, M.I.; Douglas, W.S. and Main, R.A.: Contact dermatitis attributed to ethylenediamine. British Medical Journal 1: 415 (1978).

Whyte, H.J. and Baughman, R.D.: Acute guttate psoriasis and streptococcal infection. Archives of Dermatology 89: 350 (1964).

Wilson, L.: The clinical assessment of topical corticosteroid activity. British Journal of Dermatology 94(Suppl. 12): 33 (1976).

Winter, R.J.; Kern, F. and Blizzard, R.M.: Prednisone therapy for alopecia areata. A follow-up report. Archives of Dermatology 112: 1549 (1976).

Wolff, K.; Fitzpatrick, T.B.; Parrish, J.A.; Gschnait, F.; Gilchrest, B.; Honigsmann, H.; Pathak, M.A. and Tannenbaum, L.: Photochemotherapy for psoriasis with orally administered methoxsalen. Archives of Dermatology 112: 943 (1976).

Wolff, K.; Gschnait, F.; Honigsmann, H.; Konrad, K.; Parrish, J.A. and Fitzpatrick, T.B.: Phototesting and dosimetry for photochemotherapy. British Journal of Dermatology 96: 1 (1977).

Woodward, R.K.: Acne stimulation by Ovral. Archives of Dermatology 110: 812 (1974).

Chapter XV
Obstetric and Gynaecological Disorders

I. MacGillivray and Marion H. Hall

Synopsis of Important Principles

1) Drug use in pregnancy requires a balance of judgment — a careful assessment of the risks of not giving the drug against any potential harm from its use.

2) A drug should therefore only be used in pregnancy if it is clearly indicated and of proven benefit to the mother or fetus. In the first trimester, only essential drugs should be given because of the risk of dysmorphogenesis.

3) The pathophysiological status of the mother is continually changing as pregnancy advances and as a consequence maternal absorption, distribution and elimination of drugs may be altered.

4) Administration of drugs to the mother near the time when delivery is anticipated or possible, should be cautious not only because of altered maternal disposition of drugs but also because of the immature metabolic and excretory capacity of the fetus and neonate.

5) Labour is a time of special therapeutic problems, and in the puerperium, a few drugs administered to the mother may be excreted in breast milk in sufficient amounts to cause harmful effects in the breast fed infant.

6) Fertility control by drugs has brought simple and effective contraception within the reach of millions of women. Although many side effects have been described, all are rare and most are minor, so that this form of contraception is now the method of choice for most women.

7) Infertility can be treated with drugs only when a hormonal abnormality is the cause. Careful selection of patients for induction of ovulation is essential.

8) In gynaecological disorders, hormone therapy should never be prescribed without careful assessment of the patient to exclude other pathological lesions. Even where a hormonal abnormality is undoubtedly present, hormones may not be the treatment of choice.

9) Hormones are seldom a permanent solution to any gynaecological problem and there are important contraindications and side effects associated with their use.

10) Drug induced gynaecological disorders are rare but the possibility should always be borne in mind that amenorrhoea, virilisation, galactorrhoea, gynaecomastia or endometrial cancer are due to drug administration.

A rational approach to the care of the pregnant patient requires cognisance of the potential harm to the fetus and neonate associated with drug administration, and the altered response to drugs of the mother consequent upon her continually changing pathophysiological state during pregnancy and labour and the puerperium. Continuing investigation and research has led to an improved understanding of hormonal control of the menstrual cycle, and has facilitated diagnosis of certain menstrual function disorders and made possible therapeutic advances in inhibition and induction of ovulation.

1. Clinical Pharmacological Considerations

1.1 Pregnancy and the Puerperium

The use of drugs in pregnancy and the puerperium requires special consideration for a number of reasons:

1) Dysmorphogenesis and other adverse effects on the developing embryo may occur.
2) Transplacental passage of drugs leading to adverse effects in late embryonic and fetal life may occur.
3) The metabolic and excretory capacity of the fetus and neonate is immature leading to potential problems with elimination of drugs, particularly near the time when delivery is anticipated or possible.
4) The pathophysiological status of the mother is continually changing as pregnancy advances and hence the maternal disposition of drugs may alter.
5) Pregnancy may modify the maternal response to drugs.
6) Labour is a time of special therapeutic problems.
7) Drugs administered to the mother may be excreted in breast milk.

1.1.1 Dysmorphogenesis and Other Embryopathic Effects

During the first trimester of pregnancy and especially from 4 to 8 weeks gestation (the period of organogenesis), *every* drug must be considered as potentially harmful. Given very early, in the preimplantation period, certain drugs may kill the embryo or cause abortion. During the period of organogenesis they may produce major structural abnormalities (i.e. dysmorphogenic effects). Later in fetal life, disorders produced are less striking but none the less important, for example growth retardation, virilisation, and interference with brain development (see chapters II, section 4; III, table I).

Predicting the dysmorphogenic potential of a drug is extremely difficult (Bowes, 1970; Yerushalmy, 1972). Even an established dysmorphogenic agent may not always produce a malformation: it must not only be given in the appropriate amount, but also at the appropriate time to a genetically susceptible individual and under circumstances where other environmental conditions, especially the pathophysiological state of the mother, do not prevent the effect (see further chapter II). Species differences also mean that absence of dysmorphogenicity in animal experiments does not prove that a drug is safe in humans. Nor is the converse necessarily true. For example, conventional animal tests for dysmorphogenicity would not have incriminated thalidomide (except in certain strains of rabbit) but would have incriminated aspirin which is not an established human dysmorphogen (Yaffe, 1975). It is also evident that a single dysmorphogenic agent can produce a multiplicity of malformations and conversely the same malformations can be caused by a variety of dysmorphogens. Thus, because of the lack of specificity of both cause and effect, it is difficult to establish in man a relationship between events during pregnancy and malformations seen after birth. Nevertheless, where a drug causes an unusual malformation (e.g. phocomelia) or specific combination of malformations in the majority of cases where it is administered at the critical stage of gestation, as did thalidomide, the association may become clear at a relatively early (4 years with thalidomide) stage of its use (Yaffe, 1975; Yaffe and Stern, 1976). However, where common malformations (e.g. cleft palate, harelip) occur in only a minority of patients receiving the drug, as with anticonvulsants, it may be very difficult to prove a definite cause and effect (Speidel and Meadow, 1974), especially since several other circumstances could give rise to an apparent association, for example:

a) The illness which necessitates drug consumption could be dysmorphogenic, e.g. epilepsy (Meadow, 1974; Shapiro et al., 1976)

b) The malformation may cause maternal symptoms, e.g. hydramnios or hyperemesis leading to drug consumption

c) The drug may inhibit the abortion of already malformed fetuses

d) If two drugs are taken in combination, the wrong drug may be blamed.

It is also important to remember that the harmful effect of drugs or treatment given during pregnancy may not become evident until many years later. It has been suggested that the incidence of leukaemia is increased in children whose mothers had diagnostic radiography during pregnancy (Bithell and Stewart, 1975); and a number of cases of vaginal adenocarcinoma have been reported in young girls whose mothers received the oestrogen stilboestrol as treatment for threatened abortion 15 to 20 years before (Herbst et al., 1971; 1977). Even a few doses of tetracycline in the later half of pregnancy can lead to discoloration of the deciduous teeth of the child (see chapter XIII; sect. 13.3).

1.1.2 Transplacental Passage of Drugs

As discussed in chapter III, the mother and fetus can be regarded as an integrated unit. The placenta is not a barrier to transfer of drugs from the maternal to the fetal organism and all drugs cross the placenta by simple diffusion to a greater or lesser extent. Placental transport of maternal substances to the fetus and of fetal substances to the mother is established at about the fifth week of embryonic life. Because of the changes which take place in the anatomical structure of the placenta and in uterine blood flow as pregnancy advances, the rate of drug transfer tends to be slower in early pregnancy than in the later stages and during labour (Kanto et al., 1974; Kangas et al., 1977). The transfer of some compounds is however, limited. This means that for all practical purposes some drugs do not cross the placenta, such as heparin with a molecular weight of 20,000 or drugs such as d-tubocurarine which is relatively lipid insoluble and ionised at physiological pH, but others such as thiopentone, cross the placenta so readily that the fetus has circulating levels almost as great as the mother (see further chapter III; sect. 1.2).

1.1.3 Fetal Metabolism and Excretion

During embryogenesis the fetus may of course suffer harmful effects from a drug which is quite safe for the mother, but during most of the pregnancy, even if a drug does cross the placenta, it will be eliminated by the mother on behalf of the fetus (see chapter III; fig. 1). When the time for delivery approaches, this situation alters, since a delivered fetus may be quite unable adequately to metabolise and excrete some drugs which have been administered to its mother. The more immature the fetus, the less competent its metabolic and excretory capacity, so that a baby which is unexpectedly born prematurely while its mother is receiving potent drugs which it cannot eliminate adequately, e.g. sedatives for pre-eclampsia, may be in serious difficulty.

Drugs administered to the mother at parturition may also affect the metabolic capacity of the neonate. For example, highly protein bound sulphonamides and other drugs which compete with bilirubin for plasma albumin binding sites, exacerbate neonatal jaundice, while conversely, barbiturates which enhance glucuronic acid conjugation, have been used to ameliorate neonatal jaundice, by stimulating hepatic glucuronyl transferase (see further chapter IV; sect. 2.2.2, 2.3.1).

1.1.4 Maternal Drug Disposition During Pregnancy

Pregnancy is a time of continual physiological adjustment (Assali and Brinkman, 1972; Hytten and Leitch, 1971). Such functional changes may influence the pharmacokinetics of drugs as pregnancy advances (for reviews, see Hytten, 1978; Krauer and Krauer, 1977).

Drug absorption: It has not yet been established to what extent gastrointestinal absorption of drugs (see chapter XIX; section 1.1.1) is influenced by the increased gastric and intestinal emptying time which is known to be a feature of pregnancy, or by the increase in gastric pH and buffer capacity which has been observed in early pregnancy in particular. Variable and apparent decreased absorption has however, been noted with erythromycin estolate and base, but not with clindamycin (Philipson et al., 1976). A case of malabsorption of phenytoin, which became further impaired during pregnancy, has been described (Ramsay et al., 1978). Drug absorption is more likely to be altered during labour (see section 1.1.6). Pulmonary absorption (e.g. alveolar uptake of anaesthetic gases) might be enhanced by hyperventilation and increased pulmonary blood flow. Intramuscular absorption might be increased by regional vasodilatation but from the lower limbs would tend to be slowed by venous stasis in late pregnancy.

Drug distribution might be modified during pregnancy as a consequence of the gradually decreasing plasma protein levels (Rebond et al., 1963) and increase in total body water as pregnancy advances. In addition, there are profound haemodynamic changes, as evidenced by increased circulating plasma volume and cardiac output; renal, uterine and pulmonary blood flow increasing in accordance with the increased cardiac output. Hepatic blood flow also probably increases in pregnancy (Tindall, 1975). Decreased protein binding has been demonstrated for some drugs such as salicylate, phenytoin and diazepam; the fraction of free drug increasing progressively during pregnancy and the puerperium followed by a decrease to normal by 5 to 7 weeks postpartum (Dean et al., 1977). However, plasma volume increases in late pregnancy such that the total mass of albumin in the circulation is at least as great in late pregnancy as before pregnancy (Hytten, 1978). The binding affinity of albumin for some drugs such as salicylate may nevertheless be decreased (Krasner and Yaffe, 1975). What effect a change in binding capacity of the circulation is likely to have on eventual distribution and elimination processes of particular drugs is not known. The free fraction of the local anaesthetic etidocaine is increased during delivery (Morgan et al., 1977). Although the elimination half life of diazepam is prolonged at parturition, total plasma clearance is unchanged suggesting that distribution of diazepam changes in the mother at this time (Moore and McBride, 1978). Plasma concentrations of water soluble drugs such as ampicillin and pivampicillin are markedly reduced during pregnancy, probably as a consequence of distribution into a larger volume of plasma and body water. Dosage of ampicillin needs to be doubled from 500mg to 1g to achieve therapeutic plasma concentrations (Philipson, 1977, 1978). Little data are available on alteration in distribution volumes of drugs at different stages during pregnancy or on changes in distribution of drugs as a consequence of altered regional distribution of blood flow to various organs.

Elimination of drugs is mainly by hepatic or renal mechanisms (see chapter I; sect. 3.3, 3.4). Since glomerular filtration is increased from early pregnancy onward, the elimination of drugs by this route will be increased provided there is no change in tubular reabsorption. Clearance of lithium increases during pregnancy and is reflected in an increased dose requirement during the course of pregnancy, followed by a relatively abrupt postpartum decrease in lithium requirement (Schou et al., 1973). The dose requirement of digoxin also appears to increase during pregnancy (Rogers et al., 1972). Aminoglycoside antibiotics are also eliminated by glomerular filtration and maternal plasma levels of gentamicin half of those attained in non-pregnant individuals have been reported (Weinstein et al., 1976); but no data are available on plasma concentrations attained in the same individual during pregnancy and postpartum. Renal clearance of ampicillin is increased during pregnancy and distribution altered such that therapeutic concentrations cannot be attained with normal dosage (Philipson, 1977; see also above).

Hepatic elimination mechanisms may be altered in pregnancy, particularly as a possible consequence of induction of microsomal drug metabolising enzymes by progesterone. Plasma concentrations of phenytoin decrease during pregnancy, unless dosage is increased, and rise again during the puerperium unless phenytoin dosage is reduced. Similar but less marked changes in dose requirement occur with phenobarbitone and carbamazepine and possibly ethosuximide (Eadie et al., 1977; Dam et al., 1979). Decreased plasma concentrations of phenytoin during pregnancy have been associated with an increase in seizure frequency (Mygind et al., 1976). These changes in anticonvulsant dose requirement appear to be due at least in large part to an increased rate of drug biotransformation, although other possible contributory factors such as altered folate status during pregnancy may be involved (Strauss et al., 1978). Anticonvulsant plasma levels should be monitored regularly from the outset of pregnancy and more frequently after birth (Eadie et al., 1977).

1.1.5 Maternal Response to Drugs

Most women gain 10 to 15kg during pregnancy so that in late pregnancy the dose of drugs required is greater on a weight basis. In addition, there is a disproportionate expansion in the plasma volume, so that the attainment of adequate plasma levels of drugs with relatively restricted distribution volumes (see chapter I; sect. 2.1.2) may also require larger doses for this reason (see also section 1.1.4).

The mother may be particularly sensitive to toxic effects of drugs. For example, acute yellow atrophy of the liver has been described as a result of administration of large doses of tetracycline during pregnancy (Kunelis et al., 1965).

The therapeutic efficacy of a drug can be altered by the effect of pregnancy upon the disease for which it is administered. For example, carbohydrate tolerance generally declines in pregnancy so that the insulin requirement of a diabetic can increase markedly as pregnancy advances (Plotz and Davis, 1962).

1.1.6 Problems in Labour

The absorption, distribution and elimination of drugs may be altered during labour and the puerperium. During labour, there is a delay in gastric emptying and often vomiting, which appears to be exacerbated by use of narcotic analgesics (Davison et al., 1970; Nimmo et al., 1975). Thus, the absorption of other drugs by the oral route is quite uncertain, and these should normally be administered parenterally. Plasma concentrations of ampicillin (and ampicillin from pivampicillin) and amoxycillin are considerably reduced following oral administration in labour, but adequate concentrations can be maintained with intramuscular ampicillin (Buckingham et al., 1975; Chatfield et al., 1974).

Elimination of drugs such as pethidine (meperidine) may be prolonged at the time of delivery (Morgan et al., 1978) and pathways of metabolism may be altered in labour, but any clinical implications are difficult to interpret as data are very sparse. In one series involving a non-specific assay (Morrison et al., 1973, 1976), three different patterns of maternal metabolism of pethidine were noted, with the rapid pattern of metabolism being associated with respiratory depression of the newborn infant when more than 60 minutes had elapsed following intravenous injection of pethidine (see further chapter III; sect. 3.1). The elimination of therapeutic drugs can change in the puerperium, necessitating alteration of dosage (see section 1.1.4).

Certain pathological features of pregnancy, e.g. hypertension, may change so rapidly during labour that the use of rapid acting drugs is essential to achieve control.

Where the drug is potentially harmful to the fetus, e.g. narcotic analgesics or sedatives, the dose must be kept to a minimum and wherever possible other methods of analgesia such as epidural block should be used (see chapter III, sect. 3.1, 3.3; X, sect. 8.3). If on the other hand, a drug is being used which may be essential to save the life of the fetus, such as a broad spectrum antibiotic in a case of intrauterine infection, then of course every effort must be made to use a drug which will readily cross the placenta and appear in adequate levels in liquor and fetal blood, e.g. ampicillin or cephaloridine, and not one which crosses the placenta less readily, e.g. chloramphenicol.

1.1.7 Excretion of Drugs in Breast Milk

Where a mother is suckling her infant, drugs should be administered to her with caution, since some are excreted in significant amounts in breast milk. Drugs are not selectively excreted, so that for this and other reasons relating to the physicochemical and pharmacokinetic characteristics of the particular drug, the neonate will usually receive a much smaller dose of the drug than the mother. However, the neonate may be more sensitive than the mother to the drug, as in the case of laxatives, and may also be less able to metabolise and excrete some other drugs such as those metabolised by glucuronidation (e.g. nalidixic acid). In the case of allergenic antibiotics such as penicillin, the infant may be needlessly exposed to the risk of subsequent allergy. Most drugs probably will not exert a harmful effect. However, if a potent drug is essential for the mother but of uncertain effect on the infant, it may be necessary to change to artificial feeding. This is a poorly studied area (see further chapter IV; sect. 3.1.3).

1.2 Gynaecological Disorders

Assay methods (in particular the development of radioimmunoassays of pituitary gonadotrophins, competitive protein binding and radioimmunoassays of ovarian steroids) are used to study the hormonal control of the menstrual cycle. Although it must be remembered that the biological activity of hormones does not always correspond exactly with the activity as measured by radioimmunoassays, it now seems clear that the sequence of events in the normal menstrual cycle is as follows (Short, 1972).

Basal secretion of follicle stimulating hormone (FSH) and luteinising hormone (LH), resulting from the negative feedback response, stimulate the theca interna cells of the developing graafian folli-

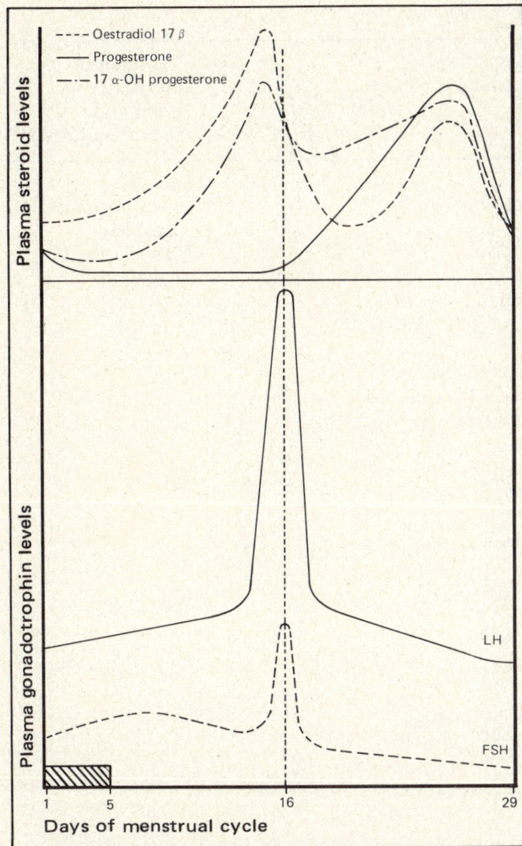

Fig. 1. Hormone changes in the human menstrual cycle (after Short: British Journal of Hospital Medicine 7: 553, 1972).

cle to produce rising levels of 17α-hydroxy-progesterone and oestradiol-17β. When an oestrogen peak is reached at mid cycle, this causes, by positive feedback, a brief surge in gonadotrophin output (especially LH) mediated by hypothalamic releasing factors. Ovulation occurs and is followed by granulosa cell hypertrophy in the developing corpus luteum, which is then invaded by theca interna cells and secretes the increased progesterone which characterises the 14 day luteal phase of the cycle.

Hormonal profiles of abnormal menstrual cycles are less complete. The elucidation of these abnormal changes has nevertheless facilitated the diagnosis of disorders of menstrual function such as unopposed oestrogen secretion in the anovulatory cycles of women with menorrhagia due to cystic glandular hyperplasia, or failure of ovulation as a cause of infertility. Many therapeutic ad-

vances have followed, such as the inhibition of ovulation for contraceptive purposes by utilising the negative feedback response of pituitary gonadotrophin output to circulating ovarian steroids, or the induction of ovulation by utilising the positive feedback response of LH release to rising levels of oestrogen, or compounds such as clomiphene which can occupy oestrogen receptor sites in the hypothalamus.

Figure 1 depicts the hormone changes in the human menstrual cycle.

2. General Principles of Prescribing and Therapy

2.1 Principles of Prescribing in Pregnancy

Administration of drugs in pregnancy requires a balance of judgment — a careful assessment of the risks of not giving the drug against any potential harm from its use. Despite this admonition drugs are widely used during pregnancy. Indeed, in one study in Edinburgh (Nelson and Forfar, 1971; Forfar and Nelson, 1973), every mother took one drug in normal daily dosage throughout 60% of her pregnancy, 2 of every 3 mothers took aspirin in full dosage for 6 weeks. Excluding iron preparations, 82% of pregnant women were prescribed drugs, and at least 65% took other drugs not prescribed by their doctors. The prevalence of consumption of drugs in pregnancy is similar in and remains so in other countries (Boethius, 1977; Brocklebank et al., 1978; Doering and Stewart, 1978). In one study in the USA, the average number of drugs taken being 6.4 prescribed and 3.2 self prescribed (Hill et al., 1977). History taking alone may not elicit the full extent of drug usage. For example, heavy aspirin users in Australia have often been identified by urine testing only (Collins and Turner, 1975).

The potential for harm would therefore seem very great, but for most drugs there is no precise information about their effects on the fetus, or for that matter, on the mother herself. Some drugs if taken by the mother can, under appropriate circumstances (see chapters II and III), affect the fetus or neonate profoundly, but most drugs probably do not affect it at all. Thus for most drugs prescribed or self administered during pregnancy, the incidence of congenital abnormalities for example, in the infants of mothers taking them appears to be only marginally above the incidence of

Table I. Drugs to be avoided or given with caution in pregnancy[1]

In early pregnancy (dysmorphogenesis)	In late(r) pregnancy (fetal and neonatal effects[2])	Throughout pregnancy (fetal and neonatal effects[2])
High Risk Cytotoxic Drugs Sex hormones Thalidomide Warfarin[8]	*Avoid* Anticoagulants (oral)[8] Aspirin (large dosage) Chloramphenicol Iodides Nitrofurantoin (in those with G6PD deficiency) Sulphonamides (highly protein bound compounds; in those with G6PD deficiency) Oral sulphonylurea hypoglycaemics (at 34 weeks)[7]	*Avoid* Sex hormones Smoking Tetracyclines Alcohol
Slightly Increased Risk[3] ?Barbiturates[5] Phenytoin[4]		
? Very Slightly Increased Risk[3] Antacids[5] Iron[5] Nicotinamide[5] Inhalational anaesthetics[5]	*Use with care[3]* Anaesthetics Narcotic analgesics Barbiturates Benzodiazepines Propranolol Rauwolfia Thiazide diuretics Lithium Phenothiazines Antithyroid drugs[9] Corticosteroids	
? Any Increased Risk[3] Co-trimoxazole Corticosteroids[6] Oral sulphonylurea hypoglycaemics[7] Aspirin Benzodiazepines		

1   See also text and chapters II, III.
2   See table I chapter III.
3   Use only when there is a clear and specific need (e.g. do not withhold barbiturates or phenytoin in epilepsy, or corticosteroids in severe asthma or ulcerative colitis). Use conservative or monitored doses wherever possible. See further, chapter III.
4   See also chapter XXV, section 4.8 and chapter III, section 3.10.2.
5   Further data needed to confirm or refute.
6   See also section 21.1 and chapter III, section 5.4.
7   See also section 21.2 and chapter III, section 5.2.
8   See also section 6 and chapter XXIII; section 3.2.6 and chapter III, section 6.
9   See also section 21.3 and chapter XVI, section 5.2.4.

abnormalities in infants born of mothers not taking these drugs. Moreover, drug ingestion is but one of many factors that may contribute to the incidence of congenital abnormalities (see also chapter II). The overall incidence of major congenital abnormalities is around 2%; thus, the majority of infants born of mothers taking 'low risk' drugs (table I) during the first trimester of pregnancy are likely to be normal (Kullander and Kallen, 1976a,b,c,d; Forfar, 1973). Nevertheless, at the present time there is sufficient evidence to warrant avoidance of use of drugs in a pregnant woman unless there are clearcut clinical indications and the drug is of proven benefit.

Another problem relates to the inadvertent or self administration of drugs in the very early weeks of pregnancy, perhaps before the woman or her doctor realises that she is pregnant. There are therefore two issues — 'drug therapy in pregnancy' and 'pregnancy in drug therapy'. The risks involved can only be prevented by a sensible prescribing policy and by the recognition that any woman of child bearing age may become pregnant (see Noble, 1974).

1) Consider the possibility of pregnancy when prescribing or caring for women of child bearing age. This means education of women to avoid self medication if they suspect that they are pregnant, and of only prescribing with assurance if the impossibility of pregnancy in an individual patient can be guaranteed.

2) Consider the possibility of drug taking when caring for pregnant women or women of child bearing age. When eliciting an obstetric drug history, ask about the ingestion of certain drugs by specific proprietary name (not generic name such as aspirin; Palmisano and Cassady, 1969), or preferably by terms that the woman will understand, for example: 'pain medication' for headache and arthritis; 'heart medicine'; 'water or fluid pills' for diuretics; 'blood pressure medicine' for antihypertensives, and 'blood thinner' for anticoagulants, and so on (Yaffe, 1975).

3) During the first trimester of pregnancy, avoid the use of any drug which is not absolutely necessary and of proven benefit. Where a drug is of significant, possibly unique therapeutic benefit to the mother, but is of some or unknown risk to the fetus there could be good reason for using it, particularly if the illness in the mother may itself harm the fetus; for example, epilepsy (Stumpf and Frost, 1978). On the other hand, where the drug is of minimum or unproven therapeutic benefit, even though it may carry only a small risk to the fetus, there might be little justification for using the drug. Thus, use of phenobarbitone would not be justified for day time sedation, but it should not be withheld when needed for the effective control of epilepsy (see also chapter XXV; sect. 4.8).

Other sections in this chapter discuss the legitimate use of drugs in obstetric practice and the treatment of medical conditions in pregnant patients.

4) After the first trimester of pregnancy, bear in mind that drugs have a potential to affect the fetus or neonate, even its later physiological and behavioural development (Stirrat, 1976; Brazelton, 1970). There is at present little reliable information on the effects of most drugs, but for some the risks have been reasonably well defined (see table I in chapter III) and for others, certain risks have been suspected (table I). Obviously, the administration of drugs to the mother near the time when delivery is anticipated or even possible, should be cautious (see section 1.1.6).

5) Bear in mind that the maternal response to drugs can be modified by pregnancy or the puerperium — a changed dose requirement of an indicated drug or an abnormal response to a drug (see section 1.1.4 and 1.1.5).

2.2 Principles of Hormone Therapy

While hormone therapy has brought great benefits to very many gynaecological patients, it is important to observe certain principles in its use.

1) Hormone therapy should never be prescribed without careful assessment of the patient — preliminary history taking, general and pelvic examination, and investigation, usually including diagnostic curettage and/or hormone assays, since carcinoma of the cervix or endometrium may masquerade as menstrual dysfunction or a pituitary tumour as hypothalamic amenorrhoea.

2) Even where a hormonal abnormality is undoubtedly present, hormones may not be the treatment of choice. For example, wedge resection of the ovaries is still an effective method of treatment in the polycystic ovary syndrome, although clomiphene is generally used. Again, in women who have completed child bearing, who are aged over 35 or in whom any other pathology such as pre-invasive cervical carcinoma or pelvic sepsis has been diagnosed, hysterectomy may be preferred to hormone therapy as treatment for menorrhagia.

3) Definite contraindications to steroid hormone therapy (e.g. oestrogens) may exist, such as a previous history of deep vein thrombosis and pulmonary embolism.

4) Most hormone preparations have side effects, so that careful supervision of patients on hormone therapy is essential.

Hormone therapy is seldom a permanent solution to any gynaecological problem even if the abnormality is primarily hormonal. However, it may be expected that the development of improved and modified hormone preparations, together with increasing knowledge of the nature of hormonal abnormalities will increase the efficacy of drugs in gynaecological practice while reducing the incidence of unwanted side effects.

3. Anaemia in Pregnancy

The diagnosis of anaemia in pregnancy is complicated by the disproportionate expansion in the plasma volume which occurs early in pregnancy, and probably persists until near term, so that a haemoglobin level which would be pathologically low in the non-pregnant state may be quite normal in pregnancy, and in fact associated with a more than adequate oxygen carrying capacity. In the diagnosis of pregnancy anaemia, it is wise, therefore, to give due attention to the packed cell volume, the mean cell haemoglobin concentration, and the morphology of the cells, as well as to the actual haemoglobin concentration, which must be measured at the time of booking, and then again at 30 and 36 weeks gestation as a minimum.

3.1 Iron Deficiency Anaemia

Iron deficiency is common in pregnancy even in 'developed' countries. Initial treatment is with oral iron, 70 to 130mg elemental iron daily (see chapter XXIII; sect. 6.1.1), which is usually acceptable and effective. Intramuscular or intravenous iron is only indicated if there is a suspicion that oral iron is not being consumed or may not be absorbed, and when anaemia is very severe or delivery imminent. Since intravenous infusion of iron dextran may be associated with collapse in pregnancy (Dawson et al., 1965), it is probably better to use intramuscular injection of iron sorbitol (iron-sorbitol-citric acid complex), 100mg daily for 7 to 10 days. This drug may occasionally cause a pyrexial response and an apparent relapse in patients with chronic pyelonephritis. Total dose iron dextran infusion may occasionally be indicated in patients with social problems, since treatment necessitates admission to hospital only for a few hours, but such treatment should be preceded by a test dose.

The necessity for and efficacy of routine oral iron prophylaxis during pregnancy in 'developed' countries is questionable (Editorial, 1978). It has certainly been shown that as many as 30% of patients will fail to consume such therapy (Bonnar et al., 1969). Most women are not in fact iron deficient, and although it is true that even in normal women the haemoglobin level will rise if iron is taken as a result of the erythropoietic effect of iron, there is no evidence that the woman feels better as a result, or that the fetus fares better (Paintin et al., 1966; Hemminki and Starfield, 1978a). Moreover, consumption of iron in the first trimester of pregnancy may possibly be associated with an increased incidence of congenital malformation (Nelson and Forfar, 1971). It seems reasonable therefore to restrict iron therapy to those patients who have been shown to suffer from genuine iron deficiency. Routine oral iron supplements should however, be prescribed in areas where iron deficiency is common (e.g. due to dietary deficiency, gastrointestinal blood loss from hookworm infestation), and possibly in the second and third trimester to women of low social class with inadequate nutrition, and those women with a history of iron deficiency anaemia (see Hall, 1974).

3.2 Folate Deficiency Anaemia

In the 'developed' countries, megaloblastic anaemia, which is due in pregnancy to folic acid deficiency, is uncommon. In the United Kingdom, for example, it occurs in only 1 to 2% of pregnancies, usually in the late third trimester but sometimes in the puerperium. Treatment is by oral folic acid 5mg 3 times daily. Since the incidence of megaloblastic anaemia is so low, the practice of administering routine folic acid supplements during pregnancy seems unnecessary. There is no good evidence that routine folate supplements will raise the haemoglobin level in those patients who do not suffer from megaloblastic anaemia (Chisholm, 1966). Neither is there any evidence of a reduction in the incidence of those pregnancy complications which were at one time attributed to folic acid deficiency (Hall, 1972a,b; Hemminki and Starfield, 1978a). Routine oral folic acid supplements (at least 300µg daily) are indicated in areas where dietary deficiency of folate is common, or where folate requirements are increased by malarial haemolysis and haemoglobinopathies (Hall, 1974).

3.3 Refractory Anaemia

Refractory anaemia in pregnancy may occasionally be due to consumption of toxic substances due to pica, when the main aim of treatment is to prevent consumption of the toxin, or to chronic infection often in the urinary tract, which inhibits the erythropoietic response to haematinics, when treatment of the infection is important. Iron is not indicated as iron stores may already be increased, but the iron is unavailable for haemoglobin synthesis.

In developed countries, anaemia is rarely sufficiently severe to require blood transfusion (Hall, 1974).

3.4 Haemoglobinopathies

In Negroes, or patients of Southeast Asian or Mediterranean descent, the possibility of haemoglobinopathies due to genetic enzyme defects should also be borne in mind (see chapter XXIII; sect. 6.2.2).

4. Urinary Infection in Pregnancy

Urinary infection is particularly likely to occur during pregnancy and the puerperium because of the ureteric dilatation and consequent stasis which appears early in pregnancy and persists for several weeks after delivery. The usual organism is *Escherichia coli,* and initial therapy with a short acting sulphonamide such as sulphafurazole (sulfisoxazole) or sulphadimidine (sulphamethazine), 1 g 6-hourly, is recommended, provided oral therapy can be tolerated. Other drugs (see chapter XXI; sect. 3.1) should be reserved for failure of clinical or bacteriological response to sulphonamide therapy, in late pregnancy when sulphonamides are best avoided (see below), or for the situation where vomiting precludes oral therapy, when ampicillin or amoxycillin may be used.

Therapy of urinary tract infection should always be preceded by urine culture and the effect checked by post-therapy culture at 10 days and then monthly, or again at 6 months if continuous treatment throughout pregnancy. Where the culture shows that the infecting organism is insensitive to the sulphonamides or ampicillin or amoxycillin, then the appropriate antibacterial drug should be administered, remembering that certain agents are relatively or completely contraindicated in pregnancy:

a) Streptomycin may cause auditory nerve damage in early pregnancy, but after 20 weeks gestation, the risk to the fetus is no greater than to the mother (see chapter XI; sect. 7.1).

b) Even a few doses of tetracycline in the later half of pregnancy can cause discoloration of unerupted teeth and possibly enamel hypoplasia (see chapter XIII; sect. 13.3). They may also impair fetal bone growth, so should never be administered in pregnancy (Cohlan et al., 1963).

c) Sulphonamides which are highly bound to plasma proteins, especially the long acting sulphonamides, should be avoided in late pregnancy because of the increased risk of kernicterus in the neonate by displacement of bilirubin from plasma protein binding sites (see chapter IV; sect. 2.2.2).

d) Nitrofurantoin and sulphonamides may cause haemolytic anaemia in glucose-6-phosphate dehydrogenase deficient infants (see chapter XXIII; sect. 8.4).

e) Co-trimoxazole (trimethoprim-sulphamethoxazole), although highly effective in bacteriuria of pregnancy (Brumfitt and Pursell, 1973), is not recommended for use during pregnancy because of the possible risk of harm to the fetus from trimethoprim (a *bacterial* folate antagonist at usual therapeutic doses) and the risk of kernicterus from the sulphonamide component when given in late pregnancy.

Asymptomatic bacteriuria occurs in about 5 to 7 % of pregnant women. It was once thought that this condition predisposed to prematurity and other complications of pregnancy. More recent study suggests that this is not so (Swapp, 1973), and there is certainly no evidence that antibacterial treatment will reduce the incidence of such complications. However, therapy may quite reasonably be given on the grounds that these patients have a 25 to 35 % risk of developing a clinical urinary tract infection during the pregnancy or puerperium (Little, 1966). This risk can be reduced, although not abolished, by therapy. Initial treatment should be with a conventional curative course of an antibacterial agent, appropriate to the organism cultured (see chapter XXI; sect. 3.1). If bacteriuria returns following initial curative treatment, the patient can usually be successfully controlled by a prophylactic regimen of 50mg nitrofurantoin or 250mg penicillin G each night until the puerperium. However, it is important to realise that these patients are more likely to have a radiological abnormality of the urinary tract, and that further postnatal investigation may be indicated, particularly where the bacteriuria persists.

5. Hypertension and Oedema in Pregnancy

5.1 Essential Hypertension

In essential hypertension, the maternal indications for the use of antihypertensive drugs are the same as in the non-pregnant state and can be used in women with a sustained diastolic blood pressure of over 110 to 115mm Hg to reduce the risk of complications such as cerebral haemorrhage (see chapter XVIII). There is some doubt as to whether one can anticipate any improvement in the perinatal mortality from the employment of antihypertensive drugs at a diastolic blood pressure lower than that which would constitute an indication for therapy in the non-pregnant woman in the reproductive age group, and certainly treatment begun after 20 weeks' gestation is ineffective (Leather et al., 1968).

Most of the antihypertensive drugs in common use may be safely employed in pregnancy, but reserpine may cause neonatal nasal stuffiness and respiratory obstruction. β-Adrenoceptor blocking drugs such as propranolol may cause a number of adverse effects including neonatal depression, bradycardia and hypoglycaemia and can increase uterine muscle tone and may alter uterine blood flow (Mitrani et al., 1975). Although propranolol is effective in controlling blood pressure in pregnancy and has been used without evidence of any adverse effects (Eliahou et al., 1978; Tcherdakoff et al., 1978), such use at present seems controversial (see further chapter III; sect. 8.2).

5.2 Pre-eclampsia

Antihypertensive drugs have also been used in the long term management of pre-eclampsia, but there are theoretical disadvantages: (a) choriodecidual blood flow may be reduced, and fetal growth impaired, and (b) the clinician may have a false sense of security because the hypertension appears to be well controlled, and may be tempted to postpone delivery beyond the optimum time for the fetus. The indications for the use of antihypertensive drugs in the antenatal management of pre-eclampsia are thus strictly limited, and most patients will respond better to bed rest with oral sedation if necessary. Barbiturates have been safely used for many years but have been superseded by chlormethiazole, 0.5 to 1g 4 times daily (a drug with hypnotic and anticonvulsant properties, which may, however, cause uncomfortable nasal stuffiness at first), or diazepam 2.5 to 5mg 4 times daily.

The oedema which so often accompanies pre-eclampsia has often been treated with oral diuretics, which may also lower the blood pressure. However, there are a number of good reasons for suggesting that the use of thiazide and similar diuretics is unwise (Gray, 1968; Lindheimer and Katz, 1973):

a) Oedema is physiological in pregnancy, and is in no way harmful to the mother or the fetus (Robertson, 1971; Thomson et al., 1967).

b) Pre-eclampsia is normally characterised by a reduced plasma volume compared with that in normal pregnancy, so it seems irrational to use a drug which will reduce it further (Palomaki and Lindheimer, 1970).

c) Oral diuretics have only a marginal hypotensive effect, and there is no evidence that lowering of the blood pressure *per se* improves the fetal outlook.

d) There is no evidence that administration of oral diuretics to 'at risk' patients — those with oedema or large weight gain — reduces the incidence of pre-eclampsia (Campbell and MacGillivray, 1975; Christianson and Page, 1976).

e) There is evidence that birthweight is reduced when diuretics are given to large weight gain women (Campbell and MacGillivray, 1975).

f) Maternal pancreatitis has been reported on rare occasions as a result of the administration of thiazide diuretics (Minkowitz et al., 1964); liver damage, as described by Fallis and Ford (1960) is a potential hazard in pre-eclampsia when liver function is already impaired.

g) Administration of thiazide diuretics to the mother has been followed by neonatal thrombocytopenia (Rodriguez et al., 1964).

Diazoxide, a non-diuretic thiazide derivative, may be of value in severe pre-eclampsia, but because of side effects with continued oral administration it should be restricted to cases where other therapy has proved unsuccessful (Pohl et al., 1972). It is given in a dosage of 100 to 200mg orally 4 times daily. The hypotensive effect is produced by generalised vasodilatation, so that maternal renal blood flow and placental perfusion may benefit, and in addition to the reduction in blood pressure, a decrease in the amount of albuminuria seems to occur. An unwanted side effect is hyperglycaemia, but this can be readily controlled by oral hypoglycaemic drugs or insulin. Delay in fetal bone growth and neonatal alopecia or hypertrichosis may occur (Milner and Chouksey, 1972).

Sodium and fluid retention may also occur and necessitate therapy with diuretics such as frusemide (furosemide).

5.3 Eclampsia

In impending eclampsia, or in patients with proteinuric pre-eclampsia in labour, when eclampsia is always a risk, intravenous chlormethiazole (0.8%) in a dose from 15 drops per minute (increasing to 50ml per minute where necessary) or diazepam 5mg intravenously, repeated twice if necessary will provide adequate hypnosis and have an anticonvulsant effect, although the mother can maintain her own airway and cooperate well. These drugs have no analgesic effect. Thus analgesia is best achieved by epidural block, which not only lowers the blood pressure, but also has no sedative effect on the baby, unlike drugs such as pethidine (meperidine) which often give rise to severe respiratory depression in the neonate, especially when used in combination with intravenous chlormethiazole, which also crosses the placenta. High doses of diazepam may cause a number of fetal and neonatal effects and care should be taken to avoid excessive dosage, particularly in view of the slow elimination of the drug and active metabolites (see chapter III; sect. 3.10.1).

If, in addition to these measures, it becomes necessary specifically to lower the blood pressure, then a rapid acting drug which can be administered parenterally is essential, such as protoveratrine (a veratrum alkaloid), bethanidine, or hydrallazine. The major problem with such drugs is sudden hypotension, and they should be used only where immediate Trendelenberg posture can be obtained, as is the case with most delivery or intensive care beds.

The above regimen can be adapted for the management of eclampsia, when a rapid intravenous infusion of chlormethiazole 0.8% or diazepam will give initial control, and may be followed by intravenous protoveratrine (or bethanidine or hydrallazine) therapy if the blood pressure is particularly high.

The use of a bolus dose of diazoxide to control blood pressure before delivery is potentially hazardous since profound hypotension, which cannot be reversed, may occur, and endanger the fetus. However, diazoxide has been successfully used in cases failing to respond adequately to magnesium sulphate and appears to stabilise the blood

Table II. Summary of management of hypertension of pregnancy

---

1. *Essential hypertension*
   a) Maternal indications for use of antihypertensive drugs are the same as in the non-pregnant state.
   b) Antihypertensives can be used when diastolic blood pressure consistently over 110 to 115mm Hg to reduce risk of complications.
   c) The outlook for the fetus *may* be improved if treatment is begun before 20 weeks.
   d) Most drugs in common use suitable; reserpine may cause respiratory obstruction in the neonate; use of β-adrenoceptor blocking drugs such as propranolol is controversial.

2. *Pre-eclampsia*
   a) Indications for use of antihypertensive drugs in antenatal management of pre-eclampsia are strictly limited.
   b) Most patients respond to bed rest and oral sedation if needed.
   c) Barbiturates have been superseded by chlormethiazole (0.5 to 1g 4 times daily) or diazepam (10 to 20mg daily in divided doses).
   d) There are many good reasons for not treating with oral diuretics the oedema which often accompanies pre-eclampsia.
   e) Oral diazoxide 100 to 200mg 4 times daily *may* be useful in severe pre-eclampsia where other therapy has proved unsuccessful.

3. *Eclampsia*
   In impending eclampsia, or in patients with proteinuric pre-eclampsia when eclampsia is always a risk:
   a) Anticonvulsant — chlormethiazole (0.8%) 15 drops per minute (increasing to 50ml/min if necessary) or diazepam (5 to 10mg/min intravenously until convulsions controlled. Do not exceed 0.5mg/kg).
   b) Antihypertensive agent —parenteral protoveratrine, bethanidine, or hydrallazine. Use only where immediate Trendelenberg position can be obtained.
   c) Analgesia — best achieved with epidural block.
   In eclampsia, use a rapid intravenous infusion of chlormethiazole or diazepam, followed by intravenous protoveratrine or alternative agents if blood pressure is particularly high.

---

pressure successfully (Morris et al., 1977). After delivery this may be a rational form of emergency treatment. β-Adrenoceptor blocking drugs such as propranolol may cause increased uterine activity, if used in labour, and may adversely affect fetal cardiac function (see sect. 5.1; chapter III, sect. 8.2). The management of hypertension in pregnancy is summarised in table II.

6. Venous Thrombosis in Pregnancy

Venous thrombosis is likely to occur during pregnancy and more commonly in the puerperium because of the mechanical effect of the gravid uterus upon venous return from the lower limbs, the effect of progesterone upon smooth muscle causing distensibility of the veins, and the increase in certain clotting factors and decrease in fibrinolysis which normally occurs from the beginning of the second trimester. Pulmonary embolism occurs rarely, although it is still a major cause of maternal mortality.

When a diagnosis of thrombosis is made, a surgical approach to treatment may be advisable because of the problems of late chronic venous insufficiency in the leg in which occlusion occurs, or because of failure of medical methods of treatment. Ileo-femoral thrombectomy cannot of course be carried out until after delivery, so that it is often necessary to treat antenatal patients with anticoagulants. Oral anticoagulants cross the placenta fairly readily. Warfarin and phenindione have been associated with multiple congenital abnormalities when used during the first trimester (Shaul and Hall, 1977) and many cases of fetal death from cerebral haemorrhage have been reported in association with oral anticoagulant therapy during the latter part of pregnancy (see Hirsh et al., 1972). It is therefore necessary to use parenteral heparin at least throughout the first trimester and if oral anticoagulants are used after this time, to switch to parenteral heparin therapy (usually intravenous but self administered subcutaneous therapy has also been used; Spearing et al., 1978) several weeks before delivery is anticipated, as heparin, a high molecular weight and electronegatively charged mucopolysaccharide, does not readily cross the placenta (see chapter III; sect. 1.2; 6). Moreover, there is also the advantage that therapy can be quickly reversed at the time of labour and delivery to reduce the risk of haemorrhage from the placental site and from other sites such as episiotomy wounds, vaginal and cervical lacerations or Caesarean section wounds.

Apart from those patients in whom a definite diagnosis of venous thrombosis has been made, prophylactic therapy may be indicated during pregnancy or particularly in the puerperium in 'at risk' patients such as older women undergoing operative delivery or postpartum sterilisation, the obese, patients with a previous history of deep vein thrombosis (Badaracco and Vessey, 1974), or with severe varicose veins. Oral anticoagulant therapy can be given in the puerperium, and even to lactating women, provided that the prothrombin time is well controlled (Orme et al., 1977; see also chapter IV; sect. 3.1.3). However, low dose subcutaneous heparin is likely to be as effective (Baskin et al., 1977; Kakkar et al., 1975) and is without the potential problems inherent in gaining initial adequate control of oral anticoagulant therapy. Intravenous infusion of high molecular weight dextran (dextran 70) may be a suitable alternative (MacIntyre et al., 1974). It is not yet absolutely clear how often it is necessary or beneficial to give the dextran infusion, but an infusion of 200ml at the time of operation (if any) followed by infusion on 3 consecutive days seems reasonable (see chapter XXIII; sect. 3.2.6).

7. Gastrointestinal Disorders of Pregnancy

7.1 Nausea and Vomiting of Pregnancy

Nausea and vomiting in the first trimester of pregnancy are common, but is due to physiological changes in most cases and most women will not require drug therapy (Biggs, 1975). When the symptoms are very troublesome, an antiemetic such as dicyclomine/doxylamine/pyridoxine may be prescribed, since there is no evidence that it is dysmorphogenic (Shapiro et al., 1977; Henderson, 1977; see also chapter III, sect. 3.9). Occasional patients will become sufficiently dehydrated to require admission to hospital, when the condition usually settles rapidly with or without intravenous fluids and parenteral antiemetics.

7.2 Heartburn of Pregnancy

This occurs in the second and third trimester of pregnancy, probably as a result of relaxation of the lower oesophageal sphincter by progesterone. Attention to diet, correction of obesity and avoidance of bending or the supine posture will usually prove helpful, but some women will also benefit from antacid therapy or from metoclopropamide (see also chapter XIX; sect. 3).

8. Threatened Abortion

For many years, progestagen therapy was given to patients with threatened or habitual abortion on the grounds that these conditions may be due to progesterone deficiency. Properly controlled trials have never shown any benefit from such therapy (Klopper and McNaughton, 1965) and in view of the possible deleterious effects of hormone therapy upon the developing fetus (e.g. virilisation of the female genital tract, disorders of the hypothalamic ovarian axis) it seems wise to eschew such therapy. In effect, there is no drug therapy for threatened abortion.

9. Premature Labour

Uterine contractions associated with inappropriate premature labour with intact membranes may be inhibited by two types of drug:

1) β-Adrenoceptor stimulants (β-mimetic agents; Ingemarsson, 1976) such as salbutamol (albuterol), fenoterol, terbutaline, ritodrine, or isoxsuprine, which are given in an intravenous infusion, the rate of infusion being that which is necessary to inhibit contractions. Unfortunately, side effects (dose related tachycardia, hypotension and vomiting) still often occur, so that effective administration cannot be continued. Metabolic changes including hyperglycaemia can occur and may cause problems in diabetics (Fredholm et al., 1978; Spellacy et al., 1978), particularly when β-adrenoceptor stimulants are used in conjunction with corticosteroids (Chapman, 1977; Kauppila et al., 1978). Provided delivery is not imminent, sedation with drugs such as pethidine may be helpful in addition. This form of treatment is relatively contraindicated by antepartum haemorrhage because hypovolaemic shock may be masked; or by ruptured membranes since contractions in the presence of ruptured membranes mean that delivery is almost inevitable, and delay may cause metabolic upset, infection and fetal distress (see also chapter III; sect. 8.1).

2) Alcohol (Zlatnik and Fuchs, 1972) — which inhibits oxytocin release (although this may not be the mechanism of action) and is administered intravenously in a dose of 1.25g absolute alcohol per kg body weight in a 10% solution in 5% dextrose, the rate of infusion again being that which is required to inhibit contractions. The side effects are similar to those which occur with oral ingestion of alcohol.

There has been no definite evidence as to which of these regimens is superior in the management of premature labour (Hemminki and Starfield, 1978b; Fuchs, 1976), but it seems wise for any particular hospital to use only one regimen so that medical and nursing staff can become familiar with the method.

The use of ritodrine to reduce fetal asphyxia in the second stage of labour has also been advocated (Humphrey et al., 1975; Campbell et al., 1978). Another measure which will reduce neonatal mortality from respiratory distress syndrome where premature delivery cannot be averted, is the antenatal administration of corticosteroids such as betamethasone 4mg 6-hourly for 48 hours; corticosteroids promote surfactant secretion and hence fetal pulmonary maturation (Liggins and Howie, 1972). It is probably effective only before 32 weeks gestation. It may, of course, be used not only in premature labour but also prior to planned premature delivery, but should be avoided in cases of pre-eclampsia where intrauterine death may result (see also chapter III, sect. 5.4).

10. Induction of Labour

Although induction of labour is usually performed by forewater rupture, and is generally successful, there has been a trend towards increased acceleration of labour by oxytocic drugs (Turnbull and Anderson, 1967). It is now realised that provided very careful (if possible continuous) monitoring of the fetal heart rate and of the uterine contractions can be carried out, there is no contraindication to the early use of large doses of synthetic oxytocin (O'Driscoll et al., 1973). Maximum control seems to be achieved if this is administered by intravenous infusion, the rate of infusion being whatever is necessary to produce regular uterine contractions of good tone and duration. The dose may be monitored manually, by mechanical pump, or in sophisticated units by a computer whose input includes intrauterine pressures and fetal heart rates. The complications of overdosage of oxytocin (uterine spasm leading to fetal anoxia and sometimes uterine rupture) still occur sufficiently often to require reiteration of the necessity for very careful continuous monitoring of any patient receiving such therapy.

There have been a number of reports of an increase in neonatal hyperbilirubinaemia following the use of oxytocin infusions in induced labour (Campbell et al., 1975), but the association seems less clear where oxytocin has been used to accelerate labour of spontaneous onset (Chew and Swann, 1977), so it remains doubtful whether there is a specific drug effect. If it exists, it is less important in causing neonatal jaundice than other factors associated with induction, such as earlier gestation.

Although uterine dysfunction is usually treated by oxytocin infusion, there are preliminary reports about the use of β-adrenoceptor blocking drugs such as propranolol (Mitrani et al., 1975).

Certain prostaglandins (substances which are found in many animal tissues and which have a wide variety of pharmacological effects) have been used in the induction of labour and have been found to be very effective (Karim and Hillier, 1974; Weekes et al., 1976). Indeed some trials have suggested that certain prostaglandins, such as E_2, have attributes which may eventually make them superior to oxytocin as an oxytocic agent (Liggins, 1974). Prostaglandins seem particularly well suited to induction of labour in women with prolonged fetal death, anencephaly or hydatidiform mole. In all of these complications of pregnancy, oxytocin is relatively ineffective and surgical intervention may be deemed unwise, whereas the uterus can usually be evacuated within 24 hours by administration of prostaglandin $F_2\alpha$ or E_2. Prostaglandins may be used to 'ripen' the unfavourable cervix prior to induction of labour (MacKenzie and Embrey, 1977).

11. Therapeutic Abortion

There are now many large series from various parts of the world in which the reported incidence of complications of therapeutic abortion is very low. Complications are much more common and serious in the second trimester than in the first.

Before the 12th week, surgical termination by the vaginal route is still the most widely used. It carries little risk of trauma, haemorrhage or sepsis, provided that reasonable precautions are taken, and particularly if it is carried out before the tenth week. The cervix need not be dilated very much and this can be done under local cervical analgesia and promazine 25mg. A plastic suction curette of the Karman type can be used and the procedure carried out on an outpatient basis.

Between 10 and 12 to 14 weeks, general anaesthesia is preferable and great care must be exercised to avoid tearing the cervix.

Recent development of prostaglandins for vaginal administration seems promising for very early abortion. Abortion is usually successful and complete; side effects do occur, but are outweighed by the advantage of self administration (MacKenzie et al., 1978).

From 14 weeks onwards, amnion infusion is usually preferred. Intra-amniotic hypertonic saline and urea give quite good results, but the use of prostaglandins ($F_{2\alpha}$ or E_2), infused transcervically between the uterine wall and the amniotic sac has emerged as an alternative method (Karim and Hillier, 1974; Brenner, 1975). It is applicable mainly in the second trimester of pregnancy. The general availability of long acting synthetic analogues of prostaglandins may make this a single injection technique (WHO Task Force, 1977a). Intra-amniotic administration has also been used and has a shorter induction-abortion interval than intra-amniotic hypertonic saline (WHO Task Force, 1976, 1977b), but hypertonic saline has been associated with fewer complications in some series (Grimes et al., 1977). Intravenous prostaglandins ($F_{2\alpha}$ and E_2) have also been successfully used, particularly when combined with an oxytocin drip or intra-amniotic hypertonic urea (Burkman et al., 1978), but side effects such as diarrhoea and vomiting are too frequent to make this a popular method. The intra-amniotic and extra-amniotic routes of administration are examples of the successful application of the principle that prostaglandins can be effective without side effects when they are delivered close to the site of action (Liggins, 1974). Another possible means of avoiding side effects is by incorporating prostaglandins into slow release drug delivery systems, e.g. for slow, predictable release of prostaglandins from sites such as the vagina.

Supplies of the synthetic prostaglandin analogues are at present limited and it has also not yet been finally determined whether an intra-amniotic, extra-amniotic, vaginal or even the oral route might prove to be the best (Brenner, 1975).

12. Lactation Suppression

Many women wish to suppress lactation in spite of the great advantages of breast feeding. For a number of years, stilboestrol was given in large doses immediately after delivery to suppress lactation, but it now seems clear that this practice is not only ineffective, since many women continue to lactate spontaneously, but also possibly dangerous.

It has been shown there may be an increased risk of venous thrombosis with stilboestrol administration, especially in women over 35 years of age who have had an assisted delivery (Jeffcoate et al., 1968).

Bromocriptine may replace the other methods of drug inhibition of lactation in the future (Roland, 1979). It appears to be specific at the pituitary level in preventing the release of prolactin, but does not seem to affect the release of any pituitary hormones (sect. 23.6). Bromocriptine 2.5mg twice daily for 2 weeks is significantly better than an oestrogen or a single dose long acting oestrogen-androgen injection, both in respect of lesser milk production and mammary congestion (Rolland and Schellekens, 1978; Utian et al., 1975). However, side effects such as nausea, headaches, and dizziness may be a problem. A further potential disadvantage is that the first ovulation will occur earlier, thus necessitating prompt attention to contraception. Bromocriptine is also expensive. Other agents being investigated for shorter course use include the antioestrogen tamoxifen (Masala et al., 1978) and the antiserotonin agent metergoline (Crosignani et al., 1978).

Lactation should be suppressed naturally, simply by not suckling the infant, with supportive measures such as binders and mild analgesics. The administration of diuretics is not contraindicated but is of no proven benefit.

13. Fertility Control

Although a number of other contraceptive techniques are available, and indeed commonly used, hormonal steroid contraception is overwhelmingly the most widely used method in developed countries. This would seem to be mainly because it is the most effective method in terms of pregnancy rates, but also because it is simple and convenient, does not interrupt the sexual act, and is taken by the woman who is naturally better motivated to adopt a method-effective contraceptive technique.

13.1 Hormonal Steroid Preparations

A variety of types of preparation have been produced and are available or under study in various countries (Seddon, 1971). These include:

a) *Continuous low dose oral progestagens* — two of these, chlormadinone as with another 17α-

hydroxyprogesterone derivative megestrol acetate, were withdrawn from the market because animal work had shown the development of nodules in the mammary glands of beagle bitches, but nor-testosterone derived progestagens norethisterone (norethindrone), ethynodiol diacetate, lynoestrenol or norgestrel are available and used, although irregular bleeding is common in early cycles of use, and pregnancy rates are slightly higher than with combined oestrogen-progestagen preparations (Brogden et al., 1973).

b) *Injectable long acting progestagens* — an intramuscular injection of an agent such as medroxyprogesterone acetate; usually 150mg once every 3 months but 450mg once every 6 months has been used (Castle et al., 1978). Norethisterone oenanthate, 200mg once every 2 months for the first 4 injections then once every 3 months, has also been used (Giwa-Osagie et al., 1978). Although effective, this method is not always accepted because of menstrual irregularities. There is also a high incidence of amenorrhoea which persists for some time after the last injection (Nash, 1975; Editorial, 1977). Menstrual irregularities and amenorrhoea appear to be less with norethisterone oenanthate than with medroxyprogesterone acetate (WHO Task Force, 1978).

c) *Intrauterine long acting progestagens* — inert T-shaped units, which release predetermined minute amounts of progestagen (e.g. 65μg a day of progesterone) over a period of 1 year. They appear to be highly effective, ovulation does not appear to be suppressed and the menstrual pattern is not disturbed (Phariss, 1978) but the incidence of ectopic pregnancy may be increased (Snowden, 1977).

d) *Sequential therapy* — cyclical administration of oestrogen only in the first part of the cycle, with added progestagen in the second half of the cycle. This type of preparation is much less popular than the combined pill because of relatively high pregnancy rates. There also appears to be an increased risk of endometrial carcinoma (Silverberg et al., 1977).

e) *Post coital contraception* — Most sexually active women require long term contraception, but there is a place for the post coital administration of hormones where a woman has already been exposed to unprotected coitus or rape. Diethylstilboestrol 50mg daily for 5 days or ethinyloestradiol 5mg for 5 days should be given (Haspels, 1976). A combination of ethinyloestradiol and norgestrel has also been used (Yuzpe and Lancee, 1977). The only side effect is nausea and vomiting. Treatment must be commenced within 48 hours of the time when conception may have occurred. Great care must be taken not to prescribe this therapy for a woman who is already in established pregnancy because of the possible risk of congenital abnormalities (Janerich et al., 1974; Nora et al., 1978; see also chapter III, sect. 5.3).

f) *Combined oestrogen-progestagens* — given usually from day 5 to day 26 of the cycle. This is by far the most widely used type of oral contraceptive. However, it has never been established that it is necessary or beneficial for administration to be cyclical, and a recent report finds continuous therapy for 84 days followed by a break of 6 days during which withdrawal bleeding usually occurs to be very acceptable to women (Loudon et al., 1977). Whether continuous therapy will have a different rate of side effects remains to be established.

The progestagen component (19-nortestosterone or 17α-hydroxyprogesterone derivatives) is in a daily dose of from 0.125 to 5mg and the oestrogen component (ethinyloestradiol or mestranol) in a daily dose of 0.02 to 0.15mg (table III). The possibility of using natural oestrogens such as oestradiol is being explored.

The contraceptive mode of action of steroidal preparations has not yet been fully elucidated, but it is likely that they act at a number of sites (Seddon, 1971). They inhibit ovulation by suppressing the mid cycle peak of luteinising hormone. Ovarian sensitivity to gonadotrophin and ovarian steroidogenesis may also be interfered with. There is not much information about the effect upon the Fallopian tube, but sperm capacitation or tubal transport rates may be affected. The endometrium is proliferative in the initial part of the cycle but then becomes atrophic so that even if ovulation did occur, implantation would be unlikely. The cervical mucus becomes thick and cellular with a high albumin content, thus unfavourable to sperm penetration. Of these effects, inhibition of ovulation seems to be the most important one with combined preparations, while the contraceptive effect of low dose oral progestagen only preparations appears to depend mainly on their effect on cervical mucus.

13.2 Acceptability

The efficacy of any contraceptive method depends upon its acceptability to the user, and upon the care with which it is used (see Liggins, 1971). Study of large populations of women using steroidal contraceptives have identified many side effects which reduce the acceptability of this method of contraception for a few users. There must always be a reasonable perspective in assessment of the problems and side effects of hormonal steroid contraception. While some side effects of hormonal steroid contraceptives are of major importance (for review, see McQueen, 1971, 1978), many of the side effects described or complained of by patients are either harmless or only minor nuisances, all are extremely uncommon, particularly since the advent of low dose preparations, and for most women seeking a reliable contraceptive, steroidal contraceptives offer a reasonable solution, although it is to be hoped that research will lead to improvements. In the meantime, combined oestrogen-progestagen oral contraceptives are the most acceptable and effective method of temporary contraception, and most women are probably safer using these preparations than using other less reliable or unreliable methods of reversible contraception. Nevertheless, intrauterine contraceptive devices challenge combination preparations in user acceptability and are preferred by some women even though they are associated with a higher risk of pregnancy and an increased risk of extrauterine pregnancy or spontaneous abortion, sometimes complicated by infection (Vessey, 1978).

It has usually been regarded as essential that hormonal steroid contraceptives be available only on prescription, and that all women using them should be subjected to repeated intensive observation during their use. However, it has been suggested that such procedures inhibit many of the women most in need from using them, and that screening should be reduced to a minimum except for selected cases, or indeed that medical intervention should occur only if the woman has a complaint. Paramedical personnel such as nurses, health visitors, midwives and pharmacists have been trained to provide oral contraception in many countries, but their use is still controversial in Western developed countries.

13.3 Minor Side Effects

There may be some symptoms which do not constitute more than a minor nuisance for most patients. Thus the oestrogen component tends to cause fluid retention, nausea, exacerbation of

Table III. Hormonal steroid contraceptive preparations

Type	Oestrogen	Progestagen	
		19-nortestosterone derivatives	17-α-hydroxy-progesterone derivatives
1. *Oral*			
Combination (20-22 day)	Ethinyloestradiol (0.02 to 0.1mg; i.e. 20 to 100µg	Ethynodiol diacetate (0.5 to 2mg) Lynoestrenol (1 to 2.5mg) Norethisterone (norethindrone) (0.5mg) Norethisterone acetate (1 to 4mg) d-Norgestrel[1] (0.125 to 0.25mg) dl-Norgestrel[1] (0.5mg) Quingestanol acetate (0.5mg)	
	Mestranol (ethinyloestradiol 3-methyl ether) 0.05 to 0.15mg; i.e. 50 to 150µg	Ethynodiol diacetate (0.5 to 1mg) Lynoestrenol (1 to 5mg) Norethisterone (1 to 2mg) Norethynodrel (2.5 to 5mg)	
Combination continuous (28 day)[2]	Ethinyloestradiol (0.05mg i.e. 50µg)	Ethynodiol diacetate (1mg) Lynoestrenol (1mg) Norethisterone acetate (1 to 2.5mg) d-Norgestrel (0.125 to 0.25mg) dl-Norgestrel (0.5mg)	
	Mestranol (0.05mg; i.e. 50µg)	Norethisterone (1mg)	
Sequential continuous (28 day)[3]	Ethinyloestradiol (0.1mg; i.e. 100µg)		Dimethisterone (25mg 5 or 6 tablets)
	Mestranol (0.08mg; i.e. 80µg)	Norethisterone (2mg 6 or 7 tablets)	
Combination[7] sequential (28 day)	Ethinyloestradiol (0.05mg; i.e. 50µg)	d-Norgestrel (0.05mg → 0.125mg)	
Progestagen only[4] continuous (28 day)		Ethynodiol diacetate (0.5mg) Lynoestrenol (0.5mg) Norethisterone (0.30 or 0.35mg) d-Norgestrel (0.03mg; i.e. 30µg) dl-Norgestrel (0.075mg; i.e. 75µg) Quingestanol acetate (0.3mg)	
2. *Injectable*			
Progestagen only[5] continuous (90 day)		Norethisterone oenanthate (200mg/ml)[6]	Medroxyprogesterone acetate (150mg/ml)

1   dl-Norgestrel (the racemate) consists of equal amounts of d-(—) [i.e. d-form, laevorotatory isomer] and l-(+) forms. Only the d-form is biologically active; 0.25mg d-norgestrel (levonorgestrel) is considered biologically equivalent to 0.5mg dl-norgestrel.

2   Employ 21 active tablets followed by 7 inert (lactose) or iron with or without vitamin B complex tablets.

3   Employ 21 to 23 active tablets followed by 5 to 7 inert (lactose) or iron with or without vitamin B complex tablets.

4   Of value for women in whom oestrogen is contraindicated or not desirable.

5   In general, for women who have completed their family (see also text for other regimens).

6   Given once every 60 days for first 4 injections, then once every 90 days.

7   Employ 11 active tablets (ethinyloestradiol 0.05mg + d-norgestrel 0.05mg) followed by 10 active tablets (ethinyloestradiol 0.05mg + d-norgestrel 0.125mg), then 7 inert tablets.

varicosities, menorrhagia, breakthrough bleeding and cervical erosion, whereas progestagens may cause acne, greasy hair, weight gain and breast fullness. The incidence of these symptoms may be reduced by switching to a different preparation with a lower ratio of the hormone thought to be responsible for the symptoms (Liggins, 1971).

It should be noted that pregnancy is more likely to occur where there is breakthrough bleeding, so that dosage should be promptly adjusted. For example, during the first cycle in which breakthrough bleeding occurs an extra tablet may be taken on days of bleeding; the patient should be prescribed a preparation with a greater progestagen-oestrogen ratio in the next cycle. Certain side effects (e.g. nausea, menstrual cramps, breast discomfort) are less common in overweight women and more so in the underweight (Talwar and Berger, 1977); body weight should therefore be taken into account when prescribing an oral contraceptive.

Beneficial side effects are reduction in the volume of menstrual flow, regularity of menstruation, and almost invariable absence of dysmenorrhoea. Functional ovarian cysts also seem to occur less often in women using oral contraceptives.

13.4 Laboratory Test Values

The results of a number of laboratory tests have been found to be altered in patients using steroidal contraceptives (Wilson, 1973). The serum iron, and the total iron binding capacity are raised, probably due to the progestagen component of the combined pill. The protein bound iodine level in the serum is raised to apparently thyrotoxic levels, which may interfere with the diagnosis of thyrotoxicosis (see chapter XVI; sect. 14.2). The incidence of disease of the thyroid, however, is reduced (Frank and Kay, 1978) probably because autoimmune processes are retarded. There is some controversy as to whether serum folate levels are reduced, as in pregnancy. α-Macroglobulin and IgG levels are increased. Absorption and metabolism of vitamins of the B group may be impaired, and vitamin C levels are also reduced, while vitamin A concentration is increased (Wynn, 1975).

The plasma concentration of dehydroepiandrosterone sulphate and androsterone sulphate is reduced, while plasma cortisol is increased. None of these effects seem to be of any clinical significance.

13.5 Drug Interactions with Oral Contraceptives

Oral contraceptives have a potential to inhibit the metabolism of other drugs (Homeida et al., 1978).

More importantly, several drugs (including barbiturates, phenytoin and rifampicin) significantly accelerate the biotransformation of oral contraceptives by induction of liver drug metabolising enzymes; hence predisposing to loss of effectiveness and unplanned pregnancy (Skolnick et al., 1976; Gelbke et al., 1977). In clinical practice, such accelerated biotransformation may be suspected if breakthrough bleeding occurs, and the oral contraceptive dose increased or another contraceptive method chosen (Hempel and Klinger, 1976; Roberton and Johnson, 1976).

13.6 Liver Function Abnormalities

After reports of cholestatic jaundice resulting from administration of the early combined oral contraceptives, many studies showed abnormalities of liver function by conventional tests in asymptomatic women on steroid contraceptives (see McQueen, 1971, 1978). Bromsulphthalein excretion was reduced, probably due to the oestrogen component, while nortestosterone derivatives with an ethinyl group at C17 are thought to cause a rise in transaminase levels. These test results do not necessarily signify liver damage, and in fact it has been shown that oral contraceptives can safely be administered to women during and following recovery from acute viral hepatitis, cholelithiasis treated surgically, liver fluke disease, or to women who have suffered from jaundice or pruritus during pregnancy (Schweitzer et al., 1975; Editorial, 1974). Cholelithiasis occurs about twice as commonly in women using oral contraceptives (Boston Collaborative Program, 1973; Howat et al., 1975). One study (Morrison et al., 1977) has suggested an increased incidence of acute hepatitis, but this is almost certainly a misleading conclusion based on inadequate control selection. Oral contraceptives should not, of course, be given to a jaundiced patient or to patients with other types of cholestatic hepatobiliary illness, since pathways of oestrogen metabolism are disturbed and under these circumstances oestrogens may be harmful (Editorial, 1974; Adlercreutz, 1974).

There have been a number of reports of benign hepatic tumours in women taking oral contraceptives, usually for prolonged periods, but it is not yet certain whether the association is one of cause and effect. Some cases have caused serious, even fatal haemorrhage, and a few have shown malignant degeneration (see McQueen, 1978).

13.7 Metabolic Effects

Progestagens seem to cause a rise in serum cholesterol levels while oestrogens lead to a rise in triglyceride levels. Oral contraceptive users have been found to show reduced high density lipoprotein cholesterol levels (Arntzenius et al., 1978; Bradley et al., 1978). Glucose tolerance has been reported as being slightly impaired by certain combination preparations (e.g. higher dose oestrogen ones). There does not seem to be any serious risk that normal women using steroid contraceptives will actually develop clinical diabetes, but caution should be exercised in their administration to at risk women such as those who have had gestational diabetes, or to women who are already diabetics (Posner et al., 1975). It should be remembered, however, that pregnancy is also diabetogenic, so that if other methods of contraception are not effective, oral hormonal contraception may be safer than a series of pregnancies (see also chapter XVI; sect. 13.1). Massive hypertriglyceridaemia leading to acute pancreatitis has very occasionally been reported (see further McQueen, 1971, 1978).

13.8 Neuro-ocular and Miscellaneous Effects

Although migraine and headaches seem to be exacerbated in some women using oral contraceptives, there is no definite evidence of a causal association (Dalton, 1976; Ryan, 1978). It seems best to treat each patient as an individual, withholding oral contraception only if headaches regularly follow hormone consumption. Oral contraception seems to exert a protective effect against rheumatoid arthritis which occurs only half as often in controls (RCGP, 1978). Chorea has been reported, with many features similar to chorea gravidarum, but seems to be uncommon (Riddoch et al., 1971). Corneal oedema rarely occurs and may constitute a nuisance in patients using contact lenses (Koetting, 1966); otherwise contact lenses appear to be well tolerated by oral contraceptive users (de Vries Reilingh et al., 1978). Women who are lactating sometimes find that the amount of milk is reduced by the use of some oestrogen containining contraceptives. Low dose oestrogen combination preparations and progestagen only oral and injectable preparations do not seem to significantly affect milk production (Buchanan, 1975; Koetsawang, 1977; Zanartu, 1976). The amount of steroid ingested by the breast fed infant is small and in the case of norgestrel is readily metabolised (Nilsson et al., 1977). Hormonal contraceptives may be responsible for induction of symptomatic hepatic porphyria or elicitation of symptoms of an underlying porphyria variegata or intermittent porphyria (Behm and Unger, 1974).

13.9 Benign Breast Neoplasia

Benign breast neoplasia is significantly less common in women using oral contraception (Sartwell et al., 1973; Li Volsi et al., 1978). There is no good evidence of any effect upon the incidence of malignancy, or upon the outcome of breast malignancy where oral contraception was in use immediately preceding diagnosis (see section 23.3). The possibility that oral hormonal contraceptives may be associated with other types of neoplasia is discussed in section 23.3.

13.10 Depression and Loss of Libido

Whether depression and loss of libido (often attributed to the progestagen component) are really due to hormonal contraception is difficult to assess (Dennerstein and Burrows, 1976), since other non-hormonal factors, such as freedom from the fear of unwanted pregnancy, or subconscious wish for pregnancy, may be involved. However, comparison of oral contraceptive users with patients using intrauterine contraceptive devices, suggests that depression and loss of libido can occur in some women, particularly those who showed some evidence of prior emotional disturbance. Some women who are depressed on oral contraception have vitamin B_6 deficiency and may respond to pyridoxine 40mg daily (Malek-Ahmadi and Behrmann, 1976).

13.11 Hypertension

Activation of the renin/angiotensin/aldosterone system occurs during oral oestrogen containing contraceptive therapy but it is doubtful whether this is of clinical significance (see McQueen, 1971; 1978; Weir, 1978). A number of women have been found to have a rise in blood pressure while using oestrogen containing oral contraceptives. The dose of and particular progestagen may contribute to the oestrogen induced rise in blood pressure (Meade et al., 1977; RCGP, 1977b). Apparently 'malignant' hypertension has been reported, regressing (sometimes slowly) after the pill was withdrawn but is usually associated with renal failure. However, a large study of normotensive women using hormonal steroid contraceptives has shown that few of them become clinically hypertensive, although there is a rise in mean systolic and diastolic pressure (Weir et al., 1974). This does not seem to be a major problem provided regular measurement of the blood pressure is made in selected cases (see Weir, 1978; also chapter XVIII; sect. 12.1).

13.12 Blood Coagulation and Circulatory Abnormalities

Various tests have shown certain abnormalities of blood clotting and fibrinolysis in women on oral contraceptives. The effect is most marked with combination preparations and is thought to be attributable to oestrogen, but may be contributed to by the progestagen component (for review, see McQueen, 1971, 1978; Vessey and Mann, 1978). Sensitive laboratory techniques appear to indicate that oral contraceptive users develop thrombotic lesions, usually of the clinically silent type, with greater frequency than non-users (Alkjaersig et al., 1975).

Clinical observation has also shown evidence of an increased risk of various forms of thrombosis. The haemolytic uraemic syndrome, possibly due to thrombotic microangiopathy, may occur more commonly in women taking oral contraceptives but is very rare (Brown et al., 1973). The risk of thrombotic strokes is increased around 4-fold in users of oral contraceptives, particularly in those who smoke cigarettes. Oral contraceptive use alone, in the absence of smoking, hypertension or migraine, also increases the risk of stroke (Collaborative Group, 1973, 1975).

Oral contraceptive usage is only one of a number of factors predisposing to myocardial infarction in women in the reproductive age group; obesity, hypercholesterolaemia, hypertension, diabetes and excessive cigarette smoking may be more important (Oliver, 1974; Ory, 1977). There is some dispute as to whether oral contraceptive usage alone augments the risk where none of these

factors is present and whether any effect is additive or synergistic (Arthes and Masi, 1976; Hennekens and MacMahon, 1977). The relative risk of death seems to be increased 3-fold in women aged between 40 and 44, and the attributable mortality is of the order of 20 per 100,000 (Mann et al., 1976) so that women in this age group certainly require careful screening before oral contraception is prescribed.

There is also an increased risk of venous thrombosis and pulmonary embolism. It seems that the risk of sustaining a clinically detectable episode of venous thrombosis is increased between 5 and 6-fold by the administration of combination oral contraceptives (RCGP, 1974) and persists if allowance is made for smoking habit (Lawson et al., 1977). The risk of developing postoperative thromboembolic complications is 3 or 4 times greater if combination oral contraceptives have been used immediately prior to operation (Vessey et al., 1970). The risk of death from thromboembolism while using combination oral contraceptives is around 7 or 8 times greater than in non-users (Inman and Vessey, 1968), although this risk may well be reduced by the use of a daily dosage of oestrogen not greater than 0.05mg (Inman et al., 1970; Committee on Safety of Drugs, 1970). In any case, it is important to emphasise that the risk is very small (only 1.5 deaths per 100,000 women aged 20 to 34 years); that the risk is much less than that of dying of cancer, or in a road accident; and that it is certainly much less than the risk of dying as a result of pregnancy, which is about 15 times greater (Inman and Vessey, 1968). It is of interest that venous thrombosis not associated with pregnancy is less likely to recur if the original episode was during oral contraceptive use than if it was not (Badaracco and Vesey, 1974), suggesting that the mechanism by which oral contraceptives predispose to venous thrombosis is dissimilar to the aetiology of idiopathic thrombosis.

The risk of death from all diseases of the circulatory system in ever users (i.e. users and ex users) of oral contraceptives is around 5 times greater than in never users; the increased death rate being concentrated in older women, in those with a long duration of oral contraceptive use and in cigarette smokers (RCGP, 1977a; table IV). It is important to emphasise that the risk of premature death from circulatory disease, in the absence of other risk factors, is very small in younger women (5 per 100,000 ever users cf 2 per

Table IV. Excess annual death rate from circulatory disease in oral contraceptive ever users related to age, duration of use and smoking habits (after Royal College General Practitioners, 1977a)

Age group	
15-34 years	1 per 20,000
35-44 years	1 per 3,000
45-49 years	1 per 700
Duration of use	
< 5 years	1 per 8,000
> 5 years	1 per 2,000
Smoking habits	
Non-smokers	1 per 10,000
Smokers	1 per 3,000

100,000 non-users aged 15 to 34 years) and that in the RCGP 1977 study, the overall risk of death was not increased since there was a deficit in other causes of death such as malignancy in the oral contraceptive users. Also, it is not known whether these risks apply to the same extent to low oestrogen dose oral contraceptives in current use. Nevertheless, there is a clear responsibility for caution and consideration of the contraceptive method in women aged 30 to 35 years and over, particularly those who have used oral contraceptives for a long time and who are cigarette smokers.

14. Infertility

Although there have been major developments in the drug treatment of infertility in women during the last 25 years, it is important to remember that this is of value only to those patients where hormonal abnormality is the cause of the infertility (at most, 15% of cases presenting at infertility clinics). Careful history taking, examination and investigation of both husband and wife are essential before embarking upon therapy, to determine, if possible, a specific hormonal cause for the infertility and to exclude other causes which would render correction of the hormonal cause ineffective (Harrison, 1977). Lesions which would contraindicate hormone therapy to the wife are, for example, azoospermia in the husband, or tubal non-patency in the wife. Treatment of infertility in the male is discussed in chapter XVI (sect. 11).

14.1 Ovulatory Infertility

Study of women who have been shown to ovulate with a luteal phase of normal length, has identified mild hyperprolactinaemia which apparently responds well to bromocriptine therapy, both in respect of reduction in the plasma production and the pregnancy rate (Lenton et al., 1977). Bromocriptine is an ergot alkaloid which acts by direct stimulation of postsynaptic dopaminergic receptors at pituitary and also hypothalamic levels, thus directly inhibiting prolactin release (Fluckiger, 1978; Mehta and Tolis, 1979). Common side effects are nausea and vomiting, dizziness and constipation. It is advisable to increase dosage gradually to the usual dose of 5mg daily, to reduce the severity of side effects. Where pregnancy does occur, it is usually recommended that therapy should be stopped as soon as pregnancy is confirmed, although there is no precise evidence of harmful effects of continuing it.

14.2 Defective Luteal Phase

If a woman is ovulating, but has been shown by temperature charting or hormone assays to have a luteal phase which is of less than 14 days duration; or is defective in that urinary pregnanediol or plasma progesterone levels are low, then it may be that infertility is due to failure of implantation of the fertilised ovum. This pattern is sometimes associated with hyperprolactinaemia. Although there is no clear evidence that hormone therapy actually improves the pregnancy rate in such women, it has been shown that plasma progesterone levels in the luteal phase are increased by administration of clomiphene 100mg daily for 5 days from the second day of the cycle, or by bromocriptine 2.5mg twice daily in cases of hyperprolactinaemia. Intramuscular injection of human chorionic gonadotrophin (which acts as a luteinising hormone) 5,000iu twice weekly during the luteal phase may also be helpful.

14.3 Failure of Ovulation

Where infertility seems to be due to failure of ovulation, or to very infrequent ovulation, but where the couple are otherwise quite normal and not too old, induction of ovulation may be tried. In addition to exclusion of other causes for the infertility investigation should also as far as possible exclude the more serious causes of failure of ovulation, which may themselves require treatment, such as pituitary tumours or adrenal cortical hyperplasia or tumour.

Induction of ovulation in normoprolactinaemic patients should normally be by clomiphene or similar compounds such as cyclofenil or tamoxifen in the first instance. Clomiphene is administered orally in a dose of from 50 to 200mg daily for 5 days. It is rather similar in structure to stilboestrol, but acts partly as an antioestrogen. It seems to be effective in ovulation induction by mimicking the oestrogen surge in the follicular phase of a normal ovulatory cycle, and possibly also stimulating ovarian steroidogenesis, and thus causing gonadotrophin release and ovulation, usually from 6 to 11 days after completion of the course (Kistner and Smith, 1960; Greenblatt, 1961). Side effects such as hot flushes are rare when small doses are used, and are not severe. Visual symptoms (scintillation and light halos) and ovarian enlargement have been reported, particularly when larger doses have been used.

The ovulation rate achieved will depend upon the type of patient to whom the drug is administered. Women with Stein-Leventhal syndrome respond very well, whereas those with prolonged amenorrhoea of hypothalamic origin, associated with very low ovarian oestrogen production, respond poorly (MacGillivray and Klopper, 1968). Overall ovulation rates of around 70% have been widely reported but not all these ovulations will result in pregnancy. Even where intercourse is correctly timed, pregnancy may only be expected to occur in about 15% of ovulations. Multiple pregnancy due to superovulation occurs more often than in women ovulating spontaneously, but is not a serious problem when small doses of the drug are used initially and are not exceeded if ovulation has occurred. Repeat courses of treatment may be given without danger, and since this form of treatment is relatively safe, very close monitoring by hormone assays is not essential. However, since it is difficult to know whether cycles produced are ovulatory or non-ovulatory (unless pregnancy occurs), serial hormone assays are advantageous in the assessment of the success of treatment and the prognosis for the patient.

In hyperprolactinaemic women treatment should, of course, be with bromocriptine, in a dose which is sufficient to lower the plasma prolactin to normal; usually 5 to 7.5mg daily (Franks, 1979; Seppala et al., 1976). Regular menstruation is usually rapidly restored but ovulation may be confirmed by luteal phase plasma progesterone assays.

Patients who have been shown to fail to ovulate on clomiphene or bromocriptine therapy may then be treated with gonadotrophins, which are much more expensive and dangerous. Two preparations are required: (a) human menopausal gonadotrophin, which contains both follicle stimulating hormone (FSH) and luteinising hormone (LH) but of these, the FSH is the important constituent, although the LH probably plays a subsidiary role; and (b) human chorionic gonadotrophin, which acts as luteinising hormone.

Human menopausal gonadotrophin is given intramuscularly in doses of from 75 to 1,500iu of FSH daily or on alternate days for 7 to 14 days. It is absolutely essential that daily oestrogen assays (in blood or urine) should be done during this phase of the treatment to assess the response of the ovaries to the drugs, since several follicles may in fact respond and be capable of ovulation (Hancock et al., 1970). Provided that an adequate but not excessive rise in oestrogen output has occurred, ovulation is then induced by the administration of human chorionic gonadotrophin in a single intramuscular injection of 5,000 to 10,000iu. Conception should be attempted within 48 hours.

The major serious side effect of this form of therapy is ovarian hyperstimulation (i.e. ovulation of several follicles), resulting in ovarian enlargement which may be massive, and sometimes associated with abdominal pain, ascites, pleural effusion, intravascular thrombosis and hypoproteinaemia. This condition may be fatal. A later sequel of non-fatal cases of ovarian hyperstimulation is the occurrence of multiple pregnancy (in 'litters' of a size never seen in pregnancy following spontaneous ovulation) with very high perinatal mortality rates. A rare sequel of gonadotrophin and bromocriptine has been rapid enlargement during pregnancy of pre-existing (though not always previously recognised) pituitary microadenoma (Bergh et al., 1978a). Frequent visual field testing offers the best chance of early diagnosis of this complication, which may be treated by reinstituting bromocriptine, by terminating pregnancy, by pituitary irradiation or surgery. Whether irradiation or sugery should preferably be undertaken prior to ovulation induction remains controversial.

Because of these serious and dangerous side effects, gonadotrophins should be administered only by specialists who have experience in this type of work, and who have access to a laboratory capable of performing urgent daily oestrogen assays with some accuracy. Improved techniques, such as radioimmunoassay of blood oestrogens, reduce the hazards of gonadotrophin therapy.

In uncomplicated cases there is no contraindication to the use of repeat courses of gonadotrophin therapy, although the cost of human menopausal gonadotrophin and the inconvenience of daily injections and assays to the patient usually limits the number of courses to around six. Gonadotrophin releasing factors are now available, and widely used in testing of ovarian-pituitary function; their place in clinical management of infertility is not yet established (Bergh et al., 1978b).

15. Disorders of Menstrual Function

15.1 Dysfunctional Uterine Haemorrhage

This is diagnosed only when history and examination (including diagnostic curettage) have shown no evidence of a specific organic condition, such as uterine fibroids, endometriosis, cervical or uterine carcinoma, or retained products of conception, to account for the haemorrhage (Beazley, 1972).

Surgical treatment, usually total hysterectomy, may be appropriate, depending upon the severity of the haemorrhage and the age and parity of the patient. However, in younger women who have not completed their family or who wish to conserve the uterus for some other reason, drug therapy may be very useful. The type of drug to be used depends upon whether investigation has shown ovulatory or anovulatory cycles.

Where menorrhagia is anovulatory, the administration of a progestagen such as norethisterone 10 to 20mg daily for 10 days from the 15th day of the cycle may achieve control. In ovulatory menorrhagia, the administration of a combined oestrogen-progestagen preparation from the 5th to the 26th day of the cycle is usually necessary. The dose of oestrogen should be as small as is compatible with control of the condition, and it is preferable not to exceed a daily dose of 0.05mg of ethinyloestradiol or mestranol (see section 13.12). It is usually wise to withdraw therapy, at least temporarily after about 3 cycles, since remission may occur.

A completely different approach to the drug therapy of menorrhagia is the use of antifibrinolytic agents such as ε-aminocaproic acid and tranexamic acid (see chapter XXIII; sect. 5.4). The rationale for the use of these preparations was the demonstration that the menstruating endometrium of women with menorrhagia (and especially those using intrauterine contraceptive devices), showed an increased content of plasminogen activators compared with that of normal women. Although controlled trials in unselected patients with dysfunctional uterine haemorrhage or excessive menstrual bleeding associated with intrauterine contraceptive devices have shown benefit from the administration of antifibrinolytic agents, their use should still be considered as experimental (Nilsson and Rybo, 1965, 1967; Kasonde and Bonnar, 1975), since it is thought that they may be thrombogenic, and there is some doubt as to whether they may be dysmorphogenic. The latter risk seems small, however, since these agents are administered only during menstruation, so that dysmorphogenesis could occur only if a threatened abortion was mistaken for a menstrual period.

The use of ethamsylate, a synthetic cyclohexadine, has been shown significantly to reduce measured menstrual blood loss. This drug acts by reducing capillary fragility. It is less effective in menorrhagia due to intrauterine contraceptive devices (Harrison and Campbell, 1976).

Recent study of women with menorrhagia has shown that treatment with prostaglandin synthetase inhibitors such as mefenamic or flufenamic acid will reduce menstrual flow in dysfunctional menorrhagia and menorrhagia due to intrauterine contraceptive devices (Guillebaud et al., 1978; Jakubowicz and Wood, 1978), suggesting that the heavy flow is associated in some way with increased endometrial prostaglandin production. The safety of this form of treatment has not been clearly established.

Another approach which shows some promise is the use of antioestrogens such as tamoxifen, to block the effect of oestrogens upon the endometrium at the endometrial level.

Clomiphene has been used to induce ovulation as a method of control in anovulatory menorrhagia, but of course the number of patients where pregnancy is desired is very limited, and its use where pregnancy was unwanted would be contraindicated.

15.2 Oligomenorrhoea

There is no indication to treat oligo- or amenorrhoea with drugs except where the patient complains of infertility, when ovulation induction may be attempted (see section 14.3). The temptation to produce regular withdrawal bleeds with cyclical oestrogen-progestagen therapy should be resisted, since the risks outweigh the marginal benefit of the emotional satisfaction for the patient of regular 'menstruation'. Such patients should of course be carefully examined and investigated to exclude serious conditions such as adrenal cortical hyperplasia or pituitary tumours which may present in this way.

15.3 Endometriosis

Extensive pelvic endometriosis, especially in an older woman, may require surgery, but the majority of patients can be treated at least for some time, with combined oestrogen-progestagen therapy, given either in a cyclical manner or continuously, in a dose sufficient to eliminate breakthrough bleeding. The aim of treatment is to produce endometrial atrophy, which is probably achieved more reliably by the continuous or 'pseudopregnancy' type of treatment. Hormone therapy inevitably prevents pregnancy, and where pregnancy is desired by the patient, therapy need not be prolonged beyond 6 months or so. An alternative, and perhaps more effective if more expensive form of therapy, is danazol, a synthetic steroid derivative of ethisterone with mild androgenic activity which may inhibit synthesis or release of gonadotrophins from the pituitary, but may act directly on the endometrium. In any event, it does produce endometrial atrophy and usually symptomatic and objective improvement (Symposium, 1977; Fraser, 1978). Usual dosage is 800mg daily initially, reduced after a month or two for a maximum course of 6 months' continuous therapy. Weight gain is common. Other less common side effects include gastrointestinal upsets, androgenic effects such as acne, oily skin, oedema and exacerbation of hirsutism, and a mild decrease in carbohydrate tolerance in diabetics.

15.4 Dysmenorrhoea

Primary dysmenorrhoea seems to occur only in ovulatory cycles, and the most rational treatment, if the condition is severe enough to require treatment, is therefore suppression of ovulation by cyclical combined oestrogen/progestagen preparations (such as oral contraceptives). However, if the patient wishes to retain her fertility during treatment, then cyclical treatment with the progestagen dydrogesterone 10mg twice daily may be tried, although it is less likely to be effective. Should cyclical hormone therapy fail to help the symptoms, menstruation may be abolished altogether by continuous therapy. It may be wise to stop this every few months to establish whether remission has occurred.

A recent development is the use of β_2-adrenoceptor stimulants such as terbutaline, salbutamol, fenoterol, etc which act by preventing or abolishing unduly high intrauterine pressures (Akerlund et al., 1976). Unfortunately, however, side effects such as tachycardia are common and distressing. The strong uterine contractions recorded may be due to prostaglandin secretion which may be inhibited by mefenamic and flufenamic acid, as in menorrhagia (Anderson et al., 1978).

Secondary dysmenorrhoea is more likely to have a specific cause, such as endometriosis and an attempt should be made to estimate the extent of this prior to therapy. Surgery may be required, but cyclical hormone therapy is often effective.

16. Menopausal Disturbances

When the ovaries are removed or become atrophied there is a marked increase in the production of FSH and LH due to the withdrawal of oestrogens. Natural loss of ovarian function usually occurs around the age of 50 years. The most dramatic and immediate changes which occur are due to the vasomotor disturbances (e.g. 'hot flushes', etc). These precede the cessation of menstruation in about 15% of women and are a transient, self limiting phenomenon, presumably associated with changes in hormone levels although the precise aetiology is not known. Many other changes occur but they develop more slowly during the postmenopausal years, when there is a stable state of very low oestrogen production. The incidence of these changes does not correlate with the degree of oestrogen 'deficiency'. Local atrophic changes in the genital tract associated with a greater predisposition to infection usually affect women after the age of 60 years. Alterations in fat and carbohydrate metabolism are most likely to occur at about the same age and this in turn possibly has an effect, not only on the higher incidence of diabetes, but also of coronary artery sclerosis. The incidence of diabetes may be related to the greater deposition of fat, but this is not necessarily dependent on oestrogen production and is probably part of the aging phenomenon. Premenopausal women are less likely than men of the same age to develop myocardial infarction, but the difference between the sexes diminishes greatly after the age of 50 (Heller and Jacobs, 1978). At the time of the menopause, oestrogen levels are reduced and it is also believed that there is a consequent increase in the resorptive activity of parathyroid hormone on bone. This results in a diminution in bone density in women aged between 50 to 65 years and in osteoporosis in women with an early or surgically induced menopause and may be responsible for the high incidence of crush fractures in this group of women. Postmenopausal bone loss can be prevented by the administration of oestrogens (Lindsay et al., 1978), calcium supplements or vitamin D, but it has not been established whether the incidence of crush fractures would be reduced (see further chapter XXII; sect. 11.2). Such treatment has no permanent effect, and would have to be continued indefinitely.

It would seem that a strong case could be made for giving oestrogens after the menopause to treat 'hot flushes' and other manifestations of vasomotor disturbance, and prophylactically to prevent atrophy not only of the genital tract but of the breasts and other tissues, and to prevent osteoporosis and loss of height. Against this are placed the risks of complications of oestrogen therapy in this age group. These are disturbances of carbohydrate metabolism, venous thrombosis (Boston Collaborative Program, 1974), hypertension, depression, and fluid retention in older patients with cardiac or renal insufficiency. There is also the problem of hormone induced uterine bleeding, which may delay the diagnosis of carcinoma of the endometrium, and the real, if remote, risk of induction of endometrial carcinoma with prolonged hormone therapy (see section 23.3). There is not too much controversy about the use of oestrogens for the treatment of vasomotor symptoms or in the treatment of atrophic ('senile') vaginitis or vulvitis, but there is doubt whether long term oestrogen therapy or oestrogen/progestagen therapy should be promoted or is justified, except in women with premature castration (see Shoemaker et al., 1977).

16.1 Vasomotor Symptoms

Hot flushes were previously treated with stilboestrol 1 to 3mg daily or ethinyloestradiol 0.1mg daily, but there may be an advantage in using natural oestrogens such as oestrone (1 to 4mg daily), oestradiol (2mg daily) or oestriol (0.5 to 2mg daily) to reduce the risk of side effects. The dose of oestrogen is regulated according to the flush count and is gradually reduced over a period of a few months. Where hot flushes are the only symptom, clonidine 50 to 75µg twice daily may be effective (Bolli and Simpson, 1975). Any other therapy is supportive. Antianxiety drugs or tricyclic antidepressants are not required for any symptoms specific to the menopause.

16.2 Atrophic Vaginitis

Atrophic vaginitis can be treated with dienoestrol vaginal cream, used night and morning for 10 to 14 days. Oral oestrogen (for 2 to 3 months) is more effective than cream in cases of atrophic vaginitis and urethritis, as indicated by symptoms of frequency and dysuria and a sterile urine.

16.3 Long Term Therapy

For long term therapy, which is advocated by some, oestriol, oestradiol, oestrone or conjugated oestrogens can be used. However, there is doubt about the safety of long term replacement oestrogen therapy (see above). There is still no practical method of selecting women most likely to benefit or of determining the minimum effective dose of oestrogen which will not produce undesirable side effects. Therapy is indicated in premature castration or gonadal dysgenesis and if the patient has a functional uterus treatment should usually be cyclical with added progestagen (see section 23.3). Prospective trials are required to establish the risks and benefits of routine therapy in postmenopausal women, but it should obviously be avoided in women with obesity, hypertension, varicose veins or a tendency to venous thrombosis, diabetes or any of the other contraindications to the use of oestrogens in this age group.

17. Hirsuties

Full investigation of women presenting with hirsuties is required, particularly if they also have oligomenorrhoea or amenorrhoea, to identify the cause. Most such women are found to have constitutional or idiopathic hirsuties, and while the response to treatment is often disappointing, some improvement can be achieved. The most effective treatment seems to be a combined oestrogen/-progestagen such as mestranol 1mg/ethynodiol diacetate 2mg, given cyclically. This acts principally by reducing ovarian steroidogenesis. The glucocorticosteroid dexamethasone 0.75mg daily has also been used (with the aim of reducing adrenocortical androgen production) and is sometimes effective. Cyproterone acetate (an anti-androgen) has not been fully evaluated but seems to be promising.

18. Gonorrhoea

Accurate diagnosis by the examination of smears and cultures is of the utmost importance in the management of gonorrhoea. Diagnosis may be particularly difficult in women, in whom the disease is often asymptomatic and infection suggested only by contact with an infected male. At the same time, the risk of serious complications, such as salpingitis, is greater in women than in men, so that diagnosis and adequate treatment is particularly important. Care should also be taken to exclude concurrent syphilis.

It is generally considered desirable that treatment should where possible be given by means of a single dose, ideally by intramuscular injection, but in any case with all treatment being administered under supervision. Penicillin is still the most effective drug in the treatment of gonorrhoea, although the dose required is very high (4.8 to 6 million units penicillin G in some communities) due to the emergence of relatively resistant gonococci. The effectiveness of therapy may be increased by the administration of probenecid 1g by mouth, half to 1 hour before the injection, and in some areas for a few doses thereafter. In cases of refusal to accept single dose injection therapy a single dose regimen of oral ampicillin or amoxycillin preceded by probenecid, can be used. Spectinomycin, a single dose by intramuscular injection, can be used in cases due to penicillinase producing strains of gonococci (see further chapter XXIX; sect. 3).

It is hoped that the rational use of drugs as outlined above and described in chapter XXIX may reduce the incidence of relative resistance of the gonococcus to penicillin, due to inefficient treatment with inappropriate penicillin regimens or other agents.

19. Vaginitis

Vaginitis is a common condition, but not every woman who presents with a complaint of vaginal discharge has vaginitis (Dennerstein, 1972). Thus management is based on the differential diagnosis of a physiological discharge from vaginitis due to infection or other pathological causes, e.g. deodorant induced, atrophic vaginitis (see section 16.2). Treatment of a physiological discharge is simple reassurance. The treatment of vaginal candidiasis or trichomoniasis is not difficult, provided that it is based on an accurate diagnosis so that an agent highly specific for the cause can be given. Preparations for which a dual spectrum of action is claimed seldom achieve the cure rate of those of more specific action for either *Candida* or *Trichomonas* spp. (see further chapter XXIX; sect. 6).

20. Malignant Disease

Drug treatment of gynaecological malignancies, with the exception of gestational choriocarcinoma, is generally disappointing, although about a third of patients with advanced or inoperable endometrial carcinoma respond to large doses of progestagens, as do some with ovarian carcinomatosis. Ovarian carcinoma often shows a good initial response to chemotherapeutic agents such as treosulphan, often rendering inoperable disease operable (Fennelly, 1977). Patients with breast cancer can be offered significant palliation by altering the hormonal milieu through additive hormone therapy or ablative surgery. Chemotherapy traditionally used when hormone manipulation is no longer effective is now being used increasingly alone or in combination with hormonal manipulation in disseminated disease and in combination with surgery in early breast cancer (Davis and Carbone, 1978; see further chapter XXIV; sect. 6.1, 6.6).

21. Medical Conditions Requiring Treatment in Pregnancy

21.1 Corticosteroid Therapy

Where the mother has an illness such as severe chronic asthma or ulcerative colitis for which she requires systemic corticosteroid therapy, certain problems arise.

Firstly, it has been suggested that when these drugs are taken in early pregnancy, an increased incidence of cleft palate occurs in the fetus (Popert, 1962). The evidence is not convincing and this hazard is not sufficient to justify withdrawal of corticosteroid therapy from a mother for whom it is necessary (Tuchmann-Duplessis, 1975a). Used in conservative dosage (e.g. 2.5 to 20mg daily prednisone or equivalent), corticosteroid therapy in pregnant asthmatics was not associated with an increase in complications (Schatz et al., 1975). No increased risk of congenital abnormalities has been observed in epidemiological studies of corticosteroid use in early pregnancy (Heinonen et al., 1977). See further chapter III, section 5.4.

Due to the high circulating cortisol levels which normally occur in pregnancy, it may be possible to reduce the therapeutic dose. Unfortunately, patients with ulcerative colitis often relapse in the puerperium and require increased doses (see chapter XIX; sect. 8.4). Most asthmatic patients can however, be managed on inhaled corticosteroids, with systemic administration reserved for exacerbations or periods of stress (see chapter XX; sect. 3.1.2).

When the mother is receiving steroid therapy, the fetal adrenal corticotrophin output is suppressed, so that the neonate may suffer from withdrawal symptoms, and should be observed very carefully. An incidental, but not harmful effect of suppression of fetal ACTH output is interference with the production of oestriol precursors from the fetal zone of the fetal adrenal, so that maternal oestriol output can not be used as an index of fetoplacental function in these patients.

21.2 Diabetes Mellitus

Insulin dependent diabetics obviously need to continue therapy during pregnancy, although the dose may well require adjustment. Control is made more difficult by such factors as renal glycosuria, hyperemesis gravidarum interfering with normal calorie intake, infection such as pyelonephritis, and the diabetogenic effect of pregnancy itself. Labour also constitutes a time of stress similar to that of surgical operation, when an adequate calorie intake must be ensured by intravenous infusion.

When a non-diabetic patient becomes a frank clinical diabetic during pregnancy, insulin therapy should be given in the normal way. However, when screening tests reveal chemical (latent) diabetes, the indications for treatment with oral hypoglycaemic agents are more doubtful. It has been suggested that sulphonylureas may be dysmorphogenic, but the balance of evidence is that this is not so (Tuchmann-Duplessis, 1975b), and large series have found the sulphonylureas to be safe (Notelovitz, 1971, 1974; Sutherland et al., 1973); although they should be stopped on the day before delivery or at least 4 days before in the case of long acting compounds such as chlorpropamide (Jackson, 1971), since prolonged neonatal hypoglycaemia has been reported following the administration of sulphonylureas to the mother (Kemball et al., 1970). There is, as yet, however, no definite evidence of any benefit resulting from treatment of gestational chemical diabetics with oral hypoglycaemic drugs in terms of reduction in perinatal mortality (see also chapter III, sect. 5.2; XVI, sect. 3.4.4).

21.3 Hyperthyroidism in Pregnancy

Thyrotoxicosis is the other common endocrine disease in pregnancy. It is treated in the same way as in the non-pregnant patient, except that radioiodine cannot be used and antithyroid drug dosage should be reduced to a minimum, especially in late pregnancy. Antithyroid drugs are withheld during lactation since they are held to be excreted in breast milk (see chapter III, sect. 5.1; XVI; sect. 5.2.4).

22. Drug Dependence in Pregnancy

Use of drugs of abuse in pregnancy has become a problem in many urban communities.

Marihuana (cannabis): There is no definite evidence as yet of any deleterious effect of cannabis smoking in pregnancy (see chapter III; sect. 3.5).

Diamorphine (heroin): Pregnancy is relatively uncommon in heroin addicts since they often have amenorrhoea, thought to be of hypothalamic origin. When addicts do become pregnant, there is a high incidence of obstetric complications, especially low birth weight and premature labour, but this may of course be due partly to the poor social background and lack of antenatal care rather than to a specific effect of the heroin. When the mother takes heroin within a week of delivery, the infant will usually suffer from withdrawal symptoms, with a 30 % mortality. There is some controversy as to whether an attempt should be made to withdraw heroin from the mother during pregnancy. This is certainly hazardous, but can be achieved in some cases, usually by methadone substitution (Blinick et al., 1976), and should be initiated as early as possible if this policy has been decided upon (see also chapter III; sect. 3.1).

Amphetamine: Dependence may be much more difficult to recognise, and although withdrawal is not particularly dangerous, it is often unacceptable to the patient. It is uncertain whether withdrawal symptoms do occur in the infant.

Barbiturates: Barbiturate withdrawal symptoms may occur in the neonate (usually rather later than heroin withdrawal symptoms) both when the mother is an addict and when barbiturates have been prescribed for the control of epilepsy.

Lysergic Acid Diethylamide (LSD): Dependence is not a problem with this drug, but it may be dysmorphogenic. There is conflicting evidence of chromosomal damage to leucocytes *in vitro,* and of dysmorphogenesis in animals and man. The birth of abnormal babies has however, followed upon the consumption of illicit LSD by both mother and father in early pregnancy, and chromatid breaks have been reported in the parents. These apparent drug related effects are hard to separate from the general effects of drug abuse.

23. Drug Induced Gynaecological and Endocrine Disorders

A variety of drugs may cause gynaecological or endocrine disorders. Patients with certain symptoms must be questioned and investigated carefully to ascertain the aetiology of their condition.

23.1 Amenorrhoea and Inhibition of Spermatogenesis

It has been reported that cytotoxic drugs (e.g. busulphan, chlorambucil, vincristine, cyclophosphamide) may commonly cause amenorrhoea in women and inhibition of spermatogenesis in men (e.g. Fairley et al., 1972; Warne et al., 1973). Such drugs are primarily used in the treatment of malignant disease, although cyclophosphamide has been widely used in the treatment of the nephrotic syndrome and various forms of glomerulonephritis, and the possibility that in any particular case the disturbance of reproductive function is due to the disease and not the drug treatment, should be borne in mind (Lendon et al., 1978). The effects on reproduction when cyclophosphamide is used in renal disease usually seem to be reversible, provided that the drug is suspended before a high total dose has been given (Buchanan et al., 1975; Etteldorf et al., 1976), although in malignant disease recovery of reproduction seems to depend on the particular chemotherapy regimen used (Roeser et al., 1978). The treatment of severe disease must of course take precedence.

By far the most common iatrogenic cause of secondary amenorrhoea in recent years has been the use of oral contraceptives (Shearman and Fraser, 1977). It is associated with galactorrhoea in about 40 % of cases and seems to be due to relatively prolonged exposure of the hypothalamic-pituitary-adrenal axis to progestagen and oestrogen with resulting low gonadotrophin output. The syndrome is in fact rare, occurring in some series in around 2 % of women using oral contraceptives (Evard et al., 1976), but is often seen because of the vast numbers of women now using these preparations. It is more likely to occur in women with a history of prior menstrual irregularity and requires investigation if lasting for a year or more, since abnormalities such as hyperprolactinaemia and microadenoma of the pituitary are found just as often as in women whose amenorrhoea was not antedated by oral contraceptive use. Fertility of both multigravid and parous women is initially impaired after stopping oral contraception, more than after stopping other methods of contraception, but after 42 months in nulliparae, and 30 months in parous women, differences are negligible, so there is no evidence of *permanent* infertility due to oral contraception (Vessey et al., 1978).

If patients complain of infertility, treatment with clomiphene or bromocriptine (or as a last resort gonadotrophins), is indicated (for details see section 14.3) and is likely to succeed in about 50 % of cases, but if they do not complain, no treatment is indicated since the condition is in itself harmless. Cases of hyperprolactinaemia should of course be kept under review. Further administration of cyclical hormone therapy should be used only if there are good reasons.

23.2 Impotence and Libido

Intensive occupational exposure to agricultural herbicides and pesticides has caused impotence in the male, with failure to achieve a satisfactory penile erection, which was gradually reversible when exposure to the chemicals was stopped (Espir et al., 1970). Lithium can also cause erectile impotence (Vinarova et al., 1972). Certain antihypertensive drugs can affect sexual function (see chapter XVIII; sect. 6.2). Methyldopa not infrequently reduces libido leading to impotence, while drugs such as guanethidine cause failure of ejaculation in the male which can sometimes lead to impotence (Bauer et al., 1973). Erectile dysfunction has occurred infrequently with propranolol (Bathen, 1978). Other drugs such as clonidine and reserpine by their side effects of drowsiness or depression may reduce sexual interest. Sedatives and antipsychotic drugs may similarly reduce sexuality, leading to reduced libido, particularly in men. Thioridazine may also cause failure of ejaculation (Kotin et al., 1976). Depending on the individual, a change to alternative therapy may be indicated. Oral contraceptives are claimed to reduce libido in some women (see section 13.10). Increased libido can occur in some patients (men and women) on levodopa. Impotence in males has been reported with cimetidine (Peden et al., 1979). Sexual side effects of drugs is a poorly understood and studied area (Renshaw, 1978; Mills, 1975).

23.3 Cancer

Prolonged exposure to high doses of unopposed synthetic oestrogen for menorrhagia or for menopausal symptoms, or as replacement therapy in gonadal dysgenesis or surgical castration, is thought to predispose to, or even to cause endometrial carcinoma, and should therefore be avoided.

Case control and mortality review studies suggest that even where the oestrogen used is a natural one in low doses, an increased risk (3 to 8-fold) of endometrial carcinoma follows (Mack et al., 1976; Smith et al., 1975; Weiss et al., 1976; Ziel and Finkle, 1975); but there has been some doubt about the selection of control cases, and about the histological diagnosis of carcinoma (Greenblatt, 1977). It seems clear that if oestrogens are given without progestagen, endometrial hyperplasia often occurs but can be prevented by simultaneous administration of progestagen for at least 10 days of each 21 day period of treatment (Sturdee et al., 1978). Whether this will actually reduce the risk of endometrial carcinoma remains to be seen. It has not yet been established whether cyclical therapy offers any ad-

vantage over continuous therapy. Sequential oral contraceptive preparations have also been suggested as being associated with an increased risk of endometrial carcinoma (Silverberg et al., 1977); sequential preparations employ a relatively large dose of oestrogen and have 2 or more weeks in every cycle of oestrogen administration unopposed by progestagen (see section 13.1).

Although there is no doubt that some breast tumours are oestrogen dependent, oestrogen containing oral contraceptives may in fact have a protective effect against breast cancer, in as much as oral contraception in early reproductive life mimics pregnancy. On the other hand, the particular oestrogens used in oral contraceptives (ethinyloestradiol and its 3-methyl ether, mestranol) are very different from those naturally occurring in high levels in pregnancy. At the present time, there is no definite evidence that oral contraceptives are harmful in this respect, and early data suggest that the use of oral contraceptives is unrelated to the risk of breast cancer (Vessey et al., 1975) or the prognosis of disease developing while using oral contraceptives (Spencer et al., 1978).

Vaginal cancer has been reported in young women whose mothers received stilboestrol in large doses in early pregnancy as a treatment for threatened abortion between 1946 and 1953 (Herbst et al., 1971; 1977) and the treated mothers themselves have now been reported as having a slightly increased incidence of breast cancer (Bibbo et al., 1978). This form of therapy is not now in use, but these cases illustrate the importance of withholding any drug during pregnancy whose value is not proven.

Some epidemiological analyses have suggested a possible association between reserpine use for hypertension and breast cancer, but studies are inconclusive (Kodlin and McCarthy, 1978; Lilienfield et al., 1976). It is very difficult to find suitable controls for studies of cervical neoplasia in women using oral contraception, so reports are inconclusive. A tendency for pre-existing dysplasia to increase in severity and progress to carcinoma *in situ,* has been noted, but the clinical significance is uncertain (Stern et al., 1977).

23.4 Virilisation

Testosterone was at one time commonly used in the treatment of menopausal disorders and of course resulted in virilisation, as evidenced by reduced menses, clitoral hypertrophy, increased libido, hirsutism or deep voice. Anabolic steroids have a similar effect when used in the management of debilitating disease. This should be considered together with the beneficial effects of these drugs in such cases, but administration may still be thought worthwhile. Masculinisation of the urogenital sinus of the female fetus has resulted from the improper use of certain progestagens in threatened abortion (sect. 8; chapter III, sect. 5.3).

23.5 Menorrhagia

Anticoagulant drugs will exacerbate menorrhagia only where there is a pre-existing cause for the condition, such as fibroids. Vaginal bleeding of pathological cause, such as endometrial or cervical cancer, will also be increased by anticoagulant therapy, but not, of course, caused by it. If possible, anticoagulants should be withdrawn.

23.6 Galactorrhoea and Gynaecomastia

Oestrogen administration often causes breast fullness in women and gynaecomastia in men (when administered as treatment for prostatic cancer, for example). Breast discomfort is a complaint of a few patients on progestagen only contraceptives. It is less widely known that a number of other drugs may be mammotrophic.

These drugs include digitalis, the aldosterone antagonist spironolactone and the antifungal agent griseofulvin, all of which have a chemical structure which resembles oestrogen (oestrone) or progesterone. The mechanism by which they exert their mammotrophic action is obscure, although inhibition of the synthesis and peripheral action of androgens seems a possible explanation in the case of spironolactone (Corvol et al., 1976). The action of digitalis has been suggested to be due to a weak oestrogenic action of digitalis aglycones (Lewinn, 1953) which because most cases of gynaecomastia have involved digitalis leaf rather than digoxin or digitoxin, may depend on the particular aglycone or combination of aglycones (digitalis leaf contains a multiplicity of cardioactive glycosides) formed by metabolism in the body.

Other drugs, such as the antituberculosis agents isoniazid, ethionamide and thiacetazone, may very rarely cause gynaecomastia, possibly by impairing the usual metabolism of oestrogen in the liver as is seen in some patients with liver disease or during severe starvation (Adlercreutz, 1974). Massive breast enlargement has been seen with isoniazid regimens containing thiacetazone or thiacetazone and ethionamide (Chunhaswasdikul, 1974; Van der Meulen, 1974), and also in patients taking penicillamine for rheumatoid arthritis (Desai, 1973; Passas and Weinstein, 1978). Breast hypertrophy is not uncommon in puberty and during pregnancy when it is apparently due to extreme sensitivity to hormone action, mainly oestrogen.

The effects of digitalis (Conn, 1964) and spironolactone (Clark, 1965; Huffman et al., 1978) are often noticed in men, especially those receiving both drugs because of heart failure, but breast enlargement is essentially seen only in women who are postmenopausal and who would otherwise expect some degree of mammary atrophy. Amenorrhoea can however occur in premenopausal women receiving spironolactone (Levitt, 1970). In men, the incidence of gynaecomastia with spironolactone is dose related, being particularly common at a dosage of 200 mg or more daily for several weeks (Huffman et al., 1978). The effects of the antituberculosis drugs have been mainly seen in women with long standing amenorrhoea and in adolescence or during pregnancy, but have also occurred in a male. Gynaecomastia after large doses of griseofulvin has been reported in children (Durand et al., 1964).

Another mechanism by which drugs may cause gynaecomastia and galactorrhoea is by interference with the hypothalamic-pituitary axis, at least in part by allowing uninhibited prolactin secretion, which is probably due to antagonism of dopaminergic receptors in the hypothalamus. [The dopaminergic receptor stimulant drug bromocriptine has been successfully used to inhibit prolactin secretion for suppression of puerperal lactation (see section 12) and inappropriate galactorrhoea associated with hypogonadism. Levodopa, a dopamine precursor, causes a fall in prolactin levels and metoclopramide a dopamine receptor antagonist, increases prolactin levels and has been associated with galactorrhoea and increased lactation (Pinder et al., 1976). It should be noted that galactorrhoea may occur with prolactin levels in the normal range and that galactorrhoea does not invariably accompany hyperprolactinaemia (Horrobin, 1975)]. Drugs which seem to act in this way include the centrally acting antihypertensive drugs methyldopa (Pettinger et al., 1963) and reserpine (Robinson, 1957), antipsychotic drugs such as phenothiazines and tricyclic antidepressants such as amitriptyline and imipramine. Young women may be affected, in whom the condition is often associated with amenorrhoea, as well as older women and men, in contrast to the effect of digitalis and spironolactone. The association seems to be quite common with the phenothiazines; galactorrhoea occurred in about 5 % of a large series of women on chlorpromazine (Khazan et al., 1962) and in 10 % of another series (Robinson, 1957), and to be one of cause and effect since withdrawal of the drug usually results in cessation of lactation (Besser and Edwards, 1972). Where the drug is absolutely essential, it is usually possible to switch to another similar drug without this side effect occurring.

Breast pain and gynaecomastia in men and galactorrhoea in women can occur with the histamine (H_2-) receptor antagonist cimetidine (Spence and Celestin, 1979; Delle Fave et al., 1977), and is not necessarily associated with hyperprolactinaemia; an antiandrogenic effect of the drug being a possible alternative mechanism (Spiegel et al., 1978). Gynaecomastia in men has also been associated with the cytotoxic drug carmustine (Schorer et al., 1978).

Most mammotrophic drugs cause a minor nuisance (except in cases of massive hypertrophy) rather than a serious problem, but this sort of breast stimulation should be avoided if possible, since it may lead to breast cancer in men and mastitis in women.

References

Adlercreutz, H.: Hepatic metabolism of estrogens in health and disease. New England Journal of Medicine 290: 1081 (1974).

Akerlund, M.; Anderson, K-E. and Ingemarsson, I.: Effects of terbutaline on myometrial activity; uterine blood flow and lower abdominal pain in women with primary dysmenorrhoea. British Journal of Obstetrics and Gynaecology 83: 673 (1976).

Alkjaersig, N.; Fletcher, A. and Burstein, R.: Association between oral contraceptive use and thromboembolism: A new approach to its investigation based on plasma fibrinogen chromatography. American Journal of Obstetrics and Gynecology 122: 199 (1975).

Anderson, A.B.M.; Haynes, P.J.; Fraser, I.S. and Turnbull, A.C.: Trial of prostaglandin-synthetase inhibitors in primary dysmenorrhoea. Lancet 1: 345 (1978).

Arntzenius, A.C.; van Gent, C.M.; van der Voort, H.; Stegerhoek, C.I. and Styblo, K.: Reduced high-density lipoprotein in women aged 40-41 using oral contraceptives. Lancet 1: 1221 (1978).

Arthes, F.G. and Masi, A.T.: Myocardial infarction in younger women. Associated clinical features and relationship to use of oral contraceptive drugs. Chest 70: 574 (1976).

Assali, N.S. and Brinkman, C.R.: Pathophysiology of Gestation, vol. 1: Maternal Disorders (Academic Press, New York 1972).

Badaracco, M.A. and Vessey, M.P.: Recurrence of venous thromboembolic disease and the use of oral contraceptives. British Medical Journal 1: 215 (1974).

Baskin, H.F.; Murray, J.M. and Harris, R.E.: Low-dose heparin for prevention of thromboembolic disease in pregnancy. American Journal of Obstetrics and Gynaecology 129: 590 (1977).

Bathen, J.: Propranolol erectile dysfunction relieved. Annals of Internal Medicine 88: 716 (1978).

Bauer, G.E.; Hull, R.D.; Stokes, G.S. and Raftos, J.: Reversibility of side effects of guanethidine. Medical Journal of Australia 1: 930 (1973).

Beazley, J.M.: Dysfunctional uterine haemorrhage. British Journal of Hospital Medicine 7: 573 (1972).

Behm, A.R. and Unger, W.P.: Oral contraceptives and porphyria cutanea tard. Canadian Medical Association Journal 110: 1052 (1974).

Bergh, T.; Nillius, S.J. and Wide, L.: Clinical course and outcome of pregnancies in amenorrhoeic women with hyperprolactinaemia and pituitary tumours. British Medical Journal 1: 875 (1978a).

Bergh, T.; Nillius, S.J. and Wide, L.: Serum prolactin and gonadotrophin levels before and after luteinising hormone-releasing hormone in the investigation of amenorrhoea. British Journal of Obstetrics and Gynaecology 85: 945 (1978).

Besser, G.M. and Edwards, C.R.W.: Galactorrhoea. British Medical Journal 2: 280 (1972).

Bibbo, M.; Haenszel, W.M.; Wied, G.L.; Hubby, M. and Herbst, A.L.: A twenty-five-year follow-up study of women exposed to diethylstilboestrol during pregnancy. New England Journal of Medicine 298: 763 (1978).

Biggs, J.S.G.: Vomiting in pregnancy: Causes and management. Drugs 9: 299 (1975).

Bithell, J.F. and Stewart, A.M.: Pre-natal irradiation and childhood malignancy: a review of British data from the Oxford survey. British Journal of Cancer 31: 271 (1975).

Blinick, G.; Wallach, R.C.; Jerez, E. and Ackerman, B.D.: Drug addiction in pregnancy and the neonate. American Journal of Obstetrics and Gynecology 125: 135 (1976).

Boethius, G.: Prescription of drugs 1970-75 in the county of Jauntland, Sweden: Epidemiological and clinical pharmacological aspects, chapter IV, PhD thesis, Department of Internal Medicine, Ostersund Hospital, Ostersund (1977).

Bolli, P. and Simpson, F.O.: Clonidine in menopausal flushing: a double-blind trial. New Zealand Medical Journal 82: 196 (1975).

Bonnar, J.; Goldberg, A. and Smith, J.: Do pregnant women take their iron? Lancet 1: 457 (1969).

Boston Collaborative Drug Surveillance Program: Oral contraceptives and venous thromboembolic disease, surgically confirmed gallbladder disease and breast tumours. Lancet 1: 1399 (1973).

Boston Collaborative Drug Surveillance Program: Surgically confirmed gallbladder disease, venous thromboembolism, and breast tumours in relation to postmenopausal estrogen therapy. New England Journal of Medicine 290: 15 (1974).

Bowes, W.A.: Obstetrical medication and infant outcome: A review of the literature. Monographs of the Society for Research in Child Development 35: 3 (1970).

Bradley, D.D.; Wingerd, J.; Petitti, D.B.; Krauss, R.M. and Ramcharan, S.: High-density-lipoprotein cholesterol and oral contraceptives. New England Journal of Medicine 299: 17 (1978).

Brazelton, B.: Effect of prenatal drugs on the behaviour of the neonate. American Journal of Psychiatry 126: 1261 (1970).

Brenner, W.E.: The current status of prostaglandins as abortifacients. American Journal of Obstetrics and Gynecology 123: 306 (1975).

Brocklebank, J.C.; Ray, W.A.; Federspiel, C.F. and Schaffner, W.: Drug prescribing during pregnancy. A controlled study of Tennessee Medicaid recipients. American Journal of Obstetrics and Gynecology 132: 235 (1978).

Brogden, R.N.; Speight, T.M. and Avery, G.S.: Progestagen-only oral contraceptives: A preliminary report of the action and clinical use of norgestrel and norethisterone. Drugs 6: 169 (1973).

Brown, C.B.; Robson, J.S.; Thomson, D.; Clarkson, A.R.; Cameron, J.S. and Ogg, C.S.: Haemolytic uraemic syndrome in women taking oral contraceptives. Lancet 2: 1479 (1973).

Brumfitt, W. and Pursell, R.: Trimethoprim-sulfamethoxazole in the treatment of bacteriuria in women. Journal of Infectious Diseases 128(Suppl.): S657-S663 (1973).

Buchanan, R.: Breast-feeding — Aid to infant health and fertility control. Population Reports Series Journal No. 4: 49 (1975).

Buchanan, J.D.; Fairley, K.F. and Barrie, J.U.: Return of spermatogenesis after stopping cyclophosphamide therapy. Lancet 2: 156 (1975).

Buckingham, M.; Welply, G.; Miller, J.F. and Elstein, M.: Gastro-intestinal absorption and transplacental transfer of amoxycillin during labour and the influence of metoclopramide. Current Medical Research and Opinion 3: 392 (1975).

Burkman, R.T.; Atienza, M.T.; King, T.M.; Tonascia, J.A.; Pang, J.C.K. and Whitmore, A.J.: Hyperosmolar urea for elective midtrimester abortion. Experience in 1,913 cases. American Journal of Obstetrics and Gynecology 131: 10 (1978).

Campbell, N.; Harvey, D. and Norman, A.P.: Increased frequency of neonatal jaundice in a maternity hospital. British Medical Journal 2: 548 (1975).

Campbell, J.; Anderson, I.; Chang, A. and Wood, C.: The use of ritodrine in the management of the fetus during the second stage of labour. Australian and New Zealand Journal of Obstetrics and Gynaecology 18: 110 (1978).

Campbell, D.M. and MacGillivray, I.: The effect of a low calorie diet or a thiazide diuretic on the incidence of pre-eclampsia and on birth weight. British Journal of Obstetrics and Gynaecology 82: 572 (1975).

Castle, W.M.; Sapire, K.E. and Howard, K.A.: Efficacy and acceptability of injectable medroxyprogesterone. A comparison of 3-monthly and 6-monthly regimens. South African Medical Journal 53: 842 (1978).

Chapman, M.G.: Salbutamol-induced acidosis in pregnant diabetes. British Medical Journal 1: 639 (1977).

Chatfield, W.R.; Schramm, B.M. and Richmond, Wendy, J.: The absorption of ampicillin in late pregnancy and labour. New Zealand Medical Journal 80: 500 (1974).

Chew, W.C. and Swann, I.L.: Influence of simultaneous low amniotomy and oxytocin infusion and other maternal factors on neonatal jaundice: a prospective study. British Medical Journal 1: 72 (1977).

Chisholm, M.: A controlled clinical trial of prophylactic folic acid and iron in pregnancy. Journal of Obstetrics and Gynaecology of the British Commonwealth 73: 191 (1966).

Christianson, R. and Page, E.W.: Diuretic drugs and pregnancy. Obstetrics and Gynecology 48: 647 (1976).

Chunhaswasdikul, B.: Gynecomastia in association with thiacetazone in the treatment of tuberculosis. Journal of the Medical Association of Thailand 57: 323 (1974).

Clark, E.: Spironolactone therapy and gynecomastia. Journal of the American Medical Association 193: 163 (1965).

Cohlan, S.Q.; Bevelander, G. and Tiamsic, T.: Growth inhibition of prematures receiving tetracycline. American Journal of Diseases of Children 105: 453 (1963).

Collaborative Group for the Study of Stroke in Young Women: Oral contraception and increased risk of cerebral ischaemia or thrombosis. New England Journal of Medicine 288: 871 (1973).

Collaborative Group for the Study of Stroke in Young Women: Oral contraceptives and stroke in young women: associated risk factors. Journal of the American Medical Association 231: 718 (1975).

Collins, E. and Turner, G.: Maternal effects of regular salicylate ingestion in pregnancy. Lancet 2: 335 (1975).

Committee on Safety of Drugs: A statement by the Committee on Safety of Drugs on combined oral contraceptives. British Medical Journal 2: 231 (1970).

Conn, H.L.: Digitalis therapy and gynecomastia. Journal of the American Medical Association 190: 1018 (1964).

Corvol, P.; Mahoudeau, J.-A.; Valcke, J.-C.; Menard, J. and Bricaire, H.: Sexual side-effects of spirolactones. Possible mechanisms of antiandrogenic action. Nouvelle Presse Medicale 11: 695 (1976).

Crosignani, P.G.; Lombroso, G.C.; Caccamo, A.; Reschini, E. and Peracchi, M.: Suppression of puerperal lactation by metergoline. Obstetrics and Gynecology 51: 113 (1978).

Dalton, K.: Migraine and oral contraceptives. Headache 15: 247 (1976).

Dam, M.; Christiansen, J.; Munck, O. and Mygind, K.I.: Antiepileptic drugs: Metabolism in pregnancy. Clinical Pharmacokinetics 4: 53 (1979).

Davis, T.E. and Carbone, P.P.: Drug treatment of breast cancer. Drugs 16: 441 (1978).

Davison, J.S.; Davison, M.C. and Hay, D.M.: Gastric emptying time in late pregnancy and labour. Journal of Obstetrics and Gynaecology of the British Commonwealth 77: 37 (1970).

Dawson, D.W.; Goldthorp, W.D. and Spencer, D.: Parenteral iron therapy in pregnancy. Journal of Obstetrics and Gynaecology 72: 89 (1965).

Dean, M.E.; Stock, B.H. and Levy, G.: Serum protein binding of drugs during and after pregnancy — studies in humans. Australasian Society of Clinical and Experimental Pharmacology, Abstract 55, Annual Meeting, Melbourne (November 1977).

DelleFave, G.F.; Tamburrano, G.; de Magistris, L.; Natoli, C.; Santoro, M.L.; Carratu, R. and Torsoli, A.: Gynaecomastia with cimetidine. Lancet 1: 1319 (1977).

Dennerstein, G.J.: Vaginitis: Diagnosis and treatment. Drugs 4: 419 (1972).

Dennerstein, L. and Burrows, G.: Oral contraception and sexuality. Medical Journal of Australia 1: 796 (1976).

Desai, S.N.: Sudden gigantism of breast: drug induced? British Journal of Plastic Surgery 26: 371 (1973).

de Vries Reilingh, A.; Reiners, H. and Vanbijsterveld, O.P.: Contact lens tolerance and oral contraceptives. Annals of Ophthalmology 10: 947 (1978).

Doering, P.L. and Stewart, R.B.: The extent and character of drug consumption during pregnancy. Journal of the American Medical Association 239: 843 (1978).

Durand, P.; Borrone, C.; Scarabicchi, S. and Razzi, A.: Hyperpigmentation of breast areolae and external genitals with gynaecomastia following griseofulvin treatment. Minerva Medica 55: 2422 (1964).

Eadie, M.J.; Lander, C.M. and Tyrer, J.H.: Plasma drug level monitoring in pregnancy. Clinical Pharmacokinetics 2: 427 (1977).

Editorial: Three-monthly depo-provera in Mexico. International Planned Parenthood Medical Bulletin 11: 2 (June 1977).

Editorial: Oral contraceptives and the liver. British Medical Journal 2: 430 (1974).

Editorial: Do all pregnant women need iron? British Medical Journal 2: 1317 (1978).

Eliahou, H.E.; Silverberg, D.S.; Reisin, E.; Romem, I.; Mashiach, S. and Serr, D.M.: Propranolol for the treatment of hypertension in pregnancy. British Journal of Obstetrics and Gynaecology 85: 431 (1978).

Espir, M.L.E.; Hall, J.W.; Shirreffs, J.G. and Stevens, D.L.: Impotence in farm workers using toxic chemicals. British Medical Journal 1: 423 (1970).

Ettledorf, J.N.; West, C.D. and Pitcock, J.A.: Gonadal function, testicular histology, and meiosis following cyclophosphamide therapy in patients with nephrotic syndrome. Journal of Pediatrics 88: 206 (1976).

Evrard, J.R.; Buxton, B.H. and Erickson, D.: Amenorrhoea following oral contraception. American Journal of Obstetrics and Gynecology 124: 88 (1976).

Fairley, K.F.; Barrie, Jean and Johnson, W.: Sterility and testicular atrophy related to cyclophosphamide therapy. Lancet 1: 568 (1972).

Fallis, N.E. and Ford, R.V.: Current concepts of therapy. Limitations in the use of thiazide diuretics. New England Journal of Medicine 263: 296 (1960).

Fennelly, J.: Treosulphan (dihydroxy busulphan) in the management of ovarian carcinoma. British Journal of Obstetrics and Gynaecology 84: 300 (1977).

Fluckiger, E.: Effects of bromocriptine on the hypothalamo-pituitary axis. Acta Endocrinologica 88(Suppl. 216): 27 (1978).

Forfar, J.O.: Drugs to be avoided during the first three months of pregnancy. Prescribers' Journal 13: 130 (1973).

Forfar, J.O. and Nelson, M.M.: Epidemiology of drugs taken by pregnant women: Drugs that may affect the fetus adversely. Clinical Pharmacology and Therapeutics 14: 632 (1973).

Frank, P. and Kay, C.R.: Incidence of thyroid disease associated with oral contraceptives. British Medical Journal 2: 1531 (1978).

Franks, S.: Use of bromocriptine in hyperprolactinaemic anovulation and related disorders. Drugs 17: 337 (1979).

Fraser, I.S.: Danazol — A new medical treatment for endometriosis. Medical Journal of Australia 1: 56 (1978).

Fredholm, B.B.; Lunell, N.O.; Persson, B. and Wager, J.: Actions of salbutamol in late pregnancy: Plasma cyclic AMP, insulin and C-peptide, carbon hydrate and lipid metabolites in diabetic and non-diabetic women. Diabetologia 14: 235 (1978).

Fuchs, F.: Prevention of prematurity. American Journal of Obstetrics and Gynecology 126: 809 (1976).

Gelbke, H.P.; Gethmann, U. and Knuppen, R.: Influence of Rifampicin treatment on the metabolic fate of (4-^{14}C) mestranol in women. Homone and Metabolic Research 9: 415 (1977).

Giwa-Osagie, O.F.; Savage, J. and Newton, J.R.: Norethisterone oenanthate as an injectable contraceptive: use of a modified dose schedule. Br. Med. J. 1: 1660 (1978).

Gray, M.J.: Use and abuse of thiazides in pregnancy. Clinical Obstetrics and Gynecology 11: 568 (1968).

Greenblatt, R.B.: Chemical induction of ovulation. Fertility and Sterility 12: 402 (1961).

Greenblatt, R.B.: Estrogens and endometrial cancer; in Beard (Ed) The Menopause. A Guide to Current Research and Practice (MTP Press, London 1977).

Grimes, D.A.; Schulz, K.F.; Cates, W. and Tyler, C.W.: Mid trimester abortion by intraamniotic prostaglandin F_{2a}. Safer than saline? Obstetrics and Gynecology 49: 612 (1977).

Guillebaud, J.; Anderson, A.B.M. and Turnbull, A.C.: Reduction by mefenamic acid of increased menstrual blood loss associated with intrauterine contraception. British Journal of Obstetrics and Gynaecology 85: 53 (1978).

Hall, M.H.: Folic acid deficiency and congenital malformation. Journal of Obstetrics and Gynaecology of the British Commonwealth 79: 159 (1972a).

Hall, M.H.: Folic acid deficiency and abruptio placentae. Journal of Obstetrics and Gynaecology of the British Commonwealth 79: 222 (1972b).

Hall, M.H.: Pregnancy anaemia. British Medical Journal 2: 661 (1974).

Hall, W.H.: Breast changes in males on cimetidine. New England Journal of Medicine 295: 841 (1976).

Hancock, K.W.; Scott, J.S.; Stitch, S.R.; Levell, M.J.; Oakey, R.E. and Ellis, F.R.: Ovarian stimulation: Problems of prediction of response to gonadotrophins. Lancet 2: 482 (1970).

Harrison, R.F.: Infertility in women. Hospital Medicine 17: 45 (1977).

Harrison, R.F. and Campbell, S.: A double-blind trial of ethamsylate in the treatment of primary and intrauterine-device menorrhagia. Lancet 2: 283 (1976).

Haspels, A.A.: Interception: post-coital estrogens in 3016 women. Contraception 14: 375 (1976).

Heinonen, O.P.; Slone, D. and Shapiro, S.: Birth Defects and Drugs in Pregnancy, p.287 (Publishing Sciences Group, Littleton 1977).

Hemminki, E. and Starfield, B.: Routine administration of iron and vitamins during pregnancy: Review of controlled clinical trials. British Journal of Obstetrics and Gynaecology 85: 404 (1978a).

Hemminki, E. and Starfield, B.: Prevention and treatment of premature labour by drugs: Review of controlled clinical trials. British Journal of Obstetrics and Gynecology 85: 411 (1978b).

Hempel, E. and Klinger, W.: Drug stimulated biotransformation of hormonal steroid contraceptives: Clinical implications. Drugs 12: 442 (1976).

Henderson, I.W.D.: Congenital deformities associated with bendectin. Canadian Medical Association Journal 117: 721 (1977).

Hennekens, C. and MacMahon, B.: Oral contraceptives and myocardial infarction. New England Journal of Medicine 296: 1166 (1977).

Herbst, A.L.; Ulfelder, H. and Poskanzer, D.C.: Adenocarcinoma of the vagina: association of maternal stilbestrol therapy with tumor appearance in young women. New England Journal of Medicine 284: 878 (1971).

Herbst, A.L.; Cole, P.; Colton, T.; Robboy, S.J. and Scully, R.C.: Age-incidence and risk of DES-related clear cell adenocarcinoma of the vagina and cervix. American Journal of Obstetrics and Gynecology 128: 43 (1977).

Hetter, R.F. and Jacobs, H.S.: Coronary heart disease in relation to age, sex, and the menopause. British Medical Journal 1: 472 (1978).

Hill, R.M.; Craig, J.P.; Chaney, M.D.; Tennyson, L.M. and McCulley, L.B.: Utilization of over the counter drugs during pregnancy. Clinical Obstetrics and Gynecology 20: 381 (1977).

Hirsh, J.; Cade, J.F. and Gallus, A.S.: Anticoagulants in pregnancy: A review of indications and complications. American Heart Journal 83: 301 (1972).

Homeida, M.; Halliwell, M. and Branch, R.A.: Effects of an oral contraceptive on hepatic size and antipyrine metabolism in premenopausal women. Clinical Pharmacology and Therapeutics 24: 228 (1978).

Horrobin, D.F.: Prolactin 1975, p.36, 142 (Eden Press, Montreal 1975).

Howat, J.M.T.; Jones, C.B. and Schofield, P.F.: Gallstones and oral contraceptives. Journal of the Institute of Medical Research 3: 59 (1975).

Huffman, D.H.; Kampmann, J.P.; Hignite, C.E. and Azarnoff, D.L.: Gynecomastia induced in normal males by spironolactone. Clinical Pharmacology and Therapeutics 24: 465 (1978).

Humphrey, M.; Chang, A.; Gilbert, M. and Wood, C.: The effect of intravenous ritodrine on the acid-base status of the fetus during the second stage of labour. British Journal of Obstetrics and Gynaecology 82: 234 (1975).

Hytten, F.E.: The handling of drugs in pregnancy. Update 17: 1097 (1978).

Hytten, F.E. and Leitch, I.: The Physiology of Human Pregnancy, 2nd Ed (Blackwell, Oxford 1971).

Ingemarsson, I.: Effect of terbutaline on premature labor. A double-blind placebo-controlled study. American Journal of Obstetrics and Gynecology 125: 520 (1976).

Inman, W.H.W. and Vessey, M.P.: Investigation of deaths from pulmonary, coronary and cerebral thrombosis and embolism in women of child-bearing age. British Medical Journal 2: 193 (1968).

Inman, W.H.W.; Vessey, M.P.; Westerholm, B. and Englund, A.: Thrombo-embolic disease and steroidal content of oral contraceptives. A report to the Committee on Safety of Drugs. British Medical Journal 2: 203 (1970).

Jackson, W.P.U.: Sulphonylurea therapy in the treatment of the pregnant diabetic. South African Medical Journal 45: 428 (1971).

Jakubowicz, D.L. and Wood, C.: The use of the prostaglandin synthetase inhibitor mefenamic acid in the treatment of menorrhagia. Australian and New Zealand Journal of Obstetrics and Gynaecology 18: 135 (1978).

Janerich, D.T.; Piper, J.M. and Glebatis, D.M.: Oral contraceptives and congenital limb reduction defects. New England Journal of Medicine 29: 697 (1974).

Jeffcoate, T.N.A.; Miller, J.; Roos, R.F. and Tindall, V.R.: Puerperal thromboembolism in relation to the inhibition of lactation by oestrogen therapy. British Medical Journal 4: 19 (1968).

Kakkar, V.V. et al.: Prevention of fatal postoperative pulmonary embolism by low doses of heparin. An international multicentre trial. Lancet 2: 45 (1975).

Kangas, L.; Kanto, J. and Erkkola, R.: Transfer of nitrazepam across the human placenta. European Journal of Clinical Pharmacology 12: 355 (1977).

Kanto, J.; Erkkola, R. and Sellman, R.: Distribution and metabolism of diazepam in early and late human pregnancy. Postnatal metabolism of diazepam. Acta Pharmacologica et Toxicologica 35(Suppl.): 36 (1974).

Karim, S.M.M. and Hillier, K.: Prostaglandins: Pharmacology and clinical application. Drugs 8: 176 (1974).

Kasonde, J.M. and Bonnar, J.: Aminocaproic acid and menstrual loss in women using intrauterine devices. British Medical Journal 4: 17 (1975).

Kauppila, A.; Tuimala, R.; Ylikorkala, O.; Haapalahti, J.; Karppanen, H. and Viinikka, L.: Effects of ritodrine and isoxsuprine with and without dexamethasone during late pregnancy. Obstetrics and Gynecology 51: 288 (1978).

Kemball, M.; McIver, C.; Milner, R.D.; Nourse, C.H.; Schiff, D. and Tiernan, J.R.: Neonatal hypoglycaemia in infants of diabetic mothers given sulphonylurea drugs in pregnancy. Archives of Disease in Childhood 45: 696 (1970).

Khazan, N.; Primo, C.; Danon, A.; Assael, M.; Sulman, F.G. and Winnik, H.Z.: The mammotropic effect of tranquillizing drugs. Archives Internationales de Pharmacodynamie et de Therapie 141: 291 (1962).

Kistner, R.W. and Smith, O.W.: Observations on use of nonsteroidal estrogen antagonist, MER-25. Surgical Forum 10: 725 (1960).

Klopper, A. and MacNaughton, M.: Hormones in recurrent abortion. Journal of Obstetrics and Gynaecology of the British Commonwealth 72: 1022 (1965).

Kodlin, D. and McCarthy, N.: Reserpine and breast cancer. Cancer 41: 761 (1978).

Koetsawang, S.: Injected long-acting medroxyprogesterone acetate: Effect on human lactation and concentrations in milk. Journal of the Medical Association of Thailand 60: 57 (1977).

Koetting, R.A.: The influence of oral contraceptives on contact lens wear. American Journal of Optometry and Archives of American Academy of Optometry 43: 268 (1966).

Kotin, J.; Wilbert, D.E.; Verburg, D. and Soldinger, S.M.: Thioridazine and sexual dysfunction. American Journal of Psychiatry 133: 82 (1976).

Krasner, J. and Yaffe, S.J.: Drug-protein binding in the neonate; in Morselli, Garattini and Sereni (Eds) Basic and Therapeutic Aspects of Perinatal Pharmacology, p. ?? (Raven Press, New York 1975).

Krauer, B. and Krauer, F.: Drug kinetics in pregnancy. Clinical Pharmacokinetics 2: 167 (1977).

Kullender, S. and Kallen, B.: A prospective study of drugs in pregnancy. I. Psychopharmaca. Acta Obstetrica et Gynaecologica Scandinavica 55: 25 (1976a).

Kullander, S. and Kallen, B.: A prospective study of drugs in pregnancy. II. Anti-emetic drugs. Acta Obstetrica et Gynaecologica Scandinavica 55: 105 (1976b).

Kullander, S. and Kallen, B.: A prospective study of drugs in pregnancy. III. Hormones. Acta Obstetrica et Gynaecologica Scandinavica 55: 221 (1976c).

Kullander, S. and Kallen, B.: A prospective study of drugs in pregnancy. IV. Miscellaneous drugs. Acta Obstetrica et Gynaecologica Scandinavica 55: 287 (1976d).

Kunelis, C.T.; Peters, J.L. and Edmondson, H.A.: Fatty liver of pregnancy and its relationship to tetracycline therapy. American Journal of Medicine 38: 359 (1965).

Lawson, D.H.; Davidson, J.F. and Jick, H.: Oral contraceptive use and venous thromboembolism: absence of an effect of smoking. British Medical Journal 2: 729 (1977).

Leather, H.M.; Humphrey, D.M.; Backer, Patricia and Chadd, M.A.: A controlled trial of hypotensive agents in hypertension in pregnancy. Lancet 2: 488 (1968).

Lendon, M.; Hann, I.M.; Palmer, M.K.; Shalet, S.M.; Morris Jones, P.H.: Testicular histology after combination chemotherapy in childhood acute lymphoblastic leukaemia. Lancet 2: 439 (1978).

Lenton, E.A.; Sobowate, O.S. and Cooper, I.D.: Prolactin concentrations in ovulatory but infertile women: Treatment with bromocryptine. British Medical Journal 2: 1179 (1977).

Levitt, J.I.: Spironolactone therapy and amenorrhoea. Journal of the American Medical Association 211: 2014 (1970).

Lewinn, E.B.: Gynecomastia during digitalis therapy. New England Journal of Medicine 248: 316 (1953).

Liggins, G.C.: Hormonal steroid contraceptives: Clinical considerations. Drugs 1: 461 (1971).

Liggins, G.C.: Prostaglandins: Current therapeutic status in obstetrics. Drugs 8: 161 (1974).

Liggins, G.C. and Howie, R.N.: A controlled trial of antepartum glucocorticoid treatment for prevention of the respiratory disease syndrome in premature infants. Pediatrics 50: 515 (1972).

Lilienfield, A.M.; Chang, L.; Thomas, D.B. and Levin, M.L.: Rauwolfia derivatives and breast cancer. Johns Hopkins Medical Journal 139: 41 (1976).

Lindheimer, M.D. and Katz, A.I.: Sodium and diuretics in pregnancy. New England Journal of Medicine 288: 891 (1973).

Lindsay, R.; MacLean, A.; Kraszewski, A.; Hart, D.M.; Clark, A.C. and Garwood, J.: Bone response to termination of oestrogen treatment. Lancet 1: 1324 (1978).

Little, P.J.: The incidence of urinary infection in 5000 pregnant women. Lancet 2: 395 (1966).

LiVolsi, V.A.; Stadel, B.V.; Kelsey, J.L.; Holford, T.R. and White, C.: Fibrocystic breast disease in oral-contraceptive users: A histopathological evaluation of epithelial atypia. New England Journal of Medicine 299: 381 (1978).

Loudon, N.B.; Foxwell, M.; Potts, D.M.; Guild, A.L. and Short, R.V.: Acceptability of an oral contraceptive that reduces the frequency of menstruation: The tricycle pill regimen. British Medical Journal 2: 487 (1977).

MacGillivray, I.: Hypertension in pregnancy and its consequences. Journal of Obstetrics and Gynaecology of the British Commonwealth 68: 557 (1963).

MacGillivray, I. and Klopper, A.: Current therapeutics — clomiphene. Practitioner 200: 727 (1968).

MacIntyre, I.M.C. et al.: Heparin versus dextran in the prevention of deep-vein thrombosis. A multi-unit controlled trial. Lancet 2: 118 (1974).

MacKenzie, I.Z. and Embrey, M.P.: Cervical ripening with intravaginal prostaglandin E_2 gel. British Medical Journal 2: 1381 (1977).

MacKenzie, I.Z.; Davies, A.J.; Embrey, M.B. and Guilleband, J.: Very early abortion by prostaglandins. Lancet 1: 1223 (1978).

McQueen, E.G.: Hormonal steroid contraceptives: Adverse reactions and management of the patient. Drugs 2: 20, 138 (1971).

McQueen, E.G.: Hormonal steroid contraceptives: A further review of adverse reactions. Drugs 16: 322 (1978).

Mack, T.M.; Pike, M.C.; Henderson, B.E.; Pfeffer, R.I.; Jerkins, V.R.; Arthur, M. and Brown, S.E.: Estrogens and endometrial cancer in a retirement community. New England Journal of Medicine 294: 1262 (1976).

Malek-Ahmadi, P. and Behrmann, P.J.: Depressive syndrome induced by oral contraceptives. Diseases of the Nervous System 37: 406 (1976).

Mann, J.I.; Inman, W.H. and Thorogood, M.: Oral contraceptive use in older women and fatal myocardial infarction. British Medical Journal 2: 445 (1976).

Masala, A.; Delitala, Lo Dico, G.; Stoppelli, I.; Alagma, S. and Devilla, L.: Inhibition of lactation and inhibition of prolactin release after mechanical breast stimulation in puerperal women given tamoxifen or placebo. British Journal of Obstetrics and Gynaecology 85: 134 (1978).

Meade, T.W.; Chakrabarti, R.; Haines, A.P.; Howarth, D.J.; North, W.R.S. and Stirling, Y.: Haemostatic, lipid, and blood-pressure profiles of women on oral contraceptives containing 50µg or 30µg oestrogen. Lancet 2: 948 (1977).

Meadow, S.R.: The teratogenicity of epilepsy. Developmental Medicine and Child Neurology 16: 375 (1974).

Mehta, A.E. and Tolis, G.: Pharmacology of bromocriptine in health and disease. Drugs 17: 313 (1979).

Mills, L.C.: Drug-induced impotence. American Family Physician 12: 104 (1975).

Milner, R.D.G. and Chouksey, S.K.: Effects of fetal exposure to diazoxide in man. Archives of Disease in Childhood 47: 537 (1972).

Minkowitz, S.; Soloway, H.B.; Hall, J.E. and Yermakow, V.: Fatal hemorrhagic pancreatitis following chlorothiazide administration in pregnancy. Obstetrics and Gynecology 24: 337 (1964).

Mitrani, A.; Dettinger, M.; Abinader, E.G.; Sharf, M. and Klein, A.: Use of propranolol in dysfunctional labour. British Journal of Obstetrics and Gynaecology 82: 651 (1975).

Moore, R.G. and McBride, W.G.: The disposition kinetics of diazepam in pregnant women at parturition. European Journal of Clinical Pharmacology 13: 275 (1978).

Morgan, D.J.; Cousins, M.J.; McQuillan, D. and Thomas, J.: Disposition and placental transfer of etidocaine in pregnancy. European Journal of Clinical Pharmacology 12: 359 (1977).

Morgan, D.; Moore, G.; Thomas, J. and Triggs, E.: Disposition of meperidine in pregnancy. Clinical Pharmacology and Therapeutics 23: 288 (1978).

Morris, J.A.; Arce, J.J.; Hamilton, C.J.; Davidson, C.; Maidman, J.E.; Clark, J.H. and Bloom, R.S.: The management of severe pre-eclampsia and eclampsia with intravenous diazoxide. Obstetrics and Gynecology 49: 675 (1977).

Morrison, A.S.; Jick, H. and Ory, H.W.: Oral contraceptives and hepatitis. Lancet 1: 1142 (1977).

Morrison, J.C.; Wiser, W.L. and Rosser, S.I.: Metabolites of meperidine related to fetal depression. American Journal of Obstetrics and Gynecology 115: 1132 (1973).

Morrison, J.C.; Whybrew, W.D.; Rosser, S.I.; Bucovaz, E.T.; Wiser, W.L. and Fish, S.A.: Metabolites of meperidine in the fetal and maternal serum. American Journal of Obstetrics and Gynecology 126: 997 (1976).

Mygind, K.I.; Dam, M. and Christiansen, J.: Phenytoin and phenobarbitone plasma clearance during pregnancy. Acta Neurologica Scandinavica 54: 160 (1976).

Nash, H.A.: Depo provera®: A review. Contraception 12: 377 (1975).

Nelson, Matilda, M. and Forfar, J.O.: Associations between drugs administered during pregnancy and congenital abnormalities of the fetus. British Medical Journal 1: 523 (1971).

Nilsson, L. and Rybo, G.: Treatment of menorrhagia with epsilon aminocaproic acid: A double blind investigation. Acta Obstetrica et Gynecologica Scandinavica 44: 467 (1965).

Nilsson, L. and Rybo, G.: Treatment of menorrhagia with an antifibrinolytic agent, tranexamic acid (AMCA). A double blind investigation. Acta Obstetrica et Gynecologica Scandinavica 46: 572 (1967).

Nilsson, S.; Nygren, K-G. and Johansson, E.D.B.: d-Norgestrel concentrations in maternal plasma, milk, and child plasma during administration of oral contraceptives to nursing women. American Journal of Obstetrics and Gynecology 129: 178 (1977).

Nimmo, W.S.; Wilson, J. and Prescott, L.F.: Narcotic analgesics and delayed gastric emptying in labour. Lancet 1: 890 (1975).

Noble, Isabel, M.: Prescribing in pregnancy. Practitioner 212: 657 (1974).

Nora, J.J.; Nora, Audrey H.; Blu, Janet; Ingram, Joy; Fountain, Agnes; Peterson, Marilyn; Lortscher, R.H. and Kimberling, W.J.: Exogenous progestogen and estrogen implicated in birth defects. Journal of the American Medical Association 240: 837 (1978).

Notelovitz, M.: Sulphonylurea therapy in the treatment of the pregnant diabetic. South African Medical Journal 45: 226 (1971).

Notelovitz, M.: Oral hypoglycaemic therapy in diabetic pregnancies. Lancet 2: 902 (1974).

O'Driscoll, K.; Stronge, J.M. and Minogue, M.: Active management of labour. British Medical Journal 3: 135 (1973).

Oliver, M.F.: Ischaemic heart disease in young women. British Medical Journal 4: 253 (1974).

Orme, M.L'E.; Lewis, P.J.; de Swiet, M.; Serlin, M.J.; Sibeon, R.; Baty, J.D. and Breckenridge, A.M.: May mothers given warfarin breast feed their infants? British Medical Journal 1: 1564 (1977).

Ory, H.W.: Association between oral contraceptives and myocardial infarction. A review. Journal of the American Medical Association 237: 2619 (1977).

Paintin, D.B.; Thomson, A.M. and Hytten, F.E.: Iron and the haemoglobin level in pregnancy. Journal of Obstetrics and Gynecology of the British Commonwealth 73: 181 (1966).

Palmisano, P.A. and Cassady, G.: Salicylate exposure in the perinate. Journal of the American Medical Association 209: 556 (1969).

Palomaki, J.F. and Lindheimer, M.D.: Sodium depletion simulating deterioration in a toxaemic pregnancy. New England Journal of Medicine 282: 88 (1970).

Passas, C. and Weinstein, A.: Breast gigantism with penicillamine therapy. Arthritis and Rheumatism 21: 167 (1978).

Peden, N.R.; Cargill, J.M.; Browning, M.C.K.; Saunders, J.H.B. and Wormsley, K.G.: Male sexual dysfunction during treatment with cimetidine. British Medical Journal 1: 659 (1979).

Pettinger, W.A.; Horwitz, D. and Sjoerdsma, A.: Lactation due to methyldopa. British Medical Journal 1: 1460 (1963).

Phariss, B.B.: Clinical experience with the intrauterine progesterone contraceptive system. Journal of Reproductive Medicine 20: 155 (1978).

Philipson, A.: Pharmacokinetics of ampicillin during pregnancy. Journal of Infectious Diseases 136: 370 (1977).

Philipson, A.: Plasma levels of ampicillin in pregnant women following administration of ampicillin and pivampicillin. American Journal of Obstetrics and Gynecology 130: 674 (1978).

Philipson, A.; Sabath, L.D. and Charles, C.: Erythromycin and clindamycin absorption and elimination in pregnant women. Clinical Pharmacology and Therapeutics 19: 68 (1976).

Pinder, R.M.; Brogden, R.N.; Sawyer, P.R.; Speight, T.M. and Avery, G.S.: Metoclopramide: A review of its pharmacological properties and clinical use. Drugs 12: 81 (1976).

Plotz, E.J. and Davis, M.E.: Endocrine patterns in pregnant diabetic women. Clinical Obstetrics and Gynecology 5: 346 (1962).

Pohl, J.E.F.; Thurston, H.; Davis, D. and Morgan, M.Y.: Successful use of oral diazoxide in the treatment of severe toxaemia of pregnancy. British Medical Journal 2: 568 (1972).

Popert, A.J.: Pregnancy and adrenocortical hormones, some aspects of their interaction in rheumatic diseases. British Medical Journal 1: 967 (1962).

Posner, N.A.; Silverstone, F.A. and Tobin, E.H.: Changes in carbohydrate tolerance during long-term oral contraception. American Journal of Obstetrics and Gynecology 123: 119 (1975).

Ramsay, R.E.; Strauss, R.G.; Wilder, B.J. and Wilmore, L.J.: Status epilepticus in pregnancy: Effect of phenytoin malabsorption on seizure control. Neurology 28: 85 (1978).

Rebond, P.; Groulade, J. and Groslambert, P.: The influence of normal pregnancy and the postpartum state on plasma proteins and lipids. American Journal of Obstetrics and Gynecology 86: 820 (1963).

Renshaw, D.C.: Sex and drugs. South African Medical Journal 54: 322 (1978).

Riddoch, D.; Jefferson, M. and Bickerstaff, E.R.: Chorea and the oral contraceptives. British Medical Journal 4: 217 (1971).

Roberton, Y.R. and Johnson, E.S.: Interactions between oral contraceptives and other drugs: a review. Current Medical Research and Opinion 3: 647 (1976).

Robinson, B.: Breast changes in male and female with chlorpromazine and reserpine. Medical Journal of Australia 2: 239 (1957).

Rodriguez, S.U.; Leiken, S.L. and Hiller, M.C.: Neonatal thrombocytopenia associated with antepartum administration of thiazide drugs. New England Journal of Medicine 270: 887 (1964).

Roeser, H.P.; Stocks, A.E. and Smith, A.J.: Testicular damage due to cytotoxic drugs and recovery after cessation of therapy. Australian and New Zealand Journal of Medicine 8: 250 (1978).

Rogers, M.C.; Willerson, J.T.; Goldblatt, A. and Smith, T.W.: Serum digoxin concentrations in the human fetus, neonate and infant. New England Journal of Medicine 287: 1010 (1972).

Rolland, R.: Use of bromocriptine in the inhibition of puerperal lactation. Drugs 17: 326 (1979).

Rolland, R. and Schellekens, L.A.: Inhibition of puerperal lactation by bromocriptine. Acta Endocrinologica 88(Suppl.

216): 119 (1978).

Royal College of General Practitioners: Oral Contraceptives and Health (Pitman, London 1974).

Royal College of General Practitioners Oral Contraception Study: Mortality among oral contraceptive users. Lancet 2: 727 (1977a).

Royal College of General Practitioners Oral Contraception Study: Effect on hypertension and benign breast disease of progestagen component in combined oral contraceptives. Lancet 1: 624 (1977b).

Royal College of General Practitioners Oral Contraception Study: Reduction in incidence of rheumatoid arthritis associated with oral contraceptives. Lancet 1: 569 (1978).

Ryan, R.F.: A controlled study of the effect of oral contraceptives on migraine. Headache 17: 250 (1978).

Sartwell, P.E.; Arthes, F.G. and Tonascia, J.A.: Epidemiology of benign breast lesions: Lack of association with oral contraceptive use. New England Journal of Medicine 288: 551 (1973).

Schatz, M.; Patterson, R.; Zeitz, S.; O'Rourke, J. and Melam, H.: Corticosteroid therapy for the pregnant asthmatic patient. Journal of the American Medical Association 233: 804 (1975).

Schorer, A.E.; Oken, M.M. and Johnson, G.J.: Gynecomastia with nitrosourea therapy. Cancer Treatment Reports 62: 574 (1978).

Schou, M.; Amdisen, A. and Steenstrup, D.R.: Lithium and pregnancy II. Hazards to women given lithium during pregnancy and delivery. British Medical Journal 2: 137 (1973).

Schweitzer, I.L.; Weiner, J.M.; McPeak, C.M. and Thursby, M.W.: Oral contraceptives in acute viral hepatitis. Journal of the American Medical Association 233: 979 (1975).

Seddon, R.J.: Hormonal steroid contraceptives: Physiological and clinical pharmacological considerations. Drugs 1: 399 (1971).

Seppala, M.; Hirvonen, E. and Ranta, T.: Bromocryptine treatment of secondary amenorrhoea. Lancet 1: 1154 (1976).

Shapiro, S.; Hartz, S.C.; Siskind, V.; Mitchell, H.A.; Slone, D.; Rosenberg, L.; Monson, R.R.; Heinonen, O.P.; Idanpaan-Heikkila, J.; Haro, S. and Saxen, L.: Anticonvulsants and parenteral epilepsy in the development of birth defects. Lancet 1: 272 (1976).

Shapiro, S.; Heinonen, O.P.; Siskind, V.; Kaufman, D.W.; Monson, R.R. and Slone, D.: Antenatal exposure to doxylamine succinate and dicyclomine hydrochloride (Bendectin) in relation to congenital malformations perinatal mortality rate, birth weight and intelligence quotient score. American Journal of Obstetrics and Gynecology 128: 480 (1977).

Shaul, W.L. and Hall, J.G.: Multiple congenital anomalies associated with oral anticoagulants. American Journal of Obstetrics and Gynecology 127: 191 (1977).

Shearman, R.P. and Fraser, I.S.: Impact of new diagnostic methods on the differential diagnosis and treatment of secondary amenorrhoea. Lancet 1: 1195 (1977).

Shoemaker, E.S.; Forney, J.P. and MacDonald, P.C.: Estrogen treatment of postmenopausal women. Benefits and risks. Journal of the American Medical Association 238: 1524 (1977).

Short, R.V.: The control of menstruation. British Journal of Hospital Medicine 7: 552 (1972).

Silverberg, S.G.; Makowski, E.L. and Roche, W.D.: Endometrial carcinoma in women under 40 years of age: Comparison of cases in oral contraceptive users and non-

users. Cancer 39: 592 (1977).

Skolnick, J.L.; Stoler, B.S.; Katz, D.B. and Anderson, W.H.: Rifampin, oral contraceptives and pregnancy. Journal of the American Medical Association 236: 1382 (1976).

Smith, D.C.; Prentice, R.; Thompson, D.J. and Herriman, W.L.: Association of exogenous estrogen and endometrial carcinoma. New England Journal of Medicine 293: 1164 (1975).

Snowden, R.: The progestasert and ectopic pregnancy. (Correspondence). British Medical Journal 2: 1600 (1977).

Spearing, G.; Fraser, I.; Turner, G. and Dixon, G.: Long-term self-administered subcutaneous heparin in pregnancy. British Medical Journal 1: 1457 (1978).

Speidel, B.D. and Meadow, S.R.: Epilepsy, anticonvulsants and congenital malformations. Drugs 8: 354 (1974).

Spellacy, W.N.; Cruz, A.C.; Buhi, W.C. and Birk, S.A.: The acute effects of ritodrine infusion on maternal metabolism: measurements of levels of glucose, insulin, glucagon, triglycerides, cholesterol, placental lactogen and chorionic gonadotrophin. American Journal of Obstetrics and Gynecology 131: 637 (1978).

Spence, R.W. and Celestin, L.R.: Gynaecomastia associated with cimetidine. Gut 20: 154 (1979).

Spencer, J.D.; Millis, R.R. and Hayward, J.L.: Contraceptive steroids and breast cancer. British Medical Journal 1: 1024 (1978).

Spiegel, A.M.; Lopatin, R.; Peikin, S. and McCarthy, D.: Serum-prolactin in patients receiving chronic oral cimetidine. Lancet 1: 881 (1978).

Stern, E.; Forsythe, A.B.; Youkeles, L. and Loffelt, C.F.: Steroid contraceptive use and cervical dysplasia: Increased risk of progression. Science 196: 1460 (1977).

Stirrat, G.M.: Prescribing problems in the second half of pregnancy and during lactation. Obstetric and Gynecologic Survey 31: 1 (1976).

Strauss, R.G.; Ramsay, R.E.; Willmore, L.J. and Wilder, B.J.: Hematologic effects of phenytoin therapy during pregnancy. Obstetrics and Gynecology 51: 682 (1978).

Stumpf, D.A. and Frost, M.: Seizures, anticonvulsants and pregnancy. American Journal of Diseases of Children 132: 746 (1978).

Sturdee, D.W.; Wade-Evans, T.; Paterson, M.E.L.; Thom, M. and Studd, J.W.W.: Relations between bleeding pattern, endometrial histology and estrogen treatment in menopausal women. British Medical Journal 1: 1575 (1978).

Sutherland, H.W.; Stowers, J.M.; Cormack, J.D. and Bewsher, P.D.: Evaluation of chlorpropamide in chemical diabetes diagnosed during pregnancy. British Medical Journal 3: 9 (1973).

Swapp, G.H.: Asymptomatic bacteriuria, birthweight and length of gestation in a defined population: in Brumfitt and Asscher (Ed) Urinary Tract Infection, p.92 (Oxford University Press, Oxford 1973).

Symposium on Danol (danazol): Journal of International Medical Research 5(Suppl. 3): 1 (1977).

Talwar, P.P. and Berger, G.S.: The relation of body weight to side effects associated with oral contraceptives. British Medical Journal 1: 1637 (1977).

Tcherdakoff, P.H.; Collard, M.; Berrard, E.; Kreft, C.; Dupay, A. and Bernaille, J.M.: Propranolol in hypertension during pregnancy. British Medical Journal 2: 670 (1978).

Thomson, A.M.; Hytten, F.E. and Billewicz, W.Z.: The epidemiology of oedema during pregnancy — a new concept of the aetiology and a rational plan of treatment. Journal of Obstetrics and Gynaecology of the British Commonwealth 74: 1-10 (1967).

Tindall, V.R.: The liver in pregnancy. Clinical Obstetrics and Gynaecology 2: 441 (1975).

Tuchmann-Duplessis, H.: Corticosteroids; in Drug Effects on the Fetus, p.219 (ADIS Press, Sydney 1975a).

Tuchmann-Duplessis, H.: Oral hypoglycaemic drugs; in Drug Effects on the Fetus, p.198 (ADIS Press, Sydney 1975b).

Turnbull, A.C. and Anderson, A.B.M.: Induction of labour. Journal of Obstetrics and Gynaecology of the British Commonwealth 74: 849 (1967).

Utian, W.H.; Begg, G.; Vinik, A.I.; Paul, M. and Shuman, L.: Effect of bromocriptine and chlorotrianisene on inhibition of lactation and serum prolactin. A comparative double-blind study. British Journal of Obstetrics and Gynaecology 82: 755 (1975).

Van der Meulen, A.J.: An unusual case of massive hypertrophy of the breasts. South African Medical Journal 48: 1465 (1974).

Vessey, M.P.: Contraceptive methods: risks and benefits. British Medical Journal 2: 721 (1978).

Vessey, M.P.; Doll, R.; Fairburn, A.S. and Glober, G.: Postoperative thrombo-embolism and use of oral contraceptives. British Medical Journal 3: 123 (1970).

Vessey, M.P.; Doll, R. and Jones, K.: Oral contraceptives and breast cancer: Progress report of an epidemiological study. Lancet 1: 941 (1975).

Vessey, M.P. and Mann, J.I.: Female sex hormones and thrombosis. Epidemiological aspects. British Medical Bulletin 34: 157 (1978).

Vessey, M.P.; Wright, N.H.; McPherson, K. and Wiggins, P.: Fertility after stopping different methods of contraception. British Medical Journal 1: 265 (1978).

Vinarova, E.; Uhlif, O.; Stika, L. and Vinar, O.: Side effects of lithium administration. Activitas Nervosa Superior 14: 105 (1972).

Warne, G.L.; Fairley, K.F.; Hobbs, J.B. and Martin, F.I.R.: Cyclophosphamide-induced ovarian failure. New England Journal of Medicine 289: 1159 (1973).

Weekes, A.R.L.; Makanji, H.H. and West, C.R.: Comparison of intravenous oxytocin and prostaglandin E_2 for accelerating labour. British Medical Journal 1: 987 (1976).

Weinstein, A.J.; Gibbs, R.S. and Gallagher, M.: Placental transfer of clindamycin and gentamicin in term pregnancy. Amer. J. Obstet. Gynec. 124: 688 (1976).

Weir, R.J.: When the pill causes a rise in blood pressure. Drugs 16: 522 (1978).

Weir, R.J.; Briggs, E.; Mack, A.; Naismith, L.; Taylor, L. and Wilson, E.: Blood pressure in women taking oral contraceptives. British Medical Journal 1: 533 (1974).

Weiss, N.; Szekely, D.R. and Austin, D.F.: Increasing incidence of endometrial cancer in the United States. New England Journal of Medicine 294: 1259 (1976).

WHO Task Force on the Use of Prostaglandins for the Regulation of Fertility: Comparison of intra-amniotic prostaglandin F_{2a} and hypertonic saline for induction of second-trimester abortion. British Medical Journal 1: 1373 (1976).

WHO Task Force on the Use of Prostaglandins for the Regulation of Fertility: Prostaglandins and abortion. II. Single extra-amniotic administration of 0.92mg of 15-methyl prostaglandin F_{2a} in Hyskon for termination of pregnancies in weeks 10 to 20 of gestation: An international multicentre study. American Journal of Obstetrics and Gynecology 129: 597 (1977b).

WHO Task Force on the Use of Prostaglandins for the Regulation of Fertility: Prostaglandins and abortion. III. Comparison of single intra-amniotic injections of 15-methyl prostaglandin F_{2a} and prostaglandin F_{2a} for termination of second-trimester pregnancy: An international multicentre study. American Journal of Obstetrics and Gynecology 129: 601 (1977b).

WHO Task Force on Long-Acting Systemic Agents for the Regulation of Fertility: Multinational comparative clinical evaluation of two long-acting injectable contraceptive steroids: norethisterone oenanthate and medroxyprogesterone acetate. 2. Bleeding patterns and side effects. Contraception 17: 395 (1978).

Wilson, L.M.: The effect of oral contraceptives on biochemistry "normal values". Canadian Journal of Medical Technology 55: 42 (Dec. 1973).

Wynn, V.: Vitamins and oral contraceptive use. Lancet 1: 561 (1975).

Yaffe, S.J.: A clinical look at the problem of drugs in pregnancy and their effects on the fetus. Canadian Medical Association Journal 112: 728 (1975).

Yaffe, S.J. and Stern, L.: Clinical implications of perinatal pharmacology; in Mirkin (Ed) Perinatal Pharmacology and Therapeutics, p. 355 (Academic Press, New York 1976).

Yerushalmy, J.: Methodologic problems encountered in investigating the teratogenic effects of drugs; in Klingberg, Abramovici, Chemke (Eds) Drugs and Fetal Development (Plenum Press, New York 1972).

Yuzpe, A.A. and Lancee, W.J.: Ethinylestradiol and dl-norgestrel as a postcoital contraceptive. Fertility and Sterility 28: 932 (1977).

Zanartu, J.; Aquilera, E. and Munoz-Pinto, C.: Maintenance of lactation by means of continuous low-dose progestogen given post-partum as a contraceptive. Contraception 13: 313 (1976).

Ziel, H.K. and Frinkle, W.D.: Increased risk of endometrial carcinoma among users of conjugated estrogens. New England Journal of Medicine 293: 1167 (1975).

Zlatnik, F.J. and Fuchs, F.: A controlled study of ethanol in threatened premature labour. American Journal of Obstetrics and Gynecology 112: 610 (1972).

Chapter XVI
Endocrine Diseases

A. Marble, H.A. Selenkow, L.I. Rose, R.G. Dluhy and G.H. Willliams

Synopsis of Important Principles

1) Precise diagnosis is a prerequisite to appropriate therapy in endocrine disorders.

2) Therapy relies upon an understanding of the normal physiological mechanisms which control endocrine function and of the factors which interfere with physiological homeostasis.

3) When feasible, treatment is directed primarily to a 'cure' of the endocrine disorder and restoration of physiological function.

4) Amelioration or correction of existing endocrine hyperfunction is used where it is not possible to restore physiological homeostasis.

5) In endocrine deficiency states, replacement therapy may be used to gain or approach physiological regulation of the endocrine disorder.

6) In some situations, endocrine therapy may only be able to approach the normal functional state.

7) Endocrine disorders such as diabetes mellitus and thyroid disease when poorly controlled or untreated, can alter the pharmacokinetics of some drugs.

8) Supportive measures and a reasonable dietary approach are the basis of an effective and prolonged weight reduction programme in those who are significantly obese; drugs have a limited role. In the obese, the dosage of some drugs (e.g. theophylline, digoxin, gentamicin) should be based on ideal body weight.

9) Some drugs may aggravate diabetes or bring latent diabetes to a clinically important state (e.g. glucocorticosteroids, diuretics). Management of the diabetic patient may occasionally be made more difficult by oral contraceptives and diuretics. The response to certain drugs (e.g. digoxin) can be altered by thyroid disease.

10) Drugs can cause endocrine disease or alter endocrine function tests, particularly those drugs which affect hypothalamic-pituitary-adrenal (e.g. glucocorticoids) or thyroid function (e.g. lithium, iodine-containing drugs).

Drug treatment of endocrine disease has advanced extensively over the recent past. These advances have been made for the most part by the identification and synthesis of many important endocrine hormones, and by the development and clinical usage of analytical methods for accurate measurements of minute quantities of hormones in serum based upon the principle of competitive binding radioimmunoassay. These now include radioimmunoassays for most polypeptide hormones (insulin, growth hormone, glucagon, somatostatin, prostaglandins, parathormone), steroids, thyroid hormones and a large group of non-endocrine substances such as vitamins, enzymes and pharmacological compounds. As in the past, and certainly for the future, precise diagnosis and an understanding of the physiological mechanisms which control endocrine function are the basis of appropriate therapy. This has been assisted greatly by application of new diagnostic methods. Identification and clinical use of hypothalamic releasing hormones have made diagnosis more precise than previously possible.

1. Clinical Pharmacological Considerations

The endocrine system provides important control mechanisms which have a broad range of regulatory functions which affect biochemical processes of all cells and tissues. Disorders of endocrine function become clinically apparent through excessive, deficient or inappropriate secretion of a hormone, either because of a primary disease of the particular endocrine gland or because of abnormal secretion by the gland in response to disease of some other organ. Thus in endocrine disease the secretion of the particular hormone is not regulated or is improperly regulated by the control mechanisms which operate under normal conditions.

The major physiological concepts involved in the regulation of carbohydrate metabolism, thyroid function and adrenal function are outlined below. Regulatory mechanisms involved in other endocrine functions are referred to in other sections in this chapter.

1.1 Carbohydrate Metabolism

Carbohydrate, which in our society accounts for a large proportion of the daily caloric intake, is utilised only after its conversion to monosaccharides (mainly glucose) and entry into cells. A number of pathways of metabolism are open to glucose following its transport into cells and its phosphorylation to form glucose-6-phosphate. Examination of these pathways shows that close inter-relationships exist between all food constituents — carbohydrate, fat and protein. Insulin, in concert with other hormones, growth hormone, glucagon, cortisol and catecholamines, affects all these pathways, either directly or indirectly, and serves a major integrative role in the intermediary metabolism of muscle and adipose tissue as well as having important effects in the liver.

Factors regulating insulin secretion are many and varied, again reflecting the extensive metabolic role of insulin. Secretion of insulin facilitates storage of food; low levels of secretion permit mobilisation of stores in periods of fasting. Although there is general agreement that the biochemical disturbance of diabetes mellitus is due to insulin deficiency, there is lack of agreement as to the exact genesis of this deficiency. Some believe that hyperglucagonaemia has an important contributory role in diabetes mellitus (Unger and Orci, 1975; Raskin and Unger, 1978). On the other hand, it has been shown that hyperglucagonaemia of the degree most frequently noted in patients with insulin requiring diabetes does not increase the requirement of insulin or decrease its effectiveness in patients receiving insulin in amounts which maintain euglycaemia (Clarke et al., 1978).

1.2 Thyroid Function

The major function of the thyroid gland is to synthesise, store and secrete two iodinated aminoacids, L-thyroxine (T_4) and L-triiodothyronine (T_3), which are necessary for body metabolism, development and growth. The thyroid gland actively extracts iodide from the plasma. The concentration of iodide within the thyroid gland and its conversion to thyroid hormones is controlled by a negative feedback mechanism in which the plasma level of pituitary thyroid stimulating hormone is determined by the plasma thyroxine and triiodothyronine levels and by hypothalamic secretion of thyrotrophin releasing hormone (figs. 1, 3). The pituitary, under stimulation by thyroid releasing hormone (TRH), releases thyroid stimulating hormone (TSH or thyrotrophin). TSH stimulates the thyroid to synthesise and release L-thyroxine

(T$_4$) and L-triiodothyronine (T$_3$). The 'free' or unbound T$_4$ and T$_3$ (FT$_4$, FT$_3$) provide negative feedback to the pituitary to inhibit release of TSH, but may provide positive feedback to the hypothalamus to activate TRH synthetase.

Ectopic thyrotrophins may 'break' into the feedback loop and cause a constant stimulus to the thyroid gland to produce T$_4$ and T$_3$ under pathological conditions. About two thirds of the circulating L-triiodothyronine (T$_3$) is derived from monodeiodination of thyroxine (T$_4$) by peripheral tissues. A portion of the deiodination of T$_4$ occurs at the 3-position, rather than at the 3'-position, producing 3,3',5'-L-triiodothyronine, designated 'reverse T$_3$' (rT$_3$). Under a variety of circumstances, a larger than normal portion of T$_4$ is deiodinated to rT$_3$ which is metabolically inert. In addition, the predominant pathway for monodeiodination of T$_4$ in the fetus is to rT$_3$ rather than T$_3$.

Circulating thyroid hormones are transported in plasma mainly bound to a globulin, thyroxine binding globulin (TBG) and much less avidly to thyroxine binding prealbumin and albumin. All but a small fraction of the thyroid hormones are bound to these serum proteins (Chopra and Solomon, 1976). Changes in TBG concentration due to drugs or disease can alter the fraction of unbound thyroxine and so interfere with thyroid function tests (see section 14.2).

The metabolic effects of thyroid hormones on peripheral tissues are complex, and there is no general agreement on a unified concept of their mechanism of action.

1.3 Adrenal Function

The adrenal cortex is essential to life and participates in responses to 'stresses' of various types. It produces glucocorticoids and other corticosteroid hormones responsible for regulating the metabolism of carbohydrate, protein, fat, water and electrolytes. Cortisol is the major corticosteroid in man. As corticosteroids are not stored in the adrenal cortex their synthesis depends on continued stimulation with corticotrophin (ACTH).

The hypothalamic-pituitary relationships which lead to the release of ACTH, and thus the synthesis and release of corticosteroids, are complex. Nevertheless humoral agents, whose detailed chemical structure has not as yet been conclusively identified, are essential for the release of ACTH. These humoral substances, also known as 'releasing factors', originate in the hypothalamus, probably in the median eminence. They are then carried in the local blood stream to the cells of the anterior pituitary.

ACTH secretion is controlled largely by a reciprocal relationship between cortisol production and ACTH release, superimposed on a basic circa-

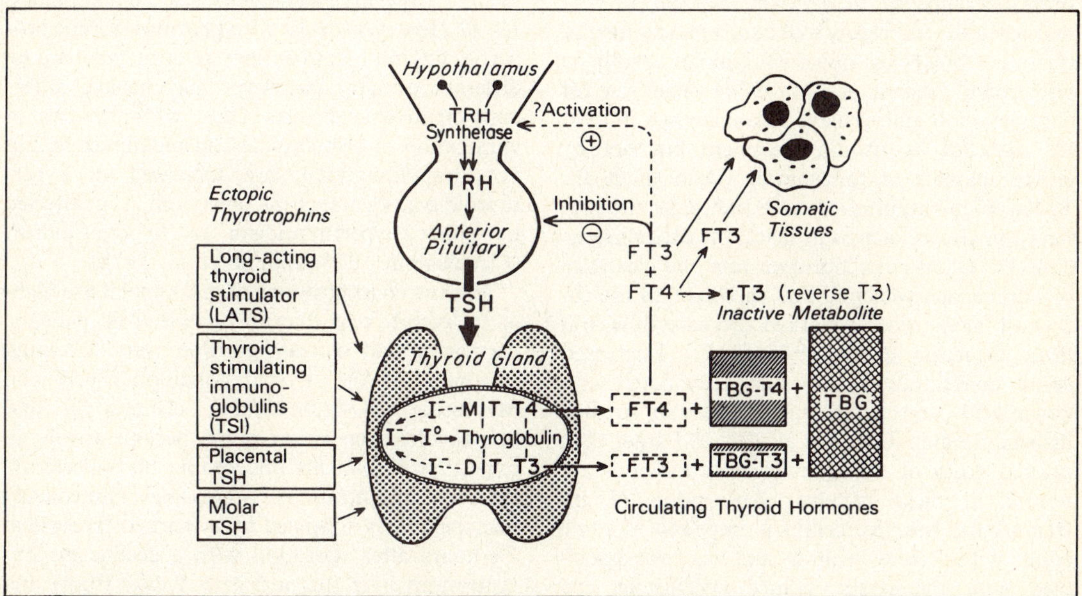

Fig. 1. Hypothalamic-pituitary-thyroid inter-relationships.

dian or 24 hour rhythm. The hypothalamic-pituitary-adrenal axis (HPA axis) is very responsive to 'feedback' inhibition in the evening or 'stress' stimulation at any given time. The plasma levels of circulating endogenous or administered corticosteroids, at the time when the morning surge of ACTH normally occurs, is of fundamental importance to the system.

Both corticotrophin and adrenal corticosteroids have a wide range of biological action when given in either physiological or pharmacological dosage. Their action may be subcellular, cellular or on the whole organs or system complexes of the body.

1.4 Drug Kinetics in Endocrine Disorders

Little definitive information is available on drug disposition in endocrine and metabolic disorders, but clearly kinetics of some drugs can be altered. In some cases, the altered disposition can be related to change in status of the endocrine disorder.

1.4.1 Influence of Diabetes Mellitus on Drug Kinetics

The untreated diabetic state and insulin treatment seem capable of altering metabolism of drugs. Thus, results in a small series of subjects suggest that the rate of conversion of phenacetin (acetophenetidin) to paracetamol (acetaminophen) and its subsequent conjugation are impaired in untreated diabetics, metabolism reverting to normal when the diabetes is well controlled by insulin treatment but being impaired again if insulin is withdrawn (Dajani et al., 1974). The rate of elimination of antipyrine is also increased in treated diabetics by insulin treatment but not by chlorpropamide or tolbutamide (Daintith et al., 1976). Elimination of drugs excreted by the kidneys can also be altered in insulin treated diabetic children. Glomerular filtration rate and clearance of intravenous penicillin and carbenicillin are increased, along with a marked decrease in serum levels (Madacsy et al., 1975, 1976). Decreased serum concentrations have also been noted with kanamycin and amikacin in insulin treated diabetic children (Garcia et al., 1977). Larger than normal doses of renally excreted antibiotics are needed in these patients. Absorption of intramuscular benzylpenicillin is impaired in some adults with diabetes mellitus and has been associated with therapeutic failure (Weinstein and Meade, 1961; Lerner and Weinstein, 1964).

1.4.2 Influence of Thyroid Disease on Drug Kinetics

Thyroid dysfunction can alter the disposition of certain drugs but whether changes occur or are important depends on the pharmacokinetic properties of the particular drug and the thyroid status of the patient at the time of using the drug (for review, see Eichelbaum, 1976). There is a need to alter dosage of some drugs as thyroid disease is treated and requirements change.

Thyroid disease is associated with disturbances of gastrointestinal motility and function which could influence absorption of orally administered drugs, but very little data are available. A number of patients with hyperthyroidism have steatorrhoea or increased intestinal motility and systemic availability of poorly soluble drugs like digoxin has been shown to be decreased in some individuals with hyperthyroidism (Huffman et al., 1977). The rate of absorption of propranolol is more rapid in hyperthyroid than hypothyroid patients (Bell et al., 1977).

Hepatic metabolism of some drugs may also be altered in untreated thyroid disease, as determined by increased clearance of antipyrine in hyperthyroidism and decreased clearance in hypothyroidism and a change to normal with effective treatment of thyroid dysfunction (Eichelbaum, 1976; Saenger et al., 1976). D-Glucaric acid excretion, a measure of hepatic microsomal glucuronidation capacity, is increased in some hyperthyroid patients (Varadi and Foldes, 1976). However, drugs with pharmacokinetic properties different from antipyrine or metabolised by different primary pathways may behave differently in thyroid disease. Thus, while the rate of elimination of tolbutamide and methimazole, but not propylthiouracil, are increased in hyperthyroidism, clearance of phenytoin is unaffected by either hyperthyroidism or hypothyroidism (Eichelbaum, 1976; Hansen et al., 1978).

Plasma concentrations of propranolol are higher in hypothyroid than in hyperthyroid patients, decreasing and increasing respectively following treatment of the thyroid condition (Feely and Stevenson, 1978a,b). Major changes in oral propranolol disposition occur perioperatively in hyperthyroid patients undergoing thyroidectomy; plasma concentrations decreasing immediately postoperatively followed by a marked increase at 24 hours after operation with a decline in concentrations over the next 3 to 5 days (Feely and Stevenson, 1978c), corresponding with the time for maximum increase in drug metabolising enzyme activity which has been observed to occur after operations (Elfstrom, 1979). Cardiac output is increased in hyperthyroidism and clearance of intravenously administered propranolol is increased, probably as a consequence of the increased liver blood flow (Rubenfeld et al., 1978). Changes in clearance and plasma concentrations of oral propranolol in thyroid disease are however, due to alteration in hepatic drug metabolising enzyme activity (see chapter XVII; sect. 6.1.5).

Renal function is also altered in thyroid disease. Thus, the rate of elimination of practolol (which is excreted by renal mechanisms) is increased in hyperthyroidism (Bell et al., 1977), presumably as a consequence of the increased glomerular filtration rate in hyperthyroidism. Glomerular filtration rate is correspondingly decreased in hypothyroidism and there is evidence of increased renal plasma flow in hyperthyroidism and decreased renal plasma flow in hypothyroidism (Bradley et al., 1974). However, apart from digoxin, there is no information available on disposition of drugs in thyroid disease which are mainly eliminated as unchanged drug in the urine (e.g. aminoglycoside antibiotics).

The response to a given dose of digitalis is influenced by the patient's thyroid status and has been attributed to both altered tissue response and altered kinetics of digitalis (Doherty and Perkins, 1966; Morrow et al., 1963). Response to a given dose is increased in hypothyroidism and decreased in hyperthyroidism. The serum concentrations of both digitoxin and digoxin are generally lower in hyperthyroidism and higher in hypothyroidism than in normal patients or when the patient is rendered euthyroid (Eichelbaum, 1976; Shenfield et al., 1977). The reasons for this are not clear. Altered distribution with changed thyroid status (Bonelli et al., 1978; Shenfield et al., 1977) seems to be contributory in the case of both digoxin and digitoxin. Digoxin is usually eliminated mainly as unchanged drug in the urine. Although changes in glomerular filtration rate correlate with renal digoxin clearance, there is not always a good correlation with renal, or extrarenal, digoxin clearance and thyroid status in individual patients (Lawrence et al., 1977; Croxson and Ibbertson, 1975). Altered metabolism and biliary excretion or malabsorption of digoxin may be contributory in some individuals (Huffman et al., 1977). Digitoxin is eliminated by hepatic metabolism and to a lesser extent as unchanged drug in the urine

and faeces (see chapter XVII; sect. 8.1.3). Apart from altered distribution, changes in metabolism as well as biliary and faecal excretion, rather than changes in renal elimination, are more likely to be the reason for altered serum concentrations of digitoxin in states of thyroid dysfunction. Whatever the mechanisms with either digoxin or digitoxin, plasma concentrations will alter as thyroid dysfunction is effectively treated. It is therefore important to monitor serum digitalis concentrations during therapy, at least until biochemical control of thyroid disease has been attained.

1.4.3 Influence of Obesity on Drug Kinetics

Obesity might be expected to alter the distribution and plasma concentration of drugs as a consequence of increased distribution into body fat or, since fat contains less extracellular fluid than other tissues, decreased distribution into extracellular fluid. However, there is very little information available and in particular on whether dosage of drugs with a low therapeutic ratio should be based on ideal body weight or actual body weight. For lipid soluble drugs such as theophylline, loading doses are best based on actual body weight, but due to increased distribution volume and prolonged half-life in obesity, maintenance dosage of theophylline should be based on ideal body weight (Gal et al., 1978). Rate of uptake of halothane and recovery time are increased in obesity, being most marked in younger subjects (Saraiva et al., 1977). Biotransformation of methoxyflurane, and to a lesser extent halothane, to ionic fluoride seems to be increased in obesity (Young et al., 1975; see chapter X, sect. 2.1.1). Obese subjects require the same dose of digoxin, a water soluble drug, to achieve similar plasma concentrations before and after weight reduction. Dosage of digoxin in obesity should therefore be based on ideal body weight and not larger doses based on actual body weight (Ewy et al., 1971). Plasma concentrations of gentamicin and tobramycin, drugs which are distributed mainly to extracellular fluid, are increased in obesity when dosage is based on actual body weight, as a consequence of a decrease in distribution volume. Dosage of these drugs should be based on ideal body weight but serum levels should be monitored to ensure that therapeutic concentrations are attained (Hull and Sarubbi, 1976; Schwartz et al., 1978).

The plasma half-life of tolbutamide, sulphafurazole (sulfisoxazole) and isoniazid are not altered in obesity or during fasting but the rate of renal excretion of sulphafurazole is decreased with fasting (Reidenberg, 1977).

Following intestinal bypass operations for gross obesity, plasma concentrations of norethisterone and to a lesser extent norgestrel in oral contraceptives are reduced, apparently as a result of decreased hepatic synthesis of steroid binding globulin (Johansson and Kral, 1976). Absorption of hydrochlorothiazide is impaired but not that of antipyrine, propylthiouracil and ampicillin. Absorption of hydrochlorothiazide is increased if intestinal transit time is delayed and since a rapid small intestine transit time has been described after intestinal bypass surgery, altered intestinal motility presumably accounts for the decreased absorption of hydrochlorothiazide (Backman et al., 1979). Steady-state plasma concentration of digoxin is not altered but the area under the plasma level-time curve is reduced in most patients after intestinal bypass operations (Marcus et al., 1976), suggesting that systemic availability might be decreased if intestinal transit time was unduly rapid (see chapter VI; sect. 5).

2. General Principles of Treatment

The major therapeutic principles upon which endocrine therapy is based can be simply stated:

1) Precise diagnosis is the cornerstone of appropriate therapy in endocrine disorders.

2) Treatment should be directed primarily to a 'cure' of the endocrine disorder and restoration of physiological function when feasible. For example, in thyrotoxicosis, through a permissive action of the antithyroid drugs in promoting a spontaneous remission; or, in hyperfunctioning tumours such as phaeochromocytoma or insulinomas, when normal physiology is restored after removal of the offending endocrine tissue.

3) Amelioration or correction of existing endocrine excess where it is not possible to restore physiological homeostasis. For example, adrenalectomy for Cushing's syndrome or ablative therapy (subtotal thyroidectomy or radioiodine) for thyrotoxicosis.

4) Replacement therapy for deficiency states. This can be physiological as in thyroid hormone treatment of hypothyroidism, or can approach the physiological — as insulin treatment of diabetes, or adrenocortical hormone therapy of Addison's disease, where physiological regulation or circadian rhythm is not restored fully despite reasonably satisfactory regulation of the endocrine disorder.

5) Certain endocrine treatment may only be able to approach the normal functional state: for example, vitamin D therapy for hypoparathyroidism.

3. Diabetes Mellitus

Although diabetes mellitus is a complex disturbance of metabolism with many ramifications, from a practical, therapeutic standpoint it is best approached as a disease of relative or absolute insulin deficiency, with probably an important role played by glucagon (Unger and Orci, 1975; Raskin and Unger, 1978). Basic to all successful treatment, whether or not drugs are involved, is a well planned diet, restricted in carbohydrate, entirely adequate although controlled in protein, and regulated in fat content so as to be appropriate in calories for the individual. The diet should also be adequate in vitamins and minerals, and should take into account the age, sex, occupation, physical activity and eating habits of the patient and his family.

In many patients with onset of diabetes above the age of 40 years, the condition can be adequately controlled by means of a restricted diet alone. Other patients with adult onset diabetes, who are unable to achieve satisfactory control with dietary restriction alone, may respond satisfactorily to the oral hypoglycaemic agents. However, practically all children and a large proportion of those with onset of diabetes under the age of 40 years, as well as many persons who develop diabetes over that age, require daily injections of insulin for adequate control. Although the diabetic state involves much more than hyperglycaemia and glycosuria, the amount of glucose in the urine and blood serve as the best and most easily determined indices of the adequacy of treatment.

3.1 Aims of Treatment

The *short term* objective is to relieve characteristic symptoms, to overcome ketoacidosis, to restore natural resistance to infection, to promote normal gain in height and weight in the growing child and to favour normal nutrition. The *long term* objective is to avoid complications or se-

Table I. Characteristics of the available insulins

Type	Appear-ance	Added protein	Zinc content (mg/100 units)	Buffer	Dura-tion of effect (hours)
Rapid					
Regular (crystalline)	Clear	None	0.016-0.04	None	5-7
Zinc suspension amorphous (semilente)	Turbid	None	0.2-0.25	Acetate	12-16
Neutral ('Actrapid'[1])	Clear	None		Acetate	4-6
Biphasic ('Rapitard'[2])	Turbid	None		Acetate	18-24
Monocomponent insulins[3]					
Neutral ('Actrapid'-MC)	Clear	None		Acetate	5-7
Amorphous-MC (semilente[1])	Turbid	None		Acetate	10-15
Intermediate					
Globin	Clear	Globin	0.25-0.35	None	12-18
Isophane (NPH)	Turbid	Protamine	0.016-0.04	Phosphate	18-24
Zinc suspension (lente; 30% amorphous, 70% crystalline)	Turbid	None	0.2-0.25	Acetate	18-24
Monocomponent insulin[3] 'Monotard' (30% amorphous; 70% crystalline)	Turbid	None		Acetate	14-22
Slow					
Protamine zinc	Turbid	Protamine	0.2-0.25	Phosphate	24-36
Zinc suspension crystalline (ultralente)	Turbid	None	0.2-0.25	Acetate	24-36

1　A clear, neutral solution of porcine insulin.
2　Neutral suspension of bovine insulin crystals (to provide long action) in a solution of 'Actrapid' (to provide rapid action).
3　Insulin obtained by further purification of crystalline insulin.

quelae, particularly those affecting the vascular and nervous systems which appear with startling frequency after 15, 20 or more years of diabetes. Although the subject is controversial there is increasing evidence to suggest that excellent chemical control of diabetes can postpone or minimise these late complications (e.g. Keiding et al., 1952; Johnsson, 1960; Pirart, 1978). Indeed, a defensible hypothesis is that if one were able to achieve throughout the life of a diabetic patient ideal chemical control in the physiological sense, complications attributable to diabetes might be prevented (Cahill et al., 1976).

The position just stated seems tenable on the basis of findings as regards microangiopathy (retinopathy and nephropathy) in both human subjects and animals with insulin requiring diabetes (Maurer et al., 1975, 1978; Engerman et al., 1977; Eschwege et al., 1979). However, in patients with stable, maturity onset diabetes not requiring insulin injections for what is commonly regarded as acceptable chemical control, it is difficult to carry out prospective studies to investigate correlation of macroangiopathy with degree of control. The difficulties include: (1) the problem of recruitment of suitable subjects who will follow over long periods of time an established protocol; (2) the fact that one never (or rarely) achieves ideal chemical control; and (3) the many factors, diabetic and non-diabetic, which influence the extent of macrovascular disease in middle aged and elderly persons. It is likely that problems of this type led to the difficulties in the interpretation of the results of the University Group Diabetes Program and the extensive controversy which has taken place over the last decade (University Group Diabetes Program, 1970, 1975, 1976; Feinstein, 1971).

3.2 Insulin

Insulin is a protein with a low molecular weight of about 6000 and consists of two peptide chains linked together by two disulphide bridges. The acidic or A chain consists of 21 amino acids and the basic or B chain of 30 amino acids. It is an anabolic hormone, promoting the synthesis of materials necessary for growth and normal metabolism. The major effects of insulin on glucose, fatty acid, and amino acid metabolism and on ion flux are apparently initiated by the attachment of the insulin molecule to a specific receptor on the cell surface.

Insulin, synthesised in the beta cell of the pancreas, induces storage of ingested food by allowing glucose to enter muscle and fat, promoting glycogen synthesis in all sensitive tissues, facilitating fat synthesis and protecting against release of energy stores in fat and protein. Insulin deficiency permits release of the stored foodstuffs for energy production and the maintenance of blood glucose levels between food intake. Anti-insulin hormones (growth hormone, adrenaline, glucagon and cortisol) probably play a part in negating the storage effect of insulin during starvation, facilitating provision of energy reserves and maintenance of blood glucose levels (Felig et al., 1971; Owen and Cahill, 1973; Aoki et al., 1974). Insulin seems to be carried with α_1-globulin and albumin in plasma. Degradation of insulin occurs in all tissues the more active being the liver and to a lesser extent the kidney, pancreas, testis and placenta (Mirsky, 1957).

The characteristics of the various insulins available are given in table I. Except for the regular (crystalline) and 'Actrapid' varieties, all insulins are modified to delay absorption from a subcutaneous or intramuscular depot and thereby to achieve a slower action of prolonged duration. Modifications are made by the addition of zinc or protein (globin or protamine) or both in the presence of a suitable buffer. Purified insulins have also been developed (Yue and Turtle, 1977; Alberti and Nattrass, 1978). The highly purified 'single peak'[1] and the even more purified monocompo-

nent and single component insulins are less contaminated by insulin fragments and appear to give less insulin resistance from IgG increments. They are indicated for trial in patients with massive insulin resistance due to high antibody titre and in the prevention and treatment of 'insulin atrophy' (atrophy of subcutaneous fat at sites of insulin injections) and insulin allergy (see section 3.2.2). In some countries, most insulins of all types are now purified to at least the 'single peak' stage.

3.2.1 Treatment Programme

The selection of a given insulin programme depends upon the individual patient and the character of his diabetes, and upon the experience and judgement of the clinician (Marble et al., 1971; Stowers, 1976). For all practical purposes, isophane insulin (NPH) and insulin zinc suspension (lente) may be used interchangeably. Rapidly acting regular insulin is the preparation of choice in the treatment of diabetic ketoacidosis and coma. Its use is often desirable, either alone or as a supplement, in the treatment of acute infections with fever, following surgery, or in other situations in which prompt action of limited duration is needed. In addition, there is great merit in a programme in which multiple doses of regular insulin alone are used in maintenance therapy. However, many patients find the routine of several injections daily unacceptable, and for this reason, programmes which utilise modified insulins with delayed absorption and prolonged action, are preferable from a practical standpoint.

Table II lists the various insulin programmes which are possible, using the types of insulin preparations currently available. Any of these insulin programmes can be made to work with greater or lesser effectiveness. Mixtures of the lente insulins are used widely and with much success. However, many clinicians find the use of NPH or lente insulin once or twice a day, either alone or with an accompanying dose of regular insulin, to be the most effective and practical. If *acid* regular and NPH (or lente) are given together, the dose of acid regular insulin is drawn into the syringe first and then the dose of modified insulin. If lente insulin is used as the modified insulin type, the dose of acid regular insulin used with it should not exceed the dose of lente insulin and preferably should be no more than one-half the dose of the lente type. Such restrictions do not apply to *neutral* regular insulin which is now the only regular insulin available in some countries.

---

1 The term 'single peak' has nothing to do with timeaction. It refers to assessment of a purification process such that on gel chromatography the insulin yields an elution profile consisting chiefly of a single peak. 'Monocomponent' and 'single component' are terms used to denote further purified insulins.

Table II. Insulin programmes

1. Multiple doses of regular insulin daily.

2. Protamine zinc insulin alone or with regular insulin (*separate* injections) before breakfast. Also, regular insulin before the evening meal often needed.

3. NPH or lente insulin before breakfast with or without regular insulin (single injection). Also, if needed, small doses of NPH or lente at bedtime (or before the evening meal, with or without a small dose of regular insulin) if needed.

4. Combinations of semilente, lente and ultralente insulins.

5. Globin insulin, 1 or 2 doses daily.

6. Programmes using neutral ('Actrapid') and biphasic ('Rapitard') insulins.

Strengths of insulin available vary in different countries, ranging from 20 to 160 units/ml (in some countries regular insulin in a strength of 500 units/ml is available for patients with marked insulin resistance). The trend in the USA and Canada is toward a single 100 unit strength whereas in Europe and Commonwealth countries strengths based on 40 units are favoured by many (Moss and Galloway, 1977; Shepherd, 1978).

3.2.2 Untoward Effects of Insulin

The untoward effects of insulin are chiefly: (1) lipodystrophy, including both atrophy and hypertrophy of the subcutaneous fat, (2) allergy to insulin, (3) insulin resistance, and (4) hypoglycaemia. However, none of these should be regarded as a reason for not employing insulin when indicated. Its beneficial effects far outweigh any disadvantages.

Lipodystrophy: Atrophy of subcutaneous fat at the site of insulin injections occurs frequently in children and women and less commonly in men. Susceptible individuals should be encouraged to make injections solely in those areas of the body not commonly exposed to public view such as the skin over the abdominal wall, flanks and buttocks. The use of purified insulins (see above) may aid in the prevention and treatment of lipoatrophy (Yue and Turtle, 1977; Alberti and Nattrass, 1978). In treatment, insulin is injected into the affected areas. Corticosteroids added to the insulin injection have also been reported to ameliorate

lipoatrophy in some patients (Kumar et al., 1977). Hypertrophy of subcutaneous fat is noticed most commonly in children and in adult males, following the repeated injection of insulin into the same area over long periods of time. When a shift is made to other sites, the hypertrophies gradually disappear. Hypertrophies are not to be confused with irregular masses of scar tissue ('insulin lumps') beneath the skin at sites in which, unwisely, injections have been made day after day.

Allergy to insulin: Hypersensitivity to insulin is common, occurring in a quarter to a third of patients at one time or another. Fortunately most untoward dermal responses are mild and transient, consisting only of stinging, burning or itching at the site of injection. This may be accompanied by some induration, increased warmth, erythema and possibly a few urticarial wheals. The signs and symptoms usually disappear gradually in 6 to 24 hours. If the reaction is severe or prolonged, transfer to a single component insulin can be made. However, dosage requirements may be much smaller in some individuals than with the standard insulins and such dose adjustment should be taken into account when transfer to single component insulin is made (Logie and Stowers, 1976; Daggett et al., 1977). Alternatively, the use of antihistamines by mouth may tide the patient over the period of hypersensitivity, and in a very few instances, an antihistamine solution may be given along with the insulin injection.

Generalised urticaria with annoying itching occurs much less frequently. Rarely, generalised responses may include angioneurotic oedema involving the eyelids, lips, and other loose tissues about the face. Generalised allergy demands prompt treatment, particularly if there is any tendency to bronchospasm. Emergency treatment consists of adrenaline (epinephrine) and corticosteroids.

Definitive treatment and prevention of future difficulty involves desensitisation, starting with minute doses (say 1/1,000 or 1/10,000 unit) of regular insulin given subcutaneously, continuing injections at 60 minute intervals, doubling the dose with each injection, until such time as evidence of allergy reappears. Dosage is then reduced a step or two for 2 or 3 times, and then increased up the scale again.

Insulin resistance: For the vast majority of patients, the true insulin requirement is less than

50 or 60 units daily, although doses administered at times reach 100 units daily if little or no attention is paid to food intake. However, true insulin requirements of over 100 units daily are uncommon, and when in the absence of ketoacidosis, infection, or other obvious complication, this reaches 200 units or more, the situation is arbitrarily referred to as one of insulin resistance. Primary insulin resistance usually does not occur until after some months of insulin therapy and is commonly associated with the development of a high titre (50 to 5,000 units/litre) of insulin antibodies in the serum (Oakley et al., 1967).

Insulin resistance is often a self limited condition which lasts from less than a month to a year or more. Recovery may be hastened by attempting to satisfy the insulin requirement daily to the fullest, short of producing hypoglycaemic episodes. Otherwise, the first and simplest step in the treatment of insulin resistance is a shift to insulin of pork origin since this differs relatively little from human insulin with respect to its amino acid composition and sequence. If this is not effective, single component (monocomponent) insulin should be tried.

Success can by no means be guaranteed by these measures and if they do not suffice, corticosteroid therapy may be instituted, starting with relatively large doses such as 40 to 80mg of prednisone (or equivalent) daily (Oakley et al., 1967). The dose of prednisone, as well as that of insulin, should be reduced promptly if and when blood glucose levels indicate the beginning of a favourable effect, lest severe hypoglycaemia be produced. If success is to be attained in lowering the insulin requirement, it will usually become evident within 2 weeks of steroid therapy, when the dose of steroids can then be reduced gradually, and finally discontinued (Shipp et al., 1965). Insulin resistance in some patients may be due to impaired absorption or excessive degradation of insulin, as continuous low dosage insulin infusions have been successfully used in patients poorly controlled on large doses of insulin who did not have insulin antibodies and did not respond to corticosteroids (Dandona et al., 1978; Schneider and Bennett, 1975).

Hypoglycaemia: Occasional episodes of mild hypoglycaemia due to insulin are difficult to prevent, particularly in the patient with unstable diabetes. There is little or no evidence to indicate that mild hypoglycaemia, even though it occurs relatively often, causes damage to the individual. However, effort should be made to prevent frequent or severe insulin reactions, and this can usually be accomplished with careful selection of the type, amount, and timing of the three controllable items — food, insulin and physical exercise. Treatment of hypoglycaemia consists of giving sugar, candy, fruit juice or liquids containing sugar orally. In patients who are unable to cooperate, glucose may be administered intravenously. Alternatively, 1mg glucagon can be given subcutaneously, repeating the dose in 5 to 10 minutes if necessary. If it is effective in restoring consciousness within a few minutes, carbohydrate should then be given promptly by mouth lest hypoglycaemia return. If glucagon is not effective, glucose (20ml of a 50% solution) should be given intravenously. Glucagon is a polypeptide produced by the alpha cells of the pancreatic islets and causes an increase in the blood glucose level by promoting the release of glucose from hepatic glycogen.

New methods of insulin delivery: Relevant to aims in achieving ideal physiological control of diabetes (see above) are the attempts in recent years to develop automatic means of delivery of insulin to the patient appropriate to the needs at any given moment. This has been accomplished to some extent on a relatively short term basis in animals and patients by transplantation of the entire pancreas or islet tissue (Kjellstrand et al., 1973; Matas, 1976; Brown et al., 1978); by a bench model of an 'artificial endocrine pancreas' (Pfeiffer et al., 1977); and by the continuous infusion of insulin through a subcutaneously implanted cannula (Pickup et al., 1978; Santiago et al., 1979). Still in the stage of development is a miniature, implantable device which embodies a glucose sensor, tiny computer, power source, pump, and an insulin reservoir refillable at long intervals (Layne et al., 1976; Colton et al., 1978). This is obviously an exciting field in which to work. All studies have in mind the goal of obtaining continuous normoglycaemia in the diabetic patient.

3.3 Oral Hypoglycaemic Agents

Oral hypoglycaemic agents can be conveniently divided into two broad classes: (1) sulphonylureas and (2) biguanides. Some of the oral hypoglycaemic agents available in various countries of the world are listed in table III.

3.3.1 Mode of Action of Oral Hypoglycaemic Drugs

There is general agreement that the sulphonylureas exert their early action, chiefly if not wholly, by stimulating the release of insulin from the beta cells of the pancreas. However, with prolonged administration of sulphonylureas, blood glucose is lowered but plasma insulin levels are unchanged. Subsequent effects on blood glucose seem to be due to improved sensitivity of the beta cells or extrapancreatic effects occurring in the liver, and on insulin sensitivity of peripheral tissues. The precise mechanism of long term sulphonylurea effect is uncertain (see Breidahl et al., 1972a; Shen and Bressler, 1977a; Olefsky and Reaven, 1976).

The chief mode of action of the biguanides remains controversial but the generally held view is that biguanides have their major effect by increasing peripheral uptake of glucose and in large doses of delaying or actually decreasing its intestinal absorption (see Breidahl et al., 1972a; Shen and Bressler, 1977a). Since the administration of biguanides may be accompanied by a rise in the serum lactic and pyruvic acids, increased anaerobic glycolysis as the mechanism of action has been postulated. Studies have yielded data which suggest decreased gluconeogenesis in the liver, an effect on the processes of electron transport and oxidative phosphorylation, an increased peripheral oxidation of glucose, and inhibition of the active transport of glucose by the intestine, thereby delaying absorption of glucose from the bowel. It has been postulated that these diverse effects may have in large part a common basis in the alteration of the physical properties of mitochondrial membranes with special reference to membrane phospholipids (Schafer, 1974). In contrast to the sulphonylureas, the hypoglycaemic action of biguanides is not demonstrable in non-diabetic subjects. The biguanides also differ in action from insulin. The mobilisation of fat is not inhibited by biguanides and they do not inhibit hepatic ketogenesis. Biguanides can therefore lower plasma glucose in diabetic patients with insufficient insulin to prevent ketoacidosis. Thus, ketoacidosis must not be overlooked in biguanide treated patients who are ketotic but have only minimal glycosuria and hyperglycaemia. The effect of biguanides on lactate metabolism is discussed in section 3.3.4.

3.3.2 Clinical Effectiveness of Oral Hypoglycaemic Drugs

The sulphonylureas are effective only in those diabetic patients who still possess some capacity for endogenous insulin production. Success may be expected only in those with the maturity onset type of diabetes with little or no tendency to ketoacidosis. In general, patients should be selected whose diabetes had its onset after the age of 40 years and who, if they were receiving insulin, would have a requirement of no more than 20, or at most 30, units of insulin daily (see further section 3.4). The sulphonylureas are contraindicated in patients with the juvenile onset type of diabetes who are classically insulin dependent and ketosis prone. They are not effective in the treatment of ketoacidosis; during acute infections, particularly with fever; nor usually in those undergoing major surgery.

The biguanides may lower the blood glucose in many patients with maturity onset type of diabetes. They are not effective clinically unless some insulin, of either endogenous or exogenous origin, is available to the patient. A specific effect on lipid metabolism has not been proved (although they may seem to aid in weight reduction), nor has

Table III. Some oral hypoglycaemic agents

Drug and class	Duration of action[1] (hours)
Sulphonylureas	
Acetohexamide	10-16h (medium)
Chlorpropamide	20-60h (progxd)
Glibenclamide (glyburide)	10-15h (medium)
Glibornuride	?12+ (medium)
Gliclazide	?12+ (medium)
Glipizide	6-12h (short)
Glisoxepide	5-10h (short)
Tolazamide	10-16h (medium)
Tolbutamide	6-10h (short)
Sulphonamide-related compounds	
Glymidine (glycodiazine)	6-12h (short)
Biguanides	
Buformin	5-6h (short[2])
Metformin	5-6h (short[2])
Phenformin[3]	6-8h (short[2])

1   Estimated total duration of effect.
2   Action may be prolonged by use of preparations providing slow release of the drug.
3   Not available or used in some countries because of increased risk of lactic acidosis (see text).

the claim that biguanides may have a 'smoothing' effect in unstable diabetes under treatment with insulin (for reviews, see Breidahl et al., 1972a; Stowers and Borthwick, 1977). Table III gives the duration of action of some of the oral hypoglycaemic compounds.

3.3.3 Pharmacokinetic Properties of Oral Hypoglycaemic Drugs

The pharmacokinetic properties of the various oral hypoglycaemic drugs are summarised in table IV. Differences which exist between the individual compounds can influence their use in some situations.

Sulphonylureas: The sulphonylureas are rapidly and reliably absorbed with the exception of tolazamide which is slowly absorbed. They are highly protein bound, some compounds more so than others (table IV). There are also differences in distribution volume between the sulphonylureas (appendix A). Those sulphonylureas such as chlorpropamide, tolbutamide and glipizide, which are highly albumin bound and have a low distribution volume, are more likely to be involved in displacement interactions with drugs which bind to the same site on albumin (table V; see chapter I, sect. 3.2.3).

All of the sulphonylureas are metabolised in the liver to some extent, although in the case of chlorpropamide a variable proportion of a dose is eliminated in the urine unchanged (6 to 60%, mean about 20%; Brotherton et al., 1969; Taylor, 1972). The various sulphonylureas differ in their rate of elimination and contribution of metabolites to hypoglycaemic activity (table IV; Shen and Bressler, 1977a; Hansen and Christensen, 1977). Chlorpropamide has a particularly long elimination half-life of about 36 hours. This means that plasma concentrations increase slowly with the once daily dose regimen and about 5 to 7 half-lives or 7 to 10 days, may be required before steady-state plasma concentrations are reached (see chapter I; sect. 2.2). Dosage should not therefore be increased before this time when making dose changes or when treatment with chlorpropamide is initiated. Plasma concentrations of the sulphonylureas vary widely between individuals given the same dose, probably because of genetically determined interindividual differences in rates of biotransformation. Plasma clearance of tolbutamide may vary 9-fold between individuals. Subjects can be categorised as slow or rapid hy-

droxylators of the drug, the trait being genetically controlled (Scott and Poffenbarger, 1979).

The particular characteristics of elimination of the sulphonylureas also influence the use of sulphonylureas in patients with impaired renal function or liver disease and the likelihood of important interactions with other drugs (see section 3.3.5; 3.4.6). Thus, with compounds which are eliminated mainly by hepatic metabolism (e.g. tolazamide, tolbutamide), the risk of symptomatic hypoglycaemia may be increased by significant liver disease, particularly if other drugs which inhibit their metabolism are given at the same time. However, with highly albumin bound drugs such as tolbutamide, clearance of unbound drugs may not change in liver disease and alteration of dosage may not be necessary (see chapter XIX; sect. 1.3). On the other hand, enzyme inducing drugs can accelerate metabolism of compounds such as tolazamide and interfere with diabetic control (Logie et al., 1976). With compounds such as chlorpropamide, which are excreted in unchanged form or acetohexamide which forms an active metabolite, the risk of accumulation and symptomatic hypoglycaemia is increased in the presence of impaired renal function or by drugs which inhibit their elimination (e.g. phenylbutazone). The plasma half-life of chlorpropamide can be as high as 200 hours in patients with renal failure, compared with 36 hours in patients with normal renal function (Petitpierre et al., 1972). Other sulphonylureas such as tolbutamide which are eliminated by hepatic metabolism and do not form active metabolites, can be used in patients with impaired renal function, but insulin may be preferable. Acetohexamide is a special case. Hydroxyhexamide, a major metabolite, has 2.5 times the hypoglycaemic activity of acetohexamide but is present in only small amounts. Concentrations are however, moderately elevated in plasma in some uraemic patients but not in others, due to further biotransformation to hydroxyhydroxyhexamide which is inactive (Cohen et al., 1967). Impairment of this latter biotransformation or renal excretion of hydroxyhexamide by phenylbutazone has however, led to episodes of severe hypoglycaemia (Field et al., 1967).

Biguanides: In contrast to the sulphonylureas, only 50% of a dose of phenformin is absorbed and it is only slightly bound to plasma proteins (about 20%). A variable proportion of a dose absorbed (from ~ one-third to two-thirds) is excreted

Table IV. Pharmacokinetic properties of oral hypoglycaemic drugs

Drug	Protein binding[1] (%)	Plasma half-life (h)	Elimination[1]	Contribution of metabolites to activity
Sulphonylureas				
Acetohexamide		3.5-11	Hepatic metabolism to hydroxyhexamide (active); then to hydroxyhydroxy-hexamide (inactive)	Hydroxyhexamide more potent than parent drug but only very small amounts remain as this metabolite
Chlorpropamide	88-96	24-42	Variable hepatic metabolism (active metabolites) and renal excretion of unchanged drug (6 to 60%)	Probably minimal (metabolites eliminated very rapidly)
Glibenclamide (glyburide)	99	10-16	Hepatic metabolism and biliary excretion	Nil (metabolites probably have little activity)
Glibornuride	95	5-12	Hepatic metabolism and biliary excretion	Probably nil
Gliclazide	94	~12	Hepatic metabolism	?
Glipizide	92-99	3-7	Hepatic metabolism	Probably nil
Glisoxepide	93	1.4-5.3	Hepatic metabolism and excretion of unchanged drug (50%, mainly in urine)	?
Glymidine[2]		2.6-5.6	Hepatic metabolism (active metabolite)	About 15 to 30% excreted as demethylated metabolite (as active as parent drug)
Tolazamide		~7	Hepatic metabolism	Small (6 major metabolites are formed, but only 3 are hypoglycaemic, and mildly so)
Tolbutamide	95-97	3-25	Hepatic metabolism	Nil (hydroxytolbutamide active but formed in small amounts)
Biguanides				
Buformin		4-6	Renal excretion of unchanged drug	
Metformin		1-2	Renal excretion of unchanged drug	
Phenformin	20	5-15	Renal excretion of unchanged drug (33 to 66% of amount absorbed); some hepatic metabolism and biliary excretion	Nil

1 For implications relating to use in liver or renal disease and interactions with other drugs, see text.
2 A sulphapyrimidine compound.

unchanged in the urine, and significant amounts are also probably excreted in the bile; hydroxylated metabolites are also formed and excreted in the urine (Alkalay et al., 1975; Beckmann, 1968). Absorption of metformin is incomplete and protein binding is negligible. Metformin and buformin are entirely excreted unchanged in the urine. Clearance of metformin approximates that of glomerular filtration rate (Pignard, 1962). Because of impaired elimination and the very real risk of lactic acidosis, biguanides must be avoided in patients with liver disease or any degree of impaired renal function (Luft et al., 1978; see section 3.3.4).

3.3.4 Adverse Effects of Oral Hypoglycaemic Drugs

In recent years, there have been relatively few reports of short term side effects or toxicity due to sulphonylureas. Published figures of frequency of side effects in large series of patients range from about 1 to 5%, with symptoms severe enough to lead to withdrawal of the drug in less than 1 to 2% (e.g. Balodimos et al., 1966; Bernhard, 1965; Cervantes-Amezena et al., 1965; O'Donovan, 1959). Adverse effects in general have been of the following types: allergic skin reactions (including photosensitivity), gastrointestinal disturbances, blood dyscrasias, hepatic dysfunction, and hypoglycaemia. Skin reactions and gastrointestinal disturbances are uncommon, mild, and usually transient. Blood dyscrasias (leucopenia, agranulocytosis, thrombocytopenic purpura, etc) are rare, and in reported cases it has been difficult to determine the role played by sulphonylureas (Balodimos et al., 1966). As for their effect upon the liver, although a slight rise of the serum alkaline phosphatase is often seen this may be transient or variable and, even if sustained, appears to have no clinical significance. Jaundice, thought to be caused by sulphonylureas, has been reported rarely, but frequently the hepatic damage has proven unrelated to diabetes or to drug administration. Jaundice due to sulphonylurea compounds is usually of the cholestatic type, and appears within 6 weeks of beginning the drug. It is often preceded by a skin rash, fever, and gastrointestinal disturbances (Lozano-Castaneda et al., 1964; Zimmerman, 1976). Water intoxication and symptomatic dilutional hyponatraemia is a well recognised complication of chlorpropamide (Weissman et al., 1971; see chapter XXI, sect. 15.4).

Symptomatic hypoglycaemia is uncommon but may occur with the use of any of the sulphonylurea compounds, chiefly in elderly, poorly nourished patients who are not eating well and whose diabetes is quite mild, and depending on the drug administered, in those with impaired renal or hepatic function (for review, see Seltzer, 1972; see also table IV). Since chlorpropamide is excreted slowly from the body and therefore has a prolonged effect, its use in the class of patient just described may be more inclined to cause hypoglycaemia unless carefully monitored, and if hypoglycaemia occurs it may persist longer and require additional feedings lest hypoglycaemia recur after initial recovery (Seltzer, 1972; Agarwal et al., 1970). Fatalities have been reported, although rarely. Similarly, clinically important interactions between the sulphonylureas and other drugs are uncommon although several cases of prolonged hypoglycaemia have occurred (see section 3.3.5).

Untoward effects of the biguanides consist of dose related gastrointestinal disturbances starting with a metallic taste, anorexia, nausea and abdominal distress, leading to actual vomiting and diarrhoea (Odell et al., 1958). Such symptoms have been the limiting factor in the use of these drugs, and some patients do not seem to tolerate even small doses. These unpleasant symptoms disappear promptly upon stopping the drug, with no recognisable residual effect.

Biguanides and Lactic Acidosis: In October, 1977 the Secretary of Health, Education and Welfare of the United States banned the marketing of phenformin, the only biguanide previously available in that country. The action was taken because of an 'unacceptably high risk' of lactic acidosis in users of the drug as interpreted from a survey made by the Food and Drug Administration. The frequency of lactic acidosis was estimated to be 0.25 to 4 cases per 1000 users per year with death in approximately 50% of cases. With about 336,000 patients taking phenformin, this was *thought* to amount to roughly 50 to 700 deaths per year.

Following the action taken in the USA, the sale of phenformin was halted in some countries but continued in others. Although metformin and buformin, available in some countries, exert metabolic effects, including those regarding lactate, similar to those produced by phenformin, the frequency of reported lactic acidosis has been lower (Alberti and Nattrass, 1977; Bergman et al.,

1978). Nevertheless, clinicians prescribing any biguanide should select patients with care, avoiding such use in those with important cardiovascular, renal or hepatic disease (Nattrass and Alberti, 1978; Luft et al., 1978). The mortality of biguanide associated lactic acidosis is high. Treatment with biguanides should be stopped immediately if gastrointestinal disturbances such as vomiting, malaise, abdominal pain or diarrhoea occur (Gale and Tattersall, 1976) or if the endogenous creatinine clearance falls below normal. Serum creatinine concentration estimation is not reliable. Patients with retinopathy and high blood lactate concentrations, for example, may have normal serum creatinine concentration but reduced creatinine clearance. Thus, minor degrees of renal impairment, which may not be revealed by serum creatinine measurement alone, can be sufficient to cause accumulation of biguanides (Alberti and Nattrass, 1977; Luft et al., 1978; see also section 3.3.3).

Effect on the Cardiovascular System: In January 1961, a long term prospective clinical study of tolbutamide and (later) phenformin was begun in 12 centres in the United States under the name of the University Group Diabetes Program (UGDP). The study included a total of 1027 older patients with stable, non-ketotic diabetes who were divided at random into 5 treatment groups: (1) tolbutamide, 1.5g daily, (2) tolbutamide placebo, (3) insulin (lente) in fixed dose of 10 to 16 units daily, (4) insulin with dosage varied in conventional fashion, and (5) phenformin 100mg daily. The results for tolbutamide were reported in 1970 and reviewed again in 1975; those with phenformin in 1971 and reviewed again in 1975 and 1976 (University Group Diabetes Program, 1970, 1975, 1976). The principal conclusions regarding tolbutamide were: (1) tolbutamide may be toxic since there were more than twice the number of cardiovascular deaths in the tolbutamide treated than in the placebo group (26 *vs* 10), and (2) treatment with tolbutamide was no more effective in controlling the blood glucose than diet alone or diet plus insulin. The conclusions reported later regarding phenformin were essentially the same. The UGDP report has led to certain cautionary pronouncements by the USA Food and Drug Administration and similar agencies in some other countries.

In the UGDP study, the number of subjects in each treatment group was relatively small and there was a very real possibility that inadvertently the selection of subjects and their distribution among the treatment groups was uneven, so that true matching did not take place. For example, most of the cardiovascular deaths took place in 4 of the 12 treatment centres, and no deaths in the tolbutamide treated group occurred in 4 centres. It is noteworthy that the same deleterious effect as regards cardiovascular mortality was reported with phenformin as with tolbutamide, despite the fact that these drugs have an unrelated mode of action. One weakness of the UGDP study is that tolbutamide was given in fixed dosage for all patients contrary to the method used in clinical practice in which the dosage of the drug is adjusted to the individual needs of the patient. Except for one group of patients on variable dose insulin, no effort was made to regulate blood glucose. Blood glucose was also ignored in tabulation of the cardiovascular complications. An analysis of the data, however, showed that the cardiovascular death rate in patients whose blood glucose was poorly controlled was significantly greater than in patients who were well controlled (Feinstein, 1976a,b).

Many criticisms have been made of the UGDP protocol and interpretation of the observed results (Feinstein, 1971, 1976a,b; Schor, 1971; Various Authors, 1975). Because of the great and continuing controversy (see Shen and Bressler, 1977b; Whitehouse et al., 1979), a committee of the Biometric Society reviewed and evaluated the tolbutamide findings. Although a suggestion of excess risk of death from cardiovascular causes (not statistically significant) appeared in certain other subgroups, such excess risk was found to be significant only in women over 53 years of age (Report, 1975).

Results obtained in a retrospective cohort study of 2167 Joslin Clinic patients showed no significant differences between insulin and tolbutamide treated patients in the percentages of those dying of all cardiovascular causes. As for deaths attributed specifically to coronary artery disease, there was no significant difference between the insulin and tolbutamide groups in females of all ages and in men who entered the study at age 60 or older. An apparent trend toward higher mortality in tolbutamide treated men who were 40 to 60 years old at first visit, was not significant when risk factors were taken into account (Kanarek et al., 1975).

To date, no convincing explanation has been

offered for the reported adverse effects of tolbutamide and phenformin on the cardiovascular system. A positive inotropic action of tolbutamide has been suggested as the mechanism of cardiovascular toxicity in experimental animals, but the critical question as to whether tolbutamide (and other oral sulphonylurea hypoglycaemic drugs) have such an effect on human hearts and whether the effect is harmful, remains to be resolved (Levey et al., 1974). Moreover, the results of many retrospective studies are not in agreement with the UGDP findings (see Shen and Bressler, 1977b) and interpretations, and many, perhaps most, clinicians throughout the world have continued to use those oral agents available in their countries; *albeit* with more caution and more strict attention to diet. The patient should be informed by the clinician of the facts in this controversial matter and given the opportunity of transferring to a daily injection of insulin if such is indicated.

3.3.5 Drug Interactions with Hypoglycaemic Drugs

Reports of interactions between hypoglycaemic agents and other drugs taken by the diabetic patient have almost always involved the sulphonylureas (for review, see Hansen and Christensen, 1977). Intolerance to alcohol, or a disulfiram-like facial flushing effect, has been reported most frequently with chlorpropamide (Logie et al., 1976; Fitzgerald et al., 1962) and is a dominantly inherited trait in non-insulin dependent diabetics (Leslie and Pyke, 1978a,b). Alcohol, itself a potential hypoglycaemic agent under conditions of prolonged fasting or malnutrition (Madison, 1968), may also increase the effect of the sulphonylureas (particularly chlorpropamide) or insulin (Arky et al., 1968; Seltzer, 1972), and may lead to a clinically significant hyperlacticacidaemia in phenformin treated diabetics (Kreisberg et al., 1972; Luft et al., 1978).

A number of drugs may increase the effect of the sulphonylureas (see table V), but in practice such interactions are relatively uncommon, although phenylbutazone is a predictable cause of enhanced effects (Hansen and Christensen, 1977; Logie et al., 1976). Only a few cases of prolonged hypoglycaemic episodes or coma thought due to interaction have been reported and in all but a very few cases, other predisposing factors (e.g. inadequate nutrition, advanced age, renal or liver impairment, etc) were also involved. Nevertheless, when the sulphonylureas are used with other drugs consideration must be given to possible changes in pharmacological activity. More importantly, drugs known to have a potential for interaction can interfere with diabetic control in patients taking sulphonylureas; e.g. barbiturates and diuretics, the effect being most marked in older patients. Poor control in patients taking barbiturates is most likely with sulphonylureas subject to extensive hepatic metabolism (see table IV; Logie et al., 1976).

Pharmacokinetic interactions (table V) have not been fully elucidated but will vary from one compound to another because of individual differences in their pharmacokinetic properties (see table IV). In some cases it is possible that more than one mechanism could be involved (e.g. phenylbutazone, sulphaphenazole), and in other cases a hypoglycaemic reaction may be more likely to occur only in the presence of associated renal or hepatic impairment (see also section 3.4.6).

3.4 Management of Therapy

To the familiar triad of items important in the treatment of patients with diabetes, namely diet, insulin, and exercise, one must add for carefully selected patients the oral hypoglycaemic agents, and for all situations, education of the patient and his family. Such instruction should be as intensive and detailed as the patient's intelligence and cooperation will permit. For the person new to diabetes, this can best be achieved during a week's stay in a hospital with a unit for ambulatory inpatients. In such a setting, instruction given individually and in classes held twice daily can proceed while the diabetes is being treated. Specially trained nurses and dietitians can take a most important part in this effort. In addition, patients learn from association with other patients. Lacking such facilities, the person with newly discovered diabetes should receive instruction on an outpatient basis with frequent visits at first. The families of patients should be encouraged to take an active part in the learning process so that they may be prepared to help in the day by day management of diabetes at home.

3.4.1 Initiation of Treatment

As indicated earlier in this chapter, diet forms the basis of all treatment of diabetes. A carefully planned diet suited to the needs of the individual is the first step in the initiation of treatment. Derivation of calories from carbohydrate, protein, and fat, respectively, varies throughout the world, depending upon the availability of food, economic status of patients, and dietary habits in the region concerned. In many parts of the world, diet prescriptions for diabetic patients are such that 40 to 50% of calories are obtained from carbohydrate, 15 to 20% from protein, and 35 to 40% from fat. In such regions, diets useful in the treatment of most middle aged and older persons with diabetes range from 150 to 200g of carbohydrate, 60 to 100g of protein, and 60 to 100g of fat daily, furnishing about 1400 to 2100 calories. For obese patients, the total caloric intake must be reduced to 1000 to 1200 calories or less. Although usually restricted in carbohydrate, the diet must be thoroughly adequate in protein, minerals and vitamins. Insofar as practicable, fat should be of the polyunsaturated type and therefore of vegetable origin.

Many middle aged and elderly persons with the maturity onset type of diabetes which is stable and relatively resistant to ketosis, may be treated successfully by dietary restriction alone, particularly if excess weight is lost and if the patient faithfully adheres to diet in a continuing effort. If after a suitable period of days or a few weeks, satisfactory control of diabetes is not obtained, then in selected patients a trial of oral hypoglycaemic agents, either a sulphonylurea or a biguanide compound (in countries where such is available), may be undertaken. If a fair, but not quite satisfactory, response is obtained, combined treatment with a sulphonylurea and a biguanide may be employed. Biguanides should be avoided in patients with significant cardiovascular, hepatic or renal disease (see section 3.3.4).

The child or any young person with newly developed diabetes as well as many persons with onset between 20 and 40 years of age and a very sizeable percentage of patients who develop diabetes after the age of 40 years, require treatment with insulin from the start, not only to prevent or treat ketoacidosis if present and to increase resistance against infection, but also in children, to provide for normal growth and development. Dietary allowances should be adjusted to the needs of the individual; for example, in the infant diabetic, one may need to provide as much as 4g of protein per kg of body weight whereas in the middle aged or older person, two thirds to a gram per kg suffices.

In all age groups, physical activity suited to the individual acts not only to increase and preserve muscle tone and promote general health, but also to enhance the effect of injected insulin. It is, therefore, an important component of treatment. A schematic outline to the treatment of diabetes is given in figure 2 (for review, see Breidahl et al., 1972b).

Insulin: For the average adult outpatient who is not acutely ill, the initial dose of NPH or lente insulin may be 12 to 16 units daily before breakfast. The dose is increased 2 to 4 units at a time until a level is found at which the urine test before the evening meal becomes satisfactory. 2 or 3 days are allowed between successive changes. When a point is reached at which the urine tests before the evening meal are satisfactory, attention is shifted to the tests just before the noon meal. If these are poor, then a small dose of regular insulin is used with the NPH or lente insulin in the morning before breakfast. Starting with only 4 or 6 units of regular insulin, the dose is increased 1 or 2 units at a time until a point is reached at which the urine tests before the noon meal become satisfactory.

In certain patients possessing little or no capacity for endogenous insulin production, particularly children and those with unstable ('brittle') diabetes, the effect of the NPH or lente insulin given before breakfast may not carry through for a full 24 hours. After about 18 to 20 hours the blood glucose may begin to rise, and by 24 hours after the time of the morning injection, may be above 200 or even above 300ml/100ml. In such a situation, it usually is not safe to increase the insulin given in the morning before breakfast, lest hypoglycaemic reactions be precipitated during the afternoon, evening, or night. Instead, a small dose of NPH or lente insulin is given at bedtime, starting with an initial dose of only 4 units. The amount is increased slowly, 1 or 2 units at a time, until the fasting blood and urine tests are satisfactory. With the institution of bedtime insulin, the requirement of regular insulin given before breakfast usually becomes less, necessitating an adjustment in dosage.

In some patients, it may be preferable to give the evening dose of NPH or lente insulin before the evening meal rather than at bedtime, and this is particularly true if the evening meal is taken late, say at 8.00 (20.00h) or 9.00pm (21.00h). In such cases, it is often advantageous to combine a small dose of regular insulin with that of the modified variety.

Table V. Potential clinically important drug interactions with sulphonylurea oral hypoglycaemic agents

Interacting drug	Reported with[1]	Mechanisms[2]	Notes/actions[3]
1. Drugs that may greatly increase sulphonylurea action			
Aspirin	Chlorpropamide	?	Prolonged hypoglycaemia has been reported. Interaction more likely with large doses of aspirin, which have slight hypoglycaemic effect in own right
Chloramphenicol	Chlorpropamide	?	Chloramphenicol markedly increases plasma half-life of chlorpropamide. No clinical reports of harmful hypoglycaemia. Best to avoid and substitute another antibacterial agent
	Tolbutamide	IM	Chloramphenicol markedly increases plasma half-life of tolbutamide. Profound hypoglycaemia, including coma reported in elderly patients. Avoid chloramphenicol, substitute another antibacterial agent
Dicoumarol	Chlorpropamide	?IM	Dicoumarol increases plasma half-life of chlorpropamide. Hypoglycaemic coma reported. (Patients were elderly, had decreased carbohydrate intake and/or congestive heart failure and renal disease). Avoid dicoumarol, substitute phenindione
	Tolbutamide	IM	Dicoumarol markedly increases plasma half-life of tolbutamide. Profound hypoglycaemia, including coma reported. (Patients were elderly, had decreased carbohydrate intake or congestive heart failure). Avoid dicoumarol, substitute phenindione, warfarin or phenprocoumon (do not prolong half-life)
Oxyphenbutazone	Tolbutamide	?DB+ ?IM	Oxyphenbutazone increases plasma half-life of tolbutamide. No clinical reports of harmful hypoglycaemia. Because of known interaction with phenylbutazone, best to avoid oxyphenbutazone, substitute indomethacin or naproxen
	Glibenclamide	?	Hypoglycaemia has been reported
Phenylbutazone	Acetohexamide	IE+ ?IM	Hypoglycaemic coma reported in one patient. Phenylbutazone inhibits renal excretion of an active metabolite (hydroxyhexamide) of acetohexamide or its further biotransformation to the inactive metabolite hydroxyhydroxyhexamide. Avoid phenylbutazone, substitute indomethacin
	Carbutamide	?	Profound hypoglycaemia reported. Avoid phenylbutazone, substitute indomethacin
	Chlorpropamide	DB+ ?IE/IM	Hypoglycaemic coma reported. Avoid phenylbutazone, substitute indomethacin
	Glibenclamide	?	Hypoglycaemia has been reported. No increase in plasma half-life of glibenclamide but decreased renal excretion of major metabolite of glibenclamide
	Tolbutamide	DB+ IM	Phenylbutazone increases plasma half-life of tolbutamide. Hypoglycaemic coma reported. Avoid phenylbutazone, substitute indomethacin or naproxen
Sulphadimidine[4] (sulphamethazine)	Chlorpropamide	?	Hypoglycaemic coma reported in a patient treated for urinary infection. Avoid sulphadimidine, substitute another antibacterial agent
Sulphafurazole[4] (sulfisoxazole)	Chlorpropamide	?	Hypoglycaemic coma in an elderly patient (also taking phenformin) with urinary infection
	Tolbutamide	?	Profound hypoglycaemia reported in a patient with uraemia. Best to avoid sulphonamides in these circumstances, substitute another antibacterial agent

Table V. (continued)

Drugs that may greatly increase sulphonylurea action (continued)

Sulphaphenazole[4]	Chlorpropamide	?DB+ ?IE	Sulphaphenazole markedly increases plasma half-life of chlorpropamide. No clinical reports of harmful hypoglycaemia. Best to avoid sulphaphenazole, substitute another antibacterial agent
	Glibenclamide	?	Sulphaphenazole decreases volume of distribution and increases plasma concentrations of glibenclamide
	Tolbutamide	DB+ IM	Sulphaphenazole markedly increases plasma half-life of tolbutamide. Profound hypoglycaemia, including coma reported. (patients were elderly; some with heart failure and pyelonephritis). Avoid sulphaphenazole, substitute another agent

2. Drugs that may possibly increase sulphonylurea action

Alcohol	Sulphonylureas[5]	PD	Intolerance (facial flushing, headache) of alcohol in some cases, particularly with chlorpropamide (see section 3.3.5). Hypoglycaemic activity may be increased with acute alcohol ingestion if food intake is restricted (e.g. malnutrition, prolonged fasting)

3. Drugs that sometimes necessitate reduced dose requirement of sulphonylurea

β-Adrenoceptor blocking drugs	Sulphonylureas[5]	PD	Reduced dose requirement of sulphonylureas in some patients, particularly when the liver contains little or no glycogen (e.g. as after prolonged fasting, in ketosis; see section 13.1)
Clofibrate	Tolbutamide	?DB+ IM	Clofibrate increases plasma half-life of tolbutamide. Hypoglycaemic activity of tolbutamide is increased. Severe hypoglycaemia has been reported
	Chlorpropamide	?	Clofibrate slightly increases plasma half-life of chlorpropamide. Some dose reduction should probably be anticipated
Levodopa	Sulphonylureas[5]	PD	?Reduced dose requirement of sulphonylureas may be needed in some patients
Monoamine oxidase inhibitors	Sulphonylureas[5]	PD	Severe and protracted hypoglycaemia with mebanazine and pheniprazine has been reported (the nonhydrazine compound pargyline is hyperglycaemic)

4. Drugs that may make diabetic control more difficult

Barbiturates Rifampicin (rifampin)	Sulphonylureas	AM	Decrease in plasma half-life. More likely to be a problem with compounds extensively metabolised in the liver (e.g. acetazolamide, glibenclamide, tolazamide, tolbutamide). Avoid occasional use of barbiturates. Substitute a benzodiazepine
Corticosteroids Oral contraceptives Diuretics	Sulphonylureas[5]	PD	See section 13.1.

---

1   The pharmacokinetic properties of the sulphonylureas in man are not identical (see table IV). An interaction reported with one of the listed sulphonylureas may not necessarily occur with another compound.

2   The mechanisms proposed in many cases have not been well elucidated, and in the case of pharmacokinetic mechanisms, vary for each compound because of differences in their individual properties (table IV).

AM = acceleration of metabolism of sulphonylurea; DB = decrease in sulphonylurea albumin binding possibly contributory; IE = inhibition of renal excretion of sulphonylurea (unchanged drug or active metabolite depending on compound); IM = inhibition of metabolism of sulphonylurea; PD = pharmacodynamic effect.

3   The reports of prolonged hypoglycaemia or hypoglycaemic coma are represented by only a few cases. In many instances other factors were also present. The risk of drug induced hypoglycaemic reactions is increased in the presence of associated renal impairment or liver dysfunction (incl. alterations induced by drugs not mentioned above, e.g. certain anabolic steroids), with restricted food intake and in the elderly (see section 3.4.6).

4   No clinical reports of harmful hypoglycaemia with other sulphonamides. Sulphadiazine, sulphamethoxazole and sulphamethizole cause a small increase in plasma half-life of tolbutamide. Sulphadimethoxine, sulfadoxine (sulformethoxine) and sulphafurazole (sulfisoxazole) do not increase the plasma half-life of tolbutamide in subjects with normal renal function.

5   This effect can also occur with insulin.

Following initial regulation of the insulin dosage, a patient may make minor adjustments at home, 2 units at a time, according to the general trend of the outcome of the urine tests before meals. At intervals, determinations of the blood glucose are indicated to evaluate the adequacy of chemical control. Such tests should be made not only before breakfast, but also in the late forenoon and during the afternoon, at 3 or more hours after food.

Oral Hypoglycaemic Agents: If oral agents are to be used successfully in the maturity onset diabetic (see section 3.3.2), the amount of carbohydrate in the diet is best limited to 150 to 160g daily. Total calories should be kept at a level which will correct or prevent obesity. The selection of the type of oral agent to be used depends upon the experience of the clinician, and there are no hard and fast rules in this regard. A case has been made for the use of a biguanide such as metformin initially in patients who remain overweight following a trial on an adequate diet (Stowers and Borthwick, 1977; Clarke and Campbell, 1977). A small dose is used at first and gradually increased as indicated by the response of the blood glucose. Table VI gives the usual range of dosage of some of the oral agents. Experience has indicated that above a certain dose, further increase is generally useless. If either the sulphonylurea or the biguanide alone is partly effective, but not to the degree desired (see below), success may often be obtained by giving the two drugs in combination. For example, 1g tolbutamide and slow release metformin (1g) twice daily may be prescribed.

At the outset of treatment, it is wise to set up arbitrary standards of control. 'Good' control may be assumed when the fasting glucose (whole blood) and that at 3 or more hours after food is 6.10mmol/L (110mg/100ml) or lower. 'Fair' control is considered to prevail when such values are 7.22mmol/L (130mg/100ml) or lower. If at

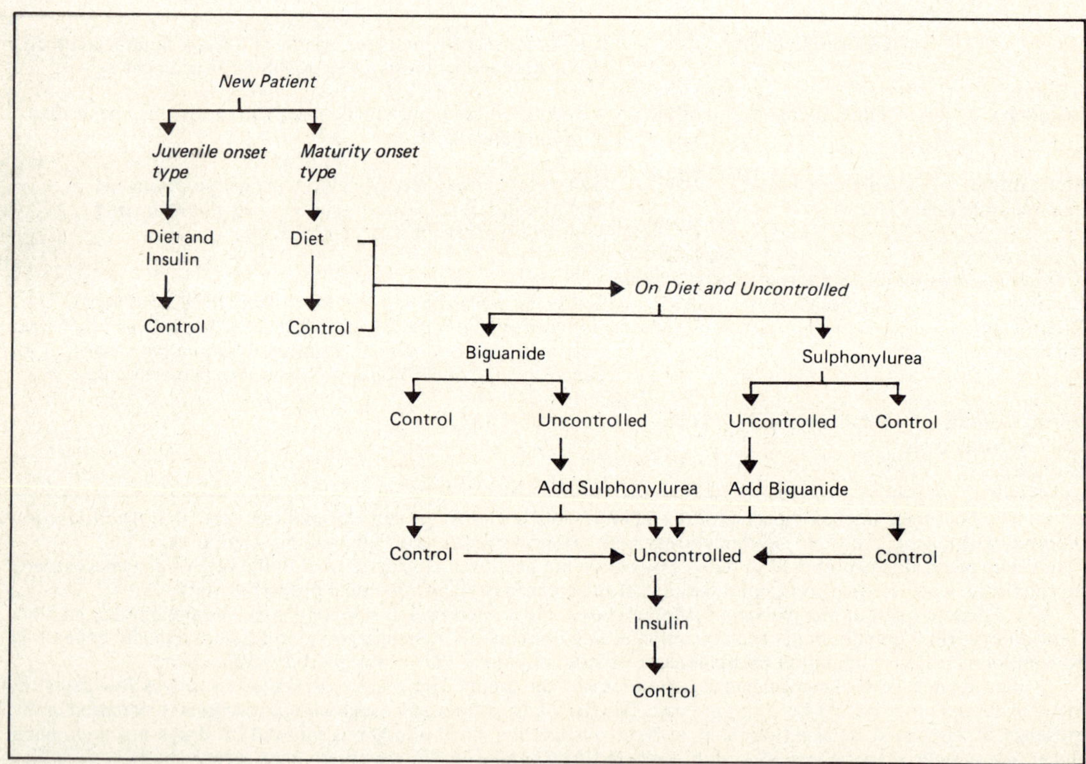

Fig. 2. Treatment flow chart of diabetes (see also text). After Breidahl et al.: Drugs 3: 204, 1972; by permission of author and editor.

Juvenile onset type: Insulin dependent, ketosis prone. May often occur in older persons. Maturity onset type: Relatively independent of injected insulin if restricted diet is followed. Relatively resistant to ketosis. May occur in a small percentage of young persons.

Table VI. Dosage of some oral hypoglycaemic agents

Compound	Strength (mg)	Daily dose range	Dosage frequency
Sulphonylureas			
Acetohexamide	250 500	0.25-1.5g	Single, or divided doses
Chlorpropamide	100 250	0.1-0.5g	Single dose
Glibenclamide	5	2.5-15mg	Single, or divided doses
Glibornuride	25	12.5-75mg	Single, or divided doses (if > 50mg daily)
Gliclazide	80	80-240mg	Single, or divided doses
Glipizide	5	2.5-30mg	Single, or divided doses (if > 10mg daily)
Glisoxepide	4	2-16mg	Divided doses
Tolazamide	100 250 500	0.1-1g	Single, or divided doses
Tolbutamide	500 1000	0.5-3g	Usually divided doses, 1-3 times daily
Biguanides			
Buformin	100	100-300mg	Usually divided doses
Metformin	500	1-1.5g	Usually divided doses[1]
Phenformin	25	50-200mg	Usually divided doses[1]

1   Preparations providing prolonged action by slow release of the drug are available.

least 70 % of the values are not within the ranges indicated, the control may be described as 'poor' and, provided that the other conditions of the selection of patients have been met, transfer should be made to insulin without hesitation. In deciding the degree of control, it is important that blood glucose values be obtained not only in the fasting state but also during the course of the day at 3 or more hours after food.

Among patients who are initially responsive to treatment with diet and sulphonylureas, there are many who, after some weeks, months or years, no longer respond. In a review of the experience of the Joslin Clinic, Balodimos et al. (1966) found that of 2555 patients treated for up to 9 years with tolbutamide, 499 or 19.5 % had experienced such a 'secondary failure'. When such 'secondary failures' occur, the clinician makes sure that the patient is following the restricted carbohydrate diet, and then either increases the dose of the sulphonylurea or changes to another compound, adds a biguanide to the treatment programme, or if these measures fail, transfers the patient to daily injections of insulin (Camerini-Davalos and Marble, 1962; Balodimos et al., 1966). The same general rules apply to the management of secondary failures with biguanides (see fig. 2).

3.4.2 Diabetes in Childhood

Some consideration has already been given to the treatment of diabetes in young persons. Two additional topics deserve discussion. The first has to do with the psychological effect of diabetes in children and adolescents. When children reach the age of 10 or 12 years, they should be encouraged to begin the assuming of control of diabetes management. They should understand and be urged to follow the principles of diet, to test the urine regularly and to record results, to give their insulin injections, and eventually to make minor adjustments in insulin dosage from time to time according to changing needs, all under the supervision of the clinician at periodic visits. These young patients should be encouraged to engage in activities common for their age, and to live in a way which is normal, insofar as practicable. It is natural that the daily routine of diabetes care with the restrictions imposed, should add to the psychological difficulties which are so common anyway in young persons, even apart from diabetes. Truly to 'accept' diabetes is often difficult for the child and adolescent and indeed for older persons. Constant support and encouragement from family and the clinician are essential.

The second item worthy of comment concerns the great frequency of vascular and nervous system complications after 15, 20 or more years of diabetes. Since there is a growing body of evidence to support the view that such complications may be postponed and lessened by careful and consistent control of diabetes (see section 3.1), it is the responsibility of the clinician to prescribe treatment with this long range view in mind, and to encourage the patient to maintain as good control of hyperglycaemia and glycosuria as is possible, short of producing frequent or severe insulin reactions (Cahill et al., 1976).

3.4.3 Diabetes in the Elderly

Diabetes may have its onset in the 60's and indeed in the 70's and 80's. It usually is of stable character and relatively easy to manage by dietary restriction either with or without oral hypoglycaemic agents (see above; also chapter V, sect. 4.3). However, in a relatively small but very definite percentage of such patients, treatment with insulin is necessary.

With advancing age, there is a gradual tendency for the level of blood glucose to rise. Opinions differ as to whether this should be regarded as simply a reflection of the aging process or as an increased frequency of diabetes. Many elderly patients do not have glycosuria even though the blood glucose may be 11.10mmol/L (200mg/100ml) or higher. One must keep in mind that patients over 60 years of age may, and sometimes do, develop diabetic ketoacidosis and coma which carries a higher mortality than in the young (Barnett et al., 1962). They may develop hyperosmolar coma with high blood glucose levels together with abnormally high levels of sodium and blood urea nitrogen (Gerich et al., 1971). Hence, diabetes in the elderly is by no means always benign.

3.4.4 Diabetes in Pregnancy

It is a good general rule that during pregnancy, insulin is the agent of choice if treatment other than diet is indicated. This is because most pregnancies occur in young women with the insulin dependent, ketosis prone type of diabetes. Furthermore, an increase in the intensity of diabetes as pregnancy progresses, is common (Greene, 1975). While some clinicians have reported the successful management of diabetes by oral agents without obvious harm to mother or fetus, these were women with stable, maturity onset type of diabetes and whose dose requirements were low (Sutherland et al., 1973; Notelovitz, 1971, 1974). Transfer to insulin is recommended after the fetus has reached viability at 34 weeks, since sulphonylureas cross the placenta and stimulate the fetal beta cells, already hypertrophied as a result of maternal diabetes.

The early reports of dysmorphogenicity associated with the use of sulphonylureas have not been confirmed. However, because of the relative frequency of congenital malformations in the offspring of diabetics treated in any manner, it is difficult to make firm conclusions in this regard (see also chapter III, sect. 5.2; XV, sect. 21.2).

3.4.5 Complications of Diabetes

The major principles of treatment of severe ketoacidosis and diabetic coma involve immediate hospitalisation, appropriate laboratory tests and prompt giving of insulin, fluid and electrolytes. Ample amounts of regular insulin must be given as dictated by determinations of the blood glucose made initially and at intervals of 2 to 3 hours. In the opinion of many clinicians, maximum success is obtained by giving large amounts of regular insulin initially, such as 100 to 200 units to adult patients (much smaller doses for young children, especially with newly diagnosed diabetes). Additional amounts of insulin are given subsequently, according to the trend of serial blood glucose determinations. The administration of insulin must be accompanied by the use of appropriate, and often large, amounts of 'normal' salt solution (full or half strength) intravenously. Within 2 or more hours in the average case, appropriate amounts of potassium must be added to the fluid being infused. Glucose is not added until a definite fall in the blood glucose is evident.

In recent years, it has become the custom in the treatment of diabetic ketoacidosis and coma in certain centres, to administer small amounts of insulin by adding such to the constant intravenous infusion. Following an initial bolus of 5 to 10 units of insulin given by vein, a constant intravenous infusion of 5 to 10 units per hour is maintained until a blood glucose level of about 13.90 mmol/litre (250mg/100ml) is attained. Usually, the insulin is administered either into an intravenous site separate from that delivering saline, or by means of an infusion pump into the main intravenous line. If frequent monitoring of the blood glucose indicates that the expected fall is not taking place, supplementary doses of insulin are given intravenously. Although prospective studies have shown no significant difference in outcome when compared with that obtained by the high dose method, certain advantages are claimed: (a) ease of administration; (b) relatively linear rate of fall of blood glucose levels; and (c) ability to discontinue insulin promptly if hypoglycaemia occurs (see Alberti, 1977; Kreisberg, 1978). Further experience is needed to determine which method is more successful in the treatment of the occasional seriously ill, high risk patient who arrives at the hospital in deep coma which has been present for some hours. Regardless of which method is used, the blood glucose *must* be monitored closely so that the amount of insulin available to the patient at any given time may equal the need.

Success in the treatment of diabetic ketoacidosis has also been reported by the intramuscular injection of insulin in dosage of 5 to 10 units per hour (Eskildsen and Nerup, 1977). However, there is always the possibility of irregular absorption initially in patients with severe ketoacidosis and dehydration. With this in mind, Sachs et al. (1979) gave an initial loading dose of insulin (0.44 units/kg body weight, half intravenously and half intramuscularly) and repeated this procedure hourly until the plasma glucose had fallen by 10% or more of the initial value. They then injected 7 units of insulin intramuscularly hourly until the plasma glucose was equal to or less than 13.9mmol/L (250mg/dl). Results were comparable with those obtained by the constant intravenous infusion method. To ensure prompt and regular absorption, the intramuscular injections of insulin should probably be given into the deltoid rather than the gluteus muscle (see Alberti, 1977). Rehydration of the patient is critical and giving of fluids intravenously from the start of treatment is essential.

The treatment of non-ketotic, hyperosmolar coma requires just as expert care and constant monitoring as that of the ketoacidotic type. Special attention is necessary as to the amount of insulin and the use of hypotonic fluid intravenously, as well as search for and treatment of complications.

3.4.6 Diabetes Associated with Other Disease

In general, the treatment of diabetes in the presence of coronary artery disease is the same as that in other patients. Great concern has been expressed by some regarding the danger of hypoglycaemia in such patients, particularly when an acute myocardial infarction has occurred. It has even been suggested that blood glucose levels of 13.90mmol/L (250mg/100ml) or higher may be beneficial. This would appear to be an illogical point of view which lacks supporting evidence. It is only common sense to avoid hypoglycaemic episodes whenever possible, but in the treatment of the patient with coronary artery disease, a happy middle road between low and high blood glucose levels can usually be attained without difficulty. The same general rules apply to patients with cerebrovascular disease. Clearly, hypoglycaemic reactions must be avoided, and the insulin dose adjusted to a level which will provide reasonably good control by common sense standards (Bradley, 1971).

In the treatment of diabetes complicated by advanced renal or hepatic disease, oral hypoglycaemic agents should in general be avoided, because of the increased risk of symptomatic hypoglycaemia with the sulphonylureas and the real risk of lactic acidosis with the biguanides (see section 3.3.3; 3.3.4). If treatment other than diet is indicated, insulin should be used carefully in type, dosage, and time of administration to maintain satisfactory control of the blood glucose level. Since in advanced renal failure insulin requirements may fall, the dosage must be carefully monitored (see chapter XXI; sect. 14.3).

4. Neonatal and Idiopathic Hypoglycaemia

Drugs have relatively little place in the treatment of hypoglycaemia. Glucagon (1mg or more, subcutaneously or intramuscularly) is used in patients who are unable to cooperate in taking readily absorbable carbohydrate by mouth. Adrenaline/epinephrine (0.3 to 0.5ml subcutaneously) may be given in place of glucagon but is not as effective and may produce side effects such as tachycardia and increase in blood pressure.

In symptomatic neonatal hypoglycaemia, glucose is the agent of choice. In persistent hypoglycaemia in the infant or child, although in many instances the identification of the cause remains elusive, nonspecific treatment measures are available (see Pagliara et al., 1973). Immediate treatment involves the administration of glucose, glucagon, or less desirably, adrenaline. For more prolonged therapy, corticotrophin gel may be given intramuscularly, starting with 10 units twice daily and then decreasing the dose gradually to 2.5 units a day. However, in patients in whom adrenal insufficiency causes the hypoglycaemia, hormonal replacement by corticosteroids is indicated. In patients with hypoglycaemia related to growth hormone deficiency, use of human growth hormone is effective, but this preparation is not available in amounts large enough to make this treatment practical. In patients in whom hyperinsulinism has been demonstrated, diazoxide should be considered in dosage of 12mg/kg per day. In infancy and childhood, functioning islet cell adenomas are not common, but must always be considered as a possibility in diagnosis. In some cases, partial pancreatectomy has been effective even though no tumour has been found in the portion removed.

In the adult with spontaneous hypoglycaemia, the causes are likewise diverse, and the first step in treatment is again identification of the aetiology, if possible. Possible causes, apart from medication (see section 14.1) which must be considered, include: reactive hypoglycaemia, either functional or secondary to early diabetes; hereditary fructose intolerance; hypofunctioning of the pituitary or adrenal cortex; ethanol in poorly nourished persons; various types of liver disease including glycogen storage disease; and finally, but importantly, functioning beta cell tumours of the pancreas, or much less commonly, certain non-pancreatic tumours. The treatment of non-malignant islet cell tumours is the most satisfying of all, because successful removal results in complete cure. If surgery has been unsuccessful or insulin producing metastases are present, various forms of drug treatment have been used, including corticotrophin, corticosteroids, adrenaline, glucagon, human growth hormone, diazoxide, mithramycin and streptozotocin (Schein et al., 1973).

5. Thyroid Disorders

Diseases of the thyroid gland can be divided for clinical purposes into those which relate only to a change in the size of the gland (non-toxic diffuse goitre, adenomatous goitre, thyroid cancer, etc.) and those which involve a change in secretion of thyroid hormones (hypothyroidism, 'T$_3$-toxicosis', thyrotoxicosis, etc.). Treatment must be based upon sound physiological and pharmacological knowledge and precepts, as well as upon predetermined therapeutic objectives. Each modality of therapy selected should be based upon the patient's individual needs, including the various modifying clinical variables such as reliability, compliance with medication instructions, of complications, social and psychiatric factors, etc (see Burrow, 1975; Selenkow, 1977).

5.1 Hypothyroidism

Two types of thyroid hormone preparations are available for physiological replacement therapy for thyroid deficiency — natural substances which are derived from the thyroid glands of domesticated animals, and synthetic compounds (see Refetoff, 1975; Selenkow and Rose, 1976).

5.1.1 Thyroid Preparations

The most useful of the natural preparations are those which have been appropriately 'standardised', such as desiccated thyroid USP, and thyroid BP. These preparations contain the two active thyroid hormones L-thyroxine and L-triiodothyronine in polypeptide form. Unfortunately, the standardisation methods are not reliable or precise, and current trends favour the use of synthetic thyroid hormone preparations such as sodium levothyroxine (T$_4$) and sodium liothyronine (T$_3$). These preparations contain measured quantities of each hormone and thus do not require 'standardisation'.

Synthetic thyroid hormones used individually, while therapeutically effective do not give the same serum thyroid hormone levels as the natural preparations (table VII). Liothyronine is more potent than thyroxine, is more completely absorbed, produces its metabolic effects more rapidly and its effects dissipate sooner after discontinuing therapy. It is useful for short term administration and when readily reversible results are desired. Thyroxine achieves more constant serum and tissue levels and allows finer dosage adjustment. Absorption of thyroxine following oral administration is however, incomplete and variable, particularly when taken with food; it should therefore be given fasting (Wenzel and Kirschsieper, 1977).

Table VII. Average maintenance dose and effect on laboratory tests of some thyroid hormone preparations (after Selenkow and Rose, 1976)

Drug	Usual dosage range (maintenance)	Thyroid tests[1] (euthyroidism)		
		T_4	resin uptake	free T_4 index
Thyroid USP, BP	90-180mg/day	$\downarrow$ N	N	$\downarrow$ N
Sodium levothyroxine USP Thyroxine sodium BP	150-300µg/day[2]	$\uparrow$ N	$\uparrow$ N	$\uparrow$ N
Sodium liothyronine USP Levotriiodothyronine BP	75-125µg/day	$\downarrow$	N	$\downarrow$
Liotrix	1-3[3] tabs/day	N	N	N

1   T_4 = serum thyroxine by displacement analysis; resin uptake = serum resin tri-iodothyronine uptake; free T_4 index = serum free thyroxine index; $\downarrow$ N = low normal; $\uparrow$ N = high normal; N = within normal limits; $\downarrow$ = decreased; $\uparrow$ = increased.

2   Some believe that a maintenance dose of 150 to 250µg daily is adequate. At this dosage T_4 and free T_4 index are usually normal.

3   Equivalent to 60-180mg (1 to 3 grains) thyroid USP, BP.

Thyroxine absorption can be reduced in malabsorption states such as coeliac disease, but the extent and clinical significance is difficult to predict (see chapter XIX; sect. 1.1.2). Thyroxine is highly (99%) protein bound, primarily to a specific thyroxine binding globulin (see section 1.2). It has a long elimination half-life of around 6 to 7 days in normal individuals, which is decreased to about 3 days in patients with hyperthyroidism and increased to around 9 to 10 days in patients with hypothyroidism (Sterling and Chodos, 1956). The long half-life means that metabolic effects of thyroxine are produced slowly and dissipate slowly. Once daily dosage is appropriate. Thyroxine is metabolised primarily to thyroacetic acid (about 45% of a dose) and thyronine (20% of a dose) with about a fifth of each metabolite present in the urine as glucuronide or sulphate conjugates (Pittman et al., 1971). The average daily rate of conversion of thyroxine to triiodothyronine is around 4% of the extrathyroidal thyroxine pool (Pittman et al., 1972).

A fixed combination of levothyroxine and liothyronine in a ratio of 4:1 has been formulated to simulate the natural thyroid hormone secretions (liotrix). It is equivalent to 60mg USP thyroid and contains 50 or 60µg thyroxine sodium and 12.5 or 15µg sodium liothyronine (liotrix Thyrolar and liotrix Euthroid). The major advantages of this preparation over individual synthetic thyroid hormones are its uniformity of chemical composition, precise dosage and predictable hormonal actions (Selenkow and Rose, 1976). Liotrix has an additional advantage: serum thyroid hormone levels increase with dosage and reflect the patient's metabolic status. Other combinations of synthetic thyroid hormones with ratios of T_4: T_3 from 9:1 to 5:1 have been marketed but do not reflect serum hormone levels as accurately as liotrix.

5.1.2 Treatment of Hypothyroidism

Treatment of patients with hypothyroidism should be initiated by using the equivalent dosage of desiccated thyroid of 15 to 30mg daily (e.g. 25 to 50µg thyroxine) for 2 to 3 weeks with gradual stepwise increments to tolerance. Dosage should be reassessed after some 8 weeks treatment and the appropriate amount needed to normalise serum thyroid hormone and TSH levels should be determined according to the patient's clinical status. Patients should be educated that treatment is life long as some discontinue therapy after months or years. In patients in whom ischaemic heart disease is suspected, initial daily dosage should not exceed 15mg thyroid (25µg thyroxine) with more gradual increments over 2 to 3 months. Maintenance dosage ranges for representative preparations are given in table VII. Anxious, thin patients generally feel best on about 120mg thyroid (or equivalent) daily, while lethargic, obese patients usually tolerate 180mg daily without symptoms. Older patients and those with cardiac

Table VIII. A guide to treatment in thyrotoxicosis

Therapy	Indications	Relative indications	Contraindications
Antithyroid drugs	Diffuse goitre (female)	Diffuse goitre (male)	Poor compliance
	Juvenile thyrotoxicosis Thyrocardiac disease	Multinodular goitre	Drug toxicity (especially haematological)
	Progressive exophthalmos Preparation for surgery		
Surgery	Failed drug treatment (under 35 years) Toxic uninodular goitre (under 35 years) Massive goitrous enlargement	Multinodular goitre not responsive to ^{131}I therapy	Uncontrolled thyrotoxicosis Post-thyroidectomy relapse Medical risks to surgery (diabetes, heart disease etc) Small thyroid
	Obstructive symptoms ?Coincident carcinoma Social factors		Thyrocardiac Severe or progressive exophthalmos
Radioiodine	Post-thyroidectomy relapse Diffuse goitre (over 35 years)	Multinodular goitre (over 35 years) Failed drug treatment (over 35 years)	Pregnancy and lactation Age under 35 years, unless special indication (e.g. severe heart disease, drug toxicity)
	Toxic uninodular goitre (over 35 years) Thyrocardiac Small thyroid		

disease should be treated cautiously to avoid sudden changes in cardiac haemodynamics. Maintenance dosage in the elderly is usually between 60 and 90mg thyroid daily (100 and 150μg thyroxine). Dosage in children aged over 1 year is now considered by some to be lower than previously; a range of 2.5 to 5μg/kg is appropriate (Abbassi and Aldige, 1977; Rezvani and DiGeorge, 1977). No drug toxicity is known for thyroid hormones when used in physiological dosages. Pharmacological overdosage (above 180mg thyroid/day) is usually well tolerated but thyrotoxicosis factitia can occur with long term dosages above 240mg daily. Nevertheless, doses used in the past have frequently been excessive (Stock et al., 1974).

5.1.3 Indications for Use of Thyroid Hormones

Indications for thyroid hormone therapy are: (a) thyroid gland insufficiency; (b) pituitary hypothyroidism, after adrenocortical therapy; (c) non-toxic goitre and thyroid cancer; (d) in combination with antithyroid drugs for thyrotoxicosis; (e) after ^{131}I therapy to prevent postradiation hypothyroidism; and (f) as a diagnostic aid in the thyroid 'suppression' test (Refetoff, 1975).

The use of thyroid hormones for non-thyroidal disorders such as gynaecological dysfunction, obesity and asthenia is not supported by sound medical evidence. There is some indication that gradual induction of mild thyroid hormone excess may be useful in patients with some forms of hyperlipidaemia (types II, III hyperlipoproteinaemia), but this use must be undertaken with great caution because of the risk of cardiotoxicity. Claims that thyroid supplements may increase the risk of breast cancer have been strongly criticised (Mustacchi and Greenspan, 1977; Gorman et al., 1977) and other studies have failed to find any association (Wallace et al., 1978).

5.2 Hyperthyroidism

There are two major approaches to the therapy of hyperthyroidism: (a) antithyroid drugs, in dosages to maintain euthyroidism when a physiological remission of the disease is anticipated, and (b) ablative procedures such as subtotal thyroidectomy or radioactive iodine therapy when a spontaneous remission cannot be induced (table VIII). For reviews, see Braverman (1978), Greffner and Hershman (1976), Irvine and Toft (1976).

5.2.1 Antithyroid Drugs

The most commonly prescribed antithyroid drugs are propylthiouracil, methimazole and its parent drug carbimazole (Selenkow and Wool, 1967). They act by blocking the intrathyroidal oxidative iodination of tyrosine to form thyroid hormones, and thus inhibit synthesis (fig. 3). Propylthiouracil is variably absorbed (Melander et al., 1977) so dosage should be individualised for this reason as well as to attain biochemical control. Antithyroid drugs are usually given in 4 divided doses (see table IX) since a more satisfactory response is obtained with divided doses than a single daily dosage (Gwinup, 1978), although once daily dosage might be possible when the condition is controlled after 4 to 6 weeks of therapy. Once euthyroidism is achieved, the dosage can be reduced to avoid consequent hypothyroidism due to drug overaction or, preferably, thyroid hormones can be added to the antithyroid programme. This ensures suppression of thyrotrophin (TSH) and prevents enlargement and vascularity of the gland which are features of overdosage. Effective control can be monitored by

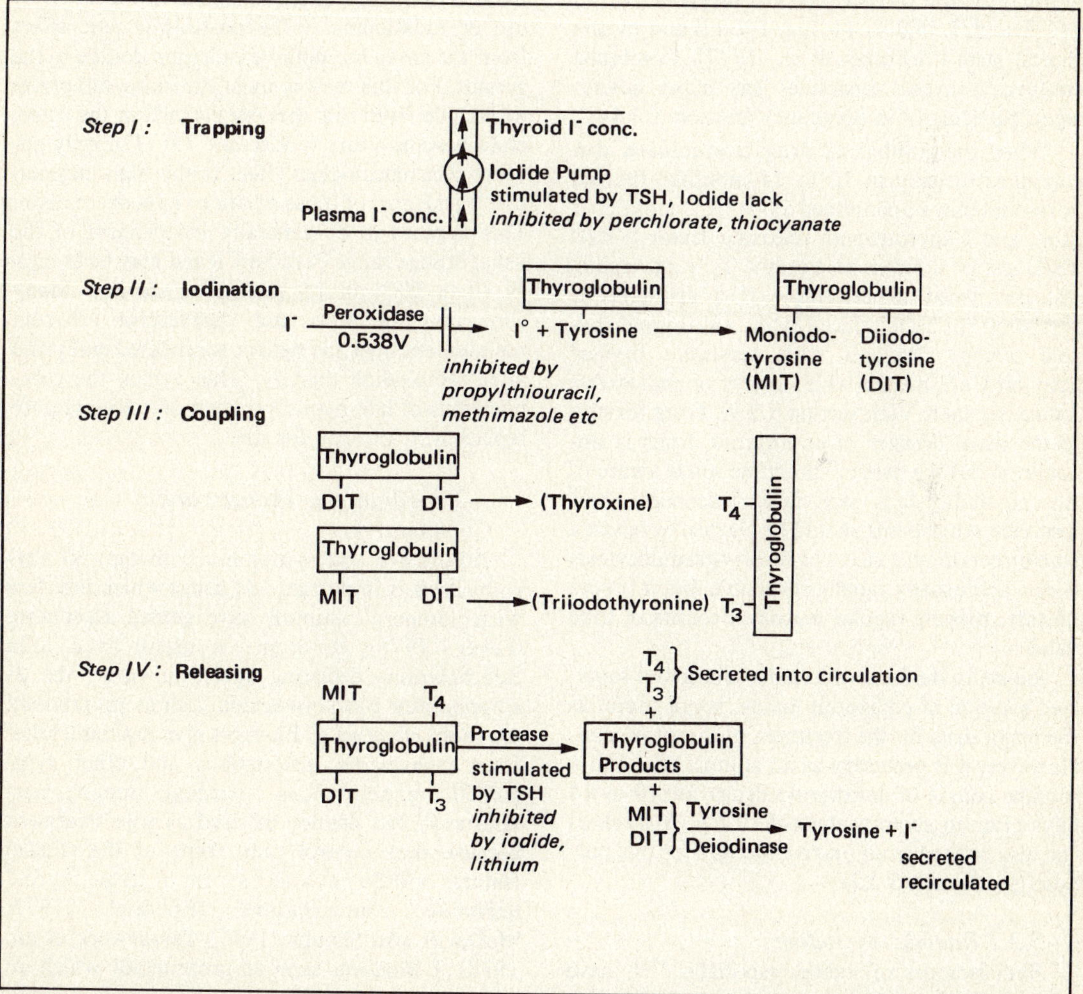

Fig. 3. Intrathyroidal iodide metabolism and the steps in thyroid hormone synthesis; showing mode of action of antithyroid and goitrogenic (section 14.2) drugs. After Selenkow et al.: Clinical Obstetrics and Gynecology 16: 66, 1973; by permission of author and editor.

Table IX. Clinical characteristics of some antithyroid drugs

Drug	Average daily dosage (mg)		Side effects (usual; all compounds)
	initial	maintenance	
Propylthiouracil	300-400	100-200	Skin rash (urticarial, miliarial,
Methimazole	30-40	10-20	morbiliform); granulocytopenia,
Carbimazole	30-40	10-20	agranulocytosis, thrombocyto-
Methylthiouracil	300-400	100-200	penia (rare); drug fever, arthralgia,
Iothiouracil[1]	150-250	100-200	SLE syndrome (rare); hair loss (carbimazole)

1   Not recommended.

serum thyroxine levels which are normally 51.5 to 142.0nmol/L (4.0 to 11.0μg/100ml) and by the clinical state (Mortimer et al., 1977). Combined antithyroid-thyroid treatment has many advantages, particularly in pregnancy (section 5.2.4).

When the antithyroid drug is eventually discontinued (usually in 12 to 24 months), thyroid hormones may be continued alone for 2 months or more and a thyrotrophin releasing factor (TRH-TSH) test or a radioactive iodine T_3 'suppression' test performed to determine if a spontaneous remission has been induced by the antithyroid-thyroid therapy. Patients with persistent thyroid autonomy are treated with surgery or radioactive iodine (see table VIII; section 5.2.2). Drug toxicity to the usual dosages of antithyroid drugs is uncommon but the patient should be made aware of this possibility (e.g. skin rash, leucopenia, hair loss, etc). All patients should be warned to report a sore throat, mouth ulcers or fever; agranulocytosis is rare and usually rapidly reversible, but it occurs quickly, making regular leucocyte counts of little value.

Iodine, in the form of Lugol's solution or saturated solution of potassium iodide, is not useful as the major drug for the treatment of thyrotoxicosis. However, it is necessary as an adjunct to a 2 to 4 months course of antithyroid drugs for 10 to 14 days prior to subtotal thyroidectomy. β-Blockers can also be used as adjunctive therapy for this purpose (see section 5.2.3).

5.2.2 Radioactive Iodine

Radioisotopes of iodine, especially ^{131}I, have been used extensively for treating hyperthyroidism. Radioiodine therapy has all the major advantages of surgical thyroidectomy without the hazards. The only disadvantage to more extensive use of radioiodine is the possible genetic effect from the small but definite radiation dosage to the gonads. For this reason, most clinicians still prefer to exclude from this therapy patients in the active child bearing years (under age 35). The only adverse pharmacological effect is the high cumulative incidence of postradiation hypothyroidism. This appears to be generally independent of the usual dosage range (4 to 8mCi) and may be as high as 40 to 50% in 15 years after therapy. Many clinicians therefore use 'preventive' thyroid replacement once the patient is rendered euthyroid after radioiodine therapy. This avoids the complications of late hypothyroidism but does require replacement therapy for life.

5.2.3 Adjunctive Therapy and Complications

Adjunctive and symptomatic therapy of thyrotoxicosis is important and drugs which interfere with adrenergic stimuli have gained acceptance (Levey, 1976). Reserpine is useful as a mild catecholamine depleting agent, however, the β-adrenoceptor blocking agents such as propranolol are more effective. β-Blockers give dramatic relief from tachycardia, palpitations and other sympathetic manifestations (sweating, tremor, 'nervousness') but cannot be used as sole treatment because they control only some of the clinical features and do not affect serum or tissue thyroid hormone concentrations (Editorial, 1977; McDevitt and Shanks, 1977; Tevaarwerk et al., 1978). β-Blockers such as propranolol which do not possess intrinsic sympathomimetic activity (see chapter XVIII; sect. 5.6.3) are more effective in hyperthyroidism than agents with this property, particularly in relation to reduction of tachycardia (McDevitt and Shanks, 1977). Propranolol is also of adjunctive benefit in preoperative preparation of the patient for subtotal thyroidectomy and has been used alone, but since the patient is not rendered euthyroid, propranolol must be given for some days after surgery to avoid the risk of thyroid crisis (Michie et al., 1974; Toft et al., 1978). Propranolol has also been added to the standard preparation regimen for a few days prior to operation and seems to provide faster relief of symptoms in minimally regulated patients. It has also been used to control symptoms after radioiodine therapy (Hadden et al., 1968; 1970).

The pathogenesis of the eye signs in Graves' disease remains unknown. A number of treatment measures can be considered if exophthalmos becomes 'malignant' (see further chapter XII; sect. 9.1).

The general principles of treatment of exaggerated manifestations of severe thyrotoxicosis or a thyroid crisis involves prompt diagnosis and treatment of any underlying illness and early institution of specific treatment — including general supportive measures, high doses of antithyroid drugs (propylthiouracil is preferred) and iodide to reduce the secretion and production of thyroid hormones, and a β-adrenoceptor blocking drug such as propranolol (orally 40 to 80mg strictly 6-hourly, or if given intravenously in an emergency 1mg/min for 2 to 10mg maximum rate and total dose, preferably after prior digitalisation) to combat the metabolic effects of thyroid hormones. With proper management of the thyrotoxic patient, the occurrence of a thyroid crisis should be rare. It is primarily seen in undiagnosed or incompletely treated hyperthyroid patients with a complication of infection, diabetic ketoacidosis, trauma or nonthyroidal surgery (Mackin et al., 1974; Rosenberg, 1976).

Potassium iodide may be required to acutely block the release of preformed thyroid hormone in the very severely thyrotoxic patient in a prethyroid crisis.

5.2.4 Hyperthyroidism in Pregnancy

The usual patient with hyperthyroidism can be managed successfully in pregnancy using a combined antithyroid-thyroid therapeutic programme (Selenkow, 1972; Selenkow et al., 1973). Since antithyroid drugs cross the placenta (potassium perchlorate and iodides are not used), the dosage in pregnancy should be kept to the minimum which will control the disorder effectively. This is usually 5 to 15mg methimazole or carbimazole daily in divided doses or 50 to 150mg propylthiouracil daily plus synthetic or natural thyroid hormone replacement therapy. Propylthiouracil is generally preferable to methimazole or carbimazole since it is less readily transferred across the placenta (Marchant et al., 1977). The patient's metabolic status should be monitored serially to avoid hypothyroidism from antithyroid drug actions. Pregnancy usually ameliorates hyperthyroidism and renders the patient more readily treated by a *low* dosage regimen so that by the third trimester, dosage of carbimazole and propylthiouracil can be as low as 2.5 to 7.5mg and 25 to 75mg daily, respectively. It is advantageous to add thyroid hormone replacement with the more complete hormones (desiccated thyroid or liotrix) so that serum free thyroid hormone levels can be determined to confirm clinical euthyroidism. There is no advantage to use of sodium liothyronine for this purpose since serum levels cannot be used to monitor the patient's metabolic status. The alternative to use of an antithyroid-thyroid drug combination in pregnancy is use of antithyroid drugs alone or to undertake subtotal thyroidectomy (Hamburger, 1972; Talbert et al., 1970). Antithyroid drugs alone can be used just as successfully, but dosage must be kept below 200mg propylthiouracil daily or equivalent and the patient monitored frequently to avoid hypothyroidism. However, despite careful observation, a high incidence of maternal hypothyroidism can still occur (Bokat, 1968). Some continue antithyroid drugs in minimum dosage until the time of delivery, while others discontinue them in the last weeks of pregnancy to reduce the possibility of neonatal goitre or hypothyroidism.

Although data are few, there is no evidence that antithyroid drugs are dysmorphogenic or, despite isolated cases of cretinism or retardation, lead to adverse effects on subsequent growth and intellectual development (Herbst and Selenkow, 1965; Burrow et al., 1968, 1978; McCarroll et al., 1976). Traditional advice is that they are withdrawn if breast feeding is elected presumably since thiouracil reaches concentrations in breast milk higher than in maternal serum (Williams et al., 1944). No specific data are available for any of the antithyroid drugs currently used in clinical practice and presumably findings with thiouracil have been extrapolated to the other drugs (see also chapter IV; sect. 3.1.3). Spontaneous remissions of hyperthyroidism occur frequently during pregnancy but relapses are common following delivery and require an increase in the antithyroid drug dosage.

Propranolol has been reported to be useful in hyperthyroidisim and pregnancy (Langer et al., 1974). It did not alter the spontaneous occurrence of labour or delivery. However, although some clinicians use small doses to control sympathetic overactivity, its use in pregnancy is not generally recommended, particularly without concomitant use of antithyroid agents, except where the seriousness of the clinical situation (e.g. thyroid crisis) justifies the possible risks of this drug (see also chapter III; sect. 8.2). For a review of hyperthyroidism in pregnancy, see Burrow (1978) and Cheron et al. (1978).

6. Parathyroid Disease

Despite remarkable advances in the pathophysiology and diagnosis of parathyroid gland function, little headway has been made in drug therapy of common parathyroid hormone diseases.

6.1 Hyperparathyroidism

Primary hyperparathyroidism is now recognised as a more common disorder than previously suspected. Development of sensitive radio-immunoassays for measurement of serum parathyroid hormone levels has greatly improved the early and more precise diagnosis of this disorder, which may be due to adenoma, hyperplasia or carcinoma of the parathyroid glands. Localisation of hypersecreting tumours is still not exact but can be assisted by measurement of differential venous serum levels of parathormone by subclavian vein catheterisation. Most parathyroid adenomas are autonomous and do not respond appreciably to fluctuations in serum calcium levels induced by challenge with the chelating agent ethylenediamine tetracetic acid (EDTA), phosphate infusion or calcium loading.

Treatment of primary hyperparathyroidism is therefore directed towards surgical removal of the hyperfunctioning parathyroid tissue, whenever this is feasible. Medical treatment may be used when this is not possible and also to alleviate symptoms due to hypercalcaemia, to restore body fluids, electrolytes and renal function toward normal, to treat hypertension and to improve the

patient's general condition prior to surgery (Coburn et al., 1972; Hoffenberg, 1972). It may also permit time while investigative procedures are being conducted to exclude other causes of hypercalcaemia. Unfortunately, the management of hypercalcaemia of any cause is a diagnostic and therapeutic problem and acute hypercalcaemia can be life threatening.

Simple measures include fluid administration, with or without intravenous saline or large doses of diuretics such as frusemide or ethacrynic acid (to enhance urinary excretion of calcium). Neutral solutions of oral or intravenous inorganic phosphate is usually an effective way of acutely lowering serum calcium levels, by causing a net movement of calcium into bone. Other agents which act similarly include corticosteroids, calcitonin and mithramycin but these drugs are of limited usefulness. Calcitonin may be of special use in the long term management of inoperable cases of parathyroid carcinoma with nephrolithiasis and renal impairment. Mithramycin could be used as an alternative in such cases. Therapy with inorganic phosphate may also be indicated in long term management of inoperable cases (without renal impairment) or of unusual cases when the abnormal parathyroid glands cannot be found. However, therapy must be monitored carefully and has complications, including metastatic calcifications in soft tissues and blood vessels, particularly with intravenous administration.

Synthetic vitamin D analogues such as 1α-hydroxycholecalciferol (alfacalcidol) have been used to control the severe and prolonged hypocalcaemia which occurs postoperatively in patients with severe bone disease (Boyle et al., 1977).

Secondary hyperparathyroidism occurs in chronic hypocalcaemic states such as malabsorption syndromes, chronic renal failure or dietary rickets. Treatment of the underlying disorder leads to reversal of the parathyroid hyperfunction except in rare cases of tertiary hyperparathyroidism, in which autonomous tumour formation is believed to derive from the stimulation of long standing hypocalcaemia.

6.2 Hypoparathyroidism

This disorder has most commonly occurred as a complication of thyroid gland surgery and is now less prevalent with the use of radioiodine therapy and thyroid hormone suppression of goitre (section 5.1). It may be a transient phenomenon after thyroidectomy and then may require only calcium salts orally until parathyroid hormone function returns. In acute hypocalcaemia, intravenous calcium is usually needed. Total absence of functional parathyroid tissue results in chronic hypoparathyroidism. Unfortunately, no direct therapy is currently available but maintenance of relatively normal levels of serum calcium can be achieved by the use of large oral doses of calcium salts (calcium chloride, lactate, or phosphate) plus carefully adjusted dosages of vitamin D (Avlioli, 1974). Symptoms can often be controlled even when serum calcium levels are in the borderline low zone. It is not uncommon for this to occur with increased renal excretion of calcium salts. The most common preparation of vitamin D in current usage is vitamin D_2 (calciferol) which is given in dosage of 50 to 100,000 units (1.25 to 2.5mg) daily. If resistance occurs, the more expensive preparation dihydrotachysterol can be tried (1.0 to 1.5mg/day is equivalent to 40 to 60,000 units of vitamin D_2).

Newer metabolites of vitamin D, such as 25-hydroxycholecalciferol (calcifediol), $1\alpha,25$-di-hydroxycholecalciferol (calcitriol) and 1α-hydroxycholecalciferol (alfacalcidol) are more active biologically than the usual vitamin D preparations in common use (see chapter XXI; section 9.6) and are useful for resistant cases or for more physiological regulation (Kooh et al., 1975; Jorgensen and Vogt, 1977). It must be emphasised that vitamin D therapy for hypoparathyroidism is pharmacological and complications of vitamin D excess must be appraised frequently during treatment (renal calcinosis; hypervitaminosis D). Thiazide diuretics plus a low salt diet have a useful hypercalcaemic effect and can maintain serum calcium levels in the normal range for prolonged periods. Such a regimen might be an alternative to vitamin D in selected patients (Porter et al., 1978). Perhaps in the near future, preparations of synthetic parathormone may become available for replacement therapy.

7. Obesity

Medical management of weight reduction in obese individuals is one of the most challenging problems in clinical practice, not only because of the indirect consequences of obesity on the coronary arteries and on mortality from other obesity related disorders, but also because its successful treatment is difficult (Goldrick, 1976; Mann, 1974). Without time and attention to detailed history taking, no understanding of the aetiology of obesity in an individual patient is possible. Thus careful understanding of the patient and his disorder are essential, but a long term contract, with motivation and psychological support, is necessary for any progress.

With certain uncommon exceptions (Cushing's syndrome, severe hypothyroidism, and rare neurological disorders of childhood), obesity is simply a result of excessive caloric intake. This basic fact is complicated by appetite control, which is an integral function of the central nervous system. Despite extensive studies, no intrinsic metabolic or biochemical abnormality has been identified to explain obesity, and the major therapeutic goal must be to limit caloric intake through disciplined appetite control and revision of poor dietary habits. The various metabolic deviations observed in the obese seem, in the light of present knowledge at least, to represent adaptations to obesity rather than its cause (Garrow, 1973; Mann, 1974).

7.1 Role of Diet and Exercise

Dietary restriction of total caloric intake is the cornerstone of any treatment programme for the obese patient and his family. This involves prescribing a diet which contains insufficient calories to maintain body weight and motivating the patient to adhere to it. Caloric requirements vary with age, sex, physical activity and body weight. Although these may be calculated from standard tables, the results in weight loss often do not agree with those expected. Most patients with moderate activity lose weight satisfactorily on a 1200 to 1500 calorie diet if it is adhered to. Some will require reduction in calories to 900 to 1000 per day. The diet should provide at least 1g of protein per kg of ideal body weight, should be well balanced and adequate in vitamins and minerals and should provide sufficient fluid and bulk to satisfy the patient's appetite. With fall in weight, revision of the prescribed calories may be necessary. Adjunctive vitamin supplements can be used for long term programmes. The weight reduction should generally be gradual, with a 2.5 to 5kg weight loss the first month and then a 2.5kg per month decrement until a first stage goal is reached (usually 10% loss of original weight). If the patient is able to maintain this for several months, a second decrement can then be attempted. The treatment programme aims to prevent development of refractory obesity, since it is extremely difficult to achieve further maintained weight reduction if this occurs. Sometimes it is unrealistic to attempt anything but prevention of weight regain. Obesity is a chronic and recurrent disease. Once the patient has lost weight, regular supervision at less frequent intervals is essential.

It is important to combine an exercise programme with the correct reduction programme. Exercise does not contribute to weight loss via caloric expenditure, but in many patients for unknown reasons decreases appetite. This exercise programme must be individualised and should emphasise aerobic principles as contrasted with muscle strengthening.

Some workers have suggested a short fasting period of 48 to 72 hours prior to embarking on a weight reduction diet. This may be performed only in relatively healthy patients under strict supervision. It must be emphasised that this is a caloric fast and not a water fast. Fluid intake has to be maintained to prevent dehydration and complications from hyperuricaemia. Prolonged fasting for weight reduction is to be avoided.

7.2 Role of Drugs as Adjunctive Treatment

The majority of patients who are obese dislike long term food restriction — certainly when it has to be sufficiently severe to lead to continuing weight loss. Thus, to achieve and maintain a therapeutic relationship an understanding of motivation is all-important and emotional support and encouragement are therefore necessary adjuncts to caloric restriction. For this reason, and because newer ideas usually tend to lose their value, drug therapy with 'anorectic' drugs is usually considered as a supportive measure to dietary restriction in patients who have a reasonable chance of responding to treatment (e.g. mild obesity, obesity of short duration, a good initial response to diet). Without strict dietary control any regimen will fail. Any drug therapy, therefore, has a very limited role but there appears to be widespread agreement on the following principles:

1) Intelligent and close dietary supervision should always be initiated before a trial of anorectic drugs which are used when the patient is having difficulty in adhering to the diet.

2) Any effective anorectic drug has some potential side effect.
3) No anorectic drug has been shown to lead to a more effective weight loss than other forms of therapy.
4) Anorectic drugs may be prescribed in some patients with the thought of helping the doctor retain patient confidence as part of a long term diet, exercise and weight control plan.

Various anorectic drugs have been used for appetite control (Craddock, 1976; Pinder et al., 1975). Possible side effects of the amphetamine derivatives, which have now been largely abandoned, include rise in blood pressure, tachycardia, central nervous system overstimulation, psychoses, impotence, diarrhoea and other sympathomimetic side effects as well as real risk of abuse and dependence. A shot gun combination of drugs including an amphetamine, thyroid, a thiazide diuretic and digitalis has been used in certain obese patients and has caused serious cardiac arrhythmias and even death (Jelliffe et al., 1969). These and other polypharmaceuticals should never be used in weight control.

Suitable anorectic agents with low abuse potential are represented by drugs such as diethylpropion, fenfluramine and mazindol. These agents produce changes in dopaminergic and serotoninergic neurotransmission and reduce appetite in short term use. Fenfluramine and mazindol have effects on glucose and lipid metabolism, but any contribution of these effects to weight loss is unclear (Pinder et al., 1975; Kirby and Turner, 1976). Diethylpropion is also a sympathomimetic amine and should be used cautiously, if at all, in patients with hypertension or cardiac disease. This restriction does not apply to fenfluramine, although dosage of antihypertensive drugs may need to be reduced. All are contraindicated in patients receiving monoamine oxidase inhibitors (see chapt. VIII; sect. 3). Side effects of drugs like diethylpropion and mazindol are similar to but less marked than with the amphetamines and are usually insomnia, dry mouth, constipation and dizziness. Fenfluramine causes drowsiness (rather than CNS stimulation), dryness of the mouth, vivid dreams and diarrhoea — particularly if large doses are used initially. Mood depression can occur during treatment and if fenfluramine is not withdrawn gradually (Steel and Briggs, 1972). It should be avoided in depressed patients.

Psyllium hydrophilic mucilloid taken prior to meals will decrease appetite in some individuals. It acts by causing an increased bulk in the stomach and thereby producing satiety. The compound is relatively safe but may cause intestinal obstruction.

7.3 Preventive Measures

Effective and prolonged weight reduction for those who are significantly obese is a challenge to both the doctor and his patient. The greatest success is achieved by supportive measures and a reasonable dietary approach. However, the generally disappointing results in the medical management of the obese patient suggest that more emphasis must be paid to the initial prevention of weight gain in the community . Particular efforts should therefore be made to prevent weight gain in those at risk — pregnant women, neonatal infants, girls around puberty, and members of families with a high rate of obesity, diabetes and premature atheroma (Brook, 1973; Mann, 1974).

Obesity is a disorder that in most cases could have and should have been prevented. Education and training of the child will help to minimise obesity in the adult. The child should be taught proper eating habits such as basic nutritional concepts, avoidance of 'junk' foods, and the importance of avoiding between meal snacks. Teaching these subjects in primary schools is helpful but only if they are practiced in the home by the parents will the desirable result be achieved. Should the child be obese, drugs should be used only with the utmost care and concern if used at all. Every effort must be made to examine the home and school environment to determine the reasons why the child is turning to food for gratification. In general, attempts to change environmental problems and low calorie diets are the treatments for obesity in the child. Obesity in the child frequently portends obesity in the adult.

8. Disorders of the Anterior and Posterior Pituitary and Hypothalamus

Replacement of trophic hormones in patients with anterior pituitary insufficiency is limited by the necessity of parenteral administration of these polypeptide hormones. Consequently, secondary adrenal, gonadal and thyroid insufficiency states are best treated with corticosteroid and thyroid hormones given daily by mouth. However, treatment with pituitary gonadotrophins, rather than replacement of testosterone or oestrogen, is necessary when infertility is a consideration. In patients with an intact anterior pituitary gland, with anovulatory cycles, or amenorrhoea without demonstrable organic cause, clomiphene or similar drugs such as tamoxifen or cyclofenil can be used to induce ovulation (see chapter XV; sect. 14).

Absence of growth hormone has no known important physiological consequences in the adult and does not require replacement therapy. Treatment is therefore reserved for growth hormone deficiency in children of short stature. Although species specificity and scarcity of supply limit the availability of human growth hormone, injections of 2mg of human growth hormone every other day will promote growth in such patients (Raben, 1959; 1962).

Central nervous system regulation of anterior pituitary function appears to be through polypeptide humoral mediators, termed releasing factors, which are synthesised in the hypothalamus and released into the hypophysial-portal circulation (American Physiology Society, 1974). These hypophysiotrophic hormones ordinarily stimulate the release and synthesis of pituitary trophic hormones, but in some instances may inhibit anterior pituitary function. The isolation, structural identification and synthesis of several releasing factors promise new applications in diagnosis and treatment of hypothalamic pituitary disorders (Fleischer et al., 1972). For example, synthetic thyrotrophin releasing hormone (TRH) is a tripeptide, active orally or intravenously in man, which can be utilised as a test of pituitary reserve of thyroid stimulating hormone (TSH) secretion. The peak TSH response following 500µg TRH given intravenously as a bolus is seen at 30 to 45 minutes. TRH is also effective in releasing prolactin in normal subjects as well as growth hormone (GH) in active acromegaly. Normally, TRH does not stimulate the release of growth hormone, ACTH or gonadotrophins. Luteinising hormone releasing hormone (LHRH) is a decapeptide which has LH and FSH releasing activity. Growth hormone release inhibiting hormone (GRIH or somatostatin) contains 14 amino acids and inhibits growth hormone secretion in physiological and pathological states. However, somatostatin is not specific for inhibiting growth hormone secretion since it also suppresses the release of other pituitary hormones; pancreatic insulin and glucagon; and gastrin and secretin.

These polypeptide neurosecretions of the hypothalamus are in turn under neurological control from higher centres and from monoaminergic neurotransmitters. Higher centre regulation of the hypophysiotrophic hormones is exemplified by the sleep rhythms of human growth hormone and ACTH and the response to stress of certain anterior pituitary hormones. Three monoamines play important roles in the neural regulation of these hypothalamic releasing hormones: the catecholamines, dopamine and serotonin. For example, α-adrenoceptor stimulation enhances, while β-adrenoceptor stimulation inhibits growth hormone secretion. Accordingly, propranolol has been used to enhance the response to stimuli of growth hormone secretion. Since growth hormone is also stimulated by the neurotransmitter dopamine, the oral administration of levodopa is a useful test of growth hormone reserve. Dopamine and other dopamine agonists (such as bromocriptine and apomorphine) also inhibit the secretion of prolactin. Since prolactin is normally under tonic inhibition by the hypothalamus, it has been postulated that hypothalamic dopaminergic receptors inhibit prolactin secretion by stimulating the release of prolactin inhibiting factor. Alternatively, it is possible that dopamine is a prolactin inhibiting factor.

This physiological action of dopamine agonists to inhibit prolactin secretion has resulted in the use of these agents in the medical management of patients with amenorrhoea-galactorrhoea syndromes (see chapter XV; sect. 14; 23). Paradoxically, dopamine agonists such as bromocriptine also inhibit growth hormone secretion in some patients with acromegaly along with symptomatic and objective clinical improvement, including improvement in hyperprolactinaemic hypogonadism (Belforte et al., 1977; Schwinn et al., 1977; Wass et al., 1977). The precise role of bromocriptine in acromegaly is not yet clear, but most believe that where tumour is present it should be used to augment the effect of the usual surgical and radiotherapeutic measures to reduce growth hormone secretion. It may be useful alone in younger patients who need to retain gonadotrophin function or for the elderly who decline or are suitable for surgical treatment. Bromocriptine has also been successfully used in patients with prolactin secreting pituitary tumours in whom hyperprolactinaemia and hypogonadism had persisted after pituitary surgery or radiotherapy (Carter et al., 1978; sect. 11). Interference with dopaminergic inhibition of prolactin secretion by certain drugs (phenothiazines, methyldopa, reserpine) may also be associated with galactorrhoea and elevated prolactin levels (see chapter XV; sect. 23.6). Serotoninergic mechanisms are also involved in the stimulation of ACTH, growth hormone and prolactin secretion. Accordingly, cyproheptadine (a potent serotonin antagonist) has been used to advantage in some patients with Cushing's and Nelson's syndromes to reduce the pituitary hypersecretion of ACTH (Editorial, 1978).

9. Adrenal Diseases and Corticosteroids

There are three principal hormones secreted by the adrenal cortex: aldosterone, cortisol and the adrenal androgens. The role of aldosterone is related primarily to sodium and potassium homeostasis since it produces sodium retention and potassium loss by a direct effect on the renal tubule (i.e. mineralocorticoid effect). The major biochemical action of cortisol is catabolic. By altering intermediary metabolism, it increases gluconeogenesis, i.e. the conversion of amino acids, proteins, and fats into glucose. Adrenal androgens are much less active than testicular androgens but do serve as the major source of androgens in the female.

Diseases of the adrenal gland may be due either to over- or underproduction of any of these compounds, particularly aldosterone and cortisol. Because both are linked via negative feedback loops with other control factors (the renin-angiotensin system for aldosterone, and ACTH for cortisol), defects in production may be primary in the adrenal gland or secondary to alterations in the secretion of these control factors. Mineralocorticoid deficiency in the absence of glucocorticoid deficiency is extremely rare. On the other hand, mineralocorticoid excess due to a tumour of the adrenal gland producing aldosterone, or to bilateral hyperplasia, is an uncommon, but curable, cause of hypertension (for reviews, see Cope, 1972; Williams et al., 1977).

9.1 Glucocorticosteroids

The widespread use of glucocorticosteroids (glucocorticoids) in clinical practice emphasises the need for a thorough understanding of their multiple actions if optimum effectiveness is to be obtained with a minimum of undesirable side effects. Before instituting corticosteroid therapy, it is necessary to carefully consider the gains that can be reasonably expected versus the potentially undesirable metabolic actions of large doses of corticosteroids. The increased incidence of hypertension, chronic infection, osteoporosis and impaired glucose tolerance as metabolic sequelae of large doses of steroids must be carefully considered before embarking on a programme of steroid administration (for reviews, see Azarnoff, 1975; Swartz and Dluhy, 1978).

9.1.1 Actions of Glucocorticoids

The physiological actions of glucocorticoids on intermediary metabolism are predominantly anti-insulin and include the regulation of protein, carbohydrate, lipid and nucleic acid metabolism. Their actions appear mainly to be catabolic in effect, with an increased protein breakdown and nitrogen excretion. Glucocorticoids increase hepatic glycogen content and promote the hepatic synthesis of glucose (gluconeogenesis). These actions of glucocorticoids are in large part explained by the mobilisation of glycogenic amino acid precursors from peripheral supporting structures, such as bone, skin, muscle and connective tissue due to protein breakdown as well as to the inhibition of protein synthesis and amino acid uptake. Glucocorticoid induced hyperaminoacidaemia also indirectly facilitates gluconeogenesis by stimulating glucagon secretion. In addition, glucocorticoids have a direct action on the liver to stimulate the synthesis of hepatic enzymes, such as tyrosine amino transferase and tryptophan pyrrolase.

Inhibition of extrahepatic protein synthesis and stimulation of hepatic enzyme synthesis is reflected in the actions of glucocorticoids on nucleic acid metabolism. Glucocorticoids inhibit the synthesis of nucleic acids in most body tissues, but in the liver ribonucleic acid (RNA) synthesis is stimulated. It is postulated that cortisol probably enters the target cell by diffusion, combines with a specific high affinity cytoplasmic receptor protein, and is transferred to a specific acceptor site on the chromatin tissue of the nucleus, which then produces an increase in RNA synthesis and later in protein synthesis (fig. 4; Feldman et al., 1972). Glucocorticoids are necessary for fatty acid mobilisation by permitting and enhancing activation of cellular lipase by lipid mobilising hormones (e.g. catecholamines and pituitary peptides).

The action of cortisol on structural protein and adipose tissue varies considerably in different parts of the body. For example, pharmacological doses

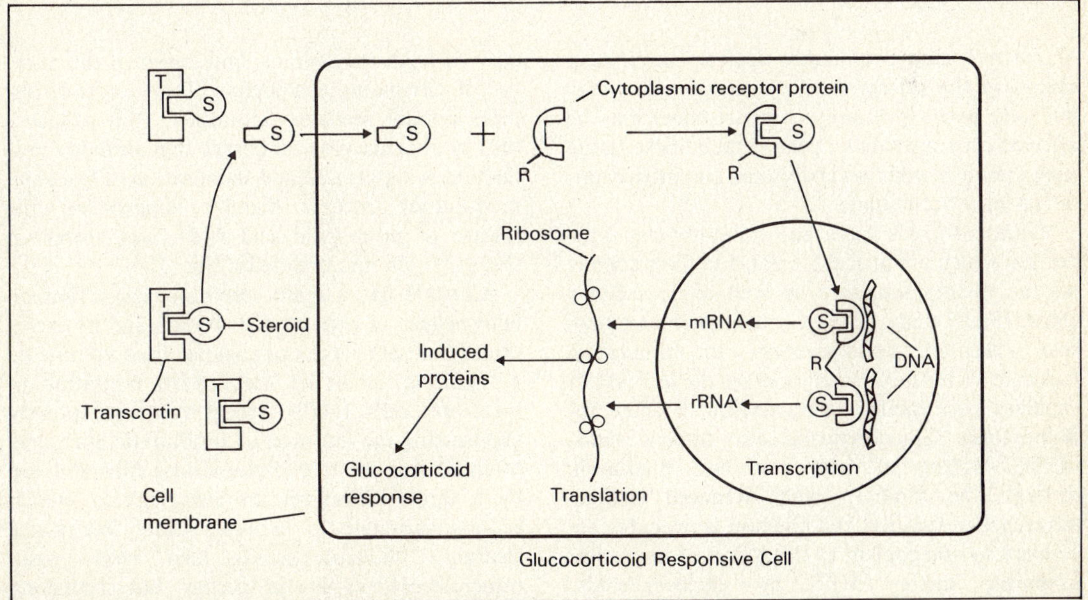

Fig. 4. Schematic representation of the mechanism of action of glucocorticosteroids (after Swartz and Dluhy: Drugs 16: 238, 1978; by permission of author and editor).

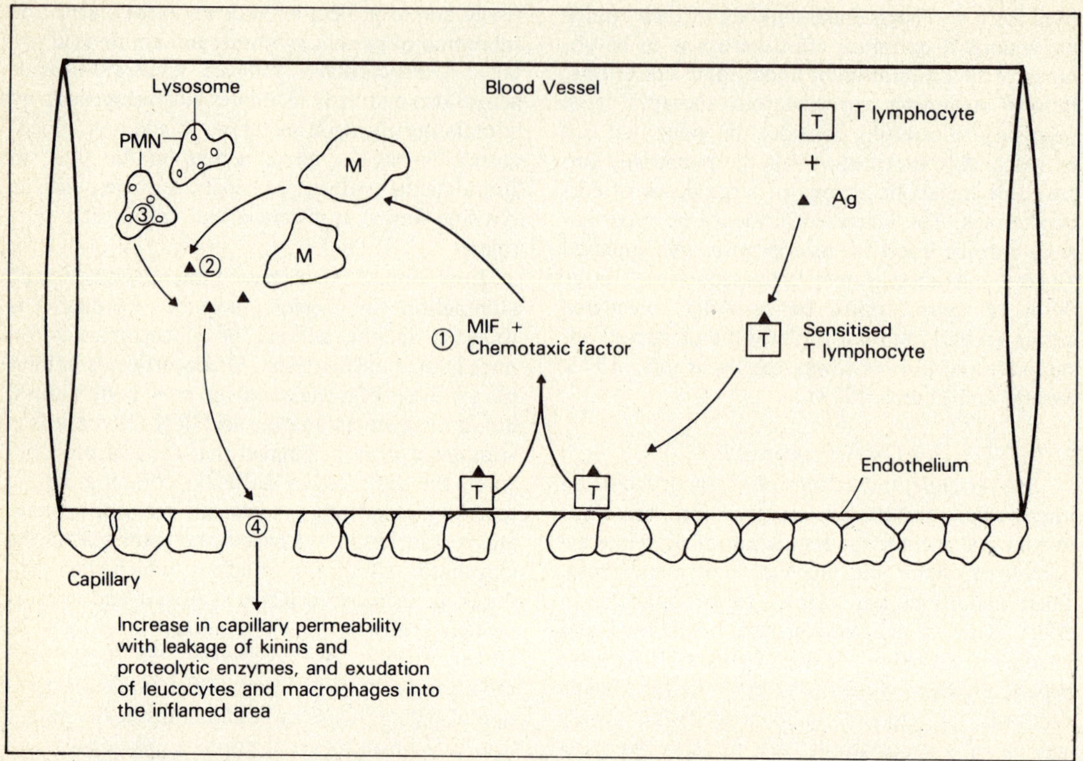

Fig. 5. Schematic representation of the inflammatory reaction. Corticosteroids (1) antagonise the action of MIF and chemotaxic factor, resulting in inhibition of endothelial sticking of leucocytes and macrophages; (2) interfere with antigen processing functions of macrophages; (3) stabilise lysosomal membranes; and (4) block the increase in capillary permeability (after Swartz and Dluhy: Drugs 16: 238, 1978; by permission of author and editor).

MIF = Migratory inhibiting factor; PMN = Polymorphonuclear cell; Ag = Antigen; M = Macrophage

of cortisol may profoundly deplete the protein matrix of the vertebral column (trabecular bone) but long bones (primarily compact bone) may be affected only minimally; peripheral adipose tissue may diminish, whereas abdominal and interscapular fat may accumulate.

Glucocorticoids have anti-inflammatory properties, which are probably related to their actions on the microvasculature as well as to cellular effects (Fauci et al., 1976). Cortisol maintains normal vascular responsiveness to circulating vasoconstrictor factors and opposes the increase in capillary permeability characteristic of acute inflammation. Glucocorticoids also impede endothelial sticking of leucocytes and diapedesis through the capillary wall. Reduced cellular adherence to vascular endothelium is probably secondary to antagonism to the action of migration inhibiting factor (MIF) by glucocorticoids. Glucocorticoids produce lysis of lymphoid tissue, specifically T cells or the small lymphocytes derived from the thymus, and diminish the number of circulating eosinophils. Thus, cortisol impairs cellular mediated immunity. It is probably only at pharmacological dosage that antibody production is suppressed and stabilisation of lysosmal membranes occurs, thereby suppressing the release of proteolytic acid hydrolases stored in these cytoplasmic organelles (fig. 5).

Cortisol has a major physiological action on body water, in both its distribution and its excretion. It subserves the extracellular fluid volume by a retarding action on the inward migration of water into cells. It affects renal water excretion by suppressing the secretion of antidiuretic hormone, by increasing the rate of glomerular filtration and by a direct action on the renal tubule, which actions summate to increase solute free water clearance. Glucocorticoids also have weak mineralocorticoid-like properties, but increasing doses will produce renal tubular sodium reabsorption and increased urine potassium excretion.

The integrity of personality is enhanced by cortisol, and emotional disorders are common with either excesses or deficits of cortisol. Lastly, another major action of cortisol is to directly suppress pituitary ACTH secretion.

9.1.2 Pharmacokinetic Properties of Glucocorticoids

Approximately 10 to 12mg of cortisol per m^2 body surface area is produced by the adrenal cortex in a normal adult each day. Although cortisol is secreted in a pulsatile or episodic fashion, the mean plasma concentration of cortisol varies predictably over a 24 hour period, with highest concentrations in the early morning and lowest levels at midnight (circadian rhythm). The normal plasma concentration at 8am is 10 to 15µg/100ml.

Half-life and Duration of Action: The plasma half-life of cortisol is approximately 90 minutes. In general, the plasma half-life of prednisone is slightly longer (3.4 to 3.8h) than that of prednisolone (2.1 to 3.5h). However, the biological half-life of corticosteroids (e.g. in terms of anti-inflammatory effect), outlasts the plasma half-life; that of cortisol lasting from 8 to 12 hours. Since the anti-inflammatory potency of synthetic or natural glucocorticoids and their suppression of the hypothalamic-pituitary-adrenal (HPA) axis, parallel each other in terms of degree and duration, biological half-lives are usually determined by the duration of suppression of the HPA axis. The duration of action and biological half-lives of the various glucocorticoids are given in table X. Duration of action influences selection of a steroid. For example, in replacement therapy, the twice daily administration of cortisol, with an 8 to 12 hour biological half-life, simulates normal daily secretion of the endogenous hormone. In alternate day therapy, the 18 to 36 hour biological half-life of prednisone allows for persistence of anti-inflammatory activity through the first half of the 'off' day, while allowing for recovery of the HPA axis during the latter part of the 'off' day (see below).

Protein Binding and Hypoalbuminaemia: Normally, approximately 90% of the cortisol is reversibly bound to plasma proteins (10% to albumin and 80% to a high affinity, low capacity α_2-globulin, transcortin or corticosteroid binding globulin); 10% circulates free or unbound. This free fraction, estimated to range between 0.7 and

1.0µg/100ml, probably determines the biological activity of the hormone, with the bound fraction serving as a reservoir. The binding capacity of transcortin is approximately 20 to 25µg of cortisol per 100ml plasma. With cortisol levels greater than 25µg/100ml, binding sites on transcortin will be saturated, and the binding of cortisol takes place increasingly to albumin, a low affinity, high capacity receptor. Thus at low or normal plasma concentrations, cortisol is largely bound to the globulin; with increasing levels, the globulin bound cortisol changes little, but the fraction of free and albumin bound cortisol increases (25% unbound and 75% albumin bound).

On the other hand, synthetic analogues of cortisol bind less avidly to transcortin (approximately 70%) and diffuse more completely into the tissues, in part explaining their propensity to produce Cushingoid side effects at low doses (Dluhy et al., 1975). Similarly, hypoalbuminaemic states, with consequent diminution in storage capacity for steroids can also, with high dose therapy, lead to unusually high concentrations of free drug and an enhanced susceptibility to steroid side effects. With high doses of prednisolone, binding decreases about 50% when serum albumin falls from 4g/100ml to 2.5g/100ml (Lewis et al., 1971; see chapter VII, sect. 5.1). The degree of binding of prednisolone determines the distribution and clearance of free pharmacologically active drug: an increase in dose leading to an increase in free (unbound) drug and an increase in volume of distribution and delayed clearance of prednisolone from plasma (Pickup, 1979). Patients with chronic active liver disease and hypoalbuminaemia are more likely to suffer major side effects of prednisone as a consequence of decreased protein binding and delayed clearance of prednisolone. Dosage in such patients should be reduced in accordance with serum albumin concentration (Uribe and Go, 1979). Corticosteroids can compete with each other for binding sites on the corticosteroid binding globulin.

Absorption and Elimination: Cortisol disappears rapidly from the circulation via hepatic metabolism and excretion in the urine as inactive glucuronide metabolites. Synthetic analogues of cortisol are metabolised in the liver more slowly than cortisol because of alterations of the steroid molecule, with the net result being a prolongation of plasma half-life. Plasma concentrations of prednisolone and prednisolone after prednisone vary

Table X. Characteristics of some adrenocorticosteroid preparations

Drug	Estimated potencies[1]		Equivalent 'anti-inflammatory' effectiveness (per nearest whole tablet)	Daily dose (mg) above which HPA axis suppression possible[2]		Approx. plasma half-life (min)	Biological half-life (h)
	gluco-corticoid	mineralo-corticoid		male	female		
Cortisol (hydrocortisone)	1	1	20mg	20-30	15-25	90	8-12
Cortisone	0.8	0.8	25mg	25-35	20-30	90	8-12
Prednisolone	4	0.25	5mg	7.5-10	7.5	200 or >	18-36
Prednisone	4	0.25	5mg	7.5-10	7.5	200 or >	18-36
Methylprednisolone	5	±	4mg	7.5-10	7.5	200 or >	18-36
Triamcinolone	5	±	4mg	7.5-10	7.5	200 or >	18-36
Paramethasone	10	±	2mg	2.5-5	2.5-5	300 or >	36-54
Dexamethasone	25	±	0.8mg	1-1.5	1-1.5	300 or >	36-54
Betamethasone	25-30	±	0.6mg	1-1.5	1-1.5	300 or >	36-54
Aldosterone	0.3	400	—	—	—	30	
Fludrocortisone (fluorohydrocortisone)	10	300	—	—	—	200 or >	18-36

1   Relative milligram comparisons to cortisol, setting the glucocorticoid and mineralocorticoid properties of cortisol as 1. Sodium retention is insignificant with usually employed doses of methylprednisolone, triamcinolone, dexamethasone, and betamethasone.
2   Intended as a guide only. The dose in an individual depends on total body surface area. The figures quoted are those which apply in general.

markedly among individuals as a consequence of interindividual differences in rates of metabolism, and possibly impaired absorption in some individuals (Green et al., 1978; Davis et al., 1978). On average, the bioavailability of prednisolone after oral prednisone is about 80% of that after prednisolone. Wide interindividual variation in plasma cortisol concentration also occurs with cortisone administration (Barbato and Landau, 1977). Cortisone and prednisone are converted in the liver (bioactivated) to their active metabolites cortisol and prednisolone; a process which can be markedly impaired in patients with or without liver disease. Although conversion of prednisone to prednisolone can be impaired in patients with severe chronic active liver disease (as evidenced by active hepatocellular necrosis), this is compensated for by a decreased rate of elimination of prednisolone from plasma and a greater fraction of unbound prednisolone in plasma (Schalm et al., 1977; Davis et al., 1978). In patients without liver disease plasma prednisolone concentration is less variable after prednisolone than after prednisone (Davis et al., 1978). Excessive effects or an inadequate response can clearly result from failure to individualise dosage of glucocorticoids due to variation in rates of metabolism (Barbato and Landau, 1977; Meikle et al., 1976). Clearance of corticosteroids may be enhanced in steroid treated patients with severe acute asthma (see chapter XX; sect. 10.2).

Drug Interactions: Hepatic metabolism of corticosteroids can be markedly influenced by enzyme inducing drugs. Thus, the rate of metabolism of corticosteroids can be enhanced by drugs such as phenobarbitone, phenytoin and rifampicin, and the therapeutic efficacy of the steroid reduced; as reflected in lack of usual response, increased steroid dose requirements, or steroid toxicity on stopping the enzyme inducing drug (Buffington et al., 1976; Brooks et al., 1972; Petereit and Meikle, 1977). The effect of enzyme inducing agents on corticosteroid metabolism may sometimes differ between compounds (Boylan et al., 1976). Corticosteroids may alter the metabolism of other drugs such as aspirin so that therapeutic salicylate concentrations may not be attained (see chapter XXII; sect. 3.2.1). On the other hand, by increasing transcortin concentrations and thus reducing binding (see above), oral contraceptives may decrease the rate of elimination of prednisolone (Kozower et al., 1974). For a review of

the clinical pharmacokinetics of prednisone and prednisolone, see Pickup (1979).

9.1.3 Principles of Glucocorticoid Therapy

The use of replacement steroid doses (that is, doses which approximate the normal daily amount of cortisol produced by the adrenal cortex) in proven primary or secondary adrenal insufficiency is straightforward (see section 9.2). Similarly, the short term, high dose administration of steroid therapy for life threatening vasculitis, status asthmaticus, or anaphylactic shock requires little hesitation. However, prolonged suppressive steroid therapy in doses which exceed the normal physiological levels (table X) in order to take advantage of the anti-inflammatory activity of the steroid, requires careful consideration. One must assess the severity of the underlying disorder and the gains that can be reasonably expected from corticosteroid therapy versus the inevitable undesirable side effects of prolonged therapy.

It is first necessary to establish a firm diagnosis of the disorder with which the patient presents, and to understand its natural course, complications, and the results of therapy with other types of agent. Then, if the decision to administer steroid therapy is made, it is important to decide in advance which signs, symptoms or laboratory tests can be used to indicate whether benefit has occurred. There are some signs which are too nonspecific to be useful (e.g. improvement in well being, fall in temperature). Signs and symptoms more specifically related to the disease being treated should be decided upon before steroid therapy is initiated. For example, when steroids are used to treat lupus nephritis, a fall in urinary protein excretion or a change in complement levels are useful parameters to follow as signs of a positive therapeutic response.

If no recognisable improvement has occurred within 7 to 10 days, the following possibilities should be considered:

1) The disorder may not be responsive to steroid therapy, implying an incorrect initial clinical diagnosis.

2) The dosage may be insufficient (this can be tested by increasing the dose).

3) Absorption of the steroid may be incomplete (this can be tested by measuring plasma cortisol levels or changing to another steroid preparation).

4) An unrecognised, concurrent problem is becoming worse, either because of the therapy or unrelated to it (e.g. reactivation of tuberculosis).

Choice of Preparation: In the treatment of acute adrenal insufficiency with decreased peripheral perfusion, intramuscular administration of steroid preparations may be ineffective. Appropriate therapy would be an intravenous bolus of the water soluble hemisuccinate or phosphate ester of cortisol (or its synthetic equivalent) followed by a continuous intravenous infusion. On the other hand, the acetates of cortisol and analogues are relatively water insoluble and intramuscular use of such repository corticosteroid preparations is suitable in the patient who requires short term, continuous therapy and for whom oral administration is either inconvenient or undesirable.

Oral glucocorticoids are preferable to ACTH therapy, particularly because oral steroids are more convenient than injections and dosage can be regulated more accurately. Although ACTH therapy suppresses hypothalamic-pituitary activity and results in active adrenal glands, whereas glucocorticoids suppress the entire HPA axis, the same degree of suppression of endogenous cortisol production ultimately results from either mode of therapy. ACTH therapy is however, useful in neuromuscular conditions such as multiple sclerosis, where the androgenic steroids released by adrenal stimulation may minimise the myopathic effects of glucocorticoids (which inhibit endogenous androgen secretion by the adrenal cortex).

Alternate Day Glucocorticoid Therapy: Alternate day steroid therapy offers effective control of a number of conditions with fewer complications than daily steroid regimens. Alternate day therapy is recommended for patients requiring high dose prolonged steroid treatment since the undesirable catabolic actions of the steroids are thereby minimised. Alternate day therapy attempts to mimic the normal cortisol diurnal cycle. A large dose of an intermediate acting steroid (e.g. one such as prednisone whose hypothalamic-pituitary suppression lasts from 18 to 36 hours; table X) is administered as a single dose in the morning when the patient's tissues would normally be exposed to the highest levels of endogenous cortisol. It may be necessary to use non-steroidal anti-inflammatory drugs (e.g. chronic active hepatitis) or to use a steroid inhaler (e.g. in severe chronic asthma) to control symptoms during those 12 hours when steroidal activity is declining. With this type of programme, HPA axis suppression, negative calcium and nitrogen balance, and Cushingoid side effects seen with continuous therapy are considerably lessened.

For alternate day therapy to be successful, daily doses of steroids usually must be given initially to achieve the desired anti-inflammatory action and bring the underlying disease under control. Then the patient can be gradually converted to an alternate day programme. The key points to remember are to have a flexible transition programme and to supplement it with supportive measures, particularly on the 'off' days when the patient is not receiving steroids. Frequently, the total dosage of steroid can also be reduced, and many patients receiving a small dosage on the 'off' day can have this dosage stopped completely. An example of a schedule designed to convert from daily to alternate day therapy is presented in table XI.

The general principles for alternate day therapy, are therefore as follows:

1) Utilise intermediate acting steroids, such as prednisone or prednisolone

2) As soon as possible, give the total daily dose as a single morning dose

3) Begin the transition to the alternate day programme as soon as feasible

4) If possible, ultimately eliminate steroid administration on the 'off' day.

Table XI. Schedule for converting to alternate day steroid therapy and then tapering the total glucocorticoid dosage[1]

Day	Prednisone (mg)	Day	Prednisone (mg)
1	60	6	20
2	40	7	90
3	70	8	10
4	30	9	95
5	80	10	5
Then, taper to:			
11	90	21	85
12	5	22	5
13	90	23	80
14	5	24	5
15	90	25	80
16	5	26	5
17	85	27	80
18	5	28	5
19	85	29	80
20	5	30	0

1   *Note:* Assume patient initially was taking 50mg prednisone every day.

Table XII. Important complications of glucocorticoid therapy

Effect	Notes
HPA axis suppression	Following doses which exceed physiological amounts (see text) or extensive use of topical steroids (see chapter XIV; sect. 6.1.3).
Linear growth retardation	Prolonged therapy. Catch-up growth in children may not be complete (see section 14.3)
Myopathy	Presents as proximal muscle weakness with marked wasting of musculature, particularly lower extremities. Not related to dosage or length of therapy (Afifi et al., 1968)
Osteoporosis	Prolonged therapy, especially in postmenopausal women, elderly patients, diabetics (see chapter XXII; sect. 11.2, 14.5)
Metabolic effects	May unmask latent diabetes mellitus or aggravate existing disease (see section 13.1)
	Hypertriglyceridaemia may occur. Dose related and reversible
Sodium retaining effects	Complicates use in patients with hypertension or cardiovascular disease. Use compound with low sodium retaining activity (e.g. triamcinolone, dexamethasone) together with dietary salt restriction, diuretics and potassium supplements
Gastrointestinal effects	Nausea and vomiting not uncommon. Susceptibility to dyspepsia increased with larger doses and prolonged therapy. Prescribe with antacids
Ocular effects	Risk of glaucoma in susceptible individuals. Other ocular complications (see chapter XII; sect. 11.1.2)
Dermatological effects	Epidermal and dermal atrophy from prolonged topical use
	Rosacea-like dermatitis from topical use on the face (see chapter XIV; sect. 6.1.3)
Psychological disturbances	Reactions range from insomnia and slight mood changes to suicide attempts (Glaser, 1953). More likely in those with prior psychological disorder
	Psychological dependence not infrequently occurs (Kimball, 1971)
Risk of infections	More likely with high dose therapy (e.g. 20 to 40mg prednisone daily) and less likely with alternate day regimens (Fauci, 1976).

Withdrawal and Termination of Glucocorticoid Therapy: The reduction from pharmacological doses (e.g. doses in excess of the amount of cortisol secreted under maximum stress, or 300mg per day) to physiological doses is limited by the activity of the underlying disease process and the rate of recovery of the endogenous hypothalamic-pituitary-adrenal axis. Suppression of the HPA axis may persist for as long as 9 to 12 or more months if steroid doses are administered in the supraphysiological range for longer than 2 weeks (Melby, 1974). As a general rule, higher doses, longer duration of use, and frequent daily administration (especially in the late evening) are all associated with the longest suppression. When glucocorticoid administration is discontinued, recovery occurs in three stages (Graber et al., 1965). Initially, plasma levels of cortisol and ACTH remain low. Plasma ACTH levels subsequently rise to normal or supranormal levels, while plasma cortisol remains low. Finally, plasma cortisol levels rise into the normal range, and function testing reveals normal HPA axis responsiveness.

The impaired release of ACTH cannot be hastened by administration of exogenous ACTH (Fleisher et al., 1967). Although repetitive administration of exogenous ACTH can rapidly restore adrenal cortical responsiveness to normal, this effect is only temporary, and adrenal cortical secretion again becomes inadequate once ACTH is stopped. Since recovery of adrenal responsiveness is normally rapid once hypothalamic-pituitary recovery has occurred, administration of ACTH to patients undergoing withdrawal of steroid therapy is unnecessary and undesirable, because recovery of the hypothalamic-pituitary function may be further delayed.

An important aspect of glucocorticoid withdrawal is to determine when the patient has satisfactorily recovered from the steroid suppression. One recommended approach (Byyny, 1976) is to first consolidate the steroid schedule into a single daily dose and then gradually taper the dose down to physiological levels.

For example, a short acting steroid, such as hydrocortisone, may be administered as a single 20mg dose each morning and then tapered by 2.5mg per day once a week to 10mg each morning. While doing this, the 8am plasma cortisol should be determined at monthly intervals; when cortisol levels rise above 10µg/100ml, the hydrocortisone therapy may be discontinued. Then adrenocortical responsiveness should be tested at monthly intervals by the administration of synthetic exogenous ACTH (0.25mg of tetracosactrin) intramuscularly; when the plasma cortisol level 1 hour after ACTH administration has increased by at least 6µg/100ml above baseline levels, adrenocortical responsiveness is considered to be normal.

At this point it can be assumed that complete recovery of the HPA axis from steroid suppression has occurred. *It is important to remember that at any point in the withdrawal programme, the steroid dose should be appropriately increased for flare ups of the underlying disease or for major stress such as infection or trauma.*

Complications of Glucocorticoid Therapy: Adverse effects are generally related to dose and duration of treatment. Some complications can nevertheless arise following small maintenance doses. Serious reactions are usually seen with prolonged therapy (for review, see David et al., 1970).

The various more important complications are summarised in table XII and appendix B.

9.2 Adrenal Insufficiency

Replacement steroid therapy for either pituitary or primary adrenal insufficiency aims at stimulating the daily secretion of cortisol. Table X lists a variety of natural and synthetic glucocorticoids and their relative potency on the basis of mineralocorticoid and glucocorticoid activity. The differences between the various preparations are usually related to the relative mineralocorticoid activity, cost and half-life. In general, daily oral replacement with 25 to 37.5mg of cortisone or 5 to 7.5mg of prednisone will approximate the normal daily rate of secretion of cortisol. However, no fixed schedule can be given, since the secretion of cortisol is related to the total body surface area. Therefore, in very large subjects, the dose of cortisone may be as high as 50mg daily for optimum response. Since cortisol is secreted in a diurnal fashion, replacement steroids are also optimally given in a similar manner: two thirds of the daily dose in the morning and one third in the afternoon.

Several important precautions need to be observed when giving glucocorticoids.

1) Because many glucocorticoids have a direct irritant effect on the gastric mucosa, patients should be advised to take the drug at meal time or with milk.

2) The dose of steroid should be reduced by 25 to 30% in patients with impaired glucose tolerance (early diabetes), in obese patients and in those with or a history of peptic ulcer.

3) In periods of physical stress, such as strenuous exercise, trauma, infection, etc., when the normal adrenal gland would increase production of cortisol, replacement therapy must also be increased. As a general rule, for infections, an additional 12.5mg of cortisone (or equivalent of other steroid) should be added to the daily programme for every degree of temperature elevation (oral) above 38.5°C. This should be continued for 1 day beyond the time when the temperature begins to return to normal.

Individual variations in systemic availability of the active steroid (Barbato and Landau, 1977) or in response to these various factors will require individualisation of the doses (see section 9.1.2).

Mineralocorticoid therapy for most persons consists of 0.05 to 0.2mg of 9-α-fluorohydrocortisone (fludrocortisone) once daily, since this is the only oral mineralocorticoid preparation available. The most convenient way of determining the necessary dose is to follow the body weight each morning. Individuals who have hypertension, congestive heart failure or a tendency to fluid retention should take smaller doses. Those who have difficulty maintaining weight and have a low serum sodium level may require larger doses. During periods of excessive sweating or high body temperature, increased dietary intake of sodium and/or increased fludrocortisone is usually necessary.

In general, patients with secondary adrenal insufficiency do not require mineralcocorticoid replacement therapy.

Table XIII. Steroid therapy schedule for Addisonian patient undergoing a major operation[1]

	Cortisone acetate (intramuscularly)		Cortisone acetate (orally)				Fludro-cortisone (orally)	Hydro-cortisone infusion)
	7am	7pm	8am	12M	4pm	8pm	8am	Continuous
Routine daily medication	—	—	25	—	12.5	—	0.1	
Day before operation	—	50	25	—	12.5	—	0.1	
Day of operation	100	50	—	—	—	—	—	200
Postoperative day　1	50	50	—	—	—	—	—	100-150
2	50	50	—	—	—	—	—	50-100
3	50	50	25	—	—	25	—	
4	50	—	25	25	25	—	0.1	
5	—	—	25	25	25	25	0.1	
6	—	—	25	25	25	—	0.2	
7	—	—	25	12.5	25	—	0.2	
8	—	—	25	12.5	25	—	0.2	
9-13	—	—	25	12.5	12.5	—	0.1	
14	—	—	25	12.5	—	—	0.1	

1　All steroid doses are given in milligrams.

9.3 Acute Adrenal Insufficiency

Acute adrenal insufficiency may occur under two different circumstances. The most common is adrenal crisis, which is a rapid and extremely marked intensification of chronic adrenal insufficiency. The other is a process which involves acute destruction of both adrenal glands by haemorrhage, usually associated with overwhelming septicaemia.

Treatment is directed primarily toward the rapid elevation of circulating adrenal corticoid hormone, in addition to repairing the sodium and water deficit that always occurs. Hence, an intravenous infusion of 1000ml of 5% glucose in normal saline solution containing 100 to 200mg of any of the soluble glucocorticoid preparations (e.g. hydrocortisone hemisuccinate; hydrocortisone phosphate) is begun rapidly, with the first 250ml infused in the first half to 1 hour, and the remaining over the ensuing 4 to 8 hours. If the condition is extreme, an immediate intravenous infusion of 100mg of hydrocortisone in a few minutes is given, followed by a rapid infusion as described above. Adrenaline (epinephrine) intravenously may also be needed. It is usually advisable to administer 100mg of cortisone acetate intramuscularly, in case the intravenous infusion is inadvertently terminated. In many cases, severe dehydration is present and large volumes of saline may be necessary for fluid repletion.

As the patient recovers from the acute situation, the dosage of hydrocortisone can be tapered gradually, from a level of 250 to 300mg daily to maintenance levels as shown in table XIII. It must be remembered that while mineralocorticoid replacement therapy is not needed with high doses of hydrocortisone, it must be added when the amount of hydrocortisone is reduced below the level of 100mg/24 hours.

Special precautions must also be taken in patients with Addison's disease who are undergoing major surgery. During this period, there will be a need for increased glucocorticoid therapy. A frequently used steroid schedule is given in table XIII.

9.4 Congenital Adrenal Hyperplasia

Some patients with adrenal disease have a genetically acquired deficiency of one of the enzymes necessary for the synthesis of cortisol. As a result, ACTH secretion is elevated in an attempt to compensate for the low cortisol production. This leads to a build up of precursors behind the enzymatic block, and diversion into the androgen biosynthetic pathway. The increased androgens lead to virilisation in the female, precocious puberty in the male, and short stature from premature epiphyseal closure.

Steroid replacement therapy to suppress ACTH is the treatment for this disease. Prednisone is often used because it has a longer half-life than cortisone. The dose varies from 2.5 to 10mg daily in divided doses, according to the age of the patient. Some patients may be controlled on a single bedtime dose of 2.5 to 5mg. The therapeutic goal is to normalise the 17-ketosteroid excretion rate (Casey, 1975).

9.5 Adrenal Glucocorticoid Hyperfunction

The causes of adrenal hyperfunction are either tumours of the adrenal gland (adenoma or carcinoma), or bilateral hyperplasia. Although the latter usually is due to hypothalamic-pituitary dysfunction, in some cases it may result from ACTH production by a pituitary or ectopic tumour. The usual form of therapy for any of these disorders is surgical removal of the adrenal lesion. However, under certain circumstances (e.g. inoperability), medical therapy is indicated. The drug that is most frequently used is mitotane (o,p'-DDD) which has been shown to be an effective drug in the treatment of adrenal carcinoma (Hutter and Kayhoe, 1966). It has also been used in patients with Cushing's disease due to bilateral hyperplasia in whom, for some reason, surgery cannot be performed.

The usual dose of mitotane is 1 to 8g daily in divided doses — in most instances, the larger the dose, the more effective the therapy. However, significant side effects (nausea, vomiting and anorexia) severely limit the use of higher doses. The effectiveness of therapy is assessed both by physical regression of metastatic lesions and by decreased steroid production. The dose of the drug is increased to tolerance and then gradually decreased if physical and biochemical parameters remain satisfactory. Because mitotane inhibits adrenal biosynthesis, replacement therapy, both glucocorticoid and mineralocorticoid, is indicated.

9.6 Adrenal Mineralocorticoid Overproduction

Inappropriate mineralocorticoid excess is also usually treated by surgery. However, the effects of hyperaldosteronism — hypokalaemia and hypertension — can be reversed by the administration of spironolactone, a specific antagonist of the metabolic action of aldosterone. Therapy is usually begun with 200 to 400mg daily in divided doses. The dose is then gradually reduced at 14 day intervals, as long as the blood pressure and serum potassium remain normal. Subjects have been maintained in good control on as little as 50mg daily for as long as 10 years. However, significant side effects (gynaecomastia, nausea, and vomiting) often limit either the dose or duration of therapy. Also, some sensitive subjects may develop hyperkalaemia, and must be watched carefully for this complication when therapy is begun, particularly if there is associated renal impairment.

9.7 Adrenal Medullary Disease

Phaeochromocytoma causes a syndrome characterised by a paroxysmal or sustained hypertension associated with symptoms of catecholamine excess (flushing, palpitation, headache and hypermetabolism). It results from hypersecretion by tumours of chromatin origin, usually located in one or both adrenals (90%), or arising from extra-adrenal paraganglionic tissue (10%).

The treatment of choice for phaeochromocytoma is surgical removal of the tumour or tumours, if possible. Because of occasional hypovolaemia and functional impairment of the neurogenic cardiovascular reflexes, surgical procedures may induce excessive discharge of pressor hormones, either during induction of anaesthesia or following manipulation of the tumour. This may cause sudden elevations in blood pressure and may precipitate cardiac arrhythmias. It is therefore advisable that patients be given an adrenolytic drug regimen for at least 1 week prior to surgery.

In the pre-operative control of hypertension, the major pharmacological agents are (Bray et al., 1972): (1) phenoxybenzamine, an α-adrenoceptor blocking drug, starting with 20 to 30mg/day orally and increasing by increments of 10 to 20mg/day to a total of 80 to 200mg/daily; (2) α-methylparatyrosine, a competitive inhibitor of tyrosine hydroxylase, 250mg every 8 hours; and (3) propranolol, a β-adrenoceptor blocking agent, to control the secondary effect of α-adrenoceptor blockade.

Adrenergic neurone blocking drugs such as guanethidine should never be used to control blood pressure because they sensitise receptors to circulating neurohumoral transmitter substances.

During the surgery, rapid injection of phentolamine intravenously (with titration to obtain the effective dosage) is the best method of treating episodic hypertension which may occur despite adequate pretreatment. Arrhythmias occurring during the surgical procedure can be treated with intravenous propranolol (1 to 3mg). Propranolol should be used pre-operatively with extreme care because of possible induction of heart failure in patients with underlying catecholamine cardiomyopathy. After surgical removal of the tumour, the blood pressure may fall to shock levels. Prophylactic or interoperative blood or plasma transfusion during the surgical procedure and before tumour removal, designed to carefully replace all fluid losses calculated during the procedure, is the best method to prevent this complication. Persistent hypotension should be treated with pressor agents (noradrenaline 4 to 12mg/L) by intravenous infusion. The likelihood of transient adrenocortical insufficiency postoperatively must be borne in mind, as a result of the removal of adrenocortical tissue with the phaeochromocytoma.

Only about 5% of cases of phaeochromocytomas are malignant. Failure of blood pressure to fall satisfactorily following removal of the phaeochromocytoma indicates the presence of other tumours. In inoperable phaeochromocytomas, phenoxybenzamine has been used on a long term basis in dosages of up to 200mg daily. α-Methylparatyrosine, 250mg every 8 hours, has also been used beneficially for long term therapy.

10. Male Hypogonadism

Before treatment of hypogonadal males is considered, every effort should be made to determine the aetiology and it is helpful to divide testicular failure into primary testicular dysfunction and secondary testicular failure (due to either a pituitary and/or hypothalamic deficiency). This separation is easily accomplished by measurement of the gonadotrophins (serum or urine). In primary testicular dysfunction, the gonadotrophins are usually elevated, whereas in secondary testicular dysfunction, they are low or may be absent.

In hypogonadotrophism, it is best to treat first with human chorionic gonadotrophin (HCG), which is usually administered in dosage of 4000μ intramuscularly twice a week (2000μ in each hip) for a period of 5 to 7 months. If desired results are

Table XIV. Some testosterone preparations

Drug	Dose	Route
Testosterone enanthate	200-400mg every 4 weeks	Intra-muscular
Testosterone cypionate	300-400mg every 3-4 weeks	Intra-muscular
Testosterone propionate	5-10mg daily	Buccal
Fluoxy-mesterone	2-10mg daily in divided doses	Oral

obtained (enlargement of the testes and rise in plasma testosterone), HCG may be continued indefinitely. Sperm counts should be monitored if fertility is desired. Side effects of HCG therapy are few and the only one encountered with any frequency is oedema from excessive salt and water retention. If it occurs, HCG should be decreased in dosage, or stopped. Frequently, because of the cost of HCG and the need for twice weekly injections, transfer to long acting testosterone, which can be given monthly, may have to be made.

In individuals with primary testicular dysfunction, HCG is not indicated and one of the many testosterone preparations which are available should be given (table XIV). Testosterone cypionate has a cotton seed oil base and is less viscous than testosterone enanthate which has a sesame oil base. Should testosterone enanthate come in contact with moisture such as a wet syringe, it may become cloudy but it still maintains its potency.

In a testosterone deficient individual it is often advisable to start the replacement therapy at 50mg intramuscularly and then increase the dosage by 50mg increments every 3 weeks until the desired dose is reached. This has the advantage of diminishing the effects of testosterone on the psyche and decreasing such distressing complications as spontaneous erections.

All testosterone preparations are contraindicated in carcinoma of the breast or prostate, prostatic hypertrophy, and nephrosis. Side effects of testosterone therapy include gynaecomastia, oedema, hypercalcaemia, hypercholesterolaemia, and urticaria. Fluoxymesterone and 17-methylated testosterone derivatives may produce increases in sulphobromophthalein (BSP) retention and elevations in serum glutamic oxaloacetic transaminase (SGOT). Cholestatic jaundice has also been reported.

11. Infertility and Impotence in the Male

Of couples with infertility problems, many will be due solely to an abnormality in the male. Thus, it is important that a thorough clinical and laboratory evaluation be performed in every male partner of an infertile marriage. Obviously, certain disorders such as germinal cell aplasia and diffuse tubular fibrosis cannot be treated with medication. Other problems such as a varicocele are best treated surgically. There does remain a large number of males in whom drug therapy may be helpful.

Testosterone rebound therapy has been used with some success in patients with low sperm counts or with morphological sperm abnormalities. In this type of therapy, the testes are 'put to rest' by administration of a long acting testosterone preparation (see section 10) every 2 to 3 weeks for 3 to 4 months. The testosterone is then discontinued and in 3 to 4 months some of the patients will 'rebound' with normal sperm (Heckel et al., 1951).

The 'syndrome of the fertile eunuch' is characterised by a prepuberal eunuch with motile sperm. Their sperm count is usually below normal limits. The aetiology of this syndrome is a relatively low luteinising hormone (LH) level. These patients are best treated with human chorionic gonadotrophin (HCG) 4000 units intramuscularly twice a week. The usual side effects encountered are due to the increased androgen output from the testes and are therefore androgen side effects (see section 10). Testosterone is not the drug of choice in this syndrome, for while it will virilise the individual it will decrease the testosterone production by the Leydig cells and therefore decrease the sperm count causing infertility.

Clomiphene citrate, an antioestrogen, has been used by some investigators in male infertility (Mellinger and Thompson, 1966). The response has usually been poor and it is not used by most clinicians. Tamoxifen, another antioestrogen but with lesser intrinsic oestrogenic activity than clomiphene, is under investigation in oligospermic men (Vermeulen and Comhaire, 1978).

Combining HCG with follicle stimulating hormone (FSH) [Pergonal] has been tried in male infertility. Results have been very disappointing and thus it is little used except experimentally.

Impotence is a distressing and frequently encountered problem in men. All cases deserve a thorough clinical and hormonal evaluation before being assigned to a psychogenic aetiology. Drug associated causes of impotence should also be excluded (see chapter XV; sect. 23.2). Patients with testicular failure are treated as described in section 10. Most investigators feel that if the hormonal levels are normal, then treatment with testosterone is not indicated.

Impotence is not uncommon in men with long term, insulin requiring diabetes. Although emotional factors must be considered, it is usually a manifestation of diabetic neuropathy and rarely is benefited by treatment with testosterone. In recent years, implants of prosthetic devices into the penis have been successful in some patients. Otherwise, psychotherapy may lead to acceptance of the situation and better adjustment to it.

A high frequency of impotence has been observed in men with prolactinomas (Carter et al., 1978; McGregor et al., 1979). Some of these patients noted improvement in their potency upon receiving bromocriptine, a dopamine receptor agonist at pituitary and hypothalamic levels, which directly inhibits prolactin secretion (see section 8). Doses ranged from 2.5mg twice a day up to 2.5mg 4 times a day. The drug should be administered with meals. Side effects noted are usually mild and include nausea, headache, dizziness, nasal congestion and alteration in bowel habits. It must be noted that usage of bromocriptine in men with prolactinomas should be considered experimental at this time, although it appears to be a very promising therapeutic approach. It has also been used in men with hypogonadotrophic hypogonadism not due to a specific neoplasm, but is of little value unless hyperprolactinaemia is a component of the disorder (March, 1979). Use of bromocriptine in treatment of female infertility is discussed in chapter XV (sect. 14).

12. Diabetes Insipidus

Diabetes insipidus is a rare disease, characterised by the passage of large quantities of dilute urine with secondary polydipsia. It results from partial or complete deficiency of vasopressin (antidiuretic hormone, ADH). The principal action of vasopressin as seen in the normal person is to render the cells of the distal renal tubules permeable to water, thereby holding in check the escape into the urine of water from the glomerular filtrate.

Deficiency of vasopressin may arise from lesions involving the hypothalamic-hypophyseal system, including brain tumours, granulomatous disorders, cranial injuries, and hypophysectomies such as that carried out for diabetic retinopathy or advanced carcinoma of the breast. In about 50% of cases, there is no discoverable cause, at least during life.

The patient must be studied carefully for active intracranial lesions, and true diabetes insipidus must be differentiated from psychogenic polydipsia. The identification of chronic nephritis or diabetes mellitus as a cause for the polyuria should present no problem.

If any remediable, underlying cause can be found, this must be treated by appropriate measures. Otherwise, therapy consists of the use of vasopressin in one form or another, as listed below:

1) Vasopressin aqueous injection, a partially purified vasopressin fraction. This is effective in doses of 0.1 to 0.3 ml (20 iμ/ml of pressor activity) intramuscularly or subcutaneously, but since the action is brief, the treatment must be repeated at intervals of 3 or 4 hours.

2) Vasopressin tannate in oil, which is given in 1 ml doses (5iμ/ml pressor activity) intramuscularly at intervals of 24 to 72 hours.

3) Posterior lobe pituitary powder may be used as snuff (or by nasal insufflation from a plastic squeeze bottle) at intervals of 3 to 6 hours or more. Such treatment is convenient but with prolonged use, patients may develop chronic inflammation of the nose and throat.

4) Synthetic lysine vasopressin solution for parenteral use is available in the same manner as aqueous vasopressin. It is also available in a strength of 50 pressor units per ml for use intranasally, as a spray or as drops, and is a convenient treatment for ambulatory patients but its duration of action is relatively short (it needs to be used 3 to 4 or more times daily) and it may also produce undesirable pressor and gastrointestinal side effects.

Another synthetic vasopressin compound, 1-desamino-8-d arginine vasopressin (dDAVP; desmopressin), an analogue of arginine vasopressin, is also available for intranasal administration as drops. It has a much longer duration of action than lysine vasopressin and markedly reduced vasopressor activity. Most adult patients can be controlled by a dosage of 0.1 to 0.2 ml (10 to 20μg) given once or twice daily. Smaller dosage is used in children (5 to 10μg) and infants (2.5 to 10μg).

Desmopressin is probably the most effective and convenient treatment for outpatients (Becker and Foley, 1978; Cobb et al., 1978), but is at present expensive for prolonged therapy.

Although thiazide diuretics may increase the reabsorption of water in the distal tubules in diabetes insipidus, their effect is not great, and patients usually require vasopressin therapy in addition. The oral hypoglycaemic drug chlorpropamide, strangely enough, may exert an antidiuretic effect in some vasopressin sensitive patients; if it is used, the possibility of symptomatic hypoglycaemia, especially in non-diabetic patients, must be borne in mind. It seems to have its greatest effect in patients in whom diabetes insipidus is secondary to some known intracranial disorder (Ehrlich and Kooh, 1970). Carbamazepine and clofibrate also have an antidiuretic effect but are not as effective or as well tolerated as desmopressin (Becker and Foley, 1978).

13. Use of Drugs in the Presence of Associated Endocrine Disorders

The relationship between the endocrine system and drug use can involve adverse drug reactions which alter endocrine function (see also section 14), modification of laboratory tests of endocrine function by drugs, and the alteration by endocrine disease of tissue sensitivity and pharmacokinetics of drugs.

13.1 Diabetes Mellitus

Certain drugs such as thiazide diuretics, frusemide (furosemide) and ethacrynic acid, oral contraceptives and glucocorticoids may influence carbohydrate metabolism adversely. The thiazide and related diuretics, frusemide and ethacrynic acid can have an aggravating influence on diabetes in occasional patients (Goldner et al., 1960; Lebacq and Marq, 1967; Walsh and O'Sullivan, 1974; Sterz, 1969). The fear of adverse effects should not lead to avoidance of their use when indicated. Some diabetic patients treated with oral hypoglycaemic drugs or insulin may however, require an increase in dosage of these agents when diuretics are added as long term therapy (Hicks et al., 1973; Cowley and Elkeles, 1978). Oral hypoglycaemic drugs have a potential for interaction with a number of other drugs, but clinically important effects are uncommon (see section 3.3.5).

The diabetogenic effect of oral contraceptives is usually slight or apparently lacking (Spellacy, 1969, 1974; Posner et al., 1975). Therefore, this consideration in itself need not be a contraindication to the use of oral contraceptives in diabetics, although management of diabetes may occasionally be made more difficult and diabetes may be precipitated in the latent diabetic. The patient with juvenile onset type diabetes, for example, must be prepared to modify the dose of insulin. The risk of an adverse effect on diabetes may be lessened by the use of low dose oestrogen combination preparations (Spellacy et al., 1977b) or oral progestagen-only preparations, but such preparations may still impair glucose tolerance in some individuals (Goldman, 1978; Spellacy et al., 1976). The long acting injectable progestagen medroxyprogesterone acetate affects carbohydrate metabolism more consistently than oral agents and may not be suitable for the diabetic patient (Spellacy et al., 1972). There is some evidence of an increased risk of vascular complications in diabetic patients taking oral contraceptives (Steel and Duncan, 1978).

Glucocorticoids promote hepatic glycogenolysis, thereby raising the level of blood glucose. The extent of the effect on the diabetic state varies from patient to patient and from situation to situation. However, not infrequently, treatment with glucocorticoids may aggravate diabetes or bring latent diabetes to a clinically important state (Thorn et al., 1953; Cope, 1972). The development of ketonuria and diabetic acidosis is rare (Alavi et al., 1971). The diabetic state is usually mild and if corticosteroid therapy is truly indicated in any clinical situation, a possible diabetogenic effect need not be a deterrent, since the situation can be managed by the judicious use of diet, and if necessary, use of appropriate amounts of insulin.

Non-selective β-adrenoceptor blocking drugs such as propranolol can impair carbohydrate tolerance of diabetics (Podolsky and Pattavina, 1973), or necessitate a reduction in dosage of insulin or oral hypoglycaemic drugs in the poorly controlled diabetic and may provoke profound hypoglycaemia in states characterised by little or no liver glycogen such as after prolonged fasting or in ketosis (Kotler et al., 1966; Skinner and Misbin, 1975). The metabolic response to hypoglycaemia is complex. Non-selective β-blockers act on both β_1 and β_2-adrenoceptors and inhibit sympathetic stimulation of hepatic and skeletal muscle glycogenolysis and gluconeogenesis due to lactate

feedback from muscles (Abramson et al., 1966; Antonis et al., 1967). Cardioselective β-blockers such as atenolol and metoprolol, which are more selective for β_1-adrenoceptors, have much less effect on metabolic, and on cardiovascular (blood pressure rise) responses to hypoglycaemia and should be less likely to cause hypoglycaemia than non-selective β-blockers in diabetic patients prone to hypoglycaemic attacks or after fasting, since the β-adrenoceptors of the liver and skeletal muscle are thought to be predominantly of the β_2-type. Membrane stabilising activity of some β-blockers such as propranolol may also contribute to metabolic consequences (Deacon et al., 1977; Waal-Manning, 1976, 1979). Both non-selective and cardioselective β-blockers nevertheless inhibit the physiological response to hypoglycaemia so that there is less awareness by the diabetic patient of some of the warning symptoms of acute hypoglycaemia such as tachycardia and palpitations, but not sweating which may be unaffected or enhanced (Abramson et al., 1966; Waal-Manning, 1979). β-Blockers can be used in diabetic patients when they are indicated, but cardioselective drugs such as atenolol or metoprolol should be used since they are less likely to aggravate hypoglycaemia or precipitate hypertensive crises during hypoglycaemia in diabetic patients liable to hypoglycaemic attacks. They are also less likely to compromise peripheral circulation in diabetics (for review, see Waal-Manning, 1979).

β_2-Adrenoceptor stimulant drugs such as salbutamol (albuterol) used to delay premature labour, can cause pronounced metabolic disturbances including hyperglycaemic ketoacidosis in diabetic patients (Fredholm et al., 1978; Thomas et al., 1977). Such use should be closely monitored (see chapter XV; sect. 9).

The insulin requirement of a diabetic is not only increased in the presence of infection (see section 3.2.1), but also the response to antibacterial therapy, for example, is slower. A temporary resistance to insulin may be observed in patients with diabetic ketoacidosis or other acute illnesses.

13.2 Thyroid Disorders

Thyroid disease can alter the response to drugs either as a result of altered tissue sensitivity or drug pharmacokinetics.

In thyrotoxicosis, the manifestations of the disease resembles sympathetic overactivity and patients may show an enhanced response to administered sympathomimetic amines. The mechanism is unclear (Levey, 1971, 1976). Patients with marked hypothyroidism are also particularly sensitive to central nervous system depressant drugs.

Thyroid dysfunction may influence the absorption and disposition of certain drugs and necessitate modification of dosage as thyroid status changes (see section 1.4). Smaller than normal doses of digitalis are needed in hypothyroid patients, since ordinary doses are associated with a much greater risk of toxicity. This is reflected (Doherty and Perkins, 1966) in higher serum digoxin and digitoxin concentrations than in the euthyroid state. The opposite effect is seen in the hyperthyroid patient but while a larger than normal dose would seem necessary, other drugs are indicated in thyrotoxicosis — propranolol is likely to be more effective in controlling the ventricular rate in atrial fibrillation or flutter and in heart failure associated with thyrotoxicosis, digoxin is unlikely to have a beneficial effect. Plasma concentrations of propranolol are also higher in patients with hypothyroidism than in those with hyperthyroidism, and as with digitalis, alter following treatment of the thyroid condition. Major changes in disposition of propranolol occur in patients with hyperthyroidism in the perioperative and postoperative period following thyroidectomy (see section 1.4).

The hypometabolic and hypermetabolic states of thyroid disease may also influence response to coumarin anticoagulants. Thus their hypoprothrombinaemic action is decreased in hypothyroid patients and enhanced in thyrotoxicosis. This appears to be reflected in the unusually slow rate of decay of the vitamin K dependent clotting proteins in hypothyroidism and in their more rapid rate of disappearance (their presence is further inhibited by the anticoagulant) in hyperthyroidism and other hypermetabolic states (Loeliger et al., 1964). Adjustment of dosage of coumarin anticoagulants may therefore be necessary in states of significant thyroid dysfunction (Self et al., 1975; Vagenakis et al., 1972).

Hypoparathyroidism may also modify the tissue response to drugs. The renal response to administered parathormone is impaired in pseudohypoparathyroidism (Lowenthal, 1974), and patients with hypoparathyroidism seem to be extremely sensitive to phenothiazines, as evidenced by acute dystonic reactions from usual doses (Schaaf and Payne, 1966).

14. Drug Induced Endocrine Disorders

Drugs can cause endocrine disease by either aggravating or precipitating the condition in a susceptible individual (see also section 13), or less commonly by producing the disease in a previously normal individual. In many cases, the reactions are a consequence of the expected pharmacodynamic action of the drug (see Dollery and Breckenridge, 1972; Evered and Yeo, 1977).

14.1 Hypoglycaemia and Hyperglycaemia

Symptomatic hypoglycaemia may occasionally arise as a consequence of overdosage of oral hypoglycaemic drugs or as a result of interaction between oral hypoglycaemic drugs and other medication (see section 3.3.4; 3.3.5). Overdosage of aspirin can cause both hypoglycaemia and hyperglycaemia (Craig et al., 1966). Hypoglycaemia is more likely to occur in children (Limbeck et al., 1965; Seltzer, 1972). Non-selective β-adrenoceptor blocking drugs such as propranolol can impair carbohydrate tolerance in diabetics and adversely affect metabolic and cardiovascular responses to hypoglycaemia, but may also provoke profound hypoglycaemia in non-diabetic subjects after prolonged fasting (Skinner and Misbin, 1975). Cardioselective β-blockers such as atenolol or metoprolol are less likely to lead to those problems (see section 13.1). A variety of chemical compounds may affect carbohydrate metabolism adversely. These include certain beta cell cytotoxic agents (alloxan, dehydroascorbic acid, oxine, dithizon) which are capable of producing permanent diabetes but which are not used clinically, and other drugs such as glucocorticoids, diuretics and hormonal steroid contraceptives, which influence carbohydrate metabolism adversely although to a lesser degree.

Diuretics such as thiazides and frusemide can very occasionally precipitate hyperosmolar nonketotic diabetic coma (e.g. Sølvsteen et al., 1968; Tasker and Mitchell-Heggs, 1976). The usual finding in non-diabetic patients treated long term with thiazides and frusemide is a progressive (within 2 years in the elderly and more than 5 years in younger subjects) slight change in blood glucose and mild impairment of glucose tolerance, but without development of clinical diabetes (Lewis et al., 1976; Amery et al., 1978). Hypokalaemia may be a contributory mechanism by which glucose intolerance is impaired. Thiazides may nevertheless, precipitate diabetes in susceptible individuals with latent disease (Breckenridge et al., 1967; Shapiro et al., 1960) and isolated cases of impaired carbohydrate tolerance or reversible diabetes in non-diabetic patients have occurred with thiazides, frusemide and ethacrynic acid (Anderson, 1971; Kohner et al., 1971; Lebacq and Marcq, 1967). Impaired carbohydrate metabolism may occur with glucocorticoids in non-diabetics, especially in those with latent diabetes (Cope, 1972). The effects are reversible and as with diuretics do not constitute a contraindication to the use of these drugs in diabetes (see section 13.1).

Oral contraceptives carry a risk of mild impairment of glucose tolerance particularly in certain susceptible individuals (e.g. women with a very strong family history of diabetes or with abnormal glucose tolerance tests during the previous pregnancy; Spellacy, 1969, 1974, 1976). Carbohydrate tolerance declines with continued long term use of oral contraceptives (Posner et al., 1975; Spellacy et al., 1977a); the impairment becoming apparent earlier with 'full dose' combination oestrogen-progestagen preparations than with progestagen alone (norethisterone, norgestrel, ethynodiol) formulations (Goldman, 1978; Spellacy et al., 1976), and probably being reduced with low dose oestrogen-progestagen combinations (Spellacy et al., 1977b). Injectable medroxyprogesterone acetate may carry a greater risk in this regard. Patients believed to be predisposed to diabetes should be followed closely when hormonal steroid contraceptives are used (see also section 13.1) but there seems to be little risk of diabetes occurring with oral contraceptive use in those not so predisposed (Wingrave et al., 1979).

Diazoxide, a thiazide derivative, can cause severe reversible hyperglycaemia if more than a few doses are given intravenously or if used orally on a continuous basis (Dollery et al., 1962; see chapter XXI; sect. 6). The hyperglycaemic effect of diazoxide has been successfully employed in decreasing or suppressing excessive insulin secretion in neonatal hypoglycaemia or from islet cell tumours, which do not lend themselves to surgical removal. Streptozotocin, another hyperglycaemic drug, has been similarly used in cases of malignant insulin secreting tumour with multiple metastases (see also section 4).

Lithium has variable effects on carbohydrate metabolism, but can impair glucose tolerance in diabetics (Waziri and Nelson, 1978) and non-

diabetic manic patients (Muller-Oerlinghausen et al., 1978). Acute onset diabetes mellitus has also been associated with lithium use in manic-depressive psychosis (Johnston, 1977; Craig et al., 1977). Obesity seems to be a risk factor. Whether the effects observed are due to the drug or the disease are not clear.

14.2 Thyroid Disorders

Thyrotoxicosis occurs in normal persons following acute or chronic ingestion of excessive pharmacological doses of any thyromimetic compound. These include the natural and synthetic thyroid hormones and their congeners and optical isomers (d-thyroxine). Thyrotrophin (TSH) or thyrotrophin releasing hormone (TRH) administration can increase thyroid gland synthesis and produce release of excessive thyroid hormones (fig. 1).

Induction of hypothyroidism by non-thyroidal drugs is much more common (Dollery and Breckenridge, 1972; Evered and Yeo, 1977). This usually occurs as a goitrogenic action of the drug (see fig. 3) and thus a palpable goitre is often present (goitrous hypothyroidism). Lithium (Schou, 1973; Lindstedt et al., 1977), and possibly sulphonylureas (Scharf et al., 1968; Burke et al., 1967) and less commonly long term use of phenylbutazone or oxyphenbutazone (Lane et al., 1977) are among the more important causes of goitre and hypothyroidism. Lithium is currently the drug most commonly associated with goitrous hypothyroidism. It can also cause hyperthyroidism in predisposed individuals (Brownlie et al., 1976). Thiocyanate and perchlorate ions similarly are goitrogenic, as are a number of lesser known or used drugs. Iodide, either alone or as a constituent of many foods and drugs in common usage, can induce goitrous hypothyroidism. This occurs in susceptible goitrous patients (chronic lymphoid thyroiditis) and with relative frequency following radioiodine therapy for thyrotoxicosis.

A number of drugs can interfere with thyroid function tests by increasing thyroxine binding globulin capacity (e.g. oestrogens and oral contraceptives), by decreasing its binding capacity as a consequence of competition for thyroxine binding sites (e.g. phenytoin, large doses of salicylates, clofibrate) or by inhibition of synthesis (e.g. testosterone and other androgens). In addition, a few drugs (e.g. glucocorticoids, antithyroid drugs) alter the metabolic pathway of T_4 to T_3 via reverse T_3 (see fig. 1) and thus reduce serum levels of T_3 and

T_4 without altering thyroxine binding globulin concentrations. A similar phenomenon occurs after surgery, in chronic illness, starvation and in the developing fetus. It is thus important to appraise the clinical status as well as the drug therapy programme of patients when assessing serum parameters of thyroid function. Iodides such as iodide containing expectorant cough mixtures, organic iodine containing radiographic contrast media, iodinated hydroxyquinolines (clioquinol) and so on, may interfere with some thyroid function tests, sometimes for years. Congenital goitre has even occurred following ingestion of expectorants containing iodide (or other goitrogenic drugs) by the pregnant mother (Carswell et al., 1970). Paradoxically, iodides can induce hyperthyroidism in susceptible goitrous subjects (Connolly et al., 1970; Gutknecht, 1977).

Increased total thyroxine concentrations can be induced by oestrogens (usually seen after oral contraceptives), during pregnancy, in certain liver diseases and in congenital thyroxine binding globulin excess, without changing the concentration of free thyroxine or the metabolic status of the patient. A decrease in serum total thyroxine concentration is seen after androgens or glucocorticoid administration, in the nephrotic syndrome and in portal cirrhosis. Serum protein bound iodine is also reduced in this case but the free thyroxine concentration is unchanged. The resin uptake test is also modified in these situations, but by calculating the free thyroxine index an allowance can be made for the change in binding protein induced by these drugs or pathophysiological states. For reviews, see Chopra and Solomon (1976) and Acland (1971).

14.3 Pituitary-Adrenal Function Disorders

Administration of glucocorticoids frequently leads to suppression of normal hypothalamic-pituitary-adrenal (HPA) axis function, and, if the dose is large enough (i.e. exceeds daily cortisol excretion rate), can cause virtually all the manifestations of Cushing's syndrome, i.e., glucose intolerance, weight gain, fluid retention, etc (David et al., 1970). The development of Cushingoid features can be prevented in part by the use of alternate day steroid administration with a drug such as prednisone if such a regimen is suited to the condition being treated. When alternate day therapy is used, the dosage should be larger than the sum of the required 2 day dosage used in daily therapy (see section 9.1.3). A patient who has been on suppressive or higher dosage of a glucocorticoid longer than 3 to 4 days must not have the medication discontinued abruptly, since adrenocortical crisis may result. In such patients, the dosage should be reduced gradually. Suppression of the HPA axis may persist for 9 to 12 or more months if supraphysiological doses have been given for more than 2 weeks (Graber et al., 1965; Melby, 1974). During this recovery period until normal adrenocortical responsiveness is attained, the patient will need to be protected with corticosteroids during exacerbation of the disease or periods of stress such as infection or trauma (see section 9.1.3). Long term ACTH administration can cause similar problems, but probably to a lesser degree than glucocorticoids (Bacon et al., 1968; Friedman and Strang, 1969).

Excessive absorption of topical fluorinated corticosteroids can lead to Cushingoid features following continued application of large amounts over a large skin surface area. Systemic absorption should be especially watched for in infants and when occlusive dressings are used (see chapter XIV; sect. 4). Adrenal suppression has also occurred with topical administration of corticosteroids to the eye, nose, mouth and by aerosol administration to the lungs (Keipert, 1971).

Long term use of systemic glucocorticoids (e.g. severe chronic childhood asthma) can interfere with normal processes of linear growth by suppressing growth hormone release from the pituitary, increased androgen secretion and also by antagonism of the action of growth promoting substances on peripheral tissues. ACTH is less likely to induce growth retardation in prepubertal children. While children exhibit increased growth rates when ACTH is substituted for oral glucocorticoids (Friedman and Strang, 1969), the improved growth rate is still suboptimal in most cases and occurs almost invariably in the individual on intermittent, low dose therapy (Editorial, 1969). Androgens and androgenic-anabolic steroids if given to prepubertal children will temporarily enhance linear growth, but will also hasten epiphyseal fusion and thus prevent them reaching their full height (Good and Bessman, 1966).

A number of other drugs can, by their action on hypothalamic-pituitary function, lead to effects such as amenorrhoea (after withdrawal of hormonal steroid contraceptives) or galactorrhoea (e.g. phenothiazines). The weight gain seen with certain psychotherapeutic drugs may possibly be due to an action on the hypothalamus (see section 14.4). Some drugs can produce disorders of reproductive or sexual function which are unrelated to effects on hypothalamic-pituitary function; for example, gynaecomastia with spironolactone, digoxin or oestrogens.

These effects are discussed in chapter XV (section 23.2, 23.6).

14.4 Weight Gain

A significant gain in weight is sometimes seen during long term use of chlorpromazine, lithium and drugs such as amitriptyline (Amdisen, 1964; Editorial, 1974). Excess weight is lost when the drugs are stopped. The weight gain could be partly due to fluid retention (although diuretics are not usually effective in combating the problem) as well as to increased appetite. The mechanism is unclear but probably involves an effect on hypothalamic function. Patients gaining weight on amitriptyline have a craving for carbohydrate foods (Paykel et al., 1973). This effect and a voracious appetite have also been noted in migraine patients on prophylactic medication with antiserotonin drugs such as pizotifen and cyproheptadine (Speight and Avery, 1972). Indeed, this effect of cyproheptadine has been dubiously employed therapeutically to induce weight gain in children. (Antiserotonin drugs reduce the release of growth hormone in the human.

Certainly, antiserotonin agents such as cyproheptadine, pizotifen and methysergide should be given with care to children in need of long term migraine prophylaxis, until more information becomes available on their effects on physical growth).

Other drugs may cause weight gain as a result of fluid retention (see further chapter XXI; section 15.4).

14.5 Disorders of Calcium Metabolism

Ingestion of excessive doses of vitamin D (more than 50,000iµ daily in a normal adult) may cause a syndrome characterised by hypercalcaemia and associated with nephrocalcinosis and calcification of other soft tissues. Renal function can be severely and irreversibly impaired (Dent, 1964; Davies and Adams, 1978). Vitamin D must be withdrawn and the condition treated promptly. There is an increased sensitivity to normal doses

of vitamin D in patients with hypoparathyroidism, sarcoidosis or metabolic disease such as renal osteodystrophy (Roe, 1966; Leeson and Fourman, 1966).

Prolonged use of therapeutic doses of calcium containing antacids in peptic ulcer patients can also cause hypercalcaemia, which in patients with pre-existing renal disease, may lead to a syndrome of hypercalcaemia, hypertension and renal failure (Burnett et al., 1949). There is no evidence of hypercalciuria and bone disease, thus distinguishing the condition from hyperparathyroidism. Long term use of diuretics may precipitate hypercalcaemia in patients taking vitamin D or in those with mild hyperparathyroidism (Parfitt, 1969). Given short term, diuretics enhance urinary excretion of calcium, an effect which can be employed in treatment of hypercalcaemia associated with primary hyperparathyroidism (see section 6.1).

Other disorders of calcium metabolism which may be induced by drugs are discussed in chapter XXI (section 15.4) and chapter XXII (section 14.5).

14.6 Diabetes Insipidus

Drugs may sometimes cause reversible nephrogenic diabetes insipidus, e.g. lithium (see chapter XXVI, table IX) and rarely demethylchlortetracycline (Castell and Sparks, 1965).

Some drugs can have an antidiuretic hormone like effect, e.g. chlorpropamide, carbamazepine, clofibrate and thiazides (see section 11; chapter XXI, sect. 15.4).

Further Reading

Bondy, P.K. and Rosenberg, L.E.: Duncan's Diseases of Metabolism, 7th Ed (Saunders, Philadelphia 1974).

Cope, C.L.: Adrenal Steroids and Disease, 2nd Ed (Pitman, London 1972).

Marble, A.; White, P.; Bradley, R.F. and Krall, L.P.: Joslin's Diabetes Mellitus, 12th Ed (Lea and Febiger, Philadelphia 1979).

Werner, S.C. and Ingbar, S.: The Thyroid, 4th Ed (Harper and Row, New York 1978).

Williams, G.H.; Dluhy, R.G. and Thorn, G.W.: Diseases of the Adrenal Cortex; in Thorn and others (Eds) Harrison's Principles of Internal Medicine, 8th Ed, p.520 (McGraw-Hill, New York 1977).

References

Abbassi, V. and Aldige, C.: Evaluation of sodium L-thyroxine (t_4) requirement in replacement therapy of hypothyroidism. Journal of Pediatrics 90: 298 (1977).

Abramson, E.A.; Arky, R.A. and Woeber, K.A.: Effects of propranolol on the hormonal and metabolic responses to insulin-induced hypoglycaemia. Lancet 2: 1386 (1966).

Acland, J.D.: The interpretation of the serum protein-bound iodine: A review. Journal of Clinical Pathology 24: 187 (1971).

Afifi, A.K.; Berman, R.A. and Harvey, M.C.: Steroid myopathy: clinical, histologic observations. Johns Hopkins Medical Journal 123: 158 (1968).

Agarwal, R.C.; Kumar, D. and Miller, L.V.: Chlorpropamide-induced hypoglycaemia. Diabetes 19(Suppl.): 376 (1970).

Alavi, I.A.; Sharma, B.K. and Pillary, V.K.: Steroid-induced diabetic ketoacidosis. American Journal of Medical Sciences 262: 15 (1971).

Alberti, K.G.M.M.: Low-dose insulin in the treatment of diabetic ketoacidosis. Archives of Internal Medicine 137: 1367 (1977).

Alberti, K.G.M.M. and Nattrass, M.: Lactic acidosis. Lancet 2: 25 (1977).

Alberti, K.G.M.M. and Nattrass, M.: Highly purified insulins. Diabetologia 15: 77 (1978).

Alkalay, D.; Khemani, L.; Wagner, W.E. and Bartlett, M.F.: Pharmacokinetics of phenformin in man. Journal of Clinical Pharmacology 15: 446 (1975).

Amdisen, A.: Drug-produced obesity: Experiences with chlorpromazine, perphenazine and clopenthixol. Danish Medical Bulletin 11: 169 (1964).

American Physiology Society: The pituitary gland and its neuroendocrine control. Part 2, secretion and regulation of adenohypophyseal hormones; in Handbook of Physiology, p.367 (American Physiology Society, Washington DC 1974).

Amery, A. and 11 others: Glucose intolerance during diuretic therapy. Results of trial by the European Working Party on Hypertension in the elderly. Lancet 1: 681 (1978).

Anderson, G.H.: Oral diuretics and carbohydrate metabolism. Journal of the Royal College of General Practitioners 21: 535 (1971).

Antonis, A.; Clark, M.L.; Hodge, R.L.; Molony, M. and Pilkington, T.R.E.: Receptor mechanisms in the hyperglycaemic response to adrenalin in man. Lancet 1: 1135 (1967).

Aoki, T.T.; Muller, W.A.; Brennan, M.F. and Cahill, G.F. Jr.: Effect of glucagon on amino acid and nitrogen metabolism in fasting man. Metabolism 23: 805 (1974).

Arky, R.A.; Veverbrants, E. and Abramson, E.A.: Irreversible hypoglycaemia, a complication of alcohol and insulin. Journal of the American Medical Association 206: 575 (1968).

Avlioli, L.V.: The therapeutic approach to hypoparathyroidism. American Journal of Medicine 57: 34 (1974).

Azarnoff, D.L.: Steroid Therapy (Saunders, Philadelphia 1975).

Backman, L.; Beerman, B.; Groschinsky-Grind, M. and Hallberg, D.: Malabsorption of hydrochlorothiazide following intestinal shunt surgery. Clinical Pharmacokinetics 4: 63 (1979).

Bacon, P.A.; Daly, J.R.; Myles, A.B. and Savage, O.: Hypothalamic-pituitary-adrenal function in patients on long-term adrenocorticotrophin therapy. Annals of Rheumatic Diseases 27: 7 (1968).

Balodimos, M.C.; Camerini-Davalos, R.A. and Marble, A.: Nine years' experience with tolbutamide in the treatment of diabetes. Metabolism 15: 957 (1966).

Barbato, A.L. and Landau, R.L.: Serum cortisol appearance-disappearance in adrenal insufficiency after oral cortisone acetate. Acta Endocrinologica 84: 600 (1977).

Barnett, D.M.; Wilcox, D.S. and Marble, A.: Diabetic coma in persons over 60. Geriatrics 17: 327 (1962).

Becker, D.J. and Foley, T.P.: 1-Deamino-8-D-arginine vasopressin in the treatment of central diabetes insipidus in childhood. Journal of Pediatrics 92: 1011 (1978).

Beckman, R.: The fate of biguanides in man. Annals of the New York Academy of Science 148: 820 (1968).

Belforte, L.; Camanni, F.; Chiodini, P.G.; Liuzzi, A.; Massara, F.; Molinatti, G.M.; Muller, E.E. and Silvestrini, F.: Long-term treatment with 2-Br-α-ergocryptine in acromegaly. Acta Endocrinologica 85: 235 (1977).

Bell, J.M.; Russell, C.J.; Nelson, J.K.; Kelly, J.G. and McDevitt, D.G.: Studies of the effect of thyroid dysfunction on the elimination of β-adrenoceptor blocking drugs. British Journal of Clinical Pharmacology 4: 79 (1977).

Bergman, U.; Boman, G. and Wiholm, B-E.: Epidemiology of adverse drug reactions to phenformin and metformin. British Medical Journal 2: 464 (1978).

Bernhard, H.: Long-term observations on oral hypoglycaemic agents in diabetes: The effect of carbutamide and tolbutamide. Diabetes 14: 59 (1965).

Bokat, M.A.: Treatment of hyperthyroidism in pregnancy; in Astwood and Cassidy (Eds), p.236 Clinical Endocrinology (Grune and Stratton, New York 1968).

Bonelli, J.; Haydl, H.; Hruby, K. and Kaik, G.: The pharmacokinetics of digoxin in patients with manifest hyperthyroidism and after normalisation of thyroid function. International Journal of Clinical Pharmacology and Therapeutics 16: 302 (1978).

Boylan, J.J.; Owen, D.S. and Chin, J.B.: Phenytoin interference with dexamethasone. Journal of the American Medical Association 235: 803 (1976).

Boyle, I.T.; Fogelman, I.; Boyce, B.; Thomson, J.E.; Beastall, G.H.; McIntosh, W.B. and McLennan, I.: 1α-Hydroxyvitamin D_3 in primary hyperparathyroidism. Clinical Endocrinology 7(Suppl.): 215s (1977).

Bradley, R.F.: Myocardial infarction and the blood sugar; in Marble et al. (Eds) Joslin's Diabetes Mellitus, 11th Ed, p.452 (Lea and Febiger, Philadelphia 1971).

Bradley, S.E.; Stephen, F.; Coelho, J.B. and Reville, P.: The thyroid and the kidney. Kidney International 6: 346 (1974).

Braverman, L.E.: Thyrotoxicos: Therapeutic considerations. Clinics in Endocrinology and Metabolism 7: 221 (1978).

Bray, G.A.; De Quattro, V.; Fisher, D.A.; Goldberg, M.A.; McIntyre, H.B.; Odell, W.D.; Sperling, M.A. and Swerdloff, R.S.: Catecholamines — a symposium. California Medicine 117: 32 (1972).

Breckenridge, A.; Dollery, C.T.; Welborn, T.A. and Fraser, R.: Glucose tolerance in hypertensive patients on long-term diuretic therapy. Lancet 1: 61 (1967).

Breidahl, H.D.; Ennis, G.C.; Martin, F.I.R.; Stawell, J.R. and Taft, P.: Insulin and oral hypoglycaemic drugs: Physiological and clinical pharmacological aspects. Drugs 3: 79 (1972a).

Breidahl, H.D.; Ennis, G.C.; Martin, F.I.R.; Stawell, J.R. and Taft, P.: Insulin and oral hypoglycaemic drugs: Clinical and therapeutic aspects. Drugs 3: 204 (1972b).

Brook, C.G.D.: Obesity. Fat children. British Journal of Hospital Medicine 10: 30 (1973).

Brooks, S.M.; Werk, E.E.; Ackerman, S.J.; Sullivan, I. and Trasher, K.: Adverse effects of phenobarbital on corticosteroid metabolism in asthmatics. New England Journal of

Medicine 286: 1125 (1972).

Brotherton,P.M.; Grievson, P. and McMartin, C.: A study of the metabolic fate of chlorpropamide in man. Clinical Pharmacology and Therapeutics 10: 505 (1969).

Brown, J.; Clark, W.R.; Molnar, I.G. and Mullen, Y.S.: Fetal pancreas transplantation for reversal of streptozotocin-induced diabetes in rats. Diabetes 25: 56 (1976).

Brown, J.; Clark, W.R.; Makoff, R.K.; Weisman, H.; Kemb, J.A. and Mullen, Y.: Pancreas transplantation for diabetes mellitus. Annals of Internal Medicine 89: 951 (1978).

Brownlie, B.E.W.; Chambers, S.T.; Sadler, W.A. and Donald, R.A.: Lithium associated thyroid disease — A report of 14 cases of hypothyroidism and 4 cases of thyrotoxicosis. Australian and New Zealand Journal of Medicine 6: 223 (1976).

Buffington, G.A.; Dominguez, H.H.; Piering, W.F.; Hebert, L.A.; Kauffman, H.M. and Lemann, J.: Interaction of rifampicin and glucocorticoids. Journal of the American Medical Association 236: 1958 (1976).

Burke, G.; Silverstein, G.E. and Sorking, A.I.: Effect of long-term sulfonylurea-therapy on thyroid function. Metabolism 16: 651 (1967).

Burnett, C.H.; Commons, R.R.; Albright, F. and Howard, J.E.: Hypercalcaemia without hypercalciuria or hyperparathyroidism calcinosis and renal insufficiency. A syndrome following prolonged intake of milk and alkali. New England Journal of Medicine 240: 787 (1949).

Burrow, G.N.: Current concepts of thyroid disease. Medical Clinics of North America 59: 1043 (1975).

Burrow, G.N.: Hyperthyroidism during pregnancy. New England Journal of Medicine 298: 150 (1978).

Burrow, G.N.; Bartsocas, C.; Klatskin, E.H. and Grunt, J.A.: Children exposed in utero to propylthiouracil: subsequent intellectual and physical development. American Journal of Diseases of Children 116: 161 (1968).

Burrow, G.N.; Klatskin, E.H. and Genel, M.: Intellectual development in children whose mothers received propylthiouracil during pregnancy. Yale Journal of Biology and Medicine 51: 151 (1978).

Byyny, R.L.: Withdrawal from glucocorticoid therapy. New England Journal of Medicine 295: 30 (1976).

Cahill, G.F., Jr.; Etzwiler, D.D. and Freinkel, N.: 'Control' and diabetes. New England Journal of Medicine 294: 1004 (1976).

Camerini-Davalos, R.A. and Marble, A.: Incidence and causes of secondary failure in treatment with tolbutamide: Experience with 2,500 patients treated up to five years. Journal of the American Medical Association 181: 1 (1962).

Carswell, F.; Kerr, M.M. and Hutchison, J.H.: Congenital goitre and hypothyroidism produced by maternal ingestion of iodides. Lancet 1: 1241 (1970).

Carter, J.N.; Tyson, J.E.; Tolis, G.; Van Vliet, S.; Faiman, C. and Friesen, H.G.: Prolactin-secreting tumors and hypogonadism in 22 men. New England Journal of Medicine 299: 847 (1978).

Casey, J.H.: Chronic treatment regimens for hirsutism in women: effect on blood production rates of testosterone and on hair growth. Clinical Endocrinology 4: 313 (1975).

Castell, D.O. and Sparks, H.A.: Nephrogenic diabetes insipidus due to demethylchlortetracycline hydrochloride. Journal of the American Medical Association 193: 237 (1965).

Cervantes-Amezena, A.; Naldjian, S.; Camerini-Davalos, R. and Marble, A.: Long term use of chlorpropamide in diabetes. Journal of the American Medical Association 193: 759 (1965).

Cheron, R.G.; Marais, H.J. and Selenkow, H.A.: Thyroid function and dysfunction: Gestational considerations. Comprehensive Therapy 4: 64 (1978).

Chopra, I.J. and Solomon, D.H.: Thyroid function tests and their alteration by drugs. Pharmacology and Therapeutics. Part C1: 367 (1976).

Clarke, B.F. and Campbell, I.W.: Comparison of metformin and chlorpropamide in non-obese, maturity-onset diabetes uncontrolled by diet. British Medical Journal 2: 1576 (1977).

Clarke, W.L.; Santiago, J.V. and Kipnis, D.M.: The effect of hyperglucagonemia on blood glucose concentrations and on insulin requirements in insulin-requiring diabetes mellitus. Diabetes 27: 649 (1978).

Cobb, W.E.; Spare, S. and Reichlin, S.: Neurogenic diabetes insipidus: management with dDAVP (1-desamino-8-D arginine vasopressin). Annals of Internal Medicine 88: 183 (1978).

Coburn, J.W.; Brickman, A.S. and Massry, S.G.: Medical treatment in primary and secondary hyperparathyroidism. Seminars in Drug Treatment 2: 117 (1972).

Cohen, B.D.; Galloway, J.A.; McMahon, R.E.; Culp, H.W.; Root, M.A. and Henriques, K.J.: Carbohydrate metabolism in uraemia: blood glucose response to sulfonylurea. Americn Journal of Medical Sciences 254: 608 (1967).

Colton, C.K.; Giner, J.; Lerner, H.; Marincic, L. and Soeldner, J.S.: Development of an implantable electrochemical glucose sensor; in Transplantation and Clinical Immunology, Vol. X., Proceedings of the Tenth International Course, p.165 (Excerpta Medica, Amsterdam 1978).

Connolly, R.J.; Vidor, G.I. and Stewart, J.C.: Increase in thyrotoxicosis in endemic goitre after iodation of bread. Lancet 1: 500 (1970).

Cope, C.L.: Adrenal Steroids and Disease (Pitman, London 1972).

Cowley, A.J. and Elkeles, R.S.: Diabetes and therapy with potent diuretics. Lancet 1: 154 (1978).

Craddock, D.: Anorectic drugs: Use in general practice. Drugs 11: 378 (1976).

Craig, J.O.; Ferguson, I.C. and Syme, J.: Infant toddlers and aspirin. British Medical Journal 1: 757 (1966).

Craig, J.; Abu-Saleh, M.; Smith, B. and Evans, I.: Diabetes mellitus in patients on lithium. Lancet 2: 1028 (1977).

Croxson, M.S. and Ibbertson, H.K.: Serum digoxin in patients with thyroid disease. British Medical Journal 3: 566 (1975).

Daggett, P.; Mustaffa, B.E. and Nabarro, J.D.N.: Effects of highly purified insulin on dosage requirements. Practitioner 218: 563 (1977).

Daintith, H.; Stevenson, I.H. and O'Malley, K.: Influence of diabetes mellitus on drug metabolism in man. International Journal of Clinical Pharmacology 13: 55 (1976).

Dajani, R.M.; Kayyali, S.; Saheb, S.E. and Birbari, A.: A study of the physiological disposition of acetophenetidin by the diabetic man. Comparative and General Pharmacology 5: 1 (1974).

Dandona, P.; Foster, M.; Healey, F.; Greenbury, E. and Beckett, A.G.: Low-dose insulin infusions in diabetic patients with high insulin requirements. Lancet 2: 283 (1978).

David, D.S.; Grieco, M.H. and Cushman, P.: Adrenal glucocorticoids after 20 years. A review of their clinically relevant consequences. Journal of Chronic Diseases 22: 637 (1970).

Davies, M. and Adams, P.H.: The continuing risk of vitamin-D intoxication. Lancet 2: 621 (1978).

Davis, M.; Williams, R.; Chakraborty, J.; English, J.; Marks, V.; Ideo, G. and Tempini, S.: Prednisone or prednisolone for the treatment of chronic active hepatitis? A comparison of plasma availability. British Journal of Clinical Pharmacology 5: 501 (1978).

Deacon, S.P.; Karunanayaka, A. and Barnett, D.: Acebutolol, atenolol and propranolol and metabolic responses to acute hypoglycaemia in diabetics. British Medical Journal 2: 1255 (1977).

Dent, C.E.: Dangers of vitamin-D intoxication. British Medical Journal 1: 834 (1964).

Dluhy, R.G.; Newmark, S.R.; Lauler, D.P. and Thorn, G.W.: Pharmacology and chemistry of adrenal glucocorticoids; in Azarnoff (Ed) Steroid Therapy, p.1 (Saunders, Philadelphia 1975).

Doherty, J.E. and Perkins, W.H.: Digoxin metabolism in hypo- and hyperthyroidism. Studies with tritiated digoxin in thyroid disease. Annals of Internal Medicine 64: 489 (1966).

Dollery, C.T. and Breckenridge, A.: Endocrine and metabolic effects of drugs; in Meyler and Peck (Eds) Drug-Induced Diseases, vol. 4, p.478 (Excerpta Medica, Amsterdam 1972).

Dollery, C.T.; Pentecost, B.L. and Samaan, N.A.: Drug-induced diabetes. Lancet 2: 735 (1962).

Editorial: Corticosteroid therapy and growth. British Medical Journal 1: 393 (1969).

Editorial: Drugs causing weight gain. British Medical Journal 1: 168 (1974).

Editorial: Beta-adrenergic blocking drugs and thyroid function. British Medical Journal 2: 1039 (1977).

Editorial: Cyproheptadine. Lancet 1: 367 (1978).

Ehrlich, R.M. and Kooh, S.W.: The use of chlorpropamide in diabetes insipidus in children. Pediatrics 45: 236 (1970).

Eichelbaum, M.: Drug metabolism in thyroid disease. Clinical Pharmacokinetics 1: 339 (1976).

Elfstrom, J.: Drug pharmacokinetics in the postoperative period. Clinical Pharmacokinetics 4: 16 (1979).

Engerman, R.; Bloodworth, J.M.B. Jr. and Nelson, S.: Relationship of microvascular disease in diabetes to metabolic control. Diabetes 26: 760 (1977).

Eschwege, E.; Job, D.; Guyot-Argenton, C.; Aubry, J.P. and Tchobroutsky, G.: Delayed progression of diabetic retinopathy by divided insulin administration: A further follow-up. Diabetologia 16: 13 (1979).

Eskildsen, P.C. and Nerup, J.: Low-dose insulin treatment of diabetic ketoacidosis. Acta Medica Scandinavica 202: 295 (1977).

Evered, D. and Yeo, P.P.B.: Drug-induced endocrine disorders. Drugs 13: 353 (1977).

Ewy, G.A.; Groves, B.M.; Ball, M.F.; Nimmo, L.; Jackson, B. and Marcus, F.: Digoxin metabolism in obesity. Circulation 44: 810 (1971).

Fauci, A.S.; Dale, D.C. and Balow, J.E.: Glucocorticosteroid therapy: mechanisms of action and clinical considerations. Annals of Internal Medicine 84: 304 (1976).

Feely, J. and Stevenson, I.H.: The effect of age and hyperthyroid on plasma propranolol steady state concentration. British Journal of Clinical Pharmacology 6: 446P (1978a).

Feely, J. and Stevenson, I.H.: Alterations in plasma propranolol steady state concentration in thyroid disease. Clinical Pharmacology and Therapeutics 23: 112 (1978b).

Feely, J. and Stevenson, I.H.: Effect of partial thyroidectomy on plasma propranolol steady state concentration. International Congress of Pharmacology, Paris, July 16-21, Abstract (1978c).

Feinstein, A.R.: An analytic appraisal of the University Group Diabetes Program (UGDP) study. Clinical Pharmacology and Therapeutics 12: 167 (1971).

Feinstein, A.R.: Clinical biostatistics. XXXV. The persistent clinical failures and fallacies of the UGDP study. Clinical Pharmacology and Therapeutics 19: 78 (1976a).

Feinstein, A.R.: Clinical biostatistics. XXXVI. The persistent biometric problems of the UGDP study. Clinical Pharmacology and Therapeutics 19: 472 (1976b).

Feldman, D.; Funder, J.W. and Edelman, J.S.: Subcellular mechanisms in the action of adrenal steroids. American Journal of Medicine 53: 545 (1972).

Felig, P.; Marliss, E.B. and Cahill, G.F.: Metabolic response to human growth hormone during prolonged starvation. Journal of Clinical Investigation 50: 411 (1971).

Field, J.B.; Ohta, M.; Boyle, C. and Remer, A.: Potentiation of acetohexamide hypoglycaemia by phenylbutazone. New England Journal of Medicine 277: 889 (1967).

Fitzgerald, M.G.; Gaddie, R.; Malins, J.M. and O'Sullivan, D.J.: Alcohol sensitivity in diabetics receiving chlorpropamide. Diabetes 11: 40 (1962).

Fleisher, N.; Ake, K.; Liddle, G.W.; Orth, D.N. and Nicholson, W.E.: ACTH antibodies in patients receiving depot porcine ACTH to hasten recovery from pituitary-adrenal suppression. Journal of Clinical Investigation 46: 196 (1967).

Fleischer, N.; Lorente, M.; Kirkland, J.; Kirkland, R.; Clayton, G. and Calderon, M.: Synthetic thyrotropin releasing factor as a test of pituitary thyrotropin reserve. Journal of Clinical Endocrinology and Metabolism 34: 617 (1972).

Fredholm, B.B.; Lunell, N.O.; Persson, B. and Wager, J.: Actions of salbutamol in late pregnancy: Plasma cyclic AMP, insulin and C-peptide, carbonhydrate and lipid metabolites in diabetic and non-diabetic women. Diabetologia 14: 235 (1978).

Friedman, M. and Strang, L.B.: The effects of corticosteroid and ACTH therapy on growth and on the hypothalamic-pituitary-adrenal axis of children. Scandinavian Journal of Respiratory Diseases 68(Suppl.): 58 (1969).

Gal, P.; Jusko, W.J.; Yurchak, A.M. and Franklin, B.A.: Theophylline disposition in obesity. Clinical Pharmacology and Therapeutics 23: 438 (1978).

Gale, E.A.M. and Tattersall, R.B.: Can phenformin-induced lactic acidosis be prevented. British Medical Journal 2: 972 (1976).

Garcia, G.; de Vidal, E.L. and Trujillo, H.: Serum levels and urinary concentrations of kanamycin, bekanamycin and amikacin (BB-K8) in diabetic children and a control group. Journal of International Medical Research 5: 322 (1977).

Garrow, J.S.: Metabolic aspects of obesity. British Journal of Hospital Medicine 10: 24 (1973).

Gerich, J.E.; Martin, M.M. and Recant, L.: Clinical and metabolic characteristics of hyperosmolar nonketotic coma. Diabetes 20: 228 (1971).

Glaser, G.H.: Psychotic reactions induced by corticotropin (ACTH) and cortisone. Psychosomatic Medicine 15: 280 (1953).

Goldman, J.A.: Intravenous glucose tolerance after 18 months on progestagen or combination-type oral contraceptive. Israel Journal of Medical Sciences 14: 324 (1978).

Goldner, M.G.; Zarowitz, H. and Akgun, S.: Hyperglycemia

and glycosuria due to thiazide derivatives administered in diabetes mellitus. New England Journal of Medicine 262: 403 (1960).

Goldrick, R.B.: The management of obesity. Drugs 12: 301 (1976).

Good, T.A. and Bessman, S.P.: Anabolic steroids in cystic fibrosis of the pancreas. American Journal of Diseases of Children 111: 272 (1966).

Gorman, C.A.; Becker, D.V.; Greenspan, F.S.; Levy, R.P.; Oppenheimer, J.H.; Rivlin, R.S.; Robbins, J. and Vanderlaan, W.P.: Breast cancer and thyroid therapy. Statement by the American Thyroid Association. Journal of the American Medical Association 237: 1459 (1977).

Graber, A.L.; Ney, R.L.; Nicholson, W.E.; Island, D.P. and Liddle, G.W.: Natural history of pituitary-adrenal recovery following long-term suppression with corticosteroids. Journal of Clinical Endocrinology and Metabolism 25: 11 (1965).

Green, O.C.; Winter, R.J.; Kawahara, F.S.; Phillips, L.S.; Lewy, P.R.; Hart, R.L. and Pachman, L.M.: Pharmacokinetic studies of prednisolone in children. Plasma levels, half-life values, and correlation with physiologic assays for growth and immunity. Journal of Pediatrics 93: 299 (1978).

Greene, J.W.: Diabetes mellitus in pregnancy. Obstetrics and Gynecology 46: 724 (1975).

Greffner, D.L. and Hershman, J.M.: Hyperthyroidism. Causes, etiology of Graves' disease, clinical features, general aspects of treatment. Pharmacology and Therapeutics Part C 1: 401 (1976).

Gutknecht, D.R.: Asthma complicated by iodine-induced thyrotoxicosis. New England Journal of Medicine 296: 1236 (1977).

Gwinup, G.: Prospective randomized comparison of propylthiouracil. Journal of the American Medical Association 239: 2457 (1978).

Hadden, D.R.; Montgomery, D.A.D.; Shanks, R.G. and Weaver, J.A.: Propranolol and iodine-131 in the management of thyrotoxicosis. Lancet 2: 852 (1968).

Hadden, D.R.; Lowe, D.C.; Montgomery, D.A.D.; Shanks, R.G. and Weaver, J.A.: Propranolol and radioactive iodine in the treatment of thyrotoxicosis. British Journal of Pharmacology 39: 198P (1970).

Hamburger, J.I.: Management of the pregnant hyperthyroid: The argument against combined antithyroid-thyroid therapy. Obstetrics and Gynecology 40: 114 (1972).

Hansen, J.M. and Christensen, L.K.: Drug interactions with oral sulphonylurea hypoglycaemic drugs. Drugs 13: 24 (1977).

Hansen, J.M.; Skovsted, J.; Lumholtz, B.I. and Siersbaek-Nielsen, K.: Unaltered metabolism of phenytoin in thyroid disorders. Acta Pharmacologica et Toxicologica 42: 343 (1978).

Heckel, N.J.; Rosso, W.A. and Kestel, L.: Spermatogenic rebound phenomenon after administration of testosterone propionate. Journal of Clinical Endocrinology 11: 235 (1951).

Herbst, A.L. and Selenkow, H.A.: Hyperthyroidism during pregnancy. New England Journal of Medicine 273: 627 (1965).

Hicks, B.H.; Ward, J.D.; Jarrett, R.J.; Keen, H. and Wise, P.: A controlled study of clopamide, clorexolone and hydrochlorothiazide in diabetics. Metabolism 22: 101 (1973).

Hoffenberg, R.: Disorders of the parathyroid glands. Practitioner 208: 360 (1972).

Huffmann, D.H.; Klaassen, C.D. and Hartman, C.R.: Digoxin in hyperthyroidism. Clinical Pharmacology and Therapeutics 22: 533 (1977).

Hull, J.H. and Sarubbi, F.A.: Gentamicin serum concentrations: pharmacokinetic predictions. Annals of Internal Medicine 85: 183 (1976).

Hutter, A.M. and Kayhoe, D.E.: Adrenal cortical carcinoma: results of treatment with o,p'DDD in 138 patients. American Journal of Medicine 41: 581 (1966).

Irvine, W.J. and Toft, A.D.: The diagnosis and treatment of thyrotoxicosis. Clinical Endocrinology 5: 687 (1976).

Jelliffe, R.W.; Hill, D.; Tatter, D. and Lewis, E.: Death from weight-control pills. A case report with objective postmortem confirmation. Journal of the American Medical Association 208: 1843 (1969).

Johansson, E.D.B. and Kral, J.G.: Oral contraceptives after intestinal bypass operations. Journal of the American Medical Association 236: 2847 (1976).

Johnsson, S.: Retinopathy and nephropathy in diabetes mellitus: Comparison of the effect of two forms of treatment. Diabetes 9: 1 (1960).

Johnston, B.B.: Diabetes mellitus in patients on lithium. Lancet 2: 935 (1977).

Jørgensen, H. and Vogt, J.H.: 1a-Hydroxycholecalciferol in the treatment of hypoparathyroidism. Acta Medica Scandinavica 201: 3 (1977).

Kanarek, P.; Balodimos, M.C. and Marble, A.: Survival and causes of death among diabetic patients treated with insulin, tolbutamide, or diet alone. Unpublished data (1975).

Keiding, N.R.; Root, H.F. and Marble, A.: Importance of control of diabetes in prevention of vascular complications. Journal of the American Medical Association 150: 964 (1952).

Keipert, J.A.: The absorption of topical corticosteroids, with particular reference to percutaneous absorption in infancy and childhood. Medical Journal of Australia 1: 1021 (1971).

Kimball, C.P.: Psychological dependency on steroids. Annals of Internal Medicine 75: 111 (1971).

Kirby, M.J. and Turner, P.: Do 'anorectic' drugs produce weight loss by appetite suppression? Lancet 1: 566 (1976).

Kjellstrand, C.M.; Simmons, R.L.; Goetz, F.C.; Buselmeier, T.J.; Shideman, J.R.; Von Hartizsch, B. and Najarian, J.S.: Renal transplantation in patients with insulin-dependent diabetes. Lancet 2: 4 (1973).

Kohner, E.M.; Dollery, C.T.; Lowy, C. and Schumer, B.: Effect of diuretic therapy on glucose tolerance in hypertensive patients. Lancet 1: 986 (1971).

Kooh, S.W.; Fraser, D.; DeLuca, H.F.; Holick, M.F.; Belsey, R.E.; Clark, M.B. and Murray, T.M.: Treatment of hypoparathyroidism and pseudoparathyroidism with metabolites of vitamin D: evidence for impaired conversion of 25-hydroxyvitamin D to 1α-, 25-dihydroxyvitamin D. New England Journal of Medicine 293: 840 (1975).

Kotler, M.N.; Berman, L. and Rubenstein, A.H.: Hypoglycaemia precipitated by propranolol. Lancet 2: 1389 (1966).

Kozower, M.; Veatch, L. and Kaplan, M.M.: Decreased clearance of prednisolone, a factor in the development of corticosteroid side-effects. Journal of Clinical Endocrinology and Metabolism 38: 407 (1974).

Kreisberg, R.A.; Owen, W.C. and Siegal, A.M.: Hyperlacticacidemia in man: Ethanol-phenformin synergism. Journal of Clinical Endocrinology and Metabolism 34: 29

(1972).

Kreisberg, R.A.: Diabetic ketoacidosis: new concepts and trends in pathogenesis and treatment. Annals of Internal Medicine 88: 681 (1978).

Kumar, D.; Miller, L.V. and Mehtalia, S.D.: Use of dexamethasone in treatment of insulin lipoatrophy. Diabetes 26: 296 (1977).

Lane, R.J.M.; Clark, F. and McCollum, J.K.: Oxyphenbutazone-induced goitre. Postgraduate Medical Journal 53: 93 (1977).

Langer, A.; Hung, C.T.; McAnulty, J.A.; Harrigan, J.T. and Washington, E.: Adrenergic blockade: A new approach to hyperthyroidism during pregnancy. Obstetrics and Gynecology 44: 181 (1974).

Lawrence, J.R.; Sumner, D.J.; Kalk, W.J.; Ratcliffe, W.A.; Whiting, B.; Gray, K. and Lindsay, M.: Digoxin kinetics in patients with thyroid dysfunction. Clinical Pharmacology and Therapeutics 22: 7 (1977).

Layne, E.C.; Schultz, R.D.; Thomas, L.J.; Slama, G.; Sayler, D.F. and Bessman, S.P.: Continuous extracorporeal monitoring of animal blood using the glucose electrode. Diabetes 25: 81 (1976).

Lebacq, E. and Marcq, M.: A study of the mechanism of ethacrynic acid induced hyperglycaemia. Revue francaise d'etudes cliniques et biologiques 12: 160 (1967).

Leeson, P.M. and Fourman, P.: Increased sensitivity to vitamin D after vitamin D poisoning. Lancet 1: 1182 (1966).

Lerner, P.I. and Weinstein, L.: Abnormalities of absorption of benzylpenicillin G and sulfisoxazole in patients with diabetes mellitus. American Journal of the Medical Sciences 248: 37 (1964).

Leslie, R.D.G. and Pyke, D.A.: Chlorpropamide-alcohol flushing: a dominantly inherited trait associated with diabetes. British Medical Journal 2: 1519 (1978a).

Leslie, R.D.G. and Pyke, D.A.: Chlorpropamide-alcohol flushing: a definition of its relation to non-insulin-dependent diabetes. British Medical Journal 2: 1521 (1978b).

Levey, G.S.: Catecholamine sensitivity, thyroid hormone and the heart. American Journal of Medicine 50: 413 (1971).

Levey, G.S.: The adrenergic nervous system in hyperthyroidism: Therapeutic role of beta adrenergic blocking drugs. Pharmacology and Therapeutics Part C 1: 31 (1976).

Levey, G.S.; Lasseter, K.C. and Palmer, R.F.: Sulphonylureas and the heart. Annual Review of Medicine 25: 69 (1974).

Lewis, G.P.; Jusko, W.J.; Burke, C.W. and Graves, L.: Prednisone side effects and serum protein levels. Lancet 2: 778 (1971).

Lewis, P.J.; Petrie, A.; Kohner, E.M. and Dollery, C.T.: Deterioration of glucose tolerance in hypertensive patients on prolonged diuretic treatment. Lancet 1: 564 (1976).

Limbeck, G.A.; Ruvalcaba, R.H.O.; Samols, E. and Kelley, V.C.: Salicylates and hypoglycemia. American Journal of Diseases of Children 109: 165 (1965).

Lindstedt, G.; Nilsson, L-A.; Walinder, J.; Skott, A. and Ohman, R.: On the prevalence, diagnosis and management of lithium-induced hypothyroidism in psychiatric patients. British Journal of Psychiatry 130: 452 (1977).

Loeliger, E.A.; van der Esch, B. and Mattern, M.J.: The biological disappearance rate of prothrombin, factors VII, IX and X from plasma in hypothyroidism, hyperthyroidism, and during fever. Thrombosis et Diathesis Haemorrhagica 11: 1 (1964).

Logie, A.W. and Stowers, J.M.: Hazards of monocomponent insulins. British Medical Journal 1: 879 (1976).

Logie, A.W.; Galloway, D.B. and Petrie, J.C.: Drug interactions and long-term antidiabetic therapy. British Journal of Clinical Pharmacology 3: 1027 (1976).

Lowenthal, D.T.: Tissue sensitivity to drugs in disease states. Medical Clinics of North America 58: 1111 (1974).

Lozano-Castaneda, O.; Camerini-Davalos, R.A.; Krall, L.P. and Marble, A.: Two years experience with acetohexamide. Metabolism 13: 99 (1964).

Luft, D.; Schmulling, R.M. and Eggstein, M.: Lactic acidosis in biguanide-treated diabetes. Diabetologia 14: 75 (1978).

McCarroll, A.M.; Hutchinson, M.; McAuley, R. and Montgomery, D.A.D.: Long-term assessment of children exposed *in utero* to carbimazole. Archives of Disease in Childhood 51: 532 (1976).

McDevitt, D.G. and Shanks, R.G.: β-Adrenoreceptor blocking drugs in hyperthyroidism; in Avery (Ed) β-Adrenoceptor Blocking Drugs, Vol 2, Cardiovascular Drugs, p.161 (ADIS Press, Sydney; University Park Press, Baltimore 1977).

McGregor, A.M.; Scanlon, M.F.; Hall, K.; Cook, D.B. and Hall, R.: Reduction in size of a pituitary tumor by bromocriptine therapy. New England Journal of Medicine 300: 291 (1979).

Mackin, J.F.; Canary, J.J. and Pittman, C.S.: Thyroid storm and its management. New England Journal of Medicine 291: 1396 (1974).

Madacsy, L.; Bokor, M. and Matusovits, L.: Penicillin clearance in diabetic children. Acta Paediatrica Academiae Scient-Hungaricae 16: 139 (1975).

Madacsy, L.; Bokor, M. and Kozocsa, G.: Carbenicillin half-life in children with early diabetes mellitus. International Journal of Clinical Pharmacology and Biopharmacy 14: 155 (1976).

Madison, L.L.: Ethanol-induced hypoglycaemia. Advances in Metabolic Disorders 3: 85 (1968).

Mann, G.V.: Influence of obesity on health. New England Journal of Medicine 291: 178, 226 (1974).

Marble, A.; White, P.; Bradley, R.F. and Krall, L.P.: Joslin's Diabetes Mellitus, 11th Ed (Lea and Febiger, Philadelphia 1971).

March, C.M.: Bromocriptine in the treatment of hypogonadism and male impotence. Drugs 17: 349 (1979).

Marchant, B.; Brownlie, B.E.W.; Hart, D.M.; Horton, P.W. and Alexander, W.D.: The placental transfer of propylthiouracil, methimazole and carbimazole. Journal of Clinical Endocrinology and Metabolism 45: 1187 (1977).

Marcus, F.I.; Horton, H.; Jacobs, S.; Pippin, S.; Stafford, M. and Zukoski, C.: The effect of jejunoileal bypass in patients with morbid obesity on the pharmacokinetics of digoxin in man. American Journal of Cardiology 37: 154 (1976).

Matas, A.J.; Sutherland, D.E.R. and Najarian, J.S.: Current status of islet and pancreas transplantation in diabetes. Diabetes 25: 785 (1976).

Mauer, S.M.; Brown, D.M.; Matas, A.J. and Steffes, M.W.: Effects of pancreatic islet transplantation on the increased urinary albumin excretion rates in intact and uninephrectomized rats with diabetes mellitus. Diabetes 27: 959 (1978).

Mauer, S.M.; Steffes, M.S.; Sutherland, D.E.R.; Najarian, J.S.; Michael, A.F. and Brown, D.M.: Studies of the rate of regression of the glomerular lesions in diabetic rats treated with pancreatic islet transplantation. Diabetes 24: 280 (1975).

Meikle, A.W.; Clarke, D.H. and Tyler, F.H.: Cushing syndrome from low doses of dexamethasone. A result of slow plasma clearance. Journal of the American Medical Association 235: 1592 (1976).

Melander, A.; Wahlin, E.; Danielson, K. and Hanson, A.: Bioavailability of propylthiouracil: interindividual variation and influence of food intake. Acta Medica Scandinavica 201: 41 (1977).

Melby, J.C.: Systemic corticosteroid therapy: Pharmacology and endocrinologic considerations. Annals of Internal Medicine 81: 505 (1974).

Mellinger, R.C. and Thompson, R.T.: The effect of clomiphene citrate in male infertility. Fertility and Sterility 17: 94 (1966).

Michie, W.; Hamer-Hodges, D.W.; Pegg, C.A.S.; Orr, F.G.G. and Bewsher, P.D.: Beta-blockade and partial thyroidectomy for thyrotoxicosis. Lancet 1: 1009 (1974).

Mirsky, I.A.: Insulinase, insulinase-inhibitors and diabetes mellitus. Recent Progress in Hormone Research 13: 429 (1957).

Morrow, D.H.; Gaffney, T.E. and Braunwald, E.: Studies on digitalis VII. Influence of hyper- and hypothyroidism on the myocardial response to ouabain. Journal of Pharmacology and Experimental Therapeutics 140: 324 (1963).

Mortimer, C.H.; Anderson, D.C.; Liendo- ch.P.; Fisher, R.; Chan, V.; Self, M. and Besser, G.M.: Thyrotoxicosis: relations between clinical state and biochemical changes during carbimazole treatment. British Medical Journal 1: 138 (1977).

Moss, J.M. and Galloway, J.A.: U-100 Insulin. A progress report. Journal of the American Medical Association 238: 1823 (1977).

Muller-Oerlinghausen, B.; Passoth, P.M.; Poser, W. and Schlecht, W.: The influence of long-term treatment with major tranquillizers or lithium salts on the carbohydrate metabolism. Arzneimittel-Forschung 28: 1522 (1978).

Mustacchi, P. and Greenspan, F.: Thyroid supplementation for hypothyroidism. An iatrogenic cause of breast cancer? Journal of the American Medical Association 237: 1446 (1977).

Nattrass, M. and Alberti, K.G.M.M.: Biguanides. Diabetologia 14: 71 (1978).

Notelovitz, M.: Sulphonylurea therapy in the treatment of the pregnant diabetic. South African Medical Journal 45: 226 (1971).

Notelovitz, M.: Oral hypoglycaemic therapy in diabetic pregnancies. Lancet 2: 902 (1974).

Oakley, W.G.; Jones, V.E. and Cunliffe, A.C.: Insulin resistance. British Medical Journal 2: 134 (1967).

Odell, W.D.; Tanner, D.C.; Steiner, D.F. and Williams, R.H.: Phenethyl-amyl and isoamylbiguanide in the treatment of diabetes mellitus. Archives of Internal Medicine 102: 520 (1958).

O'Donovan, C.J.: Analysis of long-term experience with tolbutamide (Orinase) in the management of diabetes. Current Therapeutic Research 1: 69 (1959).

Olefsky, J.M. and Reaven, G.M.: Effects of sulfonylurea therapy on insulin binding to mononuclear leukocytes of diabetic patients. American Journal of Medicine 60: 89 (1976).

Owen, C. and Cahill, G.F.: Metabolic effects of exogenous glucocorticoids in fasted man. Journal of Clinical Investigation 52: 2596 (1973).

Pagliara, A.S.; Karl, I.E.; Haymond, M. and Kipnis, D.M.: Hypoglycemia in infancy and childhood. Journal of Pediatrics 82: 365, 558 (1973).

Parfitt, A.M.: Chlorothiazide-induced hypercalcaemia in juvenile osteoporosis and hyperparathyroidism. New England Journal of Medicine 281: 55 (1969).

Paykel, E.S.; Muelter, P.S. and de la Vergne, P.M.: Amitriptyline, weight gain and carbohydrate craving: A side effect. British Journal of Psychiatry 123: 501 (1973).

Petereit, L.B. and Meikle, A.W.: Effectiveness of prednisolone during phenytoin therapy. Clinical Pharmacology and Therapeutics 22: 912 (1977).

Petitpierre, B.; Perrin, L.; Rudhart, M.; Herrera, A. and Fabre, J.: Behaviour of chlorpropamide in renal insufficiency and under the effect of associated drug therapy. International Journal of Clinical Pharmacology, Therapy and Toxicology 6: 120 (1972).

Pfeiffer, E.F.; Kerner, W. and Beischer, W.: The artificial endocrine pancreas in clinical research and practice; in Bajaj (Ed) Diabetes. Proceedings of the IX Congress of the International Diabetes Federation, p.464 (Excerpta Medica, Amsterdam 1977).

Pickup, J.C.; Keen, H.; Parsons, J.A. and Alberti, K.G.M.M.: Continuous subcutaneous insulin infusion: an approach to achieving normoglycemia. British Medical Journal 1: 204 (1978).

Pickup, M.E.: Clinical pharmacokinetics of prednisone and prednisolone. Clinical Pharmacokinetics 4: 111 (1979).

Pignard, P.: Dosage spectrophotometrique du N-N-Dimethyl biguanide dans le sang et l'urine. Annales de Biologie Clinique 20: 325 (1962).

Pinder, R.M.; Brogden, R.N.; Sawyer, P.R.; Speight, T.M. and Avery, G.S.: Fenfluramine: A review of its pharmacological properties and therapeutic efficacy in obesity. Drugs 10: 241 (1975).

Pirart, J.: Diabetes mellitus and its complications: A prospective study of 4400 patients observed between 1947 and 1973. Diabetic Care 1: 168 (1978).

Pittman, C.S.; Chambers, J.B., Jr. and Read, V.H.: The extrathyroidal conversion rate of thyroxine to triiodothyronine in normal man. Journal of Clinical Investigation 50: 1187 (1971).

Pittman, C.S.; Buck, M.S. and Chambers, J.B., Jr.: Urinary metabolites of ^{14}C-labelled thyronine in man. Journal of Clinical Investigation 51: 1759 (1972).

Podolsky, S. and Pattavina, C.G.: Hyperosmolar nonketotic diabetic coma: a complication of propranolol therapy. Metabolism 22: 685 (1973).

Porter, R.H.; Cox, B.G.; Heaney, D.; Hostetter, T.H.; Stinebaugh, B.J. and Suki, W.N.: Treatment of hypoparathyroid patients with chlorthalidone. New England Journal of Medicine 298: 577 (1978).

Posner, N.A.; Silverstone, F.A.; Tobin, E.H. and Breuer, J.: Changes in carbohydrate tolerance during long-term oral contraception. American Journal of Obstetrics and Gynecology 123: 119 (1975).

Raben, D.S.: Human growth hormone. Recent Progress in Hormone Research 15: 71 (1959).

Raben, M.S.: Growth hormone. Part 2: Clinical use of human growth hormone. New England Journal of Medicine 266: 82 (1962).

Raskin, P. and Unger, R.H.: Hyperglucagonemia and its suppression. Importance in the metabolic control of diabetes. New England Journal of Medicine 299: 433 (1978).

Refetoff, S.: Thyroid hormone therapy. Medical Clinics of North America 59: 1147 (1975).

Reidenberg, M.M.: Obesity and fasting-effects on drug metabolism and drug action in man. Clinical Pharmacology and

Therapeutics 22: 729 (1977).

Report of the Committee for the Assessment of Biometric Aspects of Controlled Trials of Hypoglycaemic Drugs. Journal of the American Medical Association 231: 583 (1975).

Rezvani, I. and DiGeorge, A.M.: Reassessment of the daily dose of oral thyroxine for replacement therapy in hypothyroid children. Journal of Pediatrics 90: 291 (1977).

Roe, D.A.: Nutrient toxicity with excessive intake. I: Vitamins. New York State Journal of Medicine 66: 689 (1966).

Rosenberg, I.N.: Thyroid storm. Pharmacology and Therapeutics Part C 1: 423 (1976).

Rubenfeld, S.; Silverman, V.E.; Welch, K.M.A.; Mallette, L.E. and Kohler, P.O.: Propranolol pharmacokinetics in thyrotoxicosis. Clinical Research 26: 295A (1978).

Sachs, H.S.; Shahshahani, M.; Kitabchi, A.E.; Fisher, J.N. and Young, R.T.: Similar responsiveness of diabetic ketoacidosis to low-dose insulin by intramuscular injection and albumin-free infusion. Annals of Internal Medicine 90: 36 (1979).

Saenger, P.; Rifkind, A.B. and New, M.I.: Changes in drug metabolism in children with thyroid disorders. Journal of Clinical Endocrinology and Metabolism 42: 155 (1976).

Santiago, J.F.; Clemens, A.H.; Clarke, W.L. and Kipnis, D.M.: Closed-loop and open-loop devices for blood glucose control in normal and diabetic subjects. Diabetes 28: 71 (1979).

Saraiva, R.A.; Lunn, J.N.; Mapleson, W.W.; Willis, B.A. and France, J.M.: Adiposity and the pharmacokinetics of halothane. The effect of adiposity on the maintenance of and recovery from halothane anaesthesia. Anaesthesia 32: 240 (1977).

Schaaf, M. and Payne, C.A.: Dystonic reactions to prochlorperazine in hypoparathyroidism. New England Journal of Medicine 275: 991 (1966).

Schafer, G.: Interaction of biguanides with mitochondrial and synthetic membranes. The role of phospholipids as natural binding sites. European Journal of Biochemistry 45: 57 (1974).

Schalm, S.W.; Summerskill, W.H.J. and Go, V.L.W.: Prednisone for chronic active liver disease: Pharmacokinetics, including conversion to prednisolone. Gastroenterology 72: 910 (1977).

Scharf, J.; Better, O.; Hemli, J. and Barzilai, D.: Tolbutamide and hypothyroidism. Lancet 1: 250 (1968).

Schein, P.S.; DeLellis, R.A.; Kahn, C.R.; Gorden, P. and Kraft, A.R.: Islet cell tumors: current concepts and management. Annals of Internal Medicine 79: 239 (1973).

Schneider, A.J. and Bennett, R.H.: Impaired absorption of insulin as a cause of insulin resistance. Diabetes 24 (Suppl. 2): 443 (1975).

Schor, S.: The University Group Diabetes Program: A statistician looks at mortality results. Journal of the American Medical Association 217: 1671 (1971).

Schou, M.: Lithium side effects and their treatment. Goitre/hyperthyroidism. Acta Psychiatrica Scandinavica Suppl. 243: 40 (1973).

Schwartz, S.N.; Pazin, G.J.; Lyon, J.A.; Ho, M. and Pasculle, A.W.: A controlled investigation of the pharmacokinetics of gentamicin and tobramycin in obese subjects. Journal of Infectious Diseases 138: 499 (1978).

Schwinn, G.; Dirks, H.; McIntosh, C. and Kobberling, J.: Metabolic and clinical studies on patients with acromegaly treated with bromocriptine over 22 months. European

Journal of Clinical Investigation 7: 101 (1977).

Scott, J. and Poffenbarger, P.L.: Pharmacogenetics of tolbutamide metabolism in humans. Diabetes 28: 41 (1979).

Selenkow, H.A.; Birnbaum, M.D. and Hollander, C.S.: Thyroid function and dysfunction during pregnancy. Clinical Obstetrics and Gynecology 16: 66 (1973).

Selenkow, H.A.: Antithyroid-thyroid therapy of thyrotoxicosis during pregnancy. Obstetrics and Gynecology 40: 117 (1972).

Selenkow, H.A. and Wool, M.S.: Thyroid hormones/Antithyroid drugs; in Rabinowitz and Myerson (Eds) Topics in Medicinal Chemistry, p.241, 273 (Wiley, New York 1967).

Selenkow, H.A. and Rose, L.I.: Comparative clinical pharmacology of thyroid hormones. Pharmacology and Therapeutics Part C 1: 331 (1976).

Selenkow, H.A.: Physiologic precepts for evaluation of thyroid function tests; in Rose and Levine (Eds) New Concepts in Endocrinology and Metabolism (Grune and Stratton, New York 1977).

Self, T.; Weisburst, M.; Wooten, E.; Straughn, A. and Oliver, J.: Warfarin-induced hypoprothrombinaemia: Potentiation by hyperthyroidism. Journal of the American Medical Association 231: 1165 (1975).

Seltzer, H.: Drug-induced hypoglycaemia: A review based on 473 cases. Diabetes 21: 955 (1972).

Shapiro, A.P.; Benedek, T.G. and Small, J.L.: Effect of thiazides on carbohydrate metabolism in patients with hypertension. New England Journal of Medicine 265: 1028 (1960).

Shen, S-W. and Bressler, R.: Clinical pharmacology of oral antidiabetic agents. New England Journal of Medicine 296: 493 (1977a).

Shen, S-W. and Bressler, R.: Clinical pharmacology of oral antidiabetic agents. New England Journal of Medicine 296: 787 (1977b).

Shenfield, G.M.; Thompson, J. and Horn, D.B.: Plasma and urinary digoxin in thyroid dysfunction. European Journal of Clinical Pharmacology 12: 437 (1977).

Shepherd, M.M.: British standard insulin syringe. British Medical Journal 1: 1140 (1978).

Shipp, J.C.; Cunningham, R.W.; Russell, R.O. and Marble, A.: Insulin resistance: clinical features, natural course, and effects of adrenal steroid treatment. Medicine 44: 165 (1965).

Skinner, D.J. and Misbin, E.I.: Uses of propranolol. New England Journal of Medicine 293: 1205 (1975).

Sølvsteen, P.; Vestergaard, V. and Hansen, E.L.: Diabetic coma without ketoacidosis. Acta Medica Scandinavica 184: 83 (1968).

Speight, T.M. and Avery, G.S.: Pizotifen (BC-105): A review of its pharmacological properties and its therapeutic efficacy in vascular headaches. Drugs 3: 159 (1972).

Spellacy, W.N.: A review of carbohydrate metabolism and oral contraceptives. American Journal of Obstetrics and Gynecology 104: 448 (1969).

Spellacy, W.N.: Metabolic effects of oral contraceptives. Clinical Obstetrics and Gynecology 17: 53 (1974).

Spellacy, W.N.: Carbohydrate metabolism in male infertility and female fertility-control patients. Fertility and Sterility 27: 1132 (1976).

Spellacy, W.N.; McLeod, A.G. and Buhi, W.C. et al.: The effects of medroxyprogesterone acetate on carbohydrate metabolism: measurements of glucose, insulin, and growth hormone after twelve months' use. Fertility and Sterility 23: 239 (1972).

Spellacy, W.N.; Buhi, W.C. and Birk, S.A.: The effects of norgestrel on carbohydrate and lipid metabolism over one year. American Journal of Obstetrics and Gynecology 125: 984 (1976).

Spellacy, W.N.; Buhi, W.C. and Birk, S.A.: Three-year prospective study of carbohydrate metabolism in women using Ovulen. Southern Medical Journal 70: 1188 (1977a).

Spellacy, W.N.; Newton, R.E.; Buhi, W.C. and Birk, S.A.: The effects of a 'low-estrogen' oral contraceptive on carbohydrate metabolism during six months of treatment: A preliminary report of blood glucose and plasma insulin values. Fertility and Sterility 28: 885 (1977b).

Spiro, R.G.: Search for a biochemical basis of diabetic microangiopathy. Diabetologia 12: 1 (1976).

Steel, J.M. and Briggs, M.: Withdrawal depression in obese patients after fenfluramine treatment. British Medical Journal 3: 26 (1972).

Steel, J.M. and Duncan, L.J.P.: Serious complications of oral contraception in insulin-dependent diabetics. Contraception 17: 291 (1978).

Sterling, K. and Chodos, R.B.: Radiothyroxine turnover studies in myxedema, thyrotoxicosis, and hypermetabolism without endocrine disease. Journal of Clinical Investigation 35: 806 (1956).

Sterz, von H.: Klinische Untersuchungen zur diuretischen Wirkung der Ethakrynsaure. Wiener Zeitschrift fur Innere Medizin 50: 34 (1969).

Stock, J.M.; Surks, M.I. and Oppenheimer, J.H.: Replacement dosage of L-thyroxine in hypothyroidism: A re-evaluation. New England Journal of Medicine 290: 529 (1974).

Stowers, J.M.: Endocrine and metabolic diseases. Modern approach to diabetes mellitus — II. British Medical Journal 1: 573 (1976).

Stowers, J.M. and Borthwick, L.J.: Oral hypoglycaemic drugs: Clinical pharmacology and therapeutic use. Drugs 14: 41 (1977).

Sutherland, H.W.; Stowers, J.M.; Cormack, I.D. and Bewsher, P.D.: Evaluation of chlorpropamide in chemical diabetes diagnosed during pregnancy. British Medical Journal 3: 9 (1973).

Swartz, S.L. and Dluhy, R.G.: Corticosteroids: Clinical pharmacology and therapeutic use. Drugs 16: 238 (1978).

Talbert, L.M.; Thomas, C.G.; Holt, W.A. and Rankin, P.: Hyperthyroidism during pregnancy. Obstetrics and Gynecology 36: 779 (1970).

Tasker, P.R.W. and Mitchell-Heggs, P.F.: Non-ketotic diabetic precoma associated with high-dose frusemide therapy. British Medical Journal 1: 626 (1976).

Taylor, J.A.: Pharmacokinetics and biotransformation of chlorpropamide in man. Clinical Pharmacology and Therapeutics 13: 710 (1972).

Tevaarwerk, G.J.M.; Malik, M.H. and Boyd, D.: Preliminary report on the use of propranolol in thyrotoxicosis: 1: Effect on serum thyroxine, triiodothyronine and reverse triiodothyronine concentrations. Canadian Medical Association Journal 119: 350 (1978).

Thomas, D.J.B.; Gill, B.; Brown, P. and Stubbs, W.A.: Salbutamol-induced diabetic ketoacidosis. British Medical Journal 2: 438 (1977).

Thorn, G.W.; Jenkins, D.; Laidlaw, J.C.; Goetz, F.C.; Dingman, J.F.; Arons, W.L.; Steeten, D.H.P. and McCracken, B.H.: Pharmacologic aspects of adrenocortical steroids and ACTH in man. New England Journal of Medicine 248: 284 (1953).

Toft, A.D.; Irvine, W.J.; Sinclair, I.; McIntosh, D.; Seth, J. and Cameron, E.H.D.: Thyroid function after surgical treatment of thyrotoxicosis. A report of 100 cases treated with propranolol before operation. New England Journal of Medicine 298: 643 (1978).

Unger, R.H. and Orci, L.: The essential role of glucagon in the pathogenesis of diabetes mellitus. Lancet 1: 14 (1975).

University Group Diabetes Program: A study of the effects of hypoglycaemic agents on vascular complications in patients with adult-onset diabetes. Diabetes 19(Suppl. 2): 747, 785 (1970).

University Group Diabetes Program: A study of the effects of hypoglycaemic agents on vascular complications in patients with adult-onset diabetes. V: Evaluation of phenformin therapy. Diabetes 24(Suppl. 1): 65 (1975).

University Group Diabetes Program: A study of the effects of hypoglycemic agents on vascular complications in patients with adult onset diabetes. VI. Supplementary reports on nonfatal events in patients treated with tolbutamide. Diabetes 25: 1129 (1976).

Uribe, M. and Go, V.L.W.: Corticosteroid pharmacokinetics in liver disease. Clinical Pharmacokinetics 4: 233 (1979).

Vagenakis, A.G.; Cote, R.; Miller, M.E.; Stohlman, F. and Braverman, L.E.: Enhancement of warfarin-induced hypoprothrombinemia by thyrotoxicosis. Johns Hopkins Medical Journal 131: 69 (1972).

Varadi, A. and Foldes, J.: Serum digoxin in patients with thyroid disease. British Medical Journal 2: 175 (1976).

Various Authors: The UGDP controversy. Journal of the American Medical Association 232: 806, 808, 813, 825, 853 (1975).

Vermeulen, A. and Comhaire, F.: Hormonal effects of an antiestrogen, tamoxifen, in normal and oligospermic men. Fertility and Sterility 29: 320 (1978).

Waal-Manning, H.J.: Metabolic effects of β-adrenoreceptor blockers. Drugs 11(Suppl. 1): 121 (1976).

Waal-Manning, H.J.: Can β-blockers be used in diabetic patients. Drugs 17: 157 (1979).

Wallace, R.B.; Sherman, B.M.; Bean, J.A. and Leeper, J.: Thyroid hormone use in patients with breast cancer. Absence of an association. Journal of the American Medical Association 239: 958 (1978).

Walsh, C.H. and O'Sullivan, D.J.: A study of the effect of frusemide on carbohydrate metabolism in diabetic subjects. Journal of the Irish Medical Association 67: 187 (1974).

Wass, J.A.H.; Thorner, M.O.; Morris, D.V.; Rees, L.H.; Mason, A.S.; Jones, A.E. and Besser, G.M.: Long-term treatment of acromegaly with bromocriptine. British Medical Journal 1: 875 (1977).

Waziri, R. and Nelson, J.: Lithium in diabetes mellitus: A paradoxical response. Journal of Clinical Psychiatry 39: 623 (1978).

Weinstein, L. and Meade, R.H.: Absorption and excretion of penicillin injected into the muscles of patients with diabetes mellitus. Nature 192: 987 (1961).

Weissman, P.N.; Shenkman, L. and Gregerman, R.I.: Chlorpropamide hyponatraemia: Drug-induced inappropriate antidiuretic hormone activity. New England Journal of Medicine 284: 65 (1971).

Wentworth, S.M.; Galloway, J.A.; Davidson, J.A.; Root, M.A.; Chance, R.E. and Haunz, E.A.: An update of results of the use of 'single peak' and 'single component' insulin in patients with complications of insulin therapy (Abstract). Diabetes 25: 326 (1976).

Wenzel, K.W. and Kirschsieper, H.E.: Aspects of the absorption of oral L-thyroxine in normal man. Metabolism 26: 1 (1977).

Whitehouse, F.W.; Arky, R.A.; Bell, D.I.; Lawrence, P.A. and Freinkel, N.: Policy statement. The UGDP controversy. Diabetes 28: 168 (1979).

Williams, G.H.; Dluhy, R.G. and Thorn, G.W.: Diseases of the Adrenal Cortex; in Thorn and others (Eds) Harrison's Principles of Internal Medicine, 8th Ed, p.520 (McGraw-Hill, New York 1977).

Williams, R.H.; Kay, G.A. and Jandorf, B.J.: Thiouracil. Its absorption, distribution and excretion. Journal of Clinical Investigation 23: 613 (1944).

Wingrave, S.J.; Kay, C.R. and Vessey, M.P.: Oral contraceptives and diabetes mellitus. British Medical Journal 1: 23 (1979).

Young, S.R.; Stoelting, R.K.; Peterson, C. and Madura, J.A.: Anesthetic biotransformation and renal function in obese patients during and after methoxyflurane or halothane anesthesia. Anesthesiology 42: 451 (1975).

Yue, D.K. and Turtle, J.R.: New forms of insulin and their use in the treatment of diabetes. Diabetes 26: 341 (1977).

Zimmerman, H.J.: Liver injury induced by chemicals and drugs; in Bockus (Ed) Gastroenterology, 3rd Ed, Vol III, Ch. 105, p.299 (Saunders, Philadelphia 1976).

Chapter XVII
Cardiovascular Diseases

J.G. Sloman and E. Manolas

Synopsis of Important Principles

1) Cardiovascular disease can modify the pharmacological response to a drug by altering its pharmacokinetics or by affecting tissue responsiveness. The disposition of many antiarrhythmic drugs is profoundly influenced by cardiac failure or low cardiac output states due to altered distribution and delayed hepatic or renal elimination.

2) Attempts to control coronary artery disease 'risk factors' will not necessarily reduce the risk of future attacks of myocardial infarction. Nor is there good evidence that atherosclerosis can be reversed once it has produced clinical manifestations.

3) In the absence of proof of benefit, the individual clinician must decide for himself whether to employ multiple preventive measures in an attempt to reduce mortality and morbidity in individual patients considered to be at 'high risk' of coronary heart disease.

4) Correction of precipitating causes is of primary importance in the treatment of angina pectoris and congestive heart failure. Other therapy is aimed at improving the quality of life.

5) Drug therapy in the early stages of acute myocardial infarction is directed at minimising the extent of myocardial damage, treating established left ventricular decompensation and preventing the occurrence of lethal arrhythmias. Prompt transfer to a coronary care unit gives the patient the best chance of survival.

6) The selection of an antiarrhythmic drug is largely empirical, but any drug chosen should be given an adequate trial before substituting or adding another agent.

7) Many factors increase the risk of toxicity to digitalis and include use of large loading doses, electrolyte and acid-base abnormalities, impaired renal function (digoxin), advancing age and small body size, hypoxia and certain types of heart disease. Dosage must be adjusted appropriately in each patient according to individual requirements and tolerance. Used in conjunction with available clinical information, estimation of plasma digitalis concentrations is a helpful guide to monitoring of therapy in special circumstances.

8) Some drugs can aggravate or precipitate heart failure (e.g. β-adrenoceptor blocking drugs, tricyclic antidepressants, phenylbutazone).

9) Many drugs can cause cardiovascular disorders, particularly disturbances of conduction and rhythm (e.g. antiarrhythmic drugs, sympathomimetic drugs, tricyclic antidepressants, thioridazine) or hypotension (e.g. guanethidine, prazosin, phenothiazines, tricyclic antidepressants). The cytotoxic drugs daunorubicin and doxorubicin (adriamycin) can cause cardiac failure by a direct action on the heart.

Patients with cardiovascular diseases present with symptoms due to circulatory insufficiency. This insufficiency may be due to a pathological process involving the heart and great blood vessels or the symptoms may be associated with pathological processes affecting the peripheral circulation. Drugs may be of value either as cardiac stimulants, directly increasing the cardiac efficiency or important in regulating the heart rate or rhythm. Drug therapy when employed in peripheral circulatory problems either causes dilatation of the blood vessels, or by a metabolic effect reduces the oxygen requirement in the peripheral tissue.

When considering the potential value of a drug for a cardiovascular condition, one must consider the drug concentration required to achieve the required pharmacological effect and this will always be influenced by the regional distribution of blood flow to various organs. Recent developments have emphasised the importance of variability in patient susceptibility and careful monitoring of the plasma concentrations of the cardioactive drug. Apart from variation in drug disposition between individual patients, variability in patient response to drugs can be due to alterations imposed by the pathological processes in cardiovascular disease.

1. Clinical Pharmacological Considerations

Cardiovascular disease can modify the pharmacological response to a drug by altering drug disposition (sections 1.2 to 1.5) or tissue responsiveness (section 1.6), thereby influencing the capacity of the heart and blood vessels to respond therapeutically and the probability that vital organs such as the brain and heart itself may react adversely.

1.1 General Considerations of Drug Pharmacokinetics in Cardiovascular Disease

The normally functioning cardiovascular system has an active role in the disposition of a drug, irrespective of its route of administration (Thomson, 1974). Absorption of an orally administered drug depends on gastrointestinal perfusion while intramuscular or subcutaneous administration depends on perfusion of the injection site for absorption. Intravenous administration avoids the uncertainties of absorption, but once absorbed, the cardiovascular system distributes the drug from the absorption site to organs or tissues where a pharmacological response may ensue. The circulation also delivers the drug to sites where metabolism and excretion occur and, as well, must support the processes involved in biotransformation and excretion.

Normally after intravenous administration, many drugs are initially distributed in proportion to the regional distribution of blood flow to various organs. There is, therefore, a tendency for organs that are highly perfused relative to their mass (e.g. heart, brain) to accumulate higher initial concentrations than other tissues. Later, there is a more uniform distribution of the drugs as circulating blood redistributes the agent from highly perfused tissues to other body tissues.

In heart failure, increased sympathetic nervous tone augments myocardial contractility and redistributes blood flow. The diminished organ perfusion results in redistribution of cardiac output; preserving flow to the heart and brain by decreasing perfusion to less vital vascular beds such as the kidney and musculoskeletal system. Blood flow may also be redistributed within organs such as the lung, liver and kidney (Benowitz and Meister, 1976; Thomson, 1974). Under conditions of decreased perfusion, a greater proportion of administered drug will initially be delivered to the heart and brain as a consequence of the increased percentage of cardiac output going to these vital organs. Toxicity may occur immediately following an initial intravenous dose if given too rapidly; as illustrated by CNS and cardiac toxicity with lignocaine (lidocaine). If vascular beds which normally participate in distribution of the drug are poorly perfused, uptake of the agent into these other tissues is delayed. This effects a smaller pool or volume of distribution and results in higher concentrations of the drug in the circulating blood. For this reason, the bolus or loading doses of drugs such as lignocaine and procainamide should be smaller.

Decreased perfusion may also result in either a diminished rate of delivery of the drug to its site of elimination, or impaired capacity of the liver or kidney to eliminate the drug. This results in a longer than normal half-life and a reduced plasma clearance of the drug. A reduced rate of elimination requires that the maintenance oral dosage or intravenous infusion rate be decreased (e.g. lignocaine, procainamide, quinidine, theophylline). Accumulation of pharmacologically active metabolites, particularly in patients with associated renal insufficiency, must also be considered (e.g. procainamide). Apart from redistribution of cardiac output, heart failure is often associated with increased pulmonary and systemic venous pressures. These pressure increases not only contribute to decreased organ perfusion, but may also result in congestion of vital organs and sodium and water retention. Secondary pathological changes such as hypoxaemia and acidosis may result from pulmonary oedema and tissue hypoperfusion.

All these disturbances have a potential to alter absorption and disposition of drugs (fig. 1), and for a number of commonly used drugs (e.g. lignocaine/lidocaine; procainamide; quinidine; theophylline) there is a clear need to modify dosage in the presence of advanced degrees of heart failure or other low cardiac output states such as shock or circulatory collapse. Variability among different patients and variable effects of the disease state make quantitative predictions for dose adjustment difficult, and measurement of plasma concentrations is required for monitoring of therapy (for review, see Benowitz and Meister, 1976).

1.2 Drug Absorption in Cardiovascular Disease

Drug absorption may be impaired in patients with low blood pressure and poor tissue perfusion; not only from the gastrointestinal tract, but also from intramuscular or subcutaneous injection sites. Decreased gastrointestinal motility and oedema of the intestinal mucosa may also contribute to impaired absorption of orally administered drugs in heart failure (Benet et al., 1976; Benowitz and Meister, 1976). An excess amount of drug might be absorbed from a given dose when the circulation improves.

After intramuscular injection, the rate of absorption of a particular drug is related to its physicochemical properties and to the characteristics of the injection site, including vascularity and blood flow (Greenblatt and Koch-Weser, 1976). Because heart failure may be associated with decreased blood flow to muscle tissue, absorption after intramuscular injection might proceed more slowly and more erratically; as proposed for procainamide (Koch-Weser, 1971).

The absorption of orally administered antiarrhythmic drugs (e.g. procainamide, mexiletine and aprindine) is very slow in patients with acute myocardial infarction (Hagemeijer, 1975; Koch-Weser, 1971; Pottage et al., 1978). There are a number of possible reasons: in particular, redistribution of blood flow from the gastrointestinal tract may interfere with uptake and narcotic analgesics used for pain relief may delay absorption by decreasing gastric emptying rate (see chapter VIII; sect. 2.3.1). Thus, if antiarrhythmic drugs are to be used for prophylaxis in the acute phase of myocardial infarction, oral administration must be avoided and the drug given intravenously, at least for the first 24 hours. Instances

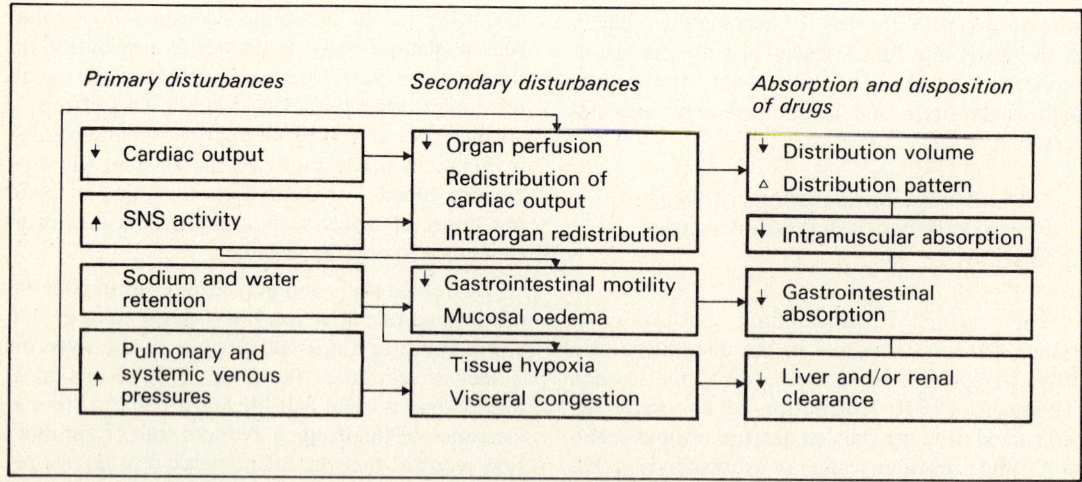

Fig. 1. Pathophysiology of cardiac failure and its potential effects on pharmacokinetics of drugs (after Benowitz and Meister: Clinical Pharmacokinetics 1: 389, 1976; by permission of author and editor).

of probable slow absorption of quinidine have been noted in patients with congestive heart failure (Bellet et al., 1971; Kessler et al., 1974). Digoxin absorption may also be delayed or reduced in some individuals with congestive heart failure (Benet et al., 1976; Benowitz and Meister, 1976). Absorption of the oral diuretic metolazone appears to be reduced in cardiac failure (Tilstone et al., 1974), but while absorption of oral frusemide (furosemide) is delayed the amount absorbed is unchanged compared with patients without heart failure (Benet et al., 1976).

The absorption of incompletely or poorly absorbed cardiovascular drugs such as digoxin and dicoumarol can also be influenced by concurrent administration of other drugs and by changes in gastrointestinal function (see table XIV; chapter XXIII, sect. 3.2.5). Cardioactive or vasoactive drugs that can change intestinal perfusion or oedema of the intestinal mucosa may also influence drug absorption (see chapter VI, sect. 5; VIII, sect. 2.3.1).

1.3 Drug Distribution in Cardiovascular Disease

The time of onset, intensity and duration of drug effect is determined by the kinetics of drug disposition and cardiovascular disease may influence regional tissue blood flow, cardiac output and the permeability of cell membranes to drugs. Changes in acid-base balance may alter uptake of drugs into cells, particularly if the pKa value of the drug is close to the blood pH of 7.4 (see chapter I; sect. 1.1). Thus, the tissue uptake and efficacy of a basic drug such as lignocaine (pKa 7.85) may be reduced in the presence of acidosis (Prescott, 1973).

An increase in total circulating proteins, with a slight decrease in concentration, is the usual finding in congestive heart failure (Seymour et al., 1942). Albumin concentration can be abnormally low in some individuals (Mokotoff et al., 1948). Whether such changes are of importance for use of highly albumin bound drugs in cardiac failure is not known.

Congestive heart failure and syndromes associated with low cardiac output can alter plasma drug concentrations by changes in drug distribution, hepatic metabolism and renal excretion (Benowitz and Meister, 1976). The volume of distribution of lignocaine, procainamide and quinidine is decreased in patients with cardiac failure,

presumably because of poor perfusion and reduced uptake of the drug by peripheral tissues. This decrease in the volume of distribution results in an increase in concentration of the drug in the plasma and adequately perfused tissues (see chapter I; sect. 2.1.2), and a decreased rate of elimination if hepatic (lignocaine) or renal (procainamide) blood flow is decreased.

The clearance of lignocaine is critically dependent on hepatic blood flow and in cardiac failure blood flow to the liver is reduced in proportion to the cardiac index (Stenson et al., 1971). Thus in patients with heart failure or other low cardiac output states, plasma concentrations of lignocaine are markedly increased when compared with normal subjects, due both to the decreased volume of distribution and the decreased rate of hepatic elimination (Thomson et al., 1973). Preservation of blood flow to the brain and heart in the presence of higher plasma concentrations of lignocaine, leads to an increased concentration of lignocaine in these organs shortly after administration, especially if the rate of administration is rapid. An increased incidence of CNS toxicity with lignocaine has occurred with use of excessive dosage in patients with congestive heart failure and syndromes associated with low cardiac output (Anderson and Pitt, 1969; Selden and Sasahara, 1967). Similarly, the plasma concentration of procainamide and quinidine is increased in patients with heart failure (Bellet et al., 1971; Koch-Weser, 1971), because of a decreased volume of distribution, and also because of delayed renal excretion (section 6.1.1 to 6.1.3). Toxicity to normal doses of procainamide and quinidine has occurred in patients with low cardiac output states (Koch-Weser and Klein, 1971; Thompson, 1956).

Patients with cardiac failure have higher plasma concentrations of thiopentone due to a decrease in adipose tissue distribution (Price et al., 1960). This may explain the observations of increased response to usual dosage of thiopentone in patients with heart failure and haemorrhagic shock.

1.4 Hepatic Metabolism in Cardiovascular Disease

Liver blood flow and hepatic microsomal drug metabolising capacity can be affected in patients with heart failure or myocardial infarction. Liver blood flow is decreased in patients with hypotension and cardiac failure and in states of shock or circulatory collapse and appears to change in proportion to cardiac index (Stenson et al., 1971). Decreased drug metabolising enzyme activity has also been demonstrated in congestive heart failure and in patients with myocardial infarction (Tokola et al., 1975; Prescott et al., 1976). Toxicity associated with high plasma concentrations of lignocaine may be largely due to decreased clearance because of reduced hepatic blood flow (see section 1.3). The plasma clearance of lignocaine is abnormally low even in patients with uncomplicated myocardial infarction (Prescott et al., 1976). Unless dosage is monitored appropriately the plasma concentration of lignocaine during continuous infusion may rise progressively to toxic levels in patients with severe cardiac failure and shock. Metabolism of lignocaine can virtually cease in patients with cardiogenic shock. Hepatic clearance of monoethylglycinexylidide (MEGX), the major pharmacologically active metabolite of lignocaine, may also be impaired in cardiac failure. CNS toxicity has been observed with lignocaine plasma concentrations in the therapeutic range, but with a markedly elevated MEGX concentration (Halkin et al., 1975a).

The clearance of propranolol is also dependent on liver blood flow. Since the β-adrenoceptor blocking effects of propranolol can result in reduced cardiac output, hepatic blood flow is decreased during administration of propranolol and the rate of hepatic elimination is reduced (Nies et al., 1976). Thus propranolol may not only decrease its own clearance but also the elimination of other drugs with a high hepatic extraction ratio, such as lignocaine (chapter VIII; sect. 2.3.5). Such haemodynamic interactions should be borne in mind in patients requiring acute intensive care with cardioactive drugs given intravenously, particularly those which influence cardiac output and the distribution of blood flow (e.g. vasopressor agents, potent diuretics, antiarrhythmic drugs).

Drugs which are dependent on hepatic microsomal drug metabolising activity for elimination are also subject to delayed clearance in patients with heart failure. Thus, clearance of theophylline is markedly decreased in patients with cardiac failure and pulmonary oedema (Piafsky et al., 1974) and toxic plasma concentrations are readily attained if initial dosage is excessive (Jenne et al., 1977). Clinical recovery is accompanied by increased clearance (Vozeh et al., 1978). Dosage of theophylline must be controlled by measurement of plasma concentrations in these patients.

1.5 Renal Excretion in Cardiovascular Disease

Cardiac failure may affect renal clearance of drugs by a number of mechanisms. Renal blood flow and glomerular filtration rate are decreased (Mokotoff et al., 1948), and there may be increased tubular reabsorption due to redistribution of intrarenal blood flow (Barger, 1966) and/or reduced urine flow. The decreased renal blood flow is correlated with the reduced cardiac output (Merrill, 1946).

Urea clearance, which is an index of both glomerular filtration and passive tubular reabsorption, may be a better predictor of clearance of certain drugs like digoxin than creatinine clearance (Halkin et al., 1975b), particularly since total clearance of digoxin in patients with severe cardiac failure is reduced beyond that which can be accounted for on the basis of reduced creatinine clearance (Benowitz and Meister, 1976). Clearance of digoxin increases with clinical improvement from overt heart failure and should obviously be considered when determining maintenance dosage (Meister et al., 1978). Procainamide is eliminated by both hepatic metabolism and renal excretion and in patients with impaired renal function due to cardiac disease, its plasma half-life is prolonged up to 2-fold compared with patients with normal renal function (Koch-Weser, 1971). Dosage of procainamide should be monitored closely to avoid accumulation (parent drug and active metabolite) and toxicity in these circumstances (sect. 6.1.2).

In patients recovering from open heart surgery, penicillin and cephaloridine, but not cephalothin, can accumulate to toxic concentrations in some patients (Benner, 1968). With improvement in cardiac output and renal function, cephaloridine and penicillin are cleared from the plasma at increased rates. Provided the antibiotic is given at the time of anaesthesia, concentrations in plasma are adequate during cardiopulmonary bypass (Williams and Steele, 1976), although for agents eliminated unchanged in the urine such as cephamandole half-life is prolonged and a supplemental dose may not be needed until the patient has been on bypass for at least 4 hours (Polk et al., 1978).

1.6 Altered Tissue Responsiveness in Cardiovascular Disease

The pathophysiological state of the heart in cardiovascular disease may also influence cardiac responsiveness to the pharmacological actions of the drug (Thomson, 1974). For example, the increased sensitivity to digitalis in acute myocardial infarction (Morrison and Killip, 1971a) and to warfarin in congestive heart failure (O'Reilly and Aggeler, 1970) and aggravation of left ventricular failure by β-adrenoceptor blocking drugs. Electrolyte and acid-base disturbances may also influence the response of a patient with cardiovascular disease to drugs. Potassium and magnesium depletion render the patient more sensitive to digitalis (Hoffman and Cranefield, 1964; Seller et al., 1970). Diuretics may lose their effectiveness in oedematous patients with severe congestive heart failure, as a consequence of electrolyte loss from previous diuretic therapy or development of secondary hyperaldosteronism. Cardiac and vascular responsiveness to endogenous and administered catecholamines such as noradrenaline (norepinephrine) is impaired in the presence of acidosis (Nash and Heath, 1967). In shock-like conditions, acidosis is very likely to occur and the full therapeutic benefit of noradrenaline may not be achieved until the acid-base disturbance is corrected.

2. General Principles of Treatment

1) *Prompt diagnosis and treatment:* Acute myocardial infarction must be diagnosed and treated as soon as it occurs. Prompt transfer to a coronary care unit probably offers the best chance of reducing mortality from infarction. Acute pulmonary oedema and acute pulmonary embolism are other examples of medical emergencies which must be diagnosed and treated promptly (see section 5.1; 8.2; 9).

2) *Remove the cause:* The first therapeutic approach in diseases such as angina pectoris, congestive heart failure and secondary hyperlipoproteinaemia is to search for and correct the precipitating causes (see sections 3.2.3; 4.1; 8.1).

3) *Individualised treatment:* In the treatment of cardiac arrhythmias, it is the patient who must be treated, not the electrocardiogram. Similarly, the dosage of antiarrhythmic drugs and digitalis must be adjusted according to individual requirements and tolerance, particularly factors which can modify the response to the drug. Plasma concentration estimations are a valuable aid to therapy with antiarrhythmic drugs and in some circum-

stances with digitalis, but are not intended to replace careful monitoring and follow-up of the patient's clinical status. Rigid adherence to a laboratory determination of what constitutes a therapeutic concentration, without evaluation of the clinical status of the patient is unwise. The aim of therapeutics is to treat the individual patient, not a plasma level (see section 6.1; 6.2; 6.3; 8.1.2; 8.1.5).

4) *Individualised judgement:* In the absence of proof of benefit from lipid lowering drugs in the prevention of coronary artery disease, the clinician must decide for himself whether to use these drugs as part of a multiple intervention approach in an individual patient considered to be at 'high risk' (see section 3.1).

5) *Review of therapy:* Heart failure may become poorly controlled because of a lessening effect of diuretics in the face of electrolyte loss or development of secondary hyperaldosteronism, or because of inadequate digitalis dosage or digitalis toxicity (see sections 8.3,10.1).

6) *Multiple drug therapy:* While concurrent use of more than one drug is often needed and of much benefit in cardiovascular therapy, adverse interaction between drugs can occasionally occur. Such adverse interactions can often be avoided or anticipated, but this requires familiarity with the pharmacokinetic properties and important therapeutic and toxic actions of each drug (see section 10.3).

3. Coronary Artery Disease

A clinical classification of the main manifestations of coronary artery disease is a help in clarifying the confusion that surrounds their treatment. Angina pectoris is generally regarded as the clinical expression of those pathological states which result in inadequate myocardial oxygenation, at rest or on exercise. Depending on the mode of presentation, angina pectoris can be subdivided into initial stable angina pectoris, progressive angina pectoris, and crescendo (or preinfarction) angina. The mechanism of the production of angina pectoris remains unclear. The clinician is therefore faced with the problem of treating a symptom complex, rather than a precise pathophysiological condition. Myocardial infarction is a clear cut clinical term reserved for the clinicopathological consequences of myocardial necrosis.

Glossary

Hyperlipidaemia: Excess cholesterol and/or triglyceride concentration in plasma.

Hyperlipoproteinaemia: Excess concentration of one or certain combinations of the lipoproteins that transport cholesterol or triglyceride in plasma.

Chylomicrons: The largest and lightest of the lipid transport particles, which serve to carry dietary (exogenous) triglycerides. The presence of chylomicrons in the fasting state, 12 to 16 hours after the last meal, is abnormal and indicates a defective handling of dietary fat.

VLDL: Very low density lipoproteins, which exist to transport triglyceride that is primarily synthesised in the liver (i.e. endogenous triglyceride).

LDL: Low density lipoproteins which normally are responsible for about a half to two thirds of the cholesterol in fasting plasma, and are probably mainly derived from VLDL degradation (catabolism).

HDL: High density lipoproteins. Like LDL they carry very little triglyceride, but about a quarter of the cholesterol in fasting plasma. High levels of HDL are associated with low rates of coronary artery disease (Gordon et al., 1977; Rhoads et al., 1976), a fact which was largely ignored until recently (Miller and Miller, 1975). HDL has a central role in lipoprotein and cholesterol metabolism and serves a carrier function clearing cholesterol from arterial tissues (Editorial, 1976; 1978).

Secondary hyperlipoproteinaemia: Elevations of lipoproteins which are secondary to various diseases.

Primary hyperlipoproteinaemia: All that is not secondary, often the result of a genetically determined disorder.

3.1 General Approach to Prophylaxis of Coronary Artery Disease

Much attention has been directed towards certain coronary heart disease 'risk factors' because of the apparent association between them and the development of coronary atheroma and generalised atherosclerosis (Stamler, 1973, 1978; Tibblin et al., 1975). However, it does not automatically follow that attempts to control 'risk factors' that predispose to the development of coronary artery disease, will reduce the risk of future attacks of myocardial infarction. Nor do the so-called 'risk factors' for coronary heart disease account for all heart attacks (Epstein, 1977). Moreover, once atherosclerosis has produced clinical manifestations, there is little evidence that the lesion can be reversed in man (Corday and Corday, 1975; Cohn et al., 1975). While it is not unreasonable to encourage widespread awareness in Western communities of the specific 'coronary risk factors' — overweight, tobacco smoking, high intake of dietary fats, especially of the saturated variety, hypertension, diabetes mellitus and physical inactivity — widespread active prophylaxis with dietary

manipulation and lipid lowering (section 3.2.4) or antiplatelet aggregating (see chapter XXIII; sect. 3.1) drugs, poses a difficult long term problem.

Until more data on the efficacy and safety of such preventive measures becomes available the practising clinician must decide for himself whether in an individual patient sufficient rationale for primary (prevention of first infarct) or secondary (prevention of reinfarction) intervention exists. In so doing, it would also seem reasonable to apply multiple intervention programmes, rather than single therapeutic manoeuvres (see Working Party, 1976; Kannel, 1974). Thus, general measures aimed at reducing the mortality and morbidity in patients considered to be 'high risk' persons, include control of hypertension and diabetes, maintenance of lean body weight and physical fitness, stopping cigarette smoking, and control of high blood cholesterol and trigylcerides.

3.2 Hyperlipidaemia and Coronary Heart Disease Risk

There is still no clear understanding of the basic nature of atherosclerosis and more particularly, of the relationships between atherosclerosis, coronary thrombosis and myocardial infarction. Although it is assumed that atherosclerosis has its beginnings in infancy and childhood, a clear understanding of the essential nature of the changes which lead to accelerated development of atherosclerosis and its complications in Western communities is still lacking. The various forms of genetic hyperlipoproteinaemias account for at the most, between 5 and 10% of a total Western population affected by atherosclerosis (Corday and Corday, 1975). Although figures vary, it is also likely that only about 25% of patients admitted to coronary care units have abnormal serum lipids, if examined adequately 2 to 3 months after an acute myocardial infarction (Scott, 1975). While there is an undoubted association between elevated cholesterol levels and the future risk of myocardial infarction in middle aged and older men (Kannel et al., 1971), a major reduction in morbidity and mortality from coronary heart disease cannot be anticipated if lowering of blood cholesterol levels in such individuals is the sole measure undertaken.

Whether control of blood lipid levels early in life would retard development of atherosclerosis in a Western population is an unresolved question although the extent of coronary atherosclerosis is related to the levels of circulating lipoproteins

Table I. Clinical considerations in the diagnosis and treatment of hyperlipoproteinaemia (summarised). After Levy and Rifkind (1973)

Type	Primary form		Secondary form	Some clinical features	Pre-mature vascular disease	Treatment[1]
	usual age of expression	familial forms				
I	Infancy and childhood	Rare and usually familial (recessive)	Disseminated lupus erythematosus Dysglobulinaemia Insulinopenic diabetes	Recurrent attacks of abdominal pain,? due to pancreatitis; hepatosplenomegaly; eruptive xanthomas; lipaemia retinalis	No	Diet[2] (low fat, 25 to 35g)
II	At birth, if genetic	Common IIa: Most obvious genetic form is expressed in heterozygote, more severe in homozygote; many mild examples are not obviously familial. IIb: Pattern alternates with IIa in families affected with 'monogenic' type II; milder defects are sporadic or due to other genetic defects	Hypothyroidism Obstructive jaundice Nephrotic syndrome Multiple myeloma Acute porphyria	Tendinous, cutaneous, ocular, arterial lipid deposits in familial forms. Mild IIb patterns tend to be accompanied by obesity, glucose intolerance	Yes	Diet[2] (low cholesterol, poly-unsaturated fat increased; restricted cal and CHO in IIb) + cholestyramine (or colestipol or probucol), sometimes with nicotinic acid as well
III	Third decade; often after menopause in women	Uncommon, frequently familial: genetic mode uncertain	Myxoedema Dysproteinaemia	Tuboeruptive, planar and less commonly tendon xanthomas; hyperuricaemia, obesity, glucose intolerance; worsened by alcohol excess	Yes	Diet[2] (low cholesterol), sometimes with clofibrate
IV	Usually third decade or later, can occur in children	Common, often half of adult close relatives will also have a type IV; number of mutants or frequency of familial involvement unknown	Nephrotic syndrome Glycogen storage disease Excess alcohol consumption Stress	Rarely eruptive xanthomas; excess caloric intake common; hyperuricaemia, obesity, glucose intolerance; worsened by alcohol excess	? Yes	Diet[2] (controlled cal, CHO; moderately restricted cholesterol), sometimes with clofibrate or nicotinic acid
V	Adulthood, very rare in children	Uncommon, when familial more than half of close relatives have either type IV or V	Alcoholism Insulin dependent diabetes Nephrosis	Similar to type I; many have severe sensory neuropathy; excess caloric intake common; obesity, hyperuricaemia, glucose intolerance, sometimes overt diabetes worsened by alcohol excess	No	Diet[2] (restricted fat, controlled CHO, moderately restricted cholesterol), sometimes with nicotinic acid, or norethisterone acetate in women or oxandrolone in men in patients who can not tolerate nicotinic acid

1 *In primary forms* drugs are only used when appropriate dietary treatment results in insufficient correction of hyperlipidaemia (i.e. as a supplement not a substitute for dietary control) or when dietary measures can not be adhered to.
   In secondary forms, Correction of lipid abnormality lies, where possible, in the treatment of the causative disorder.
2 See table III for precise details. Cal = calories; CHO = carbohydrate.

Table II. Translating hyperlipidaemia to main types of hyperlipoproteinaemia (summarised). After Levy and Rifkind (1973)

Step	1 (Detection of hyperlipidaemia)		2 (lipoprotein screening)		3 (when necessary)	
Type (incidence)	Choles-terol[1]	Trigly-ceride[2]	Appearance of plasma on cold storage[3] (chylomicron test)		Quantitation of LDL fractions[4]	
			top layer	infranatant	VLDL	LDL
I (rare)	↑	+++	Cream	Clear		
IIa (common)	↑	o	Nil	Clear		↑
IIb (common)	↑	+	Nil	Turbid	↑	↑
III (uncommon)	↑	+	Slight cream	Turbid	↑[5]	↑[5]
	↑	++	Slight cream	Turbid	↑[5]	↑[5]
IV (common)	↑	+	Nil	Turbid	↑	
	↑	++	Nil	Turbid	↑	
	o	high	Nil	Turbid	↑	
V (uncommon)	↑	++	Cream	Turbid[6]	↑	
	↑	+++	Cream	Turbid[6]	↑	

Note: For accurate diagnosis and appropriate treatment the above tests must always be interpreted in conjunction with clinical considerations. N.B. Exclude secondary cause of hyperlipidaemia.

1   Plasma cholesterol levels high (↑).
2   Plasma triglyceride levels increased + = 150 to 400mg/100ml; ++ = 400 to 1,000mg/100ml; +++ = > 1,000mg/100ml.
3   Fasting plasma allowed to stand overnight in an ordinary refrigerator — not a freezer.
4   Assistance required from a special laboratory. An adequate estimation of LDL is, however, obtainable from total cholesterol (C) and triglyceride (TG) values through the equation: LDL = C — (TG/5 + 45). ↑ = increased.
5   Abnormal composition (intermediate lipoprotein form).
6   If clear and patient a child or young adult, differentiate type V from type I by lipoprotein lipase test.

(Jenkins et al., 1978). Control of blood lipids can however, retard the development of, or lead to regression of disfiguring tendon and skin xanthomas and even xanthelasmas, in patients with genetic hyperlipoproteinaemias (Levy and Rifkind, 1973), but whether such measures also prevent the accelerated atherosclerosis in these individuals has yet to be proven. It is nevertheless logical to manipulate lipid levels in such families on this assumption (Glueck and Kwiterovich, 1978). Thus screening and prospective treatment of patients at risk is advocated rather than manipulating blood lipids in the population at large (Committee on Diet and Heart Disease, 1974). Measurement of high density lipoproteins (see glossary), high levels of which are associated with a low rate of coronary heart disease risk will probably improve the categorisation of an individual's risk. However, it is not yet known whether raising the high density lipoprotein level or the high:low density lipoprotein ratio will reduce the coronary heart disease risk in intervention programmes (Editorial, 1978).

3.2.1 Classification of the Various Types of Hyperlipoproteinaemia

Five patterns of lipoprotein increase account for the majority of hyperlipoproteinaemias (Fredrickson et al., 1967; Levy and Rifkind, 1973). Each may be the result of a primary, often genetically determined disorder, or secondary to various diseases (table I). The diagnosis of the type of hyperlipoproteinaemia can be made reasonably accurately with three tests available to most practising clinicians — the plasma cholesterol, plasma triglyceride and inspection of cold stored fasting plasma for chylomicrons (table II). A guide to the translation of primary hyperlipidaemia to hyperlipoproteinaemia is given in table II (Levy and Rifkind, 1973). Type I disease is rare, and types III and V rather uncommon; thus the great majority of patients exhibiting hyperlipidaemia in clinical practice will have type II or type IV. Type II (or IIa), as shown in table II, is characterised by a high serum cholesterol and normal triglyceride. It occurs with a genetic frequency of less than 5 %, yet, nearly half the Western male population in early middle age is hypercholesterolaemic (assuming a 'normal' value of 6.5mmol/L or 250mg/100ml). This discrepancy must surely reflect environmental causes, of which excess dietary cholesterol and animal fat are of major importance.

3.2.2 Screening of Patients for Hyperlipidaemia

On the basis of present knowledge persons who should be screened for hyperlipidaemia include:

1) Close relatives of those found or known to be hyperlipidaemic
2) Individuals with a strong family history of premature vascular disease, hyperlipidaemia or xanthomas
3) Patients with premature manifestations of atherosclerosis in any section of the arterial system
4) Patients with clinical manifestations suggesting hyperlipidaemia (e.g. xanthomas, xanthelasmas, premature corneal arcus etc)
5) Children (from age 1 year onwards), when both parents are suspected to come from families with inherited lipoprotein disorders
6) All patients under age 55 (especially men), when blood is being taken for another purpose.

Obvious hyperlipidaemia requiring strict management exists when values for cholesterol or trigylceride are well above 'normal' (generally regarded as about 6.5mmol/L or 250mg/100ml cholesterol and 1.7 to 2.3mmol/L or 150 to 200mg/100ml triglycerides). Such patients merit attention to their general health, family history and dietary habits. The younger the patient, the greater should be the attention to the abnormality. The decision on therapy lies between the clinician, the patient and his family. If therapy is deemed desirable, most patients can be managed by measures involving weight control, proper dietary change or reduced alcohol intake.

3.2.3 Treatment of Hyperlipidaemia

Primary and Secondary Hyperlipoproteinaemias: Before proceeding to treat hyperlipoproteinaemia, it is essential to exclude the possibility that the hyperlipidaemia is secondary to an underlying disease, in particular, hypothyroidism; obstructive jaundice; nephrotic syndrome; dysproteinaemia or poorly controlled diabetes mellitus sensitive to insulin. If hyperlipoproteinaemia is secondary, correction of the lipid abnormality lies, where possible, in the treatment of the causative disorder; if the disorder can be managed successfully the hyperlipidaemia should also be reduced or eliminated. When curative therapy is not available or when the disorder is primary and it is deemed necessary to reduce lipid levels, treatment directed towards the type of hyperlipoproteinaemia may be instituted (table III). Lipid lowering drugs (section 3.2.4) are used only when appropriate dietary treatment results in insufficient correction of hyperlipidaemia (i.e. as a supplement, not a substitute for dietary control) or when dietary measures can not be adhered to (Levy and Rifkind, 1973; Yeshurun and Gotto, 1976). The use of drugs with a different action and effect (see section 3.2.4) in combination is clinically more useful than single drugs alone in selected patients, especially those with increases in both cholesterol and triglycerides (Grundy and Mok, 1977) or those with more intractable familial disorders (Levy, 1976).

Primary Prevention of Coronary Heart Disease: Although diet and lipid lowering drugs have a place on their own merits in the management of primary hyperlipoproteinaemias, the question as to whether they have a place in the widespread primary prevention of coronary heart disease in the community, has still to be satisfactorily resolved (Ahrens, 1976; McMichael, 1977, 1979). In a major study, in middle aged and older men, a modest reduction in cholesterol concentrations by clofibrate was associated with a decreased incidence of non-fatal, but not fatal, myocardial infarction (WHO Trial, 1978). The reduction in non-fatal myocardial infarction was greatest in those with the highest concentrations and greatest reduction in serum cholesterol, particularly those who smoked and also had above average blood pressure levels. However, clofibrate was associated with an increased incidence of gall-stones and deaths from all causes, in particular cancer of the gall bladder, liver and intestines. A trend for increased non-car-

Table III. Summary of dietary treatment of hyperlipoproteinaemia (after Levy et al., 1972)

Factor	Type I	Type II	Type III[1]	Type IV[1]	Type V
Dietary prescription	Low-fat, 25 to 35g	Low cholesterol, polyunsaturated fat increased	Low cholesterol, approximately: 20% cal. protein 40% cal. fat 40% cal. CHO	Controlled CHO (approximately 40 to 45% calories); moderately restricted cholesterol	Restricted fat (30% calories), controlled CHO (50% calories), moderately restricted cholesterol
Calories	Not restricted	Not restricted, except in type IIb where weight reduction is often indicated	Achieve and maintain 'ideal' weight — reduction diet if necessary	Achieve and maintain 'ideal' weight — reduction diet if necessary	Achieve and maintain 'ideal' weight — reduction diet if necessary
Protein	Total protein intake not limited	Total protein intake not limited	High protein	Not limited other than control of patient's weight	High protein
Fat	Restricted to 25 to 35g; kind of fat not important	Saturated fat intake limited; polyunsaturated intake increased	Controlled to 40% to 45% calories (polyunsaturated fats recommended in preference to saturated fats)	Not limited other than control of patient's weight (polyunsaturated fats recommended in preference to saturated fats)	Restricted to 30% calories (polyunsaturated fats recommended in preference to saturated fats)
Cholesterol	Not restricted	Less than 300mg or as low as possible; only source of cholesterol is meat	Less than 300mg, only source of cholesterol is meat	Moderately restricted to 300 to 500mg	Moderately restricted to 300 to 500mg
Carbohydrates	Not restricted	Not restricted (may be controlled in type IIb)	Controlled; most concentrated sweets eliminated	Controlled; most concentrated sweets eliminated	Controlled; most concentrated sweets eliminated
Alcohol	Not recommended	May be used with discretion	Limited to 2 servings (substituted for carbohydrate)	Limited to 2 servings (substituted for carbohydrate)	Not recommended

1   Cal. = calories; CHO = carbohydrate.

diac deaths, including cancer, has also been observed in two other primary prevention trials using diets low in saturated fats and high in polyunsaturated fats (Dayton et al., 1969; Miettinen et al., 1972). In men, reduction of cholesterol concentrations by dietary intervention was associated with a decreased incidence of non-fatal but not fatal myocardial infarction in one study (Dayton et al., 1969) and of deaths from coronary artery disease in the other: benefit in women was inconclusive (Miettinen et al., 1972).

Some authorities therefore believe that lipid lowering measures should only be used as one feature of a multiple approach involving other risk factors in individual patients with a poor family history of atherosclerosis and coronary heart disease, even when blood lipid levels lie within the so-called normal range of a Western population (Scott, 1975). Their use in such a multiple intervention programme is however, based on the supposition that elevated blood lipids are a major factor intensifying the arterial reactions underlying atherosclerosis and coronary heart disease. The intensity of these reactions in individuals can not be measured at the present time, but it is a reasonable assumption that the intensity varies between one individual and another. Until the relative intensities of such reactions can be measured in individuals, it would seem logical to keep the stimuli at as low a level as possible.

Secondary Prevention of Coronary Heart Disease: There is even greater uncertainty regarding the widespread community use of diet or hypolipidaemic agents for secondary prevention of coronary heart disease in patients who have established coronary artery disease (Ahrens, 1976). Secondary prevention trials have produced no convincing information to support the hope that it would prove beneficial to administer a cholesterol lowering diet or a hypolipidaemic drug as a routine to all patients recovering from a myocardial infarction and thus prevent further attacks. The lowering of blood lipid levels by relatively small amounts does not significantly reduce morbidity and mortality from coronary heart disease. A trial in the United Kingdom (Newcastle) appeared to show a reduction in sudden deaths in patients with angina pectoris, but did not show an overall reduction in non-fatal infarcts amongst the patients taking clofibrate (Physicians of Newcastle Region, 1971). On the other hand, no sub-group in the American Coronary Drug Project Research Group trial showed a reduction in deaths amongst those taking clofibrate (Coronary Drug Project, 1975). A more recent study with colestipol did show a reduction in deaths from coronary artery disease in men, but not in women (Dorr et al., 1978). Results of studies of dietary intervention have not been convincing (Bierenbaum et al., 1973; Dayton et al., 1969).

Despite these inconclusive results, there nevertheless remains a duty for a clinician to assess the extent to which classical risk factors are present in an individual patient who has established coronary heart disease (Kannel, 1974). Thus, if it is deemed desirable to treat elevated blood pressure for example, the patient may not necessarily be protected against future myocardial infarction, although β-adrenoceptor blocking drugs seem to exert a protective effect on coronary heart disease in treated hypertensives (Berglund et al., 1978), but he will nevertheless be protected against other risks. Manipulation of elevated blood lipid levels by diet and/or drugs appears to be of benefit in those with multiple risk factors (WHO Trial, 1978). Although there are no definitive long term studies of multiple intervention measures, it does not mean that such an approach is illogical. Indeed, there is preliminary evidence that a combination of clofibrate and nicotinic acid together with dietary measures and management of other risk factors can decrease the incidence of non-fatal, but not fatal, reinfarction (Carlson et al., 1977). On the other hand, rigid adherence to the risk factor theory should not be at the expense of blinding other possibilities (Corday and Corday, 1975). The possible beneficial role of β-adrenoceptor blocking drugs (Green et al., 1977; Wilhelmsson et al., 1974) or antiplatelet aggregating agents (Sherry, 1978) also needs to be considered in individual patients (see section 5.2; chapter XXIII, sect. 3.1). The clinician must therefore decide for himself what approach he takes in an individual patient.

3.2.4 Drugs Used in Hyperlipoproteinaemia

Drugs reduce plasma lipid concentrations by decreasing plasma lipoprotein concentrations through mechanisms which either decrease lipoprotein production or increase lipoprotein clearance: a third possibility, the alteration in the distribution of lipoproteins between plasma and extravascular body compartments, may also occur (Levy and Rifkind, 1973). Figure 2 and table IV show a classification of the more commonly used hypolipidaemic drugs in terms of their effects on plasma lipoproteins. Such a classification is limited by the relatively few systematic studies which have been carried out on the effect of therapy on lipoprotein metabolism and must be regarded as tentative. For a review of the properties and indications for use of lipid lowering drugs, see Levy and Rifkind (1973) and Yeshurun and Gotto (1976).

Nicotinic Acid is an effective hypolipidaemic agent when administered in doses exceeding its daily requirements as a vitamin. Reduction in synthesis of VLDL results in a fall in level of triglycerides within 4 to 6 hours. A fall in VLDL levels results in subsequent decrease in LDL levels and there is also an immediate inhibitory effect on lipolysis of adipose tissue, resulting in a decrease in free fatty acid levels (Carlson et al., 1968; Langer and Levy, 1971). The ability of nicotinic acid to influence VLDL and LDL makes it an extremely useful drug in the treatment of hyperlipidaemia. It is chiefly used for type III, IV, V and may also be used in type IIb in combination with cholestyramine (Levy et al., 1972).

Nicotinic acid is rapidly absorbed after oral administration but with variability in time to peak plasma concentrations of 20 to 70 minutes. Elimination is rapid (half-life of around 45 minutes) and active uptake by the liver has been

demonstrated in the dog; these properties suggesting a high hepatic extraction ratio, thus low bioavailability and dependence on liver blood flow for elimination (see chapter I; sect. 3.3.3). About a third of a dose is eliminated as unchanged drug in the urine (see Gugler, 1978). The dose should be started low and gradually increased. For example, an initial dose of 100mg 3 times a day may be increased in a stepwise fashion by 300mg every 4 to 7 days up to 3 to 9g per day (in most patients the maintenance dose is 3g daily). Analogues of nicotinic acid (nicotinyl alcohol) and various esters of nicotinic acid, which are transformed in the body to nicotinic acid, and long acting forms of nicotinic acid, although more expensive than plain nicotinic acid, offer the advantage of a sustained effect. Sustained and gradual liberation of nicotinic acid is associated with a reduced incidence of flushing and free fatty acid level overshoot (initial prompt decrease at time of high peak plasma concentration of nicotinic acid, followed by an overshoot in FFA levels with rapid elimination of the drug; Carlson et al., 1968) due to a slower rise to lower longer lasting plasma concentrations of nicotinic acid (Gugler, 1978).

Side effects initially are mainly related to superficial vasodilatation producing cutaneous flushing and pruritus (usually in the upper part of the body) within 1 to 2 hours of the oral dose. This gradually diminishes after 1 to 2 weeks; however, many patients who have received the drug for a prolonged period have inexplicable episodes of flushing periodically. Gastrointestinal complications such as nausea, vomiting and diarrhoea are transient and are avoided if nicotinic acid is taken with meals. Other side effects include hepatotoxicity, glycosuria and hyperuricaemia. Therefore, caution should be exercised in use of nicotinic acid in patients with liver disease, diabetes or gout (similarly the increase in uric acid which accompanies type IV and V hyperlipidaemia may be aggravated). Periodic tests of liver function should be performed in all patients.

Clofibrate: This drug is a branched chain fatty acid ester effective in reducing elevated plasma triglyceride (VLDL) levels. The mechanism appears to be due to inhibition of production and/or release of VLDL by the liver. It is much less effective in reducing cholesterol and LDL levels. Clofibrate therapy (1.5 to 2.0g daily) is usually effective in type III hyperlipoproteinaemia, producing a considerable fall in lipid (triglyceride)

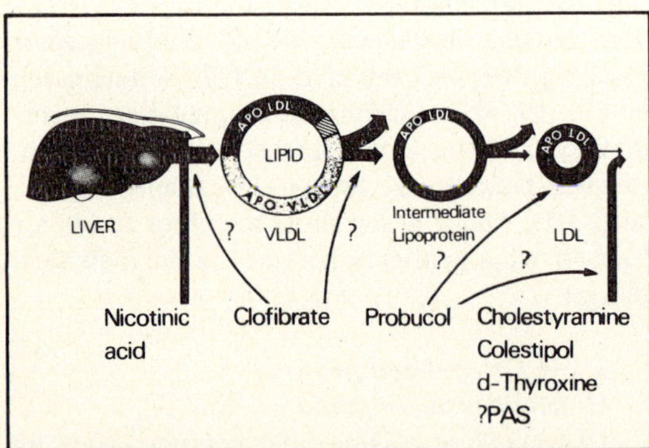

Fig. 2. Probable site of action of hypolipidaemic drugs (after Levy and Rifkind, 1973).
The hypolipidaemic drugs are classified according to whether they reduce production or increase removal of lipoproteins. Probucol may act by decreasing production of lipoproteins and/or impairing the intestinal mucosal transport of cholesterol. *Potentially useful drug combinations with complementary effects are apparent.*

Table IV. Principal side effects, and effect of commonly used hypolipidaemic drugs on lipoprotein metabolism and hyperlipoproteinaemia (after Levy and Rifkind, 1973; Gugler, 1978)

Drug	Effect on plasma lipoproteins[1]	Use[2]	Principal side effects
Cholestyramine	↓ LDL; may ↑ VLDL ↑ LDL catabolism	Type *IIa* ? IIb	Constipation, nausea; steatorrhoea
Clofibrate	↓ VLDL; effect on LDL variable	Types *III*, IV ? IIb	Nausea, diarrhoea; myositis; gall-stones; liver dysfunction; ventricular ectopy
Colestipol	↓ LDL; may ↑ VLDL ↑ LDL catabolism	Type IIa ? IIb	Constipation, nausea; steatorrhoea
Nicotinic acid	↓ VLDL; ↓ LDL; ↓ LDL synthesis	Types III, IV, V, IIb, II	Flush, pruritus; nausea, diarrhoea; glucose intolerance; hyperuricaemia; hepatotoxicity
Probucol	↓ LDL; effect on VLDL variable	Type IIa ? IIb	Diarrhoea

1   VLDL = very low density lipoproteins; LDL = low density lipoproteins.
2   Italicised copy = drug of choice.

levels. As expected from the limited effect of clofibrate on cholesterol and LDL levels, patients with type II usually show a disappointing response (Levy et al., 1972). The drug is generally held to be without effect in type I hyperlipoproteinaemia. Resolution of tuberoeruptive and planar xanthomas consistently accompanies the hypolipidaemic effects of therapy in type III patients. However, it is dependent on adequate diet control (caloric and carbohydrate restriction). Weight gain, for example, will result in worsening of lipid levels, despite clofibrate therapy in type III patients. Clofibrate may be useful in type IV patients unable to follow an appropriate diet, but is generally ineffective or produces an inadequate triglyceride fall in type V subjects (Levy and Rifkind, 1973).

Following oral administration, clofibrate undergoes hydrolysis, either in the gut lumen during absorption or during its first passage through the liver, to the active metabolite p-chlorophenoxyisobutyric acid (CPIB; clofibric acid). Absorption of clofibric acid is complete, but relatively slow with peak plasma concentrations being attained 2 to 6 hours after the dose. Clofibric acid has a low apparent volume of distribution (around 0.13L/kg) and is more than 90% bound to plasma albumin. Protein binding decreases with increasing total plasma concentrations and is also reduced in hypoalbuminaemic states such as the nephrotic syndrome, in renal failure and in cirrhosis. The rate of elimination of clofibric acid is subject to considerable interindividual variation, the elimination half-life ranging from 6 to 25 hours in patients with normal renal function, but being prolonged in patients with renal failure to between 29 and 113 hours, depending on the degree of renal impairment. The disposition of clofibric acid is altered in a number of disease states due to changes in protein binding and/or clearance of unbound drug (table V).

Clofibrate causes an increased incidence of side effects (muscle pain, malaise) in patients with impaired renal function and since clearance of unbound drug correlates with the serum creatinine concentration, dosage should be reduced accordingly (for guide, see chapter XXI; sect. 14.7). Normally, only about 10% of a dose of clofibrate is excreted in the urine as unchanged clofibric acid. The mechanism for the delayed plasma clearance in renal failure is not clear, but it appears that the glucuronide metabolite of clofibric acid accumulates to high concentrations and is constantly hydrolysed again to the active parent drug. Reduction of dose is not necessary in the nephrotic syndrome in the *absence* of impaired renal function, although the dosage interval may need to be decreased to avoid fluctuation in plasma concentrations (see chapter XXI; sect. 1.2). Dosage of clofibrate should be reduced by about a half in patients with cirrhosis. For a review of the pharmacokinetics of clofibrate, see Gugler (1978).

Clofibrate has been administered to many subjects for prolonged periods and has been found to produce relatively few and usually mild side-effects, although it increases the incidence of gall-stones and gall bladder disease (see chapter XIX; sect. 14.7). Long term use, as with cholesterol lowering diets, has also been associated with an increased incidence of mortality due to cancer, especially of the gastrointestinal tract and liver (see section 3.2.3). Gastrointestinal disturbances have been reported but may be no more frequent than during placebo therapy. Weight gain, drowsiness, weakness and giddiness are occasionally described and skin rashes, alopecia, decreased libido, and breast tenderness have been observed. Transient elevations of tests of liver function reported occasionally, are not regarded as indicating hepatic injury or contraindicating continued therapy. The significance of a puzzling increased incidence of non-fatal pulmonary embolism, angina pectoris, intermittent claudication and cardiac arrhythmias noted in the American Coronary Drug Project Research Group trial remains to be established (Coronary Drug Project, 1975). Myositis, reported occasionally, appears to be especially prone to occur in patients with impaired renal function (see above).

Subjects receiving anticoagulant therapy with coumarin or indanedione drugs also have reduced dosage requirements for these drugs when clofibrate therapy is introduced (Oliver et al., 1963; Rogen and Ferguson, 1963). It is recommended that the maintenance dose of the anticoagulants should be halved when clofibrate therapy is commenced and thereafter adjusted as the results of appropriate monitoring indicate. The early suggestion that the interaction is due to displacement of the coumarin drug from albumin binding sites can no longer be maintained. The most likely explanation is an increase in clotting factor catabolism (see chapter XXIII; sect. 3.2.5).

Cholestyramine: Cholestyramine is an ion-exchange resin that binds bile acids but acts as a lipid lowering drug by increasing the catabolism of LDL (Levy et al., 1972). It remains unchanged in the gastrointestinal tract and is unabsorbed. It is effective in type II hyperlipoproteinaemias but is ineffective, and in fact contraindicated in types III, IV and V, where it may actually boost triglyceride levels. Falls in cholesterol levels of about 15 to 25 % have been consistently obtained in various groups of type II subjects treated with 12 to 16g of cholestyramine daily (Levy and Rifkind, 1973). A single daily dose is as effective as a divided dosage regimen (Casdorph, 1975), although doses larger than 20g daily are likely to be more conveniently administered in a divided regimen. The main side effects are nausea and vomiting, abdominal cramps and distension and, most frequently, constipation. Constipation is especially liable to occur in elderly subjects, in whom the need for the drug is difficult to justify, and in predisposed individuals. It may be particularly troublesome in subjects with angina. Systemic toxicity appears to be rare with long term cholestyramine therapy and is attributable to its non-absorption. Steatorrhoea may become significant with doses > 30g daily. Cholestyramine is completely insoluble in water and is not absorbed to an appreciable extent

Table V. Effect of disease on the disposition of the active metabolite of clofibrate (clofibric acid). After Gugler (1978)

Disease	Plasma half-life	Plasma clearance		Steady state concentration	Distribution volume	Protein binding	Urinary excretion
		total drug	unbound drug				
Hyperlipidaemia	↑	o	o	↑	o	o	o
Nephrotic syndrome	↓↓	o	o	↓↓	o	↓↓	→
Renal failure	↑↑	↓	↓↓	↑↑	↑	↓	↓↓
Viral hepatitis	→	→	→	o	→	→	→
Liver cirrhosis	→	→	↓↓	o	↑	↓↓	→

→ = unchanged; ↑ = slightly increased; ↑↑ = markedly increased; ↓ = slightly decreased; ↓↓ = markedly decreased; o = no data available.

from the gastrointestinal tract. The binding properties of cholestyramine are not restricted to bile acids. As it is an anion exchange resin, cholestyramine may interfere with the absorption of any drug that is negatively charged, but also some other drugs. Such drugs, some of them in common use, are readily bound (Gallo et al., 1965) so that their absorption or enterohepatic circulation is interfered with. These include digoxin, digitoxin, warfarin and thyroxine. Any of these drugs should be administered at least 1 hour before a cholestyramine dose (thyroid drugs 4 to 5 hours before) and, where possible, their action should be appropriately monitored. In practice, it is wise to administer any other drugs at least 1 hour before the cholestyramine dose.

Colestipol is a bile sequestering polymer. It is an anion exchange resin and resembles cholestyramine in its properties and effectiveness. It is effective in reducing serum cholesterol levels with variable effects on triglyceride levels (Dujovne et al., 1974; Ryan et al., 1975). As with cholestyramine, it is not absorbed and interferes with the gastrointestinal absorption and enterohepatic circulation of other drugs. Other medication should also be given at least 1 hour before colestipol. Gastrointestinal side effects occur with a frequency similar to that seen with cholestyramine but its lack of odour and pleasant taste make colestipol more palatable. Usual dose is 4 to 5g 3 times a day, but can vary up to 25g daily.

Probucol is a lipophilic cholesterol lowering drug with a chemical structure and action which does not resemble that of any other cholesterol lowering agent (Heel et al., 1978a). It reduces serum cholesterol levels in most patients without a reduction in serum triglyceride levels (an effect similar to cholestyramine) and is thus primarily used in patients with type IIa hyperlipoproteinaemia. Reduction in serum cholesterol is not accompanied by reduction of liver cholesterol (unlike cholestyramine and colestipol) and may involve inhibition of lipoprotein formation and/or impaired intestinal mucosal transport of cholesterol. It appears to lower mainly LDL cholesterol levels. Usual dosage is 500g twice daily as tablets. Absorption appears to be limited and variable. During continued administration plasma concentrations increase gradually and a steady-state is reached only after 3 to 4 months. As expected, plasma concentrations decline very slowly after stopping the drug; by 60% after 6 weeks and by 80% after 6 months. Side effects are few, the most common being diarrhoea (around 10%). Other gastrointestinal symptoms have also been reported. Headaches, dizziness, paraesthesiae and eosinophilia have also been reported but their incidence is very small. The ease of administration and good tolerability of probucol compared with ion exchange resins may offer a considerable benefit in a group of patients in whom drug therapy once commenced is usually continued for a long time.

Other Lipid Lowering Drugs: β-Sitosterol is a plant sterol with a chemical structure similar to cholesterol. It appears to inhibit cholesterol absorption, presumably by increasing LDL clearance. It has been reported to significantly lower both the total cholesterol serum concentration and LDL concentration (Oster et al., 1976), but further evaluation is necessary to determine its usefulness. It is normally almost completely unabsorbed, but instances of significant absorption have been reported (Gugler, 1978).

Neomycin lowers cholesterol levels (by increasing bile acid and LDL clearance) in type II subjects (Samuel et al., 1970). However, the serious ototoxicity and nephrotoxicity that can be encountered during systemic neomycin administration, and the potential for emergence of multiresistant organisms (Valtonen et al., 1977), have engendered a cautious approach to its oral use over a prolonged period such as the management of primary hyperlipidaemia demands. It is not recommended for general use.

PAS is reported to be successful in lowering cholesterol and triglyceride levels (Vessby et al., 1978). Its mode of action is unclear and its gastrointestinal side effects detract from its long term use.

d-Thyroxine appears to exert its greatest effect in type II subjects and is used in a dose of 6mg daily. A major problem in the use of the drug is its cardiotoxicity (Coronary Drug Project, 1970) and it is not suitable for use in patients with coronary artery disease or arrhythmias. While it may be considered in younger patients without organic heart disease, a combination of clofibrate and nicotinic acid may also lower LDL and cholesterol levels in these subjects.

Three types of hormonal preparations have been tried. Oestrogens have little to offer in the management of hyperlipidaemia and may aggravate it. Norethisterone (norethindrone) acetate at a dose of 5mg daily may have a limited role in young women with type V hyperlipoprotein-aemia, such as in those who do not respond to clofibrate or who cannot tolerate nicotinic acid. The anabolic steroid, oxandrolone, has been reported to markedly lower serum triglyceride concentrations (Melmendier et al., 1978) and may be useful in male patients with type V hyperlipoprotein-aemia who cannot tolerate nicotinic acid. Retarded growth may occur in children by premature epiphyseal closure.

4. Angina Pectoris

When coronary artery disease causes an inadequate blood supply to the myocardium, symptoms develop. The classical manifestation of this inadequate blood supply is angina pectoris which occurs when oxygen consumption outstrips oxygen supply (Zelis et al., 1974).

The symptom complex tends to be episodic in nature and there are a number of terms used to describe various clinical syndromes of angina pectoris (Kay, 1977):

1) *Unstable angina:* Periods of change in the symptom complex:

a) Angina pectoris of recent onset either on effort or at rest.

b) Increasing frequency and severity of angina, including variant angina, in a patient with previously stable angina; the appearance of persistent angina at rest or nocturnal angina; new sites for radiation of pain or the association with new symptoms such as nausea or palpitations. The prognosis in this group is worse than in the group with recent onset of angina of effort (Plotnick, 1978).

2) *Stable angina:* Patients with stable but significant angina after the onset phase and with predictable precipitating factors.

3) *Crescendo angina:* Patients with increasing frequency and severity of attacks at rest and on exertion — a preinfarction state.

4) *Nocturnal angina:* Pain may occur with or without angina of effort — commonly due to left ventricular failure.

5) *Prinzmetal (variant) angina:* Due to coronary artery spasm. Typical ECG during attack of pain.

4.1 General Treatment of Angina of Recent Onset

The patient with recent onset of angina of effort may present within 24 hours to 6 weeks of the onset, which is often insidious. Such patients have a compromised coronary circulation and may be at risk of myocardial infarction or sudden death. Although the disease appears benign at this stage, the patient needs a period of time away from work and should have rest and relaxation. Activities which induce pain should be avoided and an anti-anxiety drug such as diazepam may be given.

Much can be done to control the underlying coronary sclerosis and reduce the number of anginal attacks (Kay, 1977; Sostman and Langou, 1978). Of first importance is the correction of obesity; weight reduction reduces cardiac work and may correct a previously abnormal blood lipid pattern (see section 3.1). Once the desired body weight has been achieved and maintained for about 2 months, serum lipids should be determined and if persistently excessive, can if deemed desirable, be treated appropriately (see section 3.2.3). After a suitable period of rest, gradual progressive physical activity should be actively encouraged in patients with stable angina.

Patients should be advised to cease smoking and instructed to avoid precipitating circumstances of angina when feasible. Patients with stable angina need to be guided towards a more relaxed style of life. Heavy meals should be avoided, as should emotional stress, sudden effort, strenuous arm activity, sudden changes in environmental temperature. Arrhythmias, hypertension, anaemia, gout, hyperthyroidism and other conditions which exacerbate angina pectoris should be sought and treated if present.

4.2 Treatment of Stable Angina

Following the onset phase there will be a group of patients with stable but significant angina who can be helped by drug therapy. Predictable precipitating factors will have been present over a period of months. The aim of long term treatment is to reduce the frequency and severity of anginal attacks, to conserve left ventricular function and prevent serious arrhythmias and sudden death due to myocardial infarction (Kay, 1977; Sostman and Langou, 1978).

In addition to relief of pain, an ideal antianginal drug would also improve exercise performance, decrease electrocardiographic evidence of myocardial ischaemia, prevent myocardial infarction and prolong life. No such agent yet exists. Anginal pain can be relieved by general measures, and by drugs that increase the threshold or alter the transmission of the pain (e.g. strong analgesics) or decrease the myocardial oxygen requirements (e.g. glyceryl trinitrate and β-blocking drugs).

4.2.1 Glyceryl Trinitrate

Glyceryl trinitrate (nitroglycerine) is the mainstay of drug treatment of angina pectoris in patients whose anginal episodes do not respond to cessation of the precipitating activity. Administered sublingually, glyceryl trinitrate acts in angina by two principal mechanisms (Kasparian et al., 1975; Zelis et al., 1974). Although it is unlikely that glyceryl trinitrate can dilate significantly sclerotic coronary arteries, it appears to be capable of inducing a dilator response in the non-ischaemic segment of collateral channels. While total myocardial blood flow does not increase there is an intramyocardial redistribution towards areas of ischaemia. Glyceryl trinitrate also acts peripherally and dilates systemic veins and to a lesser extent arterioles: left ventricular volume and pressure are reduced, leading to decreased intramyocardial wall tension and therefore myocardial oxygen requirements. Although glyceryl trinitrate does not directly increase heart rate or myocardial contractility, both may increase as a consequence of reflex changes.

Glyceryl trinitrate given sublingually is effective in 2 to 3 minutes, but its duration of action lasts for only 15 to 30 minutes due to avid and extensive hepatic first-pass metabolism (Needleman et al., 1972). Glyceryl trinitrate should be used to relieve the symptom that the patient recognises as his angina, when it does not subside promptly on cessation of the provoking circumstance. It can also be used prophylactically at the commencement of activity in anticipation of pain by those individuals who experience pain during the first minute or so of such activity (Aronow, 1972). Many of these patients can subsequently carry on at the same level of activity without recurrence. Only the patient can determine the dose required. Until this has been established the patient should start with a dose of 0.3mg. The sublingual tablet can be chewed or allowed to dissolve slowly, depending on the desired rapidity of action. The most rapid absorption through the buccal mucosa occurs after chewing. Glyceryl trinitrate can be repeated, using a larger dose, after 2 to 3 minutes. Glyceryl trinitrate loses its activity when incorrectly packaged, particularly when exposed to heat (Edelman et al., 1971). Patients should be instructed to keep their tablets in tightly stoppered glass containers and not to transfer them to polystyrene vials or pillboxes.

The patient should also be cautioned against standing still, since postural hypotension may result in syncope. This is more common in the elderly and if more than one dose is taken. Susceptibility to postural hypotension may be revealed by measuring the blood pressure lying and standing after a dose. If hypotension occurs, the patient should be instructed to sit or lie down when using glyceryl trinitrate.

Some patients prefer sublingual isosorbide dinitrate 5 to 10mg at the start of activity. Onset of action is somewhat slower, but there is no clear evidence that the effect on pain prevention is more prolonged. However, isosorbide dinitrate given orally in doses of 20 to 60mg exerts effects lasting up to 5 hours (Danahy et al., 1977). A chewable form of isosorbide combines rapid onset of action (3 to 5 minutes) with prolonged duration (3 hours), which makes this agent particularly useful in the prophylaxis of predictable anginal attacks (Mikulic et al., 1975).

Orally administered nitrates are pharmacologically active when given in high doses, which at least in part explains lack of demonstrable effect in early studies due to avid first-pass hepatic metabolism (Needleman et al., 1972). Orally administered sustained release glyceryl trinitrate in doses of 2.5 to 6.5mg twice daily is used by some for angina prophylaxis, the larger dose overcoming some of the loss of systemic drug due to hepatic first-pass metabolism. However, a more promising long acting preparation of glyceryl trinitrate is a 2% ointment, which is available in some countries. A measured amount is rubbed onto an area of thin skin (e.g. forearm or forehead) and absorption of the drug continues for some time. A consistent fall in myocardial oxygen consumption, systolic blood pressure and left ventricular ejection time for 3 to 4 hours after administration has been reported (Hardason et al., 1977; Franciosa et al., 1977). These effects were comparable with those of long acting oral nitrates. However, as with long acting oral nitrates (Zelis and Mason, 1969), tolerance may possibly occur with prolonged use of glyceryl trinitrate ointment and decrease the effect of the sublingual tablet.

The ointment would appear to be useful for nocturnal angina and other situations where a sustained prophylactic effect is desired. As with sublingual glyceryl trinitrate, headaches may occur shortly after administration. Sustained hypotension and vasodilatation can lead to salt and water retention as a result of renal underperfusion and should be recognised as a possible side effect, especially in those with poor left ventricular function or pre-existing venous insufficiency (Lee, 1978).

4.2.2 β-Adrenoceptor Blocking Drugs

Patients whose daily routine is significantly affected by angina pectoris, in spite of the use of glyceryl trinitrate, should be treated with a β-adrenoceptor blocking drug, provided there are no contraindications to its use (Warren et al., 1976; see chapter XVIII; table V). All patients can continue to take glyceryl trinitrate sublingually as required. β-Blocking drugs act in angina pectoris by decreasing heart rate, blood pressure and myocardial contractility on exercise, thereby diminishing myocardial oxygen consumption and increasing exercise tolerance (Prichard, 1974).

Small doses of a β-blocker should be used at the start of treatment (e.g. propranolol 20mg 4 times daily), increasing the dose every few days until the desired response is attained (e.g. resting heart rate under 70/min and no increase in heart rate on quiet walking). The effective therapeutic dose range of β-adrenoceptor blocking drugs in angina can vary widely. Individual variation in the metabolism of propranolol, metoprolol and alprenolol in particular causes large differences in the plasma concentrations attained after oral administration of the same dose to different patients (Vervloet et al., 1977; see section 6.1.5). For example, the effective dose of propranolol can range from 80mg to more than 2g daily, although most patients require around 160 to 320mg daily. The usual dose range with metoprolol is 150 to 300mg and with atenolol (a renally eliminated compound) 100mg daily is generally adequate. Other pharmacokinetic properties of the various β-blockers and circumstances requiring modification of usual dosage for particular compounds are discussed in chapter XVIII (sect. 5.6.6).

A combination of a β-adrenoceptor blocking drug and isosorbide is possibly synergistic, at least in providing relief of symptoms, and is worthwhile trying in patients who do not derive satisfactory symptomatic relief from a β-blocker alone

(Baxter and Lennox, 1977; Russek, 1967). Glyceryl trinitrate should continue to be taken as required. In patients with chronic obstructive airways disease, a cardioselective β-blocker such as metoprolol or atenolol can be used but cautiously (see chapter XVIII; sect. 5.6.8). Alternatively, verapamil, nifedipine or perhexiline (see section 4.2.3) may be employed. If angina pectoris remains intractable, coronary angiography is indicated, since myocardial revascularisation by saphenous vein bypass or internal mammary artery to coronary artery anastomosis may be possible (see also section 4.3).

Although specific β-adrenoceptor blockade has been shown to reduce the frequency and severity of ischaemic chest pain and improve exercise tolerance, the higher dose of β-blocker, particularly propranolol, which is required in some of these patients, may lead to symptomatic bradycardia. Such patients may benefit from simultaneous permanent transvenous pacemaker and β-blockade (Warren and Goldberg, 1976). An example would be a patient with intractable angina, severe atherosclerotic disease who is technically inoperable (e.g. poor run-off) in whom reduction of myocardial oxygen consumption becomes of primary concern.

If for any reason, β-adrenoceptor blocking drugs are discontinued in patients with severe angina pectoris, dosage reduction should be gradual. Abrupt withdrawal of propranolol in patients with advanced coronary artery disease and severe angina pectoris who received large doses (e.g. 160 to 320mg daily), may lead to recurrence of severe angina pectoris and even precipitate myocardial infarction or less commonly, sudden death (Miller et al., 1975; Mizgala and Counsell, 1976). The incidence of this so-called rebound phenomena varies in different reported series but may be of the order of 5 to 15%. If propranolol is reintroduced immediately following the increase in symptoms, the latter usually subside (Harrison and Alderman, 1976). Continuation of propranolol throughout coronary artery surgery does not necessarily complicate anaesthesia or the operative procedure and may well be less hazardous than withdrawal of propranolol 24 to 72 hours before surgery (Kopriva et al., 1978a,b; Slogoff et al., 1978).

4.2.3 Other Antianginal Drugs

There remains a small group of patients with severe angina in whom β-blockade is contraindicated or ineffective and coronary bypass grafting is not indicated. Drugs such as verapamil, perhexiline and nifedipine may be useful in these cases.

Verapamil, a calcium ion antagonist, initially developed for treatment of angina (Singh et al., 1978) and now used widely for reverting paroxysmal supraventricular tachycardias (see section 6.1.9), remains a useful drug in the angina patient in whom β-blockade may be contraindicated (e.g. patients with severe chronic obstructive airways disease). Its precise mode of action in relieving angina remains unclear, but like β-blocking drugs verapamil decreases myocardial demand for oxygen (Nayler and Szeto, 1972). Verapamil is nearly completely absorbed after oral administration but undergoes extensive first-pass metabolism in the liver, so that oral bioavailability is only about 10 to 20%; necessitating the use of large doses in angina.

Usual initial dosage is 40 to 80mg 8-hourly, which can be increased over 2 to 3 days to 120mg 8-hourly or a probable maximum of 720mg daily in patients without known contraindications (see section 6.1.9).

Perhexiline maleate appears to act as an antianginal agent by producing vasodilatation within the coronary and pulmonary vascular beds (its precise mode of action is not fully understood). There is a fall in ventricular work and consequently in myocardial oxygen consumption. Perhexiline is well absorbed after oral administration but is subject to large interindividual variation in its rate of metabolism by hydroxylation (Wright et al., 1973). Reversible peripheral neuropathy is a not uncommon side effect after some months of use of perhexiline (Fraser and Miller, 1978; Said, 1978) and occurs more readily in those who metabolise the drug slowly, in whom the parent drug tends to accumulate (Bousser et al., 1977; Singlas et al., 1978).

Other severe side effects associated with its prolonged use include hypoglycaemia, marked weight loss and liver damage resembling alcoholic hepatitis (in some cases fatal) which is associated with weight loss and also in most cases peripheral neuropathy (Paliard et al., 1978; Pessayre et al., 1979). The most common early side effect is dizziness and less often headache, nausea and vomiting. Ataxia, sometimes associated with raised intracranial pressure (Stephens et al., 1978); circumoral paraesthesiae and other central nervous system symptoms have also been reported with its use. Perhexiline is therefore limited for use in patients with intractable angina who are not suitable for coronary artery bypass surgery (Afzal Mir and Kafetzakis, 1978).

Usual recommended dosage is 100mg twice daily, increased to a maximum of 400mg daily. Clearly, dosage needs to be reduced in those who have an impaired ability to hydroxylate the drug.

Nifedipine is a newer antianginal agent. It is a potent calcium ion antagonist which results in relaxation of smooth muscle and vasodilatation, and reduces myocardial oxygen consumption. Its action as a coronary vasodilator is slower but probably more complete than that of nitrates (Ebner, 1976). Haemodynamic effects include a decrease in systolic blood pressure, increased coronary blood flow but no significant change in myocardial contractility. Heart rate and conduction velocity increase as a reflex β_1-adrenoceptor stimulant effect. Nifedipine significantly decreases the frequency of anginal attacks and the use of nitrates, and also produces a 15 to 60% reduction in the amount of ST segment depression in the electrocardiograph (Ebner, 1976). Nifedipine is almost completely absorbed following oral or sublingual administration, and is metabolised to inactive compounds before excretion in the urine (Horster, 1975; Schlossmann et al., 1975). It is highly bound to plasma proteins (greater than 90%). It may be administered orally (10 to 20mg daily), sublingually or intravenously.

The main adverse effect of nifedipine is related to vasodilatation producing flushing, headaches and postural hypotension. Severe ischaemic cardiac pain has also been noted in some patients shortly after the first dose or an increase in dosage (Jariwalla and Anderson, 1978; Rodger and Stewart, 1978); an effect which can occur with other vasodilators (see section 11.3). Mild gastrointestinal symptoms, tiredness and dizziness have also occurred. No adverse effects on respiratory, liver or renal function have been reported.

Further clinical evaluation of this drug is needed, but it may become a useful ancillary agent for treatment of intractable angina, inoperable cases or those awaiting surgery, and in Prinzmetal angina (Muller and Gunther, 1978).

4.2.4 Digitalis

Digitalis should be prescribed not as an antianginal agent but to those patients with myocardial failure, as shown by the clinical signs of congestive heart failure, nocturnal dyspnoea, or exertional dyspnoea. Whereas digitalis increases contractility and raises myocardial oxygen demands in patients without pump dysfunction, in those with heart failure it offers the potential for reducing overall myocardial oxygen requirements by decreasing myocardial wall tension (Mason et al., 1969). Digitalis is also indicated in atrial fibrillation and in most patients with cardiomegaly, and should be given a trial in patients with nocturnal angina. A diuretic should be used if signs of incipient heart failure persist following digitalis therapy. Some attacks of nocturnal angina can be prevented by either a long acting thiazide such as methyclothiazide or polythiazide in the morning or frusemide taken in the evening, at say 5pm. However, in many patients, nocturnal angina is associated with dreaming and a hypnotic such as nitrazepam or flurazepam is the best treatment. Hypertension is a proper indication for a diuretic. A diuretic should also be prescribed for those patients with a borderline blood pressure (150/90) but who show an abnormal rise (180 + /100 +) with exertion.

4.3 Crescendo Angina

This condition is characterised by an alteration in previously stable angina pectoris with an increase in frequency and/or duration of the anginal episodes, or with the appearance of new pain occurring at rest, including angina decubitus or nocturnal angina. The literature suggests that of those individuals presenting with 'crescendo angina' (depending of course upon the variable definitions of the syndrome), the majority have widespread coronary artery disease and between 10 and 30% will die within 6 months of the onset of the symptoms. Although some patients in this group have a more favourable outlook (e.g. recent onset chest pain) the overall risks of infarction and sudden death are sufficient to justify hospitalisation of all of these patients for observation in the coronary care unit. Aggravating or precipitating factors (e.g. heart failure, thyrotoxicosis or anaemia) should be corrected and a recent myocardial infarction excluded by serial enzyme studies and ECG's.

Medical treatment should include adequate patient rest (physical and emotional), the rational use of nitrates (e.g. glyceryl trinitrate sustained release tablets, isosorbide dinitrate or glyceryl trinitrate ointment) and β-blockers in adequate dosage (e.g. starting dose of propranolol of 40mg 3 times daily).

Some cardiologists advocate treatment with intravenous heparin (15,000 to 30,000 units daily) for at least 5 days, but its efficacy has not been proven.

In those patients whose pain does not subside within 24 to 48 hours, immediate coronary angiography is recommended with view to early surgery if a suitable anatomical situation exists. There is no doubt that coronary artery bypass surgery does improve quality of life (i.e. reduces incidence and severity of angina); however, definite proof of reduction of incidence of myocardial infarction or sudden death is lacking except for left main disease.

An occasional patient will suffer, at irregular and infrequent intervals, severe angina lasting up to an hour and occurring mainly at night, in the absence of a provoking factor. Glyceryl trinitrate may give partial relief after 2 or 3 doses. Between these attacks the patient is symptom-free and leads a normal life. To establish the diagnosis and to determine management, coronary angiography is essential.

If the patient persists in having disabling angina pectoris despite optimum medical management, so that the quality of his life is impaired, he should then have appropriate investigations to determine if he is a candidate for coronary artery saphenous vein bypass graft surgery.

4.4 Prinzmetal (variant) Angina

Prinzmetal angina is commonly regarded as being due to coronary artery spasm and may prove a diagnostic problem until the clinician can obtain a typical electrocardiogram during an attack of pain. However, with more experience of the condition, typical description of the pain, its episodic nature and absence of other demonstrable lesions, an accurate diagnosis may be reached. The pain may be relieved quickly by glyceryl trinitrate and the coronary artery spasm can be abolished (Higgins et al., 1976). This may be demonstrated by coronary angiography. However, some patients require morphine or equivalent for pain relief. The control of attacks by medical treatment such as vasodilator therapy with sublingual isosorbide nitrate, or β-blockers has not been particularly effective. Some success in control of symptoms has been claimed for nifedipine, a new vasodilator drug (see section 4.2.3). If the attacks of pain are frequent and severe, coronary angiography is indicated with a view to coronary bypass surgery in those patients with spasm complicating critical organic lesions.

5. Acute Myocardial Infarction

Acute myocardial infarction has its main impact on the function of the left ventricle. There is usually a decrease in cardiac output, stroke volume and systemic arterial pressure. The ejection fraction is decreased and the end diastolic pressure and the end diastolic volume in the left ventricle are elevated. Drug therapy used in the early stages of acute infarction is employed with the aim of minimising the extent of myocardial damage, treating established left ventricular decompensation and preventing the occurrence of lethal arrhythmias.

5.1 General Management

The mortality due to acute myocardial infarction is highest in the first 1 to 2 hours after the onset of the major symptom. If medical management is to reduce mortality, acute myocardial infarction must be diagnosed as soon as it occurs. Mortality can be reduced by the prompt recognition and treatment of ventricular arrhythmias. Prompt treatment in a coronary care unit probably offers the best chance of reducing mortality from infarction. Moreover, clinical experience has shown that patients are reassured by the knowledge that their heart rhythm is being watched continuously. The problems for the general practitioner in the management of acute myocardial infarction are thus 3-fold:

a) To decide whether infarction has occurred or is about to occur.
b) To relieve pain and anxiety, and to treat and prevent arrhythmias.
c) To ensure safe and rapid transfer of the patient to a coronary care unit.

5.1.1 Relief of Pain

Despite continued attempts to find a suitable non-narcotic analgesic for the relief of cardiac pain, morphine still appears to be the analgesic of choice in cardiac patients (Alderman et al., 1972; Lee et al., 1976). The amount of morphine required is variable. The initial dose of 5 to 15mg

intravenously may be repeated in 10 to 15 minutes if pain is not completely relieved. The most troublesome side effects of nausea and vomiting may be alleviated by the concomitant administration of an antiemetic such as metoclopramide or prochlorperazine.

In patients with hypotension who require continued analgesics, pentazocine may be a preferable alternative. It is best used intravenously, in a dose of either 45 or 90mg given slowly until the pain is relieved. Intramuscular administration is less effective but may have to be employed when there is intense vasoconstriction and it is not possible to insert an intravenous line. Pentazocine causes a rise in blood pressure in patients with myocardial infarction, and while it does not change cardiac output, a significant increase in pulmonary artery pressure has been noted in some studies (Jewitt et al., 1970; Lee et al., 1976), possibly because of altered left ventricular function or an increase in pulmonary vascular resistance. Nevertheless, because pentazocine is exempt from narcotic regulations, it is suitable for use by paramedical staff and mobile intensive care unit attendants, and such use in the very early prehospital management of the patient with acute infarction may outweigh its possible deleterious effect on left ventricular function.

5.1.2 Cardiac Arrhythmias

Two types of arrhythmia are characteristic of the early stage of acute myocardial infarction; ventricular arrhythmias (ventricular premature beats, ventricular tachycardia and ventricular fibrillation) and bradyarrhythmias, in which the ventricular rate falls to below 60 per minute.

Lignocaine (lidocaine) as a bolus injection given intravenously followed by a maintenance infusion (see section 6.1.3) is the drug of choice in the treatment and prevention of ventricular arrhythmias (Lie et al., 1974). As the setting up and monitoring of an intravenous drip may be impractical in the patient's home, an initial intravenous dose of 1mg/kg given over 2 to 3 minutes should be followed by an intramuscular dose of 250 or 300mg (10% solution). For ventricular arrhythmias resistant to lignocaine, procainamide 50mg/min intravenously to a total of 500mg is used. Because of the careful monitoring which is necessary with procainamide, this drug is not generally recommended for use outside hospital. The prophylactic administration of lignocaine in the absence of arrhythmia, is justified in patients transferred to hospital after a diagnosis of definite or possible cardiac infarction (Lie et al., 1977; Valentine et al., 1974). In this situation, 250 to 300mg lignocaine intramuscularly (10% solution) is advised (see further section 6.1.3).

Sinus bradycardia is common in the first hours after infarction. Although it often does not require treatment, a rate of less than 45 per minute can adversely influence cardiac output and allow 'escape' ventricular arrhythmias. In these patients, atropine 0.3 to 1mg intravenously will usually increase sinus rate and stabilise the circulation (Scheinman et al., 1975). Higher doses (1.2mg) may be effective in patients with high degree atrioventricular block and slow ventricular rate.

5.1.3 Shock

Cardiogenic shock carries a very poor prognosis despite energetic treatment. Catecholamines such as dopamine, dobutamine, adrenaline (epinephrine) and noradrenaline (norepinephrine) are widely used for their positive inotropic action and to provide circulatory support (see section 5.4). These drugs should be administered by an accurately metered power infusion pump. Frusemide (furosemide) relieves venous congestion, as well as being a powerful diuretic and can be used in high dosage — up to 500mg intravenously may be necessary to produce a diuresis. Care should be taken to administer the drug slowly. Ethacrynic acid is also effective and can be given in large intravenous doses to produce a diuresis. Vasodilators have been used as a method to contain infarct size and to improve haemodynamics and symptoms of refractory low output congestive heart failure (see further section 5.4).

5.1.4 Transfer to a Coronary Care Unit

Ideally, electrocardiographic monitoring and treatment of arrhythmias should begin in the patient's home as soon as the diagnosis of suspected myocardial infarction is made, but the necessary facilities may not be available in some centres. The patient should be kept under continuous observation until admitted to a coronary care unit.

5.2 Intensive Coronary Care

All patients with acute infarction may suffer a life threatening arrhythmia. Therefore, intensive coronary care should be available for all those patients presenting with a definite or suspected acute myocardial infarction. The concept of coronary care management starts with the stabilisation of the patient by the emergency ambulance team in the home or on the street. Pain should be relieved, oxygen administered and any rhythm disturbance controlled (see section 5.1). During transportation patients should receive oxygen and have their heart rhythm monitored. Where the rhythm diagnosis is difficult, the cardiogram should be transmitted to the parent coronary care unit for diagnosis and guidance. Prophylactic antiarrhythmic therapy with lignocaine has an important place in management (see section 5.1).

On arrival in the emergency area at the hospital a special admission procedure should apply so that 'patient delay' is minimised and the patient is taken at once to the coronary care unit without flurry or disturbance.

After a period in the coronary care area the patient may be transferred to a so-called 'step down' unit or second stage coronary area. This transfer may occur from 4 days to 10 days after admission, being decided on the basis of the clinical state of the patient and the development and control of any complications. Patients who are susceptible to late sudden death in hospital can be identified by some of the clinical manifestations seen while in the coronary care unit. Patients at increased risk have clinically severe, predominantly anterior infarction with clinical and radiological evidence of left ventricular failure, persistent sinus tachycardia and frequent ventricular arrhythmias. Certain factors are most important in identifying those patients at greatest risk. The major factors to consider are: age over 65 years, prolonged length of stay in the coronary care unit, the presence of a combined anterior and posterior infarction, the occurrence of secondary ventricular standstill while in the coronary care unit, right bundle branch block, supraventricular tachycardia or the recurrence of severe pain while in the unit. Patients with one or more of these adverse factors should have prolonged special observation in the coronary care unit and in addition, it is suggested that this observation be continued in a 'step down' type unit before return to the open ward.

Patients discharged from hospital after acute infarction appear to be at particular risk from sudden death for at least 1 year. In a group of 257 patients followed for 1 year after discharge from hospital, 29 (71%) of the total of 41 deaths occurred within 24 hours of the onset of a subsequent attack of severe chest pain. It is therefore suggested that the aim of preventing sudden dysrhythmic death in postinfarct patients after discharge from hospital remains valid. The search for a suitable long term antiarrhythmic drug continues. Preliminary studies with long term (12 to 24 months) prophylactic use of β-adrenoceptor blocking drugs in survivors of acute myocardial infarction have been promising (Green et al., 1975, 1977; Wilhelmsson et al., 1974). In the larger of these studies (over 3000 patients), a reduction in overall mortality and sudden deaths occurred particularly in patients in whom the original myocardial infarct was sited anteriorly and whose entry diastolic blood pressure was below the mean of about 78mm Hg. A combination of these characteristics resulted in the greatest difference in mortality (Green et al., 1975; 1977).

5.3 Management of Arrhythmias Occurring in Patients with Acute Myocardial Infarction

It is not possible to give a comprehensive description of the management of all arrhythmias occurring in patients with acute myocardial infarction. However, by the use of a simple classification of arrhythmias into those with a fatal outcome and those which are premonitory or warning in nature, one can gain an appreciation of the significance of rhythm disturbances in patients with infarction.

Cardiac arrhythmias may be slow or fast, intermittent or persistent, atrial or ventricular, and they may be associated with a normal relationship between atrial and ventricular contraction or on the other hand, this relationship may be severely disturbed. Almost invariably an arrhythmia has a disadvantageous effect on myocardial performance and therefore in patients with acute infarction their occurrence requires identification, classification and appropriate action.

Treatment of arrhythmias can be divided into three major categories and is discussed in section 6: (a) expectant; (b) drug therapy with antiarrhythmic drugs, and (c) electrical treatment (Julian and Oliver, 1968; Oliver and Julian, 1970).

Expectant treatment is often favoured when the patient is in good clinical condition and is being fully monitored in an intensive care cardiac unit.

Drug therapy may be used for example in a patient with premonitory arrhythmias, such as frequent multifocal ventricular ectopic beats in a patient with a myocardial infarction or a patient with frequent atrial ectopic beats and paroxysmal atrial fibrillation.

Electrical treatment can be further subdivided into the use of direct current countershock and of electrical pacemaking. Direct current countershock is used for the emergency treatment of patients with ventricular fibrillation or rapid ventricular tachycardia not responding to drug therapy. Electrical pacing is used for driving the atria or the ventricles when there is an inefficient slow heart rate, usually less than 55 beats per minute, or when overdrive of either the atrium or ventricle is used in order to suppress a recurrent atrial or ventricular arrhythmia.

When the patient with acute infarction is under intensive coronary care unit monitoring, the development of a warning or lethal arrhythmia should be treated specifically (section 6). However, under certain circumstances, a clinical cardiac arrest may occur outside the coronary care unit and diagnosis of the rhythm disturbance may not be immediately available. In such circumstances, the medical and nursing staff should institute an immediate, systematic approach to the problem. If a defibrillator is available and the patient has arrested, immediate *blind* defibrillation is used. If no defibrillator is at hand, then an effective circulation must be established using external cardiac compression, supplemented by emergency ventilation, initially with room air either from a bystander or from a breathing bag. As soon as feasible, oxygen should be used for ventilation. A sucker should be obtained and mucous secretions and solid material at the back of the throat should be immediately evacuated. If available, an electrocardiographic diagnosis may be helpful, but as soon as a defibrillator is available, a high output DC shock should be applied across the chest and the circulatory state reassessed.

In every patient sustaining a cardiac arrest, acidosis develops and it is recommended that sodium bicarbonate in a dose from 100 to 200mEq should be given initially and a further 50mEq administered during every additional 5 to 10 minutes of cardiac arrest.

When an efficient circulation has been re-established a bolus injection of an antiarrhythmic drug such as lignocaine (lidocaine), given intravenously in a dose of 1mg/kg body weight should be administered (Harrison, 1978). A continuous infusion of 4mg of lignocaine per minute should then be established for an hour and then reduced to 2-3mg/minute. Occasionally, supplementary intravenous bolus doses may be necessary before adequate plasma concentrations are attained with the continuous infusion. The dose schedule should be reduced by about half in patients with congestive heart failure, shock or liver disease (see also section 1; 6.1.3). Lignocaine is given for 24 to 36 hours after infarction or until the diagnosis of infarction is excluded in patients on the drug because of chest pain. Bradycardia should be treated with atropine sulphate and hypotension may be treated in the initial phase by the very cautious administration of a vasopressor drug. In general however, the fewer positive inotropic drugs administered the better as they all increase the myocardial oxygen requirement.

After recovery from cardiac arrest, the patient should be monitored in an intensive care ward so that any further complications whether they be cardiac, cerebral, respiratory or renal can be handled competently.

5.4 Cardiogenic Shock in Myocardial Infarction

In the WHO Technical Report Series No 441, cardiogenic shock is defined thus: 'shock in acute myocardial infarction is characterised by a marked fall of arterial blood pressure (systolic usually below 85mm Hg), cold, clammy, sweating skin, cyanosis, weak steady pulse, oliguria, mental confusion and sometimes coma. The signs correspond to acute circulatory failure with a very low cardiac output. Pulmonary congestion and elevated venous pressure when present, indicates heart failure. The term cardiogenic shock is used for such a condition'. This definition while not entirely comprehensive, covers most clinical presentations. Some of the mechanisms involved in cardiogenic shock are shown diagrammatically in figure 3.

The incidence of cardiogenic shock in acute infarction is difficult to assess because of the differing definitions. Our experience would suggest that approximately 12% of all patients admitted to a coronary care unit with acute infarction suffer from cardiogenic shock or pump perfusion failure. Dr H.J.C. Swan classified his patients with pump perfusion failure into four main groups based on bedside haemodynamic measurements. This division into four groups has merit because it gives a direct guide to the management of the patient.

a) *Low output syndrome* — characterised by a marked reduction in cardiac output and increased pulmonary vascular resistance. The blood pressure in this group may only be slightly depressed, or even maintained at normal levels, and the central venous pressure is often elevated.

b) *Low pulmonary vascular resistance syndrome* — with moderate reduction in cardiac output but severe hypotension; the pulmonary vascular resistance calculated to be low normal or normal, the central venous pressure is usually normal.

c) *Low central venous pressure syndrome* — characterised by relative or absolute hypovolaemia. The central venous pressure, cardiac output, and blood pressure are low, and pulmonary vascular resistance is variable.

d) *Mixed syndrome* — with various combinations of the above three groups.

5.4.1 Aim of Treatment
With this accurate haemodynamic information available, patients can be treated in a rational fashion. It has yet to be shown, however, that energetic treatment with a combination of drugs, mechanical devices and fluid adjustments, will lead to an improved early and late survival. Nothing can be done to save a necrotic myocardium, but other depressive factors and ischaemia can often be corrected. Severe acidosis may follow cardiac arrest and may precipitate cardiac power failure. This should be anticipated and corrected, preferably with concentrated bicarbonate solution. Excessive myocardial depression may be caused by antiarrhythmic agents; the drug should then be stopped. An overdose of a narcotic analgesic will occasionally need the specific antagonist.

Treatment should be directed at those mechanisms which reinforce causal factors. Severe hypotension, however may extend infarction and augment ischaemia and may need to be treated with a vasopressor drug or aortic balloon counterpulsation. The latter increased coronary perfusion pressure while reducing ventricular afterload. Pulmonary congestion and oedema will require a diuretic and oxygen in high concentration to maintain arterial oxygen control at a satisfactory level. Occasionally, positive pressure respiration will be desirable, if the arterial oxygen partial pressure falls below 60mm Hg.

These general principles can be applied in any hospital.

5.4.2 Counterpulsation
Aortic balloon counterpulsation is a new technique for mechanical left ventricular assistance. A

sausage shaped balloon at the end of a catheter is inserted into the femoral artery and advanced to the arch of the aorta. The balloon is inflated and deflated with each beat of the heart driven by an external pump which is timed with the patient's ECG. This technique is by far the simplest, safest and most effective method of mechanical cardiac assistance devised for long term (up to 3 weeks) use. It contrasts with the complexity of the present cardiopulmonary bypass systems which can not be continued for more than a few days.

5.4.3 Diuretics

Frusemide (furosemide) causes venous dilatation, and so relieves venous congestion as well as being a powerful diuretic. It has few side effects in patients with cardiogenic shock and can be used in very high dosage (up to 500mg intravenously), provided it is administered slowly. Ethacrynic acid is also a very useful diuretic in these patients.

5.4.4 Digitalis

Whilst some authorities consider that digitalis preparations should be avoided in patients with cardiogenic shock, at least until the acute phase has passed, others consider that treatment with digitalis is indicated in all patients with cardiogenic shock before the use of more radical forms of therapy such as assisted circulation or surgery (Karliner and Braunwald, 1972).

5.4.5 Vasopressor Drugs

Sympathomimetic amine vasopressors such as dopamine are widely used in the treatment of shock and hypotension, for their positive inotropic action and to provide circulatory support, and are combined with vasodilators in refractory congestive heart failure to improve left ventricular function and reduce myocardial ischaemia (Cohn and Franciosa, 1977; Mason, 1978).

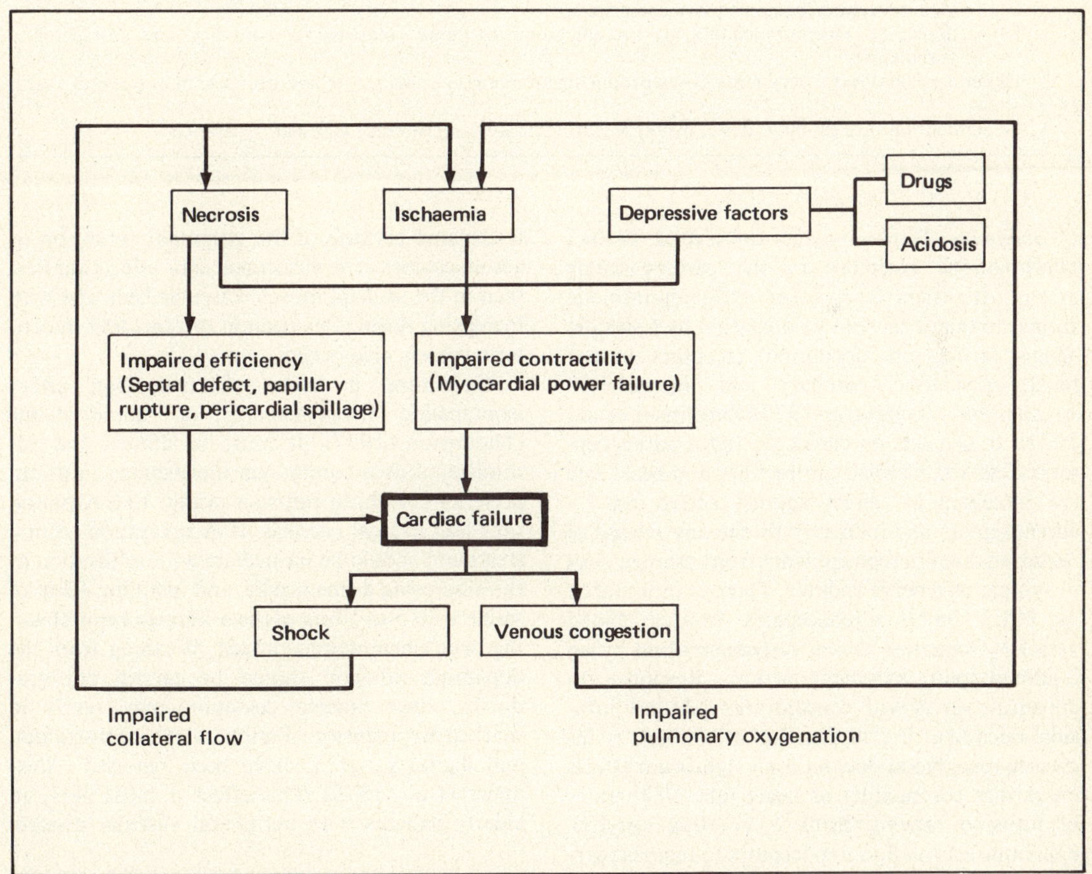

Fig. 3. Diagrammatic representation of some mechanisms involved in cardiogenic shock (after O'Rourke: Current Therapeutics 15: 31, May 1974; by permission of author and editor).

Table VI. Spectrum of activity (relative effects) of some catecholamines (after Goldberg and Hsieh, 1977; Sonnenblick et al., 1979)

Drug	Receptors stimulated[1]				Haemodynamic effects				
	β_1	β_2	α	Do	cardiac output	peripheral resistance	heart rate	renal blood flow	skeletal muscle blood flow
Isoprenaline (isoproterenol)	+	+			↑↑↑	↓↓↓	↑↑↑	↓,↔,↑	↑↑↑
Dobutamine	+	±	±		↑↑↑	↔,↓ [2]	↔,↑ [2]	↔,↑	↑
Dopamine	+		+	+	↑↑	↓,↔,↑ [3]	↑,↔,↓	↑↑↑	↓
Noradrenaline (norepinephrine)	+		+		↔,↑	↑↑↑	↔,↓	↓↓	↓↓

1 β_1 = β_1-adrenoceptor leading to cardiac stimulation (increase in contractility, heart rate, A-V conduction, cardiac excitability).
   β_2 = β_2-adrenoceptor leading to vasodilatation.
   α = α-adrenoceptor leading to vasoconstriction.
   Do = dopamine receptor leading to vasodilatation in renal, mesenteric, coronary and intracerebral vasculature.
2 Dependent on dosage, very large doses producing an increase in heart rate and decrease in peripheral vascular resistance.
3 Dependent on dosage, large doses producing an increase in peripheral vascular resistance.

Dopamine: Dopamine acts on several distinct catecholamine receptors in the cardiovascular system. It differs from other sympathomimetic amines in that it causes vasodilatation by a specific agonist action on 'dopamine' receptors in the renal, mesenteric, coronary and intracerebral vascular beds (Goldberg, 1977; Zarolinski et al., 1977). It also acts on classic β_1 and α-adrenoceptors (table VI). Cardiac contractility and heart rate are increased by direct agonist action on β_1-adrenoceptors and indirectly by causing release of noradrenaline (norepinephrine) from storage sites in sympathetic nerve endings. There is minimal or no effect on β_2-adrenoceptors (muscle blood vessels). Dopamine causes vasoconstriction by an α-adrenoceptor stimulant action. Response to dopamine varies with concentration. At low infusion rates (e.g. 0.5 to 2µg/kg/min) there is increased renal blood flow without significant effects on cardiac contractility or heart rate. With rates of infusion ranging from 2 to 10µg/kg/min, dopamine acts on β_1-adrenoceptors to increase cardiac contractility and cardiac output. With faster rates, about 10µg/kg/min, arterial blood pressure is elevated because of the stimulant action on α-adrenoceptors. The vasoconstrictor effects are first seen in the skeletal muscle vascular beds and with increasing doses, constriction of renal and mesenteric vessels also occurs.

Dopamine is more effective than either isoprenaline (isoproterenol) or noradrenaline (Thompson, 1977). It must be diluted and administered as a continuous intravenous infusion, preferably with an infusion pump. Extravasation may lead to local necrosis. If extravasation occurs, treatment should be immediate with infiltration of the area using a fine needle, and instilling 10ml of saline with 5 to 10mg of the α-adrenoceptor blocking drug phentolamine added. Weaning from the dopamine infusion should be carried out gradually, since sudden cessation may result in marked hypotension. Peripheral vasoconstriction and digital gangrene have been reported (Alexander et al., 1975). This effect is most likely in elderly patients with peripheral vascular disease.

Dobutamine is a synthetic derivative of dopamine which acts directly on the myocardium (not via release of noradrenaline) and has little chronotropic or peripheral vascular effect. It is an effective positive inotropic drug and because of comparatively little effect on heart rate and blood pressure (both major determinants of myocardial oxygen consumption) is of value in patients with a low output syndrome (Sonnenblick et al., 1979).

Isoprenaline is an agonist at both β_1 and β_2-adrenoceptors and acts to increase myocardial contractility and heart rate and to cause vasodilatation. Cardiac output is usually markedly increased but detrimental tachycardia and hypotension may occur in susceptible patients. Isoprenaline may be used with a dopamine infusion in suitable patients to minimise vasoconstriction whilst enhancing cardiac output. Conversely, vasodilatation induced by isoprenaline will be prevented by dopamine.

Adrenaline (epinephrine) and *noradrenaline* are other examples of vasopressors which have been used. Noradrenaline acts as an agonist on β_1-adrenoceptors in the heart and on α-adrenoceptors in the blood vessels. Accordingly, noradrenaline is more likely to increase blood pressure than other catecholamines. However, the intense vasoconstriction may result in ischaemic changes in skin, muscle, splanchnic and renal vascular beds.

Glucagon, which has been used in patients with cardiogenic shock, has similar theoretical disadvantages as isoprenaline and there are no studies suggesting greater benefit. Many positive inotropic drugs may have short term beneficial effects, but if myocardial functional damage is irreversible no inotropic drug is useful in the long term. Inotropic agents should not be used to flog needlessly a nearly dead heart.

5.4.6 Vasodilators

Recently, there has been considerable interest in vasodilator therapy in patients with myocardial infarction and low output states (Amsterdam et al., 1978). By reducing afterload, it was hoped that vasodilators such as glyceryl trinitrate, sodium nitroprusside and phentolamine would bring about a reduction in infarct size (Awan et al., 1976a,b). Vasodilator therapy is, however, only one of the methods used to contain infarct size (see section 5.5). In refractory low output congestive heart failure, especially in patients with increased peripheral resistance, vasodilators such as sodium nitroprusside may be more effective than vasopressor agents. The combination of dopamine and sodium nitroprusside usually produces a greater haemodynamic effect than either drug administered alone (Mikulic et al., 1977; Miller et al., 1977). Such therapy should only be carried out under close haemodynamic and electrocardiographic monitoring and is not recommended for use outside coronary care units.

5.5 Reduction of Infarct Size

Methods employed for reducing infarct size have included the use of vasodilators, β-adrenoceptor blocking drugs, hyaluronidase, and intra-aortic balloon pumping. During acute infarction there is an increase in the level of free catecholamines. Although this may represent an adequate physiological response it has potential deleterious effects, by enhancing the production of arrhythmias, increasing cardiac work, myocardial oxygen consumption and increasing infarct size. β-Adrenoceptor blockade may theoretically correct this (Singh, 1978b). The results of initial clinical trials were indefinite but all used low doses of propranolol. More recently, using propranolol 0.1mg/kg intravenously early after suspected myocardial infarction followed by 320mg orally over 27 hours, a decrease in the number of completed infarcts and a decrease in the extent of creatine kinase release has been reported (Norris et al., 1978).

Hyaluronidase, an enzyme that depolymerises mucopolysaccharides, decreases ischaemic injury following experimental acute myocardial infarction in the dog and rat. The presumed mechanism of action involves facilitation of active diffusion through poorly vascularised tissue, thus resulting in increased delivery of nutrients and also washout of potentially damaging metabolites. Because of experimental efficacy and low toxicity hyaluronidase has been tested in patients. Maroko et al. (1977) recorded a decrease in precordial ECG evidence of necrosis in 46 patients with acute myocardial infarction who received hyaluronidase for 48 hours, compared with 45 controls. A long term multicentre study of the effects of hyaluronidase in acute myocardial infarction is currently in progress.

Although glucose-insulin-potassium mixtures have been shown to have some success experimentally they have not been widely used. Intra-aortic balloon pumping may be used in patients with acute myocardial infarction to minimise the extent of infarction. Best results are achieved if pumping

Table VII. Direct electrophysiological effects and clinical application of the most commonly used and new antiarrhythmic drugs (after Singh, 1978a)

Drug	Auto-maticity	Conduction velocity	Refractory period	Clinical application
Quinidine	↓	↓	↑	Atrial and ventricular tachyarrhythmias, atrial fibrillation
Procainamide	↓	↓	↑	Atrial and ventricular tachyarrhythmias, atrial fibrillation
Lignocaine (lidocaine)	↓	– /↓	↓	Ventricular tachyarrhythmias, digitalis toxicity
Phenytoin (diphenylhydantoin)	↓	↑ /↓	↓	Refractory ventricular tachyarrhythmias, digitalis toxicity
Propranolol	↓	↓	↑	Catecholamine induced tachyarrhythmias, atrial and ventricular tachyarrhythmias, digitalis toxicity
Verapamil	↓	– /↓ *	– /↑	Paroxysmal supraventricular tachyarrhythmias
Disopyramide	↓	↓	↑	Ventricular and supraventricular tachyarrhythmias, atrial fibrillation
Mexiletine	– /↓	– /↓	– /↓	Ventricular tachyarrhythmias
Tocainide	– /↓	– /↓	↓	Ventricular tachyarrhythmias

↑ increased; ↓ decreased; – no change; – /↑ no change or slight increase; – /↓ no change or slight decrease.
* A-V conduction velocity is reduced.

is commenced early (within 6 hours) and is of most benefit in patients who continue to have pain immediately following infarction. This technique may be combined with drug therapy such as vasodilators and β-blockers.

5.6 Thromboembolism in Myocardial Infarction

Embolism, either in the lungs (section 9) or in the systemic vascular bed, is a complication of myocardial infarction responsible for a very small proportion of fatalities which occur after the first few days (Selzer, 1978). Deep leg vein thrombosis can be reduced after myocardial infarction by early ambulation. Thrombolytic agents do not add to the benefits of early treatment in a coronary care unit. Attitudes to the use of anticoagulants in acute myocardial infarction differ internationally (see chapter XXIII; sect. 4.1.3). In most American and British hospitals, anticoagulants are only used in 'poor risk' patients (e.g. after transmural infarc-tion in: those over 60, with prior infarction, large infarct, shock or congestive heart failure) and selectively or not at all for long term use following infarction.

Heparin may be given by intravenous infusion or more conveniently may be given subcutaneously in low doses (5,000u 8- or 12-hourly), and continued for 10 days or until the patient is fully ambulant. When the policy of early mobilisation is used, low dose heparin anticoagulation is the most convenient. In uncomplicated myocardial infarction, immobilisation for more than a few days is unjustified (Hayes et al., 1974; Medical Division, 1973). Rest should be advised only for patients with shock or pain.

6. Cardiac Arrhythmias

All cardiac arrhythmias influence the performance of the heart in an adverse fashion. When an arrhythmia complicates acute infarction, it is more likely to have severe consequences and the severity is closely related to the size of the infarction. Arrhythmias may be intermittent or sustained, may arise from atrial or ventricular foci and be associated with a slow or a rapid heart rate and may spread through the ventricular myocardium along either a normal or abnormal pathway. The major arrhythmias include the supraventricular and ventricular tachyarrhythmias (section 6.2) and manifestations of digitalis toxicity (section 6.3).

6.1 Drugs Used to Treat Cardiac Arrhythmias

The selection of antiarrhythmic agents in the clinical situation continues to be largely empirical. Correct and accurate identification of the arrhythmia from the surface electrocardiogram is important before therapy is commenced. However, long term ambulatory monitoring and electrophysiological studies may be necessary to provide an accurate diagnosis. Subsequent therapy should be based on careful observation of the haemodynamic consequences of the arrhythmia in the patient, a knowledge of the known pharmacological actions and pharmacokinetic properties of the antiarrhythmic agents, and familiarity with those agents which appear to be the most efffective with a given arrhythmia. The presence or absence of any underlying disease should also be considered prior to initiating antiarrhythmic treatment, particularly in relation to the need to modify usual dosage (for reviews, see Anderson et al., 1978; Mason et al., 1973).

No single drug is always successful in treating an arrhythmia, and the clinician should be familiar with alternative therapy which may be more successful when the primary drug selected does not achieve the desired results. Successful therapy of arrhythmias demands individualisation of drug dosage, which in turn requires a knowledge of how the dose to plasma concentration-therapeutic response relationship is altered by disease states, especially renal or hepatic disease and the degree of cardiac decompensation (see section 1; table IX, XI; Anderson et al., 1978; Harrison et al., 1977; Woosley and Shand, 1978).

Cardiac arrhythmias arise from abnormal patterns of automaticity and/or conduction and much information regarding these fundamental electrical properties of heart muscle has been gained through the study of cardiac cellular transmembrane potentials (Mason et al., 1973;

Singh, 1978a). It is highly reasonable to believe that antiarrhythmic agents derive their salutary actions from the electrophysiological effects they exert in normal cardiac tissue (table VII), although precise mechanisms of tachyarrhythmia termination are not definitely established in the majority of rhythm disorders in the diseased myocardium.

Dosage schedules of some commonly used antiarrhythmic drugs are given in table VIII.

6.1.1 Quinidine

Electrophysiological Properties: Quinidine reduces membrane responsiveness, decreases conduction velocity and prolongs the action potential (table VII). There is a prolongation of all ECG intervals; heart rate and AV nodal conduction are enhanced, effects mediated by a vagolytic action.

Pharmacokinetic Properties and Dosage: Oral quinidine is reasonably well absorbed and systemic bioavailability for quinidine gluconate and quinidine sulphate is relatively high, although bioavailability can vary widely (around 45 to 90%) between patients (Ueda et al., 1976). Quinidine gluconate is absorbed more slowly than the sulphate and may be associated with greater variability in steady-state plasma concentrations both within and between patients (Ochs et al., 1978a). Conventional quinidine sulphate preparations however, are not recommended because of rapid attainment of high peak serum concentrations and the attendant risk of development of unique ventricular tachycardia (quinidine syncope — usually torsades de pointes). Sustained release preparations of quinidine sulphate may overcome the high initial peak plasma concentrations and fluctuations in plasma concentrations (Eriksson et al., 1979).

Quinidine is metabolised in the liver to several compounds some of which have antiarrhythmic properties and are of clinical importance in patients with impaired renal function (Drayer et al., 1978). About 20% of a dose is excreted unchanged in the urine. Plasma concentrations of quinidine are increased in patients with cardiac failure, due to a decrease in distribution volume and plasma clearance; renal clearance being reduced by around a half (Conrad et al., 1977; Ueda and Dzindzio, 1978). Clearance of quinidine (hepatic and renal) is also reduced in the elderly; renal clearance of quinidine being decreased in accordance with reduced creatinine clearance (Ochs et al., 1978b). Dosage should be reduced and dose

Table VIII. Dosage schedules of some commonly used and new antiarrhythmic drugs

Drug	Route	Usual dose[1]
Quinidine	O or IM	0.5 to 2g daily in divided doses every 4 to 6 hours; or 2 or 3 sustained release tablets (250mg) twice daily
Procainamide	O or IM	6mg/kg every 3 hours; < 55kg — 250mgq3h; 55-90kg — 375mgq3h; > 90kg — 500mgq3h; or as 2 or 3 sustained release tablets (500mg) 8-hourly
	IV	As above. Rate: 25 to 50mg/min to total of 0.5g or continuous infusion at 2mg/kg/h
Lignocaine (lidocaine)	IM	250 to 300mg (10% solution)[2]
	IV	50 to 100mg bolus, plus additional small injections to 175mg (70kg man); then continuous infusion at 1.5 to 4mg/min, reduced by 30 to 50% after 12 to 24h[3]
Phenytoin (diphenylhydantoin)	O	200 to 400mg daily in 1 or 2 divided doses
	IV	25mg/min to total of 1g
Propranolol	O	40mg every 8 to 12 hours, increased as necessary
	IV	1 to 5mg in 1mg increments
Practolol[4]	IV	5mg slowly, repeated to a total of 20mg
Verapamil	O	120 to 160mg 2 or 3 times daily
	IV	1mg/min up to 10mg (rarely 15mg)
Disopyramide	O	300mg, then 100 to 150mg 6-hourly
	IV	1 to 2mg/kg bolus, then 0.4mg/kg/hour
Mexiletine	O	400 to 600mg, then 200 to 300mg 8-hourly
	IV	150 to 250mg bolus over 2 to 5 min, then 250mg infusion over 30 min, then 250mg in 2.5h and 500mg in 8h, followed by maintenance infusion of 500 to 1000mg over 24h[5]
Tocainide	O	400 to 600mg 2 or 3 times daily

1   In critically ill patients, plasma concentration estimations should be made early in treatment and dosage modified appropriately, particularly in presence of cardiac failure or low cardiac output states or diseases which may alter drug elimination or interpretation of plasma concentration values (see tables IX, XI, section 1, 6.1).
2   Prehospital prophylactic dosage in acute myocardial infarction (section 5.1.2).
3   See also text. For dosage schedule in acute myocardial infarction see section 5.3.
4   For intravenous use in acute coronary care units.
5   Tentative regimen only (see also text).

intervals increased when commencing therapy in the elderly or in patients with severe cardiac failure or impaired renal function. Subsequent dosage should be monitored by measurement of plasma drug concentrations (see section 1; table XI).

Therapeutic plasma concentrations are in the range of 3 to 6µg/ml (fig. 4a; table IX). Quinidine is about 80% protein bound (table X) and this binding is decreased in the presence of hypoalbuminaemia and in patients with cirrhosis (Kessler et al., 1974, 1978). Under these circumstances, the total drug concentration in plasma may decrease with an increase in the fraction of free or unbound pharmacologically active drug (see section 1.3), and the total plasma quinidine concentration therefore underestimates free quinidine concentrations. During maintenance therapy with quinidine, dosage may need to be reduced or dose intervals increased in patients with hypoalbuminaemia or cirrhosis.

Quinidine has a relatively short plasma half-life (3 to 16 hours; usually around 4 to 9 hours) and for long term use in the prevention of arrhythmias, sustained release oral preparations of quinidine gluconate or bisulphate are most useful as they permit maintenance of a desirable therapeutic plasma concentration on an 8 or 12-hourly dose regimen (Ochs et al., 1978a). Although intravenous quinidine can rapidly achieve therapeutic plasma concentrations, this route of administration can lead to severe hypotension and is *not* used.

Drug interactions with quinidine can be of potential clinical importance. By reducing cardiac output, propranolol can reduce hepatic blood flow and decrease clearance of quinidine causing a tendency to higher peak plasma concentrations with usual dosage; smaller doses of quinidine given more frequently might be indicated if such combined use was necessary (Kessler et al., 1978). Drugs which stimulate hepatic metabolism of quinidine (e.g. phenytoin, phenobarbitone) result in a clinically important reduction in quinidine plasma clearance and concentration. Plasma concentrations of quinidine can decrease to inadequate levels (Data et al., 1976). Interaction of quinidine with digoxin can also be important (see below).

Side Effects: The side effects of quinidine include nausea, vomiting, tinnitus or vertigo and idiosyncratic reactions with rash, fever, thrombocytopenia, hepatotoxicity and haemolytic anaemia. The most frequent serious side effects of quinidine are on the electrical properties of the heart. Plasma concentration of quinidine above 8mg/L may result in impaired conduction in the sinoatrial and atrioventricular nodes and the Purkinje system. Alternatively, ventricular ectopic beats leading to ventricular tachycardia (torsades de pointes) or ventricular fibrillation may occur and this may be refractory to usual treatment. Bretylium tosylate (section 6.1.6) has been tried successfully in a few patients (Vanderark et al., 1976). On the electrocardiogram the QRS duration correlates best with plasma concentrations of quinidine and the traditional approach is to decrease dosage if the QRS complex becomes prolonged to 50% or more of its predrug value. Because quinidine has a vagolytic action and enhances A-V conduction, digoxin should precede quinidine administration when the latter is used for treatment of supraventricular tachyarrhythmias (e.g. atrial flutter). However, a marked increase (up to 2-fold or more) of the plasma digoxin concentration with toxicity can occur in patients previously fully digitalised who were commenced on quinidine (Ejvinsson, 1978; Leahey et al., 1978). Where possible, the patient's plasma digoxin concentration should therefore be ascertained before commencement of quinidine therapy and after 1 or 2 days treatment. Appropriate alterations to digitalis treatment could then be made. It may well be that many of the so-called toxic effects of quinidine, particularly arrhythmias such as torsades de pointes, may in fact be manifestations of digitalis toxicity.

Clinical Use: Quinidine is used for the treatment of supraventricular and ventricular arrhythmias (e.g. to maintain sinus rhythm after reversion of atrial fibrillation or flutter), or long term treatment of ventricular ectopic beats or recurrent ventricular tachycardias.

6.1.2 Procainamide

Electrophysiological Properties: Procainamide diminishes automaticity, decreases conduction velocity, increases action potential duration and thus refractory period, and via a decrease in membrane responsiveness (table VII), increases refractory period in relation to action potential duration. Moreover, the mechanisms of action of procainamide in abolishing arrhythmias due to both disorders of impulse formation and conduction are identical to those of quinidine (Mason et

Table IX. Relation of plasma concentration to clinical effects of some of the commonly used and new antiarrhythmic drugs

Drug	Therapeutically effective concentration[1]	Toxic concentration	Notes	Principal adverse reactions[2]
Quinidine	3-6µg/ml (80% of responsive patients) > 6µg/ml (20% of responsive patients)	> 6-9µg/ml (occasionally) > 9µg/ml (usually)	Higher concentrations needed for atrial than ventricular arrhythmias	Gastrointestinal intolerance; skin rash, drug fever; tinnitus, neurological symptoms; thrombocytopenia; syncope (may be fatal), arrhythmias, heart block
Procainamide	4-8µg/ml (90% of responsive patients) 8-12µg/ml (a further 10% of patients)	> 8-12µg/ml (occasionally) > 12µg/ml (usually)	Ventricular arrhythmias occurring after myocardial infarction are usually suppressed at lower concentrations than in those with chronic coronary artery disease or other types of heart failure	Gastrointestinal intolerance; hypotension; lupus-like syndrome; arrhythmias, heart block
Lignocaine (lidocaine)	2-5µg/ml	> 5µg/ml	Knowledge of the plasma concentration is useful during sustained infusions, intramuscular use or prophylactic use	Progressive drowsiness, paraesthesiae, muscle twitching, disorientation, convulsions with progressively elevated plasma concentrations, bradycardia, conduction delays, cardiac depression (excessive doses)
Phenytoin (diphenylhydantoin)	10-20µg/ml	> 20-25µg/ml (occasionally)	About 85% of all ventricular arrhythmias which can be controlled by phenytoin respond to concentrations of between 10 and 20µg/ml	Nystagmus, ataxia, progressive drowsiness, lethargy (excessive doses); hypotension (too large or rapid IV dosage or presence severe cardiac decompensation); bradycardia, conduction delays, cardiac depression (excessive doses)
Propranolol[3]	75 to 100ng/ml[4]	?	Some patients with ventricular arrhythmias require greatly in excess of 100ng/ml. In others, exceeding 100ng/ml can be associated with recrudescence of arrhythmia	Bradycardia, aggravate heart block; heart failure (digitalise those with mild or latent cardiac insufficiency); bronchospasm (asthmatics); hypotension (IV)
Practolol[5]	1 to 3µg/ml[4]	?	No data available for arrhythmias; value given is β-blocking range	As above (propranolol). Less risk of bronchospasm and smaller reduction in cardiac output
Verapamil	?	?	80 to 100% of paroxysmal supraventricular tachycardia which will respond to verapamil, generally do so at a dose of under 10mg	Hypotension, bradycardia (particularly in those pretreated with β-blockers or with sick sinus syndrome); heart block, cardiac arrest (in presence poor myocardial function)

Disopyramide	3-6µg/ml	?	Higher concentrations needed to control ventricular than atrial arrhythmias	Cardiac depression (especially with rapid infusion); anticholinergic effects (blurred vision, urinary retention)
Mexiletine	0.75-2.5µg/ml	> 3µg/ml	Above 3µg/ml severe side effects occur frequently, but large overlap between toxic and therapeutic concentrations: some patients may tolerate and require up to 3µg/ml whereas toxicity can occur at concentrations of 1.5-3µg/ml in others	Bradycardia, hypotension, AV block (rapid IV injection, especially large doses); hand tremor, dizziness, blurred vision, progressive drowsiness, nystagmus, toxic confusional state (usually after IV administration but can occur after oral loading dosage or dose increases)
Tocainide	4-10µg/ml	> 10-15µg/ml (some patients)	Upper limit of therapeutic range and toxic concentration not yet well defined, some patients tolerating a concentration of 19µg/ml without side effects	Paraesthesiae, including hot and cold sensations; dizziness, sweats, tremor

1   Overlap exists between therapeutic and toxic concentrations (see fig. 4).
2   See text for details of cardiac disturbances (section 6.1, 10, 11).
3   Bioavailability of propranolol is low and plasma concentrations highly variable among patients after oral administration, as a consequence of individual differences in its hepatic metabolism (see section 6.1.5). Plasma concentrations after oral administration also vary much more widely than those after intravenous administration in the same subject.

4   While a relationship exists between plasma concentrations and effect in any given individual, there is some interindividual variation in the plasma concentration required to produce a given effect. Thus it is not possible to define values for a group of patients. Plasma concentration estimations are therefore only likely to be of use when desired concentration has been separately established in a particular patient.
5   For intravenous use in coronary care units.

al., 1973). Although many clinicians favour the use of procainamide for ventricular tachyarrhythmias and quinidine for rapid atrial disorders, with allowance for differences in dose, the effectiveness of the two drugs appears to be similar in either situation.

It is important to realise that the electrophysiological effects of procainamide and quinidine are additive. Therefore, the administration of procainamide after large doses of quinidine carries with it the same risk of 'toxicity' as would the administration of additional quinidine. By contrast, in certain conditions of potential or procainamide induced QRS prolongation, it may be useful to combine agents of the two different antiarrhythmic groups, for example phenytoin with procainamide.

Pharmacokinetic Properties and Dosage: Procainamide is generally well absorbed, but in occasional patients gastrointestinal absorption is quite incomplete, particularly in those with acute myocardial infarction (see section 1.1). The apparent volume of distribution is around 2L/kg but varies among normal individuals and is considerably decreased in patients with cardiac failure (Koch-Weser and Klein, 1971). Only about 15% of the drug is bound to plasma proteins. The elimination half-life of procainamide in subjects with normal cardiac, renal or liver function ranges from around 2 to 4 hours and averages 3 hours. Procainamide is mainly eliminated via the kidney, with about 50% of a dose excreted in the urine as unchanged drug. Glomerular filtration and active tubular secretion seem to be the most important mechanisms.

The major metabolite of procainamide, N-acetylprocainamide, is as active as the parent drug and accumulates in patients with impaired renal function. Because of accumulation of both unchanged drug and active metabolite, dosage reduction of procainamide should be anticipated in all patients with impaired renal function. About 7 to 34% of an oral dose is excreted in the urine as N-acetylprocainamide in normal subjects. The plasma concentration ratio of unchanged drug and acetylated metabolite formed after oral administration therefore varies greatly among patients and is genetically determined and bimodal (Karlsson, 1978). The extent of acetylation of procainamide also appears to be altered in patients with cardiac failure, chronic respiratory failure or liver disease but any clinical importance is not known (du

Souich and Erill, 1977, 1978); changes in overall clearance being of greatest importance (Koch-Weser and Klein, 1971). Drugs that diminish cardiac output (e.g. propranolol) and as a consequence renal blood flow, might also have an important effect on clearance of procainamide.

On any given dose, rapid acetylators have higher concentrations of N-acetylprocainamide and ratios of metabolite to unchanged drug in plasma than slow acetylators (Karlsson, 1978; Koch-Weser, 1977). Saturation of the acetylation mechanism in the gut wall and/or liver might also possibly occur, such that large oral doses of procainamide could result in slower clearance and unexpectedly higher plasma concentrations in slow acetylators (Tilstone et al., 1978; Lima et al., 1978). Acetylation phenotype also influences the development of the systemic lupus erythematosus-like reaction to procainamide (see below).

Cardiac failure has a marked effect on the absorption and disposition of procainamide (see section 1). Absorption of oral or intramuscularly administered drug may be slow and incomplete, particularly in patients with acute myocardial infarction. Combined with the short half-life of the drug, therapeutic plasma concentrations may never be attained. Because of its effect on renal function, clearance of procainamide is decreased and plasma concentrations markedly higher in patients with cardiac failure or low cardiac output states. Distribution volume is decreased (Koch-Weser, 1971; Lalka et al., 1978). These changes necessitate reduced dosage and a slower infusion rate when commencing therapy. It may also be necessary to reduce the dosage of oral maintenance therapy. Because accumulation of both procainamide and N-acetylprocainamide can be expected, monitoring of dosage by measurement of serum concentrations is required in patients with acute myocardial infarction.

Monitoring of serum concentrations of procainamide is in general valuable to individualise dosage, particularly when the pharmacokinetics of the drug are likely to be altered or when the clinical response to the drug is difficult to evaluate or appears to be unusual (see Koch-Weser, 1977). Like quinidine, the serum concentration of procainamide on any given dosage schedule varies widely in different individuals due to differences in pharmacokinetics and is difficult to predict in any given patient. Serum concentrations of between 4 and 10µg/ml are effective in eliminating arrhythmias in most patients and are not associated

Table X. Some pharmacokinetic properties of commonly used and new antiarrhythmic drugs[1]

Drug	Peak plasma concentration[2] (h)	Bioavailability (%)	Protein binding (%)	Distribution volume, steady-state (L/kg)	Elimination half-life (h)	Elimination[3]	Active metabolites of potential clinical importance[4]
Quinidine	1.5-2	40-90	80-90	2.1-2.6	3-16	Hepatic metabolism and some renal excretion of unchanged drug (20%)	Yes
Procainamide	1-2	75-90	15	1.7-2.2	2.2-4	Renal excretion of unchanged drug (45 to 65%) and active metabolite	Yes (major importance)
Lignocaine (lidocaine)	—	~30	70[6]	0.7-2.2[6] (1.7)	1-2[6]	Hepatic metabolism	Yes
Phenytoin (diphenylhydantoin)	4-8[5]	80-95[5]	89-91	0.5-0.8	8-60[6] (20-30)	Hepatic metabolism	No
Propranolol	1-2	~40	90-96	~4	3.5-6 (oral) 2-4 (IV)	Hepatic metabolism	Yes
Practolol[7]	—	—	<10	~1.6	9-12	Renal excretion of unchanged drug	—
Verapamil	1-2	10-20	~90	~6.5	3-7	Hepatic metabolism (metabolites exceed plasma concentration of parent drug)	?
Disopyramide	1-2	70-80	35-95[8]	0.6-1.3	4.4-8.2	Renal excretion of unchanged drug (50 to 60%)	No
Mexiletine	2-4	~90	~70	~10	~10	Hepatic metabolism and some renal excretion of unchanged drug (10 to 20%)	?
Tocainide	1-2	~100	~50	~1.4-1.6	12-15	Renal excretion of unchanged drug (20 to 70%) and hepatic metabolism	?

1   Many of these mean values or ranges in normal subjects can alter markedly in sick patients, particularly those with cardiac failure or low cardiac output states (see text and section 1).
2   Time taken in most normal subjects to attain peak plasma concentration after oral administration.
3   Predominant mechanism for elimination. Amount given in parentheses represents percentage of administered dose excreted unchanged in the urine.
4   Potential clinical importance in terms of contribution to therapeutic and/or toxic effects, particularly accumulation in patients with impaired renal function.
5   Expressed in terms of tablets with excellent dissolution and formulation characteristics. Bioavailability of phenytoin products can vary widely (see chapter VI).
6   Dose dependent (see text). Usual range given in parentheses.
7   For intravenous use in coronary care units.
8   Concentration dependent (see text).

with serious toxicity (fig. 4b; table IX). Major toxicity begins to appear above 8µg/ml, remains quite low up to 12µg/ml, but becomes progressively more frequent with higher concentrations (Koch-Weser, 1974, 1977).

In most patients it is possible to demonstrate a critical serum concentration for antiarrhythmic effectiveness and for the appearance of serious toxicity. To maintain the serum concentration within the therapeutic range, the drug should be administered every 3 to 4 hours. If therapy is begun with the maintenance dose, 4 to 5 doses are required to reach the equilibrium or steady-state concentration. When the clinical situation is urgent, a priming dose of twice the 3 hour maintenance dose or a quarter of the total daily dose should be given (table VIII). If therapeutic plasma concentrations are required in minutes, the priming dose should be given by slow intravenous infusion or in several intramuscular or intravenous injections. Sustained release tablets of procainamide have been developed to allow less frequent dosing

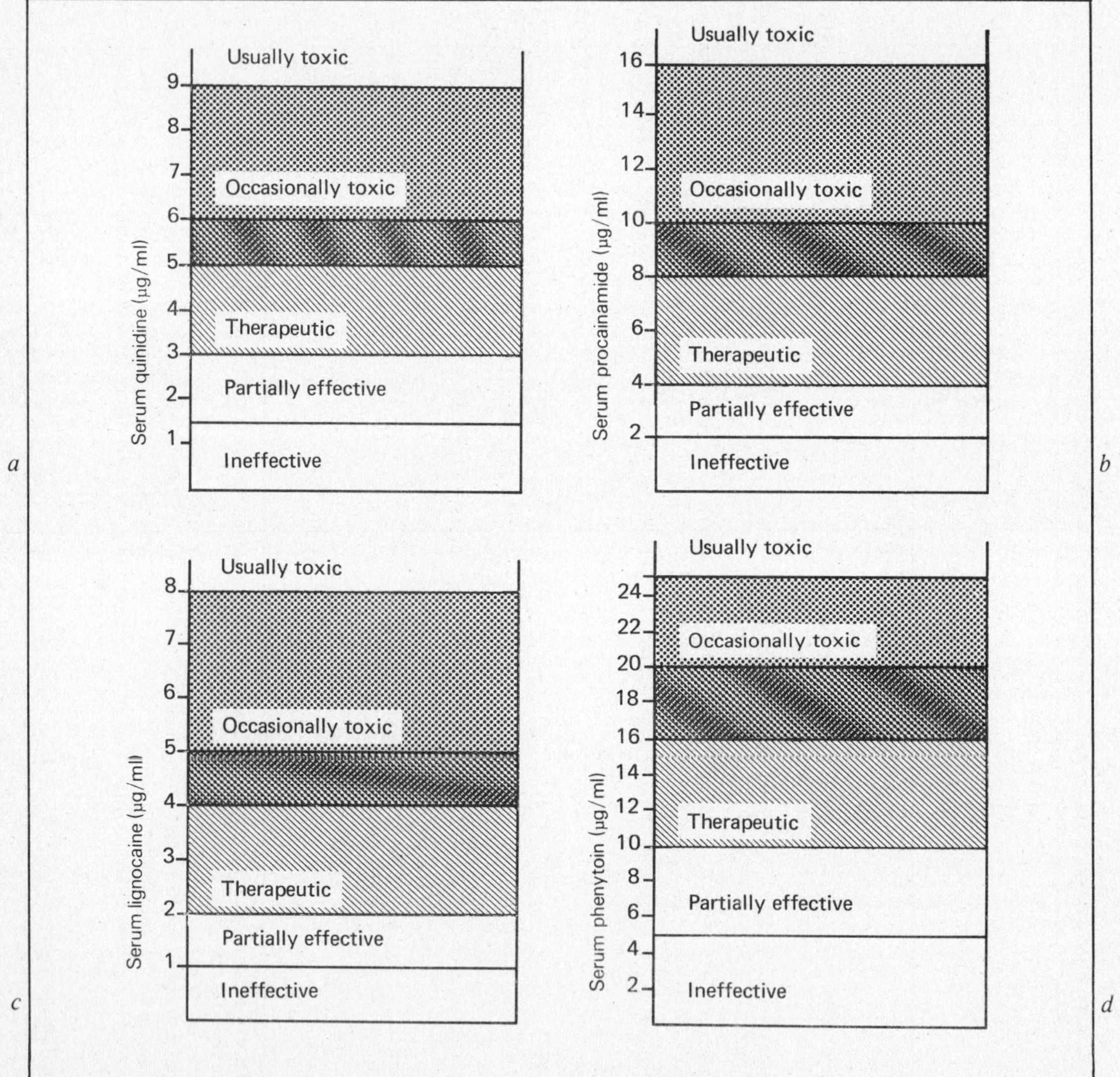

Fig. 4. Plasma concentration-effect relationship of some antiarrhythmic drugs. (a) Quinidine in various cardiac arrhythmias; (b) Procainamide in ventricular tachyarrhythmias; (c) Lignocaine in ventricular tachyarrhythmias; (d) Phenytoin in ventricular tachyarrhythmias (after Koch-Weser, 1973; by permission of author and editor).

and they appear to be effective (Cunningham et al., 1977; Karlsson, 1978). Situations requiring modification of dosage of procainamide are summarised in table XI.

Side Effects: Rapid intravenous infusion of procainamide may lead to hypotension, conduction block or arrhythmia. 'Electrical toxicity' to procainamide is, as would be expected, similar to that of quinidine. Of special note, is the syndrome resembling systemic lupus erythematosus (SLE) which has been reported to occur in some patients on prolonged procainamide therapy (Henningsen et al., 1975). In some series, development of the SLE-like syndrome has tended to be more prevalent in slow acetylators of the drug, but when dosage has been adjusted in individual patients by monitoring plasma concentrations, this tendency has not been apparent (Karlsson, 1978). However, slow acetylators do seem to develop antinuclear antibodies and the SLE reaction after a much shorter duration of therapy than rapid acetylators (Woosley et al., 1978).

Although arthralgias, fever and pleuritis occur, renal and cerebral involvement are not observed in procainamide induced SLE. Pleural and pleuropulmonary involvement are much more frequent in the procainamide disease than in spontaneous lupus (Blomgren et al., 1972). The syndrome usually resolves following withdrawal of the drug (see chapter XXII, sect.14.1).

Clinical Use: Procainamide is used as a second line drug (e.g. after lignocaine) for the treatment of acute ventricular arrhythmias and it may be useful for resistant supraventricular arrhythmias. It is not a preferred drug for long term use.

6.1.3 Lignocaine (lidocaine)

Electrophysiological Effects: Lignocaine does not differ fundamentally from quinidine and procainamide in electrophysiological properties, as was once thought to be the case (Singh, 1978a). It depresses diastolic depolarisation and automaticity in the Purkinje network and usually has no effect on, or decreases conduction velocity (table VII). Membrane responsiveness is depressed, but unlike quinidine and procainamide the effective refractory period is decreased (Rosen et al., 1976a). Lignocaine may be effective when quinidine and procainamide are not, and the reverse is also true. In as much as the electrophysiological effects of lignocaine are primarily limited to the ventricular myocardium, its major utility is in abolishing ventricular arrhythmias.

Pharmacokinetic Properties and Dosage: The pharmacokinetic properties of lignocaine are especially important in determining its use as an antiarrhythmic drug, particularly in patients with cardiac failure (see Benowitz and Meister, 1978). Lignocaine has a high hepatic extraction ratio and is subject to high first-pass hepatic metabolism (see chapter I; sect. 3.3.3) such that bioavailability after oral administration is very low. Because of this and its rapid elimination, and toxicity due to active metabolites following use of large oral doses, it is therefore only given parenterally. When administered intramuscularly, absorption is more rapid and complete after injection into the deltoid muscle than into the vastus lateralis or gluteus maximus. Volume of distribution in subjects without cardiac or liver dysfunction averages 1.3L/kg but as with clearance varies widely between subjects. The elimination half-life in normal subjects is around 1 to 2 hours.

Lignocaine is eliminated by hepatic metabolism; the rate at which the liver metabolises the drug being proportional to its blood flow. Clearance of lignocaine is therefore sensitive to disease states or drugs (e.g. propranolol) which can alter hepatic blood flow. Plasma concentrations of lignocaine after intravenous administration are increased in patients with low cardiac output in proportion with the reduction in hepatic blood flow (Stenson et al., 1971; see section 1.4). Metabolism of lignocaine is markedly impaired in patients with acute myocardial infarction, particularly those in cardiogenic shock in whom metabolism can virtually cease, and also in patients with chronic liver disease such as cirrhosis (Forrest et al., 1977; Prescott et al., 1976). CNS toxicity can readily occur if dosage is not reduced in patients with cardiac failure or liver disease. In the presence of cardiac failure, decreased volume of distribution and clearance lead to increased plasma concentrations and require reduction in loading (bolus injection) and initial maintenance infusion rate by about a half of usual (Benowitz and Meister, 1976). Severe liver disease may also require a reduction to a half of the usual infusion rate after the initial bolus injections (see also below).

Active metabolites of lignocaine may contribute to the therapeutic and/or toxic effects of the drug. Monoethylglycinexylidide (MEGX) is about as potent as lignocaine itself and is eliminated by hepatic metabolism. It appears to accumulate during prolonged intravenous administration such that toxicity can occur in patients with cardiac failure who have plasma concentrations of lignocaine within the therapeutic range but elevated concentrations of MEGX (Halkin et al., 1975a). The other major metabolite, glycinexylidide (GX), is about a quarter as active as lignocaine, and is eliminated about equally by hepatic metabolism and renal excretion but more slowly than lignocaine (Strong et al., 1975). Clearance of lignocaine does not alter in patients with impaired renal function but glycinexylidide accumulates in plasma during prolonged intravenous infusion and persists for some time after discontinuing the infusion (Collingsworth et al., 1975). The clinical importance of such accumulation is not known.

Lignocaine is usually given by initial intravenous bolus(es) followed by continuous infusion. Its distribution and clearance characteristics determine the dosing approach required to attain and maintain desirable plasma concentrations (Benowitz and Meister, 1978). Following intravenous injection, lignocaine distributes preferentially into tissues that have the highest affinity for it; the rate of accumulation depending on the blood flow to that tissue. A large proportion of the lignocaine dose is initially sequestered into the lung, followed by a rapid decline in plasma concentration due to accumulation in well perfused tissues including the brain and heart. Thus, the effects of lignocaine on the central nervous system and heart are likely to occur shortly after administration, especially in cardiac failure when preservation of blood flow to the brain and heart lead to higher concentrations in those organs (see section 1). Lignocaine then redistributes from well perfused tissues to muscle and adipose tissues from which the drug is slowly released back into the plasma and eliminated.

With continuous infusion, steady-state concentrations of lignocaine are attained after 3 to 4 hours in normal subjects and usually after 8 to 10 hours in patients with acute myocardial infarction without circulatory failure. In patients with acute myocardial infarction, especially those with cardiac failure, plasma lignocaine concentrations may continue to rise for more than 24 to 48 hours, apparently due to decreased hepatic clearance (Le Lorier et al., 1977; Prescott et al., 1976). A reduction in infusion rate by 30 to 50% should

therefore be considered after 12 to 24 hours of continuous infusion, particularly in patients with cardiac failure.

To overcome the trough in plasma concentration which occurs during the initial redistribution phase after an initial bolus intravenous injection and before adequate plasma concentrations are attained as a result of continued infusion, supplemental injections should be used. Several dosage regimens have been proposed to achieve desirable plasma concentrations (Benowitz and Meister, 1978), but because of the marked interindividual variability in disposition of lignocaine, even when cardiac and hepatic status are considered, specific dosing recommendations are a guide only and monitoring of plasma concentrations of lignocaine is the most appropriate way of adjusting dosage in an individual patient, particularly in the presence of cardiac failure or liver disease.

The predictably effective therapeutic plasma concentration of lignocaine is between 2 and 5µg/ml (fig. 4c; table IX). Cardiovascular and neurological toxicity are common at levels above 9µg/ml, but very rare at concentrations between 4 and 6µg/ml. Particular care is required in interpreting lignocaine plasma concentrations in patients with heart failure, since continued accumulation may occur for over 24 hours with prolonged infusions (see above).

Standard dosage involves initial intravenous boluses of 50 to 100mg, which should be followed by additional lignocaine preferably as small injections given several minutes apart until a total loading dose (175mg in a 70kg man) has been given over 10 to 15 minutes, followed by a continuous intravenous infusion of 1.5 to 4mg/minute. If arrhythmias recur early during therapy, an additional 25 to 50mg bolus should be given without a change in infusion rate (Harrison and Alderman, 1972). Because of decreased clearance with prolonged infusions, consideration should be given to reduction of the rate by 30 to 50% after 12 to 24 hours. In patients with cardiac failure, a 50mg initial bolus followed by infusions of 1mg/min may be adequate. Modification of usual dosage is also necessary in patients with cardiogenic shock or severe liver disease (see above; table XI).

Side Effects: Toxicity of lignocaine is essentially limited to central nervous system aberrations with progressive drowsiness, paraesthesiae, muscle twitching, disorientation and convulsions with progressively elevated plasma concentrations.

Although respiratory arrest has been reported, cardiac conduction disturbances are rare. Adverse reactions are more common in the elderly and in those with heart failure, low cardiac output states or decreased hepatic clearance (Pfeifer et al., 1976).

Clinical Use: Lignocaine is effective against ventricular arrhythmias and is usually the agent of first choice because of its efficacy, rapid action and relative safety.

6.1.4 Phenytoin

Electrophysiological Properties: Depending on the initial condition of cardiac fibre, phenytoin may either enhance or depress conduction (Rosen et al., 1976b) [table VII]. Membrane responsiveness is elevated to a relatively lesser degree than action potential duration is shortened (Mason et al., 1973). Thus, unlike quinidine and procainamide, phenytoin often enhances atrioventricular conduction and occasionally increases intraventricular conduction. Phenytoin also decreases automaticity, not only by decreasing diastolic depolarisation, but also by increasing maximum diastolic depolarisation.

Pharmacokinetic Properties and Dosage: Of all the drugs used in the treatment of cardiac arrhythmias, phenytoin shows the greatest individual differences in the relationship between dosage and plasma concentrations (Koch-Weser, 1973). These result primarily from different rates of hepatic metabolism due to genetic factors, concomitant administration of drugs which induce or inhibit hepatic microsomal drug metabolising enzymes, or disease induced impairment of plasma clearance due to changes in protein binding or metabolising capacity of the liver (Richens, 1979; see chapter XXV; sect. 3.1). Phenytoin is highly bound to plasma albumin (about 90%) and binding is decreased in patients with hypoalbuminaemia, uraemia or cirrhosis (table XI). Thus in these circumstances, as with quinidine, the unbound fraction of phenytoin in plasma can be markedly increased. There is an increase in distribution volume and plasma concentrations of total drug are lower than in patients without hypoalbuminaemia, uraemia or cirrhosis, while the concentrations of unbound drug are similar (see chapter VII, sect. 5.1; XIX, sect. 1.3; XXI, sect. 1.2). These patients therefore respond to much lower total plasma concentrations than non-

uraemic or non-cirrhotic subjects and toxicity may occur if attempts are made to raise total plasma drug concentrations to the 'normal' range. Estimation of the unbound and total plasma concentration of phenytoin is important in such situations (see chapter I; sect. 5.1.2). In addition, the half-life of phenytoin increases with its plasma concentration when hepatic metabolising capacity is saturated so that the relationship of dose and plasma concentration varies with the dose and when saturation of elimination is reached, a small increase in dose will lead to a disproportionately larger increase in plasma concentration and longer periods are required to reach the new steady-state concentration (see chapter I; sect. 2.3). Saturation of elimination can occur within the usual therapeutic concentration range in some individuals, but is more likely with toxic plasma concentrations (Richens, 1979). Thus, with high plasma concentrations and in patients with severe liver disease when clearance may be decreased (Kutt et al., 1964), dosage increments should be small and plasma concentrations must be carefully monitored to avoid toxicity during continued administration.

The rate of absorption of phenytoin following oral administration may be slow and variable. In addition, its poor water solubility leads to bioavailability problems (Neuvonen, 1979). Due to its dose dependent metabolism and narrow therapeutic plasma concentration range, even small changes in bioavailability can cause major changes in plasma concentration of phenytoin. Formulation factors (e.g. particle size, excipient) can have a marked effect on the oral absorption of phenytoin. Appropriately formulated oral products have a bioavailability of around 80 to 95%. The same very high bioavailability product should always be used (see chapter VI; sect. 8). Absorption of phenytoin given intramuscularly is slow and erratic and should be avoided.

In emergency situations, phenytoin is therefore generally given intravenously at a dose of 50 to 100mg every 5 minutes until the arrhythmia is controlled, toxicity occurs, or 1g has been given (Bigger et al., 1968). Toxicity is most likely in the elderly and in haemodynamically unstable patients, who should probably receive much lower dosage. Because of the wide interindividual variability in metabolism and dose dependent elimination, management of oral therapy can be difficult. Regular monitoring of plasma concentrations are valuable and often essential to control of

Table XI. Influence of disease states on the pharmacokinetics of some commonly used and new antiarrhythmic drugs[1]

Drug	Condition	Effect on pharmacokinetics	Therapeutic action
Quinidine	Heart failure, low cardiac output states[1]	Increased plasma concentration (decreased distribution volume and plasma clearance)	Reduce loading dose Reduced maintenance dose probably needed Monitor plasma concentration with specific assay, especially in presence of impaired renal function
	Renal impairment[2]	Increased plasma concentration (reduced renal clearance of unchanged drug and active metabolites)	Modify dosage in accordance with creatinine clearance and monitor plasma concentrations
	Hypoalbuminaemia[3] Cirrhosis[4]	Decreased protein binding	Possible reduction in maintenance dosage Monitor plasma concentrations by unbound drug concentration (see text)
Procainamide	Heart failure, low cardiac output states	Increased plasma concentration (decreased distribution volume and renal clearance)	Use smaller bolus or loading dose Reduced maintenance dose possibly needed
	Acute myocardial infarction	Impaired oral absorption, especially if narcotic analgesics given	Administer IV at least for 1st 24h of acute phase
	Renal impairment	Increased plasma concentration (reduced renal clearance of unchanged drug and active metabolite)	Modify dosage and monitor plasma concentrations of parent drug and metabolite (N-acetylprocainamide)
Lignocaine	Heart failure, low cardiac output states	Increased plasma concentration (decreased distribution volume and hepatic clearance)	Use smaller bolus or loading dose (50% usual) Reduce rate of administration (50% usual) Supplemental injections needed initially but further reduced rate infusion after 12-24h or once control attained (see text) Monitor plasma concentrations
	Cardiogenic shock Hepatic failure	Markedly increased plasma concentration (virtually no metabolism)	Use very small loading doses and maintenance infusion Monitor plasma concentrations
	Cirrhosis	Increased plasma concentration (decreased hepatic clearance)	Reduce rate maintenance infusion (50% usual) Monitor plasma concentrations

Drug	Condition	Effect	Recommendation
Phenytoin	Uraemia[2] Cirrhosis Hypoalbuminaemia	Decreased protein binding and altered total plasma concentration clinical effect relationship	Adjust dosage according to plasma concentration of unbound drug (see text)
	Liver disease[5]	Possible increased plasma concentration (decreased hepatic metabolism in severe liver disease)	Possible dose reduction. Most likely at higher plasma concentrations when elimination mechanism saturated (see text) Monitor plasma concentrations
Propranolol	Cirrhosis	Possible increased plasma concentration (decreased hepatic metabolism) Increased oral bioavailability in presence portalsystemic vascular shunts	Possible reduction of dosage
	Uraemia[2]	Bioavailability may increase (decreased hepatic first-pass metabolism)	Possible reduction of dosage when commencing therapy in those not on dialysis
Practolol[6]	Renal impairment	Increased plasma concentration (reduced renal clearance of unchanged drug)	Reduction of dosage in severely impaired renal function
Disopyramide	Heart failure, low cardiac output states	Increased plasma concentration (decreased distribution volume and renal clearance)	Possible reduction of initial and maintenance IV dose (around 30 to 50% usual) Monitor plasma concentrations, especially in presence impaired renal function
	Renal impairment	Increased plasma concentration (reduced renal clearance of unchanged drug)	Reduce dosage in accordance with creatinine clearance Monitor plasma concentrations
	Hypoalbuminaemia Uraemia Cirrhosis	Altered protein binding possible (complex; see text)	Monitor plasma concentration of unbound drug
Mexiletine	Heart failure, low cardiac output states	Increased plasma concentration (decreased hepatic clearance)	Use smaller initial and maintenance IV doses (see text)
	Acute myocardial infarction	Slow oral absorption; markedly impaired if narcotic analgesics used	Administer IV at least for 1st 24h of acute phase
Tocainide	Heart failure, low cardiac output states	Increased plasma concentration to be expected (? decreased distribution volume and renal clearance. No data yet available)	? Use smaller initial and maintenance doses Monitor plasma concentrations
	Renal impairment	Increased plasma concentration to be expected (reduced renal clearance of unchanged drug)	Modify dosage Monitor plasma concentrations

1   See section 1 and 6.1
2   See also chapter XXI (sect. 1; 14.2)
3   See also chapter VII (sect. 5.1)
4   See also chapter XIX (sect. 1; 13.4)
5   See also chapter XXV (sect. 3.1)
6   For intravenous use in coronary care units

therapy. Phenytoin has a long elimination half-life (usually around 20 to 30 hours) which means that steady-state concentrations will be slowly attained unless a loading dose is given. A suggested starting regimen to attain and maintain a desirable plasma concentration is a total of 1g on day 1 (intravenous plus oral), followed by 500mg orally on days 2 and 3, then 300 to 400mg daily for maintenance, adjusted as indicated by monitoring of plasma concentrations (Ludden et al., 1977).

Commonly used daily oral doses of 200 to 400mg can result in plasma phenytoin concentrations ranging from 3 to 50µg/ml (Koch-Weser, 1973). Not unexpectedly, the dosage of phenytoin required to control ventricular arrhythmias can vary from 0.1 to 2g daily. Moreover, plasma concentrations can vary considerably in a patient receiving a constant dose. Individual and temporal variations in the dose-plasma concentration relationship greatly complicate long term therapy, but can also be important with short term parenteral therapy.

About 85% of ventricular arrhythmias which can be controlled by phenytoin respond to serum concentrations of between 10 and 20µg/L. Levels above 25µg/L are usually toxic (fig. 4d; table IX). The therapeutic effect correlates best with the unbound phenytoin concentration. For long term administration, phenytoin has the advantage of a long plasma half-life (table X) which enables the maintenance of therapeutic serum concentrations with 1 (usually) or 2 doses a day.

Side Effects: Phenytoin toxicity is uncommon when the agent is administered carefully in small incremental doses. However, when large intravenous doses (rate greater than 50mg/min) have been given, phenytoin has exhibited the paradoxical effect of producing atrioventricular block and bradycardia and cardiac arrest have been reported apparently due to marked depression of diastolic depolarisation and automaticity (Unger and Sklaroff, 1967). Like lignocaine, phenytoin has a propensity for central nervous system toxicity in high doses or when hepatic metabolism becomes saturated and may lead to nystagmus, ataxia, progressive drowsiness and lethargy (see chapter XXV; fig 2).

Although phenytoin has produced marked hypotension, this has been attributable to too large or rapidly administered intravenous doses of the drug and diluent, or the presence of underlying severe cardiac decompensation.

Clinical Use: The use of phenytoin is mainly limited to the treatment of digitalis induced arrhythmias where it is the antiarrhythmic agent of choice.

6.1.5 Propranolol

Propranolol, the prototype β-adrenoceptor blocking agent is widely used to treat arrhythmias, since it possesses considerable efficacy in the management of many cardiac rhythm disorders (Mason et al., 1973; Singh and Jewitt, 1974).

Antiarrhythmic and Electrophysiological Properties: Its antiarrhythmic properties are considered to be principally the result of inhibition of adrenergic stimulation of the heart, since its direct membrane mediated action upon the electrophysiology of the myocardium appears of lesser importance with plasma concentrations of the drug achieved clinically (Coltart et al., 1971). Propranolol depresses myocardial contractility by blocking sympathetic drive. The β-blocking action may prolong AV nodal conduction and is of clinical importance. Combined antiadrenergic and direct effects result in decreased automaticity and conduction velocity, and refractoriness is increased, while the functional refractory period is prolonged relative to action potential duration (table VII). Since some studies with high doses have shown that the refractory period in supraventricular tissue is directly reduced by propranolol, the membrane actions of the agent are considered intermediate between those of quinidine and phenytoin.

However, membrane actions of β-adrenoceptor blocking drugs are not necessary for antiarrhythmic action, since compounds devoid of this property are clinically effective. Differences in the pharmacodynamic and pharmacokinetic properties of the various β-blockers are discussed in chapter XVIII (sect. 5.6.6).

Pharmacokinetic Properties: Propranolol is eliminated entirely by hepatic metabolism and is subject to wide variation in plasma concentrations after a given dose, particularly after oral administration (see Routledge and Shand, 1979). After intravenous administration, clearance approaches that of liver blood flow, so that its rate of elimination and variation in plasma concentrations after intravenous administration reflect differences in hepatic blood flow, as with lignocaine. Propranolol is completely absorbed after oral administration, but bioavailability is low due to its high hepatic extraction ratio or extensive hepatic first-pass metabolism (see chapter I; sect. 3.3.3). In some studies, simultaneous ingestion with food increased bioavailability. Clearance of orally administered propranolol, depends more, if not entirely, on the activity of hepatic drug metabolising enzymes rather than on liver blood flow. This occurs because alteration of hepatic blood flow produces opposite changes in hepatic extraction ratio and bioavailability (Wilkinson and Shand, 1975; Nies et al., 1976). For example, reducing blood flow will increase hepatic extraction ratio so that bioavailability is decreased. At the same time, clearance from the systemic circulation is reduced to the same extent, therefore compensating for the change in bioavailability. Factors which alter hepatic microsomal enzyme activity will therefore influence steady-state plasma concentrations after oral propranolol. Plasma concentrations vary widely (up to 20-fold) in patients given the same oral dose of propranolol, due in part to high hepatic first-pass metabolism and to genetic and individual differences in rate of metabolism. Plasma concentrations in the elderly are around twice those in younger adults. Smoking seems to decrease plasma concentrations but largely in younger people. Drugs which induce or inhibit microsomal enzyme activity (see chapter VIII; sect. 2.3.3, 2.3.4) could well affect plasma concentrations after oral propranolol.

A number of metabolites are formed after intravenous or oral administration, but for most of these their pharmacological significance is unclear. One metabolite, 4-hydroxypropranolol, is formed only after oral administration. It is present in plasma after low doses in approximately the same concentration as the parent drug and has about the same β-adrenoceptor blocking activity (Fitzgerald and O'Donnell, 1971; Paterson et al., 1970). However, the hydroxylation pathway appears to be saturable as in one study the ratio of 4-hydroxypropranolol to parent drug in plasma declined from a value of unity at 160mg daily to 0.1 at higher doses (Walle et al., 1977). The contribution of 4-hydroxypropranolol to the effects of propranolol is therefore likely to be most marked at lower doses but to differ in individual patients due to differences in extent of formation of the metabolite. Thus, the same pharmacological effect can be produced at different plasma concentrations of propranolol in different patients (Zacest and Koch-Weser, 1972).

Propranolol has a large distribution volume of around 4L/kg, reflecting its wide distribution in tissues. Although propranolol is highly bound to plasma proteins (90 to 96%), its affinity to albumin is only moderate. As with some other basic drugs, propranolol is more avidly bound to α_1-acid glycoprotein, binding showing large interindividual differences and increasing with increases in concentration of α_1-acid glycoprotein; an acute phase reactant known to increase nonspecifically in response to conditions such as infection, inflammation, cancer or trauma (Piafsky et al., 1978). The clinical implications of altered binding of propranolol are not known (see also chapter I; sect. 4.3.2).

Liver disease has a marked effect on the disposition of propranolol. In cirrhosis, clearance of propranolol is reduced and oral bioavailability markedly increased (Wood et al., 1978). The presence of portal systemic vascular shunts will greatly increase the bioavailability of oral propranolol since first-pass hepatic metabolism is bypassed (see chapter XIX; sect. 1.1). Any increase in dosage of propranolol should be made carefully in patients with liver disease. Renal disease may also influence bioavailability and clearance of propranolol but the clinical implications are not clear (see chapter XXI; sect. 14.2.4).

Disposition of propranolol can be altered by other diseases such as some gastrointestinal disorders (see chapter XIX; sect. 1.1) and thyroid disease (see chapter XVI; sect. 1.4.2), but in most situations changes in propranolol plasma concentration are not likely to be of great importance. Indeed, with oral administration changes in disposition and plasma concentration of propranolol due to any cause are probably of lesser importance than the marked variability in plasma concentration among different individuals after a given dose.

Dosage: The usual starting dose of propranolol is 40mg orally 2 or 3 times daily and this may be increased in stepwise amounts as necessary. The effective dose varies greatly due to individual differences in metabolism (see above). Failure of therapy should not be considered until doses of 640mg daily have been tried or side effects limit dose increases. Intravenous propranolol has been used with success in refractory ventricular tachycardia or fibrillation, but caution is necessary. Up to 0.1 to 0.15mg/kg (7 to 10mg total) may be given in increments of 0.5 to 0.75mg every 1 to 2 minutes with electrocardiographic and blood pressure monitoring. Smaller total doses (2 to 5mg) should be used in patients in whom left ventricular dysfunction is suspected. Plasma concentration estimations have not been as well defined and may not be as useful a guide to therapy with propranolol as with the other commonly used antiarrhythmic drugs, but a therapeutic β-blocking concentration is probably in the region of 75 to 100ng/ml (Coltart and Shand, 1970; Pine et al., 1975). However, some patients with ventricular arrhythmias require plasma concentrations greatly in excess of 100ng/ml, while some others with ventricular ectopic beats increasing concentrations beyond 100ng/ml for unexplained reasons were associated with a recrudescence of a previously controlled arrhythmia (Woosley et al., 1977). Propranolol is eliminated by hepatic metabolism and dosage may need to be reduced in patients with liver disease (see above).

Side Effects: Side effects of β-adrenoceptor blocking drugs such as propranolol include fatigue, depression, nausea, increased peripheral vascular insufficiency, impotence, nightmares and hallucinations. β-Adrenoceptor blocking drugs, because of their myocardial depressant effect, are contraindicated in the presence of uncontrolled heart failure. Propranolol, like other non-selective β-adrenoceptor blocking drugs may cause bronchospasm in asthmatic patients and others with increased bronchial reactivity. The risk is less with β_1-blockers or 'cardioselective' agents such as atenolol and metoprolol (see chapter XVIII; sect. 5.6.8).

Clinical Use: Propranolol, and other β-blockers, are useful for managing arrhythmias due to excessive catecholamine release, acute and chronic supraventricular tachycardias, and ventricular arrhythmias unresponsive to first choice agents. Propranolol can suppress digitalis induced arrhythmias but because of the potential for exacerbating bradycardia and conduction block, phenytoin is preferred. The use of β-blockers in and after acute myocardial infarction is discussed in section 5.2 and 5.5.

6.1.6 Bretylium
Bretylium tosylate, an adrenergic neurone blocking agent originally developed for use in hypertension, has been evaluated in the treatment of cardiac arrhythmias. The mechanisms of its antiarrhythmic actions are complex, but the principal

benefit of bretylium in abating tachyarrhythmias seems to be primarily due to its antiadrenergic properties, rather than to direct effects of the drug (Amsterdam et al., 1972).

Absorption after oral administration is erratic, although doses of 200 to 600mg 3 to 4 times daily have been used (Bernstein and Koch-Weser, 1972). After intramuscular administration, absorption is rapid with peak plasma concentrations attained at 1 hour. Intravenous doses of 5mg/kg by slow injection, followed by maintenance intramuscular doses of 3 to 5mg/kg every 6 to 8 hours for 48 hours (Holder et al., 1977; Romhildt et al., 1972), have been advocated for recurrent ventricular arrhythmias, particularly ventricular fibrillation resistant to conventional treatment. In the latter situation, bretylium may allow successful electrical reversion (Holder et al., 1977). As a large amount of a dose can be excreted as unchanged drug in the urine, dosage may need to be modified in patients with impaired renal function.

The relatively frequent occurrence of potentially serious side effects has hampered the elevation of parenteral bretylium to the status of a first line antiarrhythmic drug. A fall in systemic blood pressure, particularly in the upright position, is commonly observed due to the drug's antiadrenergic action, although severe hypotension requiring vasopressor therapy has not been a problem in the supine patient (Amsterdam et al., 1972). In addition, because of the early discharge of noradrenaline from sympathetic nerve endings ventricular electrical irritability is often increased prior to the onset of bretylium's prolonged antiarrhythmic effect, which ranges from 6 to 24 hours following injection.

6.1.7 Potassium
Potassium may exert antiarrhythmic effects which are useful in certain clinical settings. The electrophysiological properties of potassium are complex and often depend on the speed of administration and the serum concentration of the cation and the type of cardiac tissue involved (Fisch et al., 1966; Surawicz, 1966). Elevation of potassium concentration within the normal range reduces conduction velocity and shortens the refractory period. Further, automaticity may be diminished, especially in ectopic ventricular pacemakers, but this action is variable since the resting membrane potential is elevated while diastolic depolarisation is reduced. Potassium ad-

ministration is more likely to cause intraventricular block with widening of the QRS duration than atrioventricular block. Potassium usually exerts a mild direct depressant effect on the automaticity of the sinoatrial node which is counterbalanced by an indirect parasympathomimetic action, and thereby no change in heart rate occurs.

It is important to remember that the antiarrhythmic drugs are often ineffective in the presence of certain abnormalities of the humoral background in which the agents are administered, such as hypokalaemia, hypoxia, and disorders of acid-base regulation. Correction of these abnormalities may restore sinus rhythm even without the use of antiarrhythmic drugs. The influence of hypokalaemia predisposing to digitalis toxicity is well recognised.

Occasionally, it is advantageous to use the antiarrhythmic properties of potassium in patients in whom the serum concentration of the cation is normal. Thus, in the management of tachyarrhythmias following cardiac operations, elevation of the serum potassium concentration by 0.5 to 1.5mmol (mEq) per litre or to the upper limits of normal may be effective, with or without use of antiarrhythmic drugs. Potassium should not be used in this manner in the presence of atrioventricular block, since nodal conduction may be further impaired by the cation.

6.1.8 Digitalis

Digitalis has a place in the management of arrhythmias occurring in the early stage after acute infarction, specifically atrial fibrillation, recurrent atrial flutter or recurrent atrial tachycardia (Karliner and Braunwald, 1972). If heart failure still persists a week after a cardiac infarction, despite the use of diuretics and potassium replacement, the patient should be commenced on digitalis therapy in order to obtain a long term positive inotropic effect. For digoxin administration and dosage, see section 8.1.5.

6.1.9 Verapamil

Verapamil (iproveratrine), a papaverine derivative originally developed as an antianginal agent (see section 4.2.3), is a highly effective antiarrhythmic drug (see Singh et al., 1978).

Antiarrhythmic and Electrophysiological Properties: It acts by selectively inhibiting myocardial cell membrane transport of calcium, an action which accounts for its antiarrhythmic effects and negative inotropic propensity. Inhibition of calcium transport in vascular smooth muscle cells leads to peripheral as well as coronary vasodilatation. These actions reduce myocardial contractility and myocardial oxygen demand. The major electrophysiological effect of verapamil is depression of atrioventricular conduction. Intra-arterial conduction, H-V interval and QRS remain unchanged.

Pharmacokinetic Properties: Verapamil is well absorbed after oral administration, but bioavailability is low and plasma clearance high suggesting extensive hepatic first-pass metabolism. It is about 90 % bound to plasma proteins and has a large distribution volume of 6.5L/kg, reflecting extensive tissue uptake. There seems to be preferential uptake by the AV nodal tissues, since the duration of the depressant effect of verapamil on the AV node appears to considerably outlast the duration of the haemodynamic actions of the drug. Verapamil is eliminated by hepatic metabolism, only a small amount of a dose being excreted as unchanged drug in the urine. Other pharmacokinetic properties are summarised in table X.

Dosage and Clinical Use: Intravenous verapamil is a highly effective agent for the immediate treatment of acute paroxysmal supraventricular tachycardia (especially AV nodal re-entry tachycardia) with or without pre-excitation, in patients with normal myocardial function. It should be tried first, not only because of its high efficacy (80 to 100 % successful reversion in different series) but also because it has a shorter duration of action than other agents. Administration of verapamil should be at the rate of 1mg/min, under blood pressure and electrocardiographic monitoring. Dosage for conversion of acute supraventricular arrhythmias may range from 1 to 15mg but if the arrhythmia does not respond to a total of 10mg it seldom responds to higher dosage. Long term therapy for prophylaxis of paroxysmal supraventricular tachycardia is limited but requires high oral doses up to 120 or 160mg 2 or 3 times daily, due to low oral bioavailability. Addition of other antiarrhythmic drugs (quinidine) may be necessary.

Side Effects: The side effects of verapamil are mainly limited to bradycardia and hypotension, especially in patients who have received β-adrenoceptor blocking drugs prior to verapamil and in those with poor myocardial function or the sick sinus syndrome. Although verapamil does not depress a normal sinus node it may cause sinus node depression in those with sick sinus syndrome and marked bradycardia can develop. Immediate intravenous atropine (1.2mg) should be given to restore heart rate and blood pressure, or if this is ineffective, isoprenaline (isoproterenol) or glucagon infusion, or intravenous calcium (10 to 20ml of 10% solution).

6.1.10 Disopyramide

Antiarrhythmic and Electrophysiological Properties: Disopyramide is a new antiarrhythmic drug with actions which resemble those of quinidine and procainamide (see Heel et al., 1978b; table VII).

It decreases membrane responsiveness, prolongs the effective refractory period (ERP) and slows automaticity in cells with augmented automaticity. Effective refractory period of the atrium is lengthened, while the ERP of the AV node is shortened and conduction in accessory pathways is prolonged. Disopyramide is a myocardial depressant and has anticholinergic effects.

Pharmacokinetic Properties and Dosage: Absorption is essentially complete after oral administration but is delayed in patients with acute myocardial infarction who had received narcotic analgesics (see section 1.2). There is no significant hepatic first-pass metabolism so that bioavailability is high for both the phosphate salt or free base forms which are available. Protein binding is variable and is concentration dependent. The concentration of unbound drug increases proportionately with dose, but total drug concentration shows a less than proportionate increase. The therapeutic implications of this situation remain to be clarified. Distribution volume and elimination are reduced in patients with acute myocardial infarction suggesting that dosage should be reduced in patients with heart failure or low cardiac output states (see section 1.1). About 50 to 60% of a dose is excreted unchanged, mainly in the urine, necessitating a reduction in dosage in patients with impaired renal function in accordance with creatinine clearance. The major N-dealkylated metabolite has some antiarrhythmic activity, but less so than the parent drug. Other pharmacokinetic properties are summarised in table X and a likely desirable therapeutic plasma concentration range is given in table IX.

Oral and intravenous preparations are available. With oral administration an initial loading dose of 300mg should be followed by 100 or 150mg 6-hourly. Some patients may require doses of 150 to 300mg 6-hourly to attain therapeutic plasma concentrations. In emergency conditions, intravenous administration involves an initial bolus of 1 to 2mg/kg (but not exceeding 150mg) given over 5 to 10 minutes, followed by a maintenance infusion of 20 to 30mg/hour (0.4mg/kg/h) up to a maximum of 800mg daily. Dosage should be reduced in patients with impaired renal function and also probably in those with heart failure or low cardiac output states.

Side Effects: Disopyramide is better tolerated than quinidine. Side effects are mainly related to its anticholinergic properties (dry mouth, blurred vision, urinary retention) and it thus should be avoided in patients with prostatism or narrow angle glaucoma. The negative inotropic effect appears to be dose related. A slower rate of injection (over 10 minutes) appears to result in reduced myocardial depression compared with more rapid administration (over 2 to 5 minutes).

Clinical Use: Disopyramide is effective for both ventricular (e.g. after acute myocardial infarction) and supraventricular arrhythmias (e.g. rapid atrial fibrillation or supraventricular tachycardia).

6.1.11 Mexiletine

Antiarrhythmic and Electrophysiological Properties: Mexiletine is a new local anaesthetic antiarrhythmic agent with structural similarities and electrophysiological properties similar to lignocaine (see Chew et al., 1979; table VII).

Pharmacokinetic Properties and Dosage: Unlike lignocaine it has high bioavailability after oral administration with a plasma half-life such that it can be given 2 or 3 times daily to maintain therapeutic plasma concentrations (table IX). Oral absorption is markedly decreased in patients with acute myocardial infarction who have received narcotic analgesics (see section 1.2).

Elimination is by hepatic metabolism and appears to be reduced in patients with acute myocardial infarction; the plasma half-life in normal subjects of around 10 hours increasing to about 17-18 hours or more (Talbot et al., 1973; Prescott et al., 1977). A large proportion of a dose (up to 50%) is eliminated as unchanged drug in the urine when urinary pH is reduced to around or below pH5, but under normal conditions only about 10 to 20% is eliminated unchanged in the urine. Other pharmacokinetic properties are summarised in table X.

The distribution of mexiletine after intravenous injection follows the pattern of lignocaine (see section 6.1.3). There is therefore a rapid decline in plasma concentration due to distribution to well perfused tissues including the brain and heart, but because of the long half-life of mexiletine steady-state plasma concentrations take even longer (several days) than those of lignocaine (several hours). A combination of bolus injection (to control the acute arrhythmias) and an initial rapid but decreasing rate of infusion followed by a constant maintenance infusion has proved to be effective in practice (Prescott et al., 1977; table VIII). This regimen must be applied judiciously (particularly in the acutely ill and elderly patients) because of individual variation in response, volume of distribution and plasma clearance of mexiletine. Excessive dosage can readily lead to CNS toxicity (Campbell et al., 1977; see section 1.1). Alternatively, therapeutic plasma concentrations may be rapidly attained with an oral loading dose.

Clinical Use and Side Effects: Mexiletine is effective in treatment of ventricular arrhythmias, often when other agents have failed. It is also potentially suitable for long term oral prophylaxis of serious ventricular arrhythmias in patients with coronary heart disease. Side effects (table IX) are relatively uncommon with long term oral therapy (a fine tremor of the hands is often the first sign of CNS toxicity), but may occur during the initial loading dose phase or with an increase in dosage.

6.1.12 Tocainide

Tocainide is a new orally effective antiarrhythmic analogue of lignocaine (Danilo, 1979; table VII). As with mexiletine, oral bioavailability is high and its elimination half-life of 12 to 15 hours allows convenient dosing intervals of 2 or 3 times daily. Unlike lignocaine and mexiletine, tocainide is primarily eliminated as unchanged drug in the urine. It has been effective in ventricular arrhythmias unresponsive to other agents (Ryan et al., 1979; Winkle et al., 1978). Side effects appear to be less common than with mexiletine, although minor CNS toxicity has been reported. Intravenous tocainide is also available and under investigation. Its tentative dosage and clinical phar-

macological properties are summarised in tables VIII, IX and X.

6.1.13 Other Antiarrhythmic Drugs

N-Acetylprocainamide is an active metabolite of procainamide with comparable antiarrhythmic efficacy (Anderson et al., 1978; Lertora et al., 1979) but with a much longer elimination half-life so allowing more convenient oral administration (appendix A). It has been suggested that risk of the systemic lupus erythematosus-like syndrome associated with procainamide may be less with the acetylated metabolite (Drayer et al., 1974; Karlsson, 1978; Lertora et al., 1979).

Aprindine is a local anaesthetic with antiarrhythmic effectiveness in ventricular arrhythmias and repetitive supraventricular tachycardias. It can be given orally or intravenously. A low therapeutic index associated with troublesome neurological, cardiological and haematological side effects (including agranulocytosis, sometimes fatal) may limit its use (Anderson et al., 1978; Zipes and Troup, 1978).

Amiodarone, a benzofuran derivative introduced originally as an antianginal agent, has been effective given orally in treatment of ventricular and supraventricular arrhythmias (especially long term treatment of Wolf Parkinson White syndrome). Its main limiting side effect is a potential propensity to hypothyroidism. Reversible corneal microdeposits have also been reported on occasions. Amiodarone is very slowly eliminated from the body and administration once daily (or even on alternate days) is adequate to maintain a desirable effect (Anderson et al., 1978; Zipes and Troup, 1978).

6.2 Treatment of Tachyarrhythmias

Important principles in the treatment of arrhythmias include:

a) The clinical setting of any arrhythmia is very important, as it is the patient who must be treated, not the electrocardiogram

b) The choice of an antiarrhythmic agent is still largely empirical, but treatment must be carried out in a systematic manner — any chosen drug should be given an adequate trial without producing toxic effects before substituting or adding another agent

c) Relative toxicity of antiarrhythmic drugs tends to be increased in advanced heart disease with congestive failure (section 1).

6.2.1 Sinus Tachycardia

Sinus tachycardia exists when the heart rate is in excess of 100 per minute. This is a warning arrhythmia in that it is indicative, in most cases, of a fairly severe infarction and is taken by many to be a prelude to other clinical manifestations of heart failure. In itself, sinus tachycardia is not harmful and specific treatment is seldom indicated.

6.2.2. Atrial Premature Systoles

Atrial ectopic beats occur when the pacemaker of the heart arises in the atrium but outside the sinus node. Atrial ectopic beats usually occur prematurely and will capture the heart. They ordinarily do not require treatment in adults without apparent heart disease, but in active disease of the atrial muscle, such as following myocardial infarction, or in certain generalised metabolic disorders like thyrotoxicosis, premature atrial systoles are often premonitory of atrial fibrillation or flutter. In these abnormal situations, therapy with digitalis, propranolol or quinidine may be useful.

6.2.3 Atrial Tachycardia

This arrhythmia is present when the atrial beat increases from a rate of 150 to 250 with normal A-V conduction and normal intraventricular conduction. The arrhythmia frequently occurs in episodes and is then termed paroxysmal atrial tachycardia. This is a common arrhythmia seen in patients with the Wolf Parkinson White syndrome. Patients without organic heart disease frequently tolerate rapid ventricular rates without haemodynamic difficulty. However, in myocardial infarction, the arrhythmia is a warning arrhythmia and may precede clinical evidence of left ventricular failure. In addition, the arrhythmia may be life threatening, in that if it persists untreated, cardiac decompensation can occur quite rapidly in patients with an impaired myocardium. Expectant treatment has no place.

Verapamil, 1mg/min up to 10mg intravenously, is the drug of choice, having a high incidence of successful reversion (greater than 80%) and also a short duration of action so that other drugs may then be used if it is not effective (Singh et al., 1978; Vohra et al., 1975). A β-adrenoceptor blocking drug such as propranolol, or procainamide can also be used, but if unsuccessful,

timed direct current shock can be expected to achieve the desired result. Following successful reversion, the patient should be treated with digitalis and most would favour the addition of an antiarrhythmic drug in an attempt to prevent the arrhythmia from recurring. DC shock is the treatment of choice in a patient with marked cardiac decompensation.

6.2.4 Atrial Flutter

In this arrhythmia the ectopic atrial focus discharges at a rate of from 250 to 350 per minute. The arrhythmia may be paroxysmal or sustained and there is usually some degree of atrioventricular block which may vary from 2:1 to 4:1 block. Digitalis can be given in a patient whose general clinical state remains relatively stable despite the development of atrial flutter. However, if there is haemodynamic deterioration, treatment with verapamil or a β-adrenoceptor blocking drug may be successful. If not, immediate direct current counter shock should be administered and the patient subsequently digitalised and continued on an antiarrhythmic drug.

6.2.5 Atrial Fibrillation

Atrial fibrillation is commonly due to underlying heart disease such as rheumatic, thyrotoxic, ischaemic or alcoholic heart disease. The first goal of treatment is to control the ventricular rate and thereby improve the circulation. In most patients, oral digoxin is the drug of choice, although propranolol may be preferable in patients with thyrotoxicosis or hypertrophic cardiomyopathies. Atrial fibrillation occurs quite commonly in elderly patients suffering from acute infarction. The atrial activity is irregular and in excess of 350 impulses per minute. There is always some degree of atrioventricular block, but the ventricular rate is usually fast and this will accentuate any ventricular failure. In most cases the patient should be digitalised by a rapid method (table XII). However, if this does not improve the patient's general condition and if the fibrillation is of recent onset, direct current counter shock may be used to return to sinus rhythm. Usually, the atrial fibrillation will be paroxysmal and recurrent, however a period of return to sinus rhythm may be advantageous, giving time for digitalisation to be completed. If this is not entirely satisfactory in slowing the ventricular rate, propranolol may be added to the regimen. Alternatively, disopyramide or verapamil may be used — to both revert to sinus

Table XII. Usual average dosages and schedules of digitalis preparations in normal younger adults[1]

Drug	Oral			Parenteral (slow intravenous)
	rapid digitalisation (loading dose)	slow digitalisation (no loading dose)	maintenance[2]	
Digoxin[3]	10-15µg/kg divided into 2 or 3 equal parts 6-hourly; *or* 0.75mg single dose	0.25mg daily x 7	0.25mg	70 to 80% of oral amount in divided doses in 24h
Digitoxin	0.8 to 1.2mg as single or divided doses in 24-48h	0.1mg daily x 35	0.1mg daily	0.8 to 1.2mg in divided doses in 24h
Lanatoside C	Not Recommended	Not Recommended	0.5 to 1.5mg daily	—
Deslanoside	—	—	—	0.8mg initially; 0.2mg 2-hourly to total of up to 1.6 or 2mg in 24h
Digitalis leaf	Not Recommended	0.1g daily x 30	0.1g daily	Not Recommended
Ouabain	—	—	—	0.25-0.5mg in divided doses in 24h

1   These dosages are average amounts for younger adults with normal renal or hepatic function and no other conditions which affect the response to digitalis (see section 8.1.4). Dose requirements in individual patients may vary considerably, particularly in the elderly, those with electrolyte abnormalities or impaired ability to eliminate the particular glycoside, etc. For specific recommendations in these groups, see text.

2   Initial maintenance dose based on percentage of loading dose eliminated daily with normal excretory function (33% digoxin; 10% digitoxin). See text.

3   Assumes tablets of high bioavailability (70 to 80%) for oral dosage.

rhythm and to prevent a recurrence of atrial fibrillation.

6.2.6 *Ventricular Ectopic Beats*

Several other terms have been used to describe this phenomenon and include premature ventricular contractions, premature ventricular beats and ventricular extrasystoles. The management of ventricular extrasystoles is that of the underlying condition. In the absence of associated heart disease, ventricular extrasystoles usually do not require any treatment. Indeed, the majority of ventricular extrasystoles probably do not require therapy. If an awareness of the extrasystoles causes fear or anxiety, reassurance and treatment with small doses of propranolol will usually abolish the extrasystoles and alleviate the anxiety.

Ventricular ectopic beats occur in over 80% of patients with definite acute infarction. In the majority of patients they are benign and act only as a warning that other arrhythmias may occur. Ectopics arising from the left ventricle (RBBB pattern) are more sinister than those arising from the right ventricle (LBBB pattern). Guidelines have been laid down by many authors with respect to the ectopic beats requiring active, rather than expectant treatment.

If the ectopic activity occurs in more than 10% of all the beats, if the ectopic activity arises from varying ventricular foci or if the ectopic activity arises in the so-called vulnerable repolarisation period, so called R on T ectopic beat, then active treatment should be given. Lignocaine (1 to 2% solution) is recommended in a bolus injection of

1mg/kg body weight given over a period of 1 to 3 minutes. If this dose suppresses the ectopic activity, a further dose should be given at 15 minutes and a continuous intravenous infusion commenced at 4mg/min for 1 hour. In the patient with decreased hepatic function or cardiac reserve, a smaller total dose of lignocaine may be adequate to suppress the arrhythmia (see sect. 1.3, 1.4; 6.1.3). After an hour, the infusion can be reduced to 2 to 3mg/min. If lignocaine is ineffective, drug therapy should be changed to procainamide, in a dose of 250 to 500mg given slowly intravenously over 5 to 10 minutes. If procainamide suppresses the ectopic activity, a continuous intravenous infusion should be established (2mg/min). Whilst lignocaine and procainamide suppress ventricular ectopic beats, there is no evidence that they will prevent ventricular fibrillation. If the bolus injection of procainamide does not suppress the ectopic activity then one may change to another antiarrhythmic drug such as disopyramide, mexiletine or tocainide. If the extrasystoles are associated with digitalis intoxication, digitalis should be stopped, hypokalaemia, if present, corrected and drugs such as phenytoin or a β-adrenoceptor blocking drug used.

Although digitalis may precipitate ventricular extrasystoles it will frequently abolish ventricular ectopic beats when they occur in a non-digitalised patient. There is no reason whatsoever to withhold digitalis in a patient who presents with cardiac failure and ventricular extrasystoles, and who has not been receiving digitalis therapy.

6.2.7 Ventricular Tachycardia

Ventricular tachycardia is a life threatening and potentially lethal arrhythmia and treatment should be immediate. The ventricular rate usually varies between 150 and 250 beats per minute and although the arrhythmia may be paroxysmal it is often sustained. Sustained ventricular tachycardia should be treated with a bolus injection of 1mg/kg body weight of lignocaine (1 or 2% solution), given immediately. If the arrhythmia is not brought under control within a few minutes direct current counter shock reversion should be used. Following successful reversion, a continuous intravenous infusion of lignocaine at a minimal dose of 2mg per minute should be established, or if lignocaine does not appear to be effective, one of the other antiarrhythmic drugs such as procainamide (given intravenously) or phenytoin (250mg 4-hourly intravenously) can be used. If ventricular

tachycardia is recurrent despite treatment with these agents, prophylaxis can be attempted with propranolol, bretylium tosylate or pacemaker ventricular overdrive and suppressive drugs.

6.2.8 Ventricular Fibrillation

This lethal arrhythmia must be treated immediately. Direct current counter shock is applied with any synchroniser turned off. Following successful cardioversion an appropriate antiarrhythmic drug such as lignocaine, procainamide, phenytoin or propranolol is used. If the first defibrillator shock is not successful then one must check oxygenation, administer an appropriate dose of sodium bicarbonate to neutralise the acidosis and administer a bolus injection of an antiarrhythmic drug to facilitate cardioversion.

6.2.9 Idioventricular Tachycardia

Idioventricular tachycardia (accelerated idioventricular rhythm) is a relatively common ventricular arrhythmia in patients with cardiac infarction. It arises from an ectopic ventricular focus stimulating the ventricle at a rate of between 60 and 100 per minute. The arrhythmia is not life-threatening, and treatment can be expectant as the arrhythmia usually is paroxysmal and is not seen after about 36 hours from the commencement of the infarction. If it is associated with a slow sinus rate, atropine is the treatment of choice; given either as intravenous medication or by the intramuscular tissue spray route. It should be emphasised that antiarrhythmic drugs such as lignocaine, procainamide and propranolol should not be administered in this arrhythmia. Phenytoin can be used if there is concern about the possibility of complicating ventricular fibrillation.

6.3 Arrhythmias Due to Digitalis Toxicity

Digitalis toxicity is among the most common of adverse drug reactions (Hurwitz and Wade, 1969). In some series, digitalis has caused arrhythmias and conduction disturbances in as many as 20% or more of patients receiving the drug for congestive heart failure (Mason et al., 1971; Smith and Haber, 1973). The various digitalis preparations are equally capable of producing toxicity. Digitalis can provoke most cardiac arrhythmias, particularly ventricular ectopics and atrial tachycardia with block.

A specific antidote is not yet available. The first and obvious step in treatment is the withdrawal of the digitalis glycoside. The patient should be hospitalised if arrhythmia is present. Any hypokalaemia must be corrected by infusion of potassium (0.3 to 1.0mmol/min). Where severe potassium depletion is an important determinant of arrhythmias in a digitalised patient, infusion of potassium in 5% glucose can lead to a worsening of hypokalaemia and worsening of the arrhythmia. In this situation, potassium should be infused in physiological saline or given orally. When there is ventricular irritability, potassium should be administered even in the absence of hypokalaemia. However, elevations of plasma potassium above normal tend to impair atrioventricular (A-V) conduction and should be avoided when conduction disturbances are present and given cautiously if renal function is impaired.

Phenytoin is very useful in the treatment of digitalis toxic ectopic arrhythmias (Mason et al., 1973). 100mg of phenytoin is given slowly intravenously every 5 minutes until onset of toxicity or control of the arrhythmia. A maintenance oral dose of 400 to 600mg daily is given if the arrhythmia is controlled by the intravenous dose. Lignocaine is used in ventricular arrhythmias as for acute myocardial infarction (section 5.3). Propranolol is useful in the treatment of certain digitalis induced tachyarrhythmias and has been most successful in terminating ventricular ectopic beats (Gibson and Sowton, 1969). As propranolol may increase atrioventricular block, phenytoin is probably preferable to propranolol in the initial treatment of digitalis induced atrial tachycardia with block. In patients with digitalis induced paroxysmal supraventricular arrhythmias, with or without A-V block, propranolol can be used to slow rapid ventricular rate by decreasing the atrial rate or by reducing the conduction velocity and increasing the refractory period of the A-V node.

A new approach in the treatment of digitoxin toxicity is the use of cholestyramine or colestipol, which diminish the intestinal reabsorption and enterohepatic circulation of digitoxin (Bazzano and Bazzano, 1972; Cady et al., 1979; see chapter IX, sect. 4.7). Although a specific antidote is not clinically available at this time for reversal of digitalis intoxication, the recent development of an immunological technique for the preparation of specific antibodies to digitalis preparations offers an experimental direct approach to this problem. Thus, glycoside-induced rhythm disorders are reversed and fatal arrhythmias prevented following administration of these antibodies by the func-

tional removal of digitalis from the myocardium (Schmidt and Butler, 1971; Smith et al., 1976).

Direct current reversion has been used to reverse digitalis induced arrhythmias that have failed to respond to drug treatment, but the use of shock is generally best avoided, since there is a propensity for glycoside induced ventricular fibrillation after shock treatment. This risk may be minimised by withholding digoxin for 24 hours or digitoxin for 3 to 4 days before cardioversion, by using a small initial DC shock, and by avoiding cardioversion for arrhythmias due to excessive digitalisation.

Prevention is the best method of treatment and appropriate knowledge of the clinical pharmacology of digitalis can do much to reduce the incidence of toxicity (see section 8.1.3; 8.1.4).

7. Atrioventricular Heart Block and Resistant Tachyarrhythmias

Heart block warrants treatment if the rate is so slow as to produce Stokes-Adams attacks (syncope) or chronic symptoms (heart failure). First degree heart block very rarely, second degree block occasionally, and third degree (complete) block frequently require treatment. The heart rate may sometimes be increased by drug treatment. However, electrical stimulation is the treatment of choice for slow rates causing symptoms, provided the technical facilities for pacing are available.

In the acute situation of resuscitation in the presence of heart block, extreme bradycardia or cardiac asystole, atropine and isoprenaline (isoproterenol) are the drugs of choice. Isoprenaline is given intravenously in a dose of 10 to 100µg and may be followed by a continuous intravenous infusion, the dose ranging upwards from 1µg per minute and being 'titrated' against the rate and general circulatory state. 1mg may be added to 100ml of 5% dextrose and administered using a microdrip set. Adrenaline (epinephrine), but not noradrenaline (levarterenol) may be similarly used. β-Adrenoceptor stimulating drugs such as isoprenaline cause an increase in both the rate and the force of cardiac contraction, whereas electrical pacing increases the rate only. There can be no question, therefore, of considering electrical pacing to raise the cardiac output when the heart rate is adequate. On the other hand, if an adequate rate cannot be achieved quickly with drug treatment, especially if ectopic arrhythmias are troublesome, electrical pacing should be instituted at once.

7.1 Indications for Electrical Pacing

Artificial cardiac pacemaking may be instituted on a temporary or permanent basis. The major indications are:

1) *Stokes-Adams attacks:* Patients with high degree A-V block with episodes of syncope resulting from bradycardia, asystole, ventricular tachycardia, or ventricular fibrillation. Most patients with complete heart block will develop syncope or dizzy turns. The heart block may be intermittent and thus only diagnosed by electrocardiographic monitoring. Blocks have been described in the anterior and posterior division of the left bundle branch. A left hemi-block associated with right bundle branch block suggests that the cause of a Stokes-Adams attack is intermittent bilateral bundle branch block and complete heart block. There is usually no suggestion clinically as to the aetiology of the heart block, but histologically there may be fibrosis or degeneration of the conduction pathways.

Other causes of high degree A-V block include coronary artery disease, rheumatic heart disease (calcific aortic stenosis), cardiomyopathies and congenital heart disease, including congenital heart block. Complete heart block occasionally occurs following cardiac surgery for congenital and acquired heart disease. Pacemaker implantation should be considered in all patients with Stokes-Adams syndrome — age alone is not a contraindication.

2) *Heart Block in Acute Myocardial Infarction:* Complete heart block occurs in 5 to 7% of patients with acute myocardial infarction seen in hospital and carries an increased mortality. It usually occurs within 48 hours of onset of symptoms and is most frequently associated with inferior myocardial infarction. Because of myocardial irritability following infarction, pacing when instituted should be of the demand type.

Inferior Myocardial Infarction — usually results from right coronary artery occlusion. This vessel supplies the artery to the A-V node in 90% of people. Histologically, the A-V node exhibits only ischaemia and oedema, and therefore the heart block which results is only rarely permanent. Occasionally complete heart block appears suddenly, but usually it is preceded by first degree and then second degree heart block. The degree of block may be accentuated by digitalis, β-adrenoceptor blockers and some other antiarrhythmic drugs. In this type of block, the A-V node is directly involved and as the natural subsidiary pacemaker lies below in the bundle of His, there is a faster rate than in the chronic heart block. Stokes-Adams attacks are therefore unusual. Unless other complications develop, the mortality from inferior infarction is unaltered by the development of A-V block. However, if there is haemodynamic embarrassment due to the slow rate, demand pacing is strongly advised. Permanent pacing is rarely required but the temporary electrodes should be left *in situ* for 2 to 3 weeks.

Antero-Septal Myocardial Infarction — heart block usually results from extensive septal infarction with involvement of both the left and right bundle branches. Consequently the rate is slow, the QRS complexes are wide and complete heart block may appear suddenly. The patient may show bundle branch block prior to this. Because of the extent of the infarction, the prognosis remains poor, even if pacing is instituted early. Permanent pacing may be required if the patient survives.

3) *Other Bradyarrhythmias:* These include sinus bradycardia, nodal bradycardia, slow atrial fibrillation, sinoatrial block and the sick sinus syndromes. These often alternate with tachyarrhythmias making drug treatment difficult. Either atrial or ventricular pacing may be used.

4) *Tachyarrhythmias:* Pacemaking can be utilised to increase the cardiac rate and so suppress by overdrive, tachyarrhythmias originating from either the atrium or ventricle. High pacing rates, even 150 beats per minute or more, may be required to overdrive these arrhythmias, but the actual pacemaker rate need not always be faster than the arrhythmia. Once overdriving is achieved, the pacing rate may then be lowered. Antiarrhythmic drugs, including β-adrenoceptor blockers, may be used in conjunction with the pacemaker. Occasionally, permanent pacing is required using special high rate generators (90 to 100 per minute).

7.2 Sites of Pacing

Ventricular pacing results in the loss of the atrial boost but this is relatively unimportant unless the cardiac output is critical. Sequential pacing will overcome this problem but requires an electrode in the right atrium and another in the right ventricle. The heart is then paced sequentially to restore A-V relations. Implanted sequential pacemakers however, are cumbersome, difficult to insert and require considerable power to operate.

The majority of patients are paced from the endocardial surface of the right ventricle. There appears to be no advantage in implanting epicardial electrodes onto the surface of the heart and the procedure adds the risk of an anaesthetic and thoractomy. The newer transvenous electrodes are easy to insert and have very few complications. The indications for epicardial electrodes include the young patient, and the now rare situation where a stable transvenous electrode position can not be achieved with a satisfactory low pacing threshold. Right atrial and atrial pacing from the coronary sinus may be used in patients with intact A-V conduction for overdrive or rate control. Positioning of the transvenous electrode for this type of permanent pacing may be difficult and epicardial electrodes may have to be sutured to the atrium.

8. Heart Failure

8.1 Congestive Heart Failure

The term congestive heart failure is applied to the circulatory congestion which develops in various organs of the body as a direct result of decompensation of the heart. Therapeutic principles in the management of congestive heart failure include (Hay, 1973; Walker, 1974):

a) Determination of the nature of the underlying heart disease
b) Search for precipitating causes — e.g. hypertension, thyrotoxicosis, drugs which cause salt and fluid retention or aggravate heart failure (see section 10.1,11.4)
c) Reduction of the demands on the heart — e.g. by rest
d) Improvement of the pump — e.g. by use of the minimum effective dose of digitalis, or afterload reduction with vasodilators
e) Control of oedema — e.g. modest restriction of dietary sodium, fluid restriction in severe failure, diuretics
f) Prevention of recurrences — rehabilitate the patient

Attitudes to treatment of congestive heart failure are changing. New approaches place less emphasis on digitalis (recognising appropriate indications and need for its use), with diuretics being recommended as the first drug to use in mild to moderate congestive heart failure in patients in sinus rhythm and vasodilators as adjuncts to treatment in patients with severe congestive heart failure refractory to other therapy (Lemberg, 1978). A diuretic alone may suffice in many elderly patients with congestive heart failure (ch. V; sect. 4.1.1; Hull and MacKintosh, 1977).

A fundamental treatment in all patients with congestive heart failure is rest. Rest, which usually means chair or bed rest, reduces the work of the heart. However, the potential problems associated with bed rest (e.g. thromboembolism; chest infection; urinary retention) should be remembered and measures taken to reduce them. If necessary diazepam may be given to help provide rest during the day, whilst morphine 10 to 15mg subcutaneously may be used for the treatment of nocturnal dyspnoea. Tricyclic antidepressants when indicated, should be given with care because of their propensity to cause cardiac complications in some patients with cardiac failure (see section 10).

8.1.1 Fluid Intake

Patients with congestive heart failure can not excrete sodium as effectively as healthy subjects. In mild cases of heart failure, the capacity of the kidneys to secrete sodium may be only partly reduced and a modest restriction of dietary sodium may be all that is needed to maintain sodium balance. In more advanced failure, a diuretic may be needed. Fluid intake generally should not be restricted in moderate degrees of heart failure, provided no more than 4 to 5 litres a day are ingested. In very severe failure, with hyponatraemia, fluid intake may need to be restricted.

8.1.2 Indications and Assessment of Need for Digitalis

It is probably a sound principle to use a digitalis preparation whenever a *firm* diagnosis of cardiac failure is made, although the justification for using digitalis in the management of mild congestive heart failure in sinus rhythm is open to question. The need for digitalis and indications for its use should always be carefully assessed as continued digitalisation carries a substantial risk of toxicity, particularly in the elderly (Landahl et al., 1977; see chapter V, sect. 4.1). Digitalis should not be taken indefinitely for heart failure without regular reassessment, but evaluation of the need for continued therapy is difficult. Some patients may not actually need maintenance digitalis therapy, either because of insufficient indications for its original use or because the indication for continued use may no longer exist.

Although digitalis is of continued benefit in controlling heart rate in atrial fibrillation in those with a history of heart failure (Dobbs et al., 1977c), its value in those with sinus rhythm after an episode of heart failure is unclear. In some patients in sinus rhythm, digitalis does appear to exert a sustained effect. Overall, maintenance digitalis can be discontinued in many patients in sinus rhythm who have no clinical evidence of heart failure, particularly in those with plasma concentrations below the considered therapeutic range (Johnston and McDevitt, 1979; Liverpool Therapeutics Group, 1978). Digitalis can be much more readily withdrawn in those for whom it was given for inadequate reasons (Dall, 1970; Johnston and McDevitt, 1979).

Fear of toxicity, confusion about dosage or uncertainty about the need for digitalis should not however, lead to under prescribing when it is definitely indicated (Liverpool Therapeutics Group, 1978; Carruthers et al., 1974).

8.1.3 Clinical Pharmacology of Digitalis

A thorough knowledge of the clinical pharmacology of digitalis glycosides is essential for their effective and safe use (for reviews, see Doherty and Kane, 1973; Smith and Haber, 1973). Application of such knowledge by individual clinicians can materially reduce the incidence of digitalis toxicity (Ogilvie and Ruedy, 1972).

Actions of Digitalis: The main pharmacodynamic property of digitalis in heart failure is to increase the force of myocardial contraction (Smith and Haber, 1973). The electrophysiological effects include increased effective refractory period of the A-V node and Purkinje fibres, increased excitability of the ventricle and ventricular conducting system and a variable effect on the atria and sinus node. Automaticity of subsidiary pacemakers is enhanced. At a cellular level, digitalis inhibits Na^+ and K^+ transport. The extent of inhibition is dose related and increases with increasing cardiac glycoside concentrations. However, the role of altered Na^+ and K^+ transport in the mechanism of the positive inotropic effect of digitalis on heart muscle and in its propensity to produce cardiac arrhythmias, although intensively

investigated, is not fully understood and is controversial (Schwartz, 1977; Smith, 1978).

Digitalis Preparations: A number of glycoside preparations are available — each with different pharmacokinetic properties and onset and duration of action (table XIII), which might be exploited in individual patients. For example, when a rapid onset of effect is required (e.g. patients with severe heart failure and fast atrial fibrillation together with a rapid ventricular rate), intravenous ouabain might be an advantage, although digoxin is usually adequate. Digitoxin might be considered in a patient with renal failure. All digitalis preparations have the same type of myocardial action and same low therapeutic to toxic ratio. Digoxin is the most widely used cardiac glycoside in many countries and is the preparation of choice for routine clinical use. Medigoxin (β-methyldigoxin), a semi-synthetic glycoside, is more completely absorbed than digoxin but offers no important advantage. Because of its long elimination half-life, should toxicity occur with digitoxin, signs and symptoms may persist for weeks (Lely and van Enter, 1970). Digitoxin is highly albumin bound (97%) and is subject to altered binding in the presence of hypoalbuminaemia, cirrhosis, the nephrotic syndrome and uraemia but the clinical consequences are not yet clear (Storstein, 1977). More importantly, hepatic metabolism of digitoxin leads to large interindividual variability in rate of elimination and hence time required to attain steady-state plasma concentrations and the eventual concentration achieved (Perrier et al., 1977). Metabolism of digitoxin is not altered in cirrhosis, possibly because of excretion into the bile and faeces (see chapter XIX; sect. 1.4). Drug interactions with digitoxin are summarised in table XIV. Other preparations listed in table XII and XIII are poorly absorbed and not suitable for routine clinical use.

Pharmacokinetic Properties of Digoxin: As a consequence of its poor solubility, digoxin is incompletely absorbed and can be associated with bioavailability problems (see Greenblatt et al., 1976; Nyberg, 1977; chapter VI, sect. 2.1). About 70 to 80% of an oral dose is absorbed from well formulated (i.e. rapid dissolution) tablets, mainly from the proximal part of the small intestine. Peak plasma concentrations are attained in 0.5 to 1 hour from high bioavailability tablets. Absorption is more complete from an elixir but intramuscular injection leads to only a little better availability and

Table XIII. Pharmacokinetic properties, onset and duration of effect of the more commonly used digitalis preparations (after Iisalo, 1977; Perrier et al., 1977; Smith and Haber, 1973)

Drug	Absorption[1]	Onset of action[2]	Peak effect[2]	Half life[3]	Elimination
Ouabain (G strophanthin)	Unreliable	5-10 min	0.5-2h	~21h	Renal excretion of unchanged drug; some gastrointestinal excretion
Deslanoside (desacetyl-lanatoside C)	40-65%[4]	10-30 min	1-2h	~36h	Renal excretion of unchanged drug
Digoxin	70-80% (best tablets)	15-30 min	1.5-5h	30-40h	Renal excretion of unchanged drug; some gastrointestinal excretion (metabolism may be an important consideration in altered disposition in severe renal and cardiac failure; see text)
Digitoxin	90-100%	25-120 min	4-12h	7-8 days	Hepatic metabolism (enterohepatic cycle exists); renal excretion of unchanged drug (up to 30% in some individuals) and of active metabolites (usually quantitatively un-important)
Digitalis leaf	40% approx.	—	—	4-6 days	Similar to digitoxin

1   Amount of a dose absorbed from gastrointestinal tract after oral administration.
2   Onset of action and peak effect after intravenous administration.
3   Average value and range in persons with normal renal or liver function. Prolonged by renal impairment with digoxin, ouabain and deslanoside/lanatoside C and probably by severe liver disease with digitoxin and digitalis leaf.
4   Given orally as lanatoside C. Only trace amounts of lanatoside C appear in plasma as the parent compound (Aldous and Thomas et al., 1977); it is metabolised by gut bacteria to acetyldigoxin and digoxin which are then absorbed, giving total absorption of cardioactive compounds of 40 to 65%.

can be erratically absorbed. Food reduces the rate but not the amount of digoxin absorbed. Gastric resection does not affect absorption. However, altered intestinal motility and malabsorption syndromes can impair the absorption of digoxin (see chapter XIX; sect. 1.1), and is most likely to be a problem with tablets with slow dissolution characteristics (see chapter VI; sect. 5). Digoxin is extensively distributed in tissues, as reflected in its large volume of distribution of around 5 to 8L/kg. High concentrations are found in the heart, kidney and skeletal muscle, but not in adipose tissue. Lean body mass correlates better with digoxin dosage in obesity than total body weight (see chapter XVI; sect. 1.4.3). Protein binding is low (30 to 40%) and although variation in binding can occur in disease states (Storstein, 1977), even large changes are unlikely to be of clinical consequence (see chapter I; sect. 3.2.3).

Elimination of digoxin is mainly via the kidneys; 60 to 80% of an intravenous dose is excreted in the urine in 6 to 12 days in patients with normal renal function. About 25 to 30% of digoxin is eliminated by non-renal routes. Renal clearance correlates with creatinine clearance and hence glomerular filtration rate. In addition, some tubular secretion and possibly tubular reabsorption occurs. Some have found urea clearance, an index of both glomerular filtration rate and passive tubular reabsorption, to more accurately predict

Table XIV. Potential clinically important drug interactions which may influence response to digoxin and to digitoxin

Interacting drug	Mechanism[1]	Possible effect/action[2]
Antacid gel liquids (aluminium hydroxide or magnesium containing) Antidiarrhoeals (adsorbent type)	DA	Decreased bioavailability of digoxin. More likely to be a potential problem with slowly dissolving tablets
Anticholinergic drugs	IA	Increased risk of digoxin toxicity if bioavailability significantly increased. Only a problem with slowly dissolving tablets (see chapter VI, sect. 5; VIII, sect. 2.3.1)
Calcium	PD	Avoid intravenous calcium. If essential, do not give rapidly or in large amounts
Cholestyramine Colestipol	DA	Decreased digoxin bioavailability possible (give drugs about 8 hours after digoxin)
	DA + IE	Decreased bioavailability of digitoxin (give drugs about 8 hours after digitoxin)
Diuretics Carbenoxolone Amphotericin B	PD	Increased risk of toxicity due to electrolyte abnormalities — hypokalaemia, hypomagnesaemia. Replenish potassium stores in those on daily diuretics (see section 8.1.4). Avoid carbenoxolone
Neomycin	DA	Decreased bioavailability of digoxin. Digoxin toxicity when prolonged neomycin therapy withdrawn
PAS	DA	Decreased bioavailability of digoxin
Phenobarbitone Phenylbutazone Phenytoin (diphenyl-hydantoin) Rifampicin	AM	Accelerated metabolism of digitoxin. Marked decrease in plasma concentration of digitoxin. Increased formation of digoxin also likely (? quantitative importance). Clinical relevance of interaction not known If necessary, increase dose of digitoxin or use a substitute for phenobarbitone (e.g. diazepam) or phenylbutazone (e.g. indomethacin). Other enzyme inducing agents also likely to have same effect. Carefully watch for signs of toxicity if enzyme inducing agents withdrawn from stable digitoxin regimen (see chapter VIII, sect. 2.3.3)
Phenytoin	DA	Decreased bioavailability of digoxin
Quinidine	?IR	Marked increase in plasma concentration of digoxin with real risk of digitalis toxicity (see section 6.1.1)
Rauwolfia	PD	?Possible increased risk of toxicity. Best to avoid large parenteral doses of reserpine
Spironolactone	IR	Increase in plasma concentration of digoxin. Lower than usual loading and maintenance dose may be indicated

Table XIV. (continued)

Sulphasalazine	DA	Decreased bioavailability of digoxin in some patients
Suxamethonium (succinylcholine)	PD	Increased risk of toxicity due to release of potassium, especially in patients with trauma, burns, wounds or muscular disorders
Sympathomimetic drugs	PD	Increased risk of toxicity. Only use these drugs with caution

1   Mechanism known or thought to be most likely. Digoxin and digitoxin have different pharmacokinetic properties (table XIII).
DA   =   Decreased absorption.
IA   =   Increased absorption.
IE   =   Inhibition of enterohepatic circulation.
IR   =   Inhibition of renal clearance.
AM   =   Accelerated hepatic metabolism.
PD   =   Pharmacodynamic action (influence on tissue response).
2   Diuretics are by far the most important and likely problem. The possibility of interaction with other compounds has been suggested by a few case reports or studies.
Absorption interactions involving digoxin are generally probably of minimal clinical importance. They are most likely to be of importance with slowly dissolving tablet formulations.

digoxin clearance than creatinine clearance, particularly in patients with severe cardiac failure (Halkin et al., 1975b) in whom total clearance of digoxin seems to be reduced beyond that which can be accounted for on the basis of reduced creatinine clearance (Benowitz and Meister, 1976). A reduction in distribution volume may possibly also contribute to the higher plasma concentrations which have been observed (Dobbs et al., 1976) in patients with severe cardiac failure when dosage is determined on the basis of creatinine clearance. Initial distribution volume of digoxin is decreased in patients with advanced cor pulmonale, a condition functionally equivalent to congestive heart failure (du Souich et al., 1978). Since digitalis toxicity is more likely to occur in patients with severe heart failure (Beller et al., 1971), greater caution than usual would seem to be necessary with initial dosage in these patients. Subsequent dosage adjustment will be necessary as clinical improvement from overt heart failure leads to increased clearance of digoxin (see further section 1.5). Obviously, therefore, changing clearance, and altered distribution (see below), of digoxin should be taken into account when determining both loading and maintenance dosage.

Virtually all of the digoxin in the urine is excreted as unchanged drug, with a small proportion as active metabolites. Biliary excretion accounts for elimination of a lesser amount of a given dose; slightly more unchanged drug than active metabolites being recovered in the faeces. Enterohepatic circulation seems to be of minor importance, in contrast to digitoxin. Because the main route of excretion of digoxin is as unchanged drug in the urine and extrarenal elimination is minimal, impaired kidney function leads to a decreased rate of elimination and to accumulation of digoxin if dosage is not altered; the normal elimination half-life of around 30 to 40 hours being prolonged, in parallel with creatinine clearance, to 87-110 hours or more in anuric patients (see chapter XXI; sect. 14.2.1). Renal clearance of digoxin is also decreased in neonates and young infants, but this impairment in excretory capacity lessens rapidly as renal function develops in the first 3 months of life (see chapter IV; sect. 2.3.2). Renal function is also an important determinant of clearance and dosage of digoxin in the elderly (see chapter V; sect. 4.1). Dosage should therefore be smaller than usual in patients with impaired renal function, in the elderly and in neonates and young infants.

There is a linear relationship between the steady-state plasma concentration of digoxin and dose in patients with normal and impaired renal function such that a change in digoxin dose should result in a proportional change in digoxin plasma concentration (Okada et al., 1978b). When renal function is severely impaired (i.e. creatinine clearance below $15ml/min/1.73m^2$), minor changes in creatinine clearance result in major changes in the relationship between plasma digoxin concentration and dose and necessitates careful adjustment of the dosage of digoxin. Creatinine clearance, which correlates with *renal* clearance of digoxin, does not accurately predict *total body* excretion of digoxin, particularly in patients with severely impaired renal function. Dosing of digoxin in severe renal failure based primarily on creatinine clearance must be used with caution.

The volume of distribution of digoxin is decreased in renal failure (and in advanced cor-pulmonale; see above) and is another factor apart from decreased renal elimination which can result in higher plasma concentrations and toxicity from use of the same dose as in a patient with normal renal function (Aronson and Grahame-Smith, 1976b). This means that any loading dose should be smaller than usual (about 50%) in patients with renal failure. Similarly, a decrease in distribution volume in the elderly may also contribute to the need for smaller doses with advancing age (Cusack et al., 1978; Ewy et al., 1969). A decrease in distribution volume of digoxin may also contribute to the altered disposition of digoxin in neonates compared with older infants and children (see chapter IV; sect. 2.2.2) and in hypothyroidism (see section 8.1.4).

Occasional instances of abnormal digoxin metabolism and clearance have been reported (Fleckenstein et al., 1977; Okada et al., 1978a), emphasising the need to individualise dosage in all patients. Although only a small amount of a dose of digoxin is usually metabolised, there is wide interindividual variability in metabolic capacity. Earlier suggestions (Marcus et al., 1966b) that the amount of digoxin metabolised may increase in renal failure have not been confirmed, but requires further study, particularly since metabolism may be an important consideration in the effects of severe renal and cardiac failure on disposition of digoxin (see above). Liver disease does not influence digoxin elimination.

Breast feeding may be safely permitted in lactating mothers receiving digoxin. Although concentrations of digoxin in breast milk approach those in maternal plasma, digoxin could not be detected in the plasma of breast fed infants after usual maintenance dosage (Loughnan, 1978; see chapter IV, table VII). Digoxin is transferred across the placenta, and although uptake by fetal tissues is slow, when continued long term during pregnancy, the plasma digoxin concentration at the time of delivery is the same in the newborn as in the mother. No adverse effects have been noted on the fetus with long term use during pregnancy (see chapter III; sect. 8.4).

A number of pathophysiological conditions may change the 'sensitivity' of the myocardium to digitalis (see section 8.1.4). In some cases such as cor pulmonale and thyroid diseases, modification of the pharmacokinetics of digoxin may in part contribute to the altered response. Similarly, by far the most important drug interactions with digoxin are due to pharmacodynamic mechanisms (Binnion, 1978), but some important interactions can occur in the absorptive phase (see table XIV). For a review of the pharmacokinetics of digoxin, see Iisalo (1977) and of digitoxin, see Perrier et al. (1977).

8.1.4 Factors Affecting Digitalis Toxicity

1) *Loading dose:* The traditional concept concerning the relationship between the dose and positive action of digitalis on cardiac contractility appears to have been responsible, in part, for the high frequency of digitalis toxicity noted above. In the past, clinicians had believed that little contractile benefit was achieved until a certain digitalising dose was administered. However, it is now known that there is a linear therapeutic dose-contractile response (Lee et al., 1972). Thus, small or large amounts of the drug have the same qualitative effects and similar quantitative action proportional to the dose employed.

Only maintenance doses of the glycoside are necessary to achieve therapeutic concentrations within a period of a few days (Marcus et al., 1966a). Large loading doses are not indicated when the contractile action of the glycoside is not immediately needed. These observations are particularly important if digitalis is used to provide some salutary inotropic support in patients with cardiac dysfunction without advanced heart failure or in patients prone to digitalis intoxication. Therefore, a patient need not receive a maximally tolerated dose in a short period of time to achieve some therapeutic benefit. As the concentration of digitalis within the body accumulates slowly on a daily basis, the quantity eliminated rises until the amount excreted equals the amount taken as maintenance (Jelliffe, 1969). The body appears to eliminate daily a certain constant percentage of the quantity of systemic glycoside, about 33 % for digoxin when endogenous creatinine clearance is normal (Doherty and Kane, 1973). For example, in normal subjects taking 0.5mg digoxin orally daily, the peak concentration of digoxin in the blood obtained after 6 days is the same whether or not an initial loading dose is given (fig. 5).

2) Renal failure: Excretion of digoxin is compromised by renal insufficiency (see above). Digoxin is excreted primarily as unchanged drug by the kidney and dosage must be reduced in renal failure. Loading doses should be reduced by up to a half and maintenance dosage determined in accordance with creatinine clearance (see appendix E). Plasma concentrations should be monitored to adjust dosage in individual patients. Digitoxin however, is eliminated mainly by hepatic metabolism and to a lesser extent as unchanged drug in the

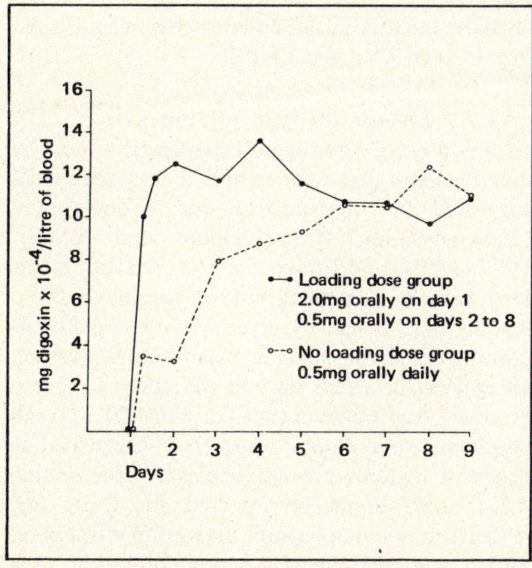

Fig. 5. Digitalisation without a loading dose (after Marcus et al., 1966a; by permission of author and editor).

Serum concentration of digoxin is plotted on the vertical axis, time on the horizontal. Closed circles (●) represent patients given 2.0mg of tritiated digoxin in a single loading dose orally with resulting blood levels. Open circles (○) represent the same patients given 0.5mg of tritiated digoxin daily for 9 days. Note similar blood level of digoxin at 6th day.

urine and faeces; in some patients up to 30 % of a dose may be excreted as unchanged drug in the urine. Although digoxin is formed from digitoxin, it usually appears to be a quantitatively unimportant metabolite (Perrier et al., 1977). Thus in most cases, digitoxin dosage probably requires no modification in renal failure, although some clinicians reduce dosage in patients with severely impaired renal function (see appendix E; see further chapter XXI, sect. 14.2.1).

3) Advanced age: Tolerance of digitalis is compromised in the elderly, perhaps because of reduced cardiac (Na$^+$—K$^+$) ATPase pump activity (Conn et al., 1972). Dosage of digoxin in the elderly should be less than in younger patients, largely because of their diminished capacity to excrete the drug and also smaller lean body size. Unless there is evidence to the contrary, renal function should be assumed to be reduced by 50 % in the elderly (Ewy et al., 1969). Loading dosage should be reduced by up to a half of usual and maintenance dosage determined on the basis of renal function and body size. Maintenance dosage may need to be as low as 0.0625mg daily, which is facilitated by the use of small strength tablets which are available (0.125 and 0.0625mg). See also chapter V (sect. 2.1.3, 4.1.1).

4) The presence of electrolyte or acid-base disturbances: Intracellular potassium, magnesium and chloride are major determinants of digitalis action, particularly potassium (Smith and Haber, 1973). Loss of these electrolytes becomes an important consideration in patients receiving diuretics. Because digitalis toxic arrhythmias may appear with hypokalaemia at normal plasma concentrations of digitalis (Aronson et al., 1978; Steiness and Olesen, 1976), replenishment of potassium stores is advised for patients on daily diuretics. Hypochloraemic alkalosis associated with intracellular potassium loss also contributes to enhanced susceptibility to digitalis toxicity whether patients are hypokalaemic, normokalaemic or hyperkalaemic (Brater and Morrelli, 1977). Potassium supplements (as potassium chloride) can be used, but they may not always be effective at restoring serum or total body potassium (see chapter XXI; sect. 7.1). A potassium sparing diuretic such as amiloride, triamterene or spironolactone, is an effective way to correct both the hypokalaemia and alkalosis. These drugs must however, be used carefully. In patients with impaired renal function, in elderly diabetics and in patients on a large daily intake of potassium (either dietary or therapeutic) hyperkalaemia may readily occur, even with small doses of the potassium-sparing diuretics. Therapeutic potassium supplements should not be used concurrently with a potassium-sparing diuretic.

Hypomagnesaemia may also increase the susceptibility to digitalis toxicity (Beller et al., 1974), and on the basis of experimental evidence, hyponatraemia and hypercalcaemia may do likewise (Harrison and Wakim, 1969; Nola et al., 1970). If hypokalaemia occurs in a patient taking digitalis it is probably best to stop therapy and correct the electrolyte abnormality. Acidosis may predispose to digitalis toxicity by causing loss of intracellular potassium.

5) *Certain types of heart disease:* Electrical toxicity is probably more frequent in acute myocardial infarction and chronic coronary artery disease than in normally perfused hearts (Smith and Haber, 1970). Patients with advanced ventricular failure from any cause are also more prone to digitalis arrhythmias than those with less severe dysfunction (Beller et al., 1971). Smaller doses (usually half those normally used) are indicated in patients with recent myocardial infarction. In normal hearts and in children with heart disease, atrioventricular conduction disturbances occur more often than tachyarrhythmias with glycoside overdose (Levine and Somlyo, 1962). In adult patients with latent disease of the atrioventricular node, digitalis can produce heart block before accelerated activity of ectopic pacemakers (Smith and Haber, 1970).

6) *Cardioversion and cardiac operations:* Excessive dosage with risk of digoxin toxicity should be avoided before cardioversion because of the risk of inducing ventricular arrhythmias. Similarly, prior to cardiac operations, digoxin dose should be reduced to below the lower limit of the accepted therapeutic range (Rose et al., 1975).

7) *Pulmonary heart disease:* Patients with pulmonary heart disease (cor pulmonale) are already prone to arrhythmias and these may be more readily provoked by digitalis, which is probably related in part to systemic arterial hypoxaemia (Morrison and Killip, 1971b). Control of the ventilatory disturbance is obviously important. Digitalis intoxication occurs at lower mean plasma

digoxin concentrations than in patients without pulmonary heart disease (Paciaroni et al., 1974). Except when necessary to control the ventricular response with atrial fibrillation, smaller doses of digoxin should be used since these patients are often elderly, thin, and sometimes have impaired renal function or coronary artery disease (Doherty et al., 1977). Advanced cor pulmonale with decreased perfusion of the kidney may lead to a reduced volume of distribution and high initial peak plasma concentration, necessitating smaller and greater caution with loading doses of digoxin (du Souich et al., 1978).

8) *Hypothyroidism:* The response to digoxin and digitoxin is enhanced in hypothyroidism and has been attributed to both altered tissue response and altered kinetics of digitalis. Disposition is altered such that patients with myxoedema have higher plasma concentrations of digoxin and digitoxin for comparable doses of the drug based on body weight. The reverse situation prevails in hyperthyroidism. Loading dosage should be reduced by up to a half in patients with untreated hypothyroidism with a proportionately smaller maintenance dosage, which will need to be adjusted as the thyroid condition is effectively treated (see chapter XVI; sect. 1.4.2).

8.1.5 Dosage of Digoxin (table XII)

The dose of any digitalis preparation must be individualised and various approaches have been suggested for digoxin (e.g. see Aronson and Grahame-Smith, 1976a; Dobbs and Mawer, 1977; Jelliffe and Brooker, 1974). Because of the long half-life of digoxin (and other glycosides) a loading dose is usually given to more rapidly attain the desired steady-state plasma concentration. Otherwise, it would take in the case of digoxin around 7 days (about 5 times its half-life), to reach steady-state (see chapter 1; sect. 2.2). Large loading doses of digitalis are not necessary (see section 8.1.4) and should be reserved for those few patients in whom a prompt maximum effect is required (e.g. extremely rapid digitalisation in a patient with fast atrial fibrillation and severe cardiac failure). Orally administered digoxin is rapidly absorbed from tablets of high bioavailability and is the route of choice. If the patient is unable to take an oral dose (e.g. vomiting, coma) or if rapid digitalisation is necessary, slow (over about 5 minutes) intravenous infusion of undiluted solution may be used, although intravenous ouabain is usually preferred for extremely rapid digitalisation. If intravenous administration of digoxin is used doses should be about 20 to 30 % lower than oral doses from high bioavailability tablets (70 to 80 % absorbed). Intramuscular administration of digoxin is painful, and it is erratically absorbed and should be avoided.

Loading dose: In normal young adults who have not been receiving digitalis, a total oral loading dose of digoxin (using high bioavailability tablets) between 10 and 15μg/kg divided into 2 or 3 equal parts and given at 6-hourly intervals (Jelliffe and Brooker, 1974), or a single smaller loading dose of 0.75mg (Dobbs and Mawer, 1977), both regimens followed by a suitable maintenance dose 6 hours later, results in plasma concentrations in the desired therapeutic range. These loading dose schedules are reduced by up to a half in the elderly and in patients with renal failure or untreated hypothyroidism (see section 8.1.4). Since digoxin renal clearance (and dosage) shows good correlation with creatinine clearance, the loading dose can be calculated and scaled down accordingly: e.g. with the single small loading dose regimen to 0.625mg at clearances of 65ml/min, with reduction to 0.5mg at 50ml/min and 0.375mg at clearances of 30ml/min (Dobbs et al., 1977b).

Either schedule is only an initial guide and adjustment of subsequent doses may be necessary according to individual response and desired therapeutic effect. Patients in atrial fibrillation tend to require larger doses than those in sinus rhythm (Chamberlain et al., 1970). In uncontrolled rapid atrial fibrillation with failure, the aim is to slow the ventricular rate, and repeated doses may be needed during the first 24 hours to achieve the desired slowing.

The clinical response is fundamental; rigid schedules of dosage are a guide only. The divided dose regimen allows a small dose to be given and the patient observed for early signs of toxicity before administration of the next dose. The single dose regimen allows more rapid attainment of the steady-state but uses a sufficiently small dose such that the patient can be observed for any evidence of toxicity before the first initial maintenance dose is given. If it is not possible or necessary to administer a loading dose, the steady-state can be attained more slowly by giving the calculated initial maintenance dose over about 7 days (i.e. 5 times the half-life of digoxin; see section 8.1.4, fig. 5).

The initial maintenance dose should be calculated on the percentage of the loading dose eliminated daily, which for digoxin depends on renal function; i.e. the maintenance dose replaces daily loss at steady-state. With normal renal function (creatinine clearance of 100ml/min) about a third of total body digoxin is eliminated daily and decreases to about 14 % when creatinine clearance falls to 0ml/min. The relationship between these two values is linear and the percentage can be readily calculated from the formula (Jelliffe, 1969):

$$\% \text{ Eliminated daily} = \frac{14 + Cl_{cr}}{5}$$

then:

$$\text{Daily maintenance dose} = \text{Loading dose} \times \% \text{ eliminated}$$

Dialysis has only a negligible effect on removal of digoxin and does not need to be considered in the calculation of dosage in patients with chronic renal failure.

In practice, the above formula means an initial maintenance dose of one third of a loading dose of 0.75mg in younger adult patients with normal renal function and electrolyte balance. This and other data (Dobbs et al., 1977a) supports the common arbitrary practice of prescribing 0.25mg digoxin daily to all adult patients, apart from the elderly and those with known renal impairment, until the clinical response can be assessed and appropriate adjustment to dose made.

The usual continuation maintenance dose of digoxin in an adult is 0.25 to 0.375mg daily, but may vary from 0.125 to 0.5mg daily. Older, smaller patients require less than younger, robust patients. The majority of patients with moderate renal function impairment (creatinine clearance < 40ml/min) require maintenance doses from 0.125 to 0.25mg daily and those with severe impairment (< 20ml/min) doses from 0.0625mg to 0.125mg daily (Dobbs et al., 1976; see also section 8.1.3 and appendix E).

Similar reductions in usual maintenance dosage of digoxin are necessary in the elderly and many require only 0.0625mg daily for maintenance (see chapter V; sect. 4.1). Small strength tablets are available to facilitate use of these dosages. Although individual dose requirements of digoxin are usually increased in neonates and young infants, this practice has been challenged (see chapter IV; sect. 2.3.2). Dosage of digoxin in obesity should be calculated on the basis of lean body weight and not larger doses based on total body weight (see chapter XVI; sect. 1.4.3).

It should be emphasised that some patients may not respond in the manner as outlined above, but the suggested approaches to calculation of loading and maintenance doses, are nevertheless a useful initial guide to treatment. Dosage of digoxin must always be adjusted according to the response of the individual patient and the presence of factors which predispose to toxicity (see section 8.1.4). Assessment of the desired response is difficult and is usually based on amelioration of the symptoms and signs of congestive heart failure. More objective tests and special procedures are available to establish the total therapeutic effect more precisely (Weintraub, 1977). Even when the desired response has been achieved, certain groups of patients require regular follow-up because of changing dose requirements; for example, those whose renal function may have altered, the elderly, and patients with thyroid disease under treatment. When adjusting maintenance dosage, it should be noted that a change in dose of digoxin will result in a proportional change in plasma concentration (see section 8.1.3).

Plasma digoxin concentrations provide a guide in an individual patient to whether a lack of response is a reflection of insufficient dosage, non-compliance with the medication regimen (in some series about a third of patients were taking less than their prescribed dose of digoxin; Johnstone and McDevitt, 1978; Weintraub et al., 1973) or poor absorption, or whether an excessive concentration might indicate digitalis intoxication (see section 8.1.7). However, multifactorial determinants of digitalis intoxication and overlap in plasma digoxin concentration between toxic and non-toxic patients, preclude the use of plasma concentrations as the sole guide to digoxin dosage. Nevertheless, reliable assays, when considered along with available clinical information can be a valuable aid to a therapeutic decision (Weintraub, 1977; see sect. 8.1.7). Drugs which may interact with digitalis in a clinical setting and increase the risk of toxicity are shown in table XIV.

8.1.6 Digitalis Intoxication and Side Effects

Although the presence of gastrointestinal, central nervous system and visual disturbances are helpful in diagnosis of digitalis intoxication, if present and elicited (Lely and van Enter, 1970), they do not always precede the more serious cardiac arrhythmias (Beller et al., 1971; Smith, 1973). Very often an intoxicated patient presents only with arrhythmia. In at least a third of cases of digitalis intoxication, disorders of cardiac rhythm (see section 6.3) are the first and sometimes only manifestation of toxicity. Gastrointestinal disturbances include anorexia, nausea, diarrhoea and abdominal pain. Fatigue and a feeling of muscular weakness are common CNS effects, but mental confusion, hallucinations, disorientation, headache, paraesthesiae and overt psychosis can also occur. Visual symptoms include blurred vision, difficulty in reading, altered colour vision and visual hallucinations. Skin rash and gynaecomastia in men (see chapter XV; sect. 23.6) are rare side effects of digoxin. Management of digitalis intoxication is discussed in section 6.3.

8.1.7 Indications for Plasma Digoxin Estimation

Estimation of the plasma level of digoxin is desirable when (Doherty, 1978; Weintraub, 1977):

a) There is suspicion of a toxic response or lack of anticipated therapeutic effect in the absence of predisposing factors
b) Renal function is markedly impaired or variable

and might be considered when:

c) There is doubt about previous absorption because of uncertain tablet reliability, suspected non-compliance with the prescribed dosage regimen, overt or suspected malabsorption including that due to interaction with other drugs (e.g. cholestyramine) or lack of adequate history
d) There is predisposition to toxicity (see section 8.1.4).

Although there are reasonable correlations between response and the plasma concentration of digoxin, it has to be appreciated that tissue response probably does not always necessarily exactly parallel the plasma concentration, particularly in the presence of hypokalaemia. Moreover, response to digoxin differs in different patients. Some patients require a higher plasma concentration for therapeutic effect, while others tolerate concentrations which would be toxic in most other patients.

Most studies have nevertheless indicated a therapeutic range for digoxin of 0.5 to 2.0ng/ml (usually about 1 to 2.0ng/ml) and a difference in plasma concentrations between toxic and non-toxic patients, but with overlap between the two groups (see Smith, 1975; fig. 6). In one definitive study, about 90% of adult patients without digitalis toxicity had plasma digoxin concentrations of less than 2.0ng/ml, while some 85% of toxic patients had concentrations above 2.0ng/ml. There was a range of overlap between the two groups from 1.6 to 3.0ng/ml (fig. 6b). Thus, in general, if a patient has a concentration much above 2.0ng/ml he is more likely to suffer toxicity, but if the concentration is below 2.0ng/ml he is much less likely to be at risk of toxicity.

This overlap can be attributed in part to individual variability but is also contributed to by various extra-cardiac factors which influence either the distribution of digoxin in the body (e.g. renal failure, elderly, neonates; see section 8.1.3) or the response of the heart to the drug (e.g. electrolyte abnormalities). Hypokalaemia in particular influences the interpretation of plasma digoxin concentrations since toxicity can occur at concentrations normally considered non-toxic. In one study (Aronson et al., 1978), virtually all patients with definite digitalis toxicity but with plasma digoxin concentrations less than 1.5ng/ml were hypokalaemic. Thus, plasma digoxin concentration estimation *alone* is of little help in the diagnosis of digitalis toxicity in patients with hypokalaemia. Plasma concentrations must therefore always be interpreted within the clinical context of the patient.

Without a loading dose, plasma must be drawn at least 1 week after starting oral therapy in a patient with normal clearance of digoxin so that values reflect steady-state concentrations. Plasma must also be drawn sufficiently after the last previous dose (generally, 6 to 8 hours is sufficient) so that the plasma concentration reflects the fully distributed concentration and not an early postdose transient high value (see further chapter I; section 5).

8.1.8 Diuretics

Diuretic therapy plays a major role in the management of heart failure by mobilising interstitial fluid, although it is still secondary to

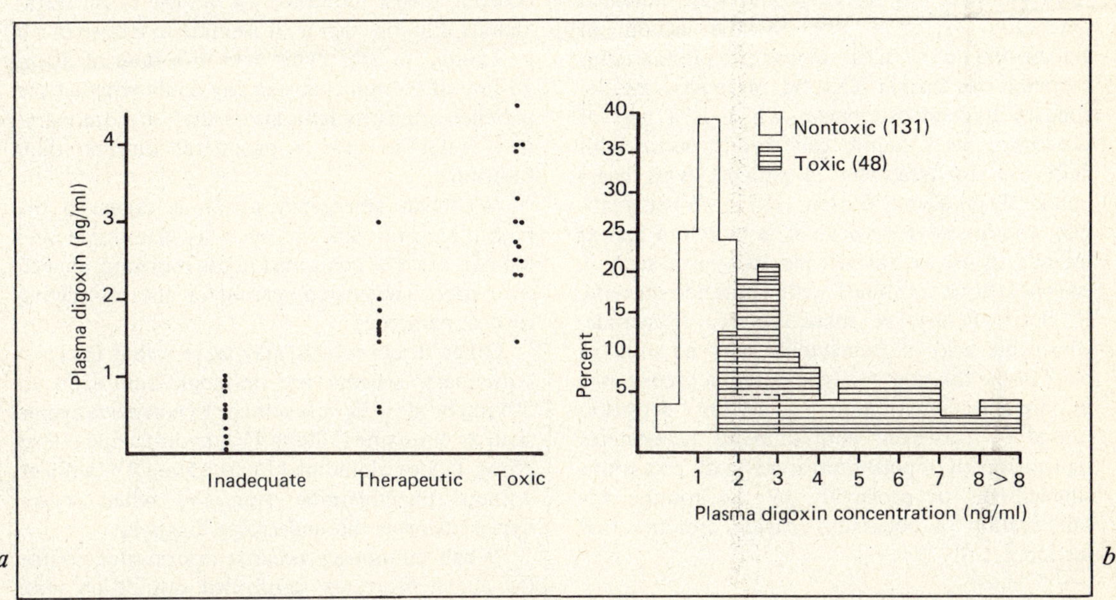

Fig. 6. Plasma digoxin concentrations and response.

(a) Plasma concentrations in patients judged inadequately digitalised, adequately digitalised, and adequately digitalised but toxic (after Oliver et al.: Amer. J. Med. 51: 186, 1971; by permission of author and editor).

(b) Frequency histogram showing plasma digoxin concentrations in non-toxic and toxic patients. The proportions in each group with concentrations in a given range are shown. 90% of patients with no evidence of digoxin intoxication had concentrations of 2.0ng/ml or below, while 87% of the toxic group had concentrations above 2.0ng/ml (after Smith and Haber: J. Clin. Invest. 49: 2377, 1970; by permission of author and editor).

measures designed to improve the performance of the pump. The object is to remove the large excess of salt from the body and to re-establish a more normal balance between the daily intake of sodium and its renal excretion. Diuretics do not cure heart failure but they may certainly relieve its symptoms and signs.

It has been argued that there is no need to use a 'mild' diuretic for mild oedema, and that it is just as reasonable to use a small dose of a 'strong' diuretic. Frusemide (furosemide) has therefore been recommended as the drug of choice, and hospital statistics bear out its popularity. However, the majority view supports a more conservative approach, and therefore the use of less potent diuretics such as thiazides (table XV) as the first line therapy in mild or moderate degrees of heart failure. More potent diuretics such as frusemide may need to be given parenterally (e.g. 4 to 16mg/hour by intravenous infusion) in patients with severe heart failure who fail to respond to large oral doses (Lawson et al., 1978).

If diuretic therapy is too precipitant, the rate of transfer of fluid into the plasma will lag behind urinary excretion and secondary hyperaldosteronism will occur. Continued diuretic therapy in such cases will meet with resistance and cause increased potassium excretion due to the action of aldosterone on the distal tubular site of potassium excretion (see chapter XXI; fig. 3). In any case, secondary hyperaldosteronism which is a part of congestive heart failure can readily occur with daily diuretic treatment in patients with heart failure (Davies and Wilson, 1975). When planning continuous treatment, it is therefore logical initially to use an aldosterone antagonist such as spironolactone combined with a thiazide diuretic. If heart failure is more severe, frusemide, ethacrynic acid or bumetanide may be used in place of the thiazide. As hypokalaemia predisposes to digitalis intoxication, potassium depletion caused by treatment with diuretics necessitates replenishment of potassium stores with potassium supplements or preferably by the routine administration of potassium-sparing diuretics (see section 8.1.4).

8.2 Acute Pulmonary Oedema

This can be a medical emergency demanding immediate therapy. Morphine given intravenously in increments up to 10 to 15mg is most important in immediate treatment. An intravenous diuretic such as frusemide 50 to 250mg should also be given slowly. Morphine relieves anxiety and respiratory distress and is said to dilate peripheral veins and thus reduce venous return, and in effect, produce a pharmacological venesection.

The patient with pulmonary oedema should be nursed upright with his legs dependent, and if oxygen is available, this should be used. Venous tourniquets on the legs applied intermittently may reduce the venous return to the heart. An intravenous digitalis preparation should be given in almost all cases, unless the patient has already been on such a drug. If digoxin is used, 0.5mg should be given intravenously and this should achieve maximal activity in 1 1/2 to 3 hours. If further digoxin is required, as in rapid atrial fibrillation, increments of 0.25mg may be repeated intravenously at 2-hourly intervals. Ouabain (G-strophanthin) has a very brief latent period of action, and in doses of 0.5mg intravenously begins to show an action within 5 minutes, which is maximal in about 1 hour.

It is usual to recommend use of a parenteral diuretic for most cases of acute pulmonary oedema. Although many patients may settle with morphine and digoxin, recurrence of pulmonary oedema is best prevented by the use of an intravenous diuretic such as frusemide in a dose of 50 to 250mg, or ethacrynic acid in a dose of 50 to 150mg. If the clinician is in any doubt whether the patient's acute problems are cardiac or pulmonary, it is safer to give a parenteral diuretic than morphine.

Whatever emergency action is taken in the night, an oral diuretic such as frusemide and digoxin must be continued in the morning, as well as a more considered search for the underlying cardiac pathology.

Other drugs which may have value in acute pulmonary oedema are aminophylline (250 to 500mg by slow IV infusion) or hypotensive agents such as diazoxide (300mg IV), hydrallazine (10 to 20mg IV) or clonidine (75 to 150µg IV with or without phentolamine 5mg IV) when severe hypertension is the underlying diagnosis.

When pulmonary oedema deteriorates despite the above measures, controlled respiration with intermittent positive pressure or continuous positive pressure ventilation may be employed. Again it will be necessary to balance the increase in oxygen saturation of arterial blood against tissue blood supply since both procedures, especially the latter, reduce cardiac output.

Table XV. Dosage of some diuretics used in heart failure

Drug	Average effective dose (daily)	Dose range (daily) in refractory heart failure
Bendrofluazide	5 to 10mg	< 20mg in combination[1]
Chlorothiazide	500 to 1,000mg	< 2g in combination[1]
Cyclopenthiazide	0.25 to 0.5mg	< 1mg in combination[1]
Hydrochlorothiazide	50 to 100mg	< 200mg in combination[1]
Frusemide	50 to 250mg	< 2.4 to 4g
Ethacrynic acid	50 to 150mg	< 16mg/kg
Bumetanide	0.5 to 10mg	< 15mg
Potassium sparing drugs		
Amiloride	5 to 20mg	5 to 20mg
Spironolactone	100 to 200mg	100 to 200mg
Triamterene	50 to 200mg	50 to 200mg

1   Best given in combination with diuretics which act on a different site on the nephron (see chapter XXI; fig. 3). See section 8.3.3.

8.3 Refractory Heart Failure

This implies that the congestion has failed to respond to the treatment or that the response is less than expected. It may be that hospital admission and a full scale cardiac investigation including catheterisation will be needed to establish a diagnosis. Heart failure should not be allowed to remain inadequately diagnosed and treated in anyone under the age of 70 years for there could well be possibilities for surgical treatment which may not be apparent to the practitioner or even to the consultant, until after full investigation has been completed.

General approaches to the management of refractory heart failure include: (a) sodium restriction; (b) a review of digitalis dosage with adjustment for inadequate dosage or toxicity (serum concentrations will help); (c) review of existing diuretic therapy and adjustment of dosage or institution of a new regimen; (d) investigation of electrolyte status and correction of any imbalance; (e) use of vasodilators if above measures prove inadequate, and (f) withdrawal of drugs which may aggravate heart failure (see section 11.4).

8.3.1 Diet

In refractory heart failure there may be justification for rigid sodium restriction, and excessive fluid intake should be discouraged (see below).

8.3.2 Digitalis Review

Heart failure may be poorly controlled because of inadequate dosage (serum digoxin concentration generally 0.5ng/ml or less) or due to digitalis toxicity. Digitalis toxicity, if present, may be secondary to hypokalaemia (see below).

8.3.3 Diuretic Review

Provided digitalis dosage is appropriate, a change in the diuretic regimen is often beneficial in refractory heart failure. Resistance may have developed due to secondary hyperaldosteronism, in which case an aldosterone antagonist such as spironolactone should be added (see section 8.1.8). The diuretics presently available act at one or more nephron segments (see chapter XXI; sect. 7.1). The earlier a diuretic acts in a nephron, the greater is its potential potency, but the expression of this may be prevented by increased reabsorption at distal sites. Consequently, the greatest diuretic effect will be achieved by combining diuretics with different sites of action (see chapter XXI; fig. 3). Thus, for example, high dose frusemide (proximal tubule and ascending limb of Henle's loop), chlorothiazide (cortical diluting segment) and amiloride (distal tubule) would give a profound diuresis. However, when transport is inhibited at so many nephron segments, the kidney is unable to regulate the relative amounts of sodium and water present in the urine. Unless great attention is paid to dietary intake of salt and water, severe hyponatraemia may result. With so many potent diuretics available, it has become unfashionable (Whight et al., 1974) to restrict salt intake, unless all other approaches have failed.

Other than using combinations of drugs which act at different sites, an adequate diuresis may be achieved by the use of more potent diuretics, by a stepwise increase in diuretic dosage (table XV) according to the response or lack of it, or by increasing the frequency of diuretic administration.

Pre-existing electrolyte disturbances may cause heart failure to be refractory to digitalis treatment (e.g. hypocalcaemia; Chopra et al., 1977), whilst conversely, the treatment of refractory heart failure with vigorous diuretic therapy can result in electrolyte disturbances (e.g. hypokalaemia, hypomagnesaemia) and increase the risk of digitalis toxicity (see section 8.1.4).

Dilutional hyponatraemia (excess body sodium with low serum sodium in the presence of oedema) requires that water intake be restricted to 600 to 800ml daily and maintained at this level until the serum sodium has risen to 135mmol/L (mEq/L) or more. Diuretics should be withdrawn until the serum sodium returns to normal limits. Rigid salt restriction is then indicated.

Hypokalaemia may result from the urinary potassium loss consequent on the diuretic action of many diuretics and as a result of the secondary hyperaldosteronism that is associated with congestive heart failure. In patients receiving digitalis it is important to avoid hypokalaemia (section 8.1.4). Hypokalaemia should be suspected when plasma potassium levels fall below 3.3mmol/L. However, it should be remembered that pH also controls the distribution of potassium between cells and interstitial fluid and in a person who is acidotic there may be potassium depletion with a serum potassium level of above 4mmol/L (Morgan, 1973).

If potassium supplements are used, potassium chloride is to be preferred and at least 20mmol potassium daily (3 slow release tablets) should be given (see chapter XXI; sect. 7.1). Potassium sparing diuretics can be used as an alternative to potassium supplements and are preferred by some clinicians. Drugs such as amiloride and triamterene have little inherent natriuretic action and usually have to be used in combination with other diuretics. In patients with cardiac disease and oedema, it is difficult to replete the total body potassium (Whight et al., 1974). Indeed, patients with heart failure do not retain potassium when

they are given it (Davidson et al., 1978). The reason for using potassium supplements or potassium sparing diuretics in heart failure is to prevent or treat a low *plasma* potassium concentration (Davidson et al., 1978; Morgan, et al., 1978). Some consider that in patients with severe cardiac failure more regular and reliable control of serum potassium is obtained with amiloride 10 to 20mg daily than with potassium chloride supplements (Morgan, 1973; Davidson and Gillebrand, 1973). Although spironolactone prevents potassium depletion, the dosage required in patients with secondary hyperaldosteronism is high and can be associated with frequent side effects such as gynaecomastia in men (see chapter XV; sect. 23.6), when used for prolonged periods.

A potential hazard with potassium sparing diuretics is the development of hyperkalaemia and when these drugs are used it is essential to ensure that renal function is normal and that potassium intake is not excessive. Potassium supplements usually should not be used in conjunction with potassium sparing diuretics.

Chronic sodium depletion is less common than dilutional hyponatraemia or hypokalaemia, but may occur in the clinical context of rigid dietary sodium restriction and vigorous diuretic therapy. In contrast to dilutional hyponatraemia, oedema is not found, and treatment consists of increasing the salt intake either orally (mild cases), or parenterally by intravenous infusion (severe cases) and withdrawal of diuretic therapy.

8.3.4 Vasodilators

In cases of congestive heart failure which remain refractory to adequate digitalis, diuretics, bed rest and sodium restriction, vasodilator drugs may be used (Cohn and Franciosa, 1977; Mason, 1978). Vasodilators (e.g. sodium nitroprusside, hydrallazine, prazosin, nitrates) have been used in a variety of clinical settings such as acute myocardial infarction, severe ischaemic cardiomyopathy and mitral regurgitation, to improve left ventricular function. Vasodilators may act by reducing impedance to left ventricular outflow or by producing venodilatation and reducing venous return. This results in an increase in cardiac output and decrease in left ventricular filling pressure, with a concomitant fall in systemic blood pressure and often a slight rise in heart rate. Sodium nitroprusside infusion has been particularly effective in rapidly improving left ventricular performance and promoting a diuresis in patients with severe refractory congestive heart failure. In some such patients the additive effects of a vasodilator and a potent inotropic agent (dopamine or dobutamine; see section 5.4) may be used to advantage (Miller et al., 1977). Haemodynamic monitoring should be used to guide the administration of vasodilators.

Nitrates are predominantly venodilators, hydrallazine produces mainly arterial vasodilatation (and also produces a greater increase in heart rate) while nitroprusside has a combined venodilator and arteriolar dilator action, but has to be given intravenously and has a short lived effect. The use of oral hydrallazine (25 to 100mg per day in divided doses) and long acting nitrates such as isosorbide dinitrate (up to 40mg 4 times daily), either alone or in combination, is often beneficial in the long term management of refractory heart failure (Cohn and Franciosa, 1977; Franciosa et al., 1978). Prazosin, a newer vasodilator, and like hydrallazine used in treatment of hypertension (see chapter XVIII; sect. 5.8), has a similar balanced venodilator and arteriolar dilator action as nitroprusside in heart failure and is an alternative oral drug to use in impedance reduction or systolic unloading and seems to be particularly suitable for long term use. A suggested initial dose is 2mg daily in divided doses, which may be increased to 4 or 5mg 4 times daily (Mehta et al., 1978). None of these vasodilators should be used indiscriminately and at present their use is best confined to specialist units (Packer and Meller, 1978).

9. Pulmonary Embolism

Impaired venous flow, alteration of the venous wall and changes in the blood coagulability are factors predisposing to thromboembolism (see chapter XXIII; section 1.1.2). Dislodgement of part of the thrombus will lead to its migration by systemic venous drainage to the right side of the heart with lodgement in the periphery of the pulmonary arteries. Although thrombosis can be initiated in any part of the peripheral venous system, significant and serious emboli arise from thrombi extending into the femoral and iliac segments. Patients over the age of 40 years who require bed rest are at greatest risk and the presence of other predisposing factors (e.g. obesity; varicose veins; heart disease; familial factors; blood diseases; certain surgical procedures, etc) add to this risk (Tibbutt and Chesterman, 1976, 1978).

Chair rest and early ambulation reduces the risk. Depending on the size of the embolus, the clinical manifestations vary from catastrophic pulmonary arterial obstruction to asymptomatic embolisation.

The type of patient presenting for diagnosis and management of pulmonary embolism usually has at least a moderate sized embolus with clinical manifestations of shortness of breath, haemoptysis, tachycardia and clinical and sometimes electrocardiographic evidence of right ventricular strain. It is also important to recognise the occurrence of small pulmonary emboli, as these may be the premonitory signs of a major embolism (MacIntyre and Ruckley, 1974). Anticoagulation may prevent recurrence of emboli, secondary thrombosis within the pulmonary vessels and extension of thrombosis at the site of origin of the embolus. The optimum period of time for which these patients should be anticoagulated has not been established but it should be several months.

About 50% of patients who suffer a major or massive pulmonary embolism die within the first hour. Energetic treatment is indicated immediately the clinical diagnosis is made (see Tibbutt and Chesterman, 1976, 1978). General measures include:

1) External cardiac compression for a patient who collapses after an acute episode.
2) Administration of oxygen at once. Some would advocate that the patient should be digitalised by the intravenous route, using an initial dose of 0.75mg digoxin in the undigitalised patient.
3) If there is bronchospasm, isoprenaline (isoproterenol) should be commenced by intravenous infusion.
4) An initial dose of heparin which will vary from 10,000 to 15,000 units should be administered.
5) If diagnostic doubt remains, the quickest, simplest screening test, when available, is an isotope lung scan, which will indicate the presence of ischaemic areas of lung parenchyma.

If the patient shows improvement after the initial therapy, then it is recommended that intravenous heparin should be continued using a constant infusion to maintain the whole blood clotting time between 2 1/2 and 3 times the normal level. The role of heparin is to prevent further thrombosis whilst autothrombolysis takes place. The alternative forms of therapy which may be considered, particularly if the patient's condition deteriorates, are thrombolytic therapy with streptokinase or surgery using cardiopulmonary bypass for pulmonary embolectomy. Although thrombolytic agents (streptokinase; urokinase) accelerate thrombolysis and reverse haemodynamic abnormalities more rapidly than heparin, the accelerated thrombolysis has not been shown to provide additional therapeutic benefit (Tibbutt et al., 1974; Urokinase Pulmonary Embolism Trial, 1973). However, the outcome of massive pulmonary embolism is unpredictable and on the basis of present knowledge it seems logical to therapeutically accelerate thrombolysis in patients with residual haemodynamic disturbance who seem likely to survive for a sufficient period to allow thrombolysis to occur.

The decision to proceed to pulmonary embolectomy is difficult and there are no categorical indications. A number of features of the clinical and haemodynamic state of the patient contribute to the decision. Certainly, if angiography shows a surgically accessible proximal pulmonary artery obstruction and if the patient's general condition is deteriorating, immediate surgery using cardiopulmonary bypass should be carried out. Similarly, if the patient deteriorates while streptokinase therapy is being used and isoprenaline fails to maintain a satisfactory circulation, immediate pulmonary embolectomy is indicated (see further chapter XXIII; sect. 4.5).

10. Use of Drugs in the Presence of Associated Heart Disease

10.1 Heart Failure and Acute Myocardial Infarction

Cardiac failure and low cardiac output states can have a marked effect on the disposition of drugs, particularly antiarrhythmic agents, by altering their distribution and hepatic or renal elimination (see section 1). Oral absorption of antiarrhythmic drugs (e.g. procainamide and mexiletine) is impaired in acute myocardial infarction, particularly if narcotic analgesics have been given. A decrease in cardiac output is of particular importance with drugs such as lignocaine (lidocaine) which are dependent on liver blood flow for elimination. Patients with congestive heart failure or shock may develop lignocaine toxicity more commonly than other patients because of higher than usual plasma concentrations after standard doses. Dosage of lignocaine must be reduced in patients with congestive heart failure or low cardiac output states if accumulation and toxicity is to be avoided. Similarly, lignocaine infusion rate must be monitored closely in patients with uncomplicated acute myocardial infarction (see further section 1.3, 1.4; 6.1.3). Lithium may accumulate to toxic levels if dosage is not adjusted to compensate for reduced renal clearance (decreased glomerular filtration rate, sodium loss due to diuretics) in patients with heart failure (see chapter XXVI; sect. 5.4).

Drugs such as corticosteroids, carbenoxolone, phenylbutazone, oxyphenbutazone and ibuprofen cause fluid and salt retention and may precipitate congestive heart failure or pulmonary oedema in individuals with borderline cardiac function (Nevins et al., 1969; Schooley et al., 1977; Odutola et al., 1978). Phenylbutazone and oxyphenbutazone have a mineralocorticoid like action on the kidney, a property which may be shared by some but not all non-steroidal anti-inflammatory analgesics (Feldman and Couropmitree, 1976).

Refractory heart failure is not uncommonly due to digitalis toxicity, as a consequence of hypokalaemia and excessive diuretic therapy. The best treatment is often to stop all drugs until toxicity lessens, usually within 2 or 3 days in the case of digoxin or 2 or 3 weeks with digitoxin. In addition, diuretics may lose their effectiveness in oedematous patients with severe congestive heart failure, as a consequence of electrolyte loss from previous diuretic therapy or development of secondary hyperaldosteronism (see section 8.1.8). The possibility that tricyclic antidepressants may aggravate heart failure should always be considered (Luke, 1971). The β-adrenoceptor blocking drugs aggravate existing heart failure or may precipitate latent heart failure. These drugs should not be used in patients with known or suspected heart failure unless they are also treated with optimum doses of digitalis. Patients in cardiac failure may respond unpredictably to central nervous system depressants or anaesthetics and the blood pressure may fall abruptly without warning.

10.2 Cardiovascular Disease

The risk of digitalis toxicity is increased in those with arrhythmias superimposed on underlying atrial fibrillation, chronic pulmonary heart disease or myocardial ischaemia (see section 8.1.4). Aminophylline and sympathomimetic amines also have an increased risk of causing cardiac arrhythmias in the presence of myocardial ischaemia.

Tricyclic antidepressant drugs such as amitriptyline and imipramine may lead to disturbances of cardiac rate, rhythm and conduction (see chapter XXVI; sect. 7.5.2), particularly in overdosage but also at therapeutic dosage in some patients with hypertension or myocardial ischaemia (Jefferson, 1975). If indicated in such patients, tricyclic antidepressants should be used cautiously and in low doses. Similarly, cardiovascular side-effects produced by emetine at dosages used in intestinal amoebiasis are more likely to be deleterious in patients with pre-existing cardiovascular disease.

Some drugs used in the treatment of cardiac arrhythmias may sometimes produce potentially serious adverse effects in patients with cardiac disease (Aviado, 1975; Deglin et al., 1977). Procainamide in large doses used in arrhythmias reduces cardiac output, and this should be borne in mind in patients with pre-existing myocardial ischaemia. Phenytoin depresses ventricular automaticity (section 6.1.4), which can be serious if it is used in patients with complete heart block. Antiarrhythmic drugs such as quinidine, procainamide or propranolol which normally cause a slowing of heart rate, may cause cardiac standstill in a patient who has an initial bradycardia or conduction abnormality.

Overzealous oxygen therapy in acute myocardial infarction may result in hyperoxaemia and vasoconstriction, or reduce coronary blood flow. Although morphine may sometimes produce considerable hypotension in patients with acute myocardial infarction, this effect may possibly be preferable to the systemic hypertension and increased cardiac work sometimes caused by pentazocine (Editorial, 1976). Nevertheless, pentazocine might be a preferable alternative to morphine where continued analgesia is required in patients with demonstrable hypotension (see section 5.1.1). Reinfarction within 6 months of an acute attack of myocardial infarction seems to be more likely to occur when such patients require general anaesthesia for surgery, particularly that involving the thorax and upper abdomen (Tarhan et al., 1972). Elective surgery should be postponed beyond 6 months of acute myocardial infarction and only life threatening emergencies should be considered for surgery before 6 months have

elapsed. Haemopericardium is a serious, though rare, complication of anticoagulant therapy, but is usually associated with some underlying condition such as myocardial infarction, pericarditis or trauma.

Alterations in plasma volume can cause marked changes in response to some cardiovascular drugs. Patients in shock, with low blood pressure and impaired tissue perfusion, secondary to or in association with a low plasma volume, and who are given an infusion of isoprenaline (isoproterenol) or a β-adrenoceptor blocking drug, invariably experience a further abrupt and sometimes fatal fall in blood pressure. This does not occur if the low plasma volume has been first corrected (Nies, 1972).

10.3 Drug Interactions in Cardiovascular Therapy

Concurrent administration of more than one drug is often necessary during cardiovascular therapy (see Dollery et al., 1974; Koch-Weser, 1975). The combined use of drugs can increase the effectiveness of treatment (e.g. propranolol and a nitrite in angina) or decrease the prevalence and severity of adverse reactions (e.g. thiazide and potassium sparing diuretic plus digitalis). Moreover, many patients need drug treatment for more than one cardiovascular problem and may also require drug therapy for non-circulatory disorders. Multiple drug therapy which is well chosen and skilfully used can be of much benefit. Concurrent administration of two or more drugs may however, occasionally lead to adverse interaction between drugs and is a potential problem with cardiovascular therapy, especially with oral anticoagulants (see chapter XXIII; sect. 3.2.5), adrenergic neurone blocking antihypertensive drugs such as guanethidine (see chapter XVIII; sect. 10.1) and digitalis glycosides (see table XIV). Antiarrhythmic drugs are often and successfully used together, but because of differences in their electrophysiological activity (table VII), one drug may sometimes counteract the effect of the other. At the same time however, the major adverse effects (depression of myocardial contractility, peripheral vasodilation, hypotension) may be additive. Combination therapy with antiarrhythmic drugs should be carefully planned and monitored closely. Interactions can also occur between antiarrhythmic drugs and other agents. These and adverse interactions with other cardiovascular drugs such as diuretics, sympathomimetic agents and adrenergic receptor blocking drugs are discussed in chapter VIII and appendix C.

Adverse drug interactions in cardiovascular therapy can largely be avoided (Koch-Weser, 1975). Drugs that are capable of adverse interaction can be given safely and effectively if the necessary dosage adjustments are anticipated or instituted promptly. Some drugs however, are best or need to be avoided (e.g. certain oral anticoagulant interactions and drugs which antagonise guanethidine). This requires familiarity with the pharmacokinetic properties and with the important therapeutic toxic actions of each drug. All clinicians should know the important cardiovascular drugs whose simultaneous administration with other drugs requires special caution (appendix C).

11. Drug Induced Cardiovascular Disease

Various drugs used in the treatment of cardiovascular disease as well as in the treatment of various non-circulatory diseases can cause cardiac disorders in some patients receiving usual therapeutic or high doses, particularly those with underlying cardiac disease (see Chung and Dean, 1972; Deglin et al., 1977). Arrhythmias and hypotension are more readily detected and occur with short term therapy, whereas other cardiac diseases are more difficult to detect or diagnose and take months or years to develop. Cardiovascular responses to drugs used in anaesthetic practice are discussed in chapter X. Drug induced hypertension is discussed in chapter XVIII (sect. 12) and drug induced thromboembolism in chapter XXIII (sect. 8.2).

11.1 Disturbance of Cardiac Rate and Rhythm

The drugs used for treatment of cardiac disease have a potential risk of causing arrhythmias (see Aviado, 1975). There are three major factors which increase the risk of arrhythmias in the drug treatment of heart disease:

a) The disease process itself may increase the sensitivity of the heart to the 'proarrhythmic' action of the cardioactive drug
b) Drugs used in the treatment of heart disease may influence autonomic innervation of the heart

c) Most cardioactive drugs directly affect the excitability, conductivity, refractoriness and automaticity of heart muscle.

Digitalis glycosides are a common cause of cardiac arrhythmias, particularly in patients who are predisposed to toxicity (see section 8.1.4). Digitalis intoxication is associated with a variety of types and combinations of cardiac arrhythmias, the treatment of which are discussed in section 6.3. The arrhythmias produced by digitalis reflect exaggerations of the pharmacological effects of the drug. The most common and characteristic arrhythmia is premature ventricular contractions (Mason et al., 1971). Complete heart block can result from both increased vagal tone and depressed refractory period of conduction tissue.

First and second degree atrioventricular block may be caused by therapeutic doses of quinidine and procainamide, and complete heart block precipitated by β-adrenoceptor blocking drugs (e.g. propranolol) and guanethidine. Quinidine and procainamide may cause both premature ventricular contractions and ventricular tachycardia. Quinidine may cause atrial flutter as well as syncopal attacks due to paroxysmal flutter and ventricular fibrillation. Quinidine can also produce a nodal rhythm, and atrioventricular dissociation can occur with quinidine and procainamide. Lignocaine (lidocaine) infusion should be stopped at the first sign of depression of cardiac conductivity as cardiac standstill has occurred. Phenytoin (diphenylhydantoin) in large intravenous doses may cause atrioventricular block, and bradycardia and cardiac arrest have also been reported.

Drugs that influence autonomic innervation to the heart may also cause disorders in cardiac rhythm. Atropine and sympathomimetic amines (bronchodilators, vasopressors except mephentermine) may cause sinus tachycardia. Adrenaline (epinephrine) induces cardiac arrhythmias by a direct effect on the electrical properties of the heart, as well as by extracardiac effects, particularly when large doses are administered. Anticholinesterase drugs (e.g. for myasthenia gravis; insecticide poisoning) increase the activity of cholinergic receptors in the heart and may cause sinus bradycardia and atrioventricular block. β-Adrenoceptor blocking drugs produce bradycardia by inhibition of cardiac β-adrenoceptors.

A number of other drugs of various pharmacological classes may cause cardiac arrhythmias. Clofibrate can cause various cardiac arrhythmias but in a major study were no more frequent than in a control group (WHO Cooperative Trial, 1978). Tricyclic antidepressant drugs such as imipramine, nortriptyline and amitriptyline cause serious ECG abnormalities in overdosage and sometimes also in therapeutic doses, particularly in elderly patients and in patients with hypertension or myocardial ischaemia (Burrows et al., 1976; Jefferson, 1975). Sinus tachycardia may be caused by phenothiazines, whilst thioridazine may cause ventricular tachycardia (see also chapter XXVI; sect. 7.5.2, 3.5.2). Sinus tachycardia may also be caused by thyroid drugs and ventricular tachycardia may also follow papaverine, potassium and intravenous mercurials. Lithium, now widely used for treatment of manic-depressive disorder (and less widely for neutropenia) can sometimes produce reversible ECG changes (T wave depression, rarely inversion, not unlike that seen in hypokalaemia) and less commonly ventricular arrhythmias. Lithium seems to deplete intracellular potassium in the myocardium. Sinus node dysfunction, prolonged sinus node recovery time, atrioventricular block and possibly myocarditis have also been reported (Jaffe, 1977; Tilkian et al., 1976a,b). Atrial fibrillation has occurred after intravenous methylphenidate. Emetine, in doses used in amoebiasis, may cause atrial tachycardia.

The cytotoxic drugs daunorubicin and doxorubicin (adriamycin) can cause ECG abnormalities and cardiac failure, sometimes fatal. Early electrographic changes include sinus tachycardia, ST-segment depression, T-wave flattening and ventricular premature beats. The early changes are slight and easily missed but are not a portent of heart failure (see section 11.4).

Levodopa and amantadine can cause a variety of cardiac arrhythmias, but their incidence is generally low (Brogden et al., 1971; Parkes et al., 1977). Transient sinus tachycardia is the most common with levodopa and usually causes palpitations, which may clear spontaneously. Atrial and ventricular extrasystoles (occasionally) and atrial flutter and fibrillation (rarely) have also been reported. The combined use of levodopa and a decarboxylase inhibitor probably decreases the incidence of cardiac arrhythmias (Desjacques et al., 1973). Dopamine itself, when used as a vasopressor drug, may also cause cardiac arrhythmias. Glucagon which has also been tried in cardiogenic shock, has caused ventricular tachycardia and fibrillation. Carbamazepine can cause bradycardia and may precipitate atrioventricular

block in those with a defective conduction system. These effects have been reported in elderly patients, usually receiving the drug for trigeminal neuralgia (Beerman and Edhag, 1978; Herzberg, 1978).

Rapid intravenous injection of large doses of lincomycin has caused bradycardia, intraventricular conduction disturbances and cardiac arrest (Paturaud and Gut, 1975); possibly due to the potential curariform action of the drug. The reaction can be avoided by giving the same dose in a larger volume by slow intravenous infusion. Rapid intravenous administration of potassium penicillin (1.7mmol K$^+$ are contained in each million units) has been associated with all types of conduction abnormalities, including asystole. Availability of the sodium salt should be remembered (Mercer and Logic, 1973). Carbenicillin on the other hand, contains 4.7mmol Na$^+$/g of drug and may cause marked hypokalaemia and alkalosis (Cabizuca and Desser, 1976) with attendant risk of arrhythmias. Hypokalaemia as a consequence of excessive liquorice ingestion has been associated with cardiac arrest (Bannister et al., 1977). A similar risk exists with liquorice derived peptic ulcer healing drug carbenoxolone (see chapter XIX; sect. 4.1).

11.2 Hypotension

Hypotension may be caused by a variety of drugs other than those used therapeutically to lower the blood pressure (Chung and Dean, 1972). Drugs normally used to lower the blood pressure may however, produce marked hypotension, particularly in patients with myocardial decompensation. Postural hypotension is a frequent side effect of the treatment of hypertension and adrenergic neurone blocking antihypertensive drugs such as guanethidine and can also occur with the peripheral vasodilator prazosin, usually with an excessive first dose or rapid dose increment (Brogden et al., 1977).

Morphine, given intravenously, may produce hypotension in patients with acute myocardial infarction. Quinidine can also produce hypotension but this is related to both dosage and route of administration and is much more frequent when the intravenous route is used. Hypotension can be associated with intravenous injections of phenytoin, and appears to be related to the speed of injection. Only occasional minor reductions in blood pressure occur with slow infusion of phenytoin. β-Adrenoceptor blocking drugs given intravenously, may cause hypotension in association with brady-cardia. This may require correction with atropine in patients with acute myocardial infarction (Stannard and Sloman, 1967). Hypovolaemia induced by potent diuretics may aggravate hypotension and low cardiac output in patients with myocardial infarction.

Glyceryl trinitrate (nitroglycerine) sometimes causes a fall in blood pressure and its combination with alcohol has led to cardiovascular collapse with marked hypotension (Shafer, 1965). Acute hypotension can occur after phenothiazine antipsychotic drugs (notably chlorpromazine) in elderly or debilitated patients or after large parenteral doses. Postural hypotension is a potential hazard with the tricyclic antidepressants in the elderly and has resulted in physical injury due to falls or possibly has precipitated myocardial infarction in those with cardiac disease (Moir et al., 1973). Levodopa commonly causes postural hypotension. It is likely to be most troublesome when levodopa dosage is being increased (Brogden et al., 1971). This reaction is possibly reduced in incidence by combined use of levodopa and a decarboxylase inhibitor (see chapter XXV; sect. 5.1).

11.3 Angina Pectoris and Acute Myocardial Infarction

Drugs which decrease myocardial perfusion by constricting coronary arteries (e.g. vasopressin, oxytocin, intramuscular ergotamine, methysergide) or by decreasing arterial blood pressure (e.g. certain antihypertensive drugs) can sometimes precipitate angina pectoris and myocardial infarction. Marked hypotensive episodes can follow an excessive first dose (or dosage increment) of prazosin and a few cases of aggravation or precipitation of angina pectoris have been reported (New Zealand Hypertension Study Group, 1977). Other peripheral vasodilators such as hydrallazine and diazoxide when given parenterally may aggravate or precipitate angina pectoris. Phentolamine when used as a diagnostic test of phaeochromocytoma has been known to precipitate myocardial infarction (Gollub, 1965). Nifedipine, a vasodilator used in angina, can cause severe ischaemic cardiac pain in some patients shortly after a first dose or increase in dosage (see section 4.2.3). Abrupt withdrawal of propranolol in patients receiving large doses for severe coronary artery disease has provoked severe angina and precipitated myocardial infarction and sudden

death (see section 4.2.2). Excessive dosage of thyroid drugs may precipitate angina and possibly myocardial infarction in patients with ischaemic heart disease. Thyroxine has been associated with an increased coronary and other cardiovascular mortality, as well as a high rate of non-fatal infarction, when used as a hypolipidaemic agent in men who had recovered from a previous myocardial infarction (Coronary Drug Project, 1970).

Oral hypoglycaemic agents may be associated with an increased risk of cardiovascular mortality according to the University Group Diabetes Program study. These findings have been vigorously questioned and the mechanism for the observed enhanced risk remains unexplained (see chapter XVI; sect. 3.3.4).

Oral contraceptive usage has been associated with acute myocardial infarction, but is only one of a number of predisposing factors. However, oral contraceptives augment the likelihood of myocardial infarction when one or more risk factors are present, particularly in women aged over 40 who smoke cigarettes (see chapter XV; sect. 13.12).

Angina and myocardial ischaemia can occur in patients who have received large doses of sympathomimetic amines such as isoprenaline (isoproterenol) and adrenaline (epinephrine), particularly in the presence of underlying cardiac disease. Acute myocarditis and diffuse myocardial fibrosis can be induced, which may largely represent ischaemic damage due to the markedly increased oxygen demand caused by the peripheral vasoconstrictor effects of these particular amines (Haft, 1974). Ischaemic chest pain can follow use of the cytotoxic drug fluorouracil (Soukop et al., 1978).

11.4 Heart Failure

β-Adrenoceptor blocking drugs (by reducing cardiac output) and drugs which cause salt and fluid retention such as corticosteroids, carbenoxolone and phenylbutazone, can precipitate or aggravate congestive heart failure (see section 10.1).

The cytotoxic drugs daunorubicin and doxorubicin (adriamycin) have a direct toxic effect on the heart, at the level of the myocardial cells.

The manifestations of cardiotoxicity are of two types — early, transient electrocardiographic changes (usually benign arrhythmias) and late appearing dose-dependent congestive heart failure (Lefrak et al., 1973; Lenaz and Page, 1976). The electrocardiographic changes are only rarely of clinical consequence and do not predict the subsequent development of cardiomyopathy. At present, there is no evidence that the cardiomyopathy is reversible. However, if the drugs are discontinued at the first signs of congestive heart failure, the complication can usually be successfully managed by conventional medical treatment (Gilladoga et al., 1976). If heart failure is allowed to develop, death follows rapidly.

The occurrence of heart failure with doxorubicin can be limited by restricting the cumulative dose to a total of 450 to 550mg/m^2; a dose above which the incidence of toxicity rises sharply (Henderson and Frei, 1979; Lefrak et al., 1973). Prior mediastinal radiotherapy increases the risk of cardiomyopathy. There does not seem to be as precise a cutoff point of total cumulative dosage for daunorubicin, but rather a continuum of increasing risk of cardiomyopathy with greater total dosage. Nevertheless, at a total cumulative dose of 600mg/m^2 the risk of heart failure is around 1% in adults and 2% in children; the difference in risk between adults and children increasing with higher total dosage (Von Hoff et al., 1977). Children also seem to be more susceptible to doxorubicin induced cardiomyopathy.

While these total dose limits can minimise the occurrence of heart failure, it seems probable that all, or almost all, patients have some degree of cardiac damage after doxorubicin and daunorubicin treatment; the extent of damage becoming progressive with larger total doses (Friedman et al., 1978). A number of tests have been devised to monitor the slowly changing cardiac function, but as yet none are clearly predictive of clinically serious heart failure, although some show some potential value (Henderson and Frei, 1979).

Concomitant administration of agents such as digoxin which are thought to compete with the same receptor sites as doxorubicin or daunorubicin and their active metabolites, have been given with the theoretical (and yet unproven) aim of decreasing the myocardial toxicity (Guthrie and Gibson, 1977).

Large doses of cyclophosphamide (>180mg/kg) can also cause cardiac failure, through direct endothelial damage (Appelbaum et al., 1976).

11.5 Myocarditis; Pericarditis

Drugs rarely implicated in causing myocarditis include PAS, sulphonamides, aspirin, phenyl-butazone, methylthiouracil, benzathine penicillin G, streptomycin and chlorpromazine (D'Arcy and Griffin, 1972). In several cases, patients have exhibited simultaneous cutaneous lesions of urticaria, angioneurotic oedema, rash or purpura, and evidence of a generalised allergic drug reaction has been present in nearly all cases. A similar situation seems to exist with methyldopa (Mullick and McAllister, 1977). Instances of pericarditis thought to be associated with the use of practolol have been reported (Dyer and Varley, 1975). Emetine, as well as causing a cardiomyopathy with electrocardiographic abnormalities has also caused premature ventricular contractions, atrial tachycardia and pericarditis. Drug induced systemic lupus erythematosus may be associated with pericarditis, for example with hydrallazine (see chapter XX, sect. 11.1.1; XXII, sect. 14.1). Haemopericardium has been rarely associated with the use of anticoagulants in myocardial infarction. The antihypertensive drug minoxidil has been associated with pericardial effusions, particularly in patients with impaired renal function (Marquez-Julio and Uldall, 1977).

11.6 Other Cardiac Diseases

Methysergide, used primarily in the preventive treatment of migraine, can cause retroperitoneal, pleuropulmonary and much less commonly constrictive pericarditis when used continuously. Some of the patients who develop retroperitoneal and pleuropulmonary fibrosis, also have endocardial fibrosis (Bana et al., 1974). The cardiac lesions have been associated with development of heart murmurs and valvular heart disease, occasionally of sufficient significance to warrant surgical correction. The lesions regress after discontinuing methysergide in some cases. The drug should only be given in courses interrupted by treatment free intervals (see chapter XXV; sect. 7.2).

Further Reading

Avery, G.S. (Ed): Cardiovascular Drugs, Vol. 1. Antiarrhythmic, Antihypertensive and Lipid Lowering Drugs; Vol. 2. β-Adrenoceptor Blocking Drugs; Vol. 3. Antithrombotic Drugs (ADIS Press, Sydney; University Park Press, Baltimore 1977, 1978).

Hurst, J.W.: The Heart, 4th ed. (McGraw-Hill, New York 1978).

Julian, D.G.: Cardiology (Bailliere, London 1973).

Melmon, K.L.: Cardiovascular Drug Therapy (Davis, Philadelphia 1974).

Various Authors: Beta-blockade in cardiovascular therapeutics. Drugs 7: 1, 426 (1974).

Whipple, G.H. et al.: Acute Coronary Care (Little Brown, Boston 1971).

References

Afzal Mir, M. and Kafetzakis, E.M.: Assessment of perhexiline maleate in angiographically proven intractable angina: A double-blind trial. American Heart Journal 96: 350 (1978).

Ahrens, E.H.: The management of hyperlipidaemia: whether, rather than how. Annals of Internal Medicine 85: 87 (1976).

Alderman, E.L.; Barry, W.H.; Graham, A.F. and Harrison, D.C.: Hemodynamic effects of morphine and pentazocine differ in cardiac patients. New England Journal of Medicine 287: 623 (1972).

Aldous, S. and Thomas, R.: Absorption and metabolism of lanatoside C II. Fate after oral administration. Clinical Pharmacology and Therapeutics 21: 647 (1977).

Alexander, C.S.; Sako, Y. and Mikulic, E.: Pedal gangrene associated with the use of dopamine. New England Journal of Medicine 293: 591 (1975).

Amsterdam, F.A.; Massumi, R.A.; Zelis, R. and Mason, D.T.: Use of bretylium tosylate in the management of cardiac arrhythmias. Heart and Lung 1: 269 (1972).

Amsterdam, E.A.; Awan, N.A.; DeMaria, A.N. and Mason, D.T.: Vasodilators in myocardial infarction: Rationale and current status. Drugs 16: 506 (1978).

Anderson, J.L.; Harrison, D.C.; Meffin, P.J. and Winkle, R.A.: Antiarrhythmic drugs: Clinical pharmacology and therapeutic use. Drugs 15: 271 (1978).

Anderson, S.T. and Pitt, A.: Lignocaine in the management of ventricular arrhythmias. Medical Journal of Australia 1: 208 (1969).

Appelbaum, F.R.; Strauchen, J.A.; Graw, R.G.; Savage, D.D.; Kent, K.M.; Ferrans, V.J. and Herzig, G.P.: Acute lethal carditis caused by high-dose combination chemotherapy. A unique clinical and pathological entity. Lancet 1: 58 (1976).

Aronow, W.S.: Medical treatment of angina pectoris IV. Nitroglycerin as an antianginal drug. Americal Heart Journal 84: 415 (1972).

Aronson, J.K. and Grahame-Smith, D.G.: Digoxin therapy: Textbooks, theory and practice. British Journal of Clinical Pharmacology 3: 639 (1976a).

Aronson, J.K. and Grahame-Smith, D.G.: Altered distribution of digoxin in renal failure — A cause of digoxin toxicity? British Journal of Clinical Pharmacology 3: 1045 (1976b).

Aronson, J.K.; Grahame-Smith, D.G. and Wigley, F.M.: Monitoring digoxin therapy: The use of plasma digoxin concentration measurements in the diagnosis of digoxin toxicity. Quarterly Journal of Medicine 47: 111 (1978).

Aviado, D.M.: Drug action, reaction, and interaction. II. Iatrogenic cardiopathies. Journal of Clinical Pharmacology 15: 641 (1975).

Awan, N.; Amsterdam, E.A.; Vera, Z.; DeMaria, A.N.; Miller, R.R. and Mason, D.T.: Reduction of ischemic injury by sublingual nitroglycerin in patients with acute myocardial infarction. Circulation 54: 761 (1976a).

Awan, N.; Miller, R.R.; Vera, Z.; DeMaria, A.N.; Amsterdam, E.A. and Mason, D.T.: Reduction of ST segment elevation with infusion of nitroprusside in patients with acute myocardial infarction. American Journal of Cardiology 36: 435 (1976b).

Bana, D.S.; MacNeal, P.S.; Le Compte, P.M.; Shah, Y. and Graham, J.R.: Cardiac murmurs and endocardial fibrosis associated with methysergide therapy. American Heart Journal 88: 640 (1974).

Bannister, B.; Ginsburg, R. and Shneerson, J.: Cardiac arrest due to liquorice-induced hypokalaemia. British Medical Journal 2: 738 (1977).

Barger, A.C.: Renal hemodynamic factors in congestive heart failure. Annals of the New York Academy of Sciences 39: 276 (1966).

Baxter, R.H. and Lennox, I.M.: Increased exercise tolerance with nitrates in beta-blocked patients with angina. British Medical Journal 2: 550 (1977).

Bazzano, G. and Bazzano, G.S.: Digitalis intoxication — treatment with a new steroid-binding resin. Journal of the American Medical Association 220: 828 (1972).

Beerman, B. and Edhag, O.: Depressive effects of carbamazepine on idioventricular rhythm in man. British Medical Journal 2: 171 (1978).

Beller, G.; Smith, T.W.; Abelmann, W.H.; Haber, E. and Hood, W.B.: Digitalis intoxication. A prospective clinical study with serum level correlations. New England Journal of Medicine 284: 989 (1971).

Beller, G.A.; Hood, W.B.; Smith, T.W.; Abelmann, W.H. and Wacker, W.E.C.: Correlation of serum magnesium levels and cardiac digitalis intoxication. American Journal of Cardiology 33: 225 (1974).

Bellet, S.; Roman, L.R. and Boza, A.: Relation between serum quinidine levels and renal function: Studies in normal subjects and patients with congestive failure and renal insufficiency. American Journal of Cardiology 27: 368 (1971).

Benet, L.Z.; Greither, A. and Meister, W.: Gastrointestinal absorption of drugs in patients with cardiac failure; in Benet (Ed) The Effects of Disease States on Pharmacokinetics, p.33 (American Pharmaceutical Association, Washington 1976).

Benner, J.E.: Metabolism of antibiotics during cardiopulmonary bypass for open-heart surgery. Antimicrobial Agents and Chemotherapy, p.373 (American Society for Microbiology, Ann Arbor 1968).

Benowitz, N.L. and Meister, W.: Pharmacokinetics in patients with cardiac failure. Clinical Pharmacokinetics 1: 389 (1976).

Benowitz, N.L. and Meister, W.: Clinical pharmacokinetics of lignocaine. Clinical Pharmacokinetics 3: 177 (1978).

Berglund, G.; Wilhelmsen, L.; Sannerstedt, R.; Hansson, L.; Anderson, O.; Sivertsson, R.; Wedel, H. and Wikstrand, J.: Coronary heart-disease after treatment of hypertension. Lancet 1: 1 (1978).

Bernstein, J.K. and Koch-Weser, J.: Effectiveness of bretylium tosylate against refractory ventricular arrhythmias. Circulation 45: 1024 (1972).

Bierenbaum, M.L.; Fleischman, A.I.; Raichelson, R.I.; Hayton, T. and Watson, P.B.: 10-Year experience of modified-fat diets on younger men with coronary heart disease. Lancet 1: 1404 (1973).

Bigger, J.T.; Schmidt, D.H. and Kutt, H.: Relationship between the plasma level of diphenylhydantoin sodium and its cardiac antiarrhythmic effects. Circulation 38: 363 (1968).

Binnion, P.F.: Drug interactions with digitalis glycosides. Drugs 15: 369 (1978).

Blomgren, S.E.; Condemi, J.J. and Vaughan, J.H.: Procainamide induced lupus erythematosus. Clinical and laboratory observations. American Journal of Medicine 52: 338 (1972).

Bousser, M.-G.; Bouche, P.; Hauw, J-J.; Singlas, E.; Touboul, P-J. and Laplane, D.: Peripheral neuropathies due to perhexiline maleate. Annales de Cardiologie et d'Angeiologie 26 (Suppl.): 493 (Nov. 1977).

Brater, D.C. and Morrelli, H.F.: Digoxin toxicity in patients with normokalaemic potassium depletion. Clinical Pharmacology and Therapeutics 22: 21 (1977).

Brogden, R.N.; Speight, T.M. and Avery, G.S.: Levodopa: A review of its pharmacological properties and therapeutic uses with particular reference to Parkinsonism. Drugs 2: 262 (1971).

Brogden, R.N.; Heel, R.C.; Speight, T.M. and Avery, G.S.: Prazosin: A review of its pharmacological properties and therapeutic efficacy. Drugs 14: 163 (1977).

Burrows, G.D.; Vohra, J.; Hunt, D.; Sloman, J.G.; Scoggins, B.A. and Davies, B.: Cardiac effects of different tricyclic antidepressant drugs. British Journal of Psychiatry 129: 335 (1976).

Cabizuca, S.V. and Desser, K.B.: Carbenicillin associated hypokalemic alkalosis. Journal of the American Medical Association 235: 956 (1976).

Cady, W.J.; Rehder, T.L. and Campbell, J.: Use of cholestyramine resin in the treatment of digitoxin toxicity. American Journal of Hospital Pharmacy 36: 92 (1979).

Campbell, N.P.S.; Pantridge, J.F. and Adgey, A.A.J.: Mexiletine in the management of ventricular dysrhythmias. European Journal of Cardiology 6: 245 (1977).

Carlson, L.A.; Oro, L. and Ostman, J.: Effect of a single dose of nicotinic acid on plasma lipids in patients with hyperlipoproteinemia. Acta Medica Scandinavica 183: 457 (1968).

Carlson, L.A.; Oro, L. and Ostman, J.: Effect of nicotinic acid on plasma lipids in patients with hyperlipoproteinemia during the first week of treatment. Journal of Atherosclerosis Research 8: 667 (1968).

Carlson, L.A.; Danielson, M.; Ekberg, I.; Klintemar, B. and Rosenhamer, G.: Preliminary report. Reduction of myocardial reinfarction by the combined treatment with clofibrate and nicotinic acid. Atherosclerosis 28: 81 (1977).

Carruthers, S.G.; Kelly, J.G. and McDevitt, D.G.: Plasma digoxin concentrations in patients on admission to hospital. British Heart Journal 36: 707 (1974).

Casdorph, H.R.: The single dose method of administering cholestyramine. Angiology 26: 671 (1975).

Chamberlain, D.A.; White, R.J.; Howard, M.R. and Smith, T.W.: Plasma digoxin concentrations in patients with atrial fibrillation. British Medical Journal 3: 429 (1970).

Chew, C.Y.C.; Collett, J. and Singh, B.N.: Mexiletine: A review of its pharmacological properties and therapeutic efficacy in arrhythmias. Drugs 17: 161 (1979).

Chopra, D.; Janson, P. and Sawin, C.T.: Insensitivity to digoxin associated with hypocalcemia. New England Journal of Medicine 296: 917 (1977).

Chung, E.K. and Dean, H.M.: Diseases of the heart and vascular system due to drugs; in Meyler and Peck (Eds) Drug-Induced Diseases, vol. 4, p.345 (Excerpta Medica, Amsterdam 1972).

Cohn, J.N. and Franciosa, J.A.: Vasodilator therapy of cardiac failure. New Eng. J. Med. 297: 27, 254 (1977).

Cohn, K.; Sakai, F.J. and Langston, M.F.: Effect of clofibrate on progression of coronary disease: A prospective angiographic study in man. American Heart Journal 89: 591 (1975).

Collingsworth, K.A.; Strong, J.M.; Atkinson, A.J.; Winkle, R.A.; Perlroth, F. and Harrison, D.C.: Pharmacokinetics and metabolism of lidocaine in patients with renal failure. Clinical Pharmacology and Therapeutics 18: 59 (1975).

Coltart, D.J. and Shand, D.G.: Plasma propranolol levels in the quantitative assessment of beta-adrenergic blockade in man. British Medical Journal 3: 731 (1970).

Coltart, D.J.; Gibson, D.G. and Shand, D.G.: Plasma propranolol levels associated with suppression of ventricular ectopic beats. British Medical Journal 1: 490 (1971).

Committee on Diet and Heart Disease of the National Heart Foundation of Australia: Dietary fat and coronary heart disease: A review. Medical Journal of Australia 1: 575, 616, 663 (1974).

Conn, H.L.; Conn, E.H. and Huang, L.: The possible role of reduced membrane ATPase activity in digitalis toxicity in the aged. American Association of University Cardiology Proceedings 11: 1 (1972).

Conrad, K.A.; Molk, B.L. and Chidsey, C.A.: Pharmacokinetic studies of quinidine in patients with arrhythmias. Circulation 55: 1 (1977).

Corday, E. and Corday, S.: Prevention of heart disease by control of risk factors: The time has come to face the facts. American Journal of Cardiology 35: 330 (1975).

Coronary Drug Project: Initial findings leading to modifications of its research protocol. Journal of the American Medical Association 214: 1303 (1970).

Coronary Drug Project Research Group: Clofibrate and niacin in coronary heart disease. Journal of the American Medical Association 231: 360 (1975).

Cunningham, T.; Sloman, G. and Nyberg, G.: Procaineamide blood levels after administration of a sustained-release preparation. Medical Journal of Australia 1: 370 (1977).

Cusack, B.; Horgan, J.; Kelly, J.G.; Lavan, J.; Noel, J. and O'Malley, K.: Pharmacokinetics of digoxin in the elderly. British Journal of Clinical Pharmacology 6: 439P (1978).

Dall, J.L.C.: Maintenance digoxin in the elderly. British Medical Journal 2: 705 (1970).

Danahy, D.T.; Burwell, D.T.; Aronow, W. and Prakash, R.: Sustained haemodynamic and antianginal effect of high dose oral isosorbide dinitrate. Circulation 55: 381 (1977).

Danilo, P.: Tocainide. Americal Heart Journal 97: 259 (1979).

D'Arcy, P.F. and Griffin, J.P.: Cardiac dysfunction; in Iatrogenic Diseases (Oxford University Press, London 1972).

Data, J.L.; Wilkinson, G.R. and Nies, A.S.: Interaction of quinidine with anticonvulsant drugs. New England Journal of Medicine 294: 699 (1976).

Davidson, C. and Gillebrand, I.M.: Use of amiloride as a potassium conserving agent in severe cardiac disease. British Heart Journal 35: 456 (1973).

Davidson, C.; Burkinshaw, L. and Morgan, D.B.: The effects of potassium supplements, spironolactone or amiloride on the potassium status of patients with heart failure. Postgraduate Medical Journal 54: 405 (1978).

Davies, D.L. and Wilson, G.M.: Diuretics: Mechanism of action and clinical application. Drugs 9: 178 (1975).

Dayton, S.; Pearce, M.L.; Hashimoto, S.; Dixon, W.J. and Tomiyasu, U.: A controlled clinical trial of a diet high in unsaturated fat in preventing complications of atherosclerosis. Circulation 39-40 (Suppl. 2): 1 (1969).

Deglin, S.M.; Deglin, J.M. and Chung, E.K.: Drug-induced cardiovascular diseases. Drugs 14: 29 (1977).

Desjacques, P.; Moret, P. and Gauthier, G.: Effets cardiovasculaire de la l-dopa et de l'inhibiteur de la decarboxylase chez les malades atteints de la maladie de Parkinson. Schweizerische Medizinische Wochenschrift 103: 1783 (1973).

Dobbs, S.M. and Mawer, G.E.: Prediction of digoxin dose requirements. Clinical Pharmacokinetics 2: 281 (1977).

Dobbs, S.M.; Mawer, G.E.; Rodgers, E.M.; Woodcock, B.G. and Lucas, S.B.: Can digoxin dose requirements be predicted. British Journal of Clinical Pharmacology 3: 231 (1976).

Dobbs, S.M.; Rodgers, E.M.; Kenyon, W.I.; Livshin, D.; Slater, E. and Godsmark, B.: Digoxin prescribing in perspective. British Journal of Clinical Pharmacology 4: 327 (1977a).

Dobbs, S.M.; Parkes, J.; Rodgers, E.M. and Kenyon, W.I.: Oral digitalisation: choice of dose. British Medical Journal 2: 168 (1977b).

Dobbs, S.M.; Kenyon, W.I. and Dobbs, R.J.: Maintenance digoxin after an episode of heart failure: a placebo-controlled trial in outpatients. British Medical Journal 1: 749 (1977c).

Doherty, J.E.: How and when to use the digitalis serum levels. Journal of the American Medical Association 239: 2594 (1978).

Doherty, J.E. and Kane, J.J.: Clinical pharmacology and therapeutic use of digitalis glycosides. Drugs 6: 182 (1973).

Doherty, J.E.; Kane, J.J.; Phillips, J.R. and Adamson, J.S.: Digitalis in pulmonary heart disease (cor pulmonale). Drugs 13: 142 (1977).

Dollery, C.T.; George, C.F. and Orme, M.I'E.: Drug interactions affecting cardiovascular therapy; in Cluff and Petrie (Eds) Clinical Effects of Interaction Between Drugs (Excerpta Medica, Amsterdam 1974).

Dorr, A.E.; Gundersen, K.; Schneider, J.C.; Spencer, T.W. and Martin, W.B.: Colestipol hydrochloride in hypercholesterolemic patients — Effect on serum cholesterol and mortality. Journal of Chronic Diseases 31: 5 (1978).

Drayer, D.E.; Reidenberg, M.M. and Levy, R.W.: N-acetylprocainamide: an active metabolite of procainamide. Proceedings of the Society for Experimental Biology and Medicine 146: 358 (1974).

Drayer, D.E.; Lowenthal, D.T.; Restivo, K.M.; Schwartz, A.; Cook, C.E. and Reidenberg, M.M.: Steady-state serum levels of quinidine and active metabolites in cardiac patients with varying degrees of renal function. Clinical Pharmacology and Therapeutics 24: 31 (1978).

Dujovne, C.A.; Hurwitz, A.; Kauffman, R.E. and Azarnoff, D.L.: Colestipol and clofibrate in hypercholesterolemia. Clinical Pharmacology and Therapeutics 16: 291 (1974).

du Souich, P. and Erill, S.: Metabolism of procainamide and p-aminobenzoic acid in patients with chronic liver disease. Clinical Pharmacology and Therapeutics 22: 588 (1977).

du Souich, P. and Erill, S.: Metabolism of procainamide in patients with chronic heart failure, chronic respiratory failure and chronic renal failure. European Journal of Clinical Pharmacology 14: 21 (1978).

du Souich, P.; McLean, A.J.; Lalka, D.; Erill, S. and Gibaldi, M.: Pulmonary disease and drug kinetics. Clinical Pharmacokinetics 3: 257 (1978).

Dyer, N.H. and Varley, C.C.: Practolol-induced pleurisy and constrictive pericarditis. British Medical Journal 2: 443 (1975).

Ebner, F. and Dunschede, H.B.: Haemodynamics, therapeutic mechanism of action and clinical findings of Adalat use based on worldwide clinical trials. Third International Adalat Symposium. New Therapy of Ischemic Heart Disease. Proceedings of the Symposium held at Rio de Janeiro, October 10-11, 1975, p.283 (Excerpta Medica, Amsterdam 1976).

Edelman, B.A.; Contractor, A.M. and Shangraw, R.F.: The stability of hypodermic tablets of nitroglycerin packaged in dispensing containers. Journal of the American Pharmaceutical Association 11: 30 (1971).

Editorial: Pentazocine in myocardial infarction. Lancet 2: 888 (1976).

Editorial: HDL — The latest in the risk factor game. Medical Journal of Australia 2: 470 (1978).

Ejvinsson, G.: Effect of quinidine in plasma concentrations of digoxin. British Medical Journal 1: 279 (1978).

Epstein, F.H.: Highlights of epidemiological research in Western countries; in Schettler, Goto, Hata and Klose (Eds) Atherosclerosis, vol. IV, p.471 (Springer Verlag, Berlin 1977).

Eriksson, J-E.; Hanson, A.; Horlin, R.; Johansson, B.W.; Ohlsson, O.; Otto, U. and Syren, G.: Evaluation of quinidine Lipettes — a sustained release preparation. Acta Medica Scandinavica 205: 53 (1979).

Ewy, G.A.; Kapadia, G.G.; Yao, L.; Lullin, M. and Marcus, F.I.: Digoxin metabolism in the elderly. Circulation 39: 449 (1969).

Feldman, D. and Couropmitree, C.: Intrinsic mineralocorticoid agonist activity of some nonsteroidal anti-inflammatory drugs. A postulated mechanism for sodium retention. Journal of Clinical Investigation 57: 1 (1976).

Fisch, C.; Knoebel, S.B.; Feigenbaum, H. and Greenspan, K.: Potassium and the monophasic action potential, electrocardiogram, conduction and arrhythmias. Progress in Cardiovascular Diseases 8: 387 (1966).

Fitzgerald, J.D. and O'Donnell, S.R.: Pharmacology and 4-hydroxy propranolol, a metabolite of propranolol. British Journal of Pharmacology 43: 222 (1971).

Fleckenstein, L.; Benet, L.Z. and Thomson, P.D.: Pharmacokinetic evaluation of a patient with unusually high digoxin requirements. Clinical Pharmacology and Therapeutics 21: 102 (1977).

Forrest, J.A.H.; Finlayson, N.D.C.; Adjepon-Yamoah, K.K. and Prescott, L.F.: Antipyrine, paracetamol, and lignocaine elimination in chronic liver disease. British Medical Journal 1: 1384 (1977).

Franciosa, J.A.; Blank, R.C.; Cohn, J.N. and Mikulic, E.: Hemodynamic effects of topical, oral and sublingual nitroglycerin in left ventricular failure. Current Therapeutic Research 22: 231 (1977).

Franciosa, J.A.; Nordstrom, L.A. and Cohn, J.N.: Nitrate therapy for congestive heart failure. Journal of the American Medical Association 240: 443 (1978).

Fraser, D.M. and Miller, H.C.: Perhexiline-induced neuropathy. British Medical Journal 1: 858 (1978).

Fredrickson, D.S.; Levy, R.I. and Lees, R.S.: Fat transport in lipoproteins: an integrated approach to mechanisms and disorders. New England Journal of Medicine 276: 32, 94, 148, 215, 273, (1967).

Friedman, M.A.; Bozdech, M.J.; Billingham, M.E. and Rider, A.K.: Doxorubicin cardiotoxicity. Serial endomyocardial biopsies and systolic time intervals. Journal of the American Medical Association 240: 1603 (1978).

Gallo, D.G.; Baily, K.R. and Schaffner, A.L.: The interaction between cholestyramine and drugs. Proceedings of the Society of Experimental Biology and Medicine 120: 60 (1965).

Gibson, D.G. and Sowton, E.: The use of beta-adrenergic receptor blocking drugs in dysrhythmias. Progress in Cardiovascular Diseases 12: 16 (1969).

Gilladoga, A.C.; Manuel, C.; Tan, C.T.C.; Wollner, N.; Sternberg, S.S. and Murphy, M.L.: The cardiotoxicity of adriamycin and daunomycin in children. Cancer 37: 1070 (1976).

Glueck, C.J. and Kwiterovich, P.O.: The lipid hypothesis. Genetic basis. Archives of Surgery 113: 35 (1978).

Goldberg, L.I.: The pharmacological basis of the clinical use of dopamine. Proceedings of the Royal Society of Medicine 70 (Suppl. 2): 7 (1977).

Goldberg, L.I. and Hsieh, Y.: Clinical use of dopamine. Rational Drug Therapy 11: 1 (Nov. 1977).

Gollub, M.J.: Myocardial infarction after the phentolamine test. New England Journal of Medicine 273: 37 (1965).

Gordon, T.; Castelli, W.P.; Hjortland, M.C.; Kannel, W.B. and Dawber, T.R.: High density lipoprotein as a protective factor against coronary heart disease. American Journal of Medicine 62: 707 (1977).

Green, K.G. et al.: Improvement in prognosis of myocardial infarction by long-term beta-adrenoreceptor blockade using practolol. British Medical Journal 3: 735 (1975).

Green, K.G. et al.: Reduction in mortality after myocardial infarction by long-term beta-adrenoceptor blockade. Multicentre international study: supplementary report. British Medical Journal 2: 419 (1977).

Greenblatt, D.J. and Koch-Weser, J.: Drug therapy: intramuscular injection of drugs: The digoxin dilemma. Clinical Pharmacokinetics 1: 36 (1976).

Grundy, S.M. and Mok, H.Y.I.: Colestipol, clofibrate, and phytosterols in combined therapy of hyperlipidemia. Journal of Laboratory and Clinical Medicine 89: 354 (1977).

Gugler, R.: Clinical pharmacokinetics of hypolipidaemic drugs. Clinical Pharmacokinetics 3: 425 (1978).

Guthrie, D. and Gibson, A.L.: Doxorubicin cardiotoxicity: possible role of digoxin in its prevention. British Medical Journal 2: 1447 (1977).

Haft, J.I.: Cardiovascular injury induced by sympathetic catecholamines. Progress in Cardiovascular Diseases 17: 73 (1974).

Hagemeijer, F.: Absorption, half-life, and toxicity of oral aprindine in patients with acute myocardial infarction. European Journal of Clinical Pharmacology 9: 21 (1975).

Hagemeijer, F. and van Houwe, E.: Tritiated energy cardioversion of patients on digitalis. British Heart Journal 37: 1303 (1975).

Halkin, H.; Meffin, P.; Melmon, K.L. and Rowland, M.: Influence of congestive heart failure on blood levels of lidocaine and its active monodeethylated metabolite. Clinical Pharmacology and Therapeutics 17: 669 (1975a).

Halkin, H.; Sheiner, L.B.; Peck, C.C. and Melmon, K.L.: Determinants of the renal clearance of digoxin. Clinical Pharmacology and Therapeutics 17: 385 (1975b).

Hardason, T.; Henning, H. and O'Rourke, R.A.: Prolonged salutary effects of isosorbide dinitrate and nitroglycerin ointment on regional left ventricular function. American Journal of Cardiology 40: 90 (1977).

Harrison, C.E. and Wakim, K.G.: Inhibition of binding of tritiated digoxin to myocardium by sodium depletion in dogs. Circulation Research 24: 263 (1969).

Harrison, D.C.: Should lidocaine be administered routinely to all patients after acute myocardial infarction? Circulation 58: 581 (1978).

Harrison, D.C. and Alderman, E.L.: The pharmacology and clinical use of lidocaine as an antiarrhythmic drug — 1972. Modern Treatment 9: 139 (1972).

Harrison, D.C. and Alderman, E.L.: Editorial: Discontinuation of propranolol therapy. Cause of rebound angina pectoris and acute coronary events. Chest 69: 1 (1976).

Harrison, D.C.; Meffin, P.J. and Winkle, R.A.: Clinical pharmacokinetics of antiarrhythmic drugs. Progress in Cardiovascular Diseases 20: 217 (1977).

Hay, D.R.: Treatment of heart failure. Drugs 5: 318 (1973).

Hayes, M.J.; Morris, G.K. and Hampton, J.R.: Comparison of mobilisation after 2 and 9 days in uncomplicated myocardial infarction. British Medical Journal 3: 10 (1974).

Heel, R.C.; Brogden, R.N.; Speight, T.M. and Avery, G.S.: Probucol: A review of its pharmacological properties and therapeutic use in patients with hypercholesterolaemia. Drugs 15: 409 (1978a).

Heel, R.C.; Brogden, R.N.; Speight, T.M. and Avery, G.S.: Disopyramide: A review of its pharmacological properties and therapeutic use in treating cardiac arrhythmias. Drugs 15: 331 (1978b).

Henderson, I.C. and Frei, E.: Adriamycin and the heart. New England Journal of Medicine 300: 310 (1979).

Henningsen, N.C.; Cederberg, A.; Hansson, A. and Johansson, B.W.: Effects of long-term treatment with procaine amide. Acta Medica Scandinavica 198: 475 (1975).

Herzberg, L.: Carbamazepine and bradycardia. Lancet 1: 1097 (1978).

Higgins, C.B.; Wexler, L.; Silverman, J.F. and Schroeder, J.S.: Clinical and arteriographic features of Prinzmetal's variant angina: documentation of etiologic factors. American Journal of Cardiology 37: 831 (1976).

Hoffman, B. and Cranefield, P.: The physiological basis of cardiac arrhythmias. American Journal of Medicine 37: 670 (1964).

Holder, D.A.; Sniderman, A.D.; Fraser, G. and Fallen, E.L.: Experience with bretylium tosylate by a hospital cardiac arrest team. Circulation 55: 541 (1977).

Horster, F.A.: Pharmacokinetics of nifedipine-^{14}C in man; in Lochner et al. (Eds) 2nd International Adalat Symposium, p.124 (Springer-Verlag, Berlin 1975).

Hull, S.M. and MacKintosh, A.: Discontinuation of maintenance digoxin therapy in general practice. Lancet 2: 1054 (1977).

Hurwitz, N. and Wade, O.L.: Intensive hospital monitoring of adverse reactions to drugs. Brit. Med. J. 1: 531 (1969).

Iisalo, E.: Clinical pharmacokientics of digoxin. Clinical Pharmacokinetics 2: 1 (1977).

Jaffe, C.M.: First-degree atrioventricular block during lithium carbonate treatment. Amer. J. Psych. 134: 88 (1977).

Jariwalla, A.G. and Anderson, E.G.: Production of ischaemic cardiac pain by nifedipine. Brit. Med. J. 1: 1181 (1978).

Jefferson, J.W.: A review of the cardiovascular effects and toxicity of tricyclic antidepressants. Psychosomatic Medicine 37: 160 (1975).

Jelliffe, R.W.: Administration of digoxin. Diseases of the Chest 56: 56 (1969).

Jelliffe, R.W. and Brooker, G.: A nomogram for digoxin therapy. American Journal of Medicine 57: 63 (1974).

Jenkins, P.J.; Harper, R.W. and Nestel, P.J.: Severity of coronary atherosclerosis related to lipoprotein concentration. British Medical Journal 2: 388 (1978).

Jenne, J.W.; Chick, T.W.; Miller, B.A. and Strickland, R.D.: Apparent theophylline half-life fluctuations during treatment of acute left ventricular failure. American Journal of Hospital Pharmacy 34: 408 (1977).

Jewitt, D.E.; Maurer, B.J. and Hubner, P.J.B.: Increased pulmonary arterial pressures after pentazocine in myocardial infarction. British Medical Journal 1: 795 (1970).

Johnson, G.D. and McDevitt, D.G.: Is maintenance digoxin necessary in patients with sinus rhythm? Lancet 1: 567 (1979).

Johnston, G.D. and McDevitt, D.G.: Digoxin compliance in patients from general practice. British Journal of Clinical Pharmacology 6: 339 (1978).

Julian, D.G. and Oliver, M.F.: Acute Myocardial Infarction (Livingstone, Edinburgh 1968).

Kannel, W.B.: Prevention of coronary heart disease by control of risk factors. Journal of the American Medical Association 227: 338 (1974).

Kannel, W.B.; Castelli, W.P.; Gordon, T. and McNamara, P.M.: Serum cholesterol, lipoproteins, and the risk of coronary heart disease. The Framingham study. Annals of Internal Medicine 74: 1 (1971).

Karliner, J. and Braunwald, E.: Present status of digitalis treatment in acute myocardial infarction. Circulation 45: 819 (1972).

Karlsson, E.: Clinical pharmacokinetics of procainamide. Clinical Pharmacokinetics 3: 97 (1978).

Kasparian, H.; Wiener, L.; Duca, P.R.; Gottlieb, R.S. and Brest, A.N.: Comparative hemodynamic effects of placebo and oral isosorbide dinitrate in patients with significant coronary artery disease. American Heart Journal 90: 68 (1975).

Kay, H.B.: Angina pectoris: Getting the most from drug therapy. Drugs 13: 276 (1977).

Kessler, K.M.; Lowenthal, D.T.; Warner, H.; Gibson, T.; Briggs, W. and Reidenberg, M.M.: Quinidine elimination in patients with congestive heart failure or poor renal function. New England Journal of Medicine 290: 706 (1974).

Kessler, K.M.; Humphries, W.C.; Black, M. and Spann, J.F.: Quinidine pharmacokinetics in patients with cirrhosis or receiving propranolol. American Heart Journal 96: 627 (1978).

Koch-Weser, J.: Pharmacokinetics of procainamide in man. Annals of the New York Academy of Sciences 179: 370 (1971).

Koch-Weser, J.: Correlation of serum concentrations and pharmacologic effects of antiarrhythmic drugs. Pharmacology and Future of Man. Proceedings of the 5th International Congress of Pharmacology, vol. 3, p.69 (Karger, Basel 1973).

Koch-Weser, J.: Clinical application of the pharmacokinetics of procainamide. Cardiovascular Clinics 6 (II): 63 (1974).

Koch-Weser, J.: Drug interactions in cardiovascular therapy. American Heart Journal 90: 93 (1975).

Koch-Weser, J.: Serum procainamide levels as therapeutic guides. Clinical Pharmacokinetics 2: 389 (1977).

Koch-Weser, J. and Klein, S.W.: Procainamide dosage schedules, plasma concentrations, and clinical effects. J. Amer. Med. Ass. 215: 1454 (1971).

Kopriva, C.J.; Brown, A.C.D. and Pappas, G.: Hemodynamics during general anesthesia in patients receiving propranolol. Anesthesiology 48: 28 (1978a).

Kopriva, C.J.; Guinazu, A. and Barash, P.G.: Massive propranolol therapy and uncomplicated cardiac surgery. Journal of the American Medical Association 239: 1157 (1978b).

Kutt, H.; Winters, W.; Scherman, R. and McDowell, F.: Diphenylhydantoin and phenobarbital toxicity. The role of liver disease. Archives of Neurology 11: 649 (1964).

Lalka, D.; Wyman, M.G.; Goldreyer, B.N.; Ludden, T.M. and Cannom, D.S.: Procainamide accumulation kinetics in the immediate postmyocardial infarction period. Journal of Clinical Pharmacology 18: 397 (1978).

Landahl, S.; Lindblad, B.; Roupe, S.; Steen, B. and Svanborg, A.: Digitalis therapy in a 70-year-old population. Acta Medica Scandinavica 202: 437 (1977).

Langer, T. and Levy, R.I.: The effect of nicotinic acid on the turnover of low density lipoproteins in type II hyperlipoproteinemia; in Gey and Carlson (Eds) Metabolic Effects of Nicotinic Acid and its Derivatives, p.641 (Huber, Stuttgart 1971).

Lawson, D.H.; Gray, J.M.B.; Henry, D.A. and Tilstone, W.J.: Continuous infusion of frusemide in refractory oedema. British Medical Journal 2: 476 (1978).

Leahey, E.B.; Reiffel, J.A.; Drusin, R.E.; Heissenbuttel, R-H.; Lovejoy, W.P. and Bigger, T.: Interaction between quinidine and digoxin. Journal of the American Medical Association 240: 533 (1978).

Lee, St. G.T.: Nitroglycerin ointment therapy and leg edema. American Heart Journal 95: 273 (1978).

Lee, G.; Peng, C.L.; Mason, D.T.; Amsterdam, E.A.; Massumi, R.A. and Zelis, R.: Demonstration of linear dose-response and quantitative attenuation by potassium of the inotropic action to digitalis. Chest 62: 367 (1972).

Lee, G.; Demaria, A.N.; Amsterdam, E.A.; Realyvasquez, F.; Angel, J.; Morrison, S. and Mason, D.T.: Comparative effects of morphine, meperidine and pentazocine on cardiocirculatory dynamics in patients with acute myocardial infarction. American Journal of Medicine 60: 949 (1976).

Lefrak, E.A.; Pitha, J.; Rosenheim, S. and Gottlieb, J.A.: A clinicopathologic analysis of adriamycin cardiotoxicity. Cancer 32: 302 (1973).

LeLorier, J.; Grenon, D.; Latour, Y.; Caille, G.; Dumont, G.; Brosseau, A. and Solignac, A.: Pharmacokinetics of lidocaine after prolonged intravenous infusions in uncomplicated myocardial infarction. Annals of Internal Medicine 87: 700 (1977).

Lely, A.H. and van Enter, E.H.J.: Large-scale digitoxin intoxication. British Medical Journal 3: 737 (1970).

Lemberg, L.: Digitalis in congestive heart failure. Fact or fancy. Archives of Internal Medicine 138: 451 (1978).

Lenaz, L. and Page, J.A.: Cardiotoxicity of adriamycin and related anthracyclines. Cancer Treatment Reviews 3: 111 (1976).

Lertora, J.L.L.; Atkinson, A.J.; Kushner, W.; Nevin, M.J.; Lee, W-K.; Jones, C. and Schmid, F.R.: Long-term antiarrhythmic therapy with N-acetylprocainamide. Clinical Pharmacology and Therapeutics 25: 273 (1979).

Levine, O.R. and Somlyo, A.P.: Digitalis intoxication in premature infants. Journal of Pediatrics 61: 70 (1962).

Levy, R.I. and Rifkind, B.M.: Lipid lowering drugs and hyperlipidaemia. Drugs 6: 12 (1973).

Levy, R.I.: Drug therapy of hyperlipoproteinemia. Journal of the American Medical Association 235: 2334 (1976).

Levy, R.I.; Fredrickson, D.S.; Shulman, R.; Bilheimer, D.W.; Breslow, J.L.; Stone, N.J.; Lux, S.E.; Sloan, H.R.; Krauss, R.M. and Herbert, P.N.: Dietary and drug treatment of primary hyperlipoproteinemia. Annals of Internal Medicine 77: 267 (1972).

Lie, K.I.; Wellens, H.J.; Van Capelle, F.J. and Durrer, D.: Lidocaine in the prevention of primary ventricular fibrillation. A double-blind, randomized study of 212 consecutive patients. New England Journal of Medicine 291: 1324 (1974).

Lie, K.I.; Liem, K.L. and Durrer, D.: A double-blind randomized study of intramuscular lidocaine in preventing primary ventricular fibrillation. American Journal of Cardiology 39: 275A (1977).

Lima, J.J.; Conti, D.R.; Goldfarb, A.L.; Golden, L.H. and Jusko, W.J.: Pharmacokinetic approach to intravenous procainamide therapy. European Journal of Clinical Pharmacology 13: 303 (1978).

Liverpool Therapeutics Group: Use of digitalis in general practice. British Medical Journal 2: 673 (1978).

Loughnan, P.M.: Digoxin excretion in human breast milk. Journal of Pediatrics 92: 1019 (1978).

Ludden, T.M.; Allen, J.P.; Valutsky, W.A.; Vicuna, A.V.; Nappi, J.M.; Hoffman, S.F.; Wallace, J.E.; Lalka, D. and McNay, J.L.: Individualisation of phenytoin dosage regimens. Clinical Pharmacology and Therapeutics 21: 287 (1977).

Luke, C.M.: Tricyclic antidepressants and heart disease. New Zealand Medical Journal 74: 345 (1971).

Macintyre, I.M.C. and Ruckley, C.V.: Pulmonary embolism — A clinical and autopsy study. Scottish Medical Journal 19: 20 (1974).

McMichael, J.: Dietetic factors in coronary disease (special article). European Journal of Cardiology 5: 447 (1977).

McMichael, J.: Fats and atheroma: an inquest. British Medical Journal 1: 173 (1979).

Marcus, F.I.; Burkhalter, L.; Cuccia, C.; Pavolovich, J. and Kapadia, G.G.: Administration of tritiated digoxin with and without a loading dose. A metabolic study. Circulation 34: 865 (1966a).

Marcus, F.I.; Peterson, A.; Salel, A.; Scully, J. and Kapadia, G.G.: The metabolism of tritiated digoxin in renal insufficiency in dogs and man. Journal of Pharmacology and Experimental Therapeutics 152: 372 (1966b).

Maroko, P.R.; Hillis, L.D.; Muller, J.E.; Tavazzi, L.; Heyndrickx, G.R.; Ray, M.; Chiariello, M.; Distante, A.; Askenazi, J.; Salerno, J.; Carpentier, J.; Reshetnaya, N.I.; Radvany, P.; Libby, P.; Raabe, D.S.; Chazov, E.I.; Bobba, P. and Braunwald, E.: Favorable effects of hyaluronidase on electrocardiographic evidence of necrosis in patients with acute myocardial infarction. New England Journal of Medicine 296: 898 (1977).

Marquez-Julio, A. and Uldall, P.R.: Pericardial effusions associated with minoxidil. Lancet 2: 816 (1977).

Mason, D.T. (Ed): Symposium on vasodilator and inotropic therapy of heart failure. American Journal of Medicine 65: 101 (1978).

Mason, D.T.; Spann, J.F. and Zelis, R.: New developments in the understanding of the action of digitalis glycosides. Progress in Cardiovascular Disease 11: 433 (1969).

Mason, D.T.; Zelis, R.; Lee, G.; Hughes, J.L.; Spann, J.F. and Amsterdam, E.A.: Current concepts and treatment of digitalis toxicity. American Journal of Cardiology 27: 546 (1971).

Mason, D.T.; DeMaria, A.N.; Amsterdam, R.; Zelis, R. and Massumi, R.A.: Antiarrhythmic agents I: Mechanisms of action and clinical pharmacology. Drugs 5: 261 (1973); Antiarrhythmic agents II. Therapeutic considerations. Drugs 5: 292 (1973).

Medical Division, Royal Infirmary, Glasgow: Early mobilisation after uncomplicated myocardial infarction. Lancet 2: 346 (1973).

Mehta, J.; Lacona, M.; Feldman, R.L.; Pepine, C.J. and Conti, C.R.: Comparative hemodynamic effects of intravenous nitroprusside and oral prazosin in refractory heart failure. American Journal of Cardiology 41: 925 (1978).

Meister, W.; Benowitz, N.L.; Melmon, K.L. and Benet, L.Z.: Influence of cardiac failure on the pharmacokinetics of digoxin. Clin. Pharm. Ther. 23: 122 (1978).

Melmendier, C.L.; Vanden Bergen, C.J.; Emplit, G. and Delcroix, C.: A long-term study of the efficacy of oxandrolone in hyperlipoproteinemias. Journal of Clinical Pharmacology 18: 42 (1978).

Mercer, C.W. and Logic, J.R.: Cardiac arrest due to hyperkalaemia following intravenous penicillin administration. Chest 64: 358 (1973).

Merrill, A.J.: Edema and decreased renal blood flow in patients with chronic congestive heart failure: evidence of 'forward failure' as the primary cause of edema. Journal of Clinical Investigation 25: 389 (1946).

Miettinen, M.; Turpeinen, O.; Karvonen, M.J.; Elosuo, R. and Paavilainen, E.: Effect of a cholesterol lowering diet on mortality from coronary heart-disease and other causes: A twelve-year clinical trial in men and women. Lancet 2: 835 (1972).

Mikulic, E.; Franciosa, J.A. and Cohn, J.N.: Comparative haemodynamic effects of chewable isosorbide dinitrate and nitroglycerin in patients with congestive heart failure. Circulation 52: 447 (1975).

Mikulic, E.; Cohn, J.N. and Franciosa, J.A.: Comparative hemodynamic effects of inotropic and vasodilator drugs in severe heart failure. Circulation 56: 528 (1977).

Miller, G.J. and Miller, N.E.: Plasma-high-density-lipoprotein concentration and development of ischaemic heart-disease. Lancet 1: 16 (1975).

Miller, R.R.; Olson, H.G.; Amsterdam, E.A. and Mason, D.T.: Propranolol-withdrawal rebound phenomenon. Exacerbation of coronary events after abrupt cessation of antianginal therapy. New England Journal of Medicine 293: 416 (1975).

Miller, R.R.; Awan, N.A.; Joye, J.A.; Maxwell, K.S.; DeMaria, A.N.; Amsterdam, E.A. and Mason, D.T.: Combined dopamine and nitroprusside therapy in congestive heart failure: Greater augmentation of cardiac performance by addition of inotropic stimulation to afterload reduction. Circulation 55: 881 (1977).

Mizgala, H.F. and Counsell, J.: Acute coronary syndromes following abrupt cessation of oral propranolol therapy. Canadian Medical Association Journal 114: 1123 (1976).

Moir, D.C.; Dingwall-Fordyce, I. and Weir, R.D.: A follow-up study of cardiac patients receiving amitriptyline. European Journal of Clinical Pharmacology 6: 98 (1973).

Mokotoff, R.; Ross, G. and Leiter, L.: Renal plasma flow and sodium reabsorption and excretion in congestive heart failure. Journal of Clinical Investigation 27: 1 (1948).

Morgan, D.B.; Burkinshaw, L. and Davidson, C.: Potassium depletion in heart failure and its relation to long-term treatment with diuretics: a review of the literature. Postgraduate Medical Journal 54: 72 (1978).

Morgan, T.O.: Clinical use of potassium supplements and potassium sparing diuretics. Drugs 6: 222 (1973).

Morrison, J. and Killip, T.: Serial serum digitalis levels in patients with acute myocardial infarction. Clinical Research 19: 353 (1971a).

Morrison, J. and Killip, T.: Hypoxemia and digitalis toxicity in patients with chronic lung disease. Circulation 44 (Suppl. II): 41 (1971b).

Muller, J.E. and Gunther, S.J.: Nifedipine therapy for Prinzmetal's angina. Circulation 57: 137 (1978)

Mullick, F.G. and McAllister, H.A.: Myocarditis associated with methyldopa therapy. Journal of the American Medical Association 237: 1699 (1977).

Nash, C. and Heath, C.: Vascular responses to catecholamines during respiratory changes in pH. American Journal of Physiology 200: 765 (1967).

Nayler, W.G. and Szeto, J.: Effect of verapamil on contractility, oxygen utilisation and calcium exchangeability in mammalian heart muscle. Cardiovascular Research 6: 120 (1972).

Needleman, P.; Lang, S. and Johnson, E.M.: Organic nitrates: Relationship between biotransformation and rational angina pectoris therapy. Journal of Pharmacology and Experimental Therapeutics 181: 489 (1972).

Neuvonen, P.J.: Bioavailability of phenytoin: Clinical pharmacokinetic and therapeutic implications. Clinical Pharmacokinetics 4: 91 (1979).

Nevins, M.; Berque, S.; Corwin, N. and Lyon, L.: Phenylbutazone and pulmonary oedema. Lancet 2: 1358 (1969).

New Zealand Hypertension Study Group: Initial experience with prazosin in New Zealand. A multicentre report. Medical Journal of Australia Special Supplement 2: 23 (1977).

Nies, A.: Cardiovascular disorders. I. Alteration of arterial pressure and regional blood flow; in Melmon and Morelli (Eds) Clinical Pharmacology, 1st ed, p.142 (Macmillan, New York 1972).

Nies, A.S.; Shand, D.G. and Wilkinson, G.R.: Altered hepatic blood flow and drug disposition. Clinical Pharmacokinetics 1: 135 (1976).

Nola, G.T.; Pope, S. and Harrison, D.C.: Assessment of the synergistic relationship between serum calcium and digitalis. American Heart Journal 79: 499 (1970).

Norris, R.M.; Clarke, E.D.; Sammel, N.L.; Smith, W.M. and Williams, B.: Protective effect of propranolol in threatened myocardial infarction. Lancet 2: 907 (1978).

Nyberg, L.: Bioavailability of digoxin in man after oral administration of preparations with different dissolution rate. Acta Pharmacologica et Toxicologica 40 (Suppl. III): 1 (1977).

Ochs, H.R.; Greenblatt, D.J.; Woo, E.; Franke, K.; Pfeifer, H.J. and Smith, T.W.: Single and multiple dose pharmacokinetics of oral quinidine sulfate and gluconate. American Journal of Cardiology 41: 770 (1978a).

Ochs, H.R.; Greenblatt, D.J.; Woo, E. and Smith, T.W.: Reduced quinidine clearance in elderly persons. American Journal of Cardiology 42: 481 (1978b).

Odutola, T.A.; Oladapo, J.M. and Falaiye, J.M.: Electrolyte status in duogastrone-treated duodenal ulcer patients. Nigerian Medical Journal 8: 337 (1978).

Ogilvie, R.I. and Ruedy, J.: An educational program in digitalis therapy. Journal of the American Medical Association 222: 50 (1972).

Okada, R.D.; Hager, W.D.; Marcus, F.I.; Perrier, D. and Graves, P.: Predicting digoxin dosage from creatinine clearance. Annals of Internal Medicine 88: 133 (1978a).

Okada, R.D.; Hager, W.D.; Graves, P.E.; Mayersohn, M.; Perrier, D.G. and Marcus, F.I.: Relationship between plasma concentration and dose of digoxin in patients with and without renal impairment. Circulation 58: 1196 (1978b).

Oliver, M.F. and Julian, D.G.: Manual on Intensive Coronary Care (WHO, Copenhagen 1970).

Oliver, M.F.; Roberts, S.D.; Hayes, D.; Pantridge, J.S.; Suzman, M.M. and Bersohn, I.: Effect of Atromid and ethyl chlorophenoxyisobutyrate on anticoagulant requirements. Lancet 1: 143 (1963).

Oliver, G.C.; Parker, B.M. and Parker, C.W.: Radioimmunoassay for digoxin: Technic and clinical application. American Journal of Medicine 51: 186 (1971).

O'Reilly, R.A. and Aggeler, P.M.: Determinants of the response to oral anticoagulants in man. Pharmacological Reviews 22: 35 (1970).

Orlando, R.C.; Moyer, P. and Barnett, T.B.: Methysergide therapy and constrictive pericarditis. Annals of Internal Medicine 88: 213 (1978).

O'Rourke, M.F.: New concepts in management of cardiogenic shock. Current Therapeutics 15 (5): 31 (1974).

Oster, P.; Schlierf, G.; Heuck, C.C.; Greten, H.; Gundert-Remy, U.; Haase, W.; Klose, G.; Nothelfer, A.; Raetzer, H.; Schellenberg, B. and Schmidt-Gayk, H.: Sitosterin bei familiarer Hyperlipoproteinamie Typ II. Eine randomisierte gekreutz Doppelblindstudie. Deutsche Medizinische Wochenschrift 101: 1308 (1976).

Paciaroni, E.; Foschi, F.; Victori, N.; Saccomanno, G. and Raspa, E.G.: Plasma digoxin levels in chronic pulmonary heart disease. Giornale di Gerontologia 22: 832 (1974).

Packer, M. and Meller, J.: Oral vasodilator therapy for chronic heart failure: A plea for caution. American Journal of Cardiology 42: 686 (1978).

Paliard, P.; Vitrey, D.; Fournier, G.; Belhadjali, J.; Patricot, L. and Berger, F.: Perhexiline maleate-induced hepatitis. Digestion 17: 419 (1978).

Parkes, J.D.; Marsden, C.D. and Price, P.: Amantadine-induced heart-failure. Lancet 1: 904 (1977).

Paterson, J.W.; Conolly, M.E.; Dollery, C.T.; Hayes, A. and Cooper, R.G.: The pharmacodynamics and metabolism of propranolol in man. Pharmacologia Clinica 2: 127 (1970).

Paturaud, J-P. and Gut, J-P.: Cardiac arrest following the rapid intravenous injection of lincomycin. Nouvelle Presse Medicale 4: 1593 (1975).

Perrier, D.; Mayersohn, M. and Marcus, F.I.: Clinical pharmacokinetics of digitoxin. Clinical Pharmacokinetics 2: 292 (1977).

Pessayre, D.; Bichera, M.; Feldmann, G.; Degott, C.; Potet, F. and Benhamou, J-P.: Perhexiline maleate-induced cirrhosis. Gastroenterology 76: 170 (1979).

Pfeifer, H.J.; Greenblatt, D.J. and Koch-Weser, J.: Clinical use and toxicity of intravenous lidocaine. A report from the Boston Collaborative Drug Surveillance Program. American Heart Journal 92: 168 (1976).

Physicians of the Newcastle Upon Tyne Region: Trial of clofibrate in the treatment of ischaemic heart disease. British Medical Journal 4: 767 (1971).

Piafsky, K.M.; Sitar, D.S.; Rangno, R.E. and Ogilvie, R.I.: Disposition of theophylline in acute pulmonary oedema. Clinical Research 22: 726A (1974).

Piafsky, K.M.; Borga, O.; Odar-Cederlof, I.; Johansson, C. and Sjoqvist, F.: Increased plasma protein binding of propranolol and chlorpromazine mediated by disease-induced elevations of plasma α_1 acid glycoprotein. New England Journal of Medicine 299: 1435 (1978).

Pine, M.; Favrot, L.; Smith, S.; McDonald, K. and Chidsey, C.A.: Correlation of plasma propranolol concentration with therapeutic response in patients with angina pectoris. Circulation 52: 886 (1975).

Plotnick, G.D.: Medical management of the patient with unstable angina. J. Amer. Med. Ass. 239: 860 (1978).

Polk, R.E.; Archer, G.L. and Lower, R.: Cefamandole kinetics during cardiopulmonary bypass. Clinical Pharmacology and Therapeutics 23: 473 (1978).

Pottage, A.; Campbell, R.W.F.; Achuff, S.C.; Murray, A.; Julian, D.G. and Prescott, L.F.: The absorption of oral mexiletine in coronary care patients. European Journal of Clinical Pharmacology 13: 393 (1978).

Prescott, L.F.: Variation in drug response due to disease: in Jouhar and Grayson (Eds) International Aspects of Drug Evaluation and Usage, p. 231 (Churchill Livingstone, Edinburgh 1973).

Prescott, L.F.; Adjepon-Yamoah, K.K. and Talbot, R.G.: Impaired lignocaine metabolism in patients with myocardial infarction and cardiac failure. British Medical Journal 1: 939 (1976).

Prescott, L.F.; Clements, J.A. and Pottage, A.: Absorption, distribution and elimination of mexiletine. Postgraduate Medical Journal 53(Suppl. 1): 50 (1977).

Price, H.L.; Kovnat, P.J. and Safrer, B.S.: The uptake of thiopental by body tissues and its relation to duration of narcosis. Clinical Pharmacology and Therapeutics 1: 16 (1960).

Prichard, B.N.C.: β-Adrenergic receptor blocking drugs in angina pectoris. Drugs 7: 55 (1974).

Rhoads, G.G.; Gulbrandsen, C.L. and Kagan, A.: Serum lipoproteins and coronary heart disease in a population study of Hawaii Japanese men. New England Journal of Medicine 294: 293 (1976).

Richens, A.: Clinical pharmacokinetics of phenytoin. Clinical Pharmacokinetics 4: 153 (1979).

Rodger, J.C. and Stewart, A.: Side effects of nifedipine. British Medical Journal 1: 1619 (1978).

Rogen, A.S. and Ferguson, J.C.: Clinical observations on patients treated with Atromid and anticoagulants. Journal of Atherosclerosis Research 3: 671 (1963).

Romhildt, D.W.; Bloomfield, S.S.; Lipicky, R.J.; Welch, R.M. and Fowler, N.O.: Evaluation of bretylium tosylate for the treatment of premature ventricular contractions. Circulation 45: 800 (1972).

Rose, M.R.; Glassman, E. and Spencer, F.C.: Arrhythmias following cardiac surgery: relation to serum digoxin levels. American Heart Journal 89: 288 (1975).

Rosen, M.R.; Merker, M. and Pippenger, C.E.: The effects of lidocaine on the ECG and electrophysiologic properties of Purkinje fibres. American Heart Journal 91: 191 (1976a).

Rosen, M.R.; Danilo, P.; Alonso, M.B. and Pippenger, C.E.: Effects of therapeutic concentrations of diphenylhydantoin on transmembrane potentials of normal and depressed Purkinje fibres. Journal of Pharmacology and Experimental Therapeutics 197: 594 (1976b).

Routledge, P.A. and Shand, D.G.: Clinical pharmacokinetics of propranolol. Clinical Pharmacokinetics 4: 73 (1979).

Russek, H.I.: Propranolol and isosorbide dinitrate synergism in angina pectoris. American Journal of the Medical Sciences 254: 406 (1967).

Ryan, J.R.; Jain, A.K. and McMahon, F.G.: Long-term treatment of hypercholesterolemia with colestipol hydrochloride. Clinical Pharmacology and Therapeutics 17: 83 (1975).

Ryan, W.; Engler, R.; Le Winter, M. and Karliner, J.S.: Efficacy of a new oral agent (Tocainide) in the acute treatment of refractory ventricular arrhythmias. American Journal of Cardiology 43: 285 (1979).

Said, G.: Perhexiline neuropathy: A clinicopathological study. Annals of Neurology 3: 259 (1978).

Samuel, P.; Holtzman, C.M.; Mielman, E. and Sekowski, I.: Reduction of serum cholesterol and triglyceride levels by the combined administration of neomycin and clofibrate. Circulation 41: 109 (1970).

Scheinman, M.M.; Thorburn, D. and Abbott, J.A.: Use of atropine in patients with acute myocardial infarction and sinus bradycardia. Circulation 52: 627 (1975).

Schlossmann, K.; Medenwald, H. and Rosenkranz, H.: Investigations on the metabolism and protein binding of nifedipine: in Lochner et al. (Eds) 2nd International Adalat Symposium, p. 124 (Springer-Verlag, Berlin 1975).

Schmidt, D.H. and Butler, V.P.: Reversal of digoxin toxicity with specific antibodies. Journal of Clinical Investigation 50: 1738 (1971).

Schooley, R.T.; Wagley, P.F. and Lietman, P.S.: Edema associated with ibuprofen therapy. Journal of the American Medical Association 237: 1716 (1977).

Schwartz, A.: New aspects of cardiac glycoside action. Federation Proceedings 36: 2207 (1977).

Scott, P.J.: Lipid lowering drugs and coronary heart disease. Drugs 10: 218 (1975).

Selden, R. and Sasahara, A.A.: Central nervous system toxicity induced by lidocaine. Report of a case in a patient with liver disease. Journal of the American Medical Association 202: 908 (1967).

Seller, R.H.; Cangiano, J.; Kim, K.; Mendelssohn, S.; Brest, A.N. and Swartz, C.: Digitalis toxicity and hypomagnesemia. American Heart Journal 79: 57 (1970).

Selzer, A.: Use of anticoagulant agents in acute myocardial infarction: Statistics or clinical judgement? American Journal of Cardiology 41: 1315 (1978).

Seymour, W.B.; Pritchard, W.H.; Longley, L.P. and Hayman, J.M.: Cardiac output, blood and interstitial fluid volumes, total circulating serum protein, and kidney function during cardiac failure and after improvement. Journal of Clinical Investigation 21: 229 (1942).

Shafer, N.: Hypotension due to nitroglycerin combined with alcohol. New England Journal of Medicine 273: 1169 (1965).

Sherry, S.: The Anturane Reinfarction Trial Research Group: Sulfinpyrazone in the prevention of cardiac death after myocardial infarction. New England Journal of Medicine 298: 289 (1978).

Singh, B.N.: Rational basis of antiarrhythmic therapy: Clinical pharmacology of commonly used antiarrhythmic drugs. Angiology 29: 206 (1978a).

Singh, B.N.: β-Adrenoceptor blocking drugs and acute myocardial infarction. Drugs 15: 218 (1978b).

Singh, B.N. and Jewitt, D.E.: β-Adrenergic receptor blocking drugs in cardiac arrhythmias. Drugs 7: 419 (1974).

Singh, B.N.; Ellrodt, G. and Peter, C.T.: Verapamil: A review of its pharmacological properties and therapeutic use. Drugs 15: 169 (1978).

Singlas, E.; Goujet, M.A. and Simon, P.: Pharmacokinetics of perhexiline maleate in anginal patients with and without peripheral neuropathy. European Journal of Clinical Pharmacology 14: 195 (1978).

Slogoff, S.; Keats, A.S. and Ott, E.: Preoperative propranolol therapy and aortocoronary bypass operation. Journal of the American Medical Association 240: 1487 (1978).

Smith, T.W.: Drug therapy. Digitalis glycosides. New England Journal of Medicine 288: 719, 942 (1973).

Smith, T.W.: Digitalis toxicity: Epidemiology and clinical use of serum concentration measurements. American Journal of Medicine 58: 470 (1975).

Smith, T.W.: Digitalis: Ions, inotropy and toxicity. New England Journal of Medicine 299: 545 (1978).

Smith, T.W. and Haber, E.: Digoxin intoxication: the relationship of clinical presentation to serum digoxin concentration. Journal of Clinical Investigation 49: 2377 (1970).

Smith, T.W. and Haber, E.: Digitalis. New England Journal of Medicine 289: 945, 1010, 1063, 1125 (1973).

Smith, T.W.; Haber, E.; Yeatman, L. and Butler, V.P.: Reversal of advanced digoxin intoxication with Fab fragments of digoxin-specific antibodies. New England Journal of Medicine 294: 797 (1976).

Sonnenblick, E.H.; Frishman, W.H. and LeJemtel, T.H.: Dobutamine: A new synthetic cardioactive sympathetic amine. New England Journal of Medicine 300: 17 (1979).

Sostman, H.D. and Langou, R.E.: Contemporary medical management of stable angina pectoris. American Heart Journal 95: 775 (1978).

Soukop, M.; McVie, J.G. and Calman, K.C.: Fluorouracil cardiotoxicity. British Medical Journal 1: 1422 (1978).

Stamler, J.: Epidemiology of coronary heart disease. Medical Clinics of North America 57: 5 (1973).

Stamler, J.: Dietary and serum lipids in the multifactorial etiology of atherosclerosis. Archives of Surgery 113: 21 (1978).

Stannard, M. and Sloman, G.: Haemodynamic effects of propranolol. British Medical Journal 1: 700 (1967).

Steiness, E. and Olesen, K.H.: Cardiac arrhythmias induced by hypokalaemia and potassium loss during maintenance digoxin therapy. British Heart Journal 38: 167 (1976).

Stenson, R.E.; Constantino, R.T. and Harrison, D.C.: Interrelationships of hepatic blood flow, cardiac output, and blood levels of lidocaine in·man. Circulation 43: 205 (1971).

Stephens, W.P.; Eddy, J.D.; Parsons, L.M. and Singh, S.P.: Raised intracranial pressue due to perhexiline maleate. British Medical Journal 1: 21 (1978).

Storstein, L.: Protein binding of cardiac glycosides in disease states. Clinical Pharmacokinetics 2: 220 (1977).

Strong, J.M.; Mayfield, D.E.; Atkinson, A.J.; Burris, B.C.; Raymon, F. and Webster, L.T.: Pharmacological activity, metabolism, and pharmacokinetics of glycinexylidide. Clinical Pharmacology and Therapeutics 17: 184 (1975).

Surawicz, B.: Role of electrolytes in etiology and management of cardiac arrhythmias. Progress in Cardiovascular Diseases 8: 364 (1966).

Talbot, R.G.; Clark, R.A.; Nimmo, J.J.; Neilson, J.M.M. and Julian, D.G.: Treatment of ventricular arrhythmias with mexiletine (Ko 1173). Lancet 2: 399 (1973).

Tarhan, S.; Moffitt, E.A.; Taylor, W.S. and Giuliani, E.R.: Myocardial infarction after general anaesthesia. Journal of the American Medical Association 220: 1451 (1972).

Thompson, G.W.: Quinidine as a cause of sudden death. Circulation 14: 757 (1956).

Thompson, W.L.: Dopamine in the management of shock. Proceedings of the Royal Society of Medicine 70(Suppl. 2): 25 (1977).

Thomson, P.D.: Alteration in pharmacologic response induced by cardiovascular disease; in Melmon (Ed) Cardiovascular Drug Therapy (Davis, Philadelphia 1974).

Thomson, P.D.; Melmon, K.L.; Richardson, J.A.; Cohn, K.; Steinbrunn, W.; Cudihee, R. and Rowland, M.: Lidocaine pharmacokinetics in advanced heart failure, liver disease, and renal failue in humans. Annals of Internal Medicine 78: 499 (1973).

Tibblin, G.; Wilhelmsen, L. and Werko, L.: Risk factors for myocardial infarction and death due to ischemic heart disease and other causes. American Journal of Cardiology 35: 514 (1975).

Tibbutt, D.A. and Chesterman, G.: Pulmonary embolism: Current therapeutic concepts. Drugs 11: 161 (1976).

Tibbutt, D.A. and Chesterman, G.: Pulmonary embolism: Current therapeutic concepts; in Avery (Ed) Cardiovascular Drugs, Vol. 2, p. 167 (ADIS Press, Sydney; University Park Press, Baltimore 1978).

Tibbutt, D.A.; Davies, J.A.; Anderson, J.A.; Fletcher, E.W.L.; Hamill, J.; Holt, J.M.; Lea Thomas, M.; Lee, G. de J.; Millar, G.A.H.; Sharp, A.A. and Sutton, G.C.: Comparison by controlled clinical trial of streptokinase and heparin in treatment of life-threatening pulmonary embolism. British Medical Journal 1: 343 (1974).

Tilkian, A.G.; Schroeder, J.S.; Kao, J.J. and Hultgren, H.N.: The cardiovascular effects of lithium in man. A review of the literature. American Journal of Medicine 61: 665 (1976a).

Tilkian, A.G.; Schroeder, J.S.; Kao, J.J. and Hutlgren, H.N.: Effect of lithium on cardiovascular performance: report on extended ambulatory monitoring and exercise testing before and during lithium therapy. American Journal of Cardiology 38: 701 (1976b).

Tilstone, W.J.; Dargie, H.; Dargie, E.N.; Morgan, H.G. and Kennedy, A.C.: Pharmacokinetics of metolazone in normal subjects and in patients with cardiac or renal failure. Clinical Pharmacology and Therapeutics 16: 322 (1974).

Tilstone, W.J.; Lawson, D.H.; Campbell, W.; Hutton, I. and Lawrie, T.D.V.: The pharmacokinetics of slow-release procainamide. European Journal of Clinical Pharmacology 14: 261 (1978).

Tokola, O.; Pelkonen, O.; Karki, N.T.; Luoma, P.; Kaltiala, E.H. and Larmi, T.K.I.: Hepatic drug-oxidizing enzyme systems and urinary D-glucaric acid excretion in patients with congestive heart failure. British Journal of Clinical Pharmacology 2: 429 (1975).

Ueda, C.T. and Dzindzio, B.S.: Quinidine kinetics in congestive heart failure. Clinical Pharmacology and Therapeutics 23: 158 (1978).

Ueda, C.T.; Williamson, B.J. and Dzindzio, B.S.: Absolute quinidine bioavailability. Clinical Pharmacology and Therapeutics 20: 260 (1976).

Unger, A.H. and Sklaroff, H.J.: Fatalities following intravenous use of sodium diphenylhydantoin for cardiac arrhythmias. Journal of the American Medical Association 200: 335 (1967).

Urokinase Pulmonary Embolism Trial: Circulation 47(Suppl. 2): 7 (1973).

Valentine, P.A.; Frew, J.L.; Mashford, M.L. and Sloman, J.G.: Lidocaine in the pre-hospital phase of acute infarction. A double blind study. New England Journal of Medicine 291: 1327 (1974).

Valtonen, M.V.; Suomalainen, R.J.; Ylikahri, R.H. and Valtonen, V.V.: Selection of multiresistant coliforms by long-term treatment of hypercholesterolaemia with neomycin. British Medical Journal 1: 683 (1977).

Vanderark, C.R.; Reynolds, E.W.; Kahn, D.R. and Tullett, G.: Qunidine syncope: A report of successful treatment with bretylium tosylate. Journal of Thoracic and Cardiovascular Surgery 72: 464 (1976).

Vervloet, E.; Pluym, B.F.M.; Cilissen, J.; Kohlen, K. and Merkus, F.W.H.M.: Propranolol serum levels during twenty-four hours. Clinical Pharmacology and Therapeutics 22: 853 (1977).

Vessby, B.; Lithell, H.; Boberg, J. and Hellsing, K.: Para-aminosalicylic acid as a lipid-lowering agent. Clinical Pharmacology and Therapeutics 23: 651 (1978).

Vohra, J.; Hunt, D. and Sloman, G.: Clinical experience with verapamil. Medical Journal of Australia 2: 417 (1975).

Von Hoff, D.D.; Rozencweig, M.; Layard, M.; Slavik, M. and Muggia, F.M.: Daunomycin-induced cardiotoxicity in children and adults: A review of 110 cases. American Journal of Medicine 62: 200 (1977).

Vozeh, S.; Powell, J.R.; Riegelman, S.; Costello, J.F.; Sheiner, L.B. and Hopewell, P.C.: Changes in theophylline clearance during acute illness. Journal of the American Medical Association 240: 1882 (1978).

Walker, W.J.: Treatment of heart failure. Journal of the American Medical Association 228: 1276 (1974).

Walle, T.; Conradi, E.; Walle, K.; Fagan, T. and Gaffney, T.E.: Steady-state kinetics of the active propranolol metabolite, 4-hydroxypropranolol and its glucuronic acid conjugate in patients with hypertension and coronary artery disease. Clinical Research 25: 10A (1977).

Warren, V. and Goldberg, E.: Intractable angina pectoris. Combined therapy with propranolol and permanent pervenous pacemaker. Journal of the American Medical Association 235: 841 (1976).

Warren, S.G.; Brewer, D.L. and Orgain, E.S.: Long-term propranolol therapy for angina pectoris. American Journal of Cardiology 37: 420 (1976).

Weintraub, M.: Interpretation of the serum digoxin concentration. Clinical Pharmacokinetics 2: 206 (1977).

Weintraub, M.; Au, W.Y. and Lasagna, L.: Compliance as a determinant of the serum digoxin concentration. Journal of the American Medical Association 224: 481 (1973).

Whight, C.; Morgan, T.; Carney, S. and Wilson, M.: Diuretics, cardiac failure and potassium depletion. A rational approach. Medical Journal of Australia 2: 831 (1974).

WHO Cooperative Trial Report. Committee of Principal Investigators: A cooperative trial in the primary prevention of ischaemic heart disease using clofibrate. British Heart Journal 40: 1069 (1978).

Wilhelmsson, C.; Vedin, J.A.; Wilhelmsen, L.; Tibblin, G. and Werko, L.: Reduction of sudden deaths after myocardial infarction by treatment with alprenolol. Preliminary results. Lancet 2: 1157 (1974).

Wilkinson, G.R. and Shand, D.G.: A physiological approach to hepatic drug clearance. Clinical Pharmacology and Therapeutics 18: 377 (1975).

Williams, D.J. and Steele, T.W.: Cephalothin prophylaxis assay during cardiopulmonary bypass. Journal of Thoracic and Cardiovascular Surgery 71: 207 (1976).

Winkle, R.A.; Meffin, P.J. and Harrison, D.C.: Long-term tocainide therapy for ventricular arrhythmias. Circulation 57: 1008 (1978).

Wood, A.J.J.; Kornhauser, D.M.; Wilkinson, G.R.; Shand, D.G. and Branch, R.A.: The influence of cirrhosis on steady-state blood concentrations of unbound propranolol after oral administration. Clinical Pharmacokinetics 3: 478 (1978).

Woosley, R.L. and Shand, D.G.: Pharmacokinetics of antiarrhythmic drugs. American Journal of Cardiology 41: 986 (1978).

Woosley, R.L.; Shand, D.G. and Kornhauser, D.M.: Relation of plasma concentration and dose of propranolol to its effect on ventricular arrhythmias. Clinical Research 25: 262A (1977).

Woosley, R.L.; Drayer, D.E.; Reidenberg, M.M.; Nies, A.S.; Carr, K. and Oates, J.A.: Effect of acetylator phenotype on the rate at which procainamide induces antinuclear antibodies and the lupus syndrome. New England Journal of Medicine 298: 1157 (1978).

Working Party Report: Prevention of coronary heart disease. British Medical Journal 1: 881 (1976).

Wright, G.J.; Leeson, G.A.; Zeiger, A.V. and Lang, J.F.: The absorption, excretion and metabolism of perhexiline maleate by the human. Postgraduate Medical Journal 49(Suppl. 3): 8 (1973).

Yeshurun, D. and Gotto, A.M.: Drug treatment of hyperlipidaemia. American Journal of Medicine 60: 379 (1976).

Zacest, R. and Koch-Weser, J.: Relation of propranolol plasma level to β-blockade during oral therapy. Pharmacology 7: 178 (1972).

Zarolinski, J.F.; Possley, L.H.; Schwartz, R.A.; Morris, R.N.; Carone, F.A. and Browne, R.K.: The pharmacology and subacute toxicology of dopamine. Proceedings of the Royal Society of Medicine 70(Suppl. 2): 2 (1977).

Zelis, R. and Mason, D.T.: Demonstration of nitrate tolerance: Attenuation of the venomotor response to nitroglycerin by the chronic administration of isosorbide dinitrate. Circulation 40 (Suppl. 3): 221 (1969).

Zelis, R.; Mason, D.T.; Amsterdam, E.A. and Green, J.F.: Current concepts in the drug management of angina pectoris; in Melmon (Ed) Cardiovascular Drug Therapy (Davis, Philadelphia 1974).

Zipes, D.P. and Troup, P.J.: New antiarrhythmic agents. Amiodarone, aprindine, disopyramide, ethmozin, mexiletine, tocainide, verapamil. American Journal of Cardiology 41: 1005 (1978).

Chapter XVIII
Hypertensive Disease

F.O. Simpson

Synopsis of Important Principles

1) The aims of antihypertensive therapy are to relieve or forestall symptoms, to prevent complications and to prolong life.

2) In severe or moderately severe hypertension the benefits of drug treatment are undoubted. For patients with mild hypertension, the potential gains have to be weighed against the inconvenience, expense and possible side effects of therapy.

3) Before drug treatment is started, factors which tend to raise the blood pressure should be eliminated — obesity, excessive salt intake, drugs which can raise blood pressure (e.g. oral contraceptives, liquorice, carbenoxolone, pressor agents and vasoconstrictors), and so on.

4) The primary aim is to find, for each patient, a drug or combination of drugs which lowers blood pressure effectively and is not contraindicated for any reason in that patient, and which may be positively helpful in other ways.

5) If a given combination of drugs is not having a satisfactory effect in a given patient, then the possibility of undesirable interactions must be considered. The main offending drugs are the sympathomimetic drugs and tricyclic antidepressants which antagonise the antihypertensive effects of adrenergic neurone blocking drugs such as guanethidine, bethanidine and debrisoquine. A number of other drugs can affect antihypertensive therapy.

6) Although hypertension of any considerable severity during pregnancy must be treated, the benefits to the mother of therapy in milder cases is uncertain.

7) Very high blood pressure, when accompanied by acute symptoms, should be treated without delay. However, the overenthusiastic use of powerful antihypertensive drugs intravenously does carry some risk, so the degree of emergency must be carefully assessed.

8) Hypertension in the elderly should be treated, but therapy must be managed with special care. Reduction of blood pressure should be gradual and postural hypotension must be avoided. Blood pressure should not be allowed to fall too low.

9) The treatment of hypertension is not just a matter of prescribing drugs. To take a regimen of tablets year in and year out is a considerable act of faith on the part of the patient, and some patients need a good deal of help along the way.

The treatment of hypertension is preventive medicine in its currently most sophisticated form, with large potential benefits but also certain problems. These problems are derived partly from the sheer number of potential patients (perhaps 5 % or more of the population), partly from the large number and complicated nature of available drugs, and partly from the sensitive endpoint of therapy: a narrow range of blood pressure at which the patient feels comfortable and the doctor feels satisfied. And there are many possible errors in the management of hypertension, as Page I.H. (1976) has pointed out.

1. Pathogenesis of Hypertension

The physiological mechanisms by which blood pressure is maintained are extremely complicated (Guyton et al., 1972). In broad terms, blood pressure is dependent on cardiac output and peripheral resistance, and these in turn are dependent on many other factors: central and peripheral sympathetic activity, suprarenal cortex and medulla, antidiuretic hormone, renal pressor and depressor mechanisms, the state of the myocardium, the state of the small resistance blood vessels, blood volume, sodium and fluid balance, blood viscosity, baroreceptor activity, etc. All of these are interwoven in an almost inextricable web of feedback mechanisms which should normally ensure that the blood pressure remains within acceptable limits. Nevertheless, the blood pressure of a significant percentage of the population rises to levels which are associated with cerebrovascular, cardiac and renal complications.

In a relatively small percentage of cases, as is well known (Berglund et al., 1976), a specific cause for hypertension can be found, e.g. primary renal disease, or an endocrine tumour (phaeochromocytoma or aldosteronism), and the mechanisms involved are at least moderately well understood. On the other hand, in the vast majority of hypertensive subjects no primary cause is detectable by present methods and the pathogenesis of the hypertension in such cases is by no means clear. In fact, hypertensive subjects differ in the balance of factors which influence their blood pressure. Consequently 'essential hypertension' cannot be looked on as a single entity. The strongest evidence for this is the large difference which is being found in plasma renin values (Buhler et al., 1975; Zanchetti et al., 1976). Plasma renin has of course to be assessed in relation to salt intake; low salt intake will cause a high plasma renin, and high intake a low plasma renin. Hypertension in a subject with inappropriately high plasma renin may be at least partly due to this, whereas hypertension in a subject with low plasma renin must have occurred in spite of the body's apparent ability to 'turn off' the production of renin. These points may have some relevance to therapy (Laragh, 1978).

20 to 30 % of patients with 'essential hypertension' have a low plasma renin (Laragh et al., 1972; Doyle et al., 1973). A possible cause for this is increased aldosterone secretion (which depresses renin secretion), but in most cases 'low renin hypertension' is not due to hyperaldosteronism (Laragh et al., 1972; Biglieri, 1972). Diuretics may be particularly effective as antihypertensive agents in subjects with 'low renin hypertension' (Spark and Melby, 1971; Karlberg et al., 1976), though not all would agree with this (Solheim et al., 1975; Woods et al., 1976).

High plasma renin levels are found in accelerated hypertension and renovascular hypertension (Brown et al., 1965; Laragh et al., 1972). In the presence of high plasma renin levels, aldosterone levels will also be high (renin generates angiotensin I which is then converted to angiotensin II which stimulates the secretion of aldosterone). Another form of hypertension with high angiotensin II levels is that associated with the use of oestrogen containing oral contraceptives which cause an increase in renin substrate (see section 12.1).

There is evidence of increased adrenergic drive in at least a proportion of hypertensives, particularly younger ones and those with labile blood pressure (Editorial, 1977b), and also a correlation between plasma catecholamines and hypertension (Louis et al., 1973; de Champlain et al., 1976), though doubt has been cast on this (Lake et al., 1977). Even if there is such a correlation, it is not yet clear whether this means that increased sympathetic activity is aetiologically responsible for the hypertension, or is simply the means whereby the blood pressure is kept at a high level in hypertension of various types.

In considering the pathogenesis of 'essential' hypertension, we must also bear in mind epidemiological aspects. If we all ate less food, took virtually no salt (Page L.B., 1976) and lived a peaceful and unhurried life, then there would undoubtedly be less hypertension. A sodium intake of, say, 200 to 250mmol/day is perhaps (Freis, 1976) enough to trigger off hypertension in some people who would remain normotensive on an intake of 25 to 50mmol/day (1gNaCl = 17mmol Na). However, within a population it is difficult to demonstrate any correlation between sodium excretion and blood pressure (Simpson et al., 1978). Obesity is certainly enough to raise the blood pressure in many people (Ramsay et al., 1978) and blood pressure can be reduced by weight reduction even though sodium intake remains unchanged (Reisin et al., 1978). The stress of modern living may raise adrenergic drive sufficiently to set off a cycle of high cardiac output and high peripheral resistance in subjects who in other circumstances would remain normotensive. Finally, people susceptible to the development of hypertension may well have some genetic predisposition to it; so far the nature of this has remained obscure.

2. Prognosis and Rationale for Treatment

2.1 Rationale for Lowering Blood Pressure in Hypertensive Patients

The aims of antihypertensive therapy are to relieve or forestall symptoms, to prevent complications and to prolong life. There is little doubt that a high blood pressure *per se,* regardless of its cause, carries with it an increased risk of cardiovascular and renal damage.

2.2 Factors Influencing Prognosis

It is of course quite possible that certain aetiological factors carry some additional risk. For instance a hypertensive patient with chronic glomerulonephritis or pyelonephritis will in general have a worse prognosis than a patient with 'essential' hypertension of similar degree, mainly because of diminishing renal function. On the other hand, excess weight appears, curiously enough, to be a favourable prognostic factor in hypertensive subjects (Simpson and Gilchrist, 1958), presumably not because it is good to be obese but because hypertension in an obese person is in some way different from that in a lean person, perhaps because it can be modified by weight

reduction, perhaps because the sphygmomanometer readings are a little exaggerated by the fat arm. Renin may be another relevant factor: there is still controversy about whether patients with a low plasma renin have less cardiovascular complications than those with a normal or high plasma renin (e.g. Laragh et al., 1972; Doyle et al., 1973; Kaplan, 1975).

Such possibilities do not alter the general thesis that high blood pressure itself causes damage. Partly this damage is a *direct* effect of the hypertension, resulting from the increased load on the heart and small vessels of the brain and kidney; antihypertensive therapy is very effective in relieving this load. However, partly the damage is an *indirect* effect of the hypertension, through an increased tendency to atheroma, and there is at present no definite evidence that antihypertensive therapy alters this tendency. Indeed it is conceivable that drugs increase the tendency a little by inducing a mild diabetic state (diuretics) or raising plasma lipids slightly (see further sections 5.1.5; 5.6.8).

2.3 Influence of Treatment on Prognosis

The prognosis of patients with accelerated hypertension is dramatically improved by effective antihypertensive drug therapy (Hodge et al., 1960; Breckenridge et al., 1970). In severe 'benign' hypertension, symptoms such as breathlessness, headache and epistaxis can be relieved, the incidence of cerebral haemorrhage and encephalopathy greatly reduced, renal damage slowed, and progression to the accelerated phase prevented. In hypertension of moderate severity also, there is evidence that the incidence of cardiovascular complications is significantly reduced by effective treatment (Veterans Administration Study, 1967, 1970).

In mild hypertension, the situation is less clear (see Perry and Smith, 1978). Life insurance data leave no doubt that even a small elevation of blood pressure carries some risk of a shortened life span (Society of Actuaries, 1959). The large scale controlled trials of treatment of mild hypertension being conducted in Great Britain, the USA and Australia are badly needed. Meantime, for patients with mild hypertension, the potential gains have to be weighed against the inconvenience, expense and possible side effects of therapy. Fortunately, antihypertensive therapy is being constantly improved.

3. Initiation of Treatment

3.1 Investigations

If a patient's hypertension is worth treating, it is worth investigating. The investigations listed in table I are intended to answer the following questions:

a) How high really is the blood pressure?
b) Is there any discoverable and remediable cause?
c) How much blood vessel and organ damage is there?
d) Is there any associated or coincidental disease (e.g. atheroma, diabetes mellitus, hyperuricaemia, emotional disorder, renal disease etc) which may affect prognosis or the choice of drugs?

3.2 When to Start Drug Therapy

Every doctor who treats patients with hypertension will have his own ideas about when to start drug therapy; those of a USA National Committee (Moser et al., 1977) and the author have recently been published (Simpson, 1978; fig. 1). The present trend is towards earlier treatment and if our drugs were perfect and very cheap, then no doubt we would aim at maintaining everyone's blood pressure at 'normal' levels. Meantime, there is general agreement that in severe or moderately severe hypertension the benefits of treatment are undoubted. If there is real doubt about the necessity or advisability of treatment in a case of hypertension, then it is usually wise to observe the patient without treatment for a period.

3.3 Other Factors to be Considered

Before starting therapy, it is best to eliminate any factors which could be tending to raise the blood pressure. The possibility of coarctation of the aorta should always be considered and occasionally hypertension is of endocrine or renovascular origin and can be cured surgically. However, in terms of numbers of patients, it is much more important to deal with obesity, the contraceptive pill and certain other drugs which can raise blood pressure (see section 12), stressful life situations, chronic urinary infection, etc.

Excessive smoking should be discouraged, not because it raises blood pressure (it does not seem to do so) but because hypertensive subjects are

Table I. Investigations which should be performed in hypertensive patients prior to starting treatment

Standard tests
History (including social and family history)

Clinical examination (including retinae, femoral and peripheral pulses and auscultation for bruits)

ECG; chest X-ray; intravenous pyelogram[1]
Urine analysis; fasting blood lipids and sugar
Serum electrolytes, urea or creatinine, uric acid
Glucose tolerance test[1]; creatinine clearance[1]; ESR; blood screen

Tests of blood pressure (e.g. repeated observations, all-day tests, or basal blood pressure tests)

Special tests (where indicated) for:
Cushing's syndrome; hyperaldosteronism; phaeochromocytoma; renovascular disease, etc.

1   Desirable but not absolutely essential in all cases.

more liable to vascular disease and therefore it is doubly important to eliminate unnecessary risk factors. Excessive salt consumption should also be discouraged, at least to the extent of reducing a patient's salt intake to the average level for his or her community. Carney et al. (1975) showed that reduction of salt intake to 70mmol/day had some effect on blood pressure but this is for most people an uncomfortably low intake. The same group (Morgan et al., 1978) have found that even a much smaller degree of salt restriction will lower blood pressure but this remains to be confirmed. In the Dunedin area of New Zealand (Simpson et al., 1978), average 24 hour urinary sodium values are 130 to 140mmol/day for women and 170 to 180mmol/day for men, both in the population at large and in patients referred to the Hypertension Clinic. However, some hypertensive subjects do take large amounts of salt, up to 300mmol daily, and they usually find it no hardship to reduce their intake to some extent.

4. Mode of Action of Antihypertensive Drugs

4.1 General Considerations

The large number of different antihypertensive drugs currently available or on clinical trial is both a blessing and a problem: a blessing because of the

Table II. Site and mode of action of main antihypertensive drugs

Site of action	Drug	Mode of Action
Cerebral cortex	Sedatives, tranquillisers	
Mid brain	Reserpine	Depletion of catecholamines and serotonin
	Methyldopa	Reduces sympathetic outflow by stimulating α-adrenoceptors
	β-Blockers	Unidentified central antihypertensive action; probably not important
	Clonidine	Reduces sympathetic outflow by stimulating α-adrenoceptors
Autonomic ganglia	Ganglion-blockers, e.g. hexamethonium, pempidine	Block sympathetic (and parasympathetic) transmission
Adrenergic axons	Rauwolfia	Depletion of axonal stores of noradrenaline
	Bretylium	Adrenergic neurone blocker, i.e. blocks release of noradrenaline (now used only for antiarrhythmic properties as it causes parotid pain)
	Bethanidine	Adrenergic neurone blocker (short action)
	Debrisoquine	Adrenergic neurone blocker (medium action)
	Guanethidine	Adrenergic neurone blocker (long action) and also depletes axonal stores of noradrenaline
	Methyldopa	Forms false transmitter α-methyl noradrenaline, causes some depletion of axonal stores of noradrenaline and has some adrenergic neurone blocking action
	Pargyline	Monoamine oxidase inhibitor; also has some adrenergic neurone blocking action
α-Adrenoceptors (mediate contraction of resistance vessels)	Phentolamine	α-Adrenoceptor blocker; short acting, used in diagnosis and management of phaeochromocytoma
	Phenoxybenzamine	α-Adrenoceptor blocker; long acting, used in management of phaeochromocytoma and in peripheral vascular disease (disappointing in essential hypertension)
	Labetalol	Combined α- and β-blocker
	Prazosin	Postjunctional α-adrenoceptor blocker; blocks vasoconstriction due to noradrenaline but possibly not by receptor occupancy
	Indoramin	α-Adrenoceptor blocker; also slows heart
β-Adrenoceptors (cardioacceleration, increased force of cardiac contraction, release of renin from renal cortex, dilatation of muscle blood vessels, relaxation of bronchioles)	Propranolol Oxprenolol Alprenolol Pindolol Timolol Sotalol	Exact mechanism of antihypertensive action remains uncertain. Reduction in cardiac output, resetting of baroreceptors or other long term adaptations, reduction in plasma renin and reduction in plasma volume may all play a part.
	Atenolol Metoprolol Acebutolol	Atenolol and metoprolol and to some extent acebutolol are cardioselective β-blockers, i.e. less effect on β_2 receptors (e.g. bronchioles and muscle blood vessels) than on β_1 receptors (heart)
	Labetalol	Combined α and β blocker

Table II. (continued)

Site of action	Drug	Mode of action
Vascular smooth muscle	Thiazide-type diuretics	May reduce Na^+ and K^+ content of smooth muscle cells
	Diazoxide Hydrallazine Minoxidil Sodium nitroprusside	Exact mode of action uncertain
	Verapamil	Ca^{++} antagonist
Extracellular water and Na	Thiazide-type diuretics Loop diuretics (frusemide) Aldosterone antagonists (spironolactone) Other K-sparing diuretics (triamterene, amiloride) Uricosuric diuretic (tienilic acid or ticrynafen)	Volume depletion
Renin-angiotensin system	β-Blockers	Inhibit renin release
	Captopril	Blocks enzyme that converts angiotensin I to angiotensin II
	Saralasin	Blocks angiotensin receptors

near certainty the blood pressure can be controlled in each patient, a problem because of the very complicated pharmacological principles involved. Antihypertensive drugs can be grouped broadly as follows:

a) Drugs that act within the CNS
b) Drugs that act on the peripheral sympathetic nervous system and the adrenoceptors
c) Diuretics
d) Drugs that act directly on vascular smooth muscle
e) Angiotensin antagonists and drugs that inhibit the enzyme which converts angiotensin I to angiotensin II.

The sites and modes of action are summarised in figures 2 and 3 and table II. Many drugs act somewhere in the sympathetic nervous system. As discussed in section 1, it seems that many patients with hypertension may have increased adrenergic activity. More than one site of action has been postulated for some drugs. There have been many detailed reviews (e.g. Page and Sidd, 1972a,b,c; Wollam et al., 1977).

The main areas of special interest at present are: the central actions of certain drugs; how diuretics lower blood pressure; the mode of action of the β-blockers; the modes of action of drugs that act directly on vascular smooth muscle; the renewed attack on α-adrenoceptors; and the inhibition of the formation of angiotensin II.

4.2 Drugs With a Central Action

Interest in the central action of antihypertensive drugs (van Zweiten, 1973) was engendered by the discovery that clonidine reduces sympathetic outflow from the central nervous system by stimulating α-adrenoceptors there (Schmitt et al., 1971). Methyldopa has been found to have a somewhat similar effect (Heise and Kroneberg, 1973; Nijkamp et al., 1975) and it seems probable that this is the main mode of action of this widely used drug. There is some evidence also of a central component to the antihypertensive action of propranolol (Conway et al., 1978), but this is in general not thought to be very important. Guanfacine is a new drug with a central action like that of clonidine (Saameli et al., 1975; MacCarthy et al., 1978a).

4.3 Diuretics

It has long been thought that there are two components to the antihypertensive action of diuretics, an initial transitory reduction in extracellular fluid volume and a slower direct vasodilator action.

The fact that diazoxide (a thiazide) lowers blood pressure, in spite of having no diuretic effect, was one point in favour of such a concept (Bartorelli et al., 1963). However, there is increasing evidence that long term use of diuretics does lead to continued restriction of body fluid volume (Shah et al., 1978) and it seems reasonable to ascribe their antihypertensive effect mainly to this, though the possibility of an additional action on vascular smooth muscle cells is not excluded. Reduction of plasma volume will of course have secondary effects such as reduced cardiac output, increased sympathetic activity, tachycardia and increased renin-angiotensin-aldosterone activity, and the patient is thereby made more sensitive to the effects of other antihypertensive drugs.

4.4 β-Adrenoceptor Blockade

The mode of action of the β-blockers in hypertension is not clear. The main possibilities are: an effect mediated through the central nervous system (see section 4.2, probably not important); a long term reduction of cardiac output as demonstrated by Lund-Johansen and Ohm (1976), possibly with subsequent baroreceptor adjustments (Prichard and Gillam, 1969); reduction of renin release from the renal cortex (Buhler et al., 1972); a slow fall (following an initial rise) in peripheral vascular resistance (Ablad et al., 1976),

Diastolic blood pressure (mm Hg)[1]			
Age < 40 years	Age 40-59 years	Age ≥ 60 years[2]	Antihypertensive treatment
130	130	130	
125	125	125	Essential
120	120	120	
115	115	115	Advisable
110	110	110	
105	105	105	Optional[3] (but if not given, then observation is essential)
100	100	100	
95	95	95	Unnecessary (nearly always)
90	90	90	

1 BP values must be based on at least three readings taken sitting, in the first place, on each of three separate occasions. The figures are intended to represent phase 5; if phase 4 is used the limits should in theory be set slightly higher.

2 Age > 70 is a factor against treatment in borderline cases (section 9).

3 *Drug treatment at these levels is advisable when any of the following are present:* definite symptoms; high systolic blood pressure; bad family history; ECG signs of left ventricular hypertrophy; enlarged heart; hyperlipidaemia; ischaemic heart disease; renal disease; or migraine.
Factors militating against drug treatment at these levels: no symptoms; low systolic blood pressure; normal ECG; normal heart size; reluctance to be treated; mental disease; physical disability; obesity; gout; diabetes; asthma, etc; and poor response to simple treatment.

Fig. 1. When to start antihypertensive treatment (after Simpson, F.O.; in Blood Pressure Screening in New Zealand, National Heart Foundation of New Zealand, Auckland 1977).

possibly due to blockade of prejunctional β-adrenoceptors mediating noradrenaline release from the sympathetic axon (Rand et al., 1976).

None of these postulated actions of the β-blockers is entirely without controversy, but the effect on renin release has been the cause of the most disagreement. As is well known, Laragh's group (Buhler et al., 1972) found a correlation be-tween the fall in plasma renin and the fall in blood pressure. Castenfors et al. (1973), using alprenolol, found a similar correlation. Others have found much less correlation or none (e.g. Stokes et al., 1974, 1976; Leonetti et al., 1975) and it seems that β-blockers are not entirely con-sistent in their effects on plasma renin, though effective in reducing blood pressure (Stokes et al.,

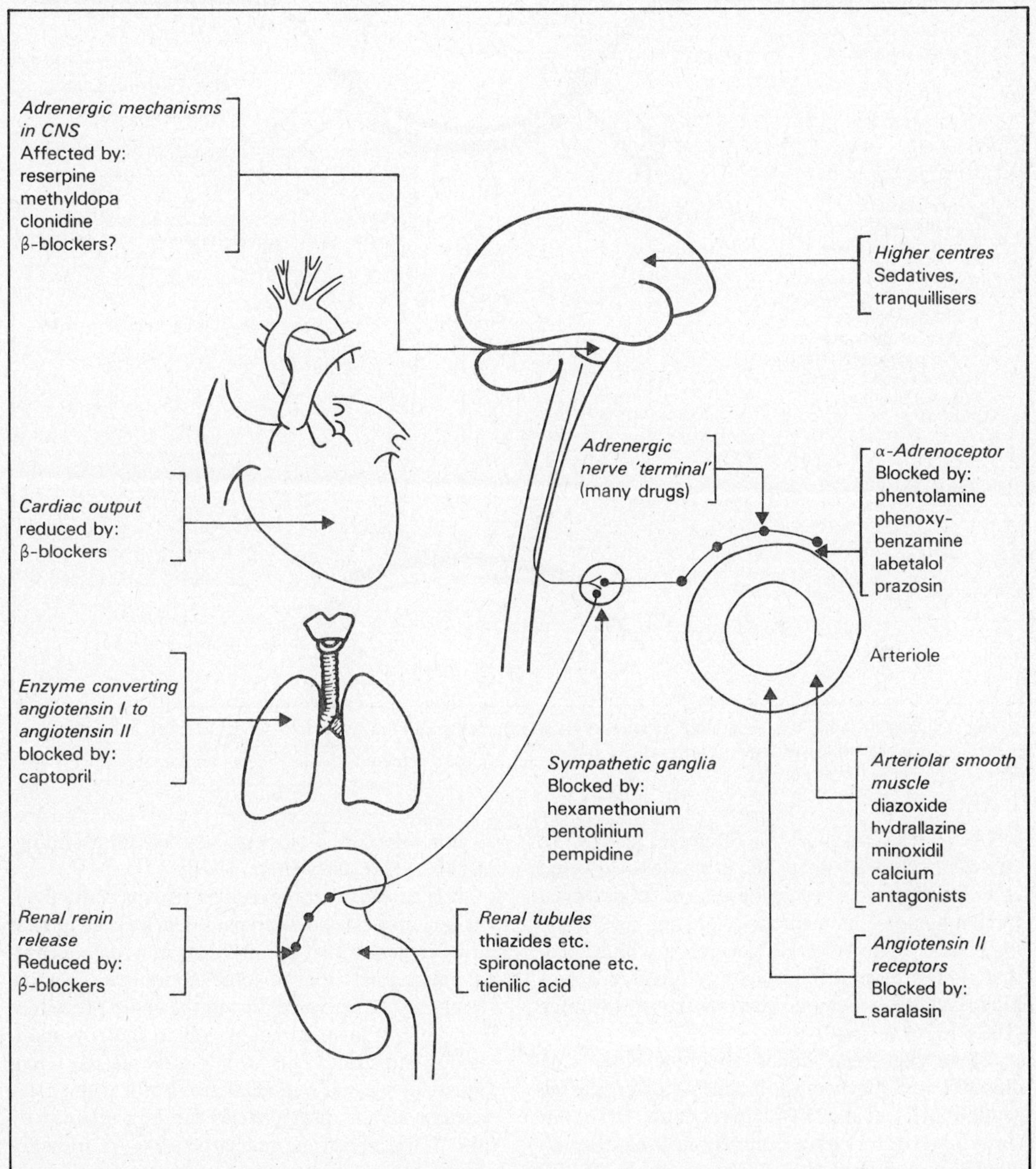

Fig. 2. Diagrammatic representation of main sites of action of antihypertensive drugs.

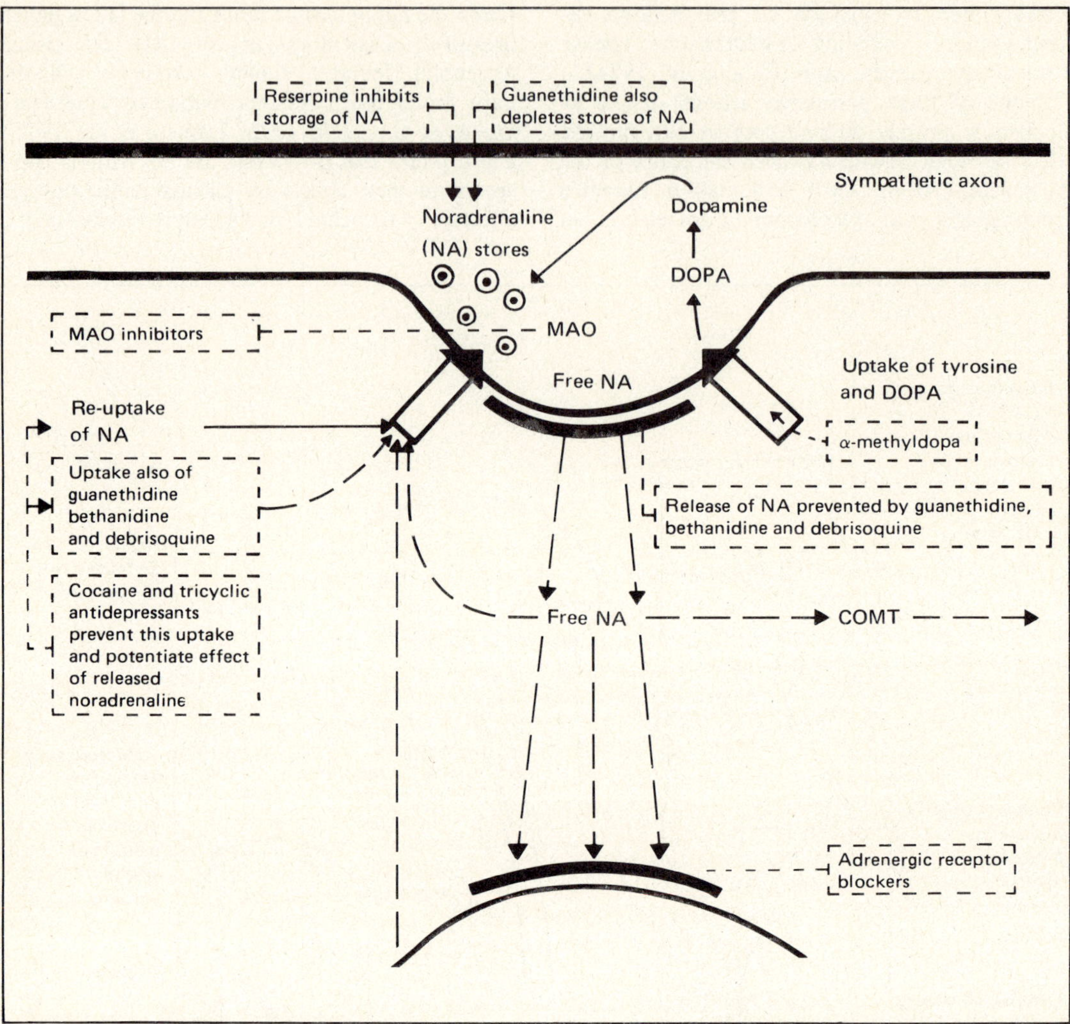

Fig. 3. Diagrammatic representation of adrenergic mechanisms and antihypertensive drug action and interaction at level of the arteriolar smooth muscle cell.

1974; 1976; Gross, 1977). Buhler et al. (1975), however, showed that all β-blockers lowered *stimulated* plasma renin levels in man, even though pindolol and oxprenolol did not lower *resting* plasma renin levels. In general, it would seem that a high plasma renin activity often reflects a high level of sympathetic nervous activity (Stumpe et al., 1976).

There has been doubt about whether cardioselective β-blockers (β₁-blockers) lower plasma renin (Amery et al., 1974; Myers et al., 1976) but some investigators have demonstrated that they do (e.g. Buhler et al., 1975; Hansson et al., 1977). Certainly, they lower blood pressure as effectively as non-selective β-blockers (e.g. Waal-Manning, 1976b,c; Davidson et al., 1976).

It is curious that the data on plasma renin from various units are so discrepant. Derkx et al. (1976) have suggested that the problem may be a technical one, namely that in some laboratories inactive renin may be activated during the assay procedure if the pH is lowered below 4.0 to destroy endogenous substrate: this would give falsely high values for plasma renin activity. But it is not clear whether all the discrepancies can be explained by this. Certainly it is not necessary to measure plasma renin before deciding whether to use a β-blocker (see Johnston, 1976).

4.5 Vasodilators

The vasodilators are a heterogenous group of drugs. Their actions at the cellular level are in most cases not well understood, though there is a large literature on their haemodynamic and general clinical effects. Sodium nitroprusside is typical in this respect, with little work done on its cellular mode of action (Palmer and Lasseter, 1975), in spite of its increasing acceptance as a valuable drug for use in hypertensive emergencies (e.g. Ahearn and Grim, 1974; Tuzel, 1974) or in patients with persistent hypertension following myocardial infarction (Franciosa et al., 1972; Mukherjee et al., 1976).

The actions of hydrallazine, diazoxide and minoxidil may well involve cyclic AMP and calcium ions within the vascular smooth muscle cell (Wohl et al., 1968; Andersson, 1973) but the details are by no means clear. The availability of calcium ions to the vascular smooth muscle cells can be prevented also by drugs such as verapamil (Krikler, 1974) which block their transport across the cell membrane. Verapamil has been variously reported to have a mild (Pedersen, 1978) or excellent (Lewis et al., 1978) antihypertensive effect; clearly this is an area for further study.

The new antihypertensive agent prazosin (see also section 5.8) was introduced as a phosphodiesterase inhibitor, with a direct effect on vascular smooth muscle, with additional α-adrenoceptor blocking properties (Constantine et al., 1973). However, it causes vasodilatation only in the presence of sympathetic innervation and its action is in fact solely α-adrenoceptor blockade (Wood et al., 1975; Cavero et al., 1978) though apparently not by receptor occupancy (Constantine et al., 1973). This blockade may be specific for the *post*synaptic α-adrenoceptors (e.g. on vascular smooth muscle) as opposed to the presynaptic α-adrenoceptors on the adrenergic neurones (Cambridge et al., 1977). Prazosin tends to reduce plasma renin (Hayes, 1977; Bolli et al., 1976) rather than to increase it, as occurs with the direct acting vasodilators or with α-adrenoceptor blockers such as phentolamine.

The place of vasodilators in antihypertensive therapy is of course not fully settled. Vasodilatation often leads to tachycardia and peripheral oedema (although much less consistently seen with prazosin) and, in susceptible subjects, angina. On this account these drugs are best used with a diuretic and a drug to slow the heart. Indeed, it is really the advent of the β-blockers which has made possible the increased use of vasodilators.

4.6 α-Adrenoceptor Blockade

α-Adrenoceptor blockade should be exactly what is needed in the treatment of hypertension because such drugs should reduce the tone of the resistance vessels, but phenoxybenzamine and phentolamine never fulfilled expectations in this respect because of various side effects, partly due to their blockade of prejunctional α-adrenoceptors (i.e. on the adrenergic neurone) thus causing increased release of noradrenaline (norepinephrine).

Now, partly because of the everwidening use of β-blockers and the realisation that some β-blocked patients have excessive α-adrenoceptor stimulation, some degree of α-blockade again appears attractive.

Prazosin, as mentioned above, is an α-blocker, but as it blocks only postjunctional α-adrenoceptors on the smooth muscle cells, it would thus not cause increased release of noradrenaline from the adrenergic neurone. Indoramin combines α-blocking and antiserotinin activity (Royds et al., 1972; Lewis et al., 1973), and has been reported to be quite effective in lowering blood pressure (Rosendorff, 1976). Labetalol (see section 5.7) combines α-blocking and β-blocking properties within the same molecule. These drugs represent most interesting developments.

4.7 Blockade of Formation of Angiotensin II

One of the most interesting new drugs is captopril (SQ 14225) which blocks the conversion of the decapeptide angiotensin I to the octapeptide angiotensin II (Ondetti et al., 1977; Rubin et al., 1978). Previous drugs with this action (e.g. SQ 20881) have been peptides and so, unlike captopril, are not active when given by mouth. Captopril is reported to be very successful in lowering blood pressure in hypertensive subjects (Gavras et al., 1978), regardless of plasma renin activity. One problem in interpreting its action is that it also blocks the breakdown in the blood of bradykinin, a naturally occurring vasodilating peptide. The relative importance of this is uncertain. Its place in therapy remains to be determined but it seems likely to find much wider use than peptide drugs such as saralasin which block the angiotensin II receptors. It is also a very powerful new tool in the investigation of the place of angiotensin in the maintenance of hypertension.

5. Pharmacodynamics and Pharmacokinetics in Practical Therapy

There is a vast mass of data about the clinical pharmacological properties of antihypertensive drugs and only the most important practical aspects can be covered here. Many of the references are to review articles (eg Wollam et al., 1977). The multiple actions and important side effects of the various drugs are summarised in tables II, III and IV. Pharmacokinetics of the individual antihypertensive drugs have in general not been systematically studied, but some characteristics are of potential relevance to their therapeutic use. Many of the antihypertensive drugs are eliminated in large part as unchanged drug in the urine, necessitating possible modification of dosage in renal failure (e.g. guanethidine, bethanidine, methyldopa, and some β-blockers such as atenolol). Some are subject to significant first-pass hepatic metabolism, such that plasma concentrations vary widely among individuals and bioavailability increases in cirrhosis (e.g. labetalol and β-blockers such as alprenolol, propranolol and metoprolol). Two are subject to important genetically determined metabolism which can affect response (debrisoquine) or occurrence of major side effects (hydrallazine). Dosage schedules of the various drugs are discussed below and summarised in table VII.

5.1 Diuretics

5.1.1 General Considerations
The best diuretics for hypertension are the medium and long acting ones; e.g. thiazides, chlorthalidone, clorexolone etc and mefruside and bumetanide (see Davies and Wilson, 1975). Frusemide (furosemide) is a very useful drug in patients who tend to have fluid retention in spite of full doses of other diuretics, but its very rapid action makes it less suitable for routine use. It is probably the best diuretic for use in subjects verging on renal failure. Ethacrynic acid is too drastic and powerful a diuretic for the long term management of hypertension.

Unless there is some urgency, it is best to start a diuretic at about half the expected maintenance dosage, for the first 2 to 3 weeks. This ensures that the patient does not get discouraged by symptoms brought on by a sudden large diuresis. The patient should also be told to expect that he may notice an increase in urine flow. The side effects of the diuretics in hypertension are largely biochemical (table IV).

5.1.2 Hypokalaemia
Hypokalaemia can be countered by increased potassium intake. If no potassium supplements are given, the proportion of patients developing hypokalaemia (serum $K < 3.5mmol/L$) becomes quite considerable and the author (like many others; e.g. Anderton and Kincaid-Smith, 1971) believes in routine use of slow release potassium chloride. However, patients vary and if as much as 6 or 8 tablets of potassium chloride are needed daily, then it is better to add a potassium-sparing diuretic instead. This not only means that the patient has to take fewer tablets but it also usually makes at least some contribution to lowering the blood pressure, something that potassium supplements do not do. However, the use of a potassium-sparing diuretic does not absolve the clinician from the need to monitor serum potassium levels. Two potassium-sparing diuretics (e.g. triamterene and spironolactone) or a potassium supplement and a potassium-sparing diuretic must never be given together, as this can cause potentially dangerous hyperkalaemia (Knight and Parkinson, 1967).

It has to be said that there is disagreement about giving potassium supplements in hypertension (see chapter XXI; sect. 7.1): they can cause minor gastrointestinal tract symptoms, they add to the cost of therapy, and it is difficult to demonstrate any effect of the thiazides on total body potassium, at least in relatively short term studies.

Of the potassium-sparing diuretics, the aldosterone antagonist spironolactone is the most interesting and it can be used in high dosage as a specific drug for high aldosterone states (Beevers et al., 1973a). It has a considerable antihypertensive effect also in essential hypertension; some have found it effective in both low renin and normal or high renin states (e.g. Bevegard et al., 1977) while others consider it is more effective in patients with low plasma renin (e.g. Carey et al., 1972). It is sometimes recommended to be used in a dose of 100mg or even 200mg daily but it can cause gynaecomastia in men and menstrual problems in women (see chapter XV; section 23.6) so it is best to keep dosage to a minimum (e.g. 25mg twice daily). Other side effects include nausea.

Amiloride (Gombos et al., 1966; Paterson et al., 1968) is probably the most widely used of the potassium-sparing diuretics, in a tablet containing 5mg in combination with 50mg hydrochlorothiazide. This is a very effective combination for hypertension but it has to be remembered that the dosage of hydrochlorothiazide is quite considerable so that a half tablet daily is sufficient in many cases, certainly for initial dosage. In our hands the combined tablet has given slightly more trouble with aggravation of diabetes than, for instance, cyclopenthiazide (Waal-Manning and Simpson, 1977). In high dosage, up to 40mg daily, it is effective even in high aldosterone states (Kremer et al., 1977) with fewer side effects than spironolactone.

Triamterene (Spiekerman et al., 1966) has much less antihypertensive effect and is best used in combination with a thiazide. It also can cause nausea.

Any of the potassium-sparing diuretics can cause hyperkalaemia, especially in the presence of impaired renal function.

5.1.3 Hyperuricaemia

Hyperuricaemia is another common side effect of the thiazide and thiazide-like diuretics. It can be overcome by the use of allopurinol or a uricosuric drug (e.g. probenecid, sulphinpyrazone) but it is best to try to do without a diuretic in patients who have high baseline levels of serum uric acid or a history of gout, unless the patient has to be on a hypouricaemic drug anyway; in such cases, the addition of a diuretic makes less difference but the dose should be kept to a minimum. In general, however, if a patient *needs* a diuretic (either because of the severity of the hypertension or because there is fluid retention), then one should be given and any resulting hyperuricaemia suitably dealt with. The new diuretic tienilic acid (ticrynafen) may well replace other diuretics in the management of the hyperuricaemic hypertensive patient (Nemati et al., 1977; Bolli et al., 1978). It is an extremely potent uricosuric agent, causing a large initial outpouring of uric acid in the urine. In theory, the water diuresis should keep the concentration of uric acid in the urine down but the initial dose should not be greater than 125mg (half a tablet); the patient should not have been dehy-

drated by other diuretics and should be encouraged to take extra fluids for the first 2 days.

5.1.4 Impairment of Glucose Tolerance

Impairment of glucose tolerance is a less common side effect of diuretics but nevertheless very real (Lewis et al., 1976; Amery et al., 1978). It can be overcome by means of suitable additional therapy (insulin or oral antidiabetic drugs) but the need to use a diuretic in patients with impaired carbohydrate tolerance must always be carefully assessed. If a diuretic *is* needed, then spironolactone should probably be tried first. Frusemide initially had the reputation of being less of a problem than the thiazides (Peltola, 1965) but this is by no means certain (Mroczek et al., 1974). Mefruside seems not to differ significantly from the thiazides in this respect (Brogden et al., 1974; Waal-Manning, 1975a). See further chapter XVI (sect. 13.1, 14.1).

5.1.5 Hypertriglyceridaemia

Thiazide diuretics have been reported to raise plasma triglycerides (Johnson et al., 1974; Ames and Hill, 1976). The clinical significance of this is not known.

5.1.6 Other Side Effects

Other side effects should not be forgotten (Dargie and Dollery, 1977). Skin rash is relatively rare but the number of patients on thiazides is so large that it is not infrequently seen. It should not be ignored as it can go on to a necrotising vasculitis. Diuretic-potassium chloride combinations should not be given to patients with ulcer-type dyspepsia. Excessive reduction of blood volume in the elderly can contribute to peripheral ischaemia (O'Rourke and Hede, 1978).

5.1.7 Pharmacokinetic Considerations

Pharmacokinetics of diuretics are discussed in chapter XXI (sect. 7.2). Apart from the possible need to modify dosage of some diuretics in severe liver disease (e.g. triamterene), there are no major pharmacokinetic problems in the use of diuretics for hypertension. Potassium-sparing diuretics should be avoided in patients with impaired renal function, not only because of the risk of hyperkalaemia but also because compounds such as spironolactone are excreted in the urine in large part as its active metabolite while amiloride is excreted in the urine unchanged.

5.2 Rauwolfia

Rauwolfia alkaloids (Schlittler and Bein, 1967; McMahon, 1978), of which reserpine is the best known, reduce the body's stores of noradrenaline, both peripherally and in the CNS. The site of their antihypertensive action is probably mainly peripheral rather than central (Nickerson and Collier, 1975). Reserpine depletes the CNS stores also of serotonin and dopamine and, possibly on this account, can cause both depression and Parkinsonism.

If drugs of this type are used (even in doses as low as 0.25mg reserpine daily), the clinician has an obligation to warn the patient beforehand of the possibility of depression and to watch for signs of depression developing, for instance after a bereavement; reserpine-induced depression can be very insidious and it does not always occur in short term trials (e.g. Gibb et al., 1970; see also chapter XXVI, sect. 15.2). Reserpine and other Rauwolfia alkaloids must *never* be given to anyone with a history of depression.

Other side effects include sedation, lassitude, nightmares, nasal congestion, ulcer-type dyspepsia and looseness of the bowels. Reserpine combines well with a diuretic and can be used with adrenergic neurone blocking agents, but its use with methyldopa is best avoided: the combination can cause much dreaming, sedation and impotence (Simpson, 1970). The relationship of reserpine to breast cancer (Armstrong et al., 1974; Boston Collaborative Drug Surveillance Program, 1974) remains uncertain (e.g. Armstrong et al., 1976; Christopher et al., 1977).

The main advantage of the Rauwolfia drugs is their cheapness. Reserpine dosage should not be higher than 0.25mg daily as the incidence of sedation and depression becomes very considerable. Reserpine can be given intramuscularly (3mg stat) in emergency situations (e.g. AMA Committee on Hypertension, 1974) and it usually leads to a smooth fall in blood pressure over several hours but the degree of sedation is often undesirable. Elimination of reserpine is prolonged in renal failure and dosage should be modified accordingly (see appendix E).

5.3 Methyldopa

This widely used drug was introduced as an inhibitor of dopa decarboxylase, thus possibly interfering with the synthesis of noradrenaline (Oates et al., 1960). Subsequently it was found that α-methyldopa is metabolised to α-methyl noradrenaline and that this is stored in the adrenergic nerve terminals (Day and Rand, 1964), where it acts as a neurotransmitter. It was thought on the basis of some animal experiments, that it was a weaker neurotransmitter than noradrenaline, but this seems to vary in different species and not to apply to man (Trinker, 1971). There is now good evidence that methyldopa, like clonidine, stimulates certain α-adrenoceptors in the CNS and that this leads to a damping down of sympathetic outflow and thus a reduction of blood pressure (see section 4.2).

Methyldopa has the advantage of being clinically easy to use. Dosage is not very critical and postural hypotension is uncommon. There are nevertheless, quite a number of side effects (Editorial, 1975; Tester-Dalderup, 1977), including such reactions as autoimmune haemolytic anaemia (see chapter XXIII; sect. 8.4), hepatic dysfunction (Rodman et al., 1976; chapter XIX, sect. 14.6), drug fever and antinuclear antibody formation (Alarcon-Segovia, 1976; chapter XXII, sect. 14.1). However, these reactions are not frequent and do not pose major problems for the use of the drug. Somnolence and lassitude can be very prominent at the start of therapy and there can be mild depression and impairment of sexual performance. Maximum practical dosage is about 3g daily but there is usually little benefit in going above 1.5g daily. Initial dosage should be kept small (e.g. 125mg twice daily) unless there is urgency, in order to avoid initial somnolence.

Methyldopa can be used intravenously, in emergency situations but it is not particularly effective (Finnerty, 1974).

As with guanethidine (section 5.4), methyldopa is variably absorbed among individuals after oral administration (8 to 62%; Kwan et al., 1976). A large proportion of an absorbed dose is eliminated unchanged in the urine and active metabolites such as methyldopa-0-sulphate are formed; dosage should probably be modified in advanced renal failure (Myhre et al., 1972a,b; appendix E). The patient who experiences drug fever with methyldopa seems to metabolise the drug to a lesser extent than others (Valnes et al., 1978). It must be remembered that patients on this drug excrete enormous amounts of α-methyl noradrenaline (norepinephrine) in their urine so that estimation of endogenous urinary catecholamines is impossible.

5.4 Adrenergic Neurone Blocking Drugs

5.4.1 Action

The adrenergic neurone blocking drugs (guanethidine, bethanidine, debrisoquine) are so called because they inhibit the release of noradrenaline at the neuroeffector junction, which occurs in response to sympathetic stimulation. All three drugs gain access to the adrenergic neurone by active transport by the 'noradrenaline pump' (Mitchell and Oates, 1970), but guanethidine differs from the other two drugs in that it causes depletion of noradrenaline stores within the nerve terminal (Chang et al., 1965). Debrisoquine has some monoamine oxidase inhibiting activity (Solomon et al., 1969) and a rise in blood pressure has been reported in some individuals who consumed tyramine rich cheese during debrisoquine therapy (Amery and Deloof, 1970; see also section 12.3).

5.4.2 Pharmacokinetics

There are pharmacokinetic differences between the 3 drugs. Guanethidine is poorly and variably absorbed (3 to 50%) after oral administration, though the extent of absorption is relatively constant in a particular individual (McMartin and Simpson, 1971), and it is variably metabolised. There are wide differences among patients in their response to the same dose of guanethidine, due to variation in absorption, rate of biotransformation and renal elimination of unchanged drug. Up to 50% of an absorbed dose of guanethidine is excreted unchanged in the urine. Bethanidine is more reliably absorbed (50 to 70%) and is not metabolised; up to 60% of a dose is excreted unchanged in the urine, renal clearance being dependent on renal plasma flow (Shen et al., 1975; Turnbull et al., 1976). If guanethidine or bethanidine are used in patients with renal failure, dosage should be reduced appropriately; accumulation (Rahn, 1971) and severe orthostatic hypotension has occurred with guanethidine in patients given usual doses (Gifford, 1973; appendix E). Debrisoquine is well absorbed (over 75%) after oral administration. A few individuals have a hereditary inability to metabolise (by hydroxylation) debrisoquine (Mahgoub et al., 1977); in general, the ability to hydroxylate the drug varies widely (Silas et al., 1977; 1978) and correlates inversely with response to it. Dose requirements thus vary considerably. As with bethanidine, renal clearance of debrisoquine is proportional to renal

plasma flow and the dose may need to be reduced in renal failure.

These properties support the well established principle that the dose of an adrenergic neurone blocking drug has to be carefully determined for each individual patient.

5.4.3 Clinical Use

These drugs (guanethidine, bethanidine, debrisoquine) became the mainstay of treatment of severe hypertension in the late 1950's and 1960's. They are effective and reliable drugs and represented a great advance on the ganglion blockers which they supplanted, and which caused uncomfortable parasympatholytic side effects. They cause postural hypotension and they tend to interfere with sexual function, so they are themselves now being supplanted. However, many patients are quite comfortable on them.

Comparisons of these drugs, among themselves or with methyldopa (e.g. Prichard et al., 1968; Talbot et al., 1975) tend to show only minor differences in effectiveness and side effects, but diarrhoea is common only with guanethidine (see table IV). All of them tend to cause fluid retention and are best given in combination with a diuretic. The latter should preferably be started first, otherwise there may be an excessive fall in blood pressure when a diuretic is added to a regimen containing an adrenergic neurone blocker. A knowledge of the speed of onset and disappearance of the therapeutic effect of these drugs is important in dose adjustment.

Guanethidine (Woosley and Nies, 1976) has the longest half-life and duration of action and the effect cumulates over 5 to 7 or more days. Unless there is urgency, therefore, it is best to keep the initial dose low (e.g. 10mg daily) and increase it at weekly intervals by 10mg steps. If the initial dose is 30 to 50mg daily, the patient may develop severe postural hypotension after 5 to 7 days and this is both dangerous and discouraging. Nocturnal or morning hypotension and exercise hypotension are very real phenomena in patients on guanethidine and the patient must be warned not to jump suddenly out of bed and then proceed immediately to the bathroom to micturate; the hard edges of bathroom fittings must have caused many head injuries in patients on adrenergic neurone blocking drugs.

Bethanidine (Bath et al., 1967) has a much shorter duration of action, which has advantages in ease of dose adjustment (table VII) but disadvantages in that it must be given 3 times a day. It is now best used as an adjunct to other therapy. The starting dose should be 5mg 3 times daily with daily increments if desired. Debrisoquine has a slightly longer duration of action than bethanidine and can be given twice daily. Neither of these drugs should be stopped abruptly as the blood pressure can rise quickly.

5.5 Clonidine

This drug stimulates α-adrenoceptors in the vasomotor centres, causing thereby a reduction in sympathetic outflow from the CNS (see section 4.2). Both cardiac output and peripheral resistance are reduced, and blood pressure is lowered in both the lying and standing positions. Postural hypotension is uncommon and renal blood flow is not significantly reduced (Lund-Johansen, 1976). These significant advantages are counterbalanced by certain disadvantages — drowsiness and dryness of mouth are common and are a very real nuisance, the drowsiness interfering with work and general enjoyment of life and leading in some cases to actual depression (Ng et al., 1967; MacDougall et al., 1970), though this is not accepted by all (Raftos et al., 1973).

Any patient being treated with clonidine must be warned that abrupt cessation of therapy can lead to a rebound hypertension with agitation and tachycardia, due to sudden increase in sympathetic outflow from the CNS (e.g. Hunyor et al., 1973; Goldberg et al., 1977). Thus, when clonidine has to be stopped, the dose should be reduced in a series of steps, the final step being no greater than 50µg. It is possible that the rebound hypertension is worse in the presence of a β-blocker (Bailey and Neale, 1976; Vanholder et al., 1977) and no patient should ever have a β-blocker started immediately when clonidine is stopped. If clonidine has unwittingly been suddenly stopped, and rebound hypertension has occurred, the best treatment is either to restart clonidine immediately (parenterally if necessary) or to use combined α- and β-adrenoceptor blockade.

Initial dosage should if possible be small, e.g. 75µg (half a tablet) twice daily, in order to avoid too much discouraging drowsiness. Sometimes it is advisable to give a considerable proportion of the dose at bedtime. In small doses (25µg tablets, 2 to 4 daily) clonidine is useful in the prevention of migraine (see chapter XXV; sect. 7.2) and can be helpful in preventing menopausal flushing. It may

be better treatment for hypertensive patients with these complaints than, for example, ergotamine and oestrogens.

Clonidine is well absorbed orally. It is excreted in large part as unchanged drug in the urine and dosage may need to be modified in renal failure (see appendix E).

5.6 β-Adrenoceptor Blocking Drugs

5.6.1 General Considerations
β-Adrenoceptor blocking drugs have revolutionised antihypertensive therapy and their use in hypertension and general pharmacological properties and side effects have been extensively reviewed (e.g. McDevitt, 1979; Simpson, 1974, 1977; Waal-Manning, 1976c). Their exact mode of action in lowering blood pressure is uncertain but there is probably a combination of reduced cardiac output and reduced renin release from the kidney. A CNS effect seemed possible but is now not thought to be important (see section 4.4).

The β-blockers vary in their subsidiary characteristics (Waal-Manning, 1976c): relative selectivity for β_1-adrenoceptors (heart) and β_2-adrenoceptors (e.g. bronchioles and muscle blood vessels), intrinsic sympathomimetic (partial agonist) activity, membrane stabilising (local anaesthetic or quinidine-like) effect and lipid solubility, as well as in their pharmacokinetic properties (see table IIIa,b). There has been a tendency, particularly in publications from the USA, to look on propranolol as typical of all β-blockers, the implication being that all other characteristics are unimportant. In practice, the latter is not correct. Other β-blockers seem to cause less gastrointestinal problems, and many of them (because of cardioselectivity or intrinsic sympathomimetic activity) have a lesser propensity than propranolol to cause bronchospasm.

5.6.2 Cardioselectivity
Cardioselectivity (greater selectivity for β_1-adrenoceptors) confers a degree of freedom from risk of causing bronchospasm (Hua et al., 1978) but this is by no means complete. Cardioselective drugs at least do not prevent the action of β_2-adrenoceptor stimulant bronchodilator drugs (Formgren, 1976; Horvath et al., 1978), but their effects in patients with chronic obstructive respiratory disease are unpredictable (see section 5.6.8). Cardioselective β-blockers are more appropriate in diabetic subjects as they are less likely

Table IIIa. Pharmacodynamic properties of β-adrenoceptor blocking drugs (after Waal-Manning, 1976c)

Drug	β-Blockade potency ratio[1]	Receptor blockade[2]		Partial agonist activity	Membrane stabilising activity
		β_1	β_2		
Acebutolol	0.3	+	±	+	+
Alprenolol	0.3	+	+	++	+
Atenolol	1	+	0	0	0
Metoprolol	1	+	0	0	±
Oxprenolol	0.5-1	+	+	++	+
Pindolol	6	+	+	+++	+
Propranolol	1	+	+	0	++
Sotalol	0.3	+	+	0	0
Timolol	6	+	+	±	0

1   Propranolol = 1.
2   Relative selectivity for β_1-adrenoceptors (heart) and β_2-adrenoceptors (e.g. bronchioles and muscle blood vessels). Selectivity is not absolute, but those compounds with relative selectivity for β_1-adrenoceptors are termed cardioselective β-blockers; the others non-selective β-blockers.

to aggravate hypoglycaemia, precipitate hypertensive crises during hypoglycaemia and compromise peripheral circulation (Waal-Manning, 1979; see chapter XVI; sect. 13.1).

5.6.3 Intrinsic Sympathomimetic Activity

Intrinsic sympathomimetic (partial agonist) activity does not appear to be very important in relation to antihypertensive effect (Cocco et al., 1978). However, pindolol which has this characteristic to a considerable degree, seems in high dosage in some individuals to be capable of actually raising the blood pressure (Waal-Manning and Simpson, 1975), although it is an effective antihypertensive agent at lower dosage (Waal-Manning and Simpson, 1974). Some confirmation of this finding has come from others (Bjerle et al., 1975; Fyhrquist et al., 1977). However, it may be that a very small proportion of patients will have a rise in blood pressure on any β-blocker (Prichard, 1977), even propranolol (Drayer et al., 1976) especially when given large doses of this drug from the start (Blum et al., 1975). The most readily recognisable effect of intrinsic sympathomimetic activity is that drugs that have it cause much less bradycardia than drugs that lack it. It may also help to minimise the likelihood of bronchospasm (Christensen et al., 1978).

5.6.4 Membrane Stabilising Effect

The local anaesthetic or membrane stabilising effect does not seem to be important clinically. Oc-casionally a patient who is not a good tablet swallower will notice the local anaesthetic effect on the tongue.

5.6.5 Lipid Solubility

Lipid solubility makes a drug more likely to be distributed into CNS tissue. This is unimportant for the basic action of the drug in lowering blood pressure, but may determine the extent to which CNS side effects occur; e.g. dreams and even nightmares, insomnia. The highly lipid soluble compounds alprenolol and propranolol are readily distributed into the brain (Johnsson and Regardh, 1976).

5.6.6 Pharmacokinetic Properties

The individual β-blockers vary considerably in their pharmacokinetic characteristics (Shand, 1974, 1977; Johnsson and Regardh, 1976; table IIIb). Propranolol, alprenolol and metoprolol undergo considerable first-pass metabolism in the liver. There is therefore wide variation in plasma concentrations achieved in different individuals and dosage may need to be reduced in cirrhosis (see chapter XIX; sect. 1.4). Food enhances the bioavailability of propranolol and metoprolol, presumably by decreasing hepatic first-pass metabolism since absorption of these drugs is virtually complete anyway and can hardly be improved (Melander et al., 1977; see chapter VI, sect. 5). Pentobarbitone reduces the bioavailability of alprenolol, presumably by inducing hepatic micro-

Table IIIb. Pharmacokinetic properties of β-adrenoceptor blocking drugs. Some differences between compounds (prepared by G.S. Avery after Johnsson and Regardh, 1976; Shand, 1974, 1977)

Drug	Oral bioavailability[1]	1st-pass hepatic metabolism	Elimination half-life (h)	Predominant route of elimination[3]	Active metabolites of potential clinical importance	Protein binding[5] (%)
Acebutolol	20-60	Yes[2b]	~ 8 (po)	Renal excretion ($\approx$ 15% unchanged; $\approx$ 28% active metabolite) and hepatic metabolism	?Yes[4]	84
Alprenolol	~ 10	Yes[2a]	2-3 (iv, po)	Hepatic metabolism	Yes[4]	85
Atenolol	50-60	No	6-9 (po)	Renal excretion ($\approx$ 40% unchanged)		< 5%
Metoprolol	40-50	Yes[2a]	3-4 (iv, po)	Hepatic metabolism	No	12
Oxprenolol	25-60	Yes[2b]	2 (po)	Hepatic metabolism		
Pindolol	~ 100	No	3-4 (iv)	Renal excretion ($\approx$ 40% unchanged) and hepatic metabolism		57
Propranolol	~ 30	Yes[2a]	2-4 (iv) 3.5-6 (po)	Hepatic metabolism	Yes[4]	93
Sotalol	$\geqslant$ 60	No	5-13 (po)	Renal excretion ($\approx$ 75% unchanged)		54
Timolol	75	No	4-5 (po)	Hepatic metabolism and renal excretion ($\approx$ 20% unchanged)		

1 Percentage of dose reaching systemic circulation as unchanged drug after oral administration.

2a The total body clearance of these drugs approaches the hepatic blood flow, indicating that they are extensively removed from the blood during its first passage through the liver (see chapter I; sect. 2.1.4, 3.3.3).

2b The total body clearance of these drugs is somewhat less than that of hepatic blood flow and they are thus only subject to moderate first-pass hepatic metabolism.

3 *Renal disease:* Compounds eliminated primarily by renal excretion accumulate in renal failure, necessitating modification of dosage. Bioavailability of propranolol increases in renal failure due to decreased hepatic first-pass metabolism (see chapter XXI; sect. 14.2.4). Bioavailability of pindolol is decreased in renal failure but is compensated by decreased renal clearance (see chapter XXI; sect. 1.1, 14.2.4). Percentages are those of the given dose.

Cirrhosis: Bioavailability of compounds subjected to significant first-pass metabolism increases due to reduced hepatic extraction. This will be particularly marked if there is significant portal systemic shunting (see chapter XIX; sect. 1.4).

4 A 4-hydroxy metabolite of alprenolol and propranolol is formed after oral, but not or to a considerably lesser extent after intravenous administration, and is about equipotent with the parent drug. 4-Hydroxypropranolol is present in about the same and 4-hydroxyalprenolol around 75% of the concentration in plasma as the parent drug. The quantitative importance of the 4-hydroxy metabolites after continued administration is not known. Propranolol also forms other active metabolites, the quantitative importance of which is unknown. Whether active metabolites of alprenolol and propranolol accumulate in renal failure is not clear.

The concentration in the plasma of the active acetyl metabolite of acebutolol exceeds that of the parent drug after oral administration but is lower after intravenous administration. The acetyl metabolite accumulates in renal failure but its contribution to the clinical effect of acebutolol is not known (see chapter XXI; sect. 14.2.4).

5 Alprenolol and propranolol are avidly bound to α_1 acid glycoprotein and have only moderate affinity to albumin. The other compounds are bound to plasma albumin. Changes in concentration of α_1 acid glycoprotein in various disease states can affect binding of alprenolol and propranolol (see chapter I; sect. 4.3.2).

somal enzyme metabolism of the drug (Alvan et al., 1977). Pindolol and timolol are partly metabolised by the liver and partly excreted by the kidneys so their dosage is less likely to be affected by disease of either organ. On the other hand, atenolol and sotalol are eliminated in the urine as unchanged drug and acebutolol as unchanged drug + active metabolite. These compounds require dose modification in patients with renal failure. Dosage of propranolol may also need to be reduced when commending therapy in patients with chronic renal failure, as a consequence of increased bioavailability. The quantitative importance of the active metabolites of propranolol and alprenolol in renal failure is not clear (see chapter XXI; sect. 14.2.4).

In general, then, these pharmacokinetic findings underline the need to titrate the dose of a β-blocking drug to the needs of the individual patient.

5.6.7 Use of β-Blockers in Hypertension

It is not necessary, for the successful use of β-blockers, to have access to plasma renin estimations. A useful rule of thumb is that in mild to moderate hypertension below the age of 45 years a β-blocker should be tried by itself first (Simpson, 1974, 1977). Others have come to the same conclusion (Buhler et al., 1978). In older subjects, or in younger people with more severe hypertension, it is usually best to start with a diuretic and then add a β-blocker if necessary. Initial dosage of any β-blocker should be small; this ensures that any symptoms produced are minor and can be dealt with at leisure. β-Blockers are not the best initial treatment in really severe hypertension (e.g. malignant); they do not have a sufficiently rapid effect in all cases and if the blood pressure fails to fall, there is a danger of precipitating left ventricular failure.

β-Blockers must never be given to a patient without first ascertaining that there is no obstructive respiratory disease, tendency to heart failure, or 2nd degree heart block.

Severe Raynaud's phenomenon is also a contraindication, as it can be aggravated by β-adrenoceptor blockade.

5.6.8 Side Effects of β-Blockade

The long term use of β-blockers is still a little under the cloud left by the practolol *oculomucocutaneous reaction* (e.g. Waal-Manning, 1975b; Behan et al., 1976). It is difficult to be certain of the significance of occasional case reports

of minor reactions to the β-blockers now in use. However, it seems wise to remain alert to possible problems and keep a watch for skin rashes and dry eyes (Editorial, 1977a). The situation with regard to antinuclear antibody activation is not yet clear (Assem, 1977; Wilson et al., 1978). Antinuclear antibodies have so far proved to be less common in subjects on β-blockers other than practolol than in those on methyldopa (Wilson et al., 1978). Haematological reactions in general are rare (Greenblatt and Koch-Weser, 1974).

Problems of withdrawal of therapy: If therapy with a β-blocker has to be stopped it should be done gradually. Blood pressure can rise quite quickly, over 2 to 3 days, in some individuals, though there is no true overshoot as can occur with clonidine (see section 5.5). But patients with severe coronary artery disease can suffer exacerbation of their angina or even myocardial infarction (Wilson et al., 1969; Miller et al., 1975). If the patient is at rest in hospital there seem to be fewer problems with β-blocker withdrawal (Shiroff et al., 1978).

Bronchospasm is a potential hazard with β-blockade in any patient, though the incidence of this side effect in patients with no history of obstructive respiratory disease is extremely small. If it occurs, then either the β-blocker should be stopped or a switch must be made to a cardioselective β-blocker. Great caution is needed, even with cardioselective compounds (β_1-blockers) in patients with chronic obstructive respiratory disease as the effects are unpredictable. Non-selective β-blockers should not be used in asthmatics but some patients may be able to be managed by cautious use of a combination of a β_1-blocker and a β_2-adrenoceptor stimulant bronchodilator such as salbutamol (albuterol) or terbutaline (see section 5.6.2; chapter XX; sect. 10.1).

Cardiac failure is a potential hazard in older patients or in those with abnormal hearts. It should be prevented, if possible, by judicious prior use of diuretics and if necessary digitalis. If it occurs, then either the β-blocker should be stopped, or else diuretic dosage should be increased and digitalis given.

Impairment of atrioventricular conduction has been unexpectedly uncommon. It is theoretically less likely to occur with drugs that have intrinsic sympathomimetic activity.

Raynaud's phenomenon, cold extremities can occur with any β-blocker but is more likely with non-selective blockers and those without intrinsic sympathomimetic activity (Marshall et al., 1976). It is probably due to lower cardiac output and increased α-adrenoceptor activity.

Muscle cramps have been reported with practolol and propranolol (Greenblatt and Koch-Weser, 1974) but in our experience occur rather more frequently with pindolol.

CNS effects include dreams, hallucinations, insomnia most often with propranolol and pindolol and depression with propranolol (Waal-Manning, 1976c). However, β-blockers often seem to have an anxiolytic effect which can be valuable (Editorial, 1976). An acute brain syndrome has been described with propranolol (Topliss and Bond, 1977; Helson and Duque, 1978).

Migraine is usually relieved by β-blockade but has been precipitated by propranolol in occasional cases (Robson, 1977).

Metabolic effects of β-blockers are complex (Waal-Manning, 1976a,c; 1979). Non-selective β-blockers can cause impairment of glucose tolerance, but in contrast can also enhance insulin-mediated hypoglycaemia (Deacon and Barnett, 1976). Although cardioselective β-blockers are less likely to have these effects, the use of β-blockers in diabetic subjects requires some caution (see chapter XVI; sect. 13.1). There are conflicting reports on the effect of β-blockers on plasma triglycerides; a slight rise being reported by some workers (Waal-Manning, 1976c; Shaw et al., 1978) but not by others (Castenfors et al., 1973; Nilsson et al., 1978).

Some long term studies have shown a significant increase in plasma triglyceride and urate concentrations, along with a decrease in plasma high density lipoprotein concentrations, in patients treated with propranolol and a thiazide compared with those treated with methyldopa and a thiazide (Helgeland et al., 1978a,b). The importance of these metabolic effects is not at present clear. β-Blockers in hypertension seem to have a protective rather than an adverse effect on coronary heart disease (Wilhelmsen, 1978; Berglund et al., 1978).

Renal function impairment has been reported after use of β-blockers in patients with pre-existing renal disease (Warren et al., 1974; Swainson and Winney, 1976) possibly due to decreased glomerular filtration (Ibsen and Sederberg-Olsen, 1973). Others have not seen this phenomenon (Kincaid-Smith and Hua, 1974). Plasma creatinine should nevertheless be monitored in such patients and dosage should be more cautious than usual (see also section 5.6.6; chapter XXI, sect. 14.2.4).

Gastrointestinal symptoms (e.g. anorexia, nausea, vomiting, diarrhoea and abdominal pain) seem to be more common with propranolol (Greenblatt and Koeh-Weser, 1974) than with other β-blockers. A case of ileus possibly due to oxprenolol has been reported (Young et al., 1977) and two rather similar cases possibly associated with atenolol have been reported to the New Zealand Committee on Adverse Drug Reactions.

Impotence on propranolol (but not on atenolol) has been reported in a few cases (e.g. Warren and Warren, 1977; Bathen, 1978). Peyronie's syndrome has been reported on propranolol (Osborne, 1977).

Weight gain can be considerable in some patients on non-selective β-blockade. Kather and Simon (1977) have found atenolol to have relatively far less antilipolytic activity than propranolol in *in vitro* experiments, but the relevance of this to weight gain is not yet clear.

5.6.9 Dosage of β-Blockers

The general rule is to start with a low dosage given as a 3 times daily regimen for the shorter acting drugs or as a twice daily regimen for the longer acting drugs (table IIIb, VII). Dosage should thereafter be increased gradually and as dosage requirement increases doses can be given less frequently or the larger dose slow release preparations used. Most β-blockers have a ceiling dose beyond which it is unlikely that further antihypertensive effect will occur. The upper limit of dosage will be greatest with those β-blockers subject to significant first-pass metabolism (table IIIb) since plasma concentrations from a given dose of these drugs varies widely among individuals. In the case of pindolol, some patients seem to show a paradoxical *increase* in blood pressure as dosage is increased, especially when the daily dose exceeds 30mg (see section 5.6.3). When the ceiling dose or maximum effective dosage has been reached and blood pressure is not adequately controlled, it is best to add another drug (see section 6.3, 6.4). Once control has been achieved by a stepwise increase in dosage and addition of other drugs, it is wise to see whether a smaller dose of β-blocker would suffice. These drugs are too expensive to be used in unnecessarily high dosage.

Once daily dosage of everything is the current vogue, and this applies to β-blockers as well as to other drugs. However, it must be seen in perspective. Twice daily dosage is no hardship on a patient and although the blood pressure lowering effect of β-blockers is much longer than predicted from their plasma half-life, the reduction in number of doses to one daily has run ahead of the development of truly long acting drugs. Atenolol is at present the drug that seems most suitable for once daily dosage (Castleden et al., 1977; Wilcox, 1978) though sustained release formulations of shorter acting drugs go some way to solving the problem. Sotalol, because of its long elimination half-life, may also be suitable for once daily dosage. If shorter acting drugs are used once a day, then the degree of β-blockade fluctuates considerably and this is probably undesirable, even though differences in blood pressure are small (Reybrouck, 1978). It is particularly undesirable in patients with angina.

5.7 Labetalol

This drug, with both α- and β-adrenoceptor blocking action is an effective antihypertensive agent (for review, see Brogden et al., 1978). It is sometimes effective in patients who have failed to respond to β-blockade alone and it has the advantage of causing less Raynaud's phenomenon than the β-blockers (Bolli et al., 1977). The α-blockade may help to protect against bronchospasm (Skinner et al., 1975). It is also often effective when given intravenously, for example in acute situations (Trust et al., 1976; Pearson and Havard, 1978a) and it is useful to have the same drug for both intravenous and subsequent oral use. It is sometimes surprisingly effective alone, i.e. without a diuretic, in severe new cases (Ghose et al., 1978). However, it has been reported to be ineffective when given intravenously to severely hypertensive patients receiving concomitant therapy with combinations of various other drugs such as large doses of β-blockers, clonidine, methyldopa and bethanidine or debrisoquine (Rosei et al., 1976a; MacCarthy et al., 1978b) and we also have the impression that labetalol is most effective in patients who are not taking a complicated regimen of drugs. Precise antagonisms have not been worked out. Variable effects of labetalol in phaeochromocytoma have been reported, with good responses in many cases but with occasional hypertensive responses (Rosei et al., 1976b; Briggs et al., 1978). It causes a number of side effects: nausea, abdominal distension, diarrhoea; tingling of the scalp; skin rash; occasional bronchospasm; and strangury and retention occasionally in men.

It has the disadvantage, compared with the β-blockers, of causing a little postural hypotension (Bolli et al., 1977), usually at higher dosages, but this is very seldom troublesome. We have the impression that in resistant cases a little more β-blockade may be advantageous.

When given orally, labetalol should be started at a dose of 100mg (half a 200mg tablet) twice daily, with increases every 2 to 7 days, depending on the degree of urgency. The average dose is about 600 to 800mg daily, but in severe hypertension about 1000 to 1200mg daily. The larger dosage is best given on a thrice daily basis.

Labetalol is extensively metabolised in the liver and undergoes a considerable first-pass effect, so that bioavailability is relatively low (Martin et al., 1976). Bioavailability is markedly increased in patients with cirrhosis, necessitating reduced dosage (Homeida et al., 1978). The dose required in patients with impaired renal function is no less than that reported for other patients (Williams et al., 1978).

5.8 Prazosin

Prazosin, a postsynaptic α-adrenoceptor blocking drug (see sections 4.5 and 4.6), lowers peripheral resistance and has little effect on cardiac output (Lund Johansen, 1974). The first dose has a curiously powerful effect on blood pressure (the 'first dose' phenomenon; Bendall et al., 1975; Graham et al., 1976) and should be as low as 0.5mg or even 0.25mg, possibly best given in the evening. Postural dizziness sometimes occurs during maintenance therapy also; usually after a rapid dose increment. Prazosin can occasionally cause fluid retention and aggravate or precipitate angina (New Zealand Hypertension Study Group, 1977). However, in spite of this it can be used to lower afterload in states of severe heart failure (Miller et al., 1977; see chapter XVII, sect. 8.3.4). In the treatment of hypertension, its main place seems to be as a third drug, to be added if a patient fails to respond adequately to a diuretic and a β-blocker (New Zealand Hypertension Study Group, 1977). It can however, be extremely effective even by itself in mild or moderate hypertension. Patients with coronary artery disease should preferably not be given prazosin without a concomitant β-blocker (Simpson et al., 1977). In patients with impaired renal function, prazosin does not cause a significant rise in blood urea or creatinine (Bailey et al.,

1976). However, the dose may need to be smaller than usual (Curtis and Bateman, 1975). The 'first-dose phenomenon' is probably a pharmaco-dynamic matter.

For a review of prazosin, see Brogden et al. (1977) and Stokes and Oates (1978).

5.9 Hydrallazine

Hydrallazine has been in use since 1950 but was difficult to use because of its side effects of tachycardia, headache and peripheral oedema and its tendency to cause a systemic lupus syndrome. The advent of the β-blockers has given it a new lease of life as a third drug to be added to the regimen of patients who fail to respond adequately to a diuretic and a β-blocker. These drugs largely counteract the side effects of hydrallazine and allow it to be used in reasonably small doses (200mg daily or less) so that systemic lupus reactions are now rare. Hydrallazine acts directly on vascular smooth muscle. It reduces peripheral resistance and causes a reflex increase in heart rate and cardiac output. It can therefore aggravate angina. For a review of hydrallazine, see Koch-Weser (1976b, 1978).

Initial dosage should be no higher than 25mg twice daily in order to avoid headache, flushing, etc which are usually most prominent at the start of therapy. The dose is then increased stepwise, up to 200mg daily if necessary; some would allow 300mg in fast acetylators (Wollam et al., 1977; Koch-Weser, 1976b). Hydrallazine is rapidly excreted and is usually given 3 times daily, though twice daily dosage has been said to be equally effective (O'Malley et al., 1975). However, the bigger the individual dose, the more likely on the whole that symptomatic side effects will occur (see below).

Hydrallazine pharmacokinetics are important (for review, see Talseth, 1977). It is subjected to polymorphic acetylation; bioavailability and plasma concentrations are higher, and half-life tending to be longer, in slow acetylators than in fast acetylators given the same dose. Dosage of hydrallazine in slow acetylators is about half that required to produce the same plasma concentration in fast acetylators. Hydrallazine is subjected to significant first-pass metabolism, with the acetylation process in the gut mucosa and liver possibly being capacity limited. Thus, an increase in dose of 25mg or more in slow acetylators or 100mg or more in fast acetylators may lead to a disproportionately large increase in the amount of unchanged drug reaching the systemic circulation. Dosage increases should probably be limited to 50mg per day.

Hydrallazine accumulates in renal failure, but despite the unusually high plasma concentrations and slower clearance, there have been no reports of an increased incidence of toxic side effects in uraemic subjects receiving usual doses of hydrallazine. The reason for the accumulation is not clear. It is possible that metabolism of hydrallazine is impaired in uraemia.

Acetylation phenotype has an important influence on the occurrence of a systemic lupus erythematosus syndrome with hydrallazine. This occurs especially in slow acetylators, most often female, who have received hydrallazine for more than 6 months. The daily dose of hydrallazine taken has varied widely: from less than 200mg to more than 400mg in different series, but there are evidently no reports of SLE at doses of less than 100mg daily (see Talseth, 1977; also chapter XXII, sect. 14.1). For the distribution of slow acetylators in different populations, see chapter VII (table VII).

5.10 Minoxidil

Minoxidil is a powerful vasodilator, acting directly on vascular smooth muscle (O'Malley et al., 1976). It causes a fall in peripheral resistance and an increase in cardiac output, and sodium and fluid retention. It is therefore almost always necessary to give a diuretic and a β-blocker along with it. At present it appears to be the most potent antihypertensive agent known. However, its use has been hampered firstly by the marked hirsutism, which can be distressing particularly in women, and secondly by doubts of its safety as it causes a haemorrhagic degeneration in the right atrium at high dosage in dogs (DuCharme et al., 1973). It is still not generally available. In the centres where it is being used, it seems to have a good reputation as a highly effective drug in patients who have been resistant to everything else, including those with very poor renal function (Dargie et al., 1977; Mitchell and Pettinger, 1978). Such patients may be prepared to put up with hirsutism and the risk of cardiac complications (table IV) may also be acceptable in this situation. Minoxidil is eliminated by hepatic metabolism.

5.11 Diazoxide

Diazoxide has structural similarities to the thiazides but has no diuretic action. The exact mechanism for its powerful vasodilating action is uncertain (for review, see Speight and Avery, 1971; Koch-Weser, 1976a). While it has been used orally for maintenance treatment in patients with malignant hypertension resistant to other agents (Fang et al., 1974), this carries a considerable risk of causing (reversible) hyperglycaemia (Dollery et al., 1962) and its use is usually restricted to hypertensive emergencies (see section 8) when it is given intravenously as a bolus within 10 to 30 seconds (Koch-Weser, 1976a; McDonald et al., 1977). It lowers blood pressure very rapidly, usually within 5 minutes, and it can cause profound hypotension with potentially disastrous results on coronary or cerebral blood flow or on renal function if dosage is excessive (Kanada et al., 1976). The usual dose suggested is 300mg but it is wise to try the effect of 150mg first. It is seldom desirable to lower blood pressure to normal in a matter of minutes. Diazoxide is highly bound to plasma albumin and its effect is related to the concentration of free drug in plasma which is greater with more rapid injection and in hypoalbuminaemic states. Binding is also reduced in renal failure and initial dosage must in this case be no higher than 150mg. Diazoxide is mainly eliminated as unchanged drug in the urine, its half-life increasing with decreasing creatinine clearance (Koch-Weser, 1976a). A potent diuretic such as frusemide (furosemide) should usually be given to patients being treated with diazoxide, to prevent sodium and water retention.

Diazoxide is a valuable drug but it has to be used with considerable care. Its pharmacological properties and side effects are discussed in chapter XXI (sect. 6.1).

5.12 Angiotensin Antagonists and Converting Enzyme Inhibitors

Saralasin is a synthetic octapeptide which is a competitive antagonist of angiotensin II. It has to be given intravenously and its use has hitherto been on a research basis. It may have a place in the identification of patients with renovascular disease (Brunner et al., 1973; Wilson et al., 1977) and in the treatment of hypertensive crises (Gavras et al., 1974) but it is itself to some degree an agonist so that in states of low endogenous angiotensin II it can have a pressor effect. While of great research interest it seems unlikely to have wide use in the treatment of hypertension.

The inactive decapeptide angiotensin I is converted to the active octapeptide angiotensin II by a 'converting enzyme' which is mainly found in pulmonary capillary endothelium. This enzyme can be blocked by the new orally active drug, SQ-14225 or captopril (see section 4.7). This represents a potential revolution in clinical antihypertensive therapy and clearly has great promise.

6. Management of Therapy

6.1 General Principles

1) *Blood pressure in the erect posture should be kept as near normal as possible.* However, a high blood pressure may have to be accepted in special cases.

a) *Impaired renal function:* blood urea may start to rise when blood pressure is kept at what would otherwise be reasonable levels.

b) *Impaired cerebral arteries:* ischaemic episodes may occur in situations when blood pressure is at its lowest. But such patients are also endangered by the blood pressure being too high, and prognosis after a stroke is improved by treatment of hypertension (Carter, 1970; Beevers et al., 1973b).

c) *Impaired coronary arteries:* angina is often relieved when blood pressure is lowered, but some extra care should be taken to lower the blood pressure gradually rather than suddenly, in order to avoid precipitating myocardial infarction.

d) *Elderly patients:* many elderly patients can take antihypertensive therapy very well, but it is important to avoid symptoms of postural hypotension, especially if the patients are living alone (see section 9).

2) *If possible, use a regimen that reduces blood pressure in the supine as well as in the erect position.* The posturally acting adrenergic neurone blocking drugs (guanethidine, bethanidine and debrisoquine) were previously the 'sheet anchor' of treatment of the more severe grades of hypertension. However, patients are usually more comfortable on non-posturally acting drugs. The β-adrenoceptor blocking drugs in particular have an advantage in this respect, and to some extent also methyldopa and clonidine.

Table IV. Principal side effects of antihypertensive drugs and their management

Drug	Side effect	Management
Diuretics	Hypokalaemia	Give KCl supplements or add potassium-sparing diuretic (also consider possibility of hyperaldosteronism)
	Hyperuricaemia, gout	Stop drug unless a diuretic is essential, in which case continue diuretic and add probenecid or allopurinol, etc., or switch to tienilic acid
	Impairment of carbohydrate metabolism	Stop drug unless a diuretic is essential, in which case treat the diabetes as required
	Rise in blood urea	Use frusemide if renal function is very poor
	Skin rash	Stop drug if it is thought to be the cause
	Necrotising vasculitis	Stop drug
Potassium-sparing diuretics	Hyperkalaemia (especially amiloride)	Reduce dose and reduce potassium intake
	Nausea (triamterene)	Reduce dose
	Gynaecomastia (spironolactone)	Change to another drug
Rauwolfia	Depression	Stop drug (essential)
	Nasal blockage Lethargy Dreams, nightmares Parkinsonism Increasing weight Diarrhoea	Stop drug (advisable)
Methyldopa	Somnolence	Increase dose more slowly. If persistent, lower the dose and add another drug
	Depression	Stop drug (essential)
	Dreams	Stop drug (advisable)
	Positive Coombs' test	Watch for haemolytic anaemia
	Haemolytic anaemia	Stop drug (essential)
	Drug fever, liver damage	Stop drug (essential)
	Fluid retention	Add a diuretic
	Lactation	Stop drug
	Reduced libido	Depends on severity. Possibly change to other therapy
Guanethidine	Diarrhoea	Change to another regimen or reduce dose and add another drug or add diphenoxylate
	Morning hypotension Exercise hypotension	Change to other therapy or encourage patient to learn to adjust, or reduce dose and add a shorter acting drug (e.g. pempidine or bethanidine)
	Fluid retention	Add a diuretic
	Failure of ejaculation	Depends on severity. Possibly change to other therapy
	Depression	Very rare. Stop drug

Table IV. (continued)

Drug	Side effect	Management
Bethanidine Debrisoquine	Postural hypotension	Adjust distribution of daily dose to take into account the time when patient is most affected
	Fluid retention Failure of ejaculation Depression	As for guanethidine
	'Cheese reaction' (debrisoquine)	Avoid large quantities of cheese and other amine-containing foods
Monoamine oxidase inhibitors	'Cheese reaction'	Reiterate food restrictions. If patient will not cooperate, change to other therapy
	Postural hypotension	Adjust dose
α-Adrenoceptor blocking drugs	Tachycardia	Make sure that the drug is having a worthwhile effect; if so, add a β-blocker; if not, stop drug
β-Adrenoceptor blocking drugs	Asthma	Stop drug (essential). Cautious transfer to a cardioselective β-blocker may be possible (see section 5.6.8)
	Cardiac failure	Add a diuretic and possibly digitalis, if continued use of β-blocker is desired. Otherwise, stop drug
	Dreams, insomnia	Avoid late evening dosage
	Raynaud's phenomenon	Keep warm; stop drug if necessary or add a vasodilator
	Tiredness	Worse with propranolol than with other β-blockers
	Depression (propranolol and possibly others also)	Stop drug (essential)
Clonidine	Drowsiness, dry mouth	Encourage to persevere. Reduce dose if possible, or change to other therapy
	Depression	Stop drug (essential)
	Fluid retention	Add diuretic
Hydrallazine	Systemic lupus erythematosus	Stop drug (essential)
	Drug fever	Stop drug (essential)
	Headache	Persevere, reducing dose temporarily
	Nausea, skin rash etc.	Depends on severity: stop drug if necessary
	Tachycardia	Use a β-blocker to prevent this
	Fluid retention	Use a diuretic to prevent this
Prazosin	Postural hypotension with first dose	Keep first dose small and warn patient of possibility
	Tachycardia	Add a β-blocker
	Angina	Rare; use a β-blocker if necessary, or stop drug
	Fluid retention	Add a diuretic
Minoxidil	Tachycardia, angina	Use a β-blocker to prevent this
	Oedema	Use a diuretic to prevent this
	Hypertrichosis	Stop drug if possible
	Pericardial effusion	Stop drug
	Pulmonary hypertension	Stop drug

3) *Do not change drugs without good cause.* Patients become discouraged with too many changes in therapy. They sometimes prefer to tolerate some minor side effect rather than change to some unfamiliar drug.

4) *Dosage changes should be gradual.* The desired endpoint of therapy is a sensitive one and there is usually no need to approach it too rapidly. Similarly, when a drug is being stopped, it is best to do this gradually in order to avoid rebound effects. This is especially important in 3 situations: with clonidine because of the rebound rise in blood pressure (see section 5.5); with β-blockers because of possible development of angina or myocardial infarction in susceptible patients with coronary artery disease (see section 5.6.8); and, in the case of patients verging on heart failure, with diuretics because of the sudden fluid retention.

5) *A single high blood pressure reading in an otherwise well controlled patient is not sufficient reason for raising the dose of drug.* Current drugs are still not able to prevent, for instance, emotionally induced rises in blood pressure.

6) *There is no place for a half-hearted trial of therapy.* Intermittent treatment of hypertension may well be worse than none. In most cases no useful purpose is achieved by withholding information about blood pressure levels from the patient. The patient must, by the doctor's interest in his blood pressure and his drugs, be made to feel that the treatment is important. Only in this way will he be persuaded to take tablets faithfully and regularly.

7) *Be alert for interactions between the various drugs and for serious side effects* (see tables IV, VIII and sections 6.2; 6.3; 10). Patients must be warned of some possible side effects: depression with reserpine, asthma or dyspnoea with β-blockers, and postural faintness with various drugs.

8) *Provide each patient with a card* on which the name and dosage schedule of each drug can be written. Changes in dosage etc must always be written on the card. The patient must be warned never to allow his supplies of tablets to run out.

9) *Patients on a powerful antihypertensive drug* should be instructed to reduce the dosage slightly if they feel faint or if the weather is very hot. Some patients like to be able to take their own blood pressure and should be allowed to do so, in order to regulate their drug dosage.

10) *Above all, get the patient's cooperation.* The patient must have the feeling that he will be listened to if he tells the doctor that the tablets do not seem to suit, or that the dosage seems to be too high.

11) *Persistent normotension* is cause for congratulation. It is also cause for reassessment of whether the patient was truly hypertensive in the first place. A cautious trial of withdrawal of therapy is often worthwhile.

12) *The frequency of visiting is a matter of judgement.* It is best to get the blood pressure under control during the first 4 to 6 weeks of outpatient treatment. If this process takes too long, the patient may become discouraged. However, if it is not convenient for him to visit the doctor or clinic frequently, some compromise will have to be reached.

In most cases, there is no advantage in seeing the patient more than twice a week during the period of increasing dosage, but a frequency of less than once a week at this stage may involve unnecessary delay in achieving control or undesirably large dose increments. Quite quickly the interval between visits can be extended; first to 1 month and then to 2 months. When it is clear that a patient's blood pressure is well controlled on a given regimen, and that side effects are not a problem, the interval between visits can be extended to 3 or even 4 months.

6.2 Side Effects of Antihypertensive Drugs

Demands on current drugs are certainly becoming more stringent. In the early days of therapy, the patient had to learn to put up with side effects. Now it is felt that no patient should have to tolerate side effects, and in addition clinicians are becoming less and less prepared to accept any significant postural fall in pressure.

All antihypertensive drugs have side effects (table IV) but judicious selection of drugs will reduce their incidence. Clearly, thiazides should not be given indiscriminately to patients with hyperuricaemia, nor reserpine to patients with depression, nor β-blockers to asthmatics, and so on. Serious side effects must be dealt with suitably and promptly, but minor symptoms attributed by patients to drugs are often difficult to assess. In such a situation it is usually best to accept that the patient may well be right. However, coincidence should be excluded as far as possible, and it must be remembered that some side effects do tend to lessen with time (e.g. somnolence with methyldopa) or are relatively so trivial that the patient should be encouraged to tolerate them.

6.3 Use of Antihypertensive Drugs in Combination

Hypertension of any considerable severity can seldom be treated successfully with a single drug. The use of two or more drugs in combination usually leads to better control of the hypertension, to lower doses of individual drugs, and to less trouble from side effects (see Gifford, 1974; Simpson, 1970).

The pharmacological principles involved in this are by no means all clear, but it is highly unlikely that they are closely associated with the multifactorial character of the pathogenesis of hypertension. Rather, it is likely that the rationale of combined therapy is based on the need to counteract secondary effects which occur with nearly all drugs and which tend to prevent single drugs being used in doses adequate to control blood pressure. These secondary events appear either as 'side effects' or as drug resistance.

The best established example of successful combined therapy is the use of a diuretic in combination with specific antihypertensive drugs in order to combat the tendency to fluid retention. Other examples include the use of a potassium-sparing diuretic in combination with a thiazide-type diuretic, and the use of a drug that slows the heart (e.g. a β-blocker) in combination with one that causes tachycardia as a side effect (e.g. hydrallazine). The simultaneous use of a diuretic, a β-blocker and a vasodilator such as hydrallazine or prazosin is a powerful combination (Koch-Weser, 1974a; Gottlieb et al., 1972).

However, it has to be remembered that many antihypertensive drugs act at more or less the same site — the vascular sympathetic neuromuscular junction (fig. 2). There are therefore opportunities for such drugs to block or antagonise the antihypertensive effect of each other, as well as to act synergistically or additively (Simpson, 1970). *If a combination of drugs is not having a satisfactory effect in a given patient, then the possibility of undesirable interactions must be considered.* In general, it is best not to permit a patient's therapy to become too complicated. Whenever a drug is added to a patient's treatment regimen, consideration should be given to withdrawing another one. Except in emergency situations, it is best to introduce (and stop) drugs one at a time, otherwise it is difficult to determine the merits or problems of the drugs for an individual patient.

The widespread use of combined therapy has in some cases led to the incorporation of two or more drugs in one tablet. This is satisfactory if the drugs in question are used in a fairly standard dosage (e.g. thiazide diuretics and Rauwolfia, with or without potassium chloride), but is highly unsatisfactory when the dose of one of the drugs is liable to differ widely from one patient to another. It is clearly a matter of pure chance whether a fixed dose ratio of guanethidine, methyldopa or β-blocker to a thiazide diuretic will coincide with an individual patient's requirements.

6.4 Selection of Drugs

Rigid schedules have been devised, linking choice of drugs to a variety of complicated classifications of 'severity' of hypertension. These schedules are (in the author's view) unhelpful, partly because response to drugs is often difficult to predict from the indices of severity and partly because there are so many factors that have to be taken into consideration apart from the hypertension itself.

The primary aim is to find for each patient a drug or combination of drugs which:
a) Lowers blood pressure effectively
b) Is not contraindicated for any reason in that patient, and
c) May be positively helpful in other ways.

At present it is easier to find contraindications (table V) than positive indications (table VI) for individual drugs. Fortunately, there are now so many different types of antihypertensive drugs that it is nearly always possible to find a regimen that suits each patient. However, the proliferation of drugs has led to a situation where it is difficult, not only for the non-specialist but also for the specialist, to keep in mind the pharmacology of the various agents (see sections 4, 5; table II). Yet it is vital that these powerful drugs should be used only with knowledge and care, if harm to a proportion of patients is to be avoided.

In a newly diagnosed patient, it will often be suitable to give only a thiazide-type diuretic initially, provided that there is no real urgency to reduce the blood pressure and no contraindication; indeed, a diuretic is often worth including in any antihypertensive regimen. After about 2 weeks (or less in severe cases), the need to add a further drug

Table V. Contraindications for various drugs and drug groups

Condition	Drugs contraindicated
Diabetes, prediabetes Hyperuricaemia Hypokalaemia	Thiazide-type diuretics and frusemide to be avoided if possible
Elderly, living alone	Posturally acting drugs to be avoided if possible
Obesity	Rauwolfia
Depression	Rauwolfia, methyldopa, clonidine and propranolol
Tricyclic anti-depressant therapy	Adrenergic neurone blocking drugs, methyldopa and possibly clonidine
Angina, tachycardia	Vasodilators (unless β-adrenoceptor blocking drug is given concomitantly)
Asthma (present or past)	β-Adrenoceptor blocking drugs (see section 5.6.8)
Cardiac impairment	β-Adrenoceptor blocking drugs (unless diuretics and digitalis are also given)
Atrioventricular conduction defects (2nd or 3rd degree)	β-Adrenoceptor blocking drugs
Raynaud's phenomenon	β-Adrenoceptor blocking drugs

has to be assessed and there are of course numerous drugs to choose from. The contra-indications to the use of the various drugs must be kept in mind (table V) and in addition, the severity of the disease must be taken into consideration. In severe cases, the adrenergic neurone blockers are reliable drugs, although a β-adrenoceptor blocking drug (β-blocker) can often with advantage be added later. Labetalol (see section 5.7) is proving to be often very effective in severe cases. In less severe cases a β-blocker or methyldopa should be tried. In mild cases, the β-blockers have emerged as the drugs of choice over Rauwolfia alkaloids and methyldopa (see Moser et al., 1977). The dosages of drugs are given in section 5 and table VII.

Various situations (e.g. hypertension in pregnancy, or in the elderly) which require special comment are discussed in sections 7 and 9. Patients with coronary artery disease should, if possible, have a β-blocker in the drug regimen.

In patients with severe renal impairment, it is best to use drugs which do not reduce renal blood flow, such as hydrallazine, methyldopa, prazosin (Fang et al., 1974; Bailey et al., 1976) or minoxidil (Wilburn et al., 1975). Frusemide is probably the most satisfactory diuretic in such cases. Diazoxide (Koch-Weser, 1976a), given intravenously, or even orally (Pohl et al., 1972) may be useful in very severe and resistant cases (see also chapter XXI; sect. 6). Some authors believe that β-blockers can cause a dramatic deterioration in renal function when this is already severely impaired. Others have not seen this phenomenon (see section 5.6.8). All are agreed that monitoring of renal function is essential in such patients during initiation or change of therapy.

6.5 Problems in Management

In many patients, antihypertensive treatment presents no particular problems. However, the presence of atheroma, renal impairment, diabetes mellitus, gout, obesity, asthma, mental disease, or severe arthritis poses undoubted problems, either because of these conditions themselves or because of their therapy, which may interfere with antihypertensive drugs. Many patients have no symptoms and may, not unreasonably, be unconvinced of the need for therapy. A few appear to have a phobia of sphygmomanometry, while occasional patients become excessively dependent on the sphygmomanometer. Some patients seem to have a very low tolerance of side effects. A few will not take tablets regularly.

Lack of intelligence is itself not too much of a problem as such patients will often adhere faithfully to a regimen arranged for them. Occasionally an uncooperative patient, particularly one with accelerated disease, may have to be told quite bluntly the likely consequences of his not persevering with treatment, but it is unwise to coerce any patient in this way unless there are very good reasons for doing so. In general, the important point is that, as in other fields of medicine, the patients are individuals and must be treated as such.

All clinicians who deal with hypertension are aware of some patients whose blood pressure is difficult to control (Gifford and Tarazi, 1978; Pearson and Havard, 1978b). It is comforting to know that even partial reduction of blood pressure confers some benefit (Taguchi and Freis, 1974) but these patients are undoubtedly a source of worry. Their numbers have become much fewer since the advent of the β-blockers, the new vasodilators and labetalol. Possible causes of poor control include failure of the patient to take the medication; drug interactions (see sections 6.3; 10.1); an undetected primary cause (e.g. phaeochromocytoma); obesity; fluid retention; mental stress; and alcoholism.

7. Antihypertensive Drugs in Pregnancy

Hypertension of any considerable severity during pregnancy must of course be treated. Similarly, a patient who becomes pregnant while on antihypertensive treatment should usually have this treatment continued. It seems reasonable also to institute therapy in milder cases of hypertension

Table VI. Positive indications for individual drugs in the treatment of hypertension

Clinical condition	Suitable drug
Oedema or dyspnoea	Diuretic
Hypokalaemia	Spironolactone, triamterene or amiloride
Sinus tachycardia (if not due to cardiac failure); paroxysmal tachycardia	β-Adrenoceptor blocking drug
Ventricular ectopics	β-Adrenoceptor blocking drug
Angina	β-Adrenoceptor blocking drug
Dissecting aneurysm aortic aneurysm	β-Adrenoceptor blocking drug (especially propranolol, which has most effect on cardiac contractility)
Severe renal impairment	Frusemide rather than a thiazide; methyldopa, prazosin or hydrallazine rather than adrenergic neurone blocking drugs

in pregnancy and there is some evidence that fetal survival is thereby enhanced (Leather et al., 1968; Redman et al., 1976).

There is no agreement at present on the best drugs to use for hypertension in pregnancy. Diuretics and methyldopa are most commonly used (Chamberlain et al., 1978), but there is increasing doubt (e.g. Gallery et al., 1978; MacGillivray, 1977) about the wisdom of using diuretics, particularly in view of the already diminished intravascular volume (see also chapter XV; sect. 5.2).

There is evidence that hypertension in pregnancy can be very satisfactorily treated by means of a β-blocker (Eliahou et al., 1978; Tcherdakoff et al., 1978) and that the dangers of such drugs on the fetus have been somewhat overemphasised (Gallery et al., 1978). However, until further evidence has accumulated, methyldopa must remain the drug of first choice, supplemented by hydrallazine if necessary (Roberts and Perloff, 1977).

The mere starting of antihypertensive therapy must not be allowed to lull one into a false sense of security and it remains necessary to keep a close watch on the behaviour of the blood pressure and on the development of oedema or albuminuria, and to make sure that the patient is resting adequately.

Hypertensive emergencies in the second half of pregnancy can present considerable problems. Management depends on the stage of pregnancy, the viability of the fetus, and the risk to the mother of allowing the pregnancy to continue. Frusemide, diazoxide (Pennington and Picker, 1972), sedatives and clonidine have a place in this situation, and intravenous hydrallazine (Joyce and Kenyon, 1972) with diazepam has also been recommended (Martin, 1974).

The need for continued antihypertensive therapy should be assessed 2 to 4 months after parturition (see further chapter XV; sect. 5).

8. The Hypertensive Crisis

By definition, a hypertensive crisis is indeed a crisis. When a patient presents with an extremely high blood pressure (e.g. 240/150mm Hg) and no acute symptoms, this is a dangerous situation but not a crisis, and there is no *immediate* need for massive doses of rapidly acting drugs. The patient may have had this sort of level of blood pressure for some weeks or longer, and it is usually safe,

Table VII. List of antihypertensive drugs and their dosages[1]

Drug	Tablet size	Frequency of dosage[2]	Increment interval	Starting dose (daily)	Mainten-ance dose (daily)	Maximum dose (daily)	Notes
Diuretics							
Chlorothiazide	0.5g	d or bd	—	0.5g	0.5 or 1g	1.5g	The smaller 'starting' dose
Hydrochlorothiazide	25, 50mg	d or bd	—	25mg	25 or 50mg	100mg	need be given for 3-5 days
Bendrofluazide	2.5, 5mg	d or bd	—	2.5mg	2.5-5mg	10mg	only. Preparations combined
Cyclopenthiazide	0.25, 0.5mg	d or bd	—	0.25mg	0.5-0.75mg	1mg	with KC1 in a non-gastric
Methyclothiazide	5mg	d	—	2.5mg	5mg	10mg	irritating form are useful
Chlorthalidone	50, 100mg	2d or d	—	25-50mg	25-50mg	100mg	(e.g. slow release forms).
Clorexolone	10mg	2d or d	—	10mg	10-20mg	20mg	It is unwise to exceed
Frusemide	40mg	d or bd	—	20-40mg	40-120mg	virtually no limit	maximum dose in long term therapy
K-Sparing Diuretics							
Spironolactone	25mg	bd or td	—	50mg	50-100mg	400mg	Large doses of spironolactone are used only in suspected primary aldosteronism
Triamterene	100mg	bd or td	—	100mg	100-200mg	300mg	
Amiloride	5mg	bd	—	5mg	5-10mg	20mg	Maximum dose of amiloride must not be exceeded
Rauwolfia							
Whole root	50mg	d	—	50mg	100mg	200mg	Maximum oral dose must not
Alseroxylon fraction	2mg	d	—	2mg	2-4mg	4mg	be exceeded. Larger
Reserpine	0.1, 0.25mg	d	—	0.125mg	0.1-0.25mg	0.25mg	intramuscular doses of
Deserpidine	0.25mg	bd	—	0.25mg	0.25-0.5mg	0.5mg	reserpine (e.g. 2.5mg) can be used once or twice in an emergency
Adrenergic neurone blockers							
Guanethidine	10, 25mg	d (or bd for large doses)	Not less than 5-7 days	20mg	Variable	120mg	Maximum dose of these drugs can be exceeded, but it is better to add some other
Bethanidine	10, 50mg	td	1-2 days	15-30mg	Variable	180mg	drug or switch drugs. Dosage
Debrisoquine	10, 20mg	bd	2-4 days	10-20mg	Variable	150mg	of debrisoquine is genetically determined (see section 5.4)
MAO inhibitor							
Pargyline	25mg	td	2-4 days	25mg	Variable	150mg	

β -Adrenoceptor blockers							
Propranolol	10, 40, 80mg	bd or td	3-7 days	30mg	Variable	960mg	Effect is partly rapid (within hours), partly delayed (weeks). No absolute upper limit to dosage; higher doses have been used but most compounds have a ceiling dose. For b d regimens give two-thirds daily dose in morning and one-third at night; give once daily doses in the morning
Oxprenolol	20, 40, 80mg	bd or td		30mg	Variable	480mg	
Alprenolol	50, 100, 200mg	bd or td		100mg	Variable	800mg	
Pindolol	5mg	bd or td		5mg	Variable	30mg	
Timolol	10mg	bd or td		10mg	Variable	40mg	
Atenolol	100mg	d or bd		50mg	Variable	200mg	
Metoprolol	50, 100mg	bd or td		50mg	Variable	450mg	
Acebutolol	100, 300mg	bd or td		200mg	Variable	800mg	
α - and β -Adrenoceptor blocker							
Labetalol	100, 200mg	bd or td	1-2 days	200mg	400-800mg	2400mg	
CNS α -adrenoceptor stimulants							
Methyldopa	125, 250, 500mg	td	3 days	250-375mg	Variable	3g	Somnolence is less troublesome if initial dose is low. Maximum can be exceeded, but it is better to reduce the dose and add some other drug
Clonidine	0.15mg	td	2-4 days	0.15mg	Variable	1.8mg	Higher doses have been used
Vasodilators							
Hydrallazine	50mg	td	7-14 days	50-75mg	150-200mg	300mg	Maximum dose should not be exceeded (risk of autoimmune disease). Dosage lower in slow acetylators (section 5.9)
Prazosin	1, 2, 5mg[3]	bd or td	3-7 days	0.5mg[3]	Variable	20mg	Higher doses have been used. First dose *must* be small

1   General note: Clearly this type of table can give general guide lines only. The 'maximum' dose must in some cases not be exceeded; in other cases it is simply a matter of deciding whether further increments in dosage are worthwhile or whether a change to, or addition of, another drug would be better.

2   Frequency of dosage: 2d = every 2nd day; d = daily; bd = twice daily; td = three times a day. Sustained release formulations of some compounds are available, allowing less frequent administration than indicated.

3   In the USA, prazosin is available as capsules. Initial dosage is 1mg twice daily. The capsule formulation in the USA results in lower peak plasma concentrations of prazosin.

and also wiser, to carry out some investigations (e.g. for phaeochromocytoma) and observations before embarking on drug treatment.

On the other hand, very high blood pressures (particularly when the rise is relatively sudden) may be accompanied by clinical features which indicate extreme danger, e.g. severe headache, seizures and other evidence of encephalopathy, massive bleeding (from nose or kidney), or left ventricular failure.

If the main problem is left ventricular failure, then combined treatment with oxygen, morphine, digitalis and intravenous frusemide (furosemide) will in most cases relieve the acute condition so that the hypertension can be dealt with in a more leisurely manner. In hypertensive encephalopathy, on the other hand, it is imperative to reduce the blood pressure quickly (though not necessarily immediately to normal levels). The drug that achieves this most effectively is diazoxide (see section 5.11), given as a bolus intravenously (Koch-Weser, 1974b, 1976a). It is advisable to start with 150mg (i.e. half an ampoule) because an initial dose of 300mg may reduce the blood pressure rather more than desired. Depending on the response, further doses of 150 to 300mg or even 450mg can be given (always as a bolus intravenously). The total daily dose should not exceed 1200mg, and hyperglycaemia (which usually responds to tolbutamide) must be watched for. As soon as possible, other antihypertensive drugs should be substituted. Other drugs worth trying include labetalol intravenously (see section 5.7) or sodium nitroprusside by intravenous infusion (see section 4.5). Intravenous ganglion blocking drugs, which are capable of bringing down the blood pressure quickly, are now little used.

It must always be remembered that a proportion of hypertensive crisis situations are due to pressor amines; endogenous in phaeochromocytoma, exogenous after the ingestion of food amines or pressor drugs by patients taking monoamine oxidase inhibitors or after the ingestion of pressor drugs by patients on adrenergic neurone blockers (see section 10.1.1; 12.3). If there is any possibility of such factors being present, it is wise first to test the response of the patient's blood pressure to phentolamine 5mg intravenously. If a dramatic response occurs, phentolamine should be infused intravenously in glucose-saline at a rate adjusted to give control of the blood pressure. Labetalol also is often effective in these situations.

9. Hypertension in the Elderly

It is some times said that hypertension in the elderly should not be treated (e.g. Whitfield, 1972), the dividing line being set even as low as 60 years of age. The reasons given are partly that hypertension in the elderly is innocuous (Fry, 1974) and partly that the patients' lives are made miserable by the drugs. Most reports of the bad results of treatment in the elderly (e.g. Jackson et al., 1976) are in fact reports of the results of bad treatment, such as grossly excessive initial doses or poorly chosen drugs or two or more drugs started simultaneously. Such events should not be taken as evidence that antihypertensive treatment is to be avoided in the elderly. Elderly patients are by no means immune from left ventricular failure, cerebral haemorrhage and severe epistaxis, not to mention headache and giddiness due to hypertension, and there seems to be no valid reason to deny them therapy. Life insurance figures (Society of Actuaries, 1959) have shown that the adverse prognostic effects of a high pressure are present even in the 60 to 70 age group, and the Veterans Administration Study (1972) showed that treatment gives greater benefit in the older than in the younger patients. For a review of hypertension and its effects in the elderly, see Dyer et al. (1977).

The suggestion that elderly patients cannot be comfortable on antihypertensive therapy is not true. In most cases the blood pressure can be kept at reasonable levels without significant side effects. Certainly, antihypertensive therapy in the elderly must be managed with special care and insight. The objectives of treatment should be defined and the blood pressure should not be allowed to fall too low, e.g. below 130mm Hg systolic. Reduction of blood pressure should, if possible, be gradual. Postural hypotension must be avoided, both because it can lead to cerebral or coronary insufficiency and also because it can lead to loss of confidence by the patient who becomes reluctant, for instance, to venture out of the house alone. Thus posturally acting drugs are not the treatment of choice in this age group, though their use is by no means excluded.

In patients on long term treatment, it sometimes happens that dosage requirements diminish with age, e.g. when the patient enters his or her late sixties or early seventies. The reason for this is not clear. It could be due to gradually diminishing renal function or to a long term change in the factors maintaining the pressure at abnormally high levels. In any event it is important to be on the alert for the phenomenon, so that the blood pressure is not allowed to fall to undesirably low levels. If the blood pressure is persistently normal or low, then a trial of gradual withdrawal of therapy should be made, the patient being kept under reasonable observation.

In the choice of drugs, the usual rules apply: avoid any drug contraindicated in a particular patient and preferably try to lower lying as well as standing pressure. A diuretic is usually beneficial as part of the regimen though hypokalaemia and other side effects must of course be watched for (Editorial, 1978). Rauwolfia drugs can be useful in the elderly but the possibility of depression, even of a mild degree, must be avoided. If some drug other than a diuretic is required, a β-blocker or methyldopa are probably best tried first (see also chapter V; sect. 4.4).

10. Use of Drugs that May Affect Antihypertensive Therapy

10.1 Drugs that Interfere with Antihypertensive Therapy

The potential for significant adverse drug interactions in this field is very considerable (for reviews see Simpson, 1970; Nies, 1975). The main offending drugs are the sympathomimetic amines and the tricyclic antidepressants. The effects of these and other commonly used drugs in the hypertensive patient are summarised in table VIII.

10.1.1 Sympathomimetic Amines
Sympathomimetic drugs are capable of inhibiting the uptake of, and later displacing, adrenergic neurone blockers (guanethidine, bethanidine and debrisoquine) from their site of action in the sympathetic neurones (Gulati et al., 1966; Flegin et al., 1970). In addition, the adrenergic neurone blockers are known to sensitise the adrenoceptors to circulating pressor agents (Boura and Green, 1962).

The effects in man are seen either as a relative or complete blockade of the antihypertensive drug (e.g. in a patient already taking an anorexiant), or as a potentially disastrous sudden rise in blood pressure in a patient who is on established antihypertensive therapy and who starts taking a pressor drug. Oral eustachian tube decongestants and

many 'cold cures' and cough mixtures contain vasoconstrictors and therefore it is best to warn patients on antihypertensive treatment to avoid such substances. Phenylpropanolamine (Misage and McDonald, 1970), phenylephrine (Aminu et al., 1970), ephedrine (Starr and Petrie, 1972) and phentermine (Simpson, 1970) have been reported to cause sudden rises in blood pressure in patients receiving adrenergic neurone blocking antihypertensive agents. A similar phenomenon has been described with phenylpropanolamine in a patient taking methyldopa and oxprenolol (McLaren, 1976).

10.1.2 Antihistamines and Phenothiazines
Antihistamines have been shown in animal experiments to have α-adrenoceptor stimulant properties and to be capable of antagonising adrenergic neurone blocking drugs (Stone et al., 1964; Gokhale et al., 1966) and their use in patients receiving antihypertensive treatment, particularly with the adrenergic neurone blocking drugs, should therefore be viewed with some suspicion. Chlorpromazine has a similar effect both in animals (Stone et al., 1964) and in man at doses of 150mg or more daily (Fann et al., 1971b; Janowsky et al., 1973). Used by themselves, the phenothiazines have α-adrenoceptor blocking activity and can, of course, cause some reduction in blood pressure.

10.1.3 Tricyclic Antidepressants and Other Tricyclic Drugs
Many hypertensive patients are in an age group in which endogenous depression is common, and some of the drugs which are prescribed for their hypertension are of course capable of inducing depression (see tables II and IV). Thus, it is not uncommon for hypertensive patients at some stage to be considered for antidepressant therapy. The tricyclic antidepressant drugs block the antihypertensive effects of guanethidine, bethanidine and debrisoquine (see Crook and Nies, 1978; Stafford and Fann, 1977). They prevent the uptake of adrenergic neurone blocking drugs into the nerve endings by inhibiting the noradrenaline (norepinephrine) pump (see fig. 3) and also potentiate the effect of any noradrenaline that is released. This drug interaction is serious and has to be guarded against.

Expresssion of the loss of blood pressure control is time- and drug-related. With guanethidine, several days are required before the effect is

Table VIII. Effect of other drugs on antihypertensive therapy

Drug	Effect on antihypertensive therapy (see also text)
Digitalis	No special effect, but if diuretics are being given long term, make sure that there is no hypokalaemia
Antidiabetic Antibiotics Antiepileptic Analgesics Antithyroid Anticoagulants	No special effect noted in clinical situations
Antianxiety agents	Little effect; may lower blood pressure slightly
Antimigraine drugs	Patients on some types of antihypertensive therapy are more sensitive to vasoconstrictors. Ergotamine should be avoided in patients with hypertension. Pizotifen may antagonise adrenergic neurone blocking drugs
Phenothiazines	May lower blood pressure considerably. Chlorpromazine may antagonise guanethidine
Tricyclic antidepressants	Antagonise adrenergic neurone blockers and probably methyldopa (cocaine-like effect, prevent uptake of the adrenergic neurone blockers into the sympathetic axons). Desipramine may antagonise clonidine
Amphetamine-like drugs	All except fenfluramine antagonise adrenergic neurone blocking drugs; some combinations can cause severe hypertensive reactions. Fenfluramine can cause a fall in blood pressure, especially in patients on Rauwolfia or methyldopa
Vasoconstrictors (e.g. in cold cures, cough mixtures, nose drops etc.)	Patients on many antihypertensive drugs are more sensitive to vasoconstrictors (e.g. phenylephrine, ephedrine, pseudoephedrine, phenylpropanolamine), and blood pressure may rise
Antihistamines	Some of these have definite α-adrenoceptor stimulant properties and can cause rises in blood pressure in patients on antihypertensive drugs; can antagonise action of adrenergic neurone blockers
Oral contraceptives	Should preferably be stopped in any patient needing antihypertensive treatment; blood pressure *may* then fall. Even if it does not fall, and antihypertensive treatment remains necessary, it still is better that the risk of pill induced vascular damage and thrombosis be avoided in patients who are already at increased risk (applies mainly to oestrogen containing preparations)
Phenylbutazone Indomethacin	May cause some fluid retention and appear sometimes to make antihypertensive therapy more difficult
Bronchodilators (mainly β-adrenoceptor stimulants)	Effect on blood pressure is variable: they appear sometimes to make antihypertensive therapy more difficult
Antianginal	Glyceryl trinitrate may cause considerable temporary falls in blood pressure. Long acting nitrates have little effect on blood pressure. Prenylamine can cause a fall in blood pressure in patients on methyldopa or adrenergic neurone blockers
Liquorice (in excess) Carbenoxolone	Aldosterone-like effect. Can cause hypertension and can make antihypertensive treatment more difficult

noticeable, whereas the effect of the interaction is seen in a few hours with bethanidine (Mitchell et al., 1970; Mitchell and Oates, 1970). Amitriptyline, imipramine and particularly desipramine have a sufficiently marked inhibitory effect on the noradrenaline pump mechanism (see chapter XXVI; sect. 1.4.2) to readily antagonise the action of the adrenergic neurone blocking drugs. Doxepin has a less marked effect on the noradrenaline pump and antagonism of guanethidine and bethanidine develops slowly and only with doses of 200mg or more daily (Fann et al., 1971a). Regain of blood pressure control after the tricyclic antidepressant is discontinued is prolonged to as much as 5 to 8 days or more and an increased antagonistic effect may occur during the first few days after withdrawal (Fann et al., 1971; Mitchell et al., 1970).

Thus, patients on guanethidine, bethanidine or debrisoquine should not be given tricyclic antidepressants as the antihypertensive effect will in nearly all cases be lost. The evidence is less clear with methyldopa (Mitchell et al., 1970) but it is our impression that such antagonism can occur (Simpson and Waal-Manning, 1971). Desipramine can antagonise the action of clonidine (Briant et al., 1973), but Raftos et al. (1973) found no evidence of this with amitriptyline or imipramine. The anorexiant drug mazindol is another tricyclic drug that antagonises adrenergic neurone blockers (Boakes, 1977), as does pizotifen (Bailey, 1976), a tricyclic drug used as a migraine prophylactic. Chlorpromazine can have a similar effect (Fann et al., 1971b).

Patients with hypertension and depression can present considerable problems in therapy (Simpson, 1973). In handling such patients, it is essential first of all to make sure that the antihypertensive drugs are not causing or aggravating the depression. Thus, any patient who shows signs of depression while on antihypertensive therapy should not simply have an antidepressant added but should have this therapy reviewed so that an offending drug can be stopped and replaced by something else. At present the best antihypertensive therapy for a patient who requires to take a tricyclic antidepressant is probably a diuretic, plus a β-blocker (preferably other than propranolol), plus perhaps hydrallazine.

10.1.4 Bronchodilators

β-Adrenoceptor stimulating drugs, as used in asthma (see chapter XX; sect. 2.3.1), do not normally have any dramatic effects on blood pressure, though they may sometimes seem to make treatment of hypertension more difficult. They are usually given for good reasons and therefore can not be withheld, but it is probably wise to keep the dosage to a minimum. Theoretically a β-adrenoceptor stimulant such as isoprenaline (isoproterenol), which acts on both β_1 and β_2-adrenoceptors, could be expected, if given in sufficient dosage, to antagonise the antihypertensive effect of the β-blockers, but the latter should of course not be used in asthmatics, except when no other drugs will adequately control blood pressure. In such cases it may be justifiable to try (cautiously) a cardioselective β-blocker (i.e. β_1-blocker; see table III) with a β_2-adrenoceptor stimulant such as salbutamol (albuterol) or terbutaline (see chapter XX; sect. 10.1).

10.1.5 Drugs that Cause Sodium and Fluid Retention

Such drugs can sometimes cause problems in controlling hypertension, though less consistently and usually much less dramatically than sympathomimetics or tricyclic antidepressants. Carbenoxolone in particular may cause problems (Pinder et al., 1976), but its effect on fluid retention and blood pressure can be counteracted, at least in part, by thiazides or by spironolactone. However, spironolactone counteracts also the ulcer healing effect of carbenoxolone (Doll et al., 1968). The fluid retaining effect of phenylbutazone and indomethacin may sometimes make it necessary to increase the dose of diuretic. These drugs have also been reported to counteract the antihypertensive effect of β-blockers (Durao et al., 1977); the mechanism of this is not clear.

10.2 Drugs that Potentiate Antihypertensive Therapy

Lowering of blood pressure is usually what is desired, but if it occurs unexpectedly the results may not always be beneficial. An increase in diuretic dosage can lead to a considerable fall in blood pressure in patients on antihypertensive therapy. Phenothiazines, tricyclic antidepressants and MAO inhibitors may cause considerable falls in blood pressure, provided that they are not given in conjunction with adrenergic neurone blocking drugs (sect. 10.1). The appetite suppressant fenfluramine can potentiate many antihypertensive drugs (Waal-Manning and Simpson, 1969).

11. General Anaesthesia in Patients on Antihypertensive Therapy

This subject was dominated by the fear that patients might go into an untreatable hypotensive state, a fear that probably dated back to the time when large doses of reserpine were used. In these circumstances, certain pressor amines were found to be ineffective in raising the blood pressure, and there was also a tendency for cardiac arrhythmias to occur. Opinion subsequently has favoured the view that the dangers of reserpine in this respect were much overemphasised (Alper et al., 1963; Ominsky and Wollman, 1969).

The reason for the lack of pressor effect seems to have been that indirectly acting amines were used, the action of which depends on the presence of tissue stores of noradrenaline (norepinephrine) which are depleted by reserpine. If noradrenaline itself (or any other directly acting pressor amine such as methoxamine or metaraminol) had been used there would probably have been no problem in restoring the blood pressure to reasonable levels, and indeed most antihypertensive drugs render the patient *more* sensitive to the blood pressure raising effects of noradrenaline. The α-adrenoceptor blocking drugs could of course cause problems in this respect, particularly phenoxybenzamine, which has a long lasting effect. There seem to have been no problems reported so far with prazosin, which has postjunctional α-adrenoceptor blocking action (see section 4.5). However, in patients treated with labetalol (which has both α- and β-blocking actions; see section 5.7), blood pressure has been reported to be very sensitive to depth of halothane anaesthesia (Scott et al., 1976).

The action of the β-blockers is a competitive blockade which can be overcome by isoprenaline (isoproterenol) in sufficient dosage. There is evidence (Prys-Roberts et al., 1973; Foex and Prys-Roberts, 1974) that β-blockers may in fact protect against marked swings in blood pressure during intubation and that they should not be stopped before general anaesthesia. Interactions between general anaesthetics and antihypertensive drugs clearly can occur, but do not seem to be too troublesome provided that the pharmacology of the drugs is borne in mind (Dingle, 1966; Grogono and Lee, 1970; see chapter X, sect. 2.1; 6).

In general, therefore, the dangers of continuing the antihypertensive drugs over a period of surgery are probably less than the dangers of stopping them altogether (Prys-Roberts et al., 1971). However, it is common experience that blood pressure often falls after major surgery. On this account it is wise to reduce the dosage of antihypertensive drugs shortly before surgery and then readjust the dosage again subsequently. Diuretics should be continued during surgery. Any patient who is suddenly taken off long term diuretic therapy is liable to gain 1.5 to 3.0kg of fluid in a few days, and consequently may go into heart failure.

12. Drug Induced Hypertension

Certain drugs and combinations of drugs can cause hypertension. Before antihypertensive treatment is started, it is obviously best to ascertain that the patient is not taking a drug, or drugs, which can cause hypertension (for review, see Stokes, 1976).

12.1 Oestrogen Containing Preparations and Contraceptives

It is well established that a small rise in blood pressure is seen in many women taking an oestrogen-containing oral contraceptive and that some women develop significant hypertension (Laragh, 1976; Weir, 1978). Malignant hypertension due to oral contraceptives has been reported (Harris, 1969; Zech et al., 1975). The mechanism of the hypertension is believed to be an increase in plasma renin substrate, leading to increased plasma renin activity, but this occurs to almost the same extent in women who take oral contraceptives but do not become hypertensive. The fault may lie in a failure (Saruta et al., 1970) of the feedback system to slow down renin release from the kidney, or in some other factor (Laragh, 1976). It seems that both the oestrogen and the progestagen content may play a part (Royal College of General Practitioners, 1977). Low dose oestrogen preparations (30μg) are not necessarily free from risk (Meade et al., 1977).

Hypertension induced by oral contraceptives is susceptible to treatment with the usual drugs (Smith, 1972), but the price (not only in money but in potential morbidity) that is then being paid for the contraception really becomes somewhat unacceptable. It seems better to advise some other form of contraception in such cases. Particularly in the latter half of the childbearing period, prolonged therapy with oral contraceptives is inadvisable in anyone with a tendency to a raised blood pressure. Some more permanent form of contraception (tubal ligation, vasectomy) is preferable in this age group once a firm decision to have no further children has been taken.

12.2 Liquorice, Carbenoxolone

When taken in considerable quantities, liquorice has an aldosterone-like effect (Epstein et al., 1977) and can cause hypertension in those who are 'addicted' to it (Borst and Borst-de-Guis, 1963; Koster and David, 1968). Carbenoxolone, used in the treatment of peptic ulceration has a similar action and can cause fluid retention or hypertension (Pinder et al., 1976; see chapter XIX, sect. 4.3.4).

12.3 Drugs which Stimulate or Mimic Adrenergic Mechanisms

These include the monoamine oxidase (MAO) inhibitors, the tricyclic antidepressants, and various pressor agents and vasoconstrictors (e.g. common cold remedies; amphetamine-type anorexiants, but not fenfluramine). The MAO inhibitors, as is well known, prevent the destruction of pressor substances like tyramine in foodstuffs during absorption across the gut wall, and they potentiate the effect of sympathomimetic amines such as phenylephrine (Boakes et al., 1973) and phenylpropanolamine (Cuthbert et al., 1969). Debrisoquine also has some MAO inhibiting effect (Solomon et al., 1969) and cheese reactions have been reported in patients on this drug (Amery and Deloof, 1970). See further chapter X (sect. 6.2.1).

The tricyclic antidepressants prolong the action of noradrenaline (norepinephrine) by preventing its re-uptake into the sympathetic nerve endings. Alone, these drugs can sometimes reduce blood pressure a little, but any combination of them with anorexiant drugs or vasoconstrictors such as phenylephrine and phenylpropanolamine, or with antihistamines or antimigraine drugs, should be considered a possible cause of hypertension (Simpson, 1970). A hypertensive crisis has been reported in a woman given levodopa, carbidopa, metoclopramide and amitriptyline (Rampton, 1977).

Patients with migraine should never simply be treated symptomatically for their migraine unless this symptom persists despite good control of blood pressure. Vasoconstrictor drugs or pressor amines should, in general, not be given to patients with raised blood pressure.

Acknowledgement

The work of the Hypertension Clinic, Dunedin Public Hospital, on which the author's personal experience is based, is supported by the Otago Hospital Board and the Medical Research Council of New Zealand.

Further Reading

Moser, M. and others: Report of the Joint National Committee on Detection, Evaluation, and Treatment of High Blood Pressure: A cooperative study. Journal of the American Medical Association 237: 255 (1977).

Page, I.H.: Egregious errors in the management of hypertension. Journal of the American Medical Association 236: 2621 (1976).

Wollam, G.L.; Gifford, R.W. Jr. and Tarazi, R.C.: Antihypertensive drugs: Clinical pharmacology and therapeutic use. Drugs 14: 420-460 (1977).

References

Ablad, B.; Ljung, B. and Sannerstedt, R.: Haemodynamic effects of β-adrenoreceptor blockers in hypertension. Drugs 11(Suppl. 1): 127 (1976).

Ahearn, D.J. and Grim, C.E.: Treatment of malignant hypertension with sodium nitroprusside. Archives of Internal Medicine 133: 187 (1974).

Alarcon-Segovia, D.: Drug-induced antinuclear antibodies and lupus syndromes. Drugs 12: 69 (1976).

Alper, M.H.; Flacke, W. and Krayer, O.: Pharmacology of reserpine and its implications for anesthesia. Anesthesiology 24: 524 (1963).

Alvan, G.; Piafsky, K.; Lind, M. and von Bahr, C.: Effect of pentobarbital on the disposition of alprenolol. Clinical Pharmacology and Therapeutics 22: 316 (1977).

AMA Committee on Hypertension: The treatment of malignant hypertension and hypertensive emergencies. Journal of the American Medical Association 228: 1673 (1974).

Amery, A. and Deloof, W.: Cheese reaction during debrisoquine treatment. Lancet 2: 613 (1970).

Amery, A.; Billiet, L. and Fagard, R.: Beta receptors and renin release. New England Journal of Medicine 290: 284 (1974).

Amery, A.; Berthaux, P.; Bulpitt, C.; Deruyttere, M.; De Schaepdryver, A.; Dollery, C.; Fagard, R.; Forette, F.; Hellemans, J.; Lund-Johansen, P.; Mutsers, A. and Tuomilehto, J.: Glucose intolerance during diuretic therapy. Lancet 1: 681 (1978).

Ames, R.P. and Hill, P.: Increase in serum lipids during treatment of hypertension with chlorthalidone. Lancet 1: 71 (1976).

Aminu, J.; D'Mello, A. and Vere, D.W.: Interaction between debrisoquine and phenylephrine. Lancet 2: 935 (1970).

Andersson, R.: Cyclic AMP as a mediator of the relaxing action of papaverine, nitroglycerine, diazoxide and hydralazine in intestinal and vascular smooth muscle. Acta Pharmacologica et Toxicologica 32: 321 (1973).

Anderton, J.L. and Kincaid-Smith, P.: Diuretics II: Clinical considerations. Drugs 1: 141 (1971).

Armstrong, B.; Stevens, N. and Doll, R.: Retrospective study of the association between use of rauwolfia derivatives and breast cancer in English women. Lancet 2: 672 (1974).

Armstrong, B.; Skegg, D.; White, G. and Doll, R.: Rauwolfia derivatives and breast cancer in hypertensive women. Lancet 2: 8 (1976).

Assem, E.S.K.: Autoimmune phenomena and autoallergy in patients treated with β-adrenoreceptor blocking drugs; in Avery (Ed) β-Adrenoceptor Blocking Drugs, Cardiovascular Drugs, Vol. 2, p.209 (ADIS Press, Sydney; University Park Press, Baltimore 1977).

Bailey, R.R.: Antagonism of debrisoquine sulphate by pizotifen (Sandomigran). New Zealand Medical Journal 83: 449 (1976).

Bailey, R.R. and Neale, T.J.: Rapid clonidine withdrawal with blood pressure overshoot exaggerated by beta-blockade. British Medical Journal 1: 942 (1976).

Bailey, R.R.; Lynn, K.L.; Neale, T.L. and Little, P.J.: Prazosin in the treatment of patients with hypertension and renal functional impairment. New Zealand Medical Journal 84: 467 (1976).

Bartorelli, C.; Gargano, N.; Leonetti, G. and Zanchetti, A.: Hypotensive and renal effects of diazoxide, a sodium-retaining benzothiadiazine compound. Circulation 27: 895 (1963).

Bath, J.; Pickering, D. and Turner, R.: Clinical experience with bethanidine in treatment of hypertension. British Medical Journal 4: 519 (1967).

Bathen, J.: Propranolol erectile dysfunction relieved. Annals of Internal Medicine 88: 716 (1978).

Beevers, D.G.; Brown, J.J.; Ferriss, J.B.; Fraser, R.; Lever, A.F. and Robertson, J.I.S.: The use of spironolactone in the diagnosis and the treatment of hypertension associated with mineralocorticoid excess. American Heart Journal 86: 404 (1973a).

Beevers, D.G.; Fairman, M.J.; Hamilton, M. and Harpur, J.E.: Antihypertensive treatment and the course of established cerebral vascular disease. Lancet 1: 1407 (1973b).

Behan, P.O.; Behan, W.M.H.; Zacharias, F.J. and Nicholls, J.T.: Immunological abnormalities in patients who had the oculomucocutaneous syndrome associated with practolol therapy. Lancet 2: 984 (1976).

Bendall, M.J.; Baloch, K.H. and Wilson, P.R.: Side effects due to treatment of hypertension with prazosin. British Medical Journal 2: 727 (1975).

Berglund, G.; Andersson, O. and Wilhelmsen, L.: Prevalence of primary and secondary hypertension: Studies in a random population sample. British Medical Journal 2: 554 (1976).

Berglund, G.; Wilhelmsen, L.; Sannerstedt, R.; Hansson, L.; Anderson, O.; Sivertsson, R.; Wedel, H. and Wikstrand, J.: Coronary heart-disease after treatment of hypertension. Lancet 1: 1 (1978).

Bevegard, S.; Castenfors, J. and Danielson, M.: The effects of four months' treatment with spironolactone on systemic blood pressure, cardiac output and plasma renin activity in hypertensive patients. Acta Medica Scandinavica 202: 373 (1977).

Biglieri, E.G.: Hypertension with primary and secondary hyperaldosteronism. Postgraduate Medicine 52: 78 (1972).

Bjerle, P.; Jacobsson, K.-A. and Agert, G.: Paradoxical effect of pindolol. British Medical Journal 4: 284 (1975).

Blum, I.; Atsmon, A.; Steiner, M. and Wysenbeck, H.: Paradoxical rise in blood pressure during propranolol treatment. British Medical Journal 4: 623 (1975).

Boakes, A.J.: Antagonism of bethanidine by mazindol. British Journal of Clinical Pharmacology 4: 486 (1977).

Boakes, A.J.; Laurence, D.R.; Teoh, P.C.; Barar, F.S.K.; Benedikter, L.T. and Prichard, B.N.C.: Interactions between sympathomimetic amines and antidepressant agents in man. British Medical Journal 1: 311 (1973).

Bolli, P. and Simpson, F.O.: Clonidine in menopausal flushing: a double-blind trial. New Zealand Medical Journal 82: 196 (1975).

Bolli, P.; Wood, A.J. and Simpson, F.O.: Effects of prazosin in patients with hypertension. Clinical Pharmacology and Therapeutics 20: 138 (1976).

Bolli, P.; Waal-Manning, H.J.; Simpson, F.O. and Seeman, H.M.I.: Treatment of hypertension with labetalol. New Zealand Medical Journal 86: 557 (1977).

Bolli, P.; Simpson, F.O. and Waal-Manning, H.J.: Comparison of tienilic acid with cyclopenthiazide in hyperuricaemic hypertensive patients. Lancet 2: 595 (1978).

Borst, J.G.G. and Borst-de-Guis, A.: Hypertension explained by Starling's theory of circulatory homeostasis. Lancet 1: 677 (1963).

Boston Collaborative Drug Surveillance Program, Boston University Medical Center: Reserpine and breast cancer. Lancet 2: 669 (1974).

Boura, A.L.A. and Green, A.F.: Comparison of bretylium and guanethidine: tolerance, and effects of adrenergic nerve function and responses to sympathomimetic amines. British Journal of Pharmacology 19: 13 (1962).

Breckenridge, A.; Dollery, C.T. and Parry, E.H.O.: Prognosis of treated hypertension. Quarterly Journal of Medicine 39: 411 (1970).

Briant, R.H.; Reid, J.L. and Dollery, C.T.: Interaction between clonidine and desipramine in man. British Medical Journal 1: 522 (1973).

Briggs, R.S.J.; Birtwell, A.J. and Pohl, J.E.F.: Hypertensive response to labetalol in phaeochromocytoma. Lancet 1: 1045 (1978).

Brogden, R.N.; Speight, T.M. and Avery, G.S.: Mefruside: A preliminary report of its pharmacological properties and therapeutic efficacy in oedema and hypertension. Drugs 7: 419 (1974).

Brogden, R.N.; Heel, R.C.; Speight, T.M. and Avery, G.S.: Prazosin: A review of its pharmacological properties and therapeutic efficacy in hypertension. Drugs 14: 163 (1977).

Brogden, R.N.; Heel, R.C.; Speight, T.M. and Avery, G.S.: Labetalol: A review of its pharmacology and therapeutic use in hypertension. Drugs 15: 251 (1978).

Brown, J.J.; Davies, D.L.; Lever, A.F. and Robertson, J.I.S.: Plasma renin concentration in human hypertension. I: Relationship between renin, sodium, and potassium. British Medical Journal 2: 144 (1965).

Brunner, H.R.; Gavras, H. and Laragh, J.H.: Angiotensin II blockade in man by sar-ala-Angiotensin II for understanding and treatment of high blood pressure. Lancet 2: 1045 (1973).

Buhler, F.R.; Laragh, J.H.; Baer, L.; Vaughan, E.D. Jr. and Brunner, H.R.: Propranolol inhibition of renin secretion. A specific approach to diagnosis and treatment of renin-dependent hypertensive diseases. New England Journal of Medicine 287: 1209 (1972).

Buhler, F.R.; Burkart, F.; Lutold, B.E.; Kung, M.; Marbet, G. and Pfisterer, M.: Antihypertensive beta blocking action as related to renin and age: A pharmacologic tool to identify pathogenetic mechanisms in essential hypertension. American Journal of Cardiology 36: 653 (1975).

Buhler, F.R.; Bertel, O. and Lutold, B.E.: Simplified and age-stratified antihypertensive therapy based on beta blockers. Cardiovascular Medicine 3: 135 (1978).

Cambridge, D.; Davey, M.J. and Massingham, R.: The pharmacology of antihypertensive drugs with special reference to vasodilators, α-adrenergic blocking agents and prazosin. Medical Journal of Australia Special Supplement 2: 2 (1977).

Carey, R.M.; Douglas, J.G.; Schweikert, R. and Liddle, G.W.: The syndrome of essential hypertension and suppressed plasma renin activity. Archives of Internal Medicine 130: 849 (1972).

Carney, S.; Morgan, T.; Wilson, M.; Matthews, G. and Roberts, R.: Sodium restriction and thiazide diuretics in the treatment of hypertension. Medical Journal of Australia 1: 803 (1975).

Carter, A.B.: Hypotensive therapy in stroke survivors. Lancet 1: 485 (1970).

Castenfors, J.; Johnsson, H. and Oro, L.: Effect of alprenolol on blood pressure and plasma renin activity in hypertensive patients. Acta Medica Scandinavica 193: 189 (1973).

Castleden, C.M.; Dathan, J.R.E. and George, C.F.: A comparison of once and twice daily atenolol in hypertension. Postgraduate Medical Journal 53: 679 (1977).

Cavero, I.; Fenard, S.; Gomeni, R.; Lefevre, F. and Roach, A.G.: Studies in the mechanism of the vasodilator effects of prazosin in dogs and rabbits. European Journal of Pharmacology 49: 259 (1978).

Chamberlain, G.V.P.; Lewis, P.J.; de Swiet, M. and Bulpitt, C.J.: How obstetricians manage hypertension in pregnancy. British Medical Journal 1: 626 (1978).

Chang, C.C.; Costa, E. and Brodie, B.B.: Interaction of guanethidine with adrenergic neurons. Journal of Pharmacology and Experimental Therapeutics 147: 303 (1965).

Christensen, C.C.; Boye, N.P.; Erikson, H. and Hansen, G.: Influence of pindolol (visken) on respiratory function in 20 asthmatic patients. European Journal of Clinical Pharmacology 13: 9 (1978).

Christopher, L.J.; Crooks, J.; Davidson, J.F.; Erskine, Z.G.; Gallon, S.C.; Moir, D.C. and Weir, R.D.: A multicentre study of rauwolfia derivatives and breast cancer. European Journal of Clinical Pharmacology 11: 409 (1977).

Cocco, G.; Burkart, F.; Chu, D. and Follath, F.: Intrinsic sympathomimetic activity of β-adrenoceptor blocking agents. European Journal of Clinical Pharmacology 13: 1 (1978).

Constantine, J.W.; McShane, W.K.; Scriabine, A. and Hess, H.J.: Analysis of the hypotensive action of prazosin; in Onesti, Kim and Moyer (Eds) Hypertension — Mechanisms and Management p.1695 (Grune and Stratton, New York 1973).

Conway, J.; Greenwood, D.T. and Middlemiss, D.N.: Central nervous actions of β-adrenoreceptor antagonists. Clinical Science and Molecular Medicine 54: 119 (1978).

Crook, J.E. and Nies, A.S.: Drug interactions with antihypertensive drugs. Drugs 15: 72 (1978).

Curtis, J.R. and Bateman, F.J.: Use of prazosin in management of hypertension in patients with chronic renal failure. British Medical Journal 4: 432 (1975).

Cuthbert, M.F.; Greenberg, M.P. and Morley, S.W.: Cough and cold remedies: a potential danger to patients on monoamine oxidase inhibitors. British Medical Journal 1: 404 (1969).

Dargie, H.J. and Dollery, C.T.: Adverse reactions to diuretic drugs; in Meyler's Side Effects of Drugs. Annual I, chapter 19 (Excerpta Medica, Amsterdam 1977).

Dargie, H.J.; Dollery, C.T. and Daniel, J.: Minoxidil in resistant hypertension. Lancet 2: 515 (1977).

Davidson, C.; Thadani, U.; Singleton, W. and Taylor, S.H.: Comparison of antihypertensive activity of beta-blocking drugs during chronic treatment. British Medical Journal 2: 7 (1976).

Davies, D.L. and Wilson, G.M.: Diuretics: Mechanism of action and clinical application. Drugs 9: 178 (1975).

Day, M.D. and Rand, M.J.: Some observations on the pharmacology of α-methyldopa. British Journal of Pharmacology 22: 72 (1964).

Deacon, S.P. and Barnett, D.: Comparison of atenolol and propranolol during insulin-induced hypoglycaemia. British Medical Journal 2: 272 (1976).

de Champlain, J.; Farley, L.; Cousineau, D. and van Ameringen, M-R.: Circulating catecholamine levels in human and experimental hypertension. Circulation Research 38: 109 (1976).

Derkx, F.H.M.; v. Gool, J.M.G.; Wenting, G.J.; Verhoeven, R.P.; Man in't Veld, A.J. and Schalekamp, M.A.D.H.: Inactive renin in human plasma. Lancet 2: 496 (1976).

Dingle, H.R.: Antihypertensive drugs and anaesthesia. Anaesthesia 21: 151 (1966).

Doll, R.; Langman, M.J.S. and Shawdon, H.H.: Treatment of gastric ulcer with carbenoxolone: antagonistic effect of spironolactone. Gut 9: 42 (1968).

Dollery, C.T.; Pentecost, B.L. and Samaan, N.A.: Drug-induced diabetes. Lancet 2: 735 (1962).

Doyle, A.E.; Jerums, G.; Johnston, C.I. and Louis, W.J.: Plasma renin levels and vascular complications in hypertension. British Medical Journal 2: 206 (1973).

Drayer, J.I.M.; Keim, H.J.; Weber, M.A.; Case, D.B. and Laragh, J.H.: Unexpected pressor responses to propranolol in essential hypertension. American Journal of Medicine 60: 897 (1976).

DuCharme, D.W.; Freyburger, W.A.; Graham, B.E. and Carlson, R.G.: Pharmacologic properties of minoxidil: A new hypotensive agent. Journal of Pharmacology and Experimental Therapeutics 184: 662 (1973).

Durao, V.; Prata, M.M. and Goncalves, L.M.P.: Modification of antihypertensive effect of β-adrenoceptor-blocking agents by inhibition of endogenous prostaglandin synthesis. Lancet 2: 1005 (1977).

Dyer, A.R.; Stamler, J.; Shekelle, R.B.; Schoenberger, J.A. and Farinaro, E.: Hypertension in the elderly. Medical Clinics of North America 61: 513 (1977).

Editorial: Side effects of methyldopa. British Medical Journal 1: 646 (1975a).

Editorial: Beta-blockers in anxiety and stress. British Medical Journal 1: 415 (1976).

Editorial: Hazards of non-practolol beta-blockers. British Medical Journal 1: 529 (1977a).

Editorial: Catecholamines in essential hypertension. Lancet 1: 1088 (1977b).

Editorial: Diuretics in the elderly. British Medical Journal 1: 1092 (1978).

Eliahou, H.E.; Silverberg, D.S.; Reisin, E.; Romem, I.; Mashiach, S. and Serr, D.M.: Propranolol for hypertension of pregnancy. British Journal of Obstetrics and Gynaecology 85: 431 (1978).

Epstein, M.T.; Espiner, E.A.; Donald, R.A. and Hughes, H.: Effect of eating liquorice on the renin-angiotensin aldosterone axis in normal subjects. British Medical Journal 1: 488 (1977).

Fang, P.; Macdonald, I.; Laver, M.; Hua, A. and Kincaid-Smith, P.: Oral diazoxide in uncontrolled malignant hypertension. Medical Journal of Australia 2: 621 (1974).

Fann, W.E.; Cavanaugh, J.H.; Kaufmann, J.S.; Griffith, J.D.; Davis, J.M.; Janowsky, D.S. and Oates, J.A.: Doxepin: effects on transport of biogenic amines in man. Psychopharmacologia 22: 111 (1971a).

Fann, W.E.; Janowsky, D.S.; Davis, J.M. and Oates, J.A.: Chlorpromazine reversal of the antihypertensive action of guanethidine. Lancet 2: 436 (1971).

Finnerty, F.A. Jr.: Hypertensive crisis. Journal of the American Medical Association 229: 1479 (1974).

Flegin, O.T.; Morgan, D.H.; Oates, J.A. and Shand, D.G.: The mechanism of the reversal of the effect of guanethidine by amphetamines in cat and man. British Journal of Pharmacology 39: 253 (1970).

Foex, P. and Prys-Roberts, C.: Anaesthesia and the hypertensive patient. British Journal of Anaesthesia 46: 575 (1974).

Formgren, H.: The effect of metoprolol and practolol on lung function and blood pressure in hypertensive asthmatics. British Journal of Clinical Pharmacology 3: 1007 (1976).

Franciosa, J.A.; Guiha, N.H.; Limas, C.J.; Rodriguera, E. and Cohn, J.N.: Improved left ventricular function during nitroprusside infusion in acute myocardial infarction. Lancet 1: 650 (1972).

Freis, E.D.: Salt, volume and the prevention of hypertension. Circulation 53: 589 (1976).

Fry, J.: Natural history of hypertension. A case for selective non-treatment. Lancet 2: 431 (1974).

Fyhrquist, F.; Kurppa, K.; Huuskonen, M. and Koistinen, A.: Blood pressure and renin during treatment with pindolol. Acta Medica Scandinavica 202: 55 (1977).

Gallery, E.D.M.; Saunders, D.M.; Hunyor, S.N. and Gyory, A.Z.: Hypertension in pregnancy. Medical Journal of Australia 1: 540 (1978).

Gavras, H.; Brunner, H.R.; Laragh, J.H.; Sealey, J.E.; Gavras, I. and Vukovich, R.A.: An angiotensin converting-enzyme inhibitor to identify and treat vasoconstrictor and volume factors in hypertensive patients. New England Journal of Medicine 291: 817 (1974).

Gavras, H.; Brunner, H.R.; Turini, G.A.; Kershaw, G.R.; Tifft, C.P.; Cuttelod, S.; Gavras, I.; Vukovich, R.A. and McKinstry, D.N.: Antihypertensive effect of the oral angiotensin converting-enzyme inhibitor SQ 14225 in man. New England Journal of Medicine 298: 991 (1978).

Ghose, R.R.; Mathur, Y.B.; Upadhyay, M.; Morgan, W.D. and Khan, S.: Treatment of hypertensive emergencies with oral labetalol. British Medical Journal 2: 96 (1978).

Gibb, W.E.; Malpas, J.S.; Turner, P. and White, R.J.: Comparison of bethanidine, α-methyldopa, and reserpine in essential hypertension. Lancet 2: 275 (1970).

Gifford, R.W.: Reserpine and guanethidine in the treatment of hypertension; in Onesti, Kim and Moyer (Eds) Hypertension: Mechanisms and Management, p.305 (Grune and Stratton, New York 1973).

Gifford, R.W.: Drug combinations as rational antihypertensive therapy. Archives of Internal Medicine 133: 1053 (1974).

Gifford, R.W. Jr. and Tarazi, R.C.: Resistant hypertension: diagnosis and management. Annals of Internal Medicine 88: 661 (1978).

Gokhale, S.D.; Gulati, O.D. and Udwadia, B.P.: Antagonism of the adrenergic neurone blocking action of guanethidine by certain antidepressant and antihistamine drugs. Archives Internationales de Pharmacodynamie et de Therapie 160: 321 (1966).

Goldberg, A.D.; Raftery, E.B. and Wilkinson, P.: Blood pressure and heart rate and withdrawal of antihypertensive drugs. British Medical Journal 1: 1243 (1977).

Gombos, E.A.; Freis, E.D. and Moghadam, A.: Effects of MK-870 in normal subjects and hypertensive patients. New England Journal of Medicine 275: 1215 (1966).

Gottlieb, T.B.; Katz, F.H. and Chidsey, C.A.: Combined therapy with vasodilator drugs and beta-adrenergic blockade in hypertension. A comparative study of minoxidil and hydralazine. Circulation 45: 571 (1972).

Graham, R.M.; Thornell, I.R.; Gain, J.M.; Bagnoli, C.; Oates, H.F. and Stokes, G.S.: Prazosin: the first-dose phenomenon. British Medical Journal 2: 1293 (1976).

Greenblatt, D.J. and Koch-Weser, J.: Adverse reactions to β-adrenergic receptor blocking drugs: A report from the Boston Collaborative Drug Surveillance Program. Drugs 7: 118 (1974).

Grogono, A.W. and Lee, P.: Danger lists for the anaesthetist. Anaesthesia 25: 518 (1970).

Gross, F.: Beta-adrenergic blockade, blood pressure, and the renin-angiotensin system. European Journal of Clinical Investigation 7: 321 (1977).

Gulati, O.D.; Dave, B.T.; Gokhale, S.D. and Shah, K.M.: Antagonism of adrenergic neuron blockade in hypertensive subjects. Clinical Pharmacology and Therapeutics 7: 510 (1966).

Guyton, A.C.; Coleman, T.G.; Cowley, A.W. Jr.; Scheel, K.W.; Manning, R.D. Jr. and Norman, R.A. Jr.: Arterial pressure regulation. Overriding dominance of the kidneys in long-term regulation and in hypertension. American Journal of Medicine 52: 584 (1972).

Hansson, B-G.; Dymling, J-F.; Manhem, P. and Hokfelt, B.: Long-term treatment of moderate hypertension with the beta₁-receptor blocking agent metoprolol. II. Effect of submaximal work and insulin-induced hypoglycaemia on plasma catecholamines and renin activity, blood pressure and pulse rate. European Journal of Clinical Pharmacology 11: 247 (1977).

Harris, P.W.R.: Malignant hypertension associated with oral contraceptives. Lancet 2: 466 (1969).

Hayes, J.M.: Prazosin in severe hypertension. Effect on blood pressure, plasma renin activity and in hypertensive emergencies. The Medical Journal of Australia Special Supplement 2: 30 (1977).

Heise, A. and Kroneberg, G.: Central nervous α-adrenergic receptors and the mode of action of α-methyldopa. Nauyn-Schmiedeberg's Archiv fur Pharmakologie 279: 285 (1973).

Helgeland, A.; Hjermann, I.; Leren, P. and Holme, I.: Possible metabolic side effects of beta-adrenergic blocking drugs. British Medical Journal 1: 828 (1978a).

Helgeland, A.; Hjermann, I.; Leren, P.; Enger, S. and Holme, I.: High-density lipoprotein cholesterol and antihypertensive drugs: the Oslo study. British Medical Journal 2: 403 (1978b).

Helson, L. and Duque, L.: Acute brain syndrome after propranolol. Lancet 2: 98 (1978).

Hodge, J.V.; McQueen, E.G. and Smirk, F.H.: Results of hypotensive therapy in arterial hypertension. Based on experience with 497 patients treated and 156 controls, observed for periods of one to eight years. British Medical Journal 1: 1 (1960).

Homeida, M.; Jackson, L. and Roberts, C.J.C.: Decreased first-pass metabolism of labetalol in chronic liver disease. British Medical Journal 2: 1048 (1978).

Horvath, J.S.; Woolcock, A.J.; Tiller, D.J.; Donnelly, P.; Armstrong, J. and Caterson, R.: A comparison of metoprolol and propranolol on blood pressure and respiratory function in patients with hypertension. Australian and New Zealand Journal of Medicine 8: 1 (1978).

Hua, A.S.P.; Assaykeen, T.A.; Nyberg, G. and Kincaid-Smith, P.S.: Results from a multicentre trial of metoprolol and a study of hypertensive patients with chronic obstructive lung disease. Medical Journal of Australia 1: 281 (1978).

Hunyor, S.N.; Hansson, L.; Harrison, T.S. and Hoobler, S.W.: Effects of clonidine withdrawal: Possible mechanisms and suggestions for management. British Medical Journal 2: 209 (1973).

Ibsen, H. and Sederberg-Olsen, P.: Changes in glomerular filtration rate during long-term treatment with propranolol in patients with arterial hypertension. Clinical Science 44: 129 (1973).

Jackson, G.; Pierscianowski, T.A.; Mahon, W. and Condon, J.: Inappropriate antihypertensive therapy in the elderly. Lancet 2: 1317 (1976).

Janowsky, D.S.; El-Yousef, M.K.; Davis, J.M. and Fann, W.E.: Antagonism of guanethidine by chlorpromazine. American Journal of Psychiatry 130: 808 (1973).

Johnson, B.F.; Bye, C.; Labrooy, J.; Munro-Faure, D. and Slack, J.: The relation of antihypertensive treatment to plasma lipids and other risk factors in hypertensives. Clinical Science and Molecular Medicine 47: 9 (1974).

Johnsson, G. and Regardh, C.-G.: Clinical pharmacokinetics of β-adrenoreceptor blocking drugs. Clinical Pharmacokinetics 1: 223 (1976).

Johnston, C.I.: Effect of antihypertensive drugs on the renin-angiotensin system. Drugs 12: 274 (1976).

Joyce, D.N. and Kenyon, V.G.: The use of diazepam and hydrallazine in the treatment of severe pre-eclampsia. Journal of Obstetrics and Gynaecology of the British Commonwealth 79: 250 (1972).

Kanada, S.A.; Kanada, D.J.; Hutchinson, R.A. and Wu, D.: Angina-like syndrome with diazoxide therapy for hypertensive crisis. Annals of Internal Medicine 84: 696 (1976).

Kaplan, N.M.: The prognostic implications of plasma renin in essential hypertension. Journal of the American Medical Association 231: 167 (1975).

Karlberg, B.E.; Kagedal, B.; Tegler, L.; Tolagen, K. and Bergman, B.: Controlled treatment of primary hypertension with propranolol and spironolactone. A crossover study with special reference to initial plasma renin activity. American Journal of Cardiology 37: 642 (1976).

Kather, H. and Simon, B.: β-adrenoceptor blocking agents and human fat cell adenylate cyclase. British Journal of Clinical Pharmacology 4: 499 (1977).

Kincaid-Smith, P. and Hua, A.S.P.: Beta-adrenergic blocking agents in renal failure. British Medical Journal 3: 520 (1974).

Koch-Weser, J.: Vasodilator drugs in the treatment of hypertension. Archives of Internal Medicine 133: 1017 (1974a).

Koch-Weser, J.: Hypertensive emergencies. New England Journal of Medicine 290: 211 (1974b).

Koch-Weser, J.: Diazoxide. New England Journal of Medicine 294: 1271 (1976a).

Koch-Weser, J.: Hydralazine. New England Journal of Medicine 295: 320 (1976b).

Koch-Weser, J.: The comeback of hydralazine. Editorial. American Heart Journal 95: 1 (1978).

Koster, M. and David, G.K.: Reversible severe hypertension due to licorice ingestion. New England Journal of Medicine 278: 1381 (1968).

Knight, A.H. and Parkinson, T.: Diuretic-induced hyperkalaemia. Lancet 1: 446 (1967).

Kremer, D.; Boddy, K.; Brown, J.J.; Davies, D.L.; Fraser, R.; Lever, A.F.; Morton, J.J. and Robertson, J.I.S.: Amiloride in the treatment of primary hyperaldosteronism and essential hypertension. Clinical Endocrinology 7: 151 (1977).

Krikler, D.: Verapamil in cardiology. European Journal of Cardiology 2: 3 (1974).

Kwan, K.C.; Foltz, E.L.; Breault, G.O.; Baer, J.E. and Totaro, J.A.: Pharmacokinetics of methyldopa in man. Journal of Pharmacology and Therapeutics 198: 264 (1976).

Lake, C.R.; Ziegler, M.G.; Coleman, M.D. and Kopin, I.J.: Age-adjusted plasma norepinephrine levels are similar in normotensive and hypertensive subjects. New England Journal of Medicine 296: 208 (1977).

Laragh, J.H.: Oral contraceptive-induced hypertension — nine years later. American Journal of Obstetrics and Gynecology 126: 141 (1976).

Laragh, J.H.: The renin system in high blood pressure, from disbelief to reality; converting enzyme blockade for analysis and treatment. Progress in Cardiovascular Diseases 31: 159 (1978).

Laragh, J.H.; Baer, L.; Brunner, H.R.; Buhler, F.R.; Sealey, J.E. and Darracott Vaughan, E. Jr.: Renin, angiotensin and aldosterone system in pathogenesis and management of hypertensive vascular disease. American Journal of Medicine 52: 633 (1972).

Leather, H.M.; Humphreys, D.M.; Baker, P. and Chadd, M.A.: A controlled trial of hypotensive agents in hypertension in pregnancy. Lancet 2: 488 (1968).

Leonetti, G.; Mayer, G.; Morganti, A.; Terzoli. L.; Zanchetti, A.; Bianchetti, G.; di Salle, E.; Morselli, P.L. and Chidsey, C.A.: Hypotensive and renin-suppressing activities of propranolol in hypertensive patients. Clinical Science and Molecular Medicine 48: 491 (1975).

Lewis, P.J.; George, C.F. and Dollery, C.T.: Clinical evaluation of indoramin, a new antihypertensive agent. European Journal of Clinical Pharmacology 6: 211 (1973).

Lewis, P.J.; Kohner, E.M.; Petrie, A. and Dollery, C.T.: Deterioration of glucose tolerance in hypertensive patients on prolonged diuretic treatment. Lancet 1: 564 (1976).

Lewis, G.R.J.; Morley, K.D.; Lewis, B.M. and Bones, P.J.: The treatment of hypertension with verapamil. New Zealand Medical Journal 87: 351 (1978).

Louis, W.J.; Doyle, A.E. and Anavekar, S.: Plasma norepinephrine levels in essential hypertension. New England Journal of Medicine 288: 599 (1973).

Lund-Johansen, P.: Haemodynamic changes at rest and during exercise in long-term prazosin therapy of essential hypertension; in Cotton (Ed) Prazosin-Evaluation of a New Antihypertensive Agent p.43 (Excerpta Medica, Amsterdam 1974).

Lund-Johansen, P.: Hemodynamic effects of clonidine in man; in Onesti, Fernandes and Kim (Eds) Regulation of Blood Pressure by the Central Nervous System p.355 (Grune and Stratton, New York 1976).

Lund-Johansen, P. and Ohm, O.J.: Haemodynamic long-term effects of β-receptor-blocking agents in hypertension: a comparison between alprenolol, atenolol, metoprolol and timolol. Clinical Science and Molecular Medicine 51: 481s (1976).

MacCarthy, P.; Isaac, P.; Frost, G.; Freeman, A. and Stokes, G.: Clinical dose-response studies with guanfacine (BS 100-141) a new antihypertensive agent. Clinical and Experimental Pharmacology and Physiology 5: 187 (1978a).

MacCarthy, E.P.; Frost, G.W. and Stokes, G.S.: Labetalol in hypertensive emergencies. Medical Journal of Australia 1: 399 (1978b).

MacDougall, A.I.; Addis, G.J.; MacKay, N.; Dymock, I.W.; Turpie, A.G.G.; Ballinghall, D.L.K.; MacLennan, W.J.; Whiting, B. and MacArthur, J.G.: Treatment of hypertension with clonidine. British Medical Journal 3: 440 (1970).

MacGillivray, I.: The current approach to hypertension in pregnancy. South African Medical Journal 51: 657 (1977).

McDevitt, D.G.: Adrenoceptor blocking drugs: Clinical pharmacology and therapeutic use. Drugs 17: 267-288 (1979).

McDonald, W.J.; Smith, G.; Woods, J.W.; Perry, H.M. and Danielson, B.D.: Intravenous diazoxide therapy in hypertensive crisis. American Journal of Cardiology 40: 409 (1977).

McLaren, E.H.: Severe hypertension produced by interaction of phenylpropanolamine with methyldopa and oxprenolol. British Medical Journal 2: 283 (1976).

McMahon, F.G.: Rauwolfia alkaloids and derivatives; in McMahon (Ed) Management of Essential Hypertension p.317 (Futura Publishing Company, New York 1978).

McMartin, C. and Simpson, P.: The absorption and metabolism of guanethidine in hypertensive patients requiring different doses of the drug. Clinical Pharmacology and Therapeutics 12: 73 (1971).

Mahgoub, A.; Idle, J.R.; Dring, L.C.; Lancaster, R. and Smith, R.L.: Polymorphic hydroxylation of debrisoquine in man. Lancet 2: 584 (1977).

Marshall, A.J.; Roberts, C.J.C. and Barritt, D.W.: Raynaud's phenomenon as side effect of beta-blockers in hypertension. British Medical Journal 1: 1498 (1976).

Martin, J.D.: A critical survey of drugs used in the treatment of hypertensive crises of pregnancy. Medical Journal of Australia 2: 252 (1974).

Martin, L.E.; Hopkins, R. and Bland, R.: Metabolism of labetalol by animals and man. British Journal of Clinical Pharmacology 3(Suppl. 3): 695 (1976).

Meade, T.W.; Chakrabarti, R.; Haines, A.P.; Howarth, D.J.; North, W.R.S. and Stirling, Y.: Haemostatic, lipid, and blood pressure profiles of women on oral contraceptives containing 50µg or 30µg oestrogen. Lancet 2: 948 (1977).

Melander, A.; Danielson, K.; Schersten, B. and Wahlin, E.: Enhancement of the bioavailability of propranolol and metoprolol by food. Clinical Pharmacology and Therapeutics 22: 108 (1977).

Miller, R.R.; Olson, H.G.; Amsterdam, E.A. and Mason, D.T.: Propranolol-withdrawal rebound phenomenon. Exacerbation of coronary events after abrupt cessation of antianginal therapy. New England Journal of Medicine 293: 416 (1975).

Miller, R.R.; Awan, N.A.; Maxwell, K.S. and Mason, D.T.: Sustained reduction of cardiac impedance and preload in congestive heart failure with the antihypertensive vasodilator prazosin. New England Journal of Medicine 297: 303 (1977).

Misage, J.R. and McDonald, R.H. Jr.: Antagonism of hypotensive action of bethanidine by "common cold" remedy. British Medical Journal 4: 347 (1970).

Mitchell, J.R. and Oates, J.A.: Guanethidine and related agents. I. Mechanism of the selective blockade of adrenergic neurons and its antagonism by drugs. Journal of Pharmacology and Experimental Therapeutics 172: 100 (1970).

Mitchell, J.R.; Cavanaugh, J.H.; Arias, L. and Oates, J.A.: Guanethidine and related agents. III. Antagonism by drugs which inhibit the norepinephrine pump in man. Journal of Clinical Investigation 49: 1596 (1970).

Mitchell, H.C. and Pettinger, W.A.: Long-term treatment of refractory hypertensive patients with minoxidil. Journal of the American Medical Association 239: 2131 (1978).

Morgan, T.; Adam, W.; Gillies, A.; Wilson, M.; Morgan, G. and Carney, S.: Hypertension treated by salt restriction. Lancet 1: 227 (1978).

Moser, M. and others: Report of the Joint National Committee on Detection, Evaluation, and Treatment of High Blood Pressure: A cooperative study. Journal of the American Medical Association 237: 255 (1977).

Mroczek, W.J.; Davidov, M.A. and Finnerty, F.A. Jr.: Large dose furosemide therapy for hypertension. Long-term use in 22 patients. American Journal of Cardiology 33: 546 (1974).

Mukherjee, D.; Feldman, M.S. and Helfant, R.H.: Nitroprusside therapy. Treatment of hypertensive patients with recurrent resting chest pain, ST-segment elevation, and ventricular arrhythmias. Journal of the American Medical Association 235: 2406 (1976).

Myers, M.G.; Lewis, G.R.J.; Steiner, J. and Dollery, C.T.: Atenolol in essential hypertension. Clinical Pharmacology and Therapeutics 19: 502 (1976).

Myhre, E.; Brodwall, E.K.; Stenbaek, O. and Hansen, T.: Plasma turnover of methyldopa in advanced renal failure. Acta Medica Scandinavica 191: 343 (1972a).

Myhre, E.; Stenbaek, O.; Brodwall, E.K. and Hansen, T.: Conjugation of methyldopa in renal failure. Scandinavian Journal of Clinical and Laboratory Investigation 29: 195 (1972b).

Nemati, M.; Kyle, M.C. and Freis, E.D.: Clinical study of ticrynafen. A new diuretic, antihypertensive, and uricosuric agent. Journal of the American Medical Association 237: 652 (1977).

New Zealand Hypertension Study Group: Initial experience with prazosin in New Zealand. A multicentre report. Medical Journal of Australia Special Supplement 2: 23 (1977).

Ng, J.; Phelan, E.L.; McGregor, D.D.; Laverty, R.; Taylor, K.M. and Smirk, F.H.: Properties of catapres, a new hypotensive drug: A preliminary report. New Zealand Medical Journal 66: 864 (1967).

Nickersen, M. and Collier, B.: Drugs inhibiting adrenergic nerves and structures innervated by them; in Goodman and Gilman (Eds) The Pharmacological Basis of Therapeutics p.557 (Macmillan Publishing Co., New York 1975).

Nies, A.S.: Adverse reactions and interactions limiting the use of antihypertensive drugs. American Journal of Medicine 58: 495 (1975).

Nijkamp, F.P.; Ezer, J. and de Jong, W.: Central inhibitory effect of α-methyldopa on blood pressure, heart rate and body temperature of renal hypertensive rats. European Journal of Pharmacology 31: 243 (1975).

Nilsson, A.; Hansson, B.-G. and Hokfelt, B.: Effect of metoprolol on blood glycerol, free fatty acids, triglycerides and glucose in relation to plasma catecholamines in hypertensive patients at rest and following submaximal work. European Journal of Clinical Pharmacology 13: 5 (1978).

Oates, J.A.; Gillespie, L.; Udenfriend, S. and Sjoerdsma, A.: Decarboxylase inhibition and blood pressure reduction by α-methyl-3,4-dihydroxy-DL-phenylalanine. Science 131: 1890 (1960).

O'Malley, K.; Segal, J.L.; Israili, Z.H.; Boles, M.; McNay, J.L. and Dayton, P.G.: Duration of hydralazine action in hypertension. Clinical Pharmacology and Therapeutics 18: 581 (1975).

O'Malley, K.; Velasco, M.; Wells, J. and McNay, J.: Mechanism of the interaction of propranolol and a potent vasodilator antihypertensive agent — minoxidil. European Journal of Clinical Pharmacology 9: 355 (1976).

Ominsky, A.J. and Wollman, H.: Hazards of general anesthesia in the reserpinized patient. Anesthesiology 30: 443 (1969).

Ondetti, M.A.; Rubin, B. and Cushman, D.W.: Design of specific inhibitors of angiotensin-converting enzyme: New class of orally active antihypertensive agents. Science 196: 441 (1977).

O'Rourke, D.A. and Hede, J.E.: Reversible leg ischaemia due to diuretics. British Medical Journal 1: 1114 (1978).

Osborne, D.R.: Propranolol and Peyronie's disease. Lancet 1: 1111 (1977).

Page, I.H.: Egregious errors in the management of hypertension. Journal of the American Medical Association 236: 2621 (1976).

Page, L.B.: Epidemiologic evidence on the etiology of human hypertension and its possible prevention. American Heart Journal 91: 527 (1976).

Page, L.B. and Sidd, J.J.: Medical management of primary hypertension (first of three parts). New England Journal of Medicine 287: 960 (1972a).

Page, L.B. and Sidd, J.J.: Medical management of primary hypertension (second of three parts). New England Journal of Medicine 287: 1018 (1972b).

Page, L.B. and Sidd, J.J.: Medical management of primary hypertension (third of three parts). New England Journal of Medicine 287: 1074 (1972c).

Palmer, R.F. and Lasseter, K.C.: Sodium nitroprusside. New England Journal of Medicine 292: 294 (1975).

Paterson, J.W.; Dollery, C.T. and Haslam, R.M.: Amiloride hydrochloride in hypertensive patients. British Medical Journal 1: 422 (1968).

Pearson, R.M. and Havard, C.W.H.: Intravenous labetalol in hypertensive patients given by fast and slow injection. British Journal of Clinical Pharmacology 5: 401 (1978a).

Pearson, R.M. and Havard, C.W.H.: Treatment of severe and resistant hypertension. British Journal of Hospital Medicine 20: 447 (1978b).

Pedersen, O.L.: Does verapamil have a clinically significant antihypertensive effect? European Journal of Clinical Pharmacology 13: 21 (1978).

Peltola, P.: Furosemide (Lasix) as a diuretic. Acta Medica Scandinavica 177: 777 (1965).

Pennington, J.C. and Picker, R.H.: Diazoxide and the treatment of the acute hypertensive emergency in obstetrics. Medical Journal of Australia 2: 1051 (1972).

Perry, H.M. and Smith, W.M. (Eds): Mild hypertension: To treat or not to treat. Annals of the New York Academy of Sciences 304: 1 (1978).

Pinder, R.M.; Brogden, R.N.; Sawyer, P.R.; Speight, T.M.; Spencer, R. and Avery, G.S.: Carbenoxolone: A review of its pharmacological properties and therapeutic efficacy in peptic ulcer disease. Drugs 11: 245 (1976).

Pohl, J.E.F.; Thurston, H. and Swales, J.D.: Oral diazepoxide in resistant hypertension with renal impairment: Review of 100 cases. International Congress of Nephrology, Mexico. Abstract p.397 (1972).

Prichard, B.N.C.: Pressor responses to beta-adrenergic-blocking drugs. Lancet 1: 536 (1977).

Prichard, B.N.C. and Gillam, P.M.S.: Treatment of hypertension with propranolol. British Medical Journal 1: 7 (1969).

Prichard, B.N.C.; Johnston, A.W.; Hill, I.D. and Rosenheim, M.L.: Bethanidine, guanethidine and methyldopa in treatment of hypertension: a within-patient comparison. British Medical Journal 1: 135 (1968).

Prys-Roberts, C.; Meloche, R. and Foex, P.: Studies of anaesthesia in relation to hypertension. I: Cardiovascular responses of treated and untreated patients. British Journal of Anaesthesia 43: 122 (1971).

Prys-Roberts, C.; Foex, P.; Biro, G.P. and Roberts, J.G.: Studies of anaesthesia in relation to hypertension v: Adrenergic beta-receptor blockade. British Journal of Anaesthesia 45: 671 (1973).

Raftos, J.; Bauer, G.E.; Lewis, R.G.; Stokes, G.S.; Mitchell, A.S. and Young, A.A.: Clonidine in the treatment of severe hypertension. Medical Journal of Australia 1: 786 (1973).

Rahn, K.H.: Plasma levels and renal excretion of guanethidine in hypertensive patients. Arzneimittel Forschung 21: 1487 (1971).

Rampton, D.S.: Side effects of drugs. Hypertensive crisis in a patient given sinemet, metoclopramide, and amitriptyline. British Medical Journal 2: 607(1977).

Ramsay, L.E.; Ramsay, M.H.; Hettiarachchi, J.; Davies, D.L. and Winchester, J.: Weight reduction in a blood pressure clinic. British Medical Journal 2: 244 (1978).

Rand, M.J.; Law, M.; Story, D.F. and McCulloch, M.W.: Effects of β-adrenoreceptor blocking drugs on adrenergic transmission. Drugs 11(Suppl. 1): 134 (1976).

Redman, C.W.G.; Beilin, L.J.; Bonnar, J. and Ounsted, M.K.: Fetal outcome in trial of antihypertensive treatment in pregnancy. Lancet 2: 753 (1976).

Reisin, E.; Abel, R.; Modan, M.; Silverberg, D.S.; Eliahou, H.E. and Modan, B.: Effect of weight loss without salt restriction on the reduction of blood pressure in overweight hypertensive patients. New England Journal of Medicine 298: 1 (1978).

Reybrouck, T.; Amery, A.; Fagard, R.; Jousten, P.; Lijnen, P. and Meulepas, E.: Beta-blockers: once or three times a day? British Medical Journal 1: 1386 (1978).

Roberts, J.M. and Perloff, D.L.: Hypertension and the obstetrician-gynecologist. American Journal of Obstetrics and Gynecology 127: 316 (1977).

Robson, R.H.: Recurrent migraine after propranolol. British Heart Journal 39: 1157 (1977).

Rodman, J.S.; Deutsch, D.J. and Gutman, S.I.: Methyldopa hepatitis. A report of six cases and review of the literature. American Journal of Medicine 60: 941 (1976).

Rosei, E.A.; Brown, J.J.; Fraser, R.; Lever, A.F.; Morton, J.J.; Robertson, J.I.S. and Trust, P.M.: Labetalol (AH5158), a competitive alpha- and beta-receptor blocking drug, in the management of hypertension. Australian and New Zealand Journal of Medicine 6: 83 (1976a).

Rosei, E.A.; Brown, A.F.; Lever, A.F.; Robertson, A.S.;

Robertson, J.I.S. and Trust, P.M.: Treatment of phaeochromocytoma and of clonidine withdrawal hypertension with labetalol. British Journal of Clinical Pharmacology 3(Suppl. 3): 809 (1976b).

Rosendorff, C.: Comparison of indoramin and methyldopa in hypertension. South African Medical Journal 50: 764 (1976).

Royal College of General Practitioners' Oral Contraception Study: Effect on hypertension and benign breast disease of progestagen component in combined oral contraceptives. Lancet 1: 624 (1977).

Royds, R.B.; Coltart, D.J. and Lockhart, J.D.F.: Pharmacologic studies of indoramin in man. Clinical Pharmacology and Therapeutics 13: 380 (1972).

Rubin, B.; Laffan, R.J.; Kotler, D.G.; O'Keefe, E.H.; Demaio, D.A. and Goldberg, M.E.: SQ 14,225 (D-3-Mercapto-2-methylpropanoyl-1-proline) a novel orally active inhibitor of angiotensinI-converting enzyme. Journal of Pharmacology and Experimental Therapeutics 204: 271 (1978).

Saameli, K.; Scholtysik, G. and Waite, R.: Pharmacology of BS 100-141, a centrally acting antihypertensive drug. Clinical and Experimental Pharmacology and Physiology Suppl. 2: 207 (1975).

Saruta, T.; Saade, G.A. and Kaplan, N.M.: A possible mechanism for hypertension induced by oral contraceptives. Archives of Internal Medicine 126: 621 (1970).

Schlittler, E. and Bein, H.J.: Rauwolfia alkaloids; in Schlittler (Ed) Antihypertensive Agents p.191 (Academic Press, New York 1967).

Schmitt, H.; Schmitt, H. Mme and Fenard, S.: Evidence for an α-sympathomimetic component in the effects of catapresan on vasomotor centres: antagonism by piperoxane. European Journal of Pharmacology 14: 98 (1971).

Scott, D.B.; Buckley, F.P.; Drummond, G.B.; Littlewood, D.G. and MacRae, W.R.: Cardiovascular effects of labetalol during halothane anaesthesia. British Journal of Clinical Pharmacology 3(Suppl. 3): 817 (1976).

Shah, S.; Khatri, I. and Freis, E.D.: Mechanism of antihypertensive effect of thiazide diuretics. American Heart Journal 95: 611 (1978).

Shand, D.G.: Pharmacokinetic properties of the β-adrenergic receptor blocking drugs. Drugs 7: 39 (1974).

Shand, D.G.: Pharmacokinetic properties of the β-adrenoreceptor blocking drugs; in Avery (Ed) Cardiovascular Drugs, Vol. 2 p.41 (ADIS Press, Sydney 1977).

Shaw, J.; England, J.D.F. and Hua, A.S.P.: Beta-blockers and plasma triglycerides. British Medical Journal 1: 986 (1978).

Shen, D.; Gibaldi, M.; Throne, M.; Bellward, G.; Cunningham, R.; Israili, Z.; Dayton, P. and McNay, J.: Pharmacokinetics of bethanidine in hypertensive patients. Clinical Pharmacology and Therapeutics 17: 363 (1975).

Shiroff, R.A.; Mathis, J.; Zelis, R.; Schneck, D.W.; Babb, J.D.; Leaman, D.M. and Hayes, A.J. Jr.: Propranolol rebound — a retrospective study. American Journal of Cardiology 41: 778 (1978).

Silas, J.H.; Lennard, M.S.; Tucker, G.T.; Smith, A.J.; Malcolm, S.L. and Marten, T.R.: Why hypertensive patients vary in their response to debrisoquine. British Medical Journal 1: 422 (1977).

Silas, J.H.; Lennard, M.S.; Tucker, G.T.; Smith, A.J.; Malcolm, S.L. and Marten, T.R.: The disposition of debrisoquine in hypertensive patients. British Journal of Clinical Pharmacology 5: 27 (1978).

Simpson, F.O.: Combination antihypertensive therapy. Cardiovascular Clinics 2: 38 (1970).

Simpson, F.O.: Hypertension and depression and their treatment. Australian and New Zealand Journal of Psychiatry 7: 1 (1973).

Simpson, F.O.: β-Adrenergic receptor blocking drugs in hypertension. Drugs 7: 85 (1974).

Simpson, F.O.: β-Adrenoreceptor blocking drugs in hypertension; in Avery (Ed) Cardiovascular Drugs p.55 (ADIS Press, Sydney 1977).

Simpson, F.O.: Hypertension. British Medical Journal 2: 882 (1978).

Simpson, F.O.; Bolli, P. and Wood, A.J.: Use of prazosin at the Dunedin Hypertension Clinic. Controlled and open studies and pharmacokinetic observations. Medical Journal of Australia, Special Supplement 2: 17 (1977).

Simpson, F.O. and Gilchrist, A.R.: Prognosis in untreated hypertensive vascular disease. Scottish Medical Journal 3: 1 (1958).

Simpson, F.O. and Waal-Manning, H.J.: Hypertension and depression: interrelated problems in therapy. Journal of the Royal College of Physicians of London 6: 14 (1971).

Simpson, F.O.; Waal-Manning, H.J.; Bolli, P.; Phelan, E.L. and Spears, G.F.S.: Relationship of blood pressure to sodium excretion in a population survey. Clinical Science and Molecular Medicine 55 (Suppl. 4): 373S (1978).

Skinner, C.; Gaddie, J. and Palmer, K.N.V.: Comparison of intravenous AH 5158 (ibidomide) and propranolol in asthma. British Medical Journal 2: 59 (1975).

Smith, R.W.: Hypertension and oral contraception. American Journal of Obstetrics and Gynaecology 113: 482 (1972).

Society of Actuaries: Build and blood pressure study 1 (1959).

Solheim, S.B.; Sundsfjord, J.A. and Giezendanner, L.: The effect of spironolactone (aldactone) and methyldopa in low and normal renin hypertension. Acta Medica Scandinavica 197: 451 (1975).

Solomon, H.M.; Ashley, C.; Spirt, N. and Abrams, W.B.: The influence of debrisoquin on the accumulation and metabolism of biogenic amines by the human platelet, in vivo and in vitro. Clinical Pharmacology and Therapeutics 10: 229 (1969).

Smith, R.W.: Hypertension and oral contraception. American Journal of Obstetrics and Gynecology 113: 482 (1972).

Spark, R.F. and Melby, J.C.: Hypertension and low plasma renin activity: Presumptive evidence for mineralocorticoid excess. Annals of Internal Medicine 75: 831 (1971).

Spiekerman, R.E.; Berge, K.C.; Thurber, D.L.; Gedge, S.W. and McGuckin, W.F.: Potassium-sparing effects of triamterene in the treatment of hypertension. Circulation 34: 524 (1966).

Speight, T.M. and Avery, G.S.: Diazoxide: A review of its pharmacological properties and therapeutic use in hypertensive crises. Drugs 2: 78 (1971).

Stafford, J.R. and Fann, W.E.: Drug interactions with guanidinium antihypertensives. Drugs 13: 57 (1977).

Starr, K.J. and Petrie, J.C.: Drug interactions in patients on long-term oral anticoagulant and antihypertensive adrenergic neuron-blocking drugs. British Medical Journal 4: 133 (1972).

Stokes, G.S.: Drug-induced hypertension: Pathogenesis and management. Drugs 12: 222 (1976).

Stokes, G.S. and Oates, H.F.: Prazosin: new alpha-adrenergic blocking agent in treatment of hypertension. Cardiovascular Medicine 3: 41 (1978).

Stokes, G.S.; Weber, M.A. and Thornell, I.R.: β-blockers and plasma renin activity in hypertension. British Medical Journal 1: 60 (1974).

Stokes, G.S.; Graham, R.M. and Weber, M.A.: The role of renin in the antihypertensive action of β-adrenoreceptor blocking agents. Drugs 11(Suppl. 1): 150 (1976).

Stone, C.A.; Porter, C.C.; Stavorski, J.M.; Ludden, C.T. and Totaro, J.A.: Antagonism of certain effects of catecholamine-depleting agents by antidepressant and related drugs. Journal of Pharmacology and Experimental Therapeutics 144: 196 (1964).

Stumpe, K.O.; Kolloch, R.; Vetter, H.; Gramann, W.; Kruck, F.; Ressel, Ch. and Higuchi, M.: Acute and long-term studies of the mechanisms of action of beta-blocking drugs in lowering blood pressure. American Journal of Medicine 60: 853 (1976).

Swainson, C.P. and Winney, R.J.: Effect of beta-blockade in chronic renal failure. British Medical Journal 1: 459 (1976).

Taguchi, J. and Freis, E.D.: Partial reduction of blood pressure and prevention of complications in hypertension. New England Journal of Medicine 291: 329 (1974).

Talbot, S.; O'Malley, B.C. and Bing, R.F.: Debrisoquine, guanethidine and bethanidine in hypertension. British Medical Journal 2: 278 (1975).

Talseth, T.: Clinical pharmacokinetics of hydrallazine. Clinical Pharmacokinetics 2: 317 (1977).

Tcherdakoff, P.H.; Colliard, M.; Berrard, E.; Kreft, C.; Dupay, A. and Bernaille, J.M.: Propranolol in hypertension during pregnancy. British Medical Journal 2: 670 (1978).

Tester-Dalderup, C.B.M.: Hypotensive drugs; in Dukes (Ed) Meyler's Side Effects of Drugs p.461 (Excerpta Medica, Amsterdam 1977).

Topliss, D. and Bond, R.: Acute brain syndrome after propranolol treatment. Lancet 2: 1133 (1977).

Trinker, F.R.: The significance of the relative potencies of noradrenaline and α-methylnoradrenaline for the mode of action of α-methyldopa. Journal of Pharmacy and Pharmacology 23: 306 (1971).

Trust, P.M.; Rosei, E.A.; Brown, J.J.; Fraser, R.; Lever, A.F.; Morton, J.J. and Robertson, J.I.S.: Effect of blood pressure, angiotensin II and aldosterone concentrations during treatment of severe hypertension with intravenous labetalol: Comparison with propranolol. British Journal of Clinical Pharmacology 3(Suppl. 3): 799 (1976).

Turnbull, L.B.; Teng, L.; Newman, J.; Chremos, A.N. and Bruce, R.B.: Disposition of bethanidine, N-benzyl-N',N''-dimethylguanidine, in the rat, dog and man. Drug Disposition and Metabolism 4: 269 (1976).

Tuzel, I.H.: Sodium nitroprusside: A review of its clinical effectiveness as a hypotensive agent. Journal of Clinical Pharmacology 14: 494 (1974).

Valnes, K.; Hillestad, L.; Hansen, T. and Arnold, E.: Alpha-methyldopa and drug fever. Acta Medica Scandinavica 204: 21 (1978).

Vanholder, R.; Carpentier, J.; Schurgers, M. and Clement, D.L.: Rebound phenomenon during gradual withdrawal of clonidine. British Medical Journal 1: 1138 (1977).

van Zwieten, P.A.: The central action of antihypertensive drugs, mediated via central α-receptors. Journal of Pharmacy and Pharmacology 25: 89 (1973).

Veterans Administration Cooperative Study Group on Antihypertensive Agents: Effects of treatment on morbidity in hypertension. Results in patients with diastolic blood pressure averaging 115 through 129mm Hg. Journal of the American Medical Association 202: 1029 (1967).

Veterans Administration Cooperative Study Group on Antihypertensive Agents: Effects of treatment on morbidity in hypertension. II. Results in patients with diastolic blood pressure averaging 90 through 114mm Hg. Journal of the American Medical Association 213: 1143 (1970).

Veterans Administration Cooperative Study Group on Antihypertensive Agents: Effects of treatment on morbidity of hypertension. III. Influence of age, diastolic pressure, and prior cardiovascular disease; further analysis of side effects. Circulation 45: 991 (1972).

Waal-Manning, H.J.: Effect of equivalent antihypertensive doses of mefruside and cyclopenthiazide on serum electrolytes, uric acid and glucose tolerance in hypertensive patients. Clinical and Experimental Pharmacology and Physiology 2: 141 (1975a).

Waal-Manning, H.J.: Problems with practolol. Drugs 10: 336 (1975b).

Waal-Manning, H.J.: Metabolic effects of β-adrenoreceptor blockers. Drugs 11(Suppl. 1): 121 (1976a).

Waal-Manning, H.J.: Experience with β-adrenoreceptor blockers in hypertension. Drugs 11(Suppl. 1): 164 (1976b).

Waal-Manning, H.J.: Hypertension: Which beta-blocker? Drugs 12: 412 (1976c).

Waal-Manning, H.J.: Can β-blockers be used in diabetic patients? Drugs 17: 157 (1979).

Waal-Manning, H.J. and Simpson, F.O.: Fenfluramine in obese patients on various antihypertensive drugs. Lancet 2: 1392 (1969).

Waal-Manning, H.J. and Simpson, F.O.: Pindolol: A comparison with other antihypertensive drugs and a double-blind placebo trial. New Zealand Medical Journal 80: 151 (1974).

Waal-Manning, H.J. and Simpson, F.O.: Paradoxical effect of pindolol. British Medical Journal 3: 155 (1975).

Waal-Manning, H.J. and Simpson, F.O.: A fixed combination of amiloride hydrochloride and hydrochlorothiazide in the treatment of hypertension: Recent studies; in Magnani (Ed) Diuresis, Kaliuresis, and Hypertension, p.48 (Futura Publishing Co., Mt. Kisco, New York 1977).

Warren, S.C. and Warren, S.G.: Propranolol and sexual impotence. Annals of Internal Medicine 86: 112 (1977).

Warren, D.J.; Swainson, C.P. and Wright, N.: Deterioration in renal function after beta-blockade in patients with chronic renal failure and hypertension. British Medical Journal 2: 193 (1974).

Weir, R.J.: When the pill causes a rise in blood pressure. Drugs 16: 522 (1978).

Whitfield, A.G.W.: Iatrogenic misadventure. British Medical Journal 1: 733 (1972).

Wilburn, R.L.; Blaufuss, A. and Bennett, C.M.: Long-term treatment of severe hypertension with minoxidil, propranolol and furosemide. Circulation 52: 706 (1975).

Wilcox, R.G.: Randomised study of six beta-blockers and a thiazide diuretic in essential hypertension. British Medical Journal 2: 383 (1978).

Wilhelmsen, L.: Beta-blockers and plasma triglycerides. British Medical Journal 1: 1348 (1978).

Williams, J.G.; de Voss, K. and Craswell, P.W.: Labetalol in the treatment of hypertensive renal patients. Medical Journal of Australia 1: 225 (1978).

Wilson, D.F.; Watson, O.F.; Peel, J.S. and Turner, A.S.: Trasicor in angina pectoris: A double-blind trial. British Medical Journal 2: 155 (1969).

Wilson, H.M.; Wilson, J.P.; Slaton, P.E.; Foster, J.H.; Liddle, G.W. and Hollifield, J.W.: Saralasin infusion in the recognition of renovascular hypertension. Annals of Internal Medicine 87: 36 (1977).

Wilson, J.D.; Bullock, J.Y.; Sutherland, D.C.; Main, C. and O'Brien, K.P.: Antinuclear antibodies in patients receiving non-practolol beta-blockers. British Medical Journal 1: 14 (1978).

Wohl, A.J.; Hausler, L.M. and Roth, F.E.: Mechanism of the antihypertensive effect of diazoxide: *in vitro* vascular studies in the hypertensive rat. Journal of Pharmacology and Experimental Therapeutics 162: 109 (1968).

Wollam, G.L.; Gifford, R.W. Jr. and Tarazo, R.C.: Antihypertensive drugs: Clinical pharmacology and therapeutic use. Drugs 14: 420 (1977).

Wood, A.J.; Phelan, E.L. and Simpson, F.O.: Cardiovascular effects of prazosin in normotensive and genetically hypertensive rats. Clinical and Experimental Pharmacology and Physiology 2: 297 (1975).

Woods, J.W.; Pittman, A.W.; Pulliam, C.C.; Werk, E.E. Jr.; Waider, W. and Allen, C.A.: Renin profiling in hypertension and its use in treatment with propranolol and chlorthalidone. New England Journal of Medicine 294: 1137 (1976).

Woosley, R.L. and Nies, A.S.: Guanethidine. New England Journal of Medicine 295: 1053 (1976).

Young, D.W.; Cottam, J. and Hoult, J.G.: Complication of oxprenolol treatment. Lancet 2: 1133 (1977).

Zanchetti, A.; Stella, A.; Leonetti, G.; Morganti, A. and Terzoli, L.: Control of renin release: A review of experimental evidence and clinical implications. American Journal of Cardiology 37: 675 (1976).

Zech, P.; Rifle, G.; Lindner, A.; Sassard, J.; Blanc-Brunat, N. and Traeger, J.: Malignant hypertension with irreversible renal failure due to oral contraceptives. British Medical Journal 4: 326 (1975).

Chapter XIX
Gastrointestinal and Hepatic Diseases

S. Bank, S.J. Saunders, I.N. Marks, B.H Novis and G.O. Barbezat

Synopsis of Important Principles

1) The absorption of some orally administered drugs can be markedly influenced by gastrointestinal disease, but malabsorption is unpredictable. Abnormal drug responses due to altered bioavailability, protein binding or delayed elimination can occur in severe liver disease with drugs mainly eliminated by the liver, particularly with drugs with a low therapeutic ratio. Liver disease may also alter the pharmacological response to some drugs.

2) Medical treatment of peptic ulcer is directed towards relief of symptoms, healing the ulcer completely and attempts to delay or prevent recurrences. Initial treatment is based on adequate physical and emotional rest; advice on stopping smoking and avoiding alcohol and caffeinated beverages; graduated bed rest, where feasible or required; and drugs to prevent or relieve symptoms, or to hasten ulcer healing.

3) Treatment of intestinal malabsorption syndromes is aimed at eradicating the primary disease and its effects, or if this is not possible, by diet or replacement therapy appropriate for the type of deficiency.

4) Diarrhoea and constipation not due to an underlying organic disease can be readily controlled by appropriate symptomatic therapy. Any persistent or severe bowel derangement must be fully investigated.

5) Acute attacks or relapses of ulcerative colitis or Crohn's disease must be managed promptly, the intensity of treatment depending on the severity of the attack. Medical treatment can reduce the number of relapses in ulcerative colitis but surgery is often necessary in Crohn's disease.

6) Treatment of pancreatitis depends on the nature of structural or functional derangement of the pancreas. Initial therapy of painful pancreatitis is based solely on clinical presentation, whereas interval therapy is based on aetiological, radiological and patho-functional considerations.

7) General management of most liver diseases involves a nutritious high protein diet and vitamin K_1 if the prothrombin index is low. Corticosteroids are valuable in chronic active hepatitis. Permanent abstinence from alcohol is the aim of treatment in alcoholic cirrhosis.

8) Many drugs can cause gastrointestinal or hepatic reactions. Few reactions are serious, but many cause much morbidity and diagnostic confusion. Diarrhoea is the most common side effect of drugs. Antibiotic induced diarrhoea must always be investigated if more than trivial. Aspirin and other 'ulcerogenic' drugs may aggravate peptic ulcer and morphine or overvigorous diuretic therapy can precipitate hepatic coma in susceptible patients with cirrhosis.

Gastrointestinal and liver diseases are major causes of morbidity and mortality with vast therapeutic implications. In 1968 in the USA, digestive diseases were responsible for 9 % of all deaths, 10 to 15 % hospital admissions, a third of all major operations and 11 % of chronic illness in the population, with a total cost of $15 billion per year. 10 years later the problem had become so vast that the Secretary of Health instituted a National Digestive Disease Commission.

When the frequency of minor gastric and colonic disorders and the proclivity of infective hepatitis, peptic ulcer, gastric, colonic and pancreatic cancer is considered, it is not surprising that gastrointestinal disease is the leading cause of industrial absenteeism, armed forces layoffs and disability and compensation claims. These statistics highlight the frequency with which the medical profession will be called upon to investigate and treat digestive diseases. The rapidly increasing exploration of physiological and psychomotor mechanisms, biochemical aberrations and even trial and error methodology, is being utilised to provide rational therapy in the large variety of major and minor gastrointestinal disorders. Thus, the combined efforts of physiology, pharmacology, psychotherapy and surgery are attempting to find a rational if not specific therapeutic treatment for peptic ulcer, whilst immunologists, dietitians and even paramedical personnel (e.g. stoma therapists) have improved the life style of patients with ulcerative colitis and Crohn's disease. The aetiology of many gastrointestinal diseases remains obscure, but even in these, symptomatic therapy is usually highly successful, and at present the high relapse rate of many of these conditions has inspired research towards lasting remission if not permanent cures.

1. Clinical Pharmacological Considerations

Although physiological and biochemical changes which can alter drug pharmacokinetics do occur in gastrointestinal and liver disease, many changes are unpredictable or of poorly defined clinical significance. Abnormal responses can occur with some drugs (section 13), because of altered sensitivity to the pharmacological action of the drug and occasionally because of altered absorption, distribution or elimination. Adjustment of dosage is needed in some of these cases, while other drugs are best avoided.

1.1 Drug Absorption and Gastrointestinal Disease

In certain circumstances it is obvious that oral administration of a drug is unreliable; for example, in repeated vomiting and intestinal obstruction. Otherwise, potential clinically significant abnormalities of drug absorption are most likely to be related to conditions associated with an altered rate of gastric emptying or gastrointestinal transit and to intestinal malabsorption syndromes (see Nimmo, 1976; Parsons, 1977).

1.1.1 Gastrointestinal Function

Physiological factors within the gut which can affect absorption of orally administered drugs include the pH of gastrointestinal secretion, gastric emptying rate and intestinal motility, the activity of gastrointestinal drug metabolising enzymes or drug metabolising bacteria and the surface area of the gut.

According to the pH partition hypothesis (see chapter I; sect. 1.1), weak acids such as aspirin should be absorbed more slowly in achlorhydric patients but studies have observed the opposite effect; plasma salicylate concentrations being higher and peak concentrations attained more rapidly (Pottage et al., 1974). Salicylamide is also absorbed more rapidly from the stomach than normal in patients with pernicious anaemia and more slowly in patients with peptic ulcer. The differences were not marked and absorption in other patients with achlorhydria without pernicious anaemia, did not differ from the normal controls (Hartiala et al., 1963). The stomach is generally not an important site of drug absorption (Prescott, 1974a,b). Drugs are absorbed more rapidly from the upper small intestine than from the stomach, probably because of the much greater surface area of the intestine (Levine, 1970). Unless absorption by the small bowel is normally very slow, the rate of gastric emptying can therefore markedly influence the rate at which orally administered drugs are absorbed, irrespective of whether they are weak acids, weak bases or neutral compounds.

Many factors affect the rate of gastric emptying (table I) and have the potential to alter the rate of absorption of orally administered drugs (Nimmo, 1976). Alteration in the gastric emptying rate or in intestinal motility, in most cases results in a change in the *rate* of absorption, but for some drugs, such as those which are poorly soluble or erratically absorbed or metabolised in the gut, the

Table 1. Some factors which influence the rate of gastric emptying (after Nimmo, 1976)

	Increased rate	Decreased rate
Gastric ulcer		+
Duodenal ulcer	+	
Pyloric stenosis		+
Migraine		+
Myocardial infarction		+
Labour		+
Trauma and pain		+
Anticholinergic drugs		+
Tricyclic antidepressants		+
Narcotic analgesics		+
Antacids		
Sodium bicarbonate	+	
Aluminium hydroxide		+
Metoclopramide	+	

amount of drug absorbed can be altered. The clinical significance of delayed or slow absorption depends on the circumstances. It may be important if a rapid onset of action is required, or if elimination is so rapid that effective plasma concentrations can not be attained (e.g. drugs with a short half-life).

In patients with delayed gastric emptying and pyloric stenosis, absorption of drugs such as paracetamol (acetaminophen)[1] and aspirin may be markedly impaired (Heading et al., 1973; Nimmo et al., 1973), and is particularly likely with enteric coated or slow release formulations (Harris, 1973; Leonards and Levy, 1965). Therapeutic failure of orally administered drugs seems inevitable in patients with gastric stasis. The absorption of effervescent aspirin is delayed in patients during an attack of migraine and this delay correlates well with the severity of headache and gastrointestinal symptoms. It seems to be due to a delay in gastric emptying during attacks of migraine since aspirin absorption and relief of symptoms is improved by intramuscular metoclopramide, which increases gastric emptying rate (Volans, 1978). Alteration in intestinal transit time can affect the amount of drug available for absorption in the case of drugs subject to gut metabolism. Levodopa may be ineffective in patients with slow gastric emptying or slow gastrointestinal transit, as large amounts of the drug can then be metabolised in the gut wall during its first passage through the intestine (chapter VI; sect. 5). Slow gastrointestinal transit can lead to a decrease in the effective plasma concentration of chlorpromazine, presumably because of increased time available for its enzymatic metabolism in the gut wall (Rivera-Calimlim et al., 1978).

Drug absorption may also be decreased by very rapid gastrointestinal transit, as in gastroenteritis. Examples of abnormal responses in gastroenteritis due to impaired drug absorption are discussed in section 13.1.2. This effect is likely to be most marked with poorly soluble drugs (e.g. digoxin), and with enteric coated and slow release formulations, absorption from which generally tends to be rather poor or variable. This could be speculated to be due in part to the reduced time available for absorption and in part because of failure of drug dissolution in the gut lumen (Prescott, 1974a). On the other hand, a decrease in gastrointestinal motility (e.g. anticholinergic drugs, period of recumbency) may lead to enhanced absorption with poorly soluble drugs, or to occasional problems with enteric coated or slow release formulations of irritant drugs (see section 13.1.2).

Although food (e.g. a large meal), pain and nausea can reduce the rate of gastric emptying, and while a rise in intragastric pH or gastrectomy increases gastric emptying rate, these effects are unpredictable. Even in fasting healthy volunteers there is usually a marked individual variation in the rate of drug absorption (Prescott, 1974a). Food intake (Melander, 1978) and antacids (Hurwitz, 1977) have variable effects on drug absorption, depending on the pharmacokinetic and formulation characteristics of the particular drug (see chapter VI; sect. 5). In general, to ensure consistent absorption, it is advisable where possible, to give other drugs at least a half to 1 hour before antacid ingestion.

Gastrointestinal surgery does not seem to have an important effect on drug absorption, unless gastrointestinal transit is increased. Absorption of digoxin is not affected by a Billroth II procedure (Ochs et al., 1975), but complete failure of absorption of another poorly soluble drug ethionamide, has occurred in some postgastrectomy patients which was attributed to rapid gastrointestinal transit (Mattila et al., 1969).

---

1 Paracetamol is used as a model for drug absorption studies since it is a weak acid (pK$_a$ 9.5) that is largely unionised in both gastric and intestinal fluids. The rate of absorption of paracetamol is directly related to the gastric emptying rate (Heading et al., 1973). Drugs with similar physicochemical properties might be expected to be absorbed similarly to paracetamol (see chapter I; sect. 1.1).

A clinically important change in drug absorption due to altered gastrointestinal function will depend on the physicochemical and pharmacokinetic properties of the particular drug. Additional variables which can affect drug absorption in patients with altered gastrointestinal function, include the confounding effects of differences in bioavailability of drug products (see chapter VI; sect. 5) and drug interaction influences on absorption (see chapter VIII; sect. 2.3.1).

1.1.2 Intestinal Malabsorption Syndromes

Frank malabsorption states, as in coeliac disease, might be expected to reduce absorption of drugs in the same way as they decrease absorption of essential foodstuffs, vitamins and trace elements. However, the effect is inconsistent, absorption being delayed (e.g. amoxycillin, lincomycin, practolol), decreased (e.g. penicillin V, pivampicillin, thyroxine), increased (e.g. co-trimoxazole, sodium fusidate, propranolol) or normal (e.g. indomethacin, aspirin, pivmecillinam) and dependent on the degree of malabsorption, the treatment being given, and on the physicochemical and pharmacokinetic properties of the individual drug (Parsons, 1977; Parsons et al., 1977). For example, in *untreated* coeliac disease the absorption of practolol (a water soluble drug) is delayed, whereas that of propranolol (a lipid soluble drug) is increased, with a resulting increase in the plasma concentration of unchanged drug (Parsons et al., 1976a). On the other hand, in patients with coeliac disease *in remission*, plasma concentrations of propranolol are not increased (Schneider et al., 1976).

Absorption of some drugs may also be altered in Crohn's disease, but as in coeliac disease is inconsistent: being decreased (e.g. lincomycin), increased (e.g. clindamycin, co-trimoxazole, sodium fusidate), slightly reduced (metronidazole) or unchanged (e.g. cephalexin, rifampicin) [Parsons et al., 1976b; Melander et al., 1977]. The reasons for altered absorption of some drugs in coeliac and Crohn's disease are not clear (Parsons, 1977). Increased plasma concentrations of propranolol in Crohn's disease are probably due to altered protein binding and decreased clearance as a consequence of impaired hepatic function rather than altered oral absorption (Routledge and Shand, 1979). Absorption of amoxycillin, ampicillin, cephalexin, co-trimoxazole, lincomycin, clindamycin and rifampicin is however, adequate in small bowel diverticulosis. The absorption of digoxin is reduced in a variety of malabsorption states due to mucosal disease, but does not seem to be altered in patients with pancreatic disease (Heizer et al., 1971). The plasma concentration of cephalexin and semi-synthetic penicillins is however, markedly reduced in patients with cystic fibrosis but at least in the case of the penicillins is due to increased renal clearance (see section 13.3). Enteropathy associated with radiotherapy may also lead to impaired absorption of drugs (Sokol et al., 1978).

The extent of these changes in drug absorption and their significance in treated patients with malabsorption problems are difficult to predict. It is likely that drug absorption will be variable depending on the particular treatment given and the clinical status of the patient. Thus a change in treatment, such as introduction of a gluten free diet in coeliac disease, may profoundly affect the ability of the intestinal mucosa to absorb certain drugs. For example, penicillin V absorption is decreased in children with untreated coeliac disease, but after 6 to 8 months of gluten free diet absorptive capacity is normal (Bolme et al., 1977). There should therefore be an awareness that dosage adjustment of some drugs may be necessary, but this cannot be done on an arbitrary basis or applied to malabsorption syndromes in general. Suspicion of poor absorption of digoxin for example, should call for plasma concentration estimation and the dosage adjusted accordingly. Reduced absorption of an orally administered antibiotic leads to a decrease in the peak plasma concentration. If the peak falls below the minimum inhibitory concentration for a particular organism then therapeutic failure may occur, if it is assumed that the peak concentration is all important for antimicrobial activity.

1.2 Drug Metabolism and Gastrointestinal Function

The bioavailability of some orally administered drugs is influenced by gut metabolism prior to absorption, such that the amount of intact drug available for absorption is reduced. Such 'first-pass' loss may be substantial and can be further influenced by altered gastric emptying rate or intestinal motility (see section 1.1.1). Gut cells are capable of a number of typical drug biotransformation and synthetic reactions, including acetylation and conjugation with sulphate and glucuronic acid (Hartiala, 1973). Sulphate conjugation in the gut mucosa greatly reduces the systemic availability of orally administered isoprenaline (isoproterenol). Hydrallazine is subject to significant first-pass loss and the polymorphic acetylation process involved in the gut mucosa and liver appears to be capacity limited (Talseth, 1977).

Some drugs are metabolised in the gut wall by nonspecific enzymes (e.g. penicillin esters; ? chlorpromazine), or by bacteria (e.g. sulphasalazine; methotrexate; levodopa, which is also metabolised by the enzyme dopa decarboxylase in the gut). Certain patients fail to absorb chlorpromazine as such (Rivera-Calimlim et al., 1973), apparently because of a marked capacity to metabolise the drug in the gut wall (Curry et al., 1971; Dahl and Strandgord, 1977). Penicillin esters such as pivampicillin, talampicillin, carindacillin and pivmecillinam are hydrolysed to their parent drug by nonspecific esterases present in the blood and tissues. Whether a deficiency of small gut esterases, which is known to occur in disorders such as coeliac disease, can influence their systemic availability is not clear. Although absorption of pivampicillin is reduced in coeliac disease that of pivmecillinam is normal (Parsons, 1977).

Other possible effects of gastrointestinal pathology on absorption of drugs metabolised in the intestinal wall are given above (section 1.1.1). In patients with an abnormal intestinal bacterial flora the amount of levodopa available for absorption is decreased (Goldman et al., 1974). The activity of sulphasalazine is also affected by the presence of colonic bacteria. Sulphasalazine is ineffective in patients with Crohn's disease who have had a relapse after colonic resection, but is effective in those with an intact colon in whom the drug is metabolised by bacteria in the large bowel to its active form (see section 8.1.2).

1.3 Drug Distribution in Liver Disease

Albumin is quantitatively the most important protein responsible for binding of acidic drugs, but some basic drugs are more avidly bound to other proteins such as α_1-acid glycoproteins (chapter I; sect. 3.2.1). Albumin concentrations are often reduced in patients with acute or chronic liver disease. The relative importance of qualitative changes in the albumin molecule or of increased concentrations of endogenous substances such as bilirubin and bile acids on binding is not clear, although the reduction in binding of highly bound acidic drugs such as phenytoin in liver disease is most marked when both hypoalbuminaemia and hyperbilirubinaemia are present (Hooper et al., 1974; Olsen et al., 1975). The concentration of α_1-acid glycoproteins does not appear to change in patients with cirrhosis (Piafsky et al., 1978), but whether altered concentrations might occur in other types of liver disease is not known. The effect of liver disease on the plasma content of other binding proteins such as ligandin is not known. Tissue binding of drugs in liver disease may also be affected by alterations in plasma or tissue pH or the presence of ascites.

A change in protein binding in liver disease will not necessarily lead to an altered pharmacological effect, although it will alter the relationship of unbound drug to total drug in plasma and therefore be of importance when plasma total drug concentrations are being monitored (see chapter I; sect. 3.2.3). A decrease in binding in liver disease will only substantially influence clearance in the case of highly albumin bound drugs with a low intrinsic clearance or hepatic extraction ratio (e.g. phenytoin and warfarin), since clearance of such drugs depends on the amount of unbound drug available for metabolism and the activity of the hepatic drug metabolising enzymes (see section 1.4). The effect of liver disease on the disposition of such drugs is nevertheless difficult to predict and complex.

A change in clearance due to altered binding is most likely to be clinically important with drugs with a low therapeutic ratio such as phenytoin and warfarin. However, in the case of warfarin the effect of liver disease on clotting factor synthesis has a greater effect on the action of the drug than altered binding and clearance (see chapter XXIII; sect. 3.2.2).

With phenytoin, which has concentration (dose) dependent elimination kinetics (see chapter I; sect. 2.1.1), the net effect of liver disease on elimination of phenytoin is reflected by a balance between any increase in the percentage of unbound drug due to decreased protein binding and a possible reduction in the capacity of the liver microsomal enzymes to metabolise the drug (Blaschke et al., 1975). The consequences of a decrease in protein binding in this situation are therefore determined by the daily dosage and the effectiveness of the drug removal process. Thus, if dosage of phenytoin is not changed and is associated with a decreased rate of elimination (e.g. at high plasma drug concentrations when the capacity of the liver to metabolise phenytoin is 'saturated'), even a

Table II. Predominant pathophysiological changes in various types of liver disease (after Blaschke, 1977)

Disease	Total hepatic blood flow	Hepato-cellular mass	Hepatocyte function	Albumin concentration	Bili-rubin
Cirrhosis					
Moderate	↓	↔ or ↑	↔	↔ or ↓	↔ or ↑
Severe	↓↓	↓	↓	↓↓	↑↑
Acute inflammatory liver disease					
Viral hepatitis	↔ or ↑	↔ or ↓	↓	↔	↔ or ↑
Alcoholic hepatitis	↔ or ↓	↑, ↔ or ↓	↓	↔ or ↓	↑↑

↓ = Decreased; ↑ = Increased; ↔ = Unchanged.

small increase in the proportion of unbound phenytoin may lead to increased plasma concentration of free drug, which may reach the toxic range in an individual patient if the ability to eliminate the drug is decreased. On the other hand, if the capacity of the liver to eliminate the drug is not 'saturated', accelerated metabolism might be expected to occur, since the larger proportion (fraction) of unbound drug makes more phenytoin available for metabolism. If dosage has not been changed, this results in a lower total drug concentration but the same concentration of free drug in plasma and thus the same intensity of pharmacological effect (see chapter I; sect. 3.2.3). Systematic studies during continued clinical use of phenytoin in liver disease have not yet been reported. However, it is known that the incidence of side effects with phenytoin is increased in cirrhotic patients with low serum albumin levels compared with patients with normal serum albumin levels (see further chapter VII, sect. 5.1; XXV, 3.1).

The incidence of major side effects with prednisone or prednisolone is increased in patients with chronic active liver disease due to reduced clearance and decreased binding in the presence of hypoalbuminaemia and hyperbilirubinaemia and dosage should be reduced accordingly (see chapter XVI; sect. 9.1).

1.4 Drug Metabolism in Liver Disease

Before they can be excreted, many lipid soluble drugs are metabolised by the mixed function oxidase system in the liver to more polar (water soluble) metabolites (see chapter I; sect. 3.3). In view of this major role of the liver in drug biotransformation, it might be expected that liver disease would have a significant effect on drug action due to an altered rate of metabolism. Although abnormal responses can occur with certain drugs (see section 13.4), these are not necessarily due to impaired metabolism. Alteration in the tissue response to drugs can also occur in the patient with severe liver disease.

The effects of liver disease on drug pharmacokinetics are complex (see Wilkinson and Schenker, 1975, 1976). In liver disease, the extent of organ damage varies with the type of liver disease and also from patient to patient in relation to parenchymal, synthetic and metabolic function, biliary excretory ability and hepatic blood flow (table II). Also, extrahepatic shunts may develop. Each of these can influence disposition of certain drugs. Other factors which influence drug kinetics are also often present in the patient with liver disease (Black, 1974; Roberts et al., 1979). For example, chronic alcohol ingestion, concomitant therapy with other drugs which may affect drug metabolising capacity, altered body water compartments, hypoalbuminaemia, hyperbilirubinaemia and other diseases such as renal impairment. Moreover, hepatic function, plasma bilirubin or albumin concentrations may fluctuate considerably over relatively short periods of time. It is not surprising therefore, that it has not been possible to predictably relate alterations in metabolism to any of the standard laboratory measurements of liver function, except perhaps with reduced serum albumin and prolonged prothrombin time, which may reflect poor protein synthesis, including the metabolising enzymes (Branch et al., 1973; Farrell et al., 1978). Further, the rate of metabolism of many drugs varies markedly between individuals with normal liver function (see chapter I; sect. 4) and may be greater than the alteration in elimination in an individual patient with liver disease.

Any alteration in the rate of drug metabolism from that normally expected depends on the nature and severity of the liver damage and on the factors which influence hepatic clearance of the drug. In fundamental terms, the importance of a change in the rate of drug metabolism in liver disease will depend on the proportion of drug which is ordinarily eliminated by hepatic metabolism. For example, about 60% of digoxin is eliminated unchanged by renal excretion and the remainder mostly by hepatic metabolism, whereas the opposite holds for methyldigoxin. Thus, in acute hepatitis the plasma concentration of methyldigoxin is increased whereas that of digoxin does not differ from normal (Zilly et al., 1975). Digitoxin is eliminated mainly by hepatic metabolism, but cirrhosis does not seem to alter the metabolism or dose requirements of digitoxin (Hamamoto et al., 1977), possibly because a significant amount of drug is excreted into the bile and the faeces (Lukas, 1976; Doherty et al., 1971).

1.4.1 High and Low Clearance Drugs

Drugs eliminated primarily by hepatic metabolism can be usefully classified into low or high clearance (extracted) compounds whose rate of elimination is largely limited by changes in hepatic blood flow or protein binding (Wilkinson and Shand, 1975; table III). High clearance drugs are those which are extracted by the liver to an extent greater than around 70% (i.e. the hepatic extraction ratio[2] is greater than 0.7) and possess 'intrinsic' clearances greater than normal liver blood flow. The intrinsic clearance is a characteristic of each drug and can be defined as the volume of liver water cleared of that drug in unit time. It is therefore an index of the total enzymatic capacity of the liver to remove drug. The rate at which the liver is able to metabolise highly extracted drugs is dependent on the amount of drug (bound and unbound) presented to the liver, which in turn is proportional to its blood flow. Hepatic clearance of such drugs is therefore sensitive to factors includ-

Table III. Pharmacokinetic classification of drugs eliminated primarily by hepatic metabolism (after Blaschke, 1977)

Drug class	Approx. hepatic extraction ratio	% Bound
High clearance (flow-limited)		
Dextropropoxyphene	0.95	78
Chlormethiazole	0.9	—
Pentazocine	0.8	60-70
Labetalol	0.7	50
Lignocaine	0.7	45-80[1]
Propranolol	0.64	93[2]
Pethidine (meperidine)	0.5	65-75
Nortriptyline	0.5	95[2]
Morphine	0.5-0.75	35
Low clearance (capacity-limited), binding sensitive		
Phenytoin	0.03	90
Diazepam	0.03	98
Tolbutamide	0.02	98
Warfarin	0.003	99
Chlorpromazine	0.22	98[2]
Clindamycin	0.23	94
Quinidine	0.27	82[2]
Digitoxin	0.005	97
Low clearance (capacity-limited), binding insensitive		
Theophylline	0.09	59
Hexobarbitone	0.16	—
Amylobarbitone	0.03	61
Antipyrine	0.07	10
Chloramphenicol	0.28	60-80
Thiopentone	0.28	72-86
Paracetamol (acetaminophen)	0.43	< 5[1]

1 Concentration dependent.
2 More avidly bound to α_1 acid glycoprotein than to albumin (see section 1.3).

---

ing certain liver diseases which can alter hepatic blood flow (see Nies et al., 1976). This class of drug is also termed as having 'high intrinsic clearance' or 'flow limited clearance'.

The rate of metabolism of poorly extracted drugs is dependent on the amount of drug available for metabolism at the hepatic enzyme receptor site, which is proportional to the concentration of free (unbound) drug in plasma. Clearance is not limited by the amount of drug brought to the liver. Such drugs have low hepatic extraction ratios, indicative of the fact that the 'intrinsic' capacity of

---

2 The hepatic extraction ratio is the fraction of drug removed from the blood during a single transit through the liver (see chapter I; sect. 3.3.3).

the liver to metabolise these compounds is small. Hepatic clearance of these drugs is therefore almost entirely determined by hepatic metabolising capacity (i.e. the activity of the liver drug metabolising enzymes). For highly albumin bound drugs the concentration of drug at the site of metabolism is proportional to the extent of plasma protein binding and is sensitive to changes in protein binding (section 1.3). This class of drug is also termed as having 'low intrinsic clearance' or 'capacity limited clearance'. When the drugs listed in table III are plotted in the diagram depicted in figure 1, the relative sensitivity of each drug to conditions in the various types and stages of liver disease which alter blood flow, hepatic enzyme metabolising capacity or protein binding can be readily appreciated (Blaschke, 1977).

1.4.2 Effect of Liver Disease on Drug Clearance

In liver disease there is a defect not only of liver function but also of the hepatic circulation (Wilkinson and Schenker, 1975; table II). Highly extracted drugs are particularly susceptible to reduced clearance and increased oral bioavailability in cirrhosis. Drugs with the largest hepatic extraction ratio will have the greatest potential for relative increases in bioavailability in cirrhotic patients due to portal systemic shunting (Neal et al., 1979; see chapter I; sect. 4.3.3).

After oral administration such drugs are subject to considerable first-pass metabolism during their passage from the gut to the systemic circulation in portal venous blood (see chapter I; sect. 3.3.3). Reduced hepatic extraction due to impaired

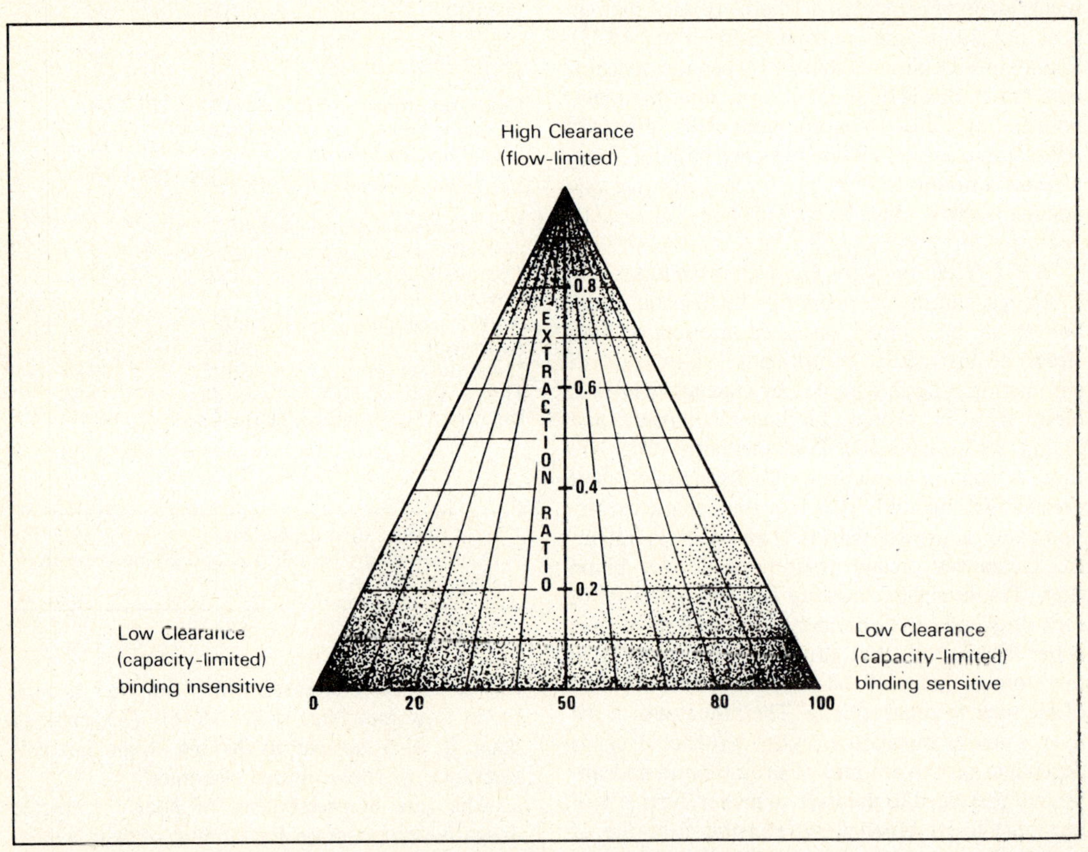

Fig. 1. This diagram illustrates the way in which two pharmacokinetic parameters (hepatic extraction ratio and percent plasma protein binding) are used to assign a drug into one of three classes of hepatic clearance (high clearance or flow-limited; low clearance or capacity-limited, binding sensitive; and low clearance or capacity-limited, binding insensitive). Any drug metabolised by the liver can be plotted on the triangular graph, but the classification is important only for those eliminated *primarily* by hepatic processes. As a drug falls closer to a corner of the triangle (shaded areas), the more likely it is to have the characteristic changes in disposition in liver disease as described for the three drug classes in the text (after Blaschke: Clinical Pharmacokinetics 2: 32, 1977; by permission).

metabolic capacity and any development of hepatic portalsystemic shunting of blood (Gugler et al., 1975), which effectively bypasses initial hepatic removal mechanisms and is one of the consequences of the pathogenesis of chronic liver disease, will lead to reduced clearance and a marked increase in systemic availability of the unchanged drug. This has been shown, for example, with drugs such as propranolol (Wood et al., 1978), pethidine (meperidine) and pentazocine (Neal et al., 1979), labetalol (Homeida et al., 1978) and chlormethiazole (Pentikainen et al., 1978) in cirrhosis. In the case of chlormethiazole, bioavailability can be increased about 10-fold and because of a real risk of toxicity, necessitates use of reduced dosage in patients with advanced cirrhosis (Pentikainen et al., 1978). Even in liver diseases in which hepatic function is relatively well maintained but in which portal systemic shunts develop (e.g. schistosomiasis), use of usual doses of the oral schistosomicide niridazole, a highly extracted drug, can lead to high plasma concentrations and an increase in adverse neuropsychiatric symptoms (Faigle and Keberle, 1969).

Clearance of intravenously administered highly extracted drugs such as lignocaine (lidocaine), propranolol, pethidine, labetalol and chlormethiazole is reduced in cirrhosis. In some patients the change in clearance may be relatively small, suggesting that hepatic blood flow is not always significantly altered and that in such cases the intrinsic clearance (i.e. hepatic metabolising capacity) is the more important factor for elimination (Branch and Shand, 1976; Pentikainen et al., 1978). Lignocaine is critically dependent on blood flow for elimination and has a low therapeutic ratio such that a relatively small increase in plasma concentration will readily lead to CNS toxicity. Its clearance is markedly impaired in chronic active hepatitis and cirrhosis (Adjepon-Yamoah et al., 1974; Thomson et al., 1973) and toxicity has resulted from usual doses (Selden and Sasahara, 1967). Clearance is less affected by acute viral hepatitis (Williams et al., 1976), possibly because although metabolism is affected by the altered hepatic function, blood flow is usually unchanged or even increased and the amount of drug delivered to the liver for metabolism is not significantly altered.

Clearance of drugs with a low hepatic extraction ratio is primarily dependent on hepatic metabolising capacity and not on changes in blood flow. For some, but not all such drugs, metabol-

ism can be impaired in liver diseases. Clearance of theophylline can be markedly reduced in cirrhosis and because of its low therapeutic ratio results in a greatly increased risk of toxicity from usual doses (Mangione et al., 1978; Piafsky et al., 1977). The stage and nature of the liver disease can obviously affect clearance. For example, in acute viral hepatitis the rate of metabolism of diazepam is decreased, with a return to normal on recovery from the illness. Clearance of diazepam is even further prolonged in patients with alcoholic cirrhosis (Klotz et al., 1975) and there is a delay in the appearance of the active metabolite desmethyldiazepam (Andreasen et al., 1976). Clearance of chlordiazepoxide is also prolonged in cirrhosis and the rate and extent of production of the active metabolite desmethylchlordiazepoxide is also reduced (Greenblatt et al., 1978). Whether active metabolites of diazepam and chlordiazepoxide will accumulate with repeated dosage in liver disease to the same extent as in healthy individuals, is not clear (Klotz et al., 1977). In contrast, the clearance of oxazepam and lorazepam, benzodiazepines which are not biotransformed but glucuronidated to inactive metabolites, does not appear to be significantly altered in either cirrhosis or acute viral hepatitis (Shull et al., 1976; Kraus et al., 1977); suggesting that glucuronidation may be relatively spared in some cases of parenchymal liver disease.

Poorly extracted acidic drugs which are sensitive to changes in protein binding illustrate a different situation in acute viral hepatitis. For example, although the clearance of tolbutamide (bound + unbound) is increased, with return to normal on recovery, protein binding is decreased due to hypoalbuminaemia and the clearance of unbound pharmacologically active drug is unaltered (Williams et al., 1977). The case with phenytoin is similar (Blaschke et al., 1975), although delayed clearance of unbound drug may occur at high plasma concentrations due to the dose dependent elimination of phenytoin (see further section 1.3). Delayed clearance and decreased albumin binding of prednisone and prednisolone occurs in chronic active liver disease and is associated with an increase in incidence of major steroid side effects (see chapter XVI; 9.1).

1.4.3 Drug Induced Liver Disease and Metabolism of Drugs

Drug induced liver disease may also affect elimination of some drugs. The rate of metabolism of barbiturates and phenytoin, even though they induce their own metabolism, can nevertheless be markedly impaired in patients with gross hepatic necrosis following paracetamol (acetaminophen) overdosage (Forrest et al., 1974). The rate of elimination of paracetamol itself is related to the extent of the liver injury (Prescott et al., 1971). Drug metabolising capacity also seems to be impaired after methyldopa induced liver damage (Sotaniemi et al., 1977). The fact that drug induced impaired liver function can lead to toxicity is well illustrated by cases of ergotamine poisoning in patients treated with triacetyloleandomycin (Hayton, 1969; Bigorie et al., 1975).

1.4.4 Disorders of Biliary Excretion and Drug Disposition

Disorders of biliary excretion may also lead to altered disposition of some drugs. Drugs such as rifampicin which are mainly excreted in the bile will accumulate in patients with cholestatic jaundice or biliary obstruction, and also in patients with chronic hepatitis, acute viral hepatitis or cirrhosis (Acocella, 1978), necessitating modification of dosage. Some drugs are eliminated by both biliary and renal excretion (e.g. ampicillin, oxytetracycline, tetracycline). With ampicillin there seems to be no need to modify dosage in cirrhosis, unless renal function is also impaired (Jusko and Lewis, 1975). The serum half-life of oxytetracycline is increased in biliary obstruction, hepatitis or cirrhosis, particularly in those with associated renal impairment (Leevy et al., 1958). As renal disease contributes to the hepatotoxicity of oxytetracycline and tetracycline, these tetracyclines should not be used in patients with renal insufficiency complicating liver disease; e.g. the 'hepatorenal syndrome' (see also chapter XXI; sect. 14.1.5). Drug metabolism can also be impaired in genetically determined disorders of bilirubin metabolism such as Gilbert's syndrome; glucuronidation capacity appears to be impaired but the reported changes in oxidation and acetylation are less certain (Macklon et al., 1979).

1.4.5 Liver Disease and Extrahepatic Drug Metabolism

Liver disease may also affect extrahepatic drug metabolism. In patients with severe liver disease a reduction in plasma pseudocholinesterase activity may be associated with prolongation of action of suxamethonium (succinylcholine), which depends on the activity of this enzyme for termination of its action (see chapter X; sect. 2.2.1).

1.4.6 Clinical Significance of Altered Disposition in Liver Disease

The clinical significance of a decrease in the rate of elimination of some of these drugs during their actual clinical use in patients with liver disease is not entirely clear due to lack of systematic study. In general, it would seem that patients with advanced cirrhosis are extremely vulnerable to the toxic effects of drugs which have a low therapeutic ratio or which have adverse effects if their action is markedly enhanced (see section 13.4). Thus, the prolonged clearance of theophylline and increased oral bioavailability of chlormethiazole necessitates use of reduced doses in cirrhosis. On the other hand, propranolol has a wide therapeutic margin and delayed elimination and increased oral bioavailability are probably not as important as the known marked variation in rate of metabolism between individual patients. Moreover, in hypertension and angina dosage can be readily titrated to a clearcut clinical endpoint.

Although the reduced clearance and increased oral bioavailability with pethidine may not lead to marked accumulation with short term use, there is evidence that drugs with sedative and respiratory depressant properties have a potential to precipitate hepatic encephalopathy in susceptible patients with liver disease. Certainly this is the case with morphine. Similarly, although the decrease in rate of elimination of diazepam is less than the variation shown between individual patients and might not be sufficient to lead to a greatly enhanced sedative effect in acute viral hepatitis, it may cause EEG abnormalities and stupor in some patients with cirrhosis (see section 13.4).

Until satisfactory predictive tests are available for individual drugs, the clinician must be guided by a knowledge that disposition of drugs primarily eliminated by hepatic metabolism may be altered in liver disease. For drugs where definite guidelines to dosage in liver disease are not at present available, dosage should be adjusted according to the patient's response and the patient observed closely (see section 13.4). A tabulation of the effect of liver diseases on disposition of various drugs is given in chapter I (tables XIV, XV).

2. General Principles of Treatment

1) *Accurate diagnosis:* Exclusion of malignancy is an essential prerequisite in management of

gastric ulcer and other gastrointestinal diseases. Many conditions and drugs can cause dyspepsia, nausea, vomiting or diarrhoea and the aim of treatment is first to establish the aetiology. As the gut is the most common area in the body to be affected by psychosomatic or functional disorder, and as the symptoms of these disorders (e.g. dyspepsia, vomiting, pain, bloating, constipation or diarrhoea) are common to functional and organic diseases, the importance of accurate diagnosis cannot be overemphasised.

Thorough examination to reach a diagnosis is also fundamental to rational treatment of constipation.

Small bowel disorders may be due to disease of the small bowel itself, postoperative bowel stasis, abnormalities and enzyme deficiencies of the intestinal mucosa and obstruction of the intestinal lymphatics. Abnormalities in the lumen of an otherwise normal small bowel may be due to pancreatic insufficiency or altered bile salt composition and, in addition, to certain worm infestations. The treatment of these conditions covers a wide range of therapeutic agents and underlines the importance of establishing a precise diagnosis. Because of the different response to treatment, particularly with regard to surgery, attempts should always be made to differentiate ulcerative colitis from Crohn's disease. A precise diagnosis of the aetiology of pancreatitis is essential for correct management.

Apart from a detailed history and examination, all consultations for a gastrointestinal disorder should include measurement of the haemoglobin, erythrocyte sedimentation rate, a rectal examination and a stool occult blood test. Other tests will depend on the symptom complex.

2) *Education of the patient:* Explanation and reassurance form an essential part of management of gastroduodenal and bowel diseases. Patients must fully understand the nature of their disease and the objectives of treatment. The clinician should assume an active supportive role in helping his patient to live with his symptoms. For example, in the irritable bowel syndrome, sympathetic explanation of the condition and strong reassurance that there is no serious organic disease is the mainstay of treatment in helping the patient to understand his symptoms. Patients with ulcerative colitis must understand that the condition relapses and that early treatment of an attack is essential. The patient with peptic ulcer must be reassured

about the satisfactory treatment available for his condition but the proclivity to relapse with stress and dietary overindulgence must be emphasised. In patients with alcoholic cirrhosis and alcohol induced pancreatitis, educational measures aimed at achieving permanent abstinence from alcohol are the most important aspects of treatment.

3) *Individualised treatment:* This means adjusting the dosage of some drugs to the needs (e.g. laxatives) or response (e.g. anticholinergics) of the individual patient and of taking into account the factors which can sometimes alter the response to certain drugs in gastrointestinal and liver disease (see section 1, 13). Drugs and diet need to be adjusted to individual needs in conditions such as chronic portal systemic encephalopathy, many intestinal malabsorption disorders and according to predominant symptoms and a host of inexplicable but definite food idiosyncrasies in the irritable bowel syndrome.

4) *Nature of diet:* Diet assumes more general importance in gastrointestinal and liver diseases than in any other area of medicine. A specific diet is the basis of treatment of many intestinal malabsorption disorders. Diet and fluids must be carefully controlled in diverticular disease. In other gastrointestinal diseases dietary restriction for specific food substances should only be instituted if the symptoms can definitely be related to that substance. Otherwise it is better to advise patients to find their own best diet by trial and error. This may mean for example, a trial of avoidance of certain foods which produce symptoms in peptic ulcer (e.g. fatty fries, spices), a milk free diet in ulcerative colitis, or a high residue diet for pain in the irritable bowel syndrome. Attention to diet to ensure an adequate intake of residue and fluid is important in management of constipation. A high protein, nutritious diet is recommended in most liver diseases, and after gastric surgery.

5) *Supportive treatment:* The nature of the symptoms of many gastrointestinal diseases often leads to or can be associated with anxiety or depression. Judicious use of antianxiety drugs and antidepressants are often helpful. A wide range of therapeutic agents is available for treatment of symptoms of gastroduodenal disease but these should not be used in place of an accurate diagnosis. Attention to electrolyte and fluid balance is the basis of treatment of most gastrointestinal in-

fections and is more important than symptomatic treatment with drugs.

3. Oesophageal Disease

3.1 Hiatal Hernia

The majority of hiatal hernias are virtually or wholly asymptomatic. The earliest symptom is usually heartburn, clinical manifestations generally being due largely to one of its complications, reflux. The aim of medical treatment of hiatus hernia is prevention of reflux of the gastric contents into the oesophagus, and of oesophagitis, oesophageal spasm and pulmonary spill over (Levine and Rubin, 1973).

Measures aimed at preventing or minimising reflux include weight reduction if the patient is obese, elevation of the head of the bed by at least 15 to 20cm (6 to 8"), avoiding stooping and bending and the wearing of tight clothing and abstinence from food or fluids for at least 2 hours before retiring at night. Sleeping propped up on pillows is contraindicated as it raises intra-abdominal pressure. Antacids are used mainly to relieve heartburn while methylpolysiloxane may be used to relieve flatulence and metoclopramide may be given 30 minutes before meals and at night to promote gastric emptying. An alginate-antacid preparation (i.e. Gaviscon) has been advocated to prevent symptoms, as it produces a soft viscous layer of floating antacid foam on the gastric contents, thus protecting the oesophagus from reflux (Stanciu and Bennett, 1974b).

Anticholinergics should probably be avoided as they reduce gastric and oesophageal motility and delay gastric emptying thereby having the potential to increase the amount of reflux (Fisher et al., 1977). Prolonged recumbency and nasogastric intubation should also be avoided, i.e. after surgical operations.

3.2 Reflux Oesophagitis

Care should be taken to exclude other gastrointestinal disease predisposing to reflux, particularly pyloric obstruction or gastric retention. The basis of therapy is to neutralise intragastric and intraoesophageal contents, to prevent reflux and to try and increase the lower oesophageal sphincter pressure (Hansky, 1973; Castell, 1978). As in hiatal hernia, the principal treatment methods consist of weight reduction; avoiding stooping and bending; sleeping with the head raised; a bland diet (frequent ingestion of small quantities); alginate-antacid preparations; and hourly antacids during waking hours, before meals and at night to neutralise intragastric and intraoesophageal contents.

The addition of a local anaesthetic such as oxethazine (e.g. as in Mucaine) may be of value in some patients. Severe intractable oesophagitis may require treatment with a continuous intraoesophageal antacid drip.

The lower oesophageal sphincter pressure (possibly under control of the hormone gastrin) is reduced in patients with oesophageal reflux, and frequent protein meals may promote gastrin release (and theoretically improve sphincter competence). Antacids may possibly do likewise by neutralising intragastric acid. Although intravenous metoclopramide increases lower oesophageal sphincter pressure, the effects of oral administration of the drug are less consistent, but it is useful at bedtime to promote gastric emptying (McCallum et al., 1977; Behar and Ramsby, 1978).

Anticholinergics are theoretically contraindicated (see section 3.1). A combination of carbenoxolone (see section 4.1) and an alginate antacid compound, as a chewing or sucking tablet, to promote the factors which may heal the oesophagetic mucosa (Reed and Davies, 1978) and cimetidine (see section 4.1), to reduce acid erosion of the lower oesophagus (Powell-Jackson et al., 1978; Wesdorp et al., 1978) are being investigated. Both provide symptomatic benefit, but oesophageal ulcer healing has only been impressive with the carbenoxolone-alginate compound.

Surgical reduction of gastric acid secretion may be required, particularly if there is associated duodenal ulceration, and recurrent endoscopically proven oesophagitis may require surgical repair of the hernia. Paraoesophageal hernia is an indication for surgical correction unless there is a contraindication to surgery.

3.3 Oesophageal Spasm, Rings and Stricture

Medical treatment of oesophageal spasm is aimed at improving retrosternal discomfort, dysphagia and preventing bolus obstruction (Levine and Rubin, 1973). If spasm is present in conjunction with hiatal hernia and oesophageal reflux, treatment should be as for these conditions in conjunction with oral antispasmodics which have *little or no* anticholinergic activity (e.g. hyoscine butylbromide, mebeverine). Any accompanying anxiety and/or depression should be treated appropriately. Care should be taken to exclude the presence of peptic ulcer and gallstones and to avoid irritative foods. Surgery or dilatations are necessary only if there is definite fibrous stricture.

3.4 Less Common Oesophageal Diseases

3.4.1 Partial Oesophageal Rupture

The aim of treatment is to elucidate the cause and prevent mediastinitis and infection. Treatment consists of sleeping with the bed elevated and avoiding postures which aggravate reflux. Nutrition is maintained by intravenous feeding, no food being taken by mouth. Small volumes of a liquid kanamycin preparation sipped hourly may be given in conjunction with an appropriate systemic antibacterial agent. As this condition represents an incomplete form of complete rupture, it usually follows severe vomiting.

3.4.2 Achalasia

Treatment of this motility disorder is directed mainly against dysphagia and the prevention of pulmonary spill over, and is usually surgical (Heller's operation), but pneumodilatation also gives good results in experienced hands (Levine and Rubin, 1973). If surgery is contraindicated the sphincter can be relaxed transiently with inhaled octyl nitrite, whilst painful spasm may be relieved with antispasmodics (e.g. hyoscine butylbromide, mebeverine).

3.4.3 Candidal (monilial) Oesophagitis

Candidal oesophagitis is an increasing complication of broad spectrum antibiotic, corticosteroid and cytotoxic drug therapy. Treatment, which is aimed at preventing stricture formation, is as for hiatus hernia, along with hourly oral administration of an appropriate antifungal agent such as nystatin or amphotericin B lozenges or oral drops (see chapter XIII; sect. 6).

3.4.4 Bolus Obstruction

Food bolus obstruction usually occurs in patients with oesophageal rings or small hiatal hernia and presents with acute aphagia. Intravenous glucagon 1mg will usually cause sufficient relaxation to permit passage of the bolus in 7 to 10 minutes in most cases (Ferrucci and Long, 1977). Oesophagoscopic removal is necessary if this fails.

4. Peptic Ulcer

Chronic peptic ulcer is a common medical problem in developed communities and is the suspected diagnosis in the majority of patients with gastroduodenal symptoms referred for barium meal, whether they present with pain or bleeding. The aim of treatment is to: (a) relieve ulcer pain; (b) heal the ulcer completely; (c) delay or prevent recurrences, and (d) prevent complications (see Piper and Heap, 1972; Isenberg, 1975).

It is generally accepted that ideally the patient should have the ulcer healed by medical means, placed on long term therapy and surgery performed if complications or intractability develop. If careful investigation and follow-up is not possible in a patient with gastric ulcer, surgery should be advised initially. As in many other gastrointestinal diseases, the clinician should take an active and supportive interest in his ulcer patient's symptoms and response to treatment. The rationale of therapy and important side effects should be thoroughly explained to him.

4.1 Pharmacological Properties of Antiulcer Drugs

Further understanding of the pathophysiological components of the time honoured equation of ulcer aetiology (acid-pepsin aggression versus mucosal resistance), the scope of initial treatment and the search for lasting maintenance therapy has provided a wide variety of potential treatments (Bank and Marks, 1973; Langman, 1977). Some of these have been proven to accelerate ulcer healing while the benefits of some others are much less certain (table IV).

4.1.1 Antacids

The three commonly used antacids, magnesium hydroxide, aluminium hydroxide and calcium carbonate all have adequate capacity to neutralise hydrochloric acid secretion. Although the neutralising effect appears to be greater with some of the combinations of these compounds than others, by and large it becomes a question of dose of antacid versus the number of H^+ ions secreted (Fordtran and Collyns, 1966; Fordtran et

Table IV. Some agents available or under investigation for ulcer healing

Drug	Action	Efficacy (promotion of healing)		Important side effects	Further notes
		duodenal ulcer	gastric ulcer		
Agents affecting acid or pepsin					
Antacids	Neutralisation of gastric juice; may also coat mucosa with protective layer, and inhibit pepsin activity	Effective	Probably effective	Diarrhoea (magnesium salts), constipation (aluminium salts), milk-alkali syndrome (calcium carbonate and milk in liberal quantities), alkalosis (excessive use of soluble antacids such as sodium bicarbonate)	Long term use to delay ulcer recurrence is not established
Amylopectin[1]	Antipepsin action, probably protects mucosa from action of pepsin	Unclear, possibly ineffective	Unclear, possibly effective	Well tolerated	Recent studies in duodenal ulcer have failed to show a statistical difference *vs* placebo, but such studies involved small patient groups. A trend for improved healing with active drug was sometimes present (Landecker et al., 1976) Long term use to delay ulcer recurrence is not established
Cimetidine	Inhibits gastric acid secretion	Effective	Effective	Gynaecomastia; mental confusion (excessive dosage in elderly, those with impaired renal function); see also text	Possibly effective in delaying ulcer recurrence when given long term, but role in this regard not clear (see section 4.2.3)
Sucralfate[1]	Unclear; inhibits gastric pepsin; may also form protective layer on mucosa	Probably effective	Probably effective	Unclear	Preliminary results in 1 study have shown sucralfate to be as effective as cimetidine in gastric or duodenal ulcers (Marks, 1979a). Long term use to delay ulcer recurrence is not established

Agents affecting mucosal resistance					
Carbenoxolone	Enhances mucus production; may also have antipepsin action and inhibit back diffusion of hydrogen ions into mucosa	Effective	Effective	Fluid retention, increased blood pressure, hypokalaemia	Side effects tend to occur more frequently in the elderly or in those with cardiovascular, respiratory or renal disease. Restricted sodium intake or concomitant use of a thiazide diuretic with a potassium supplement may permit continued treatment if side effects develop. Long term use to delay ulcer recurrence is not established
Tripotassium dicitrato bismuthate	Forms protective layer in ulcer crater	Effective	Effective	Well tolerated; faeces and occasionally tongue may take on dark discolouration	In 1 study was as effective as cimetidine in patients with gastric ulcers (antacid consumption in this study not reported; Tanner et al., 1979). Long term use to delay ulcer recurrence not established
Deglycyrrhizinised liquorice	Unclear; may affect mucus production; may also have spasmolytic action	Unclear	Effective	Well tolerated	In 1 study was as effective as cimetidine in accelerating healing of gastric ulcers (Morgan et al., 1978). Long term use to delay recurrence is not established
Gefarnate[2]	Unclear; may affect mucus production	Unclear	Probably effective	Well tolerated	Long term use to delay ulcer recurrence is not clearly established, although there is some evidence that such treatment may be effective in male patients with chronic gastric ulcers (Truelove and Rocca, 1976)
Agents affecting gastrin					
Proglumide[2]	Gastrin antagonist at receptor level; may also have spasmolytic action	Unclear, possibly effective	Probably effective	Well tolerated	Long term use to delay ulcer recurrence is not established
Sulpiride[2]	Inhibits gastrin release; may also inhibit gastric acid secretion	Unclear, possibly effective	Unclear	Unclear	Acts on the hypothalamus inducing a wide variety of hormonal effects, including increased prolactin secretion and decreased secretion of gonadotrophin and follicle stimulating hormone. Long term use to delay ulcer recurrence is not established

1 Investigational new drug.
2 Agents which require further study to clarify efficacy and role in therapy.

al., 1973). If conditions were ideal, one should really find the optimum effective antacid dose for the individual patient's capacity to secrete acid. In addition, it would appear that antacids coat the mucosa, thus providing a barrier to acid-peptic digestion and it also appears as though most acids will, in fact, combine with pepsin. Antacids relieve ulcer pain and given in adequate dosage can also accelerate ulcer healing (section 4.4). Calcium carbonate products stimulate gastrin secretion (Levant et al., 1973), but it has yet to be shown that this excellent antacid is detrimental to ulcer healing. One sulphated antacid (Altacite) has been shown to bind bile salts and may prevent bile induced gastritis. Some antacid products now contain a silicone preparation such as simethicone (methylpolysiloxane) as a defoaming agent and some a local anaesthetic in an attempt to inhibit gastrin secretion. For a review of the pharmacology of antacids in ulcer therapy, see Piper and Heap (1972) and Littman and Pine (1975).

4.1.2 Anticholinergic Drugs

Although there has been uncertainty about the value of anticholinergic drugs in ulcer disease (see Piper, 1973; Piper and Heap, 1972), their undoubted acid inhibitory-antispasmodic effect is obvious and many clinicians still find them effective as adjunctive therapy. Anticholinergic drugs should not however, be used as the sole or major basis of therapy. Many different compounds are available; the more potent in terms of inhibition of gastric acid secretion include glycopyrronium (glycopyrrolate) bromide, isopropamide iodide, oxyphencyclimine hydrochloride, poldine methylsulphate and propantheline bromide. The time of maximum action is 1 to 2 hours after oral administration and the effective duration of action is 6 to 8 hours, although this may extend up to 24 hours if large doses are used. All compounds probably have the same duration of effect if given in doses equipotent at the time of maximum action.

4.1.3 Cimetidine

Cimetidine is the newest and least toxic of a recently discovered group of specific competitive histamine H_2-receptor antagonists (see Brogden et al., 1978; Symposium, 1978). Given orally or intravenously it effectively inhibits basal, food, pentagastrin, histamine, caffeine and insulin stimulated gastric acid secretion. It reduces both volume of secretion and H^+ concentration, but the effect on pepsin output is almost totally due to reduction in volume of secretion. In studies occupying 1 year of continued therapy, there have been no persistent changes in acid secretion, serum gastrin or in the parietal cells once the drug has been discontinued (Bank et al., 1977b). The effect on acid secretion is dose related up to a dose of about 400mg and a single dose reduces stimulated acid secretion for 6 to 8 hours. It does not influence gastric emptying rate.

Cimetidine accelerates the healing of duodenal and gastric ulcer and controls peptic ulceration in some patients with the Zollinger-Ellison syndrome (see section 12.2). It would also seem to be successful in certain patients with reflux oesophagitis and in gastric bleeding from erosions, but these and the effect of long term maintenance therapy in peptic ulceration still need to be evaluated. It cannot yet be recommended for the prophylaxis of stress ulceration but clinical trials are currently in progress in the prevention of gastrointestinal bleeding. It is relatively non-toxic, but dosage needs to be reduced in patients with impaired renal function and in the elderly (see below and section 4.2.3; 4.3.3).

Cimetidine is readily absorbed after oral administration; plasma concentrations increasing with dosage up to 400mg but being disproportionately high after an 800mg oral dose (Bodemar et al., 1977; Griffiths et al., 1977). Absorption of cimetidine following oral administration is delayed when given with food, but plasma concentrations are more prolonged and the extent of inhibition of gastric acid secretion is similar whether it is given before, with or after food. Although higher concentrations are attained in the bile than plasma, very little drug is eventually eliminated in the bile. Most of an oral or intravenous dose of cimetidine is recovered in the urine within 24 hours of administration; about half (40 to 70%) of a usual dose as unchanged drug. Excretion is delayed and the plasma half-life correspondingly prolonged in patients with impaired renal function, such that peak plasma concentrations of cimetidine after 100mg orally in patients with severely impaired renal function are comparable with those after 300mg in patients with normal renal function (see Brogden et al., 1978). Although haemodialysis removes the drug from plasma, therapeutic concentrations can be maintained with doses of 200mg 12-hourly in uraemic patients with peptic lesions undergoing maintenance haemodialysis (Jones et al., 1979).

4.1.4 Carbenoxolone

Carbenoxolone, a pentacyclic triterpene derived from the hydrolysis of glycyrrhizic acid after extraction from liquorice root, has been shown to accelerate the healing of gastric and duodenal ulcer, but at the expense of a number of important mineralocorticoid-like side effects (see Pinder et al., 1976a). It should thus not be used if careful and regular monitoring of serum electrolytes, blood pressure and weight is not possible. The mode of action of carbenoxolone would appear to involve a number of effects, including an increase in the life span of proliferating mucosal cells, production of gastric mucus, protection of the mucosa against bile reflux, an antipeptic mechanism and perhaps others yet unidentified. As the symptomatic response seems to be rather slow it should be prescribed with antacids (in doses as required for pain), at least for the first few weeks. Although it has been used as maintenance therapy this should not be attempted without careful supervision, if at all. Serious side effects can occur if carbenoxolone therapy is not carefully supervised; i.e. improper monitoring by the clinician or patient default of regular check-ups (see section 4.3.4).

Carbenoxolone is absorbed directly from the gastric mucosa but to obtain a therapeutic response in the duodenum the drug is placed in a release capsule which fragments during its pyloric passage. Simultaneous administration of antacids or ingestion of carbenoxolone with food does not affect steady-state plasma concentrations of the drug (Baron et al., 1978). Carbenoxolone is highly bound to plasma proteins (mainly albumin) and has a very low apparent volume of distribution. Albumin binding is reduced in the elderly and the rate of elimination is markedly prolonged (Hayes et al., 1977). Since the incidence of side effects is higher in the elderly, this means that lower doses are desirable in the older patient as there is likely to be a higher concentration of unbound active drug as a consequence of the reduced capacity for albumin binding and delayed clearance (see further chapter I, sect. 3.2.3; V, sect. 2.1). The incidence of side effects is also increased in patients with liver or renal disease; where in conditions such as cirrhosis or uraemia there is also likely to be a reduced capacity for albumin binding (see section 1.3; chapter XXI, sect. 1.2). Carbenoxolone is not biotransformed, being conjugated in the liver and excreted almost entirely in the bile. Plasma concentrations vary markedly between patients after the same fixed dose, but are higher in the elderly and in those who develop oedema or hypokalaemia (Baron et al., 1978).

4.1.5 Colloidal Bismuth Compounds

The active ingredients in these products are stable bismuth salt complexes; available as either a bismuth citropeptide complex or tripotassium dicitrato bismuthate (see Brogden et al., 1976; Williams, 1977). The healing rate with short term use in gastric and duodenal ulcers has been impressive (e.g. Lee and Nicholson, 1977). The mode of action differs from bismuth containing antacids in that they act in an acid medium to form bismuth oxychloride and bismuth citrate, at a pH of 2.5 to 3.5 which is thought to chelate proteins and aminoacids at the ulcer base to form a protective coating against acid and pepsin (Lavy et al., 1976). Colloidal bismuth has also been shown to have pepsin binding properties. For these reasons it should be given 1 hour before meals or antacids. No toxicity has yet been reported but maintenance therapy has not been attempted (see section 4.3.5). Pharmacokinetic studies are lacking.

4.1.6 Deglycyrrhizinated Liquorice

Glycyrrhizinic acid-reduced (deglycyrrhizinated or deglycyrrhizinised) liquorice compound (Caved-S) consists of liquorice from which virtually all of the glycyrrhizinic acid has been removed, plus antacids and powdered frangula bark (Brogden et al., 1974). Carbenoxolone, another liquorice derivative, is synthesised from glycyrrhetinic acid and the aglycone of glycyrrhizinic acid. The deglycyrrhizinised liquorice compound has been shown to accelerate healing of gastric ulcer. Its efficacy in duodenal ulcer is unclear. It is well tolerated and unlike carbenoxolone has not been associated with mineralocorticoid-like side effects. It has therefore been used in elderly patients, in whom there is a high risk of side effects with carbenoxolone. The contribution of the antacids in Caved-S to the healing effect is not clear.

4.2 Dosage of Antiulcer Drugs

4.2.1 Antacids

Although many patients will have learnt that antacids taken after meals or for pain only will eventually relieve their attacks, and clinical trials have shown ulcer healing in some 30 to 60% of patients on this type of treatment, it is generally conceded that an improved rate of healing will be attained with a more intensive antacid regimen or the use of an ulcer healing drug in addition to the token doses of antacid.

In an intensive antacid regimen, an appropriate antacid should be prescribed in doses sufficient to exert a buffering effect (Fordtran et al., 1973). Although dose requirements vary between patients, in duodenal ulcer this generally means about 15 to 30ml of an aluminium hydroxide gel-magnesium hydroxide mixture or 20 to 40ml of aluminium hydroxide gel alone. Smaller doses may be adequate in patients with gastric ulcer, in whom acid secretion is less (Isenberg, 1975; Littman and Pine, 1975). Such doses are given every hour during waking hours, before bed, and during the night if symptoms demand. A reduced dosage schedule (same dose 1 and 3 hours after meals and at bedtime; Fordtran and Collyns, 1966) may be used for 4 to 6 weeks in duodenal ulcer after symptoms resolve, but in gastric ulcer intensive antacid therapy is continued until there is radiological and gastroscopic evidence of complete healing.

Although patients may find antacid tablets more convenient than liquid preparations, they are less potent buffers (Littman and Pine, 1975). While most studies showing clearly improved healing have used high dose liquid antacid regimens (e.g. Ippoliti et al., 1978; Peterson et al., 1977) there is some evidence that less intensive treatment using antacid liquids or tablets also promotes healing of duodenal (Lam et al., 1979; Marks, 1979b) and gastric ulcer (Hollander and Harlan, 1973). Most commercial antacid preparations today combine magnesium and aluminium hydroxide and some also contain simethicone in varying amounts. In practice, adequate therapy with most of these is of the order of 15 to 30ml after meals and before bed at night, together with an antacid tablet to suck hourly between doses of the liquid preparation. Calcium and sodium bicarbonate containing antacids are best avoided for long term therapy because of potential complications (see section 4.3.1). Calcium carbonate is an excellent preparation for short term treatment despite theoretical objections to its gastrin stimulating effect (Levant et al., 1973).

4.2.2 Anticholinergic Drugs

Logically, anticholinergics should be given in a pharmacologically effective dose based on individual patient response (Piper and Heap, 1972). This dose can be determined in an individual patient by commencing with small doses and increasing the dosage until the presence of minor side effects such as dry mouth and constipation. Some clinicians advocate the use of a prolonged action anticholinergic given 4 times daily, as this causes a more even inhibition of gastric acid secretion than does a twice daily dose schedule. Despite this, many prefer titrating the dose to the severity of the dyspepsia rather than to the so-called 'optimum effective dose' as determined by side effects (i.e. night dose produces side effects on waking and daytime doses minor side effects throughout the day). A long acting anticholinergic given before lunch and bedtime together with adequate antacids, is effective, as evidenced by the rapid relief of symptoms in most patients. In these cases it is doubtful whether the inconvenience of minor side effects and the hazard of urinary and visual symptoms warrants the use of larger doses. In any event, patients should be instructed about the nature of side effects and how to adjust the dose.

4.2.3 Cimetidine

A similar rate of ulcer healing has been obtained with doses of cimetidine ranging from 800mg to 2g daily (Brogden et al., 1978). In the USA and Canada (where 300mg tablets are manufactured) a dose of 300mg 4 times a day with meals and at bedtime, is recommended, while in other countries (where 200mg tablets are available) the dose schedule is 200mg 3 times daily with meals and 400mg at bedtime. Treatment should be continued for 4 to 6 weeks and ideally complete ulcer healing should be proven by endoscopy. The level of acid secretion in individual patients does not seem to influence the outcome and ulcers unhealed at 4 weeks on 1g daily may benefit from a further 4 to 6 weeks of therapy at the same or an increased dose. Preliminary evidence suggests that maintenance treatment with cimetidine 400 to 800mg daily reduces the recurrence rate of duodenal ulcer (Brogden et al., 1978; Bodemar and Walan, 1978), but its role in this regard particularly in relation to optimum dosage, asymptomatic recurrence, recurrent ulceration once maintenance treatment is discontinued, long term effect on gastric mucosa acid secretion and gastrin secretion and possible side effects with long term use, have yet to be clarified.

Cimetidine can also be used intravenously when oral therapy is contraindicated, for example, with vomiting or nasogastric suction, the intravenous dose being identical to the oral dose. As the majority of the administered dose is excreted unchanged in the urine (see section 4.1.3), dosage should be reduced in patients with impaired renal function and in the elderly (see section 4.3.3). A suggested regimen is 200 or 300mg every 12 hours in cases of moderate or severe renal impairment, with an increase in dose interval if there is a need to increase dosage (see also appendix E). Since cimetidine is dialysable, further adjustment of dosage is necessary in patients with renal failure undergoing haemodialysis (see section 4.1.3). A dosage of 200 to 300mg 12-hourly is probably adequate in elderly patients with reduced renal function. Dosage should also be reduced in patients with renal insufficiency complicating liver disease or when renal function is impaired as a consequence of cardiac failure (see section 4.3.3; chapter XVII, sect. 1.5).

4.2.4 Carbenoxolone

The dosage of carbenoxolone is a compromise between maximum rate of healing and mineralocorticoid-like side effects (Pinder et al., 1976a; see section 4.3.4). Optimum therapeutic effect in gastric ulcer with least side effects is achieved with a dosage of 100mg 3 times daily for the first week followed by 50mg 3 times daily thereafter, best taken after meals. Dosage for duodenal ulcer is 50mg 4 times daily given in the form of special 'positioned release' capsules. The capsules are designed to rupture near the pylorus and thereby deliver the drug into the duodenum. The timing of administration is critical for correct rupture of the capsules, which should be given 15 to 20 minutes before meals. Due to reduced albumin binding and delayed clearance, lower doses (of the order of 100mg daily) are desirable in the elderly, and probably also in those with cirrhosis or uraemia (see section 4.1.4).

4.2.5 Colloidal Bismuth

The dosage of colloidal bismuth preparations such as tripotassium dicitrato bismuthate is 5ml diluted with 15ml water 4 times daily, taken 30 minutes before each of the 3 main meals and 2 hours after the last meal of the day. Larger doses up to 10ml 6 times daily can be given if required, taken 30 minutes before and 2 hours after the 3 main meals.

4.2.6 Deglycyrrhizinated Liquorice

The dose of deglycyrrhizinated liquorice is 2 tablets chewed and taken with water 3 times daily

after meals. Dosage should be increased to 2 tablets 4 to 6 times daily in patients with severe duodenal ulcer symptoms.

4.3 Side Effects of Antiulcer Drugs

4.3.1 Antacids

Antacids are not innocuous, but although side effects can occur these are very seldom a problem with proper use (see Piper, 1973; Piper and Heap, 1972). A greater potential problem is the possible interference of antacids with the absorption or excretion of other drugs, particularly in intensive therapy regimens (Hurwitz, 1977; see chapter VIII, sect. 2.3.1, 2.3.8; appendix C).

The diarrhoeal and constipating effect of some antacids is well recognised. Aluminium hydroxide gels cause constipation, magnesium preparations diarrhoea and calcium carbonate may cause constipation or diarrhoea. When using a mixture of aluminium hydroxide gel and a magnesium preparation, a tendency to constipation necessitates increasing the dose of magnesium at the expense of aluminium. The converse applies if diarrhoea occurs.

Antacids taken in large doses for extended periods, especially in the presence of associated renal disease, can occasionally cause dangerous or misleading electrolyte abnormalities (hypercalcaemia or hypophosphataemia may be confused with hyperparathyroidism). The milk-alkali syndrome can occur when sodium bicarbonate containing preparations are ingested with large amounts of calcium, either as calcium containing antacids or milk (Texter and Laureta, 1966; see also chapter XVI; sect. 14.5) and phosphorus depletion and even occasional cases of osteomalacia have been noted with magnesium and aluminium containing preparations (Lotz et al., 1964, 1968; Cooke et al., 1978). Prolonged use of calcium antacids may lead to hypercalcaemia and hypercalciuria (Stiel et al., 1967; Vincent and Radcliff, 1966) and renal calculi, especially in those with a propensity to calculus formation. Sodium containing antacids may cause fluid retention which is a potential complicating problem in those with cardiac and liver disease and in those on carbenoxolone. In these situations, a low sodium antacid should be used (Barry and Ford, 1978).

4.3.2 Anticholinergic Drugs

The complications of anticholinergic drug therapy are those expected from knowledge of their pharmacological action, i.e. dry mouth, blurred vision, difficulty in micturition, and occasionally aggravation of constipation, impotence, palpitations and a confused mental state in the elderly (see chapter XXVI; sect. 15.5). All these effects can be overcome by reducing the dose. Anticholinergic drugs should not be used in patients with narrow angle glaucoma (see chapter XII; sect. 10) or prostatic hypertrophy and should be suspended for at least 3 days prior to gastric acid secretory studies. They should be omitted in pyloric stenosis, oesophageal relux and, according to some authorities, immediately after gastrointestinal haemorrhage (Piper and Heap, 1972).

By inhibiting gastrointestinal motility, anticholinergic drugs can alter the absorption of certain other orally administered drugs (see chapter VIII; sect. 2.3.1).

4.3.3 Cimetidine

On short term treatment cimetidine has been relatively free of side effects (Brogden et al., 1978). Unexplained mental confusion has occurred in a few patients, requiring withdrawal of the drug or a reduced dosage, but the remainder of the reported side effects such as diarrhoea, muscle pains, skin rash, headache, tiredness, and dizziness have occurred with similar frequency in a control placebo group. Mental confusion is most likely to occur with excessive dosage in critically ill elderly patients (particularly those with reduced renal function, cardiac failure or organic cerebral disease) and in patients with renal failure, including those with renal insufficiency complicating liver disease, in whom coma may be precipitated and confused with renal or hepatic coma (Flind and Rowley-Jones, 1979; Schentag et al., 1979). Physostigmine may be helpful in reversal of cimetidine induced stuporose states (Mogelnicki et al., 1979). Dosage must be reduced in these critically ill patients and therapy monitored closely. Gynaecomastia and galactorrhoea may occur rarely with prolonged therapy and in some cases has been associated with raised serum prolactin levels (see chapter XV; sect. 23.6). The action of warfarin may be enhanced (Silver and Bell, 1979).

There have been a few reports of rapid ulcer recurrence, haemorrhage and perforation within 2 weeks of discontinuing cimetidine therapy (Wallace et al., 1978). Although one should be aware of such a possibility it has to be interpreted in the context of the hundreds of patients in whom the drug has been discontinued without event after a course of therapy. Nevertheless, it highlights the importance of establishing complete healing (Bank et al., 1976).

Asymptomatic side effects include a temporary but unimportant rise in serum creatinine in most patients, mild neutropenia or agranulocytosis in a few patients and a few instances of rise in liver transaminases with centrilobular necrosis.

Inexplicable erosive gastritis and duodenitis during continuous treatment (Webster et al., 1978), impotence, erythema multiforme, cardiac arrhythmia, tachycardia, bradycardia, insomnia, nightmares and urinary retention must at present be placed in the anecdotal side effects list, but emphasise the importance of constant awareness that the drug is still relatively new and even anecdotal side effects should be reported. To date there have not been any significant long term effects on acid secretion, serum gastrin or changes in the gastric mucosal cells. However, because the general role of histamine and histamine H_2-receptor function is not as yet well defined in health and disease, further surveillance will be needed to monitor possible long term effects on gastric secretion and endocrine, immunological, haematological and neurological function and also the incidence of recurrence after discontinuing graduated long term therapy.

4.3.4 Carbenoxolone

The complications of carbenoxolone can be common and are due to its mineralocorticoid-like effect (fluid retention, raised blood pressure and hypokalaemia), but are only rarely a problem *if* the patient is carefully and regularly supervised at 1 to 2 week intervals (Pinder et al., 1976a). The incidence of side effects is related to dosage, especially in the elderly and in those with liver or renal disease (see section 4.1.1), and to the presence of associated diseases such as congestive heart failure and hypertension. Carbenoxolone should not be used in patients with heart failure or hypertension.

Hypokalaemia is the most serious consequence, especially if serum potassium levels are not monitored regularly and if it is allowed to develop insidiously; when pronounced it may be associated with cardiac arrhythmias, severe muscle weakness or renal tubular necrosis. Hypokalaemia tends to develop later than fluid retention or raised blood pressure. Potassium supplements should be given as indicated. Undue weight gain due to fluid retention and raised blood pressure should be treated promptly with thiazide diuretics together with potassium supplements. These drugs can be continued with carbenoxolone, provided serum potassium is measured every 3 weeks. The aldosterone antagonist spironolactone cannot be used, as although it abolishes the mineralocorticoid side effects it also interferes with ulcer healing (Doll et al., 1968).

4.3.5 Colloidal Bismuth and Other Agents

Colloidal bismuth, deglycyrrhizinated liquorice and other antiulcer agents are relatively safe. Colloidal bismuth has few side effects and thus needs little clinical or biochemical monitoring, at least for the recommended 4 to 8 week course of therapy (Brogden et al., 1976). A few patients have complained of abdominal pain soon after taking the mixture. Some find the ammoniacal odour distasteful and it may colour dentures black; and as bismuth causes black stools it may be confused with melaena. As bismuth is a heavy metal with possible but not yet reported nephrotoxicity, it should perhaps be used with care in renal disease and not be used for continuous prolonged periods.

4.4 Initial Medical Treatment of Chronic Peptic Ulcer

Initial treatment is directed towards adequate physical and emotional rest, regular feeds, relief of ulcer pain and acceleration of healing of the ulcer. Upon diagnosis (a benign gastric ulcer must be distinguished from ulcerating gastric cancer by endoscopy and biopsy), all patients should be advised to stop smoking and encouraged to avoid alcohol and caffeine containing beverages. Aspirin and other potentially 'ulcerogenic' drugs (see section 14.2.2) should be discontinued. A normal diet should be prescribed, but the patient should be instructed to avoid foods which produce symptoms (e.g. fried foods, spices). The time honoured bland diet is seldom indicated other than in patients with intractable ulcer dyspepsia.

Other aspects of treatment vary somewhat according to the severity of ulcer symptoms, occupational and home circumstances, and, of course, the attending doctor. Some prefer all patients to have an initial period of hospitalisation or bed rest to accelerate healing of the ulcer, but this is hardly feasible or desirable as the disruption of business or other important activity may in fact enhance rather than reduce emotional stress. For this reason most clinicians rely heavily on ambulatory regimens of a sensible attitude to rest, work, mental equanimity and intensive ulcer therapy.

Because of the number of drugs available for the treatment of peptic ulcer (table IV), the choice of treatment should be individualised and based on factors such as convenience and patient compliance. The choice of regimen also depends on individual experience (e.g. benefit of anticholinergic drugs) and availability of drugs in different countries (e.g. carbenoxolone, proglumide). Attitudes towards factors which contribute to relief of pain and ulcer healing are also relevant. For example, some clinicians believe that antianxiety drugs have a beneficial supportive role in initial ulcer healing. Most of the available drugs have been shown to be effective and to heal a greater proportion of ulcers more quickly and with more rapid relief of symptoms than placebo treated patients (Bank and Marks, 1973; Langman, 1977). However, it should be stressed that patients on placebo or given token antacids (i.e. as required for relief of pain) have their ulcers healed endoscopically in 4 to 6 weeks in 30 to 60 % or more of cases, reflecting the natural tendency for ulcers to undergo healing.

It is as yet uncertain whether the newer antiulcer drugs such as cimetidine and carbenoxolone are superior to an intensive antacid (or antacid/anticholinergic/antianxiety drug) regimen with regard to the speed of relief of ulcer symptoms or rate or number of ulcers healed (Englert et al., 1978; Ippoliti et al., 1978). They have, of course, the advantage of ease of administration, more tasteful to take and do not leave the lips white. However, against this must be weighed important side effects encountered with drugs such as carbenoxolone (see section 4.3.4). Antacids, which have been used succcessfully for symptoms and healing for years by eminent clinicians and their patients (Bank and Marks, 1973; Littman and Pine, 1975), have only recently been proven to have a significant advantage over placebo in accelerating healing of gastric (Hollander and Harland, 1973; as assessed radiologically) or duodenal ulcers (Ippoliti et al., 1978; Peterson et al., 1977; as assessed endoscopically). Given in adequate dosage, antacids relieve dyspepsia symptomatically in patients with uncomplicated ulcers and it is axiomatic that non-relief from suspected ulcer symptoms within 24 to 48 hours on an intensive antacid (or antacid/anticholinergic/antianxiety drug) regimen or antacid/cimetidine regimen suggests an alternate diagnosis for the symptoms or marked ulcer penetration.

Flexibility is the basis of finding the best treatment for each patient. For example, in patients who do not respond adequately to intensive antacid therapy or cimetidine alone, combination therapy may be of value. Addition of anticholinergic (Feldman et al., 1977) and/or antianxiety drugs may also be worth trying. On an effective regimen, one should achieve at least the type of response in an ambulatory patient that can be obtained with bed rest alone; e.g. symptomatic improvement and complete ulcer healing within 4 to 6 weeks in around 80 % of cases of duodenal ulcer and 70 % of cases of gastric ulcer. Larger ulcers tend to take longer to heal than small ones. Most ulcers will heal or become totally asymptomatic if treated long enough or with increased dosage of therapy, and it is likely that many of the remaining proportion not healed enter an asymptomatic but unhealed phase.

Persistent symptoms with no evidence of healing would raise the probability of surgery and persistent symptoms despite endoscopic evidence of healing should raise the question of another diagnosis (e.g. spastic bowel) or functional symptoms.

Complete ulcer healing is important. In gastric ulcer, the possibility of an underlying carcinoma lurks in every unhealed ulcer, but importantly, complete initial healing reduces the high recurrence rate when studied over a period of 4 years (Piper et al., 1978). In duodenal ulcer, there are no firm studies on the natural history of unhealed but asymptomatic ulcers, but by extrapolation from the relatively high incidence of ulcer bleeding (Novis et al., 1976) and to a lesser extent perforation and stenosis in patients with previously asymptomatic ulcers (Dent et al., 1977), it is probable that these complications will always be greater while the ulcer is not completely healed. Therefore, the aim should be to achieve complete initial healing whenever possible, but equally important to maintain healing in a disease with a very high, if not inevitable, recurrence rate (section 4.5).

Treatment is continued for an arbitrary initial period of 4 to 6 weeks. In the patient with duodenal ulcer, the ulcer will have healed, either naturally or as a result of treatment, within 8 to 12 weeks. Barium meal examination or preferably endoscopy should be used to assess ulcer healing and performed regularly in the case of gastric ulcer, and therapy continued until the ulcer is healed. Most heal in 4 and almost all by 12 weeks.

A few ulcers heal slowly and are still found to be benign lesions. Surgery is indicated for those few cases which fail to show any endoscopic evidence of healing after a proper trial of an initial 6 weeks of medical treatment.

4.5 Prevention of Recurrences

About a quarter to a half of all ulcers are finally treated surgically (Mowat et al., 1975). Even previous acceleration of ulcer healing by enforced bed rest or ulcer healing drugs does not seem to greatly change this proportion, although initial complete healing of ulcers by enforced bed rest does decrease the recurrence rate over a period of 4 years (Piper et al., 1978). The aim of long term medical treatment after ulcer healing is to further delay recurrences and hopefully also to prevent complications such as haemorrhage or perforation.

Although some clinicians continue antacids for up to 6 months in duodenal ulcer, there is no data that such use prevents recurrences. There is reasonable evidence that long term anticholinergics (Piper, 1973; Piper and Heap, 1972) and cimetidine (Brogden et al., 1978; Bodemar and Walan, 1978) can delay recurrences in duodenal ulcer and a little evidence that carbenoxolone (150mg daily) might do likewise in gastric ulcer (Pinder et al., 1976a). At present, it seems justifiable to use long term anticholinergics in an attempt to delay ulcer recurrence, assuming the dose can be adjusted without producing inconvenient side effects. Cimetidine is still under investigation for long term maintenance treatment (see section 4.2.1). Side effects of carbenoxolone (section 4.3.4) restrict its use to short term initial ulcer healing in properly supervised patients. Patients should be urged to adopt a more objective attitude to their problems and to have regular meals. Traditional advice has been to avoid regular analgesic use (particularly salicylates) or excessive alcohol intake. However, if the ulcer is initially completely healed, even regular use of large doses of analgesics or excessive alcohol intake do not adversely affect ulcer recurrence (Piper et al., 1977; 1978).

Surgery is indicated for intractable ulcers, the development of complications, or rapid or frequent recurrence after healing, for it must be considered that the patient's ulcer diathesis is so great that further medical treatment is unlikely to be of significant benefit (Piper et al., 1975).

4.6 Treatment of Complications of Chronic Peptic Ulcer

Death from peptic ulcer is usually the result of the complications of haemorrhage or perforation, but can be greatly minimised by a proper plan of management. The principles of treatment of acute upper gastrointestinal haemorrhage involve immediate hospitalisation and urgent endoscopy to diagnose the exact cause of the haemorrhage, the use of blood transfusion, careful medical observation, early ambulation (to prevent pulmonary embolism) and in selected cases (e.g. continuous or recurrent bleeding in those over age 40) skilled surgery. Two weeks hospitalisation is indicated to facilitate ulcer healing if surgery is not advisable. Other treatments that may be tried in bleeding are oral ε-aminocaproic acid, vasopressin or noradrenaline (norepinephrine), and in uncontrolled bleeding, intravenous cimetidine, massive intragastric antacid instillation and vasopressin 1 to 2u/minute given by selective arterial catheterisation. The value of laser or electrocautery coagulation at the time of endoscopy is currently being investigated. Perforation necessitates immediate oversewing of the ulcer. Conservative treatment should only be used if surgery is not available or if there has been an excessive delay in patient presentation.

The initial treatment of pyloric stenosis, which is due to either oedema, spasm or fibrous stricture, is medical. On admission, the patient should be placed on gastric suction, the tube being clamped every 2 hours and antacids given hourly or cimetidine intravenously. Anticholinergics are best discontinued because the delay in gastric emptying may accentuate the symptoms of obstruction, but an intramucosal or intravenous antispasmodic (e.g. hyoscine butylbromide), or metoclopramide may be given. Electrolyte and fluid replacement are essential. If at the end of 48 hours relief of obstruction is not significant, surgery should be advised. Ideally, one aims to allow the episode of obstruction to subside and therefore to operate at a later date, if this is then necessary.

4.7 Adjunctive Treatment in Chronic Peptic Ulcer

Although emotional factors are often associated with peptic ulcer and appear to precipitate recurrences, there is no evidence that they have a direct role in the maintenance of chronic peptic ulcer. Judicious use of antianxiety or antidepressant drugs (see chapter XXVI) may sometimes be indicated for those with genuine worries or depression or whose concern about their prognosis can not be overcome by reassurance and explanation of the good results and safety of modern medical and surgical treatment. Many of the antianxiety drugs (e.g. diazepam) reduce basal acid secretion. Insomnia and persistent nocturnal pain is particularly disturbing to the patient with peptic ulcer and a good night's sleep is essential. An effective dose of an anticholinergic drug at bedtime may be more appropriate than a hypnotic and should be tried first. If nocturnal pain or insomnia persist, both may be required. Cimetidine may come to be used in a similar manner.

5. Other Gastroduodenal Disorders

5.1 Dyspepsia

The aim of treatment is to relieve symptoms and to establish the aetiology. Antacids should be given as needed for pain until symptoms subside or the cause is found. Frequently this may be due to acute or radiologically negative peptic ulceration, but a careful search must be made for emotional factors, particularly depression, and for oesophageal, pancreatic, gall bladder, small and large bowel, pulmonary and general disease. Careful assessment should be made of irritable bowel syndrome and constipation (see section 7) which require treatment. Intestinal parasitic infestation should be treated (see section 11.4). Over or under diagnosis of functional dyspepsia should be avoided. Non-ulcer dyspepsia is frequently due to gastritis and a careful history of dietary factors (e.g. alcohol or caffeine idiosyncrasy), drugs etc is necessary. Endoscopy may show excessive bile reflux which has been claimed to cause symptomatic gastritis, and some patients appear to have poor gastric emptying. Metoclopramide (section 5.2) may be useful in both these conditions.

5.2 Nausea and Vomiting

Nausea and vomiting are common symptoms, with many causes both inside and outside the gastrointestinal tract. Rational therapy is based on identification and treatment of the cause, for example, relief of subacute intestinal or pyloric obstruction and its correction. However, sometimes this is not possible and symptomatic treatment including careful attention to fluid and electrolyte status and use of antiemetics is indicated. Antiemetics should not be used without a careful search for the cause of vomiting lest they mask an underlying disease and so delay diagnosis and corrective treatment (e.g. vomiting due to raised intracranial pressure, diabetic gastropathy, migraine or Meniere's disease). Nausea and vomiting can be inhibited by drugs acting at (Cockel, 1971):

a) The vomiting centre — anticholinergics or antihistamines (e.g. dimenhydrinate, cyclizine, meclozine, promethazine).
b) The chemoreceptor trigger zone in the fourth ventricle — phenothiazines (e.g. prochlorperazine, perphenazine, thiethylperazine) and metoclopramide.
c) The periphery — anticholinergics which delay gastrointestinal motility and metoclopramide which enhances motility and increases the rate of gastric emptying.

Metoclopramide is effective in nausea and vomiting due to gastroduodenal disease (e.g. 'gastritis'). It accelerates gastric emptying by increasing the frequency and depth of antral contractions and regularising motility between the antrum and duodenal bulb (Pinder et al., 1976b). By its very nature metoclopramide should be administered 15 to 30 minutes before a meal. It may be used orally or intramuscularly as required, a common dosage schedule being 5 to 10mg 3 times daily. Its antiemetic action may also be at the chemoreceptor trigger zone where it may act as a dopaminergic receptor antagonist. Thus, as with phenothiazines, an acute dystonic reaction can occur as an occasional but alarming side effect, especially in young children (see chapter XXV; sect. 15.5). It can be easily confused with encephalitis or tetanus. Obviously, metoclopramide should not be used with phenothiazines.

Cyclizine (50mg 3 times daily) is an effective antiemetic and may be used for the persistent nausea of infective hepatitis and for vomiting after myocardial infarction. Many drugs can cause nausea and vomiting, with digitalis the main offender (see sect. 14.2.1). Correct treatment is to withdraw the drug for a day or so and then reduce its dosage. Cyclizine (50mg 3 times daily) is frequently adequate to control the nausea and vomiting associated with cytotoxic drugs, but some patients may need a phenothiazine such as

prochlorperazine (10mg 3 times daily) or thiethylperazine (6.5mg up to 3 times daily). Phenothiazines and metoclopramide are useful in vomiting of uraemia and radiation sickness, metoclopramide being preferred when sedation is not required. Psychogenic vomiting can often be successfully managed by treatment of the emotional disturbance, without recourse to antiemetics. A phenothiazine such as chlorpromazine 25 to 100mg intramuscularly 4 to 6-hourly or as required can sometimes be effective in the control of intractable hiccup. Metoclopramide intramuscularly (10mg 4 times daily) and nasogastric intubation should be attempted if this fails (Pinder et al., 1976b). Management of pre-and postoperative vomiting is discussed in chapter X (sect. 2.7), nausea and vomiting associated with pregnancy in chapter XV (sect. 7.1) and with motion sickness and other vestibular disturbances in chapter XI (sect. 4; 5).

Administration of antiemetics orally is the most convenient in prophylaxis, but parenteral or rectal administration is necessary to control symptoms when vomiting has already started. Oral therapy can be given for continuing treatment.

5.3 Flatulence

Many carminatives (e.g. peppermint, dill) and antacids are useful in postprandial flatulence and distension. Carbohydrate restriction may be beneficial and the treatment of constipation essential. Methylpolysiloxane (simethicone, dimethicone), a silicone preparation, now present in many antacid mixtures, is reputed to coalesce gastrointestinal gas which is then thought to be more readily expelled by belching or carried on by peristaltic activity. Most dosage schedules used are probably too small; a dose of 125 to 250mg methylpolysiloxane 4 to 6 times daily is more effective. Metoclopramide is also effective in relieving flatulence (Pinder et al., 1976b).

5.4 Symptoms Resulting from Gastric Surgery

5.4.1 Dumping Syndrome
Medical therapy consists of a diet high in protein and fat and low in carbohydrate, particularly sugar, limitation or exclusion of liquids during and immediately after meals, and frequent ingestion of small meals. Only if these measures fail might tolbutamide in individualised dosage 10 to

20 minutes before main meals, or once daily chlorpropamide, be tried. If necessary, associated anxiety should be treated. Anticholinergics may also be used in an attempt to delay gastric emptying. In severe and persistent cases it may be necessary to operate again, the procedure being determined by the mechanics of the problem in each individual.

5.4.2 Diarrhoea, Steatorrhoea, Malabsorption

Investigation of a surgically or medically remedial cause is the first step to effective treatment (e.g. gastrocolic fistula, lactose intolerance). Diarrhoea may be a troublesome feature in some patients after vagotomy and is difficult to treat because of its periodic nature. Treatment is essentially symptomatic. Antimotility drugs such as codeine phosphate, (30mg), diphenoxylate (5mg) or loperamide (4mg) at night and after the first bowel action in the morning, is often of value (see section 7.2). Persistent diarrhoea, fortunately rare, may require long term treatment and antibiotics and cholestyramine occasionally help. Cholestyramine, a basic anion exchange resin, combines with intraluminal bile salts (sect. 6.1.3) and may block the cathartic effect on the colon. The usual dose is 4g 4 or more times a day (Duncombe et al., 1977).

Steatorrhoea and iron deficiency anaemia occasionally occur after the Billroth II procedure but are universal after total gastrectomy. Deficiency of vitamin B_{12} will inevitably follow total gastrectomy. Fat absorption in Billroth II patients may be improved by combined administration of pancreatic extracts and a broad spectrum antibiotic (e.g. 1g tetracycline or 1 to 2g ampicillin daily). Patients who have undergone a Billroth II procedure should receive a high calorie, protein rich diet with frequent feedings containing as much fat as is tolerable in relation to the degree of steatorrhoea/diarrhoea. Pancreatic enzymes should be given a trial.

After a total gastrectomy, 30 to 100µg of vitamin B_{12} intramuscularly must be given monthly. Calcium, iron, folic acid, and the fat soluble vitamins may be added to this regimen as needed, or when diarrhoea or steatorrhoea is so severe that deficient absorption of these substances may be anticipated.

Replacement of digestive enzymes and cautious use of insulin is important in the treatment of patients with combined pancreatic insufficiency (see section 9.3.3) and a gastric operation.

5.4.3 Gastric Retention

A slower than normal gastric emptying rate often follows truncal vagotomy and pyloroplasty. Intravenous metoclopramide accelerates gastric emptying of solid meals when it is delayed. Patients should sleep on the right side to facilitate emptying. Methylpolysiloxane may be required for flatulence and antiemetics for vomiting. Postprandial fullness is frequently due to rapid jejunal filling rather than to stasis in a gastric remnant.

5.4.4 Bilious Vomiting and Bile Gastritis

This may be due to afferent loop stasis or severe gastritis due to refluxing bile salts and presents with recurrent bile vomits or epigastric pain. Treatment should be directed at limiting vomiting, reflux and dyspepsia. An antiemetic, preferably metoclopramide, should be given along with antacids. Cholestyramine may be tried in an attempt to bind bile salts. Medical treatment is usually effective, but occasional patients with intractable symptoms will require an operation aimed at diverting the bile flow (i.e. Roux-en-Y anastomosis).

5.5 Gastroduodenal Haemorrhage

About 50% of patients presenting with upper gastrointestinal bleeding will have an ulcer. Important lesions in the other 50% are alcohol, aspirin or stress induced acute erosions or erosive gastritis, oesophageal tears and oesophageal varices. Most patients stop bleeding within 12 to 24 hours with conservative measures; antacids should be given liberally (e.g. 30ml every hour) and there is some evidence that cimetidine will be useful in erosive gastritis or acute ulceration (Brogden et al., 1978). Other methods of therapy that have been tried are oral noradrenaline (norepinephrine), vasopressin or ε-aminocaproic acid. A variety of gastroscopic techniques including laser, heat or electrical coagulation are currently being investigated and intravenous, and more effectively, angiographic infusion of vasopressin into the bleeding vessel is often successful in uncontrolled bleeding. The embolisation of such vessels has also produced excellent results. Surgery still has to be used in a number of first bleeds. The prophylaxis of stress induced bleeding after burns, trauma, surgery and in pulmonary and surgical intensive care units may be decreased by nasogastric intubation and constant acid titration to pH 7 with antacids (Hastings et al., 1978) or possibly, and still under trial, cimetidine administration or both together. Both methods remain to be proven.

6. Intestinal Malabsorption Syndromes

The vast majority of small bowel diseases may cause malabsorption of foods, vitamins, minerals and electrolytes. Therapy is directed at correcting these deficiencies and eradicating the primary disease. If the primary lesion is not correctable, replacement therapy appropriate for the type of deficiency may have to be given indefinitely. The modern concept of the intestinal malabsorption syndromes favours a luminal to serosal classification (see Bank et al., 1971a; Fordtran, 1978).

6.1 Luminal Abnormalities

6.1.1 Pancreatic Insufficiency
Postgastrectomy malabsorption and the Zollinger-Ellison syndrome, which produce pancreatic insufficiency by a delay in arrival of pancreatic juice and acidification of the duodenum respectively, require replacement therapy or surgical correction (see sect. 5.4.2, 12.2).

6.1.2 Bacterial Overgrowth
Malabsorption occurs when the normal small bowel bacteria (rarely more than 1,000 to 10,000/ml) reach concentrations of 10^6 to 10^9/ml (Gorbach and Tabaqchali, 1969). These bacteria deconjugate bile salts to unconjugated forms, resulting in inadequate micelle formation and thus defective fat absorption and steatorrhoea, and/or the bacteria utilise vitamin B_{12} or convert it into inactive cobamides, causing megaloblastic anaemia. Bacterial proliferation may be caused by: (a) dilatation and stenosis (e.g. blindloops, strictures, scleroderma), by (b) fistulae (e.g. gastrocolic or ileocolic fistulae), or (c) decreased bacterial destruction by gastric acid (e.g. postgastrectomy and pernicious anaemia).

Whatever the cause or mechanism, broad spectrum antibacterial drugs will improve the steatorrhoea and vitamin B_{12} absorption. The most commonly used antibiotic is tetracycline, a short course of 1g daily for 10 days may be adequate to relieve diarrhoea and steatorrhoea within 3 or 4 days, and the improvement may be sustained. In some patients, however, 500mg daily for a long period may be required, or co-trimoxazole (trimethoprim + sulphamethoxazole) 1 tablet daily as an alternative.

6.1.3 Choleretic Diarrhoea/Steatorrhoea
Interruption of the enterohepatic circulation by ileal disease or resection and massive small bowel resection, diminishes bile salt absorption and depletes the bile salt pool, resulting either in fat malabsorption or an irritant effect of unabsorbed bile salts on the colon with 'choleretic diarrhoea'.

A low fat diet (30g/day) is often sufficient to control the steatorrhoea and may be supplemented by antimotility drugs such as codeine phosphate, diphenoxylate or loperamide to control the diarrhoea (see section 7.2), and by vitamin B_{12} and other replacement therapy. The basic anion exchange resin cholestyramine (16g daily) has been used with some success in patients with ileal resections of under 100cm associated with mild steatorrhoea. It binds bile salts to form a non-absorbable complex, thereby increasing their faecal excretion and thus abolishing bile acid induced secretion of water and electrolytes in the colon. The effect is to control the diarrhoea in some patients, but often with an increase in steatorrhoea and fat soluble vitamin malabsorption. Nausea, vomiting and abdominal cramps are additional side effects. In those patients with severe steatorrhoea, substitution of dietary fat by medium chain triglycerides may prove helpful.

6.2 Mucosal Abnormalities

6.2.1 Gluten Induced Enteropathy (coeliac disease, coeliac sprue, idiopathic steatorrhoea, primary malabsorption)
Drug therapy plays a very small part in treatment. A strict diet which is gluten free is the basis of treatment. No food containing wheat or rye flour should be consumed. Some also include oats and barley, and recently soya has also been incriminated. Even milk products and some proteins may require deletion in unresponsive patients. As many products contain small amounts of gluten the patients should be given a comprehensive list of these. A rapid symptomatic improvement is the rule and biochemical evidence of improved absorption can also be expected, but structural recovery of the jejunal mucosa may be slow. The response is usually more complete in children than in adults.

A non-response should suggest inadvertent gluten consumption or a wrong diagnosis. In countries where coeliac disease is rare and conditions like lymphoma are more common (i.e. South Africa, Middle East) non-response is often an indication for laparotomy (Novis et al., 1971). A small number of patients fail to respond to gluten restriction and require permanent replacement therapy. Corticosteroid therapy may be indicated in the severly ill patient. Prednisone 40mg daily or corticotrophin for 6 weeks causes a rapid symptomatic improvement with a prompt but incomplete histological and metabolic improvement and in addition encourages a response to a gluten free diet.

Dietary supplements are always required. Vitamin D, potassium and calcium gluconate should be given whilst awaiting a response to dietary therapy. Iron and folate deficiency are common and should be treated with oral iron and folic acid. B group vitamins and vitamin K are necessary only if there is evidence of deficiency. The gluten-restricted diet must be maintained permanently, and a sudden change in the pattern of response should raise the possibility of a lymphomatous change in the bowel.

6.2.2 Tropical Sprue

Although the aetiology of tropical sprue is still unknown, a combination of folic acid deficiency and bowel infection appears to be the most likely cause. The results of treatment directed at these presumptive causes are usually entirely satisfactory. Apart from correction of fluid and electrolyte losses in the acute phase, and of anaemia by oral iron and parenteral vitamin B_{12}, oral or parenteral folic acid (5mg 3 times a day) produces considerable improvement in most patients, usually rapidly but occasionally only after some months. When remission has been achieved, folic acid 5mg daily is given as maintenance therapy. If absorption of vitamin B_{12} remains subnormal after remission, monthly maintenance injections should be given. Long term (6 months) broad spectrum antibiotic therapy (e.g. tetracycline 2g daily reducing to 1g daily) has produced an improvement in those patients not responding to folic acid and B_{12} and the three therapeutic measures may be tried singly or in conjunction.

6.2.3 Disaccharidase Deficiency

Treatment in these conditions consists in removing as much of the offending sugar from the diet as is necessary for a symptomatic response. This may include lactose, maltose or sucrose. In lactase deficiency a milk free diet is all that is usually required in patients with symptoms, although a diet totally free of all dairy products is required in selected patients. Lactose free nutriments are available for children with lactose intolerance and lactase enzyme may be added to milk (e.g. Lact-Aid).

6.2.4 Whipple's Disease

This rare condition which occurs predominantly in middle aged men has now been shown to be due to an atypical bacillus corresponding to periodic acid Schiff (PAS) positive inclusions seen on electron microscopy. Considered to be a lethal disease in the past, it is now completely curable with antibacterial agents. The best results have been obtained with a combination of soluble benzylpenicillin 2 mega units and streptomycin 1g daily for 2 weeks, followed by 1g tetracycline daily or phenoxymethyl penicillin 250mg 4 times daily for 6 to 12 months as maintenance therapy. If a satisfactory response is not obtained, a combination of benzylpenicillin 4 mega units and ampicillin 4g daily (or amoxycillin 2g daily) or chloramphenicol may be tried.

6.2.5 Intestinal Lymphoma and Alpha-chain Disease (immunoproliferative small bowel disease)

Intestinal lymphoma presenting with malabsorption has been described as occurring mainly in the Middle East and Mediterranean area and in the Cape Province of South Africa (Novis et al., 1972). Despite the poor prognosis, considerable short term improvement may occur after surgical resection of areas of bowel macroscopically involved by lymphoma, followed by radiotherapy to the central abdomen in a dose of 3000 rads. Chemotherapy with cytotoxic drugs and prednisone, in various doses, combinations and sequences, have also been used either initially or for relapses (Novis et al., 1971). In cases with alpha-chain disease we have achieved disappearance of the pathological alpha heavy chain by radiotherapy followed by long term prednisone 10 to 20mg daily. Another case has been reported in which the alpha-chain disappeared after therapy with prednisone 20 to 40mg daily and cyclophosphamide 900mg initially and 100 to 350mg weekly thereafter. Long term broad spectrum antibiotics have been reported to produce clinical remission in patients with plasma cell infiltration of the bowel, but who have no evidence of a malignant lymphoma. Continuous supportive therapy with low fat, high caloric diet, iron, vitamins, calcium, as needed, is frequently helpful and may result in successful maintenance of the patient's activity over a period of months.

6.2.6 *Eosinophilic Gastroenteritis*
This may require corticosteroid therapy. Long term exclusion diets have little place in the management.

6.3 Intestinal Lymphatic Obstruction

This may occur as a primary and probably congenital lymphangiectasia, or be acquired secondary to lymphoma, tuberculosis or many diseases of the bowel wall, or in congestive heart failure, which will need treatment in their own right. These abnormalities are usually associated with protein losing enteropathy, and triglyceride, cholesterol, calcium and fat soluble vitamin malabsorption.

An improvement in the serum proteins and serum lipids occurs when these patients are put onto a low fat diet and the long chain triglycerides in the diet replaced by medium chain triglycerides. Absorption of the latter directly into the portal vein reduces the lymphatic pressure and subsequent protein leakage into the bowel. These medium chain triglycerides usually contain 8 or 10 carbon fatty acids and are readily absorbed, despite insufficient bile acids or pancreatic lipase in the small bowel. Medium chain triglycerides therefore provide a source of calories, improve nutrition and diminish diarrhoea and steatorrhoea in biliary obstruction, intestinal lymphangiectasia, cystic fibrosis of the pancreas, massive small bowel resection, and a-β lipoproteinaemia. A convenient medium chain triglyceride preparation is 'Portagen'; 100g of the powder or oil supplying 463 calories, and may be used for cooking with meals or as a separate supplement.

6.4 Elemental Diets

The term 'elemental diet' is given to a food which contains an elemental protein and carbohydrate source in the form of amino acids, glucose and other easily digestible nutrients, added minerals and vitamins, together with small quantities of fat, present as triglycerides of linoleic acid and/or medium chain triglycerides. It is always worth reading the ingredients of the various elemental diets to ensure the best type for the individual patient (e.g. Vivonex, Flexical, Hycal, etc), and it is well worth starting with half or quarter strength feeds and increasing to full daily caloric requirements (e.g. 2000 to 3000 calories per day). Such a diet is also known as 'chemically defined' as the elemental components are pure chemical entities. They should not be confused with the large selection of liquid nutritional foods available (e.g. Sustacal, Precision, Compleat B, Ensure).

The principal characteristics of minimal residue and minimal digestion required, with high nutritional efficacy, leads to their potential usefulness in malabsorption and maldigestion states, as well as in the management of gastrointestinal fistulae, inflammatory bowel disease and short bowel syndrome (Russell, 1975). The main disadvantages of these diets have been their unpalatability and occasional diarrhoea due to the osmotic effects of the high sugar content. However, most manufacturers have now attempted to make them iso-osmolar. Elemental diet therapy can be given orally or via intragastric or intrajejunal tubes. In some severely ill patients with gastrointestinal disease, it may follow an initial period of parenteral nutrition (i.e. mixtures of hydrolysed protein in glucose), but in others it may replace intravenous hyperalimentation altogether. Wherever possible the oral route should be used as it is likely that the integrity of the gut mucosa may depend on intraluminal nutrients and pancreatic enzymes.

7. Large Bowel Disease

Symptoms commonly arising from the large bowel (e.g. diarrhoea and constipation) may be the first indication of organic disease. The symptoms are usually so successfully suppressed by symptomatic therapy, that nothing is done to determine the underlying pathological process. Any persistent (1 week or longer) or severe bowel derangement must be fully investigated.

7.1 Constipation

Constipation is one of the most common nonorganic symptoms, but as such may be difficult for the patient to define (Avery Jones and Godding, 1972). Many patients with 'normal' bowel function often think they are constipated. Constipation itself implies a delayed passage of faeces through the intestine, the final act of defaecation being normal, in contrast to dyschesia when the act of defaecation is deranged.

Fundamental to treatment is a thorough examination. An attempt must be made to reach a diagnosis, especially in patients past middle age, and to ensure that the patient does not have faecal impaction. Appropriate treatment of any primary condition, whether it arises in the gastrointestinal tract or not (e.g. depression, drugs, diverticulosis), may be sufficient to manage the constipation. Where a primary cause is absent (and sometimes where it is present) additional and specific help may be required (Thompson, 1976).

In general, constipation is best treated by attention to diet so that an adequate intake of residue (fibre) and fluid are maintained, encouragement of physical activity (especially in the elderly and those recovering from surgery) and emphasis on the importance of answering nature's call to stool. Cellulose, hemicellulose, pectins, gums and lignin are the main constituents of dietary fibre. These undigested products increase faecal bulk, probably holding on to water and shorten the transit time. It is possible that the water retaining properties are due to pentose containing polysaccharides. Weight for weight, fibre from unprocessed bran produces almost double the stool weight as carrot, cabbage, apple, or guar gum fibre (Cummings et al., 1978). While there is little doubt that increased dietary fibre adds bulk and softens the stool to relieve constipation, there is epidemiological support only for the many other roles ascribed to it, such as the prevention of diverticulosis, haemorrhoids, hiatal hernia, gallstones, carcinoma of the colon, heart disease and carcinoma of the breast. Clearly, much work needs to be done in these directions (Cummings, 1973; Pomare, 1977). Unprocessed bran can be bought cheaply, but may also be taken in high bulk cereals and breads. It is difficult to see why it is necessary to have bran in a tablet form or high fibre granules except for palatibility. Some patients find bran difficult to swallow and others complain of increased flatulence and abdominal distention. It is thus not a panacea for constipation. A useful regimen is to sprinkle 2 to 4 tablespoons of Miller's bran on to a conventional commercial high bulk cereal or a stewed prune compote for breakfast.

When laxatives are required they should be used in the lowest effective dosage as infrequently as possible. The patient should be told that they are being used to restore bowel function to 'normal', not to make him dependent on the drug. The long continued use of laxatives should be avoided, particularly the lubricants and cascara, but a few intractable cases may require long term treatment with an appropriate agent. The wretched colon of the elderly (presbycolon) may need drug treatment indefinitely, despite attention to the usual non-drug therapeutic measures and the pious hope that simple instruction will restore bowel function (Bank and Marks, 1977).

Laxatives can be given orally or rectally as a suppository or enema. The commonly used laxatives are classified as either stimulants or irritants, bulk producers, osmotic water retaining substances, lubricants or softening (wetting) agents (see Thompson, 1976; table V). Except for the bulk producers, strength of action is usually dose related, but response to different preparations varies markedly from patient to patient. Each patient should therefore titrate his own dose in sufficient amount such that a dose at night for example, produces one soft formed stool in the morning. Some patients prefer suppositories. Small volume disposable enemas may be useful in selected cases (e.g. faecal impaction, preparation for proctoscopy and barium enema examination) or as initial treatment of severe constipation. Otherwise oral preparations are probably most convenient or acceptable. A guide to the use of laxatives is given in table V.

Treatment of constipation in the elderly is discussed in chapter V (sect. 4.7.6).

7.2 Diarrhoea

Diarrhoea is a symptom and represents an alteration of the bowel habit of the individual. It results from the passage of stools containing excess water. Thus, diarrhoea can be explained in terms of malabsorption or hypersecretion of water and solute, and can be conveniently classified into the following categories: (a) osmotic: retardation of water absorption — e.g. malabsorption of carbohydrate or fat; (b) secretory: abnormal electrolyte and water transport — e.g. certain bacteria, bile acids; and (c) disorders of transit — e.g. hypermotility (see Phillips, 1972).

A firm diagnosis should be pursued on the basis of a thorough general physical examination and the clinical presentation of the patient, and specific treatment instituted as soon as possible

Table V. Medications used in the management of constipation

Type	Name	Potency	Usual dose	Principal side effects/Notes[1]
Stimulants or irritants	Anthraquinones			
	Cascara	++	300mg	Habitual use — especially at risk are: (a) those who begin abuse when young and continue into adulthood, (b) those requiring routine laxatives for idiopathic constipation. Melanosis coli (prolonged use); avoid in breast feeding mothers
	Senna[2]	++	0.5 to 2g	Skin eruptions; changes in bowel ganglia. Adjust dose to individual requirements and smallest effective dose
	Danthron	+	75 to 150mg	Skin eruptions; avoid in breast feeding mothers
	Rhubarb (rheum)	+	0.2 to 1g	Skin eruptions; post purge constipation
	Bisacodyl (oral)	+++	5 to 15mg	Abdominal cramps. Enteric coated tablets take 6 hours or more to exert effect
	Phenolphthalein	++	50 to 300mg	Skin eruptions (infrequent); syncope; hypersensitivity (infrequent). Activity likely due to absorbed portion of drug acting on muscle of distal colon
	Castor oil	+++	5 to 20ml	Pelvic congestion. Avoid in pregnancy and menstruation and in elderly with faecal impaction
Bulk producers[2,3]	Mucilagenous seeds, gums			All somewhat difficult to swallow; slow action
	Ispaghula (Isogel)	+	5 to 10g	
	Sterculia (Normacol)	+	5 to 10g	
	Psyllium (Metamucil)	+	7g	
	Unprocessed bran	+	1 to 4g	
	Methylcellulose	+	3 to 6g	
Osmotic	Magnesium sulphate	++	5 to 15g	Hypermagnesaemia in impaired renal function which is common in elderly
	Magnesium hydroxide[2]	+	15ml	
	Lactulose[3]	+	15 to 30ml	Abdominal cramps; diarrhoea (excessive dosage)
	Small volume enemas (phosphate; citrate)	++++	100 to 130ml	Mucosal irritation may interfere with interpretation of sigmoidoscopic findings
Lubricants	Liquid paraffin	+	10 to 30ml	Lipid pneumonia from aspiration, particularly in elderly; anal oil leak, deficiency of fat soluble vitamins. May interfere with healing of enteric fistulas. Avoid in infants or elderly patients with difficulty in swallowing, pregnancy
Wetting agents	Poloxalkol	+	200mg to 1g	Slow action
	Dioctylsodium sulphosuccinate (oral)	+	30 to 100mg	Slow action; anorexia, vomiting, diarrhoea. May facilitate absorption of other normally unabsorbed laxatives and thus should not be used in combination with such drugs
Miscellaneous	Micro dose enemas (sodium citrate, surface active agents, glycerine)	+++	5ml	

1   Habitual use of any purgative can cause severe potassium loss and accompanying muscle weakness and also impairment of homeostasis in the elderly. See also section 14.4.3.
2   Drugs most commonly used in clinical practice.
3   Suitable for long term use when indicated (see text).

(e.g. bacillary and amoebic dysentery, malabsorption diarrhoeas, gastroenteritis in children). In the interim, and where no organic or drug induced (see section 14.2.2) cause can be found, symptomatic control should be attempted (Lorber, 1971).

Attention should be paid to diet and general supportive measures and, if necessary, fluid and electrolyte replacement (e.g. gastroenteritis). Glucose added to oral fluids aids absorption in many conditions (e.g. cholera) where the primary defect is excessive secretion. Sucrose is an effective alternative to glucose (Palmer et al., 1977). Except for *Salmonella typhi, Shigella shigae* and *Sh. flexneri,* the patient should not receive antibacterial agents in acute bacterial diarrhoeas, unless there is evidence of systemic spread (see further section 11.1).

When indicated, drugs for use in symptomatic treatment of diarrhoea include adsorbents such as kaolin-pectin, and suppressants of intestinal motility such as codeine, diphenoxylate, loperamide or difenoxine, in an appropriate dosage to cover the time and severity of the stool frequency. Diphenoxylate is a derivative of pethidine (meperidine) and has, like codeine, opiate activity. Habituation, although a possibility with high doses, has not been reported with usual therapeutic doses. It is combined with atropine to discourage excessive self medication, but overdosage in young children (Penfold and Volans, 1977) has resulted in atropine poisoning and severe respiratory depression (reversed by nalorphine). Difenoxine is the active metabolite of diphenoxylate. Loperamide, is a butyramide derivative with some structural similarities to diphenoxylate, but does not have opiate activity at normal therapeutic doses. It also has a more rapid onset and more prolonged duration of effect than diphenoxylate or codeine (Heel et al., 1978).

Antimotility drugs are not a panacea for all diarrhoeas. They have been claimed to prolong antibiotic (Novak et al., 1976) and acute bacterial diarrhoeas although the evidence for the latter is rather anecdotal. Nevertheless, in bacterial diarrhoeas, associated with pathogens which invade the intestinal mucosa (e.g. *Shigella, Salmonella* species and certain strains of *Escherichia coli*); antimotility drugs by slowing intestinal transit, may delay clearance of the infecting organisms from the bowel and prolong the course of the illness (Du Pont and Hornick, 1973). Similarly, in antibiotic-associated colitis they may prolong the diarrhoea

and contribute to development of more severe colitis and should not be used in management (Pittman et al., 1974; Pittman, 1975; see section 14.4.3).

In chronic diarrhoea associated with inflammatory bowel disorders such as ulcerative colitis and Crohn's colitis, antimotility drugs are not primary therapy and are used to provide symptomatic control as an adjunct to other more specific measures. In severe acute attacks of ulcerative colitis, antimotility drugs may precipitate ileus and dilatation of the bowel ('toxic megacolon') and should be avoided. They may be used cautiously in mild or less severe attacks as an adjunct to other measures, but should be discontinued promptly if abdominal distention or other untoward symptoms occur (see further section 8.1.5).

A short course of an antianxiety agent such as diazepam, or one of the tricyclic antidepressants, may be of value in cases of mental stress and worry which lead to functional diarrhoea.

Prevention of traveller's diarrhoea is by attention to hygiene and avoidance of tap water and improperly prepared or cooked foodstuffs. Patients could be given a supply of antimotility drugs to use in the event of a bout of diarrhoea prior to seeking immediate medical advice. Although antimicrobial agents such as neomycin, sulphonamides, streptomycin plus sulphonamides and clioquinol are given prophylactically for traveller's diarrhoea, there is no convincing evidence that they are effective. There is some evidence that doxycycline can be effective in prophylaxis and might be used in selected travellers at risk (Sack et al., 1978), but efficacy is likely to depend on knowledge of the sensitivity of causative organisms, notably enterotoxigenic *Escherichia coli* in the areas of travel involved.

In some patients who have malabsorption of bile salts as a result of distal ileal disease or resection, cholestyramine may be of great benefit in reducing diarrhoea by preventing the secretory effect of bile salts on the colonic mucosa (see section 6.1.3). Steatorrhoea, if present, will be made worse by cholestyramine and is therefore a relative contraindication to its use. The minimum effective dose should be used, usually about 2 to 12g per day in divided doses. Cholestyramine is also effective in diarrhoea after vagotomy (see section 5.4.2). Aluminium hydroxide can be used in patients with bile salt diarrhoea who cannot tolerate cholestyramine (Sali et al., 1977).

7.3 Irritable Bowel Syndrome (irritable colon syndrome; spastic colon)

This is an unsatisfactory term for a symptom complex believed to result from incoordinated, abnormal motor activity of the intestinal tract (Fielding, 1977). It is characterised by recurrent abdominal pain or discomfort with a distribution of colonic pain reference, usually with disturbance in bowel habit, and occurring in the absence of demonstrable organic disease (Barbezat, 1978). The basic pathogenesis of the syndrome is unknown, so no specific treatment is possible. Great care should be taken not to label a patient with this diagnosis while overlooking remediable organic bowel disease or other organic cause for the patient's symptoms. Nor should it be thought that patients with this syndrome can never develop organic gastrointestinal disease; spastic colon has been considered by some to be the precursor of diverticular disease.

Explanation of the syndrome and strong reassurance that there is no serious organic disease are the basis of patient management. A prime aim in those with irregular bowel habits should be an attempt to achieve some bowel regularity. Treatment is directed at the predominant symptoms — pain, constipation or diarrhoea (Goulston, 1973; Fielding, 1977).

If pain is the predominant symptom, a high residue diet (e.g. unprocessed bran, high fibre breakfast cereals) is well worth trying, together with an antispasmodic/anticholinergic drug (see below), otherwise patients should find their own best diet by trial and error, at the same time correcting any dietary imbalance.

When constipation is the predominant symptom, most cases respond to exercise, fluids (particularly non-alcoholic beverages and fruit juices), prunes or bran, together with a bulk providing laxative if needed (see table V). If constipation does not respond to a combination of these simple measures, senna preparations or lactulose syrup may be used in small doses until regularisation of bowel habit occurs.

For patients in whom diarrhoea predominates, diet should be modified by restriction of fluids or foods such as prunes and stoned fruit. Antimotility agents can be used as needed. Loperamide is probably preferable to codeine, diphenoxylate or difenoxine because of its more rapid onset and prolonged duration of effect (Heel et al., 1978). Since colonic and in particular 'functional' diarrhoea tends to occur predominantly in the early hours of the morning (i.e. 5.00 to 10.00 am), appropriate doses can be taken at bedtime and after the first bowel action in the morning. Patients with the more severe 'morning rush syndrome', a variant characterised by a series of urgent bowel movements, each becoming progressively more liquid, when the patient first gets up in the morning, can be treated with antimotility agents — taken a few hours before the anticipated diarrhoea and again immediately after a loose stool, should this be passed in the morning.

Other treatment which might be helpful and which can be considered includes antispasmodics such as mebeverine, dicyclomine or hyoscine butylbromide. These can be combined with a high residue diet or antianxiety drugs if considered necessary (e.g. belladonna and phenobarbitone; clidinium bromide and chlordiazepoxide). Many patients with predominant symptoms of diarrhoea respond well to small regular doses of an antianxiety drug, while others may be depressed and respond to a tricyclic antidepressant (Hislop, 1971). In general, antianxiety and antidepressant drugs should be restricted to patients who fail to respond to other measures and should be used in short courses (see chapt. XXVI; sect. 7.3, 8.3). The clinician should be prepared to try various alternatives according to the predominant symptoms of the individual patient. Some may be helped most by a combination of a number of various treatments; for example, an antispasmodic, increased dietary fibre and an antianxiety drug with additional symptomatic control by a laxative or antidiarrhoeal drug as necessary (Ritchie and Truelove, 1979).

7.4 Diverticulosis/Diverticulitis

The pathogenesis of diverticular disease is unknown but may be related to diet and raised intracolonic pressure. Patients with diverticulosis are usually asymptomatic but those with diverticulitis, which implies inflammation, often present with pain, fever and changes in bowel habit. Careful differential diagnosis is important to permit appropriate treatment and to manage potentially dangerous complications (Barbezat, 1978). Constipation or diarrhoea should be avoided and dietary and fluid intake carefully controlled. The majority of patients can be managed by conservative medical treatment. A high residue diet (e.g. bran etc) is advised (Brodribb, 1977). If constipation remains a problem a bulk producing laxative is usually of benefit, but great care is required to avoid faecal impaction. Antimotility agents are theoretically contraindicated, but it is sometimes difficult to withhold them in patients with troublesome diarrhoea.

In acute attacks, bed rest, antibiotics (tetracycline 1g daily) a fluid diet and analgesics are indicated. In severely ill patients and where tetracycline resistant or anaerobic organisms are responsible, the appropriate antibiotic according to the causative organism will be required. Pentazocine decreases intraluminal colonic pressure and may therefore be preferable to morphine or codeine as an analgesic in the acute stages (Stanciu and Bennet, 1974a). When patients with an irritable bowel syndrome or diverticular disease have recovered from the acute phase, it seems very likely that a high residue diet will help in preventing further symptoms (see section 7.1). Surgery is considered if the condition fails to settle or if local complications (e.g. uncontrollable haemorrhage or perforation), develop.

8. Inflammatory Bowel Disease

8.1 Ulcerative Colitis

Careful diagnosis is essential to distinguish between ulcerative colitis (idiopathic proctocolitis) and amoebiasis, diverticulitis, ischaemic colitis, pseudomembranous colitis, carcinoma of the rectum or colon, and Crohn's disease (Ament, 1975; Northfield, 1977). The general principles of treatment are: (a) to control an acute attack as rapidly as possible, (b) to induce remission, and (c) to prevent relapse (Truelove, 1971). Close personal supervision by the attending clinician, and surgeon where indicated, is of utmost importance. Patients should be advised that ulcerative colitis is a relapsing disease and that a further attack may occur. It must be impressed on them that early treatment of a relapse is essential. The severity of each attack will dictate the intensity of treatment (Lennard-Jones and Ritchie, 1974).

8.1.1 Severe Attacks *(seriously ill patients)*
These demand urgent admission to hospital and immediate intensive medical treatment (Truelove and Jewell, 1974; Truelove et al., 1978). General medical measures consist of correction of dehydration and electrolyte losses, correction of

anaemia, treatment with systemic corticosteroids or corticotrophin, topical corticosteroid therapy and attention to diet. Monitoring of the patient's progress should be made by both physician and surgeon.

Correction of dehydration and electrolyte losses demands intravenous infusion with fluids such as saline or dextrose saline, and it is usually necessary to add potassium chloride to the infusion and to commence parenteral feeding. Blood transfusion is required for correction of anaemia and should be repeated as often as is necessary to maintain the haemoglobin at normal values. Iron therapy has no place during an acute attack, although it is often required afterwards to replenish the body stores of iron.

Treatment with corticosteroids is usually best begun with a water soluble compound administered in the intravenous drip (e.g. prednisolone 21-phosphate, 20mg 3 times a day, or hydrocortisone sodium succinate, 100mg 3 times a day). Intravenous corticosteroid therapy should be combined with a broad spectrum antibiotic (e.g. tetracycline, 250mg 4 times a day; supplemented by metronidazole in areas where amoebiasis is endemic), also given in the infusion, and each continued for 5 days. Oral broad spectrum antibiotics are not favoured as they may precipitate enterocolitis. Topical corticosteroid therapy may also be given and consists of a twice daily rectal drip of hydrocortisone sodium succinate (100mg in about 150mg of warm physiological saline) or retention enemas of prednisolone sodium phosphate.

During the initial phase of intensive therapy only a little water is given by mouth, but later a high calorie, high protein, low residue diet is given. If response to intensive therapy (about 5 days) is good, it is followed by resumption of normal feeding, except in the presence of a secondary lactase deficiency, when milk should be withdrawn. Oral corticosteroids (e.g. prednisolone 40 to 60mg a day in divided doses) are given and continued until the patient has been free from symptoms for about a week. The dose should then be gradually reduced over the next 4 to 8 weeks. Sulphasalazine should then be given orally as continuation therapy (see sect. 8.1.4). Surgery is indicated in patients who continue to deteriorate despite active treatment and in those who fail to respond after 5 days.

Patients with toxic megacolon should be treated as medical emergencies, preferably in an intensive care unit. They should have full treatment for severe colitis plus nasogastric aspiration. Very close monitoring (vital signs, abdominal tenderness, abdominal girth, radiology) during the first 24 to 48 hours by both physician and surgeon should decide whether the patient continues to have medical treatment or whether surgery should be performed.

8.1.2 Moderate Attacks (moderately severe disease and some systemic upset)

Admission to hospital is usually necessary. Treatment consists of oral corticosteroids (e.g. prednisolone 40 to 60mg daily in divided doses) plus topical therapy with corticosteroid retention enemas or rectal foam. The oral corticosteroid is tapered off within 4 to 8 weeks. Sulphasalazine is less effective in controlling acute attacks than corticosteroids, but can be used at a dose of 1g 3 or 4 times daily in addition to corticosteroids. Larger doses carry a considerable risk of side effects, especially nausea and vomiting, and are best avoided (see below). Sulphasalazine enemas (1g in saline or water twice daily) have been tried with success in patients with proctocolitis (Serebro et al., 1977) and are being further investigated. A high protein diet is necessary. Intravenous correction of dehydration and electrolyte depletion and/or blood transfusion is not always necessary. Failure to obtain a good response is an indication for a 5 day course of intensive intravenous steroid therapy, or corticotrophin gel (60 to 120 units) or tetracosactrin depot (1 to 2mg) as a single daily intramuscular dose for 5 days.

Sulphasalazine (salicylazosulphapyridine, azulfidine): The mode of action of sulphasalazine in ulcerative colitis is not known but effective oral treatment seems to require delivery of metabolites of sulphasalazine in the faeces to the diseased distal segment of the colon (Cowan et al., 1977). Sulphasalazine serves as a vehicle to deliver its possible active components, 5-aminosalicylic acid and sulphapyridine, to the colon in higher concentrations than could be achieved by oral administration of either alone. Sulphasalazine itself is only absorbed in small and variable amounts from the upper gastrointestinal tract and reaches the colon mostly unchanged where it is split by gut bacteria at the azo linkage, to form 5-aminosalicylic acid and sulphapyridine. 5-Aminosalicylic acid may act locally and is not absorbed to any marked extent, whereas sulphapyridine is mainly absorbed from the colon and may act both locally (during its mucosal absorption) and

systemically. Recent evidence suggests that the active forms of sulphasalazine (particularly the 5-aminosalicylic acid component) act by reducing prostaglandin synthesis in the colon (Sharon et al., 1978), raised levels of prostaglandins having previously been demonstrated in blood and colonic mucosa from patients with ulcerative colitis (Gould et al., 1977).

Both therapeutic efficacy and toxicity of sulphasalazine correlate with serum total sulphapyridine concentrations (i.e. free drug plus metabolites). Sulphapyridine is biotransformed in the liver largely by acetylation and to a lesser extent by hydroxylation; the rate of acetylation being genetically determined such that individuals can be classified as either slow or rapid acetylators in the same manner as sulphadimidine and other drugs which share the same acetylation polymorphism (see chapter VII; sect. 4.2.1). There also appears to be a genetic polymorphism in the capacity to hydroxylate sulphapyridine. Slow acetylators have higher concentrations of free sulphapyridine and lower concentrations of acetylated sulphapyridine than rapid acetylators and are more likely to experience side effects on equivalent doses of sulphasalazine. For a review of the pharmacokinetic properties and action of sulphasalazine, see Das and Dubin (1976).

The side effects of sulphasalazine illustrate important principles in clinical pharmacology. Apart from nausea and vomiting, side effects include skin rashes, intense headache, giddiness, blood dyscrasias (mainly haemolytic anaemia, but also agranulocytosis and very rarely aplastic anaemia), drug fever, 'cyanosis', and pulmonary and neurotoxicity. Side effects usually occur early in treatment and are dose related. They are observed mainly in those taking 4g or more daily, the majority of whom are slow acetylators of the drug. In all but a few cases side effects can be overcome by temporarily stopping sulphasalazine with reintroduction at a reduced dosage (Das et al., 1973). A suggested routine for the patient with nausea and vomiting is withdrawal of the drug for 5 to 7 days, and then introduction in lower dosage, say 2g per day; for patients with 'cyanosis', reduction of dose; for patients with haemolysis and transient reticulocytosis, withdrawal of the drug for 5 to 7 days, or reduction of dosage. For patients with a history of rash associated with sulphasalazine, initially 1g per day and then an increase of 2g per day after 1 week with antihistamine cover.

Patients should ideally be tested for their acetylation phenotype while receiving sulphasalazine so that dosage can be adjusted appropriately. A single serum sample for free and acetylated sulphapyridine concentration is sufficient for this purpose (Das and Eastwood, 1975). Also, haemolytic anaemia is more likely to occur in those with glucose-6-phosphate dehydrogenase deficiency and patients should also be screened for this genetic defect in areas where it is prevalent or if they develop haemolytic anaemia on the drug (see chapter XXIII, sect. 8.4; VII, sect. 4.2.2).

8.1.3 Mild Attacks (mild, usually distal disease and no systemic upset)

Corticosteroid retention enemas at night, and sulphasalazine (0.5 to 1g 3 or 4 times daily), usually control a mild attack. A few patients may require oral corticosteroid (e.g. prednisolone 20mg daily in divided doses). Some prefer to give oral steroids at this safe short term dosage from the outset, in addition to topical steroids. Even mild attacks must be controlled as rapidly as possible, since many severe attacks have begun with mild symptoms and gradually become worse (Truelove, 1971). Failure to respond within 2 weeks demands more intensive therapy. Patients with localised proctitis are often alarmed by continued rectal bleeding. These patients should be reassured of the relatively unimportant nature of the disease, despite bleeding. Corticosteroid suppositories or foam may help and slight softening of the stool may prevent traumatic bleeding in patients with proctitis and constipation.

8.1.4 Prevention of Relapse

After control of an acute attack oral corticosteroids should be tailed off completely. There is no evidence to support the use of small doses of oral steroids given continuously to prevent relapse. Patients should be placed or continued on sulphasalazine (0.5g 3 to 4 times daily), since maintenance treatment with this drug sharply reduces the relapse rate (Misiewicz et al., 1965). If the patient can tolerate sulphasalazine it should probably be continued indefinitely (Dissanayake and Truelove, 1973). Side effects of sulphasalazine during maintenance use are predominantly gastrointestinal and can be minimised by the use of enteric coated tablets or reduction of dosage. Most patients tolerate the drug well (see also section 8.1.2). Certain patients with frequent relapses not controlled by sulphasalazine can be kept well by corticosteroid retention enemas given nightly or on alternate nights. Azathioprine (2.5mg/kg daily in divided doses initially, reducing to 1.5mg/kg after 3 months) can be used cautiously in selected patients for whom all other treatment has failed and for whom surgery is not indicated. Reports of its effectiveness in maintaining remission vary and it should only be used in very carefully selected patients (Jewell and Truelove, 1974).

A milk free diet may possibly be of benefit to a small number of patients and may be worth trying on a trial and error basis. Relapses can be precipitated by gastrointestinal infection and patients should be instructed to observe good personal hygiene and eat properly prepared food when travelling to other countries. Emotional factors may also induce a relapse and this aspect should be discussed with the patient. Any abnormal psychological findings seem more likely to be a result of the disease rather than its cause, but psychological management may be helpful. A few patients will require psychiatric support.

Because of the importance of rapidly controlling an attack, patients should be given a reserve supply of corticosteroid retention enemas (or even oral steroids) so that treatment can be started immediately in the event of a relapse.

8.1.5 Supportive Drug Therapy

In general, antimotility drugs should be avoided in patients with a severe attack of colitis as they may precipitate ileus and dilatation of the bowel ('toxic megacolon'). Anticholinergic drugs are not recommended for the same reason. In mild and less severe attacks both types of drug may be cautiously used. Codeine (15mg 6-hourly), diphenoxylate (2.5mg 6-hourly) or loperamide (2 to 4mg 12-hourly) is of value in reducing the number and frequency of stools and the disturbing urgency that these patients often have. Anticholinergic drugs (e.g. propantheline 15mg 4 times daily) can be used to ameliorate abdominal cramps and nocturnal diarrhoea and to help retain enemas. Following an attack, vitamin supplements and oral iron may be indicated.

8.1.6 Complications and Failed Medical Treatment

Complications remote from the colon affect the eye (conjunctivitis and uveitis), mouth (ulceration), skin (erythema nodosum) and joints (arthritis and ankylosing spondylitis). Combinations of more than one of these not infrequently occur in the same patient. All except ankylosing spondylitis (which is usually progressive) respond to corticosteroid therapy, as does pyoderma gangrenosum which is unusual but may be dangerous. Chronic liver disease may present as fatty changes, pericholangitis or chronic active hepatitis and cirrhosis. Deep venous thrombosis of the legs is not uncommon in an attack of ulcerative colitis and is an indication for anticoagulant therapy (heparin) to minimise the risk of a fatal pulmonary embolism.

Surgery is indicated when an adequate and appropriate course of medical treatment fails to control an acute attack or disabling chronic disease, or when certain local complications develop (e.g. perforation). Suspicion or presence, or high risk of carcinoma of the colon (universal or extensive colitis of longer than 10 years duration, especially if onset in childhood or early adult life) are other indications for surgery.

8.2 Crohn's Disease (regional enteritis, granulomatous colitis)

Like ulcerative colitis, Crohn's disease (which appears to be increasing in frequency) is a chronic intermittent inflammatory bowel disease, and although usually involving the small bowel, it can affect any part of the alimentary tract from the mouth to the anus. Although sometimes difficult, it is important to distinguish between Crohn's disease and ulcerative colitis because response to treatment is different (Ament, 1975; Northfield, 1977). Patients with ulcerative colitis generally respond better to medical treatment, whereas many of those with Crohn's disease will eventually require surgery.

The aim of medical treatment of Crohn's disease is to reduce symptoms, maintain nutrition and avoid complications, without inducing major side effects. The place of surgery is controversial in the early stages of the disease and largely reserved for complications or failure of medical therapy. The extent of bowel involvement might influence how long one persists with conservative measures before resorting to surgery. The general approach to treatment is the same as for ulcerative colitis, with corticosteroids being the principal treatment in severe attacks and in those who fail to respond to more simple measures such as sulphasalazine (1g 3 or 4 times daily) in milder exacerbations. Steroids are contraindicated when there is evidence of intra-abdominal sepsis, or with asymptomatic fistulae or strictures. Prednisone in an initial oral dose of 60 to 80mg daily, gradually reduced as a clinical response is evident, frequently curtails the more severe acute exacerbation. Occasionally, corticotrophin is effective when prednisone fails; the usual dose being 60 to 120 units of ACTH gel or 1 to 2mg tetracosactrin depot daily intramuscularly. Metronidazole might be effective in some patients with colonic Crohn's disease (Blichfeldt et al., 1978), probably as a result of its activity against anaerobic organisms.

Once a remission has been induced some patients can be maintained on symptomatic treatment (see below). For those who require 'specific' treatment to reduce symptoms it is preferable to try sulphasalazine first at a dose of 0.5 to 1g 3 or 4 times daily. If symptoms are not reduced on sulphasalazine, corticosteroids can then be used, but they should not be used on a long term basis for mild symptoms or to prevent relapses. Corticotrophin, or alternate day steroid therapy (Whittington et al., 1977), should be considered in children as less growth retardation is likely to occur (see chapter XVI; sect. 14.3). The lowest possible dose of steroid to reduce symptoms must be used; not only to minimise side effects but also to prevent masking of local complications. The role of azathioprine is controversial. Used alone and for relatively short periods it appears to be of doubtful benefit in those with active disease, although some have found it to be useful in inducing remission in patients with colorectal involvement or fistulae (Brooke et al., 1976). Given in adequate dosage (2mg/kg daily) as a long term treatment it may be useful in reducing the relapse rate, especially after an initial response to corticosteroids, and may enable a reduction in corticosteroid dosage (O'Donoghue et al., 1978), but its long term benefit after surgical resection is doubtful (Brooke et al., 1976). Sulphasalazine is not effective in patients who develop recurrence of the disease after surgical resection (Anthonisen et al., 1974), presumably because it requires the presence of colonic bacteria for biotransformation to its active component (see section 8.1.2).

Supportive treatment measures include a high protein, low roughage diet supplemented by vitamin B_{12}, folic acid and iron, if evidence of malabsorption or anaemia exists. Some patients may find medium chain triglycerides more digestible than normal dietary fat. If medium chain triglycerides are used they should be introduced slowly as some patients will develop abdominal pain; 20 to 30g/day is usually tolerated by most patients. Supplementation or total replacement of normal diet for short periods may be attempted with elemental diets (section 6.4) to improve nutritional status, rest the involved bowel and to try and heal abdominal or rectal fistulae. In severe episodes and ill patients, total parenteral nutrition to a total of 3600 calories per day is frequently necessary. Abdominal cramps if present, require antispasmodics such as propantheline (15 to 30mg) or hyoscine butylbromide (10 to 20mg) 3 times a day. A non-irritant analgesic such as paracetamol (acetaminophen) or dextropropoxyphene may also be required and codeine phosphate (30 to 60mg daily), diphenoxylate (7.5 to 10mg daily) or loperamide (4 to 8mg daily) is necessary if diarrhoea is also a feature. Loperamide is at least as effective as codeine or diphenoxylate but has the advantage of apparent lack of opiate side effects and possibility of once daily dosage (Heel et al., 1978). Diarrhoea or steatorrhoea due to bacterial overgrowth in the bowel is frequently improved by prolonged courses of broad spectrum antibiotics (e.g. tetracycline 1g daily or ampicillin 1 to 2g daily), but these should not be given with sulphasalazine (see above).

8.3 Radiation Colitis, Postamoebic Colitis, Vascular Insufficiency of the Colon and Pseudomembranous Colitis

The drug therapy of these conditions is similar to that of ulcerative colitis. Reliance is usually placed on local and/or systemic corticosteroid therapy, with intensive general supportive measures. Surgery may be considered where there is a poor response to medical therapy. Pseudomembranous colitis associated with antibiotics, shock or vascular insufficiency has been shown to be due to toxin producing *Clostridia,* notably *Cl. difficile.* Treatment depends on severity and is similar to that of ulcerative colitis. Antibacterial agents active against the *Clostridia* strains and cholestyramine have been effective in some cases (see section 14.4.3).

8.4 Colitis in Pregnancy

Many patients will develop ulcerative colitis or Crohn's disease while they are still physically capable of bearing children. The colitis does not adversely affect the ability to conceive or a pregnancy *per se.* The prospect of the full term delivery of a live normal child is the same as for the general population, in spite of any medical treatment for relapse during pregnancy. The course of ulcerative colitis in pregnancy is unpredictable and a relapse in a previous pregnancy is not a useful guide to the future. However, relapses of ulcerative colitis do occur in pregnancy, usually in the first trimester or puerperium, but can generally be controlled by medical means. There is no increased incidence of relapse during pregnancy in Crohn's disease.

Colitis in pregnancy should be treated as in the non-pregnant patient, although sulphasalazine should not be given near parturition since sulphapyridine may compete with bilirubin binding to albumin and lead to kernicterus (Hensleigh and Kauffman, 1977). There should be no hesitation in using systemic corticosteroids in attacks. In moderate and severe attacks, systemic corticosteroids should be given from the outset to induce a remission as quickly as possible. Steroid dosage is gradually reduced as the colitis comes under control. It is often possible to discontinue steroids altogether during the second and third trimester. Total colectomy with ileostomy, or very occasionally ileostomy alone, will be necessary for the very rare cases of life threatening ulcerative colitis which does not respond to medical treatment. Young women who have already had ileostomies may conceive and deliver normally.

9. Pancreatic Disease

A composite classification of pancreatitis is essential for diagnosis and treatment (Marks et al., 1968; table VI). By definition, acute and acute relapsing pancreatitis denotes complete structural and functional restitution of the pancreas between attacks, while chronic and chronic relapsing pancreatitis denotes persistence of structural and functional derangement between attacks. Although gall-stones are the most common cause of acute and acute relapsing pancreatitis, normal pancreatic function may also occur after alcohol induced, idiopathic and miscellaneous pancreatitis. Alcohol ingestion and idiopathic pancreatitis are the major causes of chronic and chronic relapsing pancreatitis, but persistent abnormal histology and pancreatic function may occasionally be found in recurrent gall-stone and miscellaneous pancreatitis.

A fulminating course is common in the acute and acute relapsing varieties and mild attacks are

Table VI. Classification of pancreatitis

Clinicopathological	Aetiological	Clinical	Radiological
Acute	Alcohol induced	Fulminating	Calcific
Acute relapsing	Gall-stone	haemorrhagic	Non-calcific
Chronic	Idiopathic (cryptogenic)	oedematous	
Chronic relapsing	Miscellaneous	Severe	
	nutritional (tropical)	Mild	
	traumatic	Chronic	
	duct obstruction	pain	
	round worm infestation	insufficiency	
	metabolic		
	(e.g. hyperlipaemia; hypercalcaemia)		
	vascular		
	drug induced		
	pancreatopathy		

more common in the chronic varieties but both may occur. Calcific pancreatitis is usually alcohol induced (90 % in Cape Town) but may be due to nutritional causes in tropical areas (100 % in Indonesia), and to idiopathic pancreatitis or hyperparathyroidism (Marks and Bank, 1976).

The treatment of pancreatitis is untenable without a consideration of the 4 types of classification, as the initial treatment of painful pancreatitis is based entirely on the clinical presentation, whereas the interval treatment is based on an aetiological, radiological and pathofunctional classification (Trapnell, 1972; Bank et al., 1977a).

9.1 Fulminating and Severe Pancreatitis

Fulminating pancreatitis usually manifests with severe abdominal pain, abdominal rigidity or distension, and shock. Myocardial and cerebral instability are often prominent. Severe pancreatitis denotes an attack of sufficient severity to necessitate hospitalisation and treatment with nasogastric suction and intravenous therapy. The differentiation between haemorrhagic and oedematous pancreatitis can usually only be made at laparotomy, but the development of Grey-Turner's and Cullen's signs and methaemalbuminaemia, suggests haemorrhagic pancreatitis. The mortality rate of fulminating pancreatitis has been reduced to the order of 10 to 15 % with more enthusiastic general care, especially adequate rehydration, pulmonary care and treatment of early alcohol withdrawal. These patients should be given the benefit of treatment in an 'intensive care' ward so that the earliest signs of cardiac, cerebral, respiratory, renal or intra-abdominal complications

may be diagnosed and treated. Treatment is conventionally divided into various groups (Bank et al., 1977a; Louw et al., 1967).

9.1.1 Treatment of Shock

Fluid and electrolyte replacement are required according to overt and invisible losses and biochemical (Astrup) measurements. The vast exudation from the pancreatic bed in haemorrhagic pancreatitis necessitates plasma or blood replacement of at least 2 units and often more if the blood pressure is not maintained. However, plasma or blood replacement should only be contemplated after fluid and electrolyte abnormalities have been corrected as otherwise the hyperviscosity problems may be compounded. In severely ill patients, the volume of fluid administered is monitored by regular readings of the central venous pressure and observation of the hourly output of urine. Lost protein can be provided by plasma or human serum albumin. Intravenous isoprenaline (isoproterenol) or metaraminol should be given to maintain the circulation only if full rehydration has failed to do so, and should be used with caution and given in small doses. Intravenous steroids must be used in large doses (2g/day) if they are to be used at all, but only if the patient does not respond to all other measures.

The role of aprotinin in acute pancreatitis remains controversial (Trapnell et al., 1974; Imrie et al., 1978), but a few clinicians consider that its theoretical value in shock (see chapter XXIII; sect. 5.4) may justify its use in severe cases. If used, the drug should be administered within 12 to 24 hours of the onset of the attack in a dosage of 1 million units/day for 5 days.

9.1.2 Relief of Pain

Adequate relief of pain is customarily achieved by using pethidine (meperidine) 100mg 4 to 6 times daily in conjunction with an anticholinergic (e.g. propantheline) or antispasmodic (e.g. hyoscine butylbromide). Morphine should be avoided because of the risk of producing spasm of the sphincter of Oddi.

Pentazocine (100mg 4 to 6 times daily) may be the more appropriate strong analgesic in pancreatic disease.

9.1.3 Suppression of Pancreatic Secretion

Suppression of pancreatic secretion may be achieved by reduction of gastric acid stimulation of pancreatic secretion by efficient nasogastric suction or by cimetidine (see section 4.1.3), or by suppression of both gastric acid and pancreatic secretion with any of the injectable anticholinergic preparations (e.g. propantheline 15 to 30mg 4 to 6-hourly). Anticholinergics should not be used in patients with marked tachycardia or prolonged ileus and in these cases cimetidine, 100 to 200mg 6-hourly by intravenous injection, should perhaps be given alone. Glucagon 1mg 4-hourly by intravenous infusion has also been used for suppression of pancreatic secretion, but there is no evidence that it influences the mortality in acute pancreatitis (Durr et al., 1978; Medical Research Council, 1977).

9.1.4 Prevention of Infection

Intravenous or intramuscular broad spectrum antibiotic therapy can be used to combat pulmonary infection, Gram-negative septicaemia from gut devitalisation and cholangitis, but the use of antibiotics has been questioned by many. Some have obtained no advantage from prophylactic antibiotics.

9.1.5 Treatment of Complications

Acute diabetes should be treated only if ketosis develops and the dose of soluble insulin closely monitored because of the tendency of glucose tolerance to improve abruptly. Enzyme containing pleural effusions require repeated aspiration supplemented, possibly by aprotinin instillation. Encephalopathy may be due to delirium tremens which requires large doses of promazine, 50 to 100mg 4 times daily, diazepam 10mg 4 times daily, or chlormethiazole 40 to 100ml of 0.8% intravenously over 5 minutes, then 500 to 1000ml over 6 to 12 hours, supplemented by intravenous vitamin B complex. On the other hand, tachycardia, restlessness and confusion may be the harbinger of the respiratory distress syndrome, a serious complication in which opiates and heavy sedation is absolutely contraindicated (Ranson et al., 1973). Anoxia should always be guarded against by prevention of fluid overloading, maintenance of an adequate airway and, in severe attacks, by routine use of oxygen by mask. In more severe cases, pulmonary assist procedures will be required and a Swan-Ganz catheter inserted. Ileus will require prolonged gastric suction and the avoidance of anticholinergics. Surgery is usually indicated in patients in whom the disease is complicated by persistent cyst and abscess formation or persistent jaundice.

Hypocalcaemia requires the parenteral administration of calcium or calciferol. Peripheral fat necrosis, intraosseous fat necrosis and hyperlipaemia occurring with the acute attack rarely require specific treatment.

9.1.6 The Role of Peritoneal Lavage and Surgery in Fulminating and Severe Pancreatitis

Peritoneal lavage has apparently reduced the immediate mortality in a group of high death risk patients, but it has not reduced abscess formation (Ranson et al., 1976). If laparotomy is carried out as a diagnostic procedure or for non-response to the above therapy, the desired approach at present is to remove all overtly necrotic material, drain the pancreatic bed, abscess or cyst and remove the gall bladder if gall-stones are present. On no account should attempts be made to explore the lower common duct for possible stones unless their presence is obvious or very highly suspected. Profuse gastrointestinal bleeding and protracted ascites may require surgical intervention.

9.2 Mild Pancreatitis

Hospitalisation will depend on the severity of the attack and the availability of bed space. Outpatient treatment is generally possible, with a bland diet and initial pain relief with oral pentazocine or pethidine, followed by simple oral analgesics and antacids and anticholinergic therapy (to reduce pancreatic secretion), which will usually abate the attack in a few days. Failure to relieve the attack requires hospital admission to establish whether a cyst has developed or an associated cause of pain is present.

9.3 Chronic, Chronic Relapsing and Calcific Pancreatitis

Alcohol is the major aetiological agent of chronic pancreatitis in most western countries, and accounts for some 90% of calcific pancreatitis in these areas. Malnutrition and/or alcohol would appear to be the predisposing cause in tropical regions. The remainder of cases comprise idiopathic and, very rarely, hypercalcaemic and hyperlipaemic pancreatitis (Marks and Bank, 1976; 1977). Treatment of chronic pancreatitis is usually directed against pain, insufficiency or complications.

9.3.1 Relapsing Attacks of Pain

Patients with chronic pancreatitis rarely suffer the acute fulminating form of the disease but tend to develop mild attacks. Pain is the dominating feature and is rarely accompanied by other constitutional effects. Treatment is as outlined in section 9.2.

9.3.2 Chronic or Persistent Pain

This may be a legacy of a severe or mild attack or start *de novo,* usually in calcific pancreatitis. The causes of chronic pain include: (a) cyst formation, (b) continued alcohol intake, (c) pancreatic duct obstruction due *inter alia* to pancreatic lithiasis, (d) superadded carcinoma and (e) incidental disease such as peptic ulceration. Treatment is usually surgical if only to definitely exclude pancreatic cyst and should be preceded by retrograde pancreatography (Marks and Bornman, 1979). In intractable, non-surgically correctable cases the judicious use of strong analgesics such as pentazocine, or rarely, even a narcotic such as pethidine (meperidine), on a regular basis may convert a useless, miserable member of society to an individual who can still participate in the open labour market. A low fat diet should be given, and pork omitted. The possibility of bacterial infection beyond an obstructed duct or cholangitis should be considered and treated by antibiotics.

9.3.3 Chronic Pancreatic Insufficiency

The features of chronic insufficiency are weight loss, diabetes, steatorrhoea and peripheral neuropathy.

Weight Loss: Many patients with pancreatic insufficiency have lost 30 to 50% of their ideal weight when first seen. A high calorie diet, modified to suit diabetes and steatorrhoea is necessary, and appetite stimulants (cyproheptadine), vitamin preparations and anabolic steroids (e.g. nandrolone decanoate) may be of benefit.

Pancreatic Diabetes: The treatment of pancreatic diabetes is influenced, to some extent, by the rarity of ketosis and vasculopathy and the hazard of insulin induced hypoglycaemia probably due to inefficient growth hormone/glucagon response found in these patients (Bank et al., 1975). The tendency, therefore, is to undertreat rather than overtreat such patients (Marks and Bank, 1965). Treatment should never be undertaken without knowledge of the blood glucose level because of the occasional occurrence of marked hyperglycaemia of the order of 55.5mmol/L (1000mg/100ml) unassociated with ketosis or severe symptoms. With this proviso, asymptomatic diabetes requires little more than sugar restriction and symptomatic cases tried with oral hypoglycaemic agents such as chlorpropamide or metformin. However, insulin is often eventually needed to control symptoms in these and in more severe cases. The aim is to control hyperglycaemic symptoms and promote weight gain rather than to maintain a glycosuria free state. A liberal diabetic diet should be allowed to promote weight gain.

Pancreatic Steatorrhoea: Pancreatic replacement therapy should be given in large enough doses to reduce the diarrhoea and improve fat absorption. 4 tablets of a whole pancreas (e.g. Viokase) or pancrelipase preparation with meals and 2 with teas is a useful starting schedule, but may have to be increased to 2 to 4 tablets every hour and before, during and after meals in severe cases (DiMagno et al., 1977). A low fat, high protein diet is indicated. Addition of sodium bicarbonate has been advocated by some, on the basis of possible inactivation of enzymes by gastric acid but cimetidine in a dose of 200mg 3 times daily before meals and at night is far more effective in this regard (Regan et al., 1977), and in raising the intraduodenal pH to a level which allows adequate micellar function. As intestinal malabsorption is not a feature in pancreatic steatorrhoea, other replacement therapy is unnecessary, but the possibility of vitamin B_{12} deficiency does arise occasionally and should be treated. An antimotility agent such as codeine 30mg 2 or 3 times daily or loperamide 8 to 16mg in 1 or 2 doses daily will be required if replacement therapy is not effective in controlling the diarrhoea. A low fat diet is helpful (under 50g/day) and replacement with medium chain triglycerides may improve the total calorie intake.

Peripheral neuropathy occurs in 10 to 30% of patients with calcific pancreatitis and diabetes. Carbamazepine or phenytoin may be of value. If there is associated depression, amitriptyline should also be given.

Tuberculosis is common in calcific pancreatitis and should be excluded from time to time.

9.3.4 Removal of Aetiological Factors

When the clinical manifestations have improved, due consideration *must* then be given to correction of aetiological factors.

Alcohol induced pancreatitis is essentially a medical problem, with alcohol withdrawal the most important factor in prevention of subsequent attacks.

Conversely, gall-stone pancreatitis is a surgical condition requiring cholecystectomy and, if necessary, exploration of the common bile duct. The problem arises in the treatment of pancreatitis not obviously due to gall-stones or alcohol. Rare causes such as hyperparathyroidism and hyperlipidaemia should be excluded and, if found, treated on their merits. Piperazine or pyrantel (section 11.4) should be administered to exclude roundworms, particularly in childhood pancreatitis. Gall-stone pancreatitis may occasionally be due to small gall-stones not readily apparent on initial cholecystography. Since it is essentially an acute or acute relapsing condition, the finding of normal pancreatic function some 6 weeks after an acute attack warrants an intensification of the search for gall-stones by means of ultrasound, biliary drainage and microscopy for cholesterol crystals, repeat cholecystography and intravenous cholangiography and even endoscopic pancreatocholangiography.

9.4 Cystic Fibrosis (fibrocystic disease)

As an increasing number of these patients are reaching adulthood, therapy has assumed increasing proportions. The steatorrhoea and diabetes should be managed as outlined for pancreatitis (section 9.3.3) with the same precautions. The optimum antibiotic regimen for respiratory disease should be determined by repeated sputum culture (see chapter XX; sect. 7) and the sweat sodium loss requires sodium chloride and possibly potassium supplementation, particularly in warm climates.

10. Liver Disease

10.1 Acute Hepatitis

10.1.1 Acute Viral Hepatitis

General measures in the management of acute viral hepatitis include bed rest during the early phase of the disease which should be continued while the patient has symptoms or moderate biochemical abnormalities. Return to full activity should be planned and gradual and undue exertion and alcohol should be avoided. The diet should not be restricted once a normal diet can be tolerated and the patient should be encouraged to eat well.

There is no indication for the use of corticosteroids or immunosuppressive therapy in the management of acute viral hepatitis. Indeed, there is a suggestion that the use of corticosteroids may enhance the liability to the development of chronic liver disease such as chronic active hepatitis. Although prednisolone (10mg 3 times a day) may produce a sharp fall of serum bilirubin in severe cholestasis complicating acute viral hepatitis, it is not generally advisable to use this form of treatment. Its value as a diagnostic aid to differentiate cholestatic hepatitis from mechanical biliary obstruction is dubious and is unnecessary in the light of the development of ultrasonography, percutaneous hepatic cholangiography and endoscopic retrograde cholangiopancreatography. It should also be noted that a controlled trial showed no benefit from the use of methylprednisolone in severe viral hepatitis (Gregory et al., 1976).

In fulminant hepatitis, steroid therapy has not been shown to be of value.

10.1.2 Acute Alcoholic Hepatitis

General supportive treatment is indicated. Although some have suggested benefit from corticosteroids (Lesesne et al., 1978), most evidence supports lack of any advantage in their use (Blitzer et al., 1977; Conn, 1978).

10.2 Chronic Hepatitis

10.2.1 Chronic Persistent Hepatitis

The majority of patients with chronic persistent hepatitis recover spontaneously. Treatment is by reassurance, after the fullest possible investigations which may have to include needle biopsy of the liver. Corticosteroids or immunosuppressant therapy such as azathioprine should not be given. No specific dietary regimen is indicated.

10.2.2 Chronic Active Hepatitis
(lupoid hepatitis)

Of the various drugs used in this disease, corticosteroids and azathioprine have been shown to be the most effective even though the studies on which their benefits have been based, have shortcomings in terms of current standards and knowledge of the clinical spectrum of the disease (see Wright et al., 1977). Treatment should start with prednisolone or prednisone, in a dose of 20mg 3 times a day. Prednisone is converted in the liver to its active form prednisolone, but although this biotransformation may be impaired in some patients with active disease, bioavailability is not altered (see chapter XVI; sect. 9.1). It is important that the diagnosis should be confirmed by liver histology prior to treatment. This fairly large dose of prednisolone or prednisone may be reduced when there is clinical or biochemical evidence of improvement. Maintenance therapy is 10 to 15mg daily. To minimise side effects due to decreased albumin binding, dosage should be reduced in patients with hypoalbuminaemia in accordance with the concentration of serum albumin (Uribe and Go, 1979; see section 1.3). About 20 % of patients fail to respond, deteriorate, develop hepatocellular failure, and die (Schalm et al., 1976). In such patients, a trial of higher doses of prednisolone (50 to 60mg daily) is worth considering, but is usually ineffective.

Azathioprine is an alternative method of treatment, but it would seem wise to use azathioprine only in selected cases. It should be reserved for those in whom complications follow prednisolone therapy, when a coincidental condition such as diabetes precludes use of steroids or when control is not achieved with prednisolone alone. Because of the possibility of an increase in jaundice and development of hepatic coma with doses over 100mg per day, azathioprine should be started in small doses around 25 to 50mg daily. If there are no ill effects with this starting dose, it may gradually be increased to around 100mg per day. Whether a combination of prednisolone or prednisone and azathioprine is better than either alone, is as yet uncertain (Summerskill et al., 1975; Wright et al., 1977). Some clinicians start treatment with a low dose combination of prednisolone and azathioprine.

In hepatitis B_S antigen (HB_S-Ag) positive patients the dose of prednisolone or prednisone should be sufficient to suppress the activity of the liver cell damage, usually 10 to 20mg daily.

Therapy should be continued for 6 months after liver function tests have returned to normal. Slow withdrawal of prednisolone or prednisone should then be attempted whilst maintaining close observation for signs of relapse. However, this approach to treatment is based on limited experience, and the final therapeutic role of corticosteroids and immunosuppressant drugs generally in these patients must await further research, prolonged follow up, and prospective controlled trials (Wright et al., 1977).

General measures include a high protein nutritious diet. Alcohol and oral contraceptive drugs should be avoided. As in all liver disease, vitamin K_1 (phytomenadione) 10mg daily should be given if the prothrombin time is prolonged.

10.3 Cirrhosis

10.3.1 Alcoholic Cirrhosis

In patients with alcoholic cirrhosis, permanent abstinence from alcohol is the most important aspect of treatment. Patients who are able to abstain completely may show remarkable improvement over a period of time. Although some have suggested that the reverse may be the case (Pande et al., 1978), most evidence supports improvement following complete abstinence, as stressed by Reynolds (1978). The diet should be as nutritious as possible and a high protein diet is recommended provided that there is no evidence of hepatic precoma or coma. Patients should be given as much protein as they can tolerate and it should only be restricted if hepatic precoma occurs. If the prothrombin index is low, vitamin K_1 (phytomenadione) 10mg daily should be given by mouth. If there is no clinical improvement with such treatment a short course (1 or 2 weeks) of prednisolone 20 to 40mg daily may stimulate appetite and hasten recovery.

10.3.2 Hepatic Encephalopathy
of Cirrhosis

Any precipitating factor should be treated (see below) and in all patients with acute encephalopathy measures that lower blood ammonia concentration should be instituted.

All protein must be eliminated from the diet which should be high in calories and carbohydrates. Oral neomycin sulphate (0.5 to 1g every 6 hours) or kanamycin should be given to attempt to reduce the number of urease producing intestinal bacteria. Oral lactulose is as effective as neomycin and probably acts by acidifying the colonic contents and reducing the absorption of ammonia and possibly other toxins (Avery et al., 1972; Conn et al., 1977). The dose is increased progressively until the desired effect is obtained. Diarrhoea may result and consequently the dose may have to be reduced. In most cases the desired faecal pH is obtained with 2 to 3 soft formed, but not liquid, bowel movements per day. In acute situations requiring intravenous therapy, basic amino acids (now available commercially) may reverse the coma (see section 10.4.3).

In patients with chronic portal-systemic encephalopathy the protein content of the diet, oral neomycin and/or lactulose may be varied to meet the needs of the individual patient. The amount of neomycin absorbed is usually small. Care must be taken to avoid toxic effects, especially deafness, if neomycin is used for any length of time (see chapter XI; sect. 7.1.1). Hepatic encephalopathy is often precipitated by major gastrointestinal haemorrhage; potassium deficiency, resulting from overenthusiastic diuretic therapy (which may also initiate encephalopathy by causing shrinkage of the extracellular fluid volume); excessive dosage of strong analgesics, sedatives and hypnotics; by oral ammonium compounds and by abdominal paracentesis. Sometimes patients are agitated and they may be given promethazine 25mg as required. Chlorpromazine (25mg intramuscularly) can be used in alcoholics with impending hepatic coma. Morphine must not be used (see section 13.4).

10.3.3 Cirrhotic Oedema and Ascites

The sodium in the diet must be reduced to at least 0.5 to 2g (22 to 88mmol or mEq of sodium) in each 24 hours. The patient is often unaware that he is taking excess sodium and a list of sodium containing foods, medicines, toothpaste etc should be provided. Fluid intake should be about 1.5 litres daily, with or without diuretic therapy. Unless massive, ascites does not necessarily need to be treated with diuretics; they do not increase life expectancy and may cause severe complications.

Secondary hyperaldosteronism is almost invariably present and treatment with potent diuretics may cause increased potassium loss, electrolyte imbalance and coma (Conn, 1972; Sherlock et al., 1966). When treatment is considered, the aim is therefore to produce a slow prolonged diuresis (gauged by weight reduction at a rate of 1kg every 2 days). Spironolactone or amiloride alone, with bed rest and restricted sodium and fluid intake, is a useful starting regimen. A starting dosage of spironolactone is 50 to 200mg daily, adjusted on the basis of urinary sodium : potassium ratio (doses up to 1000mg daily have been used). If an adequate diuresis is not obtained, frusemide (furosemide) may be added with dosage increased up to 120mg daily (Eggert, 1970). Serum electrolytes should be checked as both continued hypokalaemia and hyperkalaemia can occur (potassium supplements should not be given when spironolactone or amiloride are used).

Abdominal paracentesis should only be done for diagnostic reasons, particularly to exclude unsuspected bacterial peritonitis, and the minimum amount of fluid removed. When ascites is associated with severe hypoalbuminaemia, increasing the level of the plasma albumin by intravenous salt poor human albumin may potentiate diuresis but is of little value in most instances. Resistant patients may benefit from a Le Veen peritoneal-jugular shunt.

Hyponatraemia is usually dilutional in origin and should be treated with fluid restriction. Severe hyponatraemia is treated by measures designed to remove water from the body such as mannitol infusion. Prednisolone may also be tried on a short term basis.

10.3.4 Bleeding from Oesophageal Varices

Patients with oesophageal varices often bleed from acute gastric erosions or peptic ulcer rather than their varices. If it is established at emergency endoscopy that the varices are the source of bleeding, vasopressin (20u intravenously) given in 150ml 5% dextrose over 15 minutes may sufficiently reduce portal pressure to arrest bleeding. This therapy may be repeated after 3 to 4 hours but if vasopressin is given repeatedly it tends to become less effective. However, as an intravenous infusion of vasopressin may cause intestinal contraction with abdominal colic, vomiting and also constriction of coronary arteries, vasopressin (0.1 units/ml per minute) has been infused selectively into the coeliac or left gastric artery after catheterisation of the aorta. If vasopressin fails a Sengstaken-Blakemore tube should be passed and inflated for 24 to 48 hours. However, this should be used as a secondary measure because, unless the operator is very skilled in its use, there will be a high failure rate. If other measures fail, emergency surgery aimed at lowering portal venous pressure or disconnecting the area of bleeding varices from the portal system may be performed. Bleeding in patients with varices secondary to cavernous transformation of the portal vein or portal vein thrombosis seems to be self limiting. Studies are currently in progress to see whether cimetidine will influence the incidence of recurrent bleeds in patients with varices.

Injection of varices with a sclerosing agent through a rigid oesophagoscope is an effective means of controlling acute haemorrhage from varices. Serial injections may prove to be effective in eliminating varices and preventing further bleeds (Macbeth, 1955; Terblanche, 1979).

10.4 Special Forms of Cirrhosis

10.4.1 Haemochromatosis

Treatment is regular repeated venesection, commencing initially with weekly phlebotomies of 500 to 1000ml of blood to allow mobilisation of the iron stores.

10.4.2 Primary Biliary Cirrhosis

The special treatment required is to make sure that the fat soluble vitamins are given in adequate amounts systemically. Pruritus may be treated by cholestyramine (4g 3 times daily) which lowers plasma bile acids (see section 6.1.3). Calcium infusion may help bone pain.

10.4.3 Massive Liver Cell Necrosis

The mortality is close to 90%, and these patients need intensive care. Treatment is as for chronic hepatic encephalopathy (sect. 10.3.2). In addition special attention must be paid to hypoglycaemia, which is treated by intravenous glucose, and hypokalaemia, for which the patients often require large amounts of intravenous potassium. Corticosteroids are used by some clinicians, but have largely been found to be ineffective.

The therapeutic role of heparin, based on the association of disseminated intravascular coagulation in this syndrome, has not proved to be as effective as was initially hoped, and is no longer used. Levodopa started early in the course of hepatic coma has been used with effect in a few patients, temporarily reversing the neurological abnormality (Datta et al., 1976; Fischer et al., 1976).

Exchange transfusion, isolated animal liver perfusion and cross circulation, infusion of basic amino acids only and attempts to remove an alleged toxin by charcoal and other toxin-absorbing material, have all been advocated and may all reverse the abnormal neurological state, but there is no good evidence that the survival rate is affected by these measures. The role of hyperalimentation and dialysis using a polyacrylonitride membrane is still under review (Saunders et al., 1979).

10.5 Gall-Stones

Gall-stone disease, or cholelithiasis, is a common problem in many countries. Gall-stones may be composed largely of cholesterol, bile pigments or a combination of both. Treatment for most is by surgery, but selected patients with cholesterol gall-stones can be successfully treated with a naturally occurring primary bile salt chenodeoxycholic (chenic) acid (Batey, 1977). Chenic acid, by reducing the hepatic secretory rate of cholesterol, improves the ability of bile to solubilise cholesterol; thereby providing a milieu within which cholesterol stones can gradually dissolve.

Treatment with chenic acid can be successful only for cholesterol gall-stones and only if unsaturated bile can enter the gall bladder; hence the basic requirement to select patients with radiolucent stones and functioning gall bladders. Surgery is indicated in those patients with severe symptoms or non-functioning gall bladders and those in whom chenic acid therapy has failed (e.g. calcium containing stones) or has produced intolerable side effects. Usual dosage of chenic acid is 13 to 15mg/kg, with an increase to 18 to 20mg/kg daily in obese patients (Iser et al., 1975, 1978). The daily dose can be given in divided amounts with the major fraction at night, or as a single dose at bedtime. Duration of therapy depends on stone size and is continued until stones dissolve or decrease in size and pass into the duodenum; multiple small stones dissolve more rapidly than single large stones which usually require 6 to 24 or more months of therapy. Gall-stones recur in some patients on stopping chenic acid therapy if no preventive measures are taken. Whether maintenance therapy with chenic acid will prevent recurrence is not clear. Mild diarrhoea is the only important side effect, and since it usually responds to small doses of cholestyramine (section 6.1.3) may be due to the increase in serum bile acids which occur with chenic acid therapy.

Ursodeoxycholic acid, a derivative of chenic acid, in short term experience to date is associated with a considerably smaller incidence of diarrhoea (serum bile acids do not seem to increase) and does not appear to cause the mild rise in serum transaminase seen with chenic acid (Stiehl et al., 1978; Williams et al., 1978).

11. Gastrointestinal Infections and Infestations

11.1 Acute Diarrhoeas

With the exception of bacillary dysentery, antibacterial agents are seldom indicated in acute gastroenteritis. Routine use of antibacterial drugs not only usually does not control the infection, but can also prolong the carrier state and increase the chance of subsequent relapse. However, if this approach is undertaken the patient should be carefully observed for sudden bacterial septicaemia. This applies especially at the extremes of life. Antibacterial drugs are however, indicated, if not essential, when there are signs of systemic invasion (e.g. fever) and in certain situations in children (see chapter IV; sect. 5.1.6). Treatment is therefore based on symptomatic and supportive measures, particularly fluid and electrolyte replacement. In severe diarrhoea or dehydration, parenteral fluid and electrolyte replacement is essential and is crucial to the successful management of cholera. The patient may lose body fluid up to 1.5 litres each hour and die within 6 to 8 hours after the onset of diarrhoea. Intravenous fluid supplements, as well as electrolytes, may be indicated in other forms of diarrhoea when signs of dehydration and electrolyte disturbance develop. Bed rest is also helpful. Antimotility agents such as codeine phosphate 15 to 30mg 6-hourly, diphenoxylate 2.5 to 5mg 6-hourly or loperamide 4mg followed by 2mg after each unformed stool, can be used to relieve diarrhoea (if no contraindications exist) and adsorbents such as kaolin-pectin added if necessary. Antispasmodic drugs (e.g. hyoscine butylbromide) are helpful in the relief of pain and abdominal cramps. Some consider that antimotility drugs should be avoided in infections due to invasive organisms such as *Shigella, Salmonella* and certain strains of *Escherichia coli,* since they may delay clearance of the infecting organism from the bowel and prolong the course of the illness (Du Pont and Hornick, 1973). They should be avoided in antibiotic associated colitis (see section 14.4.3).

11.1.1 Shigellosis (bacillary dysentery)

Antibacterial drugs are not indicated for simple *Sh. sonnei* infection, as the diarrhoea is self limited. However, they are indicated in cases of acute gastroenteritis or true dysentery as they shorten the duration of symptoms and duration of faecal excretion of the *Shigella* organism. In such cases, 1g ampicillin every 6 hours for 5 days is usually highly effective. Experience with amoxycillin has been very disappointing in *Shigella* infection, despite similar *in vitro* susceptibility to ampicillin. The reason for this is not clear (Nelson and Haltalin, 1974). Oxytetracycline, 250mg every 6 hours for 5 days gives similar results in terms of bacteriological and clinical cure. Co-trimoxazole, 2 or 4 tablets twice daily, has also proved effective and is the drug of choice in areas in which multiple antibiotic resistance exists (Chang et al., 1977; Nelson et al., 1976). It is desirable to perform *in vitro* drug sensitivity tests as soon as possible as a guide to the drug of choice, since the drug resistance pattern does vary from area to area and from time to time (see also chapter XXVII; sect. 5.4.3). Fluid and electrolyte replacement should be given as indicated. Antidiarrhoeal drugs are usually used to relieve diarrhoea and abdominal discomfort. Carriers should be treated with antibacterial therapy as they are a danger to another outbreak.

11.1.2 Salmonella Gastroenteritis

The most important aspect of treatment is prompt correction of dehydration and electrolyte disturbances. Antidiarrhoeal agents are usually used to relieve diarrhoea and abdominal cramps. Antibacterial drugs are not indicated or beneficial (Aserkoff and Bennett, 1969; Joint Report, 1970) in the routine case without evidence of systemic spread (but see above). When indicated, and certainly in enteric fever, chloramphenicol is given in a dose of 500mg every 6 hours. The combination of trimethoprim and sulphamethoxazole (co-trimoxazole) in a dose of 3 tablets twice a day on the first day followed by 2 tablets twice a day for 7 days is also highly recommended as an alternative and is valuable in areas where there is resistance to chloramphenicol. The convalescent carrier state is not an indication for antibacterial therapy (see also chapter XXVII; sect. 5.4.2).

11.1.3 Cholera

Fluid and electrolyte replacement is needed urgently and is the basis of therapy. Oral replacement therapy may be feasible in less severe cases, but in severely affected patients intravenous fluids are essential for survival. Antibacterial chemotherapy does not alter the course of the disease, but hastens eradication of vibrios from the faeces. Tetracycline is the drug of choice in the treatment of both El-tor and classical cholera in a dose of 40mg/kg/day in 4 divided doses. The stool culture usually becomes negative for vibrios after 4 days. Chloramphenicol 500mg 4 times a day for 7 days is also beneficial in the vibrio eradication. Co-trimoxazole in a similar dosage used in salmonellosis is also recommended (Pastore et al., 1977).

11.1.4 Staphylococcal Food Poisoning

Usually only antidiarrhoeal drugs are required. Antibacterial therapy is not indicated. Intravenous fluid replacement is necessary in cases of severe vomiting and diarrhoea.

11.1.5 Clostridium Perfringens
Food Poisoning

Fluid and electrolyte replacement and antispasmodics for abdominal pain and colic are usually adequate. Like staphylococcal food poisoning the infection is self limiting. Antidiarrhoeal drugs may be given if necessary.

11.2 Gastroenteritis in Children

Most cases of gastroenteritis in young children are due to viral infection. Antibacterial drugs are indicated in bacillary dysentery and certain cases of salmonellosis, and are traditionally given in pathogenic *Esch. coli* enteritis in infants. Treatment is aimed primarily at arresting diarrhoea by gut rest (stopping all milk and solid feeds and substitution of glucose or dextrose-saline feeds over the usual 24 to 48 hour period of acute symptoms) and replacement of fluid loss and correction of acid base and electrolyte imbalance in those with moderate and severe dehydration. Details of management are given in chapter IV (sect. 5.1.6).

11.3 Amoebiasis

The demonstration of *Entamoeba histolytica* in a specimen of warm stool, rectal scrapings or rectal biopsy demands active therapy (Juniper, 1978). In areas where this infection is endemic, treatment is recommended in patients with a suggestive clinical presentation, even if the protozoa are not found

(Bank et al., 1971b). It should be remembered that antibacterials, barium sulphate or bismuth containing compounds may interfere with the microscopic demonstration of motile forms of *E. histolytica*, but should not interfere with cyst formation.

11.3.1 Amoebic Dysentery
(acute amoebic colitis)

Treatment is directed at eradicating *E. histolytica* in both the bowel lumen and wall and protecting the liver from invasion, and in severe forms, at correction of fluid and electrolyte disturbances and anaemia. Ideally, stools should be examined monthly for 6 months and again at 1 year for proof of cure.

In patients with mild to moderate dysentery, oral metronidazole or tinidazole on an outpatient basis is the treatment of choice. These imidazole derivatives act on both intestinal and tissue forms. Efficacy is related to size of the dose and not to the duration of therapy. The usual dosage of metronidazole is 750 or 800mg 3 times daily for 5 to 10 days in adults. For children the dose is 50mg/kg in 3 divided doses for 5 to 10 days. This regimen usually provides rapid control of symptoms and can also be relied upon to control systemic spread of the disease. It achieves a parasitological cure rate of about 90%. The addition of tetracycline (250mg 6-hourly for 5 days) achieves a cure rate approaching 100%. Side effects of metronidazole include nausea and vomiting (which may necessitate a predose antiemetic), urticaria, dizziness, metallic taste and intolerance of alcohol. Tinidazole, in a dose of 600 to 800mg 3 times daily for 5 days or a single daily dose of 2g (50mg/kg for children) for 3 days also provides rapid symptomatic relief and a 90% or higher cure rate. The shorter course single daily dose regimen of tinidazole simplifies treatment and is effective against both trophozoites and cysts, whereas an equivalent single dose short course regimen of metronidazole is only effective in patients passing trophozoites and is not as well tolerated as single dose tinidazole (Bakshi et al., 1978; Misra, 1978). Patients should be instructed on the importance of completing the course of treatment as prescribed.

Alternative regimens (Hendrickse, 1972) include various combinations of tetracycline, diloxanide furoate, chloroquine or di-iodohydroxyquinoline, given in fixed combinations or used sequentially. One such regimen which has been employed is a combination of tetracycline 250mg 6-hourly for 10 days (to act against the trophozoite stage), with diloxanide furoate 0.5g 3 times daily for 10 days (to destroy any cyst forms in the lumen) and chloroquine, 600mg initially followed by 300mg 6 hours later, then 150mg twice daily for 14 to 28 days (to protect the liver from invasion). Di-iodohydroxyquinoline, 1 to 2g daily in 3 divided doses for 20 days can be substituted for diloxanide. Paromomycin (25 to 35mg/kg daily in 3 divided doses for 5 to 10 days) has also been used in such regimens, combined with or prior to di-iodohydroxyquinoline. Because of cardiotoxicity emetine and dehydroemetine cannot be recommended for use in ambulant patients. They should never be used in patients with cardiovascular disease.

In severe forms of the disease, the patient should be hospitalised with daily assessment and attention to fluid, electrolytes, diet and anaemia. Metronidazole or tinidazole should be given as before and possibly also chloroquine, in the schedule as above. Tetracycline plus diloxanide or di-iodohydroxyquinoline are alternatives for chloroquine.

Fulminating cases should receive intensive care, nasogastric suction and intravenous rehydration and electrolyte repletion. A suggested drug regimen is a combination of metronidazole or tinidazole (if an oral drug can be taken), emetine or dihydroemetine (60mg daily intramuscularly, for 3 to 10 days), chloroquine and diloxanide or di-iodohydroxyquinoline together with intravenous antibiotics. Intravenous metronidazole is now available for patients who cannot take oral drugs. Surgery is indicated in the advent of toxic megacolon unresponsive to treatment in 48 to 72 hours, perforation or uncontrolled bleeding (Bank et al., 1971b).

11.3.2 Non-Dysenteric Intestinal Amoebiasis (syndrome of chronic intestinal amoebiasis or chronic amoebic colitis)

This form of amoebiasis indicates the finding of amoebae, by chance, in patients with diarrhoea, sometimes with constipation, who have other disease such as diverticulitis, Crohn's disease or the irritable bowel syndrome. Treatment is as for mild to moderate amoebic dysentery. Some do not recommend metronidazole or tinidazole in the absence of proof that it will eradicate the infection.

11.3.3 Asymptomatic Intestinal (carrier) State

Cyst passers must be treated at once as they are a potential danger in transmission of the disease. Metronidazole and tinidazole are less effective in this situation (Spillman et al., 1976) but diloxanide furoate, 0.5 to 1g 3 times daily for 10 to 20 days, gives very good results. Alternatively di-iodohydroxyquinoline 600mg 3 times daily for 10 to 20 days, may be used. Tetracycline is advocated in addition by some. Contacts of carriers must also be treated immediately, with oral metronidazole or tinidazole as for mild amoebic dysentery.

11.3.4 Amoebic Granuloma (amoeboma)

Treatment should be conservative, as for mild amoebic dysentery. Surgery is not indicated as a primary measure but a complete response to metronidazole or tinidazole alone or with tetracycline is essential.

11.3.5 Hepatic Amoebiasis (hepatic abscess and tissue forms)

Metronidazole alone is effective in amoebic liver abscess, but the usual dosage in hepatic amoebiasis of 800mg 3 times daily for 10 days may not always eliminate the associated bowel infection and it is best to add diloxanide or di-iodochlorhydroxyquinoline. An alternative regimen is emetine or dehydroemetine combined with chloroquine. Tinidazole alone as a single daily dose of 2g (50mg/kg for children) for 2 or 3 days has given a high cure rate and appears to be superior to metronidazole as a single daily dose short course regimen (Bakshi et al., 1978; Islam and Hasan, 1978). When abscess is associated with clinical dysentery, high dose metronidazole or standard dose of tinidazole with tetracycline as for mild cases of amoebic dysentery, is most appropriate.

If liver abscess is large or pointing, needle aspiration is indicated. When the abscess is in the left lobe, open drainage is indicated. Corticosteroids appear to be a precipitating factor in some cases of amoebic liver abscess and the possibility of amoebiasis should be considered in patients who develop diarrhoea or fever during treatment with corticosteroids (El-Hennaway and Abd-Rabbo, 1978; Stuiver and Goud, 1978).

11.4 Intestinal Helminthic Infestation

Treatment is generally directed at the parasite involved by using the specific agent of choice

Table VII. Drugs for use in the treatment of some intestinal helminthic infestations

Infestation	Drug(s) of choice	Dosage	Principal side effects/Notes
Ascaris lumbricoides (roundworm)	Pyrantel	11mg/kg as a single dose	Headache, dizziness, vomiting, abdominal pain, diarrhoea — usually mild, and occur in about 20% of patients
	Mebendazole[1]	100mg twice daily for 3 days	Mild diarrhoea, abdominal pain (useful for multiple infestations)
	Piperazine	*Adults:* 4g (equivalent hydrate) as a single dose *Children:* 120mg/kg to maximum 4g as a single dose	Occasional nausea, vomiting or diarrhoea. Neurological effects are rare and usually occur in children, in renal failure or overdosage or in those with a predisposing neurological disorder (Bomb and Bedi, 1976). Ataxia is most common symptom
	Levamisole	*Adults:* 150mg as a single dose *Children:* 50mg/20kg body weight as a single dose	Transient pyrexia, nausea, vomiting, dizziness, abdominal pain (all uncommon)
Ancylostoma duodenale (hookworm)	Pyrantel	10mg/kg as a single dose	See above
	Bephenium hydroxynaphthoate	*Adults:* 5g (2.5g base) as a single dose *Children:* under 2 years: 2.5g (1.25g base) as a single dose	Nausea, vomiting, transient diarrhoea. Side effects infrequent with single dose regimen, more frequent if continued for several days (e.g. in treatment of *Necator americanus* — see below)
	Mebendazole[1]	100mg twice daily for 3 days	See above
Necator americanus (hookworm)	Pyrantel	10mg/kg single dose. For heavy infestations (over 4000 eggs/1g faeces) 20mg/kg for up to 3 consecutive days	See above
	Mebendazole[1] Tetrachloroethylene	100mg twice daily for 3 days 0.012ml/kg up to 5ml maximum as single oral dose	See above Dizziness, nausea, vomiting, abdominal cramps, diarrhoea (rest patient for 1 hour after dose). Causes *Ascaris* to migrate aberrantly and should not be used in the presence of *Ascaris* until effective *Ascaris* treatment completed
	Bitoscanate	*Adults:* 150mg after a meal as a single dose *Children:* (10 to 15 years): 100mg after a meal as a single dose	Nausea, vomiting, diarrhoea, abdominal pain, dizziness. All effects usually mild
	Bephenium hydroxynaphthoate	*Adults:* 5g (2.5g base) twice daily for 3 days	See above
Strongyloides stercoralis (dwarf threadworm)	Mebendazole[1] Thiabendazole	100mg twice daily for 3 days 25mg/kg twice daily for 2 days (maximum 3g/day)	See above Anorexia, nausea, vomiting, dizziness

Trichuris trichiura (whipworm)	Mebendazole	100mg twice daily for 3 days	See above
Enterobius vermicularis (threadworm, pinworm)	Pyrantel	10mg/kg as a single dose	See above. Treat all members of family
	Mebendazole[1]	100mg single dose	See above
	Piperazine	50 to 75mg/kg as a single dose for 7 days	See above. Treat all members of family
	Viprynium	5mg/kg as a single dose	Nausea, vomiting, stains clothing Treat all members of family
Taenia saginata (beef tapeworm)	Niclosamide	2g (4 tablets) chewed thoroughly in a single dose after a light meal	Mild colic and diarrhoea. Risk of cysticercosis with *T. solium* unless purgation (MgSO₄) brought about 1 to 2 hours after administration
	Mebendazole	300mg twice daily for 3 days	See above
Taenia solium (pork tapeworm)	Paromomycin	1g 6-hourly orally for 4 doses	Absorption minimal after oral use
	Dichlorophen	*Adults:* 6g on each of two successive days *Children:* 2 to 4g on each of two successive days	Nausea, vomiting, colic, diarrhoea. Avoid in conditions where purgation is undesirable and in liver disease
	Mebendazole	300mg twice daily for 3 days	See above
Giardia lamblia	Metronidazole	200 or 250mg 3 times daily for 5 to 7 days; 200 or 250mg twice daily for children	Anorexia, nausea, vomiting, metallic taste, tongue and urine colour changes, skin rash (infrequent). Disulfiram-like intolerance of alcohol
	Tinidazole	2g single dose (150mg twice daily for 7 days if gastrointestinal intolerance); 50mg/kg single dose in children	Anorexia, nausea, vomiting, metallic taste, skin rash (infrequent)
	Mepacrine	100mg 3 times daily for 5 to 7 days Repeat after 2 weeks	Gastrointestinal disturbances, headache, dizziness, allergic skin reactions (uncommon)

1   Mebendazole can be used as a broad spectrum agent against *Ascaris, Taenia, Enterobius vermicularis, Ancylostoma duodenale* and *Necator americanus* in endemic areas in mass therapy for helminth control (Hutchison et al., 1975).

(Katz, 1975, 1977; Marsden, 1978), but in areas where infestation is endemic, broad spectrum agents such as mebendazole are important as single agents in mass therapy for helminth control (Hutchison et al., 1975). In other areas where certain parasitic infestation is common, unexplained abdominal pain or diarrhoea may be an indication for an appropriate anthelmintic.

11.4.1 Ascariasis (roundworm)

Piperazine is widely used, and is available in elixir and tablet form for administration as a single dose (table VII). Pyrantel pamoate is also highly effective against *Ascaris lumbricoides*. It is not absorbed from the intestine and is given as a single dose. Other alternative treatments include mebendazole, a broad spectrum anthelmintic which is well tolerated and is effective against a variety of helminths (Hutchison et al., 1975). Pyrantel and mebendazole are preferred because of their efficacy, ease of administration and low incidence of side effects (Committee on Drugs, 1978). Repeat treatments may be necessary. Family members who are cyst carriers may also require treatment.

11.4.2 Enterobiasis (oxyuriasis, threadworm, pinworm)

If infection due to *Enterobius vermicularis* is to be successfully treated great emphasis should be placed on personal hygiene. It is the only intestinal nematode in which direct person to person transmission can occur. Infected individuals must be told to wash the perianal region thoroughly every morning. Bed covers and night clothes should be changed every day and all family members should preferably be treated at the same time.

Piperazine preparations, given daily for 7 days, viprynium (pyrvinium) pamoate or mebendazole or pyrantel pamoate as a single dose are effective (table VII). However, viprynium has the disadvantage of staining clothes. Quite often, single dose treatment is not sufficient to eradicate the parasite, as reinfection occurs very easily. In such cases, treatment should be repeated 2 or 3 times at weekly intervals. Pyrantel and mebendazole are preferred, as in ascariasis, although pyrantel has the advantage of being able to be given as a single dose regimen in enterobiasis as well.

11.4.3 Hookworm

There are two main species parasitic in man — *Ancylostoma duodenale* and *Necator americanus*.

Bephenium hydroxynaphthoate can be used for *Ancylostoma*, but *Necator* does not respond nearly so well and in the increased dosage schedule required side effects are more common. *Necator* can instead be treated with tetrachloroethylene. Either infection can be satisfactorily treated with pyrantel or mebendazole (table VII).

11.4.4 Trichuriasis (whipworm)

The two drugs active against *Trichuris trichiura* are thiabendazole and mebendazole. Thiabendazole however, produces only a temporary effect on the parasite. The egg count drops during the period of therapy and reverts back to the original level after the drug is withdrawn. The drug also has a characteristic effect on the morphology of the *Trichuris* eggs in that they appear deformed and irregular in shape during the period of therapy. Mebendazole has been found to be highly active. Unlike thiabendazole, the effect on the parasite is not temporary and complete cure can be achieved. Mebendazole is given twice a day for 3 days (table VII) and is well tolerated. Oxantel pamoate, an hydroxylated derivative of pyrantel, is also effective (Lee et al., 1976) and in combination with pyrantel has given good results in multiple helminth infection (Dissanaike, 1978).

11.4.5 Strongyloidiasis (dwarf threadworm)

Infestation with *Strongyloides stecoralis* is treated with mebendazole or thiabendazole (table VII). Thiabendazole acts both on the adult worm and the larval stages. It is available in chewable tablets which are pleasant tasting and generally well accepted by children. The drug can however produce nausea, and occasionally mental symptoms such as headache and drowsiness. Mebendazole is at least as effective as thiabendazole and is better tolerated. It is available in tablet form and is given twice a day for 3 days. Treatment in strongyloidiasis must aim at complete destruction of all parasites. Decrease in worm load is not sufficient as the worms can multiply and reach the pretreatment levels.

11.4.6 Trichinosis

There is no specific therapy for infestation with *Trichinella spiralis*. Limited bed rest, analgesics and antipyretics are adequate to control muscular discomfort and fever in most cases (Most, 1978). Corticotrophin or corticosteroids are best for the relief of severe acute symptoms and may be life saving. The usual dosage is 40 to 60mg prednisone or its equivalent daily for 3 to 5 days, after which the dose is reduced. In less severe cases, thiabendazole 25mg/kg twice daily is frequently given until symptoms subside or toxic effects occur. Mebendazole 100mg twice daily may be superior. There is little evidence that thiabendazole or mebendazole are effective, although it is known that thiabendazole has anti-inflammatory and analgesic properties.

11.4.7 Tapeworm

Infestation with *Taenia saginata* or *Taenia solium* is effectively treated with niclosamide, thoroughly chewed and preferably followed 2 hours later by a saline purge of magnesium sulphate (30ml). An alternative is mebendazole, dichlorophen or paromomycin (table VII). Several courses of treatment may be required.

11.4.8 Giardiasis

Infestation of the small bowel by the flagellate *Giardia lamblia* is treated with metronidazole 200 or 400mg 3 times daily for 5 to 10 days or as a single daily dose of 2g for 2 to 3 consecutive days. Tinidazole is also highly effective (Levi et al., 1977) and can be given in a single dose regimen (table VII). Mepacrine, 100mg 3 times daily for a week, is effective but unpalatable and has the disadvantage of causing yellow discolouration of the skin.

12. Hormonal Gastrointestinal Disease

The term hormonal gastrointestinal disease refers to disordered gastrointestinal physiology caused by excessive secretion of hormones which are usually derived from a tumour of the particular endocrine cell.

12.1 Carcinoid Syndrome

Therapy aims at destruction of the tumour or at preventing the synthesis and release of substance produced by the tumour, which is commonly located in the appendix or ileum. Surgery is indicated for the removal of the primary or localised metastases, although surgical removal is usually curative only in the unusual case of a solitary bronchial or ovarian carcinoid. Hypotension during surgery may be controlled by methoxamine or angiotensin, and hypotensive crisis during operation may be obviated by prior treatment with corticosteroids and serotonin antagonists (e.g. methysergide, cyproheptadine). Moderate success and temporary improvement have been obtained after oral cyclophosphamide 100 to 150mg daily (after a loading dose) or after hepatic artery perfusion with 5-fluorouracil.

Flushing may be alleviated by treatment with propranolol or methyldopa, or phenoxybenzamine 10 to 30mg daily which may also be useful for the diarrhoea or wheezing. Prednisone 5mg orally every 6 hours is useful in controlling the flushing in bronchial cases. Wheezing usually responds to aerosol bronchodilators. As tachycardia is present in the fully developed carcinoid syndrome, bronchodilators with minimal effect on the myocardial β-adrenoceptors should be used, such as salbutamol, terbutaline (see chapter XX; sect. 2.3.1). Diarrhoea may be controlled by codeine (30 to 60mg daily) or loperamide (4 to 8mg daily) or if this fails by serotonin antagonists such as cyproheptadine (4 to 12mg) or methysergide (2 to 4mg) daily.

12.2 Zollinger-Ellison Syndrome

Gastrin secreting tumours cause massive acid secretion and although the treatment of choice at present is still total gastrectomy, cimetidine may be effective, long or short term, for symptomatic management and in preparation for surgery. It also has a role in the face of a contraindication to gastrectomy, to prevent ulceration and diarrhoea in patients with multiple metastases, and in the elderly and in those who have undergone repetitive gastric surgery, in whom total gastrectomy is hazardous. However, cimetidine is not effective in all patients (Brogden et al., 1978).

12.3 WDHA Syndrome (pancreatic cholera)

The treatment of choice of the watery diarrhoea, hypokalaemia, achlorhydria (WDHA) syndrome is surgical removal of the pancreatic islet cell tumour, and hence VIP (vasoactive intestinal peptide) or prostaglandin secretion, preceded by fluid and electrolyte replacement. A remission may be obtained in a few patients with corticosteroid therapy, indomethacin (Jaffe et al., 1977), streptozotocin (Kahn et al., 1975) or combination chemotherapy (Hansen et al., 1977). However, the treatment of choice, especially with secondary deposits, is to attempt to debulk the peptide secreting tumour as much as possible, hence reducing the hormone secreting cell mass.

13. Use of Drugs in the Presence of Associated Gastrointestinal and Hepatic Disease

Abnormal drug responses can sometimes occur in patients with gastrointestinal or liver disease, because of the pharmacological effects of drugs on gastrointestinal or liver pathology and also occasionally because of altered pharmacokinetics (see section 1) of drugs.

13.1 Gastroduodenal and Small Bowel Disease

13.1.1 Peptic Ulcer

Aspirin and all the so-called ulcerogenic drugs (see section 14.2.2) should be used with caution in patients with peptic ulceration or dyspepsia and avoided during periods of therapy aimed at healing a peptic ulcer (see section 4.1.1). Paracetamol (acetaminophen) or dextropropoxyphene should always be substituted for aspirin (Ivey et al., 1978; Emmanuel and Montgomery, 1971). Regular use of aspirin does not seem to affect ulcer recurrence if the ulcer has been completely healed initially, but does influence ulcer recurrence if the ulcer is not healed (Piper et al., 1977, 1978). If phenylbutazone, indomethacin or corticosteroids are essential they should be combined with antacids and given with meals. Rectal administration of indomethacin and phenylbutazone and parenteral (intramuscular) administration of corticosteroids also lessens the risk of aggravation of existing lesions. No doubt the prophylactic role of cimetidine will be evaluated (MacKercher et al., 1977; see chapter XXII, table III).

The gastrointestinal side effects of these and other anti-inflammatory drugs is a particular problem in rheumatic disease. All anti-inflammatory drugs used in rheumatic disease cause dyspepsia, some more than others. Thus some patients with a previous history of peptic ulcer or dyspepsia can tolerate some drugs but not others (see chapter XXII; sect. 1.2). Although there is an increased incidence of peptic ulceration in rheu-

matic disease, whether this is due to the disease or to drug therapy is uncertain (Haslock and Wright, 1974).

13.1.2 Oesophageal and Gastrointestinal Dysfunction

Oesophageal stasis can lead to oesophageal ulceration and stricture following use of irritant drugs such as aspirin and potassium chloride, particularly from slow release tablet formulations (Whitney and Croxon, 1972). Potassium chloride should be avoided in patients with oesophageal, pyloric or duodenal stenosis or spasm (e.g. as associated with peptic ulcer; dysphagia caused by cardiac enlargement; cardiomegaly after cardiac surgery), for apart from the risk of local ulceration, the retention in the oesophagus or pylorus probably allows a large amount of potassium chloride to leach out from a slow release tablet matrix. Thus when the stomach empties, a high concentration of potassium chloride is suddenly released over a short segment of small bowel. Under such circumstances, small bowel ulceration can result (see section 14.2.2). A delay in gastric emptying could be speculated to be a contributing factor to small bowel ulceration with enteric coated potassium chloride tablets such that release of drug from a previously retained dose coincides with release of drug from a subsequent dose at the time of stomach emptying, as is the case with enteric coated aspirin tablets (Leonards and Levy, 1965).

Anticholinergic drugs should theoretically not be used in the presence of oesophageal reflux or pyloric stenosis as they inhibit 'clearing' of acid contents of the oesophagus (see section 3.1, 4.3.2). Pyloric stenosis is a potential cause of therapeutic failure with levodopa, since delayed gastric emptying markedly decreases the bioavailability of the drug (see chapter VI; sect. 5). Changes in gastric emptying rate and gastrointestinal transit time can also significantly affect the absorption of certain other orally administered drugs (see section 1.1.1). Very rapid gastrointestinal transit, such as in gastroenteritis and malabsorption diarrhoea, may profoundly affect absorption of some drugs. This is likely to be most marked with enteric coated or slow release formulations (Jussila et al., 1970) and with poorly soluble drugs such as digoxin (Kolibash et al., 1977). Acute gastroenteritis has been given as the reason for pregnancy following use of oral contraceptives during a bout of diarrhoea (John and Jones, 1975).

13.1.3 Intestinal Malabsorption Syndromes

Although frank malabsorption states such as coeliac disease and steatorrhoea can be associated with altered absorption of certain drugs, the therapeutic importance of such changes is far from clear (see section 1.1.2). Any modification of dosage depends on the physicochemical and pharmacokinetic properties of the particular drug, the clinical state of the patient and the treatment being given.

13.2 Large Bowel Disease

Constipation may be aggravated by opiate containing preparations (e.g. antitussive preparations, strong analgesics except perhaps pentazocine) and by certain antacids (e.g. aluminium hydroxide, calcium carbonate). If antacids are required in patients with constipation, magnesium containing preparations can be used or in magnesium-aluminium mixtures, the ratio of magnesium to aluminium increased (see section 4.3.1). In certain patients such as the elderly where the force of peristalsis is diminished, anticholinergic drugs, including tricyclic antidepressants, may precipitate ileus. Antimotility drugs should not be used in the management of antibiotic induced colitis (see section 14.4.3).

In patients with ulcerative colitis, oral broad spectrum antibiotics may increase diarrhoea and rarely precipitate enterocolitis and are best avoided. Anticoagulants are also potentially hazardous as bleeding may be aggravated. Suppositories which are potentially irritating (e.g. indomethacin) are also contraindicated. Care is required with anticholinergics and antimotility agents (and barium sulphate) as toxic dilatation of the colon has on occasion been attributed to their administration (see section 8.1.5). Similar restrictions apply to use of these drugs in patients with Crohn's disease. Broad spectrum antibiotics are however, indicated in Crohn's disease in those patients in whom diarrhoea or steatorrhoea is due to bacterial overgrowth in the bowel. Because sulphasalazine is dependent on metabolism by colonic bacteria to its active component it is not effective in ulcerative colitis patients with an ileostomy or in those with Crohn's disease who have developed recurrence after colonic resection (see section 8.1.2).

Patients known to have strictures of the alimentary tract such as occur in Crohn's disease or neoplasia (Spigelman and McNabb, 1971), should probably not receive slow release preparations. Obstruction due to retention of an unaltered matrix or mucosal damage due to sudden release of a high local concentration of irritant drugs such as iron salts or potassium chloride are both potential hazards (see section 13.1.2; 14.1).

13.3 Pancreatic Disease

Hypocalcaemia due to pancreatitis (or any other cause) prolongs the effect of neuromuscular blocking agents such as tubocurarine and also theoretically decreases the effect of cardiac glycosides on the heart. Alcohol containing proprietary preparations should be avoided in alochol induced pancreatitis, as should drugs implicated in causing pancreatitis (see section 14.5). Because of its effect on the sphincter of Oddi, morphine should be avoided in fulminating pancreatitis and also in gall-stone pancreatitis. Pethidine (meperidine) or pentazocine are suitable alternatives (see section 9.1.2). Larger or more frequent doses of penicillins such as methicillin and dicloxacillin are required in patients with cystic fibrosis, due to unusually rapid renal clearance (Yaffe et al., 1977). Plasma concentrations of cephalexin are also reduced in cystic fibrosis (Parsons and Paddock, 1975).

13.4 Liver Disease

When drugs are used in the patient with liver disease, any problem which is likely to arise depends very largely on the nature and severity of the liver disease itself and on the pharmacological action and pharmacokinetic properties of the particular drug. While an accurate assessment of the severity of liver disease is essential, unlike renal disease, there is no simple test of liver function that enables the therapeutic regimen to be easily adjusted for all drugs mainly eliminated by hepatic metabolism (see section 1.4). Although the liver has an important role in the elimination of many drugs it has a great reserve capacity and it is in severe liver disease, particularly cirrhosis, that problems in therapy are most likely to arise because of a decreased rate of metabolism or increased oral bioavailability with some drugs (see section 1.3, 1.4). Liver disease can also lead to adverse effects of drugs because of an altered pharmacological response. Adverse reactions are most likely to occur with drugs with a low therapeutic ratio or with drugs where enhancement of an effect could be dangerous. Some of the problems can be avoided by adjustment of dosage (table VIII).

Liver disease does not necessarily lead to an increased likelihood of hepatotoxicity from potentially hepatotoxic drugs, provided the hepatotoxicity is of the hypersensitivity type (see section 14.6). If hepatotoxicity is dose related, this does not apply. For example, patients with impaired liver function are much more likely to sustain liver damage from pyrazinamide and rifampicin than tuberculosis patients with normal liver function and dosage should be reduced accordingly (Accocella, 1978; Knop et al., 1977). Potentially hepatotoxic drugs should only be used in liver disease if benefits outweigh risks. Such patients already have a reduced hepatic reserve and are not only at greater risk of further hepatic damage (i.e. independently of the type of damage induced by the drug), but use of potentially hepatotoxic drugs may confuse patient management if it depends on biochemical monitoring.

The following guidelines are suggested when use of drugs is considered in patients with liver disease (James, 1975):

1) As in all therapeutic decisions, evaluate the possible benefit to risks. If risks outweigh benefits, do not prescribe the drug.
2) If possible select drugs that have no potential for hepatotoxicity, or if this cannot be done, only those which cause hypersensitivity type hepatic damage.
3) If possible select drugs that are mainly eliminated unchanged by the kidney.
4) Avoid drugs that have an effect on the central nervous system.
5) Start treatment with small doses.
6) Clinical and laboratory observations, including estimations of plasma drug concentration where feasible, provide the best means for adjusting dosage regimens in accordance with clinical response in patients with impaired or fluctuating liver function.

Most problems are likely to arise with drug use in *severe* liver disease, particularly with CNS depressants and diuretics. Patients in hepatic coma or precoma are extremely sensitive to drugs such as morphine, paraldehyde and barbiturates (Laidlaw et al., 1961; Sessions et al., 1954), presumably as a consequence of the drug induced respiratory depression and the abnormal brain metabolism in patients with liver disease. Chlorpromazine and diazepam have been used for sedation, but stupor and slowing on the EEG may occur in some patients with usual doses in chronic liver disease, particularly in those with previous episodes of encephalopathy (Read et al., 1969; Branch et al., 1976). This enhanced response is not associated with abnormally high plasma concentrations of chlorpromazine or diazepam (Maxwell et al., 1972; Branch et al., 1976). Clearance of diazepam and chlordiazepoxide is nevertheless decreased in patients with alcoholic cirrhosis. Oxazepam or lorazepam are probably the safest drugs for sedation in liver disease. Although, unlike diazepam and chlordiazepoxide, they do not form active metabolites and are not likely to accumulate with repeat doses in liver disease (see section 1.4), they should be given with care and in smaller doses because of possible increased cerebral sensitivity. Chlormethiazole is widely used for delirium tremens in patients with alcoholic cirrhosis, but prolonged sedation and intoxication may occur if dosage is not reduced. This is especially important when chlormethiazole is given orally, as bioavailability is increased markedly due to reduced hepatic first-pass metabolism (Pentikainen et al., 1978; see section 1.4).

Morphine should never be given to patients with liver disease with a history of hepatic encephalopathy or who have evidence of jaundice or ascites. Nor should it be given to patients with liver disease complicated by gastrointestinal bleeding (Laidlaw et al., 1961). Overvigorous diuretic treatment of patients with cirrhotic oedema and ascites can precipitate hepatic coma, particularly in those with prior hepatic encephalopathy (Sherlock et al., 1966; Naranjo et al., 1978a, 1979; section 10.3.3). Monoamine oxidase inhibitors are also prone to precipitate hepatic precoma in patients with cirrhosis (Morgan and Read, 1972). Small doses of a non-sedative tricyclic drug such as protriptyline may be used if an antidepressant is indicated.

Ergot poisoning, which is dramatically demonstrable, is common in the presence of acute liver disease (e.g. acute viral hepatitis) because of a reduced rate of elimination (Whelton et al., 1968). It has even occurred in the presence of drug induced liver disease due to triacetyloleandomycin (Hayton, 1969). Other abnormal drug responses due to alteration of pharmacokinetic processes are given in table VIII. Oral anticoagulants should be avoided in liver disease (due to depression of vitamin K dependent clotting factor synthesis) and in biliary obstruction (due to impaired vitamin K

Table VIII. Examples of altered response to drugs in severe liver disease[1]

Drug	Notes
Morphine Barbiturates Chlorpromazine Monoamine oxidase inhibitors	May precipitate encephalopathy in those with hepatic precoma. Due to altered brain sensitivity, respiratory depression
Diuretics	Overvigorous diuretic therapy can precipitate encephalopathy in those with cirrhotic oedema and ascites. Due to excessive potassium loss (see section 10.3.3)
Oral anticoagulants	Enhanced response due to reduced absorption of vitamin K in obstructive jaundice or decreased production of vitamin K dependent clotting factors in hepatitis, cirrhosis (see chapter XXIII; sect. 3.2.4)
Oral hypoglycaemics	Increased risk of symptomatic hypoglycaemia with sulphonylureas and of lactic acidosis with biguanides (see chapter XVI; sect. 3.4.6)
Theophylline	Increased risk of toxicity if usual dose used. Due to impaired hepatic metabolism (Piafsky et al., 1977; Mangione et al., 1978)
Chlormethiazole	Increased risk of toxicity if usual dose used. Due to impaired hepatic metabolism and increased oral bioavailability (see section 1.4)
Chloramphenicol	Increased risk of haematological toxicity. Most likely in presence of both ascites and jaundice. Due to impaired hepatic metabolism (conjugation) of drug (Surland and Weisberger, 1963)
Pyrazinamide Rifampicin	Increased risk of hepatic toxicity in those with impaired liver function if usual dose used (Di Piazza et al., 1978)
Ergotamine	Ergot poisoning has occurred in presence of acute viral hepatitis (Whelton et al., 1968), and in association with drug induced jaundice (Hayton, 1969). Due to impaired hepatic metabolism
Phenytoin (diphenylhydantoin)	Increased risk of CNS toxicity in some patients with usual dosage (Kutt et al., 1964), particularly if liver disease associated with renal impairment. Due to impaired hepatic metabolism and/or decreased albumin binding and delayed clearance. Probably dependent on dose used (see section 1.3)
Lignocaine (lidocaine)	Increased risk of severe CNS toxicity (Selden and Sasahara, 1967). Due to impaired hepatic elimination
Niridazole	Increased incidence of CNS side effects in bilharziasis patients wtih liver complications (Faigle, 1971). Due to development of portalsystemic shunts and increased bioavailability (see section 1.4)
Carbenoxolone	Increased incidence of mineralocorticoid-like side effects likely if usual dose used. Due to decreased albumin binding and delayed clearance (see section 4.1.4)
Thiopentone	Decreased protein binding may enhance activity (Shideman et al., 1949)
Tubocurarine Pancuronium Suxamethonium (succinylcholine)	Decreased serum pseudocholinesterase levels due to liver cell damage may prolong activity of suxamethonium and decrease activity of non-depolarising relaxants (e.g. tubocurarine, pancuronium). However, with pancuronium while a high initial dose is required for adequate relaxation, clearance is delayed with risk of prolonged activity if repeated doses are excessive (see chapter X; sect. 2.2.1)
Vitamin D	Failure of conventional vitamin D therapy in primary biliary cirrhosis due to impaired hepatic hydroxylation of vitamin D (Wagonfeld et al., 1976). 25-Hydroxyvitamin D is the preferred form of vitamin D in liver disease

---

1   See also discussion in section 1.4, 13.4.

absorption). In these situations there is increased and variable response to oral anticoagulants (see chapter XXIII; sect. 3.2.4).

Oral contraceptives should not be prescribed in the presence of cholestatic hepatobiliary disease of any type (see chapter XV; sect. 13.6). They are probably safe in acute viral hepatitis (Schweitzer et al., 1975), and also in those with a past history of liver disease, provided there is no history of cholestasis or pruritus during pregnancy or following use of oestrogens (Mowat and Arias, 1969); although the risk of cholestasis developing during use of oral contraceptives (usually during the first few cycles) in such patients may have been exaggerated, at least with some formulations (Rannevik et al., 1972), and is probably most likely in those populations (e.g. Chile, parts of Scandinavia) where genetic factors seem to predispose to cholestasis of pregnancy and oral contraceptive jaundice (Dalen and Westerholm, 1974; Thompson and Williams, 1969). Both are probably caused by oestrogens, but progestagens (particularly 19-nortestosterone derivatives) may be occasionally responsible and may also have an additive effect with the oestrogen (Thompson and Williams, 1969).

14. Drug Induced Gastrointestinal and Liver Disease

Because oral therapy is the most convenient form of systemic drug administration, it is not surprising that gastrointestinal reactions account for a large proportion of all adverse drug reactions (Stewart and Cluff, 1974). Some drugs are however, more often implicated than others. The liver, with its major role in the elimination of many drugs, is also not surprisingly implicated in many adverse drug reactions. Fortunately, only a few gastrointestinal and hepatic reactions are serious, but they may nevertheless cause much morbidity and diagnostic confusion (for review, see Bramble and Record, 1978; Zimmerman, 1978). Drug induced diseases of the oral cavity are discussed in chapter XIII (sect. 13).

14.1 Oesophageal Disease

Heartburn may be aggravated in patients with hiatus hernia or reflux oesophagitis by use of anticholinergic drugs (see section 3.1) or aspirin (Smith, 1978). Slow release potassium chloride tablets can lead to oesophageal ulceration when used in the presence of oesophageal stasis (see sect. 13.1.2), as may emepronium and tetracyclines if taken before retiring without adequate fluid, especially in the presence of oesophageal stasis or reflux (Crowson et al., 1976; Kobler et al., 1978). Dysphagia in patients on corticosteroids or cytotoxic drugs should raise the possibility of moniliasis. β-Adrenoceptor blocking drugs may induce oesophageal spasm (Zfass et al., 1970). Oesophageal lesions are most likely to occur with drugs with locally irritating properties, particularly in slow release formulations and in older patients who may have difficulty in swallowing or dysphagia due to cardiac enlargement (Carlborg et al., 1978; see section 13.1.2).

14.2 Gastroduodenal Disease

14.2.1 Nausea and Vomiting

All drugs are probably capable of causing nausea and vomiting in some individuals. Antibiotics, ferrous sulphate, metronidazole, sulphasalazine and opiates are common offenders. These symptoms are also common after levodopa, aminophylline, potassium chloride solutions and oestrogens. Nausea induced by oestrogens is dose related; patients who experience nausea with one oral contraceptive preparation for example, may be free of nausea on a preparation with a lower oestrogen content. Nausea and vomiting due to digitalis is an early and important symptom of overdosage (Lely and Van Enter, 1970).

14.2.2 Dyspepsia, Gastrointestinal Bleeding and Ulceration

The main causes of dyspepsia are nonsteroidal anti-inflammatory analgesics, particularly aspirin, and corticosteroids (see chapter XXII; sect. 3). These drugs may both cause dyspepsia and aggravate symptoms of peptic ulceration in those with unhealed ulcers. Caffeine in tea or coffee may also aggravate symptoms of peptic ulceration but alcohol and reserpine are not likely to do so (see Cooke, 1976; Piper et al., 1978).

Aspirin causes heartburn or dyspepsia in a small percentage of all users, in more of those with rheumatoid arthritis, in whom there is an increased incidence of peptic ulceration (see section 13.1.1), and in an even larger percentage of peptic ulcer patients (Roth, 1965; Muir and Cossar, 1955). Although aspirin causes microbleeding (Croft and Wood, 1967; Grossman et al., 1961), the relationship between severe gastrointestinal haemorrhage and aspirin ingestion is less clear cut (see Shirley, 1977). With ACTH and corticosteroids a patient's susceptibility to dyspepsia is increased with larger doses and prolonged treatment. Males over 40 appear to be most susceptible and patients with asthma or ulcerative colitis have fewer problems than those with rheumatoid arthritis, systemic lupus erythematosus or pemphigus (Benson, 1971; Roth, 1965). Symptoms may not become apparent until haemorrhage or perforation make the presence of ulceration known.

All drugs with 'ulcerogenic' properties may cause gastrointestinal bleeding, occult as well as massive in patients with active peptic ulceration, but the incidence is much greater with aspirin. Moreover, heavy aspirin intake appears to be associated with gastric ulceration in a few patients, especially women; at least in some communities (e.g. Australia; see Duggan, 1976; Piper et al., 1977) and to be associated with ulcer persistence and/or recurrence in those patients whose ulcer is not completely healed by initial treatment (see section 13.1.1; Piper et al., 1978). Multiple antral ulcers are nearly always associated with long term salicylate ingestion (Cameron, 1975). Some of the various aspirin formulations or modifications appear safer than conventional or enteric coated aspirin in terms of occult blood loss, but insufficient information is available to make firm statements about their long term effects. The only safe method of preventing aspirin damage to the stomach is to buffer the aspirin to a near neutral pH (Cooke, 1976). Such antacid buffering however, causes rapid renal excretion and these formulations are of little use in long term therapy of rheumatoid arthritis for example, as adequate plasma salicylate concentrations cannot be attained (see chapter XXII; sect. 3.2.1). On available evidence the other non-steroidal anti-inflammatory analgesics and also corticosteroids cannot be implicated as a cause of peptic ulcer (Cooke, 1976; Conn and Blitzer, 1976). With all these drugs, even the relationship between previous peptic ulceration and 'drug related' ulceration is unclear, and even drug related dyspepsia is not as common as expected when sought (Bain and Masheter, 1976). The newer propionic acid non-steroidal anti-inflammatory drugs do not cause occult bleeding and the incidence of overt bleeding appears to be less than with aspirin (Cuthbert, 1974). Despite these uncertainties, there is general agree-

ment that aspirin, other non-steroidal anti-inflammatory analgesics and corticosteroids should be avoided in the presence of an active ulcer until the ulcer is healed (see section 4.4, 13.1.1).

Other drugs are less common causes of important gastroduodenal toxicity. Gastrointestinal bleeding may nevertheless be associated with use of intravenous ethacrynic acid and with poorly controlled anticoagulant therapy (Jick and Porter, 1978).

14.3 Small Bowel Disease

Small bowel disease may be induced by a large variety of drugs. However, the frequency of complications is rare in comparison with their usage.

14.3.1 Malabsorption

Important malabsorption defects are generally dose related and usually involve multiple nutrients (Longstreth and Newcomer, 1975). Certain clinical states such as in the malnourished alcoholic, may predispose the small bowel to a drug induced absorptive defect. Drug interference with absorption of other drugs is discussed in chapter VIII.

A reversible malabsorption syndrome can be caused by cytotoxic drugs and high doses of colchicine (Race et al., 1970). These drugs inhibit mitotic activity and hence cell renewal and may induce partial villous atrophy.

Neomycin, used in doses of 3 to 12g daily to depress the growth of gut bacteria (e.g. as in chronic portal systemic encephalopathy), induces a number of effects on the small bowel and interferes with the absorption of xylose, glucose, fats and fat soluble vitamins. Neomycin, by precipitating bile salts, also leads to steatorrhoea. Similar though milder effects occur with kanamycin, paromomycin and tetracyclines. Cholestyramine, by binding bile salts in the ileum, results in steatorrhoea and malabsorption of fat soluble vitamins (see section 6.1.3). Drugs associated with mild steatorrhoea include colchicine (large doses long term), p-aminosalicylic acid (only occasionally with usual doses, but more commonly with high doses) and irritant laxatives (chronic abuse).

Impaired folic acid absorption may be induced by anticonvulsants such as phenytoin, phenobarbitone and primidone, and by p-aminosalicylic acid, oral contraceptives (rare cause of interference with dietary folate) and alcohol (Waxman et al., 1970). Other drugs can induce folate deficiency by a parenteral effect (see chapter XXIII; sect. 8.5). Interference with intestinal absorption of vitamin B_{12} is induced by neomycin, colchicine (large doses long term, phenformin, metformin, p-amino-salicylic acid and cholestyramine (Waxman et al., 1970). In most cases these changes result in only slight vitamin B_{12} or folate deficiency, but overt megaloblastic anaemia may occur, particularly in those whose vitamin or folate stores were deficient before treatment.

14.3.2 Small Bowel Ulceration

Potassium chloride may cause small bowel lesions which are nonspecific, circumferential and consist of stenosis with or without ulceration. They have most often been assoicated with enteric coated potassium chloride (Allen et al, 1965), but a few cases have been reported with slow release formulations when used in patients with oesophageal stasis or delayed gastrointestinal transit; e.g. during a period of recumbency (Farquharson-Roberts et al., 1975; Whitney and Croxson, 1972). With both enteric coated and slow release formulations the cause of the ulceration seems to be related to the sudden release of a high concentration of potassium chloride over a small segment of small bowel (see sect. 13.1.2), perhaps in some cases at least, superimposed upon chronic vascular insufficiency.

14.3.3 Peritoneal Reactions

Long term use of the β-adrenoceptor blocking drug practolol has been associated with small bowel obstruction from widespread peritoneal fibrosis ('sclerosing peritonitis'; Brown et al., 1974). The condition is usually preceded by eye and/or skin reactions (Idanpaan-Heikkila et al., 1977) and in some cases is not reversible on withdrawal of practolol, peritoneal stripping of the bowel being necessary to overcome intestinal obstruction (Thompson and Jackson, 1977). Uninterrupted use of methysergide in migraine prophylaxis may lead to retroperitoneal fibrosis, but this process is not complicated by involvement of the visceral and/or parietal peritoneum (Graham et al., 1966).

14.3.4 Ileus

Non-mechanical ileus which is either adynamic (paralytic) or dynamic (spastic) is occasionally caused by a variety of drugs. Adynamic ileus may occur on rare occasions with anticholinergic drugs such as tricyclic antidepressants (Milner and Buckler, 1964), anti-Parkinsonian drugs and chlorpromazine, the antimalarial drug mepacrine, the vinca alkaloids vinblastine and vincristine, and with the ganglion blocking agents such as mecamylamine and pempidine. The drugs with anticholinergic activity may so interfere with bowel motility, particularly in elderly patients in whom the strength of peristalsis is reduced, that a spastic ileus may result. Both spastic and adynamic ileus may follow administration of morphine. Anticoagulant overdosage may produce haemorrhage within the bowel wall which can lead to ileus.

14.3.5 Other Small Bowel Lesions

Haemorrhagic necrosis of the small and large bowel has been associated with use of digitalis, and although heart failure and poor intestinal blood flow no doubt have a role in producing this complication, digitalis does appear to have an effect on the splanchnic circulation. Corticosteroids and long term use of vasopressors may similarly produce mesenteric infarction in situations where the splanchnic circulation is already compromised. Very rarely, mesenteric vascular occlusion with infarction of the midgut has been associated with use of oral contraceptives (Nathmann et al., 1973). Long term abuse of irritant laxatives such as phenolphthalein may produce severe enteritis with systemic effects such as syncope, rash and haemorrhagic tendencies.

14.4 Large Bowel Diseases

Drugs used in the treatment of a wide range of disorders may induce several diseases which mainly affect the large bowel, including severe diarrhoea, colitis, constipation and acquired megacolon.

14.4.1 Constipation

Barium sulphate, bulk producing laxatives (if fluid intake is inadequate) and opiate containing drugs (e.g. narcotic analgesics, codeine, anti-tussives) all tend to produce constipation. Tricyclic antidepressants and anti-Parkinsonian drugs with anticholinergic activity, particularly when combined with antipsychotic drugs with marked anticholinergic activity such as chlorpromazine, can also cause constipation. Such drugs should not be given to patients prone to constipation because of the risk of faecal impaction and stercoral perforation of the colon (Cass, 1978). Certain antacids (aluminium hydroxide gel, calcium carbonate) and ferrous sulphate are constipating. The vinca alkaloids, vinblastine and vincristine may cause constipation in some patients. Patients receiving the ion exchange resin, polystyrene sodium sulphonate, often become very constipated.

14.4.2 Diarrhoea

Diarrhoea is probably the most common side effect of drugs. It is an aphorism that diarrhoea occurring while a patient is on any drug therapy be suspected to be the result of that drug. Withdrawal of the drug, if possible, will soon determine whether this is in fact so. The chronic use of laxatives may be surreptitious and should be considered in patients with ill defined diarrhoea. Large doses of magnesium containing antacids, particularly magnesium trisilicate, produce diarrhoea. Guanethidine can cause an explosive diarrhoea in some patients, but this can be avoided by use of antimotility drugs. Digitalis overdosage may result in diarrhoea as well as nausea and vomiting.

Antibiotics seem particularly likely to cause diarrhoea (Editorial, 1975; Smith and Goulston, 1975). In some instances there is a clear relationship between altered intestinal flora and diarrhoea. Withdrawal of the antibiotic, to allow recolonisation, in most cases eliminates the pathogen (e.g. *Salmonella, Shigella* spp.). In other cases diarrhoea may be due to a direct irritant effect. Staphylococcal enterocolitis is one of the most florid, albeit rare, complications affecting the intestine in antibiotic treated patients. The patients thus affected are generally elderly and may be recovering from surgery. Despite withdrawal of the offending drug, administration of oral vancomycin and resuscitation measures, this disease has a high mortality. Pruritus ani and perianal candidiasis often accompanies the use of broad spectrum antibiotics (e.g. tetracyclines) but seldom causes a true enteritis. When it does so, it may be a manifestation of systemic candidiasis in an immunosuppressed or debilitated patient. The more common mild, nonspecific diarrhoea associated with tetracycline therapy does not require concurrent use of anticandidal agents (Angel and Lacey, 1968; see also chapter XIV; sect. 2.3.1).

14.4.3 Colitis

The development of a nonspecific colitis or less commonly a more severe pseudomembranous colitis (sometimes a pseudomembranous enterocolitis) has been associated with the use of antibiotics (Smith and Goulston, 1975; Gallagher and Goulston, 1978). Histologically the nonspecific colitis is distinguishable from ulcerative colitis and the changes of pseudomembranous colitis are virtually pathognomonic. The antibiotics involved include penicillin, ampicillin, amoxycillin, cephalosporins, tetracycline, co-trimoxazole and chloramphenicol, but there have been a greater number of reports linking these conditions with lincomycin and clindamycin. No particular antibiotic or combination can be singled out as almost any antibiotic may cause colitis (Kappas et al., 1978). A toxin produced by *Clostridia* species, notably *Cl. difficile,* seems to be the most likely cause of antibiotic associated colitis (Bartlett et al., 1978a,b; George et al., 1978a,b) by causing local injury to the colonic mucosa in individuals made susceptible by previous antibiotic therapy (Larson et al., 1978). *Cl. difficile* does not appear to be a permanent resident of the gastrointestinal tract. The exact incidence of antibiotic associated colitis remains a matter of debate and with clindamycin has varied from 1 in 10 as detected sigmoidoscopically in patients followed prospectively in some series (Tedesco et al., 1974) to 1 in 100,000 on the basis of clinical experience (Hubbard, 1974). Prevalence probably depends on the care in which the condition is sought (Kappas et al., 1978) and on as yet poorly understood geographical and other factors. Deaths have mostly occurred in elderly or otherwise seriously ill patients (Price and Davies, 1977), but can also occur in children (Buts et al., 1977).

Diagnosis may be difficult, but antibiotic associated colitis should be suspected in any patient who develops moderate to profuse watery diarrhoea during or soon after antibiotic therapy. Treatment consists of stopping the antibiotic, with rehydration, correction of electrolyte disturbances and depending on severity, sometimes albumin and blood transfusion. Seriously ill patients require topical and systemic corticosteroids in a regimen similar to that used for ulcerative colitis (Goodman and Truelove, 1976). Oral vancomycin has been used successfully to treat pseudomembranous colitis in patients in whom toxigenic strains of clostridia had been isolated, but did not appear to benefit patients in whom neither toxins nor clostridia could be identified (Keighley et al., 1978). An antitoxin to *Cl. difficile* which has been developed may prove effective. Elevated concentrations of primary bile acids

Table IX. Types of drug induced hepatic injury and their clinical and biochemical characteristics (modified after Zimmerman, 1974, 1978)

Classification[1]	Clinical resemblance	Biochemical values[2]			Prototype drugs[3]
		SGOT, SGPT	alkaline phos.	cholesterol	
Hepatocellular	Viral hepatitis (severe)	++++	+	o	Halothane Isoniazid
Hepatocellular	Viral hepatitis, chronic active hepatitis	+++/ ++++	+	+	Methyldopa Oxyphenisatin
Mixed hepatocellular	Atypical viral hepatitis, obstructive jaundice	++/+++	++/+++	± /o	Sulphonamides p-Aminosalicylic acid
Steatosis, acute toxic	Fatty liver of pregnancy	++	+	o	Tetracycline
Cholestasis	Obstructive jaundice	+	++++	++++	Erythromycin estolate Chlorpromazine Anabolic steroids
Adenomas	Liver masses	—	±	—	Oral contraceptives

1   The injury may be characterised by necrosis or degeneration of the hepatic parenchyma (i.e. cytotoxic), or manifested by cholestasis, but little parenchymal injury, or may include elements of both types (i.e. mixed).

2   Degree of elevation of values: ++++ = marked; +++ = moderate; ++ = mild; + = slight; ± normal to increased; o = normal to decreased.

3   The clinical and biochemical syndrome may not be consistent in all patients.

in the colon may play a role in diarrhoea and antibiotic associated colitis, and cholestyramine (see section 6.1.3) has been useful in some cases (Hoffman, 1977). Antimotility drugs do not seem to be effective in many cases (Kappas et al., 1978). Moreover, in some series they appear to have prolonged the course of the condition (Pittman et al., 1974; Pittman, 1975) and to have been associated with the development of toxic megacolon (Boyd and Den Beston, 1976; Goodacre et al., 1976). Subtotal colectomy for such life threatening situations with deep ulceration or perforation is however, rarely necessary.

Pseudomembranous colitis need not be associated with antibiotic use, having been related to recent surgery, cardiac failure, uraemia, malignancy, cirrhosis, radiation, bowel obstruction and corticosteroids (Goulston and McGovern, 1965). A history of diarrhoea, fever and mucosal changes seen on sigmoidoscopy in a patient who has recently received an antibiotic should however, raise the possibility of colitis. Indeed, antibiotic associated diarrhoea always merits sigmoidoscopy if more than trivial.

The 'cathartic colon', which results from prolonged use (many years) of irritant purgatives in large and increasing doses, may simulate ulcerative colitis radiologically, but this diagnosis is excluded by the essentially normal appearance at sigmoidoscopy (Sladen, 1972). The patient may complain of constipation and abdominal discomfort, or alternatively diarrhoea and deny the use of laxatives. Positive diagnosis may be suggested by the mucosal pigmentation, which often accompanies prolonged consumption of anthraquinone drugs (Smith, 1968). The addition of an alkali to the stool, and often to the urine will produce a deep red colouration when phenolphthalein containing drugs have been taken. Muscle weakness and potassium deficiency is one of the most characteristic features of laxative abuse.

14.5 Pancreatic Disease

Drug induced clinically recognisable pancreatitis is rare (Nakashima and Howard, 1977). Sulphonamides such as sulphamethizole and sulphasalazine have caused rare instances of haemorrhagic pancreatitis, possibly as a result of hypersensitivity. Acute haemorrhagic pancreatitis has been reported in a few patients after large doses of thiazide and thiazide-like diuretics (e.g. chlorthalidone) and also after frusemide. In one series, a first attack of acute pancreatitis was associated with an excess use of diuretics (Bourke et al., 1978). Corticosteroids especially when given in large doses and to children have been reported to be associated with pancreatitis. In some series a causal relationship with corticosteroids has not been clearly established as the drugs implicated have been used to treat diseases which may themselves cause pancreatitis. A combination of corticosteroids and azathioprine used after organ transplantation is however, particularly liable to affect the pancreas (Nakashima and Howard, 1977). Pancreatitis has also been associated with oral contraceptives (Bank and Marks, 1970).

14.6 Liver Diseases

Since the liver is the main organ concerned with drug metabolism, particularly orally administered drugs which reach the liver via the portal vein, and is the primary site of entry for ingested foreign substances, it is not surprising that it is often associated with untoward reactions to drugs. The various mechanisms by which drugs may cause liver disease are multiple, complex and often poorly understood (for review, see Sherlock, 1969; Zimmerman, 1978). Examples of drug induced liver disease are shown in tables IX and X. Fortunately, permanent liver damage as a consequence of drugs is unusual, but prolonged illness and death may result.

14.6.1 Clinicopathological Types of Liver Disease

Drugs may produce acute liver disease which can be broadly divided into two clinicopathological types — drug induced hepatitis and drug induced cholestasis. In each group the offending drug can cause a reaction which may be either hepatotoxic, dose related and predictable, or idiosyncratic, nonpredictable and possibly due to hypersensitivity or abnormal drug metabolism. Drug induced hepatitis of the predictable type is associated with tetracyclines, methotrexate and paracetamol (acetaminophen), while idiosyncratic disease occurs with halothane, monoamine oxidase inhibitors, isoniazid, oxyphenisatin, phenytoin and methyldopa. Examples of drugs which produce cholestasis predictably are methyltestosterone and C17-alkyl substituted steroids, while chlorpromazine, erythromycin estolate, PAS and triacetyloleandomycin produce idiosyncratic reactions.

14.6.2 Diagnosis of Drug Induced Liver Disease

Diagnosis of drug induced liver disease is difficult. Thus, liver cell necrosis due to hypersensitivity (e.g. isoniazid) may often be difficult to distinguish from viral hepatitis, while cholestatic jaundice induced by drugs has to be distinguished from jaundice due to obstruction of the major bile ducts and from viral induced cholestatic jaundice. In addition to causing acute liver disease, drugs, like many other environmental agents such as viruses, alcohol, carcinogens and iron, may produce a syndrome indistinguishable from chronic liver disease; for example, methyldopa (Rodman et al., 1976), dantrolene (Utili et al., 1976) and oxyphenisatin (Reynolds et al., 1971) associated chronic active hepatitis. High doses of paracetamol used in suicide attempts produce a clinical picture similar to that of a fulminant hepatitis (Clark et al., 1973).

Interpretation of the significance of reports of drug associated liver disease is also difficult. The mere association of an hepatic reaction and drug administration is unsatisfactory as the patient is so often on multiple drug therapy, and with antituberculosis drugs it is often difficult to implicate which drug or drugs of a combination regimen are involved (see section 14.6.4). Moreover, many hepatic reactions are of unknown aetiology.

The underlying disease being treated may itself be associated with hepatic lesions. Liver abnormalities have been associated with methotrexate in psoriasis (Dahl et al., 1971, 1972), but histopathological changes do occur in severe psoriasis without treatment (Zachariae et al., 1975). However, the incidence of important changes is higher during methotrexate, particularly after prolonged treatment (Almeyda et al., 1972). Minor histological abnormalities of the liver may occur in many diseases, be part of the disease, or reflect nutritional state, hepatitis B virus, and so on. A unique lesion is more readily recognised; for example, the relatively rare hepatic cell adenomas and focal nodular hyperplasia associated with use of oral contraceptives (Klatskin, 1977).

Thus in an individual patient, even allowing for histological examination, the diagnosis of a drug reaction is only presumptive and often based on exclusion. In a carefully controlled situation (see section 14.6.4), there may be justification to use

Table X. Examples of drug induced hepatic reactions (see further Maxwell and Williams, 1971; Sherlock, 1968a, 1972; Zimmerman, 1978)

Drug class	Type of injury (clinical)	Mechanism[1]	Notes
General anaesthetics Halothane	Hepatitis-like	Liver cell necrosis due to sensitivity Unpredictable	Rare. Associated with multiple exposures. Re-exposure may be hazardous. Particular risk if repeat exposure within 7 days — warning signs not had time to develop. Very high mortality if massive necrosis. Contraindicated if unexplained jaundice or fever after previous anaesthetic (see also chapter X, sect. 2.1.1)
Monoamine oxidase inhibitors Isocarboxazid Iproniazid Phenelzine	Hepatitis-like	Liver cell necrosis due to sensitivity Unpredictable	Occurs in very small proportion of patients who receive the drug. More common after multiple exposures to the drug. Seriously affected show shrinking of liver and die of hepatic failure. Mortality high (70%) if hepatic precoma or coma reached
Analgesics Paracetamol (acetaminophen)	Hepatitis-like	Liver cell necrosis due to direct toxicity Predictable	Generally occurs with overdosage (e.g. suicide attempts) but chronic necrosis has followed long term use of low doses (Bonkowsky et al., 1978). Hepatotoxicity may also occur in those with liver disease (Johnson and Tolman, 1977; Rosenberg and Neelon, 1978)
Salicylates	—	Competitive inhibition bilirubin binding	A serious problem only in neonates (see sect. 14.6.6). In adults, jaundice enhanced in those with underlying tendency to, or actual hyperbilirubinaemia
	Hepatitis-like	Cholestasis possibly due to underlying illness Predictable	Abnormal transaminases, particularly with high doses in patients with systemic lupus erythematosus (Seaman and Plotz, 1976; Travers and Hughes, 1978) and juvenile rheumatoid arthritis (Athreya, 1975). No major toxicity
Phenacetin	Hepatitis-like	Liver cell necrosis due to sensitivity Unpredictable	Occasional occurrence, particularly in rheumatoid patients with liver disease
	Haemolytic jaundice	Increased haemolysis Unpredictable	Most likely in those with genetic defect of red cell (see chapter XXIII; sect.8.4)
Antibacterial agents Tetracycline	Fatty liver of pregnancy	Steatosis due to direct toxicity Predictable	Associated with large doses (usually intravenous) given during last trimester of pregnancy or in presence of impaired renal function. Mortality high

Table X. (continued)

Drug class	Type of injury (clinical)	Mechanism[1]	Notes
Antibacterial agents (continued)			
Erythromycin estolate Triacetyloleandomycin	Obstructive jaundice or hepatitis-like	Cholestasis due to sensitivity Unpredictable	Usually only occurs when given for periods in excess of 10 to 14 days. More common after multiple exposures. Full recovery usually follows discontinuation of the drug. Liver toxicity not seen with erythromycin base or stearate, or with oleandomycin
Sulphonamides	Generalised hypersensitivity reaction with hepatitis and jaundice	Increased haemolysis Unpredictable	In most instances increased haemolysis is combined with a generalised hypersensitivity effect or occurs in patients who have genetic defect of red cell(e.g. G6PD deficiency). Reaction usually seen within 2 weeks of beginning treatment (see sect. 14.6.6)
Sulphonamides		Competitive inhibition of bilirubin binding	Rise in serum level of unconjugated bilirubin only of clinical significance in neonates (see section 14.6.6)
Anticonvulsants			
Phenytoin	Hepatitis-like	Liver cell necrosis Unpredictable	Usually accompanied by other signs of allergy, such as rash. Clinical jaundice in about 50%. Stop drug immediately if biochemical abnormalities or symptoms suggestive of hepatic damage or hypersensitivity occur
Antituberculosis agents			
Pyrazinamide	Hepatitis-like	Liver cell necrosis Unpredictable	Incidence appears to be related to dosage, being higher on doses above 40mg/kg daily
Ethionamide	Hepatitis-like	Liver cell necrosis Unpredictable	Overt jaundice and liver damage relatively rare. Hepatitis less frequent than with pyrazinamide
Isoniazid	Hepatitis-like	Liver cell necrosis due to sensitivity[2] Unpredictable	Clinical hepatitis with jaundice seen infrequently (0.1%). Symptoms most often noted within first 3 months of treatment but may occur at 4 or 5 months. Risk increased in elderly and with regular alcohol intake (Kopanoff et al., 1978). Allergic symptoms less frequent than with PAS. Hepatitis may progress for a few weeks despite withdrawal of drug. Stop drug immediately biochemical abnormalities or symptoms suggestive of hepatic damage or hypersensitivity occur (see also chapter XX; sect. 8.1). Cross sensitivity may occur between the chemically related drugs, isoniazid pyrazinamide and ethionamide
p-Aminosalicylic acid	Atypical viral hepatitis, obstructive jaundice	Cholestasis due to sensitivity Unpredictable	Hepatic reaction is usually part of generalised hypersensitivity reaction

Table X. (continued)

Drug class	Type of injury (clinical)	Mechanism[1]	Notes
Antituberculosis drugs (continued)			
Rifampicin (rifampin)	Hepatitis-like[3]	Cholestasis due to interference with transport of bilirubin or with its conjugation Predictable	Hepatic reaction early onset (3 to 5 weeks) compared with that with isoniazid (Thompson, 1978). Possible increased susceptibility in patients also receiving isoniazid (particularly slow acetylators), in the elderly and in alcoholics and those with pre-existing disturbance of hepatobiliary function (Gronhagen-Riska et al., 1978; see also chapter XX, sect. 8.1)
Phenothiazines			
Chlorpromazine (and other phenothiazines)	Obstructive jaundice	Cholestasis due to sensitivity Unpredictable	Reaction not frequent (0.5%); not related to dosage. Onset usually in first 4 weeks of treatment. Reaction frequent (40%) upon re-exposure in sensitive individuals
Cytotoxic drugs			
Methotrexate	Cirrhosis	Liver cell necrosis due to direct toxicity Predictable	Cirrhosis has been reported most often in patients with psoriasis treated with methotrexate (Dahl et al., 1971, 1972). Histopathological changes do occur in severe psoriasis without treatment, but incidence of important changes higher during methotrexate particularly after prolonged treatment (see also chapter XIV; sect. 6.2.2)
Azathioprine	Obstructive jaundice	?	Depends on dose. When used in active chronic hepatitis, increasing jaundice may be due to primary disease or to drug. Risk of jaundice and hepatic coma with doses over 100mg daily
6-Mercaptopurine	Hepatitis-like	?	Full significance of toxicity not yet established
Antihypertensive drugs			
Methyldopa	Hepatitis-like	Liver cell necrosis due to sensitivity Unpredictable	Symptoms of hepatitis may resemble those of acute viral hepatitis. If continued some patients show manifestations of chronic active hepatitis, others cholestatic jaundice. Most reactions apparent within 3 months. Do not rechallenge patient and avoid in those with active liver disease (Rodman et al., 1976)
	Haemolytic jaundice	Increased haemolysis Unpredictable	

Table X. (continued)

Drug class	Type of injury (clinical)	Mechanism[1]	Notes
Steroidal compounds C$_{17}$-substituted steroids (e.g. methyltestosterone, norethandrolone etc.)	Cholestasis	Regular cholestasis Predictable	A dose dependent reaction which develops with orally rather than parenterally administered drugs. This reaction probably occurs with almost all orally active anabolic or androgenic agents (except nandrolone, testosterone)
Oral contraceptives	Cholestasis	Cholestasis, possibly genetically determined	Individual variation in susceptibility to jaundice; possibly genetically determined (Dalen and Westerholm, 1974). Most likely in early cycles in patients who have had cholestatic jaundice in last trimester of pregnancy or following oestrogens. Best avoided in such patients. Avoid in patients with cholestatic hepatobiliary disease, chronic active hepatitis or congenital defects in bilirubin excretion but are probably not contraindicated after, or during viral hepatitis (see section 13.4; chapter XV sect. 13.6).
	Benign tumours Hepatic cell adenomas and focal nodular hyperplasia	? Mechanism	More likely with prolonged use; ? genetic susceptibility; a few have shown malignant degeneration (Klatskin, 1977; McQueen, 1978)

1   The mechanism most often occurring is indicated. Considerable overlap may occur. *Unpredictable* (i.e. occurs in only a small proportion of individuals and not possible to predict those at risk). *Predictable* (i.e. will occur in all subjects if sufficient dose taken).

2   Liver cell necrosis not always present alone in isoniazid hepatitis. Cholestatic-hepatitic reactions have been reported.

3   In some patients histological findings are indistinguishable from viral hepatitis, but there is usually less inflammatory infiltration.

'challenge' exposures to determine whether the drug does have the potential for an idiosyncratic reaction — *provided* that the reaction involved is not serious.

14.6.3 Liver Cell Necrosis

Massive liver cell necrosis is the most serious consequence of drug induced disease and has a high mortality. In the case of halothane, massive necrosis has a mortality close to 100 % (Trey et al., 1970). Massive liver cell necrosis after halothane is a rare occurrence and only occurs after repeated exposures to this anaesthetic in sensitive individuals. Due warning is often given by unexplained pyrexia, eosinophilia and raised transaminase levels in the plasma after previous exposure, and if these should occur halothane should not be given again (Moult and Sherlock, 1975; see further chapter X; sect. 2.1.1). Fatal liver cell necrosis may follow on monoamine oxidase inhibitors (iproniazid) and when large doses of some drugs are taken in suicidal attempts (paracetamol). Fatal drug induced liver disease may also follow on the use of large doses of tetracycline; particularly when used for pyelonephritis in the last trimester of pregnancy, when acute fatty liver may develop (Kunelis et al., 1965). Pyelonephritis is probably important in potentiating the hepatotoxicity of tetracycline in this situation (Sherlock, 1968b). Drugs which produce fatal liver disease may also cause persistent liver disease if exposure is repeated (halothane).

14.6.4 Antituberculosis Drugs and the Liver

Many antituberculosis drugs, with the exception of streptomycin, are prone to cause liver toxicity (Rossouw and Saunders, 1975; table X). The wide spectrum of hepatic dysfunction ranges from slight rises of SGOT in otherwise asymptomatic patients to severe hepatocellular necrosis. PAS seems to be a common cause of drug hepatitis, but as it is generally used in regimens containing isoniazid, it is often difficult to decide which, if either, of the drugs are to blame. Some regimens seem more likely to lead to problems than others and this seems to be particularly so with isoniazid. Thus, hepatitis is generally more severe in patients receiving PAS and isoniazid than in those receiving PAS with other agents (Rossouw and Saunders, 1975). In some series, disturbed hepatic function is more common in patients taking rifampicin (rifampin) and isoniazid than in those on rifampicin and ethambutol (Lees et al., 1971), particularly in those who are slow acetylators of isoniazid (Smith et al., 1972; Lal et al., 1972). Older age, regular alcohol intake and a history of hepatobiliary disease also increase the risk of hepatitis with isoniazid-rifampicin combinations (Gronhagen-Riska et al., 1978). With isoniazid alone, it is thought that liver injury associated with isoniazid chemoprophylaxis is more likely in rapid acetylators of the drug due to a more rapid rate of formation of the highly reactive acetylhydrazine metabolite (Mitchell et al., 1975, 1976), but other studies have not observed a preponderance of either rapid or slow acetylators (Riska, 1976) and there is doubt about this for other reasons (see chapter VII, sect. 4.2.1).

To avoid hepatic complications, patients taking antituberculosis drugs should be observed carefully during the early months of therapy (the period when reactions become apparent) and all drugs stopped promptly at the first sign of fever, rash or gastrointestinal symptoms. The SGOT should be measured immediately and repeated as indicated (Rossouw and Saunders, 1975). The in-terpretation of elevated SGOT levels in the absence of other signs and symptoms of sensitivity is difficult. Very slight elevation is not necessarily a contraindication to continuing a drug such as isoniazid, but caution must be used. Elevation as high as 3 times normal levels probably mandates stopping isoniazid.

When the reaction has settled, a small single test dose of one of the agents may be given and SGOT estimations repeated at 3 days and 1 week. If no reaction occurs to a drug, it can then be introduced in full dosage for 1 week with similar precautions being taken. The procedure is then repeated in turn for each of the drugs (sensitisation may occur to more than one drug), with continued monitoring of liver function. When the causative drug(s) have been identified desensitisation, with multiple small doses of the drug, can usually be accomplished or alternative drugs which do not cross react (see below) can be introduced. Great care must be taken in reintroducing drugs in this situation and the procedure outlined above is not without risk. Each case must be judged on its merits. If the condition of the patient is such that a break in treatment would be unjustified, on no account should the same drugs be continued since the risk of precipitating fatal hepatic necrosis is high and corticosteroids provide little protection. Ethambutol and rifampicin, or even cycloserine and capreomycin may be considered as soon as the reaction settles.

Cross sensitivity may occur between the chemically related drugs isoniazid, pyrazinamide and ethionamide.

14.6.5 Oral Contraceptive Jaundice and Jaundice in Pregnancy

Oral contraceptives containing oestrogen and progestagen are potentially cholestatic and are particularly likely to cause jaundice in those communities in which there is a high incidence of idiopathic cholestatic jaundice in the last trimester of pregnancy (see also section 13.4). Drugs with potential liver toxicity should be avoided when possible, particularly during pregnancy. It is possible that sensitivity developing to drugs such as chlorpromazine in pregnancy may cause a severe and more lasting illness (Sherlock, 1968b).

14.6.6 Neonatal Jaundice

Acidic drugs such as salicylate or sulphonamides compete with and displace bilirubin from plasma albumin binding sites. In neonates, the unbound and unconjugated bilirubin then readily passes the poorly developed blood-brain barrier and may lead to kernicterus (Diamond, 1966). Some drugs may interfere with bilirubin metabolism by a haemolytic action, increasing bilirubin production from haem. Drug induced haemolysis in those with glucose-6-phosphate dehydrogenase deficiency is a common cause of neonatal jaundice in areas such as Southeast Asia where the genetically determined red cell defect is prevalent. The offending drug (e.g. sulphonamides) may be transferred to the infant via the mother's milk. Many other drugs can cause haemolysis in such susceptible individuals (see chapter XXIII; sect. 8.4) and even small quantities of these drugs if transferred in breast milk or given to the neonate could result in jaundice. Wrapping the infant in clothes stored in mothballs (naphthalene) can also cause haemolysis and lead to jaundice in susceptible neonates. Excessive dosage of water soluble vitamin K also produces haemolysis and may similarly lead to kernicterus in the neonate.

14.7 Gall-Stones

Drugs may cause gall-stones or gall-stone disease by increasing the cholesterol content in bile (Pertsemlidis et al., 1974). Thus, clofibrate is associated with an increased prevalence of gall-stones and symptomatic gall-stone disease (Bateson et al., 1978a,b; Coronary Drug Project, 1977; WHO Trial, 1978). Diets with a high polyunsaturated/saturated fat ratio have also been reported to increase the incidence of gall-stones (Sturdevant et al., 1973). Nicotinic acid also increases cholesterol saturation of bile and may increase the risk of gall-stone formation (Leijd et al., 1978). Concurrent administration of chenodeoxycholic acid (see section 10.5) with clofibrate may prevent or reduce cholesterol saturation of bile (Bateson et al., 1978a), but whether the expense of such a combination is warranted or will be effective over a long period of time is not clear. Oestrogens also lead to cholesterol rich bile, and an increased prevalence of gall-stone disease and gall-stones has been associated with use of oestrogens for either menopausal symptoms or contraception (Boston Collaborative Program, 1973; Howat et al., 1975). Whether the incidence of gall-stone disease is reduced by lower dose preparations now available is not clear (Leissner et al., 1977).

Further Reading

Bockus, H.L.: Gastroenterology, 3rd Ed, Vol. I-IV (Saunders, Philadelphia 1976).

Greenberger, N.J. and Winship, D.H.: Gastrointestinal Disorders: A Pathophysiologic Approach (Yearbook, Chicago 1977).

Janowitz, H.D. (Ed): Symposium on gastoenterology for internists. Medical Clinics of North America 62: 1 (1978).

Sherlock, S.: Diseases of the Liver and Biliary System, 5th Ed (Blackwell, Oxford 1975).

Sleisenger, M.H. and Fordtran, J.: Gastrointestinal Disease: Pathophysiology, Diagnosis, Management 2nd ed. (Saunders, Philadelphia 1978).

Truelove, S.C. and Reynell, P.C.: Diseases of the Digestive System, 2nd ed (Blackwell, Oxford 1972).

References

Acocella, G.: Clinical pharmacokinetics of rifampicin. Clinical Pharmacokinetics 3: 108 (1978).

Adjepon-Yamoah, K.K.; Nimmo, J. and Prescott, L.F.: Gross impairment of hepatic drug metabolism in a patient with chronic liver disease. British Medical Journal 4: 387 (1974).

Allen, A.A.; Boley, S.J.; Schultz, L. and Schwartz, S.: Potassium-induced lesions of the small bowel. II Pathology and pathogenesis. Journal of the American Medical Association 193: 887, 1001 (1965).

Almeyda, J.; Barnardo, D.; Baker, H.; Levene, G.M. and Landells, J.W.: Structural and functional abnormalities of the liver in psoriasis before and during methotrexate therapy. British Journal of Dermatology 87: 623 (1972).

Ament, M.E.: Inflammatory disease of the colon: Ulcerative colitis and Crohn's colitis. Journal of Pediatrics 86: 322 (1975).

Andreasen, P.B.; Hendel, J.; Greisen, G. and Hvidberg, E.F.: Pharmacokinetics of diazepam in disordered liver function. European Journal of Clinical Pharmacology 10: 115 (1976).

Angel, J.H. and Lacey, B.W.: Comparison of side-effects of tetracycline and tetracycline plus nystatin. Report to the Research Committee of the British Tuberculosis Association by the Clinical Trials Subcommittee. British Medical Journal 4: 411 (1968).

Anthonisen, P.; Barany, F.; Folkenborg, O.; Holtz, A.; Jarncum, S.; Kristensen, M.; Riis, P.; Walan, A. and Worning, H.: The clinical effect of salazosulphapyridine (salazopyrine) in Crohn's disease. A controlled double-blind study. Scandinavian Journal of Gastroenterology 9: 549 (1974).

Aserkoff, B. and Bennett, J.V.: Effect of antibiotic therapy in acute salmonellosis on the fecal excretion of salmonellae. New England Journal of Medicine 281: 636 (1969).

Athreya, B.H.: Aspirin induced hepatotoxicity in juvenile rheumatoid arthritis. A prospective study. Arthritis and Rheumatism 18: 347 (1975).

Avery, G.S.; Davies, E. and Brogden, R.N.: Lactulose: A review of its therapeutic and pharmacological properties with particular reference to ammonia metabolism and its mode of action in portal systemic encephalopathy. Drugs 4: 7 (1972).

Avery Jones, F. and Godding, E.: Management of Constipation (Blackwell, Oxford 1972).

Bain, L.S. and Masheter, H.C.: Dyspepsia and antirheumatic therapy. New England Journal of Medicine 294: 1404 (1976).

Bakshi, J.S.; Ghiara, J.M. and Nanivadekar, A.S.: How does tinidazole compare with metronidazole? A summary report of Indian trials in amoebiasis and giardiasis. Drugs 15(Suppl. 1): 33 (1978).

Bank, S. and Marks, I.N.: Hyperlipaemic pancreatitis and the pill. Postgraduate Medical Journal 46: 576 (1970).

Bank, S. and Marks, I.N.: Evaluation of new drugs for peptic ulcer. Clinics in Gastroenterology 2: 379 (1973).

Bank, S. and Marks, I.N.: The etiology and treatment of constipation and diarrhoea in geriatric patients. South African Medical Journal 51: 409 (1977).

Bank, S.; Marks, I.N. and Novis, B.H.: Progress in small bowel physiology and disease. South African Medical Journal 45: 1141 (1971a).

Bank, S.; Burns, D.G.; Marks, I.N. and Stein, D.: The clinical spectrum of amoebic colitis. South African Medical Journal 45: 219 (1971b).

Bank, S.; Marks, I.N. and Vinik, A.I.: Clinical and hormonal aspects of pancreatic diabetes. American Journal of Gastroenterology 64: 13 (1975).

Bank, S.; Barbezat, G.O.; Novis, B.H.; Ou Tim, L.; Odes, H.S.; Helman, C.: Narunsky, L.; Duys, P.J. and Marks, I.N.: Histamine H_2-receptor antagonists in the treatment of duodenal ulcers. South African Medical Journal 50: 1781 (1976).

Bank, S.; Marks, I.N. and Barbezat, G.O.: Treatment of acute and chronic pancreatitis. Drugs 13: 373 (1977a).

Bank, S.; Barbezat, G.O.; Vinik, A.I.; Halter, F. and Helman, C.A.: Cimetidine and serum gastrin levels in man; in Burland and Simkins (Eds) Cimetidine, Proceedings on the Second International Symposium on Histamine H-Receptor Antagonists, p.155 (Excerpta Medica, Amsterdam 1977b).

Barbezat, G.O.: The diagnosis and management of diverticular disease. South African Medical Journal 53: 793 (1978).

Barbezat, G.O.: Psychosomatic gastro-intestinal disease. South African Medical Journal 54: 1015 (1978).

Baron, J.H.; Gribble, R.J.N.; Rhodes, C. and Wright, P.A.: Serum carbenoxolone in patients with gastric and duodenal ulcer. Absorption, efficacy and side-effects. Gut 19: 330 (1978).

Barry, R.E. and Ford, J.: Sodium content and neutralising capacity of some commonly used antacids. British Medical Journal 1: 413 (1978).

Bartlett, J.G.; Chang, T-W.; Gurwith, M.; Gorbach, S.L. and Onderdonk, A.B.: Antibiotic-associated pseudomembranous colitis due to toxin-producing Clostridia. New England Journal of Medicine 298: 531 (1978a).

Bartlett, J.G.; Moon, N.; Chang, T.W.; Taylor, N. and Onderdonk, A.B.: Role of clostridium difficile in antibiotic-associated pseudomembranous colitis. Gastroenterology 75: 778 (1978b).

Bateson, M.C.; Maclean, D.; Ross, P.E. and Bouchier, I.A.D.: Clofibrate therapy and gallstone induction. American Journal of Digestive Diseases 23: 623 (1978b).

Bateson, M.C.; Ross, P.E.; Murison, J. and Bouchier, I.A.D.: Reversal of clofibrate-induced cholesterol oversaturation of bile with chenodeoxycholic acid. British Medical Journal 1: 1171 (1978a).

Batey, R.G.: Chenodeoxycholic acid in the management of cholesterol gallstones. Drugs 14: 116 (1977).

Behar, J. and Ramsby, G.: Gastric emptying and antral motility in reflux esophagitis. Effect of oral metoclo-pramide. Gastroenterology 74: 253 (1978).

Benson, J.A.: Gastrointestinal reactions to drugs. Digestive Diseases 16: 357 (1971).

Bigorie, B.; Aimez, P.; Soria, R-J.; Samama, F.; di Maria, G.; Guy-Grand, B. and Bour, H.: Is the combined use of triacetyloleandomycin and ergotamine tartrate dangerous? Nouvelle Presse Medicale 4: 2723 (1975).

Black, M.: Liver disease and drug therapy. Medical Clinics of North America 58: 1051 (1974).

Blaschke, T.F.: Protein binding and kinetics of drugs in liver diseases. Clinical Pharmacokinetics 2: 32 (1977).

Blaschke, T.F.; Meffin, P.J.; Melmon, K.L. and Rowland, M.: Influence of acute viral hepatitis on phenytoin kinetics and protein binding. Clinical Pharmacology and Therapeutics 17: 685 (1975).

Blichfeldt, P.; Blomhoff, J.P.; Myhre, E. and Gjone, E.: Metronidazole in Crohn's disease: A double blind cross-over clinical trial. Scandinavian Journal of Gastroenterology 13: 123 (1978).

Blitzer, B.L.; Mutchnick, M.G.; Joshi, P.H.; Phillips, M.M.; Fessel, M. and Conn, H.O.: Adrenocorticosteroid therapy in alcoholic hepatitis. American Journal of Digestive Diseases 22: 477 (1977).

Bodemar, G. and Walan, A.: Maintenance treatment of recurrent peptic ulcer by cimetidine. Lancet 1: 403 (1978).

Bodemar, G.; Norlander, B. and Walan, A.: Cimetidine in the treatment of active peptic ulcer disease; in Burland and Simkins (Eds) Cimetidine, p. 224 (Excerpta Medica, Amsterdam 1977).

Bolme, P.; Eriksson, M. and Stintzing, G.: The gastrointestinal absorption of penicillin V in children with suspected coeliac disease. Acta Paediatrica Scandinavica 66: 573 (1977).

Bomb, B.S. and Bedi, H.K.: Neurotoxic side-effects of piperazine. Transactions of the Royal Society of Tropical Medicine and Hygiene 70: 358 (1976).

Bonkowsky, H.L.; Mudge, G.H. and McMurtry, R.J.: Chronic hepatic inflammation and fibrosis due to low doses of paracetamol. Lancet 1: 1016 (1978).

Boston Collaborative Drug Surveillance Program: Oral contraceptive and venous thromboembolic disease, surgically confirmed gallbaladder disease and breast tumours. Lancet 1: 1399 (1973).

Bourke, J.B.; McIllmurray, M.B.; Mead, G.M. and Langman, M.J.S.: Drug-associated primary acute pancreatitis. Lancet 1: 706 (1978).

Boyd, W.C. and Den Beston, L.: Subtotal colectomy for refractory pseudomembranous enterocolitis. Journal of the American Medical Association 235: 181 (1976).

Bramble, M.G. and Record, C.O.: Drug-induced gastrointestinal disease. Drugs 15: 451 (1978).

Branch, R.A. and Shand, D.G.: Propranolol in chronic liver disease: A physiological approach. Clinical Pharmacokinetics 1: 264 (1976).

Branch, R.A.; Herbert, C.M. and Read, A.E.: Determinants of serum antipyrine half-lives in patients with liver disease. Gut 14: 569 (1973).

Branch, R.A.; Morgan, M.H.; James, J. and Read, A.E.: Intravenous administration of diazepam in patients with chronic liver disease. Gut 17: 975 (1976).

Brodribb, A.J.M.: Treatment of symptomatic diverticular disease with a high fibre diet. Lancet 1: 664 (1977).

Brogden, R.N.; Speight, T.M. and Avery, G.S.: Caved-S: A report of its pharmacological properties and therapeutic efficacy in peptic ulcer. Drugs 8: 330 (1974).

Brogden, R.N.; Pinder, R.M.; Sawyer, P.R.; Speight, T.M. and Avery, G.S.: Tri-potassium di-citrato bismuthate: A report of its pharmacological properties and therapeutic efficacy in peptic ulcer. Drugs 12: 401 (1976).

Brogden, R.N.; Heel, R.C.; Speight, T.M. and Avery, G.S.: Cimetidine: A review of its pharmacological properties and therapeutic efficacy in peptic ulcer disease. Drugs 15: 93 (1978).

Brooke, B.N.; Cave, D.R. and King, D.W.: Place of azathioprine for Crohn's disease. Lancet 1: 1041 (1976).

Brown, P.; Baddeley, H.; Read, A.E. and Davies, J.D.: Sclerosing peritonitis, an unusual reaction to a β-adrenergic blocking drug (practolol). Lancet 2: 1477 (1974).

Buts, J.-P.; Weber, A.M.; Roy, C.C. and Morin, C.L.: Pseudomembranous enterocolitis in childhood. Gastroenterology 73: 823 (1977).

Cameron, A.J.: Aspirin and gastric ulcer. Mayo Clinic Proceedings 50: 565 (1975).

Carlborg, B.; Kumlien, A. and Olsson, H.: Medikamentella esofagusstrikturer. Larkartidningen 75: 4609 (1978).

Cass, A.J.: Stercoral perforation: case of drug-induced impaction. British Medical Journal 2: 932 (1978).

Castell, D.O.: Medical measures that influence the gastroesophageal junction. Southern Medical Journal 71(Suppl. 1): 26 (1978).

Chang, M.J.; Dunkle, L.M.; Van Reken, D.; Anderson, D.; Wong, M.L. and Feigin, R.D.: Trimethoprim-sulfamethoxazole compared to ampicillin in the treatment of shigellosis. Pediatrics 59: 726 (1977).

Clark, R.; Thompson, R.P.H.; Borirakchanyavat, V.; Widdop, B.; Davidson, A.R.; Goulding, R. and Williams, R.: Hepatic damage and death from overdose of paracetamol. Lancet 1: 66 (1973).

Cockel, R.: Anti-emetics. Practitioner 206: 56 (1971).

Committee on Drugs: Commentary on anthelmintics. Pediatrics 62: 251 (1978).

Conn, H.O.: The rational management of ascites. Progress in Liver Disease 4: 269 (1972).

Conn, H.O.: Steroid treatment of alcoholic hepatitis: The yeas and the nays. Gastroenterology 74: 319 (1978).

Conn, H.O. and Blitzer, B.L.: Nonassociation of adrenocorticosteroid therapy and peptic ulcer. New England Journal of Medicine 294: 473 (1976).

Conn, H.O.; Leevy, C.M.; Vlahcevic, Z.R.; Rodgers, J.B.; Maddrey, W.C.; Seeff, L. and Levy, L.L.: Comparison of lactulose and neomycin in the treatment of chronic portal-systemic encephalopathy. Gastroenterology 72: 573 (1977).

Cooke, A.R.: Drugs and gastric damage. Drugs 11: 36 (1976).

Cooke, N.; Teitelbaum, S. and Avioli, L.V.: Antacid-induced osteomalacia and nephrolithiasis. Archives of Internal Medicine 138: 1007 (1978).

Coronary Drug Project Research Group: Gallbladder disease as a side effect of drugs influencing lipid metabolism. Experience in the Coronary Drug Project. New England Journal of Medicine 296: 1185 (1977).

Cowan, G.O.; Das, K.M. and Eastwood, M.A.: Further studies of sulphasalazine metabolism in the treatment of ulcerative colitis. British Medical Journal 2: 1057 (1977).

Croft, D.N. and Wood, P.H.N.: Gastric mucosa and susceptibility to occult gastrointestinal bleeding caused by aspirin. British Medical Journal 1: 137 (1967).

Crowson, T.D.; Head, L.H. and Ferrante, W.A.: Esophageal ulcers associated with tetracycline therapy. Journal of the American Medical Association 235: 2747 (1976).

Cummings, J.H.: Progress report: Dietary fibre. Gut 14: 69 (1973).

Cummings, J.H.; South Gate, D.A.T.; Branch, W.; Houston, H.; Jenkins, D.J.A. and James, W.P.T.: Colonic response to dietary fibre from carrot, cabbage, apple, bran and guar gum. Lancet 1: 5 (1978).

Curry, S.H.; D'Mello, A. and Mould, G.P.: Destruction of chlorpromazine during absorption in the rat in vitro and in vivo. British Journal of Pharmacology 42: 403 (1971).

Cuthbert, M.: Adverse reactions to non-steroidal anti-rheumatic drugs. Current Medical Research and Opinion 2: 600 (1974).

Dahl, S.G. and Strandgord, R.E.: Pharmacokinetics of chlorpromazine after single and chronic dosage. Clinical Pharmacology and Therapeutics 21: 437 (1977).

Dahl, M.G.C.; Gregory, M.M. and Scheuer, P.J.: Liver damage due to methotrexate in patients with psoriasis. British Medical Journal 1: 625 (1971).

Dahl, M.G.C.; Gregory, M.M. and Scheuer, P.J.: Methotrexate hepatotoxicity in psoriasis — Comparison of different dose regimen. British Medical Journal 1: 654 (1972).

Dalen, E. and Westerholm, B.: Occurrence of hepatic impairment in women jaundiced by oral contraceptives and in their mothers and sisters. Acta Medica Scandinavica 195: 459 (1974).

Das, K.M. and Dubin, R.: Clinical pharmacokinetics of sulphasalazine. Clinical Pharmacokinetics 1: 406 (1976).

Das, K.M. and Eastwood, M.A.: Acetylation polymorphism of sulfapyridine in patients with ulcerative colitis and Crohn's disease. Clinical Pharmacology and Therapeutics 18: 514 (1975).

Das, K.M.; Eastwood, M.A.; McManus, J.P.A. and Sircus, W.: Adverse reactions during salicylazosulphapyridine therapy and the relation with drug metabolism and acetylator phenotype. New Eng. J. Med. 298: 491 (1973).

Datta, D.V.; Maheshwari, Y.K. and Aggarwal, M.L.: Levodopa in fulminant hepatic failure: preliminary report. American Journal of the Medical Sciences 272: 95 (1976).

Dent, D.; Bank, S. and Louw, J.H.: Perforated duodenal ulcer: Is the distinction between acute and chronic valid? South African Medical Journal 51: 529 (1977).

Diamond, I.: Kernicterus: Revised concepts of pathogenesis and management. Pediatrics 38: 539 (1966).

DiMagno, E.; Malagelada, J.R.; Go. V.L.W. and Moertel, C.G.: Fate of orally ingested enzymes in pancreatic insufficiency. Comparison of two dosage schedules. New England Journal of Medicine 296: 1318 (1977).

Di Piazza, S.; Cottone, M.; Craxi, A.; Gatto, G.; Pinzello, G. and Pagliaro, L.: Severe rifampicin-associated liver failure in patients with compensated cirrhosis. Lancet 1: 774 (1978).

Dissanaike, A.S.: A comparative trial of oxantel-pyrantel and mebendazole in multiple helminth infection in school children. Drugs 15(Suppl. 1): 73 (1978).

Dissanayake, A.S. and Truelove, S.C.: A controlled therapeutic trial of long-term maintenance treatment of ulcerative colitis with sulphasalazine (Salazopyrin). Gut 14: 923 (1973).

Doherty, J.E.; Hall, W.H.; Murphy, M.L. and Beard, O.W.: New information regarding digitalis metabolism. Chest 59: 433 (1971).

Doll, R.; Langman, M.J.S. and Shawdon, H.H.: Treatment of gastric ulcer with carbenoxolone: antagonistic effect of spironolactone. Gut 9: 42 (1968).

Duggan, J.M.: Progress report. Aspirin in chronic gastric ulcer: an Australian experience. Gut 17: 378 (1976).

Duncombe, V.M.; Bolin, T.D. and Davis, A.E.: Double-blind trial of cholestyramine in post-vagotomy diarrhoea. Gut 18: 531 (1977).

Durr, H.K.; Maroske, D.; Zelder, O. and Bode, J.C.: Glucagon therapy in acute pancreatitis. Report of a double-blind trial. Gut 19: 175 (1978).

Editorial: Antibiotic diarrhoea. British Medical Journal 4: 243 (1975).

Eggert, R.C.: Spironolactone diuresis in patients with cirrhosis and ascites. British Medical Journal 4: 401 (1970).

El-Hennaway, M. and Abd-Rabbo, H.: Hazards of cortisone therapy in hepatic amoebiasis. Journal of Tropical Medicine and Hygiene 81: 71 (1978).

Emmanuel, J.H. and Montgomery, R.D.: Gastric ulcer and anti-arthritic drugs. Postgraduate Medical Journal 47: 227 (1971).

Englert, E.; Freston, J.W.; Graham, D.Y.; Finkelstein, W.; Kruss, D.M.; Priest, R.J.; Raskin, J.B.; Rhodes, J.B.; Rogers, A.I.; Wenger, J.; Wilcox, L.L. and Crossley, R.J.: Cimetidine, antacid, and hospitalisation in the treatment of benign gastric ulcer. A multicenter double blind study. Gastroenterology 74: 416 (1978).

Faigle, J.W.: Blood levels of a schistosomicide in relation to liver function and side-effects. Acta Pharmacologica et Toxicologica 29(Suppl. 3): 233 (1971).

Faigle, J.W. and Keberle, H.: Metabolism of niridazole in various species, including man. Annals of the New York Academy of Sciences 160: 544 (1969).

Farquharson-Roberts, M.A.; Giddings, A.E.B. and Nunn, A.J.: Perforation of small bowel due to slow release potassium chloride (Slow-K). British Medical Journal 3: 206 (1975).

Farrell, G.C.; Cooksley, W.G.E.; Hart, P. and Powell, L.: Drug metabolism in liver disease. Identification of patients with impaired hepatic drug metabolism. Gastroenterology 75: 580 (1978).

Feldman, M.; Richardson, C.T.; Peterson, W.L.; Walsh, J.H. and Fordtran, J.S.: Effect of low-dose propantheline on food-stimulated gastric acid secretion. Comparison with an 'Optimal Effective Dose' and interaction with cimetidine. New England Journal of Medicine 297: 1427 (1977).

Ferrucci, J.T. and Long, J.A.: Radiologic treatment of esophageal food impaction using intravenous glucagon. Radiology 125: 25 (1977).

Fielding, J.F.: The irritable bowel syndrome. Clinics in Gastroenterology 6: 607 (1977).

Fischer, J.E.; Funovics, J.M.; Falcao, H.A. and Wesdorp, R.I.C.: L-dopa in hepatic coma. Annals of Surgery 183: 386 (1976).

Fisher, R.S.; Malmud, L.S.; Roberts, G.S. and Lobis, I.F.: The lower esophageal sphincter as a barrier to gastoesophageal reflux. Gastroenterology 72: 19 (1977).

Flind, A.C. and Rowley-Jones, D.: Mental confusion and cimetidine. Lancet 1: 379 (1979).

Fordtran, J.S. and Collyns, J.A.H.: Antacid pharmacology in duodenal ulcer. New England Journal of Medicine 274: 921 (1966).

Fordtran, J.S.; Morawski, S.G. and Richardson, C.T.: *In vivo* and *in vitro* evaluation of liquid antacids. New England Journal of Medicine 288: 923 (1973).

Forrest, J.A.H.; Roscoe, P.; Prescott, L.F. and Stevenson, I.H.: Abnormal drug metabolism after barbiturate and paracetamol overdose. Brit. Med. J. 4: 499 (1974).

Gallagher, N.D. and Goulston, S.J.M.: Antibiotic associated colitis: In search of a cause and treatment. Drugs 16: 385 (1978).

George, R.H.; Symonds, J.M.; Dimock, F.; Brown, J.D.; Arabi, Y.; Shinagawa, N.; Keighley, M.R.B.; Alexander-Williams, J. and Burdon, D.W.: Identification of Clostridium difficile as a cause of pseudomembranous colitis. British Medical Journal 1: 695 (1978a).

George, W.L.; Sutter, V.L.; Goldstein, E.J.C.; Ludwig, S.L. and Finegold, S.M.: Aetiology of antimicrobial-agent-associated colitis. Lancet 1: 802 (1978b).

Goldman, P.; Peppercorn, M.A. and Goldin, B.R.: Drugs metabolised by intestinal microflora; in Morselli, Cohen and Garattini (Eds) Drug Interactions, p. 91 (Raven Press, New York 1974).

Goodacre, R.L.; Hamilton, J.D.; Mullens, J.E. and Qizilbash, A.: Persistence of proctitis in 2 cases of clindamycin-associated colitis. Gastroenterology 72: 149 (1976).

Goodman, M.J. and Truelove, S.C.: Intensive intravenous regimen for membranous colitis. British Medical Journal 2: 354 (1976).

Gould, S.R.; Brash, A.R. and Conolly, M.E.: Increased prostaglandin production in ulcerative colitis. Lancet 2: 98 (1977).

Goulston, K.: Diagnosis and treatment of the irritable bowel syndrome. Drugs 6: 237 (1973).

Goulston, S.M. and McGovern, V.J.: Pseudomembranous colitis. Gut 6: 207 (1965).

Graham, J.R.; Suby, H.I.; LeCompte, P.R. and Sadowsky, N.L.: Fibrotic disorders associated with methysergide therapy for headache. New England Journal of Medicine 274: 359 (1966).

Greenblatt, D.J.; Shader, R.I.; MacLeod, S.M. and Sellers, E.M.: Clinical pharmacokinetics of chlordiazepoxide. Clinical Pharmacokinetics 3: 381 (1978).

Gregory, P.B.; Knaner, C.M.; Kempson, R.L. and Miller, R.: Steroid therapy in severe viral hepatitis. New England Journal of Medicine 294: 681 (1976).

Griffiths, R.; Lee, R.M. and Taylor, D.C.: Kinetics of cimetidine in man and experimental animals; in Burland and Simkins (Eds) Cimetidine, Proceedings of the Second International Symposium on Histamine H_2-Receptor Antagonists, p. 38 (Excerpta Medica, Amsterdam 1977).

Gronhagen-Riska, C.; Hellstrom, P-E. and Froseth, B.: Predisposing factors in hepatitis induced by isoniazid-rifampicin treatment of tuberculosis. American Review of Respiratory Disease 118: 461 (1978).

Grossman, M.I.; Matsmoto, K.K. and Lichter, R.: Faecal blood loss produced by oral and intravenous administration of various salicylates. Gastroenterology 40: 383 (1961).

Gugler, R.; Lain, P. and Azarnoff, D.L.: Effect of portacaval shunt on the disposition of drugs with and without first-pass effect. Journal of Pharmacology and Experimental Therapeutics 195: 416 (1975).

Hamamoto, H.; Katoh, T.; Tokuoka, T.; Kitamura, K.; Nakamoto, T.; Bamba, M. and Takanashi, T.: The metabolism of digitoxin in human liver cirrhosis. Japanese Circulation Journal 41: 764 (1977).

Hansky, J.: The treatment of heartburn and oesophagitis. Drugs 5: 446 (1973).

Harris, F.C.: Pyloric stenosis. Hold-up of enteric coated aspirin tablets. British Journal of Surgery 60: 979 (1973).

Hartiala, K.: Metabolism of hormones, drugs and other substances by the gut. Physiological Reviews 53: 496 (1973).

Hartiala, K.; Kasanen, A. and Raussi, M.: The absorption of salicylamide in pernicious anaemia, gastric achylia and peptic ulcer. Annales Medicinae Experimentalis et Biologiae Fenniae 41: 549 (1963).

Haslock, I. and Wright, V.: The gut and arthritis. Rheumatology and Rehabilitation 13: 51 (1974).

Hastings, P.R.; Skillman, J.J.; Bushnell, L.S. and Silen, W.: Antacid titration in the prevention of acute gastrointestinal bleeding. New England Journal of Medicine 298: 1041 (1978).

Hayes, M.J.; Sprackling, M. and Langman, M.J.S.: Changes in the plasma clearance and protein binding of carbenoxolone with age, and their possible relationship with adverse drug effects. Gut 18: 1054 (1977).

Hayton, A.C.: Precipitation of acute ergotism by triacetyloleandomycin. New Zealand Medical Journal 69: 42 (1969).

Heading, R.C.; Nimmo, J.; Prescott, L.F. and Tothill, P.: The dependence of paracetamol absorption on the rate of gastric emptying. British Journal of Pharmacology 47: 415 (1973).

Heel, R.C.; Brogden, R.N.; Speight, T.M. and Avery, G.S.: Loperamide: A review of its pharmacological properties and therapeutic efficacy in diarrhoea. Drugs 15: 33 (1978).

Heizer, W.D.; Smith, T.W. and Goldfinger, S.E.: Absorption of digoxin in patients with malabsorption syndromes. New England Journal of Medicine 285: 257 (1971).

Hendrickse, R.G.: Dysentery including amoebiasis. British Medical Journal 1: 669 (1972).

Hensleigh, P.A. and Kauffman, R.E.: Maternal absorption and placental transfer of sulfasalazine. American Journal of Obstetrics and Gynecology 127: 443 (1977).

Hislop, I.G.: Psychological significance of the irritable colon syndrome. Gut 12: 452 (1971).

Hoffman, A.F.: Bile acids, diarrhea, and antibiotics: data, speculation and a unifying hypothesis. Journal of Infectious Diseases 135:(Suppl): S126 (March 1977).

Hollander, D. and Harlan, J.: Antacids vs placebos in peptic ulcer therapy: A controlled double-blind investigation. Journal of the American Medical Association 226: 1181 (1973).

Homeida, M.; Jackson, L. and Roberts, C.J.C.: Decreased first pass metabolism of labetalol in chronic liver disease. British Medical Journal 2: 1048 (1978).

Hooper. W.D.; Bochner, F.; Eadie, M.J. and Tyrer, J.H.: Plasma protein binding of diphenylhydantoin. Effects of sex hormones, renal and hepatic disease. Clinical Pharmacology and Therapeutics 15: 276 (1974).

Howat, J.M.T.; Jones, C.B. and Schofield, P.F.: Gallstones and oral contraceptives. Journal of the Institute of Medical Research 3: 59 (1975).

Hubbard, W.N.: Clindamycin and pseudomembranous colitis. Lancet 1: 172 (1974).

Hurwitz, A.: Antacid therapy and drug kinetics. Clinical Pharmacokinetics 2: 269 (1977).

Hutchison, J.G.P.; Johnston, N.M.; Plevey, M.V.P.; Thangkhiew, I. and Aidney, C.: Clinical trial of mebendazole, a broad-spectrum anthelmintic. British Medical Journal 2: 309 (1975).

Idanpaan-Heikkila, J.E.; Hastbacka, J. and Jarvinen, H.J.J.: Eye and skin reactions precede practolol peritonitis. Lancet 2: 1354 (1977).

Imrie, C.W.; Benjamin, I.S.; Ferguson, J.C.; Thomson, W.O.; McKay, A.J. and Blumgart, L.H.: A single-centre double-blind trial of aprotinin (Trasylol) therapy in primary acute pancreatitis. Annals of the Royal College of Surgeons of England 60: 142 (1978).

Ippoliti, A.F.; Sturdevant, R.A.L.; Isenberg, J.I.; Binder, M.; Camacho, R.; Cano, R.; Cooney, C.; Kline, M.M.; Koretz, R.L.; Meyer, J.H.; Samloff, I.M.; Schwabe, A.D.; Strom, E.A.; Valenzeuela, J.E. and Wintroub, R.H.: Cimetidine versus intensive antacid therapy for duodenal ulcer. A multicenter trial. Gastroenterology 74: 393 (1978).

Isenberg, J.I.: Therapy of peptic ulcer. Journal of the American Medical Association 233: 540 (1975).

Iser, J.H.; Dowling, R.H.; Mok, H.Y.I. and Bell, G.D.: Chenodeoxycholic acid treatment of gallstones. New England Journal of Medicine 293: 378 (1975).

Iser, J.H.; Maton, P.N.; Murphy, G.M. and Dowling, R.H.: Resistance to chenodeoxycholic acid (CDCA) treatment in obese patients with gallstones. British Medical Journal 1: 1509 (1978).

Islam, N. and Hasan, K.: Tinidazole and metronidazole in hepatic amoebiasis. Drugs 15(Suppl. 1): 26 (1978).

Ivey, K.J.; Silvoso, G.R. and Krause, W.J.: Effect of paracetamol on gastric mucosa. British Medical Journal 1: 1586 (1978).

James, I.: Prescribing in patients with liver disease. British Journal of Hospital Medicine 13(Suppl. 1): 67 (1975).

Jewell, D.P. and Truelove, S.C.: Azathioprine in ulcerative colitis: Final report on controlled clinical trial. British Medical Journal 4: 627 (1974).

Jick, H. and Porter, J.: Drug-induced gastrointestinal bleeding. Report from The Boston Collaborative Drug Surveillance Program, Boston University Medical Center. Lancet 2: 87 (1978).

John, A.H. and Jones, A.: Gastroenteritis causing failure of oral contraception. British Medical Journal 3: 207 (1975).

Johnson, G.K. and Tolman, K.G.: Chronic liver disease and acetaminophen. Annals of Internal Medicine 87: 302 (1977).

Joint Report by Members of the Association for the Study of Infectious Disease: Effect of neomycin in non-invasive Salmonella infections of the gastrointestinal tract. Lancet 2: 1159 (1970).

Jones, R.H.; Lewin, M.R. and Parsons, V.: Therapeutic effect of cimetidine in patients undergoing haemodialysis. British Medical Journal 1: 650 (1979).

Juniper, K.: Amoebiasis. Clinics in Gastroenterology 7: 3 (1978).

Jusko, W.J. and Lewis, G.P.: Pharmacokinetics of ampicillin in cirrhotic subjects. Clinical Pharmacology and Therapeutics 17: 237 (1975).

Jussila, J.; Matilla, M.J. and Takki, S.: Drug absorption during lactose-induced intestinal symptoms in patients with selective lactose malabsorption. Annales Medicinae Experimentalis et Biologiae Fenniae 48: 33 (1970).

Kahn, C.R.; Levy, A.G.; Gardner, J.D.: Miller, J.V.; Gorden, P. and Schein, S.: Pancreatic cholera: beneficial effects of treatment with streptozotocin. New England Journal of Medicine 292: 941 (1975).

Kappas, A.; Shinagawa, N.; Arabi, Y.; Thompson, H.; Burdon, D.W.; Dimock, F.; George, R.H.; Alexander-Williams, J. and Keighley, M.R.B.: Diagnosis of pseudomembranous colitis. British Medical Journal 1: 675 (1978).

Katz, M.: Parasitic infections. J. Ped. 87: 165 (1975).

Katz, M.: Anthelmintics. Drugs 13: 124 (1977).

Keighley, M.R.B.; Burdon, D.W.; Arabi, Y.; Alexander-Williams, J.; Thompson, H.; Youngs, D.; Johnson, M.;

Bentley, S.; George, R.H. and Mogg, G.A.G.: Randomised controlled trial of vancomycin for pseudomembranous colitis and postoperative diarrhoea. British Medical Journal 2: 1667 (1978).

Klatskin, G.: Hepatic tumours: possible relationship to use of oral contraceptives. Gastroenterology 73: 386 (1977).

Klotz, U.; Avant, G.R.; Hoyumpa, A.; Schenker, S. and Wilkinson, G.R.: The effects of age and liver disease on the disposition and elimination of diazepam in adult man. Journal of Clinical Investigation 55: 347 (1975).

Klotz, U.; Antonin, K.H.; Brugel, H.; and Bieck, P.R.: Disposition of diazepam and its major metabolite desmethyldiazepam in patients with liver disease. Clinical Pharmacology and Therapeutics 21: 430 (1977).

Knop, P.; Kindler, V. and Austerhoff, A.: Plasma levels of rifampicin and isoniazid and serum levels of aminotransferases in combined tuberculostatic treatment. Deutsche Medizinische Wochenschrift 102: 1913 (1977).

Kobler, E.; Buhler, H.; Nuesch, H-J. and Deyhle, P.: Drug-induced oesophageal ulcers. Deutsche Medizinische Wochenschrift 103: 1035 (1978).

Kolibash, A.J.; Kramer, W.G.; Reuning, R.H. and Caldwell, J.H.: Marked decline in serum digoxin concentrations during an episode of severe diarrhea. American Heart Journal 94: 806 (1977).

Kopanoff, D.E.; Snider, D.E. and Caras, G.J.: Isoniazid-related hepatitis. A V.S. Public Health Service Cooperative Surveillance Study. American Review of Respiratory Disease 117: 991 (1978).

Kraus, J.W.; Marshall, J.P.; Johnson, R.; Wilkinson, G.R. and Schenker, S.: Lorazepam elimination in liver disease. Gastroenterology 73: 1228 (1977).

Kunelis, C.T.; Peters, R.L. and Edmondson, H.A.: Fatty liver of pregnancy and its relationship to tetracycline therapy. American Journal of Medicine 38: 359 (1965).

Kutt, H.; Winters, W.; Scherman, R. and McDowell, F.: Diphenylhydantoin and phenobarbital toxicity. Archives of Neurology 11: 649 (1964).

Laidlaw, J.; Read, A.E. and Sherlock, S.: Morphine tolerance in hepatic cirrhosis. Gastroenterology 40: 389 (1961).

Lal, S.; Singhal, S.N.; Burley, D.M. and Crossley, G.: Effect of rifampicin and isoniazid on liver function. British Medical Journal 1: 148 (1972).

Lam, S.K.; Lam, K.C.; Lai, C.L.; Yeung, C.K.; Yam, L.Y.C. and Wong, W.S.: Treatment of duodenal ulcer with antacid and sulpiride. A double-blind controlled study. Gastroenterology 76: 315 (1979).

Landecker, K.; McCallum, E.: Fevre, D.I.; Green, P.H.; Kasumi, A. and Piper, D.W.: Effect of amylopectin (Depepsen) on the healing rate of chronic duodenal ulcer. Australian and New Zealand Journal of Medicine 6: 256 (1976).

Langman, M.J.S.: Drugs in the treatment of gastric and duodenal ulcer. Drugs 14: 105 (1977).

Larson, H.E.; Price, A.B.; Honour, P. and Borriello, S.P.: Clostridium difficile and the aetiology of pseudomembranous colitis. Lancet 1: 1063 (1978).

Lavy, U.I.; Koekkoek, P.H. and Jaitly, K.D.: Anti-ulcer activity of colloidal bismuth subcitrate in shay-rats. Archives Internationales de Pharmacodynamie et de Therapie 224: 291 (1976).

Lee, S.P. and Nicholson, G.I.: Increased healing of gastric and duodenal ulcers in a controlled trial using tripotassium dicitrato-bismuthate. Medical Journal of Australia 1: 808 (1977).

Lees, A.W.; Allan, G.W.; Smith, J.; Tyrrel, W.F. and Fallon, R.J.: Toxicity from rifampicin plus isoniazid and rifampicin plus ethambutol therapy. Tubercle 52: 182 (1971).

Leevy, C.M.; Zinke, M.R. and Chey, W.Y.: Observations on the distribution of ^{14}C oxytetracycline in man. Antibiotics Annual 1: 258 (1958).

Leijd, B.; Angelin, B. and Einarsson, K.: Biliary lipid composition during treatment with hypolipidaemic drugs; in Kritchevsky and Holmes (Eds) Proceedings of the 6th International Symposium on Drugs Affecting Lipid Metabolism (Plenum, New York 1978).

Leissner, K-H.; Wedel, H. and Schersten, T.: Comparison between the use of oral contraceptives and the incidence of surgically confirmed gallstone disease. Scandinavian Journal of Gastroenterology 12: 893 (1977).

Lely, A.H. and Van Enter, C.H.J.: Large-scale digitoxin intoxication. British Medical Journal 3: 737 (1970).

Lennard-Jones, J.E. and Ritchie, J.K.: The diagnosis and management of colitis. British Journal of Hospital Medicine 11: 180 (1974).

Leonards, J.R. and Levy, G.: Absorption and metabolism of aspirin administered in enteric-coated tablets. Journal of the American Medical Association 193: 99 (1965).

Lesesne, H.R.; Bozymski, E.M. and Fallon, H.J.: Treatment of alcoholic hepatitis with encephalopathy. Comparison of prednisolone with caloric supplements. Gastroenterology 74: 169 (1978).

Levant, J.A.; Walsh, J.H. and Isenberg, J.I.: Stimulation of gastric secretion and gastrin release by single oral doses of calcium carbonate in man. New England Journal of Medicine 289: 555 (1973).

Levi, G.C.; de Avila, C.A. and Neto, V.A.: Efficacy of various drugs for treatment of giardiasis. A comparative study. American Journal of Tropical Medicine and Hygiene 26: 564 (1977).

Levine, R.R.: Factors affecting gastrointestinal absorption of drugs. Amer. J. Dig. Dis. 15: 171 (1970).

Levine, S.M. and Rubin, W.: Benign disorders of the esophagus. Presentation, diagnosis and treatment. Medical Clinics of North America 57: 1107 (1973).

Littman, A. and Pine, B.H.: Antacids and anticholinergic drugs. Annals of Internal Medicine 82: 544 (1975).

Longstreth, G.F. and Newcomer, A.D.: Drug-induced malabsorption. Mayo Clinic Proceedings 50: 284 (1975).

Lorber, S.H.: Diarrhoea: Classification and treatment. Modern Treatment 8: 971 (1971).

Lotz, M.; Ney, R. and Bartter, F.C.: Osteomalacia and debility resulting from phosphorus depletion. Transactions of the Association of American Physicians 77: 281 (1964).

Lotz, M.; Zisman, E. and Bartter, F.C.: Evidence for a phosphorus depletion syndrome in man. New England Journal of Medicine 278: 409 (1968).

Louw, J.H.; Marks, I.N. and Bank, S.:The management of severe acute pancreatitis. Postgraduate Medical Journal 43: 31 (1967).

Lukas, D.S.: Changing concepts of digitalis therapy and toxicity; in Russek (Ed) Cardiovascular Problems, pp. 295 (University Park Press, Baltimore 1976).

Macbeth, R.: Treatment of oesophageal varices in portal hypertension by means of sclerosing injections. British Medical Journal 2: 877 (1955).

MacKercher, P.A.; Ivey, K-J.; Baskin, W.N. and Krause, W.J.: Protective effect of cimetidine on aspirin-induced gastric mucosal damage. Annals of Internal Medicine 87: 676 (1977).

Macklon, A.F.; Savage, R.L. and Rawlins, M.D.: Gilbert's syndrome and drug metabolism. Clinical Pharmacokinetics 4: 273 (1979).

McCallum, R.W.; Ippoliti, A.F.; Cooney, C. and Sturdevant, R.A.L.: A controlled trial of metoclopramide in symptomatic gastroesophageal reflux. New England Journal of Medicine 296: 354 (1977).

McQueen, E.G.: Hormonal steroid contraceptives: A further review of adverse reactions. Drugs 16: 322 (1978).

Mangione, A.; Imhoff, T.E.; Lee, R.V.; Shum, L.Y. and Jusko, W.J.: Pharmacokinetics of theophylline in hepatic disease. Chest 73: 616 (1978).

Marks, I.N.: A sceptical view of medical treatment of peptic ulcer; in Truelove and Willoughby (Eds) Topics in Gastroenterology, 7th Ed (Blackwell, Oxford 1979a).

Marks, I.N.: Healing of peptic ulcers on conventional antacid therapy with or without butriptyline. South African Medical Journal 55: 331 (1979b).

Marks, I.N. and Bank, S.: Treatment of pancratic diabetes; in Knight (Ed) Modern Treatment, Vol. 2, p.471 (Harper and Row, New York 1965).

Marks, I.N. and Bank, S.: Chronic pancreatitis, relapsing pancreatitis, calcification of the pancreas, clinical aspects; in Bockus, (Ed) Gastroenterology 3rd Ed, Vol. III, p. 1052 (Saunders, Philadelphia 1976).

Marks, I.N.; Bank, S. and Louw, J.H.: The diagnosis and management of pancreatitis; in Glass (Ed) Progress in Gastoenterology 2: 412 (Grune and Stratton, New York 1968).

Marks, I.N. and Bank, S.: Chronic pancreatitis: Classification, clinical aspects, diagnosis and management. Current Concepts in Gastroenterology 2: 21 (1977).

Marks, I.N. and Bornman, P.C.: Chronic pancreatitis; in Conn (Ed) Current Therapy 1979, p.375 (Saunders, Philadelphia 1979).

Marsden, P.D. (Ed): Symposium on intestinal parasites. Clinics in Gastroenterology 7: 1-238 (1978).

Mattila, M.J.; Friman, A.; Larmi, T.K.I. and Koskinen, R.: Absorption of ethionamid, isoniazid and aminosalicylic acid from the post resection gastrointestinal tract. Annales Medicinae Experimentalis et Biologiae Fenniae 47: 209 (1969).

Maxwell, J.D. and Williams, R.: Adverse drug reactions and the liver. Adverse Drug Reaction Bulletin No. 29: 84 (1971).

Maxwell, J.D.; Carrella, M.; Parkes, J.D.: Williams, R.; Mould, G.P. and Curry, S.H.: Plasma disappearance and cerebral effects of chlorpromazine in cirrhosis. Clinical Science 43: 143 (1972).

Medical Research Council Multicentre Trial: MRC Multicentre trial of glucagon and aprotinin. Death from acute pancreatitis. Lancet 2: 632 (1977).

Melander, A.: Influence of food on the bioavailability of drugs. Clinical Pharmacokinetics 3: 337 (1978).

Melander, A.; Kahlmeter, G.; Kamme, C. and Ursing, B.: Bioavailability of metronidazole in fasting and non-fasting healthy subjects and in patients with Crohn's disease. European Journal of Clinical Pharmacology 12: 69 (1977).

Milner, G. and Buckler, E.G.: Adynamic ileus and amitriptyline: three case reports Medical Journal of Australia 1: 921 (1964).

Misiewicz, J.J.; Lennard-Jones, J.E.; Conell, A.M.; Baron, J.H. and Jones, F.A.: Controlled trial of sulphasalazine in maintenance therapy for ulcerative colitis. Lancet 1: 185 (1965).

Misra, N.P.: A comparative study of tinidazole and metronidazole as a single daily dose for three days in symptomatic intestinal amoebiasis. Drugs 15(Suppl. 1): 19 (1978).

Mitchell, J.R.; Thorgeirsson, U.P.; Black, M.; Timbrell, J.A.; Snodgrass, W.R.; Potter, W.Z.; Jollow, D.J. and Keiser, H.R.: Increased incidence of isoniazid hepatitis in rapid acetylators: possible relation to hydrazine metabolites. Clinical Pharmacology and Therapeutics 18: 70 (1975).

Mitchell, J.R.; Zimmermann, H.J.; Ishak, K.G.; Thorgeirsson, U.P.; Timbrell, J.A.; Snodgrass, W.R. and Nelson, S.D.: Isoniazid liver injury: clinical spectrum, pathology, and possible pathogenesis. Annals of Internal Medicine 84: 181 (1976).

Mogelnicki, S.R.; Waller, J.L. and Finlayson, D.C.: Physostigmine reversal of cimetidine-induced mental confusion. Journal of the American Medical Association 241: 826 (1979).

Morgan, A.G.; McAdam, W.A.F.; Parsoo, C.; Walker, B.E. and Simmons, A.V.: Cimetidine: an advance in gastric ulcer treatment? British Medical Journal 2: 1323 (1978).

Morgan, M.H. and Read, A.E.: Antidepressants and liver disease. Gut 13: 697 (1972).

Most, H.: Current concepts in parasitology. Trichinosis — Preventable yet still with us. New England Journal of Medicine 298: 1178 (1978).

Moult, P.J.A. and Sherlock, S.: Halothane-related hepatitis. Quarterly Journal of Medicine 44(NS): 99 (1975).

Mowat, A.P. and Arias, I.M.: Liver function and oral contraceptives. Journal of Reproductive Medicine 3: 19 (1969).

Mowat, N.A.G.; Needham, C.D. and Brunt, P.W.: The natural history of gastric ulcer in a community: a four year study. Quarterly Journal of Medicine 44: 45 (1975).

Muir, A. and Cossar, I.A.: Aspirin and ulcer. British Medical Journal 2: 7 (1955).

Nakashima, Y. and Howard, J.M.: Drug-induced acute pancreatitis. Surgery, Gynecology and Obstetrics 145: 105 (1977).

Naranjo, C.A.; Gonzalez, G.; Pontigo, E.; Valdenegro, C.: Ruiz, I. and Busto. U.: Adverse reaction to furosemide in liver cirrhosis. Clinical Pharmacology and Therapeutics 23: 123 (1978a).

Naranjo, C.A.; Pontigo, E.; Valdenegro, C.; Gonzalez, G.; Ruiz, I. and Busto, U.: Furosemide-induced adverse reactions in cirrhosis of the liver. Clinical Pharmacology and Therapeutics 25: 154 (1979).

Neal, E.A.; Meffin, P.J.; Gregory, P.B. and Blaschke, T.F.: Enhanced bioavailability and decreased clearance of analgesics in paitents with cirrhosis. Gastroenterology 77: 55 (1979).

Nothmann, B.J.; Chittinand, S. and Schuster, M.M.: Reversible mesenteric vascular occlusion associated with oral contraceptives. American Journal of Digestive Diseases 18: 361 (1973).

Nelson, J.D. and Haltalin, K.C.: Amoxicillin less effective than ampicillin against Shigella in vitro and in vivo: Relationship of efficacy to activity in serum. Journal of Infectious Diseases 129(Suppl): 222 (June 1974).

Nelson, J.D.; Kusmiesz, H. and Jackson, L.H.: Comparison of trimethoprim-sulfamethoxazole and ampicillin therapy for shigellosis in ambulatory patients. Journal of Pediatrics 89: 491 (1976).

Nies, A.S.; Shand, D.G. and Wilkinson, G.R.: Altered hepatic blood flow and drug disposition. Clinical Pharmacokinetics 1: 135 (1976).

Nimmo, W.S.: Drugs, diseases and altered gastric emptying. Clinical Pharmacokinetics 1: 189 (1976).

Nimmo, J.; Heading, R.C.; Tothill, P. and Prescott, L.F.: Pharmacological modification of gastric emptying: Effects of propantheline and metoclopramide on paracetamol absorption. British Medical Journal 1: 587 (1973).

Northfield, T.C.: Ulcerative colitis and Crohn's colitis: Differential diagnosis and treatment. Drugs 14: 198 (1977).

Novak, E.; Lee, J.G.; Seckman, C.E.; Phillips, J.P. and DiSanto, A.R.: Unfavorable effect of atropine-diphenoxylate (Lomotil) therapy in lincomycin-caused diarrhoea. Journal of the American Medical Association 235: 1451 (1976).

Novis, B.H.; Bank, S.; Marks, I.N.; Selzer, G.; Kahn, L.; Sealy, R.: Abdominal lymphoma presenting with malabsorption. Quarterly Journal of Medicine 40: 521 (1971).

Novis, B.H.; Clain, J.; Barbezat, E.O. and Bank, S.: Urgent fibreoptic endoscopy in upper gastro-intestinal bleeding. South African Medical Journal 50: 93 (1976).

Ochs, H.; Bodem, G.; Kodrat, G.; Savic, B. and Baur, M.P.: Biological availability of digoxin in patients with or without gastric resection (Billroth II). Deutsche Medizinische Wochenschrift 100: 2430 (1975).

O'Donoghue, D.P.; Dawson, A.M.; Powell-Tuck, J.; Bown, R.L. and Lennard-Jones, J.E.: Double-blind withdrawal trial of azathioprine as maintenance treatment for Crohn's disease. Lancet 2: 955 (1978).

Olsen, G.D.; Bennett, W.M. and Porter, G.A.: Morphine and phenytoin binding to plasma proteins in renal and hepatic failure. Clinical Pharmacology and Therapeutics 17: 677 (1975).

Palmer, D.L.; Koster, F.T.; Rafiqul Islam, A.F.M.; Mizanur Rahman, A.S.M. and Sack, R.B.: Comparison of sucrose and glucose in the oral electrolyte therapy of cholera and other severe diarrheas. New England Journal of Medicine 297: 1107 (1977).

Pande, N.V.; Resnick, R.H.; Yee, W.; Eckhardt, V.F. and Shurberg, J.L.: Cirrhotic portal hypertension: morbidity of continued alcoholism. Gastroenterology 74: 64 (1978).

Parsons, R.L.: Drug absorption in gastrointestinal disease with particular reference to malabsorption syndromes. Clinical Pharmacokinetics 2: 45 (1977).

Parsons, R.L. and Paddock, G.M.: Absorption of two antibacterial drugs, cephalexin and co-trimoxazole in malabsorption syndromes. Journal of Antimicrobial Chemotherapy 1(Suppl.): 59 (1975).

Parsons, R.L.; Kaye, C.M.; Raymond, K.; Trounce, J.R. and Turner, P.: Absorption of propranolol and practolol in coeliac disease. Gut 17: 139 (1976a).

Parsons, R.L.; Paddock, G.M.; Hossack, G.A. and Hailey, D.M.: Antibiotic absorption in Crohn's disease; in Williams and Geddes (Eds) Chemotherapy, Vol. 4, Pharmacology of Antibiotics p. 219 (Plenum Press, New York 1976b).

Parsons, R.L.; Kaye, C.M. and Raymond, K.: Pharmacokinetics of salicylate and indomethacin in coeliac disease. European Journal of Clinical Pharmacology 11: 473 (1977).

Pastore, G.; Rizzo, G.; Fera, G. and Schiraldi, O.: Trimethoprim-sulphamethoxazole in the treatment of cholera. Comparison with tetracycline and chloramphenicol. Chemotherapy (Basel) 23: 121 (1977).

Penfold, D. and Volans, G.N.: Overdose from Lomotil. British Medical Journal 2: 1401 (1977).

Pentikainen, P.J.; Neuvonen, P.J.; Tarpila, S. and Syvalahti, E.: Effect of cirrhosis of the liver on the pharmacokinetics of chlormethiazole. British Medical Journal 2: 861 (1978).

Pertsemlidis, D.; Panveliwalla, D. and Ahrens, E.H.: Effects of clofibrate and of an estrogen-progestin combination on fasting biliary lipids and cholic acid kinetics in man. Gastroenterology 66: 565 (1974).

Peterson, W.L.; Sturdevant, R.A.L.; Frankl, H. et al.: Healing of duodenal ulcer with an antacid regimen. New England Journal of Medicine 297: 341 (1977).

Phillips, S.F.: Diarrhoea: A current view of the pathophysiology. Gastroenterology 63: 495 (1972).

Piafsky, K.M.; Sitar, D.S.; Rango, R.E. and Ogilvie, R.I.: Theophylline disposition in patients with hepatic cirrhosis. New England Journal of Medicine 296: 1495 (1977).

Piafsky, K.M.; Borga, O.; Odar-Cederloff, I.; Johansson, C. and Sjoqvist, F.: Increased plasma protein binding of propranolol and chlorpromazine mediated by disease-induced elevations of plasma α_1 acid glycoprotein. New England Journal of Medicine 299: 1435 (1978).

Pinder, R.M.; Brogden, R.N.; Sawyer, P.R.; Speight, T.M.; Spencer, R. and Avery, G.S.: Carbenoxolone: A review of its pharmacological properties and therapeutic efficacy in ulcer disease. Drugs 11: 245 (1976a).

Pinder, R.M.; Brogden, R.N.; Sawyer, P.R.; Speight, T.M. and Avery, G.S.: Metoclopramide: A review of its pharmacological properties and clinical use. Drugs 12: 81 (1976b).

Piper, D.W.: Antacid and anticholinergic drug therapy. Clinics in Gastroenterology 2: 361 (1973).

Piper, D.W. and Heap, T.R.: Medical management of peptic ulcer with reference to anti-ulcer agents in other gastrointestinal diseases. Drugs 3: 366 (1972).

Piper, D.W.; Greig, M.; Coupland, G.A.E.; Hobbin, E. and Shinners, J.: Factors relevant to the prognosis of chronic gastric ulcer. Gut 16: 714 (1975).

Piper, D.W.; Greig, M.; Landecker, K.D.; Shinners, J.; Waller, S. and Canalese, J.: Analgesic intake and chronic gastric ulcer, acute upper gastrointestinal haemorrhage, personality traits and social class. Proceedings of the Royal Society of Medicine 70(Suppl. 7): 11 (1977).

Piper, D.W.; Shinners, J.; Greig, M.; Thomas, J. and Waller, S.L.: Effect of ulcer healing on the prognosis of chronic gastric ulcer. Gut 19: 419 (1978).

Pittman, F.E.: Lomotil and antibiotic colitis. Annals of Internal Medicine 83: 124 (1975).

Pittman, F.E.; Pittman, J.C. and Humphrey, C.D.: Colitis following oral lincomycin therapy. Archives of Internal Medicine 134: 368 (1974).

Pomare, E.W.: Dietary fibre: When is it worth a trial. Drugs 14: 213 (1977).

Pottage, A.; Nimmo, J. and Prescott, L.F.: The absorption of aspirin and paracetamol in patients with achlorhydria. Journal of Pharmacy and Pharmacology 26: 144 (1974).

Powell-Jackson, P.; Barkley, H. and Northfield, T.C.: Effect of cimetidine in symptomatic gastro-oesophageal reflux. Lancet 2: 1068 (1978).

Prescott, L.F.: Gastrointestinal absorption of drugs. Medical Clinics of North America 48: 907 (1974a).

Prescott, L.F.: Drug absorption interactions — gastric emptying; in Morselli, Cohen and Garattini (Eds) Drug Interactions, p. 11 (Raven Press, New York 1974b).

Prescott, L.F.; Wright, N.; Roscoe, P. and Brown, S.S.: Plasma-paracetamol half-life and hepatic necrosis in patients with paracetamol overdosage. Lancet 1: 519 (1971).

Price, A.B. and Davies, D.R.: Pseudomembranous colitis. Journal of Clinical Pathology 30: 1 (1977).

Race, T.F.; Paes, I.C. and Faloon, W.W.: Intestinal malabsorption induced by oral colchicine: Comparison with neomycin and cathartic agents. American Journal of Medical Sciences 259: 32 (1970).

Rannevik, G.; Jeppsson, S. and Kullander, S.: Effect of oral contraceptives on the liver in women with recurrent cholestasis (hepatosis) during previous pregnancies. Journal of Obstetrics and Gynaecology of the British Commonwealth 79: 1128 (1972).

Ranson, J.H.C.; Roses, D.F. and Fink, S.D.: Early respiratory insufficiency in acute pancreatitis. Annals of Surgery 178: 75 (1973).

Ranson, J.H.C.; Rifkind, K.M. and Turner, J.W.: Prognostic signs and nonoperative peritoneal lavage in acute pancreatitis. Surgery, Gynecology and Obstetrics 143: 209 (1976).

Read, A.E.; Laidlaw, J. and McCarthy, C.F.: Effects of chlorpromazine in patients with hepatic disease. British Medical Journal 3: 497 (1969).

Reed, P.I. and Davies, W.A.: Controlled trial of a new dosage form of carbenoxolone (Pyrogastrone) in the treatment of reflux esophagitis. American Journal of Digestive Diseases 23: 161 (1978).

Regan, P.T.; Malagelada, J-R.; DiMagno, E-P.; Glanzman, S.L. and Go, V.L.W.: Comparative effects of antacids, cimetidine and enteric coating on the therapeutic response to oral enzymes in severe pancreatic insufficiency. New England Journal of Medicine 297: 854 (1977).

Reynolds, T.B.: Good news for drinkers — or is it? Gastroenterology 74: 153 (1978).

Reynolds, T.B.; Peters, R.L. and Yamada, S.: Chronic active and lupoid hepatitis caused by a laxative, oxyphenisatin. New England Journal of Medicine 285: 813 (1971).

Riska, N.: Hepatitis cases in INH treated groups and in a control group. Bulletin of the International Union against Tuberculosis 51: 203 (1976).

Ritchie, J.A. and Truelove, S.C.: Treatment of irritable bowel syndrome with lorazepam, hyoscine butylbromide, and ispaghula husk. British Medical Journal 1: 376 (1979).

Rivera-Calimlim, L.; Castaneda, L. and Lasagna, L.: Effects of mode of management on plasma chlorpromazine in psychiatric patients. Clinical Pharmacology and Therapeutics 14: 978 (1973).

Rivera-Calimlim, L.; Kerzner, B. and Karch, F.E.: Effect of lithium on plasma chlorpromazine levels. Clinical Pharmacology and Therapeutics 23: 451 (1978).

Roberts, R.K.; Desmond, P.V. and Schenker, S.: Drug prescribing in hepatobiliary disease. Drugs 17: 198-212 (1979).

Rodman, J.S.; Deutsch, D.J. and Gutman, S.I.: Methyldopa hepatitis. A report of six cases in the literature. American Journal of Medicine 60: 941 (1976).

Rosenberg, D.M. and Neelon, F.A.: Acetaminophen and liver disease. Annals of Internal Medicine 88: 129 (1978).

Rossouw, J.E. and Saunders, S.J.: Hepatic complications of antituberculous therapy. Quarterly Journal of Medicine 44: 1 (1975).

Roth, J.L.A.: Deleterious effects of drugs on the gastrointestinal tract; in Gamble and Wilbur (Eds) Current Concepts of Clinical Gastroenterology, p. 257 (Little Brown, Boston 1965).

Routledge, P.A. and Shand, D.G.: Clinical pharmacokinetics of propranolol. Clinical Pharmacokinetics 4: 73 (1979).

Russell, R.I.: Progress report: Elemental diets. Gut 16: 68 (1975).

Sack, D.A.; Kaminsky, D.C.; Sack, B.R.; Itotia, J.N.; Arthur, R.R.; Kapikian, A.Z.; Orskov, F. and Orskov, I.: Prophylactic doxycycline for traveler's diarrhoea. Results of a prospective double-blind study of Peace Corps volunteers in Kenya. New England Journal of Medicine 298: 758 (1978).

Sali, A.; Murray, W.R. and MacKay, C.: Aluminium hydroxide in bile-salt diarrhoea. Lancet 2: 1051 (1977).

Saunders, S.J.; Seagie, J.; Kirsch, R.E. and Terblanche, J.: Acute liver failure; in Wright (Ed) Liver and Biliary Disease: A Pathophysiological Approach (Saunders, Philadelphia 1979).

Schalm, S.W.; Ammon, H.V. and Summerskill, W.H.J.: Failure of customary treatment in chronic active liver disease: causes and management. Annals of Clinical Research 8: 221 (1976).

Schentag, J.J.; Cerra, F.B.; Calleri, G.; De Glopper, E.; Rose, J.Q. and Bernhard, H.: Pharmacokinetic and clinical studies in patients with cimetidine-associated mental confusion. Lancet 1: 177 (1979).

Schneider, R.E.; Babb, J.; Bishop, H.; Mitchard, M.; Hoare, A.M. and Hawkins, C.F.: Plasma levels of propranolol in treated patients with coeliac disease and patients with Crohn's disease. British Medical Journal 2: 794 (1976).

Schweitzer, I.L.; Weiner, J.M.; McPeak, C.M. and Thursby, M.W.: Oral contraceptives in acute viral hepatitis. Journal of the American Medical Association 233: 979 (1975).

Seaman, W.E. and Plotz, P.H.: Effect of aspirin on liver tests in patients with RA or SLE and in normal volunteers. Arthritis and Rheumatism 19: 155 (1976).

Selden, R. and Sasahara, A.A.: Central nervous system toxicity induced by lidocaine: Report of a case in a patient with liver disease. Journal of the American Medical Association 202: 908 (1967).

Serebro, H.; Kay, S.; Javett, S. and Abrahams, C.: Sulphasalazine rectal enemas: topical method of inducing remission of active ulcerative colitis affecting rectum and descending colon. British Medical Journal 2: 1264 (1977).

Sessions, J.T.; Minkel, H.P.; Bullard, J.C. and Ingelfinger, F.J.: The effect of barbiturates in patients with liver disease. Journal of Clinical Investigation 33: 1116 (1954).

Sharon, P.; Ligumsky, M.; Rachmilewitz, D. and Zor, U.: Role of prostaglandins in ulcerative colitis. Enhanced production during active disease and inhibition by sulphasalazine. Gastroenterology 75: 638 (1978).

Sherlock, S.: Drugs and the liver. British Medical Journal 1: 227 (1968a).

Sherlock, S.: Jaundice in pregnancy. British Medical Bulletin 24: 39 (1968b).

Sherlock, S.: Factors determining hepatic reactions to drugs. Annals of the New York Academy of Sciences 160: 775 (1969).

Sherlock, S.: Liver diseases due to drugs: in Meyler and Peck (Eds) Drug-Induced Diseases, vol. 4 p. 241 (Excerpta Medica, Amsterdam 1972).

Sherlock, S.; Senewiratne, B.; Scott, A. and Walker, J.G.: Complications of diuretic therapy in hepatic cirrhosis. Lancet 1: 1049 (1966).

Shideman, F.E.; Kelly, A.R.; Lee, L.E. et al.: The role of the liver in the detoxification of thiopental (Pentothal) by man. Anesthesiology 10: 421 (1949).

Shirley, E.: A review of papers purporting to show a cause and effect relationship between aspirin ingestion and massive gastrointestinal haemorrhage. Proceedings of the Royal Society of Medicine 70(Suppl. 7): 4 (1977).

Shull, H.J.; Wilkinson, G.R.; Johnson, R. and Schenker, S.: Normal disposition of oxazepam in acute viral hepatitis and cirrhosis. Annals of Internal Medicine 84: 420 (1976).

Silver, B.A. and Bell, W.R.: Cimetidine potentiation of the hypoprothrombinemic effect of warfarin. Annals of Internal Medicine 90: 348 (1979).

Sladen, G.E.: Effects of chronic purgative abuse. Proceedings of the Royal Society of Medicine 65: 288 (1972).

Smith, B.: Effect of irritant purgatives on the myenteric plexus in man and the mouse. Gut 9: 139 (1968).

Smith, E.R. and Goulston, S.J.M.: Antibiotic-induced diarrhoea. Drugs 10: 329 (1975).

Smith, J.; Tyrrell, W.F.; Gow, A.; Allan, G.W. and Lees, A.W.: Hepatotoxicity in rifampicin-isoniazid treated patients related to their rate of isoniazid inactivation. Chest 61: 587 (1972).

Smith, V.M.: Association of aspirin ingestion with symptomatic esophageal hiatus hernia. Southern Medical Journal 71(Suppl): 45 (Jan. 1978).

Sokol, G.H.; Greenblatt, D.J.; Lloyd, B.L.; Georgotas, A.; Allen, M.D.; Harmatz, I.S.; Smith, T.W. and Shader, R.I.: Effect of abdominal radiation therapy on drug absorption in humans. Journal of Clinical Pharmacology 18: 388 (1978).

Sotaniemi, E.A.; Hokkanen, O.T.; Ahokas, J.T.; Pelkonen, R.O. and Ahlqvist, J.: Hepatic injury and drug metabolism in patients with alpha-methyldopa-induced liver damage. European Journal of Clinical Pharmacology 12: 429 (1977).

Spiegelman, M. and McNabb, R.W.: Unusual presentation of carcinoma of the colon. British Medical Journal 4: 534 (1971).

Spillman, R.; Ayala, S.C. and de Sanchez, C.E.: Double-blind test of metronidazole and tinidazole in the treatment of asymptomatic entaboeba histolytica and entamoeba hartmanni carriers. American Journal of Tropical Medicine 25: 549 (1976).

Stanciu, C. and Bennett, J.R.: Colonic response to pentazocine. British Medical Journal 1: 312 (1974a).

Stanciu, C. and Bennett, J.R.: Alginate/antacid in the reduction of gastro-oesophageal reflux. Lancet 1: 109 (1974b).

Stewart, R.B. and Cluff, L.E.: Gastrointestinal manifestations of adverse drug reactions. American Journal of Digestive Diseases 19: 1 (1974).

Stiehl, A.; Czygan, P.; Kommerell, B.; Weis, H.J. and Holtermuller, K.H.: Ursodeoxycholic acid versus chenodeoxycholic acid. Comparison of their effects on bile acid and bile lipid composition in patients with cholesterol gallstones. Gastroenterology 75: 1016 (1978).

Stiel, J.N.; Mitchell, C.A.; Radcliff, F.J. and Piper, D.W.: Hypercalcaemia in patients with peptic ulceration receiving large doses of calcium carbonate. Gastroenterology 53: 900 (1967).

Stuiver, P.C. and Goud, Th. J.L.M.: Corticosteroids and liver amoebiasis. British Medical Journal 2: 394 (1978).

Sturdevant, R.A.L.; Pearce, M.L. and Dayton, S.: Increased prevalence of cholelithiasis in men ingesting a serum cholesterol lowering diet. New England Journal of Medicine 288: 24 (1973).

Summerskill, W.H.J.; Korman, M.G.; Ammon, H.V. and Baggenstoss, A.H.: Prednisone for chronic active liver disease: dose titration, standard dose and combination with azathioprine compared. Gut 16: 876 (1975).

Surland, L.G. and Weisberger, A.S.: Chloramphenicol toxicity in liver and renal disease. Archives of Internal Medicine 112: 161 (1963).

Symposium: Third symposium on histamine H$_2$-receptor antagonists: Clinical results with cimetidine. Gastroenterology 74: 338 (1978).

Talseth, T.: Clinical pharmacokinetics of hydrallazine. Clinical Pharmacokinetics 2: 317 (1977).

Tanner, A.R.; Cowlishaw, J.L.; Cowen, A.E. and Ward, M.: Efficacy of cimetidine and tri-potassium di-citrato bismuthate (De-nol) in chronic gastric ulceration. A comparative study. Medical Journal of Australia 1: 1 (1979).

Tedesco, F.G.; Barton, R.W. and Alpers, D.H.: Clindamycin-associated colitis. A prospective study. Annals of Internal Medicine 81: 429 (1974).

Terblanche, J.: Treatment of oesophageal varices. Journal of the Royal Society of Medicine 72: 163 (1979).

Texter, E.C. and Laureta, H.C.: The milk alkali syndrome. American Journal of Digestive Diseases 11: 413 (1966).

Thompson, J.E.: How safe is isoniazid? Medical Journal of Australia 1: 165 (1978).

Thompson, R.P.H. and Williams, R.: Developments in jaundice. Postgraduate Medical Journal 45: 196 (1969).

Thompson, R.P.H. and Jackson, B.T.: Sclerosing peritonitis due to practolol. British Medical Journal 1: 1393 (1977).

Thompson, W.G.: Constipation and catharsis. Canadian Medical Association Journal 114: 927 (1976).

Thomson, P.D.; Melmon, K.L.; Richardson, J.A.; Cohn, K.; Steinbrunn, W.; Cudihee, R. and Rowland, M.: Lidocaine pharmacokinetics in advanced heart failure, liver disease, and renal failure in humans. Annals of Internal Medicine 78: 499 (1973).

Trapnell, J.E.: The natural history and management of acute pancreatitis. Clinics in Gastroenterology 1: 147 (1972).

Trapnell, J.E.; Rigby, C.C.; Talbot, C.H. and Duncan, E.H.L.: A controlled trial of Trasylol in the treatment of acute pancreatitis. British Journal of Surgery 61: 177 (1974).

Travers, R.L. and Hughes, G.R.V.: Salicylate hepatotoxicity in systemic lupus erythematosus: a common occurrence. British Medical Journal 2: 1532 (1978).

Trey, C.; Lipworth, L. and Davidson, C.S.: Parameters influencing survival in the first 318 patients reported to the fulminant hepatic failure surveillance study. Gastroenterology 58: 306 (1970).

Truelove, S.C.: Ulcerative colitis: Medical management. British Medical Journal 1: 651 (1971).

Truelove, S.C. and Jewell, D.P.: Intensive intravenous regimen for severe attacks of ulcerative colitis. Lancet 1: 1067 (1974).

Truelove, S.C. and Rocca, M.: Treatment of chronic gastric ulcer with gefarnate: a long-term controlled therapeutic trial. Curr. Med. Res. Opin. 4: 218 (1976).

Truelove, S.C.; Willoughby, C.P.; Lee, E.G. and Kettlewell, M.G.W.: Further experience in the treatment of severe attacks of ulcerative colitis. Lancet 2: 1086 (1978).

Uribe, M. and Go, V.L.W.: Corticosteroid pharmacokinetics in liver disease. Clinical Pharmacokinetics 4: 233 (1979).

Utili, R.; Boitnott, J. and Zimmerman, H.J.: Dantrolene-associated hepatic injury. Incidence and character. Gastroenterology 72: 610 (1976).

Vincent, P.C. and Radcliff, F.J.: The effect of large doses of calcium carbonate on serum and urinary calcium. American Journal of Digestive Diseases 11: 286 (1966).

Volans, G.N.: Migraine and drug absorption. Clinical Pharmacokinetics 3: 313 (1978).

Wagonfeld, J.B.; Nemchausky, B.A.; Bolt, M.; Horst, J.V.; Boyer, J.L. and Rosenberg, I.H.: Comparison of vitamin D and 25-hydroxy-vitamin D in the therapy of primary biliary cirrhosis. Lancet 2: 391 (1976).

Wallace, W.A.; Orr, C.M.E. and Bearn, A.R.: Perforation of chronic peptic ulcers after cimetidine. British Medical Journal 11: 865 (1978).

Waxman, S.; Corcino, J.J. and Herbert, V.: Drugs, toxins and dietary amino acids affecting vitamin B_{12} or folic acid absorption or utilisation. Amer. J. Med. 48: 599 (1970).

Webster, J.; Petrie, J.C. and Mowat, N.A.G.: Erosive gastritis and duodenitis during continuous cimetidine treatment. British Medical Journal 1: 20 (1978).

Wesdorp, E.; Bartelsman, J.; Pape, K.; Dekker, W. and Tytgat, G.N.: Oral cimetidine in reflux esophagitis: A double blind controlled trial. Gastroent. 74: 821 (1978).

Whelton, M.J.; Allaway, A.; Stewart, A. and Kreel, L.: Ergot poisoning in acute hepatic necrosis. Gut 9: 287 (1968).

Whitney, B. and Croxon, R.: Dysphagia caused by cardiac enlargement. Clinical Radiology 23: 147 (1972).

WHO Trial: A co-operative trial in the primary prevention of ischaemic heart disease using clofibrate. Report from the Committee of Principal Investigators. British Heart Journal 40: 1069 (1978).

Whittington, P.F.; Barnes, H.V. and Bayless, T.M.: Medical management of Crohn's disease in adolescence. Gastroenterology 72: 1338 (1977).

Wilkinson, G.R. and Schenker, S.: Drug disposition and liver disease. Drug Metabolism Reviews 4: 139 (1975).

Wilkinson, G.R. and Schenker, S.: Effect of liver disease on drug disposition in man. Biochemical Pharmacology 25: 2675 (1976).

Wilkinson, G.R. and Shand, D.G.: A physiological approach to hepatic drug clearance. Clinical Pharmacology and Therapeutics 18: 377 (1975).

Williams, D.R.: Analytical and computer simulation studies of colloidal bismuth citrate system used as an ulcer treatment. Journal of Inorganic and Nuclear Chemistry 19: 711 (1977).

Williams, G.; Maton, P.N.; Murphy, G.M. and Dowling, R.H.: Will ursodeoxycholic acid (UDCA) replace chenodeoxycholic acid (CDCA) as the medical treatment of choice for gallstone dissolution? Gut 19: A974 (1978).

Williams, R.L.; Blaschke, T.F.; Meffin, P.J.; Melmon, K.L. and Rowland, M.: Influence of viral hepatitis on the disposition of two compounds with high hepatic clearance: lidocaine and indocyanine green. Clinical Pharmacology and Therapeutics 20: 290 (1976).

Williams, R.L.; Blaschke, T.F.; Meffin, P.J.; Melmon, K.L. and Rowland, M.: Influence of acute viral hepatitis on disposition and plasma binding of tolbutamide. Clinical Pharmacology and Therapeutics 21: 301 (1977).

Wood, A.J.J.; Kornhauser, D.M.; Wilkinson, G.R.; Shand, D.G. and Branch, R.A.: The influence of cirrhosis on steady-state blood concentrations of unbound propranolol after oral administration. Clinical Pharmacokinetics 3: 478 (1978).

Wright, E.C.; Seeff, L.B.; Berk, P.D.; Jones, E.A. and Plotz, P.H.: Treatment of chronic active hepatitis: An analysis of three controlled trials. Gastroenterology 73: 1422 (1977).

Yaffe, S.J.; Gerbracht, L.M.; Mosovich, L.L.; Mattar, M.E.; Danish, M. and Jusko, W.J.: Pharmacokinetics of methicillin in patients with cystic fibrosis. Journal of Infectious Diseases 135: 828 (1977).

Zachariae, H.; Grunnet, E. and Sogaard, H.: Liver biopsy in methotrexate-treated psoriatics — a re-evaluation. Acta Dermatovenereologica 55: 291 (1975).

Zfass, A.M.; Prince, R.; Allen, F.N.; Farrar, J.T.: Inhibitory beta adrenergic receptors in the human distal esophagus. American Journal of Digestive Diseases 15: 303 (1970).

Zilly, W.; Richter, E. and Rietbrock, N.: Pharmacokinetics and metabolism of digoxin and β-methyl-digoxin-12α-^{3}H in patients with acute hepatitis. Clinical Pharmacology and Therapeutics 17: 302 (1975).

Zimmerman, H.J.: Drug-induced hepatic disease. Israel Journal of Medical Sciences 10: 386 (1974).

Zimmerman, H.J.: Drug-induced liver disease. Drugs 16: 25 (1978).

Chapter XX
Respiratory Diseases

K.N.V. Palmer and J.C. Petrie

Synopsis of Important Principles

1) The general aims of management of respiratory tract disease are reduction of airway obstruction by improvement in airway calibre and removal of retained secretions, treatment of respiratory infection and correction of abnormal ventilation.

2) In bronchial asthma, the aim of drug treatment is to attain and maintain the best possible respiratory state for the patient and to keep him that way. This can be achieved by repeated assessment of ventilatory function, avoidance of known precipitating factors and a logical approach to the use of appropriate doses of bronchodilators, sodium cromoglycate and inhaled or oral corticosteroids — as preventive treatment and in the relief of airways obstruction.

3) If a severe attack of asthma does not respond to the patient's usual treatment, a serious medical emergency exists and the patient should be admitted to hospital for accurate assessment and intensive treatment. This is of prime importance and both doctor and patient must understand this. The major problem in asthma is the education of doctors about the disease.

4) Prompt therapy with an appropriate antibacterial agent is the basis of treatment of acute purulent exacerbations of chronic bronchitis, pneumonias, bronchiectasis and cystic fibrosis.

5) Measures aimed at removing retained secretion are also important, particularly in bronchiectasis and cystic fibrosis.

6) Rational management and early recognition of respiratory failure depends upon measurement of blood gas tensions. Oxygen therapy must be controlled with great care in cases of hypoxaemia with carbon dioxide retention (i.e. ventilatory failure).

7) The aim of treatment of pulmonary tuberculosis is to provide a combination drug regimen that is adequate for the disease and acceptable to the patient and to ensure that medication is taken regularly as prescribed.

8) Symptomatic treatment and rest are necessary in sarcoidosis. Corticosteroids are used if hypercalcaemia or extrapulmonary complications develop or if pulmonary symptoms and signs persist.

9) Some drugs may adversely affect lung function in patients with pulmonary disease. In addition, pulmonary disease or secondary complications may modify the response to drugs, particularly in the presence of hypoxia.

10) Many drugs may occasionally also induce lung reactions, especially asthmatic reactions (e.g. aspirin and β-adrenoceptor blocking drugs). Other adverse pulmonary reactions to drugs should also always be considered when the cause of a respiratory illness is not clear (e.g. nitrofurantoin, hydrallazine, procainamide, busulphan).

The rational management of respiratory disease depends upon a knowledge of the pharmacological and other factors which influence respiratory tract secretions and airway calibre and control respiration and on a knowledge of the principles of use of the drugs which can be used for treatment. Many respiratory diseases are associated or due to bacterial infection. Other chapters discuss acute viral respiratory illnesses (XXVIII; sect. 3.2), respiratory infections in children (IV; sect. 5.1.4), and upper respiratory disorders (XI; sect. 2).

1. Pharmacological Considerations

1.1 Respiratory Tract Secretions

The lower respiratory tract is sterile in patients with normal lungs (Murray, 1977). The respiratory epithelium is protected by a mucus blanket of tracheobronchial secretions (normal 10 to 100mg/day), produced principally by the mucus glands and goblet cells. There is also a small amount of transudate from serum which is increased particularly in inflammatory states. The secretions have some specific antimicrobial activity. They contain immunoglobulin A and small amounts of lysozyme.

Glycoproteins account for the physical properties of the secretions, but hydration is important as 95 % of the secretions is water. Stimulation of the vagus nerve and cholinergic drugs increase bronchial mucus gland secretory activity — atropine blocks this response. Goblet cell secretion is not under nervous control. Mucus secretion is increased by irritants such as smog or cigarette smoke, which also depress normal ciliary activity. Many other factors, including drugs and changes in the physical properties of the bronchial secretions, also lead to ciliary stasis which favours the development of infection.

Antimicrobial agents administered systemically readily penetrate purulent sputum, but with a few exceptions (e.g. amoxycillin) they do not penetrate mucoid sputum. Indeed, they do not reduce the amount of mucoid sputum.

In respiratory disease the quantity and quality of the bronchial secretions are changed, leading to the expectoration of sputum. For example, in patients with asthma, the mucoid sputum contains more sialic acid and fructose and is more viscous than the sputum in patients with chronic bronchitis, or cystic fibrosis (Charman et al., 1972).

Mucoid sputum has also more elastic recoil properties on deformation than purulent sputum (Dulfano et al., 1971). Such differences affect the ease of expectoration of sputum.

1.2. Airway Calibre

Bronchial smooth muscle tone is influenced by humoral factors and by the autonomic nervous system.

1.2.1 Humoral Factors

The humoral factors include histamine, bradykinin, slow reacting substance of anaphylaxis (SRS-A), 5-hydroxytryptamine (serotonin) and possibly also prostaglandin $F_{2\alpha}$ (Austen and Orange, 1975; Cuthbert, 1975; Turner-Warwick, 1978). These substances cause bronchoconstriction. Histamine and bradykinin also increase vascular permeability and bronchial secretions.

The influence of prostaglandins in the lung has been reviewed recently (Hyman et al., 1978). In summary, the prostaglandins (PG's) of the E series are dilators and the F series constrictors of bronchi and pulmonary vasculature. Indeed $PGF_{2\alpha}$, which is used to induce abortion (chapter XV; sect. 11) must be used with caution in asthmatic patients. However, there are exceptions to this guideline and the clinical importance of prostaglandins in control of bronchial calibre is not yet clear. The discovery of prostacyclin and its release from the pulmonary circulation, and hypotheses about its actions on local modulation of vasomotor tone (rather than PGE_2) further complicate the interpretation of the effects (Editorial, 1978). Although control of airways calibre is dominated in the healthy subject by autonomic balance and local gas tensions, humoral factors play a possible role, especially in disease. In asthma, histamine, SRS-A, eosinophil chemotactic factor of anaphylaxis (ECF-A) and serotonin are stored or elaborated in mast cells in the lung which disrupt and degranulate in response to antigen-antibody reactions and various other stimuli. The role of platelet aggregation factor (PAF), which like SRS-A is synthesised and released during the allergic response, in the causation of bronchospasm is not yet clear (Editorial, 1978; Mathe et al., 1977).

1.2.2 Autonomic Factors

The autonomic nervous system acts through the parasympathetic system (cholinergic receptors) and the sympathetic system (adrenergic receptors).

The resting state of bronchial smooth muscle is influenced by the balance between parasympathetic and sympathetic stimuli.

Stimulation of the cholinergic receptors results in increased concentrations of cyclic guanosine monophosphate (c'GMP). This results in constriction of bronchial smooth muscle. The effect is blocked by atropine and other anticholinergic compounds. Bronchospasm induced by irritants such as cold air, ozone and sulphur dioxide may be mediated by the cholinergic system.

Stimulation of adrenergic receptors leads to the following cardiopulmonary effects (Alquist, 1948; Lands et al., 1967):

a) Increased pulmonary blood flow which occurs because of an increase in heart rate and cardiac output (β_1-adrenoceptor stimulation).
b) Bronchodilatation and vasodilatation of the pulmonary and systemic circulation (β_2-adrenoceptor stimulation).
c) There are also almost certainly α-adrenergic receptors which when stimulated, as for example by histamine, lead to bronchoconstriction. In addition some sympathomimetic amines, such as ephedrine, act indirectly by releasing noradrenaline (norepinephrine) from storage sites. This stimulates both α- and β-adrenergic receptors.

In the relief of bronchoconstriction by sympathomimetic amine type drugs, the β_1-receptor stimulant effects are undesirable, because the ventilation-perfusion imbalance may be aggravated by an increase in pulmonary blood flow subsequent to the increase in cardiac output (see also section 2.3.1 and 3.1.2).

1.3 Control of Respiration

The most powerful stimulus to normal respiration is carbon dioxide, although changes in oxygen tensions and probably changes in arterial, cerebrospinal fluid and intracellular pH are also important. The complex mechanism of respiration is controlled by a sensitive feedback system which involves peripheral and central chemoreceptors (Cotes, 1975).

In disease states the respiratory centre becomes more sensitive to the depressant effect of drugs, such as sedatives, tranquillisers and opiates (see section 5.2). In addition, the respiratory centre may become insensitive to raised P_aCO_2 levels and increased intracellular H^+ ion concentration and hypoxic stimulation become an important factor in maintaining respiratory drive. It is dangerous therefore to administer inappropriate concentrations of oxygen, as this may remove the hypoxic drive to respiration.

However, in a number of circumstances pulmonary function is so disturbed that concentrations of about 60 % are needed to combat arterial hypoxaemia. A mask of 300ml volume supplied with a flow of 30 litres/minute (15L O_2; 15L air) can meet the need (Campbell and Minty, 1976).

1.4 Absorption and Metabolism of Drugs by the Lung

The majority of an inhaled dose of drug is swallowed and, depending on the drug, largely absorbed through the gastrointestinal tract (e.g. isoprenaline; Blackwell et al., 1974) or largely excreted in the faeces (e.g. sodium cromoglycate/cromolyn; Walker et al., 1972). Drug absorption by the lung, as determined by animal experiments, depends on the physicochemical properties of the drug and physiological variables. For lipid soluble drugs, absorption from rat lung is by simple diffusion at rates approximately related to their lipid/water partition coefficient at physiological pH; the greater the coefficient the more rapid the absorption. Absorption of lipid insoluble drugs from rat lung is more rapid than that from the gastrointestinal tract, depending on the molecular weight; the lower the molecular weight the more rapid the absorption. Not all drugs are absorbed by diffusion alone; for example, the fraction of the inhaled dose of sodium cromoglycate not swallowed is transported into the systemic circulation in part by a specific carrier type transport process and in part by diffusion (Enna and Schanker, 1972; Schanker, 1978). Metabolism of drugs also occurs in the lung. Human lung contains drug metabolising enzymes including catechol-O-methyl-transferase (COMT) and demethylating enzymes. Isoprenaline (isoproterenol) and isoetharine are extensively O-methylated in isolated perfused dog lung but terbutaline, which is resistant to COMT, is not metabolised in this system (Briant et al., 1973). Salmefanol and rimiterol also appear to be metabolised whereas salbutamol, not a substrate for COMT, and sodium cromoglycate are not (Shenfield et al., 1976). With some drugs a 'delay' of the drug occurs in the lung, perhaps due to uptake, but the mechanisms remain speculative.

1.5 Drug Kinetics and Pulmonary Disease

Drug kinetics may be altered by associated pulmonary disease. The clinical importance of many of the reported changes is not yet clearly established, nor can generalisations be made which apply to all drugs but the lungs must now be added to the list of organs whose dysfunction affects drug handling (for review, see du Souich et al., 1978).

Acute hypoxaemia appears to decrease intrinsic hepatic clearance and chronic hypoxaemia increase intrinsic hepatic clearance; e.g. for drugs such as tolbutamide for which the rate of metabolism is dependent on the amount of free drug in plasma (see chapter I; sect. 4.3.2). Protein binding may also be altered; α_1-acid glycoproteins are responsible for binding of basic drugs such as quinidine, binding of which is increased in pulmonary disease. Blood gas disturbances and haemodynamic changes secondary to pulmonary vascular resistance can also alter drug disposition by decreasing hepatic and renal blood flow; cor pulmonale in particular being equivalent in pathophysiological terms to congestive heart failure. Acute hypoxaemia may decrease glomerular filtration rate. Thus, drugs showing flow dependent hepatic clearance, e.g. lignocaine (lidocaine) and dextropropoxyphene, for which clearance is proportional to hepatic blood flow, or predominant renal clearance, which is proportional to glomerular filtration rate (e.g. digoxin, aminoglycosides), should also be used with caution in patients with pulmonary disease. Clearance of theophylline can be markedly decreased in severe chronic airways obstruction and in pulmonary heart disease, the mechanisms causing the reduced clearance not as yet being elucidated (table II; section 10.2). Cystic fibrosis on the other hand, can increase clearance of penicillins such as methicillin and dicloxacillin due to enhanced renal tubular secretion (see section 10.2).

2. General Principles of Treatment

The clinician must first establish the diagnosis and then assess the severity of the illness to determine the correct management. Most patients are treated outside hospital but those who require more intensive management and investigation, such as patients with status asthmaticus or respiratory failure, must be identified and referred to hospital without delay.

The assessment of the severity of the disease depends on a careful history and full clinical examination. This may include simple pulmonary function tests, such as spirometry. Most practitioners have access to facilities for sputum culture, virology studies, blood counts and radiology of the chest. Measurement of arterial (or in children, arterialised) blood gas tensions and acid base status (P_aO_2, P_aCO_2 and pH) is of great importance.

2.1 Aims of Management

The main aims of management in respiratory tract disease are to treat:
1) Reduction in airways calibre
2) Respiratory infections
3) Disorders of ventilation and control of respiration.

2.1.1 Reduction in Airways Calibre

The important aetiological factors include cigarette smoke, atmospheric pollution, cold air, fog, smog, poor working conditions, dusty occupations, exposure to substances at work, various allergens and infections. These factors are associated with abnormal sputum production and they must be avoided, removed or treated.

Expectoration of sputum must be eased by liberal fluid intake, hot drinks, regular and efficient physiotherapy including postural drainage. Abnormal sputum production results in a reduction in airways calibre but other factors, such as bronchoconstriction and respiratory tract disease, are also important and interfere with the clearing of retained secretions.

Selective β_2-adrenoceptor stimulant drugs, which are most commonly given by aerosol inhalation, are the drugs of choice to achieve bronchodilatation (see section 2.3.1). It is essential that the patient understands the technique of self administration of a bronchodilator aerosol (as also applies to cromoglycate and corticosteroid inhalers), the maximum permissible number of puffs and, most important, that a lack of response to the aerosol inhaler indicates a need for alternative therapy rather than further inhalation. Resistance and tolerance to sympathomimetic drugs are well recognised. Failure of response, or an inadequate response, can sometimes be due to a faulty aerosol or, especially in young children, to incorrect technique of inhalation. This possibility should always be considered carefully.

Optimum effects are obtained if a deep breath is taken at the same time as the aerosol is released. The breath should be held for 5 to 10 seconds at full inspiration. Greater improvements in ventilatory function are obtained when the dose is given with the mouthpiece about 3cm from the lips with the mouth open (Tuttle and Sidorov, 1977) and when inhaled at high rather than low lung volumes. For those patients who find difficulty in using the pressurised aerosol properly a powder aerosol of salbutamol may be administered from a low resistance insufflator (Rotahaler; Hetzel and Clark, 1977). This device may be of particular value to the minority of patients who cannot be taught to use conventional aerosols correctly. A nebulised aerosol is suitable for very young children who cannot use a pressurised aerosol (Bacon, 1978; Phelan and Stocks, 1974).

The value of the regular use of aerosol bronchodilators is stressed in the prevention of attacks of airflow obstruction, rather than use only for the treatment of wheezy episodes (Goldstein et al., 1978; Woolcock, 1977). Such a regimen may reduce or abolish the hyper-reactivity ('twitchiness') of the bronchi in the asthmatic to a number of stimuli such as exercise, infections, cold air, exposure to allergens and emotional upsets.

It is not rational to prescribe bronchodilator drugs unless there is evidence that a component of the airways obstruction is reversible and is influenced by the drugs. The effect of bronchodilator drugs should be assessed by spirometric measurements, e.g. an increase in the forced expiratory volume in one second (FEV_1) of more than 10%, although sometimes the only beneficial effect may be an increase in the forced vital capacity, probably indicating a reduction in lung hyperinflation.

2.1.2 Respiratory Infection

Viral infections of the respiratory tract should not be treated with antibacterial agents unless the patient is particularly susceptible to development of secondary bacterial complications. Such individuals include the very young and very old, patients with pre-existing lung disease, rheumatic heart disease or immune deficiency states (see also chapter XXVIII; sect. 3.1.2).

Established bacterial infection, however, must always be recognised early and treated promptly and effectively. Treatment, preferably with bactericidal drugs, should be started before laboratory sensitivity reports are available. The choice of drug depends on a clear understanding of the likely pathogens, usually *Streptococcus (Diplococcus) pneumoniae* and *Haemophilus influenzae* — which are usually different in patients with previously healthy lungs from those in patients with pre-existing lung disease. Before any antibacterial drug is prescribed it must be established that the patient is not hypersensitive to it or that there are no other restrictions to its use (see chapter XXVII; sect. 3.3, 4). A supply sufficient to last 7 to 10 days should be prescribed and the need to complete the course must be emphasised to the patient.

If the symptoms or fever fail to respond to the drug of first choice within 36 to 48 hours an alternative agent should be substituted, based on the results of sputum culture and sensitivity tests (see chapter XXVII; sect. 2). Treatment must continue until the patient has been afebrile for 36 to 48 hours and the sputum has become mucoid.

Any patient who shows slow resolution of fever or symptoms or signs should be carefully investigated to exclude underlying pathology, especially bronchial neoplasm, postpneumonic effusion, pulmonary tuberculosis.

The possibility of a drug fever should always be considered.

2.1.3 Disorders of Ventilation and Control of Respiration

These are discussed in section 5 on respiratory failure.

2.2 Choice of Drug Therapy

As emphasised throughout this book, the choice of a drug and its dosage depends on many different factors, all of which can be important — depending upon the circumstances of use — in particular the age of the patient, associated disease and concurrent drug therapy. For example, the tetracycline group of drugs, which are widely used in the treatment of respiratory infections, should be avoided in children (see chapter XIII; sect. 13.3) and pregnant women (see chapter XV; sect. 1.1.5) and with the exception of minocycline and doxycycline should not be used in patients with impaired renal function (chapter XXI; sect. 14.1.5).

Table I. Sympathomimetic (adrenoceptor agonist) bronchodilators

Drug	Effects on adrenoceptors	Elimination	Duration of action	Principal adverse effects
Selective β_2 agonists [1]				
Salbutamol (albuterol)	β_2 (β_1 also at high doses)	Conjugated; 50% excreted unchanged in urine; not substrate for COMT[2] or MAO[3]	Similar 1-5 hours	Tremor, cramps, cardiovascular and metabolic effects, hypokalaemia. See section 2.3.1
Orciprenaline (metaproterenol)		Oral absorption slow; not substrate for COMT		Incidence of effects related to dosage; and to patient factors
Terbutaline		Not substrate for COMT or MAO		
Isoetharine		COMT		
Fenoterol		Not substrate for COMT; conjugated		
Rimiterol		Oral, conjugated in gut wall to inactive compound; COMT	Shorter 1-3 hours especially IV	
Hexoprenaline		Slow O-methylation; active metabolite prolongs action	Longer	
Non-selective β agonist				
Isoprenaline (isoproterenol)	β_1; β_2	COMT; conjugation to inactive compound in gut wall	1-2 hours	$\beta_1 + \beta_2$ effects. See text
α and β Agonists				
Adrenaline (epinephrine)	β_1; β_2; α	Uptake 1, uptake 2[4]	Shortest	*Care:* see text. Cardiovascular, central effects, anxiety, tremor
Ephedrine	β; α Release of noradrenaline (norepinephrine) from sympathetic nerve endings	Demethylated to norephedrine; not a substrate for COMT, or MAO	Up to 4 hours	More central effects than adrenaline; tolerance; urinary retention not now recommended

1 Others include ibuterol, salfemalol, pirbuterol.
2 COMT = catechol-O-methyltransferase.
3 MAO = monoamine oxidase.
4 Uptake 1 — in sympathetic nerve endings.
   Uptake 2 — in sympathetically innervated tissues (Iversen, 1971).

If tetracyclines are taken concurrently with iron, calcium, aluminium and magnesium salts, a drug interaction can occur and the absorption of tetracycline markedly reduced (see chapter VIII, sect. 2.3.1). Many other examples of factors which influence the choice of drug are given in other chapters.

2.3 Drugs Used in the Treatment of Airways Obstruction

The principal drugs used are: bronchodilators, sodium cromoglycate (cromolyn sodium), corticosteroids, and mucolytics. Some of the more important points about their use are summarised below.

2.3.1 Bronchodilator Drugs

There are three groups: (a) sympathomimetic drugs, (b) methylxanthines, and (c) anticholinergics.

Sympathomimetic Drugs: Three groups of sympathomimetic drugs are recognised, depending on their action on adrenergic receptors (Collier and Dornhorst, 1969; Lands et al., 1967):

1) Those with so-called selective β_2-adrenoceptor agonist activity; e.g. salbutamol, terbutaline, etc. However, at high doses β_1-agonist effects are evident (Warrell et al., 1970).
2) Those with non-selective $(\beta_1 + \beta_2)$ β-adrenoceptor agonist activity; e.g. isoprenaline (isoproterenol).
3) Those with α and non-selective β-adrenoceptor agonist activity; e.g. adrenaline (epinephrine).

The *mode of action* of sympathomimetic drugs is shown in figure 1. Adrenergic receptor activation appears to be mediated by 3'5' cyclic AMP (cyclic AMP). Sympathomimetics increase adenyl cyclase activity, which in the presence of magnesium brings about the conversion of adenosine triphosphate (ATP) to the active cyclic AMP.

β_2-Adrenoceptor Agonists

The sympathomimetic agents of choice are the so-called β_2-adrenoceptor agonists such as salbutamol and terbutaline (Avery, 1971). Their β_2-agonist effects induce relaxation of smooth muscle in bronchi and vascular supply to skeletal muscle and uterus. Additional β_2-agonist effects include inhibition of reagin mediated histamine release, possibly explaining their protective effect against exercise induced asthma (Hetzel et al., 1977c); metabolic effects; muscle tremor and cramp.

In comparing different β_2 agonists the *potency, margin of safety* and *selectivity* are usually considered (Marlin and Turner, 1975). Dose-response studies are essential in comparing relative potency. Adequate and comparable dosage is essential when comparing rates of adverse reactions. Equivalent *routes of administration* are also essential when comparing the selectivity of the drugs in man because the route affects the response to the agonist greatly. For example, cardiovascular and metabolic effects can be avoided by using an aerosol formulation rather than the oral or intravenous routes (Bateman et al., 1978; Hetzel and Clark, 1976; Neville et al., 1977). The selectivity is apparently increased because the aerosol drug principally exerts a pulmonary effect on local receptors. These methodological difficulties make it difficult to make clear recommendations about the optimal β_2-agonist for use in everyday practice.

The principal drugs are shown in table I. Only a small proportion of aerosol formulations of salbutamol (about 5%) of each metered dose (100μg/puff) reaches the small bronchioles (see section 1.4). This may be increased by the use of a nebuliser. Absorption from the lungs is slow and this contributes to the longer duration of action of some aerosols relative to oral or intravenous routes, where metabolic influences may inactivate the drug reaching the systemic circulation (Blackwell et al., 1974; Hetzel and Clark, 1976).

The *indications* are discussed elsewhere. They include relief and prevention of airways obstruction, prevention and treatment of exercise induced asthma (section 3.1), and prevention of premature labour (see chapter XV; sect. 9). The *contraindications* are relative to the severity of the disease, and to the dosage and route of administration and necessity for concurrent high risk therapy. Care is required in patients with cardiovascular disease, hypertension, thyrotoxicosis, diabetes mellitus, renal and hepatic dysfunction or who are undergoing anaesthesia (e.g. halothane; see chapter X, sect. 2.1) or who are hypersensitive to sympathomimetic agents.

The principal *adverse reactions* are shown in table I. Overdosage with the so-called β_2 selective agonists unmasks the latent β_1-agonist activity which will be discussed further below. Tolerance does not occur. The metabolic effects of β_2-agonists occur particularly after parenteral and

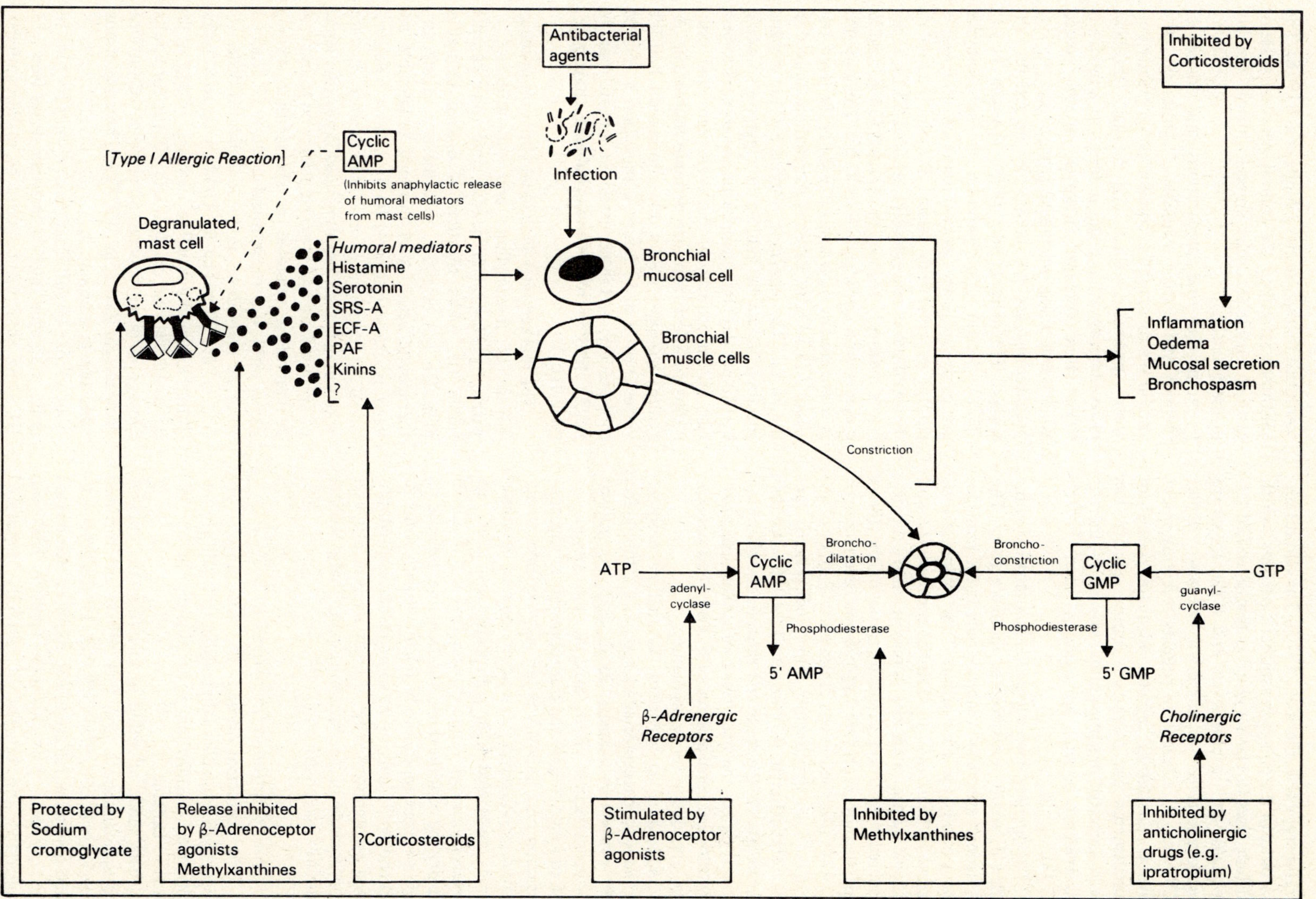

Fig. 1. Schematic representation of pharmacological mechanisms in asthma showing site and mode of action of antiasthmatic drugs (simplified).

oral therapy (Neville et al., 1977). The clinical importance of the effects in asthmatic patients, which include rises in plasma glucose, non-esterified fatty acids, and insulin levels and a fall in serum potassium levels, is unknown (see also chapter XV; sect. 9). Clearly, in patients receiving intensive corticosteroid therapy adequate potassium supplements are essential. Tumourgenicity has been suggested in some animal species but there is no evidence of such an action in man (Finkel, 1978).

Isoprenaline (isoproterenol): Isoprenaline combines β_2 and β_1-adrenoceptor agonist activity. The β_1-agonist effects are inappropriate in the management of airways obstruction. They include an increase in heart rate, myocardial contractility, and cardiac output. Such effects may intensify the disordered ventilation perfusion ratio in the lungs and thereby aggravate hypoxaemia, even though airways obstruction has diminished (Palmer et al., 1969). Such hypoxaemia may predispose to cardiac arrhythmias (Collins et al., 1969). As discussed above, the route and rate of administration greatly affect the occurrence of predictable pharmacological consequences of β_1 and β_2-adrenoceptor stimulation by isoprenaline.

Adrenaline (epinephrine): Adrenaline combines β and α-adrenoceptor agonist activity. Stimulation of α-receptors causes local and generalised vasoconstriction. Both arterial and venous α-adrenoceptors exist and disproportionate vasoconstriction may intensify pulmonary oedema. In addition, stimulation of α-adrenoceptors is sometimes associated with a bronchoconstrictor response. Although some experts find it difficult to justify the continued use of adrenaline, because its effectiveness appears to be due principally to its β-adrenoceptor activity, in some instances predominant α-adrenoceptor agonist activity is helpful as a consequence of a reduction in pulmonary oedema due to vasoconstriction.

Methylxanthines *(theophylline)*

The principal drugs of this group are theophylline and its ethylenediamine salt aminophylline. Theophylline is an alkaloid closely related to caffeine.

The mode of action is to inhibit the enzyme phosphodiesterase and this results in impaired breakdown of cyclic AMP (fig. 1). Reagin mediated histamine release is also inhibited. Combined therapy with β-adrenoceptor agonists has been suggested and benefits of carefully monitored combined therapy shown (Wolfe et al., 1978). The xanthines stimulate the central nervous system, cardiac muscle and relax smooth muscle, notably in the bronchi.

Numerous oral preparations and forms of theophylline are available. Although the anhydrous theophylline content varies greatly between products, there is similar excellent bioavailability when given in terms of anhydrous theophylline content. However, enteric coated tablets and many sustained release theophylline preparations are not completely or reliably absorbed (Hendeles et al., 1978; Spangler et al., 1978). Rectal administration as suppositories avoids troublesome gastric irritation although a painful proctitis may occur! Protein binding of theophylline is not extensive (around 53 to 65 %) but is markedly reduced in neonates (36 %) and in patients with cirrhosis (29 to 37 %). Theophylline is eliminated by biotransformation in the liver, but about 7 to 13 % of a dose is excreted unchanged in the urine. The enzymes responsible for hepatic metabolism can be induced by cigarette smoking ($>$ 10 per day) but phenobarbitone appears to be a less potent inducer of these enzymes and only seems to affect clearance in some individuals. In healthy younger adults, the elimination half-life varies from 3 to 13 hours. Elimination is delayed in the elderly and in neonates but is more rapid in young children than in adults (table II; chapter IV, table II).

The marked inter-individual variation in metabolism of theophylline, and the influence of pathophysiological or disease states on clearance (table II), make titration of dosage desirable, although not essential, to achieve a satisfactory therapeutic result with minimal predictable adverse reactions (see table II). It is nevertheless rational to commence oral maintenance therapy with smaller than recommended doses (the lesser of 400mg daily or 16mg/kg daily) and to increase at intervals as tolerated (no shorter than every 3 days) until the recommended dose is reached. Average daily doses in 4 equal divided doses (6-hourly) are 24mg/kg for children up to 9 years, 20mg/kg for children 9 to 12 years, 18mg/kg for 12 to 16 year old children and 900mg for adults. Dosage in obese patients must be based on ideal body weight (Gal et al., 1978) and because of possible slower elimination 3 equal divided doses (8-hourly) may be sufficient. Heavy smokers may require a shorter interval between doses (see table II). Dose adjustment should be made cautiously

Table II. Methylxanthine bronchodilators (after Ogilvie, 1978; Hendeles et al., 1978)

Drug	Preparations/absorption	Elimination	Principal adverse effects
Theophylline Aminophylline (theophylline ethylenediamine)	Theophylline is sometimes given as a salt, e.g. choline theophyllinate, or in a combined preparation Anhydrous theophylline content varies greatly between products. Intravenous preparations of aminophylline also vary from 75 to 85% theophylline by weight Enteric coated and many sustained release preparations not completely or reliably absorbed. Rectal absorption erratic	Hepatic metabolism: demethylation, oxidation Marked interindividual variation in elimination rate *Factors which decrease theophylline clearance* (see table III) Premature infants, neonates Elderly (> 50 years) Obesity (ideal body weight must be used to calculate maintenance dose) Dietary methylxanthines (e.g. heavy coffee intake) Hepatic cirrhosis (decreased hepatocellular function) Congestive heart failure Acute pulmonary oedema Chronic obstructive pulmonary disease with cor pulmonale Pneumonia Acute febrile episodes Troleandomycin (triacetyloleandomycin) Erythromycin *Factors which increase theophylline clearance* (see also table III) Children 1 to 16 years Heavy cigarette smoking (> 10 per day)	May be reduced by monitoring serum levels. Keep < 20μg/ml Nausea, gastric irritation, cardiovascular effects including arrhythmias, excitation, insomnia, nightmares, convulsions Rectal theophylline causes irritation and can be given in a stable form — diprophylline (dyphylline; glyphylline; dihydroxypropyl-theophylline) which does not produce theophylline *in vitro* or *in vivo*

and in small increments; because of possible dose dependent elimination kinetics a small increase in dosage may result in a disproportionate increase in serum concentration and effect. It is important to realise that because of marked interindividual variation in metabolism of theophylline, these average doses may still lead to excessive or inadequate serum concentrations in some patients. Dosage also has to be adjusted according to other factors which can alter theophylline clearance (table II), including changes in pulmonary function during acute illness (Vozeh et al., 1978).

It is imperative that in emergency therapy intravenous aminophylline is administered slowly (to allow time for distribution to be complete) or potentially serious cerebral seizures or fatal arrhythmias may occur (Piafsky et al., 1977). An initial dosage of 5 to 6mg/kg can be given over 20 to 30 minutes, but dosage must be reduced if the patient has received theophylline in the previous 12 to 24 hours. When rapid measurement of serum theophylline concentration is not possible, those who have already received theophylline may be given small loading doses of aminophylline (e.g. 2mg/kg) with caution. As with oral maintenance therapy, continued intravenous dosage must be modified for factors which alter clearance of theophylline (table II, III) and dosage in obese patients based on ideal body weight. Measurement of theophylline serum levels is now widely available and should be used to monitor therapy in difficult cases. The therapeutic range is 5 or preferably 10 to 20µg/ml. For reviews on the clinical pharmacological properties and dose guidelines of theophylline, see Ogilvie (1978a) and Hendeles et al. (1978).

Anticholinergic Drugs

Atropine-like drugs are returning to favour as adjuncts to therapy. Ipratropium bromide is available as an aerosol bronchodilator. The effect is less than salbutamol in asthmatic patients but may be superior in bronchitic patients (Petrie and Palmer, 1975) and additive with that of salbutamol (Lightbody et al., 1978). Ipratropium aerosol does not increase sputum viscosity or volume nor have an effect on heart rate (May and Palmer, 1977).

2.3.2 Disodium Cromoglycate (cromolyn sodium)

Cromoglycate is a bis-chromone derivative available in powder form for inhalation through a turbine-like inhaler 4 times daily (for review, see Brogden et al., 1974). Only a small proportion of the administered dose is absorbed from the lung (around 3% and comprising the smaller particles of < 10µm mass median diameter); the majority being swallowed and excreted in the faeces. About 2% of the administered amount following gastrointestinal absorption (0.8%) or lung absorption (3.2%) is excreted unchanged in both urine and bile.

The *mode of action* appears to be by a local action in terminal airways by inhibiting the release of chemical mediators of bronchial hyper-reactivity from mast cells, perhaps by interference with metabolic and structural changes which occur in mast cells after immunological stimulation. Cromoglycate inhibits immediate type I hypersensitivity reactions to allergen. Prior inhalation suppresses the immediate reaginic bronchial reaction to inhaled antigen. It also prevents the late (4 to 6 hour) increase in airways obstruction in patients in which immediate and late reactions occur. Membrane stabilising activity appears to be fundamental to its action. Cromoglycate does not prevent the union of antigen and specific IgE on the surface of mast cells. It has been suggested that intracellular levels of cyclic AMP are raised by interfering with calcium transport across cell walls (Foreman and Garland, 1976). Cromoglycate can inhibit α-adrenoceptor agonist induced bronchospasm but is not itself an α-adrenoceptor antagonist. Phosphodiesterase inhibition has been demonstrated *in vitro*. Cromoglycate has no intrinsic bronchodilator action.

The *indications* for use include prophylaxis against acute and late reactions to antigen challenge and exercise induced asthma in allergic and non-allergic patients. It is also used in allergic rhinitis as 2% drops given 4 times daily (see chapter XI; sect. 2.4). Because response to cromoglycate cannot be predicted, a 1 to 2 month course is recommended for individual patients with troublesome symptoms not controlled by full doses of regular bronchodilator therapy. Cromoglycate is of particular value to the younger asthmatic patient although he must be old enough to be able to use the inhaler device effectively. An alternative method of drug delivery, especially for use in children, is a 'whistle'-type system. It has also been successfully administered to very young children by nebuliser and face mask (Hiller et al., 1977; Williams and Phelan, 1973).

Table III. Maintenance intravenous doses of aminophylline in adults (after Ogilvie, 1978)[1]

Patient characteristics	Infusion rate (mg/kg/hour)[2]
Age	
< 50 years	0.9
> 50 years	0.68
Chronic obstructive lung disease[3]	0.6-0.7
Congestive heart failure	0.4-0.68
Liver dysfunction	0.25-0.45
Liver dysfunction with	
serum bilirubin > 1.5mg/100ml	0.2
serum albumin < 2.9g/100ml	0.13
cardiac dysfunction	0.1-0.3

1 *Note:* To be modified in the presence of other factors which alter theophylline clearance (table II).

2 Following an initial loading dose (see text). Given in terms of aminophylline (theophylline = aminophylline x 0.85). Final dosage may be higher or lower and should be guided by serum theophylline estimation.

3 Depending on the presence and severity of cor pulmonale, dose reduction may be required.

Few significant adverse effects have been recognised, but troublesome hypersensitivity reactions have been reported (Rosenberg et al., 1978).

2.3.3 Corticosteroids

The principal corticosteroids and routes of administration used in therapy in respiratory disease are shown in table IV.

The *mode of action* of corticosteroids in asthma is not clear. Several possible mechanisms have been postulated (Shenfield et al., 1975b). The late type III immune response, but not the type I immediate immune response, is modified. Impaired cyclic-AMP responsiveness to β-adrenoceptor agonists, present in some patients with severe asthma, may be restored. Inhibition of prostaglandin synthesis (e.g. $F_{2\alpha}$) has also been suggested.

The indications for use are discussed in section 3.1.2. Maximum benefit is not obtained until 1 to 2 weeks after starting therapy. Maintenance therapy should be attained with the minimum effective dose (e.g. beclomethasone propionate inhaler 400µg/day; prednisolone 7.5mg/day).

The adverse effects of systemic corticosteroid therapy are discussed elsewhere (see chapter XVI; sect. 9.1). Aerosol administration of surface active topical corticosteroids such as beclomethasone dipropionate minimises adverse effects due to systemic steroids (for review, see Brogden et al., 1975). Some patients (about 10%) do develop a symptomatic oropharyngeal *Candida* infection at higher doses (BTTA, 1976a). This responds readily to oral antifungal medication and only rarely necessitates withdrawal of treatment. The transfer of patients previously dependent on oral corticosteroid therapy to aerosol therapy is potentially hazardous because adrenal responsiveness to infection, trauma or stress may be impaired. In some patients, withdrawal symptoms include tiredness, aches and pains but are self limiting and disappear after about 2 to 4 weeks. Replacement of systemic steroid treatment by an aerosol may unmask allergic rhinitis or eczema previously controlled by steroid. Decrease of oral prednisolone dosage should be by 1mg per week. Special care is required until adrenal responsiveness is assured (see section 3.1.2). It is very important that the patient be educated about the gradual withdrawal of oral therapy and proper use of the aerosol. The patient must also be told that the steroid is not just another bronchodilator and that it should be used regularly.

2.3.4 Bromhexine

Bromhexine, a mucolytic agent, is a synthetic derivative of vasicine. Sputum viscosity is reduced and sputum volume is increased in patients with chronic bronchitis (Hamilton et al., 1970). Unfortunately, these changes are often not associated with an improvement in the respiratory state of the patient, especially in far advanced disease. The recommended dose is 16mg, orally, 3 times daily.

In overcoming sputum retention adequate hydration of the patient and regular physiotherapy are important.

3. Bronchial Asthma

Bronchial asthma is characterised by variable dyspnoea due to widespread narrowing of the peripheral airways, which changes in severity over short periods of time either spontaneously, or as a result of treatment. For some years this simple classification has been used (Ciba Foundation, 1959):

a) *Extrinsic asthma* — which occurs in atopic individuals (e.g. in association with eczema, hay fever, a family history of allergy) who develop non-precipitating skin sensitising antibodies or reagins to external allergens. These patients have reactive skin prick tests. Extrinsic asthma also occurs in non-atopic subjects who have precipitating antibodies, e.g. farmer's lung.

b) *Intrinsic asthma* — which often starts later in life. Antigen-antibody reactions are almost certainly involved, but their nature is as yet unknown. Prick tests are negative, but sputum and/or blood eosinophilia is often present, and indeed blood eosinophilia values tend to be higher than those commonly found in extrinsic atopic asthma.

Recently, Turner-Warwick (1977) has suggested a further clinical classification based on the patterns of serial measures of airways obstruction. The suggested clinical patterns are the so-called irreversible asthmatics, with little day to day or hour to hour variation, the 'brittle' asthmatic and the 'morning dipper' in whom early morning peak flow measurements are very low (Clark and Hetzel, 1977; Hetzel et al., 1977a). These observations have therapeutic implications in helping the clinician to 'discard drugs which are clinically ineffective and to persist usefully with others which might otherwise be abandoned' (Turner-Warwick, 1977).

It should be noted that there is no evidence that asthma is a disease exclusively based on disordered allergic mechanisms (Woolcock, 1977; Turner-Warwick, 1978). Moreover, among patients in whom clear cut allergic mechanisms can be demonstrated, attacks of asthma may be triggered by non-antigenic stimuli.

The clinical features of asthma vary depending on the severity of the attack, which ranges from a mild, easily controlled state, through to chronic semi-invalidism and severe life threatening attacks (Turner-Warwick, 1977). During attacks, airways are narrowed by oedema of the mucosa and secretion of viscid mucus, as well as by some element of contraction of smooth muscle in the bronchial tree. The treatment of the outpatient with asthma of mild to moderate severity and the patient with severe acute asthma is discussed below.

Education of the medical profession in the management and monitoring of the asthmatic patient is the major problem in therapy. In almost no other field is the gap between diagnostic and therapeutic knowledge so great (Seaton, 1978a). Asthmatics like diabetics require frequent and informed assessment. Just as no clinician would manage a diabetic without the patient or himself measuring the urine and blood sugar levels, so frequent measurement by the patient (twice daily,

especially early morning) and/or doctor of peak flow rate and its degree of reversibility are mandatory. Cheap and easy to use flow meters[1] are now available and may be issued to patients. This allows continued reassessment of ventilatory function, even in symptom free periods (Palmer and Kelman, 1975).

3.1 'Outpatient' Asthma

All asthmatic patients who are seen for the first time require full clinical assessment. This includes a clinical history, to determine precipitating factors (e.g. allergens and exercise; Anderson et al., 1975), spirometry before and after a bronchodilator, skin tests, radiology of the chest and sinuses, and examination of blood and sputum for eosinophilia. Other causes of wheezing must be excluded, particularly the accidental inhalation of foreign bodies in children. 'All is not asthma that wheezes'.

3.1.1 Allergic Factors

In so-called extrinsic asthma, allergic factors may be demonstrated. This helps to identify those atopic individuals who might benefit from more detailed assessment of hypersensitivity factors. A reactive skin prick test only indicates that reaginic antibody to that antigen is present and does not necessarily mean that the allergen is the causative factor. Attacks occurring predominantly in the summer are most often due to grass pollen, whereas autumnal attacks are often precipitated by mould allergy. Other common allergens are feathers, animal fur and chemical substances encountered at work. House dust has long been known to be an important factor and the allergenicity has been shown to be due to the house dust mite, *Dermatophagoides pteronyssinus*. Allergens must be identified by a careful history and should be avoided and removed if possible. The Radio Allergo Sorbent Test (RAST) has been introduced recently. Specific reaginic IgE antibodies which mediate atopic allergy can be identified and this may be helpful in difficult cases.

Clinical improvement may occasionally be obtained by the use of hyposensitisation vaccines in the patient who has been *properly* selected for the

---

1   For example, Mini-Wright peak flow meter: Clement Clarke International Ltd, 15 Wigmore Street, London.

therapy. These vaccines are particularly useful for grass pollen and possibly also in house dust allergies now that the house dust vaccines contain mite extract but in general hyposensitisation therapy in asthma has been unrewarding. For example, no benefit was found in a controlled trial of tyrosine adsorbed *Dermatophagoides pteronyssinus* vaccine in 45 asthmatic subjects sensitive to house dust mite (Gaddie et al., 1976). Nor have any measures to reduce exposure to dust in the home environment been shown to be effective.

The use of cromoglycate (cromolyn) is discussed below and in section 2.3.2.

3.1.2 Control of Airways Calibre

The aim of drug treatment in asthma is to attain and maintain the best possible respiratory state for the patient and to keep him like that. Relapses are likely to occur unless therapy is prolonged and intense enough to achieve maximum pulmonary function (Rebuck, 1974; Gregg, 1977).

Bronchodilator Drugs: The milder the asthma, the more likely the airway obstruction will respond to bronchodilator drugs. The sympathomimetic bronchodilator drugs of choice are the β_2-adrenoceptor stimulant drugs (see section 1.2.2 and 2.3.1) — salbutamol (albuterol), or terbutaline which are most often given by aerosol inhalation, for relief of an acute attack or for prevention (Woolcock, 1977; Goldstein et al., 1978). Their bronchodilator activity is comparable with that of isoprenaline but of longer duration, and unlike isoprenaline, there is little or no cardiostimulant effect (β_1-adrenoceptor stimulation) with usual therapeutic doses (see table I).

The high mortality from asthma in young people in the 1960's in some countries was probably due, in part, to the overuse and inappropriate use of pressurised sympathomimetic aerosols (Heaf, 1970). Patients must therefore be *carefully* instructed in the use of the metered dose aerosol inhaler (see section 2.1.1).

Bronchodilators of the methylxanthine type (aminophylline, theophylline) have a different mode of action from the sympathomimetic amine type (fig. 1; section 2.3.1). Because of this they may augment the action of the sympathomimetic bronchodilator drugs (Wolfe et al., 1978). This forms the basis for the combined use of aminophylline and β_2-agonist bronchodilators in severe acute asthma (see section 3.2). It may also be the

reason for the former popularity of oral theophylline and ephedrine combined preparations, although these have not been shown by controlled clinical trials to be as effective as the β_2-agonist bronchodilator drugs. Given alone, oral theophylline can be effective, but dosage needs to be individualised because of wide interindividual variation in metabolism and factors which can alter theophylline clearance (see section 2.3.1; table II). In such individualised dosage, theophylline is at least as effective as cromoglycate in controlling symptoms of chronic asthma in children (Hambleton et al., 1977) and in protecting against exercise induced bronchospasm in children (Pollock et al., 1977). Theophylline may also be given as rectal suppositories (aminophylline), but absorption is erratic. Aerosol ipratropium bromide, an anticholinergic compound similar to atropine (see section 2.3.1), is also effective in reducing airways obstruction, but is less effective than salbutamol (Petrie and Palmer, 1975).

Sodium Cromoglycate (Cromolyn): Cromoglycate is a prophylactic treatment and has no place whatsoever in the treatment of acute airways obstruction (see section 2.3.2).

Not all asthmatic patients respond to cromoglycate and there is, as yet, no certain way of identifying those patients likely to benefit (Brogden et al., 1974). It should certainly be tried in all asthmatic patients, and particularly those patients with perennial episodic asthma, seasonal asthma or exercise induced asthma. Some asthmatics with non-reactive skin tests also respond. Cromoglycate is especially valuable in younger, rather than older patients. The requirements/or bronchodilators may be reduced. In patients on long term steroid therapy a gradual reduction in the steroid dose may be possible, although during acute exacerbations of airway obstruction the steroid dose *must* be increased. The advent of aerosol corticosteroids has however, largely replaced cromoglycate for this purpose (see below).

Cromoglycate is well tolerated and no important toxic effects have been described. Because of this and the difficulty in identifying patients who are likely to benefit, it is worthy of a trial in all patients who cannot be adequately controlled on bronchodilators alone. One spincap should be inhaled 3 to 4 times daily. This dosage may need to be doubled to achieve an adequate response in some patients. Since cromoglycate is a prophylactic agent, the patient should be in the best possible state before therapy is started. All patients should be instructed in the proper method of use of the inhaler device and the need to continue using the drug regularly (see section 2.1.1 and 2.3.2).

Corticosteroid Drugs: Asthmatics, particularly those with sputum eosinophilia, who develop persistent and severe airways obstruction and who are unimproved significantly after bronchodilators and sodium cromoglycate, should be considered for corticosteroid therapy.

A major advance in corticosteroid therapy in asthma has been provided by the development of aerosols of topically active corticosteroids such as beclomethasone dipropionate and betamethasone valerate (Brogden et al., 1975; Cooper and Grant, 1977; section 2.3.3). Like cromoglycate, they are prophylactic agents which must be used regularly; they are not suitable for treatment of an acute attack. The main value of topical corticosteroid aerosols is to avoid the systemic side effects of oral corticosteroids in those who require steroids for the first time (e.g. patients, especially children, not adequately controlled by full doses of a bronchodilator and cromoglycate) and also to allow worthwhile dose reductions to be made in patients already receiving oral maintenance doses of steroids. While it is possible to reduce the dose of systemic steroids in most patients, complete withdrawal is generally only possible in those on moderate oral doses (i.e. up to 8 to 10mg prednisolone daily). Oral steroids should be reduced gradually when the patient is well and under careful clinical and spirometric control. Dose reductions should be made every few days and each in the order of a 1mg reduction in daily prednisolone dosage. Such patients should carry a supply of oral steroids, a warning card and a written schedule of dosage and be educated to immediately resume oral steroids (30 to 40mg prednisolone on the first day) in the event of an attack, infection or stress (Editorial, 1977; Vaisrub, 1977).

The usual dosage is 400µg daily, but patients being transferred from relatively large doses of oral steroids (e.g. 16mg prednisolone or more daily), may respond better to 800µg daily. Instruction in the correct use of the inhaler is a prerequisite to successful therapy. For those patients who have difficulty in using the pressurised aerosol, a powder aerosol of beclomethasone dipropionate may be given from a low resistance inhaler (Carmichael et al., 1978). A nebuliser and face mask can be used to deliver the drug in very young children (Freigang, 1977).

As mentioned above the aerosol route is now preferred. However, if oral therapy is also required the maintenance dose should not exceed 7.5 to 10mg prednisolone (or equivalent) per day, as with this dose there is little hypothalamic-pituitary-adrenal axis suppression; but not all patients can be adequately controlled at this dosage. An alternative is the use of corticotrophin, either as the naturally occurring or synthetic compounds such as tetracosactrin (Drever et al., 1975). The disadvantage is that both must be given by injection, but long acting preparations are available and the synthetic preparation, tetracosactrin depot can be given in a dose of 0.5 to 1mg intramuscularly once or twice weekly.

3.1.3 Bronchial Secretion

Secretions may be particularly viscid and tenacious in the asthmatic. Physiotherapy and breathing exercises are extremely valuable in removing retained secretion and in children especially, breathing exercises may help to prevent the development of thoracic deformity. Bromhexine, by mouth, may also be of some value (see section 2.3.4 and 4.2.3).

3.1.4 Other Therapy

Antihistamines are seldom useful in asthmatics despite the airway obstruction being due, at least in part, to the liberation of histamine from sensitised mast cells. If anxiety is a prominent factor or there is nocturnal wheezing, the antihistamine, promethazine, may be useful. Hypnotherapy and autohypnosis have strong advocates but do not affect the underlying disturbance of pulmonary function. Such therapy can be a serious danger to seriously ill asthmatic patients. Antibacterial drugs should be reserved for the rare occasions when there is a risk of pneumonia, or in cases of prolonged wheezing or persistent pulmonary collapse, where secondary bacterial infection may occur.

3.2 Severe Acute Asthma

In an acute attack of asthma, if the airway obstruction is unresponsive to the patient's usual treatment a serious medical emergency exists and the patient should be admitted to hospital for accurate assessment (Rebuck and Read, 1971, 1972). The gravity of the condition of these

Table IV. Corticosteroid drugs used in asthma

Drug	Route	Administration and dose	Principal adverse effects/Notes[1]
Beclomethasone dipropionate	Aerosol	100µg (50µg/puff) 4 times daily	Surface active topical corticosteroid. Symptomatic oropharyngeal Candida infection most likely at doses > 800µg/day beclomethasone
Betamethasone valerate	Aerosol	200µg (100µg/puff) 4 times daily	Activity may diminish as obstruction increases. Adverse systemic effects of exogenous steroids reduced at therapeutic doses of aerosol. *Care* during changeover from oral to aerosol therapy; see text. Requirements for β_2 agonists may diminish
Prednisolone[2]	Oral	60mg daily reducing to 10mg daily or less as one or 3 divided doses	Prednisone is metabolised to biologically active form prednisolone during passage through liver. See steroid adverse effects (chapter XVI; sect. 9.1); multiple; clinically important especially above 10mg/day. Enzyme inducers (e.g. barbiturates, rifampicin) may reduce effectiveness. Substitution by aerosol steroid desirable but *Care!*
Hydrocortisone hemisuccinate	IV	3 to 4mg/kg loading dose followed by 3mg/kg 6-hourly	See steroid adverse effects (chapter XVI; sect. 9.1)
Tetracosactrin	IM	0.5 to 1.0mg alternate days; titrate to response	See steroid adverse effects (chapter XVI; sect. 9.1). Less growth stunting not proven. Allergic reactions hazardous. Supervision for at least 30 minutes essential

1　Use corticosteroids with care in patients with active or quiescent tuberculosis (see also section 11.4).
2　The clinical pharmacological properties of systemic corticosteroids are discussed in chapter XVI (section 9). Other preparations, without proven superiority, are available; e.g. methylprednisolone, triamcinolone, betamethasone, dexamethasone.

patients is frequently not recognised. Indeed many die suddenly and unexpectedly outside hospital.

The diagnosis of status asthmaticus is not difficult: the clinical state is characteristic. However, it is not as easy to assess the severity of the attack. Unequivocal central cyanosis, dyspnoea bad enough to interfere with speech, tachycardia greater than 130/minute when the arterial oxygen tension (P_aO_2) will be 6.63kPa (50mm Hg) or less, lung over-inflation, pulsus paradoxus or disturbances of consciousness all point to a severe attack. On arrival in hospital, arterial puncture and measurement of the arterial oxygen and carbon dioxide (P_aCO_2) tensions and pH are essential for accurate assessment. Hypoxaemia is invariably present, usually with hypocapnia or normocapnia (Editorial, 1976). In the most severe cases, hypercapnia develops and these patients may have a reduction in the arterial blood pH due to an uncompensated respiratory acidosis. Specialised intensive care units have some advantages for intensive monitoring but the *identification* of patients with severe acute asthma at particular risk of sudden death, even in hospital, is difficult. An indicator of high risk of sudden death may be the pattern of wide diurnal variation in peak flow rate referred to in section 3 (Hetzel et al., 1977b).

3.2.1 Intensive Treatment Regimen

Corticosteroid drugs in adequate doses are of great importance in the management of acute severe asthma. If the patient is to be sent to hospital from an outlying district when the journey is likely to take some time, 200mg hydrocortisone sodium succinate should be given intravenously before departure. In hospital, except in the mildest cases and in those who improve markedly soon after admission, hydrocortisone, 3mg/kg/body weight 6-hourly, should be given by continuous infusion after a loading dose of 3 to 4mg/kg hydrocortisone hemisuccinate intravenously (Collins et al., 1975; see table IV).

Potassium supplements should also be prescribed (Shenfield et al., 1975a), and at the same time, oral prednisolone (30 to 120mg/day) should be given. Aminophylline, or a selective β_2-adrenoceptor agonist bronchodilator, is infused continuously over each 8-hour period. Intensive bronchodilator therapy is given at the same time as corticosteroids because of the apparent delay in onset of effect of steroids (McFadden et al., 1976). However, intravenous loading dosage of aminophylline must be given slowly and take into account any previous β-adrenoceptor agonist and/or theophylline therapy, with continued intravenous dosage based on factors which can alter theophylline clearance (section 2.3.1, table II, III; Weinberger et al., 1976). Bronchodilators of the β_2-adrenoceptor agonist type are continued by mouth, aerosol or injection, or from the nebuliser of a positive pressure respirator (e.g. 0.5% salbutamol every 2 hours unless there is pneumothorax or pneumomediastinum).

In severe acute asthma, hypercapnia is of ominous prognostic significance (Editorial, 1976). Both hypoxic and ventilatory drives are depressed in asthma and oxygen flow rates *must* be low, delivering 24 to 28% oxygen, i.e. 1 litre/minute from an MC or Edinburgh mask. Vigorous physiotherapy is given because hypercapnia is often associated with retained secretion. If the hypercapnia persists despite physiotherapy the patient must be considered, at an early stage rather than when the clinical situation is desperate, for intermittent positive pressure ventilation, with tracheal intubation (with or without tracheostomy). The use of positive pressure ventilation should also be considered in patients who are exhausted, even if they are normocapnic. Rarely, bronchial lavage, with 1% sodium bicarbonate solution, may be helpful in removing the tenacious mucus plugs before assisted ventilation.

3.2.2 Ancillary Therapy

Patients with acute severe asthma should be given a broad spectrum antibacterial agent, such as ampicillin/amoxycillin or tetracycline, and the sputum cultured, since infection, which may not be evident clinically (especially in patients on corticosteroid therapy), is a common precipitating factor.

Usually admission to hospital allays anxiety. The doctor should always allay anxiety in such patients. Barbiturates, opiates and any other sedative are absolutely contraindicated, except in the presence of assisted ventilation. No sedative can be considered safe in the severely asthmatic patient.

3.2.3 Treatment Upon Recovery

Most patients with acute attacks of severe asthma respond to the initial measures and after recovery a decision has to be made about long term corticosteroid therapy. This depends on the degree of airways obstruction, and on the extent of its reversibility with sympathomimetic drugs, and on the frequency and severity of the previous attacks.

The dose of corticosteroid used in intensive treatment should be reduced by small amounts over a period of several days and if long term maintenance steroids are necessary and the oral route is selected, the dose should wherever possible, not be more than the equivalent of 8mg of prednisolone per day. Thereby the incidence of many of the complications of long term systemic steroid therapy will be reduced. Preferably, a corticosteroid aerosol such as beclomethasone dipropionate (see section 2.3.3 and 3.1.2) may be chosen instead of oral therapy since long term control of respiratory symptoms is possible without systemic steroid-type side effects. A few patients may, however, require maintenance doses of oral steroid in addition to the corticosteroid aerosol. Patients on long term oral steroid therapy must be warned to increase the dose of steroids in the event of exacerbation of airways obstruction, infection or an operation (see also section 3.1.2). Patients on oral steroids must not be given drugs which are potent hepatic microsomal enzyme inducers (e.g. phenobarbitone, phenytoin, rifampicin), because an increase in the rate of biotransformation of the corticosteroid and consequent reduction in therapeutic effect may occur (Brooks et al., 1972; (see also section 10.2).

4. Bronchitis

4.1 Acute Bronchitis

Acute bronchitis is often preceded by an upper respiratory tract infection. The principal pathogens are viral — influenza, parainfluenza, rhinovirus and respiratory syncytial virus. *Rickettsia burneti* and *Mycoplasma pneumoniae* also cause acute bronchitis. In children, acute bronchitis or bronchiolitis, most often due to infection with respiratory syncytial virus, is often especially severe. The children wheeze, patchy atelectasis may develop and bacterial pneumonias may follow.

The treatment of acute bronchitis is essentially symptomatic. The patient should remain in bed until afebrile. 4-hourly steam inhalations or a steam kettle, and a liberal fluid intake are a help to expectoration of tenacious sputum. For myalgic symptoms and headache, paracetamol (acetaminophen) or aspirin are helpful. Antibacterial agents are not indicated in general, except in patients who have a diminished resistance to infection (Taylor et al., 1977). However, if the sputum is persistently purulent and has been cultured, the appropriate agent should be prescribed (Petersdorf and Featherstone, 1978). *Mycoplasma pneumoniae*, ornithosis or psittacosis infections are treated with tetracycline.

The study by Stott and West (1976) is salutary. Patients in general practice with cough and purulent sputum, but without abnormal chest signs were given either doxycycline or placebo. There was no advantage in speed of recovery although the 'antibiotic' group had fewer infections over the next 6 months.

4.2 Chronic Bronchitis

This common disease usually starts as a simple chronic bronchitis as the result of bronchial irritation. It is characterised by productive cough with the expectoration of mucoid sputum, mostly in the morning. A stage of mucopurulent bronchitis may follow and a number of patients go on to develop chronic obstructive bronchitis where there is permanent structural damage to the bronchial tree following episodes of bronchial infection. In addition, these patients usually have emphysema — generally of the centrilobular type. The diffuse airways obstruction is due to bronchoconstriction, swelling and oedema of the mucous membranes, and an increase in the amount of viscidity of sputum leading to sputum retention. Bronchial narrowing also occurs because of the fibrotic changes in the airways following chronic infection and the loss of elastic retraction of the peripheral airways caused by emphysema.

The criteria which determine those individuals who progress beyond simple bronchitis are not clear. The incidence is higher in men and their wives in the lower social groups, and some patients have low levels of α_1-antitrypsin. Most patients who develop chronic bronchitis smoke

cigarettes or are exposed to dust at work. The treatment of the early stage of chronic bronchitis is the avoidance and removal of irritants, especially cigarette smoke. Later the treatment of infection becomes important.

Finger clubbing does not occur in uncomplicated chronic airways obstruction. When it does, more sinister pathology must be excluded, especially bronchial neoplasm, and more rarely bronchiectasis or pulmonary tuberculosis.

4.2.1 Infection

In health, the bronchial tree is sterile below the vocal chords but in mucopurulent bronchitis, pathogenic organisms, particularly *Streptococcus (Diplococcus) pneumoniae* and *Haemophilus influenzae,* are to be found. Flare up in infection by these organisms occurs, leading to purulent bronchitis, small areas of pneumonia and segmental collapse, most commonly following an upper respiratory tract infection.

The antibacterial agents of choice are the broad spectrum drugs, such as oral ampicillin, amoxycillin or tetracycline, because *Haemophilus influenzae* is relatively insensitive to penicillin G or V. Some strains of *Str. pneumoniae* are resistant to tetracycline, but this bacteriostatic drug is effective against *Haemophilus influenzae,* as is the trimethoprim-sulphamethoxazole bactericidal combination, co-trimoxazole.

Antibacterial therapy may be given on a long term prophylactic basis in those few patients who suffer frequent acute exacerbations during the winter, or short term to treat exacerbations as soon as they begin (Hughes, 1976; Petersdorf and Featherstone, 1978). Long term prophylactic therapy does not reduce the incidence of episodes of infective exacerbations in patients with chronic bronchitis, but may reduce their duration. All patients should be given a supply of a broad spectrum drug to take as soon as the sputum becomes purulent, or when a severe upper respiratory tract infection develops. If tetracycline or ampicillin/amoxycillin fails, co-trimoxazole can be used.

In acute exacerbations, therapy should be continued for 2 days following eradication of purulent sputum — a predetermined course should not be prescribed. The doses, mode of action and important adverse reactions of the principal antibacterial agents are shown in table V (Barza and Weinstein, 1976; Craig and Welling, 1977; Ogilvie, 1978; Bint and Reeves, 1978).

Table V. Dosage and main side effects of principal antibacterial drugs in pulmonary infections

Drug	Dose — 70kg man[1] (g/day)		First choice drug[2]	Main side effects
	oral	parenteral		
Benzylpenicillin (G)	—	0.6 to 6	*Str. pneumoniae*	Hypersensitivity reactions — skin rashes, asthma serum sickness syndrome, haemolytic anaemia;
Phenoxy-methylpenicillin (V)	1 to 2	—	*Str. pneumoniae*	superinfection; neurotoxicity (convulsions) at very high doses; care with sodium salts in cardiac failure
Cloxacillin	1.5 to 3	1 to 2	*Staphylococcus aureus* (penicillinase producing)	See above; food reduces absorption; administer before meals
Dicloxacillin Flucloxacillin	1.5 to 3	—		
Ampicillin	2 to 4	1 to 3	BS[3]	See above; skin rashes, bowel upset more common especially at higher doses; skin rash — almost invariable in glandular fever
Amoxycillin	0.75 to 1.5	—	BS	See above; skin rash and bowel upset less common than ampicillin. Absorption not affected by food
Cephaloridine	—	1 to 4 (im)	BS	See above; care with renal dysfunction (appendix E), dehydration, high dose diuretics, allergy
Cephalothin	—	1 to 4 (iv)	BS	See above; effects on kidney few
Cephalexin	2 to 4	—	BS	See above; effects on kidney few, if any
Cephazolin	—	1 to 2 (im, iv)	BS (useful biliary concentration)	See above; effects on kidney few
Co-trimoxazole (trimethoprim-sulphamethoxazole)	4 to 6 tabs	—	BS	Nausea, vomiting occasional; skin reactions; ? sulphonamide side effects; ? folate deficiency (see chapter XXIII; sect. 7.2, 8.5)

Tetracyclines	1 to 3	< 1	BS *Mycoplasma*	Contraindicated — pregnancy; childhood; renal dysfunction, except minocycline and doxycycline (chapter XXI; sect. 14.1.5). Gastrointestinal upset common; super-infection Staphylococcus, Proteus, Pseudomonas, Candida; staining of teeth and enamel hypoplasia (see chapter XIII; sect. 13.3); reduced absorption by interaction with Fe,Al,Ca Mg salts if given simultaneously (see chapter VIII; sect. 2.3.1)
Doxycycline	0.1 to 0.2	0.1 to 0.2	Ornithosis Psittacosis	
Erythromycin	1 to 2	0.3 to 0.6	Penicillin allergy	Gastrointestinal disturbance (mild) common; allergic reactions uncommon; cholestatic jaundice (estolate)
Lincomycin	1.5 to 2	25mg/kg (iv)	Penicillin allergy	Diarrhoea; skin rash; cardiopulmonary arrest after rapid intravenous infusion
Gentamicin	—	5mg/kg (im or iv)	*Klebsiella pneumoniae*	Care with renal dysfunction (modify dosage; appendix E), high dose diuretics (see chapter XXI; sect. 14.1); vestibular function disturbances (see chapter XI; sect. 7.1)
Tobramycin	—	3mg/kg (im or iv)	Alternative to gentamicin	See gentamicin
Fusidic acid	1.5	< 1.5	—	Mild gastrointestinal upset; rashes occasional
Metronidazole	1.2 to 1.5	15mg/kg (iv), then 7.5mg/kg	Anaerobic infections (as in lung abscess)	Peripheral neuropathy; enhances response to warfarin (chapter XXIII, sect. 3.2.5)

1 For dosage in infants and children see chapter IV; table IX.
2 Ampicillin, amoxycillin, tetracycline and co-trimoxazole are for routine use in acute exacerbations of chronic bronchitis (see section 4.2.1). Depending on the nature and cause of the infection these and the other agents can be considered in pneumonia but the initial treatment in most pneumonias is benzylpenicillin (see section 6).
3 Broad spectrum (see also appendix D).

4.2.2 Airways Obstruction

The relief of airways obstruction in chronic obstructive bronchitis by β_2-adrenoceptor agonist drugs or by methylxanthine derivatives is much less effective than in the treatment of asthma, because of the many different factors concerned in the increased airways resistance in chronic obstructive bronchitis. There is some evidence that anticholinergic drugs such as ipratropium bromide (section 2.3.1) by aerosol may be effective (Petrie and Palmer, 1975). But in general, bronchitics respond less well to bronchodilators than asthmatics because their airways obstruction is less reversible. Corticosteroids are only indicated if they bring about an increase of FEV_1 of greater than 10%, and this usually occurs only in patients who have sputum eosinophilia.

4.2.3 Sputum Retention

Sputum retention plays an important part in the airways obstruction. Expectoration of sputum is helped by a liberal intake of fluid, steam inhalations, physiotherapy and postural drainage. Mucolytic agents may sometimes be helpful in aiding expectoration by reducing sputum viscidity (see section 2.3.4).

4.2.4 Cough

A non productive cough which is troublesome, especially at nights, may be eased by an antitussive; linctus codeine (5ml) in hot water (Hughes, 1978).

4.2.5 Treatment of Pulmonary Heart Failure

Pulmonary heart failure is right heart failure secondary to disordered function of the lungs including its blood vessels. Pulmonary hypertension occurs which eventually leads to failure of the right ventricle. There is hypoxaemia often with hypercapnia. Chronic hypoxaemia leads to secondary polycythaemia. Treatment is with rest, relief of hypoxaemia by controlled oxygen therapy, often subsequently given long term and continued in the patient's home (Leggett and Flenley, 1977), and diuretics. Digoxin is not particularly helpful unless there is a concomitant arrhythmia, such as rapid ($>120/min$) atrial fibrillation which is unusual, or congestive cardiac failure, in the presence of cor pulmonale (Doherty et al., 1977). Venesection, the avoidance of sedatives, the prompt treatment of respiratory infection are further measures (O'Donnell, 1976). Concurrent pulmonary thromboembolism is not infrequent and admission to hospital for initiation of long term anticoagulant therapy is then indicated.

4.2.6 Ancillary Measures

Many respiratory cripples benefit from domiciliary oxygen which allows them some mobility within the home (Leggett and Flenley, 1977). Vaccination against influenza is recommended. Smoking is forbidden.

5. Respiratory Failure

The early recognition of respiratory failure depends upon the measurement of the blood gas tensions (Sykes et al., 1976). There are two types:

Type 1: Hypoxaemia without carbon dioxide retention.

Type 2: Hypoxaemia with carbon dioxide retention (ventilatory failure).

5.1 Hypoxaemic Respiratory Failure

In hypoxaemic normocapnic respiratory failure (type 1) the most frequent functional abnormality is an increase in the ventilation-perfusion imbalance in the lung. The level of alveolar ventilation is normal or even increased. The common causes are pneumonia, pulmonary oedema, bronchial asthma, pulmonary embolism, cardiogenic shock, postoperative complications especially after abdominal operations, and trauma to the chest wall.

The management of type 1 respiratory failure is to treat the underlying condition and to raise the concentration of inspired oxygen to achieve P_aO_2 levels of 7.95kPa (60mm Hg); a flow rate of 8 litres/minute by MC or Polymask. There is no danger of precipitating carbon dioxide retention with these concentrations of inspired oxygen in type 1 respiratory failure.

5.2 Hypoxaemic Hypercapnic Respiratory Failure

In type 2 hypoxaemic hypercapnic (ventilatory) respiratory failure there is a reduction in the level of alveolar ventilation which leads to carbon dioxide retention. There is usually, in addition, ventilation-perfusion imbalance. This type of respiratory failure occurs in chronic bronchitis and emphysema, very severe asthma, following

Table VI. Dosage and main side-effects of respiratory stimulants (see section 5.2.2)

Drug	Dose — 70kg man		Main side effects
	intravenous (mg)	infusion (mg/min)	
Doxapram	—	2	Similar as below (? incidence less); warmth during infusion; cardiovascular stimulation
Nikethamide	50 to 250 (2 to 10ml)	20	Twitching, convulsions, anxiety, sweating at higher
Ethamivan	150 to 400	20	doses; skin irritation, gut upset

resuscitation from cardiac arrest, drug overdosage, polyneuropathy and cervical cord injuries. The injudicious use of sedatives, even so-called 'safe sedatives' such as nitrazepam or flurazepam, may be a further precipitating factor in patients with severe chronic obstructive bronchitis (Gaddie et al., 1972).

5.2.1 Diagnosis

Hypoxaemia may be diagnosed by the presence of cyanosis but this will not be detectable clinically until there has been a considerable fall in P_aO_2 (less than 7.95kPa or 60mm Hg). The classical signs of hypercapnia only appear when the P_aCO_2 is much raised. Then, flapping hand tremor, muscular twitching, overfilling of retinal veins and papilloedema may be evident.

Ventilatory failure often occurs in patients with chronic obstructive bronchitis following a severe upper respiratory tract infection. The patient becomes exhausted by coughing in his attempt to clear the airways. The level of alveolar ventilation falls and the carbon dioxide tension rises.

5.2.2 Management

The aim of management of the ventilatory failure is to improve alveolar ventilation by treatment of the infection and removal of the retained secretions as already discussed (section 4.2.3). These measures will contribute towards the relief of the severe hypoxaemia and hypercapnia (Sykes et al., 1976).

Oxygen Therapy: It is essential to control oxygen therapy with extreme care if hypercapnia is present because the P_aCO_2 may rise acutely. The lower the initial P_aO_2 the more likely is a steep rise in P_aCO_2 to occur. Masks of the high air flow oxygen enrichment principle (HAFOE) are used as their design ensures dilution of the inspired oxygen with atmospheric air. At 1 litre/minute the Edinburgh mask or Ventimask deliver inspired oxygen concentrations of approximately 24%. If the P_aCO_2 does not increase at this flow rate, or increases by only a small amount, say 5mm Hg, and the conscious level of the patient is not depressed, the flow rate may be increased gradually to achieve an inspired oxygen concentration of 28%, and after further careful assessment, up to 35%. The low flow rates of oxygen must be delivered continuously, as severe hypoxaemia may develop if oxygen is given intermittently. This is because during uncontrolled oxygen treatment the alveolar ventilation is depressed and a rise in the P_aCO_2 occurs. If the inspired oxygen is now discontinued the alveolar oxygen tension falls, because the alveolar CO_2 has risen and the hypoxaemia is intensified.

It may not be possible to achieve a P_aO_2 level of at least 7kPa (50mm Hg) without precipitating high P_aCO_2 levels. In such cases a lower PaO_2 level must be accepted, even as low as 30mm Hg. Below this level tissue damage is likely.

Occasionally, to relieve hypoxaemia, the concentration of oxygen must be at least 60% (Campbell and Minty, 1976).

Role of Respiratory Stimulants: In some patients with ventilatory respiratory failure the level of alveolar ventilation may be temporarily increased by the use of respiratory stimulant drugs (Franz, 1975; table VI). These drugs may increase the sensitivity of the respiratory centre to carbon dioxide, or they may act less specifically as central nervous system stimulants. Whatever their precise mode of action, they allow, through their arousal properties, greater co-operation by the patient with the physiotherapist in removing retained secretions.

They are suitable *only* for short term use during acute episodes of deterioration and are particularly indicated in patients with severe carbon dioxide retention and when ventilation has been depressed by sedatives or drug overdose. The therapeutic and toxic doses are close and there is interindividual variation in response. Intermittent intravenous doses are preferred because the drugs are short acting. The respiratory stimulant drugs must be used with great care in patients with epilepsy, coronary artery disease, hypertension or in patients who are on monoamine oxidase inhibitor drugs.

Assisted Ventilation: Assisted positive pressure ventilation may be used in suitable patients. This tides the patient over acute episodes until the precipitating factors — infection, sputum retention, airway obstruction and central nervous system depression are treated. Assisted ventilation is indicated only in patients whose respiratory function was adequate for a reasonable quality of life before the acute episode. The respiratory cripple in his terminal illness should not be ventilated because it may be impossible to wean him off the respirator.

6. Pneumonia

There are two groups of patients who develop pneumonia (Crofton and Douglas, 1975):

1) Those whose respiratory tract was previously healthy. These patients develop specific pneumonias due to bacterial, viral or rickettsial infections.

2) Those who have pre-existing lung disease. There is a severe breakdown of the normal defence mechanism of the lung and mixed organisms of low virulence assume pathogenic importance. These are the secondary pneumonias. Common examples are bronchopneumonia occurring in patients with chronic obstructive bronchitis and pneumonia occurring during a state of unconsciousness.

6.1 Specific Pneumonias

The most important bacterial pneumonias are due to infection with *Streptococcus (Diplococcus) pneumoniae, Streptococcus pyogenes,* or *Klebsiella pneumoniae. Str. pneumoniae* is by far the most common. Viral or rickettsial pneumonias may be suspected clinically, but these can only be confirmed when the results of laboratory tests are available.

6.1.1 Initial Treatment

When a patient is considered to have pneumonia the sputum should be stained. This enables the most likely organism to be identified. Culture of the sputum and assessment of the sensitivity of the organisms to antibacterial agents is necessary and blood is taken for culture, full blood count and measurement of the blood gas tensions.

Antibacterial therapy will be started before laboratory results are available. As most primary bacterial pneumonias are due to *Str. pneumoniae* an intramuscular injection of a long acting penicillin such as the sodium salt of penicillin G (benzylpenicillin), procaine penicillin and benethamine penicillin G is given from a single dose vial. Sputum levels bactericidal to the pneumococci are achieved for at least 3 days. At the same time the patient is started on oral penicillin V (phenoxymethylpenicillin) at a dosage given in table V.

In most cases there is a rapid fall in fever, followed by a gradual resolution of the physical signs over a few days. If this does not occur the pneumonia may be due to organisms which are insensitive to the agent first used, or the diagnosis is not correct. The patient may have a condition which simulates pneumonia, such as pulmonary infarction, or the pneumonia may be secondary to some underlying pathology, such as carinoma of the bronchus.

6.1.2 Staphylococcal Pneumonia

Staphylococcal pneumonia may be a primary infection. It may also not infrequently occur when there is an outbreak of influenza. The staphylococci are usually sensitive to penicillin G and V. However, in some instances, particularly in debilitated, hospitalised patients a penicillinase producing staphylococcus which is insensitive to penicillin G or V may be implicated. In such cases cloxacillin, dicloxacillin or flucloxacillin, or fusidic acid (table V) or methicillin by injection should be prescribed, in addition to the initial injection of depot penicillin described above. This regimen should also be used in any patient who is severely ill with pneumonia where the possibility exists that the infection may be due to a penicillinase producing staphylococcus. When the results of the sputum culture and the sensitivity of the organism are known, cloxacillin may safely be withdrawn if the organism is sensitive to penicillin G or V.

6.1.3 Klebsiella Pneumonia

Klebsiella pneumoniae is a rare cause of severe pneumonia. Early diagnosis is essential, based on sputum culture. Treatment should begin with gentamicin or with streptomycin intramuscularly combined with oral tetracycline.

6.1.4 Viral and Rickettsial Pneumonias

The viral and rickettsial pneumonias have specific clinical features which may help to differentiate them from the bacterial pneumonias. Oxytetracycline is the drug of choice for infection due to *Mycoplasma pneumoniae,* infection with *Rickettsia burneti* or Q fever, or infection with the psittacosis or ornithosis group of viruses. Erythromycin can be used as an alternative in *Mycoplasma pneumoniae* infection.

6.2 Secondary Pneumonias

In secondary pneumonias there is frequently airway obstruction and considerable impairment of bronchial drainage because of the common coexistence of chronic lung disease. Sputum retention plays an important part in the symptomatology. The treatment has been described in section 4.2.3.

The infection is assumed to be due to *Str. pneumoniae* and/or *Haemophilus influenzae,* and treatment should begin with a broad spectrum antibacterial agent such as ampicillin or amoxycillin, oxytetracycline or co-trimoxazole by mouth (table V). If improvement does not occur within 36 to 48 hours the agent to which the organisms are sensitive as shown by sputum culture should be given (see chapter XXVII, sect. 2; 3; appendix D).

Secondary pneumonias may follow infection of the upper respiratory tract and it is important to examine the sinuses, tonsils and teeth for sepsis. If repeated pneumonias occur in the same patient a barium examination of the upper gastrointestinal tract may reveal an abnormality such as achalasia. Secondary pneumonias may also develop as a postoperative complication, particularly following abdominal operations. The incidence can be reduced by stopping smoking, and vigorous physiotherapy before and after the operation.

There is no indication for prophylactic antibacterial agents in such patients.

6.3 Symptomatic Treatment

This applies to both specific and secondary pneumonias. Pleuritic pain is treated with kaolin poultices and analgesics. An antitussive such as linctus codeine (5ml) in hot water, every 3 to 4 hours, is helpful to suppress a troublesome nonproductive cough. The treatment of hypoxaemia has been discussed in section 5.2.2. If infection precipitates cardiac failure, as it may do in the aged, or in patients with pre-existing heart disease, this must be treated.

Before antibacterial therapy was available there were numerous complications of bacterial pneumonia. Nowadays complications are unusual, *provided* the patient has been treated with adequate dosage of the appropriate antibacterial agent for an adequate time.

The most common cause of a persistent mild fever in patients with pneumococcal pneumonia is a postpneumonic effusion characterised by stony dullness to percussion. Treatment consists of aspiration. Lung abscesses may complicate staphylococcal or *Klebsiella pneumoniae* or rarely, *Str. pneumoniae* infections. Most resolve with intensive antibacterial treatment, physiotherapy and postural drainage but in some, surgical resection is necessary.

A further cause of persistent pyrexia when the patient appears to have recovered is 'drug fever' which develops during the course of the antibacterial therapy. The fever falls when the drug is withdrawn. This complication occurs more frequently than is recognised.

Radiological abnormalities take longer to resolve than the clinical signs and may persist for 3 to 4 weeks. In any instance where there is delayed radiological resolution further investigation is mandatory to exclude underlying pathology such as a bronchial neoplasm. If there is a persistence of the symptomatology and clinical signs, less common pathogens must be excluded such as *Mycobacterium tuberculosis.*

7. Bronchiectasis and Cystic Fibrosis

The term bronchiectasis indicates that there are dilated bronchi, usually as a result of bronchial occlusion, either intrabronchial or extrabronchial, leading to collapse of the lung and subsequent infection. It is demonstrated by radiology of the chest. Bronchography is justified only if the patient is a candidate for surgical treatment. Bronchiectasis may occur in chronic lung disease, such as obstructive bronchitis, or it may complicate cystic fibrosis.

Cystic fibrosis is an inherited disorder (Mendelian recessive) in which there is pancreatic insufficiency and an increased secretion of highly viscid bronchial mucus. The movement by ciliary motion of the mucus blanket lining the respiratory tract is impaired. Stagnation of the mucus occurs in the smaller bronchi and bronchioles and secondary infection readily occurs, which may be followed by bronchiectasis (Wood et al., 1976).

Bronchiectasis has become less frequent since antibacterial agents have become widely available. Prevention depends upon ensuring that the bronchial infections are thoroughly treated, that upper respiratory sepsis is treated and that areas of collapse in the lung are recognised and re-expansion established. Collapse of the lung is particularly likely to occur in children. Management of established bronchiectasis is medical or surgical.

7.1 Medical Treatment

The medical treatment of bronchiectasis consists of intensive measures to bring up retained secretions and intensive chemotherapy. Postural drainage is usually taught in hospital but the patient must continue to carry this out at home, particularly first thing in the morning. Regular sputum samples should be cultured. The most important pathogens are *Haemophilus influenzae, Staphylococcus aureus* and *Streptococcus pneumoniae* and *Pseudomonas aeruginosa*. Occasionally, anaerobes complicate the infection. All patients should be given a supply of broad spectrum antibacterial drugs at home and instructed to start a course as soon as an infection threatens. Chemotherapy is not indicated when the sputum is mucoid. Smoking should be forbidden. Immunisation against influenza should be offered each autumn. Infection in the sinuses and teeth should be eradicated. Other associated conditions should be considered; e.g. hypogammaglobulinaemia.

In addition to energetic treatment for retained bronchial secretions any associated reversible airways obstruction should be treated (see section 2.3). It is particularly important to educate the parent of the child with cystic fibrosis about the importance and techniques of postural drainage and intensive physiotherapy and about antibiotic, dietary and bronchodilator regimens. With such measures there has been some improvement in life expectancy, although most patients die before the age of 40 years (Wood et al., 1976).

Most patients with cystic fibrosis (95%) also have pancreatic insufficiency and malabsorption (see chapter XIX; sect. 9.4). The diet should be high in calories, high in protein, but restricted in fat and starch. Pancreatin, the contents of 6 capsules (i.e. 6g) spinkled on the food daily, should be given with vitamin supplements, particularly vitamins A and D.

7.2 Surgical Treatment

Surgical treatment is indicated when the bronchiectatic changes are localised and when medical treatment has failed to control the symptoms.

8. Pulmonary Tuberculosis

Pulmonary tuberculosis must be diagnosed early, as prompt and effective treatment reduces the danger to the patient and the community. The presenting features classically include weight loss, night sweats, cough, sputum and haemoptysis, but atypical presentations are undoubtedly more common than in the past, e.g. unexplained fever or weight loss in the elderly.

Although patients can usually be managed outside hospital, particularly if the home circumstances are satisfactory, it is sometimes preferable to start treatment in hospital particularly if any difficulties exist such as severe infection, poor social circumstances, poor co-operation, personal home contacts with reduced immunity, resistant bacteria, hypersensitivity to drugs or associated disease of other organs. The aim of treatment is to cure the patient with the drug regimen selected for an initial intensive phase of treatment and to prevent relapse by an adequate continuation phase of treatment (Aquinas, 1975; Seaton, 1978b). This means prescribing a regimen adequate for the disease and acceptable to the patient and making sure that the patient takes it to the end of the course. In tuberculosis, more than any other disease, lack of co-operation of the patient is the principal cause of treatment failure with regimens that are otherwise 100% effective.

8.1 Drugs Used in the Treatment of Tuberculosis

The principal drugs are shown in table VII. Some of the relevant clinical pharmacological properties of the three first line drugs are discussed below.

8.1.1 Isoniazid

Isoniazid is the hydrazide of isonicotinic acid. It is invaluable as a first line drug in combination therapy with rifampicin and ethambutol. Its use as a single agent in chemoprophylaxis, particularly in older patients, is being re-evaluated because of appreciable morbidity and even mortality due to a viral hepatitis-like reaction (see section 8.6).

Isoniazid is well and rapidly absorbed (peak concentration attained in 1 to 2 hours) after oral dosing on an empty stomach. Concurrent rifampicin does not interfere with absorption of either drug. The distribution of isoniazid is extensive and it persists in caseous material. Metabolism (mainly acetylation which is genetically controlled, and hydrolysis) is extensive and 75 to 95 % of an oral dose is excreted in the urine in 24 hours, principally as acetylisoniazid and as isonicotinic acid. Patients who are 'slow' acetylators (chapter I, sect. 4.2; VII, sect. 4.2) have higher concentrations of active isoniazid and this appears to influence the occurrence of some adverse reactions (see below). On the other hand, 'rapid' acetylators respond less well to a once weekly, but not to a twice weekly, bactericidal and sterilising regimen (Ellard and Gammon, 1977; Girling et al., 1977).

The recommended dose of isoniazid is 3 to 5mg/kg/day but children tolerate much higher doses (up to 20mg/kg/day). Twice weekly and in slow acetylators, once weekly, regimens (usually combined with pyridoxine to reduce or reverse neurological and haematological adverse reactions) are also used (table VII). The dose should be reduced or therapy stopped (see section 8.6) in hepatic insufficiency because hepatic metabolism is impaired and the rate of elimination is prolonged. In severe renal insufficiency, monitoring of serum levels is indicated, particularly in patients who are slow acetylators (see appendix E).

Adverse reactions to isoniazid are infrequent if the above recommendations are followed and the benefits outweigh the risks of therapy. However, at higher dose levels (more than 6mg/kg/day) neurological reactions, particularly in slow acetylators, occur which may necessitate cessation of therapy (table VII). In addition, isoniazid induced hepatic injury is now well recognised. The aetiology of this viral hepatitis-like reaction is not understood. Metabolic products of isoniazid, immune reactions, previous liver disease, alcohol consumption, increasing age (more than 35 years), and slow acetylator status in early onset hepatic reactions and concurrent antituberculosis therapy (see chapter XIX; sect. 14.6.4), but not dose, are implicated (Grondhagen-Riska et al., 1978; Kopanoff et al., 1978).

The onset of the reaction is variable (1 week to many months) and the severity varies from a mild reversible reaction (elevation of transaminases in 10 to 20 % of patients) to severe hepatitis with considerable morbidity and mortality (see also section 8.6).

Certain neoplasms are induced by high doses of isoniazid in mice but there is no evidence of a carcinogenic effect in humans (Glassroth et al., 1977; Stott et al., 1976).

8.1.2 Rifampicin

Rifampicin is now established as a potent first line antituberculosis agent. It is a semisynthetic antibiotic and its clinical pharmacokinetics have been reviewed recently (Acocella, 1978).

Absorption is practically complete and rapid (peak levels attained with 2 to 4 hours) after dosage on an empty stomach. The presence of food causes marked variations in serum concentrations. Concurrent isoniazid (as in combined formulations) does not affect absorption. Rifampicin is subject to hepatic 'first-pass' metabolism and transferred to bile. At doses above 300 to 450mg the excretory capacity of the liver is saturated. Increases in the dose of rifampicin above these levels lead to relatively higher serum concentrations. Protein binding of rifampicin is to albumin (weak, reversible, approximately 80 %). Distribution is extensive and patients should be warned about probable red-brown colouration of body fluids (e.g. sweat, tears, urine, faeces, etc). The metabolism of rifampicin is principally by desacetylation. The metabolite is active and accounts for most of the biliary antibacterial activity. Rifampicin also stimulates its own metabolism as well as being a potent inducer of hepatic drug metabolising enzymes of certain other drugs; leading to clinically important adverse drug interactions (table VII). Rifampicin does not affect isoniazid acetylation. The excretion of rifampicin is both biliary and renal and modifications in dosage are re-

Table VII. Principal antituberculosis drugs[1]

Drugs[2]	Dose (daily)	Notes	Main adverse effects
Isoniazid	300 to 400mg 5mg/kg	Take 30 mins before food for peak levels. Bactericidal at higher doses. Active against intracellular organisms	Side effects few < 350mg/day. Hypersensitivity reactions (rare) — fever, rash, lymphadenopathy. Slow acetylators (chapter I; sect. 4.2) have greater incidence, especially peripheral neuropathy (pyridoxine responsive). Optic neuritis is rare. Occasional disturbance of liver function (see chapter XIX; sect. 14.6.4); also ataxia, euphoria, convulsions, tinnitus, restlessness, insomnia and muscle twitching. Occasional hyperglycaemia, gynaecomastia, pellagra-like state, dryness of mouth, epigastric discomfort, urinary retention
		Reduce dose in slow acetylators (chapter I; sect. 4.2)	
		Dosage in twice weekly intermittent therapy is 15mg/kg plus 10mg pyridoxine	Caution in convulsive disorders, renal and hepatic dysfunction. Contraindicated in pregnancy and manic states. Interaction with phenytoin in slow acetylators (chapter XXV; sect. 3.1)
			Rapid acetylators respond less well to once-weekly treatment, but not to a twice weekly bactericidal and sterilising regimen (Ellard and Gammon, 1977; Girling et al., 1977)
Rifampicin	450 to 600mg 10 to 20mg/kg	Take 30 mins before food. Bactericidal. If concurrent PAS essential see below	Side effects include gastrointestinal disturbance and, during initial stages of treatment, minor elevation of bilirubin and SGPT which does not preclude continuation therapy because usually reversible, transient; also orange/red urine and occasionally sputum and sweat. Erythematous reactions. Nervous system reactions including fatigue, headache, ataxia, etc
		Reduce dose in hepatobiliary disease (< 10mg/kg; see chapter XIX; sect. 1.4.4)	Few cases of purpura reported usually with intermittent therapy (see chapter VII; sect. 4.1.2). 'Flu' syndrome, less often shortness of breath, rarely acute haemolytic anaemia and renal failure with intermittent regimens, usually high doses (Girling, 1977) Enzyme induction by rifampicin reduces effects of concurrent therapy. Clinically important interactions include decreased effects of oral contraceptives, oral anticoagulant and hypoglycaemic agents (Zilly et al., 1977; see chapter XV, sect. 13.5; XVI, sect. 3.3.5; XXIII, sect. 3.2.5)
		Dosage in twice weekly intermittent therapy reduced to less than 15mg/kg	Caution in elderly, malnourished and young. Contraindicated in pregnancy (Steen and Stainton-Ellis, 1977).

Drug	Dose		
Ethambutol	15 to 25mg/kg	Absorption not significantly reduced by food. Bacteriostatic Reduce dose in renal failure (appendix E)	Side effects include optic neuritis in 1% of patients at higher doses (25mg/kg). Usually reversible. Evident as impaired visual acuity and changes in colour vision. Ophthalmological examination desirable prior to therapy but regular checks only required if on prolonged higher doses Also paraesthesiae, numbness of extremities, dermatitis, pruritus, GI symptoms, headaches, confusion, increased urate levels. Caution in renal insufficiency or pregnancy. Contraindicated in optic neuritis
Para amino-salicylic acid	10 to 12g	Well absorbed. Take with food. If concurrent rifampicin essential (not desirable), separate doses of each by 8 hours to ensure absorption, unless known that PAS preparation does not contain bentonite (see chapter I; sect. 3.1.2). No longer first choice drug Reduce dose in renal failure (appendix E)	Side effects include bitter taste, nausea, vomiting, diarrhoea, jaundice, headaches, skin rashes and hypersensitivity reactions. Also glandular fever like syndrome, reversible, Paul Bunnell test negative. Rarely goitre, myxoedema, psychosis, encephalitis, hypokalaemia, blood dyscrasia. Caution in renal insufficiency
Strepto-mycin	1g 30mg/kg in children	Intramuscular. Bactericidal in combination with pyrazinamide. Being superceded as first choice drug but remains in some short course regimens, and in developing countries Reduce dose in those > 40 years and in impaired renal function (appendix E)	Side effects are those of aminoglycosides. Include ototoxicity (vestibular > auditory) — chapter XI, sect. 7.1; renal damage; skin rashes; neuromuscular blockade (see chapter XXV; sect. 15.9); drug fever (5%). Blood levels < 2µg/ml 24 hours post dose associated with fewer adverse effects

1   Other drugs include pyrazinamide, prothionamide, ethionamide, thiacetazone and capreomycin.
2   Used in combination because of ready development of resistance to a single drug (see also section 8.2, 8.3). Exception is isoniazid for chemoprophylaxis in those with inactive disease.

quired in patients with hepatobiliary or hepato-renal insufficiency (table VII; appendix E).

Adverse reactions to rifampicin are infrequent, particularly if attention is paid to recommended dosage levels, dosage intervals, associated disease and concurrent drug therapy (Girling, 1977; also table VII). Interpretation of cause and effect relationships (e.g. hepatic dysfunction) is complicated by the fact that rifampicin is usually combined with isoniazid, which has important adverse reactions of its own.

8.1.3 Ethambutol

Ethambutol is well absorbed after oral administration (75 to 80%). Hepatic metabolism is less than with isoniazid or rifampicin and 50% of an oral dose is recovered unchanged in the urine. In renal insufficiency the dose must therefore be modified (table VII; appendix E). Adverse reactions are infrequent at recommended doses. The most important reaction is the occurrence of optic neuritis (see also table VII).

8.2 Initial Intensive Treatment

Once specimens have been obtained for culture, treatment should be started with 3 drugs to which the organism is likely to be sensitive. Triple therapy is more effective, reduces infectivity and the development of resistant strains of *Mycobacterium tuberculosis*. The three drugs of first choice are isoniazid, rifampicin and ethambutol or pyrazinamide and should be taken before food (table VII). The choice of initial drug may be influenced by other factors such as cost, availability, convenience and toxicity and in such circumstances alternative drugs may be used (table VII). The initial triple therapy regimen should be continued for at least 8 weeks and usually until the sensitivities of the organism have been established (8 to 12 weeks). During this initial phase of treatment, extrapulmonary sites should be excluded and contacts traced. The importance of adequate instruction and surveillance in tablet taking can not be overemphasised (Seaton, 1978b).

8.3 Continuation Treatment

Once the sensitivities of the organism have been established, usually within 8 to 12 weeks, continuation therapy is maintained with the 2 most appropriate drugs until the completion of the recommended 9 month course (BTTA, 1976b).

The usual drugs included in the continuation regimen are rifampicin and isoniazid. If for reason of cost or toxicity one of these first-line drugs can not be used a reserve drug (table VII) should be substituted and the course of therapy extended to 18 months. Short supervised bactericidal and sterilising courses of 6 months therapy might reduce further the duration of therapy and so increase compliance (Hong Kong Chest Service, 1978; Third East African/MRC Study, 1978).

During continuation therapy patients should be reviewed at 1 month intervals to monitor clinical and bacteriological progress and to assess compliance with drug therapy. In patients who are suspected of irregular tablet taking such as vagrants or alcoholics, a *supervised* daily or intermittent (twice weekly) regimen should be introduced, where a clinic or practice nurse watches while the medication is administered. In an intermittent regimen the dosage of both drugs must be different from that used in a daily regimen. Dosage of rifampicin is reduced to below 15mg/kg twice weekly since a high incidence of adverse reactions occurs with dosage at or above 15mg/kg twice or once weekly (Girling, 1977). The companion drug isoniazid can be tolerated in a relatively high dose (15mg/kg twice weekly), but pyridoxine 10mg needs to be given with each dose to prevent isoniazid induced peripheral neuropathy. If streptomycin is used, dosage can only be increased slightly in some patients (from 0.75 to 1g twice weekly).

8.4 Treatment of Relapse

Patients who relapse should be carefully reassessed and in some cases it may be necessary to stop the antituberculosis chemotherapy for some time to assess the sensitivities of the organism. The optimum drug therapy should be established as the careless addition of yet another agent may lead to the development of further resistance to drugs. A relapse should be treated in the same manner as for a newly diagnosed case — initially with a combination of at least 3 drugs, followed by a continuation phase with 2 drugs.

8.5 Surveillance

Until recently the general policy has been to follow up patients who have had an episode of tuberculosis at 6- to 12-monthly intervals after ceasing treatment because of the frequent recurrence of relapses. However, the introduction of newer drugs and intensive treatment regimens has led to a re-evaluation of this policy. Indeed in some countries, such as the United Kingdom, patients need not be kept under long term surveillance provided that no doubt exists that adequate chemotherapy has been prescribed and taken. If long term follow up is not to be undertaken it is essential that both the patient and the general practitioner must have clear instructions to report any symptoms suggestive of a relapse. There are important exceptions to this policy and these must be stressed. Supervision is essential in patients with 'high-risk factors' and in whom doubt exists about the compliance of the patient with adequate chemotherapy. The 'high-risk factors' include unco-operative patients (including those with personality disorders), alcoholism, diabetes mellitus, treatment with corticosteroids, partial gastrectomy, chronic debilitating disease and large residual 'opened healed cavities' (BTTA, 1975).

8.6 Management of Contacts

Close contacts of a new patient (e.g. those living in the same house) should be investigated by interview, clinical examination, chest x-ray and by tuberculin testing. If there is evidence of primary infection, the patient should be treated (see section 8.2). If the chest x-ray is normal and the tuberculin test is negative, BCG vaccination should be given (Seaton, 1978b).

If the chest x-ray is normal and the tuberculin test is positive, indicating that a preclinical infection has occurred, a 12 month course of isoniazid alone (3 to 5mg/kg body weight/day) *may* be given (see also table VII). However, there is increasing awareness of the risks of long term therapy with isoniazid, particularly in inducing liver disease, often indistinguishable from viral hepatitis (see section 8.1.1; chapter XIX, sect. 14.6.4) and the indications for chemoprophylaxis with isoniazid are being re-evaluated (Kopanoff et al., 1978). At present, chemoprophylaxis is still recommended for children (Rapp et al., 1978; Weg, 1976). In older patients (over 35 years of age), many authorities consider that isoniazid chemoprophylaxis should be restricted to patients with chest x-ray findings consistent with stable tuberculous lesions, or recently infected, or receiving prolonged corticosteroid or immunosuppressive therapy, or with a diagnosis of leukaemia, Hodgkin's disease, diabetes mellitus, silicosis or

gastrectomy (Mitchell et al., 1978). Biochemical evidence of hepatic dysfunction should be sought at regular intervals because clinical surveillance is inadequate (Byrd et al., 1977). Mitchell et al. (1976) believe that therapy with isoniazid should be stopped as soon as hepatic dysfunction is detected, particularly in older patients, unless the patient is critically ill with active, or suspected tuberculosis.

Immigrants from countries where tuberculosis is prevalent pose special problems. For example, the policy with regard to immigrants arriving in the United Kingdom has been summarised recently (BTTA, 1978a). New arrivals should be sought out, tuberculin tested, and positive reactors x-rayed. All those who are tuberculin negative should be vaccinated with BCG whatever their age. Positive reactors should undergo annual radiography and be encouraged to report symptoms early. For both new and established immigrants with strongly positive tuberculin reactions chemoprophylaxis with isoniazid is suggested. All children of immigrants, should be given BCG at birth and tuberculin tested when they start school.

Comparison of the tine and Mantoux tuberculin tests favours the latter (BTTA, 1978b), although the finding has been challenged (Caplin et al., 1978).

9. Sarcoidosis

The clinical course of sarcoidosis follows 2 principal patterns — an acute or a chronic form. The acute form of the disease usually occurs in young women and presents with erythema nodosum, hilar lymphadenopathy and only occasionally affects other organs such as the eyes (uveal tract), nerves, salivary glands, bones, spleen and liver. The Kveim test is usually positive in acute cases and biopsy of tissue (e.g. scalene node) may show non-caseating granulomata. In the acute form of the disease the prognosis is usually good and pulmonary changes generally disappear within a year. No specific treatment is needed usually.

The chronic or progressive form of sarcoidosis has a more insidious onset. The initial symptoms are of fever, cough and breathlessness. Involvement of other organs leading, for instance, to pulmonary fibrosis with prominent diffusion defect, or to nephrocalcinosis following prolonged hypercalcaemia may occur. The prognosis of chronic sarcoidosis is not as favourable as the acute form.

Symptomatic treatment and rest are necessary, particularly in the acute form of sarcoidosis. Anti-inflammatory analgesics such as aspirin, phenylbutazone or indomethacin are useful for treating the pain associated with erythema nodosum and musculoskeletal discomfort. There is some controversy about the indications for corticosteroids in the acute phase of the illness as it is often self limiting. Nevertheless, steroids are indicated if uveitis, nervous sytem involvement or hypercalcaemia develop. In chronic sarcoidosis, corticosteroids are recommended when the following indications are present: (1) active ocular sarcoidosis; (2) persisting pulmonary symptoms and signs without improvement over a 3 month period; (3) persistent hypercalcaemia or hypercalciuria; (4) involvement of the central nervous system; (5) myocardial sarcoidosis; (6) disfiguring facial lesions; (7) persistent hepatomegaly or splenomegaly; and (8) lacrimal and salivary gland enlargement. Treatment can usually be withdrawn gradually after 6 months. Oxyphenbutazone, phenylbutazone and chloroquine are also used in the treatment of chronic sarcoidosis, but they are less effective than corticosteroids, and chloroquine is more toxic (see Mitchell and Scadding, 1974).

10. Use of Drugs in the Presence of Associated Respiratory Disease

Drugs used in the treatment of non-respiratory disease may have pulmonary effects and adversely affect lung function in the patient with respiratory disease. These should be predictable as rational drug therapy depends on a knowledge of the spectrum of activity of the drugs prescribed. Alternatively, the respiratory disease itself or drugs being used to treat respiratory illnesses may modify the response to other drugs or alter their pharmacokinetic behaviour in the body.

10.1 Problems due to Mode of Action of Drugs

The pharmacological factors and drugs which influence bronchial secretions and airways calibre have been outlined in section 1 and include cholinergic and adrenergic mechanisms. β-Adrenoceptor blocking drugs such as propranolol are widely used in the treatment of cardiac arrhythmias, angina pectoris and hypertension. They may precipitate or intensify airways obstruction in susceptible subjects. Any selective β_1-adrenoceptor blocker must be used with care in asthmatics, as their effect on lung function is unpredictable (Skinner et al., 1975) and bronchoconstriction may still occur (McDevitt, 1978). Indeed, it is advisable to give a test dose and measure the effect on peak flow. Some advocate that a selective β_1-blocker only be used in asthmatics or bronchitics if it can be used in low dosage and that such use be combined with full dosage of a β_2-agonist bronchodilator (Formgren, 1976). Prostaglandin $F_{2\alpha}$ is increasingly used to induce labour and abortion, and this, too, may precipitate airways obstruction in susceptible subjects (see chapter XV; sect. 11). So too may aspirin and other analgesics in aspirin sensitive asthmatics (see section 11.3).

Cholinergic (parasympathomimetic) drugs are not widely used in general clinical practice, although carbachol is used to stimulate bladder emptying. In susceptible subjects, such drugs may precipitate airways obstruction and increase tracheobronchial secretions. Many commonly used drugs — atropine, tricyclic antidepressants, antipsychotics, some antihistamines and anti-Parkinsonian drugs — have anticholinergic (parasympathomimetic blocking) properties. The effects on airways calibre and bronchial secretions are variable and also depend on other factors (see sections 1.1 and 1.2).

Certain drugs given for respiratory illnesses may also cause problems if given concurrently with other agents (Palmer and Paterson, 1975). The action of adrenergic neurone blocking antihypertensive drugs such as bethanidine, guanethidine and debrisoquine may be antagonised if ephedrine, or nasal decongestants or proprietary common cold or cough cures containing drugs such as pseudoephedrine, phenylephrine or phenylpropanolamine are prescribed concurrently (see chapter XVIII; sect. 10.1.1). These indirectly acting sympathomimetic drugs may also interact with the monoamine oxidase inhibitor drugs, leading to an hypertensive crisis (chapter VIII; sect. 3).

10.2 Altered Response due to Changed Tissue Sensitivity or Pharmacokinetics

Pulmonary disease or secondary complications may modify the response to drugs or affect their pharmacokinetic behaviour in the body. Patients with pulmonary heart disease, particularly when accompanied by hypoxia, are extremely sensitive to the action of digitalis (Hargreave, 1965; Baum et al., 1959). These patients are seriously ill and are already prone to arrhythmias which may be more easily provoked by digitalis. Although digitalis toxicity in pulmonary heart disease occurs at lower than usual serum levels (Paciaroni et al., 1974) and a reduced distribution volume and renal clearance of digoxin have been demonstrated in cor pulmonale (Doherty et al., 1977; du Souich et al., 1978), control of the ventilatory dysfunction appears of as much importance as digitalis dosage in this situation. Smaller doses of digoxin are recommended except when it is necessary to control the ventricular response with atrial fibrillation (Doherty et al., 1977).

The hypoxic state may also alter hepatic microsomal drug metabolising enzyme activity (see section 1.5). While the clinical significance of this observation is not clear, it may explain the increased metabolic clearance rate of cortisol noted by some workers in steroid treated patients suffering a severe attack of asthma (Dwyer et al., 1967). This finding drew attention to the need for very large doses of corticosteroids to achieve adequate plasma cortisol levels and a good clinical response in a severe attack of asthma in steroid treated patients (see section 3.2). Similarly, phenobarbitone can, by its own hepatic microsomal enzyme inducing activity, contribute to an increased metabolic clearance rate of cortisol in steroid treated asthmatics, with consequent reduction in therapeutic efficacy of the steroid. This effect seems to be most likely in patients treated with larger doses of phenobarbitone, e.g. 120mg daily (Brooks et al., 1972).

Severe chronic airways obstruction causes a marked decrease in metabolic clearance of theophylline (up to 75 % but usually around 50 %) and theophylline toxicity has occurred with usual dose regimens in patients with cor pulmonale. Clearance of theophylline is also reduced in patients with acute pulmonary oedema (du Souich et al., 1978; Ogilvie, 1978). Dosage of theophylline should be modified accordingly (see section 2.3.1; table II). On the other hand, increased clearance of dicloxacillin and methicillin due to increased renal tubular secretion, has been noted in cystic fibrosis (Jusko et al., 1975; Yaffe et al., 1977). Dosage should be adjusted according to the increases in clearance demonstrated (around 25 %

for methicillin and 200 % for dicloxacillin); either by an increased dosage or more frequent dose interval.

10.3 Oxygen Therapy and Sedatives

The dangers of oxygen therapy, and of sedative, narcotic and antianxiety drugs in patients with hypercapnia have been emphasised (see section 5.2). In addition, hyperbaric oxygen therapy (at 2 atmospheres) may lead to convulsions, and when oxygen is given at atmospheric pressure at concentrations of 80 % for more than 12 hours it may be followed by adverse pulmonary effects including intra-alveolar oedema and atelectasis (Grant, 1978).

11. Drug Induced Lung Disease

Adverse pulmonary reactions to drugs are relatively uncommon, but should be considered when the aetiology of the respiratory illness is not clear. These reactions may closely resemble respiratory disease due to other causes and the diagnosis may be missed unless the possibility of drug induced disease is considered. There is little value in memorising long lists of drugs which at some time have been incriminated, although not always conclusively proven, as a cause of adverse pulmonary reactions. It is often difficult to prove that any one drug is responsible, because the majority of patients with significant illnesses tend to be given several drugs (see chapter VIII).

The nature of the pulmonary reactions varies and ranges from generalised reactions, asthma, to pulmonary infiltrates (table VIII). Differing mechanisms appear to be involved in the causation of drug induced lung disease (Cole, 1977). In most cases, a correct clinical diagnosis can be made if the clinician is aware of the drugs which can possibly be implicated and recognises the characteristic clinical and radiological features in each case. Withdrawal of the implicated drug or drugs will result in resolution of the lung disease in some cases, but in certain others steroids may also be necessary.

Recognition of drug induced lung disease may prevent further deterioration of lung function in those cases in which irreversible pathological changes have already occurred (Davies, 1969, 1976).

Table VIII. Pulmonary reactions associated with drugs (see also section 11)

Drug[1]	Generalised reactions: SLE[2]	Generalised reactions: polyarteritis	Pulmonary eosinophilia	Pulmonary alveolitis/fibrosis	Asthma ? mechanism	Asthma ? type I allergy	Asthma ? type III allergy	Mediastinal and generalised lymphadenopathy	Pulmonary oedema, acute
Antimicrobial agents									
Cephalosporins						+	+		
Erythromycin						+			
Griseofulvin	+	+				+	+		
Isoniazid	++		+						
Neomycin						+			
Nitrofurantoin			++	+					
PAS	+		+					+	
Penicillins	+	+	+			+	+		
Streptomycin	+		+			+	+		
Sulphonamides	+	+	+				+		
Tetracyclines	+	+				+			
Analgesics/anti-inflammatory agents									
Aspirin			+		++[3]				
Gold salts	+	+		+					
Phenylbutazone	+	+						+	
Opiates									+
Antineoplastic drugs									
Bleomycin				+					
Busulphan		+		+					
Chlorambucil				+					
Cyclophosphamide				+					
Melphalan				+					
Methotrexate			+	+					
Mitomycin C				+					

Table VIII. (continued)

Drug[1]	Generalised reactions: SLE[2]	Generalised reactions: polyarteritis	Pulmonary eosinophilia	Pulmonary alveolitis/fibrosis	Asthma ? mechanism	Asthma ? type I allergy	Asthma ? type III allergy	Mediastinal and generalised lymphadenopathy	Pulmonary oedema, acute
Cardiovascular drugs									
β-Adrenoceptor blocking drugs					+[4]				
Hydrallazine	++	+							
Methyldopa	+								
Procainamide	++								
Quinidine	+	+							
Anticonvulsants									
Carbamazepine	+		+						
Phenytoin	++	+						+	
Psychotherapeutic drugs									
MAO inhibitors					+				
Phenothiazines	+	+							
Imipramine			+						
Miscellaneous									
Iodides		+			+				
Iron dextran						+			
Methysergide	+			+					
Pituitary snuff				+		+	+		
Sulphasalazine			+	+					
Thiouracils	+	+					+	.	
Vaccines						+			
Parasympathomimetics					+[4]				
Paraffin, liquid				+?					

1 ++ = Most commonly implicated drug.
2 See also chapter XXII, sect. 14.1
3 The aspirin sensitive patient also reacts to other analgesics (see section 11.3).
4 Due to pharmacological mechanism (see section 10). With 'cardioselective' agents, more easily reversible.

11.1 Generalised Reactions

11.1.1 Systemic Lupus Erythematosus Like Reaction

A generalised reaction similar to systemic lupus erythematosus (SLE) with involvement of the lung has been reported following the use of many drugs (table VIII). The mechanism of these reactions may be immunological or pharmacological as some drugs produce symptoms rather than antinuclear antibodies and *vice versa*. Genetic susceptibility is important (chapt. XXII; sect. 14.1).

Drugs may be directly causative — in one series up to 20 % of cases of SLE were considered to be drug induced (Siegel et al., 1967). Alternatively, the drugs may uncover a latent tendency to develop SLE — a family history of rheumatic disease is common and the reaction occurs principally in females (Alarcon-Segovia et al., 1965). The mechanisms underlying the reaction resemble late hypersensitivity reaction (type III — Arthus). The symptoms and signs are variable and simulate a wide variety of respiratory illnesses such as pleurisy, sometimes with effusion, pericarditis, pneumonia, acute pulmonary oedema or infarction. Sometimes, onset of pleural disease may occur before any other manifestations of the lupus syndrome become apparent. An improvement usually occurs when the drug is withdrawn, or occasionally when steroid therapy is given, but occasionally may persist as in the case of hydrallazine and phenytoin (Alarcon-Segovia, 1976; see also chapter XXII, sect. 14.1).

11.1.2 Lung Involvement and Features of Polyarteritis

Generalised reactions with lung involvement and features of polyarteritis, have also been reported following the use of drugs (table VIII). The symptoms include asthmatic reactions, lesions simulating pulmonary infarction, abscess or pneumonia. The evidence of a drug cause-effect relationship is usually circumstantial rather than conclusive, but in some instances rechallenge with the drug has led to exacerbations. The mechanism of this reaction is also thought to be late hypersensitivity type reaction (type III — Arthus).

11.2 Reactions Within the Lung

11.2.1 Pulmonary Eosinophilia

Drugs associated with the development of pulmonary eosinophilia are shown in table VIII.

The most common cause is nitrofurantoin therapy (Israel and Diamond, 1962; Sovijarvi et al., 1977), but this condition has also followed PAS, sulphonamides and sulphasalazine. The general symptoms include cough, fever and severe dyspnoea often without wheeze.

The mechanism of the reaction is not known. The symptoms usually improve when the drug is withdrawn but may reappear after rechallenge of the drug.

11.2.2 Pulmonary Alveolitis and Fibrosis

Intra-alveolar fibrinous oedema which occasionally progresses to pulmonary fibrosis has sometimes occurred following the use of busulphan for myeloid leukaemia (Heard and Cooke, 1968). Other cytotoxic drugs such as cyclophosphamide, chlorambucil, methotrexate, mitomycin C, melphalan and bleomycin have also caused this reaction. Interstitial pneumonitis which can progress to pulmonary alveolitis and fibrosis is the major dose limiting toxic reaction to bleomycin, although some cases have occurred at low doses. Close observation for early signs and symptoms is imperative (Luna et al., 1972; Brown et al., 1978). A similar condition had been previously noted with the ganglion blocking drugs hexamethonium (which is chemically related to busulphan), pentolinium and mecamylamine. Gold therapy has also been associated with development of pulmonary fibrosis, initial symptoms presenting as dyspnoea and dry cough (Geddes and Brostoff, 1976).

The mechanism underlying the development of these features is not clear. Withdrawal of the drug and administration of corticosteroids has been effective in controlling progression of the disease in some cases.

Another well recognised reaction is the pleuropulmonary fibrosis which develops particularly in males following methysergide therapy for migraine; withdrawal of the drug usually brings about marked improvement (Graham, 1967; see chapter XXV; sect. 7.2).

Chronic pulmonary fibrosis may occasionally develop insidiously following prolonged nitrofurantoin therapy, although pulmonary eosinophilia is the most common respiratory reaction to this drug. In contrast to this acute reaction (see above section 11.2.1) the chronic condition may only partially resolve on withdrawal of the drug and permanent fibrosis may result (Israel et al., 1973).

11.3 Asthma

Asthma is the most common drug induced lung disease, with aspirin the most frequently implicated precipitating factor (Samter and Beers, 1967, 1968). The underlying mechanism is not known but an immunological basis is unlikely. The patients are usually non-atopic individuals who often suffer from rhinitis and nasal polyps and who develop asthma between the age of 30 and 40 years; weeks to years before aspirin sensitivity is first recognised. Thereafter, the patient experiences persistent wheezing with severe, even life threatening attacks of asthma after aspirin ingestion. Aspirin induced asthma should be treated promptly with steroids but caution is advised since such patients may also react to intravenous steroids (Partridge and Gibson, 1978). There is probably no safe analgesic for the aspirin sensitive asthmatic patient, as wheezing and sometimes severe increased obstruction to airflow may develop after ingestion of other analgesics such as indomethacin, mefenamic and flufenamic acid, phenylbutazone, ibuprofen, naproxen, diclofenac, paracetamol (acetaminophen), amidopyrine, propoxyphene and pentazocine (Szczeklik et al., 1977; Smith, 1971). Aspirin sensitive asthmatic patients are intolerant of the food colouring dye tartrazine.

Many other drugs have been associated with the development of asthma (table VIII). There are 2 main clinical patterns which appear to be induced by other drugs. The clinical features are thought to reflect the underlying mechanisms — either immediate hypersensitivity reactions (type I: reagin mediated) such as generalised anaphylactic shock or urticaria, or late hypersensitivity reactions (type III: precipitating antibody mediated) such as a drug induced serum sickness syndrome with symptoms which include fever, arthralgia, urticaria, maculopapular rash and lymphadenopathy (see Cole, 1977 and chapter VII; sect. 4.1.2).

Drugs such as β-adrenoceptor blocking agents, certain prostaglandins and cholinergic drugs may exacerbate asthma by pharmacological mechanisms (section 10.1). Ventilatory failure may occur when sedatives or narcotics are given to patients with hypercapnia (section 5.2).

11.4 Miscellaneous Types of Lung Disease

Contrast media have also been reported to cause pulmonary reactions. These may be of different types and are related either to the iodine content (acute reactions; iodism; polyarteritis nodosa) or to the lipid content of the media. Lipoid pneumonias may also occur after lymphangiography or after the aspiration of liquid paraffin or lipid containing medication, particularly in elderly patients.

Many other drugs have been reported to cause lung disease, but in particular the oral contraceptives have been associated with the development of pulmonary thromboembolism (see chapter XV; sect. 13.12). Appetite suppressants such as aminorex have been associated with the development of pulmonary hypertension (Follath et al., 1971). The mechanism of the pleural involvement associated with the oculomucocutaneous syndrome of practolol is unknown. A further presentation of drug induced lung disease is the development of prominent mediastinal and hilar lymphadenopathy, which may simulate lymphoma or glandular fever (table VIII).

Lung superinfections, particularly with fungi, may occur in patients on long term antibacterial, corticosteroid or immunosuppressive therapy. Corticosteroids do not appear to predispose to development of tuberculosis in asthmatic patients (Schatz et al., 1976) but may increase the risk of reactivation of tuberculosis in those with impaired cell mediated immunity (Sahn and Lakshminarayan, 1976). Haemorrhage into lung cysts may follow the use of anticoagulant drugs.

Further Reading

Clark, T.J.H. and Godfrey, S.: Asthma (Chapman and Hall, London 1977).
Crofton, J. and Douglas, A.: Respiratory Diseases, 2nd ed. (Blackwell, Oxford 1975).
Fletcher, C.M.; Peto, R.; Tinker, C. and Speizer, F.E.: The natural history of Chronic Bronchitis and Emphysema (Oxford University Press, Oxford 1976).
Murray, J.: The Normal Lung (Saunders, London 1977).
Sykes, M.K.; McNicol, M.W. and Campbell, E.J.M.: Respiratory Failure (Blackwell, Oxford 1976).
Turner-Warwick, M.: Immunology of the Lung (Arnold, London 1978).

References

Acocella, G.: Clinical pharmacokinetics of rifampicin. Clinical Pharmacokinetics 3: 108 (1978).
Alarcon-Segovia, D.: Drug-induced antinuclear antibodies and lupus syndromes. Drugs 12: 69 (1976).
Alarcon-Segovia, D.; Worthington, J.W.; Ward, L.E. and Wakim, K.G.: Lupus diathesis and the hydralazine syn-

drome. New England Journal of Medicine 272: 462 (1965).

Alquist, R.P.: A study of adrenotropic receptors. American Journal of Physiology 153: 586 (1948).

Anderson, S.D.; Silverman, M.; Konig, P. and Godfrey, S.: Exercise-induced asthma. British Journal of Diseases of the Chest 69: 1 (1975).

Aquinas, M.: Drug treatment of pulmonary tuberculosis. Drugs 9: 364 (1975).

Austen, K.F. and Orange, R.P.: Bronchial asthma: The possible role of the chemical mediators of immediate hypersensitivity in the pathogenesis of subacute chronic disease. American Review of Respiratory Disease 112: 423 (1975).

Avery, G.S.: Salbutamol: A review. Drugs 1: 274 (1971).

Bacon, C.J.: Nebulised salbutamol in treatment of acute asthma in children. Lancet 1: 158 (1978).

Barza, M. and Weinstein, L.: Pharmacokinetics of the penicillins in man. Clinical Pharmacokinetics 1: 297 (1976).

Bateman, S.M.; Pidgeon, J.; Spiro, S.G. and Johnson, A.J.: The metabolic effects of inhaled salbutamol. British Journal of Clinical Pharmacology 5: 127 (1978).

Baum, G.L.; Dick, M.M.; Blum, A.; Kaupe, A. and Carballo, J.: Factors involved in digitalis sensitivity in chronic pulmonary insufficiency. American Heart Journal 57: 460 (1959).

Bint, A.J. and Reeves, D.S.: A guide to new antibiotics. British Journal of Hospital Medicine 19: 335 (1978).

Blackwell, E.W.; Briant, R.H.; Conolly, M.E.; Davies, D.S. and Dollery, C.T.: Metabolism of isoprenaline after aerosol and direct intrabronchial administration in man and dog. British Journal of Pharmacology 50: 587 (1974).

Briant, R.H.; Blackwell, E.W.; Williams, F.M.; Davies, D.S. and Dollery, C.T.: The metabolism of sympathomimetic bronchodilator drugs by the isolated perfused dog lung. Xenobiotica 3: 787 (1973).

British Thoracic and Tuberculosis Association: An assessment of the need for follow-up of patients with pulmonary tuberculosis adequately treated by chemotherapy. British Medical Journal 2: 28 (1975).

British Thoracic and Tuberculosis Association: A controlled trial of inhaled corticosteroids in patients receiving prednisone tablets for asthma. British Journal of Diseases of the Chest 70: 95 (1976a).

British Thoracic and Tuberculosis Association: Short-course chemotherapy in pulmonary tuberculosis. Lancet 2: 1102 (1976b).

British Thoracic and Tuberculosis Association: Tuberculosis among immigrants in Britain. British Medical Journal 1: 1038 (1978a).

British Thoracic and Tuberculosis Association: Comparison of the tine and Mantoux tuberculin test. British Medical Journal 1: 1451 (1978b).

Brogden, R.N.; Speight, T.M. and Avery, G.S.: Sodium cromoglycate: A review of its mode of action, pharmacology, therapeutic efficacy and use. Drugs 7: 164 (1974).

Brogden, R.N.; Pinder, R.M.; Sawyer, Phyllis, R.; Speight, T.M. and Avery, G.S.: Beclomethasone dipropionate inhaler: A review of its pharmacology, therapeutic action and adverse effects. I Asthma, II Allergic rhinitis and other conditions. Drugs 10: 166 (1975).

Brooks, S.M.; Werke, E.E.; Ackerman, S.J.; Sullivan, Irene and Thrasher, Katherine: Adverse effects of phenobarbital on corticosteroid metabolism in asthmatics. New England Journal of Medicine 286: 1125 (1972).

Brown, W.G.; Hasan, F.M. and Barbee, R.A.: Reversibility of severe bleomycin-induced pneumonitis. Journal of the American Medical Association 239: 2012 (1978).

Byrd, R.B.; Horn, B.R.; Griggs, G.A. and Solomon, D.A.: Isoniazid chemoprophylaxis. Archives of Internal Medicine 137: 1130 (1977).

Campbell, E.J.M. and Minty, K.B.: Controlled oxygen therapy at 60% concentration. Lancet 1: 1199 (1976).

Caplin, M.; Capel, L.H.; Riddell, R.; Steel, S. and McCarthy, O.R.: Comparison of the tine and Mantoux tuberculin tests. British Medical Journal 2: 54 (1978).

Carmichael, J.; Duncan, D. and Crompton, G.K.: Beclomethasone dipropionate dry-powder inhalation compared with conventional aerosol in chronic asthma. British Medical Journal 2: 657 (1978).

Charman, J.; Lopez-Vidriero, M.T.; Keal, E. and Reid, L.: The physical and chemical properties of bronchial secretion. British Journal of Diseases of the Chest 68: 215 (1972).

Ciba Foundation and Guest Symposium: Terminology, definitions and classification of chronic pulmonary emphysema and related conditions. Thorax 14: 286 (1959).

Clark, T.J.H. and Hetzel, M.R.: Diurnal variation of asthma. British Journal of Diseases of the Chest 71: 87 (1977).

Cole, P.: Drug-induced lung disease. Drugs 13: 422 (1977).

Collier, J.G. and Dornhorst, A.C.: Evidence for two different types of β-receptors in man. Nature 223: 1283 (1969).

Collins, J.A.; McDevitt, D.G.; Shanks, R.G. and Swanton, J.G.: The cardiotoxicity of isoprenaline during hypoxia. British Journal of Pharmacology 36: 35 (1969).

Collins, J.V.; Clark, T.J.H.; Brown, D. and Townsend, J.: The use of corticosteroids in the treatment of acute asthma. Quarterly Journal of Medicine 44: 259 (1975).

Cooper, E.J. and Grant, I.W.B.: Beclomethasone dipropionate aerosol in treatment of chronic asthma. Quarterly Journal of Medicine 46: 295 (1977).

Cotes, J.E.: Control of respiration: in Lung Function: Assessment and Application in Medicine, p.260 (Blackwell Scientific Publications, Oxford 1975).

Craig, W.A. and Welling, D.G.: Protein-binding of antimicrobials: clinical pharmacokinetics and therapeutic implications. Clinical Pharmacokinetics 2: 252 (1977).

Crofton, J. and Douglas, A.: Pneumonia: in Crofton and Douglas (Ed) Respiratory Diseases, p.128 (Blackwell Scientific Publications, Oxford 1975).

Cuthbert, M.F.: Prostaglandins and asthma. British Journal of Clinical Pharmacology 2: 293 (1975).

Davies, P.D.B.: Drug-induced lung disease. British Journal of Diseases of the Chest 63: 57 (1969).

Davies, P.: Drug-induced lung disease. Medicine (Lond.) 22: 1074 (1976).

Doherty, J.E.; Kane, J.J.; Phillips, J.R. and Adamson, J.S.: Digitalis in pulmonary heart disease (cor pulmonale). Drugs 13: 142 (1977).

Drever, J.C.; Malone, D.N.S.; Grant, I.W.B.; Douglas, D.M. and Lutz, W.: Corticotrophin after corticosteroids in children with asthma and growth retardation. British Journal of Diseases of the Chest 69: 188 (1975).

Dulfano, M.J.; Adler, K. and Philippoft, W.: Sputum viscoelasticity in chronic bronchitis. American Review of Respiratory Disease 104: 88 (1971).

du Souich, P.; McLean, A.J.; Lalka, D.; Erill, S. and Gibaldi, M.: Pulmonary disease and drug kinetics. Clinical Pharmacokinetics 3: 257 (1978).

Dwyer, J.; Lazarus, L. and Hickie, J.B.: A study of cortisol metabolism in patients with chronic asthma. Australasian Annals of Medicine 16: 297 (1967).

Editorial: Oxygen therapy in asthma. British Medical Journal 1: 609 (1976).

Editorial: Deaths from asthma in children on aerosol corticosteroids. British Medical Journal 1: 117 (1977).

Editorial: Circulating prostacyclin. Lancet 1: 21 (1978).

Ellard, G.A. and Gammon, P.T.: Acetylator phenotyping of tuberculosis patients using matrix isoniazid or sulphadimidine and its prognostic significance for treatment with several intermittent isoniazid-containing regimens. British Journal of Clinical Pharmacology 4: 5 (1977).

Enna, S.J. and Schanker, L.S.: Absorption of drugs from the rat lung. American Journal of Physiology 223: 1227 (1972).

Finkel, M.J.: Salbutamol: Lack of evidence of tumour induction in man. British Medical Journal 1: 649 (1978).

Follath, F.; Burkart, F. and Schweizer, W.: Drug-induced pulmonary hypertension? British Medical Journal 1: 265 (1971).

Foreman, J.C. and Garland, L.G.: Cromoglycate and other antiallergic drugs: a possible mechanism of action. British Medical Journal 1: 820 (1976).

Formgren, H.: The effect of metoprolol and practolol on lung function and blood pressure in hypertensive asthmatics. British Journal of Clinical Pharmacology 3: 1007 (1976).

Franz, D.N.: Central nervous system stimulants: in Goodman and Gilman (Ed) The Pharmacological Basis of Therapeutics, p.359 (Macmillan, New York 1975).

Freigang, B.: New method of beclomethasone aerosol administration to children under 4 years of age. Canadian Medical Association Journal 117: 1308 (1977).

Gaddie, J.; Legge, J.S. and Palmer, K.N.V.: The effect of disodium cromoglycate on pulmonary function in asthma. British Journal of Diseases of the Chest 66: 254 (1972b).

Gaddie, J.; Palmer, K.N.V.; Petrie, J.C. and Wood, R.A.: Effect of nitrazepam in chronic obstructive bronchitis. British Medical Journal 2: 688 (1972a).

Gaddie, J.; Skinner, C. and Palmer, K.N.V.: Hyposensitisation with house dust mite vaccine in bronchial asthma. British Medical Journal 2: 561 (1976).

Gal, P.; Jusko, W.J.; Yurchak, A.M. and Franklin, B.A.: Theophylline disposition in obesity. Clinical Pharmacology and Therapeutics 23: 438 (1978).

Geddes, D.M. and Brostoff, J.: Pulmonary fibrosis associated with hypersensitivity to gold salts. British Medical Journal 1: 1444 (1976).

Girling, D.J.: Adverse reactions to rifampicin in antituberculosis regimens. Journal of Antimicrobial Chemotherapy 3: 115 (1977).

Girling, D.J.; Nunn, A.J.; Fox, W. and Michison, D.A.: Controlled trial of intermittent regimens of rifampicin plus isoniazid for pulmonary tuberculosis in Singapore. The results up to 30 months. American Review of Respiratory Disease 116: 807 (1977).

Glassroth, J.L.; White, M.C. and Snider, D.E.: An assessment of the possible association of isoniazid with human cancer deaths. American Review of Respiratory Disease 116: 1065 (1978).

Goldstein, R.S.; Slutsky, A.S. and Rebuck, A.S.: Severe asthma: Prevention is better than cure. Drugs 16: 256 (1978).

Graham, J.R.: Cardiac and pulmonary fibrosis during methysergide therapy for headache. American Journal of Medical Science 254: 1 (1967).

Grant, I.W.B.: Oxygen therapy and artificial pulmonary ventilation: in Girdwood and Alstead (Ed) Textbook of Medical Treatment, p.159 (Churchill Livingstone, Edinburgh 1978).

Gregg, I.: The difficult asthmatic. Drugs 13: 35 (1977).

Grondhagen-Riska, C.; Hellstrom, P.E. and Froseth, B.: Predisposing factors in hepatitis induced by isoniazid-rifampicin treatment of tuberculosis. American Review of Respiratory Disease 118: 461 (1978).

Hambleton, G.; Weinberger, M.; Taylor, J.; Cavanaugh, M.; Ginchansky, E.; Godfrey, S.; Tooley, M.; Bell, T. and Greenberg, S.: Comparison of cromoglycate (cromolyn) and theophylline in controlling symptoms of chronic asthma. A collaborative study. Lancet 1: 381 (1977).

Hamilton, W.F.D.; Palmer, K.N.V. and Gent, M.: Expectorant action of bromhexine in chronic obstructive bronchitis. British Medical Journal 3: 260 (1970).

Hargreave, F.E.: Digitalis and cor pulmonale. British Medical Journal 2: 943 (1965).

Heaf, P.J.D.: Deaths in asthma: a therapeutic misadventure. British Medical Bulletin 26: 245 (1970).

Heard, B.E. and Cooke, R.A.: Busulphan lung. Thorax 23: 187 (1968).

Hendeles, L.; Weinberger, M. and Johnson, G.: Monitoring serum theophylline levels. Clinical Pharmacokinetics 3: 294 (1978).

Hetzel, M.R. and Clark, T.J.H.: Comparison of intravenous and aerosol salbutamol. British Medical Journal 2: 919 (1976).

Hetzel, M.R. and Clark, T.J.H.: Comparison of salbutamol rotahaler with conventional pressurised aerosol. Clinical Allergy 7: 563 (1977).

Hetzel, M.R.; Clark, T.J.H. and Houston, K.: Physiological pattern in early morning asthma. Thorax 32: 418 (1977a).

Hetzel, M.R.; Clark, T.J.H. and Branthwaite, M.A.: Asthma: analysis of sudden deaths and ventilatory arrests in hospital. British Medical Journal 1: 808 (1977b).

Hetzel, M.R.; Batten, J.C. and Clark, T.J.H.: Do sympathomimetic amines prevent exercise-induced asthma by bronchodilatation alone? British Journal of Diseases of the Chest 71: 109 (1977c).

Hiller, E.J.; Milner, A.D. and Lenney, W.: Nebulized sodium cromoglycate in young asthmatic children. Double-blind trial. Archives of Disease in Childhood 52: 875 (1977).

Hong Kong Chest Service/British Medical Research Council: Controlled trial of six month and eight month regimens in the treatment of pulmonary tuberculosis. American Review of Respiratory Diseases 118: 219 (1978).

Hughes, D.: Chemoprophylaxis in chronic bronchitis. Journal of Antimicrobial Chemotherapy 2: 320 (1976).

Hughes, D.T.D.: Cough suppressants, expectorants, and mucolytic agents. British Medical Journal 1: 1202 (1978).

Hyman, A.L.; Spannhake, E.W. and Kadowitz, P.J.: Prostaglandins and the lung. American Review of Respiratory Diseases 117: 111 (1978).

Israel, H.I. and Diamond, P.: Recurrent pulmonary infiltration and pleural effusion due to nitrofurantoin. New England Journal of Medicine 266: 1024 (1962).

Israel, K.S.; Brashear, R.E.; Sharma, H.M.; Yum, M.N. and Glover, J.L.: Pulmonary fibrosis and nitrofurantoin. American Review of Respiratory Diseases 108: 353 (1973).

Iversen, L.L.: Role of transmitter uptake mechanisms in synaptic neurotransmission. British Journal of Pharmacology 41: 571 (1971).

Jusko, W.J.; Mosovich, L.L.; Gerbracht, L.M.; Mattar, M.E. and Yaffe, S.J.: Enhanced renal excretion of dicloxacillin in patients with cystic fibrosis. Pediatrics 56: 1038 (1975).

Kopanoff, D.E.; Snider, D.E. and Caras, G.J.: Isoniazid-related hepatitis. American Review of Respiratory Diseases 117: 991 (1978).

Lands, A.M.; Arnold, A.; McAuliff, J.P.; Luduena, F.P. and Brown, T.G.: Differentiation of receptor systems activated by sympathomimetic amines. Nature 214: 596 (1967).

Leggett, R.J.E. and Flenley, D.C.: Portable oxygen and exercise tolerance in patients with chronic hypoxic cor pulmonale. British Medical Journal 2: 84 (1977).

Lightbody, I.M.; Ingram, C.G.; Legge, J.S. and Johnston, R.N.: Ipratropium bromide, salbutamol and prednisolone in bronchial asthma and chronic bronchitis. British Journal of Diseases of the Chest 72: 181 (1978).

Luna, M.A.; Bedrossian, W.M.; Lichtiger, B. and Salem, P.A.: Interstitial pneumonitis associated with bleomycin therapy. American Journal of Clinical Pathology 58: 501 (1972).

Marlin, G.E. and Turner, P.: Comparison of the β_2-adrenoceptor selectivity of rimiterol, salbutamol and isoprenaline by the intravenous route in man. British Journal of Clinical Pharmacology 2: 41 (1975).

Mathe, A.; Hedgvist, P.; Strandberg, K. and Leslie, C.A.: Aspects of prostaglandin synthesis in the lung. New England Journal of Medicine 296: 850 (1977).

May, C.S. and Palmer, K.N.V.: Effect of aerosol ipratropium bromide on sputum viscosity and volume in chronic bronchitis. British Journal of Clinical Pharmacology 4: 491 (1977).

McDevitt, D.G.: β-Adrenoceptor antagonists and respiratory function. British Journal of Clinical Pharmacology 5: 97 (1978).

McFadden, E.R.; Kiser, R.; de Groot, W.J.; Holmes, B.; Kiker, R. and Viser, G.: A controlled study of the effects of single doses of hydrocortisone on the resolution of acute attacks of asthma. American Journal of Medicine 60: 52 (1976).

Mitchell, D.N. and Scadding, J.G.: Sarcoidosis. American Review of Respiratory Diseases 110: 774 (1974).

Mitchell, J.R.; Zimmerman, H.J.; Ishak, K.G.; Thorgeirsson, U.P.; Timbrell, J.A.; Snodgrass, W.R. and Nelson, S.D.: Isoniazid liver injury: clinical spectrum, pathology and possible pathogenesis. Annals of Internal Medicine 84: 181 (1976).

Murray, R.: The Normal Lung (Saunders, London 1977).

Neville, A.; Palmer, J.B.D.; Gaddie, J.; May, C.S.; Palmer, K.N.V. and Murchison, L.E.: Metabolic effects of salbutamol: comparison of aerosol and intravenous administration. British Medical Journal 1: 413 (1977).

Nicholson, D.P. and Chick, T.W.: A re-evaluation of parenteral aminophylline. American Review of Respiratory Diseases 108: 241 (1973).

O'Donnell, R.M.: The treatment of pulmonary heart failure. Drugs 11: 308 (1976).

Ogilvie, R.I.: Clinical pharmacokinetics of theophylline. Clinical Pharmacokinetics 3: 267 (1978a).

Ogilvie, C.M.: Pneumonia. British Medical Journal 1: 771 (1978b).

Paciaroni, E.; Fosch, F.; Vittori, N.; Saccomanno, G. and Raspa, E.G.: Le digoxinemia nei soggetti con cuore polmonare cronico. Giormale di Gerontologi 22: 832 (1974).

Palmer, K.N.V. and Kelman, G.R.: Pulmonary function in asthmatic patients in remission. British Medical Journal 1: 485 (1975).

Palmer, K.N.V. and Paterson, J.W.: Drug interactions in respiratory disease; in Cluff and Petrie (Eds) Clinical Effects of Interaction Between Drugs, p.154 (Excerpta Medica, Amsterdam 1975).

Palmer, K.N.V.; Legge, J.S.; Hamilton, W.F.D. and Diament, M.L.: Effect of a selective beta-adrenergic blocker in preventing falls in arterial oxygen tension following isoprenaline in asthmatic subjects. Lancet 2: 1092 (1969).

Partridge, M.R. and Gibson, G.J.: Adverse bronchial reactions to intravenous hydrocortisone in two aspirin-sensitive asthmatic patients. British Medical Journal 1: 1521 (1978).

Petersdorf, R.G. and Featherstone, H.: New antimicrobial drugs and their value in the treatment of respiratory infection. American Review of Respiratory Diseases 117: 1 (1978).

Petrie, G.R. and Palmer, K.N.V.: Comparison of aerosol ipratropium bromide and salbutamol in chronic bronchitis and asthma. British Medical Journal 1: 430 (1975).

Phelan, P.D. and Stocks, J.G.: Management of severe viral bronchiolitis and severe acute asthma. Archives of Disease in Childhood 49: 143 (1974).

Piafsky, K.M.; Sitar, D.G.; Rangno, R.E. and Ogilvie, R.I.: Theophylline kinetics in acute pulmonary oedema. Clinical Pharmacology and Therapeutics 21: 31 (1977).

Pollock, J.; Kiechel, F.; Cooper, D. and Weinberger, M.: Relationship of serum theophylline concentration to inhibition of exercise-induced bronchospasm and comparison with cromolyn. Pediatrics 60: 840 (1977).

Powell, J.R.; Thiercelin, J.F.; Vozheh, S.; Samsom, L. and Riegelman, S.: The influence of cigarette smoking and sex on theophylline disposition. American Review of Respiratory Disease 116: 17 (1977).

Powell, J.R.; Vozheh, S.; Hopewell, P.; Costello, J.; Sheiner, L.B.G. and Riegelman, S.: Theophylline disposition in acutely ill hospitalised patients; the effects of smoking, heart failure, severe airway obstruction and pneumonia. American Review of Respiratory Disease 118: 229 (1978).

Rapp, R.S.; Campbell, R.W.; Howell, R.W. and Kendig, E.L.: Isoniazid hepatotoxicity in children. American Review of Respiratory Disease 118: 794 (1978).

Rebuck, A.S.: Antiasthmatic drugs I. Pathophysiological and clinical pharmacological aspects; II: Therapeutic aspects. Drugs 7: 344, 370 (1974).

Rebuck, A.S. and Read, J.: Assessment and management of severe asthma. American Journal of Medicine 51: 788 (1971), Lancet 1: 1055 (1972).

Rosenberg, J.L.; Edlow, D. and Sneider, R.: Liver disease and vasculitis in a patient taking cromolyn. Archives of Internal Medicine 138: 989 (1978).

Sahn, S.A. and Lakshminarayan, S.: Tuberculosis after corticosteroid therapy. British Journal of Diseases of the Chest 70: 195 (1976).

Samter, M. and Beers, R.F.: Concerning the nature of intolerance to aspirin. Journal of Allergy 40: 281 (1967).

Samter, M. and Beers, R.F.: Intolerance to aspirin. Clinical studies and consideration of its pathogenesis. Annals of Internal Medicine 68: 975 (1968).

Schanker, L.S.: Drug absorption from the lung. Biochemical Pharmacology 27: 381 (1978).

Schatz, M.; Patterson, R.; Kloner, R. and Falk, J.: The prevalence of tuberculosis and positive tuberculin skin tests in a steroid-treated asthmatic population. Annals of Internal Medicine 84: 261 (1976).

Seaton, A.: Asthma — contrasts in care. Thorax 33: 1 (1978a).

Seaton, A.: Treatment of tuberculosis. British Medical Journal 1: 701 (1978b).

Shenfield, G.M.; Knowles, G.K.; Thomas, N. and Paterson, J.W.: Potassium supplements in patients treated with corticosteroids. British Journal of Diseases of the Chest 69: 171 (1975a).

Shenfield, G.M.; Hodson, M.E.; Clarke, S.W. and Paterson, J.W.: Interaction of corticosteroids and catecholamines in the treatment of asthma. Thorax 30: 430 (1975b).

Shenfield, G.M.; Evans, M.E. and Paterson, J.W.: Absorption of drugs by the lung. British Journal of Clinical Pharmacology 3: 583 (1976).

Siegel, M.; Lee, S.L. and Peres, N.S.: The epidemiology of drug-induced systemic lupus erythematosus. Arthritis and Rheumatism 10: 407 (1967).

Skinner, C.; Palmer, K.N.V. and Kerridge, D.F.: Comparison of the effects of acebutolol (Sectral) and practolol (Eraldin) on airways obstruction in asthmatics. British Journal of Clinical Pharmacology 2: 417 (1975).

Smith, A.P.: Response of aspirin-allergic patients to challenge by some analgesics in common use. British Medical Journal 2: 494 (1971).

Sovijarvi, A.R.A.; Lemola, M.; Stenius, B. and Idanpaan-Heikkila, J.: Nitrofurantoin-induced acute, subacute and chronic pulmonary reactions. A report of 66 cases. Scandinavian Journal of Respiratory Diseases 58: 41 (1977).

Spangler, D.L.; Kalof, D.D.; Bloom, F.L. and Wittig, H.J.: Theophylline bioavailability following oral administration of six sustained-release preparations. Annals of Allergy 40: 6 (1978).

Steen, J.S.M. and Stainton-Ellis, D.M.: Rifampicin in pregnancy. Lancet 2: 604 (1977).

Stott, H.; Peto, J.; Stephens, R.; Fox, W.; Sutherland, I.; Foster-Carter, A.F.; Teare, H.B. and Fenning, J.: An assessment of the carcinogenicity of isoniazid in patients with pulmonary tuberculosis. Tubercule 57: 1 (1976).

Stott, N.C.H. and West, R.R.: Randomised control trial of antibiotics in patients with cough and purulent sputum. British Medical Journal 2: 556 (1976).

Sykes, M.K.; McNicol, M.W. and Campbell, E.J.M.: in Respiratory Failure (Blackwell, Oxford 1976).

Szczeklik, A.; Gryglewski, R.J.; Czerniawska-Mysik, G. and Pieton, R.: Asthmatic attacks induced in aspirin-sensitive patients by diclofenac and naproxen. British Medical Journal 2: 231 (1977).

Taylor, G.; Abbott, E.D.; Kerr, M.M. and Ferguson, D.M.: Amoxycillin and co-trimoxazole in presumed respiratory infections of childhood. British Medical Journal 2: 552 (1977).

Third East African/British Medical Research Councils Study: Controlled clinical trial of four short-course regimens of chemotherapy for two durations in the treatment of pulmonary tuberculosis. First report. American Review of Respiratory Disease 118: 39 (1978).

Turner-Warwick, M.: On observing patterns of airflow obstruction in chronic asthma. British Journal of Diseases of the Chest 71: 73 (1977).

Tuttle, C.B. and Sidorov, J.: Correct use of aerosol inhalers. Canadian Medical Association Journal 117: 21 (1977).

Vaisrub, S.: Beclomethasone aerosol — a note of reassurance. Journal of the American Medical Association 238: 1544 (1977).

Vozeh, S.; Powell, J.R.; Riegelman, S.; Costello, J.F.; Sheiner, L.B. and Hopewell, P.C.: Changes in theophylline clearance during acute illness. Journal of the American Medical Association 240: 1882 (1978).

Walker, S.R.; Evans, M.E.; Richards, A.J. and Paterson, J.W.: The fate of [^{14}C] disodium cromoglycate in man. Journal of Pharmacy and Pharmacology 24: 525 (1972).

Warrell, D.A.; Robertson, D.G.; Newton Howes, J.; Connolly, M.E.; Paterson, J.W.; Bellin, L.J. and Dollery, C.T.: Comparison of cardiorespiratory effects of isoprenaline and salbutamol in patients with bronchial asthma. British Medical Journal 1: 65 (1970).

Weg, J.G.: Diagnostic standards of tuberculosis revised. Journal of the American Medical Association 235: 1329 (1976).

Weinberger, M.M.; Matthay, R.A.; Ginchansky, E.J.; Chidsey, C.A. and Petty, T.L.: Intravenous aminophylline dosage. Use of serum theophylline measurement for guidance. Journal of the American Medical Association 235: 2110 (1976).

Williams, H.E. and Phelan, P.D.: Administration of disodium cromoglycate to young children. British Medical Journal 2: 488 (1973).

Wolfe, J.D.; Tashkin, D.P.; Calvarese, P. and Simmons, M.: Bronchodilator effects of terbutaline and aminophylline alone and in combination in asthmatic patients. New England Journal of Medicine 298: 363 (1978).

Wood, R.E.; Boat, T.F. and Doershuk, C.F.: Cystic fibrosis. American Review of Respiratory Disease 113: 833 (1976).

Woolcock, A.J.: Inhaled drugs in the prevention of asthma. American Review of Respiratory Disease 115: 191 (1977).

Yaffe, S.J.; Gerbracht, L.M.; Mosovich, L.L.; Mattar, M.E.; Danish, M. and Jusko, W.J.: Pharmacokinetics of methicillin in patients with cystic fibrosis. Journal of Infectious Diseases 135: 828 (1977).

Zilly, W.; Breimer, D.D. and Richter, E.: Pharmacokinetic interactions with rifampicin. Clinical Pharmacokinetics 2: 61 (1977).

Chapter XXI
Renal Diseases

N. Wright and J.S. Robson

Synopsis of Important Principles

1) Ideally drugs used in renal disease should be therapeutically effective and not cause a deterioration in renal function.

2) Because kidney disorder alters the chemical composition of body fluids and hence the pharmacokinetic properties of drugs, standard regimens of some drugs may be inappropriate and need to be adjusted if adverse toxic reactions are to be avoided.

3) The activity of most drugs is usually related to the plasma concentration of unbound drug. When plasma albumin is decreased or binding of drugs altered by renal disease, the fraction of unbound drug may differ from that in individuals with normal renal function.

4) The clinical significance of a reduction in glomerular filtration rate and increased drug half-life depends on the relative importance of renal excretion and metabolism as a mode of elimination, and the therapeutic ratio of the drug.

5) Dosage of toxic drugs which are mainly excreted in active form by the kidney (i.e. as unchanged drug or active metabolites) may need to be modified to avoid accumulation — either by giving the usual dose at increased intervals or a reduced dose at the usual intervals. In renal failure, potentially toxic drugs should only be used if there is a specific indication for their use and if therapy can be monitored appropriately.

6) Treatment of disordered renal function is directed towards replacement of substances inappropriately lost and at reducing the dietary intake of those substances which are retained. Factors that place an added load on renal function should be avoided. Management of acute renal failure is supportive until intrinsic renal function recovers.

7) Asymptomatic urinary infection in adults with normal renal tracts probably does not require antibacterial therapy. However, it should be treated in infants and in children. Corticosteroids and immunosuppressive drugs are of value in a small number of specific types of glomerulonephritis. The value of antithrombotic drugs is unproven.

8) Uraemia is accompanied by many changes in the homeostatic mechanisms that in turn alter the response to drugs. There is an increased incidence of adverse reactions in patients with uraemia.

9) Many drugs can cause or exacerbate renal disease, sometimes permanently. Cephalothin, like cephaloridine, can cause acute renal failure, particularly when combined with aminoglycoside antibiotics, and methoxyflurane may occasionally do so. Tetracyclines, except doxycycline and minocycline, should be avoided in the presence of any degree of renal impairment.

The relation of the kidney and the action of drugs is important from two different points of view. The kidney is the major excretory organ for a number of drugs and their metabolic derivatives. Changes in renal function therefore exert a profound effect on the rate of excretion of these drugs or active metabolites in the urine and upon the intensity and duration of their action. In addition a number of drugs act directly on the kidney and are capable of altering glomerular and tubular function. Some of these, e.g. diuretics, are useful in correcting abnormalities in renal function which arise in the course of disease.

1. Clinical Pharmacological Principles

Diseases of the kidney cause many changes to the chemical composition of body fluid and hence alter the pharmacokinetic properties of drugs (see chapter I; sect. 4.3.2, 4.3.4). Accordingly, standard dose regimens are often inappropriate and require adjustment if adverse and toxic reactions are to be avoided. The increased incidence of adverse reactions to some drugs in patients with uraemia (see chapter VII; sect. 5.3) emphasises the need to understand the pharmacokinetic factors involved. This field remains inadequately explored and the lack of knowledge for many drugs is revealed in the following discussion (for reviews, see Fabre and Balant, 1976; Dawborn, 1974; Rubin et al., 1977).

1.1 Absorption and Bioavailability of Drugs in Renal Disease

Little is known concerning the oral absorption of drugs by patients with renal disease. Cloxacillin, chlorpropamide and pindolol are examples of drugs that do not appear to be absorbed as rapidly or as completely in patients with uraemia as in patients with normal renal function (Fabre and Balant, 1976). The individual pharmacokinetic characteristics of drugs influence their behaviour in the body. The β-adrenoceptor blocking drug pindolol is eliminated by both renal and non-renal mechanisms and while bioavailability after oral administration is decreased in patients with impaired renal function, due to reduced absorption, renal clearance is also reduced and there is probably no need to alter dosage (Lavene et al.,

1977). On the other hand, bioavailability of oral propranolol, which is eliminated by non-renal (hepatic) mechanisms, is increased in patients with chronic renal failure due to a reduced hepatic extraction and clearance (Bianchetti et al., 1976; see section 14.2.4).

1.2 Distribution of Drugs in Renal Disease

The activity of most drugs is related to available drug concentration at receptor sites. While in most instances this is not measurable, it is usually related to the plasma concentration of free or unbound drug. The latter is a function of the total drug in the body, the extent of protein binding and the body clearance. Alteration in clearance and in the plasma concentration-clinical effect relationship of drugs as a consequence of changes in plasma protein binding in renal disease mostly relate to highly albumin bound acidic drugs with a low hepatic clearance (see chapter I; sect. 4.3.2). Although extensive binding to plasma proteins limits glomerular filtration, it does not always delay clearance of drugs eliminated mainly by renal mechanisms since clearance of such drugs is influenced predominantly by tubular secretion.

In general, highly bound acidic drugs [e.g. warfarin, phenytoin, phenylbutazone, chlorophenoxyisobutyric acid (active metabolite of clofibrate), and frusemide] are less bound to albumin in plasma in patients with poor renal function as compared with those with normal renal function. Highly bound basic drugs may have normal (propranolol, quinidine, desipramine) or decreased (diazepam, triamterene) plasma albumin binding (Reidenberg, 1976, 1977a). Basic drugs such as propranolol, quinidine and desipramine are more avidly bound to α_1-acid glycoproteins in plasma than to albumin or lipoproteins (Piafsky and Borga, 1977); binding to α_1-acid glycoproteins can actually increase in patients with chronic renal failure and associated inflammatory disease (Piafsky et al., 1978). The extent of binding of acidic drugs such as phenytoin and warfarin in chronic renal failure decreases with increasing uraemia (Reidenberg et al., 1971; Bachmann et al., 1976); the impaired binding being due to the presence of endogenous competitive binding inhibitors (e.g. free fatty acids) that are not removed by dialysis and/or to molecular conformational changes which decrease the binding capacity of albumin. Hypoalbuminaemia sometimes present in uraemia is a lesser contributory factor (Reidenberg, 1977a; Sjoholm et al., 1976). Protein binding of acidic drugs returns to normal following renal transplantation, probably as a consequence of elimination of inhibitors of drug albumin binding, but is impaired again in the face of an acute rejection episode (Levy et al., 1976; Odar-Cederlof, 1977). Binding of acidic drugs is also decreased in acute renal failure but the mechanism for reduced binding is not clear; endogenous binding inhibitors do not appear to be involved since dialysis increases binding (Andreasen, 1974). Recovery from acute renal failure is also associated with increased binding of acidic drugs (Mussche et al., 1975).

In the nephrotic syndrome the plasma albumin concentration is depressed and extracellular fluid volume and albumin content is increased. The extent of binding of acidic drugs in the nephrotic syndrome is directly related to the plasma albumin concentration. In contrast to uraemia, there are no qualitative changes in albumin binding characteristics. The γ-globulin fraction may also be reduced whereas the α_2- and β-globulin fractions are usually increased. The unbound fraction of albumin bound drugs in the plasma of patients with the nephrotic syndrome may therefore differ significantly from that in an individual with normal renal function (Gugler and Azarnoff, 1976). However as in uraemia, a decrease in protein binding changes the ratio of concentrations of free to total drug in plasma and alters the distribution volume and clearance of highly bound acidic drugs with a low hepatic extraction. The clearance of such drugs is increased since elimination proceeds at rates proportional to their free fraction in plasma (Levy, 1977; Gibaldi, 1977). This is well illustrated in the case of phenytoin. In both uraemia (Odar-Cederlof and Borga, 1974) and the nephrotic syndrome (Gugler et al., 1975), there is a decrease in total drug (bound + unbound) in plasma due to a larger apparent volume of distribution and an increased rate of metabolism, but the unbound concentration of phenytoin at steady-state remains unchanged. As a result the relationship between total drug plasma level and clinical effect of phenytoin is altered and monitoring of plasma levels should involve estimation of unbound drug (see chapter I, sect. 4.3.2, 5.1.2; VII, sect. 5.1). With repeat dose administration, in the absence of factors which may delay clearance (e.g. severe liver disease, saturation of metabolism, accumulation of active metabolites), there is proba-

bly no need to change the usual daily dose in renal disease of highly albumin bound drugs eliminated by metabolism. However, a greater fluctuation of unbound drug level is observed between doses and shorter dosing intervals seem to be advisable, particularly to avoid toxicity from transient higher peak concentrations (Levy, 1976; Gugler and Azarnoff, 1976). Similar considerations appear to apply to highly bound basic drugs such as diazepam, binding of which is decreased in hypoalbuminaemic states (Greenblatt and Koch-Weser, 1974).

For highly bound acidic drugs such as frusemide (furosemide), which are eliminated about equally by renal and extrarenal mechanisms, the effects of renal disease on distribution and clearance are more complex (Rane et al., 1978).

In the nephrotic syndrome, protein binding of frusemide is reduced in proportion to the reduction in serum albumin concentration at conventional therapeutic total plasma levels. However, binding is further reduced at concentrations of $100\mu g/ml$ or more. Renal clearance of free frusemide decreases in proportion to creatinine clearance while extrarenal clearance is not appreciably altered. Thus, although the pharmacokinetics of total frusemide is only marginally influenced, the changes in binding at high total plasma concentrations and the suggestion that ototoxicity to frusemide is related to free drug concentration makes it inadvisable to use excessive doses in such cases (see chapter XI; sect. 7.1.2). In contrast in uraemia, protein binding is not decreased to the same extent and is concentration independent. However, both renal and extrarenal clearance are markedly reduced, resulting in delayed drug elimination. With a reduced nephron population it is still possible to achieve an effective diuresis if the higher portion of the dose response relationship of frusemide to diuretic response is exploited. Thus, a diuresis can be achieved in uraemic patients by using higher doses with an increase in the dose interval.

For highly tissue bound drugs such as digoxin which are eliminated by renal mechanisms, reduced clearance in renal failure can be associated with a decrease in distribution volume in some patients and increased risk of toxicity as a consequence of a greater amount of drug in plasma. Smaller than usual loading doses (up to about one half normal) of digoxin are therefore desirable in renal failure for this reason (Aronson and Grahame-Smith, 1976; chapter XVII, sect. 8.1.3).

1.3 Metabolism of Drugs in Renal Disease

Despite the extensive chemical changes of increasing uraemia, significant alterations in the rate of elimination of drugs normally biotransformed in the liver are largely confined to some minor pathways. Nevertheless, renal failure can alter the rate of biotransformation of some drugs and does decrease the rate of excretion of formed metabolites normally excreted in the urine (Reidenberg, 1977b). Accumulation of active metabolites in renal failure can be important if the metabolite is eliminated mainly by renal mechanisms, even though the rate of metabolism of the parent drug may be normal (Drayer, 1976; see section 14). Elimination rates of most drugs metabolised by microsomal oxidations (the major pathway of metabolism for many drugs) are normal in most patients with chronic renal failure (e.g. tolbutamide, quinidine). However, clearance of such drugs which are highly albumin bound (e.g. phenytoin) can be increased as a consequence of impaired protein binding in uraemia (see section 1.2). Glucuronide conjugation, another major pathway, sulphate conjugation and *O*-methylation proceed normally. Reduction of hydrocortisone to tetrahydrocortisol is however slowed in uraemia. Acetylation of sulphafurazole (sulfisoxazole), PAS, procainamide, hydrallazine (Talseth, 1977) and of isoniazid (in slow acetylators; Bowersox et al., 1973) also proceeds more slowly in uraemia. Plasma esterases exhibit diminished activity in some patients, resulting in prolongation of the effects of local anaesthetic esters such as procaine. If drugs metabolised by acetylation or esterase activity are given at usual dosage to uraemic patients, excessive accumulation may occur. The elimination of many peptides is normal. Although the metabolism of insulin is decreased in uraemia, this is offset by a dialysable insulin inhibitor which reduces tissue responsiveness (sect. 14.3.1).

1.4 Renal Excretion of Drugs

Drugs are excreted by glomerular filtration, followed in some cases by proximal tubular secretion and/or passive back diffusion which may or may not be pH dependent (see Milne, 1975; Cafruny, 1977; Weiner, 1971).

1.4.1 Filtration at the Glomerulus
The amount of drug filtered depends on the plasma drug concentration, the degree of drug protein binding and the glomerular filtration rate (GFR) as the concentration of unbound drug in plasma increases, the amount filtered increases linearly (Cafruny, 1977). A fall in GFR results in diminished excretion and often a prolonged drug half-life with a drug mainly eliminated by renal excretion. The clinical significance of this change depends on the relative importance of renal excretion compared with metabolism or other extrarenal mechanisms as a mode of elimination, and the therapeutic ratio of the drug (Fabre and Balant, 1976). For example, ampicillin is excreted mainly by glomerular filtration but the therapeutic ratio of the drug is so great that no modification of the dosage schedule need be made if the GFR is low. Moreover, ampicillin is excreted in the bile and compensatory excretion by this route becomes more important as GFR falls. Similarly, non-renal elimination of frusemide is increased in patients with low GFR compared with normals (Cutler et al., 1973). On the other hand, kanamycin has a small therapeutic ratio and is mainly eliminated by the kidneys. Accordingly, the dose of kanamycin and its pattern of use needs to be modified when the creatinine clearance falls below 35ml/min. Many nomograms have been constructed relating GFR to drug dosage in an attempt to reduce the risk of therapeutic overdosage. These assume that the drug is excreted in a manner exactly analogous to creatinine and no account is taken of passive or active processes, individual variation in clearance or rapid change in renal function of the patient (see section 14; appendix E). In addition, in some instances, accumulation occurs of an active or toxic water soluble metabolite rather than the parent drug. This is thought to be the explanation for clofibrate and nitrofurantoin toxicity in patients with poor renal function (Drayer, 1976; Gugler, 1978; see also section 14).

1.4.2 Renal Tubular Secretion
This process involves active transport of the drug into the renal tubular cells and into the tubular lumen. In contrast to drugs excreted by glomerular filtration, variations in protein binding with very few exceptions do not influence their rate of tubular secretion. There are two major pathways of tubular secretion; weak organic acids are secreted by a complex bidirectional carrier mediated process; weak bases are secreted by a similar separate system (Cafruny, 1977). These pathways are not substrate specific. Hence salicylate competes with methotrexate for the same

secretory pathway and the danger of methotrexate induced adverse effects is increased when these drugs are given together (Hendersen, 1965). The action of chlorothiazide depends on achieving an adequate concentration within the tubular cell; probenecid, a weak acid, reduces its renal clearance and prolongs its diuretic effect after intravenous administration (Brater, 1978). However, the effect of probenecid on the action of orally administered thiazides is inconsistent; an enhanced diuretic response being observed in some patients and a decreased response in others (Brater, 1978; Garcia and Yendt, 1970). The capacity of probenecid to compete for secretion with other organic acids such as the penicillins is well known and used to therapeutic advantage, as for example in gonorrhoea (see chapter XXIX; sect. 3).

1.4.3 Passive Non-Ionic Diffusion

Weak acids and bases are more rapidly reabsorbed from the renal tubules in their non-ionised relatively lipid soluble form than when ionised (see chapter I, sect. 1.1). Excretion of weak acids and bases (appendix A) can therefore be modified by altering the urinary pH and rate of urine flow. The limits of pK_a of weak bases and acids at which pH dependent excretion can occur are 3.0 to 7.5 for weak acids and 5.0 to 11.3 for weak bases (Milne, 1965; appendix A).

A forced alkaline diuresis is more effective in increasing excretion of weak acids such as salicylate than is a forced water diuresis. Similarly, the excretion of weak bases such as amphetamine is increased if a low urine pH is maintained (see also chapter I; sect. 3.4, 4.3.4; VIII, sect 2.3.8).

1.5 Drug Response in the Presence of Uraemia

Uraemia is accompanied by many changes in homeostatic mechanisms that in turn alter the response to drugs (Lowenthal, 1974; Fabre and Balant, 1976). The disturbance in coagulation renders the individual more sensitive to anticoagulants. Sodium and potassium metabolism is abnormal so the use of digoxin may be associated with increased liability to adverse reactions. Acidosis may also affect response to drugs, in particular by altering tissue penetration of some drugs. A possible explanation of the increased sensitivity to barbiturates and of reactions to other drugs including antibiotics such as colistin, in

uraemia is that the 'blood-brain' barrier is less effective (Richet et al., 1970; see also chapter VII, sect. 5.3; XXV, sect. 15). Apart from the increased risk of enhanced effects due to accumulation of renally excreted drugs or active metabolites in uraemia (section 14), the kidneys themselves have an increased susceptibility to the nephrotoxic effects of drugs (Fabre and Balant, 1976).

1.6 Renal Function, Age and Drugs

Renal blood flow in the newborn infant is low due to high renal vascular resistance; glomerular filtration is low and proximal tubular transport mechanisms are immature. Thus, overall function is less than that predicted in terms of body weight (Hook and Hewitt, 1977). Hepatic metabolism is also reduced. Prolonged drug elimination is compounded by impaired protein binding of drugs in the newborn. These factors may be the cause of unexpected accumulation of drugs or their active metabolites such as salicylates, paracetamol (acetaminophen) and penicillin. Renal vascular resistance falls rapidly in the first few months of life and tubular transport mechanisms, which are inducible, quickly develop (see also chapter IV; sect. 2.2, 2.3). At the other end of the age scale, renal function diminishes with age and reduced doses of drugs which are mainly eliminated by the kidneys are required in the elderly (see chapter V; sect. 2.1.3).

2. General Principles of Treatment

2.1 Modification of Dose Regimen

Since drugs that are mainly excreted in active form by the kidney have a prolonged half-life when given to patients with reduced renal function, cumulation occurs with resulting toxicity if the normal dose regimen is not modified. Two approaches may be made to this problem; either the same dose can be given at extended intervals or a reduced dose may be given at usual intervals (see Dettli, 1976; Fabre and Balant, 1976). If an antibiotic is given to a patient with chronic renal failure in the normal dosage, but at extended intervals, there may be considerable periods when subinhibitory concentrations of the antibiotic are present. On the other hand, more frequent but smaller doses of the antibiotic engender a greater

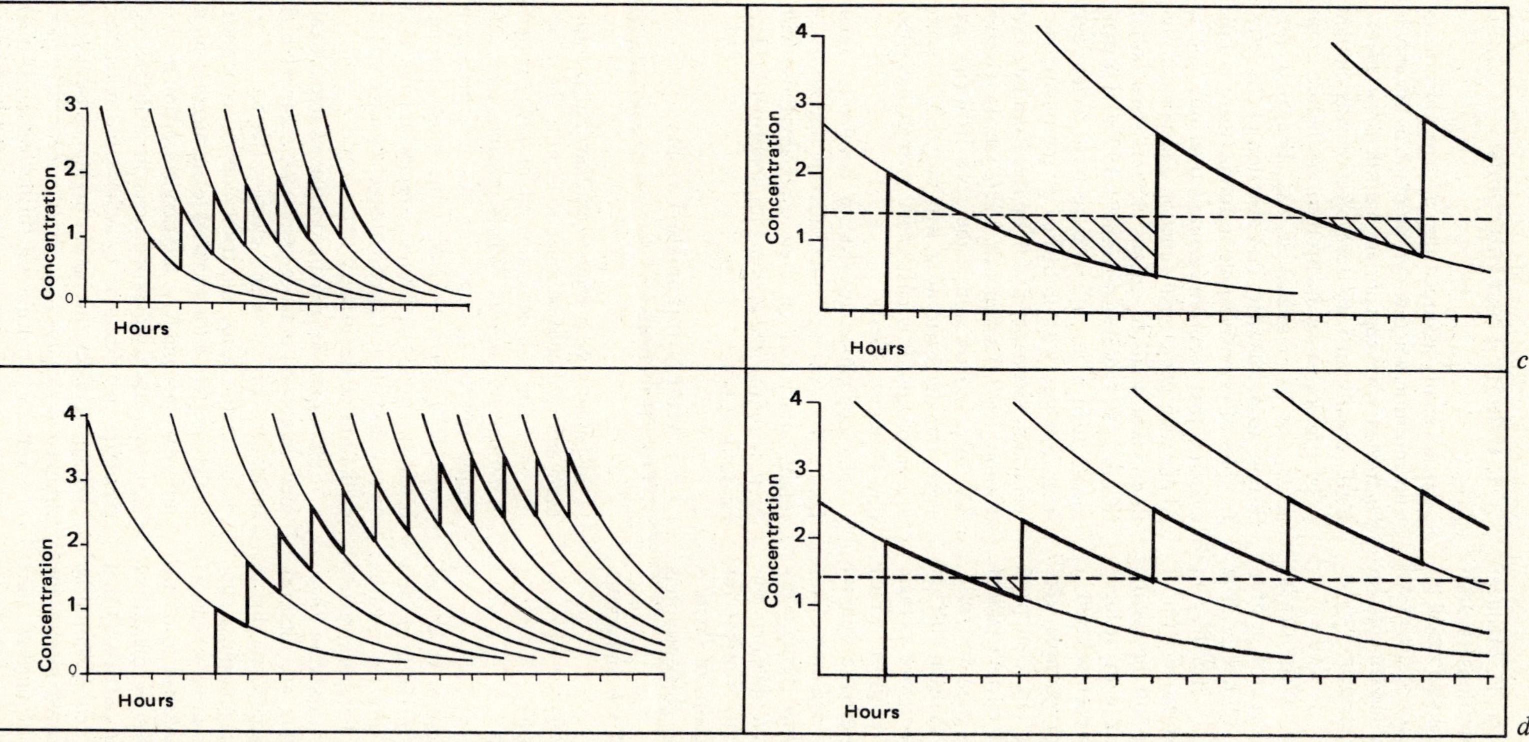

Fig. 1. Steady-state concentrations on different drug regimens and effect of dosage modification in renal failure (adapted after O'Grady: British Medical Bulletin 27: 142, 1971).

a) Normal renal function. The thin lines are identical curves showing the fall in concentration of an agent having a half-life in the patient of 1 hour. The thick line shows the effect of repeating the initial dose every half-life. After about 4 half-lives, the concentration reaches the steady-state with the concentration oscillating between 1 and 2 times that produced by the first dose.

b) Impaired capacity to excrete drug. The thin lines are identical curves showing the fall in concentration of an agent having a half-life in the patient of 2 hours. The thick line shows the effect of the same regimen as that used in *a.* The steady-state is again reached after about 4 half-lives (i.e. about 8 hours), but the concentration oscillates between about 2.5 and 3.5 times that produced by the first dose.

c) Renal failure. Reduction in dosage frequency. Hypothetical example in which the thin lines represent the fall in concentration of an agent having a half-life in the patient of approximately 8 hours; the normal half-life of the agent is 4 hours. The thick line shows the effect of doses given every 8 hours. Assuming that the agent is an antibiotic and that the dotted line represents the minimum inhibitory concentration (MIC) of the micro-organism, this method of administration in renal failure may result in prolonged periods of subinhibitory concentrations (represented by shaded portion).

d) Renal failure. Reduced dosage at normal intervals. Same hypothetical example as in *c,* except that here the thick line shows the effect of giving the same loading dose as in *c* followed by maintenance doses half this size at the normal interval of 4 hours. With this method of administration the likelihood that subinhibitory concentrations may result is lessened, but there is a greater risk of cumulation and toxicity.

risk of cumulation and toxicity (fig. 1). Frequent measurements of plasma concentrations of antibiotic are therefore necessary; these also reveal individual differences in compensatory routes of excretion (see section 1.4.1) and any sudden changes in renal function (see further chapter I; sect. 4.3.4).

The time taken to reach 90% of the steady-state concentration (equilibrium level) of a drug being given in repeated doses, is 3.3 times the drug half-life (see chapter I; sect. 2.2). Therefore in clinical situations where the cumulative level of the drug is important for attaining full therapeutic activity, and where the regimen with reduced dosage but normal frequency has been selected, a loading dose should be given. For example, gentamicin 15mg 8-hourly can be given to attain a steady state concentration of 8μg/ml in a patient with a creatinine clearance of less than 5ml/min. However, it would take 80 hours to reach 90% of the equilibrium concentration. Therefore a single loading dose of 80mg should be given which would give a peak concentration around 8μg/ml within 2 hours. If the alternative regimen of extending dosage intervals is used, then 80mg every 48 to 72 hours is given. However, plasma concentration will then be less than 4μg/ml for periods up to 24 hours. Many strains of *Pseudomonas aeruginosa* are resistant to concentrations of less than 4μg/ml.

See further chapter I; section 4.3.4; and appendix E.

2.2 Principles of Treatment of Diminished Renal Function

Disordered renal function results in an increased loss of some substances in the urine and retention of others. Treatment is directed towards replacing those substances that are inappropriately lost whilst reducing the dietary intake of those substances or their precursors that are retained. For example, familial hypophosphataemia due to hyperphosphaturia is treated with phosphate supplements. When renal function is grossly reduced then diet and fluid balance are adjusted to obtain the most favourable circumstances for maximum renal function. On the other hand, all factors that place an added load on renal function should be avoided. Infection should be treated intensively, oligaemia corrected quickly, renal outflow tract obstruction relieved, catabolic and nephrotoxic drugs avoided and cardiac failure controlled.

3. Urinary Tract Infections

It is usually assumed that all cases of urinary tract infection whether symptomatic or not should be treated with appropriate antimicrobial agents. Until recently, urinary tract infection was thought to be a major cause of chronic renal failure in the adult, and in pregnancy it was claimed to predispose to prematurity and abortion of the fetus. In spite of extensive investigations, there is little evidence that recurrent urinary tract infection in adults with good renal function and normal outflow tracts, leads to serious chronic renal failure (Kunin, 1974; Various Authors, 1975a). Furthermore, there is no difference in birth weight between mothers with untreated asymptomatic bacteriuria in pregnancy and those free from infection (Swapp, 1973; Eschenbach, 1976; see also chapter XV; sect. 4). However, as there is a 30% risk that asymptomatic bacteriuria will progress to acute pyelonephritis, it is customary to treat the infection (Whalley, 1967).

The population at risk of developing renal failure from urinary tract infection appears to be infants and young children, especially those with ureteric reflux, and adults with abnormal kidneys or outflow tracts.

3.1 Acute Symptomatic Urinary Tract Infections

In patients who require antibacterial therapy, every effort should be made to identify the infecting organism and determine its sensitivity pattern to antibacterial agents. Where possible, treatment should not be started until this information is available. *Escherichia coli* is the most common organism involved; *Proteus* species are the next most common and appear frequently after instrumentation of the urinary tract.

Sulphonamides remain popular as initial treatment in general practice despite the relatively high incidence of adverse effects (Keys, 1977). Sulphamethoxazole and trimethoprim (co-trimoxazole) interfere with bacterial folate metabolism at different sites and have a synergistic action *in vivo*. Although the fixed proportions in available preparations are designed to achieve the maximum synergistic effect, this optimum ratio is usually not attained *in vivo* due to pharmacokinetic differences between the two drugs (see further section 14.1.4). Adverse effects are similar to those of other sulphonamides when given alone, with the excep-

Table I. Suggested regimens of oral antibacterial agents (after Bailey, 1974)

Regimen	Duration of treatment	Agent[1]	Daily dosage[2]	Adequate concentrations		Principal adverse effects
				urine	blood	
Curative	5-10 days[3]	Sulphadimidine	1g 6-hly	Yes	Yes	Hypersensitivity, nausea and
		Sulphafurazole (sulfisoxazole)	1g 6-hly	Yes	Yes	vomiting, haematological abnormalities, Stevens-Johnson
		Sulphamethizole	1g 8-hly			syndrome (rare)
		Co-trimoxazole	2 tabs 12-hly	Yes	Yes	See sulphonamides
		Ampicillin	0.5g 6-hly	Yes	Yes	Skin rashes, diarrhoea, sensitivity
		Amoxycillin	0.25g 8-hly	Yes	Yes	As above (rash and diarrhoea may be less)
		Nitrofurantoin	50mg 6-8hly	Yes	No	Hypersensitivity, nausea. Pulmonary reactions, peripheral neuritis (risk > at 100mg 6-8h)
		Nalidixic acid	0.5g 6-8hly	Yes	No	Nausea, photosensitivity
		Cycloserine	250mg 6-8hly	Yes	Yes	Mood change
Preventive or prophylactic [4]	6-12 months, then re-assessment	Nitrofurantoin	50mg nocte[5]	Yes	No	See above (major reactions unlikely)
		Nalidixic acid	0.5g nocte	Yes	No	See above
		Benzylpenicillin	0.25g nocte	Yes	Yes	Hypersensitivity
		Methenamine (hexamine) hippurate	1g nocte	Yes	No	Nausea, gastric distress
		Methenamine mandelate	2g nocte[6]	Yes	No	Nausea, gastric distress
		Co-trimoxazole	1/2 tab nocte	Yes	Yes	See above
Suppressive	As long as necessary with re-assessment every 3 to 6 months	Nitrofurantoin	50-200mg	Yes	No	See above
		Nalidixic acid	0.5-2g	Yes	No	See above
		Co-trimoxazole	1-4 tabs, reducing to 2 per week	Yes	Yes	See above
		Ampicillin	500mg	Yes	Yes	See above
		Cycloserine	250mg every 2nd day	Yes	Yes	See above

1   According to results of sensitivity tests.
2   If renal function impaired see section 14.1 (table IV) and appendix E.
3   Shorter courses, including single dose regimens, of some agents are also feasible and effective (see text).
4   With drugs which do not alter the bowel flora or lead to development of resistance.
5   Some have found an immediate postintercourse dose to be almost as effective.
6   Acidifying agent given in conjunction to maintain urine pH < 5.5 (e.g. ascorbic acid, methionine, ammonium chloride).

tion that neutropenia and macrocytic anaemia are more common. Ampicillin may also be used, but maculopapular rashes occur in 10 to 15% of patients given 2g daily. The incidence of rash appears to be less with amoxycillin (Brogden et al., 1975). Nitrofurantoin and nalidixic acid are alternative drugs, but nalidixic acid is not as effective as the other antibacterial agents.

When there is systemic involvement such as fever, rigors and hypotension, parenteral agents such as the aminoglycosides kanamycin or gentamicin are indicated. Cefoxitin is a useful alternative but is not as rapidly effective as the aminoglycosides. Intensive supervised parenteral therapy is also indicated in instances of failed therapy to oral antibacterial agents; many such patients have urological abnormalities or significant renal functional impairment.

Treatment is aimed at eradicating the urinary infection with an agent most effective against the causative organism (Bailey, 1974, 1977). A 5 to 10 day course of an appropriate curative drug regimen is adequate (table I). Patients should be advised that although relief of symptoms will probably be rapid, the prescribed course of treatment must be completed. 3 day courses of amoxycillin are almost as effective as 10 days and a single dose of amoxycillin (3g adults; 100mg/kg children) or 6 tablets (adults) or 1.5 to 3 tablets (children) of co-trimoxazole give results comparable with a 5 or 7 day course (Bailey, 1979). Single dose kanamycin (500mg) also gives high cure rates (Fairley, 1978). Single dose therapy, a recent and as yet relatively untried alternative, is simple, effective, well tolerated and preferred by patients. It is also more economical and can be supervised. It also has diagnostic advantages (Bailey, 1979). If a patient fails this treatment she is more likely to have an underlying urinary tract abnormality or an infection in the kidneys, as opposed to only the bladder (Ronald et al., 1976; Fairley, 1978), and therefore justifies investigation of renal function, more intensive treatment and longer follow-up.

The volume of fluid ingested during antibacterial therapy does not appear to affect the outcome but some consider a high fluid intake is a useful adjunct because it results in more frequent bladder emptying. Although a high urine flow dilutes the drug concentration it also reduces the concentration of organisms. Alkalinising agents should not be used alone; they do not eradicate bacteriuria, although they may temporarily relieve lower urinary tract symptoms.

3.2 Recurrent Urinary Tract Infections

There are two forms of recurrence: *relapse* (20% of cases) which usually occurs within 1 month of stopping treatment and is due to infection with the same organism, and *reinfection* (80% of cases) which usually occurs after a longer interval and is due to infection with new strains or organisms (Turck et al., 1966; Kunin, 1970). The causes of relapse and reinfection are difficult to understand, but both can be due to abnormality within the urinary tract. All patients with recurrent urinary tract infection should therefore be investigated for anatomical abnormality of the renal tract and, where possible, defects should be corrected. An early relapse might be due to an inappropriate antibacterial regimen (inadequate dosage or use of an agent to which the causative organism is resistant) or to patient failure to take the prescribed course of treatment (Daschner and Marget, 1975).

In patients with a normal urinary tract, particularly women with recurrent sexual intercourse induced acute urinary infection, the great majority can be kept free of attacks by use of a long term low dose *preventive* antibacterial regimen, taken after voiding before going to bed (Bailey, 1974, 1977; Harding and Ronald, 1974; table I). Such a prophylactic regimen should be commenced after a curative course of treatment, as evidenced by bacteriological culture. Some women with recurrent infection can remain free of attacks by practising double micturition, postcoital micturition, or by applying an antiseptic cream such as 0.5% cetrimide to the periurethral area prior to sexual intercourse. It is therefore perhaps preferable to attempt these simpler measures before embarking on a prophylactic course of treatment with an antibacterial agent.

Long term *suppressive* antibacterial therapy (table I) should be considered if irremedial abnormalities in the renal tract are present, or in those few patients in whom it is impossible to eradicate infection by preventive therapy. If parenchymal infection has occurred, nitrofurantoin should not be used and only drugs which attain effective tissue and urinary concentration should be given (table I).

It would seem rational to treat on a long term basis only those patients whose recurrent infection is due to relapse, whilst giving repeated short term therapy to those who become frequently reinfected with new strains or organisms. While these two

Table II. A summary of the principles of management of symptomatic urinary tract infections (after Bailey, 1974)

---

1. *Diagnosis* (proof that bacteria are multiplying within the urinary tract)
   a) Collection of urine specimen — suprapubic aspiration of distended bladder preferable to the clean catch mid stream technique.
   b) Culture of specimen (to determine causative organism and antibacterial sensitivity).

2. *Treatment*
   a) Acute attack — 5 to 10 day course of a curative antibacterial drug regimen (see table I), but not alkalinising agents alone. Single dose regimens are as effective and have advantages (see text). Hospital use of parenteral therapy if patient severely ill or vomiting, and in cases of failed therapy to oral agents.
   b) Recurrent attacks (if no anatomical abnormality).
      i) Simple measures — in women, trial of double micturition, postcoital micturition or preintercourse application of 0.5% cetrimide cream to periurethral area; examination of sexual partner for balanitis.
      ii) Treatment of any vaginitis (e.g. OC-induced) before embarking on:
      iii) Preventive or prophylactic antibacterial regimen — 6 to 12 months course of appropriate agent (see table I), followed by trial of treatment free period.
      iv) Suppressive antibacterial regimen (see table I) — in those in whom impossible to eradicate infection (not frequently required).
   c) Special problems in men (Kunin, 1975).
      i) Careful examination — plasma creatinine, prostate, measurement residual urine, IVP.
      ii) Remove urinary obstructions.
      iii) Initial curative regimen (table I) — to eradicate infection, then follow closely.
      iv) If recurrence — co-trimoxazole for possible prostatic focus of infection (i.e. in absence of stones, obstruction).
      v) Suppressive antibacterial regimen (table I) — if above fails and recurrence continues, particularly with same organism.

3. *Investigations*
   a) Infants, children and men — at time of initial attack.
   b) Women — withold IVP if occasional infection occurs after onset of sexual activity, particularly if UTI's respond to a curative regimen (see table I) and follow up cultures are sterile.

4. *Follow-up*
   a) Culture urine at 1 week, 6 weeks and then at increasing intervals for period of 12 to 18 months (to prevent symptomatic recurrences).
   b) Reappearance of identical organism as originally within 24 to 72 hours suggests failure of eradication, likelihood of upper tract infection and need for prompt urinary tract investigation.

---

groups may be distinguished by typing the organisms involved, this is usually not possible routinely (see summary table II).

3.3 Urinary Infection in Children

Acute urinary tract infection in infants or young children should be treated, irrespective of whether they are symptomatic or asymptomatic (Heale, 1973). Studies of the natural history of the disease suggest that recurrent infections in the very young are capable of causing kidney scarring and renal failure within a few years, especially when vesicoureteric reflux and/or obstruction are present. The most important way to reduce the development of renal infection and scarring and the incidence of renal failure arising from infection is to detect and treat the patient in early childhood before the age of 5 years.

The approach to treatment is outlined in figure 2. Specific details on treatment are given in chapter IV (sect. 5.1.5).

3.4 Urinary Tract Infection in Men

Urinary tract infection in men is much less common than in women. Often it is associated with prostatitis and prostatic enlargement.

Prostatic fluid is highly acidic so basic drugs such as co-trimoxazole, erythromycin, and triacetyl-oleandomycin (troleandomycin), which distribute more readily into prostatic fluid, particularly co-trimoxazole are the drugs of choice (see Meares, 1978; table II).

3.5 Renal Tuberculosis

Renal tuberculosis should be suspected when sterile pyuria is present and may be confirmed by culturing the organism from an early morning specimen of urine. Before the sensitivity pattern of the organism is known, three antituberculosis agents should be used in treatment, otherwise two agents are sufficient when it is known that the organism is sensitive to both. When expense is not of primary importance, rifampicin, isoniazid and streptomycin are among the best available preparations. Ethambutol may be substituted for rifampicin. Treatment should be continued for 9 months. With the exception of rifampicin, dosage of common agents should be modified if renal failure is present (see table IV). Ureteric stenosis is a relatively common complication, either before treatment is begun or soon afterwards. The value of corticosteroids in relieving obstruction is controversial. In one series, 72% of 29 consecutive patients treated with prednisolone, 20mg/day, had

their ureteric obstruction relieved. Frequent assessment of progress by excretion urography or renography is essential. If corticosteroids fail, cystoscopic dilatation of the ureter may be sufficient but major reconstructive surgery may be necessary.

4. Glomerulonephritis

The term glomerulonephritis covers a number of glomerular reactions in which glomerular inflammation is either a primary reaction or a secondary consequence of a systemic disorder (Cameron, 1972; Merrill, 1974). Many diseases which affect the renal glomerulus are not precisely defined in terms of aetiology, pathogenesis, natural history and prognosis. The deposition of circulating antigen-antibody complexes in the glomerular capillary wall appears to be the main cause of the majority of the human cases of glomerulonephritis. In addition, intravascular coagulation as a primary or secondary event and the response of the mesangial cells contributes to the natural history (Davison et al., 1973). At present, treatment is aimed at these presumptive mechanisms, and in some types of glomerulonephritis, at stabilising the pathological defect in the basement membrane (Clarkson and

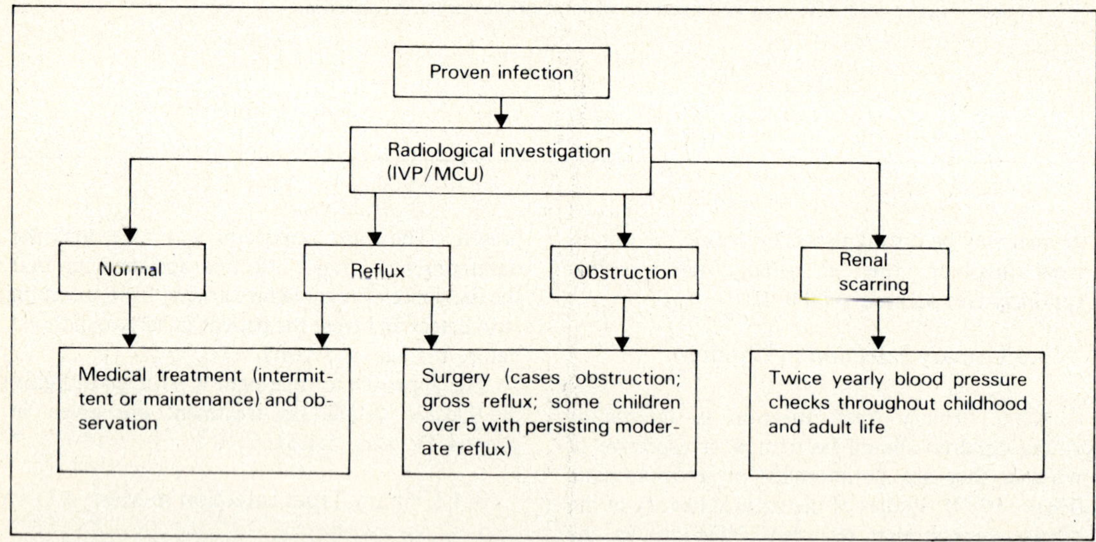

Fig. 2. The management of childhood urinary infections (following treatment of an acute proven infection). Spontaneous cessation of reflux is unlikely in children with gross reflux and in some children over 5 with persisting moderate reflux. Surgery is indicated in these children and in those with an underlying obstruction (after Heale: Drugs 6: 230, 1973).

Robson, 1972). Several types of drug have been used in an attempt to ameliorate the immunological, inflammatory and haemostatic aspects of the various forms of the disease, but in many cases results of treatment are unclear.

Another approach is with levamisole, an anthelmintic drug (see chapter XIX; sect. 11.4), which has immunostimulant properties and increases host response to antigen; it has been used experimentally in man.

4.1 Minimal Lesion (Steroid Sensitive) Glomerulonephritis

This condition commonly presents as the nephrotic syndrome with oedema, proteinuria and hypoproteinaemia. Although the glomerulus appears normal to light microscopy, fusion of the pedicels of the epithelial cells can be seen with electron microscopy. This change is probably a result rather than a cause of proteinuria. Prednisone (1mg/kg/day) for 2 to 3 weeks followed by reduced doses for 4 to 8 weeks produces a diuresis, loss of oedema, abolition or diminution in proteinuria, correction of plasma protein concentration and remission in a large majority of patients. However, studies of the natural history have shown that spontaneous remission occurs in a proportion of patients and that there is little difference in the remission rate between treated and untreated patients 2 years after presentation (Cameron, 1971a).

The mode of action of corticosteroids is uncertain; their effect may be mediated by membrane stabilisation. A significant increase in the number of patients who remit permanently can be obtained by giving the immunosuppressive drug cyclophosphamide (3mg/kg/day) for 8 weeks together with corticosteroids, or even during a steroid induced remission (Cameron, 1971b; Editorial, 1976). Adverse reactions of cyclophosphamide include alopecia, chemical cystitis, susceptibility to viral infections, leucopenia and infertility (see chapter XV; sect. 23.1). The severity of these adverse reactions together with the dangers of corticosteroids must be weighed against the advantages of treating this condition. In general it seems wise to reserve cyclophosphamide for patients who relapse after unsuccessful therapy with steroids alone. Chlorambucil is also effective in sustaining remission and can be used as an alternative to cyclophosphamide (Grupe et al., 1976; Baluarte et al., 1978).

4.2 Rapidly Progressive Glomerulonephritis

This condition is characterised by widespread inflammatory cell infiltration of the glomerulus, variable epithelial and mesangial cell proliferation and extensive crescent formation. Immunofluorescent studies show immune complexes and complement to be widely deposited in the basement membrane and electron microscopic examination reveals the presence of intra- and extraglomerular coagulation. The condition has a poor prognosis, especially in adults. Some uncontrolled studies have suggested that a few patients benefit from corticosteroids in large doses (Cameron, 1971a). Heparin by continuous infusion in amounts sufficient to maintain the clotting time between 25 and 30 minutes has also been tried (Robson et al., 1977). Most centres now use combined therapy and some have claimed success with quadruple therapy with corticosteroids, azathioprine or cyclophosphamide, the antiplatelet aggregating agent dipyridamole plus heparin followed by warfarin (Brown et al., 1974). No firm conclusions can be drawn from these uncontrolled studies at the present time.

Plasma exchange has been tried and improvement claimed in a few cases (Becker et al., 1977), but its effect is unknown.

4.3 Proliferative and Mesangiocapillary Glomerulonephritis

In the majority of cases no aetiological agent can be found. Where possible, precipitating causes such as streptococcal or staphylococcal infection should be sought and if found treated. If there is suspicion that penicillin is responsible, it should be withdrawn.

Very mild cases of diffuse proliferative glomerulonephritis may be difficult to differentiate from minimal lesion glomerulonephritis using pathological and clinical criteria; proteinuria is highly selective in both. Prednisone in doses similar to those given in minimal lesion disease appears to reduce the amount of proteinuria in some cases, but rarely abolishes it. In more severe cases of proliferative glomerulonephritis, and in mesangiocapillary glomerulonephritis the proteinuria tends to be less selective and prednisone has little effect. Large doses of prednisone also reduce the excretion of urinary fibrin degradation products (Clarkson et al., 1971, 1972). The threshold for this effect varies from patient to patient and may be due either to differences in sensitivity of the patient to the drug or variations in the rate of drug elimination. Despite these effects and the obvious immunological nature of the disease there is no evidence that corticosteroids improve the prognosis. In one controlled study morbidity in the untreated group was less than that of the treated group, the difference being due to adverse reactions to corticosteroids. The combination of azathioprine and corticosteroids has been shown to be equally ineffective (Medical Research Council Working Party, 1971).

The use of heparin has also been advised. Depot preparations of heparin may be given subcutaneously (200 to 600mg/day) to produce clotting times of 30 minutes. Although some claim a slightly improved morbidity and mortality (Kincaid-Smith et al., 1973), this view is not universal and the control of heparin dosage presents many problems. Many factors affect its activity and also independently affect coagulation.

An alternative method of possibly influencing intraglomerular coagulation is to give antiplatelet aggregating agents such as indomethacin which may act by preventing the formation of prostaglandin thromboxane. In contrast to heparin, indomethacin is relatively non-toxic. Treatment often results in an initial fall in urinary protein and in fibrin degradation products. Improvement in renal histology and function occurs in some patients but the value of indomethacin and that of other antiplatelet agents such as dipyridamole, used in combination with oral anticoagulants, has not been confirmed in controlled trials (Cameron, 1977; George et al., 1975). It may be that an inadequate dose was used. Because of the occasional induction of glomerular thromboses and the haemolytic uraemic syndrome (Boyd et al., 1975; Jackson et al., 1976), it would seem advisable to avoid the use of the contraceptive pill in patients with glomerulonephritis.

4.4 Membranous Glomerulonephritis

This condition is so named because the histological abnormality mainly consists of thickening of the basement membrane with deposits of immune material in its substance, or projecting from the epithelial surface. In about 20 % of patients the disease resolves over a period of years, but the majority of cases slowly progress, producing symptoms of the nephrotic syndrome

and leading ultimately to renal failure (Row et al., 1975). An adequately controlled multicentre trial of 2mg/kg/day prednisone given on alternate days for 2 months followed by a tapering dose for a further month is presently being undertaken in the USA. Early results (Glassock, 1978) suggest that in a number of patients the condition resolves during the period of treatment. A small controlled trial suggests that chlorambucil is effective in reducing proteinuria (Lagrue et al., 1975) but this needs to be confirmed.

5. Nephrotic Syndrome

The nephrotic syndrome describes the triad of kidney disease, proteinuria and oedema. Most cases of the nephrotic syndrome arise as a result of one or other of the primary forms of glomerulonephritis, but it is unusual for these patients to have a history of preceding acute glomerulonephritis and the precise histological diagnosis is made only after renal biopsy.

In children, minimal lesion glomerulonephritis is by far the most common form. Proliferative glomerulonephritis, followed by membranous glomerulonephritis, are most often responsible in adults (see further section 4). Many non-renal diseases (e.g. diabetes mellitus, pre-eclampsia, amyloid disease, systemic lupus erythematosus, polyarteritis and its variants) may be associated with the nephrotic syndrome and it may arise as a result of the adverse reaction to some drugs. It may also be an early manifestation of malignant disease (Robson, 1972, 1974).

5.1 Hypoproteinaemia and Proteinuria

Usually, proteinuria is of the order of 5 to 10g/day but may be as great as 40g. Though plasma protein concentrations indicate the degree of protein depletion, the deficit of body proteins may be far greater than the concentration of plasma proteins suggest. For these reasons, up to 2 to 3g/kg of dietary protein should be given each day and continued whilst there is no evidence of uraemia.

5.2 Salt and Water Retention

Hypoproteinaemia causes oligaemia and hence diminished renal blood flow. This in turn causes secondary aldosteronism, salt and water retention and potassium depletion. Bed rest improves renal blood flow. There are many diuretics which effectively reduce reabsorption in the renal tubules. Frusemide (furosemide) inhibits reabsorption of NaCl in the ascending limb of the loop of Henle and distal convoluted tubule (fig. 3). A suitable initial dose is 40mg/day orally and this may be increased up to 0.5 to 1g/daily until a diuresis is obtained. Where a satisfactory diuresis occurs there is little need to restrict the dietary content of salt. However, if the drug is only partially effective, strict dietary control with an intake of 10mmol (10mEq)/day of sodium becomes necessary. If these measures are not effective, spironolactone (100mg twice daily) may be added. This drug acts by antagonising aldosterone action in the distal tubule and should always be given with another diuretic, to ensure adequate delivery of sodium to the distal tubule. The concentration of plasma potassium should be monitored carefully to avoid potentially dangerous hyperkalaemia.

A hazard of overvigorous diuretic therapy in the nephrotic syndrome is acute renal failure. This may follow an acute fall in blood volume and can be avoided by giving a plasma expander such as salt poor albumin (Davison et al., 1974). Dextran 70 can be used when plasma proteins are not available. Plasma protein should be given daily in amounts of 20 to 40g intravenously over 1 to 2 hours. Frusemide (500mg) should be given over the last 20 to 30 minutes of the infusion. This gives an infusion rate of 25mg/min which some claim is associated with the occurrence of ototoxicity (Rupp, 1974; see chapter XI; sect. 7.1.2) but this has not been our experience. However, if tinnitus, dizziness or vertigo appear the drug should be stopped at once. Aminophylline (500mg) may also be added to the protein infusion in order to improve renal blood flow and glomerular filtration rate. Though much of the protein is lost in the urine, the regimen increases water and salt excretion and control of otherwise intractable oedema is achieved. Ethacrynic acid is an alternative to frusemide but is associated with a greater incidence of adverse effects.

5.3 Hyperlipidaemia

There is an inverse relationship between plasma cholesterol and triglyceride concentrations and plasma albumin concentration. It has therefore been claimed that the increased incidence of ischaemic heart disease in nephrotic patients is due to the hyperlipidaemia. Since cholestyramine and clofibrate lower plasma cholesterol concentration (see chapter XVII; sect. 3.2.4), these drugs may be of value in patients with persistent nephrotic syndrome. Chlorophenoxyisobutyric acid, a metabolite of clofibrate, is the active agent. High concentrations of this substance, which accumulates in the presence of impaired renal function, are associated with a toxic myopathy in the nephrotic syndrome if there is any associated renal functional impairment and dosage is not modified appropriately (Bridgman et al., 1972; Gugler, 1978; see also section 1.2, 14.7).

6. Renal Hypertension

Nephrosclerosis is probably a result of essential hypertension rather than a cause. Treatment may arrest the progress of renal damage which occurs in a small proportion of these patients. Management is described in chapter XVIII.

6.1 Accelerated Hypertension and Nephrosclerosis

This condition may arise 'de novo' or occur in association with other renal diseases such as pyelonephritis, glomerulonephritis, polyarteritis and unilateral renal artery stenosis (Ledingham, 1971). There is good evidence that adequate control of blood pressure with agents which do not reduce renal blood flow, slows the otherwise rapid decline in renal function and sometimes an improvement in GFR may occur (Various Authors, 1975b).

When severe accelerated hypertension develops and in hypertensive encephalopathy, emergency treatment with diazoxide is usually effective (Mathew and Kincaid-Smith, 1971; Finnerty, 1974). Diazoxide inhibits contraction of the smooth muscle of the arteriole. When given intravenously to adults as a single dose of 300mg over 10 seconds (5mg/kg in children and adults > 113kg), approximately 95% of patients respond within 1 to 2 minutes with a satisfactory fall in blood pressure. Diazoxide may be repeated in an hour if necessary. The fall in blood pressure is accompanied by a rise in cardiac output and a fall in peripheral resistance. A slight fall in GFR occurs but this quickly recovers to pretreatment or higher levels. The fall in blood pressure so obtained, although not as precipitous as that obtained with ganglion blockers, has been associated with cerebrovascular catastrophies (Kuman et al., 1976). Labetalol, an α and β-adrenoceptor blocking drug (see chapter XVIII; section 5.7), infusions are claimed to give a more controlled fall in blood pressure (Rosei et al., 1975).

Diazoxide has a variable duration of action of up to 4 to 12 hours or more. It has a mild salt retaining effect and expansion of the extracellular fluid volume tends to diminish its hypotensive action. Concurrent treatment with a potent diuretic such as frusemide (40mg rapidly intravenously initially) overcomes this effect. Adverse reactions include nausea, vomiting, a generalised sense of burning along the vein, angina and hyperglycaemia which can occur sometimes after beginning treatment. Hyperglycaemia may preclude its use in patients who are prediabetic or who are receiving large doses of corticosteroids, but can be readily corrected by insulin or tolbutamide. It causes skeletal deformities in animal fetuses when given in large doses to the mothers in early pregnancy (see also chapter XV; sect. 5.2, 5.3). Diazoxide has a plasma half-life of about 18 hours (i.e. greater than its hypotensive effect) and is highly protein bound. It is mainly excreted unchanged in the urine but cumulation has not been a problem in uraemic patients. However, due to reduced protein binding its action is potentiated by hypoalbuminaemia and reduced doses are probably desirable in patients with severe uraemia (Pearson, 1977). Oral diazoxide in large doses (with tolbutamide) has been successfully used in patients with uncontrolled malignant hypertension resistant to all other antihypertensive drugs (Fang et al., 1974). For a review of the pharmacology and use of diazoxide, see Speight and Avery (1971).

6.2 Renovascular Hypertension

Stenosis of the main renal artery or one of its branches is a relatively rare but important cause of hypertension. The different pathologies include atherosclerosis, fibromuscular dysplasia, renal artery thrombosis and embolism. The cause of the hypertension is obscure but it is associated with so called ischaemic changes; these include a reduced GFR and an increase in the proportion of Na^+ and H_2O reabsorbed by the tubules. Surgical correction of the abnormality should be carried out only if the patient is below 45 years, and after the specific characteristics of unilateral renal ischaemia have been demonstrated by intravenous pyelography, renography, arteriography and renal vein renin estimation. Otherwise management is medical. Propranolol reduces cardiac output and renin secretion and has been claimed to be particularly effective, whilst avoiding postural hypotension (Zacest et al., 1972). Hydrallazine, a vasodilator, is often a useful additional agent. Spironolactone may be needed to control the K^+ loss consequent upon secondary aldosteronism.

6.3 Hypertension in Chronic Haemodialysis

Regular haemodialysis is remarkably effective in controlling hypertension whatever the cause of the renal failure. Patients who adhere to dietary restriction of water and salt, but remain hypertensive, are usually secreting an inappropriately large amount of renin. If β-adrenoceptor blockade fails, bilateral nephrectomy is usually curative. Bilateral nephrectomy is particularly indicated in patients being considered for transplantation.

7. Oedema and Diuretics

7.1 Diuretic Action and Metabolic Effects

Diuretics are loosely defined as agents that increase the flow of urine. This discussion is restricted to those drugs that exert this pharmacological effect by reducing the reabsorption of NaCl and water by renal tubules, either by interfering with active transport mechanisms or by altering tubular permeability (see Anderton and Kincaid-Smith, 1971; Davies and Wilson, 1975). Benzothiadiazines and related compounds (i.e. chlorothiazide, chlorthalidone, metolazone and clopamide) are medium potency compounds which act mainly on the cortical diluting segment of the nephron (site III in fig. 3). They have a mild hypotensive action, cause a rise in plasma uric acid and are mildly diabetogenic (see chapter XVI; sect. 14.1). Tienilic acid (ticrynafen) is a nonsulphonamide diuretic which partially resembles the benzothiadiazine drugs pharmacologically, in that its primary site of diuretic action is also the cortical diluting segment of the distal tubule (see fig. 3). However, unlike the benzothiadiazines which may increase serum uric acid concentrations, tienilic acid reduces both 'normal' and elevated uric acid concentrations by inhibiting urate reabsorptive mechanisms (Bolli et al., 1978).

Frusemide, bumetanide and ethacrynic acid are more powerful diuretics which act predominantly on site II of the nephron; i.e. the ascending limb of the loop of Henle (fig. 3). By virtue of this site of action they interfere with the countercurrent multiplier system of the loop and cause the elimination of a greater volume of water for a given amount of NaCl than other diuretics. Frusemide and bumetanide are heterocyclic sulphonamyl derivatives while ethacrynic acid has an entirely different chemical structure.

Spironolactone, triamterene and amiloride are by themselves much weaker diuretics and all antagonise distal tubular sodium absorption. Whilst spironolactone is a steroid and competitively antagonises aldosterone, triamterene and amiloride, although having a similar effect on distal sodium absorption, do not mediate it through an aldosterone dependent mechanism. These diuretics cause potassium retention (a so called 'potassium sparing' effect) and thus may be hazardous in patients with impaired renal function (Greenblatt and Koch-Weser, 1973). Properties of the various diuretics in common use are summarised in table III.

In most clinical situations where oedema is present, renal perfusion is reduced resulting in a poor delivery of sodium to the distal tubule. In mild or moderately severe oedema a satisfactory diuretic response can often be achieved by using a single drug of medium potency or by giving frusemide (or bumetanide) alone. However, the response to diuretics is self limited; as the volume of the expanded extracellular fluid is reduced a number of

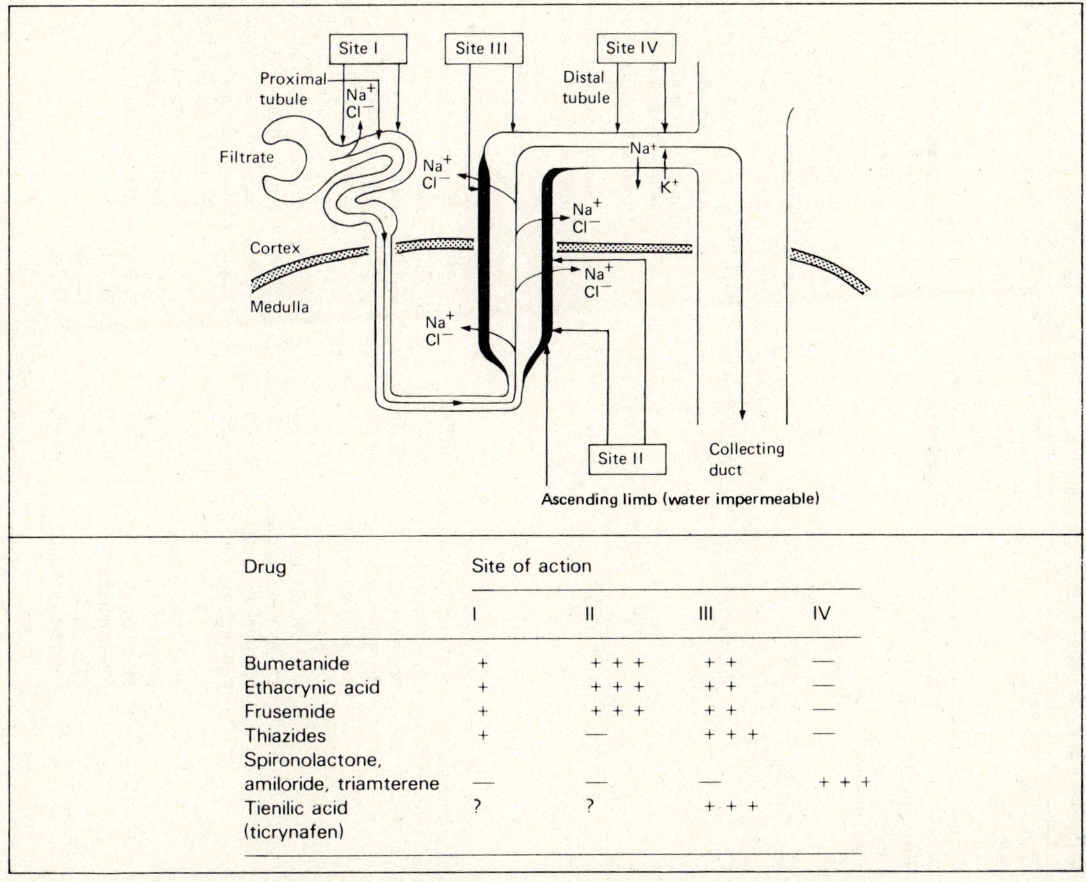

Drug	Site of action			
	I	II	III	IV
Bumetanide	+	+ + +	+ +	—
Ethacrynic acid	+	+ + +	+ +	—
Frusemide	+	+ + +	+ +	—
Thiazides	+	—	+ + +	—
Spironolactone, amiloride, triamterene	—	—	—	+ + +
Tienilic acid (ticrynafen)	?	?	+ + +	

Fig. 3. The nephron, depicting sites of diuretic action on sodium and chloride reabsorption. Site I = Proximal tubule; II = Ascending limb of Henle's loop; III = Early distal tubule (cortical diluting segment); IV = Distal tubular site of K+ secretion (after Davies and Wilson: Drugs 9: 178, 1975).

Site of action: +++ = major or sole site of action; ++ = some action at this site; + = possible action at this site.

Table III. Properties of some diuretics in common use

Primary site of action/ primary effects	Diuretic	Daily dose range in oedema (mg)	Duration of action	Important properties/notes	Main side effects
Distal tubule 'Potassium sparing' effect with acidosis and relatively small diuresis	Spirorolactone	50-800	24h	Delayed effect (up to 48 hours). Dosage required depends on amount of aldosterone present. Natriuretic and diuretic effects most pronounced in hyperaldosteronism, much lower in 'normals'. Highly protein bound. Extensively metabolised, at least 1 active metabolite. Excreted in urine and bile	Dose related gynaecomastia, menstrual irregularities; hyperkalaemia (avoid potassium supplements, check renal function and avoid in renal failure; see section 7.1)
	Triamterene	100-200 or 400	10h	Low diuretic and natriuretic potency when given alone. Activity not dependent on presence of aldosterone. Extensively metabolised and excreted mainly in urine	Hyperkalaemia (avoid potassium supplements, check renal function and avoid in renal failure)
	Amiloride	5-10	~24h	Diuretic and natriuretic activity and mechanism of action similar to triamterene; i.e. independent of aldosterone. Excreted in urine unchanged	Hyperkalaemia (avoid potassium supplements, check renal function and avoid in renal failure)
Cortical diluting segment Moderate diuresis and hypokalaemic alkalosis	*Benzothiadiazines*[1] Hydrochlorothiazide	50-200	6-12h	Benzothiadiazines and related compounds are similar pharmacologically, the duration of action being the main differing factor between drugs in this group. All benzothiadiazines and related variants have a steep dose-response curve, with little increased effect beyond upper limits shown. Reduced effectiveness in renal impairment; a 'loop' diuretic usually required in such patients. Therapeutic cross resistance occurs within this group. Excreted mainly unchanged in urine. Renal clearance of substituted benzothiadiazines is lower resulting in longer duration of action	Hyponatraemia, hyperglycaemia (see chapter XVI; sect. 13.1, 14.1), hyperuricaemia. Hypokalaemia (most clinicians use potassium replacements especially if treatment is long term or large doses of diuretics are used; of particular importance in digitalised or cirrhotic patients; see section 7.1). Concomitant use of a 'potassium sparing' diuretic with a thiazide reduces potassium loss and may increase response
	Chlorothiazide	500-2000	6-12h		
	Benzthiazide	50-200	12-18h		
	Bendrofluazide (bendroflumethiazide)	2.5-10	18-24h		
	Cyclopenthiazide	0.5-2	~12h		
	Hydroflumethiazide	25-200	18-24h		
	Trichlormethiazide	1-2 or 4	18-24h		
	Methyclothiazide	2.5-10	>24h		
	Polythiazide	0.5-8	24-48h		
	Benzothiadiazine variants Metolazone	5-20	12-24h		
	Chlorthalidone	25-100	24-72h		
	Clopamide	10-60	12-24h		
	Quinethazone	50-100	18-24h		

	Mefruside	25-100	12-24h	Resembles frusemide structurally but benzothiadiazines pharmacologically	As for benzothiadiazines
	Tienilic acid (ticrynafen)	250-500	12-24h	Non-sulphonamide derivative with uricosuric, as well as natriuretic and diuretic activity. Highly protein bound (99.5%)	Hyponatraemia, hypokalaemia (see above). Rapid uricosuric effect may cause intratubular uric acid precipitation and acute gout, especially in 'at risk' patients. Adequate fluid intake essential; colchicine and urinary alkalinisation may be indicated initially in such patients
Loop of Henle[2] Large rapid diuresis and hypokalaemic alkalosis	Frusemide IV Frusemide oral	20-100 40-1000	2h 4h	Very wide dose response curve; graded effect achieved through dosage adjustment. IV administration produces very rapid effect; useful in acute pulmonary oedema and other severe oedematous conditions. Effective in impaired renal function; higher doses but increased dosing interval may be needed (see text). Highly protein bound. Small amount metabolised. Eliminated about equally by renal and extrarenal mechanisms	Hyponatraemia, hypochloraemia, hypokalaemia, hyperuricaemia, dehydration. Ototoxicity, especially in nephrotic syndrome or excessive rate of infusion in renal impairment. Rarely dermatological and haematological reactions
	Ethacrynic acid	100-400	6h	Dose-response curve less wide than frusemide but actions similar. Highly protein bound. Partly metabolised and excreted by hepatic and renal routes	As for frusemide. Ototoxicity more likely (see chapter XI; sect. 7.1.2)
	Bumetanide	1-15	5h	Actions similar to frusemide; onset slightly slower. Highly protein bound. Mainly eliminated by renal excretion of unchanged drug	As for frusemide, but ototoxicity may be less frequent. Also myalgia, possibly dose related

1   Also exert some action in the proximal tubule (see fig. 3).
2   'Loop' diuretics also exert some action in the proximal tubule and cortical diluting segment (see fig. 3).

compensatory responses serve to stimulate the capacity of those parts of the nephron not affected by the drug to increase salt conservation and blunt the pharmacological response. If these events occur before the oedema is controlled it is rational to add spironolactone, which acts more distally (site IV) and so augments the effect of the agent which is acting more proximally.

Diuretic response to thiazides such as chlorothiazide does not increase greatly with increasing dose. However, this is not the case with those drugs which act on the loop of Henle, and with these drugs it is customary to titrate the dose of the diuretic against the desired clinical effect. In this manner, significant responses can be obtained even in advanced renal failure. The major complications of this practice are electrolyte imbalance and ototoxicity (see chapter XI; sect. 7.1).

The compensatory mechanisms described above are responsible for the major electrolyte complications that can attend diuretic therapy. Potassium depletion is a well known hazard and when severe can lead to serious adverse effects which include an enhanced response to the action of digitalis, paraesthesiae, polyuria, mental depression, sleepiness and irritability. Urinary potassium loss is promoted both by a diminution in tubular K absorption and increased distal tubular secretion consequent upon an increase in the electrical potential difference between lumen and peritubular blood. Depletion may be prevented by prescribing supplemental potassium salts by mouth or by one of the diuretics which inhibit potassium secretion. Potassium sparing diuretics are more effective than potassium supplements in the presence of hyperaldosteronism, and while potassium supplements may serve to correct diuretic induced hypokalaemia in oedematous patients with cardiac or liver disease, potassium sparing diuretics are more effective in repleting total body potassium. Potassium sparing diuretics are also probably more effective than potassium chloride in correcting both hypokalaemia and any associated metabolic alkalosis. Potassium salts are not effective in correcting hypokalaemia associated with metabolic alkalosis unless chloride is available at the same time. Alkaline salts of potassium raise blood bicarbonate levels with a consequent increase in bicarbonate flows to the distal tubule and resultant extra loss of potassium. Potassium chloride is the preferred potassium salt for general use.

The indications for routine potassium replacement in oedematous patients receiving diuretics is contentious, but most consider that replacement is indicated in all but the mildest case of oedema and when treatment is long continued, especially if large doses of diuretics are being given. When potassium supplements are used, adequate amounts must be given; for example, at least 20mmol (mEq) per day, and preferably 25 to 50mmol, in patients with nephrotic or cardiac oedema. While the risk of hyperkalaemia from potassium supplements is increased in the elderly (Lawson, 1974), small amounts of potassium can not be relied upon to prevent hypokalaemia (Krakauer and Lauritzen, 1978; see also chapter V, sect. 4.1.2). When using potassium sparing diuretics, to avoid the risk of hyperkalaemia it is necessary to ensure that dosage is not excessive, that renal function is normal and that the intake of potassium is not excessive. Regular monitoring of serum potassium is also desirable (see further Kassirer and Harrington, 1977; Morgan, 1973; Jellett, 1978).

Other electrolyte consequences of overvigorous use of diuretics are metabolic alkalosis and hyponatraemia. Hyponatraemia is liable to occur when the diuretic reduces the renal capacity to form a dilute urine, so setting a limit on the amount of solute free water that can be excreted. If the patient then ingests water in greater amounts than can be excreted, hyponatraemia is inescapable.

7.2 Pharmacokinetic Properties of Diuretics

The benzothiadiazines, the most widely used group of diuretics, are absorbed from the gastrointestinal tract, primarily from the upper small intestine (Beerman et al., 1976). Absorption of hydrochlorothiazide is dependent on intestinal transit time, being increased when intestinal transit is slowed (Beerman and Groschinsky-Grind, 1978). The thiazides are widely distributed in body fluids; bendroflumethiazide having an apparent volume of distribution of about 1.5L/kg (Beermann et al., 1977a). All members of this group (and related variants; see table III) are extensively bound to plasma proteins (mainly albumin), the substituted molecules being the most highly bound thus resulting in a lower renal clearance than the earlier compounds and a more prolonged duration of action (Davies and Wilson, 1975). Most are excreted in the urine, primarily in unchanged form; more than 95 % of hydrochlorothiazide is excreted unchanged after an oral dose (Beermann et al., 1976). However, a smaller proportion of bendroflumethiazide (about 30%; Beermann et al., 1977a) and chlorthalidone (about 50%; Riess et al., 1977) are excreted unchanged.

Spironolactone is rapidly metabolised to at least 1 active compound, canrenone, and about 50% of an oral dose is eventually excreted as canrenone and other metabolites in the urine (Karim, 1978). Although the plasma half-life may be prolonged in patients with cirrhosis or heart failure, there is no evidence of accumulation (Abshagen et al., 1977; Jackson et al., 1977), but it should be avoided in patients with renal failure because of the risk of accumulation and/or hyperkalaemia. Triamterene is extensively metabolised and excreted in the urine (Pruitt et al., 1977). Amiloride is eliminated in the urine unchanged (Weiss et al., 1969).

The 'loop' diuretics frusemide, ethacrynic acid and bumetanide are highly bound to plasma albumin (e.g. frusemide about 96%; Rane et al., 1978) and have low distribution volumes (appendix A). Frusemide and ethacrynic acid are partially metabolised and excreted in approximately equal proportions by the kidneys and the liver, while bumetanide is excreted mainly as unchanged drug in the urine and to a lesser extent as metabolites in the urine and bile (Halladay et al., 1977). In hypoalbuminaemic states such as the nephrotic syndrome, binding is decreased and the fraction of free frusemide in plasma is increased. Although the renal and extrarenal clearance of total frusemide (bound + unbound) are not altered in the nephrotic syndrome, the renal clearance of unbound drug is decreased in proportion to the creatinine clearance (Rane et al., 1978), and use of excessive doses should be avoided. In uraemia, although protein binding is reduced to a lesser extent than in the nephrotic syndrome, both renal and extrarenal clearance of frusemide are reduced (Beermann et al., 1977b; Rane et al., 1978), and use of higher doses with an increase in the dosage interval in patients with impaired renal function would seem appropriate on pharmacokinetic grounds (see section 1.2). Nevertheless, in clinical practice the dose range of frusemide is large.

Tienilic acid (ticrynafen), a diuretic with uricosuric activity, is rapidly absorbed in most subjects after oral administration. As with the benzothiadiazines, it is highly protein bound (99.5%; Wood et al., 1978). The uricosuric activity of tienilic acid is not closely related to its plasma concentration.

8. Acute Renal Failure

Drugs do not have an important role in the treatment of acute renal failure. The first priority in management is to reverse any life threatening complication. The second is to establish the cause of the renal failure and remedy any treatable one. Finally, specific therapy should be applied where indicated.

8.1 Emergency Measures

8.1.1 Initial Management of Acute Renal Failure of Ischaemic Origin

It is important to ensure that fluid deficit or blood losses are adequately replenished. This may involve the treatment of shock and the correction of acid base disorders. Central venous pressure monitoring may be useful in assessing fluid requirements and avoiding pulmonary oedema. 20% mannitol (100 to 200ml) has been advocated in the early stages of the disorder in an attempt to produce a free flow of urine, but its usefulness is not established except following major cardiovascular surgery. Whilst it is likely to act as an osmotic diuretic in patients in whom sufficient renal function remains to respond in this fashion, there is no evidence that ultimate recovery of renal function occurs more quickly than would otherwise be the case (Scheer, 1965).

Frusemide in large doses of up to 2g has also been advocated and when given in these circumstances sometimes induces a large diuresis (Cantarovich et al., 1973). For this reason it is indicated when severe pulmonary oedema is present. However, there is no evidence that it favourably influences the renal haemodynamic disorder of acute ischaemic renal failure (Epstein et al., 1975). For this reason and because of the possibility of cardiac dysrhythmias and renal damage, it is not advised as a routine measure.

8.1.2 Hyperkalaemia

Severe hyperkalaemia ($[K^+] > 7mmol/L$) is a common emergency. Calcium gluconate (1g in 10ml) intravenously, rapidly but temporarily, reverses the adverse effects of high plasma potassium concentrations on the myocardium. If acidosis is present, isotonic sodium bicarbonate should be given intravenously. 10 units of insulin subcutaneously with 25g of glucose in 50ml of water has a similar rapid but short lasting effect. Ion exchange resins such as calcium resin (30g in

30ml) given orally or by rectum have a prolonged but slower action.

Resins in the sodium cycle may exacerbate pulmonary oedema in patients who are already overloaded with fluid. Hyperkalaemia and pulmonary oedema uncontrolled by medical means are indications for emergency peritoneal or haemodialysis.

8.2 Treatment by Haemodialysis

The blood urea concentration and its rate of rise are good indications of the severity of the renal failure and the need for dialysis. Concentrations of over 35mmol/L (200mg/100ml) are associated with an increased incidence of nausea, vomiting, muscle twitching, intellectual impairment, gastrointestinal haemorrhage, pericarditis and impaired resistance to infection. Now that haemodialysis does not itself carry a significant mortality, it is best carried out if the blood urea exceeds 35mmol/L and is continuing to rise. Peritoneal dialysis is more hazardous than haemodialysis when performed repeatedly, but is useful in infants and young children and in an emergency. The energy intake during the period when renal function is supported by dialysis should be between 3,500 and 5,000 cals/day. At least 1g/kg of protein should be given. Where oral feeding is not possible, carbohydrate, fat and aminoacid solutions should be given parenterally to meet the requirements.

8.3 Treatment of Uraemia — Conservative

If dialysis is either not available or not feasible, medical management is directed towards minimising the degree of uraemia and in maintaining fluid and electrolyte balance. A low protein diet (20g/day) with potassium and sodium restriction should be given. Once adequate hydration has been attained the fluid intake should exceed the previous day's output by 500ml. Slightly more can be allowed if the patient is febrile. Any cause of increased protein catabolism such as infection should be treated.

Tetracyclines, except possibly doxycycline and minocycline, should not be used in renal failure (see section 14.1.5), and corticosteroids should be avoided unless, as is rare, they are specifically indicated.

8.4 Acute Renal Failure due to Obstruction

The diagnosis may be suggested by the presence of complete anuria in a relatively fit patient together with the absence of elevation of lactic dehydrogenase and creatinine kinase activities during the initial phase. The diagnosis should be confirmed by cystoscopy and retrograde examination. Relief of the obstruction is usually followed by a diuresis. In a minority of cases the diuresis is large and inappropriate and volumes up to 10 litre/day have been recorded. Treatment then consists of fluid and electrolyte replacement. The majority of such cases regain normal function within 2 weeks but a minority continue to excrete inappropriately large amounts of urine for up to 3 months.

9. Chronic Renal Failure

Where possible it is important to establish the cause and treat any underlying disease. However, in most cases no specific therapy is possible and the aim is to provide optimum conditions in which the diseased kidneys may function (Curtis and Williams, 1975). The clinical course of a patient with advanced renal failure is punctuated by episodes of severe uraemia. It is important to determine whether these are due to progress of the disease process or to adverse and sometimes reversible extrarenal factors. For example, nausea, vomiting and salt depletion contract the extracellular fluid volume, reduce renal blood flow and hence diminish renal function further. Dehydration, blood loss, cardiac failure, urinary or other infection, urinary tract obstruction, and hypokalaemia all aggravate renal failure in patients with chronically diseased kidneys.

The principles governing the use of therapeutic drugs in patients with chronic renal failure are discussed in sections 1; 2.1 and 14.

9.1 Water

In chronic renal failure there is an early impairment of concentrating capacity and the ability to form free water is reduced. While a high fluid intake is desirable, patients are at risk of developing water intoxication and hyponatraemia. This is best treated by water restriction; hypertonic sodium chloride is rarely if ever required and may precipitate pulmonary oedema. As renal function deteriorates, fluid requirements for each patient become fixed and the needs of each patient should be assessed individually.

9.2 Sodium

The ability to regulate sodium balance is usually well maintained but obligatory loss increases with renal failure and sometimes a salt losing state develops. The sodium intake must be adjusted for each individual patient and the amount required varies at different stages of the disease. If an excess of salt and water is given pulmonary oedema and cardiac failure develop. On the other hand, insufficient intake causes oligaemia and postural hypotension with fainting and aggravates renal failure.

9.3 Potassium

Adequate potassium excretion is usually maintained even when chronic renal failure is severe. However, the potassium excretory mechanisms operate at near maximum capacity and sudden additional loads should be avoided. Drugs such as spironolactone, triamterene and amiloride should not be given. If hyperkalaemia develops measures discussed in section 8.1.2 should be applied.

9.4 Acidosis

Renal acidosis is not life threatening in itself but is best avoided as it aggravates nausea, vomiting, potassium intoxication, uraemic osteodystrophy and pulmonary oedema. It may be treated with sodium bicarbonate when venous bicarbonate concentrations fall below 20mmol/L (20mEq/L); the dose required varies from patient to patient.

9.5 Uraemia

The protein content of a diet influences the degree of uraemia, hyperkalaemia and metabolic acidosis. A 20g protein diet of first class protein and an adequate caloric intake (2,000 cals from carbohydrate and fat) with vitamin supplements will keep a patient in nitrogen balance and reduce to a minimum the production of urea. However, lean body mass often becomes reduced in patients who take such a diet for prolonged periods. Consequently, it is probably desirable to begin intermit-

tent haemodialysis when a 30 or 40g protein diet is no longer sufficient to keep the blood urea below 35mmol/L (200mg/100ml). Some patients have benefited by the addition of essential amino acids to their diet.

9.6 Renal Osteodystrophy

Reduced intestinal absorption of calcium, hypocalcaemia with a reduced concentration of total and ionised plasma calcium are common features of renal failure. However, it is uncommon for renal osteodystrophy to cause symptoms in adults unless life is prolonged by intermittent haemodialysis. Vitamin D is the treatment of choice and in the past needed to be given in large doses (calciferol 1.25mg/day). The cause of vitamin resistance lies partly in the abnormality of vitamin D metabolism consequent upon damage to kidneys (Avioli et al., 1968). There is failure of conversion of 25-hydroxycholecalciferol to $1\alpha,25$-hydroxycholecalciferol, a metabolic step which is normally carried out in the kidneys. Before becoming physiologically active, vitamin D_3 (cholecalciferol), synthesised in the skin, is metabolised by 25-hydroxylation in the liver to 25-hydroxycholecalciferol and then by 1α-hydroxylation in the kidney to its most active form $1\alpha,25$-dihydroxycholecalciferol (1,25-dihydroxyvitamin D_3 or calcitriol). This then functions as the active form of vitamin D. Vitamin D_2 (calciferol) from the diet is also metabolised in an identical manner. A new synthetic analogue of $1\alpha,25$-dihydroxycholecalciferol, 1α-hydroxycholecalciferol (1α-hydroxyvitamin D_3 or alfacalcidol) differs from the naturally occurring active metabolite only in the absence of a 25-hydroxyl group. Since it possesses a 1α-hydroxyl group, hydroxylation in the kidney is bypassed and most or all of its biological activity probably depends on conversion in the liver to $1\alpha,25$-dihydroxycholecalciferol (see Haussler and McCain, 1977). Because they bypass metabolic conversion in the kidney, calcitriol and alfacalcidol have been used to improve bone disease in patients with chronic renal failure. Used in small doses, adjusted to avoid hypercalcaemia, both the 1α-hydroxylated vitamin D_3 preparations have been effective in promoting calcium absorption and checking bone demineralisation in some patients with renal osteodystrophy (Pierides et al., 1978). Raised plasma parathyroid hormone concentrations usually fall in those with secondary hyperparathyroidism who respond to treatment

(Brownjohn et al., 1977). The response is however, variable. Best results are obtained in those with osteitis fibrosa, with or without associated osteomalacia, whereas patients with predominantly osteomalacia generally do not respond as well (Pierides et al., 1976; Bordier et al., 1978). Some consider that calcitriol has advantages over alfacalcidol particularly in that it is the naturally occurring active form of vitamin D in the intestine and bone and as it bypasses hepatic hydroxylation (see above). Unlike alfacalcidol it is effective in uraemic patients receiving anticonvulsant therapy in whom osteomalacia can be a special problem (David, 1977; see also chapter XXII, sect. 14.5). Both calcitriol and to a lesser extent alfacalcidol have the advantage over vitamin D_2 (calciferol) of a much more rapid reversal of any inadvertent hypercalcaemia on withdrawal of treatment (Kanis and Russell, 1977). Hypercalcaemia must nevertheless be avoided, since it may lead to further deterioration in renal function (Christiansen et al., 1978).

Because of the possible development of ectopic calcification, attempts to reduce plasma phosphate should be made by giving phosphate binders such as aluminium hydroxide or aminoacetate by mouth. This curtails absorption of dietary phosphate and reduces the $[Ca^{++}] \times [PO_4^{---}]$ product. When the bone disease is predominantly that of severe hyperparathyroidism, and especially if hypercalcaemia develops, subtotal parathyroidectomy should be performed.

Following the operation, calcium supplements and vitamin D are usually required, at least for a time.

9.7 Anaemia

The anaemia of chronic renal failure is usually normocytic and normochromic in type. The cause appears to be a combination of diminished erythropoiesis due to low erythropoietin secretion and an increased rate of red cell destruction (Editorial, 1975). Iron deficiency is sometimes present because of blood loss from the gastrointestinal tract and other sites. Haemoglobin may be raised by giving androgens such as testosterone propionate injections or testosterone implants (Shahidi, 1977). Anabolic-androgenic hormones such as injections of nandrolone decanoate can be used and if given in small quantities do not have serious masculinising effects (Hendler et al., 1974). However, they increase tissue oxygen consumption and this effect will antagonise any gain from increased packed cell volume. Cobalt chloride is toxic and should be avoided. When iron deficiency is present, iron is effective. Blood transfusions should not be used routinely as their use tends to suppress erythropoiesis.

9.8 Indications for Maintenance Dialysis

Dialysis is usually started when the blood urea is over 35mmol/L (200mg/100ml) or plasma creatinine exceeds 885µmol/L (10mg/100ml) on a restricted protein diet. If dialysis is withheld, the complications of uraemia become more common and severe. Rehabilitation of a patient by dialysis in these circumstances is accompanied by a considerable morbidity and mortality.

10. Diseases of Connective Tissue of Immunological Origin

10.1 Systemic Lupus Erythematosus

Renal involvement occurs in around 45 to 70% of patients with spontaneous lupus; the incidence falls to 20% in those with hydrallazine associated disease (Alarcon-Segovia et al., 1967; see also chapter XXII, sect. 14.1). The histological picture varies from a mild to severe diffuse glomerulonephritis and glomerular necrosis. Prednisone 60mg/daily improves the prognosis, although the success of therapy seems to be inversely related to the degree of renal involvement. The diagnosis should be confirmed by renal biopsy before starting treatment. Other causes of renal failure such as diabetes mellitus, systemic sclerosis and amyloid disease are worsened by corticosteroid therapy. After symptoms have been controlled the dose of corticosteroids should be gradually reduced to the smallest dose that suppresses the activity of the disease. Azathioprine may reduce the requirements for corticosteroids and hence lessen their adverse effects. Cyclophosphamide (2mg/kg daily), has also been advised but controlled clinical trials have not shown a clear cut advantage of combined therapy over corticosteroids alone (Donadio et al., 1978). Indomethacin (25mg 3 times daily in adults), reduces fibrin degradation product excretion (see section 4.3) but whether this conveys any long term benefit has not been determined.

10.2 Polyarteritis and Wegener's Granulomatosis

Renal involvement occurs in 80% of patients. Prednisone (60 to 80mg daily) together with cyclophosphamide (2 to 3mg/kg daily) suppresses symptoms in the majority of patients but as with systemic lupus erythematosus, therapy is most successful in those with least renal involvement. Treatment is most effective if given early in the course of the disease when prolonged remissions may be obtained.

10.3 Systemic Sclerosis

Serious renal involvement is relatively uncommon, but when it occurs is of grave prognostic significance. There is no effective therapy for the disease and management is directed towards controlling complications.

11. Renal Tubular Disorders

These are metabolic disorders in which one or more tubular functions are defective but the glomerular filtration rate is normal, at least initially (Milne, 1971). They are characterised by a reduction in the tubular transport of essential substances. The ill effects which result are due to the loss of essential substances, to the presence of increased amounts of some substances such as cystine which form calculi and to the effects of H^+ retention. Many are inherited disorders but some develop as a consequence of disease or the action of drugs (table V). All are uncommon and only the less rare are discussed here.

11.1 Renal Tubular Acidosis (RTA)

This can be classified into two types:
1) Proximal RTA — where there is a low threshold for bicarbonate reabsorption in the proximal tubule so that bicarbonate excretion continues in spite of a metabolic acidosis, and
2) Distal RTA — where the lesion is in the distal tubule and consists of a reduction in the capacity to establish a hydrogen ion gradient between the interstitial fluid and tubular urine.
Patients with proximal bicarbonate wasting can acidify their urine when the plasma bicarbonate concentration is sufficiently low while patients with distal tubular acidosis are unable to do so

normally in any circumstances. The major hazards of these conditions are hypokalaemia, osteomalacia, nephrocalcinosis and nephrolithiasis. Symptomatic treatment consists of appropriate supplements of sodium, potassium and bicarbonate sufficient to make good the renal losses. It may be necessary to give vitamin D if correction of the acidosis is not sufficient to reverse the osteomalacia.

11.2 Salt Losing Nephropathy

This is almost always accompanied by irreversible chronic renal failure and is discussed in section 9.2.

11.3 Potassium Depletion Nephropathy

Severe potassium depletion from any cause reduces bicarbonate excretion and leads to metabolic alkalosis and impairs urinary concentrating ability. Treatment consists of potassium replacement and the management of the underlying disease.

11.4 Antidiuretic Hormone Resistant Diabetes Insipidus

This is a rare inherited disorder. The infant is particularly susceptible to oligaemia and mortality is high. Treatment consists of adequate fluid intake. Chlorpropamide diminishes the free water clearance and hence reduces urinary water loss.
Resistance to ADH is also induced by hypercalcaemia, K^+ depletion and lithium (see chapter XXVI; sect. 5.4).

11.5 Familial Hypophosphataemia

This is probably due to a primary defect of phosphate transport in the proximal tubular cell and also the gut (Walton, 1976). Calciferol in doses of 1.25 to 2.5mg/daily together with phosphate supplements is usually adequate therapy. $1\alpha,25$-dihydroxyvitamin D_3 is ineffective (see section 9.6).
The plasma calcium should be measured from time to time to avoid vitamin D intoxication.

11.6 Cystinuria

Cystinuria is due to a disorder of proximal tubular transport of dibasic aminoacids (Segal,

1976). A similar defect occurs in the jejunal mucosa. Four dibasic aminoacids are lost in the urine but cystine is the most insoluble and is the only one that forms stones. A high urine output should be maintained with particular attention paid to ensuring a good flow of urine during the night. Stone formation is also reduced if the urine is kept alkaline throughout the 24 hours but this is very difficult to achieve and is not practicable in the majority of cases. D-penicillamine given in doses of 500 to 750mg 3 times daily (in a few cases 1000mg tds may be needed) greatly reduces the excretion of cystine. It may slowly dissolve existing stones and is helpful in preventing new stone formation if a high fluid regimen fails. Adverse reactions include skin rash and proteinuria, sometimes accompanied by the nephrotic syndrome. The renal damage is not always reversible (Crawhall and Watts, 1968; Stephens, 1977). It is costly and should be reserved only for individuals in whom simpler methods are unsuccessful.

11.7 Adult Fanconi Syndrome

The causes of this condition include hereditary factors, plasma cell myeloma, heavy metal poisoning, Wilson's disease, gluten enteropathy, excessive ingestion of Worcester sauce and the use of degraded tetracyclines. It is characterised by proteinuria, glycosuria, general aminoaciduria, excessive bicarbonate loss leading to metabolic acidosis, hypophosphataemia, hypouricaemia and osteomalacia. Treatment is symptomatic. Sodium bicarbonate and potassium citrate supplements are required. Calciferol in doses of 1.25 to 3.75mg daily are adequate for treatment of osteomalacia, although calcium and phosphate supplements alone may be sufficient.

12. Nephrolithiasis

12.1 Calcium Oxalate and Phosphate Stones

When calcium stones are found, the patient should be investigated for the presence of hyperparathyroidism and other stone forming diseases. Enquiry should also be made into the calcium and oxalate content of the diet. However, in the majority of cases no predisposing condition is discovered and the patient may be found to suffer from idiopathic hypercalciuria. Treatment then consists of reducing any excessive dietary intake of calcium and oxalate (Robertson et al., 1976), encouraging a large fluid input and minimising overnight urine concentration (Mathew, 1974). Hypercalciuria can also be reduced by giving cellulose phosphate or a thiazide diuretic such as bendrofluazide. These regimens have been shown to reduce recurrent stone formation and the frequency of attacks of renal colic in those who are prone to suffer from them. About 10 % of patients who form calcium stones recurrently also suffer from hyperuricaemia and hyperuricosuria (Coe and Kavalach, 1974). Recent trials suggest that allopurinol given in a dose indicated below greatly reduces the incidence of recurrence (Smith, 1977).

Patients with renal stones are particularly prone to infection and this in turn predisposes to further stone formation and renal damage.

12.2 Uric Acid Stones

Uric acid is insoluble in highly concentrated acidic urine and treatment consists of avoiding these conditions by reducing the protein and purine content of the diet and ensuring a high fluid intake. Allopurinol (200 to 400mg daily) should be given to inhibit xanthine oxidase activity and uric acid formation. In the absence of stone formation, the moderation in plasma uric acid and urate production sometimes leads to improved renal function.

Xanthine oxidase is involved in the metabolism of certain cytotoxic drugs, including azathioprine and reduced dosage (to 33 % of usual) of azathioprine and 6-mercaptopurine is required when allopurinol is used to overcome urate formation as a consequence of cytotoxic therapy (see chapter VIII; sect. 2.3.4).

13. Miscellaneous Conditions

13.1 Henoch Schonlein Purpura

The clinical course of this condition, which many consider to be allergic in origin, is very variable. Renal involvement is common but causes severe damage in only a small proportion of patients. Owing to its variable course and tendency to spontaneous recovery, assessment of the value of therapy is difficult. Controlled trials are needed to assess the value of corticosteroids and immunosuppressive drugs.

13.2 Goodpasture's Disease

This condition probably has a multiplicity of causes and consists of anaemia, haemoptysis and haematuria due to glomerulonephritis. Antibodies to glomerular basement membrane have been identified in the serum and renal biopsy shows the deposition of immunoglobulins in a linear fashion along the glomerular wall. Usually, the proliferative glomerulonephritis rapidly progresses despite therapy with large doses of prednisone and in many cases it is possible to control the pulmonary lesions only by bilateral nephrectomy. Presumably this removes the stimulus to antibody production. Theoretically, renal transplantation might be expected to reactivate the disease. However, this does not appear to be the rule and several successful cases of renal transplantation have been reported. In some cases, the period of production of antibody is relatively short. Plasmaphoresis has been claimed to be effective in patients with some residual renal function but there is no clear evidence that this is so (Cove-Smith et al., 1978).

13.3 Plasma Cell Myeloma

Proteinuria occurs in well over 50 % of cases and progressive renal insufficiency with death in uraemia is a common terminal event. The causes of renal insufficiency include decreased renal blood flow, increased blood viscosity, hypercalcaemia, nephrocalcinosis, uric acid nephropathy, precipitation of protein in the tubules, accumulation of abnormal protein in the tubular epithelial cells, invasion of the kidney by myeloma cells and the deposition of amyloid. Usually, renal damage is not reversible. Increased blood viscosity should be treated by plasmaphoresis, hypercalcaemia by infusing disodium phosphate or sodium sulphate and frusemide (see also chapter XVI; sect. 6.1). Standard therapy of multiple myeloma consists of initial high dose melphalan and prednisolone followed by either high doses given every 6 weeks or continuously in low doses. Melphalan should be given in reduced doses to patients with renal failure and white cell status regularly checked. However, patients with significant renal impairment do little better than those untreated (see also chapter XXIV; sect. 5.6).

13.4 Haemolytic Uraemic Syndrome

This occurs predominantly but not exclusively in children. It is commonly related to a viral or other infection and more rarely to the use of the oral contraceptive pill (Jackson et al., 1976) and the puerperium. Thrombus formation takes place in the glomerular capillaries and may involve the afferent arterioles and interlobular arteries. Immunoreactive proteins are not deposited in significant amounts in the kidney. Approximately 50 % of cases recover completely and 10 % develop persistently diminished renal function. Various treatments have been tried, including corticosteroids, heparin, streptokinase and high molecular weight dextran, but none of the observations have been controlled. Because of the variable outcome of the disease, the value of the treatments is impossible to assess at present.

In our experience of a small number of patients, alternate treatment with heparin and placebo has not resulted in any difference between the two groups. The prognosis in individual cases probably depends on the degree of involvement of the arterioles and interlobular arteries.

13.5 Diseases of Prostate

Management of benign prostatic hypertrophy is largely surgical. There is no evidence that hormone preparations, spironolactone or bovine prostate extract has any effect on the natural history of the condition. Medical management is confined to preventing and treating infection. In the first place, catheter techniques should be scrupulously aseptic and secondly, local infection in the bladder should be treated by bladder irrigation with suitable antiseptics and only in the last resort, if infection becomes systemic, should antibiotics be used.

Treatment of carcinoma of the prostate is mainly medical. Oestrogens, usually stilboestrol, cause softening and shrinking of the prostate and even necrosis of the metastases. Dose regimens have varied between 1 mg/day and 500 mg/day. Alternative measures include castration and radiotherapy.

Treatment of chronic prostatic infection is difficult because most of the currently available antibacterial drugs fail to diffuse into prostatic fluid (see section 3.4). Co-trimoxazole is the most appropriate agent when the organism is susceptible because of its good diffusion into prostatic fluid, but even though therapy (2 tablets twice daily for 14 days) is effective initially, only about a third of patients are cured permanently. Results are better in acute prostatic infection as the intense and extensive inflammation facilitates diffusion of antibacterial drugs into infected prostatic tissue. Co-trimoxazole is again the agent of choice for initial therapy until results of sensitivity tests are known. If the clinical response is favourable, therapy should be continued for 30 days to prevent development of chronic infection (Meares, 1978). Chronic prostatitis may require long term suppressive chemotherapy.

13.6 Disorders of Bladder Function

The bladder becomes atonic during spinal shock, and in diseases such as diabetes mellitus, where the sensory pathways to the cerebral cortex are damaged, bladder muscle loses all tone and the desire to micturate is lost. Drainage should be instituted and parasympathomimetic drugs such as carbachol or bethanechol may be used to stimulate muscle activity. If the lesion in the spinal cord is above the sacral centres the bladder becomes automatic. Unfortunately, in this condition bladder emptying is incomplete and frequently there is a large residual volume. Treatment consists of regular micturition together with moderate manual compression, high fluid input and regular examination of urine for infection. If the sacral centres are destroyed the bladder becomes autonomous. Treatment is similar to that of the automatic bladder though, if micturition can not be initiated, long term drainage may be necessary. In acute retention due to obstruction, cholinergic drugs such as carbachol are potentially dangerous and should be avoided.

The antispasmodic drug, emepronium bromide has been tried in urinary frequency and incontinence. Given intramuscularly it is effective in urinary incontinence caused by an uninhibited bladder and in urge incontinence, but effectiveness after oral administration is far from convincing (Ekeland and Sander, 1976; Ritch et al., 1977a,b). By and large drug therapy has very little part in the management of disorders of bladder function.

14. Use of Drugs in Presence of Associated Renal Disease

As discussed in section 1, renal disease presents a complex situation which can modify both pharmacokinetic processes and response to pharmacological actions of drugs. The incidence of adverse reactions to some drugs is increased in patients with renal disease (Smith et al., 1966; Jick, 1977; see also chapter VII, sect. 5.3). In renal failure in particular, the response to drugs may be enhanced (see section 1.5) and there will be cumulation of those drugs or active metabolites (Drayer, 1976) which are mainly eliminated by the kidneys. Moreover, some drugs may themselves aggravate renal disease (see also section 15).

In renal failure, dose modification of such drugs and careful monitoring is required if toxic effects are to be avoided. This is particularly important with drugs with a low therapeutic ratio and which are eliminated mainly by the kidneys. Dosage should take account of changes in renal function and the effects of dialysis (Gibson and Nelson, 1977; Maher, 1977; appendix E). Drugs which are eliminated by a compensatory route (e.g. bile), which are used intermittently or have a large therapeutic ratio can generally be used safely without dose modification. Nevertheless, unexplained symptoms in seriously ill patients with renal failure may still be due to unrecognised or unexpected drug toxicity (Brater and Morrelli, 1975).

Thus there are good reasons why drugs should only be used in renal failure if there is a definite indication and if therapy can be monitored appropriately. Although nomograms have been used for dosage estimation of certain drugs in renal failure (Mawer et al., 1974), these are generally based on drug elimination as a function of glomerular filtration rate alone, and they do not take into account other possible routes of excretion or their variations in uraemia. Maximum safety of toxic drugs can only be attained by longitudinal monitoring of plasma concentrations (Noone et al., 1978). In the absence of a plasma level estimation service, dosage nomograms or other similar guides can be used (see section 2.1, appendix E). For reviews, see Fabre and Balant (1976), Cheigh (1977) and Bennett et al. (1977). A review of general considerations including dosage of drugs is given by Reidenberg (1971), Stenzel et al. (1977) and Bennett (1979).

14.1 Antimicrobial Agents

14.1.1 Penicillins

Although the penicillins are excreted mainly unchanged in the urine, their therapeutic ratio is so large that it is rarely necessary to modify their dosage in the presence of renal disease. The plasma half-life of benzylpenicillin in patients with normal

Table IV. Dosage guide of antimicrobial agents in patients with normal renal function and chronic renal failure

Agent	Normal renal function		Severe renal failure[1]		Long term therapy[2] (normal renal function)	
	dose	dose interval (hours)	dose	dose interval (hours)	dose	dose interval (hours)
Cephaloridine	500mg	6h	Avoid	Avoid	—	—
Cephalothin	500mg	6h	500mg	8-12h	—	—
Cephalexin	500mg	6h	500mg	18-24h	—	—
Clindamycin	150mg	6h	150mg	6h	—	—
Colistin	15,000u/kg	6h	15,000u/kg	36h	—	—
Co-trimoxazole	2 tabs	12h	2 tabs	24h	2 tabs	24h
Cycloserine	250mg	12h	Avoid	Avoid	250mg	48h
Erythromycin	250mg	6h	250mg	6h	—	—
Ethambutol	15mg/kg	24h	15mg/kg	48h	15mg/kg	24h
Gentamicin	80mg	8h	80mg	24-48h	—	—
Isoniazid	100mg	8h	100mg	8h	1g	60h
Kanamycin	500mg	8h	500mg	72-96h	—	—
Lincomycin	500mg	6h	500mg	12h	—	—
Nitrofurantoin	50mg	6h	Avoid	Avoid	50mg	24h
Penicillins						
Amoxycillin	250mg	8h	250mg	8h	250mg	24h
Ampicillin	500mg	6h	500mg	6h	500mg	24h
Carbenicillin	1g	6h	1g	12-16h	—	—
Cloxacillin	500mg	6h	500mg	6h	—	—
Methicillin	1g	6h	1g	12h	—	—
Benzylpenicillin	500mg	6h	500mg	6h	250mg	24h
Rifampicin	600mg	24h	600mg	24h	450mg	24h
Streptomycin	500mg	12h	500mg	72-96h	1g	60h
Tetracyclines						
Doxycycline	100mg	24h	100mg	24h[3]	—	—
Minocycline	100mg	12h	100mg	12h[3]		
Tetracycline	500mg	6h	Avoid	Avoid	—	—

1 Monitor serum concentration (see section 14.1 and appendix E).
2 Preventive or suppressive regimen for urinary tract infection (see section 3.2, 3.4).
3 See section 14.1.5.

renal function is 30 minutes and 10 hours in anephric patients. Encephalopathy has been reported when very large doses of 20 mega units or more of penicillin are given to uraemic patients (Conway et al., 1968). High dose penicillin therapy in uraemia may also lead to immune haemolytic anaemia (see chapter VII; sect. 4.1.2). Cephalothin in large doses in uraemia has also been associated with encephalopathy (Wu et al., 1978) and even relatively low doses may cause haemolytic anaemia in uraemia (see chapter VII; sect. 4.1.2). Penicillins contain a variable amount of sodium; oxacillin and carbenicillin having as much as 3.4 and 4.7mmol/g (3.4 and 4.7mEq/g) respectively. The penicillin moiety acts as a non-reabsorbable anion and may increase the negativity of the distal tubular lumen leading to the loss of K^+ (Brunner and Frick, 1968). Hypokalaemia and alkalosis may therefore occur (Klastersky et al., 1973). The potassium salt of penicillin contains 17.5mmol (mEq) potassium/10 million units, so potassium intoxication is a rare complication of therapy when very large doses are given (Tullett, 1970).

The half-lives of semi-synthetic penicillins are between 1 and 4 hours and the dose regimens with the exception of carbenicillin and methicillin do not need to be modified in uraemic patients (table IV; appendix E). Carbenicillin has a pK_a of 3.3 and contains 4.7mmol sodium/g of drug. As discussed above, hypernatraemia with hypokalaemic alkalosis may occur when large doses are given to patients with renal failure. Convulsions and an increased haemorrhagic tendency, together with granulocytopenia, have also been noted following large doses in renal failure (Hoffman et al., 1970; Waisbren et al., 1971). There is some evidence to suggest that the incidence of ampicillin rashes is dose related; a higher incidence would therefore be expected in patients with renal failure (Tourkantonis et al., 1971).

14.1.2 Aminoglycosides
Kanamycin and gentamicin are mainly excreted unchanged in the urine (appendix E). Plasma half-lives with normal renal function are 3 and 2.3 hours respectively. Unlike the penicillins, the therapeutic ratio is low. Trough concentrations over 16µg/ml of kanamycin and 10µg/ml of gentamicin are associated with a high incidence of ototoxicity (Barza and Lauermann, 1978; see chapter XI; sect. 7.1.1). After a single therapeutic dose (250mg kanamycin and 80mg gentamicin), peak concentrations are in the range of 8 and 7µg/ml. Thus the dose in chronic renal failure must be reduced (Jackson and Arcieri, 1971). If the extended interval regimen is used, the drug should be given about every second or third day. Similar modifications are appropriate for streptomycin. Other adverse effects include blockade of neuromuscular transmission (see chapter XXV; sect. (15.9) and nephrotoxicity (Appel and Neu, 1977). Excessive trough concentrations of gentamicin are associated with nephrotoxicity (Schentag et al., 1978). Similar considerations apply to the newer aminoglycoside antibiotics such as tobramycin and amikacin.

14.1.3 Lincomycin
The elimination of lincomycin is not a first order process and therefore plasma half-life determinations do not provide a useful guide to therapy (see chapter I; sect. 2.1.1, 3.3.1). Although uraemic patients accumulate the drug (Reinarz and McIntosh, 1965), this appears to result in only a slightly greater incidence of diarrhoea compared with patients with normal renal function. There is, therefore, probably no need to modify the dose.

14.1.4 Co-trimoxazole
Co-trimoxazole consists of trimethoprim 80mg and sulphamethoxazole 400mg. The optimum ratio of the two for synergistic bactericidal action

is between 1:5 and 1:40. Sulphamethoxazole clearance increases with increasing urine flow rate and pH above 7, whilst trimethoprim clearance is not affected by alteration of urine flow but increases with falling urine pH (Sharpstone, 1969). The ratio of the two drugs may range between 1:50 and 1:2 in extreme circumstances. However, in chronic renal failure urine flow and pH tend to be fixed and the ratio of the two components in urine is usually in the region of 1:6 and in plasma, 1:10. Overall excretion of both components is reduced and when creatinine clearance falls below 15ml/min the dose should be reduced to 2 tablets daily instead of twice daily (Hansen, 1978).

Trimethoprim may cause a decrease in creatinine clearance in those with normal renal function, but a decrease in glomerular filtration rate assessed by other techniques is not found (Berglund et al., 1975). Trimethoprim appears to cause this reduction in creatinine clearance through competitive inhibition of tubular creatinine clearance. It may also interfere with estimation of plasma creatinine. There have been reports of diminished overall renal function following administration of co-trimoxazole. In most of these cases renal function was restored on withdrawal of the drug (Kalowski et al., 1973; Bailey and Little, 1976). When dosage of co-trimoxazole has been reduced in patients with impaired renal function, no deterioration in renal function attributable to co-trimoxazole has been observed (Tasker et al., 1975). Animal studies have failed to support the suggestion of nephrotoxicity of co-trimoxazole in renal failure (Robinson et al., 1977). Deterioration of renal function noted may have been due to hypersensitivity to sulphamethoxazole (Richmond et al., 1979).

14.1.5 Tetracyclines
Tetracyclines apart from doxycycline and minocycline should be avoided in patients with impaired renal function because they accumulate and readily lead to further deterioration in renal function, even in patients with mild to moderate renal failure (see section 15.2.2). Doxycycline, and to a greater extent minocycline, are largely eliminated by metabolism and in renal failure their plasma half-life is not usually significantly prolonged (Heaney and Eknoyan, 1978; Sklenar et al., 1977). While they may not accumulate in the plasma in renal failure, there is evidence of accumulation in tissues, particularly with doxycycline (Mahon et al., 1976; Welling et al.,

1975). Both minocycline and doxycycline have been associated with aggravation of azotaemia in patients with severe renal failure (George et al., 1973; Kasanen et al., 1974) and doxycycline has been implicated in a case of reversible deterioration of renal function in a patient with stable chronic renal failure (Orr et al., 1978). Doxycycline has nevertheless been safely used in chronic renal failure but experience with minocycline is less. For both, while dosage does not need to be modified in patients with impaired renal function they may in some cases still aggravate azotaemia by their antianabolic effect and renal function must be carefully monitored, particularly in cases of severe renal impairment.

14.2 Drugs Affecting the Heart

14.2.1 Digitalis Glycosides

Individuals vary greatly in their response to digoxin. In the patient with normal renal function the half-life following oral administration is between 26 and 45 hours and the major route of excretion is via the kidney, which accounts for about a third or more of an oral dose each day, virtually unchanged (Iisalo, 1977; Doherty et al., 1971). The plasma half-life is 87 to 110 hours in an anephric patient, although up to 240 hours has been calculated when steady-state conditions are strictly adhered to (Gault, 1976). Clearance of digoxin (renal and extrarenal) is linearly related to creatinine clearance in renal failure (Koup et al., 1976). After an oral dose of 0.25mg, the plasma concentration of digoxin 1 hour after ingestion in the patient with normal renal function is in the region of 1ng/ml; toxic effects are associated with plasma concentrations over 2ng/ml (see chapter XVII; sect. 8.1.3). If toxic effects occur in an anephric patient concentrations fall to subtoxic levels only after several days. Dialysis does not remove significant amounts.

It is therefore necessary to give reduced amounts of the drug to patients with renal failure. A dose of 0.125 to 0.25mg 3 times a *week* is suitable for patients with a creatinine clearance of less than 5ml/min. However, it is probably not necessary to modify the normal dose regimen until the glomerular filtration rate falls below 35ml/min. Some prefer to reduce the dose size in renal failure rather than increase the dose interval (see chapter XVII; sect. 8.1.5). Until a digoxin radioimmunoassay becomes more widely available, it is probably not possible to improve standards of therapy based on precision of dosage, though careful consideration of pharmacological information in individual patients reduced the incidence of adverse reaction from 35% to 12% in one study (Jelliffe et al., 1972; see also chapter XVII; sect. 8.1.4). Nomograms relating dosage to creatinine clearance have been constructed and are of some use in the absence of facilities for monitoring plasma concentrations (Gault, 1976; see appendix E).

Other digitalis glycosides have different pharmacokinetic properties but have not been as extensively studied as digoxin in renal disease. Digitoxin is mainly eliminated by hepatic metabolism, but in some patients up to half of the administered dose can be eliminated as unchanged drug; 28% in the urine and 20% in faeces. Urinary excretion of digitoxin is decreased in renal failure, but the rate of elimination may be decreased or increased (Perrier et al., 1977). An increased clearance occurs as a consequence of decreased protein binding during haemodialysis; heparin stimulating release of free fatty acids which compete with digitoxin for albumin binding sites. Digitoxin binding is also decreased in the nephrotic syndrome, with consequent increase in distribution volume and clearance (see section 1.2). The implications of this to dose regimens during and after dialysis and in the nephrotic syndrome are not clear (Storstein, 1977). In patients not on dialysis, dose regimens are usually based on some prolongation of digitoxin elimination in renal failure (appendix E).

14.2.2 Lignocaine

Lignocaine (lidocaine) is used in the treatment of ventricular dysrhythmias. It is very rapidly metabolised and even though 20% of an intravenous dose is excreted in alkaline urine, there is usually no need to modify the dose in uraemic patients. However, accumulation of one of the two active metabolites of lignocaine can occur with prolonged infusion in uraemic patients. Increased risk of toxicity from accumulation of lignocaine or its active metabolites is most likely to occur in uraemic patients with associated cardiac failure or liver disease (Benowitz and Meister, 1978; see chapter XVII, sect. 6.1.3).

14.2.3 Procainamide

Desirable therapeutic concentrations of procainamide (4 to 8µg/ml) can be achieved with a dose of 50mg/kg daily in patients with normal renal function. The plasma half-life is approximately 3 hours and 50% of a given dose is excreted unchanged. A metabolite, N-acetylprocainamide is active (over 85% of a dose of which is excreted unchanged in the urine) and both it and procainamide accumulate in uraemic patients taking procainamide (Drayer et al., 1977). Cumulation and toxicity can occur very rapidly with drugs that have a short half-life and toxicity associated with very high plasma concentrations (15 to 25µg/ml) have occurred during the first day of therapy with procainamide (Koch-Weser, 1971). Accordingly, dosage should be reduced in patients with renal failure and therapy monitored by measurement of plasma concentrations of both procainamide and N-acetylprocainamide (Drayer et al., 1977; Koch-Weser, 1977). Adverse effects include nausea, vomiting, decreased cardiac output, conduction defects and cardiac dysrhythmias.

14.2.4 β-Adrenoceptor Blocking Drugs

The various β-blockers have different pharmacokinetic properties which determine any influence of renal disease on their elimination (Johnsson and Regardh, 1976; Shand, 1977; see also chapter XVIII, table IIIb). Propranolol, alprenolol, metoprolol and oxprenolol are eliminated almost entirely by metabolism. The first metabolic step in propranolol degradation following a single oral (but not intravenous) dose, is the production of 4-hydroxypropranolol, which is potentially as pharmacologically active as propranolol itself (see Drayer, 1976). First-pass hepatic metabolism of orally administered propranolol is markedly reduced in patients with renal failure, and peak blood concentrations and bioavailability of propranolol are thus elevated in renal failure patients. Elimination of propranolol is also reduced in chronic renal failure patients not on dialysis (Bianchetti et al., 1976; Lowenthal et al., 1974). A reduction in dose is recommended by some in uraemic patients not on dialysis who are being started on propranolol. The situation with continued administration is not clear, but dosage should be carefully monitored in view of the marked fluctuations in blood levels which can occur and the lack of knowledge about any clinical importance of the active metabolites of propranolol in renal failure (Bianchetti et al., 1976; Lowenthal, 1977). Some consider that propranolol should probably be avoided in advanced renal failure as it may reduce renal blood flow as a consequence of reduced cardiac output and cause an abrupt deterioration in renal function

(Warren et al., 1974; Swainson and Winney, 1976; Bauer and Brooks, 1979).

Alprenolol, like propranolol, also undergoes extensive hepatic first-pass metabolism and forms active metabolites such as 4-hydroxyalprenolol of potential clinical importance. Whether it behaves in a similar manner as propranolol in renal failure is not known, but might be expected. Metoprolol undergoes significant hepatic first-pass metabolism but accumulation of its active metabolites in renal failure does not appear to be of clinical importance and it does not require dose modification in renal failure. Atenolol and sotalol are however, eliminated in large part by the kidneys and their elimination half-life is significantly prolonged in patients with impaired renal function. Dosage should be adjusted accordingly (appendix E). Acebutolol is eliminated in part as unchanged drug and as an active metabolite (Meffin et al., 1976); both of which appear to accumulate in renal failure (Kaye and Dufton, 1976; Tjandramaga et al., 1978). The clinical importance of the active metabolite is not clear but dosage of acebutolol may need to be reduced in renal failure. Pindolol is eliminated about equally by the liver and kidney. Although renal clearance is reduced in patients with impaired renal function in correlation with creatinine clearance, bioavailability is decreased (Lavene et al., 1977). Accordingly, the need for dose adjustment of pindolol is probably less important. Timolol is eliminated by the liver and to a lesser extent the kidneys; as a consequence elimination is not impaired in renal failure and dose adjustment is not necessary, although timolol has caused significant hypotension during dialysis (Lowenthal et al., 1978).

14.2.5 Diuretics

Mercurial diuretics should be avoided as mercury tends to accumulate in patients with chronic renal failure and may induce acute tubular necrosis. Spironolactone, triamterene and amiloride should be avoided in renal failure because of their potassium retaining properties. Potentially fatal hyperkalaemia may develop rapidly, particularly if dietary potassium is coincidentally increased at the same time (see section 7.1). The thiazide diuretics are usually ineffective in advanced renal failure and tend to accumulate. Adverse reactions do not occur often, but include hyperuricaemia, hypercalcaemia, and the activation of latent diabetes mellitus (see chapter XVI; sect. 14.1). The risk of ototoxicity with frusemide and ethacrynic acid is increased when they are used in large doses in renal failure (see chapter XI; sect. 7.1.2).

14.3 Treatment of Diabetes in the Presence of Renal Failure

14.3.1 Insulin

Renal failure bears a complex relationship to the insulin requirements of a diabetic patient. Diminished excretion and metabolism occur but this is offset by a dialysable insulin inhibitor which reduces tissue responsiveness. However, dialysis does not completely restore insulin activity (Hampers et al., 1966). The net result is that the requirements for insulin are diminished. After successful renal transplantation the patient usually reverts to his prerenal failure insulin dose requirement.

14.3.2 Sulphonylureas

Chlorpropamide is mainly excreted unchanged in the urine so the plasma half-life in chronic renal failure is greatly prolonged (200 hours or more) compared with the normal half-life of 36 hours (Fabre and Balant, 1976). Dose requirements fall as uraemia develops. Acetohexamide is both excreted unchanged and metabolised to an active metabolite (hydroxyhexamide) in patients with normal renal function and both may accumulate in renal failure, although further biotransformation of hydroxyhexamide to an inactive metabolite reduces its contribution to the extended hypoglycaemic action (Cohen et al., 1967); dose requirements are diminished in these circumstances. However, the hypoglycaemic action of both chlorpropamide and acetohexamide is so long in renal failure that they should be avoided (appendix E). Tolbutamide is mainly metabolised to an inactive derivative, carboxytolbutamide, and dose requirements on a pharmacokinetic basis do not fall with increasing uraemia. However, in general all sulphonylureas are best avoided in renal disease (see chapter XVI; sect. 3.4.6).

14.3.3 Biguanides

Approximately one third of a dose of phenformin and two thirds of metformin is excreted as unchanged drug. Thus in theory the dosage should be reduced when renal failure develops, but since the risk of lactic acidosis is greatly increased in renal failure (Oliva, 1970) biguanides should be avoided in this situation.

14.4 Drugs Acting on the Central Nervous System

14.4.1 Benzodiazepines

Chlordiazepoxide and diazepam are extensively metabolised before being excreted. The therapeutic ratio for the drugs is large and although protein binding is decreased in uraemia (section 1.2) no major toxicity is likely, even in overdosage. Usually no modification of dose regimen is required in patients with renal failure. Similarly, the rate of elimination of oxazepam and lorazepam is not changed in patients with impaired renal function. Although the inactive glucuronide metabolites accumulate and there is evidence for enterohepatic cycling and decreased protein binding of oxazepam in uraemia, no major toxicity is likely and sedative effects are not greater than expected (Odar-Cederlof et al., 1977; Verbeeck et al., 1976).

14.4.2 Phenothiazines

These drugs are extensively tissue bound and metabolised. Renal excretion of active drug usually accounts for only a very small proportion of total elimination (chapter XXVI; sect. 1.5.1). On the other hand, isolated cases of reactions such as skin pigmentation (Murphy, 1966) and galactorrhoea (Frattini et al., 1965) in patients with renal failure receiving normal doses have been reported. The sedative effect of this group of drugs compounds the blurring of consciousness which accompanies uraemia. Cases of acute psychotic reactions have also been reported (McAllister et al., 1978).

14.4.3 Tricyclic Antidepressants

Like the phenothiazines, these drugs are highly tissue bound and extensively metabolised (chapter XXVI; sect. 1.5.2). Since renal excretion is not an important mechanism of elimination, no modification of dose regimen is usually required in patients with renal failure. However, in some patients with impaired renal function, the sedative effect may be prominent and their anticholinergic effect may precipitate acute urinary retention in the elderly patient.

The metabolic acidosis associated with chronic renal failure may increase the risk of cardiotoxicity of the tricyclics due to enhanced tissue diffusion of these basic drugs. Newer antidepressants such as mianserin or nomifensine may be safer in this respect (see chapter XXVI; sect. 7.5.2).

14.4.4 Barbiturates

With the exception of barbitone and phenobarbitone which are in part excreted unchanged by the kidneys, barbiturates used in clinical practice are eliminated by metabolism. However, sensitivity to barbiturates appears to be increased in uraemia because of reduced effectiveness of the blood-brain barrier (Richet et al., 1970; see chapter VII; sect. 5.3). An alternative explanation lies in the altered protein binding that occurs. This is probably not of importance when medium and long duration of action barbiturates are given, as most patients with chronic renal failure develop liver microsomal enzyme induction and also become habituated to the drug. The duration of anaesthesia obtained with a given dose of a short duration of action barbiturate such as thiopentone is prolonged in a uraemic patient as compared with non-uraemic individuals (see chapter X; sect. 2.1.2, 4.5).

14.4.5 Anticonvulsants

Phenytoin is less bound to plasma proteins and as a consequence, at usual therapeutic concentrations is metabolised more rapidly in uraemic patients. Full dosage should therefore be given. Monitoring of plasma levels should however, be by measurement of the unbound and total drug concentration, which are unchanged and decreased respectively in uraemia (see section 1.2; chapter I, sect. 4.3.2, 5.1.2).

14.4.6 Analgesics

Aspirin is metabolised by conjugation and excreted as free drug and conjugate. However, it is contraindicated in uraemia owing to the irritative effect on the gastric mucosa and its ability to enhance the bleeding tendency in uraemia. Paracetamol (acetaminophen) is probably the safest simple analgesic. The activity of pentazocine and morphine is not affected by uraemia except for potentiation of their sedative effects. However, the excitatory effects of pethidine (meperidine) are enhanced in patients with renal failure due to rapid accumulation of the convulsive producing metabolite norpethidine (Szeto et al., 1977). Accumulation of dextronorpropoxyphene, a potentially toxic metabolite of dextropropoxyphene, also occurs in patients with advanced renal failure (Gibson et al., 1977). Cautious use of reduced doses of pethidine and dextropropoxyphene are indicated in patients with impaired renal function. Codeine and pentazocine can be used without modification of dose in renal failure, although sedative effects may be enhanced. Although methadone is partly eliminated as unchanged drug in the urine (in some cases up to 58% of the dose), accumulation may not occur in renal failure due to elimination by the faecal route (Inturrisi, 1977). The major metabolites of methadone are inactive.

14.5 Anticoagulants

Heparin and warfarin are eliminated by non-renal mechanisms and uraemia does not result in a change in sensitivity to their action. Although albumin binding of warfarin is decreased in uraemia, it is likely that due to increased clearance, the unbound plasma concentration remains unchanged (Bachmann et al., 1977; Odar-Cederlof, 1977; see section 1.2). However, in severe uraemia the use of both warfarin and heparin is complicated by the bleeding tendency associated with the disorder and their use requires careful supervision.

14.6 Drugs used in Anaesthesia

Anaesthesia in the patient with renal disease is discussed in chapter X (sect. 4.5). A few specific examples are given below.

14.6.1 Premedication

Approximately 50% of parenteral atropine is excreted unchanged in the urine. However, as it is usually given as a single dose cumulation is not a problem.

14.6.2 Methoxyflurane

Methoxyflurane may occasionally cause acute renal failure from deposition of its metabolite (oxalate) in the tubule and the risk of this reaction appears to be increased by simultaneous use of tetracyclines (see chapter X; sect. 2.1.1). Methoxyflurane may also induce polyuria by blocking the action of vasopressin.

14.6.3 Muscle Relaxants

Tubocurarine and gallamine are eliminated by renal excretion. However, although muscle relaxation following gallamine is prolonged, that following standard doses of tubocurarine is usually normal in patients with renal failure, except when large or repeated doses are used. This apparently anomalous finding with tubocurarine is probably due to redistribution of the drug throughout the body tissues and elimination by the liver. Suxamethonium (succinylcholine) is eliminated by metabolism, but plasma cholinesterase enzyme activity which terminates its action is depressed in uraemia, hence elimination may be prolonged (see chapter X; sect. 2.2.1). It can cause a dangerous rise in plasma potassium with large (>1 mg/kg) or repeated doses and should be avoided in patients with peripheral neuropathy or preanaesthetic hyperkalaemia, or in the presence of other risk factors such as burns, trauma etc (Walton and Farman, 1973a,b; see chapter X; sect. 2.2.1) or digitalis therapy (see chapter XVII; table XIV).

14.7 Clofibrate

Clofibrate undergoes hydrolysis either during the absorption process or its first passage through the liver to its active metabolite clofibric acid which is highly bound to albumin and eliminated as the glucuronide by the kidneys. Toxic myopathy has followed use of clofibrate in patients with impaired renal function. Protein binding of clofibric acid is decreased and plasma clearance markedly reduced in correlation with serum creatinine concentration (Gugler, 1978). Clofibrate can be safely used in uraemic hypertriglyceridaemia provided dosage is reduced in accordance with serum creatinine and response monitored by serum creatine phosphokinase and triglyceride levels (Goldberg et al., 1977). Appropriate dose reduction (increased dosing interval) is 50% at a serum creatinine concentration of 5mg/100ml, 75% reduction at 8mg/100ml and in complete renal failure to about 10% of normal or 1 to 1.5g per week (Gugler, 1978). Dose reduction is not required in the nephrotic syndrome in the *absence* of impaired renal function, although dose intervals should be decreased because of fluctuation in plasma levels (see section 1.2; 5.3).

14.8 Cimetidine

Cimetidine, an histamine H_2-receptor antagonist (see chapter XIX; sect. 4.1.3), is eliminated in large part as unchanged drug in the urine. Excretion is delayed and the plasma half-life prolonged in patients with impaired renal function. Mental confusion and convulsions can readily occur in uraemic patients and in critically ill elderly patients if standard dosage is used (Edmonds et al., 1979; Schentag et al., 1979). Dosage of cimetidine should be appropriately reduced in patients with impaired renal function and in the elderly (see chapter XIX; sect. 4.2.3, 4.3.3).

15. Drug Induced Renal Disease

A large number of drugs have been implicated at one time or another in causing renal disorders, probably because many drugs are eliminated through the kidneys and because of the intrinsic nephrotoxicity of some of them. Many nephrotoxic reactions are dose related but those due to hypersensitivity are not. Some drugs are particularly likely to cause renal disease and renal function should always be monitored during their use. The more common or important reactions are listed in table V and some of these are discussed below (for review, see Curtis, 1977; Mitchell et al., 1977).

15.1 Analgesic Nephropathy

Over the last 25 years it has become clear that there is an association between chronic ingestion of large doses of analgesics and the development of papillary necrosis (Kincaid-Smith, 1978). Although initially thought to be due solely to phenacetin, all simple analgesics including aspirin, paracetamol (acetaminophen), phenazone (antipyrine), amidopyrine and phenacetin appear to be implicated. Analgesic abusers are poor historians and it is impossible to define the role of single analgesics or combinations of them from patient histories although it is generally agreed that the combination analgesics are primarily responsible. Animal studies suggest that dehydration increases toxicity. As well as causing papillary necrosis, chronic analgesic abuse is associated with a high incidence of transitional cell carcinoma of the renal pelvis and possibly bladder carcinoma (Kung, 1976; Taylor, 1972). If papillary necrosis is present, then all analgesics should be withdrawn without exception. The need for this should be carefully explained as many of the patients are psychologically addicted. If the habit is given up useful renal function returns in approximately 50% of patients. Papillary necrosis often results in a salt losing nephropathy and this should be treated appropriately.

Analgesic abuse seems to be world wide and analgesic nephropathy is an important, although sometimes underecognised cause of renal failure (Cove-Smith and Knapp, 1978; Goldberg and Murray, 1978). A detailed history of analgesic

Table V. Some renal disorders induced by drugs

Disorder	Examples	Influencing factors
Renal tubular damage and necrosis	Kanamycin Polymyxin B Colistin Streptomycin (rare) Amikacin (rare) Tobramycin (rare) Gentamicin (rare)	Large doses, excessive dose in renal failure
	Cephaloridine Cephalothin	Doses of over 4 to 6g cephaloridine daily, lower doses in renal impairment; combined use with aminoglycoside antibiotics or potent diuretics such as frusemide (furosemide). Cephalothin probably less toxic than cephaloridine
	Lithium	Long term therapy, lithium intoxication (see chapter XXVI; sect. 5.4)
	Amphotericin B	
Papillary necrosis	Analgesics	Chronic abuse of large doses. Inadequate fluid intake
Acute interstitial nephritis, arteritis, etc.	Penicillins, especially methicillin Radiographic contrast media	Very large dosage More likely in jaundiced patients and with biliary contrast media. More likely after intravenous urography in presence dehydration, diabetics with dehydration or proteinuria, myelomatosis
	Methoxyflurane	Risk increased by combination with tetracycline
	Cephalothin Phenindione Sulphonamides Phenylbutazone Rifampicin	Usually after intermittent use or reintroduction of drug
Renal tubular acidosis and other features of Fanconi syndrome	Tetracyclines	Use of degraded tetracycline (faulty dispensed and outdated preparations)
	Amphotericin B Acetazolamide	
Glomerular damage with proteinuria	Trimethadione Paramethadione D-Penicillamine Gold	
Fluid retention (with oedema)	Corticosteroids Androgenic steroids Anabolic steroids Oestrogens Diazoxide Clonidine	
	Phenylbutazone Indomethacin Carbenoxolone	Particularly with large doses and in the elderly

Table V. (continued)

Disorder	Examples	Influencing factors
Hyponatraemia due to impaired excretion of H_2O	Chlorpropamide Tolbutamide (rare) Carbamazepine Vincristine Cyclophosphamide Morphine	Patients with heart failure, impaired liver and renal function particularly susceptible
	Thiazides and chlorthalidone (rare)	Excessive dosage with sodium depletion
	Frusemide and ethacrynic acid	Excessive dosage with sodium depletion
Retroperitoneal fibrosis	Methysergide	Continuous long term therapy
Nephrocalcinosis	Acetazolamide	Long term use
	Vitamin D	Overdose leading to hypercalciuria
Crystalluria	Sulphonamides	Less soluble derivatives, low urine pH, hypo-albuminaemia
Uric acid nephropathy	Cytotoxic drugs	Use in lymphomas and leukaemia. Usually of prompt onset after starting therapy
Concentrating defect with polyuria	Vitamin D and analogues Lithium	Greater with larger doses (see chapter XXVI; sect. 5.4)
	Methoxyflurane Demeclocycline (demethylchlortetracycline) Isophosphamide Dextropropoxyphene	
K^+ depletion from increased urinary losses	Corticosteroids Diuretics (except amiloride, spironolactone and triamterene)	Long continued doses, especially in states of low cardiac output
	Carbenoxolone	Excessive doses given without supervision
	Sodium penicillin	Very large doses
	Amphotericin B Carbenicillin disodium Gentamicin Degraded tetracycline Viomycin Capreomycin	
Hyperkalaemia	Spironolactone Amiloride Trimaterene	Renal impairment
Acute ischaemic renal failure	Parenteral antihypertensive drugs	Elderly
	Low molecular weight dextran	Excessive doses in presence hypovolaemia or shock
	Excessive doses of diuretics, especially frusemide	Hypoproteinaemia

consumption should be included in the investigation of all patients with renal disease. Clinical features indicative of analgesic nephropathy are renal failure with a marked acidosis, urinary infection with renal colic and a tendency to become dehydrated easily. Papillary necrosis is the chief characteristic of analgesic nephropathy. Although there have been occasional reports of analgesic nephropathy in arthritic patients under treatment with salicylates, there is no serious suggestion that analgesic nephropathy is a frequent complication of rheumatoid arthritis or that effects on tubular function contraindicate the use of salicylates in rheumatoid arthritis (NZ Rheumatism Association, 1974; Burry et al., 1976). However, arthritic patients should be instructed to avoid compound analgesics in view of the enhanced risk of analgesic nephropathy (Cove-Smith and Knapp, 1978).

15.2 Antimicrobial Agents

Most of the antimicrobial agents in common use can damage the kidneys. Sometimes the mechanism is due to hypersensitivity, as in acute interstitial nephritis with the penicillins (especially methicillin), rifampicin (rifampin) and sulphonamides or as part of a generalised systemic reaction to sulphonamides or co-trimoxazole (see chapter VII; sect. 4.1). Some agents such as amphotericin B, the polymyxins and bacitracin are predictably toxic to the renal tubule. Others such as the tetracyclines, some cephalosporins and the aminoglycosides are potentially nephrotoxic; this possibility being enhanced by combination with other agents and in patients with existing renal damage. Dosage of antimicrobial agents mainly eliminated by the kidneys must be appropriately adjusted in patients with impaired renal function (see section 14.1).

15.2.1 Aminoglycosides and Polymyxins
Kanamycin, polymyxin B, colistin and rarely streptomycin, gentamicin, amikacin and tobramycin are capable of causing reversible damage to the proximal convoluted tubule, particularly following large doses or excessive dosage in renal failure and in combination with cephalosporins (Appel and Neu, 1977; Wade et al., 1978). Oral neomycin in patients with renal failure may do likewise. Kanamycin and gentamicin become tissue bound in the renal cortex. Cloudy swelling and acute tubular necrosis some-

times ensue, particularly if frusemide is given concurrently.

15.2.2 Tetracyclines
The tetracyclines act by interfering with protein synthesis. Transient rises in the concentration of blood urea are common as a result of the antianabolic effect (Morgan and Ribush, 1972). In patients with impaired renal function, there is a marked increase in blood urea concentration which takes some days to appear (Shils, 1963; Ribush and Morgan, 1972). Tetracyclines, other than doxycycline and minocycline, can accumulate in the serum in renal failure and when they do, anorexia, vomiting and diarrhoea are likely. These effects lead to saline depletion with progressive and sometimes rapid deterioration of renal function (Shils, 1963; Phillips et al., 1974). Doxycycline has a less marked antianabolic effect (Morgan and Ribush, 1972), but as with minocycline it can accumulate in tissues other than serum and aggravate azotaemia in those with severely impaired renal function. These tetracyclines have been safely used in chronic renal failure, but renal function should be carefully monitored, especially in those with severe impairment (see section 14.1.5). Other tetracyclines should not be used in patients with any impairment in renal function. Large doses given by infusion during which blood levels of 30 to 40µg/ml are exceeded cause acute fatty necrosis of the liver and patchy renal cortical necrosis (Davis and Kaufman, 1966). Most cases so far reported have involved pregnant women, but it is not clear whether such patients are particularly sensitive or the adverse effect reflects a former peculiarity of obstetric prescribing. Large oral doses in pregnancy have also caused hepatotoxicity (Kunelis et al., 1965).

Prolonged faulty dispensary storage of tetracyclines results in the formation of toxic degradation products which causes proximal tubular damage resembling the Fanconi syndrome (Frimpter et al., 1963). Tetracyclines given together with the anaesthetic methoxyflurane increase the risk of acute renal failure (Kuzucu, 1970).

15.2.3 Cephalosporins
Cephaloridine when given in doses of 4 to 6g or more daily, particularly if given with aminoglycoside antibiotics or potent diuretics such as frusemide (furosemide), may cause renal tubular

damage. When given to patients with some degree of renal impairment smaller doses have a similar effect. A few cases of fatal acute tubular necrosis have occurred. Now that other cephalosporins such as cephalexin and cefoxitin are available there is probably no place for the clinical use of cephaloridine. Cephalothin is probably less toxic than cephaloridine in this respect but has been incriminated as a cause of renal damage. The risk of nephrotoxicity of cephalothin is increased when used in combination with aminoglycosides, particularly in patients with impaired renal function (Apel and Neu, 1977; Wade et al., 1978). Oral cephalexin does not appear to be nephrotoxic. A positive Coombs test may occur during treatment with cephalothin. Very rarely, haemolytic anaemia has occurred with regular doses in the absence of renal disease (see chapter VII; sect. 4.1.2).

15.2.4 Miscellaneous Antimicrobial Agents

Sulphonamides are well known to be capable of inducing arteritis, crystalluria and renal colic in dehydrated patients, but not so well known are the risks of crystalluria and renal failure as a consequence of decreased binding in patients with hypoalbuminaemia (Buchanan, 1978). Amphotericin B, a polyene antifungal agent, regularly causes a fall in glomerular filtration rate and tubular dysfunction. Large doses of methicillin and rarely other penicillins cause interstitial nephritis and renal failure (Appel and Neu, 1977); the incidence of acute interstitial nephritis with methicillin may be greater than usually thought and it is advisable to monitor urinary sediment and renal excretory function in patients receiving methicillin for periods of a week or more (Nolan and Abernathy, 1977; Sarff and McCracken, 1977). Penicillin can also cause glomerulonephritis and hypersensitivity angiitis (Appel and Neu, 1977). Rifampicin has been associated with acute renal failure, usually following intermittent use or reintroduction of the drug. The reaction seems to have an immunological basis. Renal function usually returns to normal (Appel and Neu, 1977; Girling, 1977).

15.3 Miscellaneous Drugs

Phenindione has been reported to cause reversible interstitial nephritis as a result of hypersensitivity (De Baker and Williams, 1963). Trimethadione and paramethadione can cause proteinuria and the nephrotic syndrome, the time of onset of which bears no relationship to the total dose given (Heymann, 1967). D-Penicillamine may also cause the nephrotic syndrome (Bacon et al., 1976; Hill, 1977). It may induce a glomerular reaction similar to membranous glomerulonephritis (Neild et al., 1975) and in a small number of patients, Goodpasture's syndrome with severe pulmonary haemorrhage and rapidly progressive renal failure has been reported (Gibson et al., 1976). Gold may also be associated with a syndrome resembling membranous glomerulonephritis and proteinuria (Viol et al., 1977). Cyclophosphamide can cause a chemical cystitis; the severe haemorrhagic form may be fatal (Hutter et al., 1969). Some patients may develop renal failure due to radiographic contrast media, even though it is not always certain that renal failure is due to the direct action of the medium on the kidney. Biliary contrast media appear to be the most nephrotoxic, especially if the patient is jaundiced, since impairment of hepatic elimination of the contrast medium lead to increased elimination by the kidneys. Acute renal failure can also occur after intravenous urography but is uncommon (Grainger, 1972). Less severe damage may be more common (Carvello et al., 1978). Renal failure is most likely to occur in diabetic patients who are dehydrated or are proteinuric and in patients with myelomatosis and Bence Jones proteinuria (Kamdar et al., 1977; Myers and Witten, 1971). Deprivation of fluids should be avoided in patients with renal failure undergoing intravenous urography. Methysergide, used in the preventive treatment of migraine, may lead to reversible retroperitoneal fibrosis and ureteric obstruction in a few patients on continuous long term treatment (Graham et al., 1966). This complication can be avoided by a treatment free interval of 1 to 2 months every 6 months. Methyldopa, ergotamine and hydrallazine have also been claimed occasionally to exert a similar action.

15.4 Drugs Affecting Fluid and Electrolyte Balance

Corticosteroids (particularly mineralocorticoids) and androgenic and anabolic steroids cause salt and water retention. Oral steroid contraceptives (particularly high dose oestrogen formulations) and many antihypertensive drugs (if used without a diuretic) have a similar effect. Carbenoxolone has a mineralocorticoid like activity and not uncommonly leads to salt and water retention, which is commonly accompanied by a rise in blood pressure and increased urinary losses of potassium and hypokalaemia (see chapter XIX; sect. 4.3.4). Most non-steroidal anti-inflammatory analgesics have salt and water retaining activity. This is most pronounced with phenylbutazone, therapeutic doses of which may precipitate heart failure in the elderly.

Other drugs have water retaining properties which can lead to dilutional hyponatraemia resembling the syndrome of inappropriate antidiuretic hormone secretion (Moses and Miller, 1974). In this situation there is progressive weight gain but without the associated development of oedema. Drugs with this effect include the oral hypoglycaemic chlorpropamide and rarely tolbutamide, the antineoplastic drugs vincristine and cyclophosphamide, thiazide diuretics and the anticonvulsant carbamazepine (Perucca et al., 1978). The effect of chlorpropamide, and less often thiazide diuretics and carbamazepine has been used therapeutically in patients with diabetes insipidus (see also chapter XVI; sect. 12). In contrast, drugs such as lithium and rarely demeclocycline (demethylchlortetracycline) may cause reversible nephrogenic diabetes insipidus and as a consequence can be used therapeutically for treatment of the syndrome of inappropriate (excessive) secretion of antidiuretic hormone in patients who cannot tolerate severe fluid restriction (Forrest et al., 1978). The effects of lithium in impairing urine concentrating capacity during its usual use in manic-depressive disorder are important, particularly as it may be associated with development of chronic tubular atrophy and interstitial fibrosis (Hestbech et al., 1977; see chapter XXVI, sect. 5.4). Excessive dosage of oxytocin infused in a large amount of water has also caused water intoxication.

Nephrocalcinosis and nephrolithiasis with ureteral colic may occur with long term use of acetazolamide in glaucoma but can be overcome by increased fluid intake and alkalinisation of the urine (Parfitt, 1969). Vitamin D overdosage leads to hypercalcaemia, diminution in concentrating ability and polyuria. A large intake of calcium increases the risk of renal stone formation and in patients with renal disease, it may lead to hypercalcaemia, hypertension and renal failure (see also chapter XVI; sect. 14.5).

Further Reading

Black, D. and Jones, N.F.: Renal Disease, 4th ed (Blackwell, Oxford 1978).

Brenner, B.M. and Rector, F.C.: The Kidney, Vol. 1 and 2 (Saunders, Philadelphia, 1976).

Edwards, K.D.: Drugs Affecting Kidney Function and Metabolism, Progress in Biochemical Pharmacology, Vol. 7 (Karger, Basel 1972).

Edwards, K.D.: Drugs and the Kidney, Progress in Biochemical Pharmacology, Vol. 9 (Karger, Basel 1974).

Gonick, H.C.: Current Nephrology, Vol. 1 (Pinecliff, Pacific Palisades, Calif 1977).

Hamburger, J.: Advances in Nephrology, Vols. 1-7 (Year Book, Chicago 1971-1977).

McIntosh, R.M.; Guggenheim, S.J. and Schrier, R.W.: Kidney Disease: Hematologic and Vascular Problems (Wiley, New York 1977).

Strauss, M.B. and Welt, L.G.: Diseases of the Kidney, 3rd ed (Little Brown, Boston 1979).

References

Abshagen, U.; Rennekamp, H. and Luszpinski, G.: Pharmacokinetics of spironolactone in man. Naunyn-Schmiedeberg's Archives of Pharmacology 296: 37 (1976).

Alarcon-Segovia, D.; Wakim, K.G.; Worthington, J.W. and Ward, L.E.: Clinical and experimental studies on the hydralazine syndrome and its relationship to systemic lupus erythematosus. Medicine (Baltimore) 46: 1 (1967).

Anderton, J. and Kincaid-Smith, Priscilla: Diuretics I: Physiological and Pharmacological Considerations. Drugs 1: 54 (1971); II: Clinical Considerations. Drugs 1: 141 (1971).

Andreasen, F.: The effect of dialysis on the protein binding of drugs in the plasma of patients with acute renal failure. Acta Pharmacologica et Toxicologica 34: 284 (1974).

Appel, G.B. and Neu, H.C.: Nephrotoxicity of antimicrobial agents. New England Journal of Medicine 296: 663, 722, 784 (1977).

Aronson, J.K. and Grahame-Smith, D.G.: Altered distribution of digoxin in renal failure — a cause of digoxin toxicity? British Journal of Clinical Pharmacology 3: 1045 (1976).

Avioli, L.V.; Birge, S.; Lee, S.W. and Slatopolsky, E.: The metabolic fate of vitamin D_3-^3H in chronic renal failure. Journal of Clinical Investigation 47: 2239 (1968).

Bachmann, K.; Shapiro, R. and Mackiewicz, J.: Influence of renal dysfunction on warfarin plasma protein binding. Journal of Clinical Pharmacology 16: 468 (1976).

Bachmann, K.; Shapiro, R. and Mackiewicz, J.: Warfarin elimination and responsiveness in patients with renal dysfunction. Journal of Clinical Pharmacology 17: 292 (1977).

Bacon, P.A.; Tribe, C.R.; Mackenzie, J.C.; Verrier Jones, J.; Cumming, R.H. and Amer, B.: Penicillamine nephropathy in rheumatoid arthritis. A clinical, pathological and immunological study. Quarterly Journal of Medicine 45: 661 (1976).

Bailey, R.R.: The problem of recurrent urinary tract infections. Drugs 8: 54 (1974).

Bailey, R.R.: Management of cystitis in young women. Drugs 13: 137 (1977).

Bailey, R.R. and Little, P.J.: Deterioration in renal function in association with co-trimoxazole therapy. Medical Journal of Australia 1: 914 (1976).

Bailey, R.R.: Single dose antibacterial treatment for uncomplicated UTIs. Drugs 17: 219 (1979).

Baluarte, H.J.; Hiner, L. and Gruskin, A.B.: Chlorambucil dosage in frequently relapsing nephrotic syndrome: A controlled clinical trial. Journal of Pediatrics 92: 295 (1978).

Barza, M. and Lauermann, M.: Why monitor serum levels of gentamicin. Clinical Pharmacokinetics 3: 202 (1978).

Bauer, J.H. and Brooks, C.S.: The long-term effect of propranolol therapy on renal function. American Journal of Medicine 66: 405 (1979).

Becker, G.J.; d'Aspice, J.F.; Walker, R.G. and Kincaid-Smith, P.: Plasma pheresis in the treatment of glomerulonephritis. Medical Journal of Australia 2: 693 (1977).

Beermann, B.; Groschinsky-Grind, Margaretha and Lindstrom, B.: Pharmacokinetics of bendroflumethiazide. Clinical Pharmacology and Therapeutics 22: 385 (1977a).

Beermann, B.; Dalen, E. and Lindstrom, B.: Elimination of furosemide in healthy subjects and in those with renal failure. Clinical Pharmacology and Therapeutics 22: 70 (1977b).

Beermann, B. and Groschinsky-Grind, M.: Enhancement of the gastrointestinal absorption of hydrochlorothiazide by propantheline. European Journal of Clinical Pharmacology 13: 385 (1978).

Beermann, B.; Groschinsky-Grind, M. and Rosen, A.: Absorption, metabolism and excretion of ^{14}C-hydrochlorothiazide. Clinical Pharmacology and Therapeutics 19: 531 (1976).

Bennett, W.M.; Singer, I.; Golper, T.; Feig, P. and Coggins, C.J.: Guidelines for drug therapy in renal failure. Annals of Internal Medicine 86: 754 (1977).

Bennett, W.M.: Drug prescribing in renal failure. Drugs 17: 111 (1979).

Benowitz, N.L. and Meister, W.: Clinical pharmacokinetics of lignocaine. Clinical Pharmacokinetics 3: 177 (1978).

Bergeron, M.; Dubord, L. and Hausser, C.: Membrane permeability as a cause of transport defects in experimental Fanconi Syndrome. Journal of Clinical Investigation 57: 1181 (1976).

Berglund, F.; Killander, J. and Pompeius, R.: Effect of trimethoprim-sulfamethoxazole on the renal excretion of creatinine in man. Journal of Urology 114: 802 (1975).

Bianchetti, G.; Graziani, G.; Brancaccio, D.: Morganti, A.; Leonetti, G.; Manfrin, M.; Sega, R.; Gomeni, R.; Ponticelli, C. and Morselli, P.L.: Pharmacokinetics and effects of propranolol in terminal uraemic patients and in patients undergoing regular dialysis treatment. Clinical Pharmacokinetics 1: 373 (1976).

Bolli, P.; Simpson, F.O. and Waal-Manning, H.J.: Comparison of tienilic acid with cyclopenthiazide in hyperuricaemic hypertensive subjects. Lancet 2: 595 (1978).

Bordier, P.; Zingraff, J.; Gueris, J.; Jungers, P.; Marie, P.; Pechet, M. and Rasmussen, H.: The effect of $1\alpha(OH)D_3$ and $1\alpha, 25(OH)_2D_3$ on the bone in patients with renal osteodystrophy. American Journal of Medicine 64: 101 (1978).

Bowersox, D.W.; Winterbauer, R.H.; Stewart, G.L.; Orme, B. and Barron, E.: Isoniazid dosage in patients wtih renal failure. New England Journal of Medicine 289: 84 (1973).

Boyd, W.N.; Burden, R.P. and Aber, G.M.: Intrarenal vascular changes in patients receiving oestrogen-containing compounds — a clinical, histological and angiographic study. Quarterly Journal of Medicine 44: 415 (1975).

Brater, D.C. and Morrelli, H.F.: Rational drug therapy in patients with renal disease. Western Journal of Medicine 123: 393 (1975).

Brater, D.C.: Increase in diuretic effect of chlorothiazide by probenecid. Clinical Pharmacology and Therapeutics 23: 259 (1978).

Bridgman, H.F.; Rosen, S.M. and Thorp, J.M.: Complications during clofibrate treatment of nephrotic syndrome hyperlipoproteinemia. Lancet 2: 506 (1972).

Brogden, R.N.; Speight, T.M. and Avery, G.S.: Amoxycillin: A review of its antibacterial and pharmacokinetic properties and therapeutic use. Drugs 9: 88 (1975).

Brown, C.B.; Wilson, D.; Turner, D.; Cameron, J.S.; Ogg, C.S.; Chantler, C. and Gill, D.: Combined immunosuppression and anticoagulation in rapidly progressive glomerulonephritis. Lancet 2: 1166 (1974).

Brownjohn, A.M.; Goodwin, F.J.; Hately, W.; Marsh, F.P.; O'Riordan, J.L.H. and Papapoulos, S.E.: 1-alpha-hydroxycholecalciferol for renal osteodystrophy. British Medical Journal 2: 721 (1977).

Brunner, F.P. and Frick, P.G.: Hypokalaemia, metabolic alkalosis, and hypernatraemia due to 'massive' sodium penicillin therapy. British Medical Journal 4: 550 (1968).

Buchanan, N.: Sulphamethoxazole, hypoalbuminaemia, crystalluria, and renal failure. Brit. Med. J. 2: 172 (1978).

Burry, H.C.; Dieppe, P.A.; Bresnihan, F.B. and Brown, C.: Salicylates and renal function in rheumatoid arthritis. British Medical Journal 1: 613 (1976).

Cafruny, E.J.: Renal tubular handling of drugs. American Journal of Medicine 62: 491 (1977).

Cameron, J.S.: Immunosuppressant agents in the treatment of glomerulonephritis. Part I: Corticosteroid drugs. Journal of the Royal College of Physicians of London 5: 282 (1971a).

Cameron, J.S.: Immunosuppressant agents in the treatment of glomerulonephritis. Part II. Cytotoxic Drugs. Journal of the Royal College of Physicians of London 5: 301 (1971b).

Cameron, J.S.: Bright's disease today: The pathogenesis and treatment of glomerulonephritis. British Medical Journal 4: 87, 160, 217 (1972).

Cameron, J.S.: Platelets and glomerulonephritis. Nephron 18: 253 (1977).

Cantarovich, F.; Galli, C.; Benedetti, L.; Chena, C.; Castro, L.; Correa, C.; Loredo, J.P.; Fernandes, J.C.; Loatelli, A. and Tiado, J.: High dose frusemide in established actue renal failure. British Medical Journal 4: 449 (1973).

Carvello, A.; Rakowski, T.A.; Argy, W.P. and Schreiner, G.E.: Acute renal failure following drip infusion pyelography. American Journal of Medicine 65: 38 (1978).

Cheigh, J.S.: Drug administration in renal failure. American Journal of Medicine 62: 555 (1977).

Christiansen, C.; Rodbro, P.; Christensen, M.S.; Hartnack, B. and Transbol, I.: Deterioration of renal function during treatment of chronic renal failure with 1,25-dihydroxycholecalciferol. Lancet 2: 700 (1978).

Clarkson, A.R. and Robson, J.S.: The effects of drugs on immunological renal disease; in Edwards (Ed) Drugs Affecting Kidney Function and Metabolism, Progress in Biochemical Pharmacology, vol. 7, p. 427 (Karger, Basel 1972).

Clarkson, A.R.; MacDonald, M.K.; Petrie, J.J.B.; Cash, J.B. and Robson, J.S.: Serum and urinary fibrin/fibrinogen degradation products in glomerulonephritis. British Medical Journal 3: 447 (1971).

Clarkson, A.R.; MacDonald, M.K.; Cash, J.D. and Robson, J.S.: Modification by drugs of urinary fibrin/fibrinogen degradation products in glomerulonephritis. British Medical Journal 3: 255 (1972).

Coe, F.L. and Kavalach, A.G.: Hypercalciuria and hyperuricosuria in patients with calcium nephrolithiasis. New England Journal of Medicine 291: 1344 (1974).

Cohen, B.D.; Galloway, J.A.; McMahon, R.E.; Culp, J.W.; Root, M.A. and Henriques, K.J.: Carbohydrate metabolism in uraemia: blood glucose response to sulphonylurea. American Journal of the Medical Sciences 254: 608 (1967).

Conway, N.; Beck, E. and Somerville, J.: Penicillin encephalopathy. Postgraduate Medical Journal 44: 891 (1968).

Cove-Smith, J.R. and Knapp, M.S.: Analgesic nephropathy: An important cause of chronic renal failure. Quarterly Journal of Medicine 47: 49 (1978).

Cove-Smith, J.R.; McLeod, A.A.; Blainey, R.W.; Knapp, M.S.; Reeves, W.G. and Wilson, C.B.: Transplantation, immunosuppression and plasmaphoresis in Goodpasture's syndrome. Clinical Nephrology 9: 126 (1978).

Crawhall, J.C. and Watts, R.W.E.: Cystinuria. American Journal of Medicine 45: 736 (1968).

Curtis, J.R.: Drug-induced renal disorders. British Medical Journal 2: 242, 375 (1977).

Curtis, J.R. and Williams, G.B.: Clinical Management of Chronic Renal Failure (Blackwell, Oxford 1975).

Cutler, R.E.; Forrey, A.-W.; Christopher, T.G. and Kimpel, B.M.: Pharmacokinetics of furosemide in normal subjects and functionally anephric patients. Clinical Pharmacology and Therapeutics 15: 588 (1973).

Daschner, F. and Marget, W.: Treatment of recurrent urinary tract infection in children: Compliance of parents and children wtih antibiotic therapy regimen. Acta Paediatrica Scandinavica 64: 105 (1975).

David, D.S.: Clinical studies of vitamin D analogues in renal failure. American Journal of Medicine 62: 545 (1977).

Davies, D.L. and Wilson, G.M.: Diuretics: Mechanism of action and clinical application. Drugs 9: 178 (1975).

Davis, J.S. and Kaufman, R.H.: Tetracycline toxicity. American Journal of Obstetrics and Gynecology 95: 523 (1966).

Davison, A.M.; Thomson, D.; MacDonald, M.K.; Uttley, W.S. and Robson, J.S.: The role of the mesangial cell in proliferative glomerulonephritis. Journal of Clinical Pathology 26: 3, 198 (1973).

Davison, A.M.; Lambie, A.T.; Verth, A.H. and Cash, J.D.: Salt-poor human albumin in management of nephrotic syndrome. British Medical Journal 1: 481 (1974).

Dawborn, J.K.: Renal failure and drug action; in Edwards (Ed) Drugs and The Kidney, Progress in Biochemical Pharmacology, vol. 9, p. 206 (Karger, Basel 1974).

De Baker, S.B. and Williams, R.T.: Acute interstitial nephritis due to drug sensitivity. British Medical Journal 1: 1655 (1963).

Dettli, L.: Drug dosage in renal disease. Clinical Pharmacokinetics 1: 126 (1976).

Doherty, J.E.; Hall, W.H.; Murphy, M.L. and Beard, O.W.: New information regarding digitalis metabolism. Chest 59: 433 (1971).

Donadio, J.V.; Holley, K.E.; Ferguson, R.H. and Ilstrup, D.M.: Treatment of diffuse proliferative lupus nephritis with prednisone and combined prednisone and cyclophosphamide. New England Journal of Medicine 299: 1155 (1978).

Drayer, D.E.: Pharmacologically active drug metabolites: Therapeutic and toxic activities, plasma and urine data in man, accumulation in renal failure. Clinical Pharmacokinetics 1: 426 (1976).

Drayer, D.E.: Active drug metabolites and renal failure. American Journal of Medicine 62: 486 (1977).

Drayer, D.E.; Lowenthal, D.T.; Woosley, R.L.; Nies, A.S.; Schwartz, A. and Reidenberg, M.M.: Cumulation of N-acetylprocainamide, an active metabolite of procainamide, in patients with impaired renal function. Clinical Pharmacology and Therapeutics 22: 63 (1977).

Editorial: Anaemia in chronic renal failure. Lancet 1: 959 (1975).

Editorial: Immunosuppression in the nephrotic syndrome. Lancet 2: 1121 (1976).

Edmonds, M.E.; Ashford, R.F.U; Brenner, M.K. and Saunders, A.: Cimetidine: does neurotoxicity occur? Report of three cases. Journal of the Royal Society of Medicine 72: 172 (1979).

Ekeland, A. and Sander, S.: An urodynamic study of emepronium bromide in bladder dysfunction. Scandinavian Journal of Urology and Nephrology 10: 195 (1976).

Epstein, M.; Schneider, N.S. and Befeler, B.; Effect of intrarenal furosemide on renal function in acute renal failure. American Journal of Medicine 58: 510 (1975).

Eschenbach, D.A.: The kidney in pregnancy; in de Alvarez (Ed) Clinical Monographs in Obstetrics and Gynaecology, p.69 (Wiley, New York 1976).

Fabre, J. and Balant, L.: Renal failure, drug pharmacokinetics and drug action. Clinical Pharmacokinetics 1: 99 (1976).

Fairley, K.F.; Whitworth, J.A.; Kincaid-Smith, P. and Durman, O.: Single-dose therapy in management of urinary tract infection. Medical Journal of Australia 2: 75 (1978).

Fang, P.; Macdonald, I.; Laver, M.; Hua, A. and Kincaid-Smith, P.: Oral diazoxide in uncontrolled malignant hypertension. Medical Journal of Australia 2: 621 (1974).

Fillastre, J.P.; Kuhn, M.M.; Bendirdjian, J.P.;Foucher, B.; Leseur, J.P.; Rollin, P. and Vaillant, R.: Prediction of Antibiotic Nephrotoxicity, vol. 6, p. 343 (Year Book. Chicago 1976).

Finnerty, F.A.: Hypertensive crisis. Journal of the American Medical Association 229: 1479 (1974).

Forrest, J.N.; Cox, M.; Hong, C.; Morrison, G.; Bia, M. and Singer, I.: Superiority of demeclocycline over lithium in the treatment of the chronic syndrome of inappropriate secretion of antidiuretic hormone. New England Journal of Medicine 298: 173 (1978).

Frattini, G.; Mossa, R.; Rovere, C. et al.: Considerazioni sulla sindrome di amenorrea-galactorrea da chlorpromazina in donne in eta feconda. Archivio di Psicologia, Neurologia e psichiatria 26: 449 (1965).

Frimpter, G.W.; Timpanelli, A.E.; Eisenmenger, W.J.; Stein, H.S. and Ehrlich, L.I.: Reversible 'Fanconi Syndrome' by degraded tetracycline. Journal of the American Medical Association 184: 111 (1963).

Garcia, D.A. and Yendt, E.R.: The effects of probenecid and thiazides and their combination on the urinary excretion of electrolytes and on acid-base equilibrium. Canadian Medical Association Journal 12: 473 (1970).

Gault, M.H.; Jeffrey, J.R.; Chirito, E. and Ward, L.L.: Studies of digoxin dosage, kinetics and serum concentrations in renal failure and review of the literature. Nephron 17: 161 (1976).

George, C.R.P.; Guiness, M.D.G.; Lark, D.J. and Evans, R.A.: Minocycline toxicity in renal failure. Medical Journal of Australia 1: 640 (1973).

George, C.R.P.; Clark, W.F. and Cameron, J.S.: The role of platelets in glomerulonephritis. Advanced Nephrology 5: 19 (1975).

Gibaldi, M.: Drug distribution in renal failure. American Journal of Medicine 62: 471 (1977).

Gibson, T.P. and Nelson, H.A.: Drug kinetics and artificial kidneys. Clinical Pharmacokinetics 2: 403 (1977).

Gibson, T.; Burry, H.C. and Ogg, C.: Goodpasture syndrome and D-penicillamine. Annals of Internal Medicine 84: 100 (1976).

Gibson, T.P.; Giacomini, K.M.; Briggs, W.A.; Whitman, M.D. and Levy, G.: Pharmacokinetics of d-propoxyphene in anephric subjects. Clinical Pharmacology and Therapeutics 21: 103 (1977).

Girling, D.J.: Adverse reactions to rifampicin in antituberculosis regimens. Journal of Antimicrobial Chemotherapy 3: 115 (1977).

Glassock, R.J.: The treatment of idiopathic membranous nephropathy in adults; in Proceedings VIIth International Congress of Nephrology, p.425 (Karger, Basel 1978).

Goldberg, M. and Murray, T.G.: Analgesic-associated nephropathy. An important cause of renal disease in the United States? New England Journal of Medicine 299: 716 (1978).

Goldberg, A.P.; Sherrard, D.J.; Haas, L.B. and Brunzell, J.D.: Control of clofibrate toxicity in uremic hypertriglyceridemia. Clinical Pharmacology and Therapeutics 21: 317 (1977).

Graham, J.R.; Suby, H.I.; Le Compte, P.R. and Sadowsky, N.L.: Fibrotic disorders associated with methysergide therapy for headache. New England Journal of Medicine 274: 359 (1966).

Grainger, R.G.: Renal toxicity of radiological contrast media. British Medical Bulletin 28: 191 (1972).

Greenblatt, D.J. and Koch-Weser, J.: Adverse reactions to spironolactone. Journal of the American Medical Association 225: 40 (1973).

Greenblatt, D.J. and Koch-Weser, J.: Clinical toxicity of chlordiazepoxide and diazepam in relation to serum albumin concentration: A report from the Boston Collaborative Drug Surveillance Program. European Journal of Clinical Pharmacology 7: 259-262 (1974).

Grupe, W.E.; Makker, S.P. and Ingelfinger, J.R.: Chlorambucil treatment of frequently relapsing nephrotic syndrome. New England Journal of Medicine 295: 746 (1976).

Gugler, R.: Clinical pharmacokinetics of hypolipidaemic drugs. Clinical Pharmacokinetics 3: 425 (1978).

Gugler, R. and Azarnoff, D.L.: Drug protein binding and the nephrotic syndrome. Clinical Pharmacokinetics 1: 25 (1976).

Gugler, R.; Azarnoff, D.L. and Shoeman, D.W.: Diphenylhydantoin: Correlation between protein binding and albumin concentration. Klinische Wochenschrift 53: 445 (1975).

Halladay, S.C.; Sipes, I.G. and Carter, D.E.: Diuretic effect and metabolism of bumetanide in man. Clinical Pharmacology and Therapeutics 22: 179 (1977).

Hampers, C.L.; Soeldner, J.S.; Doak, P.B. and Merrill, J.P.: Effect of chronic renal failure and hemodialysis on carbohydrate metabolism. Journal of Clinical Investigation 45: 1719 (1966).

Hansen, Ib.: The combination trimethoprim-sulphamethoxazole; in Schonfeld (Ed) Antibiotics and Chemotherapy Vol. 25, Pharmacokinetics, p.217 (Karger, Basel 1978).

Harding, G.K.M. and Ronald, A.R.: A controlled study of antimicrobial prophylaxis of recurrent urinary infection in women. New England Journal of Medicine 291: 597 (1974).

Haussler, M.R. and McCain, T.A.: Vitamin D metabolism and action. New England Journal of Medicine 297: 974, 1041 (1977).

Heale, W.F.: Management of urinary infections in children. Drugs 6: 230 (1973).

Heaney, D. and Eknoyan, G.: Minocycline and doxycycline kinetics in chronic renal failure. Clinical Pharmacology and Therapeutics 24: 233 (1978).

Hendersen, E.S.; Adamson, R.H. and Olivero, V.T.: The metabolic fate of nitrated methotrexate. Cancer Research 25: 1018 (1965).

Hendler, E.D.; Goffinet, J.A.; Ross, S.; Longnecker, R.E. and Bakovic, V.: Controlled study of androgen therapy in anemia of patients on hemodialysis. New England Journal of Medicine 291: 1046 (1974).

Hestbech, J.; Hansen, H.E.; Amdisen, A. and Olsen, S.: Chronic renal lesions following long-term treatment with lithium. Kidney International 12: 205-213 (1977).

Heymann, W.: Nephrotic syndrome after use of trimethadione and paramethadione in petit mal. Journal of the American Medical Association 202: 893 (1967).

Hill, H.F.H.: Treatment of rheumatoid arthritis with penicillamine. Seminars in Arthritis and Rheumatism 6: 361 (1977).

Hoffman, T.A.; Cestero, R. and Bullock, W.E.: Pharmacodynamics of carbenicillin in hepatic and renal failure. Annals of Internal Medicine 73: 173 (1970).

Hook, J.B. and Hewitt, W.R.: Development of mechanisms for drug excretion. American Journal of Medicine 62: 497 (1977).

Hutter, A.M.; Bauman, A.W. and Frank, I.N.: Cyclophosphamide and severe haemorrhagic cystitis. New York State Journal of Medicine 69: 305 (1969).

Iisalo, E.: Clinical pharmacokinetics of digoxin. Clinical Pharmacokinetics 2: 1 (1977).

Inturrisi, C.E.: Disposition of narcotics in patients with renal disease. American Journal of Medicine 62: 528 (1977).

Jackson, G.G. and Arcieri, G.: Ototoxicity of gentamicin in man: A survey and controlled analysis of clinical experience in the United States. Journal of Infectious Diseases 124(Suppl.): S130 (1971).

Jackson, L.; Branch, R.; Levine, D. and Ramsay, L.: Elimination of canrenone in congestive heart failure and chronic liver disease. European Journal of Clinical Pharmacology 11: 177 (1977).

Jackson, B.; Clarkson, A.R. and Seymour, A.E.: The haemolytic uraemic syndrome and oral contraceptives. Aust. N.Z. J. Med. 6: 580 (1976).

Jellett, L.B.: Potassium therapy: When is it indicated. Drugs 16: 88 (1978).

Jelliffe, R.W.; Buell, J. and Kalaba, R.: Reduction of digitalis toxicity by computer-assisted glycoside dosage regimens. Annals of Internal Medicine 77: 891 (1972).

Jick, H.: Adverse drug effects in relation to renal function. American Journal of Medicine 62: 514 (1977).

Johnsson, G. and Regardh, C.-G.: Clinical pharmacokinetics of β-adrenoceptor blocking drugs. Clinical Pharmacokinetics 1: 233 (1976).

Kalowski, S.; Nanra, R.S.; Mathew, T.H. and Kincaid-Smith, P.: Deterioration in renal function in association with cotrimoxazole therapy. Lancet 1: 394 (1973).

Kamdar, A.; Weidmann, P.; Makoff, D.L. and Massry, S.G.: Acute renal failure following intravenous use of radiographic contrast dyes in patients with diabetes mellitus. Diabetes 26: 643 (1977).

Kanis, J.A. and Russell, R.G.G.: Rate of reversal of hypercalcaemia and hypercalciuria induced by vitamin D and its 1-α-hydroxylated derivatives. British Medical Journal 1: 78 (1977).

Karim, A.: Spironolactone: Disposition, metabolism, pharmacodynamics, and bioavailability. Drug Metabolism Reviews 8: 151 (1978).

Kasanen, A.; Raines, T.; Sundqvist, H. and Tikkanen, R.: Doxycycline in renal insufficiency. Current Therapeutic Research 16: 243 (1974).

Kassirer, J.P. and Harrington, J.T.: Diuretics and potassium metabolism: A reassessment of the need, effectiveness and safety of potassium therapy. Kidney International 11: 505 (1977).

Kaye, C.M. and Dufton, J.F.: Preliminary observations on the elimination of acebutolol in severe chronic renal failure. British Journal of Clinical Pharmacology 3: 198 (1976).

Keys, T.F.: Antimicrobials commonly used for urinary tract infections; sulphonamides, trimethoprim, sulfamethoxazole, nitrofurantoin, nalidixic acid. Mayo Clinic Proceedings 52: 680 (Nov 1977).

Kincaid-Smith, P. (Ed): Analgesic nephropathy. Kidney International 13: 1 (1978).

Kincaid-Smith, P.; Mathew, T.H. and Becker, E.L.: Glomerulonephritis: Morphology, Natural History and Treatment, Part 1, p.591 (Wiley, New York 1973).

Kincaid-Smith, P.; Saker, B.M. and Fairley, K.: Anticoagulants in 'irreversible' acute renal failure. Lancet 2: 1360 (1968).

Klastersky, J.; Vanderkelen, B.; Daneau, D. and Mathieu, M.: Carbenicillin and hypokalaemia. Annals of Internal Medicine 78: 774 (1973).

Koch-Weser, J.: Pharmacokinetics of procainamide in man. Annals of the New York Academy of Sciences 179: 370 (1971).

Koch-Weser, J.: Serum procainamide levels as therapeutic guides. Clinical Pharmacokinetics 2: 389 (1977).

Koup, J.R.; Jusko, W.J.; Elwood, C.M. and Kohli, R.K.: Digoxin pharmacokinetics: Role of renal failure in dosage regimen design. Clinical Pharmacology and Therapeutics 18: 9 (1976).

Krakauer, R. and Lauritzen, M.: Diuretic therapy and hypokalemia in geriatric outpatients. Danish Medical Bulletin 25: 126 (1978).

Kuman, G.K.; Dantov, F.C. and Robayo, J.R.: Side effects of diazoxide. Journal of the American Medical Association 235: 275 (1976).

Kunelis, C.T.; Peters, J.L. and Edmondson, H.A.: Fatty liver of pregnancy and its relationship to tetracycline therapy. American Journal of Medicine 38: 359 (1965).

Kung, L.G.: Hypernephroid carcinoma and carcinoma of the urinary tract associated with abuse of phenacetin. Schweizerische Medizinische Wochenschrift 106: 47 (1976).

Kunin, C.M.: The natural history of recurrent bacteriuria in schoolgirls. New England Journal of Medicine 282: 1443 (1970).

Kunin, C.M.: Detection, Prevention and Management of Urinary Tract Infections (Lea and Febiger, Philadelphia 1974).

Kunin, C.M.: Long-term therapy of urinary tract infections. Annals of Internal Medicine 83: 273 (1975).

Kuzucu, E.Y.: Methoxyflurane, tetracycline and renal failure. Journal of the American Medical Association 211: 1162 (1970).

Lagrue, G.; Bernard, D.; Bariety, J.; Druet, P. and Guenel, J.: Traitement par le chlorambucil et l'azathioprine dans les glomerulonephrites primitives. Resultats d'une etude controlee. Journal d'Urologie et de Nephrologie 81: 655 (1975).

Lavene, D.; Weiss, Y.A.; Safar, M.E.; Loria, Y.; Agorus, N.; Georges, D. and Milliez, P.L.: Pharmacokinetics and hepatic extraction ratio of pindolol in hypertensive patients with normal and impaired renal function. Journal of Clinical Pharmacology 17: 501 (1977).

Lawson, D.H.: Adverse reactions to potassium chloride. Quarterly Journal of Medicine 43: 443 (1974).

Ledingham, J.M.: Mechanisms of hypertension in renal disease. Proceedings of the Royal Society of Medicine 64: 409 (1971); Journal of the Royal College of Physicians of London 5: 103 (1971).

Levy, G.: Effect of plasma protein binding of drugs on duration and intensity of pharmacologic activity. Journal of Pharmaceutical Sciences 65: 1264 (1976).

Levy, G.: Pharmacokinetics in renal disease. American Journal of Medicine 62: 461 (1977).

Levy, G.; Baliah, T. and Procknal, J.A.: Effect of renal transplantation on protein binding of drugs in serum of donor and recipient. Clinical Pharmacology and Therapeutics 20: 512 (1976).

Lowenthal, D.T.: Tissue sensitivity to drugs in disease states. Medical Clinics of North America 58: 1111 (1974).

Lowenthal, D.T.: Pharmacokinetics of propranolol, quinidine, procainamide and lidocaine in chronic renal disease. American Journal of Medicine 62: 533 (1977).

Lowenthal, D.T.; Briggs, W.A.; Gibson, T.P.; Nelson, H. and Cirksena, W.J.: Pharmacokinetics of oral propranolol in chronic renal disease. Clinical Pharmacology and Therapeutics 16: 761 (1974).

Lowenthal, D.T.; Pitone, J.M.; Affrime, M.B.; Shirk, J.; Busby, P.; Kim, K.E.; Nancarrow, J.; Swartz, C.D. and Onesti, G.: Timolol kinetics in chronic renal insufficiency. Clinical Pharmacology and Therapeutics 23: 606 (1978).

McAllister, C.J.; Scowden, E.B. and Stone, W.J.: Toxic psychosis induced by phenothiazine administration in patients with chronic renal failure. Clinical Nephrology 10: 191 (1978).

Maher, J.F.: Principles of dialysis and dialysis of drugs. American Journal of Medicine 62: 475 (1977).

Mahon, W.A.; Johnson, G.E.; Endrenyi, L.; Kelly, M.F. and Fenton, S.S.A.: The elimination of tritiated doxycycline in normal subjects and in patient with severely impaired renal function. Scandinavian Journal of Infectious Diseases, Suppl. 9: 24 (1976).

Mathew, T.: The treatment of renal calculi. Drugs 8: 62 (1974).

Mathew, T.H. and Kincaid-Smith, P.: The use of diazoxide in hypertensive crises with particular reference to the control of hypertension in severe renal failure. Drugs 2: 73 (1971).

Mawer, G.E.; Ahmad, R.; Dobbs, Sylvia, M. and McGough, J.G.: Prescribing aids for gentamicin. British Journal of Clinical Pharmacology 1: 45 (1974).

Meares, E.M.: Prostatitis: Diagnosis and treatment. Drugs 15: 472 (1978).

Medical Research Council Working Party: Controlled trial of azathioprine and prednisone in chronic renal disease. British Medical Journal 2: 239 (1971).

Meffin, P.J.; Harapat, S.R. and Harrison, D.C.: Quantitation in plasma and urine of acebutolol and a major metabolite with preliminary observations on their disposition kinetics in man. Research Communications in Chemical Pathology and Pharmacology 15: 31 (1976).

Merrill, J.P.: Glomerulonephritis. New England Journal of Medicine 290: 257, 313, 374 (1974).

Milne, M.D.: Influence of acid-base balance on efficacy and toxicity of drugs. Proceedings of the Royal Society of Medicine 58: 961 (1965).

Milne, M.D.: Renal tubular dysfunction; in Strauss and Welt (Eds) Diseases of the Kidney (Little Brown, Boston 1971).

Milne, M.D.: Drug interactions and the kidney; in Cluff and Petrie (Eds) Clinical Effects of Interaction Between Drugs, p. 193 (Excerpta Medica, Amsterdam 1975).

Mitchell, J.R.; McMurtry, R.J.; Statham, C.N. and Nelson, S.D.: Molecular basis for several drug-induced nephropathies. American Journal of Medicine 62: 518 (1977).

Morgan, T.O.: Clinical use of potassium supplements and potassium sparing diuretics. Drugs 6: 222 (1973).

Morgan, T. and Ribush, N.: The effect of oxytetracycline and doxycycline on protein metabolism. Medical Journal of Australia 1: 55 (1972).

Moses, A.M. and Miller, M.: Drug-induced dilutional hyponatremia. New England Journal of Medicine 2911: 1234 (1974).

Murphy, K.J.: Uraemic accentuation of chlorpromazine pigmentation. Medical Journal of Australia 2: 1228 (1966).

Mussche, M.M.; Belpaire, F.M. and Bogaert, M.G.: Plasma protein binding of phenylbutazone during recovery from acute renal failure. European Journal of Clinical Pharmacology 9: 69 (1975).

Myers, G.H. and Witten, D.M.: Acute renal failure after excretory urography in multiple myeloma. American Journal of Roentgenology 113: 583 (1971).

Neild, G.H.; Gartner, H.-V. and Bohle, A.: D-penicillamine-induced membranous glomerulonephritis. Lancet 1: 1201 (1975).

New Zealand Rheumatism Association: Aspirin and the kidney. British Medical Journal 1: 593 (1974).

Nolan, C.M. and Abernathy, R.S.: Nephropathy associated with methicillin therapy. Prevalence and determinants in patients with staphylococcal bacteremia. Archives of Internal Medicine 137: 997 (1977).

Noone, P.; Beale, D.F.; Pollock, S.S.; Perera, M.R.; Amirak, I.D.; Fernando, O.N. and Moorhead, J.F.: Monitoring aminoglycoside use in patients with severely impaired renal function. British Medical Journal 2: 470 (1978).

Odar-Cederlof, I.: Plasma protein binding of phenytoin and warfarin in patients undergoing renal transplantation. Clinical Pharmacokinetics 2: 147 (1977).

Odar-Cederlof, I. and Borga, O.: Kinetics of diphenylhydantoin in uraemic patients. European Journal of Clinical Pharmacology 7: 31 (1974).

Odar-Cederlof, I.; Vessman, J.; Alvan, G. and Sjoqvist, F.: Oxazepam disposition in uraemic patients. Acta Pharmacologica et Toxicologica 40 (Suppl. I): 52 (1977).

O'Grady, F.: Antibiotics and renal failure. British Medical Bulletin 27: 142 (1971).

Oliva, P.B.: Lactic acidosis. American Journal of Medicine 48: 209 (1970).

Orr, L.H.; Rudisill, E.; Brodkin, R. and Hamilton, R.W.: Exacerbation of renal failure associated with doxycycline. Archives of Internal Medicine 138: 793 (1978).

Parfitt, A.M.: Acetazolamide and sodium bicarbonate induced nephrocalcinosis and nephrolithiasis. Archives of Internal Medicine 124: 736 (1969).

Pearson, R.M.: Pharmacokinetics and response to diazoxide in renal failure. Clinical Pharmacokinetics 2: 198 (1977).

Perrier, D.; Mayersohn, M. and Marcus, F.I.: Clinical pharmacokinetics of digitoxin. Clinical Pharmacokinetics 2: 292 (1977).

Perucca, E.; Garratt, A.; Hebdige, S. and Richens, A.: Water intoxication in epileptic patients receiving carbamazepine. Journal of Neurology, Neurosurgery, and Psychiatry 41: 713 (1978).

Phillips, M.E.; Eastwood, J.B.; Curtis, J.R.; Gower, P.E. and de Wardener, H.E.: Tetracycline poisoning in renal failure. British Medical Journal 2: 149 (1974).

Piafsky, K.M. and Borga, O.: Plasma protein binding of basic drugs. II. Importance of α_1-acid glycoprotein for interindividual variation. Clinical Pharmacology and Therapeutics 22: 545 (1977).

Piafsky, K.M.; Borga, O.; Odar-Cederlof, I.; Johansson, C. and Sjoqvist, F.: Increased plasma protein binding of propranolol and chlorpromazine mediated by disease-induced elevations of plasma α_1 acid glycoprotein. New England Journal of Medicine 299: 1435 (1978).

Pierides, A.M.; Ellis, H.A.; Simpson, W.; Dewar, J.H.; Ward, M.K. and Kerr, D.N.S.: Variable response to long-term 1α hydroxycholecalciferol in haemodialysis osteodystrophy. Lancet 1: 1092 (1976).

Pierides, A.M.; Aljama, P.; Kerr, D.N.S.; Scott, M. and Norman, A.W.: Effect of 1α-hydroxycholecalciferol, 1,25-dihydroxycholecalciferol, 3 deoxy-1α-hydroxycholecalciferol, 24R, 25-dihydroxycholecalciferol and successful renal transplantation on calcium absorption in haemodialysis patients. Nephron 20: 203 (1978).

Pollak, V.E.: Treatment of lupus nephritis: in Advances in Nephrology (Hospital Necker), vol. 6, p. 137 (Year Book, Chicago 1976).

Pruitt, A.W.; Winkel, Joan S. and Dayton, P.G.: Variations in the fate of triamterene. Clinical Pharmacology and Therapeutics 21: 610 (1977).

Rane, A.; Villeneuve, J.P.; Stone, W.J.; Nies, A.S.; Wilkinson, G.R. and Branch, R.A.: Plasma binding and disposition of furosemide in the nephrotic syndrome and in uremia. Clinical Pharmacology and Therapeutics 24: 199 (1978).

Reidenberg, M.M.: Renal function and drug action (Saunders, Philadelphia and London 1971).

Reidenberg, M.M.: The binding of drugs to plasma proteins from patients with poor renal function. Clinical Pharmacokinetics 1: 121 (1976).

Reidenberg, M.M.: The binding of drugs to plasma proteins and the interpretation of measurements of plasma concentrations of drugs in patients with poor renal function. American Journal of Medicine 62: 466 (1977a).

Reidenberg, M.M.: The biotransformation of drugs in renal failure. American Journal of Medicine 62: 482 (1977b).

Reidenberg, M.M.; Odar-Cederlof, I.; von Bahr, C.; Borga, O. and Sjoqvist, F.: Protein binding of diphenylhydantoin and desmethylimipramine in plasma from patients with poor renal function. New England Journal of Medicine 285: 264 (1971).

Reinarz, J.A. and McIntosh, D.A.: Lincomycin excretion in patients with normal renal function, severe azotemia, and with haemodialysis and peritoneal dialysis. Antimicrobial Agents and Chemotherapy pp. 232-238 (1965).

Ribush, N. and Morgan, T.: Tetracyclines and renal failure. Medical Journal of Australia 1: 53 (1972).

Richet, G.; de Novales, E.L. and Verroust, P.: Drug intoxication and neurological episodes in chronic renal failure. British Medical Journal 2: 394 (1970).

Riess, W.; Dubach, U.C.; Burckhardt, D.; Theobald, W.;

Vuillard, P. and Zimmerli, M.: Pharmacokinetic studies with chlorthalidone (Hygrofon) in man. European Journal of Clinical Pharmacology 12: 375 (1977).

Ritch, A.E.S.; Castleden, C.M.; George, C.F. and Hall, M.R.P.: A second look at emepronium bromide in urinary incontinence. Lancet 1: 504 (1977a).

Ritch, A.E.S.; Castleden, C.M.; George, C.F. and Hall, M.R.P.: Emepronium bromide in urinary incontinence. Lancet 1: 799 (1977b).

Robertson, W.G. and Peacock, M.: Risk factors in calcium stone formation; in Proceedings VIIth International Congress of Nephrology p. 363 (Karger, Basel 1978).

Robertson, W.S.; Peacock, M.; Marshall, R.W.; Marshall, D.H. and Nordin, C.: Saturation-inhibition index as a measure of the risk of calcium oxalate stone formation in the urinary tract. New England Journal of Medicine 294: 249 (1976).

Robinson, M.F.; Campbell, G.R. and Craswell, P.W.: Co-trimoxazole in chronic renal failure. A controlled experiment in Wistar rats. Clinical Toxicology 10: 411 (1977).

Robson, J.S.: The nephrotic syndrome; in Black (Ed) Renal Disease, 3rd ed, p. 331 (Blackwell, Oxford 1972).

Robson, J.S.: The nephrotic syndrome. Practitioner 212: 37 (1974).

Robson, A.M.; Cole, B.R.; Kienstra, R.A.; Kissane, J.M.; Alkjaersig, N. and Fletcher, A.P.: Severe glomerulonephritis complicated by coagulopathy: Treatment with anticoagulant and immunosuppressive drugs. Journal of Pediatrics 90: 881 (1977).

Ronald, A.R.; Boutros, P. and Mourtada, H.: Bacteriuria localisation and response to single dose therapy in women. Journal of the American Medical Association 235: 1854 (1976).

Rosei, E.A.; Trust, P.M.; Brown, J.J.; Lever, A.F. and Robertson, J.I.S.: Intravenous labetalol in severe hypertension. Lancet 2: 1093 (1975).

Row, P.G.; Cameron, J.S.; Turner, D.B.; Evans, D.J.; White, R.H.R.; Ogg, C.S.; Chantler, C. and Brown, C.B.: Membranous nephropathy. Quarterly Journal of Medicine 44: 207 (1975).

Rubin, A.L.; Stenzel, K.H. and Reidenberg, M.M. (Eds): Symposium on drug action and metabolism in renal failure. American Journal of Medicine 62: 459 (1977).

Sarff, L.D. and McCracken, G.H.: Methicillin-associated nephropathy or cystitis. Journal of Pediatrics 90: 1031 (1977).

Scheer, R.L.: The effects of hypertonic mannitol in oliguric patients. American Journal of Medical Science 250: 483 (1965).

Schentag, J.J.; Cerra, F.B.; Calleri, G.; De Glopper, E.; Rose, J.Q. and Bernhard, H.: Pharmacokinetic and clinical studies with cimetidine-associated mental confusion. Lancet 1: 177 (1979).

Schentag, J.J.; Cumbo, T.J.; Jusko, W.J. and Plant, M.E.: Gentamicin tissue accumulation and nephrotoxic reactions. Journal of the American Medical Association 240: 2067 (1978).

Segal, S.: Disorders of renal amino acid transport. New England Journal of Medicine 294: 1044 (1976).

Shahidi, N.T.: Anabolic androgenic hormones. American Journal of Medicine 62: 546 (1977).

Shand, D.G.: Pharmacokinetic properties of the β-adrenoreceptor blocking drugs; in Avery (Ed) Cardiovascular Drugs, Vol. 2, p.41 (ADIS Press, Sydney; University Park Press, Baltimore 1977).

Sharpstone, P.: The renal handling of trimethoprim and sulphamethoxazole in man. Postgraduate Medical Journal 45 (Suppl): 38 (Nov. 1969).

Shils, M.E.: Renal disease and the metabolic effects of tetracycline. Annals of Internal Medicine 58: 389 (1963).

Sjoholm, I.; Kober, A.; Odar-Cederlof, I. and Borga, O.: Protein binding of drugs in uremic and normal serum. The role of binding inhibitors. Biochemical Pharmacology 25: 1205 (1976).

Sklenar, I.; Spring, P. and Dettli, L.: One-dose and multiple-dose kinetics of minocycline in patients with renal disease. Agents and Actions 7: 369 (1977).

Smith, M.J.V.: Placebo versus allopurinol for renal calculi. Journal of Urology 117: 690 (1977).

Smith, J.W.; Seidl, L.G. and Cluff, L.E.: Studies on the epidemiology of adverse drug reactions. V. Clinical factors influencing susceptibility. Annals of Internal Medicine 65: 629 (1966).

Speight, T.M. and Avery, G.S.: Diazoxide: A review of its pharmacological properties and therapeutic use in hypertensive crises. Drugs 2: 78 (1971).

Stenzel, K.H.; Reidenberg, M.M. and Rubin, A.L.: Combined seminar on the use of drugs in renal failure: Narcotics, psychotherapeutic agents, anti-arrhythmics, antihypertensives, sorbents, vitamin D and its analogues, anabolic hormones and nutritional supplements. American Journal of Medicine 62: 527 (1977).

Stephens, A.D.: The management of cystinuria in 1976. Proceedings of the Royal Society of Medicine 70 (Suppl. 3): 24 (1977).

Storstein, L.: Protein binding of cardiac glycosides in disease states. Clinical Pharmacokinetics 2: 220 (1977).

Swainson, C.P. and Winney, R.J.: Effect of beta-blockade in chronic renal failure. British Medical Journal 1: 459 (1976).

Swapp, G.H.: Asymptomatic bacteriuria, birth weight and length of gestation; in Brumfitt and Asscher (Eds) Second National Symposium on Urinary Tract Infection p. 92 (Oxford University Press, London 1973).

Szeto, H.H.; Intrurrisi, C.E.; Houde, R.; Saal, S.; Cheigh, J. and Reidenberg, M.M.: Accumulation of normeperidine, an active metabolite of meperidine, in patients with renal failure or cancer. Annals of Internal Medicine 86: 738 (1977).

Talseth, T.: Clinical pharmacokinetics of hydrallazine. Clinical Pharmacokinetics 2: 317 (1977).

Tasker, P.R.W.: MacGregor, G.A.; de Wardener, H.E.; Thomas, R.D. and Jones, N.F.: Use of co-trimoxazole in chronic renal failure. Lancet 1: 1216 (1975).

Taylor, J.S.: Carcinoma of the urinary tract and analgesic abuse. Medical Journal of Australia 1: 407 (1972).

Tjandramaga, T.B.; Verbesselt, R.; Verbeeck, R.; Verberekmoes, R. and De Schepper, P.J.: Disposition of acebutolol and its N-acetylmetabolite in renal insufficiency. Abstract 2300 in VIIth International Congress of Pharmacology, Paris (1978).

Tourkantonis, A.; Friedrich, H. and Heinze, V.: Ampicillin-Nebenwirkungen bei Patienten mit Niereninsuffizienz. Medizinishce Klinik 66: 1154 (1971).

Tullett, G.L.: Sudden death occurring during 'massive-dose' potassium penicillin G therapy. Wisconsin Medical Journal 69: 216 (1970).

Turck, M.; Anderson, K.N. and Petersdorf, R.G.: Relapse and reinfection in chronic bacteriuria. New England Journal of Medicine 275: 70 (1966).

Various Authors: in Asscher and Brumfitt (Eds) Urinary Tract Infection. Kidney International. Suppl. No. 4 (Aug. 1975a).

Various Authors: in Kincaid-Smith and Maxwell (Eds) Hypertension and the kidney. Kidney International. Suppl. No. 5 (Sept. 1975b).

Various Authors: in David (Ed) Calcium Metabolism in Renal Failure and Nephrolithiasis. Perspectives in Nephrology and Hypertension (Wiley, New York 1977).

Various Authors: in Friedman (Ed) Strategy in Renal Failure (Wiley, New York 1978).

Various Authors: in Anderton, Parsons and Jones (Eds) Living with Renal Failure, Proceedings of Multidisciplinary Symposium, University of Stirling, July 1977 (MTP Press, Lancaster, England 1978).

Verbeeck, R.; Tjandramaga, T.B.; Verberckmoes, R. and De Schepper, P.J.: Biotransformation and excretion of lorazepam in patients with chronic renal failure. British Journal of Clinical Pharmacology 3: 1033 (1976).

Viol, G.W.; Minielly, J.A. and Bistricki, T.: Gold nephropathy. Archives of Pathology and Laboratory Medicine 101: 635 (1977).

Wade, J.C.; Smith, C.R.; Petty, B.G.; Lipsky, J.J.; Conrad, G.; Ellner, J. and Lietman, P.S.: Cephalothin plus an aminoglycoside is more nephrotoxic than methicillin plus an aminoglycoside. Lancet 2: 604 (1978).

Waisbren, B.A.; Evani, S.V. and Ziebert, A.P.: Carbenicillin and bleeding. Journal of the American Medical Association 217: 1243 (1971).

Walton, J.: Familial hypophosphataemic rickets. Clinical Paediatrics 15: 1007 (1976).

Walton, J.D. and Farman, J.V.: Suxamethonium, potassium and renal failure. Anaesthesia 28: 626 (1973a).

Walton, J.D. and Farman, J.V.: Suxamethonium hyperkalaemia in uraemic neuropathy. Anaesthesia 28: 666 (1973b).

Warren, D.J.; Swainson, C.P. and Wright, N.: Deterioration in renal function after beta-blockade in patients with chronic renal failure. British Medical Journal 2: 193 (1974).

Weiner, I.M.: Excretion of drugs by the kidney; in Brodie and Gillette (Eds) Handbook of Experimental Pharmacology, Vol. 28 Concepts in Biochemical Pharmacology, pt.1, p.328 (Springer, Berlin 1971).

Weiss, P.; Hersey, R.M.; Dujovne, C.A. and Bianchine, J.R.: The metabolism of amiloride hydrochloride in man. Clinical Pharmacology and Therapeutics 10: 401 (1969).

Welling, P.G.; Shaw, W.R.; Uman, S.J.; Tse, F.L.S. and Craig, W.A.: Pharmacokinetics of minocycline in renal failure. Antimicrobial Agents and Chemotherapy 8: 532 (1975).

Whalley, P.: Bacteriuria of pregnancy. American Journal of Obstetrics and Gynecology 97: 723 (1967).

Wood, A.J.; Bolli, P.; Waal-Manning, H.J. and Simpson, O.: Ticrynafen: kinetics protein binding and effects on serum and urinary uric acid. Clinical Pharmacology and Therapeutics 23: 697 (1978).

Wu, M.-J.; Narsete, T.A.; Hussey, J.L.; Weinstein, A.B. and Wen, S.-F.: Cephalothin neurotoxicity in renal failure. Annals of Internal Medicine 89: 429 (1978).

Zacest, R.; Gilmore, E. and Koch-Weser, J.: Treatment of essential hypertension with combined vasodilation and beta-adrenergic blockade. New Zealand Journal of Medicine 286: 617 (1972).

Chapter XXII
Rheumatic Disorders

F.D. Hart

Synopsis of Important Principles

1) Management of the rheumatic disorders is aimed at relief of pain, stiffness and joint swelling, maintenance of joint function and general health and wellbeing, control of anxiety and depression, correction of any metabolic abnormalities and prevention of deformities and crippling.

2) Drugs are used as part of a total management programme comprising patient education, specific advice on general and local rest and exercise, splintage, occupational and physiotherapy, and surgery where indicated.

3) The patient must appreciate and understand the rationale and the techniques of his own treatment for he is for much of his life his own physician and therapist, and his daily ration of drugs, though controlled by his doctor, must be varied by himself in the light of daily needs, toxic reactions and other factors.

4) Inflammation is the basis of rheumatoid arthritis and most other rheumatic disorders, but there is no agent available which can stop this inflammation progressing to erosion and destruction of joint tissues, without causing dangerous or unpleasant side effects.

5) Non-steroidal anti-inflammatory agents are the basis of drug therapy in rheumatoid arthritis. They only alleviate symptoms and should not be continued for long periods in the face of obvious and severe deterioration, when drugs such as gold and penicillamine, which often appear to alter the course of the disease, should be considered for long term use until remission or evidence of toxicity has set in.

6) Prophylactic measures are the most desirable means of management of osteoporosis since there is no established specific treatment. Adequate amounts of calcium and outdoor exercise are the basis of prevention.

7) Management of gout is directed at treatment of the acute attack, prevention of subsequent attacks, and dissolution of tophaceous deposits by reducing the serum urate to normal. Asymptomatic hyperuricaemia is sometimes due to reversible causes and only very rarely requires treatment.

8) A large number of drugs in common usage can cause aches and pains in muscles, bones and joints, and some may precipitate gout (e.g. thiazides) or exacerbate arthritis. Drug induced systemic lupus erythematosus (e.g. hydrallazine, procainamide) and the bone complications of corticosteroids and long term anticonvulsants are the most important problems.

The rheumatic diseases affect almost every person to a greater or lesser degree at some time in their life. They cause more continuous pain, more disability and more loss of time from work than any other group of disorders. They may not kill, as do neoplasms and leukaemias, but by eroding health they may shorten expectation of life, and certain of the rheumatic disorders are occasionally brutally and briskly lethal — for example Wegener's granulomatosis, polyarteritis nodosa and systemic lupus erythematosus. The therapeutic problem is therefore immense, not only because of the large numbers of persons involved in the community by the rheumatic disorders, but because of the duration of their disabilities.

1. Clinical Pharmacological Considerations and General Principles of Treatment

The study of the rheumatic disorders is essentially a study of the 'long pain', a very different therapeutic problem from episodic short term discomfort, for prolonged pain carries with it overtones of anxiety, depression and despair which call for a much more sophisticated approach than the treatment of immediate transient pain, however severe. For these reasons one does not speak of the treatment of the rheumatic disorders so much as the management of them. As many and varied as are the drugs available to the rheumatic sufferer, the number of really effective antirheumatic agents is small, and their toxic potential considerable.

The central theme throughout the rheumatic disorders is pain (Hart and Huskisson, 1972b). What drugs and what factors ease this pain and make life more endurable are all important, and the only person who knows what really works in his case is the patient. In severe pain due to trauma (e.g. road accidents), it has been shown that establishment of confidence and reassurance help make the sufferer feel that the situation is under control; his anxiety lessens, his pain diminishes and strong analgesic drugs are less often required. The same is true of pain under less dramatic circumstances. Simple analgesics do not control or relieve anxiety, and those narcotic analgesics that do, such as diamorphine (heroin), morphine and pethidine (meperidine), should not be used in the treatment of the 'long rheumatic pain' because of their dependence producing properties.

1.1 Aims of Treatment

Since the causes of most of the rheumatic diseases are unknown, treatment is aimed at relief of pain and control of inflammation in order to contain the disease process, at the same time maintaining good general and mental health. The aim of therapy in the rheumatic disorders is therefore to:

1) Relieve pain, and so enable more normal painless function at work, at home and at rest.
2) Relieve stiffness and swelling with the same aims as outlined above, to prevent contractures and deformities and to maintain as near full mobility as possible.
3) Maintain and promote general health and wellbeing, to maintain normal nutrition and prevent or treat anaemia.
4) Prevent or control depression and anxiety, to maintain mental health.
5) Correct any metabolic abnormalities.

These goals are approached by judicious use of drugs as part of a total management programme comprising patient education, specific advice on general and local rest and exercise, splintage, occupational and physiotherapy, and surgery where indicated.

1.2 Clinical Pharmacological Factors and Drug Selection

The drugs available for the treatment of the rheumatic disorders include analgesics, non-steroidal anti-inflammatory analgesics, steroidal anti-inflammatory agents, drugs which act slowly in an unknown way on the rheumatoid disease process, psychotherapeutic drugs, and drugs which improve general wellbeing (see table I). These drugs must be used judiciously and for appropriate reasons. In the relief of pain and inflammation each patient is an individual and there are no fixed rules and trial and error enter into most individual cases, with the patient knowing what suits him best (Huskisson and Hart, 1972). A few general guidelines can, however, be made about the clinical pharmacological factors which influence the selection and use of drugs (for review, see Hart, 1978b):

1) *Nature of the disease* — where a powerful anti-inflammatory action is required, as in acute gout or severe active rheumatoid arthritis or

Table I. Drugs used in the management of rheumatic disorders

---

1. Analgesic drugs without anti-inflammatory action
   a) Non-narcotic — e.g. paracetamol (acetaminophen), codeine, dihydrocodeine, dextropropoxyphene, pentazocine.
   b) Narcotic (very rarely used) — e.g. diamorphine (heroin), morphine, pethidine (meperidine), See further chapter X (table IX).

2. Anti-inflammatory drugs with analgesic and antipyretic properties — e.g. aspirin in full dosage, phenylbutazone, indomethacin, propionic acid derivatives, etc (see table II).

3. Anti-inflammatory drugs devoid of central analgesic action — e.g. corticosteroids, corticotrophin, tetracosactrin.

4. Drugs which act slowly in an unknown way on the rheumatoid disease process — gold salts, antimalarials, D-penicillamine, immunosuppressives.

5. Psychotherapeutic drugs
   a) Tricyclic antidepressant drugs — e.g. amitriptyline, imipramine, etc.
   b) Antianxiety drugs — e.g. diazepam.

6. Drugs which improve general wellbeing — iron, folic acid, vitamins.

Reiter's disease, only the truly potent anti-inflammatory agents are popular with the patient (e.g. indomethacin, phenylbutazone; see table II). When degenerative, non-inflammatory conditions (e.g. osteoarthrosis) cause intermittent pain only, quick acting simple analgesics such as small doses of aspirin (1 to 2g daily) are more appropriate, but when more severe and constant pain is present, whatever the cause, non-steroidal anti-inflammatory analgesic drugs such as phenylbutazone or indomethacin often prove superior (Hart, 1975a; Hart and Huskisson, 1972b; Huskisson and Hart, 1972).

2) The phase, stage and extent of the disease — some drugs such as non-steroidal anti-inflammatory analgesics like aspirin only alleviate symptoms; thus in rheumatoid arthritis they should not be given for long periods in the face of obvious and severe deterioration. On the other hand, corticosteroids with their considerable immediate effect on symptoms but greater side effect cost later on, should not be given as initial therapy. Where active inflammatory disease appears to be progressing, drugs such as gold and penicillamine, which can favourably affect the disease process, should be considered (Constable et al., 1975).

3) The patient's likes and dislikes — in rheumatoid arthritis the patient is the best judge of which drug provides greatest relief from symptoms with minimum side effects (Hart and Huskisson, 1972a), but inadequately instructed patients should not be allowed to dictate their own therapy against proper indications; e.g. long term use of corticosteroids (Moldofsky and Rothman, 1971).

4) The presence or absence of complications such as dyspepsia or other gastrointestinal symptoms (table III) — some patients, particularly those with a recent history of peptic ulcer, tolerate certain anti-inflammatory drugs poorly and an appropriate alternative agent should be selected. Conventional aspirin should be avoided in those with peptic ulceration (see chapter XIX; sect. 13.1.1).

5) The side effects of the drug in question (table III) — phenylbutazone is an unsuitable drug for long term use in the elderly because of an increased risk of side effects, particularly blood dyscrasias and precipitation of heart failure from fluid retention (see also chapter V, sect. 4.5), while aspirin should be avoided in those asthmatics sensitive to aspirin.

6) Possible clinically important interactions between the various drugs the patient may be taking — some of the non-steroidal anti-inflammatory drugs may modify the dose requirements of other drugs; for example, phenylbutazone may enhance the activity of oral coumarin anticoagulants while aspirin may increase the risk of bleeding complications in those on oral anticoagulants (see table IV; sect. 13; appendix C).

1.3 General Education and Instruction of the Patient

It must be emphasised that just as important as drugs, and probably more so, is the general programme of indoctrination in the rudiments of the patient's disease, whether it be gout, rheumatoid arthritis, ankylosing spondylitis or osteoarthrosis (Hart and Huskisson, 1972b).

The patient must know something of the nature of his disability, what to expect of it and what to do about it. He must be advised in the management of his life at home and at work. He must be instructed in the art of rest, relaxation, exercise and exercises. He must have talking time to ask questions about his condition and discuss his own and his family's future. He may receive different forms of physiotherapy, he may be advised to wear splints, he may have periods of hospital inpatient treatment and finally he will be given drugs and instructed in their usage and told something of their possible drawbacks.

An arthritic patient in most cases lives for many years with his disorder and is for most of this time his own doctor, nurse, dietitian and physiotherapist. Like a diabetic, he must know something of the management of his own case. His daily ration of drugs, though controlled by his clinician, must be varied by himself in the light of daily needs, side effects and other factors.

2. Rheumatic Fever

The prevention of primary rheumatic illness depends on early (within 5 days) and effective penicillin treatment of a proven β-haemolytic streptococcal pharyngitis (see chapter XI; sect. 2.7). In 'highly rheumatic regions' where bacteriological facilities are not readily available, there may well be justification for routine penicillin treatment of pharyngitis.

In the treatment of an acute attack, bed rest is the rule for as long as there is evidence of disease activity but in the absence of carditis strict bed rest is unnecessary after other acute symptoms have abated. Any β-haemolytic streptococcal carrier state, whether confirmed or not by throat culture, is treated by full doses of penicillin for 10 days; e.g. 1 mega unit benzylpenicillin by intramuscular injection daily or phenoxymethylpenicillin 250mg (young children) to 500mg 6-hourly orally. Erythromycin (250mg 4 times daily for 10 days) can be used in penicillin allergic patients. Aspirin has a profound effect on the clinical manifestations of rheumatic fever and is given in a dose of 130mg/kg of body weight, the total dosage varying from 2g daily in children to 8g in adults, the dose being that which is well tolerated and efficiently controls symptoms. Serum levels of 1.8mmol/L (25mg/100ml) or more are usually required in adults, and rather more in children; levels around 1.8 to 2.5mmol/L (25 to 35mg/100ml) giving maximum symptomatic control. There is little reason to prefer any other form of salicylate.

Salicylates appear to have no effect on the disease process or its eventual outcome, even when given in large amounts. On the credit side, pain is relieved, fever lowered or eliminated, and the clinical condition is improved. On the debit side, salicylates can precipitate heart failure and should be used only with great caution if carditis exists, or not at all if there is heart failure or cardiac deterioration (Bywaters and Thomas, 1961). Drowsiness and hyperventilation may be seen in young children.

Corticosteroids may be used in severe carditis to suppress the inflammatory reaction, prevent decompensation and generally improve the clinical condition. The usual starting dosage is about 2mg of prednisolone per kg of body weight daily in divided dosage; the dose being reduced once signs and symptoms of inflammation and carditis diminish. Corticosteroid therapy should be gradually reduced as exacerbation of disease may occur. Corticosteroids, like salicylates, do not prevent development of permanent cardiac changes (Joint Report, 1960). If congestive heart failure occurs, treatment is by conventional methods with digitalis and diuretics (see chapter XVII; sect. 8.1). Pericarditis usually calls for corticosteroid therapy.

The prevention of rheumatic fever recurrence is based essentially upon the elimination of streptococcal infection (Evans, 1950). This can be achieved by an intramuscular injection of 1 to 1.5 mega units of benzathine penicillin every month. Oral penicillin is probably slightly less effective, 250mg of phenoxymethylpenicillin being given twice daily 1 hour before food, but is only suitable for cooperative patients in whom compliance can be assured. Erythromycin 125mg twice daily can be used in cases of penicillin hypersensitivity. This preventive treatment is given to all children who have had rheumatic fever and/or evidence of rheumatic carditis. Such prophylaxis should be carried out throughout childhood, though opinions vary thereafter, prophylaxis for life being considered necessary by many investigators for those with rheumatic carditis, the risk, though less, still remaining in late middle life. Crowded living conditions, such as in armed forces barracks, schools and hospitals, carry extra risk and it is wise to continue prophylaxis throughout such periods of greater exposure. In general, only special risk groups, or patients with carditis need continue preventive therapy after the age of 25 years.

Should streptococcal infection occur in spite of this prophylactic regimen full therapeutic dosage of penicillin (or erythromycin if the patient is hypersensitive to penicillin) should be given for a minimum of 10 days. Where valvular damage has occurred, if preventive measures have been given up, to prevent bacterial endocarditis occurring, full prophylactic measures should be restarted to cover operations on teeth and tonsils and instrumentation of the genitourinary tract.

3. Rheumatoid Arthritis

Rheumatoid arthritis is a complex and variable disorder. It may last for a few days or for 50 years, affect one or 60 joints, and may be severe, painful and prostrating, or may only cause mildly annoying symptoms. It may have definite systemic effects and prove fatal, or may be merely a painful nuisance; it may be a soul destroying disorder which can precipitate suicidal attempts, or may come and go in mild palindromic form. Thus, treatment needs to be individualised and a number of different aspects of the disease need entirely different types of therapeutic attention (Hart and Huskisson, 1972b). Pain relief calls for analgesics, while inflammatory disease in the joints necessitates graded rest, splintage, exercises and the correct optimum dosage of anti-inflammatory agents. Depression calls for psychotherapeutic agents, while poor general health may be an indication for iron or vitamins (fig. 1).

Inflammation is the basis of rheumatoid arthritis and most other rheumatic disorders (Hart, 1975a), but there is no therapeutic agent which can adequately control this inflammation and stop it progressing to erosion and destruction of joint tissues (i.e. to crippling) without causing dangerous or unpleasant side effects. Nevertheless, long term treatment with potentially toxic drugs like gold or penicillamine, which do appear to act on the rheumatoid process, are necessary in certain cases of progressive disease. In general, the therapy of rheumatoid arthritis is aimed at treating symptoms as effectively as possible whilst producing a minimum of side effects.

3.1 Analgesics

The most popular analgesic is probably aspirin in its various forms. Other analgesics include paracetamol (acetaminophen), dextropropoxyphene (propoxyphene), codeine and dihydrocodeine, and others (see table II). The salicylates are

anti-inflammatory agents if used in full dosage. Salicylates in small doses such as 1 to 2g daily act essentially as analgesics and anti-inflammatory effects cannot be demonstrated, but with large doses a definite reduction in joint swelling is effected (see below).

3.2 Non-steroidal Anti-inflammatory Agents

Most of the non-steroidal anti-inflammatory agents appear to act by inhibiting the production or action of various local mediators of the inflammatory response (Paulus and Whitehouse, 1973; McQueen, 1973). These include the polypeptides of the kinin system, prostaglandins, connective tissue activating peptide, lysosomal enzymes and mediators of cellular activity such as the lymphokines. The consistent depression of prostaglandin G_2 synthesis from arachnidonic acid *in vitro* by all non-steroidal anti-inflammatory agents studied by Kuehl et al. (1977), suggests that this endoperoxide plays an important role in acute inflammation, probably as the precursor of a more potent and important inflammatory mediator. The action of these drugs is therefore essentially non-specific.

3.2.1 Salicylates

The agent most widely used, and, until the advent of newer agents such as the propionic acid derivatives (see below), usually the first to be tried in the treatment of rheumatoid arthritis, is aspirin in some form. In oral doses of 0.6 to 1g at a time it is an effective analgesic. Given every 3 hours at this dose level, with a total daily dosage of 5g or more (50 to 65mg/kg or 80 to 100mg/kg in resistant cases), it is also an effective anti-inflammatory agent (Boardman and Hart, 1967), but many patients cannot tolerate it at the higher dose level. Its mode of action in relieving pain is partly central, partly peripheral in the inflamed tissues (Lim, 1966). Salicylates inhibit the synthesis of prostaglandins in inflamed tissues and prevent sensitisation of pain receptors to the action of substances such as bradykinin that appear to mediate the pain response (Vane, 1974). Salicylates may also act by inhibiting lymphokine action or production (Morley, 1975). Aspirin has other important actions. It prolongs bleeding time and inhibits many platelet functions (Mustard and Packham, 1975), its antiplatelet aggregating action being employed in therapeutics (see chapter

Table II. Properties of analgesic and anti-inflammatory drugs used in rheumatic disorders

Drug	Analgesic efficacy (relative rating)	Anti-inflammatory efficacy (relative rating)	Dose[1] (daily)	Elimination[2]	Notes/principal side effects
1. *Analgesics*					
Aspirin	++	0	1 to 2g daily	Hepatic metabolism and renal excretion of free salicylate	Gastric irritation, bleeding
Diflunisal	++	+	250 to 375mg 12-hourly	Hepatic metabolism and renal excretion of unchanged drug	Epigastric discomfort. Reduce dose in renal failure
Paracetamol (acetaminophen)	++	0	1 to 1.5g (3 to 6-hourly intervals)	Hepatic metabolism and renal excretion (3% unchanged)	Hepatic necrosis (overdosage)
Codeine	+	0	30mg 4-hourly	Hepatic metabolism and renal excretion ($< 17\%$ unchanged)	Constipation, nausea, vomiting, dizziness
Dihydrocodeine	++	0	60mg 4-hourly	Hepatic metabolism	As for codeine (less constipating and more effective). Use with caution in asthma and those with impaired liver function. Mild sedative effect useful for pain at night
Dextropropoxyphene (propoxyphene)	++	0	65mg 4-hourly	Hepatic metabolism and renal excretion ($< 10\%$ unchanged)	Nausea, vomiting, dizziness; respiratory depression (overdosage). May need to be combined with aspirin or paracetamol
Pentazocine	++	0	50 to 75mg 4-hourly	Hepatic metabolism and renal excretion ($< 5\text{-}23\%$ unchanged)	Nausea, vomiting, dizziness, hallucinations. Low abuse potential
2. *Anti-inflammatory analgesics*					
Aspirin[1]	++	++++	5g or more (0.6 to 1g 3-hourly)	Dose related hepatic metabolism and renal excretion of free salicylate (pH dependent)	Tinnitus, nausea, gastric irritation (exacerbation of peptic ulcer). Haematemesis, melaena; asthma, sensitivity reactions (rare). Use of antacids decreases plasma levels (and efficacy) by hastening renal excretion

Table II. (continued)

Drug	Analgesic efficacy (relative rating)	Anti-inflam-matory efficacy (relative rating)	Dose[1] (daily)	Elimination[2]	Notes/principal side-effects
Phenylbutazone	++	++++	200 to 400mg (2 to 3 divided doses with food)	Slow and extensive hepatic metabolism and very slow renal excretion of active metabolites (in plasma oxyphenbutazone, ~14%; compound with uricosuric properties, ~14%)	Gastrointestinal intolerance; fluid retention (may precipitate heart failure in elderly); skin reactions, hypersensitivity (serum-sickness type), ulcerative stomatitis (stop drug if sore throat or other oral lesions); haematological complications (more common in women over 65); goitre and myxoedema (occasionally seen). Use with care in patient with severe liver disease
Oxyphenbutazone	++	++++	200 to 400mg (2 to 3 divided doses with food)	Slow hepatic metabolism and very slow excretion	As for phenylbutazone
Azapropazone	++	+++	1200mg (4 divided doses with food)	Renal excretion of unchanged drug (60%); little hepatic metabolism	Gastrointestinal intolerance, skin rash Reduce dose in patients with impaired renal function
Indomethacin	++	++++	25 to 150mg (1 to 3 divided doses with food) plus 75 to 100mg at night (for night pain)	Hepatic metabolism, entero-hepatic circulation via bile, and renal excretion (glomerular filtration and tubular secretion; 10-20% unchanged)	Gastrointestinal intolerance; headaches and unpleasant cerebral sensations (dose related); anaemia; psychotic disturbances (rare). Use with care in patients with impaired biliary function
Sulindac	++	+++	200 to 400mg (2 divided doses after food)	Hepatic metabolism, entero-hepatic circulation; faeces (active sulphide metabolite)	Gastrointestinal intolerance; headache; dizziness
Ibuprofen	++	++	1200 to 1600mg (3 or 4 divided doses with food)	Hepatic metabolism	Gastrointestinal disturbances (usually well tolerated); headache, and skin rash (uncommon)

Drug			Dose	Metabolism/excretion	Side effects
Ketoprofen	++	+++	100 to 200mg (3 to 4 divided doses with food)	Hepatic metabolism	As for ibuprofen
Fenoprofen	++	+++	1200 to 2400mg (3 or 4 divided doses with food)	Hepatic metabolism	As for ibuprofen
Flurbiprofen	++	+++	150 to 300mg (3 divided doses with food)	Hepatic metabolism and renal excretion (20 to 25% unchanged)	Gastrointestinal intolerance, headache, skin rash
Naproxen	++	+++	375 to 750mg (single dose or 2 divided doses with food)	Hepatic metabolism and renal excretion (10% unchanged drug)	As for ibuprofen
Flufenamic acid	++	++	400 to 600mg (3 divided doses with food)	Hepatic metabolism and renal excretion (up to 21% unchanged)	Gastrointestinal disturbances (espec. diarrhoea); headache, dizziness, drowsiness; skin rash (uncommon)
Mefenamic acid	++	+	750 to 1500mg (3 divided doses with food)	Hepatic metabolism and renal excretion (? % unchanged)	As for flufenamic acid; haemolytic anaemia
Alclofenac	++	+++	1.5 to 3g (3 divided doses with food)	Hepatic metabolism and renal excretion (up to 50% unchanged in some patients); faeces (some patients)	Skin rashes (often severe); gastrointestinal disturbances (unusual)
Diclofenac	++	+++	75 to 150mg (3 to 6 divided doses with food)	Hepatic metabolism	Gastrointestinal disturbances, headache, dizziness
Tolmetin	++	+++	1200 to 1800mg (3 to 4 divided doses with food)	Hepatic metabolism and renal excretion (up to 17% unchanged)	Gastrointestinal intolerance, headache, dizziness

3. *Drugs which affect the disease process*

Drug			Dose	Metabolism/excretion	Side effects
Gold (sodium aurothiomalate)	0	++++	10mg IM increased by 10mg/week to 50mg/week max. Reduce dose or increase dose intervals (to 2- to 4-weekly) once ESR falls and clinical improvement achieved (usually when around 200 to 300mg given)	Extremely slow renal excretion (60-90%; during weekly therapy patient remains in +ve gold balance with progressive increase in body stores; increased fraction dose excreted during monthly maintenance therapy, -ve balance) and faecal excretion (10-40%)	Blood dyscrasias, including aplastic anaemia (may occur with little warning, despite normal blood counts); fever, skin reactions incl. exfoliative dermatitis, mouth ulcers (stop drug immediately); haemorrhage from platelet deficiencies (give dimercaprol); proteinuria, haematuria, pulmonary reactions. *Discontinue gold as soon as toxic symptoms are reported or as soon as abnormalities appear in blood count — white cell and platelets every 3 to 4 weeks. Best used in specialist centres*

Table II. (continued)

Drug	Analgesic efficacy (relative rating)	Anti-inflammatory efficacy (relative rating)	Dose[1] (daily)	Elimination[2]	Notes/principal side effects
Chloroquine	0	+++	250mg 1 to 2 times daily, reduced for maintenance therapy to 200mg daily	Some hepatic metabolism and slow renal excretion of unchanged drug (50-70%) and metabolites; faecal excretion ($\sim 10\%$ unchanged)	Skin rashes, hair discolouration; leucopenia; peripheral neuropathy; ocular reactions which may be permanent (see chapter XII, sect. 11.1.3). Avoid in those with psoriasis. Reduce dose in renal failure
Hydroxychloroquine	0	+++	200mg 2 or 3 times daily, reduced gradually to 200 to 400mg daily		As for chloroquine
D-Penicillamine	0	+++	250mg (base) increased gradually to 750mg daily, only rarely higher to 1g or more	Some hepatic metabolism and rapid renal excretion of unchanged drug	Gastrointestinal disturbances; loss of taste; skin reactions; haematological complications (thrombocytopenia, leucopenia); proteinuria, haematuria, nephrotic syndrome; myasthenia-like syndrome. Best used in specialist centres
Azathioprine	0	+++	1 to 2.5mg/kg (in 2 or 3 divided doses)	Conversion to free 6-mercaptopurine: some hepatic metabolism and renal excretion of unchanged drug (50%) and metabolites	Haematological complications (bone marrow suppression with leucopenia, thrombocytopenia, aplastic anaemia); gastrointestinal disturbances. Reduce dose in renal failure. Use only in specialist centres in severe, active and progressive disease (see text)
Cyclophosphamide	0	++++	1 to 1.5mg/kg (in 2 or 3 divided doses)	Hepatic bioactivation and renal excretion of active metabolites and up to 25% unchanged drug; faecal excretion (17-30% unchanged) after oral administration	Haematological complications (bone marrow suppression with leucopenia, thrombocytopenia); alopecia; haemorrhagic cystitis; nausea, vomiting; ovarian (amenorrhoea) and testicular (azoospermia) toxicity (see also chapter XXIV, section 4). Reduce dose in renal failure. Use only in specialist centres in severe, active and progressive disease with risk to life (see text)

4. *Corticosteroids*					
Prednisolone	0	+++++	2mg 8-hourly (> 7.5mg daily leads to HPA axis suppression) 5mg at night (for night pain)	Hepatic metabolism	Electrolyte disturbances; gastrointestinal irritation; metabolic disturbances; osteoporosis and vertebral crush fractures Cushingoid features, HPA axis suppression (excessive dosage); growth retardation (children). See also section 3.4, 14.5 and chapter XVI, sect. 9.1, 14.1, 14.3
Corticotrophin depot gel	0	+++++	1u daily at lowest effective dose (usually 10 to 20u daily)		Corticotrophin or tetracosactrin may be used in hospital to control acute inflammatory episode
Tetracosactrin depot	0	+++++	Daily or alternate days at lowest effective dose (usually 0.1 to 0.2mg; max. 1mg per week)		
Triamcinolone acetonide, hydro-cortisone acetate, methylprednisolone acetate, etc.	0	+++++			Aspiration and intra-articular administration useful in acutely inflamed joints (repeated administration contraindicated)

1   Oral unless specified otherwise.
2   Significant impairment of renal function probably calls for modification of dosage (reduce dose or intervals) of drugs largely excreted unchanged or as active metabolites (see chapter XXI; sect. 1).
Severe liver disease probably calls for modification of dosage of drugs metabolised to a significant extent in the liver (see chapter XIX; sect. 1.4).
There is very little definitive information available on these considerations for all the above drugs.

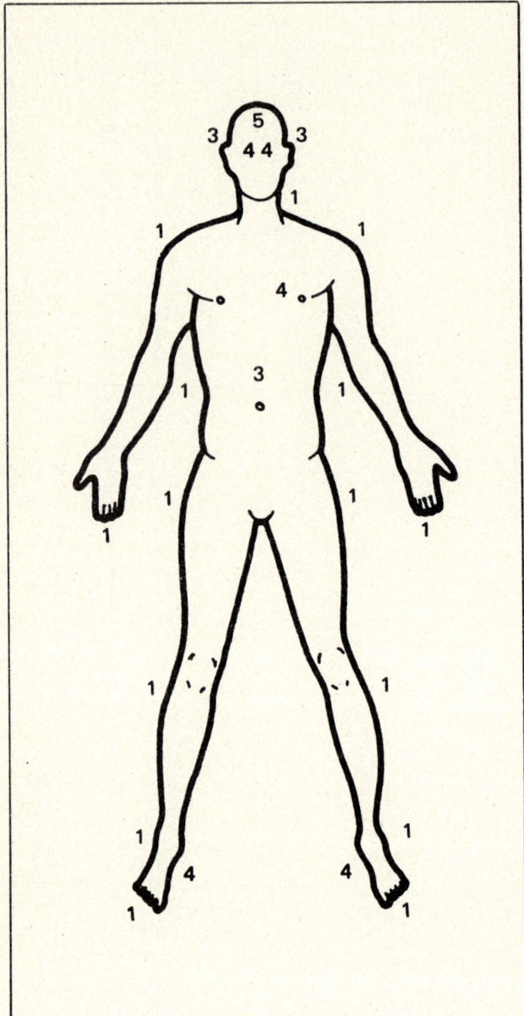

Fig. 1. The pain cocktail of rheumatoid disease.
1. Peripheral joint pain, swelling, stiffness and weakness.
2. Systemic illness — fever, anaemia, anorexia etc.
3. Iatrogenic overtones — dyspepsia, diarrhoea, nausea, tinnitus etc.
4. Extra-articular manifestations — neuropathy, pericarditis, pleurisy, scleritis, ulcerative nodules over pressure points, keratoconjunctivitis sicca etc.
5. Psychic overtones — depression, anxiety, tension.

Calling for:

1. Anti-inflammatory and analgesic agents and physical methods.
2. Iron, perhaps folic acid, vitamins, nursing, blood transfusions if anaemia severe from several factors.
3. Drug control and change of drugs.
4. Appropriate symptomatic therapy.
5. Antidepressants, antianxiety drugs, personal communication, occupation.

XXIII; sect. 3.1). In overdosage, salicylates have a depressant effect on the medulla and lead to a state of combined respiratory and metabolic acidosis (Tenney and Miller, 1955).

Simple or soluble aspirin is usually given; in doses of 0.6 to 1g every 3 to 4 hours with food. Plasma levels in adults of 1 to 2mmol/L (15 to 30mg/100ml) usually prove effective, although higher levels of 2 to 2.5mmol/L (30 to 35mg/100ml) are sometimes required in children (see section 9). Fairly constant blood levels are maintained with 4 to 6-hourly dosage, but symptomatic control is usually better achieved with drug dosage every 3 to 4 hours. Because the major pathways of metabolism of salicylate at high dosages are limited (Levy and Tsuchiya, 1972; Gibson et al., 1976), small changes in daily dose size can result in large changes in plasma concentration (Paulus et al., 1971). Thus, small adjustments in aspirin dosage may be sufficient to eliminate toxic symptoms and yet maintain therapeutic plasma levels. Plasma concentrations from a given dosage vary widely between individuals and within individuals at different times (Bardare et al., 1978; Graham et al., 1977). It is helpful, particularly in children, to monitor plasma levels but in general in adults not usually necessary as therapeutic efficacy is usually best assessed by asking the patient.

Clearance of salicylate is dependent on urine pH, being higher in alkaline than acid urine. Giving antacids at the same time to combat dyspepsia merely produces more rapid renal excretion of the drug and significantly decreased plasma levels (Levy et al., 1975). Concurrent administration of corticosteroids and aspirin also decreases plasma salicylate levels due to a more rapid rate of salicylate metabolism such that therapeutic concentrations may not be attained (Bardare et al., 1978; Graham et al., 1977). Per contra, a decrease in corticosteroid dosage, without modification of salicylate dose, may result in increased plasma salicylate levels with risk of toxicity (Klineberg and Miller, 1965). About 50 to 90% of salicylate in routine therapy is bound to plasma proteins, mostly to albumin. Decreased binding occurs at higher plasma concentrations and is an important consideration in management of overdosage, particularly in children (see chapter IV; sect. 2.2.2).

Tinnitus, which occurs at different plasma levels in different patients (Mongan et al., 1973), nausea, gastrointestinal irritation and haematemesis and melaena may occur and many patients

Table III. Risk factors and relative contraindications to the use of anti-inflammatory agents

Condition	Drugs contraindicated or increased risk of toxicity
Peptic ulcer	All the anti-inflammatory drugs (corticosteroids and non-steroidal agents) may aggravate dyspepsia of any sort, cause exacerbation of ulcer symptoms and occasionally gastrointestinal bleeding and even perforation (Cooke, 1976; see also chapter XIX; sect. 13.1.1, 14.2.2). Some drugs are better tolerated than others (see text). Cimetidine (see chapter XIX; sect. 4), by reducing gastric acid secretion heals the ulcer and allows many dyspeptic rheumatoid patients to tolerate anti-inflammatory drugs.
Gout, hyperuricaemia	Low dose salicylates, i.e. as used for analgesic effect, raise serum urate (see section 12.2.2, 12.3)
Congestive heart failure Hypertension	Avoid corticosteroids, corticotrophin and tetracosactrin, phenylbutazone and oxyphenbutazone (fluid retention)
Elderly	Increased risk of toxicity (blood dyscrasias) and precipitation of heart failure with phenylbutazone and oxyphenbutazone (see section 3.2.2; chapter V; sect. 4.5). Avoid codeine — constipation and risk faecal impaction (see chapter V; sect. 4.7.6)
Elderly females, living alone or immobile	Increased risk of osteoporotic crush fractures with corticosteroids (see section 14.5)
Severe liver disease	Risk of toxicity of some drugs may be increased — e.g. gold, phenylbutazone, oxyphenbutazone, dihydrocodeine (see table II)
Marked renal impairment	Risk of toxicity of some drugs may be increased — e.g. gold, azapropazone, alclofenac, azathioprine (see table II)
Dermatitis Atopy	Risk of serious skin reactions with gold; avoid if possible
Asthma	Avoid aspirin, dihydrocodeine (see also chapter XX; sect. 11.3)
Psoriasis	Avoid chloroquine derivatives (exacerbation of condition)
Refractory anaemia Blood dyscrasias	Risk of haematological toxicity of phenylbutazone, oxyphenbutazone, gold, D-penicillamine, immunosuppressives greatly increased
Diarrhoea (ulcerative colitis)	May be aggravated by mefenamic and flufenamic acid
Diabetes mellitus	Diabetic control made more difficult by corticosteroids (see chapter XVI; sect. 13.1)
Oral anticoagulants	Salicylates not to be used, nor phenylbutazone or oxyphenbutazone with coumarins (see table IV; also chapter XXIII, sect. 3.2.5)

cannot tolerate full dosage or will only tolerate a much smaller dosage. Most patients pass small amounts of blood in the stools on regular doses of aspirin, but this is rarely paralleled by any symptoms of dyspepsia. Rarely, aspirin may cause asthma and more serious sensitivity reactions. A pustular acneiform rash may be seen, usually after a weeks therapy. If, as often occurs, the patient cannot tolerate simple or soluble aspirin because of gastrointestinal side effects (Brooks and Buchanan, 1976), variants may be tried, and include: buffered aspirin, enteric coated aspirin, glycinated aspirin, aloxiprin, and a number of others such as aspirin/paracetamol combinations, or benorylate, a chemical combination of aspirin and paracetamol which is broken down to the active constituents after absorption and can be given 12-hourly. Slow release forms of aspirin have not been as successful as initially hoped. In general, if the gastrointestinal tract proves tolerant, other side effects of aspirin are less troublesome, but tinnitus and deafness occur frequently at high dose levels, necessitating reduction in dosage. Therapeutic overdosage may more readily occur in children, where severe acid-base (early overbreathing with respiratory alkalosis) and electrolyte disturbances may be missed, as headache and tinnitus are relatively less common; hypoglycaemia is also more common in children (see chapter IV; sect. 2.4).

Diflunisal, a salicylic acid derivative, has a long plasma half-life which permits twice daily dosage. It has analgesic activity comparable with aspirin and also has anti-inflammatory activity. It is better tolerated than aspirin and does not affect bleeding time or platelet function but may enhance the activity of coumarin anticoagulants. Dosage should be reduced in patients with impaired renal function (see chapter X; sect. 8.5.6).

3.2.2 The Pyrazolones

Phenylbutazone and oxyphenbutazone are effective anti-inflammatory analgesics. They inhibit biosynthesis of prostaglandins, uncouple oxidative phosphorylation and inhibit ATP-dependent biosynthesis of mucopolysaccharide sulphates in cartilage. At ordinary dosage, they also have a mild uricosuric effect by diminishing tubular reabsorption of uric acid, though smaller doses have the opposite effect by inhibiting tubular secretion of uric acid (Domenjoz, 1960; 1966). Phenylbutazone causes considerable sodium chloride and water retention. There is a fall in urinary output, sometimes with a considerable consequent increase in plasma volume and risk of induction of oedema. Hence the dangers of giving the drug to patients with congestive heart failure (chapt. XVII; sect. 10.1). It may reduce the uptake of iodine by the thyroid and so may inhibit synthesis of organic iodine compounds, with occasional production of goitres, or even frank myxoedema.

Phenylbutazone is highly bound to plasma proteins at usual dose levels (98 to 99 %); higher doses, by increasing plasma concentrations, may diminish the albumin bound fraction to around 90 % (Burns et al., 1953). This also means that diseases which alter total drug plasma concentrations may lead to secondary changes in protein binding. For example, certain liver diseases increase the fraction of free phenylbutazone by 400 to 500 % (Blaschke, 1977; see chapter XIX, sect. 1.3). The distribution volume of phenylbutazone is low (0.02 to 0.15L/kg); this and its high protein binding making it a candidate for binding displacement interactions with drugs such as warfarin and

tolbutamide which bind to the same primary albumin binding site (see chapter I; sect. 3.2.1). Phenylbutazone is eliminated by metabolism, only 1 % being excreted unchanged in the urine, with 10 % of a single dose in the bile as metabolites. Two of the metabolites are pharmacologically active: oxyphenbutazone, which is used as an anti-inflammatory analgesic, γ-hydroxyphenbutazone, which has a marked uricosuric but little anti-rheumatic or sodium loading effect. Elimination of phenylbutazone is slow. The plasma half-life ranges from 29 to 175 hours (mean of around 70 hours); intraindividual differences in half-life being dependent on size of the dose and interindividual differences being genetically determined. Phenylbutazone has the potential to inhibit the hepatic metabolism and renal excretion of certain drugs, which combined with its ability to displace some highly bound acidic drugs such as warfarin, tolbutamide and chlorpropamide from plasma albumin binding sites, greatly increases the risk of important drug interactions with these agents (table IV; see also chapter XVI, sect. 3.3.5; XXIII, sect. 3.2.5). For a review of the pharmacokinetic properties of phenylbutazone, see Aarbakke (1978). Oxyphenbutazone has the same general properties and the same actions, therapeutic uses, interactions and side effects as phenylbutazone.

Phenylbutazone and oxyphenbutazone are given in a daily oral dosage of 200 to 400mg and exert an even and prolonged action, and are therefore very effective in diseases such as rheumatoid arthritis where pain tends to be recurring or chronic, and inflammatory features present throughout most hours of the day and night. Gastrointestinal intolerance may occur with the pyrazolones, as may sodium retention with oedema, which is a particular risk in cardiac patients and the elderly since it may precipitate congestive heart failure (see above). The greatest risk is toxicity to the bone marrow, and a number of casualties have been reported as a result of aplastic anaemia, agranulocytosis or thrombocytopenia (Inman, 1977). Most patients who develop agranulocytosis do so within 3 months of starting treatment. Aplastic anaemia can occur early in a course, although about half of the cases develop after at least 1 years treatment (Fowler, 1967; Fowler and Faragher, 1977). Haematological complications seem to be more common in women over 65 (Inman, 1977). In spite of their toxic potential, pyrazolones continue to be in general use and are effective in the treatment of rheumatoid arthritis, but dosage should be kept at or below 300 to 400mg a day and patients asked to report any unusual symptoms (rash, fever, sore throat). Phenylbutazone may also be given by intramuscular injection, and in suppository form, 250mg per rectum. Oxyphenbutazone is also available as 250mg suppositories.

3.2.3 Indomethacin

Indomethacin is a highly effective antipyretic, anti-inflammatory analgesic (Hart and Boardman, 1963, 1964). It inhibits the biosynthesis of prostaglandins and the motility of polymorphonuclear leucocytes and uncouples oxidative phosphorylation in cartilagenous and hepatic mitochondria. Although indomethacin is highly protein bound, it has a relatively large distribution volume (0.34 to 1.57L/kg). For this and other reasons, binding displacement interactions are unlikely (see chapter I; sect. 3.2.3) and an enhanced effect of warfarin could not be demonstrated (Vessel et al., 1975). Bioavailability is good orally and rectally and there is little variation between patients in steady-state plasma levels (Alvan et al., 1975). Indomethacin is largely converted to inactive metabolites which are excreted in the urine, bile and faeces; but about 10 to 20% of a dose is excreted unchanged in the urine (Duggan et al., 1972). Enterohepatic circulation has been proposed (Kwan et al., 1976). Elimination of unchanged drug is not impaired in renal failure, but is prolonged in patients with impaired biliary function (Stein et al., 1977; Kunze et al., 1974). By reducing non-renal clearance of indomethacin (unchanged drug + metabolites), concurrent administration of probenecid increases plasma concentrations and enhances pain relief, without increasing the incidence of side effects; indeed headaches and lightheadedness may be less (Brooks et al., 1974; Baber et al., 1978). Drug interactions with indomethacin are summarised in appendix C. The effect of aspirin on indomethacin is very variable, and although an increased incidence of side effects has been reported (Brooks et al., 1975), the clinical significance of the interaction is difficult to determine; but certainly there is little point in combining two non-steroidal anti-inflammatory agents.

Indomethacin may be given orally with food, 25 to 50mg once, twice or three times a day, and for relief of night pain and early morning stiffness it may be given at night in suppository form (100mg) or by mouth 75 to 100mg with food on retiring.

The most common side effect is a dose related one — headaches and various unpleasant cerebral sensations. There are marked differences in individual tolerance of the drug, and it is advisable to initiate therapy when the patient is not going out in his car or to work. Night-time administration (see above) is usually well tolerated, headaches and similar sensations not being apparent during sleep. Gastrointestinal complications also occur and are by no means uncommon. Dyspepsia is not dose related and may appear at any time on any dosage, although it is less likely to occur with suppositories. Anaemia can also occur as a result of gastrointestinal bleeding, although the regular day to day bleeding seen with aspirin does not occur with indomethacin. Rarely, severe depression, psychosis or hallucinations may occur. Indomethacin is an indole acetic acid derivative, indoles being implicated in such CNS disturbances.

3.2.4 Sulindac

Sulindac, an indene acetic acid derivative, though less effective than indomethacin in some of the more severe cases of rheumatoid arthritis, does not cause the dose related cerebral side effects seen with indomethacin and is less irritant to the gastrointestinal tract. It also causes fewer side effects than aspirin. Sulindac itself is a sulphoxide, which once absorbed is converted in the lumen of the gut to a sulphone and sulphide compound, the sulphide metabolite being the pharmacologically active form. The sulphide metabolite, which is excreted in the faeces, has a plasma half life of around 18 hours, thus enabling twice daily administration. The usual dosage is 100 to 200mg twice daily, morning and evening (for a review, see Brogden et al., 1978a).

3.2.5 Propionic (phenylalkanoic) Acid Derivatives

A number of these anti-inflammatory, analgesic compounds are available (table II). They are relatively non-toxic but most are of lesser anti-inflammatory activity than full doses of aspirin, the pyrazolones or indomethacin. Some, such as naproxen and fenoprofen, are more active and are about as effective as aspirin as an anti-inflammatory agent but better tolerated (Huskisson et al., 1976; Hart et al., 1978). All are effective substitutes for aspirin 3.5 to 5g daily. Although the propionic acid derivatives are highly protein bound and have low distribution volumes (appendix A), they bind to a different primary albumin

Table IV. Clinically important interactions of drugs used in rheumatic diseases

Drug	May interact with	Potential result
1. *Non-steroidal anti-inflammatory agents*		
Oral anticoagulants	Aspirin	Salicylates have no clinically important effect on anticoagulant control, but should be avoided because they increase risk of bleeding by affecting platelet function
	Phenylbutazone Oxyphenbutazone	Predictable and significant prolongation of prothrombin time of coumarins and risk of haemorrhage (see chapter XXIII; sect. 3.2.5).
Oral sulphonylurea hypoglycaemic agents	Aspirin	Activity of sulphonylurea may be increased with large doses of aspirin
	Phenylbutazone Oxyphenbutazone	Probably a predictable increase in hypoglycaemic activity (see chapter XVI; sect. 3.3.5)
Phenytoin (diphenylhydantoin)	Phenylbutazone Oxyphenbutazone	In a few cases, there may be a marked increase in plasma phenytoin concentrations (see chapter XXV; sect. 3.1)
Adrenergic neurone blocking anti-hypertensive drugs (e.g. guanethidine)	Phenylbutazone Oxyphenbutazone	Antihypertensive effect may be antagonised (fluid retention) and control of blood pressure may be lost (see chapter VIII; sect. 2.2.3)
Antacids	Aspirin	Absorbable and non-absorbable antacids, markedly increase urinary excretion of salicylate so that therapeutic serum levels can not be maintained
Probenecid	Indomethacin	Increases plasma concentrations of indomethacin and enhances pain relief without increasing or less CNS effects (see text)
2. *Corticosteroids*		
Aspirin	Prednisone etc	Decreased plasma salicylate levels due to more rapid rate of salicylate metabolism; accumulation of salicylate with risk of toxicity when corticosteroid dosage decreased and salicylate dosage not modified
Barbiturates Rifampicin Phenytoin	Prednisone Dexamethasone	Metabolism of corticosteroids such as prednisone, prednisolone and dexamethasone enhanced by phenobarbitone, rifampicin, phenytoin; efficacy steroid reduced
3. *Gout drugs*		
Allopurinol	Ampicillin Azathioprine 6-Mercaptopurine	Increased incidence of skin rash. Metabolism (by xanthine oxidase) inhibited and activity of azathioprine, mercaptopurine increased (decrease dose to 33% of usual)
Probenecid Sulphinpyrazone	Salicylates (low doses) Diuretics	Therapeutic efficacy of uricosuric agent markedly inhibited (see section 12.2.2). May inhibit efficacy of uricosuric agent

binding site than warfarin and other coumarins (see chapter I; sect. 3.2.3), and can be given to patients taking oral coumarin anticoagulants. Occasional patients may show prolongation of prothrombin time which should be checked daily for the first several days of administration of any such combined therapy. Plasma concentrations of the propionic acid derivatives such as naproxen and fenoprofen can be reduced by concurrent administration of aspirin, probably insignificantly.

In any case, there is no point in giving two anti-inflammatory drugs together. The propionic acid derivatives are eliminated by hepatic biotransformation, with only small and unimportant amounts excreted unchanged in the urine (table II; see Hart et al., 1978).

Ibuprofen is a mild but well tolerated agent in the treatment of those patients who cannot tolerate the more active non-steroidal anti-inflammatory agents. Some patients with rheumatoid arthritis do extremely well on ibuprofen, but in general it is more useful in the milder cases of inflammatory or degenerative arthritis. Its anti-inflammatory action is slight at dosages up to 1200mg. At these dose levels ibuprofen has generally been well tolerated and gastrointestinal complications are relatively rare. Higher doses of ibuprofen up to 2.4g daily are used in the USA: it may well be that at higher dose levels ibuprofen will prove both more effective but possibly more toxic. Ibuprofen can be used in children in doses up to 40mg/kg daily. For a review of the early literature on ibuprofen, see Davies and Avery (1971).

Flurbiprofen, appears to be more active as an anti-inflammatory agent than ibuprofen and is usually well tolerated.

Naproxen is also more active than ibuprofen (Huskisson et al., 1976) and, although usually well tolerated, there have been a few reports of gastrointestinal intolerance, including severe haemorrhage, with its use, usually in patients who have had gastrointestinal symptoms with other agents (Hart and Matts, 1974). Some patients who tolerate ibuprofen well cannot tolerate naproxen. It has a long plasma half life (10 to 17 hours) and a long duration of action, which permits twice or once (Castles et al., 1978) daily administration. The evening dose may be doubled in those with painful nights and marked joint stiffness on awakening. Naproxen is also available as suppositories. For a review of naproxen, see Brogden et al. (1975).

Ketoprofen and fenoprofen occupy much the same place in therapeutics as naproxen although fenoprofen is the more active of the two (Huskisson et al., 1976). Ketoprofen is given 6 to 8-hourly and fenoprofen 6-hourly. Both are usually, though not invariably, well tolerated by the intestinal tract. Ketoprofen is available as suppositories. For a review of fenoprofen, see Brogden et al., (1977a) and of ketoprofen (Symposium, 1976a).

3.2.6 Other Compounds (table II)

The anthranilic acid derivatives, *mefenamic* and *flufenamic acids*, are analgesic and mild anti-inflammatory agents which may also be considered where other drugs prove ineffective or are poorly tolerated. The most common side effect is diarrhoea, though haemolytic anaemia has also been reported with mefenamic acid.

Alclofenac and *diclofenac*, phenyl acetic acid derivatives, are effective anti-inflammatory analgesics in the less severe rheumatic conditions. Skin reactions, often severe, appear to be relatively common with alclofenac tablets, but are said to be less common when used as capsules. Prolonged therapy with alclofenac appears to have a similar ameliorative effect on the course of rheumatoid arthritis as the long term agents discussed in section 3.3 (Aylward et al., 1975; Berry et al., 1978). For a review of alclofenac, see Brogden et al. (1977b) and of diclofenac, see Symposium (1978).

Fenclofenac is a similar preparation but its long plasma half-life of around 21 hours permits twice daily dosage (Goldberg and Tudor, 1977).

Azapropazone has a chemical structure resembling that of phenylbutazone, but its anti-inflammatory activity and side effects more closely resemble those of the propionic acid derivatives. It is not extensively metabolised, and is largely excreted unchanged (60%) in the urine. Dosage should therefore be reduced in patients with impaired renal function (Symposium, 1976b).

Feprazone is a similar preparation.

Tolmetin, a pyrrole acetic acid derivative, has some chemical similarities to indomethacin (but without the indole nucleus) but has anti-inflammatory activity more like the propionic acid derivatives. Side effects are less common than with aspirin or indomethacin. It is usually well tolerated by the gastrointestinal tract. Other side effects include headaches or dizziness but are usually mild. It can be used in children in doses up to 30mg/kg daily (for review, see Brogden et al., 1978b).

3.3 Drugs which Apparently Affect the Rheumatoid Disease Process

These drugs take effect slowly in an unknown way on the rheumatoid disease process, but all have a potential for dangerous toxic effects (table II) and have to be discontinued in a number of patients. Gold, chloroquine derivatives, D-penicillamine and immunosuppressives, can nevertheless be considered for careful use as long term agents in cases of active progressive and erosive disease (when the anti-inflammatory analgesics only provide symptomatic relief), but not in chronic and advanced destructive disease. The aim is to continue treatment until a remission is achieved, and to maintain that remission with prolonged suppressive therapy for many months, or usually years (Constable et al., 1975; Huskisson, 1978b). All these agents are best controlled from specialist units where closer laboratory control and observation can be kept with the collaboration of the patient's general practitioner than by the latter alone. Non-steroidal anti-inflammatory analgesics have to be used concurrently, initially in all cases (because of slow onset of effect with the long term agents), and additionally throughout the period of therapy in many cases. Agents with similar side effects should not be given together (e.g. gold and phenylbutazone).

3.3.1 Gold
The most commonly used preparation is sodium aurothiomalate (gold sodium thiomalate), dosage usually being started at 10mg intramuscularly and then increased by 10mg by weekly injections until a regular maximum of 50mg per week is given. Thereafter it is wise to treat every patient as an individual problem. Thioglucose is another gold preparation available in some countries which is equally effective and may have a lesser tendency to cause side effects (Rothermich et al., 1976). For reviews of gold therapy, see Gottlieb (1977).

Gold has a long half-life of 5 to 6 days so that the plasma level has declined to about half of its peak level after a week, when the next dose is given. After a few weeks of regular injections, a steady-state is achieved. The exact mode of excretion is not known but gold is found in both urine and faeces. It is taken up by macrophages and is identifiable in the reticuloendothelial system and in synovium, where it remains for long periods of time. The value of plasma gold estimations is unclear. Some consider that to achieve serum gold levels of 300µg/100ml or higher, early during gold therapy, may favourably influence the outcome. Patients who consistently achieve such levels before each weekly injection have in some studies fared better than those who do not, without any increase in the incidence or severity of side effects (Lorber, 1977; Lorber et al., 1973). Other studies have found no such correlation (Gottlieb et al., 1974; Billings et al., 1975). Plasma levels may fail to give warning of impending toxic reactions and do not consistently parallel clinical response. An eosinophilia may give warning of toxic effects, but by no means invariably.

Blood and platelet counts should be done repeatedly and also sedimentation rate estimations every 3 to 4 weeks for the first 8 months, then every 1 to 2 months. Changes in the blood may occur rapidly and great care should be taken, and dosage reduced or spaced more wisely, as the sedimentation rate falls to normal and the clinical condition improves. Courses may be terminated after a certain dose has been given, but most clinicians prefer to continue on small maintenance doses for many months, and usually for 2 or 3 years or more, until remission has set in. Even then most clinicians prefer to continue with monthly injections for several months longer as relapses may still occur, even at this late stage, after 5 or 6 years.

The most important aspect of gold therapy is to discontinue it as soon as toxic symptoms are reported (skin reactions, mouth ulcers, fever, any new or unusual symptoms), or as soon as abnormalities appear in the blood count. Even so, severe blood dyscrasias may occur with little warning, even though a blood count may have been done only 2 or 3 weeks previously and have been entirely normal. The urine should be tested before each injection for evidence of proteinuria and haematuria as renal damage can occur. Fatal complications have occurred as a result of haemorrhage from platelet deficiencies. In spite of these dangerous toxic effects gold salts are effective and widely used in appropriate cases (Gumpel, 1978).

3.3.2 Chloroquine Derivatives
Treatment with chloroquine or hydroxychloroquine (see table II) should be maintained for many months, but most clinicians prefer to discontinue treatment after 10 to 12 months continuous medication.

Chloroquine has a dose dependent plasma half life (chapt. XXX; sect. 6.1.1). It is mainly excreted unchanged in the urine (50 to 70%) but a small part is metabolised. Excretion occurs to some extent by non-renal mechanisms in renal failure but dosage should be modified for prolonged treatment in those with severe impairment. Chloroquine is concentrated widely in body tissues and when it is stopped, it may take months or years for the remaining drug to be excreted. Side effects are not infrequent. Skin rashes, leucopenia, peripheral neuropathy and two varieties of ocular side effects (usually after prolonged therapy) are seen: one is due to deposition of the drug in the cornea, causing haziness of vision, photophobia and the appearance of halos around lights. This is reversible. More serious are the degenerative changes in the fundus itself, which may be permanent but are not necessarily so (see chapter XII; sect. 11.1.3). Although this complication is rare, perhaps affecting 1 in 1,000 or 1 in 2,000 patients, it nevertheless has made this form of therapy less popular (Popert, 1976). Regular ophthalmological examinations are therefore essential and the drug should be stopped at the first sign of visual impairment. Gastrointestinal side effects are not common.

3.3.3 D-Penicillamine

Like gold salts, penicillamine, given over prolonged periods may after some weeks or months be accompanied by a lessening of inflammatory changes in the joints of a patient with rheumatoid arthritis. Its mode of action remains obscure. Given in a long term several year continued therapeutic programme, close watch has to be kept, as with gold salts, for side effects — dermatological, gastrointestinal, neuromuscular, haematological or renal (proteinuria, and more serious, the nephrotic syndrome).

Penicillamine does not have the rapid therapeutic action of the corticosteroids or of the nonsteroidal anti-inflammatory agents, but if tolerated, does effect improvement in the patient's clinical condition in many cases and if stopped prematurely because of side effects, is frequently followed after 1 to 3 weeks by a return of symptoms. The same type of delayed withdrawal-relapse reaction is seen with gold salts. It appears to be an effective substitute for gold therapy. Although accompanied by more side effects these tend to be milder than those seen with gold salts and treatment can more often be continued in reduced dosage and it has a more pronounced effect on progression of radiological changes (Gibson et al., 1976). Dosage tends to be more conservative than some years ago, initial therapy now starting with 125 to 250mg of the base, increases being only made very gradually by increments of 125 to 250mg every 1 to 3 months to a maximum of around 750mg or, rarely, 1g daily. Improvement may not be seen for several weeks or months; it is wise, therefore, to continue for at least 3 to 6 months before concluding that therapy has failed. In a small minority of cases, higher dosage is tolerated and is necessary to effect improvement (for review, see Lyle and Kleiman, 1977).

3.4 Corticosteroids and Corticotrophin

All the cardinal features of inflammation (local heat, redness, swelling and tenderness) are prevented or diminished by corticosteroids. How they act in rheumatic diseases is obscure; the lysosomal stabilisation hypothesis (Weisman and Thomas, 1968) popular previously, does not satisfy all investigators (Haynes, 1975). Clinically, their effect in rheumatic diseases is more on suppression of inflammation than on the course of the disease. The pharmacokinetic properties of corticosteroids are discussed in chapter XVI (sect. 9.1). The bad reputation attached to corticosteroids during the years since their introduction in 1949 may be summed up in one word — overdosage (Polley, 1970). The Cushingoid features of overdosage are seen if a dose of around 7.5mg or more of prednisolone or its equivalent is given for more than a few weeks (see chapter XVI; table X). It is wise therefore to keep daily dosage below this level — either 5mg at night on retiring for those patients with marked morning stiffness, or a small 2mg dosage 8-hourly for others. However, this will help only the milder cases, and an increased dose, although dramatically effective at the time, is later followed by the inevitable effect of hormonal overdosage and suppression of the HPA axis, along with other complications (see chapter XVI; sect. 9.1, 14.3). Corticosteroids are therefore reserved for patients with acute inflammatory disease who fail to respond to other forms of therapy including gold and penicillamine.

Corticotrophins have similar problems. They are best used for resistant cases while under close observation in hospital. An acute inflammatory episode may be controlled in this way, either by ACTH gel intramuscularly, or by the synthetic depot corticotrophin, tetracosactrin zinc phosphate complex. It is wise not to exceed a total of 1mg of tetracosactrin depot per week, whether given daily (preferably) or less frequently, and the dose in general should be kept as low as possible and discontinued in 10 to 20 days after, one hopes, the inflammatory cycle has been broken. All too often however, the patient relapses thereafter.

The intra-articular instillation of a suitable corticosteroid into a swollen joint after aspiration of fluid avoids their undesirable systemic effects and is very often followed not only by an improvement in the joint itself but also by a general systemic improvement for the next 2 to 3 days (Fitzgerald, 1976). Dosage depends on the size of the inflamed area to be injected and varies between 10 and 40mg of prednisolone or equivalent. This seems to be harmless and is not followed by any untoward events, but should not be frequently repeated. Intra-articular corticosteroid injection must be performed under strict aseptic technique and is contraindicated in the presence of infection in the joint. Patients must be instructed to return at once if the joint becomes worse because of the possibility of infection; to rest for 24 hours after injection and thereafter to avoid greatly increased activity, particularly to weight bearing joints, because of the risk of destructive changes from repeated injections.

3.5 Management of Rheumatoid Arthritis

In a disease as variable as rheumatoid arthritis with so many therapeutic agents from which to choose, which drug should one use? Treatment requires a plan and the realisation that there are two types of drug:

a) Those that can only relieve symptoms, such as analgesics and the anti-inflammatory agents, and

b) Those such as gold and penicillamine that appear to affect the course of the disease (see above).

3.5.1 Initial Management

In general one can say that where inflammatory features of the disease dominate, then non-steroidal anti-inflammatory agents should be used initially, together with a full programme of graded rest, splintage and gentle physiotherapy, with exercise and exercises designed for each individual patient. The particular non-steroidal anti-inflammatory agent selected depends upon its anti-inflammatory activity and any attributes or other considerations in an individual patient (see Huskisson, 1978a and table II, III, IV; section 3.2.1 to 3.2.6). There is marked between patient variability in response to non-steroidal anti-inflammatory drugs; differences between patients being greater than differences between drugs, so it is often necessary to try a number of compounds before finding the best in terms of efficacy and tolerance for a particular patient (Huskisson et al., 1976). The basic principle is to use the safest and best tolerated drugs first.

Aspirin in its various forms at full high dose levels (see section 3.2.1) *if tolerated*, is probably as good as any other anti-inflammatory agent in rheumatoid and similar arthropathies. Unfortunately around 50% or more of patients cannot tolerate and will not continue with this dosage, and will either discontinue the drug or reduce it to

a tolerated, but often less or even ineffective, level. It is for this reason that many clinicians now prefer to use propionic acid derivatives first. The more active compounds such as naproxen and fenoprofen are about as effective as full doses of aspirin, but with a striking reduction in the incidence of side effects and a substantial increase in the number of patients able to continue with the treatment (e.g. Huskisson et al., 1974). Agents such as tolmetin, sulindac or azapropazone could also be used first, or as an alternative to propionic acid derivatives in patients who fail to respond adequately or develop side effects. In the more severe cases of inflammatory disease, phenylbutazone or indomethacin can be substituted. The initial non-steroid anti-inflammatory agent would generally be changed only to better control symptoms, improve gastrointestinal tolerance or avoid toxic effects (see tables III, IV).

Potentially dangerous drugs should not be used unless or until the patient really needs them (see below).

In cases where inflammation is minimal, then either analgesic agents (section 3.1) spaced through the day should be given, or non-steroidal anti-inflammatory analgesic agents used for their analgesic properties rather than their anti-inflammatory ones.

3.5.2 Progressive Disease

Where the basic non-steroidal anti-inflammatory drug regimen does not prove sufficient and active disease appears to be progressing, then gold salts or penicillamine (section 3.3) should be seriously considered. Immunosuppressives or cytotoxic agents are still in the realms of experimental therapeutics; they are potentially dangerous and should preferably not be used except in specialist centres, being reserved for serious, progressive and potentially dangerous rheumatoid disease which has failed to respond to other long term agents (Currey et al., 1974; Pearson and Levy, 1975). The same can be said of levamisole (Vischer et al., 1978).

The point at which surgery is used is very much an individual decision between the patient and his physician and surgeon, as opinions differ greatly. In general, surgery is used for prevention or repair of tendon ruptures, control of aggressive synovitis, release of nerve entrapment, correction of deformity, and arthrodesis or replacement of destroyed joints (Mowat et al., 1978; Talbott, 1971).

3.5.3 Adjunctive Therapy

Depression is a part of rheumatoid arthritis in most cases and antidepressants such as amitriptyline at night, where sedation is required, or imipramine in the day when it is not, are very useful. To allay symptoms of anxiety simple 'sedatives' are often helpful, and among these diazepam is the most appropriate. It is not uncommon for anxiety to be later accompanied or replaced by depression, the clinician's attitude and the drugs used then need to be changed accordingly.

Iron by mouth or by intramuscular injection (see chapter XXIII; sect. 6.1.1) is useful to treat the anaemia of rheumatoid arthritis, and vitamin supplements are often advisable in those patients who may be relatively poorly nourished.

3.5.4 Pain Control at Night

Night time is often the worst time for the rheumatoid sufferer and some cover for this pain is often necessary (Hart et al., 1970). Otherwise the patient, restless and pain racked, wakes in the morning exhausted, in extreme pain, and unable to get out of bed because of stiffness. Indomethacin, 75 to 100mg with food on retiring, or as a 100mg suppository, is useful in this capacity and is probably the most effective agent. A nightly dose of 5mg prednisolone is an alternative, or doubling the late evening dose of the non-steroidal anti-inflammatory agent the patient is taking, particularly the longer acting compounds such as naproxen and sulindac.

3.5.5 Acute Inflammation: Swollen Joints

An acute inflammatory episode can be controlled in hospital with corticotrophin or tetracosactrin (see section 3.4). Where one particular joint is distended with fluid and is very active and retarding progress, aspiration and local instillation of a corticosteroid is obviously indicated, but such treatment frequently repeated, because of the risk of destructive changes in the joint surface, is contraindicated in most cases. Radioactive yttrium (^{90}Y) has been given with success in such resistant cases.

The knee has been the joint for which such radioactive colloids seem to be most used (Gumpel, 1977) with the aim of achieving a non-surgical or 'chemical' synovectomy. A dose of localised radiation is applied to the synovium which leads to shrinkage, fibrosis and, as a result, diminished production of synovial fluid. Total immobilisation in bivalved splints of an active joint will often cause it to settle down, and exercises can then be instituted in 2 weeks time.

Every case of rheumatoid arthritis is an individual problem and has to be treated and considered as such.

4. Osteoarthrosis

Degenerative changes in bone and joint occur in all of us, but only if symptoms occur as a result can a diagnosis of osteoarthrosis be made. Symptoms are pain, stiffness, muscle weakness and so-called cramps or muscle spasms around the affected joints. Pains are often referred to adjacent muscles and joints, an osteoarthritic hip, for instance, causing pain in thigh and knee.

The persistent and repeated recurrence of discomfort leads to physical and mental fatigue and depression, but there is not the loss of general health seen in patients with rheumatoid arthritis, although there is considerable disability. Patients have to learn to live with their disorder and they find out by practical painful experience what rest and exercise gives them the best functional results with the least pain. Several pain producing factors are present in any individual case, so that primarily one should endeavour to differentiate between the different types of pain, as this influences the nature of treatment, particularly the type and amount of rest and daily exercises and the role of drugs.

A convenient classification based on the patient's history and showing the role of drugs is as follows (see Hart, 1974a; Haslock, 1976):

1) Immobility pain — drugs not called for, unless pain interferes with sleep.
2) Pressure (weightbearing) pain — e.g. pain in lower extremities and spine on prolonged standing; positive programme of rest, exercises and graded activity assisted by analgesics as required.
3) Pain on movement — e.g. in hip; positive programme of exercises and activity assisted by analgesics by day, and sometimes at night.
4) Pain of inflammation — although osteoarthrosis is essentially a degenerative process, some inflammatory features are often present and anti-inflammatory drugs are in general more useful for pain relief than simple analgesics.

5) Pain of trauma — analgesic and anti-inflammatory drugs are useful and aspiration of affected joints and intra-articular corticosteroid may be helpful.

6) Pain due to, or aggravated by, psychogenic factors — psychotherapeutic drugs may help in some cases, but more important is a positive therapeutic attitude by doctor, and encouragement from relatives and friends.

Treatment in general is therefore based on a positive programme of activity, if necessary under suitable analgesic cover, with periods of rest and set daily exercises. Drugs are thus of secondary importance but they are indicated and needed at some time in the course of the disease in most cases. They enable the patient to get through his painful day with less discomfort and to maintain better function than would otherwise be possible. Either simple analgesics or non-steroidal anti-inflammatory agents can be used, even though the condition is not primarily an inflammatory one. Simple analgesics may be all that is necessary, but non-steroidal anti-inflammatory drugs may be of greater help in more painful cases, easing pain in the hips and cervical spine, although usually proving rather less helpful elsewhere.

In osteoarthrosis of the hip, although many patients may come eventually to operation, the daily use of an anti-inflammatory agent is often helpful. Phenylbutazone or oxyphenbutazone, because of their long even action (see section 3.2) are often effective given in doses of 200 to 400mg a day. Suppositories of 250mg are also available but because phenylbutazone and oxyphenbutazone in any form carry the rare but very real danger of causing blood dyscrasias, indomethacin is often preferred, 25 to 50mg 1, 2 or 3 times a day with meals. Many other non-steroidal anti-inflammatory agents are available and can be used as alternatives (see section 3.2.4 to 3.2.6). If the joints are painful at night, indomethacin may be given by mouth with food on retiring (50 to 75mg) or as a suppository (100mg), or the evening dose of one of the other agents can be increased; e.g. naproxen 250mg in the morning, 500mg in the evening. However, evening medication, while very effective in rheumatoid arthritis where nocturnal pain and morning stiffness are common (see section 3.5.4) is much less often required in osteoarthrosis where bed is usually the most comfortable place.

The ordinary analgesics, from aspirin to paracetamol (acetaminophen), alone or in combination (Huskisson, 1974), may be used in milder cases. Heberden's nodes rarely call for any drug treatment, and painful thumb bases are also relatively unaffected by analgesics which are only taken when the pain is particularly annoying.

Psychotherapeutic agents are needed less often in osteoarthrosis than in rheumatoid arthritis, but in the depressed or agitated housewife, often harassed and overworked, antidepressants or anti-anxiety agents are often as effective as analgesics, and sometimes even more so. Other patients need considerable psychological support from their relatives, friends or doctor to help combat the reaction due to discomfort of constant chronic pain and inability to use affected limbs in a normal manner.

5. Ankylosing Spondylitis

The essence of this disease is that it causes painful stiffness, which is at its worst in the small hours and most crippling in the early morning (Hart, 1975a). Nights are often extremely painful, as they often are in rheumatoid arthritis. To combat this early morning stiffness and nocturnal distress, 4 regimens may be tried: (1) indomethacin, either 3 or 4, 25mg capsules with food on retiring, or a 100mg suppository per rectum; (2) prednisolone, 5mg by mouth, on retiring; (3) a long acting dextropropoxyphene tablet, 150mg on retiring, or (4) doubling the evening dose of whatever anti-inflammatory agent is being given. Indomethacin is probably the most popular. It is more effective than dextropropoxyphene, and being a non-steroidal agent has not the drawbacks of the corticosteroids.

Through the day either indomethacin, 25mg 3 or 4 times daily, phenylbutazone or oxyphenbutazone, 100mg 3 times daily or one of the other non-steroidal agents, help to maintain normal function and allow the patient to remain at his normal work. Only very rarely are corticosteroids required, for patients on the whole do better on non-steroidal agents. Milder cases need only occasional doses of aspirin or some other analgesic or anti-inflammatory agent. Where regular medication is needed, most spondylitics find the pyrazolones or indomethacin preferable.

Whatever drug is given, a programme of daily exercise and exercises is essential to maintain as full mobility as possible.

6. Polymyalgia Rheumatica

In this disorder, usually based on an arteritis in an elderly subject (Mowat and Hazleman, 1974; Myles, 1975), the drug of choice is prednisolone or some other corticosteroid (Hart, 1975a). Steroids are usually dramatically effective, even in small conservative dosage such as 2.5mg prednisolone 8-hourly. If this produces dramatic relief it should be continued, and using 1mg scored tablets of prednisolone, the dosage should be very gradually reduced by 0.5mg (half tablet) every 3 to 4 weeks, the aim being to control symptoms and to normalise, or near normalise, the erythrocyte sedimentation rate. Analgesics may be used as required in addition, but an effective dose of a corticosteroid is essential.

The disease may well persist for many months and usually 3 to 4 years or more, and prednisolone will have to be continued at the lowest effective dose throughout this period, being gradually tailed off as the disease subsides (Fernandez-Herlihy, 1972; Myles, 1975). If 7.5mg is not initially effective then the daily dose may temporarily be increased up to 15mg, but gradually reduced as soon as possible to the lowest effective level. Although non-steroidal anti-inflammatory agents are useful in milder cases, prednisolone or some other corticosteroid remains the drug of choice in this condition.

If eye or cranial symptoms threaten, as there is a very real danger of blindness, partial or complete, from involvement of branches of the ophthalmic arteries, dosage of prednisolone should be immediately increased to around 50mg daily. There should be no delay in initiation of such therapy or complete loss of vision may occur (Hart, 1975b).

7. Soft Tissue Lesions

In the treatment of soft tissue lesions any of the analgesic and non-steroidal anti-inflammatory agents may be used, but not long term agents such as gold, penicillamine or the antimalarials, and certainly not systemic corticosteroids. Disorders such as periarthritis of the shoulder tend to be resistant to any agent used and continue without much relief from any therapy for many months or up to 2 years and then usually subside. Local injections of steroids may help, but wrongly sited may cause rupture of tendon or muscle fibre.

Other soft tissue lesions may occasionally be effectively attacked by the instillation of a local corticosteroid into the painful spot, either with or without a local anaesthetic agent — e.g. tennis and golfer's elbow very often respond to local injections of prednisolone, possibly with lignocaine in addition. Rubefacients locally applied, the old fashioned liniments and ointments, may occasionally help but usually do not. Many so-called 'fibrositic' pains are referred from degenerative diseases in the adjacent vertebral column or large joints: such cases may be helped by any of the anti-inflammatory or analgesic agents described in section 3.1 and 3.2. Many so-called fibrositic pains are psychogenic in origin, and thus often respond better to psychotherapeutic than to anti-inflammatory agents. Indeed, in many arthritic disorders, treatment of depression and anxiety may reduce pain and improve the patient's condition.

8. Low Back Pain

Low back pain may arise from a very large number of conditions (Huskisson and Hart, 1978). It is first essential to make sure that it is due to degenerative changes only, and is not part of a generalised metabolic or malignant disease process. Most complaints of low back pain to the primary care doctor will be due either to early disc lesions or facet syndromes. Analgesic agents (as in section 3.1) or the non-steroidal anti-inflammatory agents (as in section 3.2) may be used and are generally adequate for the common causes of back pain. Where the low back pain is very acute and causing great discomfort it may be legitimate to give a strong analgesic, but this will be very rare. Injections of the non-narcotic analgesics pentazocine 60mg, or dihydrocodeine 50 to 100mg will probably be more effective than the same substances by mouth; the latter, if given by intramuscular injection, is now classed as an addictive drug. Dipipanone or morphine, either with or without cyclizine, helps the acute episodes in many cases, but these and other narcotic analgesics should not be repeated frequently because of the fear of addiction.

Muscle relaxants have little part to play. In some cases a combination of a strong analgesic with a sedative agent such as diazepam is better in a patient confined to bed than an analgesic agent alone. Bed rest with full analgesic therapy is indicated with the acute painful back, the dosage of analgesic being gradually reduced as the patient begins to mobilise and the pain lessen.

The general management of back pain requires a confident therapeutic attitude and must take into account all the methods of treatment available and the use of them where appropriate — e.g. drugs, physical therapy (intermittent traction, manipulation, isometric exercises, heat), back supports, epidural analgesia, rest, surgery, and rehabilitation with instruction on back care and lifting techniques (Jayson, 1978).

9. Juvenile Chronic Polyarthritis (Still's disease)

In the treatment of juvenile rheumatoid arthritis the emphasis is rather more on physical treatment than drug therapy. Nevertheless, correct use of certain drugs is all important (Ansell, 1975, 1978; Bywaters, 1976; Proceedings, 1977).

Aspirin is usually the drug of first choice, not only to control pain but also pyrexia. It can, however, be a dangerous drug in childhood, especially to those under the age of 4. Drowsiness and hyperventilation are two of the earliest signs of aspirin intoxication in young children, who may later complain of tinnitus or deafness; the margin between tinnitus and acidosis is very small (see also chapter IV; sect. 2.4). The dose of aspirin in juvenile rheumatoid arthritis is usually about 80mg/kg of body weight in divided dosage daily; dosage being modified according to therapeutic response and blood levels (see section 3.2.1). Monitoring of plasma salicylate concentrations is especially helpful in children (Bardare et al., 1978; Makela et al., 1975) and when monitored should be kept in the region of 2mmol/L (30mg/100ml). Occasionally, larger dosage is necessary (up to 130mg/kg). An alternative to aspirin is benorylate, a chemical combination of aspirin and paracetamol (acetaminophen), which has the virtue of twice daily administration. A dose of 200mg/kg is necessary to effect clinical control. As plasma paracetamol levels appear to parallel salicylate concentrations, when monitored, only estimations of salicylate are necessary (Powell and Ansell, 1974).

Indomethacin is sometimes used in childhood in the United Kingdom, but is vetoed in the United States because of fear of spreading infection in a cortisone-like manner. It is used in patients who have failed to respond to aspirin and in those where reduction of corticosteroid dosage is desirable; dosage being up to a maximum total of 2.5mg/kg in divided doses daily, loading the evening dose where morning stiffness is a troublesome symptom. Other agents, which can be used in cases of lack of tolerance to aspirin, include ibuprofen (20mg/kg or more daily), naproxen suspension (10mg/kg daily) or tolmetin (30 to 50mg/kg daily). Gold therapy is often beneficial in patients with severe, persistent disease activity with clinical deterioration and to enable reduction in corticosteroid dosage in a child dependent on steroids. Dosage of sodium aurothiomalate can either be 1mg/kg body weight weekly by intramuscular injection or 10mg weekly for children of body weight up to 19kg, 20mg weekly for those with weights between 20 and 30kg. Close monitoring is necessary, as with adults; therapy being maintained for 6 or 12 months or longer depending on effect and on tolerance (see section 3.3.1 and table II). Penicillamine is under investigation in children and is usually preferred to gold by patients and parents as it is given orally. Chloroquine and hydroxychloroquine are sometimes used as long term agents, usually when gold or penicillamine cannot be used (see also section 3.3.2; 3.3.3).

Corticosteroid or corticotrophin therapy is occasionally necessary in severe systemic illness or in severe joint involvement when non-steroidal agents do not help sufficiently, and where iridocyclitis is a problem steroids may be very useful, but every effort should be made to avoid long term corticosteroid treatment. Children rapidly develop Cushingoid features, even on comparatively small dosage, and osteoporosis with vertebral collapse and fractures may occur, and stunting of growth may be even more marked than that seen in the untreated disease. Infection is also not uncommon with corticosteroids, and children are liable to develop pseudo-tumour cerebri during the administration of corticosteroids, a side effect which is not seen in adults but is seen particularly in childhood with the withdrawal of corticosteroids or with a change of dosage, boys being affected more often than girls. Clinically the child complains of headache and diplopia, and may vomit. There may be ataxia and papilloedema. This syndrome is probably due to cerebral oedema.

Intermittent corticosteroid therapy is less likely to cause stunting and growth arrest than is a regular daily dosage. Children treated with doses of prednisolone as high as 10 to 14mg on alternate days usually grow up in a normal fashion. In general, however, it is wise to keep to aspirin and simple analgesics as the main therapy, corticosteroids being avoided.

10. Miscellaneous Rheumatic Conditions

10.1 Connective Tissue Diseases of Immunological Origin

Connective tissue diseases of immunological origin include systemic lupus erythematosus, polyarteritis nodosa, progressive systemic sclerosis, polymyositis and dermatomyositis and affect many organ systems, particularly the kidney (Decker, 1975; see also chapter XXI; sect. 10).

10.1.1 Systemic Lupus Erythematosus

In systemic lupus erythematosus, in all but the mildest cases, corticosteroids are essential and often lifesaving (Urmon and Rothfield, 1977). The initial daily dose required is 20 to 60mg prednisolone, or even 100mg or more daily if necessary, depending on severity and extent of the disease; patients with severe visceral manifestations needing the higher dosage. The dosage should be tailored to the individual case, those with glomerulonephritis and involvement of the central nervous system needing usually more prolonged high dosage therapy than the others. For maintenance therapy much more modest amounts are required; 5 to 20mg being sufficient in daily divided dosage to control symptoms in less severe cases. Immunosuppressive drugs such as azathioprine can be added if corticosteroids in usual dosage are ineffective or produce unpleasant or dangerous steroid side effects, and may allow the dosage of steroid to be reduced (Decker et al., 1975). Chloroquine, hydroxychloroquine or mepacrine may help control the skin manifestations of the disease, but careful use of strong topical steroids are needed for facial lesions of discoid lupus (see chapter XIV; sect. 13.4). In using other drugs for symptomatic control (e.g. arthralgia), it should be borne in mind that these patients are notoriously prone to drug reactions (Sonnenblick and Abraham, 1978).

The main aim of treatment is to control symptoms and to prevent exacerbations and for both patient and doctor to be aware of the symptoms and signs which presage exacerbations (Estes, 1976). LE cells should lessen or disappear in the blood on adequate therapy, and sedimentation rates decrease to, or towards, normal.

10.1.2 Polyarteritis Nodosa

Treatment is essentially symptomatic. While in the early more acute inflammatory stages, large doses of corticosteroids (e.g. 40 to 60mg prednisolone daily) may be effective and helpful, later on in the disease they may not only be ineffective but actually potentially harmful, by causing Cushingoid complications and occasionally aggravating hypertension. Nevertheless, they remain the main therapeutic agents in this disorder. Other anti-inflammatory agents have little or no clear effect. Immunosuppressive drugs such as azathioprine or cyclophosphamide may be tried in resistant cases though, with the exception of Wegener's granulomatosis, their efficacy has not been clearly established in vasculitis syndromes (Christian, 1978).

10.1.3 Progressive Systemic Sclerosis (scleroderma)

Drug therapy in general is unhelpful (Siegel, 1977). Large doses of corticosteroids remain the most effective agent in acute inflammatory phases, but are otherwise potentially harmful. Aspirin in full dosage may control the arthralgia of finger joints associated with the disease. Hand care and instruction on finger exercises is vital, in order to preserve function in and prevent injury to the hands.

10.1.4 Polymyositis and Dermatomyositis

Corticosteroids (large doses initially) will improve the muscle weakness in most adult patients but not all, and side effects may be troublesome. Relapses are common if steroids are withdrawn before the first 2 to 3 years. It is important to remember that the clinical picture of dermatomyositis may be a manifestation of an underlying malignant process; such patients may deteriorate on steroid therapy. Immunosuppressive drugs have been used on empirical grounds with variable success.

10.2 Infective Arthritis

Infective arthritis is due to the presence of organisms in the joint tissues. In viraemic states, like rubella, mumps or infective mononucleosis, no therapy other than analgesics or anti-inflammatory drugs are necessary, as the condition rapidly subsides in a few days. In infections such as gonococcal, staphylococcal or streptococcal arthritis, aspiration and appropriate antibiotics are required, sometimes surgical drainage. Early diagnosis and treatment is essential for later treatment is associated with a higher mortality and cases of septic arthritis are easily missed (Hart, 1978a). It should be remembered that rheumatoid joints are more liable to infection from the bloodstream than normal joints, and a sudden flare up in one joint in a rheumatoid patient should suggest trauma or infection rather than an exacerbation of rheumatoid disease (Mitchell et al., 1976).

10.3 Postinfective Arthritis

In postinfective arthritis, as in Reiter's (Brodie's) disease, no organisms are found in the tissues and therapy of the arthritis is more on the lines of rheumatoid disease.

11. Disorders of Bone

11.1 Malignant Disease of Bone

Multiple myeloma, metastatic carcinoma, sarcoma and a number of other malignant diseases may directly affect bone or joint or be indirectly productive of an arthritis, as in pseudohypertrophic pulmonary osteoarthropathy, usually due to carcinoma of the bronchus.

Where malignant deposits cause pain in bone and joints the disease is usually metastatic and the expectation of life extremely limited. In such cases morphine or pethidine (meperidine) is probably the drug of choice, but only when the patient is in great distress, for it is not uncommon to be able to control less severe pain with the usual antirheumatic drugs such as aspirin, indomethacin or phenylbutazone. When the patient does not know of his condition, such anti-inflammatory agents do not suggest to him any sinister pathology. Injections of dihydrocodeine or pentazocine may often be helpful for some time before morphine or pethidine become necessary (Westbury, 1974).

Not all malignant deposits are painful, and it is best to treat each in its own right with either simple analgesics, more potent non-narcotic analgesics, or with pethidine or diamorphine (heroin), depending on the pain spectrum in each

case. An oral preparation which has been popular for many years is: diamorphine or morphine, 5 to 15mg; cocaine 10mg; ethyl alcohol (90%) 1.25ml; and syrup (66% sucrose in water) 2.5ml, with chloroform water up to 10ml (diamorphine and cocaine elixir BPC 1973). This may be given as often as is required, and if the pain is severe it is best to give it regularly every few hours, the amount of morphine or diamorphine being gradually increased as required. By thus overcoming the pain and anticipating and preventing its return many of these patients can be maintained on such an oral preparation without the need of injections. In some cases however, diamorphine in gradually increasing dosage from 5mg subcutaneously every 4 to 6 hours (or morphine from 10mg subcutaneously) is the only therapy that enables the patient to have any relief from his incessant pain. Cocaine may be eliminated if it causes nightmares and mental confusion. If nausea, vomiting or agitation occurs, chlorpromazine or prochlorperazine elixir can replace the syrup. It is important to note that the shelf life of such elixirs is around 6 weeks, after which time they should be discarded.

It is of interest that excision of the malignant lesion (as, for example, a carcinoma of the bronchus) may be followed by rapid improvement in the joints in pseudohypertrophic pulmonary osteoarthropathy.

11.2 Osteoporosis

It is important to look for an identifiable cause of osteoporosis whenever this diagnosis is established, so that corrective treatment can be given where possible. A number of factors can cause osteoporosis and include endocrine disorders, early menopause (see chapter XV; section 16), nutritional deficiency, drugs (see section 14.5), immobility, and certain chronic diseases (e.g. renal disease in children and adolescents).

Osteoporosis is usually only acutely painful after a spinal compression fracture, when bed rest is essential until the pain subsides. Treatment is directed at arresting and stabilising the condition and at symptomatic relief of pain, back support initially, with exercise as soon as possible, rehabilitation, and education of the patient to avoid further fractures.

There is no established specific therapy to increase bone mass, but calcium supplements at night (1,000mg elemental Ca as effervescent tablets) and small doses (1,000u daily) of vitamin D, or its analogues, if adequate exposure to sunlight is not possible, are given to raise the serum calcium level and thus suppress the normal nocturnal rise of parathyroid hormone with its resorptive activity on bone (Mundy and Raisz, 1974; Ingham, 1974). Concomitant fluoride therapy (40 to 60mg daily) to stimulate bone formation (Jowsey et al., 1972), may be considered but the value of additional fluoride has not been proven. Similarly, reports on the effect of calcitonin therapy in senile osteoporosis are contradictory.

Analgesic agents of one sort or another are indicated initially, preferably the non-narcotic variety such as pentazocine or dihydrocodeine, or the simple oral preparations such as paracetamol (acetaminophen) or aspirin. As soon as pain is adequately controlled it is wise to mobilise the patient, as prolonged immobility only aggravates the osteoporosis. Injection or oral administration of anabolic agents is of only limited assistance and is unlikely to affect the acutely painful episode. Such therapy is of unproven benefit in established osteoporosis.

Prophylactic measures are the most desirable means of management of osteoporosis (Ingham, 1974; Editorial, 1978a). Young people should have an adequate diet with appropriate amounts of calcium (800 to 1,000mg daily) and encouraged to partake in regular outdoor exercise, which should be continued throughout life to provide sufficient vitamin D to stimulate osteoblastic cells. Patients at risk of developing osteoporosis (e.g. the elderly female with a poor diet; women who have had an early menopause) may be offered prophylactic therapy. Calcium can be given at night (500 to 1,000mg as effervescent calcium) to those with normal calcium absorption. Oestrogens can also delay or prevent postmenopausal bone loss (Horsman et al., 1977; Lindsay et al., 1978) and may be expected (but not established) to reduce the incidence of multiple crush fractures, but the routine use of prophylactic oestrogen immediately after the menopause is more controversial (see chapter XV; sect. 16.3). Anabolic and progestational hormones have a similar effect to oestrogen (fig. 2) but androgenic side effects of anabolic agents limit acceptance of this therapy by some patients. Older women tend to absorb calcium less efficiently and although synthetic vitamin D analogues can be used in small doses to raise calcium absorption, hypercalcaemia may occur and much of the increased calcium absorbed is excreted in the urine (Nordin et al., 1976; Marshall and Nordin, 1977).

11.3 Osteomalacia

Vitamin D deficiency is relatively rare in developed countries, especially those with plentiful sunlight. Nevertheless, abnormalities of vitamin D metabolism do occur in patients with renal disease and malabsorption syndromes, and sometimes as a consequence of anticonvulsant therapy (see section 14.5). The patient may complain of bone pain or muscular weakness or may dismiss the symp-

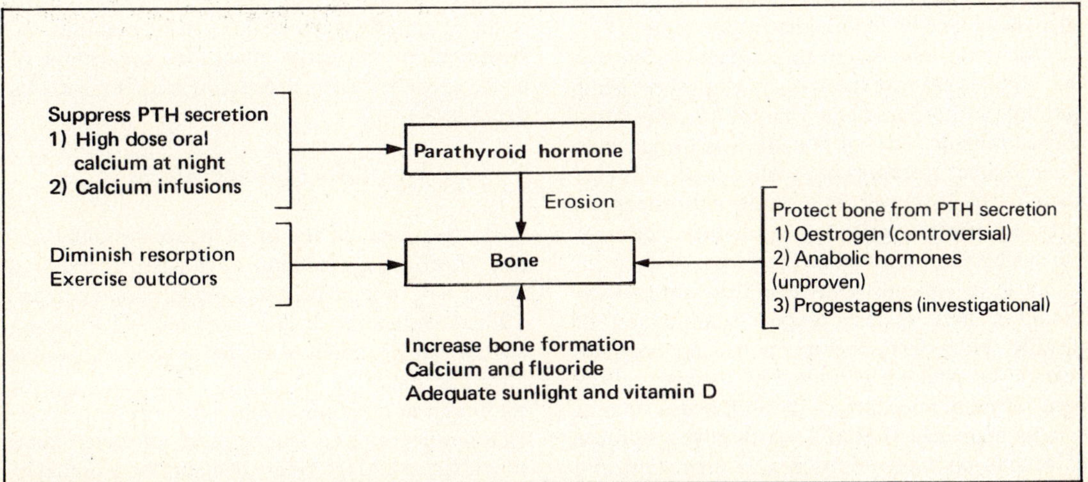

Fig. 2. Putative action of drugs used in osteoporosis (after Ingham: Drugs 8: 290, 1974; by permission of author and editor).

toms because of the more severe manifestations of the underlying disease. The condition of these patients is greatly improved by vitamin D therapy. Analogues of vitamin D or large doses may be needed in 'resistant' cases (Brooks et al., 1978; see also chapter XVI; sect. 6.2). Osteomalacia may be present in 25% of postgastrectomy patients (Eddy, 1971).

11.4 Paget's Disease of Bone

Paget's disease of bone affects over 10% of the population by age 80 years. It may cause considerable suffering and disability and is predominantly due to a greatly accelerated bone resorption rate, but in many cases the disorder is entirely symptomless and no treatment is necessary. In others it causes extreme pain for a period — often for many weeks or months. For no apparent reason it may then subside and again be painless. Such painful episodes may be associated with small bony fractures, often incomplete.

During the painful episode almost any of the current analgesics may be used, but often with limited success. It is wise, therefore only to use narcotic analgesics when there is definite evidence of the condition having become malignant, Paget's sarcoma being amongst the most painful of all conditions of bone. When this has developed, diamorphine (heroin), pethidine or a similar drug may be used as required. In mild cases, simple analgesics such as salicylates, paracetamol (acetaminophen) and dextropropoxyphene may be tried, and for more severe pains one of the non-steroidal anti-inflammatory analgesics such as phenylbutazone or indomethacin (see table II).

Calcitonin, one of the three major substances that regulate calcium metabolism (the others being parathyroid hormone and vitamin D), may bring about dramatic relief of bone (but not joint) pain when simpler measures have failed to provide adequate relief. Moreover, in a significant proportion of mildly affected patients it can induce biochemical evidence of remission. The remission is incomplete in patients with severe disease and the condition may relapse despite continuation of therapy. Long term therapy with calcitonin appears to be safe, but is limited by its cost and the need for daily injections. Diphosphonates such as sodium etidronate (EHDP), which have a number of actions on mineralisation and formation and resorption of bone, also bring about symptomatic and biochemical improvement in Paget's disease

and can be given orally. Remissions appear to last longer than after calcitonin, but radiological evidence of bone healing has not yet been reported and, with the possibility of osteomalacia developing, its long term prophylactic use is debatable. Mithramycin, a cytotoxic agent, has also been used with some success, particularly in patients with severe and generalised osseous Paget's disease, but its toxic effects limit its general use (see further, Haddad, 1972; Mundy and Raisz, 1974; Editorial 1978b). It must be re-emphasised that most patients with Paget's disease have few or no symptoms and need no treatment.

12. Gout

In gout, there is an abnormality in urate metabolism which results in high and sustained serum urate levels. In a minority of cases of primary gout there is evidence of overproduction, and in a majority underexcretion. In a few cases both mechanisms operate. In most cases of primary gout there appears to be an isolated defect in the renal handling of urate, the main feature of which is that higher levels of plasma urate are needed to achieve the same values of urate clearance as in normal subjects (Nuki, 1976). Precipitation of urate crystals into joints, renal tubules and other tissues may result in acute arthritis, renal (uric acid) calculi and tophi. Renal calculi occur in some patients and may actually precede the acute attack, whereas tophi are usually late manifestations of gout occurring some years after the initial acute arthritis (Fessel, 1972; Hall et al., 1967). Treatment of gout falls under three main headings: (a) treatment of the acute attack, (b) prevention of acute episodes, and (c) dissolution of tophaceous deposits.

12.1 Treatment of Acute Attack

In treatment of the acute attack a rapidly acting, effective anti-inflammatory agent is required which will relieve pain as soon as possible (Hart, 1975a). Whatever drug is used (table V) it is essential that treatment be started as soon as possible after the onset of symptoms. Treatment started within an hour of onset may often prevent the attack developing and will be more effective than a much larger dosage taken 24 hours or more later. The essential aim is for the patient to find by trial and error which drug suits him best and to take it in adequate dosage at the very beginning of an attack.

A most effective approach is to give 25 to 50mg indomethacin with meals 3 times a day, plus 3 or 4 capsules with food (75 to 100mg) or an indomethacin suppository (100mg) on retiring. The daily dose should be gradually reduced as the attack comes under control. Indomethacin acts rapidly and is usually effective, but a number of patients prefer and obtain better results with the pyrazolones, phenylbutazone or oxyphenbutazone.

Treatment on the day of onset should start with 600 to 800mg phenylbutazone or oxyphenbutazone orally in divided dosage with food. The dose is then gradually reduced by 100 to 200mg every day, the period of treatment depending on the relief obtained, but usually lasting for 5 to 8 days. If therapy is withdrawn too rapidly acute symptoms may recur. Alternatives are naproxen, sulindac, azapropazone or ketoprofen given in full dosage.

Colchicine is less regularly effective than indomethacin or the pyrazolones (Boardman and Hart, 1965) and frequently causes diarrhoea, but some patients undoubtedly derive more benefit from stable preparations of colchicine (it is degraded by exposure to light) than from anything else — 1mg is given immediately, as soon as possible after the onset of the acute attack, followed by 0.5mg every hour for 4 further doses, and then 0.5mg every 2 to 3 hours until relief has been obtained, diarrhoea has set in or a total of 6mg has been given (Wallace, 1974).

Only in cases where the above drugs have proved ineffective need corticosteroids or corticotrophin be considered, but some acute cases do not settle until these agents are given. In such cases it may be necessary to give 30 to 40mg of prednisolone on day 1, the dosage then being reduced by 5 to 10mg daily. Alternatively, corticotrophin, 50 to 60 units may be given on day 1, the dosage then being reduced by 5 to 10 units every day. The equivalent dosage of tetracosactrin depot is 0.4 to 0.5mg on day 1, the dosage then being reduced by 0.05mg every day. On the whole it is best to avoid corticosteroids or corticotrophins as they are endocrine substances with a wide effect on tissues other than the inflamed joint, and rebound attacks are common if the agent is withdrawn or reduced rapidly. Happily, the resistant case with acute symptoms persisting for several weeks for which corticosteroid therapy was formerly occasionally necessary is rarely seen today.

12.2 Prevention of Acute Episodes

Once the attack has subsided there are two alternatives to prevent further attacks of gouty arthritis. Each is aimed at preventing hyperuricaemia:

1) Conservative treatment — education of the patient to avoid excessive dietary intake of purines (e.g. 3 meat meals a day) or alcohol, gradual correction of obesity, treatment of hyperlipoproteinaemia (type IV) and maintenance of a high urine output.
2) Drug treatment — use of urate altering drugs to lower serum urate levels.

The conservative approach is preferable since the patient's history is not predictable and he may never develop further episodes of gout, or not for some years. Urate altering drugs should be reserved essentially for:

1) Those patients with isolated or infrequent attacks but with high maintained serum urate levels — above 0.54 to 0.65mmol/L (9 to 11mg/100ml), depending on the method used 1.5 times the maximum normal laboratory value.
2) Patients with hyperuricaemia at lower levels who have 2 or more episodes of gout a year.
3) Patients with tophi and elevated serum urate levels.

12.2.1 Prophylaxis of Recurrent Attacks

When acute attacks fail to settle completely and recrudescences occur intermittently, colchicine (0.5 to 1mg daily), indomethacin (25mg 2 or 3 times daily) or phenylbutazone (200 to 300mg daily in divided doses) or one of the other nonsteroidal anti-inflammatory agents such as naproxen or sulindac, may be used as preventive agents, especially if the recurrent attacks are particularly severe. Dosage of these agents is temporarily increased to the higher level if an acute attack does occur (see section 12.1). Alternatively, urate altering drugs may be used as discussed below.

12.2.2 Persistent Hyperuricaemia: Tophi

Action of Urate Altering Drugs: There are two types of urate altering drugs: (a) uricosuric agents such as probenecid, sulphinpyrazone and benzbromarone, and (b) the xanthine oxidase inhibitor allopurinol. Normally a high percentage of

Table V. Properties of drugs used in gout

Drug	Action	Dosage	Elimination	Notes/principal side effects
1. *Drugs used in acute attack*				
Indomethacin	Anti-inflammatory, antipyretic	25 to 50mg 3 times daily with food plus 75 to 100mg (orally) or 100mg (rectal) at night; dose gradually reduced as attack comes under control (usually 2 or 3 days)	See table II	Gastrointestinal irritation; headaches, cerebral sensations
Phenylbutazone Oxyphenbutazone	Anti-inflammatory, antipyretic	600 to 800mg in 3 divided doses with food, reduced gradually by 100 to 200mg each day until attack comes under adequate control (usually 3 to 4 days)	See table II	Gastrointestinal irritation; fluid retention
Colchicine	Anti-inflammatory, (?inhibition of leucocyte motility necessary for urate crystal induced inflammation; interferes with formation of kinins)	1mg immediately at onset of attack; then 0.5mg every hour for 4 further doses; then 0.5mg every 2 to 3 hours until relief, diarrhoea or total 6mg given. 3mg IV as single dose	Partial hepatic metabolism, biliary and renal excretion of unchanged drug and metabolites	Abdominal cramps, nausea, vomiting, diarrhoea. Reduce dose in patients with severe liver disease or significant renal impairment. Degraded by exposure to light, rapidly losing therapeutic effectiveness Venous irritation
Naproxen	Anti-inflammatory, antipyretic	500 to 750mg, then 250mg 250mg 8-hourly	See table II	Gastrointestinal irritation
2. *Drugs used in interval treatment to prevent attacks*				
Indomethacin	Anti-inflammatory prophylaxis	25mg 2 or 3 times daily with food	See table II	Used when acute attacks fail to settle completely and symptoms occur intermittently (see section 12.2.1)
Phenylbutazone	Anti-inflammatory prophylaxis	200 to 300mg in divided doses with food	See table II	As above
Colchicine	Anti-inflammatory prophylaxis	0.5 to 1mg daily	See above	Gastrointestinal disturbances; haematological abnormalities, myopathy, alopecia (infrequent)

3. Drugs used to prevent further acute episodes, to normalise serum uric acid levels and to prevent or eliminate tophi

Probenecid	Uricosuric agent (increases renal excretion of urate by inhibiting its tubular reabsorption)	0.25g 2 or 3 times daily for 1 week, gradually increased to 1 to 2g daily in week 2 or 3	Hepatic metabolism and little renal excretion of unchanged drug	Gastrointestinal irritation (dose related); skin rash; fever (rare). Not effective in presence moderate to marked impaired renal function. Colchicine may be used in first months of therapy (see section 12.2.2)
Sulphinpyrazone	Uricosuric agent (increases renal excretion of urate by inhibiting its tubular reabsorption)	100mg 2 times daily for 1 week, gradually increased to 300 to 600mg daily in week 2 or 3 if necessary	Some hepatic metabolism and renal excretion of unchanged drug and active metabolite	Gastrointestinal irritation (more common than with probenecid); skin rash; fever (rare). Not effective in presence moderate to marked impaired renal function. Colchicine may be used in first months of therapy (see section 12.2.2)
Benzbromarone	Uricosuric agent (as above + ?extrarenal action)	50mg once daily for 1 week, gradually increased to 100 to 200mg daily in week 2 or 3. Given once daily	Hepatic metabolism and excretion of active metabolites in bile, faeces; little renal excretion	Gastrointestinal irritation (diarrhoea). Increased dosage effective when renal function moderately impaired; ineffective in severe renal impairment. Colchicine may be used in first months of therapy (see section 12.2.2)
Allopurinol	Reduces formation of urate (inhibits enzyme xanthine oxidase conversion of hypoxanthine to xanthine and xanthine to uric acid; also inhibits early steps in *de novo* purine synthesis)	200mg daily for 1 week gradually increased to 400 to 600mg daily in week 2 or 3 if necessary. Up to 400mg may be given once daily	Hepatic metabolism and renal excretion of active metabolite	Gastrointestinal irritation; rash, pruritus, fever; leucopenia, reversible hepatotoxicity (rare). Effective in patients with impaired renal function. Colchicine may be used in first months of therapy (see section 12.2.2)

uric acid filtered by the glomerulus is reabsorbed by the proximal tubule, and this is so when plasma levels are very much elevated. The proximal tubule also probably secretes uric acid in man. Small doses of uricosuric agents (including agents such as the salicylates and phenylbutazone) actually depress the excretion of uric acid presumably by inhibiting the secretion but not reabsorbtive transport. Large doses, however, depress the reabsorption of uric acid in the renal tubules and lead to increased excretion and a fall in serum levels. Allopurinol, on the other hand, reduces production of uric acid by inhibiting the conversion of hypoxanthine to xanthine and xanthine to uric acid. The xanthines pass into solution in the urine and are removed in non-crystalline form (fig. 3; for review, see Rastegar and Thier, 1972).

Pharmacokinetic Properties of Urate Altering Drugs: The pharmacokinetic properties of the urate altering drugs have important implications in their use; the interaction of the uricosuric drugs with renal excretory mechanisms, and pathways of metabolism and elimination of allopurinol, being of significance. Aspirin in low doses inhibits the uricosuric action of probenecid and probenecid also reduces the renal excretion of salicylates. Pro-

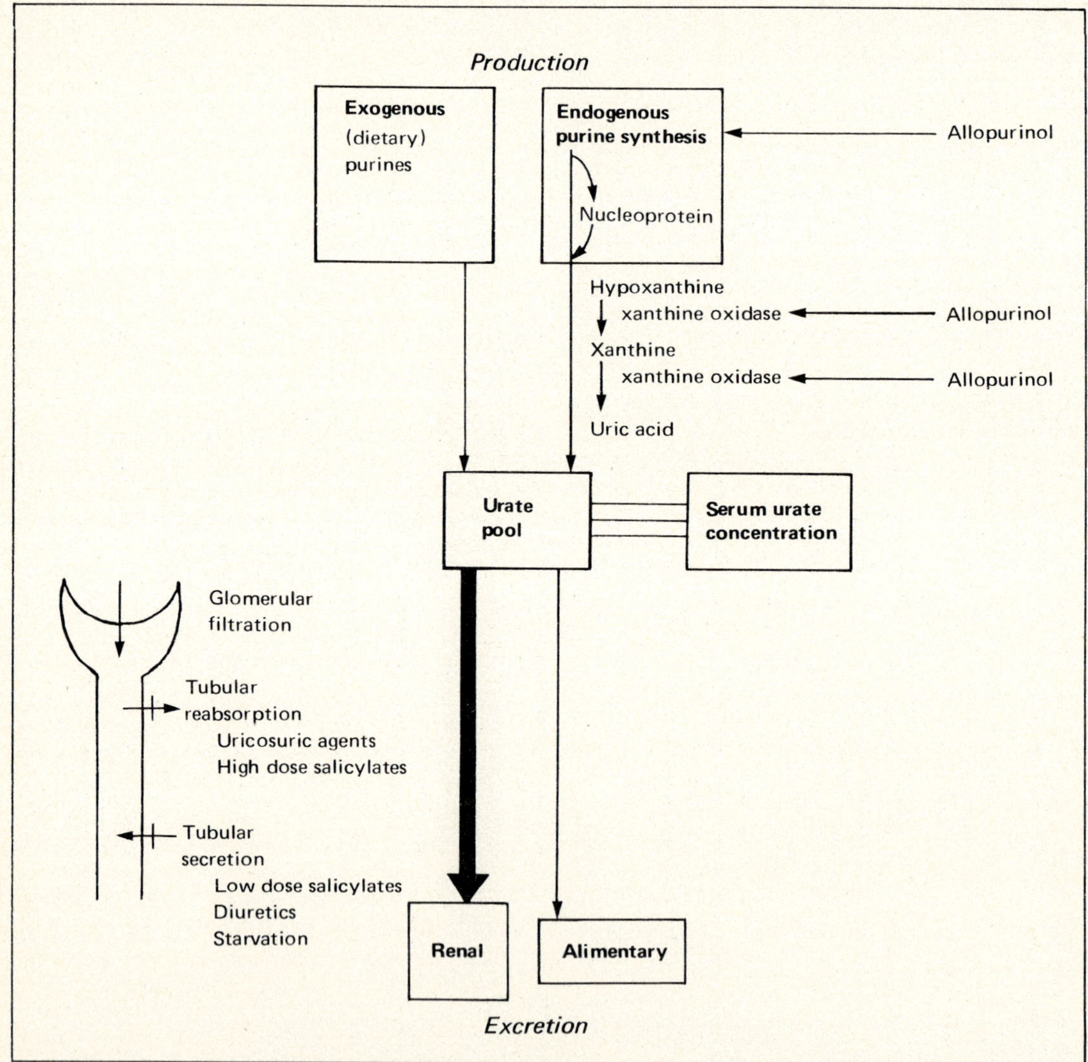

Fig. 3. Schematic representation of the urate pool (a balance between urate production and excretion) and its modification by urate altering drugs (after Emmerson: Drugs 9: 141, 1975; by permission of author and editor).

benecid also inhibits the renal tubular secretion of a variety of weak organic acids (see chapter VIII; sect. 2.3.7); use of which is made in enhancing serum levels of penicillin in treatment of gonorrhoea (see chapter XXIX; sect. 3). As with probenecid, low doses of aspirin inhibit the uricosuric effect of sulphinpyrazone and sulphinpyrazone blocks the uricosuric effect of salicylates (Yu et al., 1963). Probenecid is eliminated by hepatic metabolism, but a large proportion of a dose of sulphinpyrazone is eliminated unchanged in the urine together with metabolites with uricosuric activity (Dieterle et al., 1975). This plus the fact that probenecid markedly inhibits the renal excretion of sulphinpyrazone and its metabolites (Perel et al., 1969) probably accounts for the enhanced effect when the two drugs are used together (see below). Benzbromarone has a longer duration of action than probenecid or sulphinpyrazone, probably due to a slow rate of biotransformation or renal excretion of active metabolites so formed, enabling it to be given once daily. It also differs from these other uricosuric agents in that its action seems to be little affected by concomitant administration of analgesic doses of aspirin (Heel et al., 1977).

The elimination of allopurinol is also important in its use. Following absorption, allopurinol is converted to its major active metabolite oxypurinol, much of which remains unchanged. Oxypurinol has a much longer plasma half-life (around 14 hours) than allopurinol (around 40 minutes) [Hande et al., 1978], which makes it possible for allopurinol to be given once daily. The renal handling of oxypurinol is similar to that of uric acid and probenecid accelerates the renal excretion and reduces the efficacy of allopurinol if given concurrently (Elion et al., 1966). More importantly, elimination of oxypurinol is delayed in patients with renal impairment and plasma levels become markedly increased, necessitating use of reduced dosage (Elion et al., 1968). The incidence of skin reactions to allopurinol may rise to around 15% in patients with impaired renal function (Chan et al., 1977; Frisch et al., 1974). Some drugs are normally metabolised by xanthine oxidase (which is inhibited by allopurinol) and therefore the action of drugs such as 6-mercaptopurine and its precursor azathioprine is markedly potentiated by concurrent use of allopurinol. In such cases of combined use, the dose of mercaptopurine and azathioprine should be reduced to 33% of the usual (Rundles et al., 1963). The pharmacokinetic properties of urate

altering drugs are summarised in table V and appendix A, and their important drug interactions in table IV.

Clinical Use of the Urate Altering Drugs: Whenever allopurinol or uricosuric agents are used it must be made clear to the patient that he must continue for the rest of his life, or at least for many years, regularly on daily doses of the chosen drug. Stop/start treatment is not only useless but harmful, as stopping and starting tends to provoke fresh acute episodes. The patient must therefore agree to cooperate completely; he must understand that certain other drugs may not be given at the same time (table IV), and must also understand that freedom from acute attacks will take a little time to achieve. Although the serum urate level may be normal within a few days, the tendency to have acute attacks may not diminish until 2 or 3 months have passed.

Therapy with any urate altering drug should be started in small dosage; not during or just after an acute episode, as acute attacks of gout are particularly prone to follow the start of this treatment. If, for instance, probenecid is used, 0.25g 2 or 3 times daily is given for a week, and the dose is gradually increased to the full maintenance dose of 1 to 1.5g daily in the second or third week. Colchicine may be given at the same time, 0.5mg twice daily, to prevent any acute episode occurring at this time and should be continued prophylactically for some weeks or months, and in those with tophi, for longer periods. Sulphinpyrazone, if used, should also be introduced at low dosage (100mg once or twice daily) increasing to 300 to 600mg later as found necessary. Benzbromarone is given once daily in a dose of 100 to 200mg, range 50 to 600mg (Heel et al., 1977).

If a patient's tolerance of full dosage of sulphinpyrazone or probenecid is poor, smaller doses of the two drugs used together may work better with less side effects (see above). In general, allopurinol and the uricosuric agents are well tolerated and they have an acceptable incidence of side effects (table V) to justify long term use when indicated.

With any of the uricosuric agents an increased passage of uratic material may produce renal and ureteric symptoms, but this can be minimised by ensuring a high fluid intake and maintaining urine pH above 6 (e.g. by use of alkalinisers such as sodium citro-tartrate). Great care should be taken with any uricosuric agent if there is impaired renal function, and these agents should not be used if the glomerular filtration rate is less than

20ml/minute. In general, uricosuric agents are contraindicated: (1) in patients who are over-producers, passing more than 3.6mmol (600mg) urate per day in the urine on a purine free diet, or more than 4.8mmol (800mg) on any diet; (2) in patients with a persistently poor urinary volume; or (3) patients who have suffered from renal calculi of any type. Uricosuric agents will be ineffective in patients with a moderate or marked degree of renal insufficiency (Emmerson, 1978; Hart and Emmerson, 1978), although benzbromarone (in increased dosage) can be effective in those with moderately impaired renal function (Heel et al., 1977). Their use logically is in those patients with reduced renal excretion of urate (i.e. underexcretors) with daily urate in the urine less than 2.4mmol (400mg) when uricosuric agents will correct the essential defect.

Allopurinol, which reduces urate production, is logically indicated in patients who are over-producers of urate (i.e. > 3.6mmol/day on a purine free diet), but can also be used in those with daily urate in the urine above 2.4mmol. It is also indicated in those with uric acid calculi and in the presence of impaired renal function. In general, apart from these considerations, there is little to choose between the different urate altering drugs although allopurinol is the drug of choice with most clinicians. It is effective in lowering urate concentration in underexcretors as well as over-producers, although it will not be primarily directed towards correction of the basic defect if, in a particular patient, it is underexcretion. Dosage of allopurinol is usually 200 to 400mg daily; given as one dose or in divided dosage appears to matter little, but it is best introduced at initial low dosage to prevent precipitation of acute crises. Dosage should be reduced in renal impairment (see above).

The presence of renal calculi and extensive tophaceous deposits generally suggests urate over-production and high urate excretion. Isolated attacks of renal calculi can be managed with a high fluid intake and urinary alkalinisation, but more extensive disease should be treated with allopurinol. Surgical excision of tophi is indicated if a proper trial of drugs and dietary restriction have failed and there is persistent ulceration or infection.

12.3 Asymptomatic Hyperuricaemia

Hyperuricaemia in the absence of gouty arthritis is a finding rather than a disease (Emmerson, 1975). Transient hyperuricaemia can occur in many physiological situations and does not necessarily have serious implications. When persistent, hyperuricaemia can be due to a number of potentially reversible causes such as drug ingestion (e.g. thiazide diuretics, analgesic doses of salicylates), regular consumption of alcohol, a high purine diet (e.g. 3 meat meals daily, and especially organ meats; sardines etc), obesity, hypertension, hypertriglyceridaemia (type IV hyperlipoproteinaemia), diseases causing overproduction of urate (e.g. myeloproliferative and lymphoproliferative disorders) or underexcretion of urate (e.g. renal disease).

Indications for treating asymptomatic hyperuricaemia are not compelling. Serious clinical consequences, other than gout or renal calculi, have not been established. Even if serum urate levels are consistently moderately elevated (up to 0.54 mmol/L or 9mg/100ml) one would not treat the condition with a lifetime ingestion of drugs, since an attack of gouty arthritis might never occur. Only a few hyperuricaemic individuals develop gout, and then after an average period of about 20 years to the first attack. It is difficult to justify the use of drugs to prevent renal calculi, since the ability to predict those at risk is so indefinite. Any risk of insidious development of irreversible renal disease or hypertension, presumably related to urate crystal deposition within the kidney, is very rare. In a large series of patients, there was no increase of renal disease in patients with asymptomatic hyperuricaemia compared with a normouricaemic population (Fessel et al., 1973). Risk of developing renal disease or hypertension is chiefly a concern when serum urate is persistently elevated (of the order of 1.5 times the top normal figure by the laboratory method used), or if the patient is an overexcretor of urate (Emmerson, 1976). Overexcretors are also more likely to develop renal calculi, but even then the risk can be minimised by maintaining a high urine volume.

Drug treatment for asymptomatic hyperuricaemia is therefore justified if all three of the following criteria are met:

1) When hyperuricaemia appears to be primary, persistent and not reversible by simple measures such as restriction of calories, high purine foods and alcohol consumption.
2) When serum urate is persistently in the range of 1.5 times the maximum normal value by the laboratory method used. Such a finding would justify careful observation

and full assessment of basal urate metabolism (see below) before any urate altering drugs were prescribed.

3) When the patient is well motivated to continue long term therapy and understands the benefits and risks involved.

Study of basal urate metabolism is made by assessing the effect of purine restriction on serum urate over a 7 day period and measuring the mean 24 hour urinary urate on the last 2 days. If this consistently exceeds 3.6mmol (600mg/day), the patient can be considered to be an overproducer of urate. If the mean 24 hour urinary urate is less than 1.8mmol (300mg per 24h), underexcretion of urate due to renal factors could be inferred and a search made for correctible conditions. Development of severe hyperuricaemia in such patients would be an indication for urate lowering drugs.

12.4 Acute Crystal Deposition Syndromes (Pseudogout)

Pseudogout from the deposition of calcium pyrophosphate crystals rather than urate in the joint fluid, mainly occurs in the elderly and may present as an acute or chronic arthritis (Angevine and Jacox, 1973). The acute inflammatory response resembles gout but usually involves the knee joint rather than the big toe. Indomethacin, or some other non-steroidal anti-inflammatory analgesics, but not phenylbutazone in the elderly (see table III), can be used. Colchicine may not be effective, although the calcium hydroxyapatite pseudogout of renal failure patients on haemodialysis will often respond to colchicine. Intra-articular corticosteroid injection at the time of aspiration is also effective for acute knee involvement. There is no known method of preventing the pyrophosphate crystal deposition, which can be distinguished from urate crystals by polarised light microscopy of synovial fluid.

13. Use of Drugs in the Presence of Associated Rheumatic Disease

Arthritis may be exacerbated, although not induced, by certain drugs (Hart, 1974b). Total dose infusion of iron dextran may produce an acute exacerbation of rheumatoid arthritis, but may also produce a mild arthralgia in those without rheumatic disease. Oral contraceptives may appear to cause an exacerbation of pre-existing rheumatoid disease, though this occurrence is very rare. There have also been reports of dramatic worsening of the condition of patients with systemic lupus erythematosus while they were taking oral contraceptives, with improvement when these were withdrawn (Chapel and Burns, 1971). Drug-tissue sensitivity is not clearly understood in individuals prone to drug reactions in general. Thiazide diuretics may precipitate an attack of gout in a hyperuricaemic individual (see section 14.4), as may any briskly effective diuretic or cytotoxic drugs or radiotherapy given for leukaemia, ^{32}P for polycythemia, pyrazinamide for tuberculosis, or nicotinic acid for hyperlipidaemias.

A full pre-operative assessment, and in patients who have recently had or who are still taking large doses of corticosteroids, pre- and postoperative cover with hydrocortisone hemisuccinate (see chapter X; sect. 6.2.4) is essential in the anaesthetic management of the patient with rheumatoid arthritis (Jenkins and McGraw, 1969).

Certain other drugs given concurrently, especially oral anticoagulants, may interact with some non-steroidal anti-inflammatory agents used in rheumatic diseases, particularly aspirin and phenylbutazone (table IV) but clinically important reactions seem to be relatively uncommon, perhaps because problem combinations are avoided. Nevertheless, fatalities have occurred (see chapter VIII, sect. 2.3.2, 2.3.4; XXIII, sect. 3.2.5). This also seems to be so in gout. The xanthine oxidase inhibitor allopurinol is a special case. 6-Mercaptopurine and azathioprine (which is converted in the body to 6-mercaptopurine) are metabolised by xanthine oxidase and the dose of these drugs must be reduced to 33% of usual when allopurinol is used to combat the increased nucleoprotein breakdown and consequent urate overproduction which can follow cytotoxic chemotherapy (see section 12.2.2). The incidence of ampicillin rashes appears to be higher in hyperuricaemic patients treated with allopurinol (Boston Collaborative Drug Surveillance Program, 1972).

14. Drug Induced Rheumatic and Bone Disorders

A large number of drugs in common usage can cause aches and pains in muscles, bone and joints (table VI). When a patient presents with an obscure 'rheumatism' which does not fall into any

Table VI. Rheumatic diseases and disorders of bone induced by drugs (after Hart, 1974b; Au and Raisz, 1972)

Condition	Examples	Notes
Systemic lupus erythematosus-like syndrome	Procainamide Hydrallazine Isoniazid Phenytoin	Development may depend on genetic susceptibility (see section 14.1). See also table VII
Arthritis, arthralgia	Drug hypersensitivity Sulphonamides Corticosteroids ?Oral contraceptives Isoniazid Pyrazinamide Ethionamide Rubella vaccine	Generalised skin reactions; 'serum sickness'-type reaction. Manifestation of a polyarteritis. Symptoms of arteritis if dose or preparation changed. Aches and pains, myalgia in calves on walking; arthritis of hands. Joint swelling common with pyrazinamide + isoniazid More prominent in females
Muscle pain, cramps	Clofibrate Corticosteroids Oral contraceptives Oestrogens Diuretics Corticosteroids Carbenoxolone Suxamethonium	Excessive dosage in nephrotic syndrome Fluid retention Sodium and potassium depletion Hypokalaemia (if marked severe muscle weakness can occur; see also text) Delayed muscle pains common
Acute gout	Diuretics Pyrazinamide Cytotoxic drugs (espec. leukaemia)	Thiazides, frusemide etc raise serum urate; tienilic acid lowers serum urate but initial marked uricosuria may precipitate gout in the predisposed patient (Lelievre et al., 1978) Increased breakdown of nucleoprotein and urate over-production
Haemarthrosis	Anticoagulants	Misdiagnosed as acute gout
Osteoporosis	Corticosteroids Heparin Methotrexate	High doses and in partly immobilised females over 50. Long term high doses. Prepubertal children on long term treatment
Osteomalacia	Anticonvulsants Non-absorbable antacids Diphosphonates Fluorides	Long term high dose therapy in institutionalised children Long term therapy and activation of condition at time of partial gastrectomy Inhibit mineralisation of bone. If used alone in osteoporosis (combined with calcium + vitamin D)
Aseptic necrosis	Corticosteroids	Unpredictable and not duration or dose related
Tooth discoloration	Tetracyclines	See chapter XIII (sect. 13.3)
Inhibition bone growth	Tetracyclines	Prematures or use in pregnancy. Reversible if short courses given
Osteosclerosis Fluorosis	Fluorides	Excessive dosage

of the usual disease patterns a drug induced arthropathy should be considered (for review, see Hart, 1974b).

14.1 Systemic Lupus Erythematosus Syndrome

Some individuals when exposed to certain drugs develop a systemic lupus erythematosus-like syndrome (Alarcon-Segovia, 1969, 1976). These patients complain of aching joints and muscles, and there are rashes, fever, pleural and pulmonary involvement and a number of other lupus-like symptoms. Arthralgia is more common than arthritis but both may occur and joint effusions are present in about 10% of cases. Hepatomegaly and splenomegaly may be present. LE cells are usually present and tests for antinuclear factor positive. In comparison with the 'spontaneously' appearing disease, the drug reactions appear to be associated with more fever, rashes, and in the case of procainamide more pleuropulmonary involvement, but with a relative lack of serious renal involvement. The syndrome as a whole is less severe and can disappear completely, within a few weeks of stopping the causative drug, but some cases may persist for several months and need corticosteroid therapy for a few weeks, while others can persist for years after withdrawal of the eliciting drug. In some cases the drug can be reintroduced many months later without exacerbation of the condition.

The drugs most often involved are procainamide, hydrallazine, isoniazid and phenytoin (diphenylhydantoin). These drugs by pharmacological properties of their own elicit antinuclear antibodies in a large proportion of individuals who receive them for some time, but only cause lupus in a small percentage of patients. Allergic mechanisms do not seem to be involved with these drugs. The development of systemic lupus erythematosus may therefore depend on a genetic susceptibility to environmental factors, including certain drugs. Other genetic factors seem to be involved in drug related cases, since a genetically determined slow rate of drug metabolism (acetylation) appears to be a determinant in the development of the lupus syndrome induced by hydrallazine and isoniazid and also in the earlier development of the syndrome with procainamide (Woosley et al., 1978). Most patients who develop spontaneous systemic lupus erythematosus also appear to be slow drug acetylators. The questions posed by these proposals are as

Table VII. Drugs reported to induce or activate systemic lupus erythematosus (after Alarcon-Segovia, 1976)[1]

Group I (by pharmacological action)	Group II (by allergic reaction)
Hydrallazine	Aminosalicylic acid
Procainamide	Chlorthalidone[2]
Anticonvulsants	Griseofulvin
mephenytoin	Guanoxan
phenytoin	Isoquinazepon
primidone	Levodopa
trimethadione	Methyldopa[2]
ethosuximide	Methysergide
carbamazepine	Methylthiouracil
pheneturide	Oral contraceptives
Isoniazid	Oxyphenisatin
Chlorpromazine	D-Penicillamine
	Penicillin
	Phenylbutazone
	Practolol
	Propylthiouracil
	Quinidine
	Reserpine
	Streptomycin
	Sulphonamides and sulphasalazine
	Tetracycline
	Tolazamide

1   Drugs most often implicated are in italics.
2   May belong to group I.

yet unanswered. A number of other drugs such as tetracycline, sulphonamides and propylthiouracil, have been implicated in causing lupus (table VII). In contrast to the drugs above, these drugs appear to trigger the syndrome after only brief periods of use and often seem to do so by an allergic reaction, which may be quite dramatic. Moreover, they cause lupus only rarely and do not often elicit antinuclear antibodies in patients receiving them (Alarcon-Segovia, 1976).

14.2 Arthritis and Arthralgia

Arthralgia may accompany any of the generalised skin reactions caused by drugs (see chapter XIV; section 22) and joint swellings are features of the 'serum sickness' type of reaction, seen most often with penicillin and the barbiturates, but also with a large number of other drugs. Development of the skin eruption usually makes diagnosis of the condition obvious.

Arthritis and arthralgia may be manifestations of a polyarteritis induced by certain drugs, most commonly by sulphonamides. Changes in dosage or type of corticosteroid in the treatment of rheumatoid arthritis may precipitate acute symptoms of an arteritis. On present evidence, giant cell arteritis or polymyalgia rheumatica does not appear to be induced or exacerbated by drugs.

Although oral contraceptives seem to exert a protective effect against rheumatoid arthritis (RCGP, 1978), aches and pains occurring in women on oral contraceptives may disappear on stopping them, but cause and effect usually remain uncertain and non-proven. Pains in the legs in patients on oral contraceptives should always arouse suspicion of venous thrombosis, but myalgia affecting the calves on walking may also occur, making the patient fear venous thrombosis when none is present (Spiera and Plotz, 1969). A syndrome of myalgia, arthralgia and swelling of the hands has also been attributed to oral contraceptives (Davies and Lund, 1965).

Arthralgia has also been attributed to treatment with the barbiturates, sometimes accompanied by contractions (rheumatisme barbiturique). It is possible that some cases of shoulder-hand syndrome may also be due to barbiturate therapy.

The antituberculosis drugs isoniazid, pyrazinamide and ethionamide can cause arthritis and arthralgia, sometimes with joint swelling. Joint pain of the shoulders, elbows and knees is common with pyrazinamide, especially when combined with isoniazid (Schneeweiss and Poole, 1960).

Rubella vaccination, as in rubella itself, may result in arthralgia and arthritis, the incidence of which increases with age and is more prominent in females than males (Katz, 1972).

14.3 Muscle Pain, Cramps

Myalgia, with or without cramps, may be an early symptom of a drug induced polyneuropathy. Myalgia is also seen after corticosteroid manipulation in established cases of rheumatoid arthritis. Excessive dosage of clofibrate in patients with the nephrotic syndrome and associated impaired renal function, or in those with chronic renal failure, can cause severe myalgia, with muscle stiffness and weakness (Bridgman et al., 1972; Kijima et al., 1977; see chapter XXI; sect. 14.7). Drug induced myopathy or parkinsonism can also be associated with muscle pains, stiffness and cramps, but as in the myalgia of polyneuropathy is usually overshadowed by other features of the

disease. Similarly, aching in legs and back may be early features of vascular compression retroperitoneal fibrosis induced by methysergide, but usually more obvious signs of peripheral vascular insufficiency occur soon afterwards (see further chapter XXV; sect. 15).

Drugs which cause fluid retention may cause aches in muscles and extremities, examples being the corticosteroids, corticotrophin or tetracosactrin, oral contraceptives, oestrogens and (less often) androgens. The fluid retention induced in some patients by phenylbutazone is usually painless, but elderly cardiacs may be precipitated into congestive heart failure (see section 3.2.2).

Sodium depletion following prolonged diuretic therapy may cause muscular pains and cramps. Similarly, potassium depletion may lead to muscle aching, and can be caused by carbenoxolone or crude liquorice extracts; corticotrophin, tetracosactrin or corticosteroids (this complication may add to the muscle weakness sometimes induced by steroids); long term diuretic therapy or chronic and excessive use of purgatives (see further chapter XXV; sect. 15.9). Severe muscle weakness can occur with carbenoxolone if marked hypokalaemia is allowed to develop (Pinder et al., 1976). Delayed onset of severe muscle pain commonly occurs after administration of the depolarising muscle relaxant suxamethonium (succinylcholine [Collier, 1978].

14.4 Acute Gout

Acute gout may be precipitated in susceptible individuals by drugs which raise serum urate levels such as certain diuretics (e.g. thiazides and frusemide; Manuel and Steele, 1974), nicotinic acid in hyperlipaemias, radioactive phosphorus in polycythaemia, and cytotoxic drugs, particularly in the treatment of leukaemia. The uricosuric drugs and allopurinol may precipitate acute attacks in the early days of therapy (see section 12.2.2). A moderate rise in serum urate levels occurs with small doses of salicylates, the antituberculosis drug pyrazinamide (sometimes a steep rise leading to acute gout may occur), and with large doses of nicotinic acid. Different types of alcohol may precipitate gout in different individuals.

Anticoagulant induced haemarthrosis is not uncommon, despite few published reports (Wild and Zvaifler, 1976). It leads to a condition sometimes misdiagnosed as acute gout, as the patient may complain of severe pain and swelling of rapid onset in the offending joint. Haemarthrosis treatment induced pseudogout is by no means uncommon, the knee being usually affected.

14.5 Bone Disorders

Pain may arise from osteoporotic crush fractures and from osteomalacia. Osteomalacic pain differs from osteoporotic pain, in being more diffuse and more readily eased by bed rest. Corticosteroids are often aggravating factors in spinal osteoporosis (Saville, 1970). Acute pain after collapse of a vertebral body is not uncommon, particularly where high steroid dosage has been used in rheumatoid arthritis, but it is also seen in other disorders, especially in partly immobilised females over the age of 50. Peripheral changes in the small joints, however, are not seen.

Long term treatment (6 months or more) with large doses of heparin has led to osteoporosis and spontaneous fractures of the vertebrae or ribs (Griffith et al., 1965). Severe osteoporosis, associated with fractures and bone pain, has been noted in prepubertal children with acute leukaemia in remission on long term methotrexate therapy. Remineralisation of bone occurred within 6 months of withdrawing methotrexate (Ragab et al., 1970).

Pain from osteomalacia can be caused or aggravated, although rarely, by long term treatment with excessive doses of aluminium or magnesium hydroxides (which impair phosphorus absorption and lead to increased bone resorption) or by chronic overuse of laxatives (Lotz et al., 1964; Frame et al., 1971). Such pains usually arise diffusely in the spine, though they are associated with aching in other parts of the body. In patients treated long term with normal doses of the non-absorbable antacids, symptoms may remain quiescent until partial gastrectomy performed for gastric ulceration aggravates and exacerbates the whole condition.

A more important problem is the osteomalacia and rickets which can arise in some patients, particularly institutionalised children, who have received prolonged anticonvulsant therapy (Hahn, 1976; Richens and Rowe, 1970). The severity of the bone changes seems to be particularly correlated with the dose and duration of therapy and amount of sunlight exposure and degree of physical activity, and appears most marked with a combined regimen of phenytoin (diphenylhydantoin) and phenobarbitone. The most likely cause of this adverse effect is a disturbance of calcium and vitamin D metabolism, particularly biotransformation of vitamin D in the liver and possibly elsewhere, or of effects of vitamin D metabolites on receptor cells (Mosekilde et al., 1977). Appropriate vitamin D supplementation (around 10,000 iu weekly) can significantly reduce the clinical manifestations of the disorder in those at risk of complications (e.g. institutionalised patients who have been on therapy for 6 months or longer). Non-institutionalised patients on lower dose levels probably do not require prophylactic vitamin D therapy, provided they have adequate exposure to sunlight. Serum calcium, phosphorus and alkaline phosphatase estimations should be made periodically and X-rays where indicated among other investigations. Large doses of vitamin D ($50,000 iu/m^2$ body area per week in 2 to 3 divided doses) and calcium 500mg daily are required for treatment of rickets, with care to avoid intoxication. Osteomalacia, if present, should be treated with vitamin D and calcium and adequate prophylaxis given. Serum and urinary calcium levels should be monitored periodically (e.g. at least every 2 to 3 months) in all patients maintained on vitamin D and calcium supplements, so that dosage can be adjusted to individual requirements and inadvertent vitamin D overdosage avoided.

Corticosteroid therapy can cause aseptic necrosis, generally of the femoral head although the humeral head may also be involved (Au and Raisz, 1972). This adverse effect is unpredictable and does not appear to be correlated with duration of treatment or dosage. Bone necrosis may also occur after steroid therapy has been discontinued. Patients on steroid therapy should be instructed to report and stop ambulation at the first suggestion of hip pain in order to prevent any further destruction. Long term corticosteroid therapy in children leads to a retardation of linear growth (Blodgett et al., 1956; see chapter XVI; sect. 14.3). Osteonecrosis of the femoral head has occurred as an infrequent long term complication of combination chemotherapy in lymphoma (Ihde and DeVita, 1975).

The tetracyclines are avid bone seekers, particularly for areas of new bone formation (Au and Raisz, 1972). Tooth discolouration and enamel hypoplasia following use of tetracyclines in pregnancy, the neonatal period and early childhood are discussed in chapter XIII (sect. 13.3). Tetracycline may also have a generalised effect on skeletal bone growth. Decreased linear growth of long bones can occur in premature infants treated with tetracyclines and effects on the fetal skeleton have also been noted following use of tetracycline in pregnancy (Cohlan et al., 1963). The effect on inhibition of bone growth is reversible if short courses of therapy have been given. It is not known whether permanent effects on skeletal growth result from long term administration.

Drugs used in the treatment of bone disease such as fluorides, diphosphonates and mithramycin, can themselves cause adverse effects on bone (Au and Raisz, 1972; Mundy and Raisz, 1974). Diphosphonates may lead to osteomalacia or rickets because they limit mineralisation of normal bone. Mithramycin can cause marked hypocalcaemia and should be reserved for resistant cases of severe hypercalcaemia due to increased bone resorption. Fluorides have complex effects on bone and chronic ingestion of excessive doses can lead to mottled teeth, osteosclerosis and 'crippling fluorosis'. Given alone in osteoporosis, fluoride can lead to osteomalacia, but this can be prevented by concomitant use of calcium and vitamin D (see further section 11.2, 11.3). Other disorders of calcium metabolism due to drugs are discussed in chapter XVI (sect. 15.5) and chapter XXI (sect. 15.4).

Further Reading

Hart, F.D.: Drug Treatment of the Rheumatic Diseases (ADIS Press, Sydney 1978).
Huskisson, E.C. and Hart, F.D.: Joint Diseases, 3rd ed (John Wright, Bristol 1978).
McCarthy, D.J.: Arthritis and Allied Conditions, 9th ed (Lea and Febiger, Philadelphia 1979).
Scott, J.T.: Textbook of the Rheumatic Diseases, 5th ed (Livingstone, Edinburgh 1978).

References

Aarbakke, J.: Clinical pharmacokinetics of phenylbutazone. Clinical Pharmacokinetics 3: 369 (1978).
Alarcon-Segovia, D.: Drug-induced lupus syndromes. Mayo Clinic Proceedings 44: 664 (1969).
Alarcon-Segovia, D.: Drug-induced antinuclear antibodies and lupus syndromes. Drugs 12: 69 (1976).
Alvan, G.; Orme, M.; Bertilsson, L.; Ekstrand, R. and Palmer, L.: Pharmacokinetics of indomethacin. Clinical Pharmacology and Therapeutics 18: 364 (1975).
Angevine, C.D. and Jacox, R.F.: Pseudogout in the elderly. Archives of Internal Medicine 131: 693 (1973).
Ansell, Barbara M.: Treatment of juvenile chronic polyarthritis. Clinics in Rheumatic Diseases 1: 443 (1975).
Ansell, Barbara M.: Juvenile chronic polyarthritis; in Hart (Ed) Drug Treatment of the Rheumatic Diseases, p.170 (ADIS Press, Sydney 1978).
Au, W.Y.W. and Raisz, L.G.: Drugs toxic to bone. Seminars in Drug Treatment 2: 137 (1972).
Aylward, M.; Maddock, J.; Wheeldon, R. and Parker, R.J.: A study of the influence of various antirheumatic drug regimens on serum acute-phase proteins, plasma tryptophan and erythrocyte sedimentation rate in rheumatoid arthritis. Rheumatology and Rehabilitation 14: 101 (1975).
Baber, N.; Halliday, L.; Sibeon, R.; Littler, T. and Orme, M.L'E.: The interaction between indomethacin and probenecid: A clinical and pharmacokinetic study. Clinical Pharmacology and Therapeutics 24: 298 (1978).
Bardare, M.; Cislaghi, G.U.; Mandelli, M. and Sereni, F.: Value of monitoring plasma salicylate levels in treating juvenile rheumatoid arthritis: observations in 42 cases. Archives of Disease in Childhood 53: 381 (1978).
Berry, H.; Fernandes, L.; Ford-Hutchinson, A.W.; Evans, S.J.W. and Hamilton, E.B.D.: Alclofenac and D-penicillamine. Annals of the Rheumatic Diseases 37: 93 (1978).
Billings, R.; Grahame, R.; Marks, V.; Wood, P.J. and Taylor, A.: Blood and urine gold levels during chrysotherapy for rheumatoid arthritis. Rheumatology and Rehabilitation 14: 13 (1975).
Blaschke, T.F.: Protein binding and kinetics of drugs in liver diseases. Clinical Pharmacokinetics 2: 32 (1977).
Blodgett, F.M.; Burgin, L.; Iezzoni, D.; Gribetz, D. and Talbot, N.B.: Effects of prolonged cortisone therapy on the statural growth, skeletal maturation and metabolic status of children. New England Journal of Medicine 254: 636 (1956).
Boardman, P.L. and Hart, F.D.: Clinical measurement of the anti-inflammatory effects of salicylates in rheumatoid arthritis. British Medical Journal 4: 264 (1967).
Boardman, P.J. and Hart, F.D.: Indomethacin in the treatment of acute gout. Practitioner 194: 560 (1965).
Boston Collaborative Drug Surveillance Program: Excess of ampicillin rashes associated with allopurinol or hyperuricaemia. New England Journal of Medicine 286: 505 (1972).
Bridgman, H.F.; Rosen, S.M. and Thorp, J.M.: Complications during clofibrate treatment of nephrotic syndrome hyperlipoproteinaemia. Lancet 2: 506 (1972).
Brogden, R.N.; Pinder, R.M.; Speight, T.M. and Avery, G.S.: Fenoprofen: A review of its pharmacological properties and therapeutic efficacy in rheumatic diseases. Drugs 13: 241 (1977a).
Brogden, R.N.; Pinder, R.M.; Speight, T.M. and Avery, G.S.: Fenoprofen: A review of its pharmacological properties and therapeutic efficacy in rheumatic diseases. Drugs 13: 241 (1977a).
Brogden, R.N.; Heel, R.C.; Speight, T.M. and Avery, G.S.: Sulindac: A review of its pharmacological properties and therapeutic efficacy in rheumatic diseases. Drugs 16: 97 (1978a).
Brogden, R.N.; Heel, R.C.; Speight, T.M. and Avery, G.S.: Sulindac: A review of its pharmacological properties and therapeutic efficacy in rheumatic diseases. Drugs 16: 97 (1978a).
Brogden, R.N.; Heel, R.C.; Speight, T.M. and Avery, G.S.: Tolmetin: A review of its pharmacological properties and therapeutic efficacy in rheumatic diseases. Drugs 15: 429 (1978b).

Brooks, P.M. and Buchanan, W.W.: in Buchanan and Dick (Eds) Recent Advances in Rheumatology, Part 2 (Churchill Livingstone, Edinburgh 1976).

Brooks, P.M.; Bell, M.A.; Sturrock, R.D.; Famaey, J.P. and Dick, W.C.: The clinical significance of indomethacin-probenecid interaction. British Journal of Clinical Pharmacology 1: 287 (1974).

Brooks, P.M.; Walker, J.J.; Bell, M.A.; Buchanan, W.W. and Thymer, A.R.: Indomethacin-aspirin interaction: a clinical appraisal. British Medical Journal 3: 69 (1975).

Brooks, M.H.; Bell, N.H.; Love, L.; Stern, P.H.; Orfei, E.; Queener, S.F.; Hamstra, A.J. and DeLuca, H.F.: Vitamin-D-dependent rickets type II. Resistance of target organs to 1,25-dihydroxyvitamin D. New England Journal of Medicine 298: 996 (1978).

Burns, J.J.; Rose, R.K.; Chenkin, T.; Goldman, A.; Schulert, A. and Brodie, B.: The physiological disposition of phenylbutazone (Butazolidin) in man and a method for its estimation in biological material. Journal of Pharmacology and Experimental Therapeutics 109: 346 (1953).

Bywaters, E.G.L.: The management of juvenile chronic polyarthritis. Bulletin on the Rheumatic Diseases 27: 882 (1976-1977).

Bywaters, E.G.L. and Thomas, G.T.: Bed rest, salicylate and steroid in rheumatic fever. British Medical Journal 1: 1628 (1961).

Castles, J.J.; Moore, T.L.; Vaughan, J.H.; Bolzan, J.A.; Lee, M.; Lidsky, M.D.; Caldwell, J.R.; Ehrlich, G.E.; Sharp, J.T. and Kaye, R.: Multicentre comparison of naproxen and indomethacin in rheumatoid arthritis. Archives of Internal Medicine 138: 362 (1978).

Chan, H.L.; Ku, G. and Khoo, O.T.: Allopurinol associated hypersensitivity reactions: cutaneous and renal manifestations. Australian and New Zealand Journal of Medicine 7: 518 (1977).

Chapel, T.A. and Burns, R.E.: Oral contraceptives and exacerbation of lupus erythematosus. American Journal of Obstetrics and Gynaecology 110: 366 (1971).

Christian, C.L.: Vasculitis syndromes; in Hart (Ed) Drug Treatment of the Rheumatic Diseases, p.147 (ADIS Press, Sydney 1978).

Cohlan, S.Q.; Bevelander, G. and Tiamsic, T.: Growth inhibition of prematures receiving tetracycline. American Journal of Diseases of Childhood 105: 453 (1963).

Constable, T.J.; Crockson, R.A.; Crockson, A.P. and McConkey, B.: Drug treatment of rheumatoid arthritis. Lancet 1: 1176 (1975).

Cooke, A.R.: Drugs and gastric damage. Drugs 11: 36 (1976).

Currey, H.L.F.; Harris, J.; Mason, R.M.; Woodland, J.; Beveridge, T.; Roberts, C.J.; Vere, D.W.; Dixon, A.St. J.; Davies, J. and Owen-Smith, B.: Comparison of azathioprine, cyclophosphamide, and gold in treatment of rheumatoid arthritis. British Medical Journal 3: 763 (1974).

Davies, E.F. and Avery, G.S.: Ibuprofen: A review of its pharmacological properties and therapeutic efficacy in rheumatic disorders. Drugs 2: 416 (1971).

Davies, D.M. and Lund, J.F.: Myalgia and an oral contraceptive. Lancet 2: 1187 (1965).

Decker, J.L.: Systemic lupus erythematosus. Contrasts and comparisons. Annals of Internal Medicine 82: 391 (1975).

Decker, J.L.; Klippel, J.H.; Plotz, P.H. and Steinberg, A.D.: Cyclophosphamide or azathioprine in lupus glomerulonephritis. A controlled trial: Results at 28 months. Annals of Internal Medicine 83: 606 (1975).

Dieterle, W.; Faigle, J.W.; Mory, H.; Richter, W.J. and Theobald, W.: Biotransformation and pharmacokinetics of sulphinpyrazone in man. European Journal of Clinical Pharmacology 9: 135 (1975).

Domenjoz, R.: The pharmacology of phenylbutazone analogues. Annals of the New York Academy of Sciences 86: 263 (1960).

Domenjoz, R.: Synthetic anti-inflammatory drugs: Concepts on their mode of action. Advances in Pharmacology 4: 143 (1966).

Duggan, D.E.; Hogans, A.F.; Kwan, K.C. and McMahon, F.G.: The metabolicm of indomethacin in man. Journal of Pharmacology and Experimental Therapeutics 181: 563 (1972).

Eddy, R.L.: Metabolic bone disease after gastrectomy. American Journal of Medicine 50: 442 (1971).

Editorial: Treatment of osteoporosis. British Medical Journal 1: 1303 (1978a).

Editorial: Ten years' treatment for Paget's disease. Lancet 1: 914 (1978b).

Elion, G.B.; Kovensky, A.; Hitchings, G.H.; Metz, E. and Rundles, R.W.: Metabolic studies of allopurinol, an inhibitor of xanthine oxidase. Biochemical Pharmacology 15: 863 (1966).

Elion, G.B.; Yu, T.F.; Gutman, A.B. and Hitchings, G.H.: Renal clearance of oxipurinol the chief metabolite of allopurinol. American Journal of Medicine 45: 69 (1968).

Emmerson, B.T.: Hyperuricaemia — To treat or not? Drugs 9: 141 (1975).

Emmerson, B.T.: Gout, uric acid and renal disease. Medical Journal of Australia 1: 403 (1976).

Emmerson, B.T.: Drug control of gout and hyperuricaemia. Drugs 16: 158 (1978).

Estes, D.: Clinical aspects of systemic lupus erythematosus, in Hughes (Ed) Modern Topics in Rheumatology, p.85 (Heinemann, London 1976).

Evans, J.A.P.: Oral penicillin in prophylaxis of streptococcal and rheumatic fever relapse. Proceedings of the Royal Society of Medicine 43: 206 (1950).

Fernandez-Herlihy, L.: Polymyalgia rheumatica. Seminars in Arthritis and Rheumatism 1: 236 (1972).

Fessel, W.J.: Hyperuricaemia in health and disease. Seminars in Arthritis and Rheumatism 1: 275 (1972).

Fessel, W.J.; Siegelaub, A.B. and Johnson, S.E.: Correlates and consequences of asymptomatic hyperuricaemia. Archives of Internal Medicine 132: 44 (1973).

Fitzgerald, R.H.: Intrasynovial injection of steroids. Mayo Clinic Proceedings 51: 655 (1976).

Fowler, P.D.: Marrow toxicity of the pyrazoles. Annals of the Rheumatic Diseases 26: 344 (1967).

Fowler, P.D. and Faragher, E.B.: Drug and non-drug factors influencing adverse reactions to pyrazoles. Journal of International Medical Research 5(Suppl. 2): 108 (1977).

Frame, B.; Guiang, H.L.; Frost, H.M. and Reynolds, W.A.: Osteomalacia induced by laxative (phenolphthalein) ingestion. Archives of Internal Medicine 128: 794 (1971).

Frisch, J.M.; Lovatt, G.E.; Sproit, A.R.M. and Turner, P.: The adverse reaction profile of allopurinol. Proceedings of the 12th International Congress of Internal Medicine 412 (1974).

Gibson, T.; Zaphiropoulos, G.; Grove, J.; Widdop, B. and Berry, D.: Kinetics of salicylate metabolism. British Journal of Clinical Pharmacology 2: 233 (1975).

Gibson, T.J.; Huskisson, E.C.; Wojtulewski, J.A.; Scott, P.J.; Balme, H.W.; Burry, H.C.; Grahame, R. and Hart, F.D.:

Evidence that D-penicillamine alters the course of rheumatoid arthritis. Rheumatology and Rehabilitation 15: 211 (1976).

Goldberg, A.A.J. and Tudor, R.: A seminar on fenclofenac. Proceedings of the Royal Society of Medicine 70(Suppl. 6): 1 (1977).

Gottlieb, N.L.: Chrysotherapy. Bulletin on the Rheumatic Diseases 27: 912 (1976-1977).

Gottlieb, N.L.; Smith, P.M. and Smith, E.M.: Pharmacodynamics of ^{197}Au and ^{197}Au labelled aurothiomalate in blood: Correlation with course of rheumatoid arthritis, gold toxicity and gold excretion. Arthritis and Rheumatism 17: 171 (1974).

Graham, G.G.; Champion, G.D.; Day, R.D. and Paull, P.D.: Patterns of plasma concentrations and urinary excretion of salicylate in rheumatoid arthritis. Clinical Pharmacology and Therapeutics 22: 410 (1977).

Griffith, G.C.; Nichols, G.; Asher, J. and Flanagan, B.: Heparin osteoporosis. Journal of the American Medical Association 193: 91 (1965).

Gumpel, J.M.: Irradiation of knee with yttrium 90: Results 3 years after treatment. Annals of Rheumatic Diseases 36: 285 (1977).

Gumpel, J.M.: Deaths associated with gold treatment: a reassessment. British Medical Journal 1: 215 (1978).

Haddad, J.G.: Paget's disease of bone: Problems and management. Orthopedic Clinics of North America 3: 775 (1972).

Hahn, T.J.: Bone complications of anticonvulsants. Drugs 12: 201 (1976).

Hall, A.P.; Barry, P.E.; Dawber, T.R. and McNamara, P.M.: Epidemiology of gout and hyperuricaemia. American Journal of Medicine 42: 27 (1967).

Hande, K.; Reed, E. and Chabner, B.: Allopurinol kinetics. Clinical Pharmacology and Therapeutics 23: 598 (1978).

Hart, F.D.: Pain in osteoarthrosis. Practitioner 212: 244 (1974a).

Hart, F.D.: Drug-induced arthritis. Current Medical Research and Opinion 2: 505 (1974b).

Hart, F.D.: Inflammatory disease and its control in rheumatic disorders. British Medical Journal 4: 191 (1975a).

Hart, F.D.: Visual complications of polymyalgia rheumatica (polymyalgia arteritica). Practitioner 215: 763 (1975b).

Hart, F.D.: Infective arthropathies; in Hart (Ed) Drug Treatment of the Rheumatic Diseases, p.162 (ADIS Press, Sydney 1978a).

Hart, F.D.: Drug Treatment of the Rheumatic Diseases (ADIS Press, Sydney 1978b).

Hart, F.D. and Bordman, P.L.: Indomethacin: a new non-steroid anti-inflammatory agent. British Medical Journal 2: 965 (1963).

Hart, F.D. and Boardman, P.L.: Indomethacin. Practitioner 192: 828 (1964).

Hart, F.D. and Huskisson, E.C.: Measurement in rheumatoid arthritis. Lancet 1: 28 (1972a).

Hart, F.D. and Huskisson, E.C.: Pain patterns in the rheumatic disorders. British Medical Journal 4: 213 (1972b).

Hart, F.D. and Matts, S.G.F.: Naproxen (Naprosyn) and gastrointestinal haemorrhage. British Medical Journal 2: 51 (1974).

Hart, F.D. and Emmerson, B.T.: Gout; in Hart (Ed) Drug Treatment of the Rheumatic Diseases p.117 (ADIS Press, Sydney 1978).

Hart, F.D.; Taylor, R.T. and Huskisson, E.C.: Pain at night. Lancet 1: 881 (1970).

Hart, F.D.; Huskisson, E.C. and Ansell, B.M.: Non-steroidal anti-inflammatory analgesics; in Hart (Ed) Drug Treatment of the Rheumatic Diseases, p.8 (ADIS Press, Sydney 1978).

Haslock, I.: Medical treatment of osteoarthrosis. Clinics in Rheumatic Diseases 2: 615 (1976).

Haynes, R.C.: Biochemical mechanisms of steroid effects in Azarnoff (Ed) Steroid Therapy, p.19 (Saunders, Philadelphia 1975).

Heel, R.C.; Brogden, R.N.; Speight, T.M. and Avery, G.S.: Benzbromarone: A review of its pharmacological properties and therapeutic use in gout and hyperuricaemia. Drugs 14: 349 (1977).

Horsman, A.; Gallagher, J.C.; Simpson, M. and Nordin, B.E.C.: Prospective trial of oestrogen and calcium in postmenopausal women. Brit. Med. J. 2: 789 (1977).

Huskisson, E.C.: Simple analgesic for arthritis. British Medical Journal 4: 196 (1974).

Huskisson, E.C.: Non-steroidal anti-imflammatory analgesics: Basic clinical pharmacology and therapeutic use. Drugs 15: 387 (1978a).

Huskisson, E.C.: Drugs which apparently affect the rheumatoid disease process; in Hart (Ed) Drug Treatment of the Rheumatic Diseases, p.44 (ADIS Press, Sydney 1978b).

Huskisson, E.C. and Hart, F.D.: Pain threshold and arthritis. British Medical Journal 4: 193 (1972).

Huskisson, E.C. and Hart, F.D.: Joint Disease, 3rd ed., p.15 (John Wright, Bristol 1978).

Huskisson, E.C.; Wojtulewski, J.A.; Berry, H.; Scott, Jane; Hart, F.D. and Balme, H.W.: Treatment of rheumatoid arthritis with fenoprofen: Comparison with aspirin. British Medical Journal 1: 176 (1974).

Huskisson, E.C.; Woolf, D.L.; Balme, H.W.; Scott, Jane and Franklyn, Sue: Four new anti-inflammatory drugs: responses and variations. British Medical Journal 1: 1048 (1976).

Ihde, D.C. and DeVita, V.T.: Osteonecrosis of the femoral head in patients with lymphoma treated with intermittent combination chemotherapy (including corticosteroids). Cancer 36: 1585 (1975).

Ingham, J.: Osteoporosis: Diagnosis and treatment. Drugs 8: 290 (1974).

Inman, W.H.: Study of fatal bone marrow depression with special reference to phenylbutazone and oxyphenbutazone. British Medical Journal 1: 1500 (1977).

Jayson, M.I.V.: Back pain, spondylosis and disc disorders; in Scott (Ed) Copeman's Textbook of the Rheumatic Diseases, p.960 (Churchill Livingstone, Edinburgh 1978).

Jenkins, L.C. and McGraw, R.W.: Anaesthetic management of the patient with rheumatoid arthritis. Canadian Anaesthetists' Society Journal 16: 407 (1969).

Joint Report: The evolution of rheumatic heart disease in children. Five year report of a co-operative clinical trial of ACTH, cortisone and aspirin. A joint report by the Rheumatic Fever Working Party of the Medical Research Council of Great Britain and the Subcommittee of Principal Investigators of the American Council on Rheumatic Fever and Congenital Heart Disease, American Heart Association. Circulation 22: 503 (1960).

Jowsey, J.; Riggs, B.L.; Kelly, P.J. and Hoffman, D.L.: Effect of combined therapy with sodium fluoride, vitamin D and calcium in osteoporosis. American Journal of Medicine 53: 43 (1972).

Katz, S.L.: Experience with rubella vaccines in the USA, 1969-1971. Scandinavian Journal of Infectious Diseases 6(Suppl.): 14 (1972).

Kijima, Y.; Sasaoka, T.; Kanayama, M. and Kubota, S.: Untoward effects of clofibrate in hemodialyzed patients. New England Journal of Medicine 296: 515 (1977).

Klineberg, J.R. and Miller, R.: Effect of corticosteroids on blood salicylate concentrations. Journal of the American Medical Association 194: 601 (1965).

Kuehl, F.A.; Egan, R.W.; Humes, J.L.; Beverage, G.C. and van Arman, C.G.: Biochemical Aspects of Prostaglandins and Thromboxanes, p.55 (Academic Press, New York 1977).

Kunze, M.; Stein, G.; Kunze, E. and Traeger, A.: Zur Pharmakokinetik von Indomethazin in Abhangigkeit vom Lebensalter, bei Patienten mit Gallenwegsverschluβ, Nierenfunktionseinschrankung und Unvertraglichkeitsercheinungen. Deutsche Gesundheitwesen 29: 351 (1974).

Kwan, K.C.; Breault, G.O.; Umbenhauer, E.R.; McMahon, F.G. and Duggan, D.E.: Kinetics of indomethacin absorption, elimination, and enterohepatic circulation in man. Journal of Pharmacokinetics and Biopharmaceutics 4: 255 (1976).

Lelievre, G.; Raviart, B.; Lepoutre, E. and Tacquet, A.: Acute renal failure during the administration of a hypo-uricaemic diuretic: tienilic acid. Nouvelle Presse Medicale 7: 2654 (1978).

Levy, G. and Tsuchiya, T.: Salicylate accumulation kinetics in man. New England Journal of Medicine 287: 430 (1972).

Levy, G.; Lampman, T.; Kamath, B.L. and Garrettson, L.K.: Decreased serum salicylate concentrations in children with rheumatic fever treated with antacid. New England Journal of Medicine 293: 323 (1975).

Lim, R.K.S.: Salicylate analgesia; in Smith and Smith (Eds) The Salicylates: A Critical Bibliographic Review (Wiley, New York 1966).

Lindsay, R.; Hart, D.M.; MacLean, A.; Clark, A.C.; Kraszewski, A. and Garwood, J.: Bone response to treatment of oestrogen treatment. Lancet 1: 1325 (1978).

Lorber, A.: Monitoring gold plasma levels in rheumatoid arthritis. Clinical Pharmacokinetics 2: 127 (1977).

Lorber, A.; Atkins, C.J.; Chang, C.C.; Lee, Y.B.; Starrs, J. and Bovy, R.A.: Monitoring serum gold values in rheumatoid arthritis. Annals of Rheumatic Diseases 32: 133 (1973).

Lotz, M.; Ney, R. and Bartter, F.C.: Osteomalacia and debility resulting from phosphorus depletion. Transactions of the Association of American Physicians 77: 281 (1964).

Lyle, W.H. and Kleiman, R.L. (Eds): Penicillamine at 21: Its place in therapeutics now. Proceedings of the Royal Society of Medicine 70: Suppl. 3 (1977).

McQueen, E.G.: Anti-inflammatory drug mechanisms. Drugs 6: 104 (1973).

Makela, A.-L.; Yrjana, T. and Haapasaari, J.: Dosage of salicylates for children with juvenile rheumatoid arthritis, a preliminary report. Scandinavian Journal of Rheumatology 4: 250 (1975).

Manuel, M.A. and Steele, T.H.: Changes in renal urate handling after prolonged thiazide treatment. American Journal of Medicine 57: 741 (1974).

Marshall, D.H. and Nordin, B.E.C.: The effect of 1α-hydroxyvitamin D3 with and without oestrogen on calcium balance in post-menopausal women. Clinical Endocrinology 7: 159S (1977).

Mitchell, W.S.; Brooks, P.M.; Stevenson, R.D. and Buchanan, W.W.: Septic arthritis in patients with rheumatoid disease: a still underdiagnosed complication. Journal of Rheumatology 3: 124 (1976).

Moldofsy, H. and Rothman, A.I.: Personality, disease parameters and medication in rheumatoid arthritis. Journal of Chronic Diseases 24: 363 (1971).

Mongan, E.; Kelly, P.; Nies, K.; Porter, W.W. and Paulus, H.E.: Tinnitus as an indication of therapeutic serum salicylate levels. Journal of the American Medical Association 226: 142 (1973).

Morley, J.: Proceedings of the Aspirin Symposium, p.19 (Royal College of Surgeons, London 1975).

Mosekilde, L.; Melsen, F.; Christensen, M.S.; Lund, B. and Sørensen, O.H.: Effect of long-term vitamin D_2 treatment on bone morphometry and biochemical values in anticonvulsant osteomalacia. Acta Medica Scandinavica 201: 303 (1977).

Mowat, A.G.: Surgical management of rheumatoid arthritis. Clinics in Rheumatic Diseases 4: 249 (1978).

Mowat, A.G. and Hazleman, B.L.: Polymyalgia rheumatica — a clinical study with particular reference to arterial disease. Journal of Rheumatology 1: 190 (1974).

Mundy, G.R. and Raisz, L.G.: Drugs for disorders of bone. Drugs 8: 250 (1974).

Mustard, J.F. and Packham, M.A.: Platelets, thrombosis and drugs. Drugs 9: 19 (1975).

Myles, A.B.: Polymyalgia rheumatica and giant cell arteritis. A seven-year survey. Rheumatology and Rehabilitation 14: 231 (1975).

Nordin, B.E.C.; Wilkinson, R.; Marshall, D.H.; Gallagher, J.C.; Williams, A. and Peacock, M.: Calcium absorption in the elderly. Calcified Tissue Research 21(Suppl.): 442 (1976).

Nuki, G.: Gout and purine metabolism in Hughes (Ed) Modern Topics in Rheumatology, p.164 (Heinemann, London 1976).

Paulus, H.E. and Whitehouse, M.W.: Nonsteroid anti-inflammatory agents. Annual Review of Pharmacology 13: 107 (1973).

Paulus, H.E.; Siegel, M.; Mongan, E.; Okun, R. and Calabro, J.J.: Variations of serum concentrations and half-life of salicylate in patients with rheumatoid arthritis. Arthritis and Rheumatism 14: 527 (1971).

Pearson, C.M. and Levy, J.: Immunosuppressive drugs: Mechanism of action, toxicity and clinical effects. Clinics of Rheumatic Diseases 1: 459 (1975).

Perel, J.M.; Dayton, P.G.; Snell, M.M.; Yu, T-F. and Gutman, A.B.: Studies of interactions among drugs in man at the renal level: Probenecid and sulphinpyrazone. Clinical Pharmacology and Therapeutics 10: 834 (1969).

Pinder, R.M.; Brogden, R.N.; Sawyer, P.R.; Speight, T.M.; Spencer, R. and Avery, G.S.: Carbenoxolone: A review of its pharmacological properties and therapeutic efficacy in peptic ulcer disease. Drugs 11: 245 (1976).

Polley, H.F.: Evolution of steroids and their value in the control of rheumatic disease. Mayo Clinic Proceedings 45: 1 (1970).

Popert, A.J.: Chloroquine: A review. Rheumatology and Rehabilitation 15: 235 (1976).

Powell, R.H. and Ansell, B.M.: Benorylate in the management of Still's disease. British Medical Journal 1: 145 (1974).

Proceedings of the ARA Conference on the Rheumatic Diseases of Childhood: Arthritis and Rheumatism 20(Suppl.): 510 (Mar 1977).

Ragab, A.H.; Frech, R.S. and Vietti, T.J.: Osteoporotic fractures secondary to methotrexate therapy of acute leukaemia in remission. Cancer 25: 580 (1970).

Rastegar, A. and Thier, S.O.: The physiologic approach to hyperuricaemia. New Engl. J. Med. 286: 470 (1972).

Richens, A. and Rowe, D.J.F.: Disturbance of calcium metabolism by anticonvulsant drugs. British Medical Journal 3: 73 (1970).

Rothermich, N.O.; Philips, V.K.; Bergen, W. and Thomas, M.H.: Chrysotherapy. A prospective study. Arthritis and Rheumatism 19: 1321 (1976).

Royal College of General Practitioners' Oral Contraception Study: Reduction in incidence of rheumatoid arthritis associated with oral contraceptives. Lancet 1: 569 (1978).

Rundles, R.W.; Wyngaarden, J.B.; Hitchings, G.H.; Elion, G.B. and Silberman, H.R.: Effects of a xanthine oxidase inhibitor on thiopurine metabolism, hyperuricaemia and gout. Transactions of the Association of American Physicians 76: 126 (1963).

Saville, P.D.: Osteoporosis and corticoid drugs. Annals of Internal Medicine 73: 1038 (1970).

Schneeweis, J. and Poole, G.W.: Hyperuricaemia due to pyrazinamide. British Medical Journal 2: 830 (1960).

Siegel, R.C.: Scleroderma. Medical Clinics of North America 61: 283 (1977).

Sonnenblick, M. and Abraham, A.S.: Ibuprofen hypersensitivity in systemic lupus erythematosus. British Medical Journal 1: 619 (1978).

Spiera, H. and Plotz, C.M.: Rheumatic symptoms and oral contraceptives. Lancet 1: 571 (1969).

Stein, G.; Kunze, M.; Zaumseil, J. and Traeger, A.: Zur Pharmacokinetik von Indomethazin und Indomethazin-metaboliten bei wiederholter Applikation an nierengesunden und nierengeschadigten Patienten. International Journal of Clinical Pharmacology 15: 470 (1977).

Symposium on Ketoprofen: Rheumatology and Rehabilitation Suppl. 1: (1976a).

Symposium: Recent advances in rheumatology: A review and clinical assessment of azapropazone. Current Medical Research and Opinion 4(Suppl. 1): 3 (1976b).

Symposium: Diclofenac sodium: Antirheumatic, anti-inflammatory, and analgesic agent. Pharmacological, pharmacokinetic and clinical studies. Scandinavian Journal of Rheumatology Suppl. 22 (1978).

Talbott, J.H.: Surgical treatment in rheumatology. Seminars in Arthritis and Rheumatism 1: 1 (1971).

Tenney, S.M. and Miller, R.M.: The respiratory and circulatory actions of salicylate. American Journal of Medicine 19: 498 (1955).

Urmon, J.D. and Rothfield, N.F.: Corticosteroid treatment in systemic lupus erythematosus. Journal of the American Medical Association 238: 2272 (1977).

Vane, J.R.: in Robinson and Vane (Eds) Prostaglandin Synthetase Inhibitors, p.159 (Raven Press, New York 1974).

Vessel, E.S.; Passananti, G.T. and Johnson, Alice, O.: Failure of indomethacin and warfarin to interact in normal human volunteers. Journal of Clinical Pharmacology 15: 486 (1975).

Vischer, T.L. et al.: Levamisole in rheumatoid arthritis. A randomised double-blind study comparing two dosage regimens of levamisole with placebo. Lancet 2: 1007 (1978).

Wallace, S.L.: Colchicine. Seminars in Arthritis and Rheumatism 3: 369 (1974).

Weissmann, G. and Thomas, L.: The effects of corticosteroids upon connective tissue and lysosomes. Recent Progress in Hormone Research 20: 215 (1964).

Westbury, G.: The management of pain in incurable malignant disease in Hart (Ed) The Treatment of Chronic Pain, p.97 (MTP, Lancaster 1974).

Wild, J.H. and Zvaifler, N.J.: Hemarthrosis associated with sodium warfarin therapy. Arthritis and Rheumatism 19: 98 (1976).

Woosley, R.L.; Drayer, D.E.; Reidenberg, M.M.; Nies, A.S.; Carr, K. and Oates, J.A.: Effect of acetylator phenotype on the rate at which procainamide induces antinuclear antibodies and the lupus syndrome. New England Journal of Medicine 298: 1157 (1978).

Yu, T-F.; Dayton, P.G. and Gutman, A.B.: Mutual suppression of the uricosuric effects of sulfinpyrazone and salicylate: A study in interactions between drugs. Journal of Clinical Investigation 42: 1330 (1963).

Chapter XXIII
Haematological Disorders

M. Verstraete and R. Verwilghen

Synopsis of Important Principles

1) The basic aim of antithrombotic and thrombolytic drug therapy in thromboembolic disorders is to reduce morbidity and mortality. In some situations (e.g. myocardial infarction) the therapeutic gain is real but small. In others (e.g. pulmonary embolism) the drugs, while being highly effective, sometimes may not be able to be given soon enough or may not act quickly enough.

2) The benefit from antithrombotic drugs in the treatment of thrombosis and embolism is greater and better documented in the venous than in the arterial circulation. Anticoagulant therapy is primarily prophylactic and can only prevent deposition of a thrombus or limit its extension and fragmentation (embolisation). Thrombolytic drugs, if given early enough, can hasten the lysis of preformed thrombi. Agents affecting platelet function, when used in certain combinations, are of potential use in attempts to prevent thrombus formation in the arterial and venous circulation.

3) Despite the availability of effective prophylactic therapy for venous thrombosis, considerable emphasis must still be placed on the recognition of thrombosis-prone patients, and on early diagnosis and prompt treatment of established deep vein thrombosis.

4) Effective and safe use of oral anticoagulant drugs depends on careful regulation of the intensity of pharmacological response, the margin between adequate therapy and haemorrhage being relatively narrow. Dosage varies from patient to patient and depends not only on individual differences in rate of elimination, but also on the numerous factors affecting vitamin K availability or clotting factor synthesis and which can influence the response or increase the risk of complications.

5) The treatment of a patient with a defect of the haemostatic mechanism is very specific and is determined by the type of abnormality and its pathogenesis. Accurate diagnosis is essential. In every anaemic patient, a correct diagnosis must precede the use of haematinics, with identification and elimination, if possible, of any underlying cause. There is no place for 'shot gun' therapy.

6) Some drugs can increase the risk of haematological complications when used in patients with disorders of the blood — for example aspirin in those with bleeding disorders or in those on anticoagulants, co-trimoxazole in those with megaloblastic anaemia.

7) The haematopoietic system is particularly sensitive to the action of drugs and many drugs are regularly associated with idiosyncratic haematological reactions in susceptible individuals. Bleeding disorders and coagulation disturbances are not infrequently caused by drugs.

Disorders of the blood are of major importance in therapeutics. This is not only because of the high morbidity and mortality associated with conditions like thromboembolic occlusive vascular disease and blood dyscrasias such as aplastic anaemia, but also because they illustrate more than any other area of medicine, the application of clinical pharmacological principles to individualisation of therapy. This is possible not only because the blood is an easily sampled tissue and individualised therapy is necessary for effective treatment, but also because excessive drug effects on the blood can be disastrous.

1. Clinical Pharmacological Considerations

Drugs used in haematological diseases include agents for the management of haemorrhagic disease, anaemias and white cell disorders, and drugs for the prevention and treatment of thromboembolic disorders. An understanding of the pathophysiology of haemostasis is fundamental to the individualised therapy of both haemorrhagic disease and thromboembolic disorders, and awareness of the clinical pharmacological factors which can modify the response of antithrombotic drugs is essential in the control of anticoagulant therapy.

1.1 Haemostasis and Thrombosis

Physiological haemostasis, or the spontaneous arrest of bleeding, takes place following the severing of a blood vessel and results in the formation of a haemostatic plug and is largely extravascular. Thrombosis occurs most readily where there is local damage to the vascular endothelium and slowing of the blood flow, and results in the formation of an intravascular thrombus. Haemostasis and thrombosis are generally considered to be similar processes and although formation of a haemostatic plug and a thrombus are not identical, a platelet-fibrin mass is common to both formations (fig. 1).

1.1.1 Haemostatic Mechanism

Blood loss after injury is minimised by a complex series of inter-related reactions involving vascular constriction (transient and probably of relatively minor importance), the production of a platelet plug, and the formation of fibrin through the coagulation mechanism.

Platelet Function: The co-ordinated series of events leading to the formation of a haemostatic platelet plug essentially involve: (a) contact of blood with a surface other than normal endothelium, such as collagen or some types of basement membrane; (b) a platelet adhesion-aggregation reaction to form a platelet plug to seal the breech in the vessel wall; and (c) via activation of the coagulation mechanism, generation of thrombin and formation of fibrin to reinforce the platelet plug (see Mustard and Packham, 1975, 1977; Weiss, 1975a). Although aggregation of platelets and formation of a platelet plug is sufficient to effect haemostasis in injured venules and capillaries, the higher rate of blood flow in larger vessels necessitates the formation of fibrin to reinforce the platelet aggregate and form an efficient haemostatic plug at the site of injury (fig. 1a). During organisation of the platelet-fibrin mass recanalisation of the vessel may occur.

Platelet adhesion and aggregation can be affected by several types of drug, but the clinical use of most is still largely investigational (see section 3.1).

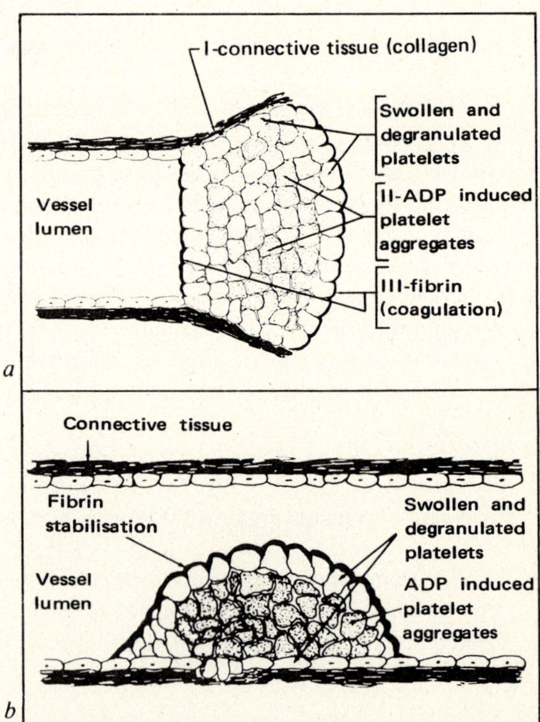

Fig. 1. Diagrammatic representation of: (a) haemostatic plug; (b) thrombus (after Mustard and Packham: Drugs 9: 19, 1975; by permission of authors and editor).

Coagulation Mechanism: The coagulation mechanism depends on the conversion of the soluble protein fibrinogen to insoluble fibrin, through the action of thrombin (for review, see Bennett and Douglas, 1973; Esnouf, 1977; Ogston and Bennett, 1978). Free thrombin is not present in normal circulating blood, but may be formed from its circulating precursor prothrombin through two principal mechanisms, the intrinsic (blood) and extrinsic (tissue) activating pathways of coagulation. Both pathways are thought to involve a series of reactions in which an enzyme precursor is converted to its active form in sequence, the activated form then converting the next enzyme precursor in the sequence to its active state. The precise sequence of reactions is not finally established, but a widely accepted scheme is presented diagrammatically in figure 2.

The components of the intrinsic system are all present within the blood and are activated by injury to blood vessels or by contact of the blood with a foreign surface (e.g. prosthetic heart valve) or even with modified endothelium. When extravascular injury occurs and the vascular endothelium is disrupted, blood comes in contact with tissue and the extrinsic pathway of coagulation is initiated. It needs both tissue and plasma clotting factors. These react to form a complex capable of converting prothrombin to thrombin, with the eventual formation, via the splitting of fibrinogen, of an insoluble and firm clot composed of not yet stable fibrin strands, platelets and enmeshed cells, which is haemostatically efficient. A further enzymatic step reinforces the fibrin, which becomes more stable.

Some of the blood clotting factors (prothrombin, VII, IX and X) require vitamin K for their synthesis in the liver and their formation is inhibited by oral anticoagulant drugs (see section 3.2.2). Several plasma clotting factors participating in the extrinsic system are measured for the control of anticoagulant therapy (see section 3.5). Naturally occurring inhibitors of the coagulation mechanism have a role in physiological haemostasis, and one of these, antithrombin III (an α_2-globulin) the natural inhibitor of activated factor X, is influenced by low doses of heparin (see section 3.2.1). Heparin complexes with antithrombin III in plasma, markedly potentiating the rate of its serine protease neutralising activity (Rosenberg, 1975); activated factors XII, XI, X, IX and thrombin have a serine active centre. Certain snake venoms catalyse removal of fibrinopeptide A from

fibrinogen (and not both the peptides A and B as thrombin does) and thus affect the coagulation mechanism by depleting plasma fibrinogen (Ewart et al., 1969; see section 3.2.3). The fibrin monomer so formed is then removed by the fibrinolytic enzyme system.

Fibrinolytic Enzyme System: The precise physiological function of the fibrinolytic enzyme system has not been established but it is probably complementary to the coagulation mechanism in view of its proposed action of limiting the persistence of unwanted fibrin (fig. 2; for review, see Kernoff and McNicol, 1977; Schmutzler and Koller, 1969). The system also has the potential to dissolve fibrin deposits and various approaches have been made to develop drugs which stimulate natural fibrinolysis (see section 3.4) or which lyse preformed thrombi (see section 3.3). Agents which inhibit fibrinolytic activity (fig. 2) have also been developed for use in management of haemorrhagic disorders (see section 5.4).

The basis of the system is the formation of a rather specific proteolytic enzyme, plasmin, from an inactive precursor termed plasminogen. Physiological activation of the system, is achieved by natural activators of plasminogen which can be found in the blood, in body fluids, in tissues (except the liver) and in platelets.

Inhibitors of the fibrinolytic enzyme system may act at the stage of activation of plasminogen (either by inhibiting activators or on the process of activation) or on formed plasmin. The principal circulating antiplasmins which have been characterised are antiplasmin to which plasmin is preferentially bound, α_1-antitrypsin and α_2-macroglobulin, which neutralises plasmin once the antiplasmin is saturated, but there are others, such as C'1 esterase inhibitor (Collen, 1976). In plasma there is more antiplasmin activity ($10\mu M$) than potential plasmin (plasminogen $1\mu M$). Rarely, when plasmin is formed rapidly in excess of the ability of antiplasmins to neutralise it, does hyperplasminaemia occur (e.g. in certain patients with cirrhosis, prostatic carcinoma and metastases, after major thoracic surgery), but it is a potential problem during thrombolytic therapy (sect. 3.3). Hyperplasminaemia results in degradation of fibrinogen and other coagulation factors as a consequence of the proteolytic activity of plasmin. If the effect is sustained severe bleeding may result.

The mechanism of action of the fibrinolytic enzyme system is not finally established (see

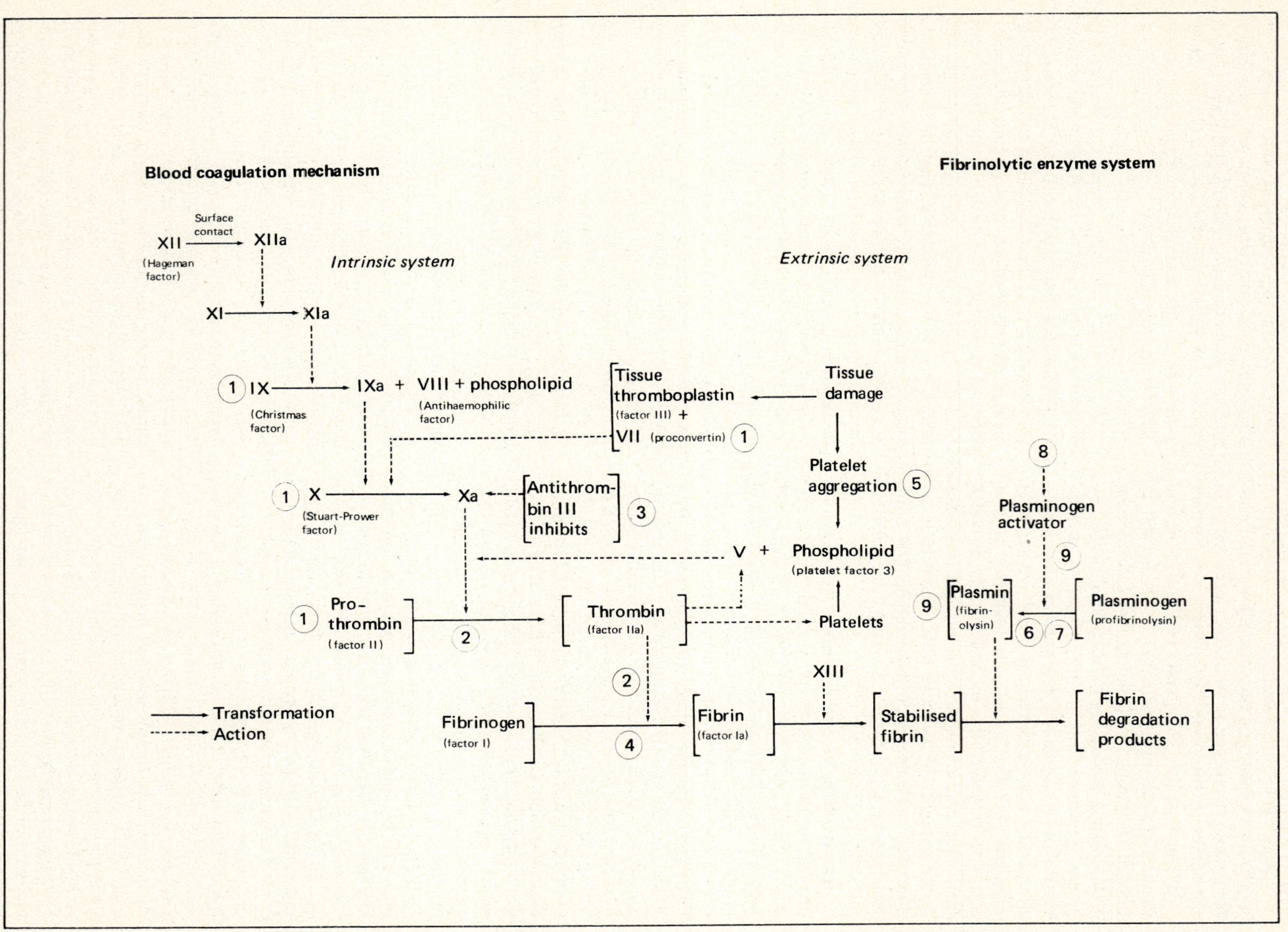

Blood coagulation mechanism
Fibrinolytic enzyme system
Intrinsic system
Extrinsic system
XII
(Hageman factor)
Surface contact
XIIa
XI
XIa
1 IX
(Christmas factor)
IXa + VIII + phospholipid
(Antihaemophilic factor)
Tissue thromboplastin
(factor III) +
VII (proconvertin) 1
Tissue damage
Platelet aggregation 5
1 X
(Stuart-Prower factor)
Xa
Antithrombin III inhibits 3
V + Phospholipid
(platelet factor 3)
Platelets
1 Pro-thrombin
(factor II)
2
Thrombin
(factor IIa)
2
8
Plasminogen activator
9
9 Plasmin
(fibrin-olysin)
6 7
Plasminogen
(profibrinolysin)
Transformation
Action
Fibrinogen
(factor I)
4
Fibrin
(factor Ia)
XIII
Stabilised fibrin
Fibrin degradation products

Brogden et al., 1973; Verstraete, 1978b), but most evidence favours the view that plasminogen activator and plasminogen which are adsorbed onto fibrin during clotting, rather than plasmin-antiplasmin complexes, has the major role in induced thrombolysis. The occurrence of systemic fibrinolysis depends on depletion of the circulating antiplasmin pool (Wiman and Collen, 1978).

1.1.2 Intravascular Thrombosis

Intravascular thrombosis probably requires the participation of platelets and activation of the coagulation mechanism (fig. 1b), but in view of the difference in structure of arterial and venous thrombi, the relative roles of platelet adhesion and aggregation and fibrin formation seem to differ, depending on whether the vascular occlusion occurs in the arterial or venous system. The major difference is the presence of endothelial damage and a high rate of blood flow in arteries, as opposed to the less prominent endothelial damage and low rate of blood flow in the venous system (Sevitt, 1969, 1974; Mustard and Packham, 1970).

Structure of Thrombi: Venous thrombi are composed of a small platelet head with a large tail consisting mainly of fibrin and entrapped red cells (i.e. red thrombus) and the structure closely resembles that of a blood coagulum formed under static conditions in a test tube. Arterial thrombi are composed of a large platelet head surrounded by leucocytes and a small fibrin tail with few entrapped red cells (i.e. white thrombus) but as they grow to occlusive proportions, local stasis occurs and a fibrin mesh with entrapped red cells is more readily formed and results in a fibrin mass over a period of days. Despite these structural differences, it is not known whether venous thrombosis starts with the formation of a small platelet nidus, which then activates the coagulation mechanism by the altered platelet surface, or whether the activation of the coagulation mechanism with minute amounts of thrombin formation is independent of platelet adhesion and aggregation. Platelet aggregates in the turbulence of valve pockets of veins may be involved initially (Paterson, 1969), but since fibrin rather than platelets forms the major part of venous thrombi, blood coagulation is likely to be the predominant mechanism. In the arterial system however, the major part in initiation of the thrombus does appear to be played by platelets since arterial thrombi consist principally of a platelet mass at a site of vascular injury (Mustard and Packham, 1975, 1978; White and Heptinstall, 1978). Thus, in the case of arterial thrombi related to atheromatous plaques or to autoimmune reactions (e.g. after organ transplantation), presumably platelets adhere to the damaged or modified endothelium of the vessel wall and initiate thrombosis.

Both venous and arterial thrombi can be detached and carried onward in the blood stream and are of importance in major veins, when pulmonary embolism results.

Fig. 2. Diagrammatic representation (simplified) of the human blood coagulation mechanism and fibrinolytic enzyme system. For clarity, the role of calcium in the activation reactions of coagulation factors is not included in this diagram. Calcium is not required for the activation of factor XII and for action on factor XI.

Anticoagulants

1. Coumarin and indanedione anticoagulants — reduce the activity of vitamin K dependent clotting factors II, VII, IX and X.
2. Heparin — inhibits the generation and activity of thrombin.
3. Low dose heparin — increases the activity of antithrombin III and potentiates this naturally occurring plasma inhibitor of activated factor X, IX, XI, XII and of plasmin.
4. Ancrod — converts fibrinogen to an unstable form of fibrin, the plasma fibrinogen level being markedly reduced.

Antiplatelet agents

5. Drugs which inhibit some platelet functions (e.g. aspirin, indomethacin, sulphinpyrazone, dipyridamole, ?dextran).

Thrombolytic agents

6. Streptokinase — activates plasminogen to form plasmin indirectly (via the formation of an activator complex with plasminogen or plasmin).
7. Urokinase — activates plasminogen to form plasmin directly.

Fibrinolytic stimulants

8. Ethyloestrenol, stanozolol + phenformin — enhance plasma fibrinolytic activity (possibly by increasing activator content of the walls of veins).

Antifibrinolytic agents

9. ε-Aminocaproic acid, tranexamic acid, aprotinin — competitively inhibit plasminogen activation and non-competitively inhibit plasmin; aprotinin also has vasoactive properties.

Composition of Thrombi and Drug Action:
Drugs available for the management of thromboembolic disorders include those which may prevent the deposition of fibrin (anticoagulant drugs), promote an increased rate of removal of deposited fibrin (thrombolytic drugs) or prevent deposition of platelets (antiplatelet drugs). On theoretical grounds it might seem more logical to use anticoagulant drugs to prevent venous thrombosis and antiplatelet agents for prophylaxis of arterial thrombosis, and in part this seems to be borne out in clinical practice. Thus, anticoagulants have a limited clinical effect on the predominantly platelet-rich arterial thrombi, in contrast to their significant effect on the fibrin mass of venous thrombi and pulmonary emboli (see section 3.2; 4). Oral drugs affecting platelet function when used in combination and in appropriate doses have been shown to prevent postoperative deep vein thrombosis, and when used with anticoagulants to be effective in reducing the incidence of arterial thromboembolism in patients with a substitute valve, and when used alone in preventing closure of artificial vessels such as arteriovenous shunts. Aspirin, but not other antiplatelet drugs given alone, can reduce cerebral ischaemia and mortality in patients with cerebrovascular disease. Platelet function among other changes in the blood, is also affected when dextran is infused and dextran has been shown to be effective in the prevention of postoperative deep vein thrombosis (see sections 3.1; 4).

The age and site of thrombus formation are major factors in the outcome of therapy with the thrombolytic agents. Thus, recently formed thrombi are more easily lysed than thrombi of more than 6 to 7 days duration, which may be partially or completely resistant to lysis. In general, venous thrombi are easier to lyse than arterial thrombi, and those in the limbs respond better than those elsewhere (Brogden et al., 1973).

An ideal scheme of indications for the various types of antithrombotic drug based on the putative phases of thrombus formation and dissolution is given in figure 3.

1.2 Factors Influencing Anticoagulant Therapy

Numerous clinical and pharmacological factors influence the choice of and response to anticoagulants and are particularly important in view of the risk of haemorrhage from poorly controlled

therapy or from a changed response to previously stable therapy. The dosage of anticoagulants must be individualised. Differences exist in the pharmacokinetic properties between oral anticoagulant compounds and these differences influence both the selection of an oral agent and its use (see sections 3.2.2 to 3.2.6).

1.3 Haematopoiesis

Constant levels of erythrocytes, leucocytes and thrombocytes (platelets) are necessary for adequate blood formation but are only maintained if their production and destruction are in equilibrium. The body is unable to influence significantly the loss or destruction of these elements and has to regulate, within a narrow margin, the production of cells according to its needs. Haematopoiesis is regulated by a feedback system in which different hormones, the 'poietins' are responsible for the

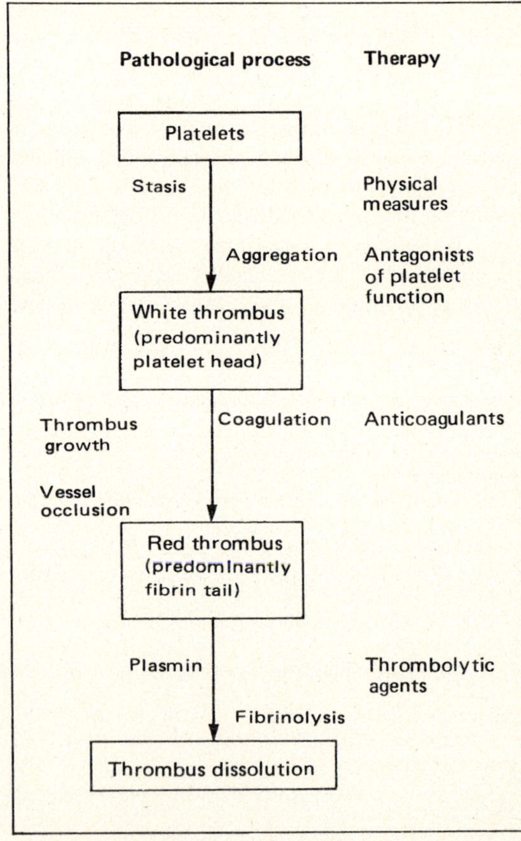

Fig. 3. Therapeutic approaches corresponding to putative phases of thrombus formation and dissolution (after Marder: Medical Clinics of North America 58: 1121, 1974; by permission of author and editor).

modulation of the haematopoietic response. A sufficient haematopoietic stem cell pool and a normal bone marrow stroma are essential for an adequate haematopoietic response. The haematopoietic system, as one of the metabolically most active tissues of the adult, has appreciable needs. Dietary factors, particularly iron, vitamin B_{12} and folate, are important for normal haematopoiesis.

A large number of drugs can adversely affect the blood (see section 8). Haematopoietic tissues are one of the rare organs where, even in adults, high mitotic activity persists. This makes the haematopoietic system particularly sensitive to agents interfering with DNA synthesis and mitosis. The erythrocyte is an enucleated structure, particularly well adapted to haemoglobin and oxygen transport. This makes the red cells sensitive to oxidation and unable to synthesise enzymes needed to counteract this aggression. All blood cells are in intimate contact with plasma, plasma immunoglobulins and complement, and are thus exposed to immune destruction by drugs.

1.4 Anaemias and Drug Disposition

Anaemias may alter drug disposition, apparently as a consequence of changes in distribution. Iron deficiency anaemia tends to increase the distribution volume and increase the plasma clearance of antipyrine (Langman and Smithard, 1977). Similar changes in antipyrine distribution and elimination rate occur in patients with thalassaemia major (Rifkind et al., 1976), and with both antipyrine and more noticeably phenylbutazone, a highly protein bound drug, in patients with sickle cell anaemia (Anderson et al., 1977). Response to enzyme inducing drugs is normal in sickle cell anaemia. Low haemoglobin levels, for unknown reasons, can increase the duration of thiopentone anaesthesia (Dundee, 1956).

2. General Principles of Treatment

Rational treatment of haematological disorders is based on an accurate diagnosis, individualisation of therapy, and with antithrombotic drugs, on an awareness of the many factors which can modify the response to therapy or increase the risk of complications.

1) *Correct diagnosis* — effective treatment of haemorrhagic disorders and anaemias requires ac-

curate diagnosis so that highly specific treatment can be given or the causative factor removed or treated (see section 5, 6).

2) *Early diagnosis* — in thromboembolic disorders, screening techniques are important to identify potential thrombi in patients at risk of postoperative deep vein thrombosis (see section 4.6). Early and accurate diagnosis is vital to the success of treatment in pulmonary embolism (see section 4.5).

Early detection of drug induced blood dyscrasias can be crucial to the chance of success of initial therapy (e.g. aplastic anaemia) or recovery (e.g. phenothiazine agranulocytosis).

3) *Prevention* — since aplastic anaemia and severe episodes of acute haemolytic anaemia carry a poor prognosis and there is no effective treatment, drugs which are known to cause these reactions should not be used for trivial indications or in patients known to be at risk (see section 8).

4) *Basic aim* — the basic premise of antithrombotic therapy in thromboembolic disorders is to reduce or prevent morbidity and mortality. In some cases the therapeutic gains are real but small (e.g. anticoagulants in myocardial infarction; see section 4.1), while in others they are significant (e.g. acute major pulmonary embolism).

5) *Individualised therapy* — in thromboembolic disorders effective and safe therapy with oral anticoagulants depends on careful regulation of the intensity of pharmacological response. The margin between adequate therapy and undue haemorrhage is relatively narrow and varies from patient to patient and depends not only on dosage, but also on the numerous factors which can influence the response or increase the risk of complications (see section 3.2.2; 3.2.4; 3.2.5).

6) *Patient co-operation* — in thromboembolic disorders, because of the ever present risk of haemorrhage and the importance of tight anticoagulant control for effective but safe therapy, patients should be educated in the aims and expectations of treatment and made aware of those factors which may alter their response to anticoagulants.

Anticoagulants should not be used for inadequately established indications if full co-operation or supervision of the patient cannot be achieved. Long term therapy should not be given to patients who cannot understand instructions about therapy, particularly dosage, or who do not attend regularly for control of dosage. Patients should be given written instructions about the nature of

Table I. Properties and uses of antithrombotic drugs

Drug	Clinical effect (mechanism action)	Indications[1] (see also text)	Side effects/notes	Antagonist
1. Anticoagulant drugs Heparin	Prevents formation of thrombus or limits its extension (inhibits generation and activity of thrombin; low doses enhance activity of antithrombin III)	Rapid induction of anticoagulant effect before oral agents take effect (acute pulmonary embolism***, recent deep vein thrombosis***, acute myocardial infarction**) Acute peripheral artery occlusion** Disseminated intravascular coagulation* Situations requiring extracorporeal circulation*** (e.g. haemodialysis, cardiac surgery) Prophylaxis of deep vein thrombosis and pulmonary embolism (low doses***) Prophylaxis of puerperal thrombosis (full doses***; low doses**)	Haemorrhage (risk greatest in females over 60 and with intermittent intravenous administration; see text); thrombocytopenia Hypersensitivity (rare; give test dose 1,000u in those with history allergy) Minor bleeding only	1 to 1.5mg protamine (by slow intravenous injection) for each 100u heparin
Coumarins Indanediones	As for heparin (inhibit synthesis vitamin K dependent clotting factors)	*Short term therapy* Acute pulmonary embolism*** Recent deep vein thrombosis*** Prevention of postoperative deep vein thrombosis*** Acute myocardial infarction** Recent arterial occlusion** Extensive superficial thrombophlebitis* (if patient is immobile) Elective cardioversion* (1 week before, 2 weeks after) *Long term therapy* Atrial fibrillation with rheumatic heart disease*** Transient cerebral ischaemic attacks*** Recent myocardial infarction** (to prevent recurrence) Idiopathic recurrent venous thrombosis** Acute coronary insufficiency* (preinfarction angina) Pulmonary hypertension due to emboli* Mitral valve disease* Prosthetic heart valves* Patients with vascular grafts* Occlusive arterial disease in the limbs*	Haemorrhage (overdosage) NB intercurrent illness, other drugs and risk increased in elderly and patient in poor general health Red discolouration of urine; severe skin rash, hepatitis, nephropathy (indanediones) Rash, transient alopecia (uncommon); rarely necrosis skin (coumarins)	Vitamin K_1 (phytomenadione) Severe bleeding and therapy to be discontinued (25 to 50mg) Severe bleeding and therapy to be continued (15mg) Overdosage and no bleeding (5mg)

Ancrod Defibrase	As for heparin (convert fibrinogen to unstable fibrin)	Alternative to heparin in acute peripheral arterial occlusion	Haemorrhage (overdosage) Sensitivity Antibodies (prevents retreatment within 6 months) Do not use concurrently with drugs which inhibit the reticulo-endothelial system (e.g. dextrans) or the physiological fibrinolytic system (e.g. ε-amino-caproic acid, tranexamic acid)	Fibrinogen and fresh blood
2. Antiplatelet agents Aspirin Indomethacin Dipyridamole Sulphinpyrazone	Prevent thrombus formation (inhibit platelet function)	Prosthetic heart valves*** Arteriovenous shunts*** Prevention of transient ischaemic attacks (aspirin)** Proliferative and membranoproliferative glomerulonephritis* Renal or cardiac allografts* (thrombosis due to rejection phenomena) Prophylaxis of arterial thromboembolism* Prevention of postoperative deep vein thrombosis (aspirin + dipyridamole)* Recurrent venous thrombosis* Primary or secondary prevention of myocardial infarction* Peripheral arterial insufficiency* Patients with vascular grafts*	Increased risk of bleeding if used with anticoagulants Gastric intolerance (aspirin, sulphinpyrazone); headache (indomethacin, dipyridamole)	
Dextran 70	Prevent thrombus formation (inhibits platelet function as well as coagulability of blood)	Prevention of postoperative deep vein thrombosis** Prophylaxis of puerperal thrombosis**	Increased risk of bleeding if used with anticoagulants	
3. Thrombolytic drugs Streptokinase Urokinase	Hasten lysis of pre-formed thrombi (activate fibrinolytic enzyme system by activation of plasminogen)	Acute major pulmonary embolism*** Acute deep vein thrombosis*** Acute thrombosis of peripheral artery** Chronic occlusion of peripheral artery* Thrombosis of sinus cavernosus and renal vein or artery thrombosis* Priapism* Anterior chamber hyphaemia* (local) Occlusion of arteriovenous shunt (local)**	Haemorrhage from prolonged hyperplasminaemia (avoid too large dose on initial infusion) Hypersensitivity with streptokinase (give corticosteroid concomitantly) Antibodies with streptokinase (prevents retreatment within 3 months)	Fibrinolytic inhibitors if excessive bleeding cannot be controlled by withdrawal of drug and administration of fibrinogen or fresh blood

1 *** = Definite indications; ** = less definite indications; * = indications limited to certain cases.

therapy, the dangers of abnormal bleeding or symptoms of recurring thromboembolism, the times to contact their clinician, the danger of relying on memory for the frequency and size of the dose, the value of keeping a diary of the amount of anticoagulant drug and all other medication actually taken, and the need to record any authorised changes in therapy.

Patients who genuinely require replacement therapy for deficiency anaemias should be encouraged to take their medication as prescribed. Many patients with iron deficiency anaemia do not take or complete their course of iron tablets.

Patients receiving drugs which regularly cause idiosyncratic blood dyscrasias should always be instructed about warning symptoms and the need to report these, particularly any unusual minor bleeding.

3. Thromboembolic Disorders and Antithrombotic Drugs

The high morbidity and mortality from thromboembolic occlusive vascular disease has prompted the continuing search for effective methods for its prevention and treatment. The drugs now available (table I) for management of thromboembolism can be divided into three types: (1) those affecting platelet aggregation or adhesiveness (antiplatelet agents); (2) those preventing fibrin formation (anticoagulants); and (3) those drugs which will digest fibrin (thrombolytic agents) or stimulate natural lysis of fibrin (fibrinolytic stimulants). Anticoagulant and antiplatelet therapy is primarily prophylactic, and while these drugs can prevent the deposition of a thrombus, once it is formed they can only limit its extension (see section 1.1). Fibrinolytic stimulant drugs are also only of potential prophylactic value in patients prone to occlusive vascular disease. The thrombolytic drugs on the other hand, are not prophylactic but if given early enough can hasten the lysis of preformed thrombi (for review, see Gallus and Hirsh, 1976a,c; 1978).

3.1 Antiplatelet Agents

Several compounds which inhibit platelet adhesion and aggregation *in vitro* have been evaluated with regard to the prevention of thromboembolic disorders in man (Mustard and Packham, 1975, 1978; Weiss, 1978). Most have not been en-

couraging, particularly because the *in vitro* tests of platelet function may not be relevant to thrombosis in man. Drugs which affect platelet function *in vitro* tests do not necessarily influence *ex vivo* tests of platelet function and are ineffective in certain clinical situations, while other drugs which do not affect *in vitro* tests, may have a favourable clinical effect. In most cases, the mechanism by which these drugs affect platelet function is unknown. Moreover, the precise role of platelets in thromboembolic disorders is not clear. It is therefore not surprising that the clinical effects of antiplatelet aggregating drugs are somewhat unpredictable. In addition, the efficacy of combinations of some antiplatelet drugs depends critically on the doses used (see below). Clearly, the ultimate proof of the clinical usefulness of oral antiplatelet agents such as aspirin, sulphinpyrazone, dipyridamole, suloctidil, hydroxychloroquine, clofibrate, dextrans and indomethacin must be demonstrated in controlled clinical trials having vascular thromboembolism as the end point by which to judge the drug effect.

Action of Antiplatelet Drugs: The mechanism of attachment of platelets to surfaces (e.g. adhesion) and to each other (e.g. aggregation) is not completely understood. Platelets that have adhered to damaged vessel walls or other surfaces, or that have aggregated in response to various stimuli (fig. 4) are activated to secrete (the so-called release reaction) some of the contents of their storage granules. Among these released substances is adenosine diphosphate (ADP), which causes platelets in the vicinity of the aggregate to swell and adhere to each other, further accelerating platelet aggregation. The platelet release reaction appears to be mediated by synthesis (via platelet microsomes) of prostaglandins and in particular thromboxane A_2; whereas limitation of platelet aggregation and thrombus formation seems to be controlled by another prostaglandin metabolite, prostacyclin, generated by the vessel walls of arteries and veins and released from the lung into the circulating blood, especially on the arterial side (see Editorial, 1978a; Dollery and Hensby, 1978). In some circumstances, for example high concentrations of thrombin or collagen, the initial platelet release reaction can occur by mechanisms which are independent of thromboxane A_2 (fig. 4).

That platelet aggregation is controlled by a delicate balance between formation of thromboxanes and prostacyclin is illustrated by the dose related interaction between the antiplatelet drugs aspirin

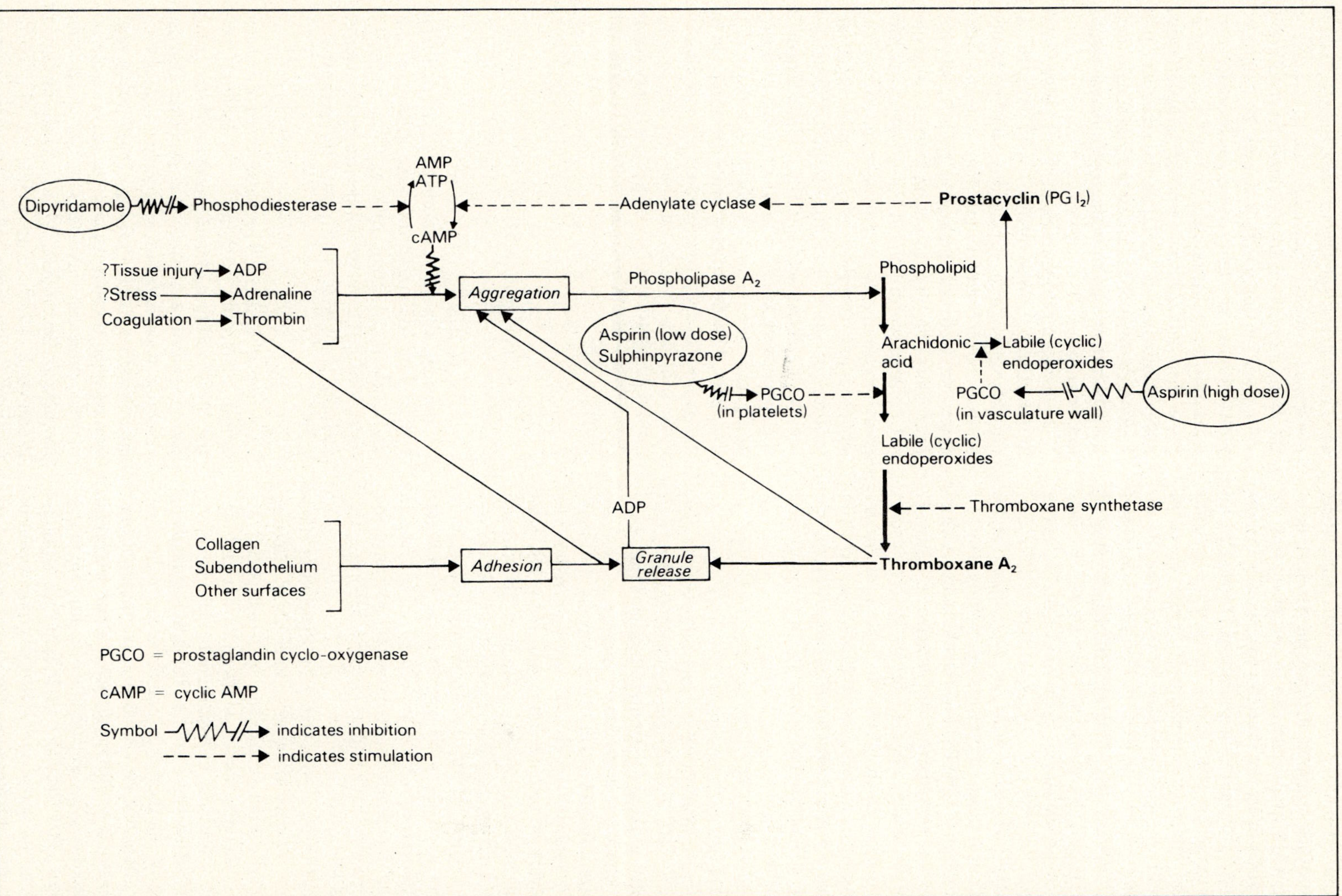

Fig. 4. Schematic representation of platelet reactions showing mechanisms controlling release and aggregation (modified from Weis: New England Journal of Medicine 298: 1344, 1978; Didisheim and Fuster: Seminars in Hematology 15: 55, 1978).

and dipyridamole in the rabbit. The antiplatelet action of dipyridamole depends on stimulation of cyclic AMP by prostacyclin in the blood (fig. 4). Low doses of aspirin prevent generation of thromboxane A_2 (by inhibiting the enzyme prostaglandin cyclo-oxygenase in platelets) and enhance the antiplatelet effect of dipyridamole. High doses of aspirin also inhibit prostacyclin formation (by inhibiting prostaglandin cyclo-oxygenase in vessel walls), thereby abolishing the antiplatelet effect of dipyridamole (Moncada and Korbutt, 1978). Since platelet prostaglandin cyclo-oxygenase is more sensitive to inhibition by aspirin than the cyclo-oxygenase in vessel walls, it is possible that by using small doses of aspirin (e.g. 500mg daily), a more selective inhibition of thromboxane A_2 formation can be obtained. As depicted in figure 4, drugs can inhibit platelet aggregation by various mechanisms which prevent formation of thromboxane A_2 or increase the level of cyclic AMP in platelets, or potentiate circulating prostacyclin (see further, Moncada and Vane, 1978; O'Grady and Moncada, 1978).

Clinical Use of Antiplatelet Drugs: Of the drugs affecting platelet function, low molecular weight dextrans (40, 70, 75) are the best studied, particularly in the postoperative state, but they have other effects on blood which may be as or more important in prevention of thrombosis. In orthopaedic surgery, dextran 70 administered before and every second day after operation, has been shown most convincingly to reduce the incidence of phlebographically determined deep vein thrombosis (Harris et al., 1974). Major orthopaedic surgery is precisely the type of surgery in which the effectiveness of low dose heparin is much in doubt and in which the effectiveness of aspirin and dipyridamole have still to be confirmed (see section 4.6).

There is no good evidence for the clinical effectiveness of aspirin or any other drug affecting platelet function in patients with peripheral arterial obliterative disease or after vascular grafting. In cerebrovascular disease there is reasonable evidence that aspirin can reduce cerebral ischaemia or mortality, but there is no convincing evidence that other antiplatelet drugs, such as sulphinpyrazone, dipyridamole or clofibrate, given alone are useful (see section 4.3). Similarly there is no convincing evidence that aspirin, clofibrate or sulphinpyrazone are useful in the primary prevention of myocardial infarction in apparently healthy or

aged individuals. In patients with angina, there is reasonable evidence that clofibrate is effective in the prevention of a fatal and non-fatal myocardial infarction, but long term use may be associated with a higher mortality from causes other than ischaemic heart disease (see section 4.1.2). Nor as yet is there any certainty whether drugs affecting platelet function are useful in the secondary prevention of myocardial infarction; although there have been some encouraging preliminary results (see section 4.1.2).

In patients with prosthetic heart valves, oral anticoagulants supplemented with aspirin or dipyridamole offer a significantly better protection against thromboembolism than anticoagulants alone, but aspirin used alone is less effective than in combination with coumarin drugs (see section 4.1.4). Aspirin can prevent the symptoms of peripheral ischaemia in thrombocytosis and so can sulphinpyrazone prevent the occlusion of an arteriovenous shunt used for chronic dialysis (for review, see Verstraete, 1976b, 1978a). There is still much uncertainty as to whether indomethacin or dipyridamole, given in addition to conventional treatment, benefit patients with membranous or mesangiocapillary glomerulonephritis (see chapter XXI; sect. 4.3). The same holds for use of antiplatelet drugs after kidney or heart transplantation (for review, see Verstraete, 1976b; Turpie and Hirsh, 1978).

3.2 Anticoagulant Drugs

3.2.1 Heparin

Heparin, a mucopolysaccharide extracted from bovine lung tissue and intestinal mucosa of pigs and cattle is a natural anticoagulant, whose activity is related to its strong electronegative charge, forming complexes with positively charged proteins.

Action of Heparin: The most important mechanism of action of heparin is binding with the ε-lysyl residues of antithrombin III, the cofactor of heparin in plasma. It is proposed that the resulting heparin-cofactor complex undergoes a special reorientation allowing a more ready reaction between the heparin and the active serine site of the proteases involved in the coagulation mechanism (factor XII, XI, IX, X and thrombin) [Rosenberg, 1975; Barrowcliffe et al., 1978]. Compared with thrombin, the complex preferentially inhibits activated factor X. This is not only the best studied, but probably also the most important inhibitor, in view of the central role of factor X in thrombogenesis. Moreover, the coagulation is an amplification system with positive feedback; an early inhibition in the activating system will prevent the generation of a greater amount of thrombin than the same quantity of inhibitor could do in neutralising thrombin. The property of the heparin-antithrombin III complex to neutralise previously formed thrombin will decrease the autocatalytic effect of thrombin in the coagulation cascade (fig. 2). As the inhibition of factor X by the heparin-antithrombin III complex is attained at very low concentrations of heparin, this action provides the rationale for low dose subcutaneous heparin in the prophylaxis of deep vein thrombosis (see section 4.6). Once a thrombus is formed, full doses of heparin, administered intravenously, are required to prevent its extension.

Pharmacokinetic Properties of Heparin: Heparin is not bound to plasma albumin but is bound extensively to low density lipoproteins, globulins (including the α-globulin antithrombin III) and to fibrinogen (Marciniak, 1974). Clearance of heparin varies widely between individuals and is dose dependent; higher doses leading to more prolonged elimination from the plasma (Simon et al., 1978; Estes and Poulin, 1975). Clearance also varies with the condition treated; being much more rapid in patients with pulmonary embolism than in normal subjects or patients with venous thrombosis, thus supporting the need for larger initial doses of heparin in acute pulmonary embolism (Simon et al., 1978; Hirsh et al., 1976). The pathways of elimination of heparin are not clear. Uptake by the reticuloendothelial system has been proposed as an important mechanism of removal of heparin from plasma (Estes and Poulin, 1975). It is not known whether heparin is metabolised or otherwise biotransformed in man, and the effect of liver disease or impaired renal function on elimination of heparin is not clear (Simon et al., 1978; Teien, 1977). Elimination might be prolonged after larger doses in patients with chronic renal failure or severe liver disease (Teien and Bjornson, 1976; Teien, 1977), but the clinical importance of any alteration in clearance is not known. Variability in clearance between patients is however, sufficiently marked to make laboratory control of dosage desirable (Simon et al., 1978).

Administration of Heparin: Heparin is not absorbed when given by mouth and must be given parenterally. Absorption from intramuscular sites is variable. Intravenous heparin may be given by continuous infusion or by intermittent injection. Major bleeding seems to be less frequent with continuous infusion, and it is as effective for prevention of thromboembolism (Salzman et al., 1975; Glazier and Crowell, 1976). Moreover, continuous infusion reduces the dosage of the drug and accelerated clearance in pulmonary embolism (see above) makes it more difficult to attain adequate concentrations for any duration with usual intermittent regimens. It is not certain how intense the anticoagulant effect of heparin must be to prevent thrombosis in man, and the relationship of the degree of effect to bleeding complications is also uncertain (Basu et al., 1972; Pitney et al., 1970). When given by continuous intravenous infusion, a loading dose of 5,000 (sometimes 10,000) units given as bolus, followed by 20,000 to 30,000 units in a litre of normal saline or 5% dextrose over 24 hours is usual practice; the rate of the infusion is subsequently regulated to keep the activated partial thromboplastin time around twice the baseline level. Given intermittently, the usual dose is 10,000 units 6-hourly or 15,000 units 8-hourly. Some use 5,000 to 10,000 units 4-hourly. Intermittent injection is preferred by some because laboratory monitoring can be ignored but, in the experience of most, at the risk of more major bleeding. There is a wide variation between individuals in the anticoagulant response to a given dose of heparin (Hirsh et al., 1976) or of the dose required to produce a particular anticoagulant response (Basu et al., 1972). The wide variation in clearance of heparin between individuals and different types of patient (see above), also suggests the desirability of monitoring therapy so that dosage can be adjusted appropriately.

Concentrated aqueous heparin usually contains 20,000 units/ml and is given subcutaneously in a skinfold raised from the abdominal wall. The 'full' dose of this slow release heparin is 20,000 to 30,000 units per 24 hours, administered in 1 or 2 injections. In the 'low dose' regimen, 5,000 units of concentrated heparin are given subcutaneously 8- or 12-hourly for the prophylaxis of deep vein thrombosis (see section 4.6). In most cases it causes only slight, if any, prolongation of clotting times and no clinically significant bleeding, except in a few cases after major orthopaedic surgery when 5,000 units are given 8-hourly.

Clinical Use of Heparin: The indications for heparin are given in table I and its use in the management of thromboembolic disorders is discussed in section 4. Bleeding is the major complication of heparin and is a direct extension of its therapeutic action. Spontaneous bleeding is most likely in elderly patients, especially females (Jick et al., 1968; Viewig et al., 1970) or in those with a haemostatic defect (Pitney et al., 1970). Postoperative or post-traumatic bleeding is more common than spontaneous bleeding (Basu et al., 1972). Other complications are uncommon but osteoporosis can occur with full doses continued for 6 months or more (Sackler and Lin, 1973). Thrombocytopenia is being increasingly reconised (Babcock et al., 1976; Bell et al., 1976).

3.2.2 Oral Anticoagulants

The oral anticoagulants are synthetic compounds of two chemical types — coumarin and inanedione derivatives (Douglas, 1971).

Action of Oral Anticoagulants: Both types act by inhibiting the synthesis of biologically active prothrombin, and factors VII, IX and X (fig. 2). The normal synthesis of these four coagulation factors requires vitamin K (Suttie et al., 1974). Oral anticoagulants inhibit the normal action of vitamin K, resulting in the accumulation of biologically inactive derivatives of clotting factors (Hemker and Loeliger, 1968; Larrieu and Meyer, 1970; Esmon et al., 1975). These derivatives may represent a common precursor or incomplete individual factors. Active clotting factors are formed by carboxylation of their precursor proteins during which vitamin K is oxidised to a vitamin K epoxide. Oral anticoagulants prevent the reduction of this biologically inactive epoxide back into active vitamin K. There is a resultant accumulation of the epoxide, a depletion of vitamin K and a reduced rate of formation of 'complete' clotting factors (O'Reilly, 1976a).

Oral anticoagulants are therefore indirect acting drugs and all require a delay before their action is seen. The delay of their effect depends on the clearance from the circulation of the four coagulation factors whose synthesis is inhibited, and on the extent of this inhibition, which in turn depends on the induction dose. The usual practice is to give a loading (induction) dose of the drug followed by progressively smaller doses until the daily maintenance level for desired control (see section 3.5) is reached.

Pharmacokinetic Properties of Oral Anticoagulants (see Bachmann and Shapiro, 1977; Kelly and O'Malley, 1979): All oral anticoagulants with the exception of dicoumarol (bishydroxycoumarin) are reliably absorbed. All coumarins are highly protein bound; that of ethylbiscoumacetate being somewhat less so. Virtually all of the binding is to plasma albumin. Distribution volumes are low (see appendix A). Major differences between compounds exist in the rate of hepatic metabolism and the effect of dose on elimination rate (table II). Pathways of metabolism can also differ for some compounds. Oral anticoagulants are extensively metabolised by the enzymes of the hepatic reticulum, and genetically determined individual variations in enzyme activity leads to marked differences in rate of elimination between individuals. Other drugs can also influence the activity of these drug metabolising enzymes (see section 3.2.5). Along with variation in vitamin K availability and clotting factor turnover (see section 3.2.4), these differences in rate of elimination cause marked variation in dose requirements of oral anticoagulants in individual patients; 10 or even 20-fold differences being common (see Breckenridge, 1977). The long elimination half-life of some of the coumarins means that there will be a slow approach to a new steady-state concentration. For example, after a change in maintenance dose of phenprocoumon it can take 23 days to complete 90 % and 46 days to complete 99 % of the change to the new steady-state plasma concentration (see chapter I; sect. 2.2). Rare instances of abnormal sensitivity to warfarin apparently due to a defect in metabolism have occurred (Bochner et al., 1975), as have rare instances of resistance due to a genetically determined defect in hepatic receptor site affinity for vitamin K and warfarin (O'Reilly, 1971).

Dicoumarol and ethylbiscoumacetate have two coumarin ring systems and both have dose dependent elimination half-lives, which increase with increasing dose. This does not occur with the other coumarins which are single ring compounds. This dose dependent elimination means that small dose increases may result in disproportionately larger increases in plasma concentration, making initial anticoagulant control and subsequent dose adjustment more difficult (see chapter I; sect. 2.1.1; 3.3), so increasing the risk of bleeding episodes (Husted and Andreasen, 1976). The ring system of the coumarins also influences pathways of metabolism due to differences in kinetics of the optical

Table II. Pharmacokinetic properties of some anticoagulants[1]

Drug	Absorption	Protein binding (%)	Half-life (h)	Elimination	Important excretion in breast milk	Placental transfer
Heparin	Nil	Yes[2]	1 to 2[3] (iv bolus)	Plasma clearance is dose dependent; ? biotransformation	No	No
Coumarins						
Dicoumarol (bishydroxycoumarin)	Poor and erratic	> 99	60 to 100	Hepatic metabolism (dose dependent)	No	Yes
Ethylbiscoumacetate	Good	90	2 to 5	Hepatic metabolism (dose dependent)	?	Yes
Phenprocoumon	Good	> 99	65 to 170	Hepatic metabolism	No	Yes
Warfarin sodium	Good	⩾ 99	35 to 45	Hepatic metabolism	No	Yes
Indanediones						
Phenindione	Good	?	5 to 10	Hepatic metabolism	?Yes	Yes

1 See also text discussion.
2 Not to plasma albumin.
3 Determined by bioassay of heparin concentration (standard dose).

isomers (enantiomers) of the single ring compounds. Warfarin, a racemic mixture of two isomers, R and S warfarin, has been studied in most detail (Lewis et al., 1974). The two major metabolites of warfarin are R-warfarin and S-warfarin; both are pharmacologically active, although of differing and lesser potency than the parent drug, and are metabolised at different rates and by different pathways: S warfarin forming 7-hydroxywarfarin as the major metabolite and R warfarin forming RS warfarin alcohol and 6-hydroxywarfarin. This has important potential implications for metabolic interaction with certain other drugs. Thus, phenylbutazone inhibits the clearance of the usually more rapidly eliminated S isomer of warfarin but does not affect or induces the metabolism of the 3 to 5 times less active R warfarin. Metronidazole also inhibits metabolism of the more potent S isomer of warfarin (O'Reilly, 1976b). Other single ring coumarins also have optical isomers with differences in potency and pharmacokinetic properties; the S isomer of phenprocoumon being around 2 times more potent, and because of higher protein binding, also having a slower plasma clearance than the R isomer. Potency, binding and clearance of the racemic mixture, as used clinically, is between that of the enantiomers (Jahnchen et al., 1976).

Protein binding of coumarins has an important influence on their elimination from the body, since with acidic drugs which are highly albumin bound and have capacity limited metabolism, there is a correlation between the fraction of free (unbound) drug in the plasma and hepatic clearance (see chapter I; sect. 3.2.3). Thus, an increase in the free fraction of a coumarin such as warfarin will result in an increased clearance rate, as more drug is available for metabolism. Differences in extent of protein binding of coumarins also exist between individuals and will be an important contribution to interindividual variations in rate of elimination (Yacobi et al., 1976a,b). A decrease in binding of coumarins as a consequence of displacement by other drugs from its specific binding site on albumin (see chapter I; sect. 3.2.1), or in uraemia, largely as a consequence of the presence of an endogenous binding inhibitor, does not however, lead to an enhanced effect (Bachmann et al., 1977), since as a consequence of increased clearance the concentration of unbound drug in plasma is the same (see chapter I; sect. 3.2.3); although before the new steady-state is reached, there may be a significant temporary increase in plasma concentration of unbound active drug (see section 3.2.5).

Enhancement of the response to warfarin in liver disease appears to be largely associated with altered clotting factor synthesis rather than to decreased binding or metabolism. Similarly, with thyroid disease (Bachmann and Shapiro, 1977; see also section 3.2.4). Also the increased effect of warfarin in the elderly is not due to altered pharmacokinetics, but seems to result from a greater inhibition of vitamin K dependent clotting factor synthesis at the same plasma concentration (Shepherd et al., 1977).

Warfarin is not found in breast milk (Orme et al., 1977). The other coumarins also do not seem to be excreted in significant amounts. Ethylbiscoumacetate might be an exception. Although it can be detected in only very small amounts in breast milk (Illingworth and Finch, 1959), it has been suggested that it seems to be converted to a pharmacologically active compound with haemorrhagic properties (i.e. unrelated to vitamin K dependent clotting factors) and which rapidly attains higher concentrations in breast milk than in plasma of the mother. It has caused spontaneous bleeding in breast fed infants with evidence of previous vascular damage (Gostof et al., 1952). Phenindione can be detected in breast milk and has caused bleeding problems in a breast fed infant undergoing surgery. Warfarin, dicoumarol and phenprocoumon have been used safely in breast feeding mothers, but many prefer to use heparin in the puerperium (see further section 3.2.6).

The relationship between plasma concentrations of oral anticoagulants and their pharmacological effect is complex. Their primary effect is due to inhibition of the *synthesis* of vitamin K dependent clotting factors (see above) and the observed effect a function of both synthesis rate of clotting factors and their degradation rates (Levy, 1973; Koch-Weser and Sellers, 1971). There is therefore no simple correlation between plasma concentration and anticoagulant effect, but if the response is defined in terms of a change in the rate of clotting factor synthesis, there is a direct relationship between the logarithm of plasma warfarin concentration and its effect (Nagashima et al., 1969). Individual differences in vitamin K activity at the hepatic receptor site (Zieve and Solomon, 1969) or in receptor affinity for the oral anticoagulant may also affect the plasma concentration-effect relationship, since patients with a similar rate of elimination and plasma concentration of dicoumarol have widely different concentrations of plasma prothrombin (Solomon and Schrogie, 1967). For these reasons, plasma concentration estimation is not of value for monitoring routine therapeutic use of oral anticoagulants. Pharmacokinetic interactions with oral anticoagulants are discussed in section 3.2.5. For reviews of the clinical pharmacokinetics of coumarin anticoagulants, see Bachmann and Shapiro (1977) and Kelly and O'Malley (1979).

3.2.3 Choice and Clinical Use of Oral Anticoagulants

Selection of a particular oral anticoagulant is generally based on side effects (indanedione compounds can cause serious and even fatal sensitivity reactions; table III) and personal experience (where familiarity with a coumarin compound is probably more important than its duration of action), but pharmacokinetic considerations should also be taken into account. Dicoumarol (bishydroxycoumarin) is poorly and erratically absorbed. It and ethylbiscoumacetate have concentration dependent elimination kinetics which as discussed above makes dose adjustment more difficult. Other coumarin derivatives do not have these drawbacks and selection is mainly based on a personal preference to use a drug with a short or long plasma half-life (see above). The pharmacokinetic properties of some compounds such as dicoumarol also influence the type and likelihood of interaction with other drugs. Its absorption is increased by drugs which decrease gastric emptying rate or intestinal transit and it is also capable of inhibiting the metabolism of drugs such as phenytoin, tolbutamide and chlorpropamide (table IV).

Many factors can influence the response to oral anticoagulants and necessitate modification or individualisation of dosage. The dosage of any oral anticoagulant required to depress prothrombin complex synthesis and to prolong the prothrombin time at any given level therefore varies widely among individual patients (see section 3.2.2; 3.2.4). Principles in the use of oral anticoagulants are discussed in section 3.5 and their use in treatment in section 4. A guide to induction and maintenance doses, onset and duration of effect and important side effects is given in table III. The indications for use of oral anticoagulants are summarised in table I. In contrast to venous thrombosis, their use in arterial disease has not been a particular success, as discussed in sections 1.1.2 and 4, and in some areas of arterial disease, therapy with antiplatelet drugs or oral anticoagulants plus antiplatelet drugs may be more promising (Mackie and Douglas, 1978).

Table III. Anticoagulant drugs for oral use

Drug	Induction dose (mg first 24h)	Maintenance dose (mg/24h)[1]	Time to produce 'therapeutic levels' (hours)[2]	Duration of effect	Side effects[3]
Coumarin compounds					
Dicoumarol (bishydroxycoumarin)	200-300	25-150	36-72	Long	Rash and transient alopecia (uncommon); skin necrosis (rare)
Ethyl biscoumacetate	1,800-2,400	150-900	18-36	Short	
Ethylidene dicoumarin	500-1,000	100-200	72	Intermediate	
Nicoumalone (acenocoumarol)	36-52	2-12	24-42	Short	
Phenprocoumon	18-30	0.75-6	30-48	Long	
Warfarin sodium	30-50	2.5-25	36-48	Intermediate	
Indanedione compounds					
Anisindione	800-900	25-300	36-60	Intermediate	Red discolouration of urine; sensitivity reactions (rash, fever, leucopenia, hepatitis, renal failure, diarrhoea and steatorrhoea)
Chlorphenylindanedione	12-18	2-8	36-60	Intermediate	
Diphenadione	30-45	3-5	48-60	Long	
Phenindione	200-300	25-200	36-48	Intermediate	

1   Average only. Varies widely and must be determined for each individual patient.
2   Therapeutic level means doubling the normal value of the one stage prothrombin time.
3   Bleeding is major undesirable side effect of all oral anticoagulants. Risk of spontaneous bleeding from excessive dosage most likely in the elderly and in patient in poor general health. During well controlled therapy, bleeding usually due to surgery or other forms of trauma.

3.2.4 Factors Affecting Response to Oral Anticoagulants

Since relatively small decreases or increases in the intensity of action of oral anticoagulants can lead to an inadequate therapeutic effect or haemorrhagic reactions, optimum therapy depends on careful regulation of the intensity of pharmacological response in an individual patient. Oral anticoagulants act by inhibiting the action of vitamin K on several coagulation factors synthesised in the liver (see section 3.2.2). The magnitude of this effect at any given time depends on the plasma concentration of the oral anticoagulant concerned (Nagashima et al., 1969; Husted and Andreasen, 1977a). Many factors, particularly those which alter the amount of vitamin K available at the site of synthesis or which alter the plasma concentration of anticoagulant, can influence the response to oral anticoagulants (table IV; for review, see O'Reilly and Aggeler, 1970; Breckenridge, 1977).

With proper control, most patients are relatively stable in respect of the individualised dosage needed to produce a desirable anticoagulant effect but some are difficult to control, and others who have been stable for a long time may suddenly present with haemorrhage. Lack of understanding of dosage or erratic ingestion of tablets is

Table IV. Factors which can alter the response to the usual dose of oral anticoagulant drugs (after O'Reilly and Aggeler, 1970)

Condition	Mechanism
Increased responsiveness[1] Obstructive jaundice Biliary fistula (particularly in patients with associated pancreatitis)	These disorders hinder delivery of bile to the small bowel and reduce absorption of the lipid soluble vitamin K, and may also inhibit biliary excretion
Steatorrhoea	Reduced absorption of vitamin K
Periods of starvation	Reduced dietary intake of vitamin K
Liver disease Acute viral hepatitis	Decreased production of vitamin K dependent clotting factors
Onset of congestive heart failure	Increased response to anticoagulant as hepatic congestion develops (i.e. decreased clotting factor synthesis) with decreased responsiveness on relief of the congestion by diuretics (i.e. increased clotting factor synthesis)
Hyperthyroidism Fever	Increased rate of decay of vitamin K dependent clotting factors
Bleeding tendency (many conditions)	See table VII
Other drugs	Some drugs (i.e. 17α-alkylated anabolic steroids) may cause liver dysfunction and increase the response to oral anticoagulants. Others do so by affecting platelet function (e.g. aspirin) or by pharmacokinetic mechanisms (see section 3.2.5, table V)
Decreased responsiveness Nephrotic syndrome	Decreased protein binding and marked increase in plasma clearance of warfarin. Dosage requirements increased
Hereditary resistance (autosomal dominant)	Marked increase in affinity for vitamin K and anticoagulant (warfarin) at its receptor site (two human kindreds identified). Major increase in dose requirements

1   In many of these conditions the increased response is variable, and the clinical significance difficult to predict.

responsible for a number of these cases, but intercurrent diseases, a change in diet, the commencement or cessation of other drug therapy may also interfere with anticoagulant response (e.g. Husted and Andreasen, 1976; Williams et al., 1976). The risk of anticoagulant induced bleeding is increased in the patient in poor general health and in the elderly, in whom dosage requirements of warfarin are also less than in a younger patient (Shepherd et al., 1977; Husted and Andreasen, 1977b; chapter V; sect. 4.6). The onset of congestive heart failure or a deterioration in cardiac status is a frequent cause of increased response to oral anticoagulants, necessitating changes in digitalis and diuretic therapy. Increased response is also seen in hepatic disease including onset of acute viral hepatitis, in hyperthyroidism, following surgery, and in the postcardiotomy syndrome. Periods of starvation, conditions impairing bile delivery to the bowel (e.g. obstructive jaundice, biliary fistula), gastrointestinal disturbances (e.g. steatorrhoea) and fever due to infections of any sort, also lead to a reduction in oral anticoagulant dose requirements (table IV).

A number of drugs have a potential to modify the response to coumarin anticoagulants and other drugs such as aspirin markedly increase the risk of bleeding. Changes of therapy in patients on anticoagulants must be kept to a minimum and with certain drugs need to be made under careful laboratory control. The use of other drugs with oral anticoagulants and the ways in which potential problems can be avoided are discussed in section 3.2.5.

3.2.5 Drug Interactions with Oral Anticoagulants

The effects of interaction between drugs are well known in the case of oral coumarin anticoagulants because the pharmacological effect is easily and routinely checked by measuring the 'prothrombin time', and also because the patient becomes aware of prolonged bleeding in cases of enhancement of the activity of the coumarin anticoagulant. Drug interaction is a particular problem with oral anticoagulants since they can be used for prolonged periods and because of the nature of the diseases for which they are given, numerous other drugs are often given concurrently. The need for modification of anticoagulant dosage for proper control increases with the number of drugs given (Williams et al., 1976). In practice, although the potential for interaction is considerable, clinically harmful interactions are not that common (Kleinman and Griner, 1970; Starr and Petrie, 1972) and predictable effects are largely confined to a few drugs such as phenylbutazone, oxyphenbutazone, clofibrate and barbiturates (see table V; Husted and Andreasen, 1976; Williams et al., 1976). Nevertheless, several fatalities have resulted from severe bleeding (Koch-Weser and Sellers, 1971) and, conversely, many patients taking potentially interacting drugs may not achieve desirable anticoagulant control if seen only irregularly (Williams et al., 1976; O'Malley et al., 1977). Some coumarin anticoagulants (dicoumarol) can affect the metabolism of other drugs such as phenytoin (see chapter XXV; sect. 3.1), tolbutamide and chlorpropamide (see chapter XVI; sect. 3.3.5). Phenindione has only rarely been implicated in clinically important interactions with other drugs but is also much less used. For reviews, see Dollery et al. (1975); Koch-Weser and Sellers (1971) and MacLeod and Sellers (1976).

Determinants of Interactions: Apart from the effect of pathophysiological conditions (e.g. liver disease, congestive heart failure, renal dysfunction) which in themselves can alter the response to oral anticoagulants (see section 3.2.4), other determinants which make a clinically important interaction more likely to occur have not been well defined. A change in concurrent therapy in a patient on a stable anticoagulant regimen can however, be important. Drugs which are capable of altering oral anticoagulant response can be used concurrently, provided dosage of the anticoagulant has been modified appropriately. Thus, in an already stable regimen, barbiturates taken regularly as anticonvulsants do not affect anticoagulant control, but barbiturates used occasionally as hypnotics can affect anticoagulant control. Introduction of hypnotic drugs such as barbiturates and dichloralphenazone, which in some patients can significantly induce drug metabolising enzymes in the hepatic endoplasmatic reticulum, may increase over a period of some days the rate of metabolism of coumarins and thus lead to a marked increase in anticoagulant dose requirements to regain the desired level of anticoagulation (Breckenridge et al., 1973). Sudden withdrawal of the inducing drug (e.g. at time of or shortly after discharge from hospital) without corresponding reduction of the dose of anticoagulant can have disastrous effects. Such interactions are difficult to

Table V. Potential clinically important drug interactions with oral anticoagulants

Interacting drug	Reported with[1]	Mechanism[2] (see also fig. 5)	Notes/action[3]
1. Drugs that are known to increase anticoagulant action clinically			
Anabolic steroids (methandrostenolone, norethandrolone, ethylestrenol)	Warfarin Dicoumarol	?	Marked potentiation. Adjust dose of anticoagulant. ? Avoid by use of non C-17 alkylated agents such as nandrolone
Benziodarone	Warfarin Nicoumalone Ethylbiscoumacetate Diphenadione	?	In many patients (all patients with warfarin), markedly potentiates effect of these coumarins and diphenadione. Reduced dose of anticoagulant when 300mg benziodarone added (e.g. by 50% with warfarin, 40% diphenadione, 25% nicoumalone, 20% ethylbiscoumacetate)
	Phenprocoumon Phenindione Clorindione	—	No effect on anticoagulant control with these compounds in one study when anticoagulant dose requirements expressed as a mean for the group. In another study of phenprocoumon, some patients required a reduced dosage because of enhanced coumarin action (e.g. by 20% at 300mg benziodarone, 50% at 600mg)
Clofibrate	Warfarin Ethylbiscoumacetate	IC	In many patients markedly potentiates effect of coumarins. Reduced dose of coumarin (e.g. by 25 to 30% with warfarin) when clofibrate added. Monitor degree hypoprothrombinaemia daily for a few days or more
D-Thyroxine	Warfarin Dicoumarol	IC	In virtually all patients markedly potentiates effect of warfarin and dicoumarol. Reduced dose of coumarin (e.g. by one third with warfarin) when D-thyroxine added. Monitor degree hypoprothrombinaemia daily for a few days or more
Glucagon	Warfarin	?	Doses greater than 24mg daily in most patients markedly potentiate effect of warfarin. Avoid. Use other treatment for refractory heart failure
Metronidazole	Warfarin	IM	Markedly potentiates effect of warfarin. Reduce dose of warfarin and monitor anticoagulant control, or substitute alternative agent (effect of other imidazole derivatives on warfarin unknown)
Phenylbutazone Oxyphenbutazone	Warfarin Ethylbiscoumacetate Phenprocoumon Dicoumarol	DB+IM	Predictably and markedly potentiates effect of warfarin and may reduce dose requirement of warfarin by 50 to 75%. Same phenomenon reported with ethylbiscoumacetate, phenprocoumon and dicoumarol Avoid. Substitute indomethacin, ibuprofen or naproxen with care
Phenyramidol	Warfarin Dicoumarol Phenindione	IM	Markedly potentiates effect of warfarin, dicoumarol and phenindione. Avoid. Substitute other analgesic (paracetamol) or muscle relaxant (diazepam)
Quinidine	Warfarin	?	Markedly potentiates effect of warfarin in some patients. Avoid. Substitute procainamide

2. Drugs that may possibly increase anticoagulant action

Chloral hydrate Triclofos	Warfarin	DB	Some reports of a limited potentiation of effect and small change in anticoagulant control with warfarin but others have detected no change. Probably only a transient enhancement of warfarin effect in some patients (Udall, 1969; 1975). May be desirable to substitute a benzodiazepine
Salicylates	Coumarins	PD	No effect on anticoagulant control but increased risk of bleeding due to effect on platelet function and haemorrhagic action on gastric mucosa. Avoid. Substitute paracetamol (analgesic) or indomethacin, ibuprofen or naproxen with care (anti-inflammatory analgesic)
Antibiotics, oral (neomycin, chlortetracycline, oxytetracycline)	Warfarin	DK	A few reports of slight potentiation of coumarins in some patients. Significant interference with control only likely if dietary intake vitamin K grossly deficient
Allopurinol	Dicoumarol	IM	Prolongs plasma half-life of dicoumarol (at least in some patients). No clinical reports of harmful hypoprothrombinaemia with dicoumarol
	Phenprocoumon	IM	Prolongation of plasma half-life and enhanced activity has been reported
	Warfarin	—	No effect on warfarin metabolism but a case report of enhanced activity with a combination of allopurinol and indomethacin
Cimetidine	Warfarin	?	Clinically harmful hypoprothrombinaemia has been reported. Reduced dose requirement should be anticipated
Dextropropoxyphene + paracetamol (acetaminophen)	Warfarin	?IM	Prolongation of plasma half-life and clinically harmful hypoprothrombinaemia has been reported. Substitute paracetamol alone
Co-trimoxazole	Warfarin	DB+ ?IM	Can increase action of warfarin
Isoniazid	Warfarin	?IM	Can apparently increase action of warfarin (case report)
Chloramphenicol Disulfiram	Dicoumarol Dicoumarol Warfarin	IM	Prolongs plasma half-life of coumarin. No clinical reports of harmful hypoprothrombinaemia
Amitriptyline Nortriptyline	Dicoumarol	?IA	Increased bioavailability of dicoumarol in many patients. No effect on dicoumarol metabolism. No clinical reports of harmful hypoprothrombinaemia
	Warfarin	—	No effect on bioavailability or plasma half-life of warfarin
Thyroid drugs		IC	Increase in clotting factor catabolism. No clinical reports of harmful hypoprothrombinaemia

Table V. (continued)

Interacting drug	Reported with[1]	Mechanism[2] (see also fig. 5)	Notes/action[3]
Sulphonamides (sulphaphenazole; sulphafurazole/ sulfisoxazole; sulphamethizole)	Warfarin Phenprocoumon	?DB + IM	Some highly protein bound compounds (e.g. sulphafurazole) may displace warfarin and phenprocoumon from human albumin and others (e.g. sulphaphenazole; sulphamethizole) may inhibit the metabolism of warfarin. Avoid sulphaphenazole. Watch for any potentiation (probably slight or transient) with others

3. Drugs that are known to decrease anticoagulant action clinically

Interacting drug	Reported with[1]	Mechanism[2]	Notes/action[3]
Barbiturates	Nicoumalone Dicoumarol Ethylbiscoumacetate Phenprocoumon Warfarin	AM	A marked decrease in effect of coumarin anticoagulant in many patients. Dose requirement may increase many-fold (even up to 10x). Avoid. Substitute a benzodiazepine
Chloral hydrate	Dicoumarol	?AM	Apparent inhibition of effect of dicoumarol. Avoid with dicoumarol. Substitute a benzodiazepine
Cholestyramine	Warfarin	DA	Markedly reduces absorption of warfarin when given with cholestyramine or up to 3 hours after it. Likely to be more marked with dicoumarol. Enterohepatic circulation of warfarin is also inhibited. Give warfarin 2 hours or more before cholestyramine, but monitor therapy as an increase in dosage may still be required
Dichloral phenazone Ethchlorvynol	Warfarin Warfarin Dicoumarol	AM	Can antagonise effect of coumarin. Avoid. Substitute a benzodiazepine
Glutethimide	Warfarin ?Ethylbiscoumacetate	AM	
Griseofulvin	Warfarin	DA	Can in some patients antagonise effect of warfarin. Monitor closely and adjust dose of anticoagulant carefully
6-Mercaptopurine	Warfarin	?	Increased warfarin dose requirement (2-fold) during mercaptopurine phase of treatment of a patient with chronic granulocytic leukaemia
Rifampicin	Warfarin Nicoumalone Phenprocoumon	AM	Can markedly antagonise action of warfarin, phenprocoumon and nicoumalone. Plasma concentration of a fixed dose of warfarin often falls to zero and prothrombin activity returns to 100% (O'Reilly, 1974, 1975). Monitor anticoagulant control and adjust dose of coumarin, or avoid rifampicin in anti-tuberculosis regimen (e.g. if compliance with regimen cannot be guaranteed)

4. Drugs that may possibly decrease anticoagulant action

Carbamazepine	Warfarin	AM	No clinical reports of adverse effects on anticoagulant control

5. Anticoagulant effect on other drugs

Chlorpropamide	Dicoumarol	?	Dicoumarol markedly potentiates effect of chlorpropamide and tolbutamide in elderly patients with
Tolbutamide	Dicoumarol	IM	decreased carbohydrate intake or congestive heart failure. Avoid dicoumarol. Warfarin and phenindione do not inhibit metabolism of tolbutamide. These can be substituted but with careful watch on dosage of oral hypoglycaemic, renal function and nutrition (see also chapter XVI; sect. 3.3.5)
Phenytoin (diphenylhydantoin)	Dicoumarol	IM	Dicoumarol in some patients can significantly increase plasma concentration of phenytoin. Reduced dose of phenytoin may be needed (see chapter XXV; sect. 3.1). ?Substitution of warfarin

1   The pharmacokinetic properties of coumarins in man are similar but not identical (see table I). Thus, drug effects on absorption or metabolism are most likely to be more significant with dicoumarol, and interactions involving plasma albumin binding least likely to be significant with ethylbiscoumacetate. Other coumarins not listed may therefore interact on basis of their individual pharmacokinetic properties.

2   The mechanism shown, or in some cases thought, most likely to be involved.

DA   =   Decrease in anticoagulant absorption.
IA   =   Increase in anticoagulant absorption.
DB   =   Decrease in anticoagulant albumin binding.
DK   =   Decrease in vitamin K availability.
AM   =   Acceleration of anticoagulant metabolism.
IM   =   Inhibition of anticoagulant metabolism.
IC   =   Increase in clotting factor catabolism.
PD   =   Additive pharmacodynamic effect.

3   Time course and extent of interaction vary with the individual, the mechanism of the interaction, with the specific drug and its dose (see section 3.2.5). Careful and frequent monitoring of prothrombin time is essential if known interacting drugs have to be added or withdrawn from therapy.

recognise because the enhanced anticoagulant effect develops gradually over a period of some days or weeks and the interindividual variation in effect is marked (see chapter VIII; sect. 2.3.4).

Mechanisms of Interaction and Time Course of Interaction Effect: There are many possible mechanisms for interaction (fig. 5). These include either interference with clotting factor synthesis (e.g. ?anabolic steroids, ?quinidine), alteration of vitamin K availability (hypolipidaemic drugs) or interference with the rate of decay of clotting factors (e.g. thyroid drugs), and pharmacokinetic mechanisms such as interference with absorption (e.g. cholestyramine), displacement of coumarin from plasma albumin (e.g. chloral hydrate), acceleration of coumarin metabolism (e.g. barbiturates, rifampicin) or inhibition of coumarin metabolism (e.g. chloramphenicol). In some cases, more than one mechanism is probably involved, such as decreased binding and inhibition of metabolism (e.g. phenylbutazone; Aarbakke, 1978).

The time course of onset and also the extent of the interaction effect vary considerably among patients and depend on the mechanism involved, with the specific drug, its dose, and duration of administration (Dollery et al., 1975; Koch-Weser and Sellers, 1971).

Displacement interactions: With repeated daily doses of a displacing drug, potentiation of the hypoprothrombinaemic effect is always transient and will only be significant for other highly albumin bound drugs with a small apparent volume of distribution and which share the same albumin binding site as coumarins (see chapter I; section 3.2.1). The time required for the potentiation and for the subsequent return to previous values is complex and depends on several factors, particularly the rate of plasma clearance of the individual coumarin and the displacing drug.

In general, usual daily doses of a strongly potentiating drug can be expected to potentiate warfarin within 24 hours, with the prothrombin time returning to previous values within 2 weeks or more. Unless an alteration of the prothrombin time is looked for in this period of time, it may be missed (see also chapter VIII; sect. 2.3.2).

Acceleration of metabolism (enzyme induction) interactions: The degree of inducibility varies considerably among individuals and in part is genetically determined and is dependent on the specific inducing drug, its dosage and duration of exposure. A potent inducing drug (e.g. phenobarbitone, rifampicin) introduced to a stable regimen might accelerate coumarin metabolism with a single dose or one day's therapy (2 days in most cases), but up to 3 weeks may be required for maximum induction intensity to be reached (Breckenridge et al., 1973; Breckenridge, 1976). On withdrawal of the inducing drug, return to the original rate of coumarin metabolism takes place gradually over several weeks (even as long as 4 to 5 weeks or more). The increase in rate of metabolism can be very large (even up to 10-fold reduction in warfarin dose requirements on withdrawal of inducing drug), but the extent of change is impossible to predict in an individual patient. Even with careful monitoring, optimum anticoagulant control may be difficult with strong inducing drugs and they should be avoided and alternatives used.

Inhibition of metabolism (biotransformation) interactions: In contrast to hepatic microsomal enzyme induction, interference with coumarin metabolism may become apparent within hours of administration of the inhibiting drug. When such a drug (e.g. phenylbutazone) is given to a patient stabilised on long term anticoagulant therapy, the maintenance dose of coumarin must be reduced to avoid excessive hypoprothrombinaemia and bleeding. However, the extent of enhancement cannot be predicted and dose adjustment must be made on the basis of results of careful monitoring of prothrombin time.

Avoiding Interactions: Adverse clinical events due to interactions with coumarin anticoagulants can be prevented by following a few simple rules (Koch-Weser, 1975):

1) Before prescribing, know all medications the patient is taking and instruct him not to change or add to his intake of medication, either prescribed or self prescribed, without first communicating with his doctor.

2) Drug therapy should always be kept as simple as possible and restricted to those drugs genuinely indicated and of proven benefit.

3) Occasional use of predictably interacting drugs should be avoided and alternatives prescribed (see table V).

4) Changes of drug therapy should be kept to a minimum. If changes are necessary and involve known interacting drugs, some alteration in coumarin dosage can be anticipated, but dose adjustment should only be made on the basis of results of close monitoring of anticoagulant control over a period of some weeks after the change. The time course and extent of interaction can vary

considerably among individual patients (see also above).

3.2.6 Anticoagulants in Pregnancy and the Puerperium

Venous thromboembolism in pregnancy and the puerperium poses a number of therapeutic dilemmas. Apart from minor pulmonary embolism, when heparin is generally the emergency treatment of choice and the thrombolytic or surgical approach for massive pulmonary embolism, surgery is sometimes considered for an iliofemoral thrombosis but has often to be postponed until after delivery. In the meantime and in all patients at high risk of thromboembolism (e.g. history of previous thromboembolism, mitral valve disease with atrial fibrillation, varicose veins) it is recommended to use anticoagulants during pregnancy.

Because of its physiochemical properties, heparin does not readily cross the placenta and if necessary its effects can be neutralised more quickly (with protamine) than can excessive hypoprothrombinaemia of oral anticoagulants, but there are problems associated with its long term administration. Oral anticoagulants readily cross the placenta and when used in the first trimester of pregnancy there is a real risk of congenital abnormalities very similar to the rare inherited syndrome chondrodystrophia fetalis hypoplastica (Shaul and Hall, 1977). Moreover, CNS anomalies, stillbirths and fetal wastage secondary to fetal bleeding may result following use of excessive dosage of oral anticoagulants during the second and third trimester of pregnancy (Hall, 1976). Their use in the period prior to delivery may predispose to fetal and neonatal haemorrhage (Hirsh et al., 1970a; 1972). When anticoagulation is absolutely required, heparin is probably a safer alternative as it does not cross the placenta. Dosage requirements of heparin increase as preg-

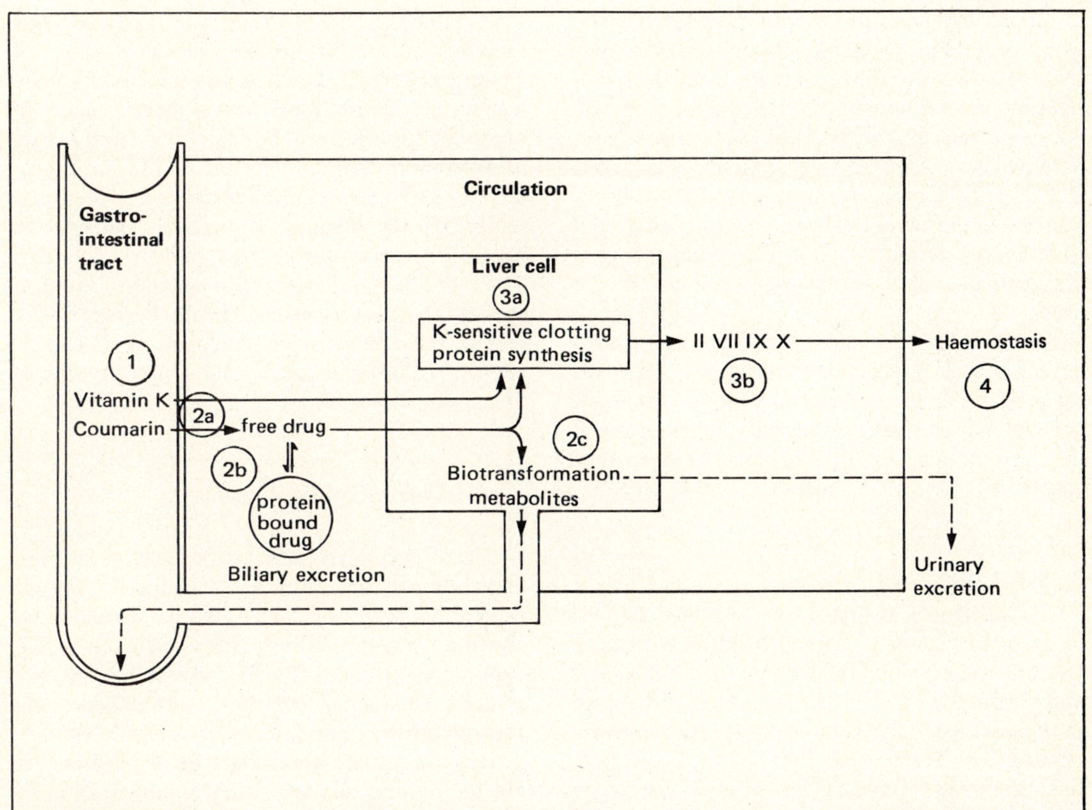

Fig. 5. Possible sites of drug interactions with action of oral coumarin anticoagulants. (1) vitamin K bioavailability; (2a) coumarin absorption; (2b) coumarin binding to plasma albumin; (2c) coumarin metabolism. (3a) prothrombin-complex synthesis; (3b) prothrombin-complex catabolism; (4) haemostasis (after Koch-Weser: American Heart Journal 90: 93, 1975; by permission of author and editor).

nancy advances (see chapter XV; sect. 1.1.4). Appropriately instructed patients can successfully manage self administration of subcutaneous heparin (Spearing et al., 1978).

Use of anticoagulants in the puerperium is not a contraindication to breast feeding. While excessive haematoma formation following surgery has been noted with phenindione (Eckstein and Jack, 1970), no evidence of spontaneous bleeding has been detected in breast fed infants of mothers on warfarin (Orme et al., 1977), phenprocoumon (Fries et al., 1957) or dicoumarol (Bramble and Hunter, 1950). Although ethylbiscoumacetate has also been used without event (Illingworth and Finch, 1959), instances of spontaneous haemorrhagic episodes have been noted in breast fed infants with evidence of previous vascular damage (see section 3.2.2). Warfarin has been studied best; a sensitive and specific assay not being able to detect warfarin in breast milk of mothers or in the plasma of their breast fed infants (Orme et al., 1977). Although the pharmacokinetic properties of most compounds allow them to be safely given to breast feeding women (it would seem sensible that therapy is carefully and well controlled), it is not easy to gain initial adequate control with oral anticoagulants and particularly with dicoumarol or ethylbiscoumacetate (see section 3.2.2). Thus also during the puerperium, heparin (which is not excreted in breast milk) is probably to be preferred in mothers desiring to breast feed. After this time oral anticoagulants except phenindione can be used.

Dextran 70 or low dose subcutaneous heparin are likely to be as effective as full doses of heparin for prophylaxis of puerperal thrombosis in at risk patients, but adequately designed studies to prove this assumption are not available (see further chapter III, sect. 6; IV, sect. 3.1.3; XV, sect. 6).

3.2.7 Defibrinating Agents

Those agents available are enzymes derived from snake venom — ancrod from the venom of the Malayan pit viper *Agkistrodon rhodostoma boie* and Defibrase from the *Bothrops atrox* and *Bothrops jararaca* snakes. Both agents remove a peptide from fibrinogen converting the latter to an unstable form of fibrin, the plasma fibrinogen level being markedly reduced. As the snake venoms do not activate factor XII which cross links the fibrin, the unstable fibrin 'microclots' are probably removed by activation of the endogenous

fibrinolytic enzyme system (fig. 2) and through phagocytosis by the reticuloendothelial system. As the two snake venoms under discussion affect only fibrinogen, the entire anticoagulant effect is therefore due to the resulting fibrinogen depletion and their effect is easy to measure. Provided the drug is administered slowly, intravascular fibrin can be cleared as it is formed and the effect is termed therapeutic defibrination (Bell et al., 1968; Dormandy et al., 1977). Ancrod and Defibrase are foreign proteins and induce formation of antibodies which can neutralise their effect. This can be overcome by increasing the dose when the antibodies appear, but this is only effective for 2 or 3 weeks, after which time treatment becomes ineffective. Antibodies disappear within 6 months and prevent retreatment before this time.

The commonly used defibrinating initial dose of ancrod is 2 to 3 units per kg body weight in 100ml 0.9% saline over a 4- to 6-hour period using a constant infusion pump; followed by 1 unit per kg body weight given in 20ml over 10 minutes at the end of the first infusion and this repeated every 12 hours. The daily dose of Defibrase is about 1 batroxobin unit per kg body weight in 100ml 0.9% saline over 1 hour. If necessary the effect can be rapidly reversed by use of antivenom and transfusion of fibrinogen. So far, no convincing clinical evidence has been presented that therapeutic defibrination is superior to heparin in venous thrombosis, even when used in a dose providing intense anticoagulation (Davies et al., 1972), but it may theoretically be superior in arterial thrombosis since peripheral blood flow is helped by the reduction in blood viscosity due to fibrinogen depletion.

3.3 Thrombolytic Agents

These agents include: (a) proteolytic enzymes acting directly on fibrin, e.g. plasmin, trypsin and aspergillus proteases, and (b) drugs capable of activating plasminogen, either directly (e.g. urokinase) or indirectly (e.g. streptokinase), and thereby enhancing enzymatic fibrinolysis. The proteolytic enzymes are too nonspecific in their action and to date, the activators of plasminogen are the only agents which have shown effectiveness in hastening lysis of thrombi from both the venous and arterial circulations (see section 4). Both drugs are able to increase activator activity in man several hundred times baseline levels. The principal aim of thrombolytic therapy is the removal of pathological intravascular fibrin deposits which have not been dissolved by spontaneous fibrinolysis. If a venous thrombus is lysed before it becomes adherent to the vein wall the valves may possibly be saved. The usefulness of thrombolytic agents is limited by the speed with which they need to be given after vascular occlusion (Kakkar and Scully, 1978).

Streptokinase: Streptokinase is a metabolic product of group C β-haemolytic streptococci; it is a non-enzymatic protein with a molecular weight of 47,000. Highly purified preparations are commercially available and are usually well tolerated. Therapeutic plasma levels are rapidly achieved and can be sustained for several days if necessary (Fletcher et al., 1959). The antigenicity of streptokinase in man is its major disadvantage and prevents retreatment within the first 3 months of a previous course, as a consequence of a sustained rise of antistreptokinase antibodies induced during treatment.

Since antibodies from prior streptococcal infection also exist in all patients in varying amounts, an initial dose must be given which is adequate to neutralise their effect; the streptokinase-antibody complex thus formed being rapidly cleared from the circulation. The initial dose for an individual patient can be either determined by the streptokinase resistance test, if the laboratory facilities are available or time permits, or a standard initial intravenous dose ranging from 250,000 to 600,000 units can be given over a period of 10 to 30 minutes (not more rapidly); followed by a continuous intravenous infusion maintenance dose of 100,000 units hourly. Such a fixed dosage regimen will produce a satisfactory thrombolytic effect in the vast majority of patients (Verstraete et al., 1966; Hirsh et al., 1970b). Moreover, laboratory control is simplified and thrombolytic treatment can be started quickly after thromboembolism; this is an important matter as it is relatively ineffective in lysing thrombi more than 3 days old.

Apart from the age of the thrombus, the site of occlusion also influences response. Venous thrombi are apparently easier to lyse than arterial thrombi, and those in the limbs respond better than do those elsewhere. Clinical success also depends in large part on the extent of occlusion, and the ability of the tissue to survive temporary restriction of its blood supply. To prevent the formation of new thrombi containing non-lysable fibrin, anticoagulant therapy should be started as soon as streptokinase administration stops. Even then late rethrombosis and post-thrombotic symptoms can still occur in some cases.

Complications are usually confined to bleeding from sites of vascular puncture, recent surgical incisions or some other trauma and to reactions consequent upon its antigenicity. Bleeding complications are due to an induced state of hyperplasminaemia (see section 1.1.1), and can be minimised by using a scheme aiming at a high activator and low plasmin levels. A high activator level may however, still digest the fibrin in haemostatic plugs and cause rebleeding, even when the coagulation system is only mildly affected. It is advisable to give a corticosteroid (e.g. 25 to 50mg prednisone orally or 100mg hydrocortisone intravenously) before the start of infusion to control any febrile or anaphylactic reaction.

The principal indications for streptokinase are treatment of selected cases of acute massive or major pulmonary embolism, recent arterial occlusion and deep vein thrombosis involving the iliofemoral and peripheral venous segments (for review, see Brogden et al., 1973; Kakkar and Scully, 1978).

Urokinase: Urokinase is a trypsin-like enzyme consisting of a single polypeptide chain with a molecular weight of 54,000. This naturally occurring plasminogen activator is excreted in human urine. Purified urokinase preparations are non-antigenic, non-pyrogenic and their proper use is associated with a milder coagulation defect than that with streptokinase, but with a similar incidence of bleeding to that shown for streptokinase treated patients (Urokinase-Streptokinase Embolism Trial, 1974). As the level of inhibitors in plasma is relatively constant, a fixed dosage regimen can readily be used. In practice, an initial intravenous dose of 4,000 units/kg body weight over 10 minutes followed by the same maintenance dose per kg hourly is used. Further experience to establish the efficacy of differing dosage schedules is needed, but delayed because of the high cost of the drug and its lack of widespread availability.

The principal indications for urokinase are probably similar to those for streptokinase. It has been shown to be effective in acute major pulmonary embolism and deep vein thrombosis (for review, see Kakkar and Scully, 1978).

3.4 Fibrinolytic Stimulants

A number of drugs have been found to increase the natural fibrinolytic activity of blood but the response obtained is either so mild that no dissolution of preformed thrombi can be expected (e.g. testosterone), or is marked but too brief to be thrombolytic and is followed by a period of refractoriness (e.g. biguanides, nicotinic acid). The oral anabolic steroids ethyloestrenol and stanozolol have a moderate stimulating effect on fibrinolysis but resistance tends to develop later (ethyloestrenol) or not at all (stanozolol). A combination of anabolic steroids with a biguanide, which are active fibrinolytic agents when used alone, may possibly prove to be useful in the medium to long term. Promising results have been achieved with ethyloestrenol + phenformin (8mg + 100mg daily) in reducing the frequency of thrombotic episodes in patients with recurrent occlusive vascular disease (Nilsson et al., 1975), but in view of the risk of lactic acidosis, phenformin can no longer be recommended. Stanozolol alone may be an alternative (Jarrett et al., 1977). The mode of action of fibrinolytic stimulants is depicted in figure 2.

3.5 Principles of Use of Antithrombotic and Thrombolytic Drugs

The antithrombotic drugs illustrate the application of clinical pharmacological principles to therapeutics in their most practical form. Antithrombotic drugs, particularly the oral anticoagulants, have a narrow therapeutic ratio and many factors can modify their response. Thus dosage must be carefully adjusted to produce a precise pharmacological effect without causing unwanted coagulation disturbances. The following specific considerations should guide the use of antithrombotic drugs.

1) *Speed of response* — in general, heparin is mainly used for its immediate anticoagulant effect in the first 48 hours before oral agents have induced an appreciable effect. In some circumstances rapid introduction of *deep* anticoagulation may be unwise; e.g. the first days after major surgery, and makes it sensible to allow a period of 36 to 48 hours before a deep anticoagulant effect is established. On the other hand, a rapid effect is desirable in pulmonary embolism, recent thrombosis in a deep vein or limb artery, and in certain cases of disseminated intravascular coagulation (see section 5.2.2).

2) *Desirable dosage* — the dose schedule of anticoagulant drugs should not only be optimum for control to avoid bleeding, but also should relate to the most beneficial arbitrary level in a particular indication — e.g. a thrombotest range of 5 to 10 % is aimed at for oral antithrombotic prophylaxis in myocardial infarction, but rather a value up to 15 % (Loeliger et al., 1964; Sevitt and Innes, 1964) for prophylaxis in deep vein thrombosis (see also 6 below).

3) *Duration of therapy* — anticoagulants should only be given for as long as benefits are expected to outweigh hazards. However, the number of patients at risk from thromboembolism following an acute myocardial infarction is sufficiently great and the favourable clinical impressions are sufficiently strong so that the possibility of benefit can not be excluded; a relative reduction of the mean fatality rates of 21 % (Chalmers et al., 1977). However, thromboembolic complications are no longer an important cause of mortality following infarction with the advent of treatment regimens directed at early mobilisation and ambulation (Selzer, 1978). In this therapeutic dilemma, some believe (a policy in Europe) an acceptable course is to use oral anticoagulants to treat all patients having proved acute myocardial infarction while they are hospitalised, unless there are contraindications. Many such clinicians continue anticoagulation for 3 to 18 months thereafter, but the well organised Dutch Thrombosis Services have presented impressive evidence in 2 controlled trials to show that further continuation of anticoagulants until there are definite contraindications, results in a statistically greater benefit in terms of mortality and morbidity (cardiovascular events) when compared with a control group (Loeliger et al., 1967; Meeuwissen et al., 1969). Few British and American hospitals use anticoagulants routinely for or following acute myocardial infarction (see section 4.1.3). In special situations, such as a hip fracture, anticoagulants are continued until the patient is ambulatory, whereas in patients with prosthetic heart valves their use is justified indefinitely (see further table VI).

The duration of therapy with thrombolytic drugs is best assessed by the clinical result. In lesions subjected to serial angiography, therapy should continue until the desired angiographic vessel clearing is achieved and is associated with a significant clinical gain. In most cases however, at

Table VI. Some indications and approximate duration of treatment for anticoagulant therapy

Condition	Heparin	Oral anticoagulants (started 48 hours before heparin withdrawn)
Pulmonary embolism	3 days	3 months after full mobilisation
Deep vein thrombosis	7 days	2 months after full mobilisation
Acute peripheral arterial emboli	3 days	Depends if atrial fibrillation can be corrected. If not, continue indefinitely
Acute myocardial infarction	2 days	Controversial (see text). If anticoagulants are used heparin to start is optional. In principle, continue oral anticoagulants for 2 years after infarction, certainly in those less than 65 years of age
Hip fracture	2 days (low dose)	Until patient is mobile
Cerebral emboli after myocardial infarction	—	As for acute myocardial infarction
Transient ischaemic attacks due to stenosis of extracranial arteries	—	Indefinitely
Prosthetic heart valve	—	Indefinitely with presently available valves
Atrial fibrillation with rheumatic heart disease	—	Indefinitely, even if no cerebral or peripheral emboli occurred
Cerebral emboli with rheumatic heart disease	—	Indefinitely, even if atrial fibrillation can be corrected because of large left atrium

least with streptokinase, therapy should in principle not be continued for longer than 72 hours.

4) *Patients at risk of complications* — anticoagulant drugs should not be used in unreliable outpatients, or in patients in whom there is a definite risk of haemorrhage which cannot be avoided by careful adjustment of dosage, particularly when the bleeding could occur in certain tissues (eyes, brain, central nervous system, etc). The presence of a haemostatic defect obviously contraindicates the start of anticoagulant therapy. Similar precautions apply to the use of thrombolytic drugs (see table VII).

Many surgical procedures can be conducted in patients on oral anticoagulant therapy without risk of undue bleeding, provided the anticoagulant effect is well controlled (Storm, 1958). In certain operative situations (e.g. surgery involving the central nervous system or eye or prostatectomy where a large raw surface must be left), oral anticoagulants should be stopped beforehand for suffi-

ciently long to allow the clotting factors to return to near normal, or if surgery is urgent, vitamin K_1 (phytomenadione) can be given. The missing clotting factors can be replaced in certain very urgent situations (e.g. sudden availability of a donor kidney for a recipient on anticoagulants).

5) *Factors which modify response* — a number of factors related to the patient necessitate a reduction of dosage of oral anticoagulants and these must always be borne in mind. The elderly are particularly sensitive to the effects of oral anticoagulants (see section 3.2.3 to 3.2.5).

6) *Monitoring of therapy* — with all antithrombotic drugs response can be measured, and therefore therapy can be governed by appropriate laboratory control of the desired anticoagulant or thrombolytic effect, but it is not always required. Certainly, monitoring of oral anticoagulants is mandatory (e.g. one stage prothrombin time, thrombotest); some monitoring is desirable with continuous infusion of heparin (e.g. whole blood

glass clotting time or preferably the activated partial thromboplastin time), particularly when elimination is accelerated in the presence of liver disease (see section 3.2.1) but is not essential for short term intermittent intravenous administration or with long term low dose subcutaneous administration. The relationship between monitoring heparin therapy and bleeding rate or recurrent thromboembolism is unfortunately less striking than was anticipated (Basu et al., 1972; Pitney et al., 1970). The major therapeutic usefulness of laboratory control is to ensure the presence of at least some anticoagulant effect at all times during treatment, since coagulation must be inhibited continuously to inhibit fibrin deposition or impede

Table VII. Risk factors and contraindications to anticoagulants and thrombolytic drugs

Condition	Risk
Haemorrhagic disorder or diathesis Potentially bleeding lesions (e.g. active peptic ulcer)	Danger of severe haemorrhage with anticoagulants and thrombolytic drugs (contraindications)
Severe hypertension Recent cerebrovascular accident	Cerebral bleeding
Recent trauma or surgery to CNS	Bleeding at operative site
Subacute bacterial endocarditis	Risk of haemorrhage in areas infarcted by emboli, particularly in the brain
Chronic renal failure	Increased risk of bleeding
Recent operation or trauma	Risk of bleeding from recent wounds with thrombolytic drugs
Full doses of salicylates (e.g. rheumatoid arthritis)	Increased risk of bleeding with long term anticoagulants
Early pregnancy	Risk of fetal abnormalities with oral anticoagulants Risk of premature separation of the placenta with thrombolytic drugs
Late pregnancy	Risk of fetal and neonatal haemorrhage with oral anticoagulants
Unreliable or uncooperative patient, including chronic alcoholics	Increased risk of bleeding from poorly controlled oral anticoagulant therapy

extension of the thrombus, but the ideal test and intensity of anticoagulant effect have not been established (Loeliger et al., 1970). Some suggested desirable ranges of clotting tests are given in table VIII. With oral anticoagulants, the initial clotting time should be made 48 hours after the first dose and then checked every alternate day until a stable response at the desired level of anticoagulation is attained.

Although monitoring of streptokinase therapy can be ignored with a standard dosage regimen (see section 3.3), adjustment of the maintenance dose according to the degree of plasma thrombolytic activity and to the degree of haemostatic impairment produced, is usually recommended. However, tests of plasminogen activator (to measure thrombolytic activity) are outside the scope of most routine laboratories and even then there is no general agreement on which tests should be used. Many consider that twice daily measurements of the plasma thrombin time (2 to 3 times of control value) to assess the coagulation defect, is the primary guide.

7) *Other treatment* — sometimes antithrombotic drugs may not be the most appropriate or beneficial form of treatment. For example, surgical embolectomy is indicated in certain cases of massive pulmonary embolism (see section 4.5) and is the treatment of choice in cases of limb threatening recent peripheral emboli in non-atheromatotic arteries (see section 4.2.2).

4. Treatment and Prevention of Thromboembolic Disorders

The aim of treatment of a thromboembolic occlusion is prompt restoration of blood flow. Ideal treatment of thrombosis is therefore to remove the obstruction. If this is not possible, treatment should ensure that the thrombus does not extend or generate an embolus.

Prevention of thromboembolism is at present easier to achieve in most situations than treatment of pre-formed thrombi (Morris and Mitchell, 1978a). In treating *established* thrombosis, antithrombotic drugs can at best only prevent extension of thrombi and emboli formation and these limitations should be borne in mind. Since fibrin formation appears to play a predominant role in venous thrombi, agents which inhibit fibrin deposition (i.e. anticoagulants) are expected to be more valuable in *prevention* of venous occlusion.

On the same theoretical grounds, antiplatelet agents, especially when combined with anticoagulants, are likely to be more promising in attempts to *prevent* arterial occlusion (see section 1.1.2).

4.1 Coronary Artery Disease

4.1.1 Treatment of Angina and Impending Infarction

There is only one well designed study on the long term use (2.5 years) of oral anticoagulants in patients under 70 years with a history of angina of less than 2 years in which significantly less patients developed or died from myocardial infarction in the anticoagulant group (Borchgrevink, 1960; 1962). There is no satisfactory evidence that anticoagulants are of major benefit in patients with 'crescendo' or unstable angina (impending infarction). However, there is some evidence (to be confirmed), that in patients with unstable angina, a streptokinase infusion for 24 hours followed by oral anticoagulation is associated with a significant reduction in myocardial infarction and sudden death compared with oral anticoagulation alone (Lawrence et al., 1978).

4.1.2 Prevention of Myocardial Infarction

Antithrombotic drugs might be used to prevent a first myocardial infarction or to prevent reinfarction or reduce cardiac mortality following a prior infarction. Several large scale prospective trials have been conducted with agents which affect platelet function, either in *healthy* or in aged individuals, to evaluate their usefulness in the primary prevention of myocardial infarction. The evidence available at present does not allow the recommendation for use of clofibrate, aspirin or sulphinpyrazone in healthy or in elderly individuals for the prevention of a first myocardial infarction (Verstraete, 1978a). There is, however, reasonable evidence that patients *with angina* but without prior infarction may benefit from treatment with clofibrate; as reflected in a reduced incidence of fatal and non-fatal myocardial infarction (Scottish Physicians, 1971; Newcastle Physicians, 1971). Nevertheless, it is necessary to emphasise the importance of proper patient selection if clofibrate is recommended for the *primary prevention* of an infarction, since it cannot be recommended as a prophylactic agent in those with a prior infarct, either with or without angina. Moreover, the long term use of clofibrate in

Table VIII. Tests used to monitor anticoagulant therapy

Test	Suggested value[1] (prolongation of clotting time)
Heparin	
Whole blood clotting time (WBCT)[2]	1.5 to 2.5 times control value (just prior to bolus iv or throughout continuous infusion)
Activated partial thromboplastin time (APTT)[2]	1.5 to 2.5 times control value
Thrombin clotting time	3 to 4 times control value
Oral anticoagulants (coumarin/indanediones)	
One-stage prothrombin time (Quick)	2 to 2.5 times control value (with saline extract of brain)
Prothrombin and pro convertin test (Owren)	5 to 15% of control value
Thrombotest	5 to 10% of control value

1 Unfortunately, wide differences still exist between laboratories in techniques and methods of expressing results. This means that uniform standards for the optimum degree of anticoagulation are difficult to define. Nevertheless, the upper value is probably necessary when full anticoagulation is required to completely prevent thrombus formation or extension.

2 Although the values in these two tests are the same they do not equate with each other; e.g. an APPT assay of 1.5 times control may equate with a WBCT assay of 2 times control value.

patients without angina or prior myocardial infarction may be associated with serious pathological consequences and increased mortality from causes other than ischaemic heart disease, even though the incidence of non-fatal, but not fatal, infarction is reduced (Committee of Principal Investigators, 1978). Thus, clofibrate cannot be recommended as a lipid lowering agent for general use (Editorial, 1978b,c).

Until recently, there was no certainty whether drugs affecting platelet function such as clofibrate, aspirin and dipyridamole are useful in the prevention of *recurrent* myocardial infarction, although a positive trend has been observed in some trials which used a higher dose of aspirin or dipyridamole alone or in combination (Verstraete, 1978a). In an interim report of the first large scale trial with sulphinpyrazone, a reduction in cardiac deaths of 48.5% was observed in the first 8.4 months of the trial (Anturane Reinfarction Trial, 1978).

Long term anticoagulant therapy after myocardial infarction has been evaluated in a number of well designed trials which have been critically reanalysed (International Anticoagulant Review Group, 1970). The results taken together, point to a small but real reduction in cardiac mortality from anticoagulant therapy; at all age groups in males and probably also in females who had prolonged angina and/or a previous infarction (see also section 4.1.3).

4.1.3 Treatment of Acute Myocardial Infarction

On present evidence, there appears to be only a slight reduction in hospital mortality by using thrombolytic agents in the first 48 hours after acute myocardial infarction. Several studies in non-coronary care unit settings have shown that streptokinase provides a significant reduction of mortality compared with heparin or no anti-coagulation, in patients treated within 12 hours of onset of an acute myocardial infarction. Studies conducted in coronary care units have failed to reveal a significant benefit. Although these different results cannot yet be fully explained, the lack of a major benefit is not surprising. Not all such patients have a coronary occlusion and those who do, may also have an atherogenic narrowing with or without a thrombus composed largely of platelets. Moreover, the myocardium survives severe hypoxaemia for a shorter time than is required to induce and achieve thrombolysis, thus limiting the chance of success. Nevertheless, the possibility remains that the prompt restoration of blood flow through the peripheral zone of partial ischaemia will diminish the risk of ventricular arrhythmias and result in a smaller infarct and a better cardiac output (Verstraete, 1978b).

The place of antithrombotic drugs as part of the overall management of myocardial infarction has still to be clearly defined (see chapter XVII; sect. 5.6). Although acute myocardial infarction is the most common form of heart disease for which anticoagulants are sometimes given, it is still the most controversial with regard to the degree of benefits achieved (see Selzer, 1978). Considering that there is often failure to find a thrombotic occlusion of a coronary artery as the primary causal event in acute myocardial infarction, it is not surprising that any attempt to remove thrombi or prevent their formation is liable to meet with only limited success. The recommendation to use anticoagulants in acute myocardial infarction is based on a well established conviction of a reduction in thromboembolic complications, rather than on any firm proof of an effect on the mortality rate. However, thromboembolic complications are no longer an important presumed cause of mortality in acute myocardial infarction, presumably because of current treatment approaches directed at early mobilisation and ambulation (Selzer, 1978). Long term use of anticoagulants in patients who have recovered from acute myocardial infarction does however, provide a small benefit against another infarct (see section 4.1.2). Men under the age of 55 years appear to derive most benefit, but it is not limited to this group.

Attitudes to use of anticoagulants in acute myocardial infarction differ internationally (Bassan and Rogel, 1976). In most European hospitals, an acceptable approach to use of anticoagulants in acute myocardial infarction, bearing in mind the limited long term benefits to be achieved, is that most patients with proven acute myocardial infarction should be treated with anticoagulants whilst in hospital and for up to 12 to 18 months after myocardial infarction, unless there are contraindications or other risks with the therapy (see table VII). There is supporting evidence for extending the administration of anticoagulants in younger patients until they have reached the age of 65 years, provided no contraindications intervene in the meantime (Loeliger et al., 1967; Meeuwissen et al., 1969). On the other hand, in the majority of American and British hospitals, anticoagulants are used selectively for acute myocardial infarction in 'poor risk' patients (e.g. after transmural infarction in: those over 60, with prior infarction, large infarct, shock or congestive heart failure) and selectively or not at all for long term use following infarction (Bassan and Rogel, 1976; Rogers and Sherry, 1976). Whatever decision is taken, clinicians and patients should recognise that anticoagulant treatment is not a panacea for prophylaxis of ischaemic myocardial disease. Most investigators now believe that anticoagulation with oral anticoagulants need not be complemented with heparin at the start of prophylactic therapy. Anticoagulants should be withheld as long as the diagnosis of acute myocardial infarction is not fully proven, in order not to anticoagulate patients later shown to have pericarditis, dissecting aneurysm, pancreatitis or gastrointestinal abnormalities.

4.1.4 Prevention of Thromboembolism in Patients With Prosthetic Heart Valves

Patients with valvular disease of the heart have a high incidence of thromboembolism, especially if the mitral valve is stenosed. Valvular repair improves the heart function but operated patients with substituted valve(s) are still susceptible to thromboembolic complications. The combination of oral anticoagulants and either dipyridamole (450mg daily) or aspirin (1g daily) is significantly more effective in preventing arterial embolism in these patients than anticoagulants alone. Aspirin alone does not appear to offer the desired protection; whether the same dose of aspirin combined with dipyridamole would be as effective in preventing systemic embolism as oral anticoagulants supplemented with either one of these antiplatelet aggregating drugs has still to be demonstrated (Taguchi et al., 1975).

4.1.5 Prevention of Graft Occlusion After Aortocoronary Bypass Surgery

The place of aspirin and/or dipyridamole in the prevention of graft occlusion after aortocoronary bypass surgery is not yet clear. The combination of one of these drugs with oral anticoagulants is superior in this respect than anticoagulants alone (Hall et al., 1974). Whether the combined use of large doses of dipyridamole and aspirin is as effective as either of these plus anticoagulants remains to be confirmed (Levine et al., 1975).

4.2 Peripheral Arterial Occlusion

4.2.1 Prevention of Arterial Occlusions in Patients with Obliterative Arteriopathy in the Limbs

There is no good evidence for the clinical effectiveness of aspirin or any other drug affecting platelet function in patients with peripheral arterial insufficiency due to arteriosclerosis or after vascular grafting. A similar uncertainty still prevails concerning the use of oral anticoagulants in the same group of patients (Verstraete, 1976c).

4.2.2 Treatment of Recent Arterial Occlusions in the Limbs

Surgery has developed greatly in recent years and results obtained with the Fogarty catheter with emboli in large arteries have definitely surpassed those achieved by thrombolysis. Thrombolytic agents such as streptokinase, however, may be useful in the management of acute (less than 72 hours) thromboembolism in arteries distal to the knee and in occlusions in larger arteries with extensive atherosclerosis, provided reconstructive surgical repair is not either desirable or feasible (Brogden et al., 1973).

4.2.3 Treatment of Chronic Arterial Occlusions in the Limbs

Streptokinase can improve blood flow in patients with chronic (weeks or months) arterial occlusion and stenosis (Brogden et al., 1973). As only unorganised thrombi can be lysed, these results suggest that in some cases organisation of thrombi in larger arteries may be delayed for months and proceed more slowly than in more distal arteries. An explanation for this surprising phenomenon may be that calcified atherosclerotic lesions of the vessel wall may form a mechanical barrier for the ingrowth of fibroblast involved in thrombus organisation. However, streptokinase should be reserved for patients with severe symptoms not requiring rapid relief, in whom vascular surgery is not feasible or undesirable, and with occlusions of the main arteries less than 10cm in length. Reocclusion can nevertheless occur, even with use of anticoagulants.

4.3 Cerebral Vascular Disease

4.3.1 Prevention of Transient Ischaemic Attacks

Some evidence that the administration of sulphinpyrazone could significantly reduce the frequency of transient neurological episodes, has not been confirmed by more extensive controlled trials with this drug or with dipyridamole or clofibrate. On the other hand, aspirin (1.2g daily) has been shown to produce a substantial reduction in risk for continuing transient ischaemic attacks, stroke or death in men but not women in a large scale Canadian trial (Canadian Cooperative Study Group, 1978), confirming the favourable trend observed in an earlier American trial (Fields et al., 1977). Aspirin (1.3g daily) has also been shown to reduce the incidence of transient ischaemic attacks and to have a beneficial effect on stroke related deaths in patients who have had reconstructive operations of the carotid artery (Fields et al.,

1978). There is also clear evidence that long term use of oral anticoagulants can significantly reduce the incidence of transient ischaemic attacks and of subsequent cerebral infarction (Whisnant et al., 1973). See further chapter XXV (sect. 8.2).

4.3.2 Treatment of Established Stroke

Antiplatelet aggregating agents, anticoagulants and thrombolytic drugs have so far not been shown to have a beneficial clinical effect in patients with an acute or subacute cerebral thromboembolism, probably because the ischaemic brain necrosis was already irreversible. Furthermore, the ischaemic damage of the cerebral vessels may more readily bleed even when the systemic coagulation is only mildly affected (Fletcher et al., 1976). See further chapter XXV (sect. 8.1).

4.4 Deep Vein Thrombosis

Not all forms of deep vein thrombosis are associated with the same risk of pulmonary embolism (Beckering and Titus, 1969; Walker, 1972). Although there is agreement on the much higher risk of pulmonary embolism in thrombosis in iliofemoral segments, there is no agreement on the need to routinely treat deep vein thrombosis confined to the calf, particularly in asymptomatic cases detected by fibrinogen scanning or ultrasound. The majority of venous thrombi beginning in the calf do not propagate proximally, and when the thrombus remains confined to the calf, emboli, essentially, do not occur. However, some peripheral venous thrombi do propagate and this must be prevented, because the larger the thrombus, the greater the risk should it break free and become an embolus. Thus, some treat all cases of deep vein thrombosis, regardless of the site and irrespective of the presence of clinical symptoms or signs.

The most important aspect is the early detection of deep vein thrombosis. Clinical diagnosis alone is unreliable and detection should be complemented by ultrasound and radiolabelled fibrinogen screening, and ideally the location and extent of the thrombus confirmed by phlebography (Gallus et al., 1976; Browse, 1978). Such diagnostic accuracy permits individualisation of treatment according to the site and extent of the thrombus. Treatment is either aimed at preventing extension of the thrombus with anticoagulants, or at removal of the thrombus by thrombectomy or thrombolysis (Adar and Salzman, 1975; Morris and Mitchell, 1978).

4.4.1 Treatment of Thrombosis in Calf Veins

Although anticoagulants are probably sufficient to prevent extension of a thrombus confined to calf veins they do not enhance its removal. Streptokinase however, can lyse fresh thrombi and restore vessel patency in approximately 50% of patients and was shown to preserve venous valve function a year after treatment (Kakkar et al., 1969; Rosch et al., 1976; Widmer et al., 1978). As with the other forms of treatment, rethrombosis and post-thrombotic symptoms can occur after successful thrombolysis. Streptokinase is probably best reserved for patients with extensive thrombi involving calf and more proximal veins, provided that clinical features have not been present for longer than 96 hours (see section 1.1.2). It is given for up to 3 days and then followed by anticoagulants (see section 3.3). In cases in which a short segment of calf vein(s) is occluded, full doses of heparin can be instituted along with oral anticoagulants and continued for 5 to 7 days after the desirable level of oral anticoagulant control has been achieved (Brogden et al., 1973).

Treatment with oral anticoagulants is continued for several months; 3 months is long enough, provided the patient is fully ambulatory. Patients with recurrent embolism and a permanent thrombotic tendency may require anticoagulants, unless oral fibrinolytic stimulants such as stanozolol or antiplatelet aggregating drugs are shown to prevent rethrombosis, indefinitely.

4.4.2 Treatment of Iliofemoral Thrombosis

Because of the greater morbidity and mortality associated with iliofemoral thrombosis, therapy must be more definitive. In patients with non-occlusive or 'floating' iliofemoral thrombosis, bilateral phlebography should be performed routinely and once located, the thrombus surgically removed and clearance confirmed radiologically. In occlusive iliofemoral thrombosis, therapy is aimed at preventing pulmonary emboli as well as chronic venous insufficiency of the lower leg, and at restoring patency of the vessel. Venous thrombectomy or preferably thrombolytic therapy may be used, provided clinical signs have been present for less than 96 hours. Both forms of treatment are less effective when older thrombi are involved and both are associated with rethrombosis. Other factors, particularly contraindications and surgical experience, will determine which of the two forms of treatment should be used. Following treatment oral anticoagulants are given for several months as discussed above.

4.4.3 Treatment of Superficial Thrombophlebitis

In the absence of deep vein thrombosis, it is probable that symptomatic treatment with certain non-steroidal anti-inflammatory agents (e.g. indomethacin but not phenylbutazone; see section 3.2.5) suffices for superficial phlebitis of limited extent below the knee. For cases which progress despite 24 to 48 hours of simple treatment, the choice lies between anticoagulants and vein ligation, with or without excision of the involved vein. To avoid the risk of pulmonary embolism, saphenous thrombosis in the upper half of the thigh deserves prompt anticoagulant treatment, even with emergency saphenofemoral ligation, according to some surgeons, if the process ascends despite treatment, and thrombectomy or thrombolysis if the thrombus extends into the femoral vein (Adar and Salzman, 1975).

4.5 Treatment of Acute Pulmonary Embolism

Pulmonary embolism is a form of arterial obstruction due to a thrombus from a peripheral vein. For treatment purposes it may be considered in 4 different clinical categories (for review, see Tibbutt and Chesterman, 1976, 1978):

1) The emboli may be large and immediately fatal, when of course no form of treatment is of value
2) The emboli may be large and cause collapse, hypotension, progressive deterioration and death, or
3) May cause collapse followed by partial recovery but residual major haemodynamic problems
4) The emboli may be small and produce no lasting haemodynamic effects.

Heparin (40,000 to 60,000 units per 24 hours) is the emergency treatment for pulmonary embolism immediately the diagnosis is suspected. The duration of treatment depends on assessment of the duration of risk. It is the treatment of choice in category 4 patients, supplemented by investigation of the peripheral veins, and prior to discharge, oral anticoagulants for 3 to 6 months to prevent further embolism. In the relatively small group in category 3, the choice is between surgical embolectomy and thrombolytic therapy. As the necessary highly skilled surgical facilities are often not available, streptokinase or urokinase (if available) most often will be used, even more so in those patients with underlying cardiac or respiratory disease. The rapidly deteriorating patient (category 2) needs immediate relief from pulmonary artery obstruction and is best treated by surgical embolectomy, but if not available, or in the meantime, thrombolytic agents can be tried. With streptokinase, clinical improvement is seen in 2 to 4 hours, but measurable haemodynamic change is not seen for 6 to 8 hours after the start of treatment (Brogden et al., 1973).

The difference in the haemodynamic improvement achieved with heparin or thrombolysis (urokinase or streptokinase) clearly favours the latter at 72 hours. Patients treated with heparin alone show similar improvement within 2 weeks (Urokinase Pulmonary Embolism Trial, 1973; Urokinase-Streptokinase Embolism Trial, 1974). Therefore, thrombolytic treatment is indicated. A suggested regimen is 600,000 units of streptokinase in the first half hour and 100,000 units per hour for 72 hours, together with hydrocortisone 100mg 6-hourly during the infusion (Tibbutt et al., 1974). Patients in shock seem to have the most favourable response to streptokinase. It is not known whether the initial accelerated thrombolysis by streptokinase is of greater value in terms of long term resolution and survival. Other aspects and the general management of pulmonary embolism are discussed in chapter XVII (sect. 9).

4.6 Prophylaxis of Postoperative Deep Vein Thrombosis

The three important causes of thrombosis are abnormalities in the vessel wall, changes in the coagulability of blood, and stasis. Most arterial thrombosis is secondary to atheroma in the artery wall. This stimulus cannot be fully overcome by anticoagulants, so it is highly unlikely that their long term use will prevent the eventual formation of arterial thrombosis. In contrast, venous thrombosis (e.g. associated with major surgery or childbirth) is due to a change in the coagulability of the blood, superimposed in many instances by changes in the rate of blood flow. In this situation, short term prophylaxis with antithrombotic drugs or mechanical measures can often prevent venous thrombosis in patients at high risk. These groups include patients with fractured neck of femur, and puerperal and postoperative patients. Risk factors include severe varicose veins, history of previous episodes of deep vein thrombosis, marked obesity, malignancy, age over 40, lengthy surgery or patients whose mobilisation is to be delayed (Kakkar et al., 1970). The risk is also high in the paralysed limb of patients who have suffered a stroke. Management of puerperal thrombosis is discussed in chapter XV (sect. 6).

The aim of prophylaxis of postoperative deep vein thrombosis is to prevent thromboembolism by stimulating the blood flow in the leg or by decreasing the coagulability of the blood, but there is currently no universally accepted prophylactic method (see Gallus and Hirsh, 1976b). Two effective mechanical measures for preventing stasis are intermittent electrical stimulation of the calf muscles and calf compression with pneumatic leggings. These can be used during surgery and in the case of pneumatic leggings continued afterwards. Both reduce calf vein thrombosis, but it is not known whether the incidence of pulmonary embolism is reduced (Browse et al., 1974, 1976; Clark et al., 1974), and do not appear to add to the benefits of low dose heparin or dextran 70 (Roberts and Cotton, 1975; Smith et al., 1978). They are impractical when the patient is in the lithotomy position or the operation is on a lower limb.

Low dose subcutaneous heparin can effectively reduce the incidence of deep vein thrombosis and pulmonary embolism and this protective effect has been particularly well demonstrated in general and gynaecological surgery (Multicentre Trial, 1975; 1977). In orthopaedic and urological surgery the complications are greater and desired effects are less marked with low doses of heparin and the prophylaxis of postoperative deep vein thrombosis appears to be better secured with dextran 70 (Verstraete, 1976a). It is presently accepted by most experts that 500ml of dextran 70 during the operation followed by 500ml every second day decreases the incidence of fatal and non-fatal pulmonary embolism. It is the method of choice in patients with an average or high risk of embolism associated with an average or high risk of bleeding. Occasional fluid overload and right heart strain are disadvantages and dextran can damage the kidney if there is coincident hypotension and oliguria.

Bleeding and wound complications are generally not a serious problem when 5,000 units of heparin are administered subcutaneously at 12-hourly intervals but can result in larger haematoma formation and minor bleeding particularly when given 8-hourly. This suggests that perhaps the routine use of low dose heparin should be reserved for those patients with preoperative factors indicating an increased risk from thromboembolism (Pachter and Riles, 1977).

Oral anticoagulants (properly employed) are also effective but have the disadvantages of risk of serious bleeding and need for strict laboratory control. Nevertheless, oral anticoagulants are the only regimen proven to prevent death from pulmonary embolism in elderly patients with hip fractures (Morris and Mitchell, 1978b) and appear to be superior to dextran 70 in patients undergoing total hip replacement (Barber et al., 1977).

The position of antiplatelet aggregating drugs is not yet clear. A combination of aspirin (300mg) and dipyridamole (100mg) given 8-hourly has successfully prevented deep vein thrombosis following hip or knee surgery, but this combination seems to be ineffective in elderly patients with hip fracture (Morris and Mitchell, 1977), as is aspirin alone (600mg 12-hourly) in patients undergoing total hip replacement surgery (Stamatakis et al., 1978).

It is not entirely clear how often or for how long it is necessary or beneficial to give either low dose subcutaneous heparin or intravenous dextran 70. A suggested regimen for low dose heparin in major surgery is 5,000 units 2 hours before the operation and every 8 to 12 hours thereafter for 7 days. A high concentration solution (5,000-units/0.2ml) in single dose ampoules appears to be essential to get a correct dose administered in a routine prophylaxis. Lower doses (2,500u 6-hourly) have been used but might not be as effective, although the incidence of minor bleeding may be less. Dextran 70 is given in isotonic saline; the currently recommended regimen is 500 to 1,000ml of a 6% solution started before surgery, and 500ml the following and next 3 alternate days.

As in clinical practice it is not possible to treat prophylactically all operated patients, considerable emphasis should be placed on selection of patients at risk and on the early detection and treatment of deep vein thrombosis (see section 4.4).

4.7 Miscellaneous Thromboembolic Conditions

4.7.1 Thrombus Formation on Artificial Surfaces

Anticoagulants and also antiplatelet agents have been effective in reducing the incidence of thrombus formation on non-biological surfaces such as prosthetic heart valves and arteriovenous shunts and on the walls of the heart-lung machine. Thrombi occluding arteriovenous shunts can be cleared by local treatment with thrombolytic agents (Forbes and Prentice, 1978).

4.7.2 Microcirculatory Thrombosis

The prevention of cerebral emboli and transient ischaemic attacks is discussed in section 4.3 and chapter XXV (sect. 8.2, 8.3). The use of anticoagulants and antiplatelet drugs to prevent intraglomerular coagulation in proliferative glomerulonephritis is discussed in chapter XXI (sect. 4.3).

5. Bleeding Disorders

Effective treatment of the numerous bleeding disorders depends on accurate diagnosis. A haemorrhagic tendency can be due to an abnormality of any of the three major components of the haemostatic mechanism — vascular defects, platelet abnormality or clotting factor deficiency — and can be congenital or acquired. Bleeding following surgery or trauma is most often directly attributable to injury of blood vessels and is not, or only to a very small extent, influenced by systemic treatment with drugs. The treatment of a patient with a defect of the haemostatic mechanism is very specific and is determined by the nature of the defect and its pathogenesis (see Forbes and Davidson, 1973). A precise diagnosis is therefore essential; the large variety of causes of abnormal bleeding, however, requires a large range of laboratory procedures.

Many agents are available for the treatment of specific types of bleeding, but none of these is a haemostatic substance in the strict sense of the term. For instance vitamin C is a most effective drug in the treatment of scurvy, a bleeding disorder which in most countries is limited to dietary deficiency (e.g. bottle fed infants and elderly men living alone). Ascorbic acid is of no value in all the other bleeding disorders for which it is prescribed.

The same holds true for the practice of giving vitamin K to patients with a normal prothrombin level. When topical measures are not feasible or are inadequate, and no specific treatment is available, synthetic haemostatic drugs are used, usually with more hope than certainty of efficacy (Verstraete, 1977).

5.1 Treatment of Congenital Bleeding Disorders

Classical haemophilia (haemophilia A), Christmas disease (haemophilia B) and von Willebrand's disease (angiohaemophilia) are the most common hereditary haemorrhagic states which result from a deficiency of specific clotting factors. Discussion of treatment of these and other congenital bleeding disorders is confined to the use of drugs including blood components, and does not include mention of general measures for the prevention of bleeding (see Brinkhous and Heinker, 1975). Patients with a deficiency of a specific clotting factor tend to have a delayed but persistent bleeding, even after minor injury. The aim of replacement therapy is to raise the concentration of the deficient clotting factor activity in the patient's blood to a level which will bring about haemostasis and to maintain this level until healing of the injury is adequately advanced. Administration of fibrinolytic inhibitors such as ε-aminocaproic acid and tranexamic acid (section 5.4) significantly reduces the incidence and severity of bleeding, as does synthetic vasopressin, desmopressin (Manucci et al., 1977; Kobayashi et al., 1978). Desmopressin raises factor VIII activity, but also enhances fibrinolytic activity, and is thus used in combination with an antifibrinolytic drug such as tranexamic acid.

5.1.1 Classical Haemophilia (haemophilia A)

Administration of human plasma or concentrates of factor VIII (AHF) is the only effective treatment of major bleeding in classical haemophilia (Rizza, 1977). A significant reduction both in blood lost postoperatively and in the requirements of factor VIII (or factor IX) can be obtained by the simultaneous use of the fibrinolytic inhibitors ε-aminocaproic acid or the 10 times more potent tranexamic acid (section 5.4; table IX).

At present the only source of factor VIII available for the routine treatment and prophylaxis of haemophilia is human blood. Transfusion of whole blood should be used only to replace blood loss, not to supply factor VIII. Fresh plasma contains more factor VIII than whole blood and is useful for haemorrhages requiring factor VIII levels of less than 20 % of normal (table IX). More concentrated forms of factor VIII include cryoprecipitate, obtained by rapid freezing and subsequent thawing of plasma, which contains about 40 % of the original factor VIII activity in plasma, and lyophilised concentrates of factor VIII obtained from human plasma by precipitation. Cryoprecipitate contains about 60 units (1 unit of factor VIII activity is the amount present in 1 ml of fresh citrated normal plasma) per bag, whilst lyophilised concentrates of factor VIII contain variable but labelled amounts of factor VIII per ml. After transfusion, the half-life of factor VIII in the blood of a haemophiliac, without inhibitor, is about 12 hours. In the past, animal factor VIII has been used occasionally in patients with high titre antibodies to human factor VIII. At present, high potency human factor VIII is used to 'overcome' the inhibitor, but this is not always successful. More recently concentrates of activated clotting factors have been used to treat patients who have a high titre of antibodies to human factor VIII but thromboembolic complications have occurred. A factor VIII inhibitor bypass activity (Feiba) has been prepared from human blood which is useful in this circumstance (Preston et al., 1977), and this benefit is not due to thrombin or the activated clotting factors IX and X.

Early spontaneous haemarthrosis and intramuscular haematoma will be controlled by increasing the level of factor VIII to 15 to 20 % of normal and can be achieved with a dose of 10 to 15 units of factor VIII per kg body weight (table IX). Severe haematomas and haemarthrosis may require factor VIII levels of about 20 to 30 %, whilst levels of over 40 % of normal are required in haemophilic patients who are to undergo major surgery.

Minor surgical procedures such as dental extraction can be performed with minimal requirement of factor VIII replacement therapy, provided that fibrinolytic inhibitors (see section 5.4) such as epsilon aminocaproic acid or tranexamic acid are also given during (100mg EACA/kg body weight per day or 25mg tranexamic acid/kg body weight per day) and after the procedure (oral intake of 100mg EACA/kg 6-hourly or 25mg tranexamic acid/kg 6-hourly) [Forbes et al., 1972; Walsh et al., 1971; table IX]. Because of the possible complication of intrarenal obstruction, fibrinolytic inhibitors should not be given in the presence of haematuria (Gebauer and Heigel, 1969).

Other preparations such as oestrogens, oral contraceptives and so-called haemostatic substances (e.g. peanut extracts) have been used in haemophilia but have no place in treatment. Prednisone, 2mg/kg daily in 2 divided doses for 3 days, followed by half this dose for the next 2 days, can significantly decrease the amount of replacement therapy required in acute haemarthrosis (Kisker and Burke, 1970), but continuous steroids, even in low doses, are not recommended. In haematuria, the value of corticosteroids in reducing the amount of replacement therapy is not convincing and conflicting (Rizza et al., 1977).

5.1.2 Christmas Disease (haemophilia B)

The general principles of replacement of factor IX in Christmas disease are the same as for that of factor VIII in haemophilia A. The same level of factor IX as for factor VIII in the classic haemophiliac are required for haemostasis in the same clinical situation (see table IX).

Fresh or stored plasma at a dose of about 20ml/5kg body weight administered over 60 minutes raises the factor IX level by 5 to 10 %, which is adequate for minor haemorrhage. Ordinary blood bank plasma is adequate, preferably given in individual blood donation units to decrease the risk of serum hepatitis. A more concentrated factor IX preparation will be needed for severe bleeding. The half-life of factor IX in the blood is 18 to 36 hours but the *in vivo* recovery is less complete than after factor VIII administration in classic haemophilia, a still not satisfactorily explained finding. It is assumed that because of its smaller molecular weight, factor IX is distributed throughout the intravascular and extravascular fluid spaces (which are 2 to 7 times larger than the plasma volume) whereas factor VIII is largely retained within the circulation.

As in classical haemophilia the amount of factor IX required by transfusion for dental surgery can be reduced by the concomitant use of epsilon aminocaproic acid or tranexamic acid. Concomitant use of systemic corticosteroids may reduce the amount of infused factor IX required to relieve the pain of acute haemarthrosis but evidence for their value in haematuria is not convincing (see above).

Table IX. Levels of factor VIII in the blood and doses of different materials used for treatment of different lesions in haemophilia

Lesion	Level of factor VIII desirable in patient's blood immediately after transfusion	Therapeutic material	Factor VIII dose (units per kg)[1]	Duration of therapy
Spontaneous bleeding Early haemarthrosis	5-20 (0-5)[2]	Human factor VIII concentrate	10-15	1 to 2 doses
Dangerous haematomas Multiple dental extraction	20-40 (5-10)	Human factor VIII concentrate	15-30	*Haematoma:* daily for 2-4 days, immobilise limb. *Dental extraction:* single dose morning of procedure plus IV amino-caproic acid 0.lg/kg over 24h and also 0.lg/kg orally 6-hourly for 7 to 10 days. For tranexamic acid: 25mg/kg IV over the first day and 25mg/kg orally every 6 hours for 7 to 10 days
Major surgery Serious accidents	80-100 (20-25)	Human factor VIII concentrate	55-70	Preoperative dose, followed by 12-hourly infusions of 30µg/kg for 6 to 10 days, then daily until wound healing well advanced

1   A unit factor of VIII is the amount of factor VIII present in 1ml of fresh average normal citrated plasma.
2   The figures in brackets are the approximate levels to which the patient's factor VIII level will have fallen in 24 hours after transfusion.

5.1.3 Von Willebrand's Disease

This disease is an autosomally inherited bleeding disorder, probably dominant with varying expressivity, although not everyone accepts this view. These patients have a moderate decrease of factor VIII (10 to 40 %) but in contradistinction to classical haemophilia, the factor VIII level rises after a few hours above that expected from the amount infused.

From presently available data, the following concept of factor VIII seems to emerge. 'Factor VIII' actually consists of a non-covalently bound asymmetric complex of a low molecular weight factor VIII (LMW FVIII C) carrying the procoagulant activity, and a high molecular weight fragment responsible for the interaction of factor VIII with platelets (HMW FVIII RAG). The latter subunit carries the major antigens, reacting with rabbit antibody against human factor VIII. The gene responsible for synthesis of the subunit carrying the procoagulant activity would be located on the X-chromosome and the gene-product absent or defective in haemophilia A.

The gene responsible for synthesis of the subunit interacting with platelets would be located on an autosome and the gene-product absent or defective in von Willebrand's disease. The possibility that in many instances a defective gene-product exists, is suggested by the description of patients with von Willebrand's disease but with normal levels of factor VIII-related antigen (F VIII RAG) or normal levels of ristocetin-cofactor.[1] In haemophilia A, this autosomal gene product would be synthesised normally, explaining the normal bleeding time in this disorder.

Post-traumatic bleeding can usually be readily controlled by transfusion therapy and packing and suturing of the wound. As the level of factor VIII remains raised much longer than in haemophiliacs it is easier to maintain a haemostatic level of factor VIII in patients with von Willebrand's disease. A

1   The antibiotic ristocetin induces platelet aggregation in normal and haemophilic A plasma but not in von Willebrand plasma; a ristocetin cofactor is almost always missing in the latter patients.

priming dose of 5ml/kg body weight of fresh plasma or the corresponding dose of factor VIII cryoprecipitate or lyophilised human factor VIII, is usually effective in preventing or arresting bleeding and can be given on alternate days as maintenance therapy. Oral contraceptives apparently decrease menstrual bleeding in affected individuals.

5.1.4 Congenital Afibrinogenaemia

Effective haemostasis is usually obtained by a concentration of fibrinogen of 100mg per 100ml plasma. This level is easily obtained with 4g of commercial fibrinogen preparations. The half-life of fibrinogen in the blood is about 4 days so that injection of 1 or 2g every second day is usually satisfactory (table X).

5.1.5 Congenital Deficiency of Factor II, VII and X

These rather rare hereditary deficiencies do not respond to the administration of even large doses of vitamin K, despite the fact that it is required for the synthesis of the factors II, VII and X (see section 1.1.1). Stored blood contains factors II, VII and IX and is therefore convenient for the treatment of these patients. The same dose regimen as in classical haemophilia is used because the half-life of factor VII is also short (4 to 6 hours; the corresponding value for factor X is about 40 hours and for factor II 3 to 5 days).

5.1.6 Factor V Deficiency

The hereditary deficiency of factor V or parahaemophilia requires fresh frozen plasma, as factor V is unstable upon storage, even at 4°C. The same doses are used as in classical haemophilia, but because the half-life of factor V is 12 to 36 hours, only one infusion daily is required.

5.2 Acquired Defects of Coagulation

In contrast to the common congenital haemorrhagic states, acquired disorders are due to multiple clotting factor deficiency (Bowie and Owren, 1977).

5.2.1 Prothrombin Complex Deficiency

The three distinguishable causes for prothrombin complex deficiencies are: (a) severe liver disease, which primarily affects factor V but also the factors II, VII, IX and X may be low; (b) vitamin K deficiency, characterised by a reduction of factors II, VII and X, and (c) excessive utilisation of factor V and to a lesser extent of factors II and X.

In the presence of liver disease, a poor response to vitamin K is obtained and replacement therapy with fresh plasma is required, because of the lability of factor V in stored plasma and as this coagulation factor is often decreased in patients with liver disease. The administration of a fibrinogen preparation or concentrated prothrombin complex may be required if surgery is contemplated in these patients.

Major vitamin K deficiency may be caused by interference with the flow of bile salts in the gastrointestinal tract (e.g. obstructive jaundice, biliary fistula), any conditions with impaired absorption from the intestine following extensive surgical

Table X. Stability of blood factors in stored plasma and their dosage in the treatment of congenital bleeding disorders

Congenital deficiency of	Half-life of deficient factor (hours)	Assumed haemostatic level in plasma	Stability in plasma	Recommended initial dose	Maintenance dose
Factor I (fibrinogen)	96-120	100mg/100ml	yes	4g/l	1-2g every 2nd day
Factor II (prothrombin)	72-120	40%	yes		
Factor V	12-36	20%	no	20ml plasma/kg	10ml/kg every 12h
Factor VII	4-6	20%	yes	25u/kg	10u/kg every 12h
Factor VIII	10-12	15%	no	15u/kg	10u/kg
Factor IX	18-36		yes		
Factor X	16-72	20%	yes		
Factor XI	60-84	?	—		
Factor XIII	96-168	1%	yes		
Von Willebrand		20%	yes	5ml plasma/kg	5ml/kg every 2nd day

resection of the intestinal tract, dietary deprivation, sterilisation of the intestinal tract and therapeutic or surreptitious intake of oral anticoagulants. In adults, 5mg per day of vitamin K given orally raises and maintains a normal prothrombin level. In patients with obstructive jaundice or biliary fistula, oral treatment should be confined to water soluble vitamin K (i.e. not phytomenadione). In all situations, any vitamin K preparation will be adequate if given parenterally. With normal liver function, safe therapeutic levels are obtained in 4 to 6 hours. In patients receiving oral anticoagulant therapy, the same dose of 5mg is usually sufficient, but if haemorrhage is actually present, 25 to 50mg should be given parenterally and repeated every 12 hours for the first 2 days if a coumarin drug of prolonged action has been used (see table III).

The daily vitamin K requirement of infants of mothers not receiving oral anticoagulants is 25µg, because there is no bacterial synthesis during the neonatal period. Cow's milk contains approximately 6µg of vitamin K per 100ml but normal human milk only 1 to 5µg per 100ml. Parenteral administration of 1mg phytomenadione is usually sufficient, but may be repeated after 6 hours. Excessive amounts, especially of water soluble vitamin K analogues, can produce haemolytic anaemia with its consequences, particularly in premature infants.

5.2.2 Disseminated Intravascular Coagulation

Disseminated intravascular coagulation, the defibrination syndrome or consumption coagulopathy all refer to a haemorrhagic diathesis due to a consumption of fibrinogen, platelets and clotting factors, which becomes more dominant than their synthesis (Sharp, 1977). A heterogeneous group of rare conditions (table XI) can lead to an acute process, with production of a severe haemorrhagic state, or a subacute or chronic form, with mild or no bleeding features. In both situations, small vessel obstruction by fibrin and/or platelets, tissue necrosis and single or multiple organ dysfunction may occur. The intravascular presence of fibrin normally stimulates secondary development of local fibrinolytic activity but may on very rare occasions, be accompanied by an increase in systemic fibrinolytic enzyme activity. The correct diagnosis is often difficult to make in time because the pattern of abnormalities may be continually changing and even have disappeared by the time of

blood sampling. Useful clues are a low platelet count, decreased levels of factor V and VIII, fibrinogen and plasminogen, associated with fibrin degradation products which cause a prolongation of the thrombin time.

Treatment must first be directed at termination of the underlying disease (e.g. antibiotics in sepsis; emptying of the uterus in abruptio placentae and dead fetus syndrome) and this may be the only therapy necessary in chronic defibrination states. In acute defibrination, supportive therapy (expansion of blood volume, if depleted, control of acidosis and electrolyte imbalance) is the first step. In case of bleeding with serious anaemia, fresh whole blood is indicated with replacement of depleted coagulation factors. If the clinical situation further deteriorates and/or the laboratory tests are becoming worse, heparin treatment must be seriously considered. About 1,000 units heparin (about 10mg) are administered per hour by continuous intravenous infusion. In this situation, oral anticoagulants cannot be used because their onset of action is too slow. In more urgent situations fibrinogen (4 to 6g) can also be administered under cover of the heparin infusion. In some instances, the results of serial laboratory tests may lead to an increase in the rate of the heparin infusion by a factor of 1.5 or 2. If the diagnosis is correct the factor V and fibrinogen level should rise within 12 hours. There is growing evidence that heparin should be administered without any delay in disseminated intravascular coagulation secondary to amniotic fluid embolism, severe incompatible transfusion reactions, acute leukaemia and carcinoma with multiple metastases (Sharp, 1977).

5.2.3 Transfusion Induced Bleeding

Massive transfusion of citrated blood can cause hypocalcaemia and induce cardiac standstill, especially in patients in prolonged shock. Citrate overdosage is rare because the liver can metabolise 0.03 to 0.04mmol per kg per minute, which allows the safe transfusion of 2 litres of citrated blood in 20 minutes. If more than 10 units of blood or plasma per hour are administered, 0.25g of calcium chloride should be administered after each unit. If bleeding occurs, this is not because of hypocalcaemia but due to massive transfusion of stored blood low in platelets and factors V and VIII. When more than 10 units of blood are required on the same day, 1 of every 3 units should be less than 6 hours old.

Table XI. Conditions leading to intravascular coagulation

Acute	Subacute	Chronic
Abruptio placentae	Septic abortion	Haemangiomata
Amniotic fluid embolism	Toxaemia of pregnancy	Falciparum malaria
Haemolytic transfusion	Acute leukaemia	Cirrhosis
Purpura fulminans	Rhabdomyosarcoma	(decompensated)
Septicaemia (Gram-negative)	Carcinomatosis (including,	Dead fetus (> 3 wks)
Snake bite	lung, prostate)	Congenital
Waterhouse-Friderichsen syndrome	Neuroblastoma	haemangioma
Lung surgery	Haemolytic-uraemic	(Kasabach-Merritt
Some allergic reactions	syndrome (Gasser-syndrome)	syndrome)
Burns	Eclampsia	Hydatidiform mole
Heat stroke	Sickle cell disease	
Acute promyelocytic leukaemia		
Dengue		
Psittacosis		
Ebola virus		
Rocky mountain spotted fever		
Fat embolism		
Head injury		
Trauma (massive)		

5.2.4 Uraemia

The cause of the bleeding tendency observed in uraemic patients is unclear and there is no satisfactory treatment. High levels of prostacyclin-like activity, capable of inhibiting platelet aggregation generated by the vessel wall, was found in uraemic patients with a prolonged bleeding and normal platelet count (Remuzzi et al., 1977)

5.2.5 Myeloproliferative Disorders

The bleeding observed in polycythaemia vera, acute or chronic leukaemia and thrombocythaemia may have several causes, including intravascular coagulation. Although treatment of the primary disease is essential, heparin and fibrinogen (if depleted) may be helpful when disseminated intravascular coagulation is present.

5.3 Disorders of Platelet Function

These disorders may be divided into three groups — abnormal bleeding due to (a) a thrombocytopenia, which is due to failure of platelet production, a reduction in platelet survival or sequestration, and is the most common form; (b) thrombocythaemia; and (c) functionally abnormal platelets (O'Brien, 1972; Weiss, 1975b).

5.3.1 Idiopathic Thrombocytopenia (ITP)

In life threatening situations or before surgery, platelet rich plasma (as a rule of thumb concentrates of 1 or 2 units of blood per 10kg body weight) is administered, although there is increasing awareness that the life span of transfused platelets can be very short (1 to 2 hours) in these patients. Subsequently, oral prednisolone (10 to 20mg 4 times daily), is given until cessation of bleeding and the return to normal of the platelets, when the dose is gradually decreased. Corticosteroids may merely tide patients over an acute period until a natural remission develops. Some patients have a remarkably long remission, others relapse within months and the dosage of steroids should be maintained at the lowest level compatible with reasonable control of bleeding. Splenectomy is considered if this treatment fails or if the dose of prednisolone required is too high or poorly tolerated, particularly if the spleen shows an increased sequestration of platelets. Vincristine or immunosuppressive agents may be tried in those patients who fail to respond to prednisolone and/or splenectomy (Ries, 1976; Ahn et al., 1978).

Thrombocytopenia which develops after a viral infection or results from a hypersensitivity to a drug (see section 8.1.1) is self limiting, if recognised early enough. Thrombotic thrombocytopenic purpura is a puzzling syndrome characterised by thrombocytopenic purpura, haemolytic anaemia and fleeting neurological symptoms. No rational therapy is available and empirical treatment with heparin, dextran or large doses of corticosteroids is still investigational.

5.3.2 Neonatal Thrombocytopenic Purpura

This condition occurs not infrequently in newborn infants of mothers who have ITP or disseminated lupus erythematosus. Agglutinins crossing the placenta have been demonstrated. Iso-immune neonatal thrombocytopenic purpura due to incompatible platelet groups is another rather rare cause of severe bleeding and a self limiting condition. The management of thrombocytopenia associated with disseminated lupus erythematosus is the same as for ITP and as difficult.

5.3.3 Thrombocythaemia

This condition can be associated with myeloproliferative disorders or considered as primary. Overt bleeding is common when the platelet count exceeds 800,000 per mm^3. Suppression of platelet production by busulphan (4 to 6mg/day) or radioactive phosphorus are the usual treatments with more hesitation for the latter in view of the risk of delayed leukaemia.

5.3.4 Functional Platelet Disorders

Various haemorrhagic congenital bleeding disorders have been ascribed to defective platelet function in the presence of adequate numbers of platelets. Hereditary disorders of platelet function may be due to disorders of connective tissue with which platelets interact, of plasma proteins necessary for this interaction or due to a defect of the platelets themselves.

Acquired disorders of platelet function can be associated with other conditions (e.g. myeloproliferative or renal diseases, fibrin degradation products) or occur after intake of drugs which affect platelet function (e.g. aspirin and other non-steroidal anti-inflammatory agents, antihistamines, penicillins, etc; see also section 8.1.1). For a review, see Hardisty (1977).

5.4 Antifibrinolytic Drugs and Blood Loss

A few types of blood loss can be controlled by drugs which inhibit the fibrinolytic enzyme system. Synthetic inhibitors of fibrinolysis include epsilon aminocaproic acid (EACA) and tranexamic acid (AMCA) and p-aminomethyl benzoic acid (PAMBA). At appropriate concentrations, these drugs are competitive inhibitors of plasminogen activator and non-competitive inhibitors of plasmin (fig. 2). It is however, generally claimed that the concentration of aminocaproic acid and the cyclic inhibitors of fibrinolysis necess-ary to inhibit plasmin are 10 to 100 times higher than those necessary for inhibition of activation of plasminogen (Verstraete, 1977). Tranexamic acid is about 10 times more potent than aminocaproic acid and it persists longer in the tissues. They are also inhibitors of C'1 esterase which is deficient in patients with familial angio-oedema and have been used as long term prophylaxis to control spontaneous attacks (see chapter XIV; sect. 10.4) and have enabled these patients to undergo dental and general surgery (Sheffer et al., 1977).

Aprotinin, a polypeptide isolated and purified from bovine lung and liver, inhibits serine proteases including plasmin and kallikrein, the proteinase which liberates vasoactive peptides from the α_2-globulin fraction of plasma. In contrast to the synthetic fibrinolysis inhibitors, aprotinin also has anticoagulant and vasoactive properties (Cantin et al., 1975). It is known that uninhibited vasoactivity with resultant widespread vasodilatation and pooling of blood, mainly in the splanchnic bed, is an important factor in several forms of shock. Aprotinin has been shown experimentally to reduce mortality and prolong survival in shock due to endotoxin, trauma, anaphylaxis, and peritonitis, but its benefits in shock due to acute fulminating pancreatitis are controversial (see chapter XIX; sect. 9.1.1). It has to be administered by continuous infusion, its plasma half-life being only 37 to 100 minutes, and the dose has to exceed 100,000 units/hour.

5.4.1 Blood Loss Associated with Surgery

In prostatic surgery and operations on the urinary bladder, prophylactic aminocaproic acid (100mg/kg per day intravenously or orally 4 to 6 times daily, or by continuous infusion) or tranexamic acid (25mg/kg/day intravenously or 25mg/kg orally 4 to 6 times daily) can reduce measured blood loss after transurethral or transvesical prostatectomy by about 50% (Hedlund, 1969; Ro et al., 1970). This treatment also has a favourable effect on drainage of the urinary bladder, thereby reducing the risk of bleeding. Antifibrinolytic treatment in association with prostatectomy does not increase the frequency of postoperative thromboembolism. Aprotinin does not have a useful effect, even when 500,000 units/day are administered.

As discussed in section 5.1.1, aminocaproic acid and tranexamic acid, by reducing the fibrinolytic activity in the alveolar tooth sockets, can significantly decrease the risk of bleeding (and requirements of replacement clotting factors) after tooth extraction in haemophiliacs. They have also been used to reduce blood loss in normal children undergoing adenotonsillectomy.

5.4.2 Essential Menorrhagia

Oral administration of tranexamic acid, in a dosage of 3g daily from the first day of menstruation onwards, significantly decreases menstrual blood loss (by 40 to 50%) in women with so-called essential menorrhagia which cannot be controlled by other means (Vermylen et al., 1968). These agents can also be used to control menorrhagia associated with aplastic anaemia (see section 6.3) and haemorrhagic complications after insertion of intrauterine contraceptive devices (see further chapter XV; sect. 15.1).

5.4.3 Ruptured Intracranial Aneurysm

Once an intracranial aneurysm is ruptured, neurosurgery is usually deferred but in the meantime rebleeding must be prevented. Antifibrinolytic agents may prolong the duration of the naturally occurring blood clot within and about the wall of a cerebral aneurysm, thus promoting a condition for surgical repair of the ruptured site (Fodstad et al., 1978). Prolonged administration of tranexamic acid also appears to be effective in actually preventing rebleeding without operation (Maurice-Williams, 1978). Tranexamic acid is given intravenously for the first few days and then orally in a dose of 1.5g 6-hourly.

6. Anaemias

Anaemias can be conveniently classified as follows: (a) anaemias due to a deficiency of factors essential for normal blood formation; iron, vitamin B_{12}, folic acid; (b) anaemias due to excessive blood destruction; haemolytic anaemias; (c) anaemias due to loss of cells in the bone marrow; e.g. aplastic anaemia, and (d) anaemias of uncertain origin; e.g. uraemia, rheumatoid arthritis, chronic infection, disseminated malignancy. Success in the treatment of patients with anaemia depends on a correct diagnosis with identification and elimination, if possible, of any underlying cause. While the aetiology of many anaemias, such as idiopathic haemolytic and aplastic anaemia remains unknown, most of the commonly occurring anaemias arise as a result of blood loss or nutritional, toxic or hereditary factors which can be defined.

6.1 Deficiency Anaemias

Appropriate treatment is extremely rewarding in these conditions. A correct diagnosis is however, essential. For example, iron deficiency anaemia may be due to blood loss from a malignant gastrointestinal lesion. There is no place for blind treatment of the anaemia without a thorough search for an underlying cause. This is not only wasteful, but may also delay or mask the correct diagnosis. The treatment of deficiency anaemias consists of the administration of the deficient substance and there is no justification for 'shotgun' treatment with mixtures of haematinics (see Beal, 1971).

6.1.1 Iron Deficiency Anaemia

Iron deficiency is a symptom and not a disease. In infants and children it usually results from inadequate dietary intake, but in adults the most common causes of iron deficiency are disorders due to blood loss (e.g. excessive menstrual flow, gastrointestinal bleeding, hookworm infestation) and pregnancy. Although adequate therapy may be given either orally or parenterally, the treatment of choice is oral iron, given in a sufficient dose and for a sufficient time to restore the body iron stores to normal. Oral iron therapy is usually effective and has none of the dangers of the parenteral administration of iron. Gastrointestinal intolerance of oral iron preparations has often been given as a reason for preference of parenteral administration, but this is not correct. Gastric discomfort, constipation or diarrhoea can occur when oral treatment is started, and the psychological impact is reinforced by the black discoloration of the stools, but the importance of these complaints have been grossly exaggerated (Beutler et al., 1963; O'Sullivan et al., 1955). They can be kept to a minimum if treatment is started with a low dose and progressively increased.

Oral Iron Preparations: Ingested iron must be reduced to the ferrous form in the stomach and intestine before it is absorbed. Absorption is greatest in the upper part of the small intestine and progressively less in the distal segments. It is transferred across the mucosal cell as part of an active metabolic process. Ferritin in the intestinal mucous membrane regulates iron absorption. When iron passes into plasma, it is oxidised to the ferric state and transported in combination with transferrin. Iron is stored in liver and spleen as ferritin and haemosiderin. Both are mobilised for haemoglobin synthesis.

Simple reduced forms of iron like ferrous sulphate and ferrous gluconate are commonly used. Ferrous sulphate is administered in doses of 200 to 300mg from which an iron deficient patient will absorb 20 to 30mg of iron. This will be enough to allow doubling of the rate of erythropoiesis. Administration of larger daily doses is of no value. Absorption of iron will decrease as anaemia improves. Duration of oral therapy will depend on the severity of anaemia and tissue depletion of iron stores. By keeping iron in the ferrous form, reducing agents like ascorbic acid promote iron absorption. Monosodium succinate also enhances iron absorption. Plant phytates, phosphates and tannic acid (tea) form insoluble complexes with iron; the administration of iron together with meals can improve tolerance but, inclusion of some food compounds will interfere with absorption. If acceptable to the patient, iron is best given between meals. Iron medication should not be taken simultaneously with tetracyclines, since there is a mutual decrease in absorption of both drugs. This effect is no longer apparent when the drugs are given about 3 hours apart (Neuvonen, 1976).

Slow release preparations offer no real advantage over conventional preparations (Elwood and Williams, 1970). Their better tolerance is mainly due to their low iron content and there is no justification for the higher cost. All oral iron preparations produce some side effects and hence the aim of therapy should be to administer a form of iron which gives maximal absorption with minimal side effects. The main iron preparations (ferrous sulphate, gluconate, succinate and fumarate) do give similar results (Brise and Hallberg, 1962) and selection of one or other compound will be mainly based on the prescriber's choice and patient's taste; the only important factor being the administration of an adequate dose of bivalent iron for a sufficient period of time (table XII). Most patients will respond readily to the cheapest preparation, ferrous sulphate. The main problem with oral iron therapy is that to replace the deficit, treatment has to last 3 to 6 months and patients may soon feel better and not complete the course as required (Porter, 1969).

Parenteral Iron: Indications for iron injections are limited to genuine and severe gastrointestinal intolerance or clearly demonstrable malabsorption (as in coeliac disease, postgastrectomy patients, ulcerative colitis, Crohn's disease), to chronic and intractable blood loss which cannot be corrected by other measures or to conditions where the iron stores have to be replenished rapidly (e.g. severe anaemia in last trimester of pregnancy, urgent major surgery), and where self medication of oral iron is unreliable. Blood transfusion is not a suitable form of treatment for iron deficiency anaemia.

Parenteral iron dextran or iron sorbitol treatment is given in a dose appropriate to the iron deficit. In the absence of chronic blood loss, the needed dose is computed by a formula on the basis of the haemoglobin deficit and the size of the patient. Excretion of an excess dose is not possible and a haemosiderosis-like syndrome may develop after repeated administration. Local effects are not uncommon with intramuscular iron and systemic reactions may occur occasionally. After intravenous administration or large intramuscular doses serious reactions (including anaphylaxis) may occur. The treatment of iron deficiency anaemia in pregnancy is discussed in chapter XV (sect. 3.1).

Iron Toxicity and Overload: Excessive dosage of iron (or as haemoglobin iron in transfused blood) can result in iron overload and haemochromatosis. Intravenous or subcutaneous infusion of the iron chelating agent desferrioxamine together with vitamin C is effective in treating iron overload in anaemic patients receiving regular blood transfusions, particularly in children with thalassaemia major (Hussain et al., 1977; Graziano et al., 1978), but the treatment is very expensive. Acute iron toxicity, mainly in children, can occur after accidental intake of oral iron preparations (as little as 1g ferrous sulphate may be fatal in a young child) and needs urgent treatment, including intensive administration (intragastric and systemic) of desferrioxamine (see chapter IX; sect. 6.4).

6.1.2 Vitamin B_{12} Deficiency Anaemia

Vitamin B_{12} deficiency is due mainly to defective absorption. In pernicious anaemia, the main form of megaloblastic anaemia in Caucasians, defective absorption of vitamin B_{12} results from the absence of intrinsic factor normally secreted by the gastric mucosa. More than half of all patients with pernicious anaemia have intrinsic factor antibodies. Other mechanisms can also result in inadequate vitamin B_{12} absorption. Disorders of the nervous system and of the tissues with a high

Table XII. Iron content and dosage of some oral and parenteral iron preparations (after Beal, 1971)

Salt	Iron content [1]	Daily adult dose [2]	Side-effects
Oral Preparations — Conventional			
Sodium iron edetate	27.5mg/5ml	5-10ml, tds	Nausea, diarrhoea
Ferrous gluconate	35mg	1-2, tds	and/or constipation
Iron aminoate	35mg	1-2, tds	
Ferrous succinate	37mg	1-2, tds	
Iron polymaltose	40mg	1-2, tds	
Ferrous aminoacetosulphate	50mg	1-2, bd-tds	
Ferrous carbonate	50mg	1-2, bd-tds	
Ferrous sulphate	60mg	1-2, bd-tds	
Ferrous fumarate	65mg	1-2, bd-tds	
Oral Preparations — Slow or Sustained Release			
Ferrous sulphate	50mg	2-4, once daily	As above
	100mg	1-2, once daily	
	105mg		
Parenteral Preparations			
Sodium-ferric gluconate complex	12.5mg/ml	5ml slow ivi	*Intravenous:*
Dextri-ferron	20mg/ml	1.5-5ml slow ivi	venous spasm; syste-
		Not for im use	mic chills, fever,
Iron dextran	50mg/ml	2-5ml deep imi; also	nausea; chest, lumbar
		by iv infusion	and loin pain
Iron polymaltose	50mg/ml	2-5ml deep imi; also	*Intramuscular:*
		by iv infusion	local pain and inflam-
Iron sorbitol (iron sorbitol	50mg/ml	2-5ml deep imi	mation; skin staining
citric acid complex)		Not for iv use	(if admin. not cor-
			rect); systemic reac-
			tions; metallic taste

1   As elemental iron per tablet, capsule or specified volume of liquid.
2   The daily therapeutic adult dose for optimum haemoglobin response is usually in the range 180 to 270mg elemental iron. The daily prophylactic dose (e.g. pregnancy) is about 60 to 100mg elemental iron.

Parenteral dosage can be calculated by a formula based on the severity of the anaemia and size of the patient. One formula which has been used to calculate the approximate total amount is:
Total ml to be injected = body weight in kg × haemoglobin deficiency (100% − actual concentration) × 0.0132.

An empirical intramuscular dosage is to give an initial 1ml trial dose, followed by 2 to 5ml daily into alternate buttocks. In practice a course of 1.5 to 3g elemental iron will be required.

mitotic rate are main abnormalities observed in vitamin B_{12} deficiency.

Intramuscular vitamin B_{12} is the treatment of choice. Although hydroxocobalamin has some clear advantages when given in low doses, cyanocobalamin given in a sufficient amount and at appropriate intervals, gives satisfactory results. Treatment is aimed at achieving a haematological remission and at replacing body stores of vitamin B_{12}. The dose regimen therefore takes into account an initial need to replace vitamin B_{12} stores and a subsequent daily maintenance need of 1 to 2µg vitamin B_{12}. If the response to vitamin B_{12} therapy is poor or absent, it is likely that the megaloblastic anaemia is due to folate deficiency.

Several different initial dosage regimens are in use. They include intramuscular injection of cyanocobalamin 30µg daily for 5 to 10 days, 50 to 100µg weekly or 5 doses of 1,000µg over a period of 2 to 3 weeks, or hydroxocobalamin 1,000µg weekly for 4 weeks. Maintenance therapy requires cyanocobalamin or hydroxocobalamin 100 to 250µg monthly or the two-monthly administration of a higher dose of hydroxocobalamin. The 'shotgun' treatment with combinations of 'all-known' haematinics must be condemned. Oral treatment with hog intrinsic factor can give unsatisfactory results when antibodies are produced. Other forms of treatment (long acting vitamin B_{12} preparations; high dosage oral administration bypassing the intrinsic factor dependent resorption mechanism) have no clearcut advantage. Oral vitamin B_{12} is only indicated in the patient in whom injections are undesirable (e.g. bleeding disorder). As with iron deficiency anaemia (section 6.1.1), blood transfusion in the patient with vitamin B_{12} deficiency should be avoided, except in exceptional circumstances (e.g. a patient dyspnoeic at rest who has not responded to B_{12} and who has a haemoglobin of 2 to 3g/100ml), when packed cells should be used. Side effects to vitamin B_{12} include very occasional allergic reactions and rarely, anaphylactic type reactions. Antibody production against long acting vitamin B_{12} preparations has been reported (Olesen et al., 1968).

6.1.3 Folate Deficiency Anaemia

Folate deficiency states are relatively frequent and result mainly from several coexisting causes, such as inadequate dietary intake, poor absorption, increased requirements or loss, and use of drugs which interfere with folate metabolism or utilisation (see section 8.5).

Oral treatment with folic acid will give satisfactory results, even in patients suffering from malabsorption. In the normal adult, daily requirement of folic acid amounts to about 0.1 to 0.2mg. Until recently a daily oral dose of 5mg folic acid was generally used for prophylaxis. This amount when given erroneously to vitamin B_{12} deficient patients for prolonged periods, can precipitate vitamin B_{12} neuropathy. It has also been suspected of inducing mild psychological disorders in normal subjects (Hunter et al., 1970). For these reasons some clinicians prefer to administer a 'physiological' daily dose of 0.1 to 0.3mg folate for long term therapy (e.g. in some elderly patients who are unlikely to alter their dietary habits). Folinic acid administration is useful in patients overtreated with folic acid antagonists (e.g. methotrexate, pyrimethamine, trimethoprim), but it has no use in other states of folate deficiency. There is no case for the routine prophylactic administration of folate during pregnancy, except in areas where dietary deficiency of folate is common or where folate requirements are increased by malarial haemolysis and haemoglobinopathies (see chapter XV; sect. 3.2).

6.2 Haemolytic Anaemias

In these anaemias there is evidence of excessive blood destruction. Haemolytic anaemias may be caused by an intrinsic red cell defect, such as occurs in certain hereditary (e.g. hereditary spherocytosis) and racial (hereditary haemoglobinopathies) forms, or acquired by extrinsic mechanisms (e.g. idiopathic autoimmune haemolytic anaemia; haemolytic disorders due to drugs, infections; haemolytic disease of the newborn). In these forms, therapy will often be restricted to treatment or removal of the underlying cause (Girdwood, 1971). Preventive measures are clearly of importance in the acquired or 'extrinsic' haemolytic anaemias.

6.2.1 Hereditary Spherocytosis (congenital haemolytic anaemia)

Treatment centres around whether or not to perform splenectomy, which invariably cures the anaemia and stops the increased haemolysis, although the intrinsic red cell defect still remains. The condition is due to the production of abnormal erythrocytes. Even though patients with mild forms of this disease may be able to lead normal occupational lives with little ill health, it is probably best to perform the operation in all cases while the patient is well, rather than risk biliary complications at a later date. Splenectomy should probably be postponed to childhood when the disease commences in infancy or early childhood. There should be no hesitation in performing splenectomy if the disease is affecting physical or mental health, if there is a history of severe haemolytic or aplastic crises, or if there is a history of the disease in severe forms in relatives. Because problems may arise during pregnancy, a stronger case exists for splenectomy in the female, who may also suffer from iron deficiency anaemia or from megaloblastic anaemia due to folate deficiency when pregnant.

Corticosteroids are ineffective in this type of haemolytic anaemia. Severe haemolytic and aplastic crises are treated by carefully matched and administered transfusion of blood. Splenectomy may be useful in selected cases of other forms of hereditary haemolytic anaemia (e.g. pyruvatekinase deficiency, congenital dyserythropoietic anaemia; Verwilghen et al., 1973).

6.2.2 Hereditary Haemoglobinopathies (racial haemolytic anaemias)

In some of these diseases there is excessive haemolysis and in others apparent iron deficiency anaemia which does not respond to iron therapy.

Thalassaemia and sickle cell disease are important examples of the condition, which is due to the production of abnormal haemoglobins.

Thalassaemia is frequently encountered among people of Mediterranean or Southeast Asian origin and the hypochromic anaemia of both β-thalassaemia minor and heterozygous α-thalassaemia may be confused with iron deficiency. In general, thalassaemia minor requires no treatment, but in patients with thalassaemia major (homozygous form), haemoglobin H disease and other more severe haemoglobinopathies, red cell transfusions, iron chelating agents (see section 6.1.1) and splenectomy (where there is a marked haemolytic element) may be necessary.

Sickle cell anaemia is common in Negroes, but rare in other races, although is also seen in some Mediterranean, Arab and Indian populations. Definitive therapy involving use of agents such as urea, cyanate and carbamyl phosphate has proved disappointing (Dean and Schechter, 1978) and present treatment is directed at prevention of crises by good general medical care including folate supplements and prompt treatment of any infections, even if minor. Antimalarial prophylaxis should be given to children with the disease in areas where malaria is endemic. Patients with a crisis or severe infection should be managed in hospital, with prompt treatment of infection and supportive care including analgesics and hydration plus blood transfusion for prolonged painful crises and anaemic crises. Folic acid should be given routinely in anaemic crises (Sheehy and Plumb, 1977).

6.2.3 Acquired Haemolytic Anaemia

The so-called idiopathic form occurs mainly in adults and is mostly due to circulating antibodies to which the patient's erythrocytes are sensitive. Acute forms of autoimmune haemolytic anaemia require blood transfusion. There is a danger of propagating the haemolytic process during a haemolytic crisis, but this may be minimised by careful matching of donor and recipient blood and by slow administration. Corticosteroids (prednisone 60mg daily) should be tried for 3 to 4 weeks before splenectomy is considered, and also the possibility that haemolytic anaemia is not secondary to lymphadenoma or leukaemia must be excluded. If corticosteroids and splenectomy fail to control the disease, the immunosuppressive drugs 6-mercaptopurine and azathioprine may be worthy of trial (Dacie and Worlledge, 1969).

In secondary forms of haemolytic anaemia accompanying certain neoplastic diseases and disseminated lupus erythematosus, treatment is that of the primary condition, supplemented by blood transfusion. In haemolytic anaemia due to drugs, other chemicals or plants, the causative agent should be stopped and treatment with corticosteroids or possibly blood transfusion instituted. Glucose-6-phosphate dehydrogenase (G6PD) deficiency is a common hereditary defect of the erythrocyte in Africans, Negroes, Oriental and Sephardic Jews, Northwest Indians, and some Mediterranean and Asian peoples, and this should be excluded in such patients presenting with acute haemolysis and less commonly, a chronic haemolytic state. Many factors, including fava beans, certain drugs, infections and metabolic disorders such as diabetic ketoacidosis can precipitate haemolysis in the enzyme deficient subject (Beutler, 1969, 1971). The haemolysis may be severe and may lead to haemoglobinuria and death, and since there is no effective treatment, it is important that patients are screened for this defect before they are given drugs known to provoke haemolysis (see section 8.4). Individuals with abnormal haemoglobins also have an increased propensity to haemolysis if given oxidising agents (e.g. nitrites, certain sulphonamides, phenacetin in patients with haemoglobin H, and sulphonamides and primaquine in those with haemoglobin Zurich). See further chapter VII (sect. 4.2.2).

6.3 Aplastic Anaemia

Aplastic anaemia is a disease with a grave prognosis. While idiopathic, constitutional and postinfective (notably following viral hepatitis) aetiologies are well documented, in a large proportion of patients the disease must be regarded as induced by drugs, chemicals or radiation and is thus potentially preventable. A large number of drugs and chemicals may be causally related to aplastic anaemia, but the actual risk in each case is difficult to assess (see section 8.3). Chloramphenicol is the drug most commonly incriminated; the development of irreversible marrow aplasia is unpredictable and is believed to represent a form of idiosyncrasy. Phenylbutazone, oxyphenbutazone, sulphonamides and gold are other common drug related causes (see section 8.3).

The mainstay of therapy is supportive care directed towards the control of bleeding and infection, as these are the commonest causes of death. Antibacterial agents for specific infections, and red cell and platelet (or sometimes granulocytes) transfusion when indicated, play an important role in maintaining life till spontaneous or drug induced remissions are achieved. The dangerous menorrhagia which is common in female patients can be controlled by the fibrinolysis inhibitors epsilon aminocaproic acid and tranexamic acid (see section 5.4.2) together with an oral contraceptive, preferably containing a large dose of norethisterone (norethindrone) since such oral contraceptives usually decrease menstrual blood loss. Androgenic-anabolic steroids given for 3 to 6 months have been used to stimulate erythropoiesis (Shahidi, 1973) and so induce remissions and while these are frequently employed, definite proof of their effectiveness in properly designed trials is lacking (Branda et al., 1977). Nevertheless, many believe that early use of androgenic-anabolic steroids, together with supporting transfusions and antibacterial drugs, represents the best readily available treatment at present, even though they do not appear to alter the outcome of the disease (Davis and Rubin, 1972; Tso et al., 1977). There is probably little to choose between the many different preparations, but the most commonly used agent is oxymetholone (2mg/kg daily, sometimes up to 6mg/kg; with dosage gradually reduced at evidence of remission). It is a 17α-alkylated compound and liver function abnormalities, including cholestatic jaundice, are common (Sanchez-Medal et al., 1969). Virilisation is common and nausea and epigastric discomfort may also be troublesome. From 30 to 50% of patients surviving long enough to receive adequate treatment with one of these anabolic steroids may respond. However, such responses are often incomplete and thrombocytopenia is usually the least responsive (Tso et al., 1977).

Recently, an altered outlook has been obtained with transplantation of bone marrow from histocompatible sibs. The exceedingly demanding and expensive technique decreases early mortality and significantly improves the prospect for long term recovery (Storb et al., 1976; Camitta et al., 1976). Treatment with immunosuppressive drugs or antilymphocyte globulin is needed to prevent graft versus host reaction. In some patients, recovery of the recipient's bone marrow in the absence of a take of the donor's graft has been observed.

Recovery has even been obtained in patients treated only with antilymphocyte globulin without subsequent bone marrow graft (Speck et al., 1977), suggesting that immune phenomena are involved in the aetiology of at least some cases of aplastic anaemia.

6.4 Anaemias of Unknown Origin

In these forms of anaemia, therapy will often be restricted to attempts to control the primary condition (chronic infection, uraemia, malignant condition, liver disease) or to symptomatic measures (e.g. iron in uraemia and rheumatoid arthritis). Blood transfusion may be required. Androgenic-anabolic steroids have also been used. Management of the anaemia of chronic renal failure is discussed in chapter XXI (sect. 9.7) and that of rheumatoid arthritis in chapter XXII (sect. 3.5.3).

7. Use of Drugs in the Presence of Associated Haematological Disorders

Drugs used in the treatment of non-haematological disease may have haematological side effects and cause serious toxicity in patients with blood diseases. A knowledge of the spectrum of activity of the drugs prescribed is obviously essential for their safe use. Alternatively, the haematological disease itself may influence the response to other drugs. Interactions with certain groups of drugs used in haematological disorders can also be important.

7.1 Thromboembolic Disorders

Many drugs have a potential to modify the response to oral coumarin anticoagulants and although clinically harmful effects are not that common, fatalities from severe bleeding have occurred. Predictably interacting drugs such as phenylbutazone and enzyme inducing drugs such as barbiturates should be avoided. Most adverse interactions may be prevented if a few simple precautions are followed (Koch-Weser, 1975; see section 3.2.5). Oral contraceptives of the oestrogen-progestagen type, especially high dose preparations, should be avoided in those with thrombotic lesions or a thrombotic tendency of any kind (see chapter XV; sect. 13.12).

7.2 Anaemias

In patients with iron deficiency anaemia, simultaneous administration of oral iron preparations (ferrous sulphate, fumarate, succinate, tartrate) and oral tetracyclines can markedly inhibit the absorption of the tetracycline. Iron absorption (from supplements but not food) is inhibited as well. If such combined therapy is indicated, the interaction can be avoided (except in the case of doxycycline and minocycline) by giving the drugs 3 hours apart. The affect of slow release iron preparations on absorption of tetracyclines is less (Neuvonen, 1976). Anaemias can affect the rate of elimination of some drugs (see section 1.4).

Patients with megaloblastic anaemia given cotrimoxazole not only show a poor response to specific haematinic therapy, but the antifolate effect of the drug can also increase the severity of the megaloblastic changes and cause significant haematopoietic depression (Chanarin and England, 1972). In patients with pernicious anaemia and achlorhydria the absorption of drugs such as cephalexin can be impaired in some patients, but the clinical significance of this is far from clear (see also chapter XIX; sect. 1.1.1).

Individuals with inherited abnormalities of erythrocyte (e.g. G6PD deficiency) or haemoglobin (haemoglobin H, Zurich) function are particularly susceptible to oxidising agents (e.g. nitrites) and certain other drugs (see section 8.4). Such drugs also cause an increase in methaemoglobinaemia in those with hereditary methaemoglobinaemia (see also chapter VII; sect. 4.2.2).

7.3 Bleeding Disorders

Ingestion of usual therapeutic dosages of aspirin produces a marked prolongation of bleeding time in some patients with haemophilia A or B, or with von Willebrand's disease (see section 5.1). Aspirin and other drugs which affect platelet function (section 3.1) should be avoided in those with functional platelet disorders, and also in the presence of even a mild haemostatic defect; e.g. a history of even slightly prolonged bleeding after tooth extraction (Editorial, 1974). Paracetamol (acetaminophen) is a suitable alternative analgesic (Miekle et al., 1976). Fibrinolytic inhibitors such as epsilon aminocaproic acid and tranexamic acid can lead to temporary kidney blockade if used in patients with haematuria (Van Itterbeek et al., 1968).

8. Drug Induced Haematological Disorders

Many drugs can adversely affect the blood, sometimes with disastrous results. The haematopoietic system is particularly susceptible to drug action (see section 1.3) and toxic effects can be exerted on the formed elements of blood, on haemoglobin or on the bone marrow. Certain drugs are regularly associated with idiosyncratic haematological reactions in susceptible individuals. Most reactions are due to either increased destruction or a decreased production of blood elements. Some drugs can very rapidly and extensively eradicate an enormous cell pool such as the granulocyte series. Bleeding disorders and coagulation disturbances can also be induced by drugs.

The more serious reactions can be prevented: by careful monitoring of therapy (e.g. repeated blood counts with gold), sometimes with adjustment of dosage (e.g. oral anticoagulants); by avoiding certain drugs if they are not indicated (e.g. chloramphenicol) or if they have an increased likelihood of precipitating reactions in susceptible subjects (e.g. sulphonamides and nitrofurantoin in those with G6PD deficiency; phenylbutazone in those on oral coumarin anticoagulants); and by careful instruction of the patient to immediately report warning symptoms (e.g. rash, sore throat, unusual bleeding with gold and phenylbutazone). The large range of drugs most often implicated or presumed to have been implicated are summarised in table XIII. For review, see Girdwood (1973a) and Symposium (1973).

As the blood is an easily sampled tissue, drug-induced blood disorders seem to be better known and more frequently reported than are drug induced diseases of most other organs. It should also be remembered that an adverse effect on the blood may be a sign of a systemic reaction to a drug (e.g. LE cells and positive ANF in systemic lupus erythematosus syndrome (chapter XXII; sect. 14.1). Drug induced malignant disorders of blood are discussed in chapter XXIV (sect. 9).

8.1 Bleeding Disorders

Drugs may cause bleeding disorders by affecting platelet function, the coagulation mechanism or by causing increased vascular fragility (e.g. large doses of corticosteroids). Aspirin, apart from effects on the blood (platelet function, bleeding time), causes bleeding by its erosive effects on the gastrointestinal mucosa (see chapter XIX; sect. 14.2.2).

8.1.1 Thrombocytopenia

The mechanisms by which drugs cause thrombocytopenia are platelet destruction and bone marrow suppression (see Gyn et al., 1972; Miescher, 1973).

The so called 'allergic' drug induced thrombocytopenia has been described for many drugs (table XIII) and consists of the appearance of thrombocytopenia during the first hours after intake of a drug to which there has been prior exposure. Patients usually develop an acute bleeding syndrome with bleeding from mucous membranes (e.g. oozing after brushing of teeth), appearance of petechiae, and eventually more severe bleeding. Thrombocytopenia disappears a few hours or days after withdrawal of the drug. It is generally accepted that in these patients, drug related antibodies of both IgB and IgM immunoglobulin classes are present.

Thrombocytopenia is believed to occur through one of two mechanisms. In the first, the drug is bound to the platelet membrane and the antibody is directed against the drug-membrane complex. As a result, complement is activated and the platelet membrane damaged. In the second, circulating antigen-antibody complexes are formed; the platelet being more or less an 'innocent bystander'. Platelets phagocytose certain immune complexes and as a consequence release some of their constituents. This so called 'release reaction' may lead to intravascular platelet aggregation and thrombocytopenia. It is to be expected that immune complex thrombocytopenia would be associated with systemic symptoms and this appears to be so for rifampicin, thiazides, thiouracils, apronal ('Sedormid'), quinidine and quinine.

With drug induced thrombocytopenia, the erythrocyte and leucocyte counts in general remain normal, but pancytopenia and suppression of platelet formation may occur in response to bone marrow suppression. Thus thrombocytopenia can occur from dose related toxic effects of cytotoxic drugs (see chapter XXIV; section 4), or as a reaction to chloramphenicol or other drugs which cause aplastic anaemia. It can also occur in association with megaloblastic anaemia due to drugs such as phenytoin (diphenylhydantoin), co-trimoxazole and methotrexate.

8.1.2 Bleeding Due to Coagulation and Platelet Defects

A bleeding disorder characterised by blood coagulation disturbances may result from the administration of excessive dosage of an anticoagulant or too rapid administration of a thrombolytic drug, from the failure to modify dosage in the presence of the many conditions which can increase the response to oral anticoagulants, or from a significant interaction between oral coumarin anticoagulants and another drug (see sections 3.2.3, 3.2.4, 3.2.5). In the case of significant drug interactions, bleeding results from failure to modify dosage following administration of a drug which potentiates the action of the coumarin anticoagulant or from the sudden withdrawal of a drug which inhibits its action. The problem and significance of drug interactions which affect the response to the coumarins are discussed in section 3.2.5.

Aspirin, by its effects on platelet function and prolongation of bleeding time, increases the risk of bleeding in patients on oral anticoagulants and should be avoided (O'Reilly et al., 1971). It also increases the risk of surgical bleeding in non-anticoagulated patients and may be implicated in some cases of unexpected severe bleeding (Davies and Steward, 1977). The risk of postoperative bleeding complications is also increased (Hepso et al., 1976). Paracetamol (acetaminophen) is a suitable simple analgesic for postoperative pain as it does not affect platelet function or prolong bleeding time (Skjelbred et al., 1977). Carbenicillin causes platelet dysfunction and prolongs bleeding time and increases the risk of severe bleeding following surgery or in uraemia (Woodruff et al., 1976; Andrassy et al., 1976a). Large doses of penicillin G and sodium valproate also affect platelet function and prolong bleeding time (Andrassy, 1976b; Von Voss et al., 1976). Thrombocytopenia and spontaneous bruising can occur with sodium valproate (Winfield et al., 1976).

8.2 Thromboembolism

Large doses of oestrogens appear to increase the risk of thromboembolism in the puerperium when used to suppress lactation and also in men with carcinoma of the prostate. High dose oestrogen-containing oral contraceptives increase the risk of venous thrombosis and pulmonary embolism, as well as coronary and cerebral thrombosis and also, though less significantly, postoperative thromboembolic complications. There is general agreement that oral contraceptives cause a hypercoagulable state but an associated impairment of fibrinolytic activity may also contribute to produce clinically relevant thromboembolism (see McQueen, 1978; chapter XV; sect. 12, 13.12). The overall risk of thromboembolism from oral contraceptives is very small but care should be taken in potential users who have a family or personal history of hypertension, diabetes, obesity, heart disease, varicose veins and other factors predisposing to thromboembolism or who are older than 35, have been taking the pill continuously for a long time and who smoke cigarettes. It seems that low dose progestagen-only oral contraceptives and progestagen-only injectable contraceptives have no clinically harmful effect on blood coagulation mechanisms. Deep vein thrombosis has been associated with use of the antioestrogen tamoxifen in advanced breast cancer in women with risk factors for thrombosis (Nevassaari et al., 1978).

8.3 Aplastic Anaemia

Although aplastic anaemia is an uncommon complication of therapy with some drugs, it is unpredictable and the haematological and clinical manifestations are severe and not infrequently fatal (see section 6.3). About half or more of all cases of aplastic anaemia are associated with use of drugs. Many drugs have been implicated, but the most important frequently implicated drugs known to be associated with aplastic anaemia are chloramphenicol, phenylbutazone, oxyphenbutazone, sulphonamides and gold (Bottiger and Westerholm, 1973; Williams et al., 1973; Inman, 1977; table XIII). Organic chemicals, inhaled agents such as benzene or glue solvents, and insecticides can also cause aplastic anaemia (Williams et al., 1973).

Chloramphenicol accounts for the greatest number of cases. However, as the frequency of its use varies in different countries so does the frequency of aplastic anaemia associated with its use. It has a mortality rate of between 50 and 100%. There are two forms of chloramphenicol induced bone marrow suppression (Yunis and Bloomberg, 1964). One type is a dose related erythroid suppression of early onset, associated with anaemia, leucopenia and mild thrombocytopenia and is reversible on stopping the drug. The second form is less common but much more serious and results in true marrow aplasia which is often irreversible. This effect is not clearly related to dosage or duration of administration but usually arises some weeks or months after cessation of treatment. Aplastic anaemia can nevertheless occur soon after a single and very small dose of chloramphenicol, while in other cases the aplasia occurs only after a long lasting course or after repeated administration spread over many years. The incidence is said to be from 1 in 24,000 to 1 in 40,000 (Clarke, 1967). A genetically determined basis for this 'idiosyncratic response' has been suggested but conclusive proof is lacking (Yunis, 1973). Chloramphenicol has been associated with aplastic anaemia in identical twins (Nagao and Mauer, 1969).

Hepatitis has been associated with aplastic anaemia in which many drugs have been implicated, but the relationship between the diseases is not clearly understood (Williams et al., 1973). It seems possible that impaired or abnormal metabolism of some drugs could result in a higher than normal incidence of aplastic anaemia in patients with significant liver disease than in those with normal liver function. Delayed clearance of acetanilide has been noted in cases of hypoplastic anaemia due to phenylbutazone, but not in patients with idiopathic aplastic anaemia (Cunningham et al., 1974). Both drugs are metabolised by the same primary pathway. Allergic mechanisms have also been proposed for some drugs (Nieweg, 1973). The mechanism whereby drugs cause aplastic anaemia is seldom understood. Leukaemia very occasionally supervenes and this may indicate an action on chromosomes (Girdwood, 1976).

Therapy consists of immediately stopping all drugs. Platelet and red cell or granulocyte transfusion may be needed in some cases, but whole blood transfusion should be used only to prevent symptoms of severe anaemia. Antibiotics should be given immediately in the event of infection. The use of androgen-anabolic steroids has been associated with remission in some cases (see section 6.3). Despite standard readily available treatment, drug induced aplastic anaemia is a very serious disorder with an anticipated 5-year mortality of about 70%, a partial recovery rate of 20%, and a complete recovery rate of only 10% (Williams et al., 1973). A much improved outlook has been made possible by the demanding technique of bone marrow transplantation, and possibly by use of antilymphocyte globulin (see section 6.3).

Prevention is clearly very important. Chlor-

Table XIII. Haematological abnormalities associated or presumed to be associated with drugs

Drug[1]	Thrombo-cytopenia	Aplastic anaemia	Haemo-lytic anaemia[2]	Megalo-blastic anaemia	Agranulo-cytosis
Cytotoxic Drugs					
Alkylating agents (e.g. cyclophosphamide)	++		+(mel-phalan)		+
Antibiotics (e.g. adriamycin)	++				+
Antipurines (e.g. 6-mercaptopurine)	++			+	+
Antipyrimidines (e.g. 5-fluorouracil)	++			+	+
Folate antagonists (e.g. methotrexate)	++			+	+
L-asparaginase (colaspase)	++			+	+
Antibacterial Agents					
Cephalothin	+		+		+
Chloramphenicol	+	++	± (G6PD)		+
Co-trimoxazole	+	+	± (G6PD)	+	++
Cycloserine				+	
Erythromycin	+				
Furazolidone			+G6PD)		
Isoniazid	+		+		+
Nalidixic acid			+(G6PD)		
Nitrofurantoin			+(G6PD)		+
PAS	+		+ ± (G6PD)	+	+
Penicillins	+		++		+
Rifampicin	++		+		
Streptomycin	+	+	+		
Sulphonamides	+	+	+ +(G6PD)		++
Sulphones (e.g. dapsone)			+(G6PD)		+
Tetracyclines	+	+			
Thiamphenicol		+			+
Anticonvulsants					
Carbamazepine	+	+			
Ethosuximide	+				+
Mephenytoin (methoin)	+	++	+		+
Methsuximide and phensuximide	+				
Paramethadione	+				
Phenytoin (diphenylhydantoin)	+	+		+	+
Primidone		+		+	
Trimethadione	+	++			+
Valproate sodium	++				

Table XIII. (continued)

Drug[1]	Thrombo-cytopenia	Aplastic anaemia	Haemo-lytic anaemia[2]	Megalo-blastic anaemia	Agranulo-cytosis
Antirheumatic Drugs/Analgesics					
Acetylsalicylic acid	+	+	± (G6PD)		+
Allopurinol		+			
Amidopyrine (aminopyrine)		+	+ +(G6PD)		++
Colchicine	+	+		+	
Gold	+	++			+
Indomethacin	+	+	+		
Levamisole					++
Mefenamic acid			+(AIHA)		
Oxyphenbutazone	+	++			+
Paracetamol (acetaminophen)	+				+
Penicillamine	+	+			+
Phenacetin	+	+	+ ± (G6PD)		+
Phenylbutazone	+	++			+
Probenecid			± (G6PD)		
Cardiovascular Drugs					
Ajmaline					+
Aprindine					++
Digitoxin	+				
Hydrallazine	+				
Methyldopa	+	+	++(AIHA)		+
Phenindione					++
Procainamide			± (G6PD)		+
Propranolol					+
Quinidine	+		+ +(G6PD)		+
Diuretics					
Acetazolamide	+	+			+
Ethacrynic acid					+
Frusemide (furosemide)	+				+
Mercurials	+				+
Spironolactone	+				
Thiazides	+				+
Triamterene				+	
Hypoglycaemic agents					
Carbutamide	+	+			++
Chlorpropamide	+	+	+		+
Insulin	+		+		
Metformin				+	
Tolbutamide	+	+	+		+
Antimalarials					
Chloroquine	+	+	± (G6PD)		+
Mepacrine (quinacrine)	+	+	+(G6PD)		+
Pamaquine			+(G6PD)		+
Pentaquine			+(G6PD)		
Primaquine			+(G6PD)		+
Quinine	+		+ +(G6PD)		+
Quinocide			+(G6PD)		
Hydroxychloroquine	+		± (G6PD)		+

Table XIII. (continued)

Drug[1]	Thrombo-cytopenia	Aplastic anaemia	Haemo-lytic anaemia[2]	Megalo-blastic anaemia	Agranulo-cytosis
Psychotherapeutic Drugs					
Apronal	+				
Carbromal	+		+		
Barbiturates	+			+	+
Chlordiazepoxide		+			+
Chlorpromazine	+	+	+		++
Clonazepam	+				
Clozapine	+				+
Diazepam	+				
Lithium		+			
Meprobamate	+	+			+
Phenothiazines	+	+			+
Promazine	+	+			++
Tricyclic antidepressants					+
Miscellaneous Drugs					
Amphotericin B		+	+		
Antihistamines (some compounds)	+	+			+
Arsenicals	+	+			+
BAL (dimercaprol)			± (G6PD)		
Carbimazole	+	+			+
Dinitrophenol					+
Levodopa	+		+(AIHA)		
Methimazole	+	+			+
Oral contraceptives				+	
Prednisolone/prednisone	+				+
Stibophen	+		++		
Thiouracils	+	+			++
Vitamin K (aqueous preparations)	+		± (G6PD) (neonates)		

1	++	=	Most frequently implicated drug.
2	+	=	Immune haemolytic anaemia.
	+(AIHA)	=	Autoimmune haemolytic anaemia.
	+(G6PD)	=	Haemolytic anaemia in those with glucose-6-phosphate dehydrogenase deficiency.
	± (G6PD)	=	Haemolytic anaemia in those with glucose-6-phosphate dehydrogenase deficiency, usually in conjunction with other factors such as infection, acidosis, renal failure, neonates but can occur in the absence of such factors in those with the Mediterranean variant of enzyme deficiency (see chapter VII; sect. 4.2.2).

amphenicol should never be used unless truly indicated (e.g. typhoid fever, *Haemophilus influenzae* meningitis). With other drugs, all that can be done is to keep a watch for early signs of minor haemorrhage and the patient instructed accordingly. Regular monitoring by repeated blood counts is not effective. However, with phenyl-butazone for example, a blood count at the first time the patient reports a rash, sore mouth or unusual bleeding, will soon reveal any important change (platelet deficiency being the most common). Treatment can then be stopped while there is still time to avert irreversible aplasia of the marrow.

8.4 Haemolytic Anaemia

Haemolytic anaemia due to drugs can be caused by direct cytotoxicity or by immunological mechanisms.

Non-immune haemolysis is relatively rare except in persons with G6PD deficiency or other more rare erythrocyte metabolic abnormalities, or with unstable haemoglobins such as haemoglobin H or Zurich (see Beutler, 1969; 1972). Metabolic abnormalities of the erythrocytes render the cells more sensitive to drugs and are the main predisposing cause of drug induced haemolytic anaemia. In normal individuals, much higher doses of the involved drugs (table XIII) are needed to cause erythrocyte destruction. Patients with G6PD deficiency with infection, acidosis, or impaired renal function (with consequent delay in drug elimination) may be even more susceptible to haemolysis from a given dose of one of the involved drugs. The condition is generally self limiting, but with some variants of G6PD deficiency, it can be severe and may lead to haemoglobinuria and death (see chapter VII; sect. 4.2.2). Methaemoglobinaemia with Heinz body formation is observed during the haemolytic episode and hyperbilirubinaemia and jaundice often supervene.

Many drugs can cause a positive direct antiglobulin (Coombs) test and in some cases, usually after repeat administration, immune haemolytic anaemia, but methyldopa and less often penicillin are by far the most common (see Garratty and Petz, 1975; Worlledge, 1969, 1973). Development of antibodies can be of two types: (a) those apparently directed against the drug or its metabolites (penicillin), and (b) those apparently directed against body constituents (methyldopa).

Drug induced immune haemolytic anaemia in which the antibody is apparently directed against the drug or its metabolite and in which the drug is firmly bound to red cells, is caused by penicillin, cephalothin and possibly carbromal. The antibody will only react with erythrocytes in the presence of the drug. Penicillin induced haemolytic anaemia usually occurs in patients taking large doses (10 to 20 mega units daily), particularly when renal function is impaired, and its occurrence is rare relative to the frequency of its administration. Patients with cephalothin induced haemolysis have not necessarily received high doses.

Haemolysis induced by drugs which bind less to red cells *in vitro* (e.g. quinine, quinidine, PAS, phenacetin, sulphonamides, rifampicin) usually occurs when the drug is given for the second or subsequent time, and the dose is not large. These patients develop antibodies that will react with the drug. These drug-antibody complexes are bound to the red cell (the 'innocent bystander') and induce complement fixation and lysis of the erythrocyte. This very exceptional disorder will often appear as a massive haemolytic crisis complicated by severe renal symptoms.

Methyldopa is the most commonly involved drug in autoimmune haemolytic anaemia, in which the antibody is apparently directed against intrinsic red cell antigens (Worlledge et al., 1966; Worlledge, 1969). Although a dose related positive direct antiglobulin test occurs in about 10 to 30 % of patients on long term therapy, overt haemolysis occurs in only a few patients (about 1 %) and development of a positive direct antiglobulin test is therefore not always an indication to stop methyldopa. The incidence of a positive direct antiglobulin test seems to vary between racial groups, being highest in Caucasians, lower in Chinese and almost absent in black races. Levodopa and mefenamic acid appear to act in a similar manner to methyldopa. Immediate withdrawal of the drug in the event of haemolytic anaemia results in the rapid disappearance of clinical symptoms, but in contrast to penicillin the antibody is active in the absence of the drug and the antiglobulin test may remain positive for some months after stopping methyldopa.

8.5 Megaloblastic Anaemia

Megaloblastosis most frequently results from inhibition of vitamin B_{12} or folic acid metabolism, but blockade in synthesis of any of the components of deoxyribonucleoprotein (purine, pyrimidine or protein) may produce megaloblastosis. Drug induced megaloblastic anaemias frequently represent interference with folic acid utilisation or availability (see Waxman et al., 1970; Stebbins and Bertino, 1976).

Therapy with the purine antagonists, 6-mercaptopurine, thioguanine or azathioprine may produce megaloblastic anaemia with normal serum folate and vitamin B_{12} levels which is unresponsive to vitamin B_{12} or folic acid therapy. Such anaemia is also produced by cytarabine and hydroxyurea. Interference with folate metabolism by folate antagonists (methotrexate), pyrimethamine, trimethoprim (co-trimoxazole) and triamterene can also cause megaloblastic anaemia, particularly when excessive or large doses are used in patients with a dietary deficiency of folate or who are likely to have a megaloblastic bone marrow, e.g. chronic alcoholism (see also section 7.2). This is well illustrated with co-trimoxazole (Girdwood, 1973b; Blackwell et al., 1978). Folinic acid can be used to reverse the anaemia if it is essential that the drug be continued. Such an effect can be enhanced by combined therapy with drugs which themselves can sometimes cause megaloblastic anaemia due to impaired absorption and/or utilisation of folic acid (phenytoin, cycloserine, primidone, barbiturates, oral contraceptives, metformin, chronic alcoholism), or to impaired absorption and/or utilisation of vitamin B_{12} (colchicine, neomycin, metformin, chronic alcoholism). The effects and inter-relationships between epilepsy, long term anticonvulsant therapy, enzyme induction and folate deficiency is not well understood (Norris and Pratt, 1974; Labadarios et al., 1978).

8.6 Pyridoxine and Iron Deficiency Anaemia

Some antituberculosis drugs (isoniazid, pyrazinamide, para aminosalicylate, cycloserine), phenacetin, paracetamol (acetaminophen), chloramphenicol and chronic alcohol ingestion can interfere with early stages of haem synthesis and cause a sideroblastic anaemia due to induced pyridoxine deficiency (Verwilghen et al., 1965; Girdwood, 1976). The clinical picture is of a hypochromic anaemia with ringed sideroblasts in the marrow. Treatment is difficult. Large doses of pyridoxine (e.g 0.5 to 1g daily for 3 months) or pyridoxal-5-phosphate do not always achieve a response. Associated folate deficiency may require treatment and blood transfusion may be necessary.

Drugs such as aspirin, large doses of corticosteroids and poorly controlled oral anticoagulant therapy can produce blood loss and iron deficiency anaemia.

8.7 Agranulocytosis

Agranulocytosis occurs during treatment with the drug rather than appearing after the drug has been discontinued as in some cases of drug induced aplastic anaemia. At least three types of agranulocytosis are distinguishable (see Pisciotta, 1973, 1978): one marked by peripheral damage due to an immune mechanism and another by direct damage to marrow cells. The former is ex-

emplified by sensitivity to amidopyrine (aminopyrine) and the latter to phenothiazine derivatives. A third type involves agranulocytosis associated with development of antinuclear antibodies or a drug induced lupus-like syndrome; e.g. procainamide (see chapter XXII; sect. 14.1). Agranulocytosis can also occur as part of the bone marrow suppressant effects of some drugs (e.g. cytotoxic drugs, chloramphenicol). Population factors can sometimes apparently contribute to the toxic effects of drugs, as illustrated by the markedly higher (21-fold) incidence of agranulocytosis to the antipsychotic drug clozapine in some areas of Finland (Anderman and Griffith, 1977; Idanpaan-Heikkila et al., 1977). No genetic or environmental factor has yet been identified, but the clinical features and characteristics are similar to phenothiazine agranulocytosis (Amsler et al., 1977; de la Chapelle et al., 1977). A similar clustering of cases has been suggested in Switzerland (Jungi et al., 1977).

The first of these types of agranulocytosis might be manifested by sudden onset of violent chills, fever, bone aches, and collapse in a patient receiving amidopyrine continuously or intermittently. It occurs a short time after ingestion of a small amount of drug in a previously sensitised individual. The peripheral blood would show leucopenia with granulocytopenia. Complete recovery can be expected after stopping the drug, but subsequent administration of even very small amounts of the drug would precipitate a recurrence. In this type of agranulocytosis, leucocyte antibodies are demonstrable in the blood for a short time after administration of the offending drug. A variety of drugs are capable of causing agranulocytosis through an immune mechanism. These include sulphonamides, tolbutamide, chlorpropamide, phenylbutazone, carbimazole, propylthiouracil and aprindine (Van Leeuwen and Meyboom, 1976) and levamisole (Rosenthal et al., 1977).

The phenothiazines appear to act via a toxic mechanism by interference with bone marrow granulocyte production in individuals in whom the marrow is unable to replenish the damaged cells because of a limited proliferative potential of bone marrow cells. Chlorpromazine has most often been implicated of the phenothiazines. Leucopenia also occurs suddenly but in contrast to the immune mediated type of agranulocytosis, is frequently asymptomatic at onset and only occurs after a period of some 20 to 40 days with a large cumulative dose (e.g. 10 to 20g chlorpromazine). Any patient who receives 3 or more months of treatment with chlorpromazine for example and does not develop agranulocytosis, is usually not likely to do so. Sore throat with mucosal ulcerations, chills, fever are among the early symptoms and generally signify bacterial infection. Phenothiazine induced agranulocytosis is particularly liable to occur in females aged over 40. In a patient who has recovered from such a reaction, retreatment with a lower dose of phenothiazine is not usually associated with an immediate recurrence, but this is likely if dosage exceeds a certain minimal amount for a length of time.

In cases of agranulocytosis, the causative drug must be withdrawn immediately as there is a not inconsiderable mortality rate, usually due to infection, if the condition is not diagnosed soon enough or any infection not successfully contained. With early diagnosis, granulocyte recovery takes place in a week or more.

Further Reading

Biggs, R: Human Blood Coagulation, Haemostasis and Thrombosis 2nd ed (Blackwell, Oxford 1976).

de Gruchy, G.C.: Drug-Induced Blood Disorders, 1st ed (Blackwell, Oxford 1975).

Douglas, A.S.: Blood coagulation and fibrinolysis in clinical practice. Clinics in Haematology 2: 1 (1973).

Kakkar, V.V. and Jouhar, A.J.: Thromboembolism: Diagnosis and Treatment (Churchill Livingstone, Edinburgh 1972).

Penington, D.; Rush, B. and Castaldi, P.: de Gruchy's Clinical Haematology in Medical Practice, 4th ed (Blackwell, Oxford 1977).

Thomas, D.: Haemostasis. British Medical Bulletin 33: 183 (1977).

Thomas, D.: Thrombosis. British Medical Bulletin 34: 101 (1978).

Wintrobe, M.M. et al.: Clinical Hematology, 7th ed (Lea and Febiger, Philadelphia 1974).

References

Aarbakke, J.: Clinical pharmacokinetics of phenylbutazone. Clinical Pharmacokinetics 3: 369 (1978).

Adar, R. and Salzman, E.W.: Treatment of thrombosis of veins of the lower extremities. New England Journal of Medicine 292: 348 (1975).

Ahn, Y.S.; Byrnes, J.J.; Harrington, W.J.; Cayer, M.L.; Smith, D.B.; Brunskill, D.E. amd Pall, L.M.: The treatment of idiopathic thrombocytopenia with vinblastine-loaded platelets. New England Journal of Medicine 298: 1101 (1978).

Amsler, H.A.; Teerenhovi, L.; Barth, E.; Harjula, K. and Vuopio, P.: Agranulocytosis in patients treated with clozapine. A study of the Finnish epidemic. Acta Psychiatrica Scandinavica 56: 241 (1977).

Anderman, B. and Griffith, R.W.: Clozapine-induced agranulocytosis: A situation report up to August 1976. European Journal of Clinical Pharmacology 11: 199 (1977).

Anderson, K.E.; Peterson, C.M.; Alvares, A.P. and Kappas, A.: Oxidative drug metabolism and inducibility by phenobarbital in sickle cell anemia, Clinical Pharmacology and Therapeutics 22: 580 (1977).

Andrassy, K; Weischedel, E.; Ritz, E. and Andrassy, T.: Bleeding in uremic patients after carbenicillin. Thrombosis and Haemostasis 36: 115 (1976a).

Andrassy, K.; Scherz, M.; Ritz, E.; Walter, E.; Hasper, B.; Storch, H. and Vomel, W.: Pencillin-induced coagulation disorder. Lancet 2: 1039 (1976b).

Anturane Reinfarction Trial Research Group: Sulfinpyrazone in the prevention of cardiac death after myocardial infarction. New England Journal of Medicine 298: 289 (1978).

Babcock, R.B.; Dumper, C.W. and Scharfman, W.B.: Heparin-induced thrombocytopenia. New England Journal of Medicine 295: 237 (1976).

Bachmann, K. and Shapiro, R.: Protein binding of coumarin anticoagulants in disease states. Clinical Pharmacokinetics 2: 110 (1977).

Bachmann, K.; Shapiro, R. and Mackiewicz, J.: Warfarin elimination and responsiveness in patients with renal dysfunction. Journal of Clinical Pharmacology 17: 292 (1977).

Barber, H.M.; Feil, E.J.; Galasko, C.S.B.; Edwards, D.H.; Sutton, R.A.; Haynes, D.W. and Bentley, G.: A comparative study of dextran-70, warfarin and low-dose heparin for the prophylaxis of thrombo-embolism following total hip replacement. Postgraduate Medical Journal 53: 130 (1977).

Barrowcliffe, T.W.; Johnson, E.A. and Thomas, D.: Antithrombin III and heparin. British Medical Bulletin 34: 143 (1978).

Bassan, M.M. and Rogel, S.: Current practice in the use of anticoagulants for ischemic heart disease. Heart and Lung 5: 742 (1976).

Basu, D.; Gallus, A.; Hirsh, J. and Cade, J.: A prospective study of the value of monitoring heparin treatment with the activated partial thromboplastin time. New England Journal of Medicine 287: 324 (1972).

Beal, R.W.: Haematinics I: Patho-physiological and clinical aspects. Drugs 2: 190 (1971); II: Clinical pharmacological and therapeutic aspects. Drugs 2: 207 (1971).

Beckering, R.E. and Titus, J.L.: Femoral-popliteal venous thrombosis and pulmonary embolism. American Journal of Clinical Pathology 52: 530 (1969).

Bell, W.R.; Pitney, W.R. and Goodwin, J.F.: Therapeutic defibrination in the treatment of thrombotic disease. Lancet 1: 490 (1968).

Bell, W.; Tomasulo, P.A.; Alving, B.M. and Duffy, T.P.: Thrombocytopenia occurring during the administration of heparin. A prospective study in 52 patients. Annals of Internal Medicine 85: 155 (1976).

Bennett, B. and Douglas, A.S.: Blood coagulation mechanism. Clinics in Haematology 2:3 (1973).

Beutler, E.: Drug-induced haemolytic anaemia. Pharmacological Reviews 21: 73 (1969).

Beutler, E.: Abnormalities of the hexose monophosphate shunt. Seminars in Hematology 8: 311 (1971).

Beutler, E.: Drug-induced anaemia. Federation Proceedings

31: 141 (1972).

Beutler, E.; Fairbanks, V.F. and Fahey, J.I.: Clinical Disorders of Iron Metabolism (Grune and Stratton, New York 1963).

Blackwell, E.A.; Hawson, G.A.T.; Leer, J. and Bain, B.: Acute pancytopenia due to megaloblastic arrest in association with co-trimoxazole. Medical Journal of Australia 2: 38 (1978).

Bochner, F.; Hooper, W.D.; Eadie, M.J. and Tyrer, J.H.: Decreased capacity to metabolize diphenylhydantoin in a patient with hypersensitivity to warfarin. Australia and New Zealand Journal of Medicine 5: 462 (1975).

Borchgrevink, C.F.: Long-term anticoagulant therapy in angina pectoris and myocardial infarction. A clinical trial between intensive and moderate treatment. Acta Medica Scandinavica, Suppl. 359 (1960).

Borchgrevink, C.F.: Long term anticoagulant therapy in angina pectoris. Lancet 1: 449 (1962).

Bottiger, L.E. and Westerholm, B.: Drug-induced blood dyscrasias in Sweden. British Medical Journal 3: 339 (1973).

Bowie, E.J.W. and Owren, C.A.: Hemostatic failure in clinical medicine. Seminars in Hematology 14: 341 (1977).

Bramble, C.E. and Hunter, R.E.: Effect of dicoumarol on the nursing infant. American Journal of Obstetrics and Gynecology 59: 1153 (1950).

Branda, R.F.; Amsden, T.W. and Jacob, H.S.: Randomized study of nandrolene therapy for anemias due to bone marrow failure. Archives of Internal Medicine 137: 65 (1977).

Breckenridge, A.: Oral anticoagulants - the totem and the taboo. British Medical Journal 1: 419 (1976).

Breckenridge, A.M.: Interindividual differences in the response to oral anticoagulants. Drugs 14: 367 (1977).

Breckenridge, A.; Orme, M.; Davis, L.; Thorgeirson, S.S. and Davis, D.S.: Dose dependent enzyme induction. Clinical Pharmacology and Therapeutics 14: 514 (1973).

Brinkhous, K.M. and Hemker, H.C.: Handbook of Hemophilia (Excerpta Medica, Amsterdam 1975).

Brise, H. and Hallberg, L.: A method for comparative studies on iron absorption in man using two radio iron isotopes. Acta Medica Scandinavica 171 (Suppl. 376): 7 (1962).

Brogden, R.N.; Speight, T.M. and Avery, G.S.: Streptokinase: A review of its clinical pharmacology, mechanism of action and therapeutic uses. Drugs 5: 357 (1973).

Browse, N.: Diagnosis of deep-vein thrombosis. British Medical Bulletin 34: 163 (1978).

Browse, N.L.; Jackson, B.T.; Majo, M.E. and Negus, D.: The value of mechanical methods of preventing postoperative calf vein thrombosis. British Journal of Surgery 61: 219 (1974).

Browse, N.L.; Clemenson, G.; Batteman, N.T.; Gaunt, J.I. and Croft, D.N.: Effect of intravenous dextran 70 and pneumatic leg compression in incidence of postoperative pulmonary embolism. British Medical Journal 2: 1281 (1976).

Camitla, B.M.; Thomas, E.D.; Nathan, D.G.; Santos, G.; Gordon-Smith, E.C.; Gale, R.P.; Rappeport, J.M. and Storb, R.: Severe aplastic anemia: A prospective study of the effect of early marrow transplantation on acute mortality. Blood 48: 63 (1976).

Canadian Cooperative Study Group: A randomised trial of aspirin and sulfinpyrazone in threatened stroke. New England Journal of Medicine 299: 53 (1978).

Cantin, M.; Haberland, G.L.; Schnells, G. and Seleye, H. (Ed): New Aspects of Trasylol Therapy. Experimental Myocardial Infarction (F.K. Schattauer Verlag, Stuttgart 1975).

Chalmers, T.C.; Matta, R.J.; Smith, H. and Kunzler, A.M.: Evidence favoring the use of anticoagulants in the hospital phase of acute myocardial infarction. New England Journal of Medicine 297: 1091 (1977).

Chanarin, I. and England, J.M.: Toxicity of trimethoprim-sulphamethoxazole in patients with megaloblastic haemopoiesis. British Medical Journal 1: 651 (1972).

Clark, W.B.; McGregor, A.B.; Prescott, R.J. and Ruckley, C.V.: Pneumatic compression of the calf and postoperative deep vein thrombosis. Lancet 2: 5 (1974).

Clarke, W.T.W.: Fatal aplastic anemia and chloramphenicol. Canadian Medical Association Journal 97: 815 (1967).

Collen, D.: Identification and some properties of a new fast-reacting plasmin inhibitor in human plasma. European Journal of Biochemistry 69: 209 (1976).

Committee of Principal Investigators: A co-operative trial in the primary prevention of ischaemic heart disease using clofibrate. British Heart Journal 40: 1069 (1978).

Cunningham, J.L.; Leyland, M.J.; Delamore, I.W. and Price Evans, D.A.: Acetanilide oxidation in phenylbutazone-associated hypoplastic anaemia. British Medical Journal 3: 313 (1974).

Dacie, J.V. and Worlledge, S.M.: Auto-immune hemolytic anemias. Progress in Hematology 6: 82 (1969).

Davies, D.W. and Steward, D.J.: Unexpected excessive bleeding during operation: Role of acetylsalicylic acid. Canadian Anesthetist's Society Journal 24: 452 (1977).

Davies, J.A.; Merrick, M.V.; Sharp, A.A. and Holt, J.M.: Controlled trial of Ancrod and heparin in treatment of deep-vein thrombosis of lower limb. Lancet 1: 113 (1972).

Davis, S. and Rubin, A.: Treatment and prognosis in aplastic anaemia. Lancet 1: 871 (1972).

de la Chapelle, A.; Kari, C.; Nurminen, M. and Hernberg, S.: Clozapine-induced agranulocytosis. A genetic and epidemiologic study. Human Genetics 37: 183 (1977).

Dean, J. and Schechter, N.: Sickle-cell anemia: Molecular and cellular basis of therapeutic approaches. New England Journal of Medicine 299: 804, 863 (1978).

Dollery, C.T. and Hensby, C.N.: Is prostacyclin a circulating anti-coagulant. Nature 273: 706 (1978).

Dollery, C.T.; George, C.F. and Orme, M.l'E.: Drug interactions affecting cardiovascular therapy; in Cluff and Petrie (Eds) Clinical Effects of Interaction Between Drugs, p. 117 (Excerpta Medica, Amsterdam 1975).

Dormandy, J.A.; Goyle, K.B. and Reid, H.L.: Treatment of severe intermittent claudication by controlled defibrination. Lancet 1: 625 (1977).

Douglas, A.S.: Management of thrombotic diseases. Seminars in Hematology 8: 95 (1971).

Dundee, J.W.: Thiopentone and Other Barbiturates, p. 137 (Livingstone, Edinburgh 1956).

Eckstein, H.B. and Jack, B.: Breast-feeding and anticoagulant therapy. Lancet 1: 672 (1970).

Editorial: Aspirin and what else? British Medical Journal 3: 5 (1974).

Editorial: Circulating prostacyclin. Lancet 2: 21 (1978a).

Editorial: Clofibrate: A final verdict? Lancet 2: 1131 (1978b).

Editorial: Clofibrate and the primary prevention of ischaemic heart disease: British Medical Journal 2: 1585 (1978c).

Elwood, P.C. and Williams, G.: A comparative trial of slow-release and conventional iron preparations. Practioner 204: 812 (1970).

Esmon, C.T.; Suttie, J.W. and Jackson, C.M.: The functional significance of vitamin-K action. Difference in phospholipid binding between normal and abnormal prothrombin. Journal of Biological Chemistry 250: 4095 (1975).

Esnouf, M.P.: Biochemistry of blood coagulation. British Medical Bulletin 33: 213 (1977).

Estes, J.W. and Poulin, P.F.: Pharmacokinetics of heparin distribution and elimination. Thrombosis et Diathesis Haemorrhagica 33: 26 (1975).

Ewart, M.R.; Hatton, M.; Basford, J.M. and Dodgson, K.S.: The proteolytic action of arvin on human fibrinogen, Biochemical Journal 115: 17 (1969).

Fields, W.S.; Lemak, N.A.; Frankowski, R.F. and Hardy, R.J.: Controlled trial of aspirin in cerebral ischemia. Stroke 8: 301 (1977).

Fields, W.S.; Lemak, N.A.; Frankowski, R.F. and Hardy, R.J.: Controlled trial of aspirin in cerebral ischemia. Part II: Surgical group. Stroke 9: 309 (1978).

Fletcher, A.P.; Alkjaersig, N. and Sherry, S.: The maintenance of a sustained thrombolytic state in man. I. Induction and effects. Journal of Clinical Investigation 38: 1096 (1959).

Fletcher, A.P.; Alkjaersig, N.; Lewis, M.; Tulevski, V; Davies, A.; Brooks, J.E.; Hardin, W.B.; Landau, W.M. and Raichle, M.E.: A pilot study of urokinase therapy in cerebral infarction. Stroke 7: 135 (1976).

Folstad, H.; Liliequist, B.; Schanning, M. and Thulin, C.A.: Tranexamic acid in the preoperative management of ruptured intracranial aneurysms. Surgical Neurology 9: 9 (1978).

Forbes, C.D. and Davidson, J.F.: Management of coagulation defects. Clinics in Haematology 2: 101 (1973).

Forbes, C.D. and Prentice, C.R.M.: Thrombus formation and artificial surfaces. British Medical Bulletin 34: 201 (1978).

Forbes, C.D.; Barr, R.D.; Reid, G.; Thomson, C.; Prentice, E.R.M.; McNicol, G.P. and Douglas, A.S.: Tranexamic acid in control of haemorrhage after dental extraction in haemophilia and Christmas disease. British Medicial Journal 1: 311 (1972).

Fries, K.; Konig, F.E. and Reich, T.: Einfluss der Marcoumar-Therapie bei voll gestillten kindern. Schweizerische Medizinische Wochenschrift 87: 615 (1957).

Gallus, A.S. and Hirsh, J.: Antithrombotic drugs. Drugs 12: 41, 132 (1976a).

Gallus, A.S. and Hirsh, J.: Prevention of venous thromboembolism. Seminars in Thrombosis and Hemostasis 2: 232 (1976b).

Gallus, A.S. and Hirsh, J.: Treatment of venous thromboembolic disease. Seminars in Thrombosis and Hemostasis 2: 291 (1976c).

Gallus, A.S. and Hirsh, J.: Antithrombotic drugs; in Avery (Ed) Cardiovascular Drugs, Vol. 3 Antithrombotic Drugs, p. 85 (ADIS Press, Sydney; University Park Press, Baltimore 1978).

Gallus, A.S.; Hirsh, J.; Hull, R. and van Aken, W.G.: Diagnosis of venous thromboembolism. Seminars in Thrombosis and Hemostasis 2: 203 (1976).

Garratty, G. and Petz, L.D.: Drug-induced immune hemolytic anemia. American Journal of Medicine 58: 398 (1975).

Gebauer, D. and Heigel, K.: Therapeutische Beeinflussung der Hamophilie durch AMCHA. Medizinische Klinik 64: 378 (1969).

Girdwood, R.H.: Disorders of the blood; in Alstead, Macgregor and Girdwood (Eds) Textbook of Medical Treatment, p. 142, 12th ed (Churchill Livingstone, Edinburgh 1971).

Girdwood, R.H.: Blood Disorders Due to Drugs and Other Agents (Excerpta Medica, Amsterdan 1973a).

Girdwood, R.H.: Trimethoprim/sulphamethoxazole: Long-term therapy and folate levels. Medical Journal of Australia. Suppl. 1: 34 (1973b).

Girdwood, R.H.: Drug-induced anaemias. Drugs 11: 394 (1976).

Glazier, R.L. and Crowell, E.B.: Continuous heparin therapy appears significantly safer than intermittent use. Journal of the American Medical Association 236: 1365 (1976).

Gostof, P.: Les substances derivees du tromexane dans le lait maternel et leurs actions paradoxales sur la prothrombine. Schweizerische Medizinishe Wochenschrift 82: 764 (1952).

Graziano, J.H.; Markenson, A.; Miller, D.R.; Chang, H.; Bestak, M.; Meyers, P.; Pisciotto, P. and Rifkind, A.: Chelation therapy in β-thalassemia major. I. Intravenous and subcutaneous deferoxamine. Journal of Pediatrics 92: 648 (1978).

Gyn, T.N.; Messmore, H.L. and Friedman, I.A.: Drug-induced thrombocytopenia. Medical Clinics of North America 56: 65 (1972).

Hall, J.G.: Warfarin and fetal embryopathy. Lancet 1: 1127 (1976).

Hall, R.J.; Garcia, E.; Al-Bassam, M.C. and Dawson, J.T.: Aortocoronary bypass surgery, 1969-1973, review of 2566 patients. Cardiovascular Diseases Bulletin 1: 74 (1974).

Hardisty, R.M.: Disorders of platelet function. British Medical Bulletin 33: 207 (1977).

Harris, W.H.; Salzman, E.W.; Athanasoulis, C.; Waltman, A.C.; Baum, S. and De Sanctis, R.W.: Comparison of warfarin, low-molecular-weight dextran, aspirin, and subcutaneous heparin in prevention of venous thromboembolism following total hip replacement. Journal of Bone and Joint Surgery, American Volume 56: 1552 (1974).

Hedlund, P.O.: Antifibrinolytic therapy with Cyclokapron in connection with prostatectomy. A double-blind study. Scandinavian Journal of Urology and Nephrology 3: 177 (1969).

Hemker, H.C. and Loeliger, E.A.: Kinetic aspects of the interaction of blood-clotting enzymes. Demonstration of the existence of an inhibitor of prothrombin conversion in vitamin K-deficiency. Thrombosis et Diathesis haemorrhagica 19: 346 (1968).

Hepso, H.U.; Lokken, P.; Bjornson, J. and Godal, H.C.: Double-blind crossover study of the effect of acetylsalicylic acid on bleeding and post-operative course after bilateral oral surgery. European Journal of Clinical Pharmacology 10: 217 (1976).

Hirch, J.; Cade, J.F. and Gallus, A.S.: Fetal effects of coumarin administered during pregnancy. Blood 36: 623 (1970a).

Hirsh, J.; O'Sullivan, E.F. and Martin, M.: Evaluation of a standard dosage schedule with streptokinase. Blood 35: 341 (1970b).

Hirsh, J.; Cade, J.F. and Gallus, A.S.: Anticoagulants in pregnancy: A review of indications and complications. American Heart Journal 83: 301 (1972).

Hirsh, J.; van Aken, W.G.; Gallus, A.S.; Dollery, C.T.; Cade, J.F. and Yung, W.L.: Heparin kinetics in venous thrombosis and pulmonary embolism. Circulation 53: 691 (1976).

Hunter, R.; Barnes, J.; Oakeley, H.F. and Mathews, D.M.: Toxicity of folic acid given in pharmacological doses to healthy volunteers. Lancet 1: 61 (1970).

Hussain, M.A.M.; Flynn, D.M.; Green, N. and Hoffbrand,

A.V.: Effect of dose, time and ascorbate on iron excretion after subcutaneous desferrioxamine. Lancet 1: 977 (1977).

Husted, S. and Andreasen, F.: Problems encountered in long-term treatment with anticoagulants. Acta Medica Scandinavica 200: 379 (1976).

Husted, S. and Andreasen, F.: Individual variation in the response to phenprocoumon. European Journal of Clinical Pharmacology 11: 351 (1977a).

Husted, S. and Andreasen, F.: The influence of age on the response to anticoagulants. British Journal of Clinical Pharmacology 4: 559 (1977b).

Idanpaan-Heikkila, J.; Alhava, E,; Olkinuora, M. and Palva, I.P.: Agranulocytosis during treatment with clozapine. European Journal of Clinical Pharmacology 11: 193 (1977).

Illingworth, R.S. and Finch, E.: Ethyl biscoumacetate (tromexan) in human milk. Journal of Obstetrics and Gynaecology of the British Commonwealth 66: 487 (1959).

Inman, W.H.W.: Study of fatal bone marrow depression with special reference to phenylbutazone and oxyphenbutazone. British Medical Journal 1: 1500 (1977).

International Anticoagulant Review Group: Collaborative analysis of long-term anticoagulation administration after acute myocardial infarction. Lancet 1: 203 (1970).

Jahnchen, E.; Meinertz, T.: Gilfrich, H.J.; Groth, U. and Martini, A.: The enantiomers of phenprocoumon: Pharmacodynamic and pharmacokinetic studies. Clinical Pharmacology and Therapeutics 20: 342 (1976).

Jarret, P.E.M.; Moreland, M. and Browse, N.L.: Idiopathic recurrent superficial thrombophlebitis: treatment with fibrinolytic enhancement. British Medical Journal 1: 933 (1977).

Jick, H.; Slone, D.; Borda, I.T. and Shapiro, S.: Efficacy and toxicity of heparin in relation to age and sex. New England Journal of Medicine 279: 284 (1968).

Jungi, W.F.; Fischer, J.; Senn, H.J.; Hartlapp, J.; Poldinger, W.; Kunz, H. and Krupp, P.: Clustering of clozapine-induced agranulocytosis in Eastern Switzerland. Schweizerische Medizinische Wochenschrift 107: 1861 (1977).

Kakkar, V.V. and Scully, M.F.: Thrombolytic therapy. British Medical Bulletin 34: 191 (1978).

Kakkar, V.V.; Howe, C.T.; Laws, J.W. and Flanc, C.: Late results of treatment of deep vein thrombosis. British Medical Journal 1: 810 (1969).

Kakkar, V.V.; Howe, C.T.; Nicolaides, A.N.; Renney, J.J.G. and Clarke, M.B.: Deep vein thrombosis of the leg — is there a 'high risk' group? American Journal of Surgery 120: 527 (1970).

Kelly, J.G. and O'Malley, K.: Clinical pharmacokinetics of oral anticoagulants. Clinical Pharmacokinetics 4: 1 (1979).

Kernoff, P.B.A. and McNicol, G.P.: Normal and abnormal fibrinolysis. British Medical Bulletin 33: 239 (1977).

Kisker, C.T. and Burke, C.: Double-blind studies on the use of steroids in the treatment of acute haemarthrosis in patients with hemophilia. New England Journal of Medicine 282: 639 (1970).

Kleinman, P.D. and Griner, P.F.: Studies of the epidemiology of anticoagulant-drug interactions. Archives of Internal Medicine 126: 522 (1970).

Kobayashi, I.; Ito, M. and Shibata, A.: D.D.A.V.P. in haemophilia B. Lancet 1: 615 (1978).

Koch-Weser, J.: Drug interactions in cardiovascular therapy. American Heart Journal 90: 93 (1975).

Koch-Weser, J. and Sellers, E.M.: Drug interactions with coumarin anticoagulants. New England Journal of Medicine 285: 487, 547 (1971).

Labadarios, D.; Dickerson, J.W.T.; Parke, D.V.; Lucas, E.G. and Obuwa, G.H.; The effects of chronic drug administration on hepatic enzyme induction and folate metabolism. British Journal of Clinical Pharmacology 5: 167 (1978).

Langman, M.J.S. and Smithard, D.J.: Antipyrine metabolism in iron deficiency. British Journal of Clinical Pharmacology 4: 631P (1977).

Larrieu, M.J. and Meyer, D.: Abnormal factor IX during anticoagulant treatment. Lancet 2: 1085 (1970).

Lawrence, J.R.; Shepherd, J.T.; Bone, I.; Rogen, A.S. and Fulton, W.F.: Fibrinolytic therapy in unstable angina pectoris: a controlled clinical trial. British Heart Journal. In press (1979).

Levine, J.A.; Bechtel, D.J.; Gorlin, R.; Cohn, P.F.; Herman, M.V.; Cohn, L.H. and Collins, J.J.: Coronary artery anatomy before and after direct revascularization surgery: clinical and cinearteriographic studies in 67 selected patients. American Heart Journal 89: 561 (1975).

Levy, G.: Relationship between pharmacological effects and plasma or tissue concentration of drugs in man; in Davies and Prichard (Eds) Biological Effects of Drugs in Relation to Their Plasma Concentrations, p. 83 (Macmillan, London 1973).

Lewis, R.J.; Trager, W.F.; Chan, K.K.; Breckenridge, A.; Orme, M.; Rowland, M. and Schary, W.: Warfarin: Stereochemical aspects of its metabolism and the interaction with phenylbutazone. Journal of Clinical Investigation 53: 1607 (1974).

Loeliger, E.A.; Hensen, A.; Mattern, M.J. and Hemker, H.C.: Behaviour of Factors II,VII,IX and X in bleeding complications during long-term treatment with coumarin. Thrombosis et Diathesis Haemorrhagica 10: 278 (1964).

Loeliger, E.A.; Hensen, A.; Kroes, F.; Van Dijk, L.; Fekkes, M.; de Jonge, H. and Hemker, H.C.: A double blind trial of long-term anticoagulant treatment after myocardial infarction. Acta Medica Scandinavica 182: 549 (1967).

Loeliger, E.A.; Meuwisse-Braun, J.B.; Muis, H.; Buitendijk, F.J.J.; Veltkamp, J.J. and Hemker, H.C.: Laboratory control of oral anticoagulants. Definition of therapeutic range in terms of different thromboplastin preparations. Thrombosis et Diathesis Haemorrhagica (Stuttgart) 23: 499 (1970).

MacLeod, S.M. and Sellers, E.M.: Pharmacodynamic and pharmacokinetic drug interactions with coumarin anticoagulants. Drugs 11: 461 (1976).

McQueen, E.G.: Hormonal steroid contraceptives: A further review of adverse reactions. Drugs 16: 322 (1978).

Mackie, M.J. and Douglas, A.S.: Oral anticoagulants in arterial disease. British Medical Bulletin 34: 177 (1978).

Mannucci, P.M.; Ruggeri, Z.; Pareti, F.I. and Capitanio, A.: 1-Desamino-8-D-Arginine Vasopressin: a new pharmacological approach to the management of haemophilia and von Willebrand's disease. Lancet 1: 869 (1977).

Marciniak, E.: Binding of heparin in vitro and in vivo to plasma proteins. Journal of Laboratory and Clinical Medicine 84: 344 (1974).

Maurice-Williams, R.S.: Prolonged antifibrinolysis: an effective non-surgical treatment for ruptured intracranial aneurysms? British Medical Journal 1: 945 (1978).

Meeuwissen, A.J.A.Th.; Vervoon, A.C.; Cohen, O.; Jordan, F.L. and Nelemans, F.A.: Double blind trial of long-term anticoagulant treatment after myocardial infarction. Acta Medica Scandinavica 186: 361 (1969).

Miekle, C.H.; Heiden, D.; Britten, A.F.; Ramos, J. and Flavell, P: Hemostasis, antipyretics and mild analgesics. Acetaminophen vs aspirin. Journal of the American Medical Association 235: 613 (1976).

Miescher, P.A.: Drug-induced thrombocytopenia. Seminars in Hematology 10: 311 (1973).

Moncada, S. and Korbutt, R.: Dipyridamole and other phosphodiesterase inhibitors act as antithrombotic agents by potentiating endogenous prostacyclin. Lancet 1: 1286 (1978).

Moncada, S. and Vane, J.R.: Unstable metabolites of arachidonic acid and their role in haemostasis and thrombosis. British Medical Bulletin 34: 129 (1978).

Morris, G.K. and Mitchell, J.R.A.: Preventing venous thromboembolism in elderly patients with hip fractures: studies of low dose heparin, dipyridamole, aspirin, and flurbiprofen. British Medical Journal 1: 535 (1977).

Morris, G.K. and Mitchell, J.R.A.: Clinical management of venous thromboembolism. British Medical Bulletin 34: 169 (1978a).

Morris, G.K. and Mitchell, J.R.A.: Can death from venous thromboembolism be prevented in elderly patients with hip fractures. American Heart Journal 95: 139 (1978b).

Multicentre Trial: Prevention of fatal postoperative pulmonary embolism by low doses of heparin. Lancet 2: 45 (1975).

Multicentre Trial: Prevention of fatal postoperative pulmonary embolism by low doses of heparin. Lancet 1: 567 (1977).

Mustard, J.F. and Packham, M.A.: Thromboembolism: A manifestation of the response of blood to injury. Circulation 42: 1 (1970).

Mustard, J.F. and Packham, Marian A.: Platelets, thrombosis and drugs. Drugs 9: 19 (1975).

Mustard, J.F. and Packham, M.A.: Normal and abnormal haemostasis. British Medical Bulletin 33: 187 (1977).

Mustard, J.F. and Packham, M.A.: Platelets, thrombosis and drugs; in Avery (Ed) Cardiovascular Drugs, Vol. 3 Antithrombotic Drugs, p. 1 (ADIS Press, Sydney 1978).

Nagao, T. and Mauer, A.M.: Concordance for drug-induced aplastic anaemia in identical twins. New England Journal of Medicine 281: 7 (1969).

Nagashima, R.; O'Reilly, R.A. and Levy, G.: Kinetics of pharmacological effects in man: the anticoagulant action of warfarin. Clinical Pharmacology and Therapeutics 10: 22 (1969).

Neuvonen, P.J.: Interactions with the absorption of tetracyclines. Drugs 11: 45 (1976).

Nevasaari, K.; Heikkinen, M. and Taskinen, P.J.: Tamoxifen and thrombosis. Lancet 2: 946 (1978).

Newcastle upon Tyne Physicians: Trial of clofibrate in the treatment of ischemic heart disease. British Medical Journal 4: 767 (1971).

Nieweg, H.O.: Aplastic anaemia (panmyelopathy); in Girdwood (Ed) Blood Disorders Due to Drugs and Other Agents, p. 49 (Excerpta Medica, Amsterdam 1973).

Nilsson, I.M.; Hedner, V. and Isacson, S.: Phenformin ethyloestranol in recurrent venous thrombosis. Acta Medica Scandinavica 198: 107 (1975).

Norris, J.W. and Pratt, R.F.: Folic acid deficiency and epilepsy. Drugs 8: 366 (1974).

O'Brien, J.R.: Platelet disorders. Clinics in Haematology 1: 231 (1972).

O'Grady, J. and Moncada, S.: Aspirin: A paradoxical effect on bleeding-time. Lancet 2: 780 (1978).

Ogston, D. and Bennett, B.: Surface-mediated reactions in the formation of thrombin, plasmin and kallikrein. British Medical Bulletin 34: 107 (1978).

Olesen, H.; Hom, B.L. and Schwartz, M.: Antibody to transcobalamin II in patients treated with long acting vitamin B_{12} preparations. Scandinavian Journal of Haematology 5: 5 (1968).

O'Malley, K.; Stevenson, I.H.; Ward, C.A.; Wood, A.J.J. and Crooks, J.: Determinants of anticoagulant control in patients receiving warfarin. British Journal of Clinical Pharmacology 4: 309 (1977).

O'Reilly, R.A.: Vitamin K in hereditary resistance to oral anticoagulant drugs. American Journal of Physiology 221: 1327 (1971).

O'Reilly, R.A.: Interactions of sodium warfarin and rifampin. Studies in man. Annals of Internal Medicine 81: 337 (1974).

O'Reilly, R.A.: Interaction of chronic daily warfarin therapy and rifampin. Annals of Internal Medicine 83: 506 (1975).

O'Reilly, R.A.: Vitamin K and the oral anticoagulant drugs. Annual Review of Medicine 27: 245 (1976a).

O'Reilly, R.A.: The stereoselective interaction of warfarin and metronidazole in man. New England Journal of Medicine 295: 354 (1976b).

O'Reilly, R.A. and Aggeler, P.A.: Determinants of the response to oral anticoagulant drugs in man. Pharmacological Reviews 22: 35 (1970).

O'Reilly, R.A.; Sahud, M.A. and Aggeler, P.M.: Impact of aspirin and chlorthalidone on the pharmacodynamics of oral anticoagulant drugs in man. Annals of the New York Academy of Sciences 179: 173 (1971).

Orme, M.L.'E.; Lewis, P.J.; de Swiet, M.; Serlin, M.J.; Sibeon, R.; Baty, J.D. and Breckenridge, A.M.: May mothers given warfarin breast-feed their infants? British Medical Journal 1: 1564 (1977).

O'Sullivan, D.J.; Higgins, P.G. and Wilkinson, J.E.: Oral iron compounds, a therapeutic comparison. Lancet 2: 482 (1955).

Pachter, H.L. and Riles, T.S.: Low dose heparin: bleeding and wound complications in the surgical patient. A prospective randomized study. Annals of Surgery 186: 669 (1977).

Paterson, J.C.: The pathology of venous thrombi; in Sherry, Brinkhous, Genton and Stengle (Eds) Thrombosis, p. 321 (National Academy of Sciences, Washington DC 1969).

Pisciotta, A.V.: Immune and toxic mechanisms and drug-induced agranulocytosis. Seminars in Hematology 10: 279 (1973).

Pisciotta, A.V.: Drug-induced agranulocytosis. Drugs 15: 132 (1978).

Pitney, W.R.; Pettit, J.E. and Armstrong, L.: Control of heparin therapy. British Medical Journal 4: 139 (1970).

Porter, A.M.W.: Drug defaulting in a general practice. British Medical Journal 1: 218 (1969).

Preston, F.E.; Dinsdale, R.C.W.; Sutcliffe, D.J.; Bardham, G.; Wyld, P.J. and Hamlyn, J.F.: Factor VIII inhibitor bypassing activity (FEIBA) in the management of patients with factor VIII inhibitors. Thrombosis Research 11: 643 (1977).

Remuzzi, G.; Cavenaghi, A.E. and Mecca, G.: Prostacyclin-like activity and bleeding in renal failure. Lancet 2: 1195 (1977).

Ries, C.A.: Vincristine for treatment of refractory autoimmune thrombocytopenia. New England Journal of Medicine 295: 1136 (1976).

Rifkind, A.B.; Canale, V. and New, M.I.: Antipyrine clearance in homozygous β-thalassemia. Clinical Pharmacology and Therapeutics 20: 476 (1976).

Rizza, C.R.: Clinical management of haemophilia. British Medical Bulletin 33: 225 (1977).

Rizza, C.R.; Kernoff, P.B.A.; Mathews, J.M.; McLennan, C.R. and Rainsford, S.G.: A comparison of coagulation factor replacement therapy with and without prednisolone in the treatment of haematuria in haemophilia and Christmas disease. Thrombosis and Haemostasis 37: 86 (1977).

Ro, J.S.; Knutro, O.; Stormorken, H.: Antifibrinolytic treatment with tranexamic acid (AMCA) in pediatric urinary tract surgery. Journal of Pediatric Surgery 5: 315 (1970).

Roberts, V.C. and Cotton, L.T.: Failure of low-dose heparin to improve efficacy of peroperative intermittent calf compression in preventing postoperative deep vein thrombosis. British Medical Journal 3: 458 (1975).

Rogers, P.H. and Sherry, S.: Current status of antithrombotic therapy in cardiovascular disease. Progress in Cardiovascular Diseases 19: 235 (1976).

Rosch, J.; Dotter, C.T.; Seaman, A.J.; Porter, J.M. and Cimmon, H.H.: Healing of deep venous thrombosis; venographic findings in a randomized study comparing streptokinase and heparin. American Journal of Roentgenology 127: 553 (1976).

Rosenberg, R.D.: Actions and interactions of antithrombin and heparin. New England Journal of Medicine 292: 146 (1975).

Rosenthal, M.; Breysse, Y.; Dixon, A.St.J.; Franchimont, P.; Huskisson, E.C.; Schmidt, K.L.; Schuermans, Y.; Veys, E.; Vischer, T.L.; Janssen, P.A.J.; Amery, W.K.; Brugmans, J.; De Crepe, J.; Symoens, J. and MacNair, A.L.: Levamisole and agranulocytosis. Lancet 1: 904 (1977).

Sackler, J.P. and Lin, L.: Heparin-induced osteoporosis. British Journal of Radiology 46: 548 (1973).

Salzman, E.W.; Deykin, D.; Shapiro, Ruth, M. and Rosenberg, R.: Management of heparin therapy. Controlled prospective trial, New England Journal of Medicine 292: 1046 (1975).

Sanchez-Medal, L.; Gomez-Leal, A.; Duarte, L. and Rico, M.G.: Anabolic androgenic steroids in the treatment of acquired aplastic anaemia. Blood 34: 283 (1969).

Schmutzler, R. and Koller, F. Thrombolytic therapy; in Poller (Ed) Recent Advances in Blood Coagulation, p. 324 (Churchill, London 1969).

Scottish Society of Physicians: Ischemic heart disease: A secondary prevention trial using clofibrate. British Medical Journal 2: 775 (1971).

Selzer, A.: Use of anticoagulant agents in acute myocardial infarction: Statistics or clinical judgement. American Journal of Cardiology 41: 1315 (1978).

Sevitt, S.: Venous thrombosis in injured patients (with some observations on pathogenesis); in Sherry, Brinkhous, Genton and Stengle (Eds) Thrombosis, p. 29 (National Academy of Sciences, Washington DC 1969).

Sevitt, S.: Organization of valve pocket thrombi and the anomalies of double thrombi and valve cusp involvement. British Journal of Surgery 61: 641 (1974).

Shahidi, N.T.: Androgens and erythropoiesis. New England Journal of Medicine 289: 72 (1973).

Sharp, A.A.: Diagnosis and management of disseminated intravascular coagulation. British Medical Bulletin 33: 193 (1977).

Shaul, W.L. and Hall, J.G.: Multiple congenital anomalies associated with oral anticoagulants. American Journal of Obstetrics and Gynecology 127: 191 (1977).

Sheehy, T.W. and Plumb, V.J.: Treatment of sickle cell disease. Archives of Internal Medicine 137: 779 (1977).

Sheffer, A.L.; Fearon, D.T.; Austen, K.F. and Rosen, F.S.: Tranexamic acid: Preoperative prophylactic therapy for patients with hereditary angioneurotic edema. Journal of Allergy and Clinical Immunology 60: 38 (1977).

Shepherd, A.M.M.; Hewick, D.S.; Moreland, T.A. and Stevenson, I.H.: Age as a determinant of sensitivity to warfarin. British Journal of Clinical Pharmacology 4: 315 (1977).

Simon, T.L.; Hyers, T.M.; Gaston, J.P. and Harker, L.A.: Heparin pharmacokinetics: Increased requirements in pulmonary embolism. British Journal of Haematology 39: 111 (1978).

Skjelbred, P.; Album, B and Lokken, P.: Acetylsalicylic acid vs paracetamol; Effects on post-operative course. European Journal of Clinical Pharmacology 12: 257 (1977).

Smith, R.C.; Elton, R.A.; Orr, J.D.; Hart, A.J.L.; Graham, D.F.; Fuller, G.A.G.; Rundle, J.S.H.; MacPherson, A.I.S. and Ruckley, C.V.: Dextran and intermittent pneumatic compression in prevention of postoperative deep vein thrombosis: multiunit trial. Brit. med. J. 1: 952 (1978).

Solomon, H.M. and Schrogie, J.J.: The anticoagulant response to bishydroxycoumarin I. The role of individual variation. Clinical Pharmacology and Therapeutics 8: 65 (1967).

Spearing, G.; Fraser, I.; Turner, G. and Dixon, G.: Long-term self-administered subcutaneous heparin in pregnancy. British Medical Journal 1: 1457 (1978).

Speck, B.; Gluckman, E.; Haak, H.L. and van Rood, J.J.: Treatment of aplastic anaemia by antilymphocyte globulin with and without allogeneic bone marrow infusions. Lancet 2: 1145 (1977).

Stamatakis, J.D.; Kakkar, V.V.; Lawrence, D.; Bentley, P.G.; Nairn, D. and Ward, V.: Failure of aspirin to prevent postoperative deep vein thrombosis in patients undergoing total hip replacement. British Medical Journal 1: 1031 (1978).

Starr, K.J. and Petrie, J.C.: Drug interactions in patients on long-term oral anticoagulant and antihypertensive adrenergic neurone-blocking drugs. British Medical Journal 4: 133 (1972).

Stebbins, R. and Bertino, J.R.: Megaloblastic anaemia produced by drugs. Clinics in Haematology 5: 619 (1976).

Storb, R.; Thomas, E.D.; Buckner, C.D.; Clift, R.A.; Fefer, A.; Fernando, L.P.; Giblett, E.R.; Johnson, F.L. and Neiman, P.E.: Allogenic marrow grafting for treatment of aplastic anemia: A follow-up on long-term survivors. Blood 48: 485 (1976).

Storm, O.: Anticoagulant protection in surgery. Thrombosis et Diathesis Haemorrhagica 2: 484 (1958).

Suttie, J.W.; Grant. G.A.; Esmon, C.T. and Shah, D.V.: Postribosomal function of vitamin K in prothrombin synthesis. Mayo Clinic Proceedings 49: 933 (1974).

Symposium: Drug-induced blood dyscrasias. Seminars in Haematology 10: 179-268, 269-352 (1973).

Taguchi, K.; Matsumba, H.; Washizu, T.; Hirao, M.; Kato, K.; Kato, E.; Mochizuki, T.; Takamura, K.; Mashimo, I.; Morifuji, K.; Nakagaki, M. and Suma, T.: Effect of athrombogenic therapy, especially high dose therapy of dipyridamole, after prosthetic valve replacement. Journal of Cardiovascular Surgery 16: 8 (1975).

Teien, A.N.: Heparin elimination in patients with liver cirrhosis. Thrombosis and Haemostasis 38: 701 (1977).

Teien, A.N. and Bjornson, J.: Heparin elimination in uraemic patients on haemo-dialysis. Scandinavian Journal of Haematology 17: 29 (1976).

Tibbut, D.A.; Davies, J.A.; Anderson, J.A.;Fletcher, E.W.L.; Howell, J.A.; Holt, J.M.; Lea Thomas, M.; De J. Lee, G.; Miller, G.A.H.; Sharp, A.A. and Sutton, G.C.: Comparison by controlled clinical trial of streptokinase and heparin in treatment of life-threatening pulmonary embolism. British Medical Journal 1: 343 (1974).

Tibbutt, D.A. and Chesterman, C.N.: Pulmonary embolism: Current therapeutic concepts. Drugs 11: 161 (1976).

Tibbutt, D.A. and Chesterman, C.N.: Pulmonary embolism: Current therapuetic concepts; in Avery (Ed) Cardiovascular Drugs, Vol. 1 Antithrombotic Drugs, p. 167 (ADIS Press, Sydney; University Park Press, Baltimore 1978).

Tso, S.C.; Chan, T.K. and Todd, D.: Aplastic anaemia: A study of prognosis and the effect of androgen therapy. Quarterly Journal of Medicine 46: 513 (1977).

Turpie, A.G.G. and Hirsh, J.: Platelet suppressive therapy. British Medical Bulletin 34: 183 (1978).

Udall, J.: Drug interference with warfarin. American Journal of Cardiology 23: 143 (1969).

Udall, J.A.: Clinical implivations of warfarin interactions with five sedatives. Amer. J. Card. 35: 67 (1975).

Urokinase Pulmonary Embolism Trial: A national cooperative study. Circulation 47 (Suppl. 11): 1-108 (1973).

Urokinase-Streptokinase Embolism Trial: Phase 2 results. A cooperative study. Journal of the American Medical Association 229: 1606 (1974).

Van Itterbeek, H.; Vermylen, J. and Verstraete, M.: High obstruction of urine flow as a complication of the treatment with fibrinolysis inhibitors of haematuria in haemophiliacs. Acta Haematologica 39: 237 (1968).

Van Leeuwen, V. and Meyboom, R.H.B.: Agranulocytosis and aprindine. Lancet 2: 1137 (1976).

Vermylen, J.; Verhaegen-Declercq, M.L.; Verstraete, M. and Fierens, F.: A double-blind study of the effect of tranexamic acid in essential menorrhagia. Thrombosis et Diathesis Haemorrhagica 20: 583 (1968).

Verstraete, M.; Vermylen, J.; Amery, A. and Vermylen, C.: Thrombolytic therapy with streptokinase using a standard dosage scheme. British Medical Journal 1: 454 (1966).

Verstraete, M.: The prevention of postoperative deep vein thrombosis and pulmonary embolism with low dose subcutaneous heparin and dextran. Surgery, Gynecology and Obstetrics 143: 981 (1976a).

Verstraete, M.: Are agents affecting the platelet functions clinically useful? Amer. J. Med. 61: 897 (1976b).

Verstraete, M.: Haemostatic Drugs. A Critical Appraisal, p. 155 (Martinus Nijhoff, The Hague 1977).

Verstraete, M.: Antiplatelet agents in coronary disease: Are they of prophylactic value? Drugs 15: 464 (1978a).

Verstraete, M.: Biochemical and clinical aspects of thrombolysis. Seminars in Hematology 7: 135 (1978b).

Verwilghen, R.; Reybrouck, G.; Callens, L.; Cosemans, J.: Antituberculous drugs and sideroblastic anaemia. British Journal of Haematology 11: 92 (1965).

Verwilghen, R.L.; Lewis, S.M.; Dacie, J.V.; Crookston, J.H. and Crookston, M.: HEMPAS: Congenital dyserythropoietic anaemia (Type II). Quarterly Journal of Medicine 42: 237 (1973).

Viewig, W.V.R.; Piscatelli, P.L.; Houser, J.J. and Proulx, R.A.: Complications of intravenous administration of heparin in elderly women. Journal of the American Medical Association 213: 1303 (1970).

Von Voss, H.; Petrich, C.; Karch, D.; Schulz, H-V. and Gobel, V.: Sodium valproate and platelet function. British Medical Journal 2: 179 (1976).

Walker, M.G.: The natural history of venous thromboembolism. British Journal of Surgery 124: 169 (1972).

Walsh, P.N.; Rizza, C.R. and Matthews, J.M.: Epsilonaminocaproic acid therapy for dental extraction in haemophilia and Christmas disease. British Journal of Haematology 20: 463 (1971).

Waxman, S.; Corcino, J.J. and Herbert, V.: Drugs, toxins and dietary amino acids affecting vitamin B_{12} or folic acid absorption or utilisation. American Journal of Medicine 48: 599 (1970).

Weiss, H.J.: Platelet physiology and abnormalities of platelet function, Part 1. New England Journal of Medicine 293: 531 (1975a).

Weiss, H.J.: Platelet physiology and abnormalities of platelet function. Part II. New England Journal of Medicine 293: 580 (1975b).

Weiss, H.J.: Antiplatelet therapy. New England Journal of Medicine 298: 1344, 1403 (1978).

Whisnant, J.P.; Matsumoto, N. and Elveback, L.R.: The effect of anticoagulant therapy on the prognosis of patients with transient cerebral ischemic attacks in a community - Rochester 1955-1969. Mayo Clin. Proc. 48: 844 (1973).

White, A.M. and Heptinstall, S.: Contribution of platelets to thrombus formation. Brit. med. Bull. 34: 123 (1978).

Widmer, M. Th.; Madar, G. and Widmer, L.K.: Incidence of post-thrombotic syndrome. Follow-up on 99 patients with a deep venous thrombosis and thrombolytic or heparin treatment. Aktuelle Probleme in der Angiologie 37: 191 (1978).

Williams, D.M.; Lynch, R.E. and Cartwright, G.E.: Drug-induced aplastic anaemia. Seminars in Haematology 10: 195 (1973).

Williams, J.R.B.; Griffin, J.P. and Parkins, A.: Effect of concomitantly administered drugs on the control of long-term anticoagulant therapy. Quarterly Journal of Medicine 45: 63 (1976).

Wiman, B. and Collen, D.: On the kinetics of the reaction between human antiplasmin and plasmin. European Journal of Biochemistry 84: 573 (1978).

Winfield, D.A.; Benton, P.; Espir, M.L.E. and Arthur, L.J.H.: Sodium valproate and thrombocytopenia. British Medical Journal 2: 981 (1976).

Woodruff, R.K.; Bell, W.R. and Castaldi, P.A.: Carbenicillin danger. Medical Journal of Australia 1: 278 (1976).

Worlledge, S.M.: Immune drug-induced hemolytic anemias. Seminars in Hematology 6: 181 (1969).

Worlledge, S.M.: Immune drug-induced hemolytic anemias. Seminars in Hematology 10: 327 (1973).

Worlledge, S.M.; Carstairs, K.C. and Dacie, J.V.: Autoimmune haemolytic anaemia associated with α-methyldopa therapy. Lancet 2: 135 (1966).

Yacobi, A.; Udall, J. and Levy, G.: Serum protein binding as a determinant of warfarin body clearance and anticoagulant effect. Clin. Pharm. Ther. 19: 552 (1976a).

Yacobi, A.; Udall, J.A. and Levy, G.: Intrasubject variation of warfarin binding to protein in serum of patients with cardiovascular disease. Clin. Pharm. 20: 300 (1976b).

Yunis, A.A.: Chloramphenicol-induced bone marrow suppression. Seminars in Hematology 10: 225 (1973).

Yunis, A.A. and Bloomberg, G.R.: Chloramphenicol toxicity: Clinical features and pathogenesis. Progress in Haematology 4: 138 (1964).

Zieve, P.D. and Solomon, H.M.: Variation in the response of human beings to vitamin K_1. Journal of Laboratory and Clinical Medicine 73: 103 (1969).

Chapter XXIV
Malignant Diseases

S.K. Carter and G. Mathé

Synopsis of Important Principles

1) The goal of cancer treatment is to obtain a cure by eradicating 'the last neoplastic cell'. Surgery, radiotherapy and chemotherapy all have their specific role in the general strategy employed against malignant diseases.

2) Cytotoxic drugs act on cellular proliferation by interfering with the protein and nucleoprotein synthesis of mitosis. The various classes of antineoplastic drugs are prescribed in doses and schedules to obtain maximum tumour cell kill with minimum damage to the normal tissues of the host, especially the haematopoietic and immunocompetent cells.

3) The final outcome of the administration of an antineoplastic drug is determined by the dynamic interplay of drug, tumour cell and patient characteristics.

4) Treatment should be started early when it is postulated that the tumour cell burden is smallest with a high growth fraction and a rapid doubling time.

5) For the most responsive tumours, combination chemotherapy is more effective than single agent therapy. Effective combinations include drugs which are active when used alone against the specific tumour type.

6) High dose intermittent schedules are more effective and less immunosuppressive than low dose daily administration. Succeeding doses of therapy are given as soon as the host recovers from the previous course.

7) It is in the treatment of acute leukaemias, especially acute lymphoid leukaemia in childhood and Hodgkin's disease, that the application of these treatment principles has achieved its most impressive results.

8) It is anticipated that chemotherapy will be more useful when used as an adjuvant to surgery and radiotherapy of localised tumours that are at high risk of relapse or dissemination.

9) Cytotoxic agents are not specific for tumour cells and affect all cells of the host, especially of rapidly proliferating tissues such as bone marrow, lymphoid system, oral and gastrointestinal epithelium, skin and hair roots, germinal epithelium of the gonads and embryonic structures. Paradoxically, antineoplastic drugs can be carcinogenic.

Cancer is a group of diseases of unknown (and probably multiple) causes which occurs in all human and animal populations and arises in all tissues composed of potentially dividing cells. There is a wide range of definitions of cancer which reflect current lack of understanding of the basic process which underlies the problem.

More than 270 types of human neoplasms have been recognised and defined histologically and the degrees of variation within a single tumour type can be infinite. Therefore, the often made statement that cancer is not one but a hundred different diseases is, in truth, an understatement. The clinical spectrum of these various disease entities can also be infinite, since the neoplastic process has to be viewed within the framework of a host with various potentials for intrinsic host response and co-morbid processes which can affect the tumour's development and response to therapy.

1. Principles of Cancer Therapy

1.1 Basic Concepts in Cancer Therapy

The fundamental concept in the treatment of cancer is to eradicate or remove the last neoplastic cell. The basic principle in therapy is to achieve this eradication or removal (cure) with minimal structural impairment. Since this almost always involves intensive and potentially dangerous approaches, therapy should only be undertaken by trained oncologists within a proper structure of adequate laboratory, nursing, social and psychological support.

The decision concerning the individual treatment for a given patient should be made on a multidisciplinary basis — by a team involving surgical oncologist, radiation oncologist, medical oncologist, and pathologist; all working within an understanding of the social and psychological framework of treatment.

Simply stated, the long term goal of cancer treatment is to achieve normal life expectancy in cancer patients. On a shorter time scale, the goal is to increase the number of patients responding to treatment, to prolong the period of disease free remission and to improve the quality of life. To achieve either goal, new experimental treatment strategies should be designed, based not only upon research and development efforts to improve the curative potential of individual treatment methods, but also upon detailed understanding of relevant factors in cancer biology, in host biology, and in individual tumour behaviour. Moreover, clinical results must be continually collected and analysed to delineate whether or not each new strategy is superior to the best conventional therapy.

The basic assumption in cancer treatment is that all malignant cells should be destroyed, removed, or neutralised to achieve cure. In practice, five forms of treatment may do this — surgery, radiotherapy, chemotherapy, endocrinotherapy and possibly immunotherapy. Some methods are more successful than others, but all are incompletely understood and all need more study.

For some tumours, a specific therapeutic procedure may represent the only choice of treatment while for others a number of satisfactory alternatives may exist. In the latter case, optimum therapy is determined not only by the nature and extent of the disease but also by the experience of the attending clinician and the facilities available for treatment. Surgery is the most frequently used method of treatment. The proper application of surgical techniques is responsible, for example, for achieving 5 year survival (although not necessarily achieving cure) in about 50 % of women with breast cancer in approximately 30 to 40 % of patients with cancer of the colon.

Radiotherapy is also important as a means of controlling a wide variety of local or regional solid tumours. It is used either in combination with surgery or alone. Radiotherapy is successful in curing local disease in at least 90 % of men with seminoma of the testis, in at least 80 % of children with retinoblastoma, and in about 50 % of patients with local squamous cell carcinoma of the nasopharynx.

Chemotherapy is the utilisation of drugs to treat cancer. It is sometimes limited in its definition to chemicals which are cytotoxic in action, but can include hormonal additive therapy within its scope, as well as any other drugs which can affect cancer in any way that is therapeutically beneficial.

Endocrine treatment involves the manipulation of hormonal function in the patient and is designed to influence the behaviour of tumours growing in hormone dependent organs such as the breast and prostate. Particularly important is the concept that endocrinotherapy is relatively non-toxic to normal tissues. For the purpose of this chapter, endocrinotherapy will be considered as part of cancer chemotherapy.

In theory, immunotherapy could be useful in treating both localised and, in combination with other therapy, disseminated disease, but in terms of practical results it is still in its early phase of development (see Gutterman, 1978; Morton and Goodnight, 1978).

1.2 Factors Limiting Curative Potential of Applied Therapy

Cancer can be classified into two major categories: solid tumours and haematological malignancies. Solid tumours are initially confined to specific tissue or organ sites. In time, however, cancer cells break off from the original tumour mass, enter the blood or lymph system, reach distant parts of the body, and start secondary growth there (metastasis). When this occurs, the disease is in the disseminated stage. Conversely, haematological malignancies involve the blood and lymph systems, and for this reason, they are frequently disseminated at the time of initial presentation.

For solid tumours, surgery and/or radiotherapy are the traditional initial treatments. Neither method is curative once the disease has metastasised beyond the local region (primary site and nearby lymph nodes) or has involved a vital organ extensively. Chemotherapy has been relegated almost exclusively to secondary or tertiary treatment of solid tumours; i.e. it is used when surgery and radiotherapy fail.

Since the highest curative potential for solid tumours exists when the tumour is both small and localised, early detection offers the best opportunity for control. However, at the time of initial diagnosis, a number of patients already have extensive disease which local treatment methods can not cure. Alternatively, by the time of primary therapy, some other patients have established microscopic foci of metastatic disease which available diagnostic techniques cannot detect and local treatment methods cannot remove or destroy. In this case, it erroneously appears that the tumour is still localised. Relapses after surgery and/or radiotherapy are largely attributable to metastatic spread prior to treatment. This is not to deny, however, that in certain situations development of additional primary tumour growths at other anatomical sites could be responsible for the reappearance of the disease.

Extensive local involvement of a vital organ and metastatic spread are factors limiting the curative potential of surgery and radiotherapy, so that eradication of the last neoplastic cell requires systemic treatment. However, systemic methods used for secondary or tertiary treatment, are rarely successful in curing any tumours, including haematological malignancies. It is understandable, therefore, that chemotherapy as now used in patients with solid tumours is often not curative, despite the fact that some tumour regression, some subjective benefit and some increases in survival are being achieved.

Each type of cancer has a unique therapeutic flow which is influenced by the location of the primary tumour, its patterns of spread, responsiveness to therapy and relapse patterns. The flow begins with the diagnosis and the initial staging of the patient. In many cases, the initial staging is clinical and has as its major aim, determination of whether the patient is amenable to therapy directed at cure. In tumours involving organs such as breast, colorectum and lung, the clinical staging defines whether the patient is operable or not. It is well known that clinical staging has its imperfections as many patients deemed 'operable' are found to be beyond the hope of a curative resection after laparotomy or thoracotomy is performed. In some tumours, pathological staging has been attempted through staging laparotomies first popularised in Hodgkin's disease. In tumours such as prostate cancer and cervix cancer this has been tried as an investigational tool but has not been proven to have a positive cost vs benefit ratio. The techniques of peritoneoscopy, fiberoptic bronchoscopy and colonoscopy are helping to delineate the extent of disease to a better degree prior to the initiation of major therapeutic intervention.

In many tumours, pathological staging is used after surgical resection. This staging has as its major aim prognostic grouping and a means of comparing research data and results between major investigational groups and countries. Pathological staging plays a crucial role in the design of combined therapy strategies. Pathological staging allows investigators to focus on a subset of patients who are at a high risk for recurrence based on past experience. This past experience not only tells who is likely to relapse but also determines the most likely relapse patterns so that appropriate strategies can be developed. If the major recurrence pattern is local and/or regional, as in head and neck cancers, then radiation as an adjuvant to surgery can be contemplated. If the major relapse pattern is metastatic, as in breast and colon, then chemotherapy becomes the most appropriate form of adjuvant therapy.

The form of therapy for each type of cancer is therefore based on a study of pathological staging and its prognostic implications, along with the relapse pattern. This identifies a subset of patients who are prime candidates for adjuvant therapy as well as what type of adjuvant therapy might be indicated. In breast cancer it has been shown that involvement of the axillary lymph nodes is a potent prognostic variable for relapse after curative resection (Carter, 1976a). In addition, the major failure pattern is a metastatic one. Therefore, current research is directed at studying chemotherapy as a surgical adjuvant therapy in women with positive axillary lymph nodes.

In colon cancer, patients whose tumour penetrates through the entire bowel wall and involves the regional nodes, have been shown to have a high relapse rate in metastatic sites. Chemotherapy adjuvant studies in Dukes C lesions are now being widely studied. In rectal cancer, the prognostic indicators are the same but the relapse patterns differ. In these low lying bowel lesions failures often occur locally and regionally and so radiation therapy becomes an important variable in study design.

2. Clinical Pharmacological Considerations

2.1 Basic Concepts of Cancer Chemotherapy

All living organisms have an inherent capacity to multiply and they cease multiplication for a variety of reasons. In complex cellular organisms, such as man, a cellular 'brake' is required to prevent overgrowth for the benefit of the community of cells. This appears to be controlled by an unknown feedback mechanism, probably resulting from contact phenomena when cells are crowded together. In cancerous growth, cells no longer cease multiplying when they reach a critical mass and the uncontrolled growth leads to the death of the host. In the early phases of growth, tumour cells grow exponentially but, as tumour mass increases, the time it takes a tumour to double its volume increases with it (fig. 1). Three mechanisms have been postulated to explain broadly the prolonged volume-doubling time: (1) an increase in cell cycle time (the time from one mitosis to the next); (2) a decrease in the growth fraction (cells participating in cell division in the tumour); and (3) an increase in cell loss from tumour cells with consequent loss of nutrients and vascular supply.

2.1.1 Rationale for Use of Drugs

The rationale for the use of drugs in the treatment of cancer is to achieve the selective killing of tumour cells. Underlying this rationale are the principles of the 'cell kill hypothesis' as elucidated by Skipper and his colleagues (Skipper et al., 1964). The principles are based on the following considerations:

1) The survival of an animal (with L1210 leukaemia) is inversely related to either the number of leukaemic cells inoculated or the number remaining after treatment

2) A single leukaemic cell is capable of multiplying and eventually killing the host

3) For most drugs, a clear relationship exists between the dose of drug and its ability to eradicate tumour cells

4) A given dose of a drug kills a constant fraction of cells, not a constant number, regardless of the cell numbers present at the time of therapy. This means that cell destruction by drugs follows first order kinetics. For example, treatment which reduces a population from 1,000,000 to 10 cells should reduce a population of 100,000 to 1 cell. The clinical implication of first order cell destruction is that to eradicate a tumour population effectively, it is necessary either to increase the dose of drug or drugs to the maximum limits tolerated by the host or to start treatment when the number of

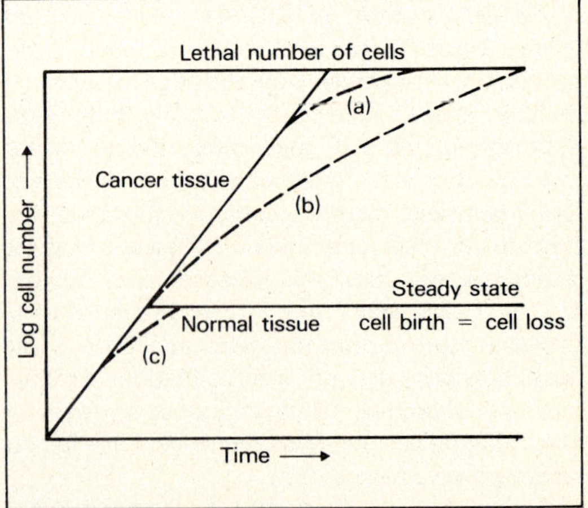

Fig. 1. Comparison of normal and cancerous growth (a) expanding; (b) renewing; (c) static.

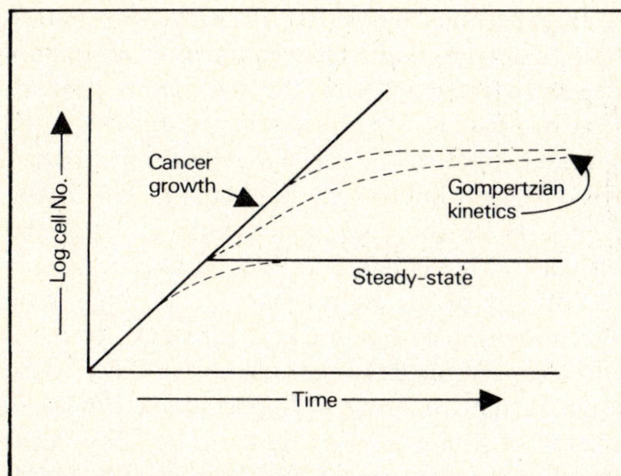

Fig. 2a. Gompertzian curve.

cells is small enough to allow the destruction of tumour at doses of drug that are reasonably tolerated. The logical conclusion derived from the above hypothesis is that the maximum opportunity for achieving cure exists during the early disease stage. It is more difficult to eradicate disseminated disease than localised cancer, and much easier to control small tumours than larger ones.

2.1.2 Growth of Tumour Mass and Drug Action

The experimental model view of the growth curve of a cancer is that it follows a Gompertzian function. This means that growth at every instant is exponential but with a growth constant which is simultaneously exponentially slowing (fig. 2a). Therefore, as a tumour mass increases in size, its mass doubling time becomes progressively longer. It needs to be recognised that the Gompertzian aspect of tumour growth is only recognisable when a tumour is measured in its clinically palpable range. It is assumed that in the clinically indetectable period the growth is exponential. While this may be true in rodent models there are no data that prove that this obtains in the human situation.

If the Gompertzian model would be clinically relevant it would have significant clinical implications and these have guided a good deal of clinical chemotherapy research over the last decade. As a tumour mass responds to treatment, i.e. gets smaller, it would be assumed that the doubling time would increase as a consequence of a greater number of cells moving into cycle. This larger percentage of metabolically active cells would therefore increase the sensitivity of the neoplastic population to cell cycle specific agents. This has led to the sequential use of cell cycle nonspecific agents (e.g. cyclophosphamide) to reduce the size of the mass, to be followed by cell cycle specific agents such as cytarabine or methotrexate. While these sequential combinations have been theoretically attractive, none have proven clearly superior in clinical trials to other approaches.

Another implication of the Gompertzian growth concept is that metastasis would be expected to be more sensitive to chemotherapy in general, and to cell cycle specific agents in particular, than the primary tumour from which they arise. The smaller the size of the metastatic focus the greater the differential sensitivity will be. Therefore, the insensitivity of a primary tumour to a given drug regimen might not necessarily predict the response of its metastasis to the same regimen. This theoretical construct has made 'adjuvant' chemotherapy highly attractive. It has been assumed that regimens that could shrink clinically evident metastatic growth would be that much more effective against minimal residual disease left after surgical removal of the primary tumour. However, this assumption may not hold in clinical practice. There is evidence in stage III breast cancer (DeLena et al., 1978) that chemotherapy can shrink the primary tumour to a higher degree than it can metastatic masses. Yet the same kind of chemotherapy is not effective against microscopic residual disease in postmenopausal women. Chemotherapy can shrink a primary osteogenic sarcoma in nearly every case tried and yet in the adjuvant situation many relapses are still observed (Rosen et al., 1976). In head and neck cancer, preoperative drug treatment can shrink the primary (Carter, 1977a), but data on adjuvant treatment postsurgery are still not available. There is therefore some evidence from clinical experience to indicate that either the classic Gompertzian construct is not clinically relevant or that other factors, besides kinetics, are causing chemotherapy to be less effective in the adjuvant situation than would be expected.

2.1.3 Tumour Burden and Drug Action

A sine qua non of the cell kill hypothesis and the Gompertzian growth concept is an inverse relationship between sensitivity to chemotherapy and the tumour burden. This is based not only on a purely kinetic construct but on the basis of biochemical resistance as well. This means that the larger the total malignant mass the higher will be the proportion of the permanently drug resistant variants to any given compound or regimen. This has been estimated to be one in 10^6 to 10^7 cells (Hutchinson and Schmid, 1973). It takes only 5 to 6 doses of cyclophosphamide to induce significant resistance in L1210 leukaemia (Skipper et al., 1964) and as few as 2 to 3 doses of semustine (methyl CCNU) doing the same in rodent solid tumours (Skipper, 1971).

2.1.4 Pharmacological Factors and Number of Viable Cells

Pharmacological factors can also explain why clinical results can differ from those predicted from experimental models. The higher the cell number, the greater the chances will exist for the existence of sites, either within the tumour, or in selected organs, where tumour cells will be protected from exposure to adequate concentrations of cytotoxic drugs.

One assumption built into clinical studies is that the period to tumour recurrence is directly related to the number of viable cells which have escaped surgery of the primary. It assumes that these cells are acting consistently with the early part of the Gompertzian growth curve. In experimental tumours, it is possible to obtain estimates of the metastatic tumour exterior present at diagnosis. From data of this kind, Skipper (1978) has attempted to make such an analysis for human breast carcinoma and osteogenic sarcoma. The basis of the analysis is the clinically observed recurrence rates after surgery plus available data indicating that the median doubling time of some metastatic lesions in breast cancer is 30 to 40 days. The analysis assumes that the limit to clinical detection of a recurrence is 10^9 cells, which corresponds to a spherical mass of 10mm in diameter. It also assumes exponential growth until this size, which is probably the most unproven assumption in the analysis. The analysis indicates that in women with four or more positives nodes, about 85% could be expected to have 10^8 residual cells or less but only about half could be expected to have 10^5 residual cells or less. In node negative women, on the other hand, 86 to 90% could be expected to have 10^4 residual cells or less. This calculation is very dependent on the assumed doubling time of cells. In osteogenic sarcoma, when the estimate is 10 to 20 days, the estimated residual tumour cell burden after amputation would be 10^5 or less in 69% if the doubling time is 10 days. If it is 20 days, however, the estimate falls to 38%.

In experimental systems a steep dose-response relationship has been observed for most anticancer drugs. In these systems the maximum dose of drug compatible with host survival appears to be optimum in terms of achieving maximum reduction of the tumour cell population. For many agents, twice the dose which kills 10% of the animals (LD_{10}) is lethal to 90% (LD_{90}).

For almost all antitumour agents, high dose intermittent drug treatment is substantially more effective antitumor treatment than low dose equitoxic daily treatment (Skipper et al., 1964). As a result of studies such as these in the USA, most cytotoxic drug treatment uses high dose intermittent scheduling. It is worth noting that the superiority of such high dose intermittent therapy is not clearly established by review of existing clinical data.

Controlled comparisons of continuous daily dosing of a drug with a high dose intermittent schedule of the same drug in the same tumour are hard to find. Some drugs do not appear to show a classic dose-response effect. For example, low doses of bleomycin in lymphomas appear equivalent to high doses in terms of response rate (Friedman, 1978). The same is true for L-asparaginase (colaspase) in childhood leukaemia (Rausen and Glidewell, 1970). The Eastern Cooperative Oncology Group showed that 2.0mg/kg/day for 5 days of dacarbazine was equivalent to 4.5mg/kg/day for 5 days in a melanoma trial that has generally been ignored (Nathanson et al., 1971). In patients with advanced ovarian cancer, the response rates to low dose oral melphalan were equivalent to those of very large parenteral doses of cyclophosphamide, but the toxicity of cyclophosphamide was greater (Young et al., 1974a). Low doses of cyclophosphamide, methotrexate and 5-fluorouracil (CMF) for breast cancer are equally effective and less toxic, when compared with the usual high dose approach (Creech et al., 1975).

A recent hypothesis has been proposed which assumes that human tumours grow in a Gompertzian fashion; that is, there is an initial exponential growth phase followed by a slowing in the rate of growth (Norton and Simon; cited in DeVita, 1977). This hypothesis runs counter to some older assumptions. In Gompertzian growth, tumour volume increases until it reaches a plateau. The growth rate is expressed as the increase in tumour volume per unit of time. The instantaneous growth rate decreases as the volume of tumour increases. In the mathematical model proposed, cell production is slowest at either the beginning or the end of the Gompertz curve, even though the fraction of cells proliferating at any instant will be large at the beginning of the curve. It is postulated that the maximum growth rate (and therefore the maximum sensitivity to drugs) will occur when the tumour mass is approximately 37% of its eventual maximum size (fig. 2b). Therefore, the most intensive drug treatment would be indicated when the tumour cell burden is very low. As DeVita (1977) has pointed out, the Gompertzian model predicts that a therapeutic regimen which causes regression of an advanced tumour will only be as effective when the foci of tumour are microscopic, if doses are not reduced. In fact, the highest doses of drug may be required to eradicate the residual cells in microscopic foci. The very highest doses might be needed toward the end of a regimen. The concept is equivalent to a chemotherapeutic 'booster'. Contrary to the Gompertzian model, in most studies of adjuvant therapy, the doses of drugs in therapeutic regimens which are effective in advanced disease have been decreased for patients with less advanced disease in order to make the concept of therapy more palliative to both patient and primary care clinician.

Since the kinetics of microscopic residual tumour cells in man cannot be measured and the concentration versus time of exposure of these

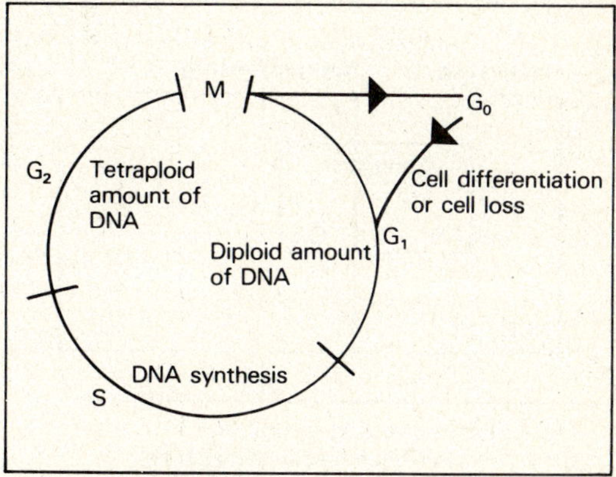

Fig. 3. The cell cycle.
G_1 First gap period. Variable in duration, may be extremely long: prolonged G_1 or G_0 = temporarily nondividing cells. These cells can however return to a proliferative state.
G_0 Second gap period; relatively short and fairly fixed in duration.
G_2 Premitotic phase.
M Mitosis or cell division.
S Period of DNA synthesis and chromosome replication.

cells to drugs cannot be quantified, the choice and dose schedule of drugs used in adjuvant treatment must be empirical. The choice of drugs, until recently, has been based on the activity the drugs have had against advanced disease. What is currently unknown is whether the level of activity of drugs for advanced disease is correlated with a positive therapeutic effect when the drugs are used as adjuvant therapy (Carter, 1977b).

2.2 Cell Kinetics

It is now well established that all renewing cells that are synthesising DNA go through a series of phases known as the cell cycle, which is shown in figure 3. At the completion of mitosis (M) the cell spends a variable period of time in a resting phase (G_1); the synthesis of DNA for cell replication is apparently absent while the synthesis of RNA and protein continues normally. In late G_1 phase (the G-S conversion) an unknown signal initiates a burst of RNA synthesis and shortly thereafter the period of DNA synthesis (S phase) begins and the cell is committed to undergo division or remain polyploid. Next, the cell ceases DNA synthesis during the G_2 phase before entry into mitosis, although RNA and protein synthesis continue. In mitosis the rates of protein and RNA synthesis

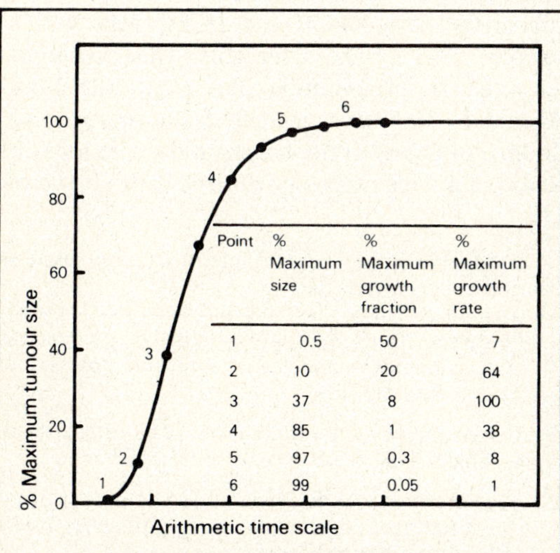

Point	% Maximum size	% Maximum growth fraction	% Maximum growth rate
1	0.5	50	7
2	10	20	64
3	37	8	100
4	85	1	38
5	97	0.3	8
6	99	0.05	1

Fig. 2b. Relationship, for Gompertzian growth, between tumour size, instantaneous growth fraction and growth rate presented in tabular form.

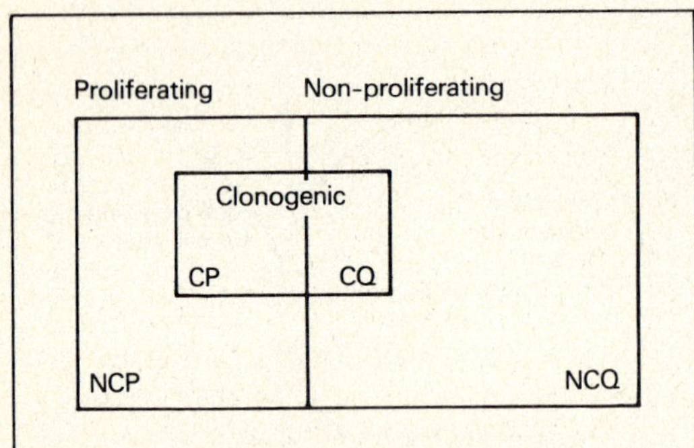

Fig. 4. Types of cell in a tumour.
CP　　= clonogenic proliferating cells.
CQ　　= clonogenic non-proliferating cells (G_0 cells).
NCP　= non-clonogenic proliferating cells (doomed cells).
NCQ　= non-clonogenic non-proliferating cells (end cells).

diminish abruptly while the genetic material is segregated into daughter cells. An additional resting phase (G_0) of the cell cycle has also been described. G_0 cells are cells which although not in cycle are capable of proliferation; they constitute the cells which are for the most part refractory to cancer chemotherapeutic agents.

Tumour growth is dependent on the proliferating pool (growth fraction) of cells in the tumour. This concept of the proliferation pool or growth fraction was first developed by radiobiologists and was later intensively followed up by experimental chemotherapists. The experimental data can briefly be summarised as follows (Mendelsohn, 1962; Schabel, 1975). The rate of growth and the doubling time of small tumours depends largely, but not entirely, on the percentage of cells in the mitotic cycle. Particularly in larger tumours, the rate of growth is also contingent on the number of tumour cells spontaneously dying or perhaps becoming differentiated.

The cell types in any individual tumour can be represented as though in 4 compartments (fig. 4). Tumour cell populations probably resemble a renewing population of normal cells. Some cell differentiation may be associated with inability to divide beyond 1 or 2 cell divisions, and tumour cells would be continually renewed from the tumour stem cell or clonogenic pool. Such a model would explain current cytokinetic information and would suggest that cancer cells are not totally unresponsive to growth control mechanisms. Cell population kinetics provides one approach to understanding drug susceptibility in some tumours. Tumour cells may be proliferating more or less rapidly than normal cell populations and they may have more cells in the drug sensitive phases of the cell cycle. This does not, however, explain all successes and failures of drug therapy.

Differences in cell kinetics between normal and malignant cells have been demonstrated in a spleen colony assay technique applied to the AKR lymphoma (LCFU) and normal haematopoietic stem cells (NFCU) [Bruce et al., 1966]. Based on studies in these systems, cytotoxic drugs have been classified into three classes. Class I, or non-phase specific agents are equally toxic for both proliferating and resting (G_0) cells and equally affect LCFU and NFCU cells. Dose survival curves for both cell lines are exponential. Examples of class I drugs are nitrogen mustard or gamma irradiation. Class II drugs are phase specific agents and kill cells only during a specific part of the cell cycle. They do not affect G_0 cells if the exposure time is short. These drugs generate dose-survival curves which reach plateau levels. The difference in sensitivity between LCFU and NFCU cells can be attributed to differences in the proliferative states of these cell populations. Class II drugs include vinblastine, methotrexate and azaserine.

Class III drugs are called cycle specific agents. They damage both proliferating and resting cells but cycling cells are more sensitive than G_0 cells. Cycling cells are killed throughout the cell cycle. These drugs produce exponential dose-survival curves for both NFCU and LCFU cells with a steeper curve for the latter cells. This can be interpreted as proliferation dependent selectivity. Agents in this class include 5-fluorouracil, actinomycin D and cyclophosphamide. The locus of action of a wide range of cytotoxic drugs based on

Table I. Principles of drug administration based on murine experimental data

1. Phase specific agents (fig. 5) should be administered in fractionated schedules or infusions unless they have a long half-life.

2. Cycle specific agents (fig. 5) should be administered as single, large doses in intermittent schedules.

3. Treatment should be repeated for a number of cycles if tumour cell populations of significance ($> 10^4$ cells) are to be eradicated.

4. Courses should be spaced widely enough to allow recovery of normal tissues.

action on the cell cycle is summarised in figure 5 (Hill and Baserga, 1975).

The administration scheduling of anticancer drugs can be rationalised using the 3 class concept (table I). Both phase and cycle specific drugs are usually given in short intensive courses using the maximum tolerated dose with retreatment initiated as soon as toxicity recovery permits. Class II agents should be given repeatedly, or as an infusion, in order to expose all tumour cells as they arrive in the sensitive phase of the cycle. This will also expose normal cells to an increasing degree. The schedule dependency of cytarabine in L1210 leukaemia and the need for prolonged exposure in man with these agents is the best example of this rationale.

The effective administration schedule of a drug will obviously depend on a lot more than tumour cell kinetic factors (fig. 6). There must be a complex interaction of the kinetics of tumour and normal tissues, pharmacological and host factors.

2.3 Pharmacokinetics of Antineoplastic Drugs

Another reason for success or failure of chemotherapy may be related to the disposition of drugs in a patient. A drug cannot influence the tumour in a favourable way unless it reaches the tumour site and remains there in tumouricidal concentration for a sufficiently long period to kill the tumour cells. (e.g. see Sadee and Wong, 1977; Zaharko and Dedrick, 1973).

2.3.1 General Kinetic Considerations and Characteristics of the Drug

In general, the purpose of clinical pharmacological studies is to devise dose regimens which

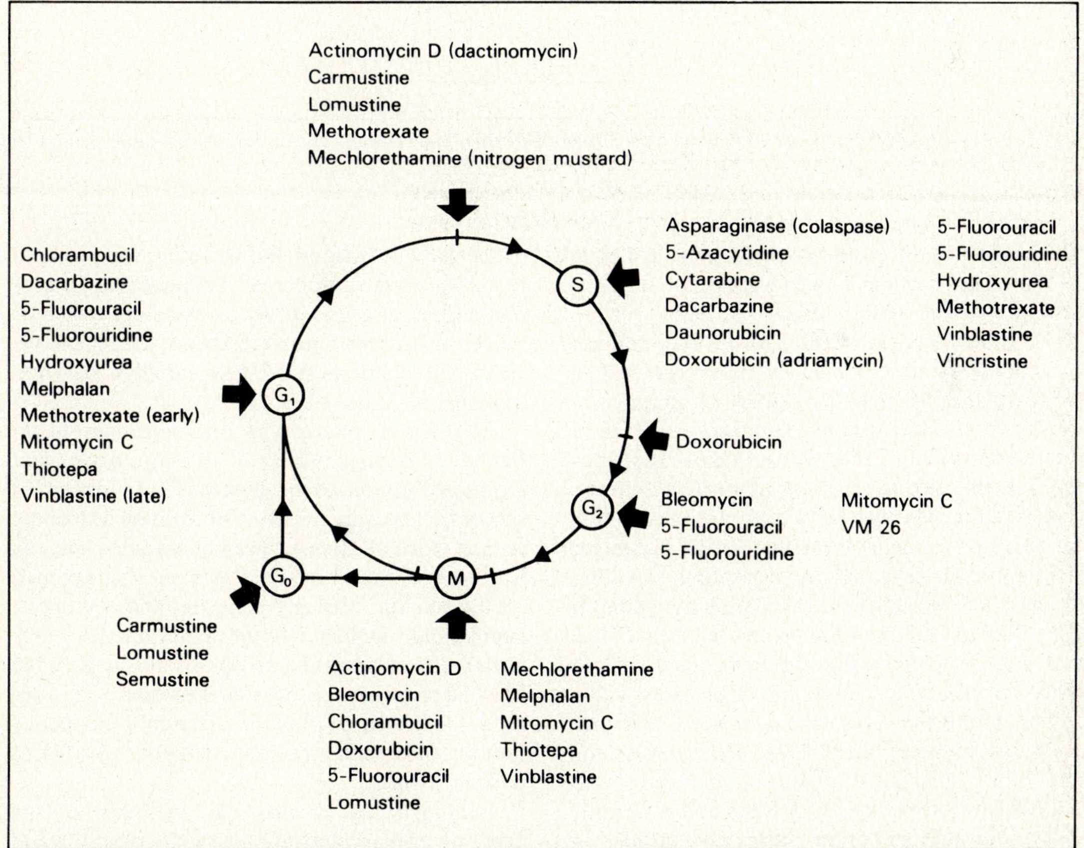

Fig. 5. The phases of the cell cycle where antitumour agents exert their lethal effects (after Hill and Baserga: Cancer Treatment Reviews 2: 159, 1975; by permission of author and editor).

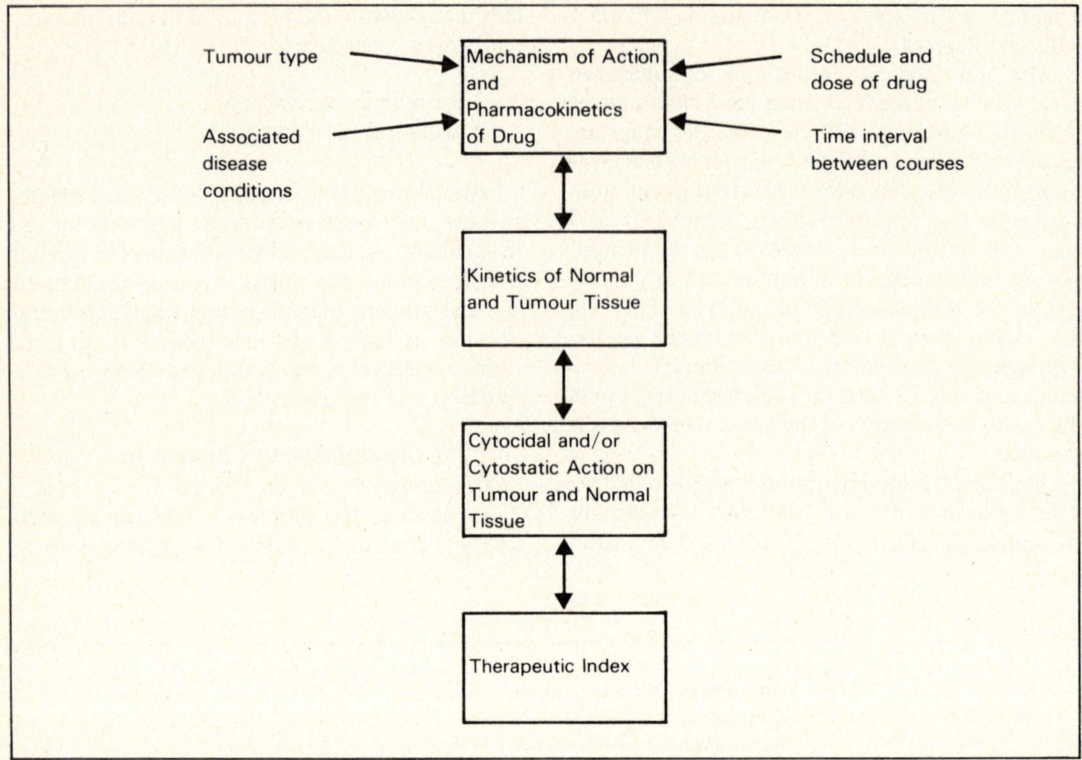

Fig. 6. Factors contributing to effective administration schedule and effect of antitumour drugs (after Capizzi et al., 1977).

will achieve an effective concentration (C) of drug to the target site for a long enough time (T) to bring about the desired effect (see Bender et al., 1978; Chabner et al., 1975). This is often referred to as the optimum C x T and in most cases can be approximated for man by studies of animals on the delivery of the drug to the organs or tissue of interest (Sartorelli, 1969). What makes cancer different is the need to relate optimum C x T to the phases of the cell cycle. Firstly, the optimum C x T for the tumour may be estimated for the real target — the tumour cells that are susceptible to killing by the drug. Secondly, the calculation of optimum C x T for the safety of the patient (e.g. the C x T that will be tolerable for the bone marrow and other normal target tissues in most cases) must compute with the percentage of normal cells that are at risk by being in DNA synthesis, mitosis, or any other susceptible phase of the cell cycle (Zaharko and Dedrick, 1973; Shen and Azarnoff, 1978). Another important factor to consider is that the cells are perturbed as a result of drug administration so that after the perturbation the size

of the growth fraction and therefore the potential for drug effect are altered. An understanding of the failures of active drugs to cause regression of cancer will depend to a significant extent on the successful delineation of this complex pharmacological basis of effect.

The above interactions are summarised in figure 7. The effectiveness of an antitumour agent is markedly affected by dose and administration schedule. The tumour cell, and to some degree the critical normal tissues, present variable targets. Knowledge of cell kinetics of normal tissue (which should remain relatively constant) and of tumour populations can help to determine the most effective means of obtaining an optimum C x T by the most appropriate doses and schedules. The optimum C x T should kill the maximum number of tumour cells with minimum lethality to cells of normal tissue.

Although the biochemical reactivity of the drug, its primary and secondary site of action and its effect on the cell cycle traverse relate most directly to kill of cells, the drug must first pass a

Table II. Some pharmacokinetic properties of cytotoxic drugs (after Adamson, 1971; Bender et al., 1978; Spreafico and Rossi, 1977)

Drug	Route	Predominant route of elimination[1,2]	Notes[3]
Actinomycin D (dactinomycin)	IV	Biliary (50 to 90%) and renal excretion (up to 20%) of unchanged drug	
L-Asparaginase (colaspase)	IV	Slow sequestration by reticuloendothelial system	Being a bacterial protein can induce antibody response which then influences plasma clearance (considerable interindividual variation in elimination kinetics)
Azacytidine	IV	Rapid hepatic metabolism (and possibly spontaneous decomposition) and execretion in urine	Plasma concentration of parent drug remains higher for longer periods with continuous infusion rather than IV bolus doses
Bleomycin	IV, IM	Renal excretion (60% unchanged in urine); remainder probably undergoes hepatic metabolism	Elimination markedly prolonged in renal impairment; extreme caution needed in patients currently receiving nephrotoxic drugs (e.g. high dose methotrexate, aminoglycosides)
Busulphan	Oral	Hepatic metabolism (metabolites inactive)	
Carmustine (BCNU)	IV	Hepatic metabolism (metabolites active)	Readily penetrates CSF
Chlorambucil	Oral	Hepatic metabolism	
Cyclophosphamide	IV, Oral	Hepatic metabolism (microsomal bioactivation) and renal excretion of active metabolites and up to 25% unchanged drug; faecal excretion (17 to 30% unchanged drug) after oral administration	Incompletely absorbed orally; active metabolites $\sim$ 50% protein bound, parent drug not bound. Bioactivation and elimination enhanced by enzyme inducing agents but influence on therapeutic activity not clear. Delayed elimination of active metabolites in impaired renal function; active metabolites cause chemical cystitis
Cytarabine	IV, SC	Hepatic metabolism (partly activation by kinases and partly inactivation by deamination), renal metabolism (deamination) and excretion of active drug	Continuous infusion or short dose interval needed due to rapid elimination ($t_{1/2\beta} \simeq 0.5\text{-}3h$). Penetrates into CSF to some extent
Dacarbazine	IV	Hepatic metabolism and renal excretion ($\sim$ 50% unchanged drug and $\sim$ 50% active metabolite in urine)	
Daunorubicin (daunomycin)	IV	Hepatic metabolism, biliary and renal excretion ($\sim$ 25% unchanged drug and active metabolite in urine)	High hepatic clearance; dose reduction needed in liver disease to avoid severe toxicity

Table II. (continued)

Drug	Route	Predominant route of elimination[1],[2]	Notes[3]
Dibromannitol	Oral	Hepatic metabolism and renal excretion ($\sim$ 25% unchanged drug in urine)	
Doxorubicin (adriamycin)	IV	Hepatic metabolism and biliary excretion	High hepatic clearance; dose reduction needed in liver disease to avoid severe toxicity
Fluorouracil	IV, Oral	Hepatic metabolism (initial pathway saturable) and renal excretion (20% unchanged in urine)	Oral bioavailability variable due to high hepatic first-pass metabolism Readily penetrates into CSF Intracellular bioactivation and catabolism
Hydroxyurea	Oral	Hepatic metabolism and renal metabolism to urea	
Lomustine (CCNU)	Oral	Hepatic metabolism (metabolites active)	Readily penetrates CSF
Melphalan	Oral, IV	Some hepatic metabolism (extent unknown) and renal excretion (?% unchanged)	Oral bioavailability variable
Mercaptopurine	Oral	Hepatic metabolism (xanthine oxidase); faecal excretion (50%) after oral administration and renal excretion (20% unchanged after IV dose)	Incomplete oral absorption Concurrent use of allopurinol (xanthine oxidase inhibitor) requires reduction of dose to about a third of usual
Methotrexate	IV, IM, Oral	Renal excretion (up to 90% unchanged); in general parallels creatinine clearance About 30% oral dose metabolised by gut bacteria during absorption (i.e. high first-pass absorption loss)	Saturable oral absorption (large doses $\sim$ 10mg/kg or 80mg/m^2 incompletely absorbed); up to 70% protein bound, primarily albumin Marked accumulation in impaired renal function Renal clearance decreased by weak organic acids such as salicylate
Mitomycin C	IV	Probably about 30% unchanged in urine; insufficient data on remaining portion	Oral bioavailability variable
Nitrogen mustard (mustine; mechlorethamine)	IV	Very rapid chemical transformation to inactivate drug in body fluids	Rapid degradation makes it possible to protect a given tissue from drug action by interrupting blood flow for a few minutes after administration
Procarbazine	Oral	Hepatic metabolism (metabolites inactive)	
Semustine (methyl-CCNU)	Oral	Hepatic metabolism (metabolites active)	Readily penetrates CSF
Thioguanine	Oral	Hepatic metabolism (metabolite inactive)	

Table II. (continued)

Drug	Route	Predominant route of elimination[1,2]	Notes[3]
Thio-TEPA	IV, IM	Hepatic metabolism (metabolites inactive)	Intramuscular absorption is variable
Vinblastine	IV	Hepatic metabolism, biliary and renal excretion ($\sim 20\%$ unchanged in urine)	Extensive binding to formed blood elements
Vincristine	IV	Hepatic metabolism and biliary excretion ($\sim 40\%$ unchanged in faeces)	Extensive binding to formed blood elements
VP-16213 (etoposide)	IV, Oral	Renal (30% unchanged in urine) and faecal ($< 16\%$) excretion; fate other portion not known	
VM-26 (teniposide)	IV	Hepatic metabolism; lesser faecal ($< 10\%$) and renal excretion ($\sim 9\%$ unchanged) than VP-16	$> 90\%$ protein bound

1   Amounts given as unchanged drug relate to % of administered dose.

2   Dosage of drugs excreted in significant quantities as active metabolite or unchanged drug (e.g. bleomycin, cyclophosphamide, cytarabine, dibromomannitol, dacarbazine, methotrexate, mitomycin C, carmustine, lomustine, semustine, VP-16213) may need to be reduced in the presence of impaired renal function. See also appendix E.

Dosage of drugs subject to significant hepatobiliary elimination (e.g. actinomycin D, cyclophosphamide, cytarabine, daunorubicin, doxorubicin, fluorouracil, vinblastine, vincristine) may need to be reduced in the presence of liver or hepatobiliary diseases.

3   For elimination half-lives and other pharmacokinetic data, see appendix A.

number of physiological 'barriers' before it reaches its intracellular site of action (Walker, 1973). Such kinetic processes govern not only the availability of the antineoplastic drug for tumour cell kill but also its toxicity.

The drug, administered by whatever route (orally, SC, IM, IV, intra-arterial), traverses various compartments of the body before reaching the site of action and the ease with which it does this depends on its particular physicochemical and pharmacokinetic properties (see chapter I; sect. 1). Taken orally, the drug must pass via the stomach, intestine and hepatic circulation and attain an adequate concentration in the systemic circulation. From here it traverses the capillary wall into the extracellular space, where the cell membrane forms a last barrier to the intracellular space and the site of action. Along this route considerable changes can occur that may alter the final critical intracellular concentration and time relationships. While in the circulation a particular drug can be bound to plasma proteins, metabolised within the liver or other tissues, or excreted via biliary or renal routes. The importance of such pharma-

cokinetic properties varies with the individual drug (table II) and can be influenced by a number of factors relating to the patient (see section 2.3.3). When it reaches the target cell, the final series of drug-cell interactions occur: drug transport, intracellular drug metabolism, binding and inactivation of target molecules, compensatory cell reactions and, most importantly the final critical drug induced biochemical derangement required to kill the cell.

For drugs which are highly ionised, molecular size influences transport across cell membranes; larger molecules requiring longer exposure times. Therapy with highly ionised drugs of large molecular size such as L-asparaginase may be hampered by poor distribution and tissue penetration. Many cytotoxic agents such as methotrexate are water soluble and highly ionised and fail to attain effective concentration in the CSF. Only the lipid soluble nitrosoureas cross the blood-brain barrier sufficiently to be useful with usual routes of administration in the treatment of brain tumours; although agents such as methotrexate can be given intrathecally. Solubility (influenced by pH) and tissue tolerance qualities determine feasible routes for administration. The local tissue reactions caused by extravasation of nitrogen mustard, actinomycin D, daunorubicin, doxorubicin (adriamycin), vincristine and vinblastine are well known. Less irritating drugs can be injected intramuscularly (e.g. bleomycin, methotrexate), subcutaneously (e.g. bleomycin, cytarabine) or intrathecally (e.g. cytarabine, methotrexate).

2.3.2 Characteristics of the Target Cell

Tumour cell membrane characteristics may influence the uptake of and sensitivity or resistance to cytotoxic drugs. For example, the intracellular penetration of methotrexate can be inhibited by other drugs such as certain antibiotics (cephalothin, gentamicin) or L-asparaginase, while vincristine increases penetration of methotrexate (Garattini et al., 1973; Bender et al., 1978).

Metabolic functions of the cell are equally important. Hormone sensitive breast tumours contain in the cytoplasm specific hormone binding receptor proteins (Jensen et al., 1967; McGuire et al., 1975). A certain degree of tumour selectivity has been attempted by developing drugs with selective bioactivation in target tissue; for example, diethylstilboestrol diphosphate is hydrolysed and activated in prostatic tumours rich in acid phosphatase (Flocks et al., 1955). Cyclophosphamide

was originally developed in the hope that a phosphamidase or phosphatase within tumour cells would hydrolyse the inactive parent drug to an active antitumour compound (Arnold and Bourseaux, 1958).

Certain metabolites required by tumour cells, and presumably accumulated in tumours, have been used as transport forms for cytotoxic drugs; for example phenylalanine-, uracil-, and mannitol mustard.

Certain anatomical locations may protect tumour cells against cytotoxic therapy. The most important of these 'sanctuaries' is the central nervous system. Tumour cells located close to a blood vessel are more likely to be exposed to high drug concentrations. Furthermore, higher growth fractions are found closer to a blood vessel than at some distance from it.

2.3.3 Characteristics of the Patient

A number of characteristics of the patient influence the response to cancer chemotherapy (Brule et al., 1973). Examples of age, sex and racial influence are occasionally cited in the literature: younger patients generally tolerate larger doses of chemotherapy than older ones. Female patients with melanoma treated with dacarbazine show higher response rates than males. Negro children with acute lymphoid

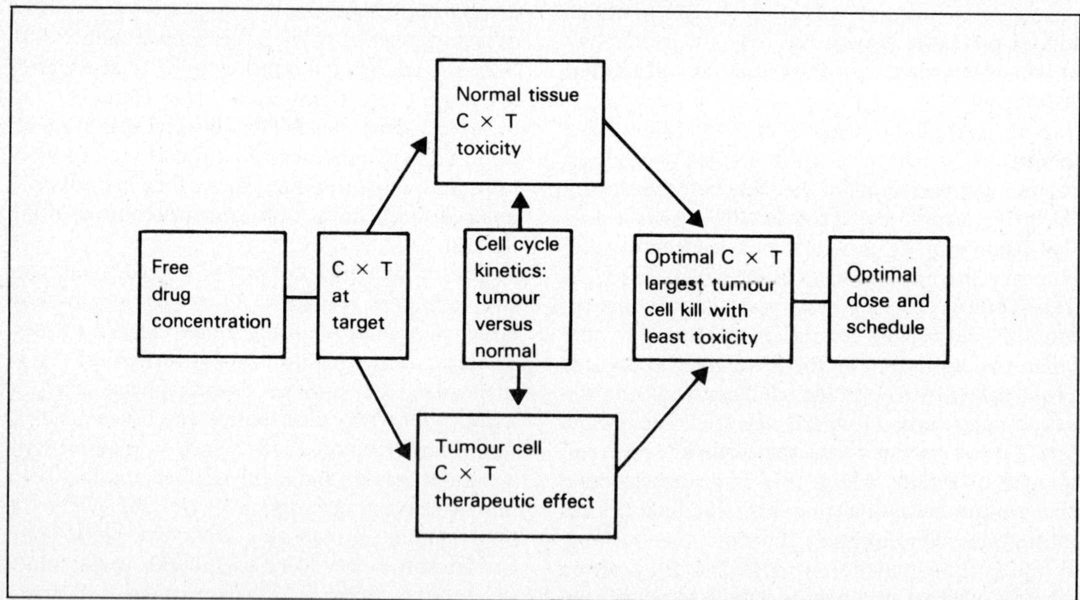

Fig. 7. Schematic relationship between cellular kinetics of normal and tumour tissue and effective plasma concentrations of antitumour agents.

leukaemia are far less responsive to identical chemotherapy than are their age matched and socioeconomically equivalent white counterparts. On the other hand, African children with Burkitt's lymphoma tolerate higher doses of cyclophosphamide than white children, so that their superior regression rates may be partially racial in origin.

A number of factors relating to the patient can modify the metabolic fate of individual cytotoxic drugs. Such changes not only affect the systemic availability of the drug but also necessitate dosage adjustment to avoid undue toxicity. Cyclophosphamide requires activation in the liver by microsomal enzyme hydrolysis of the parent compound, while many drugs including cyclophosphamide (further metabolites), procarbazine, nitrosoureas, nitrogen mustard, 5-fluorouracil and some steroids are metabolised by liver microsomal enzymes. Methotrexate and cyclophosphamide are excreted via the kidneys, doxorubicin and vinca alkaloids via the liver (table II). Thus, pre-existing diseases or metastatic involvement of liver or kidneys calls for an appropriate dosage adjustment to avoid undue toxicity. The renal clearance of methotrexate is correlated with endogenous creatinine clearance which may be used to provide a guideline to dosage adjustment according to renal function and age (Shen and Azarnoff, 1978). Plasma concentrations of cytotoxic drugs may also be altered by drugs prescribed to the patient for conditions other than the malignant process. Therapy with microsomal enzyme inducing agents such as barbiturates and rifampicin may alter the rate of metabolism of agents that require hepatic biotransformation for activation (e.g. cyclophosphamide) or which are eliminated by hepatobiliary excretion; e.g. doxorubicin (Bender et al., 1978; Garattini et al., 1973). Aspirin and other organic acids can possibly inhibit the urinary excretion of methotrexate and necessitate a reduction in its dosage (Liegler et al., 1969). Biotransformation of 6-mercaptopurine is inhibited by concomitant ingestion of allopurinol, necessitating a 3-fold reduction of usual dosage (Rundles et al., 1963).

Other aspects of treatment can affect the response to treatment. Prior cancer treatment with either radiation or cytotoxic drugs frequently reduces the patient's ability to tolerate subsequent doses of myelosuppressive agents, while the host's immune reactivity against tumour antigens may be interfered with by concomitant cytotoxic (immunosuppressive) therapy.

2.4 Biochemical Mechanism of Action of Antineoplastic Drugs

The cancer therapist has acquired in the past 30 years several classes of antineoplastic drug: cytotoxic agents such as antimetabolites, alkylating agents, antitumour antibiotics, mitotic inhibitors, and the miscellaneous group of synthetic agents, enzymes and hormones (Bender et al., 1978; Chabner et al. 1975). Cytotoxic drugs, like ionising rays, do not kill tumour cells directly, but prevent cell division and thereby cell proliferation. A number of fundamental molecular processes must continue to take place for cells to proliferate. The genetic material, DNA, must be replicated without error once every cycle. This requires an adequate supply of purine and pyrimidine nucleotides as building blocks, the enzyme DNA polymerase, and last an intact DNA template to direct the synthesis of new DNA. DNA also acts as a template for the synthesis of complementary RNA, a process catalysed by RNA polymerase. RNA is then translated into proteins through a complex polymerisation reaction that takes place on the ribosomes in the cell cytoplasm. The sequence of nucleotides of the messenger RNA determines the sequence whereby amino acids, attached to their specific transfer RNA, are positioned in the growing protein. After the cells have replicated their DNA, thereby having a double complement of genetic material, they undergo mitosis. The various chemotherapeutic agents interfere with one or the other of these essential cellular processes (fig. 8).

Antimetabolites interfere with the synthesis of building blocks for nucleic acids. Methotrexate, a folic acid antagonist; 6-mercaptopurine and 6-thioguanine, purine analogues; and 5-fluorouracil (5-FU) and cytarabine or cytosine arabinoside, pyrimidine analogues; are the best known examples. Cytarabine is also a competitive inhibitor of DNA polymerase. Dacarbazine (imidazole carboxamide; DIC) is a structural analogue of 5-aminoimidazole-4-carboxamide, a precursor in the *de novo* synthesis of purine bases. Other agents besides purine and pyrimidine analogues can inhibit the synthesis of these bases or their nucleotides. Hydroxyurea may interfere with the conversion of ribonucleotides into deoxyribonucleotides. The nitrosoureas, carmustine (BCNU), lomustine (CCNU) and semustine (methyl CCNU), interfere with the insertion of carbon fragments in the purine ring. Procarbazine

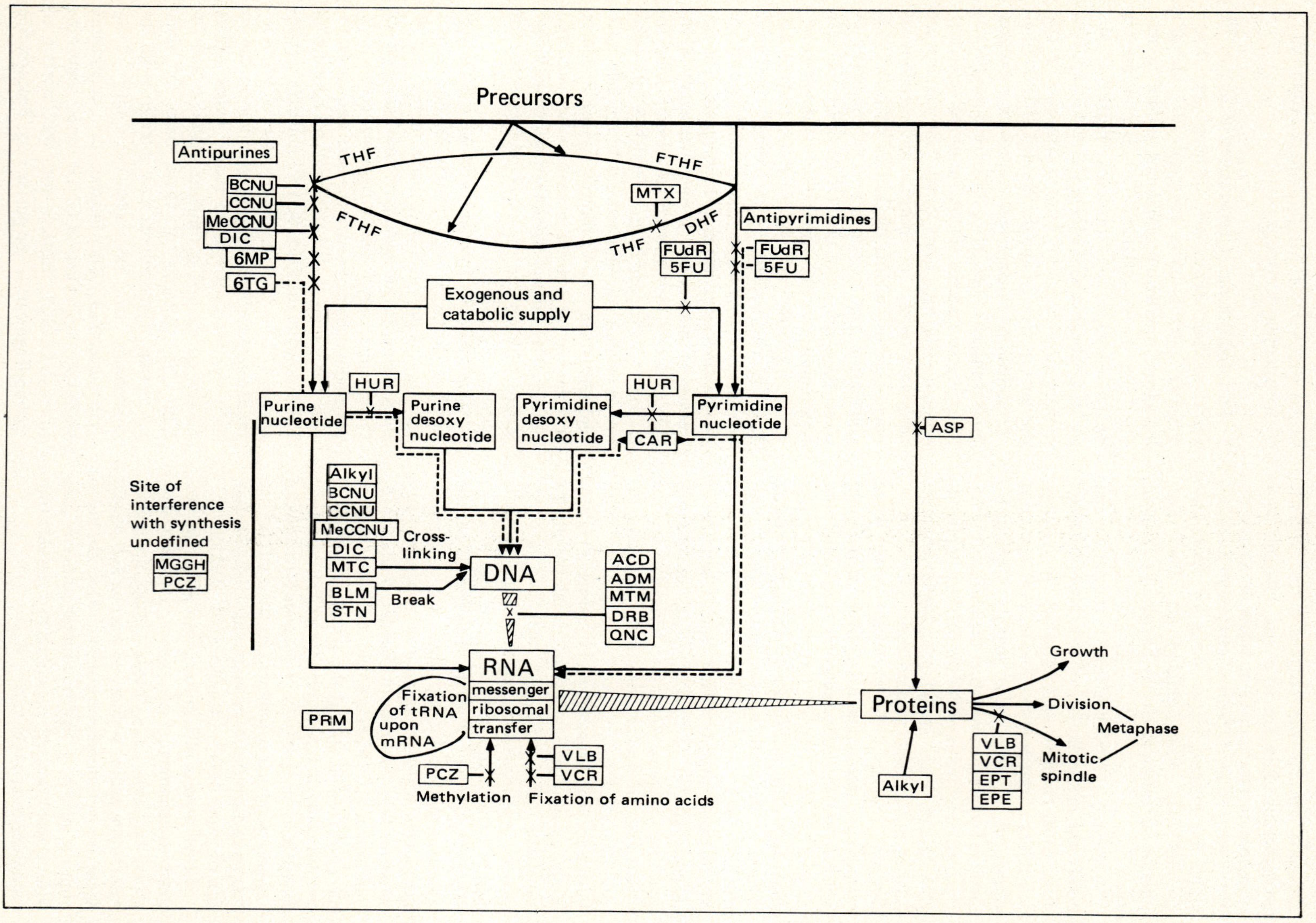

Precursors
Antipurines
THF
FTHF
MTX
BCNU
CCNU
FTHF
MeCCNU
DIC
6MP
6TG
THF
DHF
Antipyrimidines
FUdR
5FU
FUdR
5FU
ASP
Exogenous and catabolic supply
HUR
HUR
Purine nucleotide
Purine desoxy nucleotide
Pyrimidine desoxy nucleotide
Pyrimidine nucleotide
CAR
Site of interference with synthesis undefined
MGGH
PCZ
Alkyl
BCNU
CCNU
MeCCNU
Cross-linking
DIC
MTC
BLM
STN
Break
DNA
ACD
ADM
MTM
DRB
QNC
RNA
messenger
ribosomal
transfer
Fixation of tRNA upon mRNA
PRM
PCZ
Methylation
VLB
VCR
Fixation of amino acids
Proteins
Alkyl
Growth
Division
Metaphase
Mitotic spindle
VLB
VCR
EPT
EPE

is capable of inhibiting biosynthesis of DNA, RNA and protein.

Alkylating agents contain highly reactive alkyl groups and have a complex action. They damage the DNA template and cross-link the two strands of the double helix preventing replication (fig. 9). The most common of these drugs in clinical use are: nitrogen mustard, chlorambucil, cyclophosphamide, melphalan, triethylene thiophosphoramide (thiotepa), and busulphan. Some agents have complex modes of action, one of which is alkylation: mitomycin C, nitrosoureas, and dacarbazine.

Antibiotics: Many of the 'antibiotic' type antitumour agents bind selectively with DNA forming complexes that block the formation of DNA-dependent RNA; e.g. actinomycin D, daunorubicin, doxorubicin (adriamycin) and mithramycin.

Enzymes: The enzyme L-asparaginase causes depletion of endogenous asparagine. This amino acid is non-essential for normal cells, but some malignant cells require an exogenous source of asparagine for protein synthesis.

Mitotic inhibitors: The principal mitotic inhibitors are the vinca alkaloids, vincristine and vinblastine and the semisynthetic epipodophyllotoxin derivatives, VM-26 and VP-16213. They produce metaphase arrest by their action against the microtubules of the mitotic spindle apparatus.

Hormones may inhibit certain cancers originating in the organs that are normally sensitive to their suppressant action or their maturing effect. They may also have an indirect effect through inhibition of certain pituitary secretions that may stimulate the growth of malignancies derived from tissues sensitive to pituitary hormones.

Corticosteroids inhibit poorly differentiated lymphoid cells, probably by a direct action. They retard the growth of breast cancers, most likely through inhibition of pituitary secretions. By a similar mode of action, androgens may be effective in breast cancer in premenopausal women. Oestrogens also cause tumour regressions in prostatic carcinoma by a double mechanism of direct tumour inhibition and indirect pituitary influence. The maturing effect of progesterone on the normal endometrium and the sensitivity of this tissue to hormonal stimuli prompted the use of progestagens in the treatment of advanced endometrial carcinoma.

2.5 Resistance

Resistance to cancer chemotherapy may be either natural (innate), or acquired. Natural resistance means that the tumour is resistant from the outset of treatment. Acquired resistance occurs after therapy has begun as a result of epigenetic or genetic phenomena. Either types of resistance may be brought to clinical attention as a result of the selective pressure exerted by the therapy. What occurs is that the treatment selectively destroys the sensitive population with subsequent overgrowth of the resistant population. In advanced tumour situations where the neoplastic cell burden is high, heterogeneity as regards sensitivity is most likely. For example, a human melanoma nodule can give four permanent varied cell lines each with differing sensitivity to cytarabine (Barranco et al., 1972).

Spontaneous mutants have been shown to arise to various antimetabolites in mammalian cells

---

Fig. 8. Biochemical mechanisms of action of the main drugs used in cancer chemotherapy.

ACD	Actinomycin D		HUR	Hydroxyurea
ADM	Adriamycin (doxorubicin)		MeC-	
Alkyl	Alkylating agents		CNU	Chloroethyl-methyl
ASP	L-asparaginase (colaspase)			cyclohexyl nitrosourea (semustine)
BCNU	Bis-chloroethyl nitrosourea (carmustine)		MGGH	Methyl-gag
BLM	Bleomycin		6-MP	6-Mercaptopurine
CAR	Cytosine arabinoside (cytarabine)		MTC	Mitomycin C
CCNU	Chloroethyl-cyclohexyl nitrosourea		MTM	Mithramycin
	(lomustine)		MTX	Methotrexate
DHF	Dihydrofolic acid		PCZ	Procarbazine
DIC	Imidazole carboxamide (dacarbazine)		PRM	Puromycin
DRB	Daunorubicin		QNC	Quinacrine
EPE	Epipodophyllotoxin-ethylidene (VP-16213)		STN	Streptonigrin
EPT	Epipodophyllotoxin-thenylidene (VM-26)		6-TG	6-Thioguanine
FTHF	Formyltetrahydrofolic acid		THF	Tetrahydrofolic acid
5-FU	5-Fluorouracil		VCR	Vincristine
FUdR	5-Fluorodeoxyuridine		VLB	Vinblastine

(Fischer, 1971). Considering that acute leukaemia in relapse has been estimated to contain 10^{12} cells this would mean a significant number of resistant mutants to any given antimetabolite. Other factors which contribute to natural drug resistance include the low growth fraction and long generation time of the tumour and the failure of drugs to enter pharmacological sanctuaries (see section 2.3.1).

Clinical resistance has to combine inputs not only from the tumour but also from the host as well. The toxicity of normal tissues, such as the bone marrow, limit the doses of drugs which can be administered. Many drugs are highly active *in vitro* at concentrations which could never be achieved in man because of normal tissue damage. In order to fully understand clinical resistance, comparisons should be made between drug effects on tumour and on normal host systems, and of the different responses of sensitive and resistant tumour.

Some of the factors that may explain at a cellular level why some tumours cells are resistant and others sensitive include (Hall, 1977):

1) Transmembrane transport of drug into the cell
2) Extent of phosphorylation of purine and pyrimidine analogues
3) Extent of catabolism, e.g. deamination, decarboxylation, phosphorolysis, hydrolysis, reduction, oxidation, or esterification of drug to inactive forms
4) Altered affinity of target enzymes for inhibiting drugs
5) Different pathways of precursor utilisation for DNA synthesis by tumour cells
6) Extent of repair of drug induced damage
7) Drug induction of enzymatic activity in tumour or normal tissue
8) Distribution of drug receptors in cell surfaces, cytoplasm, or nucleus
9) Immune inactivation of antigenic drugs
10) Fraction of cell population in drug sensitive phases of the mitotic cycle.

In any given case of acquired resistance more than one of these factors may be involved. Each drug class tends to exhibit the influence of certain primary factors. With a few exceptions (e.g. hair follicles and cyclophosphamide), normal tissue resistance or the lack thereof stays stable and so strategies to predict sensitivity can concentrate on the tumour cells.

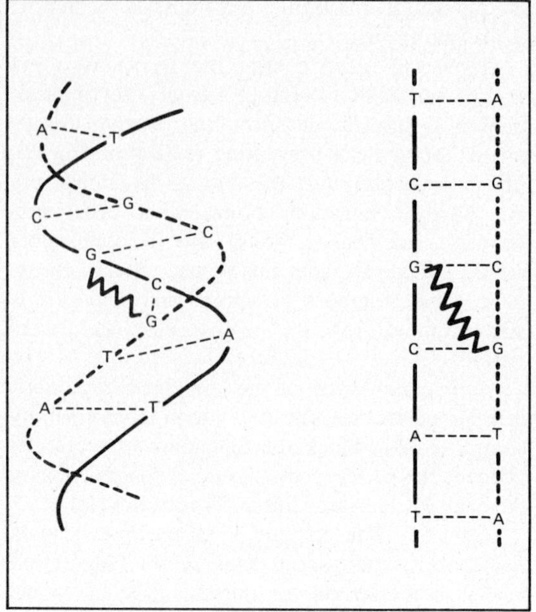

Fig. 9. Schematic representation of the mechanism of action of alkylating agents (cross-linkage).

3. Factors Affecting Choice of Chemotherapy Regimen

3.1 General Considerations

These include: (1) general sensitivity of the tumour to chemotherapy, (2) specific sensitivity of an individual's tumour to individual agents, (3) the likelihood of response and clinical improvement vs serious toxicity (assessment of therapeutic index), and (4) whether chemotherapy is to be used in the setting of advanced disease as a single method of therapy (modality), in a combined modality setting (e.g. with radiation therapy for regional disease), or in the adjuvant setting after potentially curative surgery.

Since acute leukaemia, lymphomas, paediatric solid tumours, breast and ovarian cancer, and small cell lung cancer are generally sensitive to chemotherapy, the choice of antineoplastic drug treatment is generally an appropriate one, even if the patient is bedfast from his disease. In tumours where chemotherapy has given low response rates (e.g. renal, pancreatic, oesophageal, colorectal and non-small cell lung), routine drug treatment is not recommended by many oncologists. This is especially true for non-ambulatory patients who have only a minimal possibility of achieving benefit. Whether to treat the ambulatory patient with dissemination of one of these cancers depends on several factors, including the patient's own informed desire for treatment, the availability of adequate facilities, and the possibility of contributing toward an eventual solution through involvement in a therapeutic research protocol.

To be able to determine the specific sensitivity (or lack of it), of an individual patient's tumour to chemotherapeutic agents is a long sought, but frustratingly distant goal. The importance of the oestrogen receptor content of a mammary tumour in determining whether endocrine therapy should be employed is the most significant advance yet made (McGuire, 1978). Recent work with effects of chemotherapeutic agents on clonability of human tumour cells *in vitro* (Salmon et al., 1978), and on the labelling index of tumour cells *in vitro* (Livingston, 1979) is promising, but still short of routine clinical usefulness.

Assessment of the therapeutic index may be vastly different, depending on the patient. For example, a 60 year old debilitated man with head and neck cancer, is a less suitable candidate for cisplatinum than a relatively healthy, 30 year old woman with ovarian cancer. Although the likelihood of a partial response may be the same, the young woman with ovarian cancer is much less likely to have disastrous side effects.

The setting in which chemotherapy is to be used is an extremely important variable. For example, in disseminated breast cancer, many oncologists would choose doxorubicin (adriamycin) as a component of initial treatment. Its use in simultaneous combination with radiation therapy to the chest wall in a patient with stage III disease can produce severe local toxicity as a result of their interaction, and necessitates at least a reduction in dosage. In the treatment of patients with disease which may have been eradicated by surgery, in many communities the majority of surgeons are unwilling to expose the patient to the risks of even a 'little bit' of doxorubicin (Bristow et al., 1978).

3.2 Combination Chemotherapy

The potential circumvention of resistance to treatment has probably been the most important factor prompting studies of use of combinations of antineoplastic drugs. Several conceptual approaches to the design of clinical combinations have been described.

1) One approach is biochemical. Combinations of drugs can be designed, using agents that produce different biochemical lesions, to attack multiple sites in biosynthetic pathways or to inhibit several processes involved in the maintenance and function of essential macromolecules. The common goal is to decrease the production and availability of a specific endproduct vital for tumour cell growth and replication.

Three basic schemes have been described. The inhibition of different enzymatic steps in a biochemical pathway leading to the production of an essential metabolite has been designated 'sequential blockade'. The simultaneous inhibition of parallel metabolic pathways involved in the synthesis of a common endproduct has been termed 'concurrent blockade'. The production of biochemical lesions at different loci in the synthesis of polymeric macromolecules is called 'complementary inhibition'.

Although the biochemical approach to the design of drug combinations is intellectually satisfying, it is complex and difficult to apply in human systems and it does not lead to an estimation of the degree of depletion of the specific endproduct required for tumour cell destruction. It also assumes selective toxicity for the tumour tissue. None of the successful combinations in use today have been developed purely as a result of this approach, but it is quite possible that some of them owe their effectiveness in part to the synergistic mechanisms envisaged in the biochemical approach.

2) Another approach to combination chemotherapy is cytokinetic. Most chemotherapeutic agents are not effective against non-proliferating cells (cells in G_0), but some agents (such as the nitrosoureas) that are effective in G_0 phase are now being developed (fig. 5). The existence of this particular population of cells is considered as a major obstacle to curative chemotherapy. It has been shown that reduction of the tumour mass (by surgery or other means) increases the growth fraction of the remaining cells, thus rendering them more sensitive to chemotherapy (Schabel, 1975). Intermittent chemotherapy may achieve the same results. One refinement is to try to synchronise the cells by giving an agent (e.g. vincristine) that arrests cells in one particular phase (mitosis in the case of vincristine). Cells not killed by the drug then enter a new cycle (see section 2.2) more or less synchronously, and when the majority are estimated to be in the S-phase, an S-phase specific

agent such as methotrexate or cytarabine is given (fig. 3, 5). Different combinations based on this principle have been used and found effective but their superiority over other types of combinations is not established.

3) The third and most successful approach to combination chemotherapy has been empirical and has involved the use of drugs that are known to be individually active against the particular tumour when used alone. In line with this, the tumours successfully treated with combinations have generally been the ones regarded as 'drug sensitive', meaning that they are amenable to treatment by several drugs that act by different mechanisms (see section 2.4). Examples from haematological malignancies would be the use of vincristine and prednisolone in acute lymphoblastic leukaemia and the use of mechlorethamine, vincristine, prednisone, and procarbazine (the so-called MOPP combination) for the treatment of Hodgkins' disease. When several choices of drugs are available within a class of agents, drug selection is guided by the type of dose limiting toxicity likely to be produced by other agents employed in the combination. Selections made in this manner have allowed antineoplastic agents to be used in combination at nearly full tolerated dosage.

Another facet of successful combination chemotherapy has been the application of intermittent treatment schedules, which permit treatment of greater intensity (see also section 2). One theoretical advantage of this is that if the combination exerts a more highly selective killing effect on tumour cells, an interval 2 to 3 weeks between courses is usually sufficient to allow recovery of the normal tissues to their pretreatment condition. An additional advantage of intermittent scheduling is the potential recovery of the host's immunological mechanism between exposures to chemotherapy.

3.3 Combined Modality Treatment

As discussed in section 1.2, surgical and radiotherapeutic interventions are successful only if metastatic spread from the primary tumour has not yet occurred. Since many malignant tumours in man have metastasised prior to clinical recognition, they may be beyond the reach of surgical and radiotherapeutic treatment when they initially present. Metastatic tumour cell foci of 10^8 or fewer cells, particularly if widely disseminated, are generally undetectable and therefore a target for chemotherapy. The utilisation of chemotherapy to eradicate these microscopic metastatic foci remaining after surgery and/or irradiation, is the cornerstone of the new combined modality approach to solid tumour therapy (Carter and Soper, 1974; Carter and Wasserman, 1975b; Schabel, 1975).

3.3.1 Tumour Cell Burden and Drug Kill

Estimations have been made of the likely total body burden of viable tumour remaining after surgery and/or radiation therapy has removed all clinically visible or detectable tumour foci. These estimates are based on the indicated probability that each gram of tumour may contain as many as 10^9 cells. A single metastatic focus 1mm in diameter may contain 10^5 to 10^6 tumour cells, and this number will range downwards to a few cells for still smaller foci. The number and size of the micrometastases will determine the likely requirements for the cure of the patient. The total tumour cell population in unrecognised metastases is highly variable and may often be formidable, especially if reduction to small numbers (perhaps zero) is required for cure. The conceptual design of chemotherapy in this situation is based on first order kinetics; namely, that a given dose of drug kills a given fraction of tumour cells and not a given number of cells. It has been repeatedly shown that the time duration of the division cycle (Tc) of tumour cells in a wide range of systems is related to tumour mass — i.e. the larger the tumour cell population, the longer the division cycle time.

A reduction of the total body burden of tumour cells by any effective but non-curative treatment has been shown to shorten the division cycle time of the remaining cells in both acute lymphoblastic leukaemia and ovarian cancer (Schabel, 1975). In experimental systems, it has been shown that the division cycle time of micrometastases is significantly shorter than that of cells in the primary tumour (in the same host). Reduction in the total body burden of tumour cells has been shown to decrease the doubling time of the tumour mass with sarcoma 180 and adenocarcinoma 755 in mice. All this implies that drugs will achieve increased cell kill in residual tumour cell populations as the tumour burden is reduced (see also section 2.1.3).

Tumour population kinetics and the first order kinetics of drug kill indicate that:

1) Drugs capable of killing tumour cells in the advanced state should be even more effective when used to treat micrometastatic disease, and

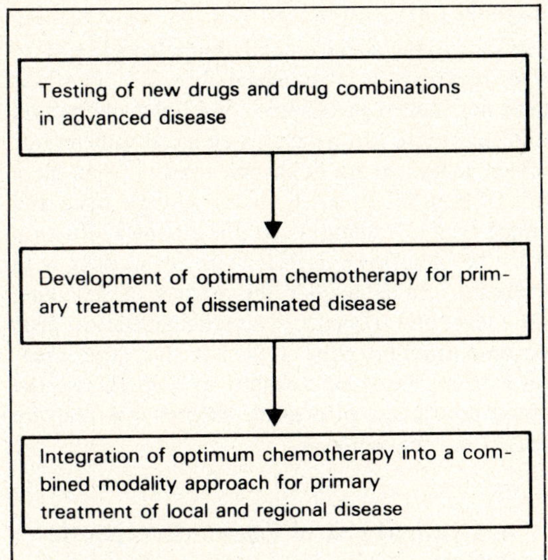

Fig. 10. Strategy adopted in development of a chemotherapy regimen.

2) Where there is a high probability of micrometastatic disease, chemotherapy is best started as soon as possible after the primary treatment as an adjuvant to surgical or radiological therapy.

To increase cure rates in patients with solid tumours, research workers are developing a broad overall strategy in which chemotherapy is integrated with other kinds of treatment. The single drugs or drug combinations showing positive results in advanced cancer will be used in the initial treatment of disseminated disease. Then, the optimum drug regimens developed, in this situation will be integrated with other modalities into combined treatments of local and regional disease (fig. 10).

3.3.2 Interaction of Radiotherapy and Chemotherapy

When radiation therapy and chemotherapy are combined the situation is more complicated than with surgery and drugs. The reason for this is that drugs can potentially interact with radiation in 2 ways regarding tumour cells. Drugs can kill tumour cells that radiation cannot kill and thus function as adjuvant to radiation cell kill. In addition, drugs can sensitise cells to the killing effect of radiation and therefore increase the therapeutic ratio for radiation through a sensitisation effect (Elkind, 1969). Many drugs which are used to

effectively treat disseminated disease have been shown experimentally to sensitise cells to radiation cell kill (Goffinet and Bagshaw, 1974). When drugs such as actinomycin D, bleomycin and doxorubicin are given in combination with radiation, there exists the possibility that there may be a combination of adjuvant cell kill and sensitisation which is taking place. To the same degree that this can be true for tumour cell kill, it may also occur with normal tissue damage. Therefore, the interaction of radiation therapy and chemotherapy has to be viewed as a balance of two general effects (table III).

In the early days of cancer chemotherapy, the major aim was to achieve some level of response and the major toxicological emphasis was on the price in terms of acute toxicity that the patient had to pay for the benefit of tumour regression. As chemotherapy has become more successful, long term disease free survival after the achievement of complete remission has become commonplace for some tumours (Karle et al., 1973). However, in association with these therapeutic triumphs has come an increased awareness of the chronic toxicities of anticancer drugs. It is now recognised that for diseases such as childhood leukaemia, Hodgkins's disease, non-Hodgkin's lymphoma, choriocarcinoma, disseminated testicular carcinoma and Burkitt's tumour, the final endpoint for evaluation of chemotherapy will be survival compared with chronic toxicity. Similarly, as studies are undertaken testing combined modality approaches such as radiation therapy and chemotherapy, chronic toxicity will be an endpoint to measure as against survival gain.

The chronic toxicity of radiation and drugs can be viewed from three conceptual aspects (table IV). Many drugs cause chronic organ damage. Some examples are the cardiac toxicity of doxorubicin, (Carter, 1975), the pulmonary toxicity of bleomycin, the renal toxicity of cis-platinum and mitomycin C and the hepatic toxicity of 6-mercaptopurine and methotrexate (Carter et al., 1977).

Table III. The interaction of radiation therapy and chemotherapy is a balance of two general effects

1. Antitumour action
   a) Adjuvant effect
   b) Sensitisation effect

2. Toxicity
   a) Acute
   b) Chronic

Table IV. Chronic toxicities of radiation therapy and chemotherapy

1. Organ and tissue damage
   a) Heart
   b) Lung
   c) CNS
   d) Kidney
   e) Liver
   f) Gonads
   g) Mucous membranes
   h) Hair roots

2. Immunosuppression

3. Carcinogenicity

Many other examples could be cited. Chronic organ damage from radiation is a well established fact. When radiation and drugs are combined, there is the possibility of an enhanced chronic organ site toxicity.

Immunosuppresion is another side effect of both radiation and cytotoxic chemotherapy (Hersh et al., 1966). It is a well known fact that cancer patients can be made more susceptible to infection through the reduction of the functioning leucocyte count as a consequence of the immunosuppressive effect of cytotoxic therapy. Stjernsward (1974) has documented the immunosuppressive effects of radiation and has postulated an increase of failure of response of metastatic disease to therapy due to this immunosuppression in women with stage II breast cancer given postoperative radiation. There is therefore the possibility that combined radiation and cytotoxic drugs will lead to a synergism of immunosuppressive effects with resultant chronic toxicities of either infection, increased incidence of failure of metastatic disease to respond or the development of second primary neoplasms.

Radiation therapy and most cytotoxic chemotherapy regimens are carcinogenic in potential (Sieber et al., 1975). This has been well established in rodent systems and with radiation in a variety of clinical situations. When the 2 modalities are used together there is the risk that an enhancement of the carcinogenic effects will occur. Indeed, there is preliminary evidence from Hodgkin's disease studies that this may be in fact a reality (Williams et al., 1977).

At any cellular level, four possibilities for the interaction of radiation and drugs exist (table V). The two may act independently at different sites and not interact at all $(2 + 2 = 2)$. The two may have an additive effect $(2 + 2 = 4)$ or a subaddi-

tive effect $(2 + 2 = 3)$. The two may be synergistic, giving a true potentiation effect $(2 + 2 = 5)$ or they may be antagonistic $(2 + 2 = 1)$. If one assumes these 4 possibilities of cellular interaction and that these can be expressed as an antitumour effect, acute toxicity or chronic toxicity, then there are 64 possible interactions for a single drug and single type of radiation. To this complex situation must be added the variables of using one drug with radiation which include the aspects of schedule, dose level and sequence. The possible clinical tests become mind boggling. It is clear that experimental systems must be designed to help choose the small percentage of possible interactions that are feasible to test clinically.

4. Clinical Use of Chemotherapeutic Agents

The generally available antineoplastic drugs that are considered useful in cancer therapy today are listed in table VI, along with their dosages, acute and chronic toxic effects and precautions in use. Table VI also lists investigational drugs that have shown definite antitumour activity. In the USA, these are usually available only from the National Cancer Institute under US Food and Drug Administration regulations governing the use of experimental drugs. The drugs currently preferred or used for chemotherapeutic approaches to the treatment of the major types of cancer are listed in table VII.

The dosages indicated are those most commonly used when the drugs are employed as single agents in patients less than 65 years of age with good performance status, intact bone marrow and normal liver and kidney function. In patients with disseminated bone metastases and/or extensive prior radiothcrapy to thorax, spine and pelvis, the initial drug dosage should be reduced to about two-thirds of the conventional dose. The disposition of the drug must also be considered (see sec-

Table V. Possibilities for the interaction of radiation therapy and chemotherapy

1. Independent action

2. Additive effect

3. Synergistic effect

4. Antagonistic effect

tion 2.3; table II) and dosage reduced to about half in case of impairment of the organ primarily responsible for elimination of the drug (e.g. kidney for methotrexate and liver for doxorubicin).

For the large majority of anticancer drugs, administered either singly or in combination, bone marrow suppression represents the most important dose limiting factor. Therefore, as a minimum requirement, complete blood counts should be determined immediately before each course when intermittent chemotherapy is used. Table VIII presents a simple guide for a dose reduction schedule. Since single agent as well as combination chemotherapy is most effective when administered in full dosage, it is advisable, whenever possible, to prolong the interval between courses rather than reduce the dosage.

Severe marrow suppression may require adequate supportive measures, and sophisticated techniques are still available in only a limited number of centres. Repeated platelet transfusions are usually considered necessary in case of petechiae or bleeding tendency or when the platelet level is below $25,000/mm^3$. In patients with severe granulocytopenia (less than $1,000/mm^3$), Gram-negative septicaemia often occurs and specific antibiotics such as gentamicin plus carbenicillin are indicated, especially when the temperature rises to over 38°C. In this situation, repeated granulocyte transfusions have proved to be very helpful in the control of infection in more than 80% of patients (McCredie and Freireich, 1975).

In susceptible tumours, a rapid destruction of bulky tumour masses can produce, through an increased purine and pyrimidine breakdown, uric acid nephropathy. To prevent this important complication, adequate fluid intake, alkalinisation of the urine and administration of allopurinol (300 to 350mg/day by mouth) are indicated during the first period of induction chemotherapy. Allopurinol inhibits the metabolism of azathioprine and 6-mercaptopurine and dosage of these must be reduced to about a third of usual when used with allopurinol (Boston Collaborative Program, 1974; see chapter VIII; sect. 2.3.4).

5. Haematological Malignancies

5.1 Acute Lymphoid Leukaemia

It is in the treatment of childhood acute lymphoid leukaemia (ALL) that cancer chemotherapy,

based on the principles outlined above, has achieved some of its most impressive results (Carter, 1978; table IX).

The first remissions were obtained in 1948 with single agent therapy. It was soon learned that these were of short duration if no complementary therapy was given following the induction treatment. This led to the introduction of 'maintenance' therapy, initially with the same agents used for induction, and later, as more agents became available, with different drugs, so called maintenance agents. This was followed by trials using intensive combination chemotherapy not only for induction but also for maintenance of remission as well as protocols integrating 'consolidation' and 'periodic re-inducer' therapy.

As the number of long term remissions increased it was appreciated that the CNS represents an important tumour sanctuary that calls for special therapy. Resting cells (G_0), which are not affected by most cytotoxic agents (section 2.2; fig. 5) are also a possible source of relapse. Current protocols concern themselves with this fraction of the leukaemic cell population.

Significant progress has also been made in supportive care to combat both the consequences of the disease and the side effects of the drugs, especially the development of pathogen free environments and techniques to replace essential blood components. Such advances have been made in the management of acute lymphoid leukaemia in the past 2 decades that a treatment should no longer be undertaken with the simple aim of palliation (i.e. prolongation of comfortable survival), while accepting relapse and death as inevitable. Instead, treatment must be planned from the outset for cure; i.e. total disease eradication. With current protocols in specialised leukaemia centres, more than 50% of children affected have a leukaemia free survival of 5 years. It is hoped and anticipated that a considerable percentage, if not most of these, will be permanent cures. The best way to treat leukaemia is to refer the patient to a leukaemia centre.

5.2 Acute Myeloid Leukaemia

Most of the treatment principles outlined for acute lymphoid leukaemia apply to the management of acute myeloid leukaemia (Clarkson et al., 1975; Woodruff, 1978). The treatment must result in the destruction of the leukaemic cell population and permit the restoration of normal

Table VI. Toxicity, precautions and dosage of antineoplastic drugs

Drug	Major toxicity		Some precautions	Dosage and route of administration
	acute	delayed		
Alkylating Agents				
5-Azacytidine[1]	Nausea and vomiting; diarrhoea; fever	Leucopenia (may be prolonged); thrombocytopenia; hepatic damage; unrelated to dosage[2]	Change infusion solution every 3 to 4 hours to avoid loss of potency	150-300mg/m^2 per day IV x 5; or 150-200mg/m^2 2 x/weeks for 2-8 weeks
Busulphan	Nausea and vomiting diarrhoea	Bone marrow depression; pulmonary fibrosis; hyper-pigmentation of skin; alopecia; gynaecomastia; impotence, sterility (see chapter XV; sect. 23.1)		2-10mg/day PO for 2-3 weeks maintenance with 1-3mg daily
Chlorambucil		Bone marrow depression; sterility (see chapter XV; sect. 23.1)		0.1-0.2mg/kg per day; PO dose decreased if severe bone marrow depression develops; only 2-4mg daily may be necessary in chronic lymphoid leukaemia
Cyclophosphamide	Nausea and vomiting	Bone marrow depression; alopecia; haemorrhagic cystitis; possible secondary malignancy; sterility (may be temporary; see chapter XV, sect. 23.1) pulmonary fibrosis; hyperpigmentation	Maintain adequate fluid intake to avoid cystitis	500-1500mg/m^2 as a single IV dose; 60-120mg/m^2 per day PO; dose decreased if severe leucopenia develops
Hexamethyl-melamine[1]	Nausea and vomiting	Bone marrow depression; CNS depression; peripheral neuritis[2]		4-15mg/kg per day PO for 21-90 days; usually limited by gastrointestinal toxicity
Mechlorethamine (nitrogen mustard; HN2)	Severe nausea and vomiting; local reaction and phlebitis	Bone marrow depression; alopecia	Unstable (use immediately after reconstitution); strong local irritant, administer through a running IV infusion; protect eyes and skin of person administering the drug	0.4mg/kg as a single dose IV or in 2 divided doses
Melphalan (L-phenyl-alanine mustard)	Mild nausea	Bone marrow depression (especially platelets)	Check platelets before each dose	0.2mg/kg per day PO x 4 q 6 weeks (myeloma); or 0.1 mg/kg per day PO for 2-3 weeks; maintenance with 2-4mg/day when bone marrow has recovered

Alkylating Agents (continued)				
Thiotepa (triethylene-thiophosphor-amide)	Nausea and vomiting; local pain	Bone marrow depression; anorexia		0.2mg/kg per day IV x 5
Antimetabolites				
Cytarabine (cytosine arabinoside)	Nausea and vomiting; diarrhoea	Bone marrow depression; megaloblastosis; oral ulceration; hepatic damage	Use with special caution in hepatic disease	Leukaemia: 3mg/kg per day IV for 1-3 weeks; or 2.5mg/kg q 12h IV for 1-3 weeks with 6-thioguanine); or intrathecally, 20-30mg/m^2
Fluorouracil (5-FU)	Nausea and vomiting; diarrhoea; may precipitate angina	Oral and gastrointestinal ulceration; stomatitis; bone marrow depression; neurological defects, usually cerebellar; pigmentation; alopecia; dermatitis	Decrease dose in patients with impaired hepatic or renal function, or after adrenalectomy; do not exceed daily dose of 800mg; contraindicated in poor nutritional state	12mg/kg per day IV x 4, then alternate days at 6mg/kg x 4 or or until toxicity; repeat course monthly or give weekly IV dose of 12-15mg/kg maximum dose 1g for either regimen
Mercaptopurine (6-MP)	Occasional nausea and vomiting, usually well tolerated	Bone marrow depression; hepatic damage	Since allopurinol potentiates mercaptopurine, if it is given to prevent hyperuricaemia dosage of mercaptopurine should be reduced to no more than one-third of usual dose (see chapter VIII; sect. 2.3.4)	2.5mg/kg per day PO
Methotrexate	Nausea; diarrhoea	Oral and gastrointestinal ulceration; bone marrow depression; hepatic toxicity, including cirrhosis (see chapter XIX; sect. 14.6) renal toxicity; pulmonary infiltration (see chapter XX; sect. 11.2) osteoporosis	Normal renal function should be present and urine output must be maintained. Adjust dosage according to creatinine clearance in cases of impaired renal function and in the elderly	Choriocarcinoma 10-30mg/day PO or IM x 5 Acute leukaemia maintenance; child 1.25-5mg/day PO; adult, 5-10mg/day PO; or both, 30mg/m^2 IM or PO twice weekly Meningeal leukaemia 0.2-0.4mg/kg intrathecally
Thioguanine (6-TG)	Occasional nausea and vomiting, usually well tolerated	Bone marrow depression; possible hepatic damage	Use lower doses in patients with impaired renal or hepatic function	100mg/m^2 PO q 12h for 8 days, often in combination with cytarabine Head and neck 50mg/day intra-arterially with concomitant or sequential systemic antidote (calcium folinate)

Table VI. (continued)

Drug	Major toxicity		Some precautions	Dosage and route of administration
	acute	delayed		
Natural Products (plant alkaloids and antibiotics)				
Actinomycin D (dactinomycin)	Nausea and vomiting; diarrhoea; local reaction and phlebitis	Stomatitis; oral ulceration; alopecia; foliculitis; bone marrow depression	Administer through a running IV infusion; use with special caution in hepatic disease	15-40µg/kg per week IV for 3-5 weeks in adults; 15µg/kg per day IV x 5 in children
Bleomycin	Nausea and vomiting; fever	Pneumonitis and pulmonary fibrosis (see chapter XX; sect. 11.2); cutaneous reactions; stomatitis; alopecia; anorexia (may be prolonged)	Anaphylactic reactions may occur in patients with lymphoma — two 2 unit test doses are recommended; use with extreme caution in renal or pulmonary disease; do not exceed total dosage of 400 units	10-20 units/m^2 IV or IM 1-2 x/week; start with 5 units for first 2 doses in lymphoma
Daunorubicin[1] (daunomycin)	Nausea and vomiting; fever, red urine (not haematuria)	Bone marrow depression; cardio-toxicity (see chapter XVII; sect. 11.4) alopecia[2]	Administer through a running IV infusion; avoid giving to patients with heart disease	1mg/kg per day IV x 5; or 30-60mg/m^2 per day IV x 3; or 30-60mg/m^2 per week IV
Doxorubicin (adriamycin)	Nausea and vomiting; red urine (not haematuria), severe local tissue damage at infiltration site; diarrhoea	Bone marrow depression; cardiotoxicity (may be irreversible see chapter XVII; sect. 11.4) alopecia; stomatitis; hepatic damage; cutaneous toxicity; renal damage	Administer through a running IV infusion; special caution in patients with heart disease; reduce dose if hepatic function is impaired; do not exceed total dosage of 550mg/m^2	60-90mg/m^2 IV q 3 weeks
Mithramycin	Nausea and vomiting; diarrhoea	Haemorrhagic diathesis, probably related to abnormalities of clotting factors; bone marrow depression (thrombocytopenia); hepatic damage; hypocalcaemia and hypokalaemia; stomatitis	Very toxic drug; strict adherence to monitoring of LDH, BUN, prothrombin time and platelet count before each dose; contraindicated in hepatic and kidney dysfunction and in patients with coagulation disorders	25-50µg/kg IV on alternate days for 3-8 doses or until toxicity develops
Mitomycin C	Nausea and vomiting; local reaction if extravasation; fever	Bone marrow depression (cumulative); stomatitis; renal toxicity; alopecia	Administer through a running IV infusion (acts as alkylating agent)	0.05mg/kg IV per day x 6, then alternate days until 50mg total dose

Natural Products (plant alkaloids and antibiotics) [continued]

Streptozocin[1] (strepto-zotocin)	Nausea and vomiting; local pain	Renal damage[2]	Slow infusion rate to prevent local pain; contraindicated in patients with renal disease; albuminuria used to monitor toxicity; do not repeat dose until renal function recovers	1g/m^2 per week for 5-6 weeks
Vinblastine	Nausea and vomiting; local reaction and phlebitis	Bone marrow depression; alopecia; stomatitis; loss of deep tendon reflexes	Administer through a running IV infusion or inject with great care to prevent extravasation	0.10-0.15mg/kg per week IV
Vincristine	Local reaction if extravasation	Peripheral neuropathy; neuritic pain; alopecia; bone marrow depression (leucopenia); constipation leading to paralytic ileus; sterility (see chapter XV; sect. 23.1)	Administer through a running IV infusion or inject with great care to prevent extravasation; omit or decrease dose if reflexes diminish or paraesthesiae appear; patients with underlying neurological problems may be more susceptible to neuro-toxicity; hyperuricaemia can be treated with allopurinol; prophylactic laxatives may be helpful	0.4-1.4mg/m^2 IV weekly in adults; 2mg/m^2 weekly in children
VM-26[4] (etoposide)	Nausea and vomiting	Bone marrow depression; alopecia[2]		
VP-16213[1] (teniposide)	Nausea and vomiting	Bone marrow depression; alopecia[2]		

Table VI. (continued)

Drug	Major toxicity		Some precautions	Dosage and route of administration
	acute	delayed		
Other Synthetic Agents				
Asparaginase[1] (colaspase)	Nausea, fever, and possible anaphylaxis; abdominal pain: diabetes leading to coma	Hepatic damage; pancreatitis; CNS depression; coagulation defects[2]	Adrenaline (epinephrine) should be available; rise in BUN and ammonia is due to action of the enzyme and is not evidence of toxicity	10-500IU/kg per day IV x 2-20; or 100-500 IU/kg 3 x/week
Carmustine (BCNU)	Nausea and vomiting; local phlebitis	Delayed leucopenia and thrombo-cytopenia (may be prolonged)	Slow infusion rate to prevent local pain	75-100mg/m^2 per day IV x 2; repeat course in 6-8 weeks
Cis-platinum diammine dichloride[1]	Nausea and vomiting	Bone marrow depression; renal damage; ototoxicity[2]	Maintain adequate fluid intake; use lower dose in patients with impaired renal function; do not repeat until recovery of baseline renal function	
Dacarbazine (DTIC; DIC)	Severe nausea and vomiting	Bone marrow depression; flu-like syndrome; alopecia; renal impairment; liver damage		150-250mg/m^2 per day IV x 5; or 950-1200mg/m^2 IV once
Estramustine phosphate	Nausea, vomiting, phlebitis, urticaria	Thrombocytopenia (rare), gynaeco-mastia (rare) or breast tenderness[2]	Early nausea and vomiting are controllable with phenothiazines	600-1000mg PO daily; or 300-450mg IV daily
Hydroxyurea	Mild nausea and vomiting	Bone marrow depression; hyperkeratosis and hyper-pigmentation; stomatitis	Decrease dose in patients with renal dysfunction	80mg/kg q 3 days PO; or 20-30mg/kg per day
Lomustine (CCNU)	Nausea and vomiting	Delayed (4 to 6 weeks) leucopenia and thrombocytopenia (may be prolonged); stomatitis; alopecia		130mg/m^2 PO; repeat in 6-8 weeks
Mitotane (o,p'-DDD)	Nausea and vomiting: diarrhoea	CNS toxicity, mental depression visual disturbances; dermatitis; adrenal insufficiency	Low dose should be used initially with gradual build-up to maximum tolerated dose (usually 8-10 grams per day); discontinue following shock or severe trauma; decrease dose in patients with hepatic disease	8-10g/day PO in 3-4 divided doses; tolerated dose varies from 2 to 16g/day

Other Synthetic Agents (continued)

Procarbazine	Nausea and vomiting; CNS depression	Bone marrow depression; stomatitis; dermatitis	Decrease dose in patients receiving CNS depressants (phenothiazines, barbiturates); mental disturbances may occur as well as a disulfiram-like reaction with ethanol; acts as mild MAO inhibitor — sympathomimetic drugs and foods with high tyramine or dopamine content should be avoided (chapter VIII, sect. 3)	50-300mg/day PO with slow build-up in dose
Semustine[1] (methyl-CCNU)	Nausea and vomiting	Delayed leucopenia and thrombo-cytopenia (may be prolonged)[2]		$175\text{-}200\text{mg/m}^2$ PO; repeat in 6-8 weeks
Hormones				
Diethylstilboestrol (DES)	Nausea and vomiting; cramps	Fluid retention; hypercalcaemia; feminisation; uterine bleeding; if given during pregnancy, may cause vaginal carcinoma in offspring; increased frequency of vascular accidents (see chapter XV; sect. 13.12, 23.3)	Use low doses in patients with prostate cancer; do not use in premenopausal breast cancer patients; serum calcium can rise rapidly in breast cancer patients shortly after therapy is started, especially with bone disease	Diethylstilboestrol Prostate cancer: up to 1mg/day PO Breast cancer: up to 15mg/day PO in divided doses
Fluoxymesterone		Fluid retention; masculinisation; cholestatic jaundice; hypercalcaemia	Contraindicated in patients with prostate cancer; immobilised patients are especially likely to develop hypercalcaemia; use with care in patients with cardiac, hepatic, or renal disease	20-30mg/day PO
Hydroxypro-gesterone caproate	Local abscess, pain	Hypercalcaemia; cholestatic jaundice	Contraindicated in patients with impaired hepatic function, breast cancer	1000mg IM twice weekly
Medroxypro-gesterone acetate	Orally, nausea (rare); IM, local pain, abscess at site of injection	Fluid retention; hypercalcaemia	Use with care in hepatic dysfunction	400-800mg/week IM or PO

Table VI. (continued)

Drug	Major toxicity		Some precautions	Dosage and route of administration
	acute	delayed		
Hormones (continued)				
Megestrol acetate		None reported		20mg bid PO
Prednisone or Prednisolone		Hyperadrenocorticism (see chapter XVI; sect. 9.1)		40-100mg daily PO of prednisone or equivalent; maintain at lower doses, if possible
Testosterone propionate		Fluid retention; masculinisation; hypercalcaemia	Contraindicated in cancer of prostate and hepatic disease; immobilised patients are especially likely to develop hypercalcaemia	50-100mg 3 x/week IM
Tamoxifen	Nausea and vomiting	Hot flushes; pruritus vulvae; vaginal bleeding; hypercalcaemia; ? ocular toxicity	Can induce ovulation — use with mechanical contraceptive in premenopausal patients	10-20mg bid PO

1   Classed as an investigational drug in the USA. Asparaginase and daunorubicin are generally available in most other countries.
2   Information is preliminary; additional or more severe adverse effects may be reported.

haematopoiesis. Acute myeloid leukaemia is much less sensitive to chemotherapy. Only 4 drugs: cytarabine, daunorubicin, doxorubicin (adriamycin) and 5-azacytidine result in at least 25 % responses. Doxorubicin and daunorubicin are cross resistant. Methyl GAG which is also active is rarely used. All 4 drugs are myelosuppressive, in contrast to the 'selective' toxicity of the agents used for induction of remission in acute lymphoid leukaemia. It seems that marrow aplasia must be induced before a remission can be expected in acute myeloid leukaemia. The cost in toxicity is thus very high and one must be equipped to administer adequate supportive care.

Remissions can be obtained in about 50 % of patients with various combinations of 2, 3, 4 or more drugs; generally administered in intermittent courses at 2 to 3 week intervals. No one particular regimen is clearly superior to another one. Cytarabine plus thioguanine (rate of remission: 65 to 15 %) or cytarabine plus daunorubicin (77 to 21 % remission) are the two most popular drug combinations in the USA at the present time.

To maintain a remission one can either: (1) continue at greater intervals the same agents that were used to induce the remission, (2) switch to different agents or (3) rely on immunotherapy. Remissions do not last as long as in acute lymphoid leukaemia. The median duration ranges between 6 to 12 months. Preliminary reports indicate that immunotherapy may be capable of prolonging the duration of remission (McCredie and Freireich, 1975).

5.3 Chronic Leukaemias

5.3.1 Chronic Myeloid Leukaemia

Chronic myeloid leukaemia is characterised by an increase in the total granulocyte mass (TGM). 90 % of cases have the Philadelphia chromosome (Ph'), which can be found in the myeloid precursors, erythroblasts and megakaryocytes, and indicates that they are all derived from the same abnormal stem cell. Chemotherapy, splenic irradiation or radioactive isotopes can reduce the expanded TGM (Spiers, 1974). However, they seem unable to eradicate the abnormal population since the Ph' chromosome persists during such remission. 'Total cell kill' cannot be attempted until it is known whether or not there is a normal haematopoietic stem cell besides the abnormal one (Ph'). If there is none, a successful technique of bone marrow transplantation would have to be avail-

able before total cell kill can be attempted. Combination chemotherapy as employed in acute lymphoid leukaemia is therefore rarely used and prolonged suppression rather than cure is all that can be hoped for at the present time.

Busulphan is the most commonly used treatment. It is superior to splenic irradiation, but neither treatment can prevent the·occurrence of blastic transformation. Busulphan is given initially in relatively large doses. Once the TGM is reduced, which is reflected in a return of the peripheral blood count to normal, it can be kept under control by either continuous or intermittent maintenance therapy. Such therapy has improved the quality of life but affects only slightly the survival; median 2.5 to 3 years. Dibromomannitol and hydroxyurea are equally effective but the remissions are of shorter duration, especially with hydroxyurea. The effect of splenectomy early in the disease is being studied.

Chronic myeloid leukaemia generally terminates in an acute blastic transformation, which is refractory to most of the treatment programmes effective in acute leukaemia.

5.3.2 Chronic Lymphoid Leukaemia

Chronic lymphoid leukaemia seems to result from the accumulation of long lived, probably functionally inert B lymphocytes[1]. It is therefore not surprising that alkylating agents have given the best response rate (Huguley, 1977). Chlorambucil is the drug of choice and achieves a response rate of 60 %, but regressions are rarely complete. Continuous and intermittent maintenance therapy seem equally effective. Cyclophosphamide is second choice, achieving a 40 % response rate. Corticosteroids, although lympholytic, are mainly indicated for haemolytic anaemia, thrombocytopenia, or severe marrow insufficiency. Splenectomy may be necessary for intractable haemolytic anaemia. Radiotherapy can reduce painfully enlarged lymph nodes or spleen.

---

1   Lymphocytes in normal subjects can be divided into two main groups. T-lymphocytes originate as stem cells in the bone marrow but mature in the thymus. They constitute the lymphocyte populations functioning in cell mediated immune reactions. B-lymphocytes also originate from stem cells in the bone marrow but, unlike T-lymphocytes, mature in the bone marrow and possibly in the wall of the intestinal tract or spleen of mammals. When stimulated by antigen, B-lymphocytes proliferate and differentiate into plasma cells, which are the major source of immunoglobulins.

Table VII. Drugs commonly used for treatment of major types of cancer

Cancer type	Drugs currently preferred	Alternative or secondary drugs	Other drugs with reported activity
Haematologic Malignancies			
Acute lymphoid leukaemia	Induction: vincristine + prednisone	Daunorubicin[1] Doxorubicin (adriamycin) Asparaginase[1] Cyclophosphamide Cytarabine	Thioguanine
	Prophylaxis of CNS disease with intrathecal methotrexate and/or radiotherapy		
	Maintenance: combination chemotherapy with methotrexate + mercaptopurine, or other combinations		
Acute granulocytic leukaemia	Doxorubicin or daunorubicin[1] + cytarabine; *or* Cytarabine + thioguanine; *or* Cytarabine, vincristine + prednisone		5-Azacytidine[1] Mercaptopurine
Acute myelomonocytic or monocytic leukaemia	Doxorubicin or daunorubicin[1] + cytarabine; *or* Cytarabine + thioguanine; *or* Cytarabine, vincristine + prednisone		VP-16213[1]
Chronic granulocytic leukaemia	Busulphan	Dibromomannitol[1] Hydroxyurea	Mercaptopurine
Chronic lymphoid leukaemia	Chlorambucil or cyclophosphamide	Prednisone	
Multiple myeloma	Melphalan or cyclophosphamide + prednisone	Cyclophosphamide if melphalan used first Carmustine	Doxorubicin Chlorambucil
Hodgkin's disease	MOPP (mechlorethamine, vincristine, procarbazine, prednisone)	ABVD (doxorubicin, or adriamycin, bleomycin, vinblastine, dacarbazine)	Lomustine Carmustine Chlorambucil Thiotepa Hexamethylmelamine[1]
Nodular lymphomas	CVP (cyclophosphamide, vincristine, prednisone)	ABP (doxorubicin, bleomycin, prednisone)	Lomustine Carmustine Hexamethylmelamine[1]
Diffuse histiocytic lymphoma	CHOP (cyclophosphamide, doxorubicin, vincristine, prednisone); *or* BACOP (bleomycin, doxorubicin, cyclophosphamide, vincristine, prednisone); *or* COMA (cyclophosphamide, vincristine, methotrexate, cytarabine)		Lomustine Carmustine[1] Cytarabine Hexamethylmelamine[1]
Burkitt's tumour	Cyclophosphamide	Carmustine[1]	Methotrexate
Mycosis fungoides	Methotrexate	Mechlorethamine	Vinblastine Cyclophosphamide

Table VII. (continued)

Cancer type	Drugs currently preferred	Alternative or secondary drugs	Other drugs with reported activity
Paediatric Solid Tumours			
Wilms' tumor	Dactinomycin (actinomycin D) + vincristine	Doxorubicin	
Ewing's sarcoma	Cyclophosphamide or dactinomycin[2] or vincristine	Doxorubicin	
Embryonal rhabdomyosarcoma	Cyclophosphamide or dactinomycin or vincristine	Doxorubicin	Thiotepa Methotrexate
Retinoblastoma	Cyclophosphamide		
Neuroblastoma	Cyclophosphamide or vincristine	Doxorubicin	Daunorubicin[1] Dacarbazine[2] Vinblastine Prednisone
Osteogenic sarcoma	Doxorubicin or high dose methotrexate + folinic acid 'rescue'	Drug not used for primary treatment	Melphalan Mitomycin Cis-platinum[1]
Solid Tumours			
Adrenocortical carcinoma	Mitotane		
Bladder	Cis-platinum or doxorubicin Thiotepa bladder instillation where indicated	Other drug not used, mitomycin bladder instillation	Fluorouracil Cyclophosphamide
Breast	CMF ± P Cyclophosphamide Methotrexate Fluorouracil Prednisone; *or* Doxorubicin Cyclophosphamide	Doxorubicin + vincristine if CMF ± P used as primary otherwise combination or single agent regimen made up from preferred drugs not previously used (including vincristine)	Vinblastine Thiotepa Melphalan
	Additive (where hormones indicated): diethylstilboestrol, testotactone, tamoxifen, megestrol, depending on menopausal status and tumour hormone receptor studies	Dependent upon response to initial treatment and location of recurrent disease	Ethinyloestradiol Fluoxymesterone
Bronchogenic carcinoma small cell or 'oat cell'	Doxorubicin + cyclophosphamide + vincristine; *or* Cyclophosphamide + lomustine + methotrexate	VP-16 or combination or single agent regimen made up from preferred drugs not previously used	Procarbazine Hexamethylmel-amine[1]
Squamous cell, large cell anaplastic, and adenocarcinoma[3]	Doxorubicin; *or* Cyclophosphamide; *or* Methotrexate	A preferred drug not previously used	
Cervix squamous cell	Mitomycin	Bleomycin	Methotrexate Fluorouracil Vincristine Cyclophosphamide

Table VII. (continued)

Cancer type	Drugs currently preferred	Alternative or secondary drugs	Other drugs with reported activity
Solid Tumours (continued)			
Colon carcinoma	Fluorouracil	Semustine; *or* Mitomycin	Ftorafur[1]
Endometrial carcinoma	Megestrol *or* Hydroxyprogesterone caproate *or* Medroxyprogesterone	Doxorubicin	Fluorouracil[2] Cyclophosphamide
Gastric adenocarcinoma	FAM (fluorouracil, doxorubicin, mitomycin) *or* Fluorouracil + Semustine	Semustine or mitomycin if not used in primary combination	Ftorafur[1]
Head and neck squamous cell	Cis-platinum + bleomycin or methotrexate	Single agent not used in primary treatment	Vinblastine Cyclophosphamide Fluorouracil
Hepatocellular carcinoma, primary[3]	Fluorouracil[2]; *or* Fluorouracil[2] + lomustine[2]	Doxorubicin	Ftorafur[1]
Malignant insulinoma	Streptozocin[1]		
Malignant melanoma	Dacarbazine or semustine[1]		Hydroxyurea
Ovary	Melphalan; *or* Doxorubicin + cyclophosphamide	Doxorubicin; *or* Cis-platinum; *or* Hexamethylmelamine depending upon primary treatment	Fluorouracil Chlorambucil Thiotepa
Pancreatic adenocarcinoma[3]	Fluorouracil	Mitomycin	Ftorafur[1]
Prostate	Diethylstilboestrol	Cyclophosphamide Doxorubicin	Ethinyloestradiol
Sarcomas, miscellaneous	Doxorubicin + dacarbazine[2]	Dactinomycin[2] Cyclophosphamide Vincristine	Methotrexate
Testicular	Vinblastine + bleomycin + cis-platinum; *or* VAB IV (above three plus doxorubicin, dactinomycin, cyclophosphamide)	Mithramycin; *or* Dactinomycin + chlorambucil + methotrexate	Melphalan
Brain neoplasms, primary	Carmustine; *or* Lomustine	Procarbazine[2]	Semustine[1] Mithramycin[2]
Choriocarcinoma	Methotrexate	Dactinomycin Vinblastine Chlorambucil	VP16213[1]
Renal cell[3]	Medroxyprogesterone	Vinblastine	Lomustine

1 Available only for investigational use in the USA.
2 Not approved for this indication by the U.S. Food and Drug Administration.
3 Chemotherapy considered ineffective by some authorities.

Table VIII. Recommended dose reductions in presence of myelosuppression on the day of drug administration

Grade of toxicity	Leucocytes per mm^3	Platelets per mm^3	Percentage of the initial dose that can be administered
0	$\geqslant 4000$	$\geqslant 120,000$	100%: All drugs
1	3999-2500	119,000-80,000	100%: Bleomycin, vincristine, streptozocin 50%: All other drugs
2	< 2500	< 80,000	100%: Bleomycin, all other drugs being withheld until at least grade 1 toxicity is reached

Radioisotopes, although effective, are less readily available. Fractionated total body irradiation, extracorporeal irradiation of the blood, and anti-lymphocyte serum and lymphocytophoresis are experimental treatment methods. Treatment has not significantly influenced the length of survival; the median being 3 years. When to start treating early asymptomatic, so called 'indolent' chronic lymphoid leukaemia is still a matter of debate. It is generally agreed, however, that 'active' disease or complications should be treated.

5.4 Polycythaemia Vera

It is essential to differentiate polycythaemia vera (PV) from stress polycythaemia and secondary erythrocytosis caused by inappropriate or compensatory erythropoietin elaboration. Therapy can be either symptomatic, through the removal of the end product of marrow proliferation by phlebotomy, or more corrective panmyelosis by means of myelosuppressive agents (Gilbert, 1973). Since polycythaemia vera runs a relatively benign and prolonged course, therapy must not be aggressive and should be applicable over extended periods. Radioactive phosphorus (^{32}P) and chemotherapy can probably equally well control the disease. Alkylating agents, including busulphan, chlorambucil, cyclophosphamide, melphalan, and the new agents dibromomannitol and pipobroman are all capable of inducing remissions, but there are few appropriately designed trials comparing the relative merits of these agents. They control the excessive proliferation of all three haematopoietic cell lines in 80 to 90% of cases. ^{32}P is easy to use, its effect is predictable in most cases, its side effects are few and much fewer patient visits are required than for chemotherapy. However, a major concern of its opponents is the risk of leukaemogenic action of ionising irradiation (Huguley, 1972).

Long term studies comparing phlebotomy, alkylating agents and ^{32}P are in progress.

5.5 Myelosclerosis With Myeloid Metaplasia

The management of myelosclerosis with myeloid metaplasia is highly controversial, reflecting the lack of a uniformly effective therapy (Gilbert, 1973). Many asymptomatic patients are better off untreated. Splenectomy has both its proponents and opponents. It may be indicated in selected cases where it can be demonstrated that the spleen is more harmful than beneficial in maintaining normal blood counts. Splenic irradiation, ^{32}P and alkylating agents can reduce spleen size and the peripheral white cell and platelet count, but this is rarely associated with clinical improvement or any prolongation of survival and these measures may precipitate severe cytopenias. Corticosteroids rarely improve haemolytic anaemia. Androgenic anabolic steroids have been useful in some patients to stimulate erythropoiesis (see also chapter XXIII; sect. 6.3).

5.6 Myeloma

Alkylating agents are the only compounds consistently effective in myeloma (Farhangi and Osserman, 1973). Melphalan and cyclophosphamide are equally effective in producing objective improvement (30 to 50%) and in prolonging survival. There is a significant difference in survival between responders (median survival 48 months) and non-responders (9 months). Improved survival is accounted for by time spent in remission. The question of the best schedule, intermittent or continuous, with or without a loading dose, remains unsettled. Patients who have become resistant to melphalan may still respond to cyclophosphamide. Doxorubicin (adriamycin), nitrosoureas, procarbazine and prednisone seem to have a limited effect.

Combination chemotherapy has not been evaluated extensively in myeloma since the choice of effective drugs is limited. Several preliminary reports refer to higher remission rates (60 to 100%) obtained with combinations of 3 to 5 drugs, including several alkylating agents (Salmon, 1976). Cell kinetic studies indicate that recruitment occurs following a good response to alkylating agents. It would be logical to try phase dependent agents at this point in the course of the disease.

Myeloma offers a unique opportunity to monitor the cell kill by following the concentration of M-protein in the serum of 24 hour urine, since these measurements reflect the plasma cell tumour mass. In approximately 10% of patients the M-protein[2] will disappear. These patients are clinically considered to be in complete remission. Such an apparent compete remission caused by alkylating agents is brought about by a reduction in tumour cells of not more than 1 or 2 log. Thus, as in leukaemia, a large number of tumour cells may survive in patients who appear to be in remission. Yet this limited degree of tumour shrinkage may be associated with marked improvement in survival because of the slow growth rate of myeloma.

An increasing number of cases of myeloma are being seen which terminate in an acute leukaemia (Salmon, 1976). It is not known whether these are the result of a terminal dedifferentiation of the plasma cell tumour, or of the carcinogenic effect of the alkylating agents or radiotherapy.

5.7 Malignant Lymphomas

There are at least 10 major variables which need to be considered in attempting to analyse results of lymphoma trials. Pathology is one of the most critical. There is much debate about the optimum pathological classification for the non-Hodgkin's lymphomas in the USA. The Rappaport (Rappaport, 1966) classification has now achieved wide acceptance and for the first time

Table IX. Effectiveness of current chemotherapy

Condition	Response rate[1] (%)
1. *Curative* (in high % of cases)	
Gestational trophoblastic tumours	
Burkitt's tumour	
Hodgkin's disease	
Diffuse histiocytic lymphoma	
Testicular cancer	
2. *Very sensitive to chemotherapy* (high % of responses, long term remissions, prolongation of survival and some cures, even in advanced stages often in combination with surgery and/or radiotherapy)	
Childhood acute lymphoid leukaemia	> 90
Chronic myeloid leukaemia	90
Retinoblastoma	85
Polycythaemia vera	80
Wilms' tumour	80
Childhood rhabdomyosarcoma	65
Chronic lymphoid leukaemia	60
Ewing's sarcoma	60
Oat cell lung cancer	60-75
3. *Moderately sensitive to chemotherapy* (frequent tumour regressions, possibly with prolongation of survival)	
Breast cancer	60
Myeloma	60
Soft tissue sarcomas	60
Osteogenic sarcoma	25-50
Acute myeloid leukaemia	50
Neuroblastoma	50
Myelosclerosis with myeloid metaplasia	30-50
Ovarian cancer	50-60
Head and neck cancer	50-60
Cervix cancer	30-50
Brain tumours	30-50
Bladder	30-50
4. *Relatively resistant to chemotherapy* (tumour regressions in less than one-third; no prolongation of survival)	
Non-oat cell bronchus cancer	30-50
Melanoma	25-40
Gastrointestinal cancer	20-40
Endometrium cancer	30
Renal cancer	20

---

2   M-protein is a 'monoclonal' immunoglobulin or immunoglobulin fragment of uniform antigenicity, mobility and size in serum or urine and is characterised by a sharp homogeneous peak on protein electrophoresis.

---

1   Estimates based on the more effective cytotoxic therapy.

some consistency can be seen in this aspect of clinical trial reporting. It is fervently to be hoped that the current National Cancer Institute (NCI) sponsored study at Stanford University, which is reviewing case material and correlating classifications with clinical results, will lead to an internationally consistent classification.

Another important aspect of pathology in analysing trials is adequate pathology review. In the USA, lymphoma review panels exist which review the slides on study cases to confirm the pathology reported. It has been consistently shown that these panels change a significant number of histological subtype classifications (Lukes and Collins, 1975).

Staging is another critical factor. The Ann Arbor classification is utilised for both Hodgkin's disease and non-Hodgkin's lymphoma. While adequate for Hodgkin's disease, the Ann Arbor staging is suboptimal for the other lymphomas since the stages do not give fully defined prognostic groupings. At some point in the future thought will have to be given to a better staging system for the non-Hodgkin's lymphomas.

With the success of cancer chemotherapy, the importance of the complete remission has been highlighted. The complete remission has a significant implication for long term disease free survival while the partial regression is of minimal impact when survival is examined. Definitions of complete response are becoming more stringent. In comparing clinical trial data, it will be essential to delineate the criteria of complete remission including the 'restaging' procedures which might have been done. Until 'restaging' for delineation of complete remission is widely accepted this will be a complicating factor in analysing clinical trial results from various centres.

5.7.1 Hodgkin's Disease

In evaluating the impact of a therapeutic regimen, the complete response rate is only the beginning of the analysis. It is absolutely essential to have data on disease free remission and survival before a definitive analysis can be made. One of the major complicating factors in this area is the fact that excellent salvage therapy exists after chemotherapy failure, radiation therapy failure or combined modality treatment failure. Recently, the National Cancer Institute in the USA (DeVita et al., 1978) has reported that a significant number of MOPP (table VII) failures can be reinduced into complete remission with MOPP again and that

some have long disease free remissions. In one series, the salvage rate after failure with radiation therapy alone or radiation + MOPP is 45% (Rosenberg et al., 1978). It is higher in those treated with radiation alone as compared with radiation + MOPP, where only nodal relapse could be salvaged. The implication of this is that a regimen might seem superior to another in terms of relapse free survival but show no difference in overall survival because of the ability to salvage patients with relapse.

An example of this can be seen in the study of Rosenberg et al. (1978) in which total nodal radiation (TNR) alone was compared with TNR + MOPP for stage I-III disease. The results with long follow-up showed that the relapse free survival overall was 81% for TNR + MOPP and 61% for TNR alone, but the survival rate was 88% for TNR + MOPP vs 78% for TNR alone; which is not significant. Therefore, while the study could be called positive for adjuvant MOPP in terms of relapse free survival it was negative in terms of overall survival. This is particularly true when it is considered that 61% of the TNR alone group was exposed to MOPP, which was not necessary since TNR alone was curative.

With the increasing data indicating that combined TNR and drugs leads to a significant incidence of secondary acute myeloid leukaemia (section 9) this aspect of chronic toxicity will bear watching in the final analysis.

One of the important emerging concepts coming from combined modality adjuvant trials in general, is that there are two phases of risk vs benefit analysis. The first is relapse vs acute toxicity, while the second is survival vs chronic toxicity. Too great a reliance on the first, especially early in the trial history, can lead to interpretations which will not stand the test of long term follow-up. It will be necessary to alter thinking about long term analysis, by giving thought to how to follow-up on chronic organ damage and the development of second malignancies.

Chemotherapy for advanced stage lymphoma is at a plateau currently in Hodgkin's disease. No regimen has been shown to be clearly superior to the MOPP regimen originally developed at the National Cancer Institute. The Southwest Oncology Group has added bleomycin and is now evaluating a 6 drug approach of MOPP + bleomycin and doxorubicin (adriamycin). While the complete remission rate with MOPP + bleomycin appears higher than with MOPP alone the long term analysis data are not as yet available. The same is

Table X. Attempts to improve on initial induction potential of MOPP (mechlorethamine, vincristine, procarbazine, prednisone)

1. *Additive*
   a) MOPP + bleomycin
   b) MOPP + bleomycin + doxorubicin (adriamycin)

2. *Substitution*
   a) Lomustine, vinblastine, procarbazine, prednisone
   b) Carmustine, vinblastine, procarbazine, prednisone, cyclophosphamide (BCVPP)

3. *Non-cross resistant combinations*
   a) Doxorubicin, bleomycin, vinblastine, dacarbazine (ABVD)
   b) Doxorubicin, bleomycin, vinblastine, streptozocin (ABVS)

true for substitution approaches such as lomustine (CCNU), vinblastine, procarbazine, prednisone of the Cancer and Leukemia Group and the BCVPP (carmustine or BCNU, cyclophosphamide, vinblastine, procarbazine, prednisone) of the Eastern and Southeastern groups in the USA. The newest approach is the integration of non-cross resistant combinations with MOPP, as exemplified by the ABVD regimen of Bonadonna (table X).

The problem of maintenance therapy still remains unresolved. There is no clear evidence that any maintenance therapy evaluated to date is superior to 6 courses of MOPP with no maintenance and salvage therapy upon relapse. Immunotherapy in the maintenance phase is being evaluated by several groups.

5.7.2 Non-Hodgkin's Lymphomas

The chemotherapy of the non-Hodgkin's lymphomas is a complicated picture since there is a need to separate these diseases minimally into a good and poor risk category. The seminal combination regimen for non-Hodgkin's lymphoma is cyclophosphamide, vincristine and prednisone which is called either CVP or COP depending upon how the alkylating agent is given (table XI). For the diffuse histiocytic group of lesions, the addition of doxorubicin alone, or with bleomycin, to COP in regimens such as CHOP and BACOP (table XI) has led to a significant number of long term disease free complete remissions which appear to be cures (Bonadonna and Monfardini, 1974). It is worth noting, however, that C-MOPP

(cyclophosphamide substituted for nitrogen mustard) at the US National Cancer Institute has given results as good as any reported with combinations containing doxorubicin. Little data are currently available on long term complications due to doxorubicin cardiac damage or bleomycin pulmonary damage in this group of patients.

For the good risk categories, the Stanford group (Rosenberg, et al., 1975) has shown that conservative approaches utilising single agent chemotherapy, and occasionally even no initial therapy, can give results equivalent to more intensive combinations. The NCI, however, has recently reported (Schein et al., 1975) what appear to be high cure rates for the nodular lymphoma with combination chemotherapy and it will be of interest to see if this can be confirmed.

As in Hodgkin's disease there is no clear cut evidence that combined radiation and chemotherapy gives superior results to either method used alone as appropriate to stage. There is one positive study at the NCI in Milan (Bonadonna et al., 1975), but other studies are negative and the issue remains to be resolved. One of the current enigmas in cancer treatment is why the combination of drugs and radiation has not been more successful in the lymphomas, since they are both so effective when used alone.

5.7.3 Burkitt's Lymphoma

Burkitt's lymphoma, a highly undifferentiated blastic (immunoblast-like) tumour with a rapid growth rate, is distinguished from other haematosarcomas by its unique sensitivity to single agent therapy, at least in localised stages (Ziegler, 1979). This unusual responsiveness is thought to be related to favourable cell kinetics (rapid proliferation

Table XI. Attempts to improve on initial induction potential of COP/CVP (cyclophosphamide, vincristine, prednisone)

1. *Additive*
   a) COP + bleomycin
   b) COP + doxorubicin/adriamycin (CHOP)
   c) COP + bleomycin + doxorubicin (BACOP)

2. *Substitution*
   a) Doxorubicin, vincristine, prednisone (HOP)
   b) Streptonigrin, vincristine, prednisone
   c) Carmustine, vincristine, prednisone

3. *Non-cross resistant combinations*
   a) Doxorubicin, bleomycin, vinblastine

rate and a high growth fraction) and the participation of the host's immune defenses. A single dose of cyclophosphamide, 40mg/kg intravenously, is capable of inducing long term remission (Ziegler, 1972). More sustained therapy is recommended for more advanced stages. 90% remissions have been obtained in patients relapsing after cyclophosphamide with the sequential use of vincristine, methotrexate and cytarabine (Ziegler, 1979). CNS involvement, as in childhood acute lymphoid leukaemia, is a frequent problem.

6. Solid Tumours

The results of chemotherapy of solid tumours in general have not been as dramatic, with a few exceptions, as in haematological malignancies (table IX). Most solid tumours have a low growth fraction and are therefore less sensitive to cycle- or phase specific agents. Attempts are made to convert the malignant cells making up solid tumours to logarithmic growth (recruitment), by treatment with non-cycle dependent agents or by reducing the tumour load by preliminary surgery or radiotherapy. The current trend is to explore combination chemotherapy in most solid tumours. Some investigators attempt to exploit synchronisation and potentiation phenomena in the hope of augmenting cell kill (Carter et al., 1977).

Reports on solid tumour chemotherapy are generally difficult to evaluate and especially to compare. There are few controlled studies. Patient selection may be different with respect to the extent of the disease or histological variants. Different criteria are used to evaluate the responses: survival, tumour regression, performance status, or subjective response. Some investigators require tumour regression to last for a minimum of 3 months, while others accept a regression of not more than 2 weeks as a response. This explains, for instance, how a response rate ranging from 8 to 85% has been reported for 5-fluorouracil in colon cancer.

Until 1950 there was essentially no effective treatment for disseminated malignancies. Since that time significant progress has been made in cancer chemotherapy. Today, a normal life expectancy, thus hopefully a cure, can be obtained with chemotherapy alone in Burkitt's tumour and gestational choriocarcinoma; two disseminated malignancies. A normal life expectancy is nowadays also possible in several other haematological malignancies and solid tumours, by combining chemotherapy with surgery and/or radiotherapy. Most of these tumours are relatively rare and occur predominantly in children and young adults. However, before the advent of chemotherapy, normal life expectancy was negligible in these malignancies.

In some of the more common solid tumours, for instance of the breast, prostate and ovary, significant palliation and some prolongation of survival is obtained. Unfortunately, the majority of patients with inoperable cancer fall into the category where chemotherapy produces tumour regressions in fewer than one third of patients. These regressions are usually of short duration and do not improve survival substantially.

6.1 Breast Cancer

The treatment of advanced breast cancer is a sequential mixture of hormonal and cytotoxic therapy which varies from patient to patient depending upon: (1) menstrual status; (2) age; (3) disease free interval after surgical treatment; (4) extent and location of metastases; (5) rapidity of tumour growth; and (6) previous response of metastatic disease to hormonal manipulation or positive assay for oestrogen receptors (Davis and Carbone, 1978; Kennedy, 1974). No standard regimen exists for treating every patient with disseminated breast cancer. Most clinicians divide women into three broad categories based on menopausal status and proceed on to treatment sequences which utilise initial hormonal therapy of some type unless the disease involves lymphangitic pulmonary metastases, symptomatic liver metastases or some evidence of rapid growth.

6.1.1 Initial Therapy in Advanced Breast Cancer

Castration is the usual therapy for the premenopausal woman. In most treatment centres surgical oophorectomy is preferred over radiation castration. This approach yields responses of 20 to 40%. The best responses occur in women from 35 to 45 years of age. Younger women and those with rapidly progressive disease should be treated initially with chemotherapy (i.e. cytotoxic drugs) since they are less likely to benefit from castration. The premenopausal women who respond to castration have a reasonable likelihood of responding to a second hormonal treatment. Some clinicians prefer the additive use of androgens while others lean toward the surgical ablative procedures of either bilateral adrenalectomy or hypophysectomy. A cogent argument can also be made to utilise chemotherapy at this time since the response rates reported are higher than those for secondary hormonal treatment. The premenopausal women who fail to respond to oophorectomy have a poor prognosis and chemotherapy should be the next therapy attempted.

Women 6 months to 5 years postmenopausal are a difficult group in which to prescribe treatment. Castration gives a low response rate as does additive hormonal treatment. The utilisation of chemotherapy for initial treatment is one valid alternative in this situation. The major ablative procedures can be done initially, with castration added to adrenalectomy, and the reported response rate is about 30%. Chemotherapy gives comparable to higher response rates, although with a somewhat shorter duration of remission. Patients with liver metastases do poorly with ablative procedures and should go initially to chemotherapy. The best group in which to consider this approach is women who have relatively slow growing bone metastases or advanced local disease with a free interval of more than 2 years duration.

The traditional approach to women more than five years postmenopausal is therapy with oestrogens. The older the patient the higher the potential response, and in women over 70 with predominant cutaneous or lymph node metastases the response rate may approach 50%. Androgens can also be used and for women with bone metastases may be equal in efficacy to oestrogens. In this group of patients, chemotherapy response rates are also higher and a valid approach could be to utilise chemotherapy from the initial point of relapse.

Several general points concerning the therapy of recurrent breast cancer are as follows:

1) Local disease can be treated with radiotherapy only, which can be highly effective for symptomatic relief.

2) A second 'withdrawal response' sometimes occurs after hormonal treatment is stopped because the patients have ceased to respond. Therefore, further therapy should be withheld whenever possible until it is decided that a withdrawal remission is unlikely.

3) Major endocrine ablation (hypophysectomy or adrenalectomy) should not be performed in patients with lymphangitic lung metastases, brain metastases or hepatic metastases with jaundice.

4) Patients should be watched carefully for the first few weeks of androgen or oestrogen treatment because these hormones occasionally exacerbate the tumour. Fulminant hypercalcaemia, although uncommon, may lead to death if untreated. Other adverse effects are increased bone pain or rapid development of new skin metastases.

A new approach involves the utilisation of antioestrogens, such as tamoxifen, especially in postmenopausal women (Heel, et al., 1978). Response rates close to 50% can be achieved with durations of response of more than a year. Tamoxifen is rapidly replacing oestrogens as the preferred initial hormonal therapy for postmenopausal women.

6.1.2 Role of Chemotherapy in Breast Cancer

Breast cancer is a disease which is in the forefront of much that is happening with chemotherapy and can be viewed as the solid tumour for which the most data exists in which to evaluate the various roles for drug treatment. The traditional role of chemotherapy in the treatment of breast cancer has been for the palliation of patients with disseminated disease who have failed hormonal manipulation or for whom surgery would not be applicable. Much of the available literature describes results of chemotherapy in patients treated only after primary or secondary hormone treatments had failed and thus were far advanced, often with poor performance abilities, heavily pretreated and with a large tumour burden. Despite this, a wide range of chemotherapeutic agents have been shown to be active (Carter, 1972) and have served as the basis for the development of successful combination approaches.

5-Fluorouracil has been the most extensively studied drug and has probably been the most commonly used non-hormonal agent for breast cancer study. Among the alkylating agents, all of which have similar activity rates, cyclophosphamide is the most commonly used agent and has been the alkylating agent used in almost all combinations. Doxorubicin (adriamycin) is perhaps the most active of all the single agents. Methotrexate and the *Vinca* alkaloids have been less commonly used as single agents by practicing oncologists but their clear cut activity has led to their inclusion in combination studies.

The common denominator in the development of almost all successful combination chemotherapy regimens, such as those for leukaemia, lymphoma, and testicular tumours, has been the availability of drugs active as single agents, with different mechanisms of action and without completely overlapping toxicity patterns. This potential has existed for breast cancer for a long period of time (Greenspan, 1966). A five drug combination (cyclophosphamide, methotrexate, fluorouracil, vincristine, prednisone; CMFVP) originally developed by Cooper, has been shown subsequently to be effective in about half the cases treated (Broder and Tormey, 1974). Dissection of the CMFVP regimen has involved removing 1 or 2 drugs and most of these 3 or 4 drug combinations have achieved response rates similar to those reported for the 5 drug approach. Some such regimens have dropped vincristine, while others have dropped both vincristine and prednisone. This latter regimen (CMF) also has activity in excess of 50% and is now one of the major commonly used combinations.

Doxorubicin still appears to be the most active of the single agents for the treatment of advanced breast cancer with a reported cumulative response rate of 43% for previously untreated patients. The rate falls to 26% for previously treated patients (Carter, 1974). When pretherapeutic variables are looked at, the site of the dominant lesion appears to be the most critical. Thus the response rate is 60% for soft tissue, 42% for visceral and only 10% for bone. In comparison, cyclophosphamide gives a 24% response rate in bone and 5-fluorouracil a 28% response rate. The chemotherapy of advanced disease breast cancer appears to have reached a temporary plateau. The promise of the 5 drug Cooper regimen and doxorubicin have been confirmed, but the ability to increase response rates beyond 50 to 65% appears to be stalled. More importantly, the complete response rate has not risen and the survival figures in most series tend to be very similar. It is hard to understand why, with 6 active drug classes to manipulate, oncologists treating advanced breast cancer have not been able to improve results in the last 5 years.

Today, the exciting new development is adjuvant drug treatment after mastectomy.

In 1972, the National Cancer Institute in the USA launched a large scale controlled trial of the use of chemotherapy as an adjuvant to surgical operation in women in whom cancer had already spread. This study was carried out by the National Surgical Adjuvant Breast Project (NSABP). Half of the women were given L-phenylalanine mustard (L-PAM) after radical mastectomy and half were given a placebo (Fisher et al., 1975). Treatment failures occurred in 22% of 108 patients receiving placebo and in 9.3% of 103 women given L-phenylalanine mustard. This difference was only statistically significant for premenopausal women and continued follow-up has shown no meaningful difference for postmenopausal women.

In 1973, Bonadonna at the National Cancer Institute of Milan began a study identical to Fisher's except that the chemotherapy was CMF (cyclophosphamide, methotrexate, fluorouracil), which had been found to be superior to L-PAM in advanced disease (Bonadonna et al., 1976). At the time of this first report, only 5.3% of 207 women who received the CMF regimen had recurrence of cancer, as opposed to 24% of 179 women who had surgery only. However, the patients in the study had been followed for an average of only 14 months. In the most recent analysis of these data (3 years after mastectomy), the total failure rate was 45.7% in control patients compared with 26.3% in women given CMF (Bonadonna et al., 1977). New disease manifestations were higher in the subgroup having 4 or more nodes (37.9% vs 19.1%). After 12 months of analysis, however, there was no difference in the recurrence rate for postmenopausal women. At 3 years, the failure rate in postmenopausal women was 40.1% in control vs 36.2% in the CMF group. When the control group is analysed, it is seen that premenopausal patients show a higher incidence of early recurrence compared with postmenopausal patients. In the CMF treated women, the failure rate was comparable in both the pre and postmenopausal groups.

Most patients receiving the CMF regimen complained of various degrees of nausea and vomiting within a few hours after the drug injection. In more than two thirds of the patients, the daily administration of cyclophosphamide caused prolonged nausea and loss of appetite. Some patients showed a repeated tendency to discontinue treatment or diminish the dose to decrease the abdominal discomfort.

In the large majority of patients, myelosuppression has been the signal to limit the dose. Severe leucopenia and/or thrombocytopenia were rare and no one required transfusion of white blood cells or platelets. Stomatitis was observed in 19% of patients, but was mild and promptly reversible. Some degree of alopecia occurred in 69% of the women, but only 5% required a wig. Cystitis secondary to cyclophosphamide occurred in 30% but haemorrhagic cystitis was documented in only 2 cases.

Despite the variety of toxic manifestations, CMF was, in general, fairly well tolerated. All patients were treated as outpatients and the large majority continued to work while on therapy.

The updated results of the CMF study leave us in a difficult position. On the one hand, the overall study in terms of relapse rate still favours the CMF regimen over the control in a statistically significant manner.

The same is true of Fisher's L-PAM study (Fisher and Redmund, 1977). On the other hand when post-menopausal women with positive nodes are looked at separately, there is no evidence to support adjunctive chemotherapy, at least as prescribed to date. If one reads Bonadonna's original paper carefully, it can be seen that he stated that the 'results should be considered with caution, since, at present the effects of this therapy on survival and possible long-term side effects remain unknown'. He indicated that, while the results were 'promising,' the optimism should be tempered by the consideration that it is too early to tell whether CMF therapy was merely delaying recurrence or actually lengthening survival. Since breast cancer is a chronic disease which may reappear as many as 20 years after initial surgical operation, there is validity to the above statement. Fisher also cautioned about the preliminary nature of his study. Unfortunately, these cautions were not heeded and the studies were highly publicised in a manner which suggested that a clearcut therapeutic triumph had occurred.

It is clear that we cannot meaningfully analyse adjuvant studies for at least several years in terms of making therapeutic recommendations to the public. In the CMF update, there is no statistically significant survival gain overall for the treated group and it will be years before the definitive analysis can be undertaken.

6.2 Large Bowel Cancer

5-Fluorouracil (5-FU) is the standard single agent for the therapy of advanced large bowel cancer. An overall response rate of 20 % has been observed (Carter, 1976b). The most commonly utilised approach to administering fluorouracil is the loading course schedule in which the drug is given daily for 5 days and then possibly every other day for several additional doses. A wide range of additional approaches have been devised for administering the drug, including 2-, 8-, and 24-hour infusions, administration by weekly injection or by an intensive course followed by weekly injection administration in 5 % or 10 % dextrose, and oral use in capsules or liquid form. There is considerable evidence that a change in the duration of frequency of administration alters the intensity of the overall pharmacological effect of fluorouracil (Moertel and Reitemeier, 1969), but no definitive evidence that this is accompanied by tolerance superior to that of the loading course approach.

One of the latest approaches to fluorouracil therapy has involved a resurgence of interest in oral administration (Hahn et al., 1975). With the oral route, twice the dose is required to reach a degree of marrow toxicity equal to that induced by rapid intravenous injection. Oral administration also produces a higher incidence of gastrointestinal toxicity. More importantly, the response rate with oral therapy is much less than with parenteral administration. The duration of response is also significantly shorter with the oral drug, even in patients with metastatic disease in the liver. Plasma concentrations of fluorouracil after oral administration are substantially more erratic than after intravenous administration and bioavailability also varies widely among patients, generally being low (Christophidis et al., 1978). Bioavailability increases markedly with the size of the oral dose, suggesting saturation of the 'first-pass' hepatic metabolism of the drug and the need for study of individualised dosage of orally administered drug (Christophidis et al., 1978; Sadee and Wong, 1977). At this time, the oral approach to therapy with fluorouracil cannot be recommended for routine use.

Another drug with evidence of activity in colorectal cancer, is mitomycin C, which was originally isolated and developed in Japan. A review of the Japanese literature has shown 50 regressions in 154 patients with gastrointestinal cancer (Frank and Osterberg, 1960). At the Mayo Clinic in the USA, only 6 objective regressions in 56 patients with large bowel cancer were observed and these were of short duration. Although the drug is capable of inducing regressions in large bowel cancer, its marked potential for marrow toxicity and the hazard of infiltration ulcers limits its use.

Among newer agents, the nitrosoureas developed in the USA, have shown some level of activity. Studies at the Mayo Clinic have shown response rates of 12.5 % with carmustine, 10 % with lomustine and 17.5 % with semustine (Moertel, 1973). Semustine appears to be at least equal to, or perhaps slightly better, than fluorouracil (Moertel et al., 1975). Another compound, razoxane (ICRF-159), has also shown a response rate of 12 % in US studies (Carter et al., 1977).

In the past few years various drug combinations have been tested in the search for more effective chemotherapy of gastrointestinal cancer. None have been shown to be clearly superior to single agent fluorouracil therapy. Studies utilising fluorouracil as an adjuvant to surgery in the hope of eradicating the microscopic foci of metastatic disease remaining after surgery, have not been significantly successful and this approach cannot be routinely recommended.

6.3 Gastric Cancer

The two major drugs which are commonly utilised to treat gastric cancer are fluorouracil and mitomycin C (Comis and Carter, 1974b). Fluorouracil is the most extensively studied single agent for the treatment of gastric carcinoma.

Studies have shown that fluorouracil added to radiotherapy can enhance survival in patients with locally unresectable disease. The overall objective response rate with fluorouracil is 20 to 25%, with an average 4 to 5 month duration of response. In spite of the relatively large number of patients treated with fluorouracil, there has rarely been a systematic analysis of factors such as age, sex, disease free interval, histological grade of the tumour, or sites of metastasis, which might predispose to a favourable or unfavourable response.

In Japan, the most commonly utilised drug is mitomycin C and it has been the second most frequently used drug in the United States. The daily schedule of administration has proven to have marked toxicity, a narrow therapeutic index and a potential for delayed and persistent haematopoietic toxicity.

Mitomycin C generally causes delayed cumulative toxicity, which probably explains the difficulty in giving prolonged courses and favours use of a high intermittent schedule where the toxicity observed in one course can be used to adjust the dose in subsequent courses. Renal toxicity has been described and may be more pronounced with the high intermittent dose schedule.

The overall objective response rate is between 20 to 30% with the higher response rates being reported in Japanese data. The average duration of response ranges from 1 to 3 months.

The nitrosoureas (carmustine, lomustine, semustine) have shown some evidence of activity. Carmustine has yielded an objective response rate of near 20% and an average duration of response of 4.5 months in gastric cancer patients, most of whom had no prior therapy (Moertel, 1975). Recently, evidence of activity has been seen with doxorubicin (adriamycin), with an approximate response rate of 25% (Comis and Carter, 1974b).

Combination approaches have been more successful in stomach cancer than in any other gastro-intestinal neoplasm (Comis and Carter, 1974a). Higher response rates than single agent therapy have been achieved with a combination of fluorouracil, mitomycin C and cytarabine. A response rate of around 40% can be attained with the combination of fluorouracil + carmustine; with survival superior to either agent alone. More recently, the combination of fluorouracil and semustine has achieved these high response rates (Moertel, 1975).

The utilisation of chemotherapy as an adjuvant to surgery has been extensively evaluated in Japan, the USSR and the USA. The Japanese have studied predominantly mitomycin C alone or in combination. While a few results are positive, most studies have not shown a meaningful survival gain.

In the United States, studies with thiotepa and 5-fluorouridine, an analogue of fluorouracil, have all been negative but all utilised short term regimens of chemotherapy. Current trials involve long term administration of semustine plus fluorouracil (Comis and Carter, 1974a).

6.4 Lung Cancer

Bronchogenic carcinoma is now the most common malignancy among men in many countries and the leading cause of death from cancer in that group. The data in over 22,000 cases analysed in the USA from 1955 to 1964 show that only 21% of the patients could receive a surgical resection at the time of diagnosis (Selawry and Hansen, 1973). In this group, the overall 5 year survival rate was 7% with an observed median survival time of 0.4 years. For 4193 cases that were localised at diagnosis, the 5 year survival was 24% with a 1.1 year median survival time. Unfortunately, the percentage of cases with localised disease at diagnosis has remained stable since 1940.

The situation is truly dismal in patients who are considered inoperable at the time of diagnosis. The Veterans Administration Lung Cancer Study Group of the US, has reported an analysis by extent of disease, as well as histological type, in a series of inoperable patients who received only supportive therapy (Roswit et al., 1968). Patients with tumour clinically confined to one hemithorax (i.e. within the confines of a single radiotherapy portal) were termed as having 'limited' disease and all others as 'extensive' disease. In 130 patients with limited disease, the median survival time was 15.7 weeks from the time the patient was deemed inoperable, while in extensive disease the median survival time was only 9.4 weeks.

Efforts to improve these dismal results by radiotherapy and chemotherapy have so far met with very limited success. Patients with limited disease may experience some improvement in survival from radiotherapy alone. A large scale randomised study of radiation therapy versus placebo, showed that treated patients survived about 20 % longer than untreated controls (Roswit et al., 1968). The effect of radiotherapy on limited disease may be particularly true for the squamous cell types, with a median survival time of 60 weeks in such patients, versus 25 weeks in a group receiving single drug therapy in one study (Green et al., 1969). However, other studies have failed to demonstrate improved survival, even in limited disease, for patients receiving radiotherapy.

Small cell carcinoma of the lung is a single bright spot in what is otherwise a dismal picture of lung cancer treatment. This type of lung cancer accounts for 15 % to 20 % of all tumours diagnosed. The results of therapy for small cell are so dramatically superior to those for the other cell types that it is now commonplace for clinical trials to be specifically designed for this cell type. The rest of the cell types are now described in negative terminology as 'non-oat' cell or 'non-small cell'. Small cell is the preferred terminology over oat cell by many because the oat shaped cell is only one of several configurations which can be seen in tumours of this kind.

Small cell carcinoma of the lung is characterised by rapidity of growth and a very high potential for extrapulmonary metastatic spread. In one series (Broder et al., 1977), extrathoracic metastases were diagnosed in 84 % of cases at the time of initial diagnosis and the rarity of surgical cure indicates that microscopic dissemination has occurred in nearly every case.

Common metastatic sites of spread for small cell lung cancer include mediastinal and supraclavicular lymph nodes, liver, bone marrow, brain and adrenals. Liver metastases have been seen in up to 42 % of patients when an extensive pretreatment review, including peritoneoscopy, is performed. Bone marrow involvement, as demonstrated by bone marrow biopsy, has been reported to be as high as 45 %. Clinically apparent brain metastases were observed in 30 % of one large series and at autopsy were seen in 45 % in another series (Broder et al., 1977).

The diagnosis of small cell lung cancer is now considered a contraindication to surgical resection and in the American Joint Committee staging, the diagnosis automatically places the patient into a stage III category. Radiotherapy is an effective treatment for producing palliative remissions, particularly when bronchial, tracheal or superior vena caval obstructions or painful bone lesions are present. The optimum dose and fractionation schedule of radiation has not been well delineated. The range of doses for so called radical radiotherapy has varied from 3000 rads delivered in 2 weeks to 6500 rads in 7 weeks. Objective evidence of tumour shrinkage can be seen with effective radiation in up to 90 % of cases treated (Broder et al., 1977).

Small cell lung cancer is a tumour which is sensitive to a wide range of anticancer drugs. There are 8 drugs which are considered to be active in this tumour — cyclophosphamide; doxorubicin (adriamycin), lomustine; methotrexate; vincristine; procarbazine; etoposide (VP16213); and hexamethylmelamine. While all of these drugs can shrink tumour masses to some degree, their impact on survival when used alone is minimal. They do however, offer a significant basis for developing combination chemotherapy regimens and many have been shown to be superior to single agent therapy (Broder et al., 1977).

While all small cell lung cancer is AJC stage III by definition, staging is still important in this tumour. The critical separation performed by staging involves 'limited' vs 'extensive' disease. Limited disease is disease which clinically involves only one hemithorax inclusive of the ipsilateral supraclavicular lymph node. The percentage of patients in any series defined as having limited disease will depend to some degree upon how thorough staging has been. The major therapeutic implication of staging is the indication for the administration of radiation with meaningful benefit when routinely done for extensive disease patients. The common approach in most centres today is to treat limited disease patients with an intensive combined modality approach, while extensive disease falls mainly to combination chemotherapy alone, with radiation used for CNS prophylaxis.

When the extensively studied combinations are examined (Broder et al., 1977), cyclophosphamide appears to be a nearly universal component. This is followed closely by vincristine which is included because it combines activity with lack of myelosuppression. The most commonly reported combinations are the three drug approaches in which either methotrexate or doxorubicin (adriamycin) are added to the basic regimen of cyclophosphamide plus vincristine (e.g. Livingston et al., 1978). In terms of overall response rate, there is little basis for choice of one over the other. The ultimate analysis in this disease will involve the complete response rate, its duration and overall survival.

This type of therapy involving combinations of drugs and radiotherapy is not without its risks and requires a team approach involving an experienced medical oncologist or radiation oncologist. It is not therapy to be undertaken by a practitioner with only casual experience in cancer therapy. Moreover, treatment schedules are exacting, since there are so many variables to consider. These include the radiation dose and fractionation schedule, the radiation ports, drugs used and their dose schedules as well as the sequence of drugs and radiation. Other considerations in programming treatment include extent of disease, performance status, prior therapy, associated disease conditions and all the other prognostic variables.

At this time, no single approach can be recommended as definitive. It appears that intensive therapy with a combination of drugs and radiation offers a significant potential for induction of complete remission. The drug combinations all include cyclophosphamide and the additional drugs can be vincristine and methotrexate, or vincristine and doxorubicin or lomustine, and methotrexate or some other combination. Continued research is needed so that the complete remission rate can be maximised and then maintenance therapy developed which will optimise long term disease free control.

There appear to be several major obstacles to further progress in the treatment of small cell lung cancer, in spite of its sensitivity to drugs and radiation. Perhaps most importantly, resistance to a given drug regimen develops rather rapidly. Once the patient has relapsed, it is unusual to see a response to subsequent chemotherapy, with the possible exception of vincristine (Broder et al., 1977). Thus, survival beyond the point of disease progression usually approximates that of an untreated patient — about 6 to 8 weeks.

Small cell lung cancer is a disease which should be treated as intensively as possible with complete remission as the goal. Those patients who attain complete remission can obtain a significant survival prolongation. Disease free remissions in excess of 2 years are no longer uncommon (Broder et

al., 1977). This tumour should be approached in a similar fashion as acute leukaemia in adults where intensive therapy and intensive supportive care are standard approaches.

6.5 Malignant Melanoma

Dacarbazine (DTIC) has been the most extensively studied single agent in malignant melanoma (Comis and Carter, 1974c). The overall response rate for this drug is 25 % in over 800 cases recently reviewed, with great consistency in many large series. Complete response rates of 5 to 6 % have been consistently observed. In the reports on all major series, responders have lived longer than non-responders, as might be expected. In view of the propensity of malignant melanoma to metastasise to the brain, the nitrosourea class of antitumour compounds are of particular interest because of their relatively high lipid solubility and ability to cross the blood-brain barrier. The first generation nitrosourea, carmustine (BCNU), has undergone extensive clinical trials. Published data, relating only to objective response rate, are currently available for 122 patients showing a response rate of 13 %. Lomustine (CCNU), the first oral congener of carmustine, has achieved an objective response rate of 13 % in 133 patients with disseminated malignant melanoma. Semustine (methyl CCNU), which is the newest nitrosourea to enter clinical trials, has shown response rates in excess of 20 % and appears to be as clinically effective as dacarbazine (Wittes et al., 1977b).

While combination chemotherapy has been extensively investigated, no regimen is clearly superior to single agents and this approach can not be recommended.

Malignant melanoma is a complex disease in which not only the clinical stage, but also the level of invasion of the primary lesion, and possibly patient immunocompetence, strongly affect prognosis. The vast majority of patients die from disseminated disease, which at presentation is already beyond the scope of the primary local treatment method. Chemotherapy is the only systemic method of treatment possessing a well documented potential for tumour cell kill in advanced disease. Immunotherapy, although less well documented, may be capable of controlling subclinical disease, occasionally widespread subcutaneous disease, and possibly enhancing the effect of chemotherapy in advanced disease. The integration of these treatment methods in a multifaceted adjuvant attack on disease in high risk patients might lead to greater control or actual eradication of the subclinical disease to which these patients ultimately succumb (Comis and Carter, 1974c).

6.6 Ovarian Cancer

Alkylating agents have been utilised more extensively in patients with advanced ovarian cancer than any other class of chemotherapeutic agents. The initial response rates for various drugs in this class are around 30 to 65%, with 5 to 15% of all treated patients continuing to respond 2 years after initiation of therapy (Young et al., 1974b).

Available information does not suggest particular advantages for one alkylating agent over another and all appear to have approximately equal activity. Furthermore, no particular dose or schedule has been shown to be superior as similar response rates have been achieved with daily oral doses, oral loading doses, and intermittent intravenous doses.

Intraperitoneal administration of alkylating agents has been frequently advocated, although there is little evidence that it is effective or even equivalent to the effect of the same agent administered systemically. Generally, the intraperitoneal use of alkylating agents has been reported to be less effective than the intravenous use of the same drug and dosage.

Patients with ovarian carcinoma who have received previous therapy will be less responsive to subsequent treatment with alkylating agents. In a large series where cyclophosphamide was used, there was a 75% response rate in previously untreated patients but only a 42% response rate in those relapsing after, or refractory to radiotherapy (DeVita et al., 1976).

Alkylating agent chemotherapy as an adjuvant to initial surgery or radiotherapy in localised disease is currently of considerable interest, although few such studies have been published (Young, 1975). At this time one cannot make definite conclusions but further exploration of adjuvant chemotherapy in stage I disease is warranted and is in progress in several randomised clinical trials.

Drugs other than the alkylating agents have been investigated much less completely in ovarian carcinoma. In such cases, patients have often failed therapy with alkylating agents, as well as radiation therapy, and might therefore be expected to respond poorly to subsequent chemotherapy.

The antimetabolite 5-fluorouracil has been the most extensively studied of the non-alkylating agents and, regardless of schedule, appears to achieve a response rate of approximately 32% (Young, 1975). Because of the extensive prior chemotherapy and/or radiotherapy that many of the patients received, direct comparison of the activity of fluorouracil with that of the alkylating agents is not possible from the retrospective data.

Hexamethylmelamine has shown consistent activity in several trials against ovarian cancer (Wampler et al., 1972). It is a derivative of the alkylating agent triethylenemelamine but is not felt to act primarily as an alkylating agent and has dose limiting gastrointestinal and neurotoxicity, rather than causing bone marrow suppression. Furthermore, it is now clear that the drug is active in some patients with ovarian carcinoma who have become refractory to conventional alkylating agents.

The only antitumour antibiotic which has been studied in any detail is doxorubicin (adriamycin). In a number of studies it is active as a single agent in both previously untreated patients and in those who have failed to respond to alkylating agent therapy. The overall response rate collected from the literature is around 33% (Carter et al., 1977). Only a small number of studies of combination chemotherapy have been published in which more than a few patients with ovarian carcinoma were included. There are no data to support routine use of any combination at this time.

6.7 Head and Neck Cancer

The prognosis for patients with recurrent or disseminated head and neck cancer is generally dismal. Survival data for such patients are not readily available, but survival is often less than 6 months. This occurs despite the ability of several drugs to shrink tumour measurably. The reason for the lack of much impact of single agents on survival, even in responders, probably lies in the shortness of response duration; which is generally of the order of 8 weeks or less with the two most active agents, methotrexate and bleomycin (Bertino et al., 1975).

The major difficulty in evaluating data for chemotherapy in head and neck cancer is that the data tend to ignore the heterogeneity of sites and histologies which comprise this group of tumours. In those series in which response by site is analysed, the large number of sites comprising head and neck cancer results in fragmentation of the data into numbers too small to be meaningful (Bertino et al., 1973). When one considers that for each site there are important subcategories such as stage, histology, prior therapy, nutritional status, and performance status, then the numbers available for analysis with any given regimen become considerably smaller.

The fact that single agent chemotherapy has not been more extensively studied in head and neck cancer is partially accounted for by the generally debilitated state of these patients at the time when initiation of systemic chemotherapy is contemplated. This limitation is further enhanced by the general inability of these patients to sustain their nutritional status during therapy because of local tumour, radiation induced fibrosis, surgical defects, and orocutaneous fistulas. Such factors, coupled with the common side effects of most anticancer drugs, account for the general decline of these patients even when significant tumour regression is accomplished.

Methotrexate is the drug which has been most extensively studied in head and neck cancer (Goldsmith and Carter, 1975). While the data are extensive there is controversy about how best to give the drug. Variables which can be found in the literature include the route of administration, the schedule of administration, the dose level and the use of 'rescue' with calcium folinate.

When all the data are analysed, intermittent parenteral methotrexate appears to be at least as good as any other approach. The intra-arterial approach results in no higher a response rate, despite careful patient selection inherent in the procedure. In addition, the toxicity of treatment is greater. The high dose methotrexate approach with folinic acid 'rescue' does not result in higher response rates (Goldsmith and Carter, 1975). The toxicity of this approach may be less in very experienced hands, but the morbidity factor is still highly significant.

Bleomycin is the second most studied agent in head and neck cancer. It is the generic name for a group of antibiotics isolated in Japan from *Streptomyces verticillus* (Goldsmith and Carter, 1975). The optimum dosage is 0.25 to 0.50 unit/kg administered twice weekly or weekly, either intravenously or intramuscularly. Cis-platinum diammine dichloride (DDP) is a new investigational agent which has demonstrated activity in head and neck cancer. Structurally, it is an inorganic complex formed by a central atom of platinum sur-

rounded by chlorine and ammonia ions in the cis position in the horizontal plane. The mechanism of antitumour action of cis-platinum has not been fully elucidated (Rosencweig et al., 1977). In the early studies with the drug in which it was given by intravenous push, toxicities observed included dose related renal damage, myelosuppression, nausea and vomiting and hearing loss. While activity was observed in a range of solid tumours, the renal toxicity in particular appeared to limit the usefulness of the drug. Recently, it has been shown that, in most patients, even high doses of platinum are tolerated without significant renal impairment, provided care is taken to maintain adequate hydration before the drug is administered and if a vigorous osmotic diuresis with mannitol and half normal saline is maintained during and after platinum administration (Wittes et al., 1975, 1977a). However, hearing loss including total deafness can occur (Wittes et al., 1975).

It is quite apparent from the available data to date that there has not yet been a clear delineation of the role of chemotherapy in combination with surgery and radiotherapy in the treatment of early head and neck cancer. There is evidence suggesting that therapeutic enhancement by chemotherapy can be obtained in tumours at specific sites such as the oral cavity and the maxillary sinuses. However, there has been no demonstration that intra-arterial perfusion affords better results than those obtained by systemic administration of the same drug. Similarly, no judgements can be made of the relative efficacy of one drug over another as an adjuvant to surgery and radiotherapy.

6.8 Sarcomas

Considerable progress has been made in recent years in the treatment of both soft tissue and bony sarcomas. This has been due to the introduction of new drugs, more effective ways of using established drugs and better integration of combined methods of treatment.

Although for localised tumours surgery is still the most effective treatment, it may require mutilating ablations to reach all of the tumour. Where less radical surgery is employed, recurrences are frequent as they are with radiotherapy used alone, but stage, type and site of presentation of the tumour influence results. Soft tissue sarcomas are a group of tumours consisting of a variety of malignancies derived from mesenchymal tissue, and their histological appearance frequently presents histopathological difficulties so that no definitive diagnosis can be made.

Until the advent of doxorubicin (adriamycin), the use of chemotherapy for bone or soft tissue sarcomas, after the failure of primary therapy with surgery or radiotherapy, had not been very successful. Jacobs (1970), in a review of the literature, noted that treatment with an alkylating agent (usually cyclophosphamide), actinomycin D (dactinomycin) and vincristine given alone or in combination yeilded an objective response rate in about 25 % of patients. When childhood rhabdomyosarcomas, which are relatively sensitive to chemotherapeuitc agents, are removed from consideration, the response rate is only about 20 %. There were few long term remissions on these regimens.

Doxorubicin has been active against sarcomas in both adults and children. The overall response rate is 25 % for sarcomas of all types and is roughly equivalent for soft tissue sarcomas and bone and joint sarcomas (Carter, 1975). However, a combination of doxorubicin and dacarbazine is more effective; an objective response being achieved in around 40 % of patients (Gottlieb et al., 1972). Although there are some minor differences in response rates by cell type, the number of cases per cell type is not sufficient to demonstrate significant differences. Both drugs can be given in combined doses nearly equivalent to those used for each as a single agent. The addition of vincristine to this combination does not improve the induction rate but may increase survival (Gottlieb et al., 1974).

The response may however, be increased to around 60 % by a regimen of doxorubicin, dacarbazine, vincristine and cyclophosphamide (Gottlieb et al., 1974). The regimen is given intravenously in courses every 21 days as follows: doxorubicin $50mg/m^2$, day 1; cyclophosphamide, $500mg/m^2$, day 1; dacarbazine, $250mg/m^2$, days 1-5; and vincristine, $1mg/m^2$, days 1-5. Dose limiting toxicity has been transient leucopenia in a third of patients, but serious infections have been rare.

This combination regimen appears to represent a significant advance in the therapy of those with metastatic sarcoma.

Currently, a wide range of combinations with doxorubicin is being investigated, and only time will tell which combination, if any, will be superior to the 2 drug combination of doxorubicin plus dacarbazine.

6.9 Testicular Cancer

Testicular malignancy represents approximately 1 to 2 % of all malignant tumours of males. It is the most common malignant tumour among men between the ages of 29 to 35 years and most tumours occur between the ages of 20 and 40 (Rubin, 1970). As these tumours generally occur in men in the prime of life, the psychological impact of the disease is great. Chemotherapy however, offers an exciting new curative potential in testicular tumours.

Testicular tumours are sensitive to a wide range of anticancer drugs. In fact, there has been no drug given an adequate evaluation which has not shown some evidence of activity (Carter and Wasserman, 1975a). The concept of combining antitumour drugs, which has proven so valuable in the haematological malignancies, had one of its first applications more than a decade ago in testicular tumours; a regimen of chlorambucil, methotrexate, and actinomycin D being used (Li et al., 1960; Li, 1966). For a long time this combination remained the chemotherapeutic regimen of choice until the advent of bleomycin and its incorporation into combinations with vinblastine and other drugs. Regimens studied include intermittent or continuous bleomycin plus vinblastine (Blum et al., 1973; Samuels, 1975; Samuels et al., 1973, 1976) and bleomycin-vinblastine plus actinomycin D (Silvay et al., 1973). More recently, bleomycin has been used in combination with cis-platinum (Cvitkovic et al., 1975); some regimens also including vinblastine (Einhorn et al., 1976) or cyclophosphamide plus actinomycin D (Cvitkovic et al., 1976). Pulmonary toxicity (interstitial pneumonitis) secondary to bleomycin has occurred in all regimens and stomatitis has been another dose limiting toxic reaction. Haematological reactions including severe leucopenia, thrombocytopenia and haemolytic anaemia have also occurred and in some cases have necessitated hospitalisation for presumed sepsis and granulocytopenic fever. Alopecia and weight loss are also common. Renal toxicity with cis-platinum has been minimised by ensuring adequate hydration of the patient.

In the past with chemotherapy, complete remission has been associated with cure, although the complete remission rate was not high. In some series, cure has been seen in 50 % of these who achieved complete remission. In general, most relapses after complete remission have occurred within 2 years of initiation of therapy. This would bode well for an increased cure rate with the newer combinations which have achieved very high remission rates. Some investigators follow patients postoperatively once a month for the first year with chest x-rays and β-HCG and α-fetoprotein determinations (Einhorn et al., 1976). This allows relapses to be detected with minimal disease being present. In such patients, complete remission has been achieved in around 90% of cases. There is now ample evidence that metastatic testicular cancer is potentially curable with intensive combination chemotherapy. The regimens used are toxic and should only be administered by trained oncologists within a therapeutic setting of ample supportive care. It would seem realistic to approach metastatic testicular cancer at least as intensively as is done with acute myelocytic leukaemia where the cure potential is less. Clinicians who diagnose testicular cancer should be sure to consult with, or refer to, oncology treatment centres so as to give every patient the optimum chance for cure.

Testicular cancer raises complex issues concerning the strategy for utilising chemotherapy within a combined treatment approach setting. A major problem centres around the curative potential for drug treatment against metastatic disseminated disease. Two approaches have to be balanced. There is on the one hand the total cure potential from primary therapy with surgery and/or irradiation; utilising chemotherapy at the first sign of relapse. On the other hand, there is the cure potential of drug treatment as adjuvant to surgery and/or irradiation; with secondary chemotherapy used at the time of relapse should it occur. Each approach needs to include assessment of toxicity risks which include the acute morbidity and mortality as well as chronic toxicity. When adjuvant chemotherapy is given to patients with microscopic tumour in the abdominal lymph nodes, more than half will be exposed to the risks of systemic therapy for no reason since they would be cured by their primary therapy. Since the combinations most effective against testicular cancer are highly intensive, the toxicity risks are not insignificant. Attenuation of the doses in adjuvant usage, to diminish the toxicity potential, runs the risk of impinging upon the ability to achieve the total tumour cell kill required for cure. The hypothesis of Norton and Simon (cited in De Vita, 1977), if valid, would indicate that reduction of drug doses is exactly what should not be done (see section 2.1.4).

Another problem revolves around being able to accrue significant numbers to prove the worth of adjuvant chemotherapy for stage II disease. If for example 70% of a subset of patients would be cured by surgery and 30% of those who relapse would be cured by drugs, then 80% would be the total cure rate. To demonstrate that a 95% cure rate with say the newer chemotherapy regimens alone (see above) was statistically significantly better than 80% at the 0.05 level would require a large number of patients (more than 1000). This number would be extremely difficult to accrue in a clinical trial.

6.10 Bladder Cancer

Cancer of the bladder ranks seventh among the causes of death due to cancer in males and thirteenth in females. Estimates of new cancer cases in the United States show that bladder cancer is the fifth most prevalent malignancy in males and the eleventh as a cause of cancer among females. It is a disease of elderly men and the incidence in men is about 3 times higher than in women; over 60% of patients are between ages of 50 and 70 years.

Three active drugs seem to have been studied for the treatment of advanced bladder cancer. These are doxorubicin or adriamycin (DeKernion, 1977), cis-platinum (Yagoda et al., 1977) and 5-fluorouracil. At this time, platinum seems to be the most active, but doxorubicin has been the most studied. Response rate achieved with all 3 drugs has been up to around 35%. Consistent with the history of chemotherapy for all kinds of cancer, as the numbers increase, the overall response rate falls. A large number of additional cases with platinum alone may not be seen because of the fact that combinations now seem to be the order of the day.

When the available data or combinations are looked at, what stands out is the impression, still based on very small numbers, that combinations including platinum and doxorubicin may lead to a significant increase in response rate. If the higher response rates can be confirmed, then cell kill potential in the advanced disease condition will be available to indicate that adjuvant studies to surgery and x-ray should be initiated.

6.11 CNS Tumours

Evaluation of objective response to chemotherapy in brain tumour patients is exceedingly difficult when survival statistics are not available. So-called objective measurements of tumour size, as determined by brain scan or angiogram, are notoriously inaccurate. The brain scan cannot distinguish tumour from surrounding cerebral oedema, nor viable from necrotic tumour. In one series, a brain scan did not agree with the clinical assessment of patient improvement or deterioriation in 27 % of 150 sequential scans (Walker, 1973). There was positive correlation of parallel carotid arteriograms in only 42 % of cases. This, then, would leave the objective evaluation of response mainly to the clinical assessment of the patient. Given the vagaries of cerebral oedema, especially where the use of corticosteroids is uncontrolled, one must be sceptical about the critical evaluation of an objective response.

The nitrosoureas are probably the only drugs that are genuinely active in this disease. Carmustine (BCNU) produces a response rate of 26 % with a definitive prolongation of survival over no therapy following surgery (Goldsmith and Carter, 1974). When combined with radiotherapy, the survival exceeds that of either method alone. Fewer patients have been studied with lomustine (CCNU) and semustine (MeCCNU), but the response rates are roughly similar. These drugs are highly lipid soluble, which explains their activity in glioblastoma. Assuming this is the case, further attention should be directed to cytotoxic drugs possessing this property.

In the miscellaneous class of antitumour agents, 3 drugs are interesting. Procarbazine has CNS toxicity and may also exert a cytotoxic effect but the data, although promising, are as yet not sufficient for a definitive statement. VM-26 (teniposide) is active against intracerebral L1210 leukaemia in mice and preliminary studies indicate it may be an active agent against glioblastoma (Goldsmith and Carter, 1973).

7. Tumours in Children as Examples of Successful Adjuvant Therapy

Cancers in children have been in the forefront of many innovative treatments, including approaches that use combinations of different types of therapy. Since chemotherapy has been particularly effective against a wide variety of aggressive neoplasms in children (table IX), these diseases have proven to be an appropriate model for the study of adjuvant chemotherapy.

7.1 Wilms' Tumour

Wilms' tumour is one of the earliest examples of chemotherapy being effective as an adjuvant to surgery and radiation. Surgery alone gives a 2 year relapse free survival rate of 30 % (Cross and Neuhauser, 1950), which in this tumour is considered to be equivalent to cure. The addition of postoperative radiation increased the 2 year relapse free survival rate to 47 % (Cross and Neuhauser, 1950). In 1959, when Klapproth (1959) analysed the world literature, the 2 year survival rate was only 21 % with surgery and 25 % with surgery plus radiation. Actinomycin D and vincristine are active in Wilms' tumour and a 2 year disease free survival of around 80 to 90 % has been achieved with actinomycin D alone (Farber, 1966) or a combination of actinomycin D and vincristine (D'Angio et al., 1976) as adjuvant therapy to surgery plus radiation.

Current investigators are attempting to improve these results by adding the highly active agent doxorubicin (adriamycin) to the adjuvant regimens.

7.2 Ewing's Sarcoma

Ewing's sarcoma had a dismal prognosis before the utilisation of chemotherapy as adjuvant therapy. When clinically localised disease was treated only with surgery and/or radiation, the 5 year survival was 4 to 19 % (Dahlin et al., 1961; Falk and Alpert, 1967). Metastatic recurrence in lungs and bone occurred frequently and 75 to 85 % of patients were dead within 2 years. Since the first report on the success of a combination of radiotherapy and chemotherapy (Pinkel, 1962), cyclophosphamide, vincristine, actinomycin D and, most recently, doxorubicin (adriamycin), have been used singly or usually in combination in a variety of adjuvant studies. Surgery is no longer employed (Boyer et al., 1967) and radiotherapy is the major treatment method for local control, with new approaches being evaluated (Suit et al., 1973). Adjuvant chemotherapy regimens employing doxorubicin, cyclophosphamide and vincristine have achieved a 2 year disease free survival of more than 50 to 65 % and a 5 year survival of around 50 % (Pomeroy and Johnson, 1975; Fossati-Bellani et al., 1977), while a regimen of radiation plus doxorubicin, cyclophosphamide, vincristine and actinomycin D has attained a 2 year disease free survival of 80 % (Tefft et al., 1977a). Chemotherapy is not only diminishing relapses due to metastatic disease, but is also having a positive effect on the local control achieved with radiation (Tefft et al., 1977a).

Newer approaches to Ewing's sarcoma include irradiation of both lungs.

7.3 Embryonal Rhabdomyosarcoma

Embryonal rhabdomyosarcoma is the most common soft tissue sarcoma which afflicts children. The embryonal type is only one of four known histological types (Horn and Enterline, 1958; Ivins et al., 1976). The tumour can be found in sites as diverse as the head and neck area, pelvis, limbs, and retroperitoneum. At the time of initial diagnosis, only 20 to 30% of children are amenable to radical surgery (Heyn, 1975), and the cure by this approach appears to range from 10 to 50% with only a slight increase in long term survival when radiation is added to surgery (Johnson, 1975; Heyn and Holland, 1970). However, the addition of a regimen of actinomycin D and vincristine to surgery and radiotherapy has achieved a 5 year survival of around 70%, with survival approaching 90% in those children whose tumour was 'completely resectable' (Kilman et al., 1973). Similar responses have been achieved by others using actinomycin and vincristine (Heyn and Holland, 1970) or a combination of doxorubicin (adriamycin), cyclophosphamide, vincristine and actinomycin D (Ghavimi et al., 1975).

One of the benefits of the use of drugs for rhabdomyosarcoma is that less mutilating surgery than was practised in the past can now be contemplated (Tefft et al., 1977b). Heyn (1975) has reported a 2 year survival rate of around 70% in patients with microscopic residual disease in whom radical surgery was not technically feasible. Even when residual disease was gross, the 2 year survival rate was still about 40%.

Currently, all of the cooperative research study groups in the United States who treat solid tumours in children have joined an intergroup study of rhabdomyosarcoma. Their protocol is designed to answer the following questions: (1) is postoperative radiotherapy routinely indicated in surgically resectable tumours?; (2) is actinomycin D plus cyclophosphamide plus vincristine superior to actinomycin D plus vincristine? and (3) is the optimum duration of chemotherapy in the adjuvant situation 1 or 2 years?

8. Use of Drugs in the Presence of Associated Malignant Disease

In animals, the presence of a tumour can modify the metabolic capacity of the host, resulting in alterations in the distribution and elimination and consequent pharmacological activity of the drug administered (Garattini et al., 1973; Boulos and Sirtori, 1971). The implications in man are not clear (Tschanz et al., 1977). Interactions can also occur between antineoplastic agents and other classes of drug (section 2.3.3; Bender et al., 1978) and between different antineoplastic agents (section 2.4). The latter may be additive or synergistic or antagonistic, due to modification of the distribution and elimination of other anticancer drugs or through mechanisms not involving pharmacokinetic drug handling (Garattini et al., 1973).

Drugs that may cause anaemia, leucopenia or thrombocytopenia, or immunosuppressive agents are best avoided in cancer patients who tend to be cytopenic and immunosuppressed as a result of their disease or its treatment.

9. Drug Induced Neoplasia

Several drugs have been associated with cancer in man (table XII; Hoover and Fraumeni, 1975). Radioisotopes owe their carcinogenic properties to ionising radiation at the site of deposition in the body. Radioactive phosphorus appears to increase the risk of leukaemia in patients with polycythaemia vera. Immunosuppressive therapy has been blamed for a higher cancer risk, especially lymphomas, in renal transplant recipients.

There is a considerable amount of experimental data which reveals the carcinogenic potential of anticancer agents, especially the alkylating agents, procarbazine and the nitrosoureas. Immunosuppression caused by anticancer drugs may also be a factor in second tumour development and the lymphomas and squamous cell carcinomas associated with purine antimetabolites such as azathioprine may well be due to that effect (Sieber and Adamson, 1975).

Acute myeloid leukaemia, acute lymphoid leukaemia, chronic myeloid leukaemia and chronic lymphoid leukaemia have been reported in patients with Hodgkin's disease (Rosner, 1976). Many of the chronic leukaemias and acute lym-

Table XII. Cancers related to drug exposures in man (after Hoover and Fraumeni, 1975)

Drug	Condition
Radioisotopes	
Phosphorus (^{32}p)	Acute leukaemia
Radium, mesothorium	Osteosarcoma, sinus carcinoma
Thorotrast	Haemangioendothelioma of the liver
Immunosuppressive drugs	
Antilymphocyte serum	Reticulosarcoma
Antimetabolites	?Other cancers (skin,
Corticosteroids	liver, soft tissue sarcoma)
(high cancer risk experienced by renal transplant patients)	
Cytotoxic drugs	
Chlornapnazine	Bladder cancer
Cyclophosphamide	
Alkylating agents	Acute and chronic leukaemias (see text)
Hormones	
Synthetic oestrogens	
prenatal	Vaginal and cervical adenocarcinoma (clear cell type)
postnatal	Endometrial carcinoma (adenosquamous type)
Androgenic-anabolic steroids (for aplastic anaemia)	Hepatocellular carcinoma
Other	
Arsenic	Skin cancer
Phenacetin containing drugs	Renal pelvis carcinoma
Coal tar ointments	Skin cancer
?Phenytoin	Lymphoma
?Chloramphenicol	Leukaemia
?Phenylbutazone	
?Amphetamines	Hodgkin's disease

phoid leukaemias occurred simultaneously with an antedated lymphoma. It is hard to know in this series if this occurrence is part of the natural history of the disease or is due to therapy since the treatment was not, in this series, given in a systematic way according to current standards. Others have however, reported cases of a second malignant tumour, including cases of acute myelogenous leukaemia in patients with Hodgkin's disease treated with drugs and radiation (Canellos, 1975; Canellos et al., 1975). An earlier estimate was of a 21-fold increase of second

tumours in patients with Hodgkin's disease treated with total nodal irradiation and combination chemotherapy (Arseneau et al., 1972). The exact incidence is difficult to determine. In one study of 680 patients with Hodgkin's disease treated from 1968 through 1975, 6 cases of leukaemia occurred in patients in clinical remission with the longest being 7.5 years after diagnosis (Coleman et al., 1977). 2 additional cases occurred in patients with active Hodgkin's disease. In 320 cases treated only with radiation, no cases of leukaemia were observed and the same was true for 30 patients treated with drugs only. The cases occurred in the group receiving combined radiation and drugs. The actuarial probability of developing leukaemia at 5 and 7 years is 1.5 and 2.0 % for the whole group and 2.9 and 3.9 % for the 330 patients treated with combined radiation and chemotherapy.

Acute myelocytic leukaemia has been reported in a small series of women with breast cancer who received long term adjuvant chlorambucil therapy (Lerner, 1977). A survey of 70 institutions in which alkylating agents were used to treat ovarian cancer in 5455 women, has specifically sought evidence of second tumours developing (Reimer et al., 1977). It would be expected that 0.62 cases of acute non-lymphoid leukaemia might occur in a population of that size. 13 cases were found for a 21-fold increase in relative risk. 12 of these 13 cases occurred in women who were followed for more than 2 years. The relative risk for patients given chemotherapy was 36.1 and rose to 171.4 for those surviving for 2 years with the rate being 13.75 per 1000 patients per year.

The fact that we now are concerned about such long term complications is a manifestation of the great success of cancer chemotherapy in prolonging life. In many situations treatment aims at cure and no therapy is without associated risk. The risk of second malignancies is now a fact that will have to be included in the final interpretation of many studies.

Bladder cancers are seen following prolonged cyclophosphamide therapy (Wall and Clausen, 1975). Prenatal exposure to synthetic oestrogens has been linked to clear cell carcinomas of the vagina and cervix in young women, and patients receiving oestrogens postnatally for gonadal dysgenesis have developed endometrial carcinoma (see chapter XV; sect. 23.3). The occurrence of hepatocellular carcinomas following treatment of aplastic anaemias with androgens, primarily oxymetholone, necessitates further evaluation of these compounds (Meadows et al., 1974). Patients with nephropathy resulting from continued use of large doses of phenacetin containing analgesics are at risk of developing transitional cell tumours of the renal pelvis (Johansson et al., 1974). Phenytoin (diphenylhydantoin) therapy can induce lymphoid hyperplasia that rarely transforms into malignant lymphoma (Gams et al., 1968; see chapter XXV, sect. 4.7.3). Chloramphenicol and phenylbutazone depress bone marrow function and have been suspected, by case reports, of inducing leukaemia (Fraumeni, 1967, 1969; Jensen and Roll, 1965).

Some drugs in clinical use have induced tumours in experimental studies but thus far no carcinogenicity has been demonstrated for man (e.g. isoniazid) or the carcinogenic potential has not been evaluated in man (e.g. oral contraceptives). Isoniazid induces pulmonary adenomas in mice but it does not appear to be carcinogenic in man (Glassroth et al., 1977; Stott et al., 1976). Reports of an increased risk of benign tumours of the liver, some showing malignant degeneration, and *in situ* cervix carcinoma in users of oral contraceptives stress the need for further studies (see chapter XV; sect. 13.6, 23.3).

Further Reading

Brule, G.; Eckhardt, S.J.; Hall, T.C. and Winkler, A.: Drug Therapy of Cancer (World Health Organisation, Geneva 1973).
Carter, S.K.; Bakowski, M. and Hellman, K.: Chemotherapy of Cancer (Wiley, New York 1977).
Clarysse, A.; Kenis, Y. and Mathe, G.: Cancer Chemotherapy (Springer-Verlag, Berlin 1976).

References

Adamson, R.H.: Metabolism of anticancer drugs in man. Annals of the New York Academy of Sciences 179: 432 (1971).
Arnold, H. and Bourseaux, F.: Neuartige Krebschemotherapeutika aus der Gruppe der zyklischen N-Lost-Phosphamidester. Naturwissenschaften 45: 64 (1958).
Arseneau, J.C.; Sponzo, R.W.; Levin, D.L.; Schnipper, L.E.; Bonner, H.; Young, R.C.; Canellos, G.P.; Johnson, R.E. and DeVita, V.T.: Nonlymphomatous malignant tumours complicating Hodgkin's disease: Possible association with intensive therapy. New England Journal of Medicine 287: 1119 (1972).
Barranco, S.C.; Ho, D.H.W.; Drewinko, B.; Romsdahl, M.M. and Humphrey, R.M.: Differential sensitivities of human melanoma cells grown in vitro to arabinosylcytosine. Cancer Research 32: 1218 (1972).
Bender, R.A.; Zwelling, L.A.; Doroshow, J.H.; Locker, G.Y.; Hande, K.R.; Murinson, D.S.; Cohen, M.; Myers, C.E. and Chabner, B.A.: Antineoplastic drugs: Clinical pharmacology and therapeutic use. Drugs 16: 46 (1978).
Bertino, J.R.; Boston, B. and Capizzi, R.L.: The role of chemotherapy in the management of cancer of the head and neck: a review. Cancer 36: 752 (1975).
Bertino, J.R.; Mosher, M.B.; DeConti, R.C. et al.: Chemotherapy of cancer of the head and neck. Cancer 31: 1141 (1973).
Blum, R.H.; Carter, S.K. and Agre, K.: A clinical review of bleomycin — a new antineoplastic agent. Cancer 31: 90 (1973).
Bonadonna, G. and Monfardini, S.: Chemotherapy of non-Hodgkin's lymphomas. Cancer Treatment Reviews 1: 167 (1974).
Bonadonna, G.; Brusamolino, E.; Valagussa, P.; Rossi, A.; Brugnatelli, L.; Brambilla, C.; DeLena, M.; Tancini, G.; Bajetta, E.; Musumeci, R. and Veronesi, U.: Combination chemotherapy as an adjuvant in operable breast cancer. New England Journal of Medicine 294: 405 (1976).
Bonadonna, G; De Lena, M.; Lattuada, A.; Milani, F.; Monfardini, S. and Beretta, G.: Combination chemotherapy and radiotherapy in non-Hodgkin's lymphomata. British Journal of Cancer 31(Suppl. 2): 481 (1975).
Bonadonna, G.; Rossi, A.; Valagussa, P.; Banfi, A. and Veronesi, U.: Adjuvant chemotherapy with CMF in breast cancer with positive axillary nodes; in Salmon and Jones (Eds) Adjuvant Therapy of Cancer (North-Holland, Amsterdam 1977).
Boston Collaborative Drug Surveillance Program: Allopurinol and cytotoxic drugs: Interaction in relation to bone marrow depression. Journal of the American Medical Association 227: 1036 (1974).
Boulos, B.M. and Sirtori, C.: Barbiturate metabolism as affected by neoplastic disease. Clin. Toxi. 4: 361 (1971).
Boyer, C.W.; Brickner, T.J. and Perry, R.H.: Ewing's sarcoma — case against surgery. Cancer 20: 1602 (1967).
Bristow, M.R.; Mason, J.W.; Billingham, M.E. and Daniels, J.R.: Doxorubicin cardiomyopathy: evaluation by phonocardiography, endomyocardial biopsy and cardiac catheterization. Annals of Internal Medicine 88: 168 (1978).
Broder, L.E. and Tormey, D.C.: Combination chemotherapy of carcinoma of the breast. Cancer Treatment Reviews 1: 183 (1974).
Broder, L.E.; Cohen, M.H. and Selaway, O.S.: Treatment of bronchogenic carcinoma II small cell. Cancer Treatment Reviews 4: 219 (1977).
Bruce, W.R.; Meeker, B.E. and Valeriote, F.A.: Comparison of the sensitivity of normal hematopoietic and transplanted lymphoma colony-forming cells to chemotherapeutic agents administered in vivo. Journal of the National Cancer Institute 37: 233 (1966).
Brule, G.; Eckhardt, S.J.; Hall, T.C. and Winkler, A.: Drug Therapy of Cancer (World Health Organisation, Geneva 1973).
Canellos, G.P.: Second malignancies complicating Hodgkin's disease in remission. Lancet 1: 1294 (1975).
Canellos, G.P.; DeVita, V.T.; Arseneau, J.C.; Whang-Peng, J. and Johnson, R.E.C.: Second malignancies complicating Hodgkin's disease in remission. Lancet 1: 947 (1975).
Capizzi, R.L.; Keiser, L.W. and Sartorelli, A.C.: Combination chemotherapy: theory and practice. Seminars in Oncology 4: 227 (1977).

Carter, S.K.: Single and combination nonhormonal chemotherapy in breast cancer. Cancer 30: 1543 (1972).

Carter, S.K.: The chemical therapy of breast cancer. Seminars in Oncology 1: 131 (1974).

Carter, S.K.: Adriamycin — a review. Journal of the National Cancer Institute 55: 1265 (1975).

Carter, S.K.: Integration of chemotherapy into combined modality treatment of solid tumors. VII: Adenocarcinoma of the breast. Cancer Treatment Review 3: 141 (1976a).

Carter, S.K.: Large bowel cancer — the current status of treatment. Journal of the National Cancer Institute 56: 3 (1976b).

Carter, S.K.: The chemotherapy of head and neck cancer. Seminars in Oncology 4: 413 (1977a).

Carter, S.K.: Correlation of chemotherapy activity in advanced disease with adjuvant results; in Salmon and Jones (Eds) Adjuvant Therapy of Cancer (North-Holland, Amsterdam 1977b).

Carter, S.K.: Acute lymphocytic leukemia; in Staquet (Ed) Randomized Trials in Cancer: A Critical Review by Sites (Raven Press, New York 1978).

Carter, S.K. and Soper, W.T.: The integration of chemotherapy into combined modality treatment of solid tumors. I. The overall strategy. Cancer Treatment Reviews 1: 1 (1974).

Carter, S.K. and Wasserman, T.H.: The chemotherapy of urologic cancer. Cancer 36: 729 (1975a).

Carter, S.K. and Wasserman, T.H.: Interaction of experimental and clinical studies in combined modality treatment. Cancer Chemotherapy Report 5(pt 2): 235 (1975b).

Carter, S.K.; Bakowski, M. and Hellman, K.: Chemotherapy of Cancer (Wiley, New York 1977).

Chabner, B.A.; Myers, C.E.; Coleman, C.H. and Johns, D.G.: The clinical pharmacology of antineoplastic agents. New England Journal of Medicine 292: 1107, 1159 (1975).

Christophidis, N.; Vajda, F.J.E.; Lucas, I.; Drummer, O.; Moon, W.J. and Louis, W.J.: Fluorouracil therapy in patients with carcinoma of the large bowel: A pharmacokinetic comparison of various rates and routes of administration. Clinical Pharmacokinetics 3: 330 (1978).

Clarkson, B.D.; Dowling, M.D.; Gee, T.S.; Cunningham, I.B. and Burchenal, J.H.: Treatment of acute leukemia in adults. Cancer 36: 775 (1975).

Coleman, C.N.; Williams, C.J.; Flint, A.; Glatstein, E.J.; Rosenberg, S.A. and Kaplan, H.A.: Hematologic neoplasia in patients treated for Hodgkin's disease. New England Journal of Medicine 297: 1249 (1977).

Comis, R.L. and Carter, S.K.: Integration of chemotherapy into a combined modality treatment of solid tumors III. Gastric cancer. Cancer Treatment Reviews 1: 221 (1974a).

Comis, R.L. and Carter, S.K.: A review of chemotherapy in gastric cancer. Cancer 34: 1576 (1974b).

Comis, R.L. and Carter, S.K.: Integration of chemotherapy into combined modality treatment of solid tumors. IV. Malignant melanoma. Cancer Treatment Reviews 1: 285 (1974c).

Creech, R.H.; Catalano, R.B.; Mastrangelo, M.J. and Engstrom, P.F.: An effective low-dose intermittent cyclophosphamide methotrexate and 5-fluourouracil treatment for metastatic breast cancer. Cancer 35: 1101 (1975).

Cross, R.E. and Neuhauser, E.B.D.: Treatment of mixed tumors of the kidney in childhood. Pediatrics 6: 843 (1950).

Cvitkovic, E.; Currie, V.; Krakoff, I.H. and Golbey, R.: Bleomycin infusion with cis-platinum diammine dichloride as secondary chemotherapy for germinal cell tumors. American Society of Clinical Oncology Abstract No. 1023. Proceedings of the American Association of Cancer Research 16: 273 (1975).

Cvitkovic, E.; Hayes, D. and Golbey, R.: Primary combination chemotherapy (VAB III) for metastatic or unresectable germ cell tumors. Proceedings of the American Association for Cancer Research 17: 296 (1976).

D'Angio, G.J.; Evans, A.E.; Breslow, N.; Beckwith, B.; Bishop, H.; Faigl, P.; Goodwin, W.; Leape, L.L.; Sinks, L.F.; Sutow, W.W.; Tefft, M. and Wolff, J.: The treatment of Wilm's tumor. Cancer 38: 633 (1976).

Dahlin, D.C.; Coventry, M.B. and Scanlon, P.W.: Ewing's sarcoma. A critical analysis of 165 cases. Journal of Bone Joint Surgery 43(A): 186 (1961).

Davis, T.E. and Carbone, P.P.: Drug treatment of breast cancer. Drugs 16: 441 (1978).

DeKernion, J.B.: The chemotherapy of advanced bladder cancer. Cancer Research 37: 2771 (1977).

DeLena, M.; Zucali, R.; Viganotti, G.; Valagussa, P. and Bonadonna, G.: Combined chemotherapy-radiotherapy approach in locally advanced (T_{3b}-T_4) breast cancer. Cancer Chemotherapy and Pharmacology 1: 53 (1978).

DeVita, V.T.: Adjuvant therapy — an overview; in Salmon and Jones (Eds) Adjuvant Therapy of Cancer (North-Holland, Amsterdam 1977).

DeVita, V.T.; Lewis, B.J.; Rozenweig, M. and Muggla, F.M.: The chemotherapy of Hodgkin's disease: Past experiences and future directions. Cancer 42: 979 (1978).

DeVita, V.T.; Wasserman, T.H.; Young, R.C. et al.: Perspectives on research in gynecologic oncology. Treatment protocols. Cancer 38: 161 (1976).

Einhorn, L.H.; Furnas, B.E. and Powell, N.: Combination chemotherapy of disseminated testicular carcinoma with cis-platinum diammine dichloride, vinblastine and bleomycin. Proceedings of the American Association of Cancer Research 17: 240 (1976).

Elkind, M.M.: Some principles for rational cell based development of combined radiation-drug therapy. Frontiers of Radiation Therapy and Oncology 4: 76 (1969).

Falk, S. and Alpert, M.: Five year survival of patients with Ewing's sarcoma. Surgery, Gynecology and Obstetrics 124: 319 (1967).

Farber, S.: Chemotherapy in the treatment of leukemia and Wilm's tumor. Journal of the American Medical Association 198: 826 (1966).

Farhangi, M. and Osserman, E.F.: The treatment of multiple myeloma. Seminars in Hematology 10: 149 (1973).

Fischer, G.A.: Predictive tests in culture of drug resistant mutants selected in vivo. National Cancer Institute Monograph 34: 131 (1971).

Fisher, B. and Redmund, C.: Studies of the national surgical adjuvant breast project in Salmon and Jones (Eds) Adjuvant Therapy of Cancer (North-Holland, Amsterdam 1977).

Fisher, B.; Carbone, P. and Economou, E.: L-phenylalanine mustard (L-PAM) in the management of primary breast cancer: A report of early findings. New England Journal of Medicine 292: 177 (1975).

Flocks, R.H.; Marberger, H.; Begley, B.J. and Prendergast, L.J.: Prostatic carcinoma: Treatment of advanced cases with intravenous diethylstilbestrol diphosphate. Journal of Urology 74: 549 (1955).

Fossati-Ballani, F.; Barni, S.; Gasparini, M.; Lombardi, F.;

Lattuada, A. and Bonadonna, G.: in Salmon and Jones (Eds) Adjuvant Therapy of Cancer, p.646 (North-Holland, Amsterdam 1977).

Frank, W. and Osterberg, A.E.: Mitomycin C (NSC-26980) — An evaluation of the Japanese reports. Cancer Chemotherapy Reports 9: 114 (1960).

Fraumeni, J.F.Jr.: Bone marrow depression induced by chloramphenicol or phenylbutazone. Leukemia and other sequelae. Journal of the American Medical Association 201: 828 (1967).

Fraumeni, J.F.Jr.: Clinical epidemiology of leukemia. Seminars of Hematology 6: 250 (1969).

Friedman, M.A.: A reveiw of the bleomycin experience in the United States. Recent Results in Cancer Research 63: 152 (1978).

Gams, R.A.; Neal, J.A. and Conrad, F.G.: Hydantoin-induced pseudo-pseudolymphoma. Annals of Internal Medicine 69: 557 (1968).

Garattini, S.; Donelli, M.G. and Spreafico, F.: Specific problems in cancer chemotherapy — drug interaction; in Proceedings 5th International Congress of Pharmacology, San Francisco, vol. 3, p.393 (Karger, Basel 1973).

Ghavimi, F.; Exelby, P.R.; D'Angio, G.J.; Cham, W.; Lieberman, P.H.; Tan, C.; Mike, V. and Murphy, M.L.: Multidisciplinary treatment of embryonal rhabdomyosarcoma in children. Cancer 35: 67 (1975).

Gilbert, H.S.: The spectrum of myeloproliferative disorders. Medical Clinics of North America 57: 355 (1973).

Glassroth, J.L.; White, M.C. and Snider, D.E.: An assessment of the possible association of isoniazid with human cancer deaths. American Review of Respiratory Disease 116: 1065 (1978).

Goffinet, D.R. and Bagshaw, M.A.: Clinical use of radiation sensitizing agents. Cancer Treatment Reviews 1: 15 (1974).

Goldsmith, M.A. and Carter, S.K.: Glioblastoma multiforme: A review of therapy. Cancer Treatment Reviews 1: 153 (1973).

Goldsmith, M.A. and Carter, S.K.: Glioblastoma multiforme — a review of therapy. Cancer Treatment Reviews 1: 153 (1974).

Goldsmith, M.A. and Carter, S.K.: The integration of chemotherapy into a combined modality approach to cancer therapy — V: Squamous cell cancer of the head and neck. Cancer Treatment Reviews 2: 137 (1975).

Gottlieb, J.A.; Baker, L.H.; Quagliana, J.M.; Luce, J.K.; Whitecar, J.P.; Sinkovics, J.G.; Rivkin, S.E.; Brownlee, R. and Frei, III, E.: Chemotherapy of sarcomas with a combination of adriamycin and dimethyl triazeno imidazole carboxamide. Cancer 30: 1632 (1972).

Gottlieb, J.A.; Bodey, G.; Sinkovics, J.; Rodriguez, V. and Burgess, M.A.: An effective new 4-drug combination (CY-VA-DIC) for metastatic sarcomas. Proceedings of the American Society of Clinical Oncology, (Abstract No. 713). Proceedings of the American Association of Cancer Research 15: 162 (1974).

Green, R.A.; Humphrey, E.; Close, H. et al.: Alkylating agents in bronchogenic carcinoma. American Journal of Medicine 46: 516 (1969).

Greenspan, E.: Combination cytotoxic chemotherapy in advanced disseminated breast cancer. Journal of Mt. Sinai Hospital 33: 1 (1966).

Gutterman, J.U.: Chemoimmunotherapy of human cancer: The need for a unified drug development program. Cancer Immunology and Immunotherapy 3: 153 (1978).

Hahn, R.G.; Moertel, C.G.; Schutt, A.J. et al.: A double blind comparison of intensive 5-fluorouracil by oral vs intravenous route in the treatment of colorectal carcinoma. Cancer 35: 1031 (1975).

Hall, T.C.: Prediction of responses to therapy mechanisms of resistance. Seminars in Oncology 4: 193 (1977).

Heel, R.C.; Brogden, R.N.; Speight, T.M. and Avery, G.S.: Tamoxifen: A review of its pharmacological properties and therapeutic use in the treatment of breast cancer. Drugs 16: 1 (1978).

Hersh, E.M.; Carbone, P.P.; Freireich, E.J.: Recovery of immune responsiveness after drug suppression in man. Journal of Laboratory and Clinical Medicine 67: 566 (1966).

Heyn, R.M.: The role of chemotherapy in the management of soft tissue sarcomas. Cancer 35: 291 (1975).

Heyn, R.M. and Holland, R.: Treatment of rhabdomyosarcoma in children. Proceedings of the American Association of Cancer Research 11: 36 (1970).

Hill, B.T. and Baserga, R.: The cell cycle and its significance for cancer treatment. Cancer Treatment Reviews 2: 159 (1975).

Hoover, R. and Fraumeni, J.F. Jr.: Drugs in clinical use which cause cancer. Journal of Clinical Pharmacology 15: 16 (1975).

Horn, R.C. and Enterline, H.T.: Rhabdomyosarcoma. A clinico-pathological study and classification of 39 cases. Cancer 11: 181 (1958).

Huguley, C.M.: Chronic myelocytic and chronic lymphocytic leukemia. Cancer 30: 1583 (1972).

Huguley, C.M.: Treatment of chronic lymphocytic leukemia. Cancer Treatment Reviews 4: 261 (1977).

Hutchinson, D.J. and Schmid, F.A.: In Minich (Ed) Drug Resistance and Selectivity, p.73 (Academic Press, New York 1973).

Ivins, J.E.; Ritts, R.E.; Pritchard, D.J.; Gilchrist, G.S.; Miller, G.C. and Taylor, W.F.: Transfer factor versus combination chemotherapy. A preliminary report of a randomized postsurgical adjuvant treatment study in osteogenic sarcoma. Annals of the New York Academy of Science 277: 558 (1976).

Jacobs, E.: Combination chemotherapy of metastatic testicular terminal cell tumors and soft part sarcomas. Cancer 25: 234 (1970).

Jensen, M.K. and Roll, K.: Phenylbutazone and leukaemia. Acta Medica Scandinavica 178: 505 (1965).

Jensen, E.V.; De Sombre, E.R. and Jungblut, P.W.: Estrogen receptors in hormone responsive tissues and tumors; in Wissler, Dao and Wood (Eds) Endogenous Factors Influencing Host-Tumor Balance (University Press, Chicago 1967).

Johansson, S.; Angervall, L.; Bengtsson, U. and Wahlqvist, L.: Uroepithelial tumors of the renal pelvis associated with abuse of phenacetin-containing analgesics. Cancer 33: 743 (1974).

Johnson, D.G.: Trends in surgery for childhood rhabdomyosarcoma. Cancer 35: 916 (1975).

Karle, H.; Ernst, P. and Killman, S.A.: Changing cytokinetic patterns of human leukemic lymphoblasts during the course of the disease studied in vivo. British Journal of Haematology 24: 231 (1973).

Kennedy, B.J.: Hormonal therapies in breast cancer. Seminars in Oncology 1: 119 (1974).

Kilman, J.W.; Clatworthy, H.W.; Newton, W.A. and Grosfeld, J.L.: Reasonable surgery for rhabdomyosarcoma: a study of 67 cases. Ann. Surg. 178: 346 (1973).

Klapproth, H.J.: Wilm's tumor. A report of 56 cases and analysis of 1,351 cases reported in the world literature from 1940 to 1958. Journal of Urology 81: 633 (1959).

Lerner, H.: Second malignancies diagnosed in breast cancer patients while receiving adjuvant chemotherapy at the Pennsylvania Hospital. Proceedings of the American Association of Cancer Research 18: 340 (1977).

Li, M.C.: Management of choriocarcinoma and related tumors of uterus and testis. Medical Clinics of North America 45: 667 (1966).

Li, M.C.; Whitmore, W.F.; Golbey, R. and Grabstald, H.: Effects of combined drug therapy on metastatic cancer of the testis. Journal of the American Medical Association 174: 1297 (1960).

Liegler, D.G.,: Henderson, E.S.; Hahn, M.A. and Oliverio, V.T.: The effect of organic acids on renal clearance of methotrexate in man. Clinical Pharmacology and Therapeutics 10: 849 (1969).

Livingston, R.B.: Unpublished observations.

Livingston, R.B.; More, T.N.; Heilbrun, L.; Bottomley, R.; Lehane, D.; Rivkin, S.E. and Thigpen, T.: Small cell carcinoma of the lung. Combined chemotherapy and radiation. Annals of Internal Medicine 88: 194 (1978).

Lukes, R.J. and Collins, R.D.: New approaches to the classification of the lymphomata. British Journal of Cancer 31 (Suppl. 2): 1 (1975).

McCredie, K.B. and Freireich, E.J.: Acute leukemia: Chemotherapy and management; in Greenspan (Ed) Clinical Cancer Chemotherapy, p.71 (Raven Press, New York 1975).

McGuire, W.L.: Hormone receptors. Their role in predicting prognosis and response to endocrine therapy. Seminars in Oncology 5: 428 (1978).

McGuire, W.L.; Carbone, P.P.; Sears, M.E. and Escher, G.C.: Estrogen receptors in human breast cancer: An overview; in McGuire, Carbone and Vollmer (Eds) Estrogen Receptors in Human Breast Cancer, p.1 (Raven Press, New York 1975).

Manni, A.; Trujillo, J.E.; Marshall, J.S.; Brodkey, J. and Pearson, O.H.: Antihormone treatment of stage IV breast cancer. Cancer 43: 44-450 (1979).

Meadows, A.T.; Naiman, J.L. and Valdes-Dapena, M.: Hepatoma associated with androgen therapy for aplastic anemia. Journal of Pediatrics 84: 109 (1974).

Mendelsohn, M.L.: Autoradiographic analysis of cell proliferation in spontaneous breast cancer of C3H mouse III. The growth fraction. Journal of the National Cancer Institute 28: 1015 (1962).

Moertel, C.G.: Therapy of advanced gastrointestinal cancer with the nitrosoureas. Cancer Chemotherapy Reports 4: 27 (1973).

Moertel, C.G.: Clinical management of advanced gastrointestinal cancer. Cancer 36: 675 (1975).

Moertel, C.G. and Reitemeier, R.J.: Advanced Gastrointestinal Cancer. Clinical Management and Chemotherapy (Harper and Row, New York 1969).

Moertel, C.G.; Schutt, A.J.; Hahn, R.G. et al.: Therapy of advanced colorectal cancer with a combination of 5-fluorouracil, methyl-l-3-cis(2-chloroethyl)-l-nitrosourea, and vincristine. Journal of the National Cancer Institute 54: 69 (1975).

Moore, J.; Bull, J.; Jones, S. et al.: Sequential radiotherapy and chemotherapy in the treatment of Hodgkin's disease. Annals of Internal Medicine 77: 1 (1972).

Morton, D.L. and Goodnight, J.E.: Clinical trials of immunotherapy. Present status. Cancer 42: 2224 (1978).

Nathanson, L.; Wolter, J.; Horton, J.; Colsky, J.; Shnider, B.I. and Schilling, A.: Characteristics of prognosis and response to imidazole carboxamide in melanoma. Clinical Pharmacology and Therapeutics 12: 955 (1971).

Pinkel, D.: Cyclophosphamide in children with cancer. Cancer 15: 42 (1962).

Pomeroy, T.C. and Johnson, R.E.: Combined modality therapy for Ewing's sarcomas. Cancer 35: 36 (1975).

Rappaport, H.: Tumors of the hemopoietic systems; in Atlas of Tumor Pathology, Section III, Fascicle 8, Washington, DC, Armed Forces Institute of Pathology (1966).

Rausen, A. and Glidewell, O.: L-asparaginase in advanced childhood leukemia. Comparative trial of drug schedules singly and in combination. Proceedings of the American Association of Cancer Research 11: 66 (1970).

Reimer, R.R.; Hoover, R.; Fraumeni, J.F. and Young, R.C.: Acute leukemia after alkylating-agent therapy of ovarian cancer. New England Journal of Medicine 297: 177 (1977).

Rosen, G.; Murphy, M.L.; Huvos, A.G.; Guiterriz, M. and Marcove, R.C.: Chemotherapy in block resection and prosthetic bone replacement in the treatment of osteogenic sarcoma. Cancer 37: 1 (1976).

Rosenberg, S.A.; Dorfman, R.F. and Kaplan, H.S.: A summary of results of a review of 405 patients with non-Hodgkin's lymphoma at Stanford University. British Journal of Cancer 31 (Suppl. 2): 168 (1975).

Rosenberg, S.A.; Kaplan, H.S. and Glatstein, E.J.: Combined modality therapy of Hodgkin's disease. A report on the Stanford trials. Cancer 42: 991 (1978).

Rosner, F.: Acute leukemia as a delayed consequence of cancer chemotherapy. Cancer 37: 1033 (1976).

Roswit, B.; Patno, M.E.; Rapp, R. et al.: The survival of patients with inoperable lung cancer: A large-scale randomized study of radiation therapy versus placebo. Radiology 90: 688 (1968).

Rozencweig, M.; Von Hoff, D.D. and Slavik, M.: Cis-dimine dichloro platinum (II). A new anticancer drug. Annals of Internal Medicine 86: 803 (1977).

Rubin, P.: Cancer of the urogenital tract. Testicular tumor. Journal of the American Medical Association 213: 89 (1970).

Rundles, R.W.; Wyngaarden, J.B.; Hitchings, G.H.; Elion, G.B. and Silberman, H.R.: Effects of a xanthine oxidase inhibitor on thiopurine metabolism, hyperuricaemia and gout. Transactions of the Association of American Physicians 76: 126 (1963).

Sadee, W. and Wong, C.G.: Pharmacokinetics of 5-fluorouracil: Inter-relationship with biochemical kinetics in monitoring therapy. Clinical Pharmacokinetics 2: 437 (1977).

Salmon, S.E.: Nitrosoureas in multiple myeloma. Cancer Treatment Reports 60: 789 (1976).

Salmon, S.E.; Hamburger, A.W.; Soehnlen, B.; Durie, B.G.M.; Alberts, D.S. and Moon, T.E.: Quantitation of differential sensitivity of human-tumor stem cells to anticancer drugs. New England Journal of Medicine 298: 1321 (1978).

Samuels, M.L.: Continuous intravenous bleomycin therapy with vinblastine in testicular and extragonadal germinal tumors. Proceedings of the Americal Association of Cancer Research 16: 112 (1975).

Samuels, M.L.; Johnson, D.E. and Holoye, P.Y.: The treatment of stage III metastatic germinal cell neoplasia of the testis with bleomycin combination chemotherapy. Proceedings of the American Association of Cancer Research 14: 23 (1973).

Samuels, M.L.; Bayle, L.E.; Holoye, P.V. and Johnson, D.E.: Intermittent versus continuous infusion bleomycin in testicular cancer. Proceedings of the American Association of Cancer Research 17: 98 (1976).

Sartorelli, A.C.: Some approaches to the therapeutic exploitation of metabolic sites of vulnerability of neoplastic cells. Cancer Research 29: 2292 (1969).

Schabel, F.M.: Concepts of systemic treatment of micro metastases. Cancer 35: 15 (1975).

Schein, P.S.; Chabner, B.A.; Canellos, G.P. et al.: Results of combination chemotherapy of non-Hodgkin's lymphoma. British Journal of Cancer 31 (Suppl. 2): 465 (1975).

Selawry, O.S. and Hansen, H.H.: Lung cancer; in Holland and Frei (Eds): Cancer Medicine, p.1473 (Lea and Febiger, Philadelphia 1973).

Shen, D.D. and Azarnoff, D.L.: Clinical pharmacokinetics of methotrexate. Clinical Pharmacokinetics 3: 1 (1978).

Sieber, S.M. and Adamson, R.H.: Toxicity of antineoplastic agents in man. Chromosomal aberrations, effects, congenital malformations and carcinogenic potential. Advances in Cancer Research 22: 57 (1975).

Silvay, O.; Yagoda, A.; Wittes, R.; Whitmore, W. and Golbey, R.: Treatment of germ cell carcinomas with a combination of actinomycin D, vinblastine and bleomycin. Proc. Amer. Ass. Cancer Res. 14: 68 (1973).

Skipper, H.E.: Clowes Memorial Lecture. Cancer Research 31: 1173 (1971).

Skipper, H.: Booklet 7 of 1975 from Southern Research Institute quoted in Spreafico and Garattini. Chemotherapy of experimental metastasis; in Baldwin (Ed) Secondary Spread of Cancer, p.101 (Academic Press, London 1978).

Skipper, H.E.; Schabel, F.M. and Wilcox, W.S.: Experimental evaluation of potential anticancer agents XIII on the criteria and kinetics associated with curability of experimental leukemia. Cancer Chemotherapy Reports 35: 1 (1964).

Spiers, A.S.D.: Blood and neoplastic diseases. Chronic granulocytic leukemia and chronic lymphocytic leukemia. British Medical Journal 4: 460 (1974).

Spreafico, F. and Rossi, M.S.: Antineoplastic agents; in Morselli (Ed) Drug Disposition During Development, p.101 (Spectrum, New York 1977).

Stjernsward, J.: Decreased survival related to irradiation postoperatively in early operable breast cancer. Lancet 2: 1285 (1974).

Stott, H.; Peto, J.; Stephens, R.; Fox, W.; Sutherland, I.; Foster-Carter, A.F.; Teare, H.B. and Fenning, J.: An assessment of the carcinogenicity of isoniazid in patients with pulmonary tuberculosis. Tubercule 57: 1 (1976).

Suit, H.D.; Martin, R.G. and Sutow, W.W.: In Sutow, Vietti and Fernbach (Eds) Medical Pediatric Oncology, p.473, 602 (CV Mosby, St Louis 1973).

Tefft, M.; Chabora, B.M. and Rosen, G.: Radiation in bone sarcomas: A re-evaluation in the era of intensive systemic chemotherapy. Cancer 39: 806 (1977a).

Tefft, M.; Fernandez, C.H. and Moon, T.E.: Rhabdomyosarcoma response with chemotherapy prior to radiation in patients with gross residual disease. Cancer 39: 665 (1977b).

Tschanz, C.; Hignite, C.E.; Huffman, D.H. and Azarnoff, D.L.: Metabolic disposition of antipyrine in patients with lung cancer. Cancer Research 37: 3881 (1977).

Walker, M.D.: Physiologic barriers to pharmacologic efficacy; in Proceedings 5th International Congress of Pharmacology, San Francisco, vol. 3, p.354 (Karger, Basel 1973).

Walker, M.D.: Brain and peripheral nervous system tumours; In Holland and Frei (Eds): Cancer Medicine, p.1385 (Lea and Febiger, Philadelphia 1973).

Wall, R.L. and Clausen, K.P.: Carcinoma of the urinary bladder in patients receiving cyclophosphamide. New England Journal of Medicine 293: 271 (1975).

Wampler, G.L.; Mellette, S.J.; Kuperminc, M. et al.: Hexamethylmelamine (NSC 13875) in the treatment of advanced cancer. Cancer Chemotherapy Reports 56: 505 (1972).

Williams, C.J.; Coleman, C.N.; Glatstein, E.J.; Rosenberg, S.A. and Kaplan, H.S.: Hematologic malignancies in remission of Hodgkin's disease. Proceedings of the American Association of Cancer Research 18: 288 (1977).

Wittes, R.E.; Brescia, F. and Young, C.W.: Combination chemotherapy with Cis-diamine dichloro platinum (II) and bleomycin in tumors of the head and neck. Oncology 32: 202 (1975).

Wittes, R.E.; Cvitkovic, E. and Shah, J.: Cis-dichloro diamine platinum (II) in the treatment of epidermoid carcinoma of the head and neck. Cancer Treatment Reports 61: 359 (1977a).

Wittes, R.E.; KiHong, W.; Gatchell, L.; Krakoff, I.H. and Golbey, R.: Methyl-CCNU in malignant melanoma — a divided dose schedule of administration. Oncology 34: 45 (1977b).

Woodruff, R.: Management of adult acute lymphoblastic leukemia. Cancer Treatment Reviews 5: 95 (1978).

Yagoda, A.; Watson, R.C.; Gonzalez-Vitale, J.C.; Grabstalo, H. and Whitmore, W.: Cis-diamine dichloro platinum (II) in advanced bladder cancer. Cancer Treatment Reports 60: 917 (1977).

Young, R.C.: Chemotherapy of ovarian cancer: past and present. Seminars in Oncology 2: 267 (1975).

Young, R.C.; Canellos, G.P.; Chabner, B.A.; Schein, P.S.; Hubbard, S.P. and DeVita, V.T.: Chemotherapy of advanced ovarian cancer. A prospective randomized comparison of phenylalanine mustard and high dose cyclophosphamide. Gynecology and Oncology 2: 489 (1974a).

Young, R.C.; Hubbard, S.P. and DeVita, V.T.: The chemotherapy of ovarian carcinoma. Cancer Treatment Reviews 1: 99 (1974b).

Zaharko, D.S. and Dedrick, D.L.: Applications of pharmacokinetics to cancer chemotherapy; in Proceedings 5th International Congress of Pharmacology, San Francisco, vol. 3, p.316 (Karger, Basel 1973).

Ziegler, J.L.: Chemotherapy of Burkitt's lymphoma. Cancer 30: 1534 (1972).

Ziegler, J.L.: Management of Burkitt's lymphoma: an update. Cancer Treatment Reviews 6: In Press (1979).

Chapter XXV
Neurological Diseases

H. Kutt and F.H. McDowell

Synopsis of Important Principles

1) In all but a few instances, drug treatment of neurological disorders is limited to prevention or amelioration of signs and symptoms.

2) In those diseases where the long term administration of drugs produces symptomatic relief, the doses of drugs need to be individualised — in patients with severe disease a compromise dosage between the greatest benefit and least intoxication is often necessary.

3) Epileptic seizures can be reduced in frequency or abolished in about two thirds of the patients. Monitoring drug plasma concentrations is extremely useful in adjusting the dosage and confirming the proper intake or the presence of intoxication.

4) Drug treatment is also effective in symptomatic relief of facial pain, migraine headaches, extrapyramidal syndromes, and in myasthenic or spastic states. Long term treatment has not proven of value in multiple sclerosis.

5) Prevention or reduction of transient cerebral ischaemic attacks and cerebral embolism can be achieved with anticoagulants or antiplatelet drugs such as aspirin. Stroke in evolution should be treated with anticoagulants to reduce mortality and morbidity. Anticoagulants are ineffective in completed stroke.

6) Bacterial meningitis may be cured by prompt diagnosis and treatment with adequate CSF concentrations of an appropriate antibacterial agent. Tuberculosis or fungal meningitis requires prolonged treatment, which can reduce mortality significantly.

7) The potential neurotoxicity of drugs must always be considered when prescribing drugs for the patient with neurological disease. Certain drugs may aggravate neurological disease — e.g. aminoglycoside and polymyxin antibiotics may aggravate symptoms in myasthenic patients and oral contraceptives may increase the severity of migraine attacks.

8) Drugs may also induce neurological diseases, particularly in the elderly and in the presence of impaired renal function. Drug induced toxic delirium is the most frequent drug induced neurological disorder and is most commonly found when sedatives and some tranquillisers or anticholinergic agents are given to elderly or brain damaged patients.

Effective drug treatment of neurological diseases is limited to a relatively few entities. Cures may be achieved with vitamins in some nutritional or metabolic neuropathies, or with antimicrobial agents in nervous system infections. Frequently, dramatic symptomatic relief of facial pain, migraine headaches, seizures, extrapyramidal syndromes, myasthenic or spastic states can be effected with drugs. Drug treatment is less effective in cerebral vascular disease and multiple sclerosis, and is least effective in the degenerative and/or hereditary diseases, such as amyotrophic lateral sclerosis, Friedreich's ataxia, muscular dystrophies; or in brain tumour. Continuing research efforts may improve this situation, but because of the poor regenerative potential of nervous tissue, emphasis should be on preventive rather than curative programmes.

1. General Principles of Treatment

1.1 Pharmacodynamic Considerations

In most neurological disorders, long term administration of drugs renders symptomatic relief such as in seizure disorders, extrapyramidal syndromes, myasthenia, or facial neuralgias. Appropriate agents must be given then in sufficient amounts to control symptoms. Because the severity of the disease process varies among individual patients, the doses of drugs need to be individualised. In patients with severe neurological diseases, high doses producing some intoxication may be required, if complete control of symptoms is desired. A compromise dosage producing the greatest benefit and least intoxication is frequently settled for in these patients. Achievement of optimum results is aided by knowledge of some pharmacokinetic aspects of the agents being used.

1.2 Pharmacokinetic Considerations

1.2.1 Absorption of Drugs

Most drugs used in the treatment of disorders of the nervous system are well absorbed. These include the majority of the antiepileptic drugs (phenytoin is a notable exception), anticholinergic drugs and antimicrobial agents. Anticholinesterases and some antimigraine drugs, on the other hand, are incompletely absorbed or bioavailable and the oral dose greatly exceeds the parenteral dose.

The absorption of one drug can be enhanced or inhibited by the previously or simultaneously ingested other substances (see chapter VIII; section 2.3.1). For example, in the treatment of acute migraine, the absorption of ergotamine is enhanced by caffeine (Schmidt and Fanchamps, 1974). Gastric emptying rate is delayed during a migraine attack and metoclopramide, which increases gastric emptying (see chapter XIX; sect. 5.2), enhances the rate of absorption of aspirin and relief from the attack (Volans, 1978). In epilepsy, the absorption of phenytoin may be inhibited by simultaneously ingested antacids. Thus, a treatment failure with an agent can result from poor absorption. Food has a complex effect on absorption of drugs, such that depending on the drug, the amount absorbed may be increased, decreased or not affected (see also chapter VI; sect. 5).

1.2.2 Distribution of Drugs

It is important for the majority of drugs used in the treatment of disorders of the nervous system that they penetrate into the nervous tissue. Most antiepileptic drugs are lipid soluble and reach the brain readily in concentrations that equal that of blood or even higher. Diazepam concentration in the brain reaches the maximum within 5 minutes after intravenous injection, phenytoin in 10 to 20 minutes, while phenobarbitone concentration reaches the maximum in about 30 minutes. This is relevant when treating status epilepticus. Many antimicrobial agents on the other hand are less lipophilic and pass the blood-brain or spinal fluid barrier modestly or poorly, although that passage may be enhanced considerably by inflammation. Those agents that penetrate poorly, even in the presence of inflammation, need to be given intrathecally or intraventricularly (see sect. 13).

Slow penetration to the central nervous system may, however, be an advantage; as in the case of anticholinesterases. They can be given to patients with myasthenia gravis in large amounts without causing central nervous system related side effects.

Entry of levodopa into the brain is only modest. This necessitates a relatively high dose and blood concentration to achieve a therapeutic effect, and systemic side effects from the peripheral dopamine produced by peripheral dopa decarboxylase may become prominent. Using dopa decarboxylase inhibitors, which do not enter the brain and thus prevent only excessive systemic dopamine formation, alleviates this situation (see section 5.1).

Plasma protein binding has an important effect on distribution of some drugs. For instance, of the total phenytoin concentration in plasma normally 90 % is bound, leaving 10 % free to penetrate into the tissues. A decrease of phenytoin binding to 80 %, as is often seen in patients with chronic uraemia or liver disease, will double the fraction of free drug in plasma and available to enter the brain. In such cases, it would be desirable to monitor unbound as well as total drug concentration in the plasma (see chapter I, sect. 5.1.2).

1.2.3 Elimination of Drugs

Many drugs such as the majority of antiepileptic drugs must undergo extensive and nearly complete biotransformation before they can be eliminated. The rate of elimination of the active drug determines the duration of the effect of a single dose and influences the extent of accumulation of the drug in the body during continued administration. The elimination rate parallels the plasma half-life if there is no change in distribution of the drug (see chapter I; sect. 2.1.3, 3.3.1). Drugs with a short half-life such as anticholinesterases need to be given frequently, if a continuous effective plasma concentration is to be maintained. Several antiepileptic drugs have long half-lives and can be given once a day. Following the commencement of multiple dose administration of drugs, there is a progressive rise of drug concentration in the body until the intake and output are in balance and a plateau or steady-state is achieved (see chapter I; sect. 2.2). Empirically, it has been proven that the time to reach the steady-state with a given dose is around 4 to 6 times the duration of half-life. For instance, the half-life of phenobarbitone is approximately 3 days; thus attainment of the steady-state takes over 2 weeks following initial dosage or a change of maintenance dosage. This means that further dose alteration should not be made within this time with such drugs. Although the half-life of a drug in the majority of patients falls into a definable range of values, it is important to recognise that there can be considerable interindividual variation (see chapter I; sect. 4.2). Furthermore, the half-life of a drug can change with progression of age in the same individual (see chapter IV, sect. 2.3; V, sect. 2.1.3).

The half-life and the rate of elimination of a drug are influenced by a variety of factors. Thus alkalinisation enhances the elimination of phenobarbitone, while phenobarbitone in turn can enhance the elimination of other drugs by inducing enzymes that are involved in their biotransformation. Biotransformation of drugs is carried out mostly in the liver by the microsomal enzyme system (see chapter I; sect. 3.3; 4.2). The rate of activity of these enzymes is determined in part by genetic make-up of the patient, but it may be influenced also by environmental factors. These include other drugs that can either enhance or inhibit the enzymes involved in the biotransformation of the primary drug. Drug interactions at the drug biotransformation stage are seen with some antiepileptic drugs and with coumarin anticoagulants, leading to a change of the rate of elimination and change in dosage requirement (see section 3; chapter VIII, sect. 2.3.3, 2.3.4; appendix C).

2. Seizure Disorders

2.1 Clinical Considerations

Convulsions may result from systemic abnormalities such as hypocalcaemia, hypoglycaemia, pyridoxine deficiencies or toxic states. The majority of patients with seizure disorders, however, fall into the category of: (1) 'idiopathic' or epilepsy of unknown origin, and (2) epilepsy secondary to known brain lesions; both of which require long term treatment with antiepileptic drugs.

Epileptic seizures originate from groups of hyperexcitable cells (epileptic neurons) from which discharges periodically build up and spread, either to limited areas resulting in focal seizures, or to large areas resulting in generalised seizures (Ward, 1969).

2.2 Seizure Classification

The terminology of seizures has undergone changes in the past decade. The conventional terms grand mal, petit mal, minor motor, focal and psychomotor epilepsies are being replaced by terms that allow definition of seizures more precisely. It appears that since the publication of the International League Against Epilepsy Classification of seizures about a decade ago (Gastaut, 1970), its terminology is often being used in communications and texts dealing with epilepsy. The clinical relevance of proper seizure classification lies in the observation that some seizure types respond best to treatment with certain antiepileptic drugs. The International Classification considers the site of origin of the seizure and the extent of spread of seizure discharges. There are 4 major groups of seizures, including: (1) generalised seizures, (2) partial seizures, (3) unilateral seizures, and (4) unclassified seizures (see table I).

1) *Generalised Seizures:* This group contains 8 subcategories and covers manifestations in which activation of widespread areas of brain occur suddenly. The major subgroups are the following:

a) Generalised tonic-clonic seizures, which correspond to the traditional term of grand mal seizures.

b) Absence seizures, either simple or complex. This category comes nearest to the traditional pure petit mal definition.

c) Myoclonic and akinetic attacks with brief prominent jerking movements or sudden loss of muscle tone and falling. These were included in the category of 'minor motor' in the previous terminologies.

d) Infantile spasms with the characteristic nodding movements clinically and the 'hypsarrhythmia' in the electroencephalogram.

2) *Partial Seizures:* Partial seizures are often associated with acquired focal lesions in the brain. The major subcategories in this group are the following:

a) Partial seizures with elementary symptomatology; i.e. limited focal seizures without loss of consciousness.

b) Partial seizures with complex symptomatology which involve impairment of consciousness and disturbances of cognitive, affective and psychomotor or psychosensory functions. These manifestations were mostly covered by the terms psychomotor and temporal lobe epilepsies.

c) Partial seizures secondary generalised which correspond to grand mal seizures with focal onset.

3) *Unilateral Seizures:* This is a group of rarely occurring manifestations where the epileptic discharges appear over one of the hemispheres predominantly.

4) *Unclassified Seizures:* A group to include those seizures that do not fit into any other group.

2.3 Pharmacological Considerations

2.3.1 General Considerations

The choice of an antiepileptic drug should be made according to the type of seizure as defined by

Table I. International League Against Epilepsy Classification of Seizures (Gastaut, 1970)

---

1. Partial seizures (begin locally) with elementary symptomatology (usually without impairment of consciousness)
     With motor symptoms (include Jacksonian)
     With sensory or somato-sensory symptoms
     With autonomic symptoms
     Compound forms

   Partial seizures with complex symptomatology (usually with impairment of consciousness)
     With cognitive symptomatology
     With affective symptomatology
     With psychosensory symptomatology
     With psychomotor symptomatology
     Compound forms

   Partial seizures secondarily generalised

2. Generalised seizures (bilaterally symmetrical and without local onset)
     Absence (petit mal), simple or complex
     Bilateral massive epileptic myoclonus
     Infantile spasms
     Clonic seizures
     Tonic-clonic seizures (grand mal)
     Atonic seizures
     Akinetic seizures
     Tonic seizures

3. Unilateral seizures (or predominantly)

4. Unclassified epileptic seizures (due to incomplete data)

---

clinical manifestations and EEG patterns. Good control of seizures can be achieved with average non-toxic doses of single or combined antiepileptic drugs in over two-thirds of patients. For patients with a severe seizure process, higher doses have been used at the expense of some intoxication and/or side effects.

The antiepileptic drug, particularly the barbiturates, should not be stopped suddenly; change over should be effected gradually over several days or weeks to avoid exacerbations of seizures or withdrawal status epilepticus (Schmidt and Wilder, 1968). When starting a new drug, the patient should be told about its possible untoward effects.

2.3.2 Mechanism of Action

Antiepileptic drugs act by depressing the neural excitability by stabilising the cell membrane and also prevent the spread of seizure discharges by modifying the synaptic transmission. These effects

Table II. Important pharmacokinetic properties of some antiepileptic drugs (after Hvidberg and Dam, 1976)

Drug	Systemic bioavail-ability (%)	Protein binding (%)	Plasma half-life (hours)	Elimination	Active metabolites	Notes
Phenytoin	80-95	87-93	~ 20-30*	Hepatic metabolism (saturable); 1-5% unchanged in urine	No	Bioavailability may vary markedly between brands. Value given is for tablets of high quality *Half-life may vary many fold between individuals (e.g. 8 to 60h) and is dose dependent (at higher plasma concentrations dose increases must be small)
Phenobarbitone	~ 80	50-60	48-120+	Hepatic metabolism (about 50-80%) and renal excretion of unchanged drug (about 20-50%)	No	Half-life is shorter in children (~ 36-72 hours); proportion of dose metabolised subject to interindividual variation Induces metabolism of other drugs
Carbamazepine	70+	70-80	10-20*	Hepatic metabolism; < 1-2% unchanged in urine	Yes**	Food increases bioavailability *Induces own metabolism (half-life shown is after repeat doses) **Ratio of active epoxide metabolite to parent drug varies from 5 to 81% (see text) Plasma concentrations can fluctuate during day, particularly when combined with phenytoin and/or phenobarbitone
Primidone	?	Little or none	6-12*	Hepatic metabolism to phenobarbitone and phenyl-ethyl-malon-amide (PEMA)	Yes (both metabolites)	*Half-life shown is for parent drug; half-life for derived phenobarbitone is about 3-5 days and for PEMA about 40-60 hours
Ethosuximide	100	None	~ 60*	Hepatic metabolism; 10-20% unchanged in urine	Probably not	*Half-life is shorter in children (~ 30 hours)

Trimethadione (troxidone)	?	Little or none	~ 16*	Hepatic metabolism; about 1% unchanged in urine	Yes	*Half-life shown is for parent drug; half-life for active metabolite (dimethadione) about 10 days Plasma concentrations can fluctuate considerably during day Half-life decreased by phenytoin, phenobarbitone, primidone and carbamazepine
Sodium valproate	?	~ 90	13-21	Hepatic metabolism	No	Reduces phenobarbitone elimination
Diazepam	~ 75	97-99	~ 24-48*	Hepatic metabolism; about 2% unchanged in urine	Yes	*Half-life shown is approximate half-life of parent drug; half-life of major active metabolite (desmethyldiazepam) is about 51-120h
Nitrazepam	53-94	~ 90	21-25	Hepatic metabolism; about 5% unchanged in urine	No	
Clonazepam	?	~ 80	20-60	Hepatic metabolism; about 1-2% or less unchanged in urine	No	Half-life is shorter in children (22-33 hours)
Methsuximide	?	Little or none	~ 36-45*	Hepatic metabolism; < 1% unchanged in urine	Yes	*Half-life shown is for active N-desmethyl metabolite
Phensuximide	?	Little or none	5-12	Hepatic metabolism; negligible excretion of unchanged drug in urine	Probably	Half-life shown is for parent drug; desmethyl metabolite has similar short half-life

are believed to be related to modification by anti-convulsants of the movements of Na, K and Ca ions across the cell membrane and/or the release, uptake or recycling of neural transmitters. Continued presence of the drug is necessary for maintenance of these effects (see Kutt and Louis, 1972; Woodbury et al., 1979).

2.3.3 Pharmacokinetic Aspects

Almost all effective antiepileptic drugs are eliminated slowly and accumulate during long term administration (table II), thus allowing relatively stable plasma and tissue concentrations to be achieved and maintained.

The plasma and tissue concentrations of an antiepileptic drug are generally dependent upon its dosage, but the concentrations achieved with a dose are subject to variations among patients, mainly due to individual differences in the pharmacokinetic processes such as absorption, rate of drug metabolism and/or elimination (Hvidberg and Dam, 1976). Increases of the dose generally produce relatively proportionate rises in plasma concentration until for some drugs, the elimination mechanisms become saturated. Such dose dependent elimination (see chapter I; sect. 2.1.1) is relevant with phenytoin and although the saturation point for elimination generally occurs at higher plasma concentrations (fig. 2), it may be quite low in some individuals (Houghton and Richens, 1974). This means that a small increase in dosage may lead to a relatively larger increase in plasma concentration when elimination mechanisms are saturated in an individual patient. Other antiepileptic drugs such as carbamazepine stimulate their own metabolism (Eichelbaum et al., 1975) and again means disproportionate changes in plasma concentration with alteration of maintenance dosage. A decrease in protein binding of highly albumin bound drugs such as phenytoin in uraemia or liver disease leads to an increase in the fraction of unbound drug in plasma. Adjustment of dosage to achieve a given plasma concentration of total drug in this situation, underestimates the amount of free pharmacologically active drug. The therapeutic implications of these and other pharmacokinetic properties of antiepileptic drugs are summarised in table II and discussed further in section 3 (see Hvidberg and Dam, 1976).

2.3.4 Pharmacodynamic Aspects

The degree of seizure control is generally related to drug concentration in the blood and to the intensity of the seizure process. Because the intensity of the seizure process varies among individuals, the effective drug doses and plasma concentrations vary. The signs and symptoms of intoxication are also related to drug concentration, but their intensity with the same plasma concentrations may vary among individuals, depending at least in part upon the acquired tolerance (Kutt and Louis, 1972).

2.3.5 Monitoring of Plasma Concentrations

Monitoring of drug plasma concentrations has revealed that in a majority of patients with a given dose of antiepileptic drug, concentrations are achieved which fall into certain expected ranges (Kutt and Louis, 1972; Eadie, 1976). Plasma concentrations far below the expected range indicate most frequently that the patient is taking less than the prescribed dose. Confronting the patient with plasma concentration data may improve his attitude towards taking medication. Less frequent causes of low concentrations are incomplete absorption or unusually rapid elimination; in both cases higher than average doses need to be used. High plasma concentrations relative to a dose may result from greater than the prescribed intake. Other causes of high plasma concentrations include impairment of drug elimination by other concomitantly administered drugs (table III; Kutt, 1975; Richens, 1977), or rarely, by inborn or acquired abnormal patterns of drug metabolism (Kutt, 1971).

There is also a relationship between the antiepileptic drug blood concentration and clinical effects. With most drugs plasma concentration ranges can be defined above which the seizures in the majority of patients are controlled; i.e. the effective concentration range. Similarly, drug concentration ranges can be defined above which intoxication and/or dose related side effects are expected to start to occur in the majority of patients; i.e. potentially 'toxic' concentration range (Eadie, 1976; Hvidberg and Dam, 1976). These empirically derived expected concentration, effective concentration and toxic concentration ranges are best used as general guidelines along with careful clinical observation in making decisions to achieve optimum therapeutic results. Used in this way, monitoring of plasma concentrations can greatly improve control of seizures (Lund, 1974; Sherwin et al., 1973). Better control from the start of therapy in previously untreated patients also offers the possibility of avoiding multiple drug regimens in many patients (Reynolds et al., 1976; Shorvon et al., 1978).

3. Major Antiepileptic Drugs

3.1 Phenytoin (diphenylhydantoin)

Action: Phenytoin acts mainly by reducing afterdischarges and diminishing the post-tetanic potentiation. Thus, it prevents the spread of seizure discharges by a somewhat selective action at the hyperactive synapses (Kutt and Louis, 1972; Woodbury et al., 1979).

Pharmacokinetic Properties: Phenytoin is poorly water soluble and is slowly and variably absorbed from the small intestine, depending on the particle size and other characteristics of the particular formulation; peak plasma concentrations occurring 4 to 6 or sometimes 24 hours after ingestion. Bioavailability of phenytoin from tablets of different makers can differ markedly. As a result, a change of brand or even batch, might cause considerable changes in the plasma concentration of phenytoin and toxicity has resulted (Neuvonen, 1979). The same brand, and particularly tablets with good dissolution characteristics, should always be used (see chapter VI). Bioavailability is of the order of 80 to 95% from tablets of high quality. The elimination of phenytoin is almost entirely dependent upon its biotransformation which is subject to saturation kinetics (see section 3.1; fig. 2). The major metabolic product is p-hydroxyphenyl-phenylhydantoin which has little or no pharmacological activity. About 90% of phenytoin is bound to plasma proteins (mainly albumin); less in the very young and elderly and in patients with chronic uraemia or liver disease (see chapter IV, sect. 2.2.2; V, sect. 2.1.2; XXI, sect. 1.2; XIX, sect. 1.3). The plasma half-life is dose dependent but generally in the range of 20 to 30 hours in adults, and shorter in children. The concentration of phenytoin in breast milk is less than that in maternal plasma and is probably not of clinical significance in breast feeding when the maternal plasma concentrations are within the therapeutic range.

Dosage: The usual dose of phenytoin in adult patients is 300mg, 6 to 8mg/kg in children, given daily as a single or in 2 or 3 divided doses. The decision to use a single or divided dose regimen must be made separately for each patient. A maximum plasma phenytoin concentration is reached within 5 to 15 days; thus onset of full benefit is delayed. The lag time can be reduced by giving a loading dose of 1000mg. Absorption of phenytoin from intramuscular injection sites is usually erratic and lower than that after oral administration; thus, it is the least satisfactory route of administration (Wilder and Ramsay, 1976). In the majority of patients, 300mg orally will produce plasma concentrations ranging from 20 to 60µmol/L (5 to 15µg/ml), average 40µmol/L (10µg/ml). Upon increase of the dose, there is a rise of the blood concentration, but because of the saturation elimination kinetics which may occur within the therapeutic range of plasma concentrations (Richens, 1979), dosage increases in patients with blood concentrations near 80µmol/L (20µg/ml) are best made in small (25mg) increments. Concomitant use of other medications known to interfere with phenytoin metabolism and elimination (Kutt, 1975; Richens, 1977; see table III) may cause a higher than expected plasma concentration with the possibility of intoxication. This is found particularly with disulfiram and often with sulthiame. With isoniazid, phenytoin accumulation takes place only in the very slow isoniazid acetylators (inactivators) which in the USA comprise about 10% of the patients receiving the combined medication (Kutt et al., 1970; see fig. 1a,b).

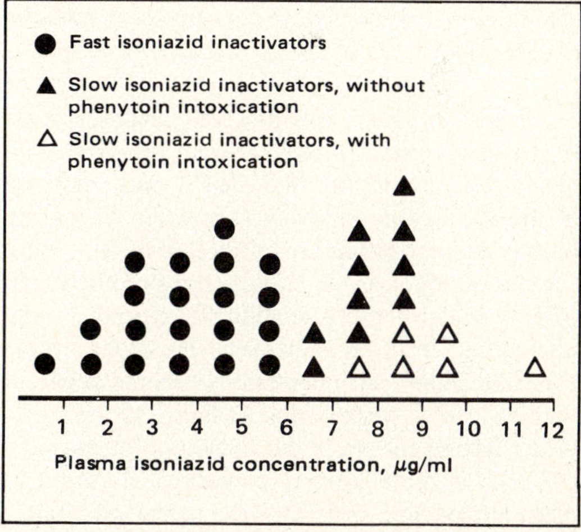

Fig. 1a. Isoniazid plasma concentrations of 36 patients 3 hours after a test dose of 10mg/kg isoniazid. All patients in whom phenytoin intoxication developed had high isoniazid plasma concentrations (open triangles). After Kutt et al.: American Review of Respiratory Diseases 101: 377, 1970; by permission.

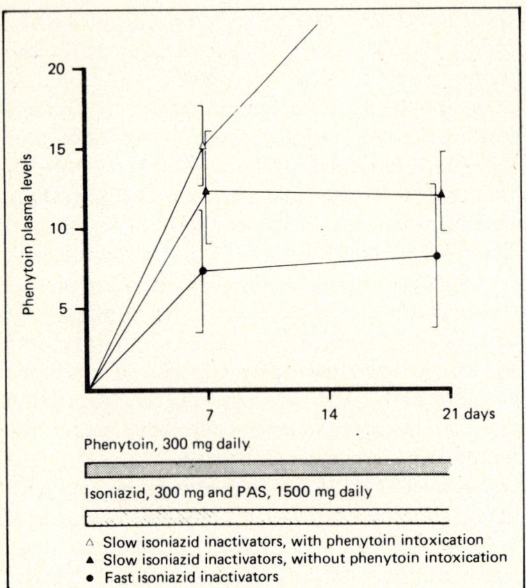

Fig. 1b. Phenytoin blood concentrations of patients who were fast, moderately slow, and very slow isoniazid acetylators (inactivators). There was a rapid rise to the toxic range without stabilisation in the very slow acetylators and the average level in the moderately slow acetylators was higher than in the fast acetylators (after Kutt et al.: American Review of Respiratory Diseases 101: 377, 1970; by permission).

A reduction of phenytoin dose to 100 to 200mg daily circumvents the problem. Liver disease or rarely an inborn error of drug metabolism may also cause a high phenytoin concentration in some patients (Kutt, 1971).

Drug Interactions: For practical purposes, most of the drugs listed in table III can be given with phenytoin, if clinically indicated. Concurrent use of these drugs is relatively safe when phenytoin plasma concentrations are monitored (Kutt, 1975). Careful observation for clinical signs of phenytoin toxicity initially after the addition of a potentially interacting drug is however, in order. Most clinically significant interactions become apparent within 1 to 6 weeks after addition of the other drug; beyond that time the likelihood of their occurrence is quite low. If a marked elevation of plasma phenytoin concentration to the toxic range does occur, the interacting drug may be eliminated, but if this cannot be done, as in the case of isoniazid or dicoumarol, the phenytoin dose has to be reduced and a new dosage titrated while monitoring plasma concentrations.

The extent of change of plasma concentration with the same interacting drugs and the same dosages show considerable variation among individual patients, suggesting that some patients are more susceptible to significant interactions than others. The interaction may not always be detrimental; thus, modest elevation of an initially low plasma concentration of phenytoin may actually improve seizure control, whereas modest elevation of a plasma concentration initially in the upper therapeutic range may lead to toxicity. Phenytoin elimination can be enhanced by phenobarbitone and some other drugs, but this is rarely of clinical consequence (Kutt, 1975, Kutt and Louis, 1972).

Toxicity and Desirable Plasma Concentration Range: Signs and symptoms of intoxication (nystagmus, ataxia of gait, and sedation) usually appear with plasma concentrations of over 80 to 120µmol/L (20 to 30µg/ml; fig. 2). Reduction or control of seizures is usually achieved with concentrations of over 20µmol/L (5µg/ml) in children and over 40µmol/L (10µg/ml) in adults. Therefore, a desirable phenytoin plasma concentration range would be between 20 and 80µmol/L for children, and between 40 and 120µmol/L for adults. Higher plasma concentrations may be needed in patients with a more severe seizure process, despite ensuing intoxication. Some

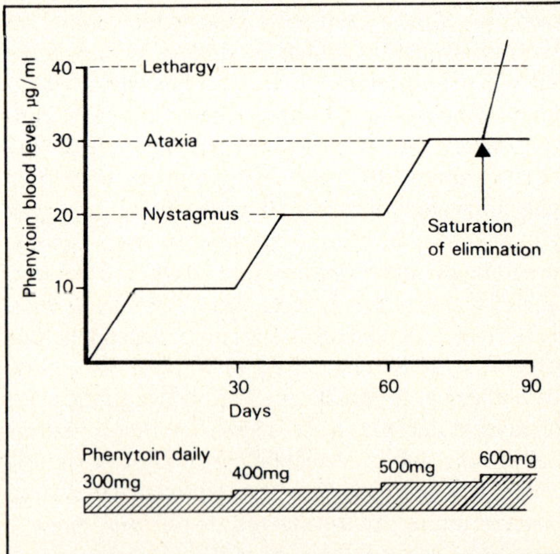

Fig. 2. Relationship of phenytoin blood concentrations to various dosages, and the evidence of intoxication in adults (after Kutt and McDowell: Journal of the American Medical Association 203: 969, 1968; by permission).

Table III. Drugs which cause changes in phenytoin plasma concentration (after Kutt, 1975; Richens, 1977)

Incidence	Increase in plasma concentration		Decrease in plasma concentration	
	marked	small	marked	small
High	Sulthiame Disulfiram Isoniazid (slow acetylators)	Valproate sodium		Valproate sodium
Low	Diazepam Chlordiazepoxide Dicoumarol Methylphenidate Phenylbutazone Phenyramidol Sulphaphenazole Chloramphenicol	Pheneturide Phenobarbitone Primidone Phenprocoumon Alcohol Chlorpromazine Prochlorperazine Halothane Sulphamethizole	Diazoxide	Phenobarbitone Primidone Carbamazepine Diazepam ?Clonazepam Tolbutamide Alcohol

Note: The clinical significance of these interactions varies. See section 3.1 for discussion of implications of a change in plasma phenytoin concentration. Appendix C and section 3 provide information on important interactions with other antiepileptic drugs.

tolerance to toxic effects develops frequently. Prolonged very high concentrations should be avoided since permanent cerebellar damage has been reported in this situation (Selhorst et al., 1972). For a review of the clinical pharmacokinetics of phenytoin, see Richens (1979).

3.2 Phenobarbitone

Phenobarbitone acts primarily by non-selective depression of synaptic transmission; thus some sedation with higher doses may occur (Kutt and Louis, 1972; Woodbury et al., 1979).

Phenobarbitone is nearly completely, but somewhat slowly, absorbed after oral administration; peak blood level occurring in 6 to 12 or 18 hours. About 20 to 50% of the dose is excreted unchanged in the urine; excretion being enhanced by alkalinisation of the urine. The major metabolic product is p-hydroxyphenobarbitone which is inactive. Plasma protein binding of phenobarbitone is about 50%. The plasma half-life varies from 2 to 5 or more days; lower in children, 1.5 to 3 days (Hvidberg and Dam, 1976). Phenobarbitone is an inducer of hepatic microsomal drug metabolising enzymes and may thus alter the dosage requirements of other metabolised drugs (see chapter VIII; sect. 2.3.3). This is of clinical consequence mostly in the use of oral coumarin anticoagulants (see chapter XXIII; sect. 3.2.5).

The average dose of phenobarbitone is 180mg in adults (2 to 5mg/kg in children) given in a single or divided dose, and produces a maximum plasma concentration of 45 to 135μmol/L (10 to 30μg/ml) within 2 to 3 weeks. These concentrations are usually effective (Buchthal and Lennox-Buchthal, 1972). Higher doses produce proportionally higher levels; saturation elimination kinetics have not been observed. Concentrations over 180 to 270μmol/L (40 to 60μg/ml) tend to produce excessive sedation, but tolerance to this side effect develops in many patients. Phenobarbitone is often used together with phenytoin in doses of 45 to 90mg daily and frequently results in better seizure control with fewer side effects. Phenobarbitone should not be discontinued suddenly because withdrawal seizures may ensue (Schmidt and Wilder, 1968).

3.3 Primidone

The mechanism of action of primidone is complex. The parent compound yields 2 active metabolites, phenobarbitone and phenyl-ethyl-malonamide (PEMA). The major factor probably is phenobarbitone.

Primidone is well absorbed; peak blood concentrations occurring in 2 to 4 hours following oral ingestion. The biotransformation products mentioned above are eliminated slowly. The half-life of derived phenobarbitone is 3 to 5 days, that of PEMA 40 to 60 hours. The half-life of primidone itself is 6 to 12 hours. About a half of the dose is excreted as the unchanged parent compound in the urine (Zavadil and Gallagher, 1976). Plasma protein binding of primidone is negligible.

The dose of primidone in adults is 750mg daily, which will produce a plasma concentration of around 44μmol/L (10μg/ml); PEMA appears in plasma a few hours after a dose of primidone and concentrations eventually attained equal that or are somewhat higher than the parent drug. Phenobarbitone appears in the plasma about 4 days after continuous therapy has been started and concentrations reach values 2 to 3 times that of the parent drug in 2 to 3 weeks from the onset of therapy (Olesen and Dam, 1967).

3.4 Carbamazepine

Carbamazepine, like phenytoin, reduces post-tetanic potentiation and modifies selectively the synaptic transmission resulting in prevention of seizure spread (Fincham et al., 1974).

Absorption of carbamazepine is not complete as about 20 to 30 % of the oral dose is excreted in the faeces. Bioavailability is decreased when given on an empty stomach but increased when given with food. Peak plasma concentrations occur in 4 to 10 hours. Biotransformation of carbamazepine yields up to 8 metabolites, one of which (carbamazepine 10,11-epoxide) is active and is found in the blood in important but variable amounts. The ratio of epoxide metabolite to parent drug in plasma varies from 15 to 55 % in adults and 5 to 81 % in children. Carbamazepine induces its own metabolism and the plasma half-life of 18 to 65 hours after single doses is decreased to 10 to 20 hours after continuous administration. This means that with continued therapy an increase in dose may not lead to a proportional rise in plasma concentration. The half-life of the epoxide metabolite after continuous administration is slightly shorter than that of the parent drug. Plasma half-lives in newborns exposed to the drug in fetal life and in children are similar to those in adults. Carbamazepine metabolism is induced by phenytoin and phenobarbitone which lowers the parent compound concentration in the plasma and alters the parent compound to metabolite ratio (Dam et al., 1975). Protein binding of parent compound and the metabolite is 70 to 80 % and 50 % respectively (for review, see Bertilsson, 1978).

Clinically effective doses range from 800 to 1200mg daily; 2 divided doses are appropriate in most cases, but due to fluctuations of plasma concentrations some patients may benefit from more frequent dosing to 3 or 4 times a day to avoid side effects. A 4 times a day schedule is required when carbamazepine is used with phenytoin and/or phenobarbitone. The above doses render blood concentrations of 16 to 50μmol/L (4 to 12μg/ml) of the parent compound and 1 to 4μg/ml of carbamazepine 10,11-epoxide. Concentrations over 50μmol/L of the parent drug may cause side effects which include headache, unsteadiness and drowsiness. Plasma concentrations of carbamazepine also fluctuate widely in patients on combination therapy compared with carbamazepine alone; necessitating 4 daily doses, with the largest dose of the day given as late as possible in the evening (Hvidberg and Dam, 1976).

Carbamazepine may induce the metabolism of phenytoin and coumarin anticoagulants such as warfarin to some extent (Hansen et al., 1971). See further chapter XXIII (sect. 3.2.5) and appendix C.

3.5 Ethosuximide

Ethosuximide prevents pentylenetetrazole induced seizures. It reduces synaptic transmission to low frequency electrical stimulation which is in accordance with its effectiveness against absence seizures accompanied by three per second discharges.

The drug is readily absorbed; peak blood concentrations occur within 4 hours following oral ingestion. It is extensively metabolised to inactive products with about 10 to 20 % of a dose excreted in the urine unchanged. Plasma half-life is about 60 hours in adults, 30 hours in children. Protein binding is negligible (Hvidberg and Dam, 1976).

The effective doses of ethosuximide range from 15 to 30mg/kg; higher doses are needed in younger children, lower in older children and in adults. Effective blood concentrations range from 300 to 750μmol/L (40 to 100μg/ml); dose related toxic effects are poorly defined.

3.6 Clonazepam

Clonazepam acts probably as do other benzodiazepines by influencing the after discharge threshold, synaptic transmission and the seizure spread. On a molecular level, alteration of monoamine transmitter balance appears to be involved. Clinically, it has a wide spectrum of effect but it is mostly used in the treatment of childhood seizures, such as myoclonic, infantile spasms and absences (see Pinder et al., 1976c; Browne, 1978a).

The drug is quickly and completely absorbed; peak blood concentrations occurring in 2 to 4 hours following oral ingestion. Several metabolites have been identified which are pharmacologically inactive. Plasma half-life of clonazepam is 20 to 60 hours; shorter in children. About 80% of the drug is bound to plasma proteins (Hvidberg and Dam, 1976; Pinder et al., 1976c).

Effective doses in children range from 0.1 to 0.2mg/kg daily; in adults 10 to 15mg per day. These are built up gradually from 0.01 to 0.03mg/kg daily in children and 1.5mg daily or less in adults. The plasma concentrations in patients who benefitted from clonazepam have ranged from 70 to 230nmol/L (20 to 70ng/ml). High doses and plasma concentrations are associated with drowsiness. Clonazepam may reduce phenytoin and primidone plasma concentrations in some patients, but this effect is rarely marked (Pinder et al., 1976c).

3.7 Diazepam

Diazepam is effective against experimental seizures induced either by electrical stimulation or pentylenetetrazole. It limits the spread of seizure discharges from penicillin foci and raises the after-discharge threshold in subcortical nuclei. The molecular mechanism probably involves alteration of monoamine transmitter balance and turnover (Woodbury et al., 1979).

The drug is well absorbed from the intestinal tract; the peak blood concentration occurring in 1 to 2 hours. Following intravenous administration, blood-brain penetration is rapid. The plasma half-life of diazepam is around 24 to 48 hours. The drug is rapidly metabolised to desmethyldiazepam, which is pharmacologically active and has a half-life of 51 to 120 hours (see further chapter XXVI; sect. 1.4.3).

Diazepam given intravenously is one of the major agents used in treatment of status epilepticus. A dose of 5 to 10mg given over 3 to 5 minutes stops the seizures, but the effect may not last longer than 20 to 30 minutes; the dose is then repeated (Duffy and Lombroso, 1978).

Diazepam is sometimes also used orally to treat minor motor seizures in doses of 10 to 30mg daily. Effective blood concentrations during continued therapy vary in the range of 335 to 670nmol/L (100 to 200ng/ml) of diazepam and 200 to 300ng/ml of desmethyldiazepam. Marked interindividual variation in tolerance to sedative effects of diazepam has been noted (Eadie and Tyrer, 1974).

3.8 Sodium Valproate (valproic acid)

Sodium valproate may act at least in part by elevating γ-aminobutyric acid concentration in the brain. Clinically, it is most effective against absence seizures and other childhood 'spike and wave' epilepsies (Pinder et al., 1977b).

Sodium valproate is rapidly absorbed; peak blood concentrations occurring in 1 to 2 hours following oral ingestion. The metabolites found in the urine include 2-n-propyl-5-hydroxypentanoic acid and 2-n-propylglutaric acid which are inactive. The plasma half-life is quoted as ranging between 8 and 15 hours but the half-life reflecting the true elimination phase from plasma is 13 to 21 hours. Protein binding is approximately 90% (Gugler et al., 1977). Binding is reduced in patients with chronic uraemia. The half-life is shortened in patients receiving phenytoin, phenobarbitone, primidone or carbamazepine, suggesting induction of metabolism of sodium valproate. Prolongation of half-life up to 30 hours in cases of overdosage, suggests saturation of elimination mechanisms. Enterohepatic elimination has been suggested in the rat (Pinder et al., 1977b).

Effective doses in patients with absence seizures have ranged from 15 to 30mg/kg daily, taken in 3 to 4 divided doses. Diurnal variations of blood concentrations are considerable (Schobben et al., 1975). The effective plasma concentrations have ranged from 280 to 840μmol/L (40 to 120μg/ml). High dose related side effects are vague and include sedation and gastrointestinal complaints. Tolerance develops to the gastric irritation which can also be alleviated by taking the drug with meals.

Sodium valproate alters phenobarbitone elimination, causing a rise of the phenobarbitone plasma concentration. Thus, in patients taking phenobarbitone or drugs producing phenobarbitone such as primidone and methylphenobarbitone, the barbiturate dose often needs to be reduced after sodium valproate has been added. The effect of sodium valproate on phenytoin plasma concentration is variable and usually not marked (Pinder et al., 1977b). Sodium valproate is a fatty acid and has the potential to displace highly albumin bound drugs such as phenytoin from protein binding sites. Such displacement when sodium valproate is added to the regimen, is only likely to lead to a marked increase in plasma phenytoin concentration if concentrations were initially high and/or in the range in an individual patient when the capacity of the liver to eliminate the drug becomes saturated. Otherwise, a modest lowering of phenytoin plasma concentrations may occur (see chapter I; sect. 3.2.3).

3.9 Adverse Effects of Antiepileptic Drugs

The untoward effects of antiepileptic drugs can be divided into (a) signs and symptoms of intoxication; (b) side effects; and (c) idiosyncratic phenomena.

3.9.1 Signs and Symptoms of Intoxication (overdosage)

Sedation, nystagmus or disturbances of equilibrium and co-ordination will occur in every patient with excessive dosage (barbiturates, hydantoins and benzodiazepines) or with usual dosage when interfering factors lead to high plasma concentrations (see sections 3.1 to 3.8).

3.9.2 Side Effects

A number of side effects have been observed following the prolonged use of antiepileptic drugs (Reynolds, 1975; 1978). With phenytoin, gum hypertrophy is frequent (over 30%), particularly when the drug is started in very young patients (see chapter XIII; sect. 13.2); hirsutism and acne are not infrequent and peripheral neuropathies may occur in some patients after years of therapy. Depression of serum calcium and elevated serum alkaline phosphatase occur often, but rickets or osteomalacia is usually seen in patients with limited exposure to sunlight or with diet low in vitamin D (see chapter XXII; sect. 14.5). Depression of serum folate levels (rarely leading to megaloblastic anaemia, and responsive to folic acid 5mg daily) has been observed in patients treated with phenytoin, phenobarbitone or primidone (see chapter XXIII; sect. 8.5). Carbamazepine has a membrane stabilising effect similar to quinidine and procainamide and can suppress idioventricular

rhythm in those with a defective conduction system (Beerman and Edhag, 1978). Bradycardia or conduction disturbances are most likely to occur with excessive doses in elderly patients receiving the drug for trigeminal neuralgia, which often occurs at an age when cardiovascular disturbances first appear (Hamilton, 1978; Herzberg, 1978).

A further discussion of these and other side effects with antiepileptic drugs is given in section 4.

3.9.3 Idiosyncratic Phenomena

Idiosyncratic reactions occur rarely, but may be serious. Skin eruptions have occurred with all antiepileptic drugs. With a benign morbilliform rash, the drug may be cautiously tried again with a chance that the rash may not recur. Vesicobullous eruptions, however, may lead to fatal exfoliative dermatitis and the offending drug should not be used again. Blood dyscrasias are rare but must always be taken seriously; if the white cell count is below $4000 \times 10^6/L$ ($4000/mm^{-3}$), the drug should be discontinued. Lupus erythematosus, the Stevens-Johnson syndrome, liver and kidney damage occur rarely with most antiepileptic drugs, and a lymphoma-like picture is a rare observation with hydantoins (Charlesworth, 1977; Wilden and Scott, 1978). Periodic yearly blood counts and liver function tests should be obtained in all patients on antiepileptic drugs.

4. Treatment of Seizure Disorders

All patients presenting with seizures must have a thorough diagnostic work-up to establish that episodes are really seizures that would respond to antiepileptic drugs, and to exclude brain lesions that require specific treatment, such as brain tumour or abscess. The selection of the drug is based upon the seizure type (see Eadie and Tyrer, 1974; Richens, 1976). It is always wise to start therapy with one drug and use combinations only if single drug therapy fails. More than 3 drugs at a time is rarely practical. The importance of regular drug intake should be emphasised to the patient: 'the insurance policy becomes void if premiums are not paid.'

4.1 Tonic-Clonic Seizures (primary or secondary generalised)

Since generalised tonic-clonic seizures are potentially life endangering, they should be treated after diagnosis is made. Effective agents include phenytoin, phenobarbitone, primidone and carbamazepine. Phenytoin is usually the first choice because of its long relative safety record and lack of sedation. Maximum effect of a selected dose is expected within a week unless a loading dose is used. The dosage requirement of phenytoin may vary among individuals and the common starting dose of 300mg daily is adjusted accordingly (see section 3.1). When plasma concentrations reach near 20µg/ml, dose increases in small amounts (e.g. 25mg daily) will avoid a marked upswing of plasma concentration in those individuals whose hepatic metabolic capacity to eliminate the drug is readily saturated (see section 2.3.3). Gingival hyperplasia frequently occurs with phenytoin, particularly when the drug is started at an early age (see chapter XIII; sect. 13.2). If phenytoin alone is not providing sufficient seizure control with near toxic doses and plasma concentrations, its dosage should be reduced and phenobarbitone or primidone added (table IV; section 3.2, 3.3). It is best to start the barbiturate drug with low doses such as phenobarbitone 45mg a day or primidone 250mg daily and increase the dose slowly to avoid excessive initial sedation. Carbamazepine may be considered as the third drug, if needed. Some clinicians, particularly in paediatric practice, prefer phenobarbitone as the drug of first choice. Once the effective dosage regimen has been established, patients are followed at 1 to 3 month intervals, less often if good control is maintained.

Patients with focal features should remain as brain tumour suspects and re-evaluated periodically, since a small tumour may escape the initial work-up.

If the above mentioned regimens are ineffective, methoin (mephenytoin), sulthiame (200 to 1200mg daily) or benzodiazepines (table IV) may be used. Addition of acetazolamide (500 to 1000mg daily) has been helpful, particularly if the seizures tend to occur around the time of menstrual periods.

4.2 Partial Seizures with Complex Symptomatology (psychomotor)

These disorders have been traditionally treated with phenytoin and/or primidone, but in more recent years carbamazepine is considered the drug of first choice by many clinicians. If carbamazepine is used, it is best to build up the dose slowly (table IV; section 3.4). Plasma concentrations over 21µmol/L (5µg/ml) may be effective. Since carbamazepine induces its own metabolism to some extent, the rise of plasma concentration is often not proportional to the increase of dosage. Concentrations over 50µmol/L (12µg/ml) usually cause side effects, but lower concentrations may also do so if used together with high doses of phenytoin or primidone (see section 3.4). Blood counts and liver function should be monitored monthly after onset of carbamazepine therapy; less often later if found stable. Because of its water retaining properties, excessive intake of fluids should be discouraged in patients taking carbamazepine (Perucca et al., 1978).

Complete control of partial complex seizures is sometimes difficult to achieve. Since the seizure manifestations are often not too disruptive, the patient may prefer incomplete control over the side effects of high doses of medication. Further drugs sometimes helpful in patients with hard to control partial complex seizures include phensuximide, methoin, a benzodiazepine and sodium valproate.

4.3 Absence Seizures

Ethosuximide has been the drug of first choice (table IV; section 3.5). Gastric irritation may be a problem in some patients, but is alleviated by taking the drug with meals. A syrup rendering 250mg per 5ml is available for use in young children. Blood counts should be monitored during ethosuximide therapy because of the risk of leucopenia in particular. Sodium valproate is a good alternative or add-on drug in patients with absence seizures. It also causes gastric irritation; therefore, the dose (table IV; section 3.8) is best increased slowly and given initially with meals. Sedation from sodium valproate alone is rare, and usually occurs if the patient is also taking phenobarbitone (see section 3.8). Haematological complications from sodium valproate are extremely rare and include isolated instances of prolonged bleeding times and thrombocytopenia due to disturbances of platelet function, but impairment of liver function may occur (Pinder et al., 1977b). Liver and platelet function should be monitored.

Trimethadione, the first effective antiabsence agent is now used sparingly because of its relatively high toxicity. Benzodiazepines and acetazolamide may be of use in difficult to control patients.

Table IV. Commonly used drugs for treatment of convulsive disorders. Dosage and desirable plasma concentrations

Drug	Use	Usual daily maintenance dose range		Therapeutic plasma concentration[1]		Notes
		adult	paediatric	μg/ml	μmol/L	
Phenytoin (diphenyl-hydantoin)	Tonic-clonic and partial seizures with complex symptomatology (psychomotor)	200-600mg*	6-8mg/kg*	10-20	40-80	*Dosage adjustments should be in small (25mg) increments at near upper range of therapeutic blood concentration. Since bioavailability may vary markedly, do not change brands
Phenobarbitone	As above	60-400mg	2-5mg/kg	10-30	45-135	
Carbamazepine	As above	400-1600mg	~ 100-600*	4-12**	16-50	*Up to 1000mg in older children. In combination regimens give in 4 divided doses with major portion at night time **Plasma concentration active epoxide metabolite should also probably be monitored
Primidone	As above	500-1500mg	5-20mg/kg	5-10*	20-40	*Metabolised to phenobarbitone (see table II) which may accumulate; phenobarbitone levels should also be monitored
Methoin (mephenytoin)	As above	300-800mg	3-10mg/kg			
Ethosuximide	Absence seizures	15-30mg/kg	20-60mg/kg	40-100	300-750	
Trimethadione	As above	600-1800mg	20-60mg/kg	> 700*	> 5000*	*As dimethadione, the active metabolite
Paramethadione	As above	600-1800mg	20-60mg/kg			
Sodium valproate	As above; also myoclonic and akinetic seizures, infantile spasms	1000-2000mg	15-40mg/kg	40-120	280-840	

Drug	Indications	Dose	Dose	Therapeutic level (ng/ml)	Therapeutic level (nmol/L)	Notes
Diazepam	Myoclonic and akinetic seizures, infantile spasms; also tonic-clonic seizures	5-30mg	0.1-1mg/kg	100-200 (ng/ml)	335-670 (nmol/L)	
Nitrazepam	As above		0.15-2mg/kg			
Clonazepam	As above	10-15mg	0.1-0.2mg/kg*	20-70 (ng/ml)	70-230 (nmol/L)	*Lower starting doses to minimise sedation (see text)
ACTH	Myoclonic and akinetic seizures, infantile spasms		0.15-2mg/kg			
Methsuximide	Partial complex seizures	600-2400mg	20-60mg/kg	10-40*	50-200*	*As the desmethyl metabolite
Phensuximide	As above	1000-4000mg				

1 Values based on findings in the majority of patients. However, considerable variation among individual patients regarding these figures occur (see section 3).

4.4 Myoclonic and Akinetic Seizures and Infantile Spasms

These disorders have been and still are difficult to treat (Solomon and Plum, 1976). For infantile spasms, a trial with pyridoxine is sometimes undertaken. If unsuccessful, ACTH 20 to 40 units daily for 4 to 6 weeks or prednisone 2mg/kg for 1 to 2 months may be beneficial. Benzodiazepines have also been effective in some instances. The benzodiazepines are mostly used in patients with myoclonic and akinetic seizures. Nitrazepam in doses of 0.15 to 2mg/kg and diazepam 5 to 30mg per day were used prior to the availability of clonazepam. The latter is often effective in doses of 0.1 to 0.2mg/kg daily, but the starting dose should be lower to avoid extreme sedation at the onset of therapy (see section 3.6). Clonazepam, although reducing myoclonic seizures, has caused major generalised seizure manifestations in some patients (Pinder et al., 1976c; Browne, 1978). The beneficial effects of benzodiazepines are often not long lasting. Sodium valproate also deserves a try in patients with myoclonic seizures. A ketogenic diet is used as a last resort.

4.5 Status Epilepticus

Status epilepticus of the generalised tonic-clonic type is a medical emergency. It may be caused by head trauma, brain abscess or other infections, or sudden stopping of antiepileptic drugs, particularly the barbiturates.

In the treatment of status epilepticus, the immediate goals are: (1) to secure adequate pulmonary ventilation; (2) to stop the seizures as soon as possible, and (3) to identify and treat precipitating factors (Browne, 1978b; Duffy and Lombroso, 1978). Antiepileptic drugs are given intravenously. Phenytoin provides definitive, long term control of generalised tonic-clonic seizures but must be given slowly and takes time to attain desirable concentrations in the brain. Intravenous diazepam achieves therapeutic concentrations more rapidly. A practical regimen is to give 10mg of diazepam intravenously over 5 minutes, which often stops the seizures by the time the injection is completed. Paediatric doses are 1mg every 2 to 5 minutes to maximum of 10mg in children over 5 years and half these doses in those under 5 years. The effect of diazepam may be of short duration, then the dose should be repeated and followed by an infusion of phenytoin in a loading dose of 25mg/kg in children; 20mg/kg in adults. Phenytoin should be infused at a rate of 50mg per minute or less while monitoring respiration, blood pressure, and ECG to avoid respiratory or cardiac depression (Cranford et al., 1978). Clonazepam in a dose of 1 to 4mg intravenously is also highly and rapidly effective and appears to have a longer duration of effect than diazepam, but respiratory depression and sedation may be more prominent than with diazepam (Pinder et al., 1976c).

If the above regimens are ineffective in stopping status epilepticus, ether or short acting barbiturate anaesthesia may have to be used. In some patients with refractory status epilepticus, success has been achieved with chlormethiazole (Harvey et al., 1975). When used for the treatment of status epilepticus, it may be given intravenously as an 0.8% solution at a rate of 0.3 to 0.7g per hour for a total dose of 3 to 5g per day. Side effects include drowsiness, depression of respiration, increased bronchial secretions and nasal stuffiness.

Usually, status epilepticus of absence and partial seizures also responds to intravenously given diazepam or clonazepam. However, in the case of partial seizures, phenytoin or phenobarbitone may have to be used as well.

4.6 Use of Plasma Drug Concentrations

The rationale of application of plasma concentrations in clinical management of seizures was discussed in section 2.3.5. When ordering plasma concentration estimations, it should be kept in mind that most antiepileptic drugs reach steady-state slowly. A plasma concentration determination ordered too soon following onset of therapy or change of dosage may indicate whether a low or high steady-state is forthcoming, but not the maximum concentration to be achieved. In office practice, ordering plasma concentrations has proven to be useful in the following instances:

1) After starting therapy to ascertain what concentration the patient will achieve with the prescribed dose; and if therapy is effective, to reveal the patient's effective concentration.

2) When seizure control is inadequate.

3) After a change of dosage.

4) After addition of new drugs, either antiepileptic drugs or other medication, particularly, if the addition is a potentially interacting drug (table III; appendix C).

5) In the presence of signs and symptoms of intoxication, particularly, if several drugs are taken.

6) Periodically during the course of therapy; the patient now knows that his compliance can be checked by a blood test.

What plasma concentrations to order: With phenytoin, phenobarbitone, ethosuximide, and sodium valproate the parent compound is the active principle. Active metabolites, which are more important than the rapidly metabolised parent compound, are produced by trimethadione, methoin (mephenytoin), methylphenobarbitone (mephobarbital), and methsuximide. Primidone produces two active metabolites: phenylethyl-malonamide and phenobarbitone (see section 3.3). Carbamazepine also produces an active metabolite which can influence interpretation of plasma concentrations (see section 3.4).

When to draw blood: One should try to obtain the samples about the same time of day, if serial follow-up is planned, since some diurnal variations may occur. An early morning sample drawn before the first dose will represent the lowest point of the plasma concentration-time curve.

There is no difference in the drug concentration between serum and plasma, but severe haemolysis tends to reduce the values for most drugs. For short term storage, 4°C is adequate; refrigeration is not necessary when mailing samples.

4.7 Antiepileptic Drugs in Pregnancy

Use of antiepileptic drugs has to be continued in pregnancy, particularly if the mother is subject to frequent seizures (Stumpf and Frost, 1978). Apart from the usual side effects, problems related to the baby exist — sedation of the neonate and withdrawal seizures may occur with barbiturates (see chapter III; sect. 3.3); and neonatal bleeding, which is responsive to vitamin K_1, has occurred as a complication of phenytoin and barbiturate use (Mountain et al., 1970). Congenital malformations in babies born to mothers taking antiepileptic drugs (including phenytoin and trimethadione) occur 2 to 3 times more often than in the general population (6.5% vs 2.5%; Speidel and Meadow, 1974; Janz, 1975). Nevertheless, at the present time there is not a clear indication for altering the antiepileptic drug regimen of the mother or choosing one drug over another. The presence of epilepsy in either parent may contribute to an increased occurrence of congenital abnormalities (Meadow, 1974; Shapiro et al., 1976).

In some patients, the rate of elimination of phenytoin, phenobarbitone and carbamazepine (and possibly also ethosuximide) may change as pregnancy advances; the plasma concentration may fall and the seizure frequency increase, particularly in the second and third trimester. After delivery, the dose requirement declines to the equivalent of that of the prepregnancy period. Plasma concentrations should be monitored frequently during pregnancy and in the puerperium (Eadie et al., 1977; Dam et al., 1979).

Most antiepileptic drugs are found in the breast milk in low concentrations. Only phenobarbitone (or that derived from primidone) may be of clinical concern in nursing if the mother's plasma concentration of phenobarbitone is high, since phenobarbitone is excreted in breast milk in moderate amounts (Tyson et al., 1938). The capacity of the newborn to eliminate phenobarbitone is nevertheless adequate (Boreus et al., 1978).

5. Extrapyramidal Syndromes

5.1 Parkinson's Disease

The symptomatic control of Parkinson's disease was greatly improved by the introduction of levodopa, following the observation that most of the dopamine in the central nervous system is concentrated in the extrapyramidal system, and that in the brains of patients with Parkinson's disease, there is a deficiency of dopamine. In addition to the deficiency of dopamine, subsequently, deficiencies in other neurotransmitters in patients with Parkinson's disease have been recognised and include γ-aminobutyric acid, serotonin, noradrenaline (norepinephrine) and others. It is now postulated that a balance between normal neurotransmitter activity has been interrupted in patients with Parkinson's disease (Calne, 1977).

5.1.1 Levodopa
Levodopa is the therapy of choice in Parkinson's disease. Levodopa replacement therapy (fig. 3), in an effort to increase the quantity of dopamine in the basal ganglia, has been effective in eliminating many of the major symptoms of Parkinson's disease, including hypokinesia and rigidity, and in many patients, it significantly eliminates tremor. Levodopa is less effective in eliminating such signs of Parkinson's disease as

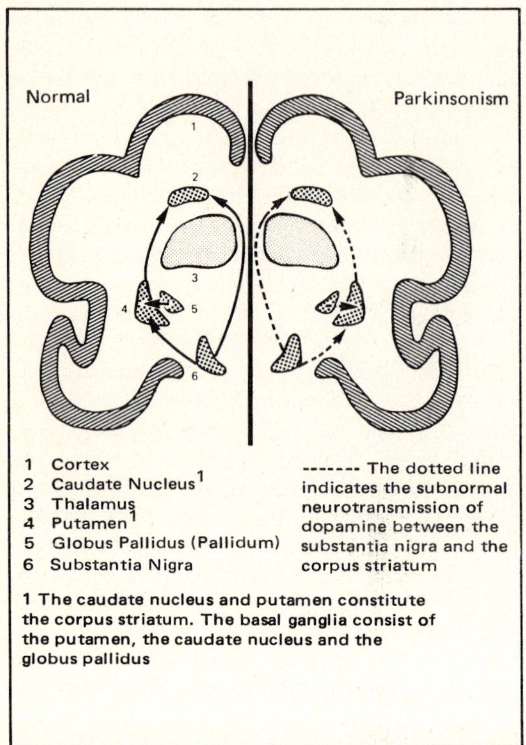

Fig. 3. Diagrammatic representation of the basal ganglia, substantia nigra and the nigrostriatal dopaminergic pathways (after Brogden et al.: Drugs 2: 262, 1971).

postural instability. Most patients respond well to levodopa therapy, and only a few patients do not respond at all (see Brogden et al., 1971). The agent does not however, affect the cause of the disease, and the condition continues to progress in every patient. However, many patients have 2 to 5 or more years of excellent sustained improvement following the beginning of use of levodopa (Barbeau, 1975; Markham et al., 1974; Sweet and McDowell, 1975). Parkinson's syndrome induced by antipsychotic agents such as phenothiazines or butyrophenone drugs is refractory to levodopa because these drugs block dopamine receptors.

Metabolism and Absorption: Levodopa is able to cross the blood-brain barrier and reach the parenchyma where it is converted to dopamine by the enzyme aromatic L-amino acid decarboxylase (dopa decarboxylase). However, the enzyme is found in many areas outside the brain in such structures as the stomach, intestinal wall, liver, kidneys and heart, and only a small amount of the administered dose of levodopa actually reaches the neurons deficient in dopamine (fig. 4a). Owing to the rapid extracerebral metabolism of levodopa, large doses are needed to replenish brain dopamine stores.

Levodopa is taken orally, and is absorbed by an active transport mechanism in the small intestine. In addition to auto-oxidation and other loss within the lumen of the intestinal tract, dopa decarboxylase is present in the intestinal tract, stomach and small intestine, and much of the levodopa that is administered is decarboxylated before it passes from the intestinal tract into the systemic circulation. The availability of levodopa is therefore very variable and critically dependent on gastric emptying rate. Conditions which delay gastric emptying such as hyperacidity reduce the amount of levodopa available for absorption (see chapter VI, sect. 5; XIX, sect. 1.1.1). This reduction in effective doses of levodopa can be altered by decreasing gastric acidity and increasing the rapidity of gastric emptying, by the reduction of amino acids competing for dopa absorption, or by the use of dopa decarboxylase inhibitors (Bianchine and Shaw, 1976). In practice, it has been found that the efficiency of levodopa can be increased by a combination of levodopa with a selective peripheral decarboxylase inhibitor such as α-methyldopa hydrazine (carbidopa) or benserazide, both of which almost completely abolish extracerebral metabolism of levodopa and increase the availability of levodopa to the brain (fig. 4b). Without administration of a dopa decarboxylase inhibitor, due to loss during the absorption process, it is estimated that approximately only 0.1 % of the total levodopa administered arrives at the central nervous system. The plasma concentration achieved with the administration of levodopa is low; generally only 1 µg/ml.

Combination with a Decarboxylase Inhibitor and Side Effects: The regimen of levodopa, combined with a peripheral dopa decarboxylase inhibitor (see Pinder et al., 1976a), reduces the dose of levodopa required for optimum therapeutic benefit by approximately 80 %. It also reduces the incidence of nausea and vomiting, the most conspicuous early side effects of levodopa administration. The use of a dopa decarboxylase inhibitor with levodopa also allows a much more rapid institution of treatment because of the absence of nausea and vomiting and a more rapid onset of a therapeutic effect. Combined therapy may also reduce the risk of cardiac arrhythmias in patients with associated heart disease. Combined therapy has generally been shown to reduce the incidence of postural hypotension, which has been a side effect in up to 20 % of the patients receiving levodopa alone (Desjacques et al., 1973). Hypotension however, is rarely symptomatic, and generally decreases in severity with continued treatment. When hypotension is present, elastic stockings are useful in counteracting it, and in instances where hypotension is marked, small amounts of ephedrine (25mg taken twice daily) can sometimes be effective. Other side effects associated with levodopa alone, such as abnormal involuntary movements and psychiatric disturbances, may however, become more severe with long term use of levodopa and a dopa decarboxylase inhibitor (Yahr et al., 1971).

Approximately 25 % of the patients who take levodopa alone develop trouble in thinking or an acute drug intoxication delirium, manifested by confusion, hallucinations, anxiety and mental clouding. Reduction of the dose is usually suffi-cient to eliminate the symptoms, but a few patients require total cessation of levodopa to overcome this side effect.

Long Term Effectiveness and Complications: With appropriate doses, levodopa has shown sustained effectiveness without major difficulties from side effects in patients treated for up to 10 years (Barbeau, 1975; Markham et al., 1974; Sweet and McDowell, 1975, 1979). Long term use of levodopa therapy has not been associated with significant abnormalities of renal, liver or haematological function.

A new involuntary disorder or dyskinesia may develop in up to 50 % or more of patients treated for long periods of time (Barbeau, 1973; Brogden et al., 1971). The appearance of these movements, which are chorea-athetoid in nature, usually involving the face, tongue, or neck, and sometimes the extremities, has been used as evidence of a peak dose of levodopa. This motor disturbance has always been eliminated by dose reduction or cessation of levodopa. In some instances, however, the

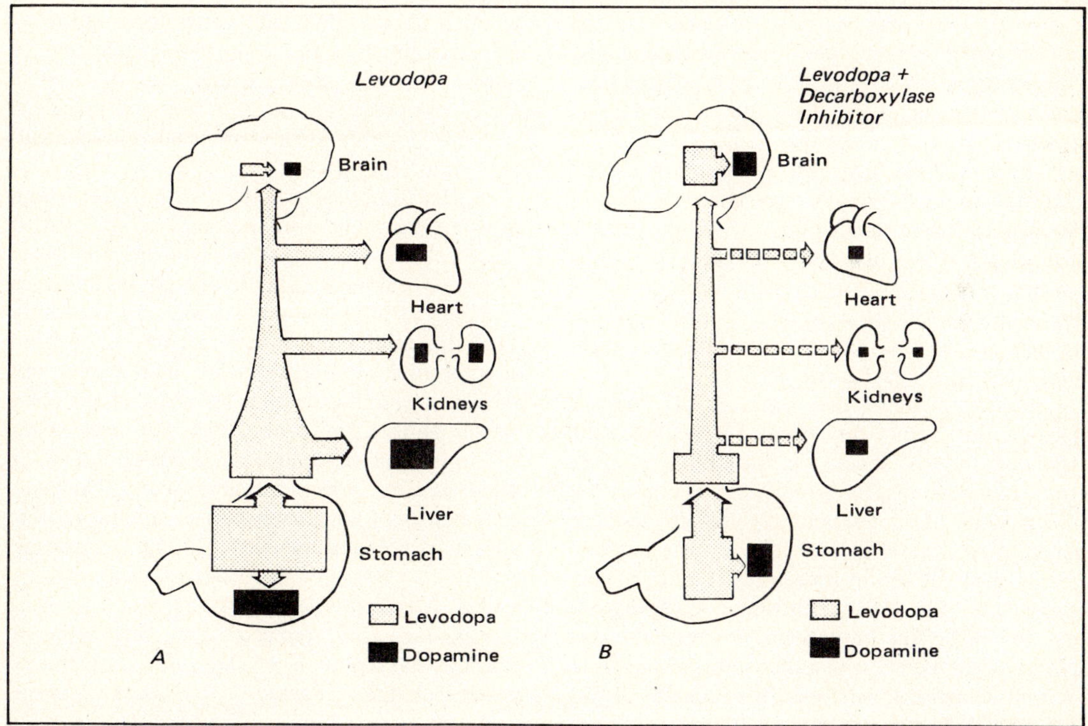

Fig. 4. Diagrammatic representation of the peripheral decarboxylation of levodopa to form dopamine (A) and the inhibition of this by the administration of a decarboxylase inhibitor (B). The concurrent administration of levodopa and a decarboxylase inhibitor decreases the amount of levodopa required to elicit a therapeutic response in Parkinsonism (after Brogden et al.: Drugs 2: 262, 1971).

development of dyskinetic movements has limited an effective intake of levodopa. Generally, these movements appear 1 to 2.5 hours after the ingestion of the dose, and when they occur, most evidence of Parkinson's disease has been eliminated. In some patients, new involuntary movements have tended to reappear with progressively lower doses of levodopa.

A conspicuous long term complication has been the 'on-off' effect or fluctuation in the patient's response to the medication (Barbeau, 1975; McDowell and Sweet, 1976; Sweet and McDowell, 1974a). In this situation, periods of nearly normal function ('on') alternate abruptly with periods of akinesia or increased tremor ('off'). This phenomenon has generally appeared 2 or more years after straight levodopa therapy, and has appeared a little earlier after using levodopa plus a decarboxylase inhibitor (Marsden and Parkes, 1976). The evidence to date indicates that 'on' periods are associated with relatively high serum concentrations of dopa, and that 'off' periods are associated with exceedingly low or undetectable amounts of dopa in the serum; reflecting end of dose deterioration (Chase et al., 1976). Generally, those patients who do not exhibit an 'off-on' phenomenon have relatively stable low concentrations of dopa in their blood throughout the day. Patients who show the phenomenon, develop widely fluctuating concentrations of serum dopa (Bianchine and Shaw, 1976; Sweet and McDowell, 1974b). A more complex form of fluctuating disability is termed 'yo-yo-ing' and is characterised by 'on' and 'off' periods which swing from one to the other within minutes. It is extremely difficult to treat and is apparently not related to levodopa intake or plasma concentrations (Marsden and Parkes, 1976).

The treatment of the common 'off and on' phenomenon has not been very successful. Initially, patients should be tried on a multiple small dose regimen, spreading the total intake over a period of 12 to 16 hours, given in relatively small doses, as it has been demonstrated that maintaining the serum concentration of dopa constant by an intravenous infusion will abolish the 'on and off' effect. In patients where this is not effective, the addition of other anti-Parkinsonian agents sometimes smooths the course of the patient's treatment programme. Earlier, this included dopa decarboxylase inhibitors (Sweet et al., 1975), and more recently, it has included the addition of such other agents as amantadine, piribedil

or bromocriptine (Kartzinel and Calne, 1976). If the addition of other anti-Parkinsonian agents is not effective, the patient should be tried on a low protein intake, as a number of amino acids compete with levodopa for absorption (Bianchine and Shaw, 1976). Low protein diets, 20 to 30mg of protein per day, are often associated with alleviation of the 'off-on' phenomenon, although unfortunately, not for very long periods. It is extremely difficult to maintain an individual for long periods on a low protein intake.

Dosage: It is mandatory that the dosage of levodopa and levodopa with decarboxylase inhibitors be titrated for each individual patient, until either maximum therapeutic response is observed or side effects preclude further dose increases. When levodopa is given alone, initial doses are usually 0.5 to 1g daily in 2 to 4 divided doses, with an increase in dose of 0.5g every 4 to 5 days (for frail patients these doses may be halved). On average, the patient begins to show some evidence of effect from levodopa at doses of 2.5g daily and the average sustaining dose of levodopa is approximately 5g. The range of dosage for producing benefit without side effects varies from as low as 0.5g to as much as 10 or 11g in a few patients. In general, the daily dosage usually does not exceed 8g. To minimise the risk of nausea and vomiting, levodopa alone should always be taken with meals or with a light snack.

When levodopa is given with a peripheral decarboxylase inhibitor, initial doses are approximately 100 to 125mg 4 times a day and 10 to 12.5mg of inhibitor. The dosage can be increased by 10mg of inhibitor and 100mg levodopa every other day until a maximum response is obtained or side effects prevent further increments. The average sustaining dose of levodopa in the combined regimen is about 25% of that when levodopa is used alone, with a maximum of 2g levodopa and 200mg of inhibitor daily. The usual daily dosage of the decarboxylase inhibitor is 50 to 200mg of carbidopa or 100 to 200mg benserazide.

5.1.2 Anticholinergic Agents

Levodopa has replaced the anticholinergic drugs as the treatment of choice for idiopathic or postencephalitic Parkinson's disease. Anticholinergic drugs however, because of their ability to inhibit the effects of acetylcholine in the central nervous system, and perhaps restore the balance of neurotransmitter activity, act synergistically with

Table V. Dosage of some commonly used anticholinergic drugs in Parkinsonism (after Calne and Reid, 1972)

Drug	Presentation	Starting dose	Usual daily dose
Benzhexol	Tablets	1-2mg bd	6-30mg
(trihexphenidyl)	Elixir		
Benztropine	Tablets	2mg at night	4-8mg
	IM or IV	2mg	—
Biperiden	Tablets	1mg bd	5-20mg
	IM or IV	5mg	—
Chlorphenoxamine	Tablets	50mg tds	200-400mg
Cycrimine	Tablets	1.25mg tds	5-20mg
Ethopropazine	Tablets	10mg qds	600-800mg
Methixine	Tablets	2.5mg tds	15-20mg
Procyclidine	Tablets	2.5mg tds	45-60mg
Orphenadrine	Tablets	50mg tds	200-400mg

levodopa (Hughes et al., 1971; see fig. 5). Existing therapy with anticholinergic drugs usually can be continued with benefit. These agents are also of value in patients who fail to respond to levodopa therapy, and in those in whom levodopa is considered to be contraindicated (e.g. presence of cardiac arrhythmia or cardiac failure, recent myocardial infarction). The dosage of some commonly used anticholinergic drugs is given in table V. Side effects from anticholinergic medication include dry mouth, blurred vision, mental clouding and occasionally urinary retention. The appearance of urinary retention and mental confusion and clouding usually requires cessation of the medication. The development of mental confusion in any patient taking levodopa and an anticholinergic agent should be treated first by elimination of the anticholinergic drug, as these drugs have a much higher incidence of this side effect than does levodopa alone.

5.1.3 Amantadine

Amantadine, which was originally used as an antiviral agent (see chapter XXVIII; sect. 4.4), was fortuitously discovered to have a potentially beneficial effect in Parkinson's disease (Schwab et al., 1969). It is believed to act by augmenting dopaminergic function (Stromberg et al., 1970). Although it causes fewer side effects than levodopa it is a much less powerful therapeutic agent (Hunter et al., 1970). Frequently a combination of levodopa and amantadine does however, act synergistically and amantadine may be very useful in patients who tolerate only small doses of levodopa. The most important side effects of amantadine are ankle oedema (which responds to salt restriction and/or diuretics) and livedo

reticularis (Parkes et al., 1971). Very infrequent, but disturbing complications, are intermittent confusion, nightmares, hallucinations, restlessness and giddiness. Dosage should be individualised, but the initial dosage is usually 100mg once or twice daily, increased to 200mg after a few days. Many patients tolerate 300mg daily, but few need more than this. In over half of the patients treated the effect of amantadine tends to wear off after 6 weeks or more of treatment. The effectiveness of amantadine can be restored by giving the patient a 2 to 3 week period off the drug and beginning it again.

5.1.4 Role of Other Anti-Parkinsonian Drugs

Since the introduction of levodopa, a number of agents have been discovered which have a direct dopaminergic action. The first of these was *piribedil,* which stimulates dopaminergic receptors, and produces improvement in patients with Parkinson's disease. This agent is not as effective as levodopa, but is occasionally a useful adjunct to levodopa therapy (Feigenson et al., 1976). Dosages again should be individualised, and can be started with 20 to 40mg 3 times a day. The maximum dose should not exceed 300mg daily. The side effects associated with piribedil therapy are abnormal involuntary movements or dyskinesia, and a relatively high incidence of mental clouding and confusion.

Other agents which have been discovered to have a direct dopaminergic stimulating effect are derivatives of ergot and include *bromocriptine* and *lergotrile.* Both stimulate dopaminergic receptors, and have been tried extensively in the United States and in Europe for their anti-Parkinson effects (Lieberman et al., 1976; Teychenne et al., 1978). Bromocriptine has been demonstrated to be beneficial in patients who have developed adverse effects from levodopa therapies such as the 'on-off' response. In general, neurological improvement occurs when daily dose levels are reached of 80 to 100mg. Bromocriptine and lergotrile are most effective when combined with levodopa plus a decarboxylase inhibitor. Adverse effects of both are more common when dosage exceeds 100mg a day. Distressing side effects of bromocriptine and lergotrile include a high incidence of nausea and vomiting, postural hypotension (Teychenne et al., 1978), and a high incidence of mental clouding and confusion, especially in patients who show any evidence of loss of higher integrative function or dementia. Unfortunately, lergotrile has been shown to produce, in addition to severe transient hypotension and moderate amounts of dyskinesia, some evidence of liver damage. Because of this, it is still considered an experimental drug. Bromocriptine, is available in most countries and it is an agent that can be tried when levodopa therapy is not providing the desired benefits or has caused the 'on-off' phenomenon (Calne et al., 1978; Parkes, 1979).

5.2 Athetosis

Athetotic movements are common in patients with cerebral palsy. They are characteristically

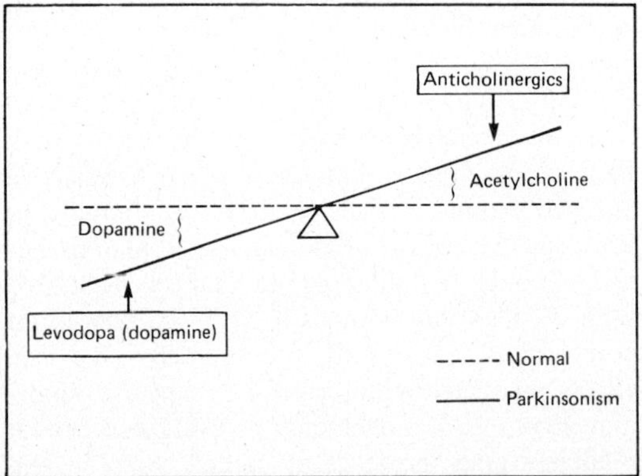

Fig. 5. Simplified schematic representation of the proposed imbalance between the excitatory neurotransmitter, acetylcholine, and the inhibitory neurotransmitter, dopamine, in the basal ganglia of Parkinsonian patients, thus suggesting a possible rationale for the synergistic effect of levodopa and anticholinergic drugs in Parkinsonism (after Brogden et al.: Drugs 2: 262, 1971).

twisting, writhing movements of the trunk or extremities which may make it impossible for a patient to function in any effective way, and are generally unaffected by medications other than muscle relaxants and sedatives given in such large amounts that the patient is oversedated. Levodopa is helpful in reducing the athetoid movements, and although its effect on athetosis is not dramatic, it appears to be better than most agents used so far (Rosenthal et al., 1972). As with Parkinson's disease, the levodopa dose must be started as low as 500mg once a day, and gradually increased until the symptoms are abolished or until the patient develops evidence of toxicity.

5.3 Sydenham's and Huntington's Chorea

Both Sydenham's and Huntington's chorea produce similar movement disorders. Sydenham's chorea is a self limiting disorder so medication need be given for chorea movement for a period of only a few weeks to a few months. Agents used are those which are dopamine antagonists. Chlorpromazine has been used in initial doses of 10mg 3 or 4 times. If this is not sufficient to control chorea, the dose is gradually increased until movements are brought under control. At times, doses up to 75mg 3 or 4 times a day are necessary for control of chorea. Tetrabenazine may also be used in initial doses of 25mg twice daily, gradually increased by 25mg daily every 2 to 4 days up to a maximum of 200mg daily (McLellan et al., 1974). Thiopropazate, 10mg gradually increased to 30mg daily, pimozide (2 to 6mg daily), haloperidol (1 to 4.5mg daily) and reserpine (2.5 to 10mg daily) have also been reported to be effective in the control of chorea. All patients should be observed closely for evidence of excessive or unwanted side effects.

Huntington's chorea, in addition to choreiform movements, is accompanied by progressive fall off in intellectual capacity or dementia. The brains of patients with Huntington's chorea have markedly reduced levels of γ-aminobutyric acid and glutamic acid decarboxylase. These reduced levels are generally confined to the basal ganglia, especially the caudate nucleus. Choline acetyltransferase levels have also been found to be lower than controls in these same areas (Bird and Iverson, 1974).

Control of choreiform movements in Huntington's chorea can be achieved by the use of dopamine antagonist drugs as outlined for

Sydenham's chorea. More recently, Huntington's chorea has been treated with agents which increase the amount of γ-aminobutyric acid in the central nervous system. Isoniazid, which inhibits γ-aminotransferase when given in large doses, will elevate the γ-aminobutyric acid content of the brain. Patients have been treated with 10 to 21mg/kg body weight together with pyridoxine, for 2 to 16 months with marked amelioration of symptoms (Perry et al., 1977). Patients placed on such high dosage of isoniazid should be carefully observed for evidence of hepatic dysfunction.

Bromocriptine, a dopaminergic agonist (section 5.1.4), has also been reported to be useful in the treatment of Huntington's chorea. When given in relatively small doses (10mg daily), it acts as a dopaminergic antagonist and it has been reported to decrease symptoms when given in this manner (Frattola et al., 1977). Levodopa accentuates the abnormal movements of Huntington's chorea and has been used as a means of identifying individuals at risk with a family history of Huntington's chorea. Those at risk of developing Huntington's chorea appear much more sensitive to induction of chorea by levodopa than individuals not at risk.

5.4 Muscular Dystonia and Wilson's Disease

Treatment of muscular dystonia has usually relied on muscle relaxants and sedatives which have been only moderately effective. Some patients, especially those with a clear hereditary factor in their dystonia have been reputed to benefit from levodopa. With violent dystonia, heavy doses of sedatives or muscle relaxants are resorted to.

The aim of treatment in Wilson's disease is to reduce the intake of copper as much as possible and to increase the output of copper in the patient's urine. Effective reduction of copper in the diet is impractical, and the mainstay of treatment is to improve urinary copper elimination. Two agents, D-penicillamine and dimercaprol, are available for increasing copper output. Penicillamine is the drug of choice; the size of the dose depends on the age and size of the patient and the severity of the illness, but in an adult it is usually given in doses of 1.5 to 2g orally daily in 3 divided doses before meals and should be continued for the duration of the patient's life (Walshe, 1977). D-penicillamine causes relatively few toxic reactions but the nephrotic syndrome, muscle weakness and myasthenic signs, and instances of leucopenia, urticaria and thrombocytopenia have been reported. Dimercaprol may be used in addition to penicillamine.

6. Facial Pain

Facial pain will be discussed in 3 categories: (a) the typical neuralgias, (b) postherpetic neuralgia, and (c) atypical facial pain.

6.1 Typical Neuralgias (trigeminal neuralgia)

Trigeminal neuralgia is characterised by sudden brief bouts of high intensity excruciating pain in the sensory distribution of the branches of the trigeminal nerve. Pain is usually elicited by stimulation of 'trigger zones'.

Based on the paroxysmal nature of this disorder, antiepileptic drugs have been tried and frequently proven to be successful in relieving pain. Carbamazepine is the drug of first choice in a dose of 200mg, 3 to 6 times daily (Killian and Fromm, 1968). Patients should start with the lower dose and increase it as needed until the pain is eliminated. Pain from these neuralgias is subject to remissions, thus continuous medication is not always required. Phenytoin (diphenylhydantoin) 300 to 600mg daily is also beneficial in many patients, but the effect is usually less dramatic and complete than with carbamazepine.

In refractory cases, alcohol injection of the involved nerve branch or ganglion may give relief for periods of months. In the most refractory cases retroganglionic surgical section of the involved nerve may have to be performed.

Dose related side effects of carbamazepine and phenytoin include blurred vision, nystagmus, unsteadiness and sedation; vomiting and anorexia may also occur. Idiosyncratic reactions such as skin rashes and bone marrow depression with rare fatal outcome have been reported. The side effects tend to be more frequent in elderly patients and in patients receiving carbamazepine in whom cardiac conduction disturbances should also be watched for (see section 4.7.2).

6.2 Postherpetic Neuralgias

Following herpes zoster infections (see chapter XXVIII; sect. 3.8) continuous burning pain may occur without stimulation in the skin supplied by the involved nerve branches. Antiepileptic drugs are rarely effective in the treatment of this problem, but analgesics such as propoxyphene, codeine, or pentazocine may be helpful. Their action can be potentiated with tranquillisers (chlorpromazine 100 to 500mg daily; chlordiazepoxide 10 to 30mg daily or diazepam 5 to 20mg daily). Spontaneous improvement may sometimes occur after several months. Depression is often a contributing factor to the discomfort, particularly in patients with prolonged intractable pain, and supportive measures and tricyclic antidepressant drugs may be of benefit in such cases (see chapter X; sect. 8).

6.3 Atypical Facial Pain

Patients with atypical facial pain have episodes of pain in various areas of the face, head or neck lasting hours or days. No apparent trigger zones or precipitating factors are present. Drug treatment is generally unsatisfactory. Limited or temporary success may be achieved with antiepileptic drugs, antimigraine agents, tranquillisers and analgesics, indicating the primary suggestive value of these agents. Psychiatric disorders, particularly depression and delusional psychoses, are frequent among these patients and antidepressant agents or electroshock therapy may be of benefit in some.

7. Migraine

A typical migraine attack is characterised by an aura, usually visual, which is related to vasoconstriction of intracranial vessels. The aura is followed by hemicranial headache which is related to dilatation of extracranial vessels and an oedema of the vessel wall. Migraine attacks are episodic in nature with intervals of variable duration of freedom from headache between attacks (Friedman, 1978). Drugs which prevent vasodilatation, particularly in the external carotid artery bed, or maintain the tone of the extracranial arteries, are the most effective in treatment or preventive therapy of this disorder (Lance, 1978; Fanchamps, 1975).

7.1 Treatment of an Acute Migraine Attack

Treatment of an acute migraine should begin with the use of simple analgesics such as aspirin, paracetamol (acetaminophen) or propoxyphene. Frequently, these prove to be effective (Wilkinson, 1976). Their efficacy can be enhanced and the nausea and vomiting and gastrointestinal stasis associated with an acute attack (Lance and Anthony, 1966; Carstairs, 1958), relieved by use of metoclopramide (see section 1.2.1). In those instances when simple analgesics prove ineffective, ergotamine tartrate can be used (Bradfield, 1976). Ergotamine is a vasoconstrictor and as such is specific for the attack, but is most effective when given at the onset of a headache. Absorption of ergotamine is incomplete (60% of the dose) but is relatively rapid (Aellig and Nuesch, 1977). 2 to 3mg should be given at the onset of a headache, followed by 2mg every hour until the headache has disappeared or a total dose of 6mg has been taken. For patients who have severe nausea and vomiting with their headache, 0.5mg of ergotamine can be given intramuscularly at the onset of the attack. Other routes of administration of ergotamine are an aerosol inhaler delivering 0.36mg per application, or rectal suppositories. With adequate doses of ergotamine, relief of attacks can be expected in 70 to 80% of patients. Ergotamine tartrate is probably more effective when used in combination with caffeine, which enhances its absorption (Schmidt and Fanchamps, 1974). Combination preparations containing 1 to 2mg ergotamine with 50 to 100mg of caffeine are available. Dihydroergotamine is also effective but is poorly absorbed (Aellig and Nuesch, 1977) and therefore is given parenterally in doses of 1 to 2mg.

When a migraine attack continues despite a maximum dose of ergotamine, strong analgesics such as pentazocine should be used. Sedation with barbiturates may be helpful; inducing sleep with pentobarbitone (pentobarbital) 100 to 200mg has terminated many attacks. Nitrazepam 5 to 10mg or flurazepam 15 to 30mg could also be used for sedation. Long term use of strong analgesics such as pentazocine, pethidine (meperidine) or morphine should be avoided. If nausea and vomiting continue, phenothiazine antiemetics such as prochlorperazine 5 to 10mg or thiethylperazine 6.5mg, either parenterally or as suppositories, may be used for relief; or alternatively metoclopramide (10mg intramuscularly), which relieves the nausea and vomiting and the gastrointestinal stasis associated with an attack (Volans, 1978).

Side effects of ergotamine occur in up to a third of patients and include muscle cramps, stiffness, tiredness, numbness and paraesthesiae of the extremities and precordial distress. Side effects are less frequent and less severe with lower doses. Prolonged overdosage may lead to ergotism with gangrene of toes and fingers (Hokkanen et al., 1978). Ergotamine should not be used in patients with severe hypertension or with peripheral, cerebral or coronary vascular disease, or impaired liver or renal function or sepsis.

Ergotamine habituation may occasionally be a problem. This is a state characterised by daily rebound headache when the effect of ergotamine ceases a few hours after it is taken. The vicious circle of continued daily medication can be broken by a carefully supervised 'weaning-off' period during which time headaches are treated with pentazocine 30 to 45mg intramuscularly or codeine 30 to 45mg orally, repeated 4 hourly if necessary.

7.2 Preventive Therapy of Migraine

Preventive treatment is indicated in patients with two or more attacks per month. The aim is to achieve a 50% reduction in the previous incidence of headaches (Anthony and Lance, 1972). Before embarking on such interval therapy, aggravating factors should be excluded or if found, treated appropriately. These include arterial hypertension, cervical spondylosis, mental depression or anxiety, oral contraceptive medication, oestrogen therapy, or excessive use of ergotamine (see section 7.1).

A number of effective drugs are available for interval therapy. The least toxic drugs should be tried first and those commonly used for initiating therapy include pizotifen and cyproheptadine (Speight and Avery, 1972).

Pizotifen and Cyproheptadine: Both act as competitive inhibitors of serotonin; antagonising many effects of the amine on several organ systems, and simulating the action of serotonin in maintaining constriction of scalp arteries. They are effective in about half of the patients treated. Side effects include drowsiness and weight gain due to increased appetite. Drowsiness can be overcome by starting with a small dose and increasing gradually over a week — 0.5mg pizotifen or 4mg cyproheptadine 3 times daily increased to 1mg pizotifen or 8mg cyproheptadine after a week. Effectiveness of the drug should be assessed after 1 or preferably 2 months. A change to another drug can then be made at the end of that period if there has been less than a 50% reduction in the frequency of attacks.

Pizotifen and cyproheptadine should probably not be used in children as they reduce growth hormone release and their long term effect on growth is not known (see chapter XVI; sect. 13.4).

β-Adrenoceptor blocking drugs such as propranolol are also effective in reducing the frequency of headaches by 50% in about two-thirds of patients (Diamond and Medina, 1976; Forssman et al., 1976). Propranolol probably acts by creating a peripheral vasoconstrictive bias and preventing the dilatation of extracranial arteries. It may also have some effect upon serotonin mechanisms as it has been shown to reduce serotonin uptake by platelets and increase the amount of extracellular serotonin, which promotes vasoconstriction. Dosage of propranolol in interval therapy of migraine ranges from 80 to 240mg daily (average 160mg). Treatment may be started with 20mg twice a day and the dose increased as needed. Dosage should be kept below that level which would lower the heart rate to less than 60 per minute. Side effects are relatively common but rarely a problem; the most frequent being sensations of fatigue and insomnia. As hypertension is one of the aggravating factors of migraine, propranolol which is an effective antihypertensive drug, is probably the most suitable drug for prevention of headache in hypertensive migraineurs. Propranolol should not be used in patients with heart failure (unless they are receiving digitalis) or asthma (see chapter XVIII; sect. 5.6.8).

Clonidine, another antihypertensive drug (see chapter XVIII; section 5.5), is used in a strength one-eighth of that for hypertension for prevention of migraine headache, but it is probably effective in only a small proportion of patients (Mondrup and Moller, 1977). Its precise mode of action in migraine is obscure. Dosage ranges from 0.025mg twice daily to 0.05mg 3 times a day. Side effects include drowsiness and dry mouth.

Methysergide maleate is one of the most effective drugs for general use but is much more toxic than the other preventive agents, which should be tried first. It acts as a competitive inhibitor of serotonin, in a similar manner as pizotifen and cyproheptadine (see above). Methysergide reduces the frequency of attacks in almost two thirds of patients treated and when the attacks do recur, less ergotamine is usually needed to abate an attack.

The dose should be built up slowly — a test dose of 0.5mg can be given initially to exclude idiosyncrasy and then increased from 1mg daily to 1mg 3 times daily or 2mg 3 times daily over 1 week. Treatment may be continued for a 3 to 6 month period but then it must be withdrawn for 1 to 2 months to forestall the development of retroperitoneal, pleuropulmonary and cardiac valvular fibrosis, which have occurred as a rare side effect in patients on continuous long term methysergide therapy (Graham et al., 1966; see also chapter XVII, sect. 11.6).

Dose related early side effects of methysergide occur in up to 45% of patients treated and include nausea, epigastric discomfort, and circulatory disturbances such as muscle cramps and paraesthesiae due to its peripheral vasoconstrictor activity. These symptoms may disappear during continued therapy or after reduction of the dose. About 10% of patients are however, unable to continue on methysergide. In all patients continuous close supervision is mandatory. Methysergide should not be used during pregnancy or in the presence of active peptic ulcer, peripheral vascular disease, severe hypertension, ischaemic heart disease, thrombophlebitis or renal disease.

Lisuride hydrogen maleate is similar in structure to methysergide and has a similar action. It has been utilised in the prevention of migraine headache and is about as effective as methysergide in preventing attacks but appears to be better tolerated (Hermann et al., 1977). The dosage required is 25mg 3 times a day. Side effects include weakness, coldness of the extremities and dizziness, but it is not yet known whether it causes fibrotic complications with continuous use.

A number of other preparations have been used, including a combination of phenobarbitone, belladonna and ergotamine (in children); methdilazine; and as a last resort in resistant cases, monoamine oxidase inhibitors.

Other drugs: Barbiturates, phenothiazines and benzodiazepines may be beneficial in migraine prophylaxis by reducing anxiety and modifying reactions to frustration. In some patients tricyclic antidepressant drugs are more effective than anti-anxiety agents, as depression frequently accompanies chronic migraine.

Oral hormonal steroid contraceptive agents may reduce the incidence of migraine attacks in some patients, but in others they have provoked the attacks or caused headache *de novo* (Dalton, 1975; Ryan, 1978); therefore they should be used with caution, as the effect is unpredictable.

7.3 Migrainous Neuralgia (cluster headache)

Cluster headaches are typically attacks of severe pain, mostly retro-orbital, associated with lacrymation and blockage of the nostril on the same side. They occur in bouts of days or weeks with each episode lasting for less than an hour to several hours. Between bouts there may be free intervals of months to years (Graham, 1972). The drug of choice is methysergide given regularly throughout the bout in doses of 2mg 3 times daily at the onset of the headache, with additional doses up to 12mg daily, if needed. Medication can then be stopped until the next bout appears. The dose related side effects of methysergide (see section 7.2) occur frequently with these relatively high doses, but since the clusters are limited to a few weeks, long term complications are not expected.

Subcutaneous ergotamine tartrate 0.25mg 3 to 6 times daily, which was used before the introduction of methysergide, may still be useful in refractory cases. Lisuride (section 7.2) can also be considered in prevention of cluster headaches in a dose of 25mg 3 times daily. If these drugs prove ineffective, prednisone (40 to 60mg daily) can be tried (Couch and Ziegler, 1978). Histamine has a causative role in cluster headache and corticosteroids probably act in the condition by inhibiting the formation of histamine. Histamine H_1 and H_2 receptor antagonists are not effective in cluster headache (Anthony et al., 1978). Lithium has been used in patients with chronic symptoms who have failed to respond to all other medication including methysergide and prednisone (Kudrow, 1977).

8. Cerebral Vascular Diseases

Rational treatment of cerebral vascular disease depends on the type of cerebral vascular accident. The most commonly occurring cerebral vascular accident is cerebral infarction due to embolism or thrombosis and this is followed in prevalence by primary subarachnoid haemorrhage and primary intracerebral haemorrhage.

8.1 Treatment of Cerebral Infarction

Treatment of cerebral infarction can be divided in two phases: (1) immediate treatment, and (2) preventive treatment. Usually there is little that can be done immediately to reduce the size or extent of a cerebral infarction. Therapeutic attempts directed at this phase of the illness have generally included agents which dilate cerebral vessels and presumably improve blood flow to the region of infarction. Suggested therapeutic agents have been carbon dioxide inhalation and papaverine hydrochloride by injection. With both, one can demonstrate an increased cerebral blood flow but as yet this has not been demonstrated to clearly improve patients clinically. A variety of agents said to dilate cerebral vessels are under investigation. At present, there is no agent known to improve cerebral blood flow which clinically clearly benefits patients with cerebral vascular disease.

In stroke there is always some cerebral oedema. With massive cerebral infarctions, oedema is extensive and may be life threatening. Corticosteroids, mannitol and glycerol have been recommended for the treatment of a patient with an acute stroke to reduce cerebral oedema. The use of cerebral dehydrating agents such as mannitol and glycerol may temporarily relieve the situation by dehydrating normal brain and alleviating the threat of tentorial herniation (Meyer et al., 1972). However, there is no evidence that corticosteroids reduce oedema of cerebral infarction (Mulley et al., 1978). Nor is there any clearly demonstrable evidence that agents which reduce cerebral oedema improve the long term outlook for a patient with stroke (Study Group, 1977).

8.2 Prophylactic Treatment of Stroke

The most logical and effective means of treatment of patients with cerebral infarction, is that designed to prevent a stroke initially or to prevent catastrophic stroke in a patient with a mild deficit following the first stroke. Treatment is largely limited to those individuals who have transient ischaemic attacks, since in up to 50% of cases these herald a stroke (Acheson and Hutchison, 1971; Millikan and McDowell, 1978), and a few patients who have evidence of progressive cerebral infarction while under observation by a clinician. Reducing the chances for a patient with a severe completed stroke of having another cerebral infarction has limited therapeutic merit.

8.2.1 Transient Ischaemic Attacks

Each patient's clinical picture must be considered for treatment on its own merits. Before starting treatment, a number of causes of, or conditions which mimic transient cerebral ischaemic attacks should be excluded. These include conditions such as severe hypertension, syncope, episodes of cardiac arrhythmia or seizures (Fisher, 1965; McAllen and Marshall, 1973). When discovered, these should be treated with suitable medical therapy (Millikan and McDowell, 1978).

Two forms of medical therapy are available at present which have been shown to reduce the frequency of transient ischaemic attacks and to reduce the future chances of cerebral infarction. Oral anticoagulants were shown to reduce the frequency of transient ischaemic attacks almost 25 years ago. In patients with evidence of transient ischaemic attacks continuously treated with oral anticoagulants, the frequency of transient ischaemic attacks is reduced and the chances of having a future stroke have been shown to be reduced (Millikan, 1971). Anticoagulants are given in a dose large enough to keep the prothrombin time at least 2 to 2.5 times its normal level. Therapy should be continued for approximately 6 months, as this is the period of the greatest chance of cerebral infarction following the onset of transient ischaemic attacks. Following this, a gradual withdrawal from the medication is indicated (Marshall and Reynolds, 1965). Anticoagulants are started again if attacks recur.

The most recently developed therapy which has been shown to reduce the incidence of transient ischaemic attacks and the incidence of a future stroke, primarily in males, is use of antiplatelet aggregating agents such as aspirin (see chapter XXIII; sect. 3.1). Platelet emboli released from ulcerated endothelium over atherosclerotic plaques have been found to cause some transient ischaemic attacks and strokes (Genton et al., 1977). Preventing platelets from adhering to those surfaces, has been found to prevent transient ischaemic attacks. Evidence from both the United States (Fields et al., 1977) and Canadian (Barnett et al., 1978) studies indicates that approximately 1.3g of aspirin per day reduces the frequency of transient ischaemic attacks in patients with atherosclerotic vascular disease; including after reconstructive operations (Fields et al., 1978). Only the Canadian study provided evidence that regular use of aspirin was of value in the prevention of future stroke in patients with transient ischaemic attacks. This protection was confined to males, for reasons which are not entirely clear. It is likely, with the evidence, that drugs such as aspirin, which produce a reduction of transient ischaemic attacks and their serious long term adverse consequences, will replace oral anticoagulants as the treatment of choice in male patients. Female patients who have frequent transient ischaemic attacks, after careful evaluation, should be treated with oral anticoagulants.

8.2.2 Progressive Stroke

Individuals who are developing increasing symptoms and signs of stroke while under the observation of a clinician are in considerable jeopardy and deserve emergency treatment. The most effective treatment is heparin, which should be given initially for 4 to 6 days. Heparin should be administered initially intravenously, in doses of 5 000 to 10 000 units every 6 hours. The partial thromboplastin time is used to monitor heparin therapy, and enough heparin should be given to keep it at 1.5 times control. After approximately 3 to 4 days, heparin can be discontinued. If oral anticoagulants have been started when heparin is first administered, oral anticoagulation should be continued for 4 to 6 weeks. This programme markedly reduces the mortality rate from progressive brain stem infarction and reduces the disability and morbidity from hemisphere infarction.

8.3 Cerebral Embolisation

If cerebral emboli are of cardiac origin in patients with rheumatic heart disease, anticoagulants should be given continuously to reduce the chances of recurrent emboli. Oral coumarin anticoagulants are the drugs of choice and should be given indefinitely to keep the prothrombin time at 2 to 2.5 times normal.

8.4 Subarachnoid Haemorrhage

Medical treatment of subarachnoid haemorrhage consists in offering life saving measures for the patient during the period of depressed consciousness. Other medical therapy consists of bedrest and reduction of elevated blood pressure to normal levels or slightly below normal levels. Methyldopa 250mg 3 to 4 times a day given orally or 250mg intravenously is often effective. Reserpine in doses of 0.25mg 2 to 3 times a day may also be useful, or a combination of a variety of drugs which effectively reduce blood pressure may

be used. Blood pressure should be maintained at normal or lower than normal levels during the acute phase of the illness and to prevent recurrence or haemorrhage; longer treatment should be given if blood pressure remains elevated 3 to 4 weeks after the recovery. Prevention of recurrent bleeding in subarachnoid haemorrhage by blocking the enhancement of spinal fluid thrombolysis with the antifibrinolytic agent aminocaproic acid (see chapter XXIII; sect. 5.4) has been found useful by some workers. It is believed that the enhanced thrombolytic activity of spinal fluid following subarachnoid haemorrhage may lyse the clot plugging the aneurysmal sac. Studies indicate that this is a useful treatment (Nibbelink and Cooperative Aneurysm Study, 1975). The doses of aminocaproic acid required are large and range from 20 to 30g daily intravenously given for approximately a week to 10 days.

8.5 Primary Intracerebral Haemorrhage

Primary intracerebral haemorrhage carries with it a mortality of approximately 70 to 80% and with unconsciousness at the onset, a mortality of nearly 90 to 100%. The only effective means of treatment which in any way alters the outcome of the disorder, other than the acute care for a patient in coma, is to reduce elevated blood pressure. This generally requires emergency treatment with hydrallazine or trimetaphan. Hydrallazine 50 to 100mg in a 1 litre infusion is given by slow intravenous drip. Trimetaphan 1000mg/litre can be used in refractory cases and is given by a slow intravenous drip. Both are given at a rate which will keep the blood pressure at a desirable level.

8.6 Hypertensive Encephalopathy

Hypertensive encephalopathy, which is often found in individuals with hypertension who have a sudden rise in blood pressure, is associated with marked cerebral vessel spasm which results in mental confusion, visual disturbances and often convulsions. Immediate reduction of the blood pressure to normal and near normal levels is an emergency procedure (see chapter XVIII; sect. 8).

9. Myasthenia Gravis

Myasthenia gravis is clinically characterised by weakness of muscles. The age of onset varies.

Women are more often inflicted than men. Babies born to myasthenic mothers may show transient myasthenia and require temporary treatment. The incidence of myasthenia gravis in the general population is 0.01 to 0.05%. Familial incidence, however, is 3 to 5%, suggesting hereditary disposition to susceptibility to myasthenia gravis. Abnormalities of the thymus are frequent among patients suffering from myasthenia gravis and surgical removal of the thymus has often alleviated the myasthenic symptoms (Mann et al., 1976). The crises in myasthenia are medical emergencies.

9.1 Pathophysiology of Myasthenia Gravis

The basic defect in myasthenia gravis appears to be impaired neuromuscular transmission (Elmqvist et al., 1964). The exact mechanism of this defect is not yet entirely clear. Investigators looking for a presynaptic defect have postulated a disturbance in the transmitter; i.e. in acetylcholine (AcCh) production, release, or recycling. Investigators looking for a postsynaptic defect have postulated decreased responsiveness to the transmitter at the endplate. Still others have considered the existence of circulating inhibitor substance(s) that may act either pre- or postsynaptically (Engel et al., 1974).

Currently accepted by the majority of investigators as a key finding is the reduction of the miniature endplate potentials at the myasthenic myoneural junction (Elmqvist et al., 1964). This may result from the fact that the postsynaptic acetylcholine receptor substance (AcChR) is defective in the myasthenic endplate. Autoradiographic studies, using as a marker labelled α-bungarotoxin which binds irreversibly with AcChR, have shown marked diminution of AcChR in the myasthenic endplates (Keesey et al., 1976). Furthermore, circulating antibodies contained in the immunoglobulin G fractions, which react with the AcChR, have been found in the serum of the majority of myasthenic patients thus studied. It appears then that a major factor in the genesis of myasthenia gravis is damage to AcChR caused by the circulating antibodies against AcChR; an autoimmune mechanism (Simpson, 1978; Harvard, 1977). The antibodies against AcChR are thought to be produced in the thymus. However, what sets off the production of antibodies remains to be elucidated.

9.2 General Treatment of Myasthenia Gravis

Generally, two therapeutic approaches are being used to overcome the block of neuromuscular transmission (Engel et al., 1974; Flacke, 1973). The first approach is to administer agents with anticholinesterase action which increase and/or prolong the activity of the acetylcholine at the myoneural junction. The second approach is to suppress the autoimmune response by administering corticosteroids or by thymectomy. Both approaches may be used in combination. The first approach is usually used in milder cases, the second or the combination in the more severe forms.

9.2.1 Anticholinesterase Therapy of Myasthenia Gravis

The agents displaying anticholinesterase effects act by competing for the enzyme with acetylcholine at the cholinergic synapses. They are hydrolysed by acetylcholine esterase at a relatively lower rate than acetylcholine. Therefore, sufficient concentration of the drug must be present for effective competition. Preferable are agents that do not enter significantly into the central nervous system, thus minimising the central side effects.

Currently used anticholinesterases include neostigmine, pyridostigmine and ambenonium (Flacke, 1973; Harvard, 1977). Edrophonium serves as a diagnostic aid (Engel et al., 1974). Atropine in doses of 0.3 to 0.6mg is often used to alleviate the systemic peripheral muscarinic side effects of anticholinesterases. It has little effect on nicotinic receptors; i.e. it does not counteract the anticholinesterases at myoneural junctions.

Neostigmine has a relatively short half-life as it is rapidly inactivated. The inactivation starts in the intestinal tract which explains the marked differences in the size of the effective parenteral and oral doses. The short half-life also necessitates frequent administration of doses, every 2 to 6 hours in maintenance therapy.

The starting oral dose is usually 15mg administered 3 times daily. Starting with low dosages alleviates the intensity of its muscarinic side effects. The dose is then built up according to the individual patient's need; reaching on the average 120 to 180mg daily, taken in 15 or 30mg installments every 2 to 6 (average 4) hour intervals.

Parenterally, 0.5 to 1.0mg is usually equivalent to 15mg taken orally. The parenteral route is mostly used in treating the myasthenic crises.

The common muscarinic side effects of neostigmine are nausea, vomiting, diarrhoea, and intestinal cramps; increased perspiration, salivation, lacrimation, and bronchial secretion; less often hypotension. With gross overdose, cholinergic crisis will ensue and enough neostigmine may enter the central nervous system to cause agitation, mental clouding, and coma.

Pyridostigmine is longer acting than neostigmine; thus, doses need to be given every 3 to 8 hours. The oral dose of pyridostigmine equivalent to 15mg of neostigmine is 60mg. Plasma concentrations of 20 to 60ng/ml have been observed in patients receiving effective doses of pyridostigmine. Dosage must be individualised and varies widely, not only because of the variable severity of the disease but also because of marked interindividual differences in absorption of the drug (Calvey and Chan, 1977; Cohan et al., 1977). Moreover, in some patients increasing the dose may lead to a disproportionately greater increase in plasma concentration (Calvey and Chan, 1977). Parenterally, 1.0mg of pyridostigmine usually has the same effect as 0.5mg of neostigmine. The side effects of the two drugs are similar.

Ambenonium is effective for longer than pyridostigmine or neostigmine, allowing longer intervals between doses. The oral dose equivalent to 15mg of neostigmine is 5mg of ambenonium. The side effects are similar to those of other anticholinesterases but ambenonium appears to penetrate the blood-brain barrier to a somewhat greater extent than neostigmine and pyridostigmine.

Edrophonium, due to its very brief action, is impractical for maintenance therapy but is useful primarily as a diagnostic agent. Given intravenously in a dose of 10mg, it reduces markedly the myasthenic weakness within seconds, for a few minutes. Non-myasthenic weak muscles may also respond but the effect is still briefer and much less dramatic than in myasthenic muscles. Cholinergic crises can be differentiated from myasthenic crises (in an intensive care unit) by injecting 2 or 5mg of edrophonium. The patient in myasthenic crisis improves dramatically; the patient in cholinergic crisis either does not change or becomes worse for a short period.

9.2.2 Immunosuppressive Therapy of Myasthenia Gravis

The use of immunosuppressive agents such as prednisone and corticotrophin has become an important supplement to anticholinesterase therapy in selected myasthenic patients (Engel et al., 1974; Brunner et al., 1976). The initial worsening of myasthenic symptoms from immunosuppressive agents can be minimised by appropriate dosing schedules and by the preparedness to cope with transient worsenings. A marked long term improvement of myasthenia often follows; allowing substantial reductions from the previous anticholinesterase dose requirements. The selection of immunosuppressive agents and the administration schedules are still in flux and are likely to be modified as the general experience grows.

Patients selected for treatment with immunosuppressive agents usually are those with generalised myasthenia, who do not respond well to the average doses of anticholinesterases. Excluded are usually patients to whom the common side effects of steroid treatment (gastrointestinal bleeding, electrolyte disturbances, impaired resistance to infection etc) are likely to pose undue risks. These include patients with peptic ulcers, diabetes mellitus and cardiovascular diseases.

The initiation of steroid treatment is best carried out in facilities where the potential initial worsening of myasthenic symptoms can be quickly and expertly coped with, such as intensive care units or neurology inpatient wards. The common steroid side effects are minimised by reducing sodium intake and supplementing potassium intake, as well as by administration of antacids.

Corticotrophin: On the average, 100 units can be infused intravenously over an 8 hour period or 160 units given intramuscularly for 8 to 14 days. More than one course at intervals of 7 to 10 days may be given if no improvement occurs or only transient effect is seen. The maintenance doses of 100 units weekly are then continued for months, as indicated. This form of treatment is nowadays generally used when all other forms of therapy have failed.

Corticosteroids: Prednisone, a synthetic glucocorticoid, which has a short plasma half-life, undergoes biotransformation to prednisolone and is eliminated in the urine (see chapter XVI; sect. 9.1). It is well absorbed following oral intake. The dosages of prednisone used successfully have ranged from 50 to 100mg; given as a single oral dose every other day. The alternate day schedule seems to reduce the hypothalamic-pituitary-adrenal axis suppression. Starting with a low (25mg) dose, followed by increases might minimise the occurrence of the initial worsening of myasthenic symptoms. Improvement on this high alternate day dosage schedule is usually seen in a couple of months. Later, the maintenance dose can be reduced very gradually (2.5 to 5.0mg per month) to near one half or less from the earlier maximum.

The anticholinesterase drugs may be withdrawn at the onset of prednisone therapy, but more often it may be practical to continue them. The amount of anticholinesterase drug needed, however, diminishes considerably, if prednisone becomes effective.

Plasmapheresis: Another way to remove circulating immunoactive material from the organism is plasmapheresis. This has been used experimentally in conjunction with immunosuppressive drugs and has resulted in improvement of myasthenic symptoms for variable periods (Dau et al., 1977; Newsom-Davis et al., 1979).

The complexity and cost of this procedure, however, limit its general clinical application at the present time.

9.3 Myasthenia of Newborns

Babies born to mothers with myasthenia gravis may show myasthenic symptoms and need anticholinesterase therapy in order to survive (Fenichel, 1978). This is probably a reflection of passively transferred immunoactive agents from the mother that affect acetylcholine receptors in the newborn. Repeated 0.1mg intramuscular doses of neostigmine may be needed in the first days of life. The condition usually improves in the following days and abates in a week or two.

9.4 Treatment of Crises

Sometimes a rapid increase of muscle weakness to the extreme, including respiratory muscles, occurs in patients with myasthenia gravis. Two mechanisms are recognised: (1) myasthenic crises (undermedication) and (2) cholinergic crises (overmedication). The myasthenic crises occur when the patient has not taken or has no supplies of medication, or there is an increased need of anti-

cholinesterase drug. Cholinergic crises are caused by an excess of acetylcholine at the myoneural junction; usually from excessive intake of anticholinesterase drugs. Both are medical emergencies. Differential diagnosis is made with the use of edrophonium as described in section 9.2.1.

9.4.1 Myasthenic Crises

Treatment is carried out in an intensive care unit and consists of maintaining adequate respiratory ventilation and giving anticholinesterase drugs parenterally. Neostigmine (0.5mg) intramuscularly or subcutaneously is given every 15 to 30 minutes until the desired response is seen. After the required dose to maintain adequate function has been established, pyridostigmine may be substituted as it has a longer action. Later, when the patient has completely stabilised, oral medication can be resumed.

9.4.2 Cholinergic Crises

The cholinergic crises are best treated by stopping medication and waiting, to allow excess medication to be hydrolysed *in situ*. It would seem that logical chemotherapeutic agents in this situation would be antidotes such as pralidoxime, which act by regeneration of cholinesterase, and are used for the treatment of excessive exposure to insecticides containing organophosphorus (see chapter IX; sect. 6.2). However, these agents are rarely needed. Supportive measures are used; primarily to maintain adequate pulmonary ventilation. Atropine may be administered to alleviate the muscarinic side effects.

10. Spasticity

Spasticity generally develops following lesions of the corticospinal tract. It is characterised by increased resistance to passive stretching of limbs and exaggerated deep tendon reflexes; clonus may be present also. The pathophysiology of spasticity is not well understood but it may be related to alterations of transmitter balance at synapses and changes in the muscle spindle sensitivity.

Patients presenting with spasticity as subjects for treatment are most often those who have suffered a spinal cord injury, have a spinal cord tumour, or degenerative cord disease; or have multiple sclerosis. For the patient with established cerebral infarction and neurological disability with hemiparesis or hemiplegia, spasticity of the paralysed arm and leg is frequently a distressing late complication. The treatment of spasticity is often unsatisfactory. Drugs that have been used with some success are diazepam, baclofen and dantrolene (Burke, 1975).

Diazepam is thought to relieve spasticity by suppressing activity in interneuronal and spinal reflex pathways. It is of little value in patients with cerebral lesions. Clinically, small doses are sometimes effective in reducing spasticity. A reasonable starting dose is 2mg twice a day. A sedative effect at the onset of therapy is not unusual but the tolerance to diazepam varies considerably among patients. The dose is then increased in 2 or 5mg increments until a beneficial effect is seen, and many patients tolerate 30 or 40mg daily without side effects. Unfortunately, the effect of diazepam on spasticity is often not long lasting. It is advisable then to stop the medication and rest the patient for a few weeks or months. Restarting later may produce another period of relief. The pharmacokinetic properties of diazepam are discussed in chapter XXVI (sect. 1.5.3).

Side effects with diazepam other than sedation rarely pose problems. Dermatological, renal, hepatic, and haematological complications are extremely infrequent but habituation may develop. Discontinuation of diazepam in patients who have received high doses should not be abrupt.

Baclofen is an analogue of γ-aminobutyric acid (Brogden et al., 1974). Whereas diazepam acts mainly on supraspinal pathways, baclofen acts predominantly at a spinal level where it inhibits monosynaptic and polysynaptic transmission. Baclofen has become the drug of choice for spinal spasticity, including multiple sclerosis, but also has some effect in spasticity resulting from a cerebral vascular lesion. It is well absorbed from the intestinal tract; peak plasma concentrations occurring in about 2 hours following oral ingestion. Biotransformation of baclofen is not extensive; over 75% of the dose is excreted unchanged in the urine, necessitating reduction of dosage in patients with impaired renal function. The plasma half-life is 3 to 4 hours. Baclofen does not penetrate the blood-brain barrier easily; nevertheless, it reaches an effective concentration in the spinal cord with adequate doses.

The effective dose varies among patients. It is advisable to start with 5mg 3 times daily and in-

crease slowly over weeks until a beneficial effect is seen. In multiple sclerosis, 70 to 80mg daily in divided doses seems to be adequate in over 75% of patients who benefitted from the drug (Sachais et al., 1977). A dosage of up to 80mg daily maximum, in divided doses, often considerably reduces the disability associated from hemiparesis or hemiplegia and its attendant spasticity. Side effects of baclofen include nausea and somnolence; less often headache, constipation, increased weakness, vertigo and insomnia.

Dantrolene, a nitrophenyl amino hydantoin derivative, is thought to act by directly blocking muscle contraction through interference with the calcium mechanism in the muscle cell. It has no effect on neural pathways (Pinder et al., 1977a). Dantrolene is of benefit in spasticity of both spinal or cerebral origin, but appears to be much less effective than baclofen in multiple sclerosis. It is effective in some children and adults with spasticity associated with cerebral palsy. Dantrolene is incompletely absorbed (only about 20% of an oral dose), extensively metabolised and excreted in the urine; principally as the 5-hydroxy derivative and in lesser amounts (around 20% of the urinary recovery) as the 5-acetamino metabolite. The amino metabolite precursor is pharmacologically active but much less so than the parent drug. Whether subsequent acetylation of this amino metabolite is subject to genetically controlled polymorphism is not known (see chapter VII; sect. 4.2.1). Plasma concentrations of dantrolene show marked interindividual variation. It has a plasma half-life of around 9 hours.

The starting dose of dantrolene in adults is 12.5 or 25mg once daily, increased to 25mg 2 or 3 times daily; with further increments over 4 to 7 day periods until effective or a maximum of 600 to 800mg is reached. Dosage in children is similarly built up gradually commencing with 1mg/kg once or twice daily to a maximum of 400mg daily. The common side effects are drowsiness, diarrhoea and nausea; and muscle weakness, which may be the principal limiting side effect in ambulant patients and is most prevalent in patients with multiple sclerosis. Less common but most important is potential serious liver damage, heralded by abnormal liver function tests, which may culminate in a fatal toxic hepatitis (Utili et al., 1977). Onset of hepatic injury is delayed for at least 45 days after starting the drug, with serious toxicity even more delayed. Patients over 30 years

Table VI. Choice of drugs for the treatment of meningitis according to causative organism

Organism	Drug(s) of choice[1]	Alternative(s)
Neisseria meningitidis	Benzylpenicillin[1] Ampicillin[3]	Chloramphenicol Sulphonamide Cephaloridine
Streptococcus pneumoniae	Benzylpenicillin[1] Ampicillin	Chloramphenicol Erythromycin Lincomycin Vancomycin
Haemophilus influenzae	Chloramphenicol[1] (β-lactamase producing strains) Ampicillin[1] (non β-lactamase producing strains)	Tetracycline Sulphonamide with streptomycin
Streptococcus pyogenes	Benzylpenicillin[1] Ampicillin	Erythromycin Lincomycin
Streptococcus faecalis	Benzylpenicillin Ampicillin	Streptomycin Vancomycin
Group B β-haemolytic streptococcus	Benzylpenicillin[1]	Ampicillin
Staphylococcus aureus	Benzylpenicillin[1] Ampicillin	Erythromycin Cephaloridine Lincomycin
Staphylococcus aureus (penicillinase-producing)	Methicillin[1] Cloxacillin (or flu(di)cloxacillin, nafcillin, oxacillin)	Fusidic acid Vancomycin Cephaloridine
Listeria monocytogenes	Ampicillin, alone or with gentamicin[1]	Benzylpenicillin Erythromycin Tetracycline
Escherichia coli[4]	Chloramphenicol Ampicillin	Gentamicin Kanamycin Co-trimoxazole Carbenicillin
Klebsiella Enterobacter[4] spp. *Serratia* spp.	Chloramphenicol Gentamicin	Kanamycin Colistin
Pseudomonas aeruginosa	Gentamicin Tobramycin Carbenicillin	Colistin
Proteus spp.	Kanamycin Gentamicin Carbenicillin	Ampicillin
Salmonella spp.	Chloramphenicol[1]	Ampicillin Co-trimoxazole
Shigella spp.	Ampicillin	Co-trimoxazole
Bacteroides spp.	Chloramphenicol Metronidazole	Carbenicillin
Mycobacterium tuberculosis	Isoniazid[5] Rifampicin[5] Ethambutol[5]	Streptomycin[5] PAS[5]
Candida, Cryptococcus, Coccidioides spp.	Amphotericin B[5] Fluorocytosine[5]	Miconazole

1   Drug of first choice. Local sensitivity patterns should also be taken into account, particularly where no indication of drug of first choice is made.
2   If pseudomonas infection is suspected the alternative choice should be used.
3   Parenteral amoxycillin can be used instead.
4   The most common causative organisms in the neonatal period. Many other organisms which cause meningitis in this period are not listed, but can be covered by chloramphenicol alone or the combination of ampicillin and gentamicin (or tobramycin).
5   Given in combination.

of age who have received daily doses of 300mg or more seem most susceptible, as do females. Only patients who show important benefit after a 45 day trial should be allowed to continue with the drug.

All patients who receive dantrolene should have regular monitoring of SGOT and SGPT levels and the drug stopped if liver dysfunction develops. In some patients it may be possible to readminister dantrolene without recurrence of liver dysfunction, but if it does recur it should not be given again.

In patients who do not respond to drug therapy and in whom spontaneous improvement is not expected to take place, instillation of phenol intrathecally or rhizotomy may have to be resorted to.

11. Multiple Sclerosis

A number of agents have been tried in the treatment of multiple sclerosis and include isoniazid, tolbutamide, clofibrate, heparin and vitamin B_{12}. Though they were all once thought to be promising, none of these is now considered to have therapeutic value. Long term low dose therapy with corticosteroids or ACTH has been recommended, but it has not proven effective in preventing progression or improving the basic condition of patients with multiple sclerosis.

Short term high dose treatment with ACTH may hasten improvement in patients with symptoms of recent exacerbation, but it has little or no effect on the extent of improvement (Rose et al., 1968, 1970; Henderson et al., 1978). The dosage recommended in patients with acute exacerbation is 60 units ACTH twice daily for the first week, 40 units daily for 4 days and 20 units daily for 3 days, for a total of 14 days. Also, high dose (50 to 100mg per day) short term (4 to 7 days) steroid therapy (prednisone and prednisolone) has been found by some to be of value in the treatment of an acute exacerbation (Calne, 1974). Long term steroid treatment has caused exacerbation of peptic ulcer, psychoses and septicaemia, besides cushingoid features, in some patients.

Disability due to spasticity may be reduced in some patients with diazepam 6 to 20mg or baclofen 70 to 80mg daily (see section 10), or with intrathecal phenol injections. Development of faecal impaction in sedentary patients must be avoided by use of laxatives.

12. Bell's Palsy

Bell's palsy is peripheral facial paralysis of unknown aetiology. If the patient is seen within a few days of the onset, high dose corticosteroid therapy has been recommended for 7 to 10 days to reduce oedema in the facial nerve (Taverner et al., 1971). An effective regimen is prednisolone 80mg daily concluding with 10mg daily. After the acute phase has passed, nerve stimulation together with facial exercises to keep facial muscle from atrophing during nerve regeneration, may be beneficial. Recovery may be complete but frequently some weakness or altered facial motility may persist.

13. Infections of the Central Nervous System

Bacterial infections of the nervous system are extremely serious life threatening situations which develop either by spread of organism from adjacent infected structures or by haematogenous dissemination. Bacterial meningitis has its greatest incidence in early childhood and is responsible for a variable mortality and morbidity, despite the range of antibacterial drugs available (see Hambleton and Davies, 1974, 1975; Mathies and Wehrle, 1968). Early diagnosis is the single most important factor in determining final outcome, especially in very young children, and delay may be associated with significant CNS handicap in survivors. *Haemophilis influenzae, Neisseria meningitidis* and *Streptococcus (Diplococcus) pneumoniae,* are the most common causative organisms after the first weeks of life. A wide variety of bacteria may cause meningitis in the neonatal period, but Gram-negative organisms predominate (see further chapter IV; sect. 5.1.2).

For purulent meningitides, the first choice drugs indicated in table VI are the most effective and ones to which organisms are least likely to be resistant. However, sensitivity studies should always be carried out and following proper interpretation of the Gram stain of CSF may lead to a change of the agents. The treatment should be continued until the patient is afebrile for at least 5 to 10 days and until the spinal fluid cell counts have returned to normal. This usually takes 10 to 14 days. Dosage should *not* be decreased with clinical improvement, as CSF levels are dependent on the degree of meningeal inflammation. Indeed, with ampicillin at least, dosage should theo-

Table VII. Data relating to the administration of some antimicrobial agents in the treatment of meningitis (after Barling and Selkon, 1978; Hambleton and Davies, 1974; 1975)

	Dose[1] (mg/kg/day)	Peak serum levels[2] (μg/ml)	CSF/serum ratio[3] (%)	MIC[4] (μg/ml)	IT[5] therapy	IT[6] dose
Benzylpenicillin	150-300	1.2-12	1-6	0.003-0.06	No	1-6mg
Ampicillin	150-400	6-38	10-50	2	Yes	10mg
Cloxacillin	50	8-17	Nil	0.25-0.5	Yes	3-10mg
Methicillin	100	$\geqslant$ 4-36	8-24	0.5-4	Yes[6]	5-40mg[6]
Carbenicillin	50-600	50-400	Nil	2.5-125.0	Yes	10-20mg
Chloramphenicol	100	10-40	10-60	8-10	No	
Sulphadiazine Sulphadimidine	200	4-20	50-80	4-20	No	
Erythromycin	10	20-80	Nil	0.1-1.6	No	
Lincomycin	100	5-18	40	2-2.8	No	
Cephaloridine	100	10-80	6-50	1-8	No	
Gentamicin[7]	6	5-7	Nil	0.3-1.0	Yes	1-2mg
Kanamycin[7]	15-50	10-20	20-40	0.5-5.0	No	2-10mg
Tobramycin	3-5	4-11	Nil	0.1-5.0	Yes[6]	5mg[6]
Colistin[7]	2.5-5	5-25	20-40	0.1-10.0	No	
Co-trimoxazole	6-8/30-40[8]	1-2/30-50[8]	~ 50-200/35-90[8]	0.03-0.5[9]	No	
Metronidazole	15	21-48	~ 90-100	0.8-16	No	
Isoniazid	10 → 5[10]	~ 5-10	~ 100	0.02-0.05	No	
Ethambutol	15-30	4-5	10-55	0.8-1.5	No	
Rifampicin	8	5-30	10-20	0.1-0.5	No	
Amphotericin B	0.6-1.0	0.5-2.0	2-10	0.01-0.5	Yes[11]	0.5-1mg
Flucytosine	150-200	50-100	50-80	0.5-16	No	
Miconazole	30	2-8	< 3-50	0.4-1.0	Yes[11]	20mg

　　1　Dose: The dosage stated should normally give adequate therapeutic effect. Larger doses may be required if serum or cerebrospinal fluid levels and minimum inhibitory concentration estimations so indicate. Drugs should be given intramuscularly or intravenously. Larger doses are required in hydrocephalus.
　　For dosage schedules in newborn infants, see chapter IV (sect. 5.1.2).
　　2　Peak serum levels: Ranges are given according to those published in the literature. They are obviously dependent on dosage and route of administration and use of probenecid (e.g. carbenicillin).
　　3　Cerebrospinal fluid/serum ratio: Ranges are given according to those published in the literature.
　　4　Minimum inhibitory concentration: The ranges given cover the organisms referred to in table VI. If the minimum inhibitory concentration of an antibiotic against a particular strain of a species, against which it is the drug of choice or suitable alternative, is greater than the figure given, then use of the drug is possibly inappropriate.
　　5　Intrathecal therapy: this column indicates whether this route of administration is required in normal circumstances. The dose depends on the patient's age. Intrathecal (or intraventricular) therapy is almost always required in hydrocephalus.
　　6　Intrathecal dose: It is advisable to refer to the literature before deciding on the dose. The doses listed for penicillin and kanamycin are appropriate when this mode of therapy is used. The lower doses in the ranges are for infants, the upper doses for adults. Caution is in order with intrathecal penicillin since convulsions may occur with high doses. Intrathecal dose of methicillin and tobramycin not well established.
　　7　Monitoring of plasma concentrations of gentamicin, tobramycin, kanamycin and colistin is advisable in patients with proven Gram-negative infection, especially if renal function is compromised.
　　8　Trimethoprim/sulphamethoxazole.
　　9　Trimethoprim.
　　10　In children, 15 to 20mg/kg daily reduced by half after 4 weeks. Use in conjunction with pyridoxine (see text).
　　11　Only needed in coccidioidomycoses.

retically be increased as the patient improves, for the penetration of ampicillin is directly related to the cell and protein content of the CSF (Taber et al., 1967).

The aim of treatment is to maintain a blood level which will result in a CSF concentration well above the minimum inhibitory concentration for the causative organism. The intramuscular or intravenous routes are to be preferred as absorption is assured and high blood concentrations can be attained. Most antibacterial agents penetrate the CSF adequately in meningitis, provided they are given in sufficient parenteral dosage. If the agent chosen (table VI) does not penetrate the CSF, then intrathecal or intraventricular administration is mandatory (see table VII). When hydrocephalus is present, large intrathecal doses are needed in addition to larger than usual systemic doses.

If immediate diagnosis is not possible or uncertain, treatment must be started at once to cover the most likely causative organisms — *H. influenzae, N. meningitidis* and *Str. pneumoniae* — and ampicillin (or chloramphenicol) alone in adults, or chloramphenicol alone (or preferably with ampicillin) in children less than 5 years, can be used for this purpose. In the neonatal period when the causative organism is not known, chloramphenicol alone or a combination of ampicillin and gentamicin (or tobramycin) is desirable; intravenously initially and then intramuscularly. Intraventricular administration of aminoglycosides (when ampicillin plus gentamicin or tobramycin is used) will be needed in addition in most cases of Gram-negative neonatal meningitis. Specific dosage schedules for antibacterial drugs in the neonatal period are given in chapter IV (table XIII).

Tuberculous meningitis untreated is uniformly fatal. Because of its ready penetration into CSF fluid, treatment must include isoniazid daily 10mg/kg in adults, 15 to 20mg/kg in children for the first 4 weeks; then reduced by half and continued for a total of 1 year. This is supported by ethambutol 15 to 25mg/kg and rifampicin (rifampin) 600mg daily. Rifampicin will be given for the same length of time as isoniazid; ethambutol may be discontinued after the first 2 or 3 months of therapy. Some prefer to combine ethambutol with streptomycin (1g daily intramuscularly) or to add pyrazinamide (0.5g 3 times daily) plus streptomycin to rifampicin-isoniazid in the initial 2 to 3 month phase (Fallon, 1978). Pyridoxine 100mg daily will reduce the incidence of isoniazid induced neuropathies.

Fungal meningitides and encephalitides (cryptococcus, coccidioidomycoses) can be treated with amphotericin B intravenously, starting with a test dose of 0.25mg/kg and gradually increasing to 1mg/kg per day until 2 to 3g total has been given. The drug has also been given intrathecally 0.5mg dissolved in 5ml of CSF 3 times a week until 15mg total has been given, particularly in patients with coccidioidomycoses. Amphotericin B is quite toxic; anaphylaxis, thrombocytopenia, anaemia and impairment of renal or liver function may occur. Fever and chills occur with each injection in 50% of patients. Flucytosine (150 to 200mg/kg day orally) can be used as an alternative to amphotericin B in cryptococcal and coccidioidal meningitis. Amphotericin B and flucytosine act synergistically and such a combination is now the preferred method of treatment. Not only is the combination more effective than either drug alone, but dosage of amphotericin B can be reduced with a corresponding decrease in incidence of toxicity (Jimbrow et al., 1978; Utz et al., 1975). Dosage is 0.35mg/kg daily amphotericin B intravenously and 150mg/kg daily flucytosine orally given for at least 6 weeks. An alternative regimen is miconazole 30mg/kg daily intravenously for 4 to 8 weeks or in coccidioidal meningitis 20mg intrathecally (Deresinski et al., 1977; Sung et al., 1978).

Constant examination of the patient with meningitis is essential during the course of the illness if complications are to be recognised and treated early. Follow-up is also important, particularly expert tests of hearing in the very young.

Luetic (syphilitic) infections of the nervous system include general paresis, tabes dorsalis and gumma. These are all treated with high doses of penicillin G. Procaine penicillin G 600 000 units daily for 2 to 3 weeks for a total of 20 million units, or benzathine penicillin G 2.4 million units weekly for a total of 10 to 20 million units. Erythromycin 2g daily for 20 to 30 days or tetracycline 3g daily for 30 days are used in patients sensitive to penicillin. The return of CSF protein and white cell count values to normal are criteria by which success of treatment is gauged.

14. Use of Drugs in the Presence of Associated Neurological Disease

A large number of drugs can induce (see also section 15) or aggravate neurological disorders.

Thus one must always consider the potential neurotoxicity of drugs prescribed for the patient with neurological disease.

14.1 Myasthenia Gravis and Other Neuromuscular Diseases

In patients with myasthenia gravis, certain drugs may aggravate muscle weakness, especially in those with serious and generalised involvement (Flacke, 1973; Lane and Mastalgia, 1978). The drugs most likely to be implicated include the polymyxin antibiotics, colistin and polymyxin B and the aminoglycoside antibiotics streptomycin, kanamycin, gentamicin, tobramycin and amikacin. A difficult dilemma frequently exists in patients with myasthenia gravis; severe infection is a threat to the patient but antibiotics may be a hazard as well. Avoidance of unnecessarily high antibiotic doses, close observation and preparedness for extreme weakness and respiratory failure are helpful in avoiding serious complications. Further drugs which should be used with great caution in myasthenic patients are quinine, quinidine, procainamide, lignocaine, propranolol, phenytoin, chlorpromazine and parenteral tetracyclines, notably rolitetracycline. Patients with myasthenia gravis also seem to be especially sensitive to CNS depressants such as morphine, barbiturates and tranquillisers (Flacke, 1973).

Suxamethonium (succinylcholine) may lead to a dangerous rise in serum potassium levels, as well as a risk of triggering malignant hyperpyrexia, in patients with neuromuscular disease (muscle paralysis, multiple sclerosis, muscular dystrophy etc) who are undergoing general anaesthesia (Cooperman, 1970). It should be avoided (see chapter X; sect. 2.2.1).

14.2 Cerebral Vascular Disease

In patients with advanced cerebrovascular disease, ergotamine, a powerful vasoconstrictor, should be used with extreme caution, if at all, as ischaemic episodes may ensue. Antihypertensive drugs and other drugs that can cause a sudden fall in blood pressure (e.g. tricyclic antidepressants, phenothiazines) can also cause ischaemic episodes in elderly patients with marked cerebral atherosclerosis or in those who have had a recent stroke, and must be used judiciously (see also section 8.2; chapter XVIII, sect. 9). While the effect of sedative drugs seems to be much greater in patients with cerebral vascular disease, the therapeutic (but not toxic) effects of tricyclic antidepressants often appear to be diminished in depressed patients with cerebral arteriosclerosis (James, 1974; see also section 15.1; chapter V, sect. 4.7.2).

14.3 Migraine, Epilepsy and Other Disorders

In patients with migraine headaches, the use of progestagen-oestrogen contraceptive agents may sometimes aggravate the attacks and should be used with caution (Dalton, 1975; Ryan, 1978).

Respiratory depressant drugs (e.g. barbiturates, strong analgesics) are particularly hazardous in the presence of raised intracranial pressure due to cerebral tumours or trauma; the intracranial pressure being raised even further as a consequence of cerebral vasodilatation secondary to the carbon dioxide retention (see also chapter XX; sect. 5.2).

It is possible for a number of drugs to aggravate seizures in epileptic patients, but such an occurrence is rare (see section 15.3). Toxic delirium however, is often induced by drugs in patients with degenerative neurological disorders (see section 15.1).

15. Drug Induced Neurological Diseases

Neurological diseases induced by drugs may involve both the central and peripheral nervous system (see De Jong, 1970; Hollister, 1972). The clinical manifestations include diffuse encephalopathies, cerebrovascular syndromes, convulsions, extrapyramidal and cerebellar syndromes, myelopathies, peripheral neuropathies and neuromuscular syndromes. Drug induced neurological disorders are particularly prone to occur in the elderly and in patients with impaired renal function (Richet et al., 1970; see chapter VII; sect. 5.3).

15.1 Confusion: Toxic Delirium

The most frequent neurological disorder induced by drugs is toxic delirium. This is characterised by disorientation, confusion, anxiety, delusions and hallucinations. It is common in older patients, patients with dementia and cerebral atrophy or in patients with degenerative CNS diseases. The offending drugs include sedatives, reserpine, methyldopa, alcohol, digitalis, anticholinergics, tricyclic antidepressants, antianxiety and antipsychotic drugs and cimetidine. Stopping the causative medication usually suffices to reverse the process. It may however, take as long as 2 weeks before mental processes fully recover (see also chapter V, sect. 4.7.2; XXVI, sect. 15.5).

15.2 Complications Related to Cerebral Circulation

Complications related to the cerebral circulation include intracerebral or subarachnoidal haemorrhages following hypertensive crises caused by monoamine oxidase inhibitors, when these drugs are given together with tyramine-rich foods or sympathomimetic drugs (see chapter X; sect. 6.2.1). Intracerebral bleeding may also occur following poorly controlled anticoagulant therapy (Petrov and Bonnal, 1975) or with the administration of pressor amines such as adrenaline and noradrenaline (epinephrine, levarterenol), particularly in patients with intracerebral aneurysms or clotting defects. Cerebral infarcts have been reported after a sudden fall of blood pressure induced by ganglion blocking antihypertensive drugs such as pentolinium and hexamethonium.

Oral contraceptives have been associated with reports of intracranial arterial thrombosis or embolus, as well as sinus thrombosis (Masi and Dugdale, 1970). Oral contraceptives used alone, in the absence of smoking, hypertension or migraine, significantly increases the risk of stroke in young women (Collaborative Group, 1975). There seems to be a peculiar predilection to thrombosis of the right cerebral artery when contraceptives are involved (Ask-Upmark, 1976). Pseudotumor cerebri has also been reported as a possible association with use of oral contraceptives (Weisberg, 1977).

15.3 Convulsive States

Convulsions may be induced by CNS stimulants and analeptics (amphetamines, bemegride). Antibiotics, particularly penicillin G, when applied intrathecally or intracerebrally, will cause convulsions with relatively small amounts, i.e, 50 000 units, in some patients. Massive daily doses of penicillin (over 20 million units) given intravenously may cause penicillin encephalopathy characterised by confusion, stupor and multifocal myoclonus and may culminate in the generalised convulsion, particularly in elderly patients with

impaired renal function (Bloomer et al., 1967) or those undergoing cardiac surgery with cardiopulmonary by-pass (Seamans et al., 1968; Smith et al., 1967). Myoclonic seizures have also been noted in patients with impaired renal function treated with moderate intravenous doses of cephalosporins (Bloomer et al., 1967; Yost et al., 1977). Other antimicrobial agents that may cause convulsions are metronidazole in large doses (Frytak et al., 1978), cycloserine and isoniazid. Convulsions with isoniazid are probably due to pyridoxine deficiency and most likely to occur in those who are genetically slow acetylators of the drug or are epileptics or have a history of brain trauma (Goldman and Braman, 1972). Nalidixic acid has been reported to exacerbate seizures in epileptics or cause convulsions in non-epileptics usually after excessive doses (Fraser and Harrower, 1977); renal impairment may make this complication more likely to occur since nalidixic acid accumulates in such patients (see appendix E). Cimetidine can cause confusion and convulsions with excessive dosage in the elderly and in uraemic patients (see chapter XX; sect. 14.8).

Anaesthetics such as procaine, lignocaine or amethocaine (lidocaine, tetracaine) applied locally (mucosa) in high concentrations or accidentally injected intravenously have caused seizures, as have excessive doses of lignocaine and phenytoin when used in cardiac arrhythmias (Crampton and Oriscello, 1968; Russell and Bousvaros, 1968) or aminophylline in acute severe asthma (Yarnell and Chu, 1975). Other agents that rarely cause convulsions or aggravate seizures in epileptic patients include insulin, phenothiazines, MAO inhibitors, antihistamines, tricyclic antidepressants, chloroquine, vincristine and oral contraceptives.

15.4 Encephalopathy and Other Brain Syndromes

Vaccines and antisera are the most common cause of encephalomyelitis, particularly smallpox and pertussis vaccine and tetanus antitoxin. Excessive dosage of lithium carbonate may lead to severe neurological reactions (coma, spasticity, convulsions), particularly in the presence of impaired renal function (see chapter XXVI; sect. 5.4).

Coma and dysarthria have occurred following usual doses of lignocaine in patients with severe liver impairment (Selden and Sasahara, 1967). In patients with liver failure, encephalopathy may be precipitated or aggravated by morphine or over-vigorous diuretic therapy (see chapter XIX; sect. 13.4). Encephalopathy can occur with methotrexate and l-asparaginase (Weiss et al., 1974), disulfiram (Hotson and Lanston, 1976), aluminium antacids in chronic uraemic patients on dialysis (Ulmer, 1976) and after long term use of bismuth subnitrate for constipation (Supino-Viterbo et al., 1977).

Indomethacin produces a cerebral syndrome manifested by headaches, mental 'muzziness', drowsiness and vertigo (Hart and Boardman, 1963). A range of drugs can lead to the syndrome of pseudotumor cerebri which is characterised by headache, blurred vision, papilloedema and increased intracranial pressure. Corticosteroids, especially in children and usually when the dose of steroid is decreased, but also after high doses in adults, and excessive dosage of vitamin A, are most commonly implicated (Sternberg and Bierman, 1965; Ivey and Den Besten, 1969). Oral contraceptives (Weisberg, 1977), and use of nalidixic acid (Duffau et al., 1971) and tetracyclines (Opfer, 1963) in infants, have also been incriminated on a few occasions. Tetracyclines have also caused raised intracranial pressure in isolated instances when used long term in low doses in adolescents with acne (Hall Stuart and Litt, 1978; Monaco et al., 1978). Perhexiline also seems to occasionally cause raised intracranial pressure (Stephens et al., 1978).

15.5 Extrapyramidal Syndromes

Extrapyramidal syndromes may be caused by agents that block or deplete brain catecholamines or serotonin (Ayd, 1961; Hollister, 1972). These include phenothiazines, Rauwolfia alkaloids and other antipsychotic drugs such as the butyrophenones (haloperidol) and thioxanthenes (thiothixene). A frequent clinical manifestation is akathisia or motor restlessness causing the patient to pace about or tap his feet and shift the legs while sitting. Grimacing, smacking of lips and tongue and chewing movements are often present. A Parkinsonian-like state is also frequent, usually starting with tremor, followed by rigidity and motor retardation. Dyskinesias mostly of the dystonic type with twisting, writhing movements, torticollis and oculogyric crises are not infrequent.

The clinical manifestations tend to be more severe in patients receiving higher doses and occur more frequently in females than in males, but some patients seem to be inherently more susceptible than others. Older patients tend to develop a Parkinsonian-like state and younger patients a dystonic picture, which can be confused with encephalitis or tetanus in children who have taken overdoses of phenothiazines (see chapter XXVI; sect. 3.5.3). The antiemetic metoclopramide can also cause acute dystonic reactions, particularly in children after large doses (Cochlin, 1974). Very prolonged (years) use of antihistamines has been associated with facial dyskinesia (Davis, 1976; Thach et al., 1975).

The extrapyramidal signs and symptoms, with rare exceptions, are reversible after discontinuation or reduction of the dosage of the causative agent, but permanent or tardive dyskinesias have been reported (see further chapter XXVI; sect. 3.4, 3.5.1).

15.6 Cerebellar Syndromes

Reversible drug related cerebellar signs and symptoms occur with high dose anticonvulsant therapy (see section 3) and permanent cerebellar dysfunction has been suspected as a result of prolonged overdosage of phenytoin (Selhorst et al., 1972).

A reversible acute cerebellar syndrome can occur with 5-flurorouracil (Weiss et al., 1974).

15.7 Myelopathy

Myeloradiculopathy and arachnoid adhesions may rarely occur as a result of radiographic contrast media instilled into the subarachnoid space of the spinal cord for myelography.

15.8 Peripheral Neuropathy

Peripheral neuropathy has been caused by a variety of drugs and both motor and sensory loss may occur (Argov and Mastalgia, 1979; Hollister, 1972). Drugs implicated include antimicrobial agents such as nitrofurantoin, chloramphenicol, sulphonamides, kanamycin, streptomycin, isoniazid (due to pyridoxine deficiency and most likely in slow acetylators; Devadatta, 1965), ethambutol, ethionamide, polymyxin B, colistin and long term high dose metronidazole for Crohn's disease. Further drugs which can cause peripheral neuropathy include MAO inhibitors, tricyclic antidepressants, methaqualone, indomethacin (Eade et al., 1975), chloroquine, disulfiram, arsenicals, emetine, vincristine and procarbazine (Weiss et al., 1974), and the anticonvulsant phenytoin. Individuals who are genetically slow metabolisers of dapsone (Gutman et al., 1976; Koller et al., 1977) or perhexiline (see chapter XVII; sect. 4.2.3) seem to be more likely to suffer peripheral neuropathy from these drugs. Halogenated hydroxyquinolines such as clioquinol have been implicated as a cause of subacute myelo-optico-neuropathy (SMON) and of a major epidemic of the condition in Japan, but whether clioquinol was the sole factor involved is far from clear (Meade, 1975).

Paraesthesiae may be an early feature of drug induced peripheral neuropathy and patients should always be examined for other evidence of neuropathy such as sensory loss and so on. It is probably best to stop the suspected drug if paraesthesiae are severe and persistent — it is essential to stop nitrofurantoin (Toole and Parrish, 1973) and metronidazole (Karlsson and Hamlyn, 1977) and any other drug which can cause severe neuropathy.

15.9 Neuromuscular Syndromes

A wide variety of drugs can cause myopathies or muscular syndromes (Lane and Mastalgia, 1978). Muscle weakness due to myopathy with vacuolar and/or hyaline degeneration in biopsy material has been observed following treatment with corticosteroids, particularly fluorinated compounds such as triamcinolone, usually following prolonged high dose treatment of severe rheumatoid arthritis or collagen disease (Editorial, 1965; Kalyanaraman, 1977). Long term chloroquine treatment of rheumatoid arthritis may be complicated by a neuromyopathy affecting the pelvic girdle muscles (Whisnant et al., 1963). Tremor and muscle weakness is a frequent sign of toxicity with lithium therapy. Muscle pain and stiffness are common after suxamethonium (succinylcholine; Usubiaga et al., 1967) and myoglobinuria has been observed when used in conjunction with halothane anaesthesia (Airaksinen and Tammisto, 1966; Bennike and Jarnum, 1964). Prolonged paralysis may occur in those individuals with an atypical pseudocholinesterase who cannot metabolise suxamethonium rapidly enough following usual doses (see chapter X; sect. 2.2.1). Muscle damage and profound muscle weakness can occur with carbenoxolone if severe

hypokalaemia is allowed to develop (Pinder et al., 1976b) and similarly with amphotericin B.

The polymyxin and aminoglycoside antibiotics can lead to neuromuscular blockade and respiratory paralysis, particularly with high doses or in the presence of impaired renal function (McQuillen et al., 1968; Pittinger et al., 1970). The reaction resembles the myasthenia gravis syndrome and can usually be reversed by neostigmine or calcium in the case of aminoglycosides and by withdrawal of the antibiotic in the case of polymyxins. These agents should therefore be used with great care in patients with myasthenia gravis (see section 14) and in bowel surgery when used in conjunction with skeletal muscle relaxants (see chapter X; sect. 6.2.5). Muscle weakness and myasthenic signs have been noted in some patients taking penicillamine for rheumatoid arthritis or Wilson's disease (Bucknall, 1977). Other drugs which can cause muscle pain or cramps are discussed in chapter XXII (sect. 14.3).

Further Reading

Calne, D.B.: Progress in the Treatment of Parkinsonism. Advances in Neurology, vol. 3 (Raven Press, New York 1973).

Calne, D.B.: Therapeutics in Neurology (Blackwell Scientific Publications, Oxford 1975).

Carpi, A.: Pharmacology of the Cerebral Circulation (Pergamon, Oxford 1972)

Eadie, M.J. and Tyrer, J.H.: Anticonvulsant Therapy: Pharmacological Basis and Practice (Churchill Livingstone, Edinburgh 1974).

Laidlaw, J. and Richens, A.: A Textbook of Epilepsy (Churchill Livingstone, Edinburgh 1976).

Lance, J.W.: The Mechanism and Management of Headache, 3rd ed (Butterworths, London 1978).

Merritt, H.: A Textbook of Neurology, 6th ed (Lea & Febiger, Philadelphia 1979).

Richens, A.: Drug Treatment of Epilepsy (Year Book, Chicago 1976).

Woodbury, D.M.; Penry, J.K. and Glaser, G.H.: Mechanisms of Action of Antiepileptic Drugs (Raven Press, New York 1979).

Woodbury, D.M.; Penry, J.K. and Schmidt, R.P.: Antiepileptic Drugs (Raven Press, New York 1972).

References

Acheson, J. and Hutchinson, E.C.: The natural history of "focal cerebral vascular disease". Quarterly Journal of Medicine 40: 15 (1971).

Aellig, W.H. and Nuesch, E.: Comparative pharmacokinetic investigations with tritium-labelled ergot alkaloids after oral and intravenous administration in man. International Journal of Clinical Pharmacology 15: 106 (1977).

Airaksinew, M. and Tammisto, T.: Myoglobinuria after intermittent administration of succinylcholine during halothane anesthesia. Clinical Pharmacology and Therapeutics 7: 583 (1966).

Anthony, M. and Lance, J.W.: Current concepts in the pathogenesis and interval treatment of migraine. Drugs 3: 153 (1972).

Anthony, M.; Lord, G.D.A. and Lance, J.W.: Controlled trials of cimetidine in migraine and cluster headache. Headache 18: 261 (1978).

Argov, Z. and Mastalgia, F.L.: Drug-induced peripheral neuropathies. British Medical Journal 1: 663 (1979).

Ask-Upmark, E.: Strokes in young women caused by oral contraceptives. Folia Clinica Internationale 26: 391 (1976).

Ayd, F.J.: A survey of drug-induced extrapyramidal reactions. Journal of the American Medical Association 175: 1054 (1961).

Barbeau, A.: Treatment of Parkinson's disease with 1-dopa and Ro 4-4602: Review and present status. Advances in Neurology 2: 173 (1973).

Barbeau, A.: Long-term assessment of levodopa therapy in Parkinson's disease. Canadian Medical Association Journal 112: 1379 (1975).

Barling, R.W.A. and Selkon, J.B.: The penetration of antibiotics into cerebrospinal fluid and brain tissue. Journal of Antimicrobial Chemotherapy 4: 203 (1978).

Barnett, H.J.M. and the Canadian Cooperative Study Group: A randomized trial of aspirin and sulfinpyrazone in threatened stroke. New England Journal of Medicine 299: 53 (1978).

Beerman, B. and Edhag, O.: Depressive effects of carbamazepine on idioventricular rhythm in man. Lancet 2: 171 (1978).

Bennike, K-A. and Jarnum, S.: Myoglobinuria with acute renal failure possibly induced by suxamethonium. British Journal of Anaesthesia 36: 730 (1964).

Bertilsson, L.: Clinical pharmacokinetics of carbamazepine. Clinical Pharmacokinetics 3: 128 (1978).

Bianchine, J.D. and Shaw, G.M.: Clinical pharmacokinetics of levodopa in Parkinson's disease. Clinical Pharmacokinetics 1: 313 (1976).

Bird, E.D. and Iverson, L.L.: Huntington's chorea, postmortem measurement of glutamic acid decarboxylase, choline acetyl transferase and dopamine in basal ganglia. Brain 97: 457 (1974).

Bloomer, H.A.; Barton, L.J. and Maddock, R.K.: Penicillin-induced encephalopathy in uremic patients. Journal of the American Medical Association 200 (2): 121 (1967).

Boreus, L.O.; Jalling B. and Kallberg, N.: Phenobarbital metabolism in adults and in newborn infants. Acta Paediatrica Scandinavica 67: 193 (1978).

Bradfield, J.M.: A new look at the use of ergotamine. Drugs 12: 449 (1976).

Brogden, R.N.; Speight, T.M. and Avery, G.S.: Levodopa: A review of its pharmacological properties and therapeutic uses with particular reference to parkinsonism. Drugs 2: 262 (1971).

Brogden, R.N.; Speight, T.M. and Avery, G.S.: Baclofen: A preliminary report of its pharmacological properties and therapeutic efficacy in spasticity. Drugs 8: 1 (1974).

Browne, T.R.: Clonazepam. New England Journal of Medicine 299: 812 (1978a).

Browne, T.R.: Drug therapy of status epilepticus. Journal of the Maine Medical Association 69: 199 (1978b).

Brunner, N.G.; Berger, C.L.; Namba, T. and Grob, D.: Corticotrophin and corticosteroids in generalized myasthenia gravis: Comparative studies and role in management. Annals of the New York Academy of Science 274: 577 (1976).

Buchthal, F. and Lennox-Buchthal, M.A.: Phenobarbital. Relation of serum concentration to control of seizures; in Woodbury, Penry and Schmidt (Eds) Antiepileptic Drugs, p.335 (Raven Press, New York; North-Holland, Amsterdam 1972).

Bucknall, R.C.: Myasthenia associated with D-penicillamine therapy in rheumatoid arthritis. Proceedings of the Royal Society of Medicine 70 (Suppl. 3): 114 (1977).

Burke, D.J.: An approach to the treatment of spasticity. Drugs 10: 112 (1975).

Calne, D.B.: Therapeutics in Neurology (Blackwell Scientific Publications, Oxford 1974).

Calne, D.B.: Developments in the pharmacology and therapeutics of parkinsonism. Annals of Neurology 1: 111 (1977).

Calne, D.B. and Reid, J.L.: Antiparkinsonian drugs: Pharmacological and therapeutic aspects. Drugs 4: 49 (1972).

Calne, D.B.; Plotkin, C.; Williams, A.C.; Nutt, J.G.; Neophytides, A. and Teychene, P.F.: Long-term treatment of Parkinsonism with bromocriptine. Lancet 1: 735 (1978).

Calvey, T.N. and Chan, K.: Plasma pyridostigmine levels in patients with myasthenia gravis. Clinical Pharmacology and Therapeutics 21: 187 (1977).

Carstairs, L.S.: Headache and gastric emptying time. Proceedings of the Royal Society of Medicine 51: 790 (1958).

Charlesworth, E.N.: Phenytoin induced pseudolymphoma syndrome. An immunologic study. Archives of Dermatology 113: 477 (1977).

Chase, T.N.; Glaubiger, G.A. and Shoulson, I.: Clinical and pharmacological studies of the 'on-off' response in L-dopa treated parkinsonian patients; in Birkmayer and Hornykiewicz (Eds) Advances in Parkinsonism, p.613 (Editiones Roche, Basel 1976).

Cochlin, D.L.: Dystonic reactions due to metoclopramide and phenothiazines resembling tetanus. British Journal of Clinical Practice 28: 201 (1974).

Cohan, S.L.; Dretchen, K.L. and Neal, A.: Malabsorption of pyridostigmine in patients with myasthenia gravis. Neurology 27: 299 (1977).

Collaborative Group for the Study of Stroke in Young Women: Oral contraceptives and stroke in young women. Associated risk factors. Journal of the American Medical Association 231: 718 (1975).

Cooperman, L.H.: Succinylcholine-induced hyperkalaemia in neuromuscular disease. Journal of the American Medical Association 213: 1867 (1970).

Couch, J.R. and Ziegler, D.K.: Prednisone therapy for cluster headache. Headache 18: 219 (1978).

Crampton, R. and Oriscello, R.: Petit and grand mal convulsions during lidocaine hydrochloride treatment of ventricular tachycardia. Journal of the American Medical Association 204: 202 (1968).

Cranford, R.E.; Leppik, I.E.; Pattrick, B.; Anderson, C.B. and Kostick, B.: Intravenous phenytoin: clinical and pharmacokinetic aspects. Neurology 28: 874 (1978).

Dalton, K.: Migraine and oral contraceptives. Headache 15: 247 (1975).

Dam, M.; Jensen, A. and Christiansen, J.: Plasma level and effect of carbamazepine in grand mal and psychomotor epilepsy. Acta Neur. Scand. Suppl. 60: 33 (1975).

Dam, M.; Christiansen, J.; Munck, O. and Mygind, K.I.: Antiepileptic drugs: Metabolism in pregnancy. Clinical Pharmacokinetics 4: 53 (1979).

Dau, P.C.; Lindstrom, J.M.; Cassell, C.K.; Denys, E.H.; Shev, E.E. and Spitler, L.E.: Plasmapheresis and immunosuppressive drug therapy in myasthenia gravis. New England Journal of Medicine 297: 1134 (1977).

Davis, W.A.: Dyskinesia associated with chronic antihistamine use. New England Journal of Medicine 294: 113 (1976).

De Jong, R.: Neurological complications of drugs with primary action on the nervous system. New York State Journal of Medicine 70: 1857 (1970).

Deresinski, S.C.; Lilly, R.B.; Levine, H.B.; Galgiani, J.N. and Stevens, D.A.: Treatment of fungal meningitis with miconazole. Archives of Internal Medicine 137: 1180 (1977).

Desjacques, P.; Moret, P. and Gauthier, G.: Effects cardiovasculaire de la l-dopa et de l'inhibiteur de la decarboxylase chez les malades atteints de la maladie de Parkinson. Schweizerische Medizinische Wochenschrift 103: 1783 (1973).

Devadatta, S.: Isoniazid-induced encephalopathy. Lancet 2: 440 (1965).

Diamond, S. and Medina, J.L.: Double-blind study of propranolol for migraine prophylaxis. Headache 16: 24 (1976).

Duffau, G.T.; Emilfork, M.; Llorente, J. and Soza, G.: Acido nalidixicoe hipertension intracraneana. Pediatria (Santiago) 14 (2): 83 (1971).

Duffy, F.H. and Lambroso, C.T.: Treatment of status epilepticus; in Klawans (Ed) Clinical Neuropharmacology, pp.41-56 (Raven Press, New York 1978).

Eade, O.E.; Acheson, E.D.; Cuthbert, M.F. and Hawkes, C.H.: Peripheral neuropathy and indomethacin. British Medical Journal 2: 66 (1975).

Eadie, M.J.: Plasma level monitoring of anticonvulsants. Clinical Pharmacokinetics 1: 52 (1976).

Eadie, M.J. and Tyrer, J.H.: Anticonvulsant therapy: Pharmacological Basis and Practice (Churchill Livingstone, Edinburgh 1974).

Eadie, M.J.; Lander, C.M. and Tyrer, J.H.: Plasma drug level monitoring in pregnancy. Clinical Pharmacokinetics 2: 427 (1977).

Editorial: Corticosteroid myopathy. Lancet 2: 1118 (1965).

Eichelbaum, M.; Ekbom, K.; Bertilsson, L.; Ringberger, V.A. and Rane, A.: Plasma kinetics of carbamazepine and its epoxide metabolite in man after single and multiple doses. European Journal of Clinical Pharmacology 8: 337 (1975).

Elmqvist, D.; Hofmann, W.W.; Kugelberg, J. and Quastel, D.M.J.: An electrophysiological investigation on neuromuscular transmission in myasthenia gravis. Journal of Physiology 174: 417 (1964).

Engel, W.K.; Festoff, B.W.; Patten, B.M.; Swerdlow, M.L.; Newball, H.H. and Thompson, M.D.: Myasthenia gravis. Annals of Internal Medicine 81: 225 (1974).

Fallon, R.J.: The treatment of tuberculous meningitis. Journal of Antimicrobial Chemotherapy 4: 1 (1978).

Fanchamps, A.: Pharmacodynamic principles of antimigraine therapy. Headache 15: 79 (1975).

Feigenson, J.S.; Sweet, R.D. and McDowell, F.H.: Piribedil: Its synergistic effect in multidrug regimens for parkinsonism. Neurology 26: 430 (1976).

Fenichel, G.M.: Clinical syndromes of myasthenia in infancy and childhood. A review. Archives of Neurology 35: 97 (1978).

Fields, W.S.; Lemak, N.A.; Frankowski, R.F. and Hardy, R.J.: Controlled trial of aspirin in cerebral ischemia. Stroke 4: 301 (1977).

Fields, W.S.; Lemak, N.A.; Frankowski, R.F. and Hardy, R.J.: Controlled trial of aspirin in cerebral ischemia. Part II: Surgical group. Stroke 9: 309 (1978).

Fincham, R.W.; Schottelius, D.D. and Sahs, A.L.: The influence of diphenylhydantoin on primidone metabolism. Archives of Neurology 30: 259 (1974).

Fisher, C.M.: Lacunes: small, deep cerebral infarcts. Neurology 15: 774 (1965).

Flacke, W.: Treatment of myasthenia gravis. New England Journal of Medicine 288: 27 (1973).

Forssman, B.; Henriksson, K-G; Johannsson, V.; Lindvall, L. and Lundin, H.: Propranolol for migraine prophylaxis. Headache 16: 238 (1976).

Fraser, A.G. and Harrower, A.D.B.: Convulsions and hyperglycaemia associated with nalidixic acid. British Medical Journal 2: 1518 (1977).

Frattola, L.; Albizzate, M.G. and Spano, P.F.: Treatment of Huntington's chorea with bromocriptine. Acta Neurologica Scandinavica 56: 33 (1977).

Friedman, A.P.: Symposium on headache and related pain syndromes. Migraine. Medical Clinics of North America 62: 481 (1978).

Frytak, S.; Childs, D.S. and Albers, J.W.: Neurologic toxicity associated with high-dose metronidazole therapy. Annals of Internal Medicine 88: 361 (1978).

Gastaut, H.: Clinical and electroencephalographic classification of epileptic seizures. Epilepsia 1: 102 (1970).

Genton, E.; Barnett, H.J.M.; Fields, W.S.; Gent, M. and Hoak, J.C.: Cerebral ischemia: role of thrombosis and of antithrombotic therapy. Stroke 8: 150 (1977).

Goldman, A.L. and Braman, S.S.: Isoniazid, a review with emphasis on adverse effects. Chest 62: 71 (1972).

Graham, J.R.: Cluster headaches. Headache 11: 175 (1972).

Graham, J.R.; Suby, H.L.; Le Compte, P.R. and Sadowsky, N.L.: Fibrotic disorders associated with methysergide therapy for headache. New England Journal of Medicine 274: 359 (1966).

Gugler, R.; Schell, A.; Eichelbaum, M.; Froscher, W. and Schulz, H.-U.: Disposition of valproic acid in man. European Journal of Clinical Pharmacology 12: 125 (1977).

Gutman, L.; Martin, J.D. and Welton, W.: Dapsone motor neuropathy — an axonal disease. Neurology 26: 514 (1976).

Hall Stuart, B. and Litt, I.F.: Tetracycline-associated intracranial hypertension in an adolescent: A complication of systemic acne therapy. Journal of Pediatrics 92: 679 (1978).

Hambleton, G. and Davies, P.A.: Diagnosis and management of bacterial meningitis. Drugs 8: 15 (1974).

Hambleton, G. and Davies, P.: Bacterial meningitis: Some aspects of diagnosis and treatment. Archives of Disease in Childhood 50: 674 (1975).

Hamilton, D.V.: Carbamazepine and heart block. Lancet 1: 1365 (1978).

Hansen, J.M.; Siersbaek-Nielsen, K. and Skovsted, L.: Carbamazepine-induced acceleration of diphenylhydantoin and warfarin metabolism in man. Clinical Pharmacology and Therapeutics 12: 539 (1971).

Hart, F.D. and Boardman, P.L.: Indomethacin: A new nonsteroid anti-inflammatory agent. British Medical Journal 2:

965 (1963).

Harvard, C.W.H.: Progress in myasthenia gravis. British Medical Journal 2: 1008 (1977).

Harvey, P.K.; Higenbottom, T.W. and Loh, L.: Chlormethiazole in treatment of status epilepticus. British Medical Journal 2: 603 (1975).

Henderson, W.G.; Tourtellotte, W.W.; Potvin, A.R. and Rose, A.S.: Methodology for analyzing clinical neurological data: ACTH in multiple sclerosis. Clinical Pharmacology and Therapeutics 24: 146 (1978).

Herrman, W.N.; Horowski, R.; Dannehl, K.; Kramer, V. and Lurati, K.: Clinical effectiveness of lysuride hydrogen maleate, a double-blind trial versus methysergide. Headache 17: 54 (1977).

Herzberg, L.: Carbamazepine and bradycardia. British Medical Journal 1: 1097 (1978).

Hokkanen, E.; Waltims, O. and Kallanranta, T.: Toxic effects of ergotamine used for migraine. Headache 18: 95 (1978).

Hollister, L.E.: Disorders of the nervous system due to drugs; in Meyler and Peck (Eds) Drug-Induced Diseases, vol. 4, p.549 (Excerpta Medica, Amsterdam 1972).

Hotson, J.R. and Lanston, J.W.: Disulfiram-induced encephalopathy. Archives of Neurology 33: 141 (1976).

Houghton, G.W. and Richens, A.: Rate of elimination of tracer doses of phenytoin at different steady-state serum phenytoin concentrations in epileptic patients. British Journal of Clinical Pharmacology 1: 155 (1974).

Hughes, R.C.; Polgar, J.G.; Weightman, D. and Walton, J.N.: Levodopa in Parkinsonism. The effects of withdrawal of anticholinergic drugs. British Medical Journal 2: 487 (1971).

Hunter, K.R.; Stern, G.M.; Laurence, D.R. and Armitage, P.: Amantadine in Parkinsonism. Lancet 1: 1127 (1970).

Hvidberg, E.F. and Dam, M.: Clinical pharmacokinetics of anticonvulsants. Clinical Pharmacokinetics 1: 161 (1976).

Ivey, K. and DenBesten, L.: Pseudotumor cerebri associated with corticosteroid therapy in an adult. Journal of the American Medical Association 208: 1698 (1969).

James, I.M.: Diseases affecting drug responses. British Journal of Hospital Medicine 12: 823 (1974).

Janz, D.: The teratogenic risk of antiepileptic drugs. Epilepsia 16: 159 (1975).

Jimbow, T.; Tejima, Y. and Ikemoto, H.: Comparison between 5-fluorocytosine, amphotericin B and the combined administration of these agents in the therapeutic effectiveness for cryptococcal meningitis. Chemotherapy (Basel) 24: 374 (1978).

Kalyanaraman, K.: Iatrogenic myopathies and disorders of neuromuscular transmission. New York State Journal of Medicine 77: 1102 (1977).

Karlsson, I.J. and Hamlyn, A.N.: Metronidazole neuropathy. British Medical Journal 2: 832 (1977).

Kartzinel, R. and Calne, D.B.: Studies with bromocriptine. Part 1. "On-off" Phenomena. Neurology 26: 508 (1976).

Keesey, J.; Shaikh, I.; Wolfgram, F. and Chao, L.P.: Studies on the ability of acetylcholine receptors to bind alpha-bungarotoxin after exposure to myasthenic serum. Annals of the New York Academy of Sciences 274: 244 (1976).

Killian, J.M. and Fromm, G.H.: Carbamazepine in the treatment of neuralgia. Archives of Neurology 19: 129 (1968).

Koller, W.C.; Gehlmann, L.K.; Malkinson, F.D. and Davis, F.A.: Dapsone-induced peripheral neuropathy. Archives of Neurology 34: 644 (1977).

Kudrow, L.: Lithium prophylaxis for chronic cluster headache. Headache 17: 15 (1977).

Kutt, H.: Biochemical and genetic factors regulating Dilantin metabolism in man. Annals of the New York Academy of Sciences 179: 704 (1971).

Kutt, H.: Interactions of antiepileptic drugs. Epilepsia 16: 393 (1975).

Kutt, H. and Louis, S.: Anticonvulsant drugs I: Pathophysiological and pharmacological aspects; II: Clinical pharmacological and therapeutic aspects. Drugs 4: 227, 256 (1972).

Kutt, H.; Brennan, R.; Dehejia, H. and Verebely, K.: Diphenylhydantoin intoxication. A complication of isoniazid therapy. American Review of Respiratory Disease 101: 377 (1970).

Kutt, H.; Solomon, G.; Wasterlain, C.; Peterson, H.; Louis, S. and Carruthers, R.: Carbamazepine in difficult to control epileptic out-patients. Acta Neurologica Scandinavica Suppl. 60: 27 (1975).

Laidlaw, J. and Richens, A.: A Textbook of Epilepsy (Churchill Livingstone, Edinburgh 1976).

Lance, J.W.: The Mechanism and Management of Headache, 3rd ed (Butterworths, London 1978).

Lance, J.W. and Anthony, M.: Some clinical aspects of migraine. Archives of Neurology 15: 356 (1966).

Lane, R.J.M. and Mastalgia, F.L.: Drug-induced myopathies in man. Lancet 2: 562 (1978).

Lieberman, A.; Zolfaghari, M.; Boal, O.; Hassouri, H.; Vogel, B.; Battista, A.; Fuze, K. and Goldstein, M.: The antiparkinsonian efficacy of bromocriptine. Neurology 25: 405 (1976).

Lund, L.: Anticonvulsant effect of diphenylhydantoin relative to plasma levels. A prospective three-year study in ambulant patients with generalised seizures. Archives of Neurology 31: 289 (1974).

McAllen, P.M. and Marshall, J.: Cardiac dysrhythmia and transient cerebral ischaemic attacks. Lancet 1: 1212 (1973).

McDowell, F.H. and Sweet, R.D.: The "on-off" phenomenon in advances in parkinsonism; in Birkmayer and Hornykiewicz (Eds) Advances in Parkinsonism, p.603 (Editiones Roche, Basel 1976).

McLellan, D.L.; Chalmers, R.J. and Johnson, R.H.: A double-blind trial of tetrabenazine, thiopropazate and placebo in patients with chorea. Lancet 1: 104 (1974).

McQuillen, M.P.; Cantor, H.E. and O'Rourke, J.R.: Myasthenic syndrome associated with antibiotics. Archives of Neurology 18: 402 (1968).

Mann, J.D.; Johns, T.R.; Campa, J.F. and Muller, W.H.: Longterm prednisone followed by thymectomy in myasthenia gravis. Annals of the New York Academy of Sciences 274: 608 (1976).

Markham, C.H.; Treciokas, L.J. and Diamond, S.G.: Parkinson's disease and levodopa. A five-year follow-up and review. Western Journal of Medicine 121: 188 (1974).

Marsden, C.D. and Parkes, J.D.: "On-off" effects in patients with Parkinson's disease on chronic levodopa therapy. Lancet 1: 292 (1976).

Marshall, J. and Reynolds, E.H.: Withdrawal of anticoagulants from patients with transient ischaemic attacks. Lancet 1: 5 (1965).

Masi, A. and Dugdale, M.: Cerebrovascular disease associated with the use of oral contraceptives. A review of the English-language literature. Annals of Internal Medicine 72: 111 (1970).

Mathies, A.W. and Wehrle, P.F.: Management of bacterial meningitis in children. Pediatric Clinics of North America 15: 185 (1968).

Meade, T.W.: Subacute myelo-optic neuropathy and dioquinol. An epidemiological case history for diagnosis. British Journal of Preventive and Social Medicine 29: 157 (1975).

Meadow, S.R.: The teratogenicity of epilepsy. Developmental Medicine and Child Neurology 16: 375 (1974).

Meyer, J.S.; Fukuuchi, Y.; Shimazu, K.; Onuchi, T. and Ericsson, A.D.: Effect of intravenous infusion of glycerol on hemispheric blood flow and metabolism in patients with acute cerebral infarction. Stroke 3: 168 (1972).

Millikan, C.H.: Reassessment of anticoagulant therapy in various types of occlusive cerebrovascular disease. Stroke 2: 201 (1971).

Millikan, C.H. and McDowell, F.H.: Progress in cerebrovascular disease, treatment of transient attacks. Stroke 9: 299 (1978).

Monaco, F.; Agnetti, V. and Mutani, R.: Benign intracranial hypertension after minocycline therapy. European Neurology 17: 48 (1978).

Mondrup, K. and Moller, C.E.: Prophylactic treatment of migraine with clonidine. Acta Neurologica Scandinavica 56: 405 (1977).

Mountain, K.R.; Hirsh, J. and Gallus, A.S.: Neonatal coagulation defect due to anticonvulsant drug treatment in pregnancy. Lancet 1: 265 (1970).

Mulley, G.; Wilcox, R.G. and Mitchell, J.R.A.: Dexamethasone in acute stroke. British Medical Journal 2: 994 (1978).

Neuvonen, P.J.: Bioavailability of phenytoin: Pharmacokinetic and therapeutic implications. Clinical Pharmacokinetics 4: 91 (1979).

Newsom-Davis, J.; Wilson, G.; Vincent, A. and Ward, C.D.: Long-term effects of repeated plasma exchange in myasthenia gravis. Lancet 1: 464 (1979).

Nibbelink, D.W. and Cooperative Aneurysm Study: Antihypertensive and antifibrinolytic therapy following subarachnoid hemorrhage from ruptured intracranial aneurysm in cerebral vascular diseases; in Whisnant and Sandok (Eds) Cerebral Vascular Diseases 9th Conference. (Grune and Stratton, New York 1975).

Olesen, O.V. and Dam, M.: The metabolic conversion of primidone (Mysoline) to phenobarbital in patients under long-term treatment. Acta Neurologica Scandinavica 43: 348 (1967).

Opfer, K.: The bulging fontanelle. Lancet 1: 116 (1963).

Parkes, J.D.: Bromocriptine in the treatment of Parkinsonism. Drugs 17: 365 (1979).

Parkes, J.D.; Baxter, R.C.H.; Curson, G.; Knill-Jones, R.P.; Knott, P.J.; Marsden, C.D.; Tattersall, R. and Vollum, D.: Treatment of Parkinson's disease with amantadine and levodopa. Lancet 1: 1183 (1971).

Perry, T.L.; MacLeod, P.M. and Hansen, S.: Treatment of Huntington's chorea with isoniazid. New England Journal of Medicine 297: 840 (1977).

Perucca, E.; Garratt, A.; Hebdige, S. and Richens, A.: Water intoxication in epileptic patients receiving carbamazepine. Journal of Neurology, Neurosurgery and Psychiatry 41: 713 (1978).

Petrov, V. and Bonnal, J.: Neurological complications of anticoagulants. Acta Neurologica Belgica 75: 205 (1975).

Pinder, R.M.; Brogden, R.N.; Sawyer, P.R.; Speight, T.M. and Avery, G.S.: Levodopa and decarboxylase inhibitors: A review of their clinical pharmacology and use in the treatment of parkinsonism. Drugs 11: 329 (1976a).

Pinder, R.M.; Brogden, R.N.; Sawyer, P.R.; Speight, T.M.; Spencer, R. and Avery, G.S.: Carbenoxolone: A review of its pharmacological properties and therapeutic efficacy in peptic ulcer disease. Drugs 11: 245 (1976b).

Pinder, R.M.; Brogden, R.N.; Speight, T.M. and Avery, G.S.: Clonazepam: A review of its pharmacological properties and therapeutic efficacy in epilepsy. Drugs 12: 321 (1976c).

Pinder, R.M.; Brogden, R.N.; Speight, T.M. and Avery, G.S.: Dantrolene sodium: A review of its pharmacological properties and therapeutic efficacy in spasticity. Drugs 13: 3 (1977a).

Pinder, R.M.; Brogden, R.N.; Speight, T.M. and Avery, G.S.: Sodium valproate: A review of its pharmacological properties and therapeutic efficacy in epilepsy. Drugs 13: 81 (1977b).

Pittinger, C.B.; Eryasa, Y. and Adamson, R.: Antibiotic-induced paralysis. Anesthesia and Analgesics 49: 487 (1970).

Reynolds, E.H.: Chronic antiepileptic toxicity: A review. Epilepsia 16: 319 (1975).

Reynolds, E.H.: Drug treatment of epilepsy. Lancet 2: 721 (1978).

Reynolds, E.H.; Chadwick, D. and Galbraith, A.W.: One drug (phenytoin) in the treatment of epilepsy. Lancet 1: 923 (1976).

Richens, A.: Drug Treatment of Epilepsy (Year Book, Chicago 1976).

Richens, A.: Interactions with antiepileptic drugs. Drugs 13: 266 (1977).

Richens, A.: Clinical pharmacokinetics of phenytoin. Clinical Pharmacokinetics 4: 153 (1979).

Richet, G.; de Novales, E.L. and Verroust, P.: Drug intoxication and neurological episodes in chronic renal failure. British Medical Journal 2: 394 (1970).

Rose, A.S.; Kuzma, J.W.; Kurtzke, J.F. et al.: Cooperative study in the evaluation of therapy in multiple sclerosis: ACTH vs placebo in acute exacerbations. Preliminary report. Neurology 18 (pt. 2): 1 (May 1968).

Rose, A.S.; Kuzma, J.W.; Kurtzke, J.F. et al.: Cooperative study in the evaluation of therapy in multiple sclerosis: ACTH vs placebo. Final report. Neurology 20 (pt. 2): 1 (May 1970).

Rosenthal, R.K.; McDowell, F.H. and Cooper, W.: Levodopa therapy in athetoid cerebral palsy: a preliminary report. Neurology 22: 1 (1972).

Russell, M. and Bousvaros, G.: Fatal results from diphenylhydantoin administered intravenously. Journal of the American Medical Association 206: 2118 (1968).

Ryan, R.F.: A controlled study of the effect of oral contraceptives on migraine. Headache 17: 250 (1978).

Sachais, B.A.; Logue, I.N. and Carey, M.S.: Baclofen, a new antispastic drug. A controlled multicenter trial in patients with multiple sclerosis. Archives of Neurology 34: 422 (1977).

Schobben, F.; van der Klein, E. and Gabreels, F.J.M.: Pharmacokinetics of di-n-propylacetate in epileptic patients. European Journal of Clinical Pharmacology 8: 97 (1975).

Schmidt, R. and Fanchamps, A.: Effect of caffeine on intestinal absorption of ergotamine in man. European Journal of Clinical Pharmacology 7: 213 (1974).

Schmidt, R.P. and Wilder, B.J.: Epilepsy, p.178 (F.A. Davis Company, Philadelphia 1968).

Schwab, R.S.; England, A.C.; Poskanzer, D.C. and Young, R.R.: Amantadine in the treatment of Parkinson's disease. Journal of the American Medical Association 208: 1168 (1969).

Seamens, K.B.; Gloor, P.; Dobell, A.R.C. and Wyant, J.D.: Penicillin-induced seizures during cardiopulmonary bypass. A clinical and electroencephalographic study. New England Journal of Medicine 278: 861 (1968).

Selden, R. and Sasahara, A.A.: Central nervous system toxicity induced by lidocaine: Report of a case in a patient with liver disease. Journal of the American Medical Association 202: 908 (1967).

Selhorst, J.B.; Kaufman, B. and Horwitz, S.J.: Diphenylhydantoin-induced cerebellar degeneration. Archives of Neurology 27: 453 (1972).

Shapiro, S.; Hartz, S.C.; Siskind, V.; Mitchell, H.A.; Slone, D.; Rosenberg, L.; Monson, R.R.; Heinonen, O.P.; Indanpaan-Heikkila, J.; Haro, S. and Saxen, L.: Anticonvulsants and parental epilepsy in the development of birth defects. Lancet 1: 272 (1976).

Sherwin, A.L.; Robb, J.P. and Lechter, M.: Improved control of epilepsy by monitoring plasma ethosuximide. Archives of Neurology 28: 178 (1973).

Shorvon, S.D.; Chadwick, D.; Galbraith, A.W. and Reynolds, E.H.: One drug for epilepsy. British Medical Journal 1: 474 (1978).

Simpson, J.A.: Myasthenia gravis: A personal view of pathogenesis and mechanism. Muscle and Nerve 1: 151 (1978).

Smith, H.; Lerner, P.I. and Weinstein, L.: Neurotoxicity and 'massive' intravenous therapy with penicillin. Archives of Internal Medicine 120: 49 (1967).

Solomon, G.E. and Plum, F.: Clinical Management of Seizures (W.B. Saunders Company, Philadelphia 1976).

Speidel, B.D. and Meadow, S.R.: Epilepsy, anticonvulsants and congenital malformations. Drugs 8: 354 (1974).

Speight, T.M. and Avery, G.S.: Pizotifen (BC-105): A review of its pharmacological properties and its therapeutic efficacy in vascular headaches. Drugs 3: 159 (1972).

Stephens, W.P.; Eddy, J.D.; Parsons, L.M. and Singh, S.P.: Raised intracranial pressure due to perhexiline maleate. British Medical Journal 1: 21 (1978).

Sternberg, T.H. and Bierman, S.M.: Corticosteroids. Pseudotumor cerebri. Archives of Dermatology 92: 746 (1965).

Stromberg, U.; Svensson, T.H. and Waldeck, B.: On the mode of action of amantadine. Journal of Pharmacy and Pharmacology 22: 959 (1970).

Study Group, Joint Committee for Stroke Resources: Brain, edema and stroke. Stroke 8: 512 (1977).

Stumpf, D.A. and Frost, M.: Seizures, anticonvulsants and pregnancy. American Journal of Diseases of Children 132: 746 (1978).

Sung, J.P.; Campbell, G.D. and Grendahl, J.G.: Miconazole therapy for fungal meningitis. Archives of Neurology 35: 443 (1978).

Supino-Viterbo, V.; Sicard, C.; Risvegliato, M.; Rancurel, G. and Buge, A.: Toxic encephalopathy due to ingestion of bismuth salts: clinical and EEG studies of 45 patients. Journal of Neurology, Neurosurgery and Psychiatry 40: 748 (1977).

Sweet, R.D. and McDowell, F.H.: The 'on-off' response to chronic L-dopa treatment of Parkinsonism. Advances in Neurology 5: 331 (1974a).

Sweet, R.D. and McDowell, F.H.: Plasma dopa concentrations and the 'on-off' effect after chronic treatment of Parkinson's disease. Neurology 24: 953 (1974b).

Sweet, R.D. and McDowell, F.H.: Five years' treatment of Parkinson's disease with levodopa. Therapeutic results and survival of 100 patients. Annals of Internal Medicine 83: 456 (1975).

Sweet, R.D. and McDowell, F.H.: In press (1979).

Sweet, R.D.; McDowell, F.H.; Wasterlain, C.G. and Stern, T.H.: Treatment of 'on-off effect' with a dopa decarboxylase inhibitor. Archives of Neurology 32: 560 (1975).

Taber, L.H.; Yew, M.D. and Nieberg, F.G.: The penetration of broad spectrum antibiotics into the cerebrospinal fluid. Annals of the New York Academy of Sciences 145: 473 (1967).

Taverner, D.; Cohen, S.B. and Hutchinson, B.C.: Comparison of corticotrophin and prednisolone in treatment of idiopathic facial paralysis (Bell's palsy). British Medical Journal 4: 20 (1971).

Teychenne, P.F.; Pfeiffer, R.F.; Bern, S.M.; McInturff, D. and Calne, D.B.: Comparison between lergotrile and bromocriptine in Parkinsonism. Annals of Neurology 3: 319 (1978).

Thach, B.T.; Chase, T.N. and Bosma, J.F.: Oral facial dyskinesia associated with prolonged use of antihistaminic decongestants. New England Journal of Medicine 293: 486 (1975).

Toole, J.F. and Parrish, M.L.: Nitrofurantoin polyneuropathy. Neurology 23: 554 (1973).

Tyson, R.M.; Schrader, E.A. and Perlman, H.H.: Drugs transmitted through breast milk II. Barbiturates. Journal of Pediatrics 14: 86 (1938).

Ulmer, D.D.: Toxicity from aluminum antacids. New England Journal of Medicine 294: 218 (1976).

Usubiaga, J.E.; Wikinski, J.A.; Usubiaga, L.E. and Molina, F.: Intravenous lidocaine in the prevention of postoperative muscle pain caused by succinylcholine administration. Anesthesia Analgesia 46: 225 (1967).

Utili, R.; Boitnott, J.K. and Zimmerman, H.J.: Dantrolene-associated hepatic injury. Incidence and character. Gastroenterology 72: 610 (1977).

Utz, J.P.; Garriques, I.L.; Sande, M.A.; Warner, J.F.; Mandell, G.L.; McGehee, R.F.; Duma, R.J. and Shadomy, S.: Therapy of cryptococcosis with a combination of flucytosine and amphotericin B. Journal of Infectious Diseases 132: 368 (1975).

Volans, G.N.: Migraine and drug absorption. Clinical Pharmacokinetics 3: 313 (1978).

Walshe, J.M.: Brief observations on the management of Wilson's disease. Proceedings of the Royal Society of Medicine 70 (Suppl. 3): 1 (1977).

Ward, A.A.: The epileptic neuron: chronic foci in animals and man; in Jasper et al. (Eds) Basic Mechanisms of the Epilepsies, pp.263-274 (Little, Brown and Company, Boston 1969).

Weisberg, L.A.: Intracranial hypertension associated with oral progestational agents. Neurology 27: 406 (1977).

Weiss, H.D.; Walker, M.D. and Wiernik, P.H.: Neurotoxicity of commonly used antineoplastic agents. New England Journal of Medicine 291: 75, 127 (1974).

Whisnant, J.P.; Espinosa, R.E.; Kierland, R.R. and Lambert, E.H.: Chlorquine neuromyopathy. Proceedings of the Staff Meetings of the Mayo Clinic 38: 501 (1963).

Wilden, J.N. and Scott, C.A.: A pseudolymphomatous reaction in soft tissue associated with phenytoin sodium. Journal of Clinical Pathology 31: 761 (1978).

Wilder, B.J. and Ramsay, R.E.: Oral and intramuscular phenytoin. Clinical Pharmacology and Therapeutics 19: 360 (1976).

Wilkinson, M.: Editorial: The treatment of acute migraine attacks. Headache 15: 291 (1976).

Woodbury, D.M.; Penry, J.K. and Glaser, G.H.: Mechanisms of Action of Antiepileptic Drugs (Raven Press, New York 1979).

Woodbury, D.M.; Penry, J.K. and Schmidt, R.P.: Antiepileptic Drugs (Raven Press, New York 1972).

Yahr, M.D.; Duvoisin, R.C.; Mendoza, M.R. et al.: Modification of l-dopa therapy of Parkinsonism by alpha-methyl dopa-hydrazine. Transactions of the American Neurological Association 96: 55 (1971).

Yarnell, P.R. and Chu, N-S.: Focal seizures and aminophylline. Neurology 25: 819 (1975).

Yost, R.L.; Lee, J.D. and O'Leary, J.P.: Convulsions associated with sodium cefazolin: A case report. American Surgery 43: 417 (1977).

Zavadil, P. and Gallagher, B.B.: Metabolism and excretion of ^{14}C-primidone in epileptic patients; in Janz (Ed) Epileptology, pp.129-139 (Georg Thieme, Stuttgart 1976).

Chapter XXVI
Psychiatric Disorders

L.E. Hollister

Synopsis of Important Principles

1) Psychotherapeutic drugs are not curative, but many drugs are available to ameliorate the course of schizophrenic or manic psychoses or depressive illness and for short term symptomatic adjunctive treatment in anxiety and insomnia.

2) The indications for antipsychotic drugs are best for major psychiatric illnesses; they should never be used for trivial indications or where simpler drugs do equally well. Drug treatment is not indicated for everyone who is depressed, anxious or complaining of poor sleep. Excessive reliance on drugs to the exclusion of concomitant treatments may do more harm than good.

3) In prescribing psychotherapeutic drugs, learn to use a few drugs well, rather than all poorly. The differences in clinical response between the proper and improper use of a drug will probably exceed any actual differences between drugs.

4) Most psychotherapeutic drugs in common use are intrinsically long acting and can therefore generally be given with much advantage as a single daily dose, once the optimum dose for an individual patient has been established. Lithium is the outstanding exception, divided doses being needed to avoid gastrointestinal irritation and excessive peak concentrations. Because of marked interindividual differences in metabolism there is no such thing as a standard dose of a psychotherapeutic drug.

5) When starting treatment with psychotherapeutic drugs, small doses are generally used initially. These minimise the impact of side effects and increase flexibility in determining the optimum dose. Doses should be much smaller and dose increases more gradual in the elderly.

6) Duration of treatment depends on the natural history of the disorder. Most patients with chronic schizophrenia require indefinite treatment. Some patients with frequent or increasingly severe episodes of depression or manic-depressive disorder may require long term therapy, but treatment of anxiety and insomnia is limited to short courses.

7) A few drugs can unmask or aggravate psychiatric disorders. The combined effects of drugs with sedative properties is one of the most common drug interactions. The additive effect of alcohol can be especially dangerous with barbiturates and in those driving motor vehicles.

8) Many drugs can induce psychiatric syndromes; either associated with the therapeutic use of a drug or abuse of a drug. The elderly are particularly sensitive to mental effects of drugs. Depression due to centrally acting antihypertensive drugs, deliria due to overdosage with centrally acting anticholinergic drugs and oversedation with antianxiety drugs are the most common and important. Excessive caffeine intake can cause symptoms resembling anxiety and also interfere with sleep.

Psychiatric thinking and practice were drastically altered by the introduction of new psychotherapeutic drugs 25 years ago. The possibility that a great many 'functional' psychiatric disorders have a genetic, and therefore biochemical, cause has become more and more likely. We think more of genes and amines in seeking to explain schizophrenia than we do of dreams and schemes of the unconscious. The case for a biochemical substrate of serious mental depressions is even more advanced. These disorders also seem to have a pattern of genetic transmission. One might envisage that depressive illness represents an interaction between environmental stress and some biochemical alteration in a specific individual.

The hospital practice of psychiatry has changed remarkably in the past 25 years. Although antipsychotic drugs have neither cured schizophrenia nor altered its prognosis, they have significantly ameliorated its course. The number of hospital beds occupied by psychiatric patients has steadily declined over the past 25 years, such that some hospitals have only one-quarter to one-tenth the bed occupancy of 25 years ago. Proposals have even been made to eliminate many mental hospitals and to transfer almost entirely the care of mentally ill patients to the community. Such trends would have been unthinkable without the availability of drugs which curb the course of serious mental disorders. Unfortunately, good as drugs have been, they are not good enough. Although there are many patients who are better, there are too few who are well.

Simultaneous with these developments are concerns about possible overuse of psychotherapeutic drugs, especially the antianxiety agents. Worldwide, these are the most widely prescribed of all drugs, relief of anxiety now having surpassed relief of pain as the prime reason for prescribing. If such overuse occurs, as seems likely, it may reflect less overprescription of these drugs for individual patients than prescribing too long for those patients in whom they are used. We shall suggest ways in which this source of overuse may be limited. On the other hand, it is probable that many patients with depression are undertreated, either because of failure to recognise the nature of their disorder, or hesitancy in using adequate drug treatment. Questions of over or underuse of psychotherapeutic drugs are more pertinent, therefore, when addressed to specific classes of drugs rather than to the whole lot (see Hollister, 1975).

1. Clinical Pharmacological Considerations

1.1 Nomenclature of Psychotherapeutic Drugs

The most realistic and clinically relevant nomenclature is based on the putative clinical uses of the various drugs. Drugs used for treating anxiety, in all its many clinical guises, are referred to as antianxiety drugs; those for mental depressions, as antidepressants; and those used for treating schizophrenia and other psychoses are termed antipsychotic drugs; while drugs for treating mania are spoken of as antimanic drugs. Even such a nomenclature has defects; each of the drug types may, under certain circumstances, be used for the other purposes. Nonetheless, the 'anti' system of nomenclature has greater simplicity and more clinical relevance than any of the others proposed.

While the term tranquilliser has some pertinence to the antianxiety drugs, it is inappropriate in the case of antipsychotic drugs, which are 'liberating' rather than 'constricting' agents, and the confusion caused by the term is still widespread. Attempts to differentiate 'tranquillisers' from conventional sedatives by introducing the divisions, 'major' and 'minor', or by coining Greek root neologisms such as 'ataractic', 'neuroleptic', 'psycholeptic' or 'psychoinhibitor', also suffer from some implicit assumptions about the modes of action of the drugs so labelled, as well as the relevance to their clinical use. Similarly, one had for so long associated an 'antidepressant' drug with a stimulant, that even today tricyclic antidepressants are often referred to as stimulants, something they clearly are not.

1.2 Chemical Classes of Psychotherapeutic Drugs

Within each broad category of drugs, a number of chemical classes may be represented (see tables III, XII, XIII). The different chemical classes of drug types have no bearing on total therapeutic efficacy, but in some instances can determine certain pharmacological actions or the side effect profile and thereby influence the selection of a drug; for example, antianxiety drugs (see section 8.1). Differences in pharmacological effects within a chemical class are less than differences between them. Nevertheless, individual patients sometimes fail to respond to one drug but may respond well to one from another chemical class, making chemical distinctions important in this situation. This phenomenon may possibly be due to differences in pathways of metabolism.

1.3 Potency of Different Psychotherapeutic Drugs

The potency of drugs (i.e. dose on a weight-for-weight basis) should never be confused with efficacy, as despite greater potency, 'low dose' antipsychotic drugs for example, offer no advantages in terms of total efficacy. They do however, offer a generally higher ratio between the desired effects and some other undesired pharmacological effects. Thus the aliphatic side-chain phenothiazines such as chlorpromazine are relatively low in potency and high in sedative effects. On the other hand, piperazine phenothiazines such as perphenazine are high in potency and low in sedative effects (see table IV).

1.4 Multiple Actions of Psychotherapeutic Drugs

Most drugs have multiple pharmacological effects rather than the single one we think is important. This is especially so with psychotherapeutic drugs.

1.4.1 Antipsychotic Drugs

All of the many chemical classes of antipsychotic drugs in clinical use (table III) share two novel pharmacological actions which were unknown prior to their advent: (a) the ability to ameliorate the course of schizophrenia, and (b) the ability to evoke in many patients extrapyramidal syndromes of various types, including one that mimics naturally occurring Parkinson's disease. Both effects appear to be mediated through the same biochemical mechanism, a decreased dopaminergic transmission in those pathways in the brain that use this neurotransmitter (Carlsson, 1978). Thus antipsychotic drugs, by blocking dopaminergic receptors in both the mesolimbic area of the brain and in the globus pallidus and corpus striatum, produce the desired therapeutic effect as well as an unwanted effect. They also block dopaminergic receptors in the hypothalamus and can thereby cause unwanted pituitary-endocrine effects (see chapter XV; section 23.6). The ideal antipsychotic drug would localise only in the mesolimbic system of the brain and therefore produce solely the desired effect (Hollister, 1973).

Antipsychotic drugs also have an anticholinergic action. Ordinarily, this effect is relatively weak at therapeutic doses, although it may account for many minor side effects such as dry mouth, blurred vision, constipation and so on, but with massive doses it dominates such that in this situation most antipsychotic drugs produce few, if any, extrapyramidal reactions. It seems that antipsychotic drugs have anticholinergic actions in proportion to their relative lack of propensity to evoke extrapyramidal reactions. Thus the reason that thioridazine evokes so few extrapyramidal reactions is that it is clearly the most potent drug in terms of anticholinergic effects. The action of antipsychotic drugs is therefore probably related to effects on the balance of neurotransmitters in the brain, rather than the state of one (Antelman and Caggiula, 1977; McGeer and McGeer, 1977). Parkinson's disease, as well as the drug induced syndrome, provides an excellent example of how the balance of neurotransmitters in the brain may be more important than their actual levels (see chapter XXV; sect. 5.1). According to current theory, the catecholamine neurotransmitters, dopamine and noradrenaline (norepinephrine), are counterbalanced by serotonin and acetylcholine.

All antipsychotics are sedative, which led to the early use of the erroneous term 'tranquilliser'. Although some such as trifluoperazine have a reputation clinically as 'activating' drugs, they are by no means stimulants. Rather, this reputation is based on an increased motor activity as well as a lesser sedative : antipsychotic ratio. Most antipsychotics are α-adrenoreceptor blocking drugs; some, such as chlorpromazine and thioridazine, being especially so. With the conspicuous exception of thioridazine, all are antiemetic drugs, which is an additional clinical use.

1.4.2 Antidepressant Drugs

The tricyclic and newer drugs and the monoamine oxidase (MAO) inhibitors, as well as the older sympathomimetic stimulants, may be considered as antidepressants (table XII). As discussed in section 7, other drug classes may also vie for this description. The tricyclics are the most important and most widely used agents.

Tricyclic antidepressants possess varying degrees of 3 major pharmacological actions (table XIIa). Firstly, they are sedatives, not stimulants. The quality of sedation resembles that produced by the phenothiazines more than that produced by more conventional sedatives, such as the benzodiazepines. Tertiary amines (the nitrogen of the side-chain is fully substituted), such as doxepin, amitriptyline, imipramine and trimipramine are most sedative, the secondary amine tricyclics such as nortriptyline and desipramine (the demethylated active metabolites) are somewhat less sedating; protriptyline is virtually devoid of this action. This difference in drugs may be pertinent to their choice for avoiding side effects, but apparently is unrelated to their clinical efficacy.

Secondly, tricyclics have both a peripheral and central anticholinergic action. Theoretically, it could be argued that this action contributes to the antidepressant effect, but if so any contribution must be minor. The anticholinergic action leads to the most common unwanted effects of the tricyclic antidepressant drugs. Amitriptyline is the strongest anticholinergic and desipramine the weakest, with the others in between. These differences may sometimes affect one's choice of drug (Snyder and Yamamura, 1977; see section 7, 11).

Thirdly, tricyclics block the amine pump. This epithet has been given to an active transport system located in the synapse which recaptures released amine neurotransmitters into the presynaptic nerve ending (Axelrod, 1971; fig. 1). One may construe it as the most important off-switch for terminating aminergic synaptic transmission, comparable with the role of acetylcholinesterase in cholinergic neurotransmission. This action is presently thought to be most related to the antidepressant effects of tricyclics (Schildkraut, 1973; Baldaressini, 1975).

Soon after the introduction of reserpine in the early 1950s, it became apparent that the drug could induce depression in patients being treated for hypertension and schizophrenia as well as in normal subjects. Within the next few years, pharmacological studies revealed that the principal mechanism of action of reserpine was to inhibit the storage of amine neurotransmitters, such as 5-hydroxytryptamine (serotonin) and noradrenaline (norepinephrine), in synaptic vesicles at presynaptic nerve endings. Reserpine induced depression; reserpine depleted stores of aminergic neurotransmitters; therefore, depression must be associated with decreased functional aminergic transmission. This simple syllogism provided the basis for what became known as the amine hypothesis of depression. Just how the postulated decreased aminergic function is mediated in

depressed patients is not yet clear, although it is currently believed to be a gentically transmitted biochemical defect (Weil-Malherbe and Szara, 1971). The relative importance of serotonin versus noradrenaline has also been debated, although present theories accommodate both neurotransmitters (Maas, 1975).

The amine hypothesis was further supported by studies on the mechanism of action of various types of antidepressant drugs. As mentioned earlier, tricyclics block the amine pump, which presumably permits a longer sojourn of neurotransmitter in the synapse. Monoamine oxidase inhibitors block a major degradative pathway for the amine neurotransmitters, which presumably permits more amines to accumulate presynaptically and more to be released. Sympathomimetics, among other actions, also block the amine pump. Thus, the 3 major classes of antidepressant drugs might remedy a deficiency in aminergic neurotransmission, although by somewhat different mechanisms.

The action of tricyclics on the amine pump is not the same for all drugs (table XIIa). Pharmacological studies indicate that tertiary amines such as amitriptyline and imipramine more markedly block the amine pump for serotonin, while secondary amines such as desipramine and nortriptyline more selectively block it for noradrenaline (Carlsson et al., 1969, Sjoqvist, 1975). Some newer antidepressants such as the bicyclic compound zimelidine or the tricyclic clomipramine are highly selective in this regard (Siwers et al., 1977; Bertilsson et al., 1974); defining their clinical utility may help clarify the issue of whether or not these differences in pharmacological action are of clinical importance.

The amine hypothesis of depression, as is the fate of all hypotheses, is currently under some attack. Not all effective antidepressants block the amine pump. For most tests, doxepin is relatively weak in this action (Pinder et al., 1977) and iprindole and the tetracyclic compound mianserin have little or no effect on noradrenaline or serotonin uptake mechanisms, influencing the action of biogenic amines in other ways. Mianserin combines presynaptic α-adrenoceptor blocking activity with antihistamine activity and has no central anticholinergic activity (Brogden et al., 1978). Nomifensine, another new antidepressant, like desipramine more selectively inhibits the amine pump for noradrenaline uptake than for serotonin uptake and like the amphetamines, inhibits the

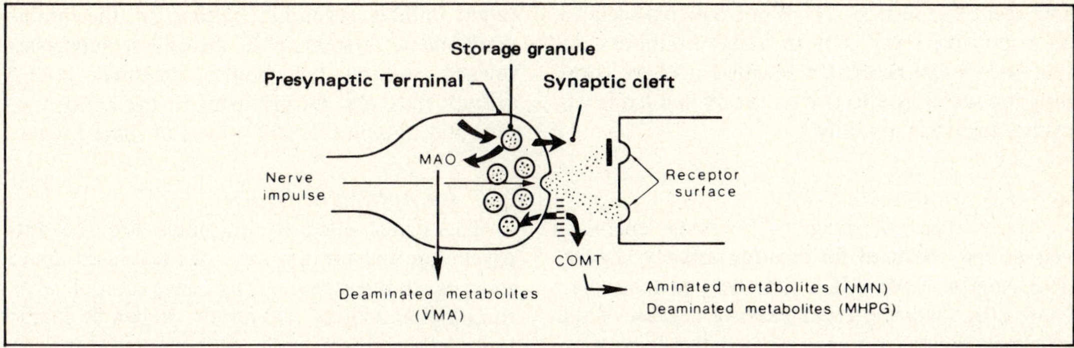

Fig. 1. Model of central noradrenergic synapse. Constant intraneuronal synthesis, storage and catabolism (via monoamine oxidase, MAO) to deaminated metabolites (vanilmandelic acid, VMA). Neural transmission releases noradrenaline into synaptic cleft where postsynaptic receptor is activated. Transmission is limited by enzymatic catabolism of transmitter (via COMT, catechol-*O*-methyltransferase) to aminated metabolites (NMN, 3-*O*-methylnoradrenaline or normetanephrine) or deaminated, decarboxylated metabolites (MHPG or MOPEG, 3-methoxy, 4-hydroxyphenylglycol).

Major limit of synaptic transmission is via specific amine pump which reabsorbs transmitter back into nerve ending; tricyclic antidepressants and amphetamine block this pump (vertical cross hatched lines). Monoamine oxidase inhibitors block enzyme MAO, allowing for greater accumulation of transmitter in storage. Chlorpromazine and other antipsychotic drugs block postsynaptic receptor (vertical solid line). For interactions of drugs at adrenergic neuron, see chapter X (fig. 2).

amine pump for uptake of dopamine, but unlike amphetamine does not release stores of dopamine (Brogden et al., 1979). In common with mianserin, nomifensine has negligible central anticholinergic activity. Although block of the amine pump is immediate, clinical response to tricyclic antidepressant drugs tends to be delayed by days or weeks. The use of precursors for serotonin, such as tryptophan and 5-hydroxytryptophan, has not been especially effective for treating depression. Increased serotonin in brain may therefore reflect more the sedative than the antidepressant properties of these drugs. Possibly too much emphasis has been placed on individual amines, and the dynamic balance between aminergic systems (noradrenaline and serotonin; noradrenaline and dopamine; noradrenaline and histamine) or that between aminergic and non-aminergic systems (noradrenaline and acetylcholine) may be of greater importance than the state of any single neurotransmitter, as is probably the case with the antipsychotic drugs (see section 1.4.1). These are only some of the questions now being raised about the amine hypothesis of depression and antidepressant drug action, but it still remains the most viable one available.

One of the implications of the amine hypothesis currently under investigation is that it might be possible to define by biochemical tests subtypes of depression and to predict the best drug for treating them. Many metabolites of noradrenaline excreted in urine originate largely from peripheral rather than central adrenergic activity. One particular metabolite, 3-methoxy-4-hydroxyphenylglycol (also designated MHPG or MOPEG) is considered to derive in substantial amount from central adrenergic activity. If the amount of MHPG excreted in urine is 'low', the biochemical defect is surmised to be a deficiency of noradrenergic neurotransmission; the proper drug to use would be one somewhat selective in blocking uptake of noradrenaline, such as nortriptyline or desipramine. Conversely, 'normal' or 'high' excretion of MHPG would be construed as indicating a deficiency of serotonin, indicating a tricyclic somewhat selective in blocking uptake of serotonin, such as amitriptyline. Current evidence suggests that these predictions might hold, but much more work needs to be done to validate it (Schildkraut, 1974; Beckman and Goodwin, 1975).

Monoamine oxidase inhibitors, such as tranylcypromine and phenelzine, or sympathomimetic stimulants, such as dextroamphetamine and methylphenidate, are rarely first choice antidepressant drugs. They may be used either in combination with or in place of tricyclics when treatment with the latter drugs has failed (see section 7). As failure of tricyclics is not uncommon, interest has been renewed in the idea of using MAO inhibitors in combination with tricyclics or as a sole agent (see section 7.1). Some patients seem to be responsive specifically to MAO inhibitors, so that one cannot be certain whether it is the combination which is effective or the switch from tricyclics to MAO inhibitors.

1.4.3 Antianxiety Drugs

Many types of drugs of varying chemical classes may be used for treating anxiety (Lader, 1975, 1976; table XIII). On the one hand, are those drugs which possess varying degrees of the pharmacological actions of sedative-hypnotics: sedation proceeding to hypnosis; muscle relaxation; anticonvulsant action; development of tolerance; and potential for habituation and physical dependence. These include the barbiturates, mainly phenobarbitone (phenobarbital) or amylobarbitone (amobarbital) sodium, meprobamate and its congeners, and the benzodiazepine derivatives, chlordiazepoxide, diazepam, oxazepam, lorazepam etc. On the other hand, are those drugs which might be termed 'sedative-autonomic', which unlike the others, affect the peripheral autonomic nervous system. They also differ in increasing muscle tone, lowering convulsive thresholds and lacking the potential for habituation and physical dependence. Drugs in this class include sedative antihistaminics, such as hydroxyzine or diphenhydramine; small doses of antipsychotics such as trifluoperazine or haloperidol, and the more sedative tricyclic antidepressants, such as doxepin or amitriptyline.

One can get into many arguments about the various similarities and differences among the pharmacological properties of sedative-hypnotic antianxiety drugs, but to the clinician the similarities outweigh the differences, with exceptions to be noted in section 8.1 and table XV. Both the site and mechanism of action of the benzodiazepines are unclear at the present time (Greenblatt and Shader, 1974). Various proposed sites have included the reticular activating system (reducing sensory input), the limbic system (changing affect), the median forebrain bundle (involving reward and punishment systems), and the hypothalamus (reducing the effector components of anxiety). There is evidence that these drugs may affect levels and turnover rates of various neurotransmitters, such as dopamine, noradrenaline and serotonin (Wise et al., 1972). For the most part, the evidence is contradictory and most persuasive only for increased gamma-aminobutyric acid (GABA) activity. Such an increase might inhibit serotonin release in the brain's punishment system and disinhibit suppressed reward seeking behaviour. Increased GABA activity may also be pertinent to the anticonvulsant and muscle relaxant effects of these agents.

1.4.4 Antimanic Drugs

The drugs effective in mania are the antipsychotics and lithium salts. As discussed above, most psychotherapeutic drugs have multiple pharmacological actions, and almost all can be characterised somewhere in the sedative-stimulant continuum. Lithium ion seems to be devoid of any specific sedative or stimulant effects, its presence in normal subjects being virtually undetectable. Neither does it have any other major pharmacological effects such as adrenergic blocking actions or anticholinergic effects. It is generally regarded as a specific treatment for manic-depressive disorder.

As yet no pathogenetic mechanism of this disorder is known and no single mechanism has been accepted as an explanation for the therapeutic effect of lithium in it (Cade, 1975). Lithium has many effects that might be pertinent to its use in mania (Singer and Rotenberg, 1973). It tends to decrease the effects of various neurotransmitters by a variety of mechanisms. It probably interacts with cell membranes to increase permeability. It alters the ionic composition of water in the body and alters the relationship between sodium and potassium. It abolishes the abnormal daily rhythm of corticosteroid secretion found in manics, but this might be an epiphenomenon. At present, its mode of action is unclear.

1.5 Pharmacokinetic Properties of Psychotherapeutic Drugs

The pharmacokinetic properties of the various classes of psychotherapeutic drugs have been studied extensively, but data for most compounds are still inadequate. Although some important differences in pharmacokinetic behaviour exist between compounds in the various classes, all psychotherapeutic drugs show a marked difference in rate of elimination between individual patients. Thus, steady-state plasma concentrations can be expected to differ widely among individuals, necessitating individualisation of dosage. Some similarities and differences in pharmacokinetic properties of psychotherapeutic drugs are summarised in table I and appendix A.

Table I. Some pharmacokinetic characteristics of some psychotherapeutic drugs

Drug	Plasma half-life (hours)	Elimination	Notes (see also section 1.5)
Antipsychotics			
Chlorpromazine	16-30	Hepatic metabolism with entero-hepatic recirculation; very little renal excretion of unchanged drug. Possible metabolism in gut wall. Many metabolites possible (some active, others inactive)	Oral absorption variable. Effective plasma levels decreased in presence of delayed gastric emptying and by use of drugs which decrease gastrointestinal motility (see chapter VI, sect. 5; VIII, sect. 2.3.1).
Thioridazine	26-36	Hepatic metabolism (active metabolite), little renal excretion of unchanged drug	
Perphenazine	∼21	Hepatic metabolism, possibly enterohepatic circulation; some renal excretion of unchanged drug	Significant first-pass hepatic metabolism after oral administration
Thiothixene	∼34	Hepatic metabolism, some renal excretion of unchanged drug	
Haloperidol	13-35	Hepatic metabolism	
Pimozide	∼29	Hepatic metabolism	
Antimanic drugs			
Lithium	8-35	Renal excretion	Renal excretion dependent on sodium balance and urine volume. Elimination delayed in the elderly (see section 1.5.4; 5.4). Patients with long half-lives ($> 20h$) presumably reflect delayed clearance due to impaired renal function or decreased sodium balance (see section 1.5.4; table VIII).
Antidepressants			
Amitriptyline	32-40	Hepatic metabolism (active metabolite)	Active metabolite (nortriptyline) may accumulate and eventually attain greater concentration than parent drug.
Imipramine	6-20	Hepatic metabolism and renal excretion of active metabolite and small amounts of unchanged drug	Active metabolite (desipramine) may accumulate and eventually attain greater concentration than parent drug. Subject to significant hepatic first-pass metabolism after oral administration. Plasma half-life prolonged in the elderly.
Nortriptyline	15-90	Hepatic metabolism	Significant first-pass hepatic metabolism after oral administration.
Desipramine	12-54	Hepatic metabolism	
Clomipramine	17-28	Hepatic metabolism	Probable significant hepatic first-pass metabolism after oral administration.
Doxepin	8-25	Hepatic metabolism, little renal excretion of unchanged drug	Significant hepatic first-pass metabolism after oral administration.
Maprotiline	27-58	Hepatic metabolism (active metabolites)	
Mianserin	8-19	Hepatic metabolism, renal excretion of small amount of unchanged drug (4-7%)	
Nomifensine	3-5	Hepatic metabolism; renal excretion of active metabolite and unchanged drug*	Plasma half-life prolonged to 46h in anuric patients *15-22% of total drug plasma levels

Table I. (continued)

Drug	Plasma half-life (hours)	Elimination	Notes (see also section 1.5)
Antidepressants (continued)			
Viloxazine	2-3	Hepatic metabolism, some renal excretion of unchanged drug (12-15%)	
Antianxiety drugs/Hypnotics			
Chlordiaze-poxide	5-30	Hepatic metabolism (active metabolites)	Plasma clearance decreased in the elderly and in severe liver disease. Active metabolites (desmethylchlordiazepoxide, demoxepam) metabolised more slowly than parent drug and can accumulate on repeated dosage (see section 1.5.3).
Diazepam	24-48	Hepatic metabolism (active metabolites)	Plasma half-life is age dependent: 20h at age 20, 90h at age 80 but due to change in distribution volume, plasma clearance not altered in elderly. Severe liver disease decreases plasma clearance. Active metabolites are desmethyldiazepam (major metabolite) and oxazepam. Desmethyldiazepam metabolised more slowly than parent drug and can accumulate on repeated dosage (see section 1.5.3).
Oxazepam	6-25	Hepatic metabolism to inactive glucuronide	Plasma half-life not affected by severe liver disease or in the elderly.
Lorazepam	9-16	Hepatic metabolism to inactive glucuronide	Plasma half-life not affected by severe liver disease or in the elderly
Flunitrazepam	~13-19	Hepatic metabolism (active metabolites); possible metabolism in gut wall	Plasma half-life of active metabolites about 25-30 hours.
Flurazepam	47-100	Hepatic metabolism (active metabolite)	Plasma half-life very short. Figure shown is for principal active metabolite desalkylflurazepam, which can accumulate on repeated dosage (see section 1.5.5).
Nitrazepam	18-34	Hepatic metabolism (? activity of metabolites)	Acetylation of amine metabolite subject to genetic polymorphism (see section 1.5.5).
Temazepam	5-8	Hepatic metabolism (active metabolites)	
Prazepam	~78	Hepatic metabolism (active metabolites)	Half-life shown is for drug and active metabolites.
Medazepam	~1-2*	Hepatic metabolism (active metabolites)	*Plasma half-life short; rapidly metabolised to active compounds with longer half-lives, including diazepam.
Bromazepam	8-19	Hepatic metabolism	
Clobazam	~50	Hepatic metabolism (desmethyl metabolite presumably active)	
Ketazolam	~1.5*	Hepatic metabolism (active metabolites)	*Plasma half-life short, rapidly metabolised to active compounds with longer half-lives, including diazepam.
Triazolam	~5	Hepatic metabolism; small amounts excreted unchanged in urine	Probable significant first-pass hepatic metabolism after oral administration
Meprobamate	6-17	Hepatic metabolism and renal excretion of unchanged drug (8-19%)	Induces hepatic drug metabolising enzymes (see chapter I, sect. 3.3; VIII, sect. 2.3.3).

Table I. (continued)

Drug	Plasma half-life (hours)	Elimination	Notes (see also section 1.5)
Antianxiety drugs/Hypnotics (continued)			
Pentobarbitone	23-30	Hepatic metabolism and renal excretion of unchanged drug (20%)	Induces hepatic drug metabolising enzymes
Phenobarbitone	48-144	Hepatic metabolism and renal excretion of unchanged drug (27 to 50%)	Induces hepatic drug metabolising enzymes. Clearance greater in alkaline urine.
Methaqualone	20-60	Hepatic metabolism; about 2% excreted unchanged in urine	Induces hepatic drug metabolising enzymes.
Glutethimide	5-22	Hepatic metabolism (active metabolite); enterohepatic circulation; < 2% excreted unchanged in urine	Active metabolite 4-hydroxyglutethimide accumulates on overdosage and is eliminated more slowly than the parent drug Oral absorption erratic. Induces hepatic drug metabolising enzymes.
Chloral hydrate	7-10	Hepatic metabolism (active metabolite)	Plasma half-life very short; figure shown is for active metabolite trichlorethanol; second major metabolite trichloracetic acid has half-life of 4-5 days (see text).
Chlormethiazole	3-9	Hepatic metabolism (active metabolites)	Significant first-pass hepatic metabolism after oral administration. Bioavailability increased and clearance decreased in the elderly and in cirrhosis.

1.5.1 Antipsychotic Drugs

The metabolism of chlorpromazine has been studied most extensively, because it was the prototype drug and because of the substantial doses used, making measurement in biological fluids and tissues easier. Over 160 different metabolites of chlorpromazine have been postulated, of which only a minority have yet been identified and still fewer tested for pharmacological activity. Thioridazine undergoes ring sulphoxidation similar to chlorpromazine, with production of an inactive metabolite. The thiomethyl ring substituent undergoes 2 sulphoxidations — to sulphoxide (one oxygen) and sulphone (two oxygen atoms) forms. Both are active. The side-chain sulphoxide metabolite is used as a separate antipsychotic drug — mesoridazine (Muusze, 1975). The piperazine phenothiazines such as butaperazine form most major metabolites through the same metabolic pathways as for chlorpromazine, with ring or ring substituent alterations predominating (Bruce et al., 1974). Side-chain alterations may include opening of the piperazine ring. Metabolic transformations of the thioxanthenes, which are closely related to the phenothiazines, are similar, but no hydroxylation occurs. The metabolism of the buty-

rophenone, haloperidol, involves a primary step of N-dealkylation that results in a series of metabolites with no activity (Forsman et al., 1977).

Chlorpromazine

Plasma concentrations of chlorpromazine reach their peak in 2 to 4 hours after most forms of administration. Following almost any oral dosage form, one is likely to get some instances of extremely poor absorption (Hollister et al., 1970; Curry et al., 1970). Bioavailability after oral administration in fact varies from 27 to 67% and is possibly due to metabolism by nonspecific enzymes in the gut wall (Curry et al., 1971; Dahl and Standgord, 1977). Systemic availability of orally administered chlorpromazine may therefore be reduced by delayed gastric emptying or drugs which decrease gastrointestinal motility (Rivera-Calimlim et al., 1976, 1978; see also chapter VIII, sect. 2.3.1; XIX, sect. 1.1). Intramuscular administration almost always provides prompt and probably total systemic availability of the drug, with measurable plasma levels evident in 15 minutes. It also provides plasma concentrations approximately 3 to 4 times as high as equivalent oral doses of the drug (Hollister et al., 1963; 1970).

Plasma disappearance rates of chlorpromazine following single doses have shown a 2-phase curve of the type characteristic of highly lipid soluble drugs. An initial rapid or distributive phase, with a half-life of 2 hours, is followed by a slow elimination phase of about 16 hours. Even in the presence of definite liver damage, as in patients with compensated Laennec's cirrhosis, these rates of disposition still hold (Maxwell et al., 1972), but there is a wide interpatient variability in the rate of elimination of chlorpromazine (Curry et al., 1970; Green et al., 1965). Chlorpromazine is highly protein bound (98 to 99%) and localised in tissues to a marked extent (as reflected in its large distribution volume of 32 to 150L/kg), so that final residues of drug may not disappear for months.

When chlorpromazine is administered in an ordinary divided dose schedule, diurnal variations of 5- to 10-fold may be observed in plasma concentrations within a single patient, even in steady-state conditions (24 and 53 days of treatment). Such variations in plasma concentrations might be related more to side effects, such as drowsiness, than to the desired clinical effects (Cooper et al., 1973). Moreover, almost all investigators have observed a marked variability between patients in plasma concentrations attained during long term treatment with equal doses of chlorpromazine (see Cooper, 1978). Such interindividual variations, which can be up to 50-fold or more, are due to a variety of influences, including different biotransformation pathways and genetic patterns of drug metabolism (see chapter I; sect. 3.3.4, 4) and different prior histories of drug exposure. Because of its long half-life, steady-state plasma concentrations are maintained throughout the day following single daily dosage (Rivera-Calimlim et al., 1976).

Thioridazine

The data available for thioridazine suggest that the time span of plasma concentrations following oral doses is similar to that for chlorpromazine, peak levels being attained in 1.5 to 4 hours. The drug appears to be metabolised as extensively; only small amounts being recovered unchanged in the urine, and the principal metabolites are either ring or side-chain sulphoxide derivatives or their combinations (Buyze et al., 1973). The elimination half-life varies between individuals but in most cases is around 26 to 36 hours. Plasma concentrations from a given dose as a consequence show wide interindividual variation and are higher in the elderly (Axelsson and Martensson, 1976,

1977). Protein binding is 96 to 99% and the volume of distribution large (18L/kg).

Perphenazine

The elimination half-life of perphenazine from plasma is variously reported as between 8 and 12 hours, and around 21 hours. Like chlorpromazine, volumes of distribution are large and vary between 10 and 35L/kg. Perphenazine is found in blood following oral doses only after repeat dose administration and with a high ratio of the sulphoxide metabolite to the parent compound. A large hepatic first-pass metabolism (see chapter I; sect. 3.3.3) is likely following oral doses. Clearance shows a 3-fold interindividual variation (Hansen et al., 1976).

Haloperidol

Systemic availability of haloperidol after oral administration is around 60 to 70% (Forsman and Ohman, 1977). Following intramuscular injection, haloperidol is absorbed rapidly; peak levels being attained in 20 minutes. Variation in peak plasma levels attained in different subjects are scarcely more than 2-fold by this route of administration (Cressman et al., 1974) but steady-state plasma levels vary up to 30-fold or more between individuals given the same oral dose (Forsman and Ohman, 1977). The terminal elimination half life is approximately 21 hours after intramuscular administration (Cressman et al., 1974), and approximately 20 hours after oral administration (Forsman and Ohman, 1977). Haloperidol is about 92% protein bound, binding being higher at higher plasma concentrations, and has a distribution volume of 18 to 30L/kg. The long elimination half-life of haloperidol, as with other antipsychotic drugs, means that steady-state plasma levels are not attained for several days after commencing treatment.

1.5.2 Tricyclic Antidepressants

The tricyclic antidepressants are metabolised in much the same fashion as the phenothiazines. Side-chain transformations are most important, especially the initial demethylation step, which produces active metabolites (desipramine from imipramine; nortriptyline from amitriptyline). Ring hydroxylation leads to formation of glucuronide conjugates. The activity of ring hydroxylated metabolites is not certain. Nortriptyline is preferentially hydroxylated at the 10-position rather than the 2-position. Relatively little is known about the metabolism of protriptyline or doxepin, although it may be assumed to be somewhat similar to that of the other tricyclics.

The ratio between the parent drug, imipramine, and its major active metabolite, desipramine, varies markedly; the desipramine:imipramine ratio ranging from 0.3 to 15.0 (Nagy and Treiber, 1973). Available evidence suggests that both compounds possess pharmacological activity, so it has generally been the custom in plasma level monitoring (see section 1.6.3) to measure both and use the sum of the two. The same considerations apply in the case of amitriptyline and its metabolite, nortriptyline. The different rates of formation of desipramine versus retention of imipramine may be clinically important due to possible differences in their pharmacological effects.

The elimination half-life of the tricyclic antidepressants, as with phenothiazines, varies markedly between individuals; for example, imipramine 6 to 20 hours and nortriptyline 15 to 90 hours (Gram, 1977; see appendix A). Half-life is prolonged in the elderly and steady-state plasma concentrations are correspondingly increased: for example, with imipramine, mean steady-state levels in the elderly are over twice those of younger patients on the same dose (imipramine 84 cf 32ng/ml; desipramine 57 cf 21ng/ml) [Nies et al., 1977]. Steady-state plasma levels are usually attained within 1 to 4 weeks, depending on the drug and patient characteristics but can show some variation during treatment in an individual patient. However, such intraindividual variation is much less than the interindividual variation in steady-state plasma concentrations: for example, 48 to 238μg nortriptyline; imipramine 6 to 356μg/L and of its active metabolite desipramine formed following imipramine administration, 28 to 659μg/L (Gram, 1977; Gram et al., 1977). There is no difference in this variability between once daily and divided (tds) daily dose administration (Zeigler et al., 1977).

Tricyclics are lipid soluble in their non-ionised forms and consequently are readily absorbed from the gut and easily diffused to all tissues. However, bioavailability of orally administered nortriptyline varies between 56 and 79% and of imipramine from between 29 and 77%. More desipramine is formed after orally administered imipramine than when it is given parenterally. These differences in availability are assumed to represent hepatic first-pass metabolism (Gram and Christiansen, 1975).

Protein binding of tricyclics is high and volume of distribution large, as with phenothiazines (see appendix A), and varies between individuals (Gram, 1977). Tricyclic antidepressants are basic drugs and binding to α_1-acid glycoproteins is important in determining the degree and interindividual variation in protein binding (Piafsky and Borga, 1977). This interindividual variation in binding may explain in part some of the difficulties encountered in trying to make correlations between plasma concentrations and clinical response. Little is known about the actual tissue distribution of tricyclics in humans. One study focused primarily on cardiac uptake in rabbits, because of the cardiotoxicity of tricyclics on overdosage (see section 7.4.2). Following infusions of 5mg doses, concentration in the heart was 40 to 200 times higher than measured in plasma. It was highest for protriptyline and did not correlate with reported toxicity (Elonen et al., 1975). Entry of imipramine into human erythrocytes in patients treated long term is less than desipramine, but the significance of this difference is not clear (Kragh-Sorenson et al., 1976).

1.5.3 Antianxiety Drugs

Both chlordiazepoxide and diazepam form a number of active metabolites, some of which (N-desmethylchlordiazepoxide; N-desmethyldiazepam) are more slowly eliminated than the parent compounds. Two of the active metabolites of both chlordiazepoxide and diazepam; desmethyldiazepam, and as its dipotassium acetate salt (clorazepate), and oxazepam, are marketed as separate drugs, which is a rare situation in therapeutics. Oxazepam needs only to be conjugated to be disposed of; the same is true of lorazepam, the glucuronide conjugates of both being inactive. Clorazepate is the prodrug for desmethyldiazepam, as the dipotassium acetate salt is hydrolysed on exposure to normal stomach acidity; if gastric acid is not present, the active form of the drug is not achieved. Antacids may therefore decrease the rate of conversion and decrease the amount of drug absorbed and the effects of the active agent (Shader et al., 1978). The biotransformation pathways of the benzodiazepines and the inter-relationships between compounds is shown in figure 2.

Both chlordiazepoxide and diazepam are slowly and erratically absorbed after intramuscular administration and as a consequence clinical effects are delayed and unpredictable (Gamble et al., 1975). It is wiser to avoid this route entirely.

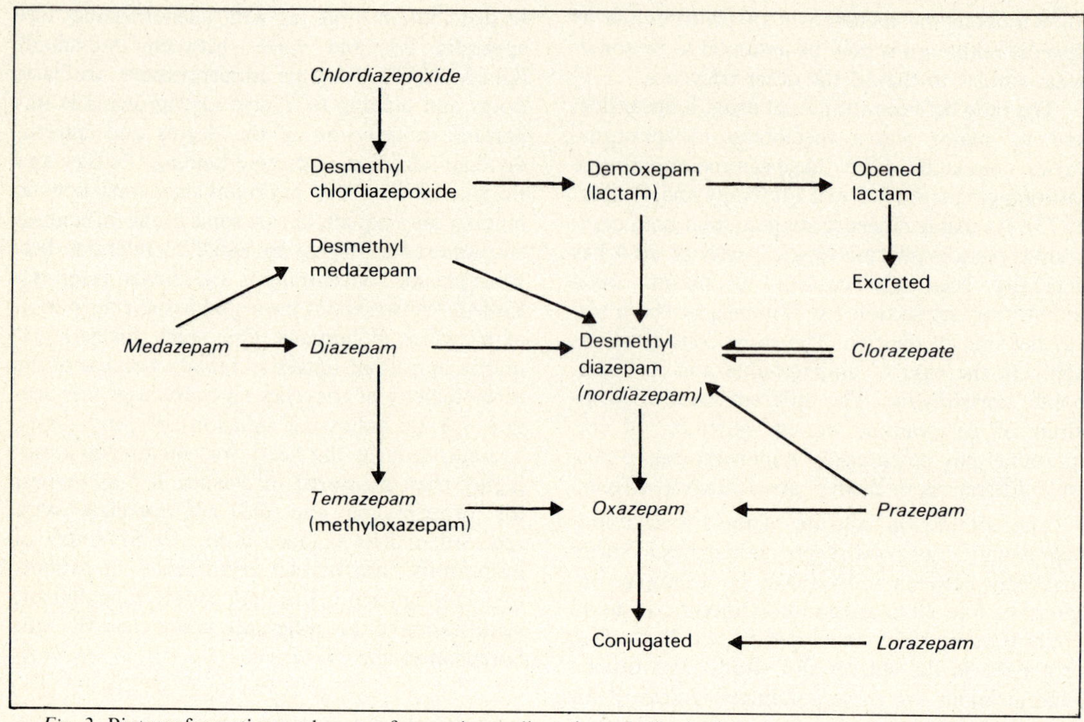

Fig. 2. Biotransformation pathways of some benzodiazepines. Italics indicates compound marketed as separate drug.

Great variation between individuals in pharmacokinetic properties have been noted with chlordiazepoxide, diazepam and other benzodiazepines. Thus, it is impossible to provide a single value that is characteristic, although a range can be defined.

Chlordiazepoxide

Following multiple doses, chlordiazepoxide disappears from plasma fairly rapidly, but desmethylchlordiazepoxide and demoxepam and the even later formed desmethyldiazepam are more slowly eliminated. The elimination half-life of chlordiazepoxide has been estimated to range from 5 to 30 hours, but more slowly eliminated metabolites may prolong the biological half-life (Dixon et al., 1976; Greenblatt et al., 1978a). Accumulation of chlordiazepoxide to steady-state is reached within 3 days, but that of the metabolites is less rapid; desmethyldiazepam accumulating over 2 or more weeks (Boxenbaum et al., 1977) and elimination of the drug after treatment correspondingly prolonged. The rate and extent of accumulation varies markedly between individuals. When steady-state is attained, chlordiazepoxide and its active metabolites persist throughout the day on a once daily dosage basis (Greenblatt et al., 1978a).

The rate of elimination of chlordiazepoxide is prolonged in the elderly; clearance being about half that of young adults in those over 60 years of age. The elderly are also more 'sensitive' to the CNS effects of chlordiazepoxide, thus indicating the need for smaller doses. Clearance of chlordiazepoxide is also reduced in patients with cirrhosis, as is the rate and extent of formation of desmethylchlordiazepoxide. Disulfiram also inhibits the rate of metabolism of chlordiazepoxide (Greenblatt et al., 1978a).

Chlordiazepoxide is about 94 to 97 % bound to plasma proteins and has a distribution volume of 0.3 to 0.4 L/kg in males and a somewhat larger volume in females. For a review of the pharmacokinetic properties of chlordiazepoxide, see Greenblatt et al. (1978a).

Diazepam

Diazepam is absorbed more rapidly than oxazepam and produces discernible sedative effects (Bliding, 1974). Such rapid absorption (peak levels are attained in 1 hour) could account for its vast popularity but could also predispose one to abuse of it. Bioavailability of oral diazepam is between 70 to 100% whereas that of oxazepam is about 50 to 70% (Greenblatt et al., 1975a). Despite some conflicting reports, intravenous administration of diazepam leads to higher plasma concentrations than oral doses, which in turn lead to higher concentrations than intramuscularly administered doses (Hillestad et al., 1974b; Gamble et al., 1975). Alcohol·in social concentrations (10% by volume) decreases the rate of absorption of orally administered diazepam given at the same time, but not the amount absorbed; higher concentrations of alcohol (50% by volume) may increase diazepam absorption (Greenblatt et al., 1978b).

It is likely that the initial effects of diazepam are terminated by redistribution, probably to a lipid compartment. The plasma half-life of diazepam shows two phases — a rapid, distributive phase and a second, slower elimination phase. The elimination half-life varies between individuals and with age; interindividual variation in half-life is less after repeat dose treatment and a value of 24 to 48 hours is a good reference for clinical application in younger adults (Mandelli et al., 1978). At age 80 years the half-life is 90 hours compared with 20 hours at age 20. Due to an increase in distribution volume, plasma clearance does not change with age (Klotz et al., 1975). As with chlordiazepoxide, dosage of diazepam should be less in the elderly (initial dose about half the usual), not only because of these pharmacokinetic differences but also because accumulation of parent drug and active metabolites is more likely to lead to muddled confusion and muscle weakness in the elderly. Further, the elderly seem to be more sensitive to the depressant effects of diazepam than younger patients (Reidenberg et al., 1978; see also chapter X, sect. 2.1.2).

Peak plasma levels at steady-state show a 2-fold interindividual variation both for diazepam and its major active metabolite, desmethyldiazepam (Berlin et al., 1972), and the ratio of diazepam to desmethyldiazepam plasma levels can show up to an 8-fold variation between individuals; ranging from 0.21 to 1.7 (Bond et al., 1977). Of more importance is the difference in their rate of elimination. Because of the longer half-life of desmethyldiazepam (51 to 120h) than diazepam, accumulation of desmethyldiazepam to steady-state can continue over 3 or more weeks. Moreover, accumulation of desmethyldiazepam may have an inhibitory influence on the rate of

diazepam metabolism (Klotz et al., 1976) and also, dose dependent elimination kinetics of desmethyldiazepam have been suggested (Tognoni et al., 1975). The effects of these elimination patterns with repeated doses, are difficult to predict in an individual case, but they do mean that no significant accumulation of diazepam and particularly desmethyldiazepam or excessive duration of effect following discontinuation of treatment, should occur with an individualised dose given once daily at night (see also section 8.2). Only small amounts of diazepam or desmethyldiazepam are excreted in the bile and enterohepatic circulation is not responsible for the slow rate of elimination of the unchanged drug and active metabolites (Mandelli et al., 1978).

Plasma protein binding of diazepam is about 97 to 99% in adults, regardless of age, but the distribution volume of around 1L/kg is larger in the elderly and also in females (Klotz et al., 1975; MacLeod et al., 1977a). Hypoalbuminaemia leads to an increase in the fraction of unbound drug in plasma and a faster rate of elimination, since more drug is available for metabolism (Klotz et al., 1975). However, the temporary increase in plasma concentration of free drug may lead to an increase in clinical effects. Thus, in 1 study when serum albumin levels were lower than 3.0g/100ml oversedation occurred in 9.3% of patients compared with 2.9% in those with albumin levels of 4.0g/100ml or more (Greenblatt and Koch-Weser, 1974). Clearance of diazepam by the liver is also sensitive to altered protein binding. Thus, a decrease in binding in alcoholic cirrhosis, for example, is reflected in an increased volume of distribution and diminished plasma clearance (Klotz et al., 1975). A delay in the appearance of desmethyldiazepam also occurs in cirrhotics (Andreasen et al., 1976). The influence of acute viral hepatitis on the rate of diazepam elimination is less marked (Klotz et al., 1975). Precise guidelines for dose adjustment of diazepam (or chlordiazepoxide) in liver diseases cannot be given at this time and clinicians so using these drugs should titrate dosage on the basis of both careful patient observation and available kinetic findings. An initial dose of both might be one third the usual. However, oxazepam or lorazepam should be considered in these patients since their clearance is not influenced by liver disease. Renal disease does not appear to affect the rate of elimination of diazepam, but disulfiram does inhibit the rate of metabolism of diazepam (Martin et al., 1977).

Diazepam readily crosses the placenta, particularly in the later stages of pregnancy and during labour: its pathways of metabolism are altered in the fetus and newborn and elimination of both diazepam and desmethyldiazepam are prolonged. Diazepam must therefore be used judiciously in pregnancy and labour (see chapter III, sect. 3.10.1; IV, sect. 2.3; XV; sect. 5.3). Diazepam and desmethyldiazepam appear in breast milk and in plasma of breast fed infants, but adverse effects are only likely to be a problem if doses greater than 10mg daily need to be given repeatedly (chapt. IV; sect. 3.1.3). For a review of the pharmacokinetics of diazepam, see Mandelli et al. (1978).

Oxazepam

Oxazepam is absorbed less rapidly after oral administration than diazepam (Bliding, 1974; Wretlind et al., 1977), limiting its usefulness in insomnia. As occurs with diazepam, alcohol administered concurrently slows the rate of oxazepam absorption (Mallach et al., 1975), but food does not affect either the rate or extent of absorption (Melander et al., 1977). In healthy subjects oxazepam is relatively highly protein bound (about 90 to 95%) like other benzodiazepines. Unlike chlordiazepoxide and diazepam, the biotransformation of oxazepam involves only simple glucuronidation to an inactive metabolite (Greenblatt et al., 1975a). The elimination half-life of oxazepam varies between individuals (5.9 to 25 hours; Alvan et al., 1977) but is shorter than that of diazepam. In healthy subjects, the plasma clearance is low (0.050 to 0.171L/kg/hour) after a single oral dose, indicating an hepatic extraction ratio of less than 10% (Alvan et al., 1977). In contrast to chlordiazepoxide and diazepam, neither age nor liver disease alter the elimination half-life or plasma clearance of oxazepam (Shull et al., 1976). Renal impairment does not affect plasma clearance of oxazepam, but the renal clearance of the inactive conjugated metabolites is closely related to the creatinine clearance, and the elimination half-life is prolonged (24 to 91 hours; Odar-Cederlof et al., 1977).

Lorazepam

Lorazepam is absorbed from the gastrointestinal tract at a rate similar to that of oxazepam; peak plasma concentrations occurring about 2 hours after a single oral dose (Verbeeck et al., 1976). Steady-state plasma levels as with other benzodiazepines may vary considerably between individuals during repeated dosing, but age has no effect on steady-state concentrations attained (Greenblatt et al., 1977a). Unlike diazepam or chlordiazepoxide, absorption of lorazepam from intramuscular injection sites is predictable, producing a pattern of absorption similar to that with an oral dose (Dundee et al., 1978). Like other benzodiazepines, lorazepam has a relatively large volume of distribution; 0.9L/kg (Greenblatt et al., 1977b). More than 90% of circulating lorazepam is bound to plasma proteins (Kraus et al., 1978). As with oxazepam, glucuronidation to an inactive metabolite is the primary metabolic pathway of lorazepam, although very small amounts of other metabolites (hydroxylorazepam and quinazolinone derivatives) have been identified in man (Greenblatt et al., 1976). As with oxazepam, age or liver disease do not appreciably alter either the elimination half-life (probably about 12 hours) or the plasma clearance of lorazepam (Kraus et al., 1978). Similarly, in severe renal impairment the elimination half-life of unchanged lorazepam is not altered, but as might be expected accumulation of the inactive lorazepam glucuronide occurs (Verbeeck et al., 1976).

1.5.4 Lithium

Absorption of lithium is rapid following an oral dose and is virtually complete within 6 to 8 hours. Less than 1% of the oral dose is recoverable in the stool. Peak plasma levels occur within 30 minutes to 2 hours after the dose. Absorption depends on gastrointestinal function and is more variable following conventional than sustained release tablets (Amdisen, 1977). Plasma concentrations of lithium in patients on a 3 times daily dose schedule may vary over a 2-fold range. Levels rise as successive doses are absorbed and then fall due to elimination during the period in which doses are not given. Clinical monitoring of plasma levels uses those obtained at the nadir; that is, approximately 12 hours after the last dose (Amdisen, 1975, 1977).

Lithium is not protein bound and is distributed in the total body water, shifting slowly into cells. The slow entry into cells accounts for the delay of several days before full clinical responses are noted; exit from cells is likewise slow. Various tissues concentrate lithium to various degrees. Lithium levels in the cerebrospinal fluid peak 24 hours later than those in the extracellular fluid, and generally reach a concentration only 50% of that in plasma. Passage into the brain is slow, but some areas contain levels higher than those in plasma. Apparent volumes of distribution range widely between individuals; from 40 to 140% of body weight (0.4 to 1.4L/kg), somewhat higher than the actual body content of water, which is 50 to 55% (Mason et al., 1978).

No metabolism of lithium occurs, as virtually all of the ion is excreted unchanged by the kidney. From one third to two thirds of single oral doses appears in the urine after 6 to 12 hours; the remaining lithium is excreted slowly over a period of 10 to 14 days. Eventually, over 95% of systemically available lithium can be accounted for by urinary excretion. Appreciable amounts of lithium might be excreted in sweat during hot weather. Renal clearance of lithium varies between 10 and 40ml/min and is correlated with renal creatinine clearance (Amdisen, 1977; Mason et al., 1978). Clearance is characterised by high and potentially toxic concentrations in the distal tubules and in the lumen of the collecting tubules, particularly during the periods of peak serum concentration which occur during the course of daily administration (Amdisen, 1977).

Lithium clearance is reduced by sodium depletion and may be decreased by 24% in the presence of long term treatment with thiazide diuretics. Under such conditions, a compensatory increase of sodium reabsorption occurs in the proximal tubules of the kidney. Lithium is also absorbed with sodium in the proximal tubules, where thiazides exert little effect. Thus, lithium may be reabsorbed more rapidly, with a consequent decrease in its clearance (Petersen et al., 1974). Lithium can be safely used with thiazide diuretics but dosage must be reduced (see section 5.4).

The elimination half-life varies markedly between individuals, but for those with normal renal function is between 7 and 20 hours but appreciably longer in patients with impaired renal function. Steady-state concentrations should be attained within 2 to 6 days in those with normal renal function but will take longer in those with renal impairment and will be much higher than in patients with normal renal function after the same dose (Amdisen, 1975, 1977). Steady-state plasma concentrations of lithium are also higher in the elderly (Hewick et al., 1977) due to a decreased distribution volume and reduced rate of renal clearance (Lehmann and Merten, 1974). Although lithium has a sufficiently long half-life for single dose administration, daily dosage needs to be on a divided basis in order to avoid gastrointestinal ir-

ritation and excessive peak concentrations which follow single daily dose administration (Amdisen, 1975, 1977; see section 5.4).

1.5.5 Hypnotics

In insomnia, duration of drug action should be restricted to the night and residual effects should be absent during daytime, and there should be no accumulation of drug during the day. A rapid rate of elimination is therefore probably of advantage for a hypnotic, although qualitative effects on sleep are also important. The rate of absorption of the drug must be rapid. Of the various hypnotics available, benzodiazepines such as nitrazepam and flurazepam and chloral derivatives come closest to fulfilling ideal requirements (see section 9). However, little information is available on their pharmacokinetic properties in man.

Oral bioavailability of nitrazepam and time to peak plasma concentrations varies between individuals, but the implications to its use are not clear. It has an elimination half-life of between 18 and 34 hours (Breimer, 1977), explaining why residual sedative effects can occur on the day following administration. Nitrazepam is metabolised in part by nitro reduction to an amine metabolite followed by acetylation; the acetylation pathway being genetically determined into a slow or rapid phenotype (Karim and Price Evans, 1976; see chapter VII, sect. 4.2.1). Nitrazepam is highly protein bound ($\sim 90\%$).

Flurazepam is so rapidly biotransformed after oral administration that unchanged drug is barely detectable in blood. A number of metabolites are formed and the principal active metabolite desalkylflurazepam attains peak plasma concentrations 1 hour after an oral dose (Greenblatt et al., 1975c). This metabolite in turn undergoes slow metabolism (elimination half-life of 47 to 100h) and accumulates during continuous administration (Kaplan et al., 1973), which correlates with onset of maximum effectiveness until 2 to 3 nights of administration (Kales et al., 1976) and residual effects after single doses. Flurazepam is probably only weakly albumin bound.

The metabolite trichlorethanol is responsible for the hypnotic action of chloral hydrate after oral administration, peak levels of which are attained within 1 hour of administration of an aqueous solution. Availability may not be as rapid after some capsule and tablet formulations of chloral hydrate. The elimination of trichlorethanol is quite rapid (half-life of 7 to 10h), but another important metabolite trichloracetic acid has a half-life of 4 to 5 days and accumulates during repeated administration. This metabolite can displace highly bound acidic drugs such as warfarin from albumin binding sites, but in practice interactions are not usually important (see chapter XXIII; sect. 3.2.5). However trichlorethanol and alcohol do interact to an important extent, leading to enhanced sedation as a result of a mutual increase in blood levels. For a review of the pharmacokinetic properties of hypnotics, see Breimer (1977).

1.6 Pharmacokinetic Considerations in Use of Psychotherapeutic Drugs

1.6.1 Drug Dosage and Dose Frequency

As discussed in section 1.5, the psychotherapeutic drugs in common use show vast differences in steady-state plasma concentrations between different patients treated with similar daily doses, and are due principally to genetically determined differences in metabolism (see chapter I; sect. 4.2). The wide variation in plasma concentration means that dosage needs to be individualised and this is reflected in the wide range of doses used in clinical practice. There is no such thing as a standard dose of a psychotherapeutic drug. Using the same dose for all patients is pharmacological nonsense. Because of altered pharmacokinetics, the dosage of many psychotherapeutic drugs, but particularly chlordiazepoxide and diazepam, lithium and the tricyclic antidepressants, should be reduced in the elderly. The elderly also appear more 'sensitive' to the CNS depressant effects of benzodiazepines such as chlordiazepoxide, diazepam and nitrazepam (Greenblatt and Allen, 1978). In general, dosage should be reduced for many drugs in the elderly (see chapter V; sect. 2). Associated diseases or other drugs may influence the disposition of some of the psychotherapeutic drugs and necessitate individualisation or adjustment of dosage; for example, altered intestinal transit time with chlorpromazine, reduced renal function or diuretic therapy with lithium or cirrhosis with chlordiazepoxide and diazepam (see further section 1.5).

The pharmacokinetic properties of a drug also determine the frequency of drug dosage (see chapter I; sect. 3.3.1). Thus, most psychotherapeutic drugs in common use are intrinsically long acting because of their slow rate of disappearance from plasma (see section 1.5; table I) and can therefore generally be given with much advantage as a single daily dose once the optimum dose has been established. Lithium is a notable exception (see section 3.2, 7.1, 8.2).

1.6.2 Dosage Form of Drug

The dosage form of the drug can be an important consideration (Hollister et al., 1970). Thus, absorption of an orally administered antipsychotic drug is usually best from liquid concentrates, next best from coated tablets and least from capsuled pellets (see section 1.5; chapter VI, sect. 4). Plasma levels following some extended release preparations are often very low. Intramuscular administration of antipsychotic drugs generally achieves much higher plasma levels than after oral administration and doses should be adjusted on this basis.

1.6.3 Relationship of Plasma Concentrations and Clinical Effects

During the past 10 years, advances in chemical technology have made it easier to measure plasma concentrations of drugs. Sometimes such monitoring has proven to be essential to effective clinical use, as in the case of anticonvulsant and antiarrhythmic drugs (see chapters XXV, sect. 2.3.5; XVII, sect. 6.1). At present, it is technically possible to measure plasma concentrations of almost all psychotherapeutic drugs. The major questions we must answer is when such measurements should be done and what we may expect from them.

No one has yet reported on clinical experience with routine monitoring of antipsychotic drugs for the treatment of schizophrenic patients. With the exception of some evidence of a possible relationship between plasma concentrations of chlorpromazine or the ratio of active drug and metabolites to inactive metabolites and therapeutic outcome, it has not been possible to define a good relationship between plasma drug concentrations and clinical effects with any antipsychotic drug. Current practice is not to monitor plasma concentrations of these drugs, which seems to be reasonable in view of the uncertainties (for reviews, see Kane et al., 1976; Cooper, 1978).

A great amount of work has been done during the past several years to define therapeutic plasma concentrations for tricyclic antidepressants. Nortriptyline, which for technical reasons has been most frequently studied in relation to plasma concentrations, tends to show an inverted U-shaped relationship between plasma concentrations and clinical response. Patients with levels below 40 to 50ng/ml show little response to the drug; when levels exceed 140 to 170ng/ml, therapeutic results tend to decline. Thus, a range of therapeutic levels for this drug has been proposed (Asberg, 1974). A number of studies have failed to find such a relationship between plasma concentrations of nortriptyline and therapeutic results, but unlike the positive studies, they have not used exclusively patients with endogenous depressions (Reisby et al., 1977). Measurement of plasma concentrations following use of amitriptyline or imipramine must also account for the active secondary amine metabolites. Usually one expresses the combined value for levels of amitriptyline/nortriptyline or of imipramine/desipramine. The pattern of response is different from nortriptyline. For imipramine, most patients respond well when plasma concentrations of imipramine plus desipramine are above 200 to 240ng/ml, whereas for amitriptyline, the corresponding level seems to be about 80 to 120ng/ml of amitriptyline plus nortriptyline.

The evidence presently available indicates that in patients with endogenous depression, clinical response is correlated with plasma concentrations of drug (for review, see Gram, 1977). Determination of plasma concentrations might be of value in detecting or confirming occasional patients who fail to comply with treatment or in deciding whether or not an increase in dose is warranted due to inadequate or suboptimum dosage. Another use of such determinations would be to elucidate unwanted or unexpected effects that are not clearly due to the drugs. Arguments for routine monitoring of plasma concentrations of tricyclics are neither compelling clinically nor on the basis of any cost-benefit analysis.

Routine monitoring of plasma concentrations of lithium however, is such established practice that it is difficult to imagine using the drug without it (Amdisen, 1975, 1977). Unlike most of those drugs discussed previously, lithium has a remarkably low therapeutic margin. Symptoms and signs that may occur from therapeutic doses merge with those that herald toxicity. Clinical guides to toxicity are not adequate.

The usual plasma concentrations of lithium sought for therapeutic purposes are from 0.9 to 1.4mEq/L, and for maintenance purposes, 0.8 to 1.0mmol (mEq)/L (see section 5.1, 5.2). It should be emphasised that these concentrations are not absolute. If a patient does well at lower concentrations, rejoice. On the other hand, if an unrespon-

sive patient has no remarkable toxic effects even though the plasma concentration is at the upper end of this range, one might feel free to increase the dose. Finally, if a patient has clearly toxic symptoms, the dose should be reduced no matter what the plasma concentration may be. Laboratory tests are not meant to supplant good clinical judgment (Strayhorn and Nash, 1977).

The values quoted are nadir values in the postabsorptive state, meaning the blood samples should be taken approximately 12 hours after the last dose. If samples are drawn too close to the last dose, values may be factitiously high.

Measurement of erythrocyte concentrations of lithium have not been widely adopted. Initially, these concentrations were assumed to correlate better with clinical response than those from plasma, but proof of that assumption has been lacking. Past experience has shown that plasma concentrations are adequate for most purposes. Lithium concentrations in saliva can be measured, but no doubt most clinicians would prefer to use the more rapidly available blood.

For practical purposes, the class of antianxiety drugs is subsumed by the benzodiazepines. Measurements of plasma concentrations of these drugs have been directed at elucidating their kinetics in man, never for routine monitoring of treatment (see Greenblatt et al., 1978a; Mandelli et al., 1978). As treatment both of anxiety and insomnia is purely symptomatic, and the complaints are largely subjective, one could scarcely tell an anxious patient that she should feel better because her plasma concentrations of diazepam were in the therapeutic range. Further, measurement of anxiety has really not been good enough to make fine correlations between plasma concentrations and clinical effects, even if they were desirable. One can measure sedation more accurately, plasma levels correlating well with this effect. One would scarcely want to measure the plasma concentrations of hypnotics during the night when the desired effects occur.

2. General Principles of Treatment

1) *Diagnosis and assessment of response to psychotherapeutic drugs:* Throughout this book much emphasis has been given to the need for accurate diagnosis as a prerequisite to the selection and effective use of drugs. In psychiatric disorders not only do we lack the ability to verify diagnosis by

the ultimate demonstration of some pathological change, but also we have little concept of the pathogenesis of the illnesses we are treating. This makes measurement and evaluation of the symptoms and signs more difficult than usual. Psychiatric diagnosis is almost completely based on inference. With the exception of those acute and chronic brain syndromes associated with neuropathological abnormalities, the data upon which diagnostic inferences are made are soft, being based on what patients tell us, either by reporting on their symptoms and feelings without our intervention (self reports) or with it (interviews), or on what other people tell us about them. Despite these difficulties, clinical data of the type mentioned can at least be handled in a standardised fashion. Experience with the numerous psychiatric rating scales indicates that these assessments approach the validity and the level of consensual agreement between raters that one might expect from interpretations of abnormal electrocardiograms or chest x-rays. Such assessments, although time consuming, should be used more widely in routine clinical practice if psychotherapeutic drugs are to be used more rationally and effectively.

Theories of pathogenesis for the functional psychiatric disorders abound, but evidence for any of these is relatively scanty. Due to uncertainty regarding pathogenesis, multifaceted treatment programmes are used with most emotional disorders. While no one could argue against any measures which help patients, it is obvious that the many treatments offered confound the problem of drug effects to varying degrees. Besides the influence of concurrent treatments, the course of many emotional disorders is variable, with some spontaneous improvement or remission. Not every anxious patient is always so; environmental influences play a considerable role in determining the degree of anxicty. The same is true of depression, a fact which has been documented repeatedly during controlled studies of antidepressant drugs. Schizophrenic reactions also may remit spontaneously, although apparently not as often as thought. They may also become worse in the absence of effective treatment.

2) *Correct indications for use of drugs:* The indications for antipsychotic drugs are best for major psychiatric illnesses. To use antipsychotic drugs for inducing sleep, rather than hypnotics, is completely unjustified in normal persons. They are not especially good hypnotics, and are generally more dangerous and more expensive than usual hypnotics. Often, one may wish to exploit the sleep producing effects of these drugs in schizophrenics, or in some patients with disordered sleep associated with psychoses of old age, but hypnosis is never a primary indication. Drug treatment is not indicated for everyone who is depressed. Some patients require no specific treatment with drugs, while all who do probably require other treatments as well. To use antianxiety and hypnotic drugs less may be the better way to use them. Unless clinicians use these drugs with restraint, political pressures stemming from the growing problem of drug abuse may lead to unwise constraints.

3) *Concomitant non-drug treatment:* While the antipsychotic drugs are the foundation for an effective total treatment programme of psychosis, they do not prevent any benefits from other therapies, and vice versa. Realistic efforts must be made to help the patient so that he can live and work in the community despite his handicap. Many depressions are mild and clearly related to life experiences. Excessive reliance on drug therapy to the exclusion of 'psychotherapy' or attempts to change the environment of the depressed patient, may do more harm than good. Treatment of these disorders requires a combination of all methods of therapy available. The benefits of ECT in severe depression should not be neglected. In many clinics this treatment is underutilised. It is no longer a fearful or traumatic experience. Anxiety is clearly related to life experiences. 'Psychotherapy' and altering the environment may be more to the point. Use of drugs, at least in our present understanding, should be considered no more than symptomatic, adjunctive treatment. Anxious patients and patients suffering from insomnia tend to respond favourably to any attention and drugs may interact favourably with the personality of the prescriber (Rickels, 1978). Thus, if antianxiety drugs or hypnotics are to be prescribed, try to work up some enthusiasm for them and try to communicate this to patients.

4) *Rational selection of drugs:* Learn to use a few drugs well rather than all poorly. The differences in clinical response between the proper and improper use of a drug will probably exceed any actual differences between drugs. Nevertheless, with antipsychotic drugs individual patients can

respond differently to different drugs, doing poorly on some and better on others. A rational approach is to master the use of one of each of the chemical types of drug when one should be able to exploit the full range of pharmacological differences between the various compounds (see section 3.1). In depression one should be prepared to use a whole array of drugs, depending on the presenting depressive syndrome (see section 7). In anxiety and insomnia, the extensive popularity of the benzodiazepines probably stems from a few important pharmacological differences (see section 8, 9.1).

The over-riding consideration with all psychotherapeutic drugs is the patient's previous response to a drug, if that information is available. One would be loth to change a patient from a drug which he has found to be acceptable and beneficial, even though it might not be one's ordinary first choice.

5) Doses and dose schedule: Patients vary widely in their dose requirements for psychotherapeutic drugs, not only because of marked interindividual differences in rates of metabolism (see section 1.5.1) but also because of tolerance of side effects. Few drugs have such a wide range of therapeutic doses as the antipsychotic drugs (table III). Similar ranges exist with the antidepressant (table XII) and antianxiety drugs (table XIII).

When starting treatment with antipsychotics and tricyclic antidepressants, divided doses are usually given. These minimise the initial impact of many of the unwanted pharmacological effects (sedation and α-adrenoceptor blocking activity with antipsychotics; sedation and anticholinergic effects with tricyclics) and increase the flexibility in determining the optimum dose. The elderly are especially prone to unwanted pharmacological effects of psychotherapeutic drugs (see section 11; chapter V, sect. 4.7) and doses of antipsychotic and antidepressant drugs in particular must be very low initially and adjusted with great care. Tolerance of the sedative effects of antianxiety drugs can be assessed by giving the initial doses when the patient is at home in the evening hours (not as he is about to leave home to drive his car to work). If he gets sleepy, then little harm is done. Traditional divided dose schedules of the tid or qid type make little sense with most of the psychotherapeutic drugs (see section 1.5), especially once a patient has reached a satisfactory maintenance dose; lithium being a notable exception. A single night-time dose may be used with the antipsychotics, tricyclic antidepressants and antianxiety drugs, whereas a single morning dose can be used with the MAO inhibitor and sympathomimetic antidepressants. In short, using the pharmacological attributes of these drugs, the traditional treatment programme of equally divided doses can be largely abandoned. Moreover, in schizophrenia and manic-depressive disorder where compliance of the patient is essential, a single daily dose regimen when feasible is very much more convenient. Divided doses are necessary with lithium to avoid gastrointestinal irritation and excessive peak concentrations which follow single dose administration.

6) Combinations of drugs: There is no good evidence to support the superiority of any combinations of psychotherapeutic drugs over the proper use of a single drug. In depression accompanied by obvious psychotic symptoms, a combination of antipsychotic and tricyclic antidepressant drug may be used to assist in making the correct diagnosis (see section 7). In schizophrenia and in some moderately severe depressions, antianxiety drugs may be used adjunctively with other agents when required (see section 3.3, 7). Anti-Parkinsonian drugs should be given when clear indications for their use exist, and not routinely in the absence of any extrapyramidal symptoms. They can however, be used prophylactically when extrapyramidal reactions are to be expected in the initial course of parenteral medication or when high doses are given orally (see section 3.4).

7) Duration of treatment: The natural history of a disorder is the best guide to prognosis. Thus the antipsychotic drugs may be discontinued after brief periods in acute psychotic disturbances but need to be continued indefinitely in chronic conditions. Chronic schizophrenic patients at home on weekend passes may not *need* the drug, but should still adhere to their dosage regimen to prevent the assumption that once they are discharged their need for medication is ended. The value of antipsychotic drugs in preventing readmission must be appreciated (see further section 3.2).

The decision of whether or not to undertake maintenance therapy in mania and depression is also determined by the past course of the illness. For example, if the attack being treated was the patient's first, it is usual to discontinue treatment after remission has been attained, whereas if attacks were becoming more frequent and more severe, long term treatment can then be considered (see section 5.2, 7.4).

Treatment of anxiety is limited to short courses and drugs are not given indefinitely, although a few patients with chronic symptoms may require small doses of an antianxiety drug indefinitely (see section 8.3). Management of insomnia should always be limited to short courses (see section 9.1).

3. Schizophrenia

Antipsychotic drugs have been clearly established as the primary treatment of schizophrenics, but not all patients treated with antipsychotics are helped, and many who are, still leave much to be desired (for review, see Davis and Casper, 1977). The effects of drug therapy on the natural course of schizophrenia are unknown since few good studies were done prior to the drug era. Antipsychotic drugs therefore do not cure schizophrenia. The aim of treatment is to curb the course of the illness — by achieving sufficient initial improvement following the acute psychosis to discharge the patient from hospital and by maintenance therapy to reduce the need for re-admission due to relapse.

The benefits from antipsychotics are not due simply to sedation. Disturbed thinking, paranoid symptoms, delusions, emotional and social withdrawal, and personal neglect improve as well as anxiety and agitation, symptoms which might be expected to respond to conventional sedatives, but which do not. Improvement from drugs approximates the familiar learning curve. There is rapid change in the first few weeks, a slowing of improvement in the 6th to 12th weeks of treatment, and very slow change thereafter. There is often an unevenness in rate of symptom change; hyperactivity may disappear after only a few doses of a phenothiazine, while delusions and hallucinations may persist, with lessened affect, for weeks. Abnormal thinking and interpersonal relationships in catatonic patients may improve weeks before the pathological motor pattern is altered. Changes for the better are more apt to occur in women than in men.

Although antipsychotic drugs are a primary treatment, this does not necessarily mean that they should be given indiscriminately to all patients. Some schizophrenic patients have rather good pre-

morbid adjustments and their psychosis has relatively clear precipitants (e.g. 'reactive' schizophrenia, or in European literature, schizophreniform psychosis). They may present explosively, but the course may be self limiting and a relatively full remission obtained. Many have responded to treatment without drugs (these probably represent the handful of cases reported to respond to psychoanalysis or to 'crazy therapists'). Drugs may be useful for these patients during the acute episode, but are probably not required for maintenance after resolution of the acute psychosis. Another group of patients for whom drug therapy might be questioned are those with exceedingly chronic schizophrenia and long term hospitalisation. Often such patients show only meaningless improvement from drug therapy, which is more often given for the benefit of the hospital staff than for that of the patient. The need of such patients for drug treatment has been questioned, especially as this group seems most vulnerable for developing tardive dyskinesia (see section 3.5.1). This latter complication should lead to the most conservative use of these drugs. Even patients with acute schizophrenia, where drugs are most clearly indicated, may be overtreated in the zeal to reduce hospital stay or even to avoid hospitalisation. Not all chronically psychotic patients require large doses of these drugs or prolonged, *uninterrupted* treatment (see section 3.2). The risks for some may outweigh the benefits. Principles in the use of antipsychotic drugs are summarised in table II and discussed further below.

3.1 Initial Treatment and Choice of Drug

A completely rational choice between the many antipsychotic drugs (table III) cannot currently be made for individual patients. While the target symptom approach to evaluation of antipsychotic drugs remains valid, to use it as a basis for choosing drugs in clinical practice is an error. Antipsychotic drugs do not treat specific symptoms; they treat an illness.

An old therapeutic axiom is that 'it is better to learn to use a few drugs well than to use many poorly'. To narrow the choice among the numerous available antipsychotic drugs, one might make two assumptions: (a) that chemical differences denote differences in the spectrum of pharmacological actions of drugs; and (b) that differences within members of a chemical class or subclass are negligible (Hollister, 1972a; Davis

Table II. Summary of principles of use of antipsychotic drugs

---

1. Treat schizophrenia, not lesser symptoms
    a) Agitation — use barbiturate, often with antipsychotic
    b) Insomnia — use chloral hydrate or a benzodiazepine, major antipsychotic dose at night

2. Carefully select dosage form
    a) Initial treatment may start with parenteral dosage form followed by oral maintenance doses; assures delivery of drug
    b) If only oral doses used, and results not adequate, consider brief course of parenteral drug followed by oral liquid concentrates

3. Tailor dose to patient's needs
    a) Clinically, doses that are effective have varied over a wide range
    b) Two clinical indicators of somewhat adequate dose
       i) amelioration of schizophrenia
       ii) extrapyramidal syndromes

4. Dosage schedules
    a) Initially, all doses divided, but not necessarily equal throughout the day
    b) Later, shift major burden of dose to evening hours, possibly only to a single bedtime dose

5. Maintenance treatment
    a) Indefinite for many. May still be interrupted such as 'weekends off' (impossible to predict those who will not relapse on longer 'holidays')
    b) Long acting drugs useful for those who default oral regimen

6. Indications other than schizophrenia; no trivial indications
    a) Schizoaffective disorders (section 6)
    b) Acute mania (section 5.1).
    c) Depression accompanied by agitation (section 3.3, 7)
    d) Psychoses associated with old age (section 11)
    e) Gilles de la Tourette syndrome (rare)
    f) Severe vomiting

---

and Casper, 1977). Therefore one might choose an exemplar from each of the various chemical classes as shown in table III. Such a basis for choice might select, for example, the following drugs: chlorpromazine, thioridazine, fluphenazine, thiothixene, haloperidol, pimozide, loxapine and molindone. Chlorpromazine may properly be considered to be obsolete, but is still included as it is generally much cheaper than the others. Thioridazine has limitations due to a low ceiling dose and lack of a parenteral dosage form, but is included for those patients in whom extrapyramidal reactions may be a formidable problem. Pimozide, loxapine and molindone would be second-echelon drugs, to be tried where the others may have failed or may have produced excessive side effects.

The degree of sedative, anticholinergic and α-adrenoceptor blocking action varies among different drugs, so that those with less of these properties may be preferred as being more specific in their antipsychotic action (see table IV). The sedative property of a drug is not in itself a suitable basis for choice; it now seems quite clear that adequate doses of drugs with low sedative properties, such as fluphenazine, haloperidol or thiothixene, may be highly effective for controlling excited or combative patients. These drugs also may be safely used parenterally.

Over-riding all other considerations is the patient's past history of response to a drug, if that information is available. The importance of various side effects to the patient should also be a guide to choosing his specific treatment. Unless a patient tolerates a drug well, he is not likely to maintain treatment faithfully. A patient who is made unbearably restless by a drug may much prefer no drug (see section 3.2). On the other hand, some patients may prefer restlessness rather than impairment of their sexual capacity.

When starting treatment, divided doses are usually given. These minimise the initial impact of many of the unwanted pharmacological effects (sedation and α-adrenoceptor blocking activity) and allow better titration of dose. Unfortunately, this eminently sensible practice in initiating treatment is seldom changed, and patients may unnecessarily stay on divided doses for years (see section 3.2). Dosage of the antipsychotic drugs needs to be individualised (see section 1.5.1) and the doses shown in table III are only rough guides. While no patient should be considered a drug failure without an intensive course of therapy, high doses should not become a routine for all patients. With the exception of thioridazine, where a maximum daily dose of 800mg is recommended to avoid retinal pigmentary changes (see chapter XII; sect. 11.1.1), no specific maximum doses have been set for any antipsychotic drug.

The response to an antipsychotic drug is assessed by either an improved mental state or the appearance of an extrapyramidal reaction. These are the two unique pharmacological actions, which bear somewhat on each other (see section 1.4.1). If neither outcome is evident, then more

Table III. Chemical classes and dosage relationship among antipsychotics

Drug and class	Relative potency in mg	Range of total daily dose (mg)[1]	
		outpatient	inpatient
Phenothiazines			
Aliphatic			
Chlorpromazine	100	50-400	200-1600
Piperidine			
Thioridazine	100	50-400	200-800
Mesoridazine	50	25-200	100-400
Piperacetazine	10	10-40	20-160
Piperazine			
Carphenazine	25	50-150	75-400
Acetophenazine	20	40-80	60-100
Prochlorperazine	15	20-60	60-200
Perphenazine	10	8-24	12-64
Butaperazine	10	10-30	10-100
Trifluoperazine	5	4-10	10-60
Fluphenazine	2	1-5	2-60
Thioxanthenes			
Thiothixene	5	6-30	10-120
Butyrophenones			
Haloperidol	2	2-6	4-100
Diphenylbutylpiperidines			
Pimozide	2	2-8	5-30
Dibenzoxazepines			
Loxapine	10	15-40	40-160
Indolics			
Molindone	10	15-60	40-225

1   Rough guide only (see section 1.5.1, 3.1).

drug is needed. Neither outcome necessarily indicates that the optimum dose has been attained. Exploration of the upper limits of effective dose should be based on other considerations such as tolerance of side effects (e.g. oversedation, cardiovascular complications). Obviously, routine use of an anti-Parkinson drug at the outset of treatment may deny the clinician one of these two clinical criteria for assessing the adequacy of dose.

Rapid 'neuroleptisation' is a current vogue (Ayd, 1977), based on the erroneous pharmacological assumption that these drugs exert an all-or-none effect, something previously believed to be the case for digitalis. Just as is now known to be the case with digitalis, antipsychotic drugs produce graded effects that are often time dependent. An erroneous social assumption is that it is vitally important to avoid hospitalisation for schizophrenia or to reduce it to a minimum; often hospitalisation is required for elucidating social problems that may have contributed to the exacerbation of psychosis. The danger of routine use of rapid intensive treatment programmes is that many patients may be overtreated for the dubious gain of shortening hospitalisation for a few.

An oral dosage form (see section 1.6.2) is normally used to commence treatment, reserving parenteral forms for disturbed, excited or hyperactive patients, but there is a good case to start all patients on intramuscular doses for several days and then begin oral therapy. One might then be far more certain of not under dosing the patient due to some vagary in absorption or first-pass metabolism of the drug, or due to his covert refusal of the medication when given by mouth. A patient who shows less therapeutic effect than desired should not be switched immediately to another drug. A brief trial of intramuscular drug followed by oral doses with liquid concentrate, even without changing the previous ineffective doses, may enhance the clinical response. Parenteral haloperidol has been used effectively for treating acute schizophrenics. Other of the more potent drugs, such as fluphenazine or thiothixene, might be used in a similar way. It should be remembered that antipsychotic drugs administered intramuscularly are usually 3 to 4 times more potent than when given orally and doses should be adjusted on this basis (see section 1.5.1).

The doses shown in table III somewhat reflect the current practice towards using higher doses of antipsychotics. Enthusiasm for using 'mega doses' of highly potent antipsychotics, such as 1200mg daily of fluphenazine or haloperidol, has waned as the number of patients salvaged has been few and the potential dangers are still uncertain. A controlled attempt to replicate previously encouraging results with 1200mg daily doses of fluphenazine in treatment-refractory patients showed that those who received the standard dose had greater improvement than those receiving the 'mega dose'. The latter had more akinesia, which may have contributed to the lack of benefit (Quitkin et al., 1975). The paradox of why these large doses of drug are less likely than smaller ones to produce the Parkinson syndrome may be explained on the basis of the concomitant anticholinergic actions that most of these drugs also have: as one reaches the flat portion of the dose-response curve, the block of dopamine receptors is no longer a great deal more than block of muscarinic cholinergic receptors.

3.2 Maintenance Treatment

Antipsychotic drugs may be discontinued after brief periods of treatment of acute brain syndromes, some manic episodes and some acute schizophrenic disturbances. Acute responses of patients newly treated with drugs are variable, ranging from days to weeks. Most clinicians would feel that failure of acute or newly admitted schizophrenics to improve after 6 to 8 weeks of adequate treatment with a drug would be reason to try another. Newly treated chronic patients might require 12 to 24 weeks of treatment before a change of medication would be warranted. Im-

Table IV. Choice among some selected antipsychotic drugs according to pharmacological profile[1] (adapted after Byck, 1975)[1]

Drug and class	Extra-pyramidal effects	Sedative effects[2]	Hypotensive effects[2]
Aliphatic phenothiazine			
Chlorpromazine	++	+++	+++
Piperidine phenothiazine			
Mesoridazine	±	+++	++
Thioridazine	±	+++	++
Piperazine phenothiazine			
Fluphenazine	+++	++	+
Perphenazine	+++	+	+
Trifluoperazine	+++	+	+
Thioxanthenes			
Thiothixene	+++	+	+
Butyrophenone			
Haloperidol	+++	+	+
Diphenylbutylpiperidines			
Pimozide	+	+	+
Dibenzoxazepines			
Loxapine	++	+	+
Dibenzodiazepines			
Clozapine	0	++	+++
Indolics			
Molindone	+++	+	+

1 Patient's previous response major guide (see section 3.1).
2 Relative incidence usually encountered: (0) negligible; (±) minimal; (+) low; (++) moderate; (+++) high.

provement tends to be more rapid earlier than later on.

As a rule, to decrease the extent of relapse following resolution of acute symptoms (Hogarty and Goldberg, 1973), schizophrenic patients are placed on maintenance doses which should be as low as possible for retaining therapeutic gains, but dosage should remain flexible to permit management of the inevitable periods of increased emotional difficulty (Davis, 1975; Davis and Casper, 1977). The initially used dosage should be reduced gradually to avoid a sudden recrudescence of symptoms. As the antipsychotic drugs are intrinsically long acting (table I), no pharmacokinetic basis for divided doses obtains. Thus, once a patient reaches a satisfactory daily maintenance dose, it is feasible also to reduce the dose frequency. Many clinicians aim for a single daily dose to be given just before retiring, and even when they use divided doses, tend to give the major dose of the day at this time. Two advantages accrue. The patient sleeps when he should, not because he is oversedated during the day. Second, he is less likely to suffer disabling extrapyramidal symptoms if the major impact of the drug occurs while he is sleeping. For reasons still not clear, manifestations of Parkinson's disease are ameliorated by sleep.

The technique of reducing doses may vary. Some prefer to eliminate the morning dose first, consolidating it with one given later in the day and then progressively doing the same to the noon and afternoon dose. If very large amounts of drug are required for maintenance treatment, one may still prefer to divide the total daily dose, giving perhaps one-third in the late afternoon and the remainder before bedtime. In most cases, however, the goal of a single daily maintenance dose can be attained. Many drugs are now available in larger single dose units to meet the growing acceptance of the single daily dose.

The minimum maintenance dose at which the patient functions best is preferred to an arbitrarily imposed maintenance dose such as one-third or one-fourth of the peak dose. Reduction of doses for maintenance treatment is of considerable importance. Many instances of so-called 'postschizophrenic depression' are probably due to overtreatment with antipsychotic drugs. Patients tolerate very well reductions in the maintenance doses of drug, for example by eliminating drugs on 2 or 3 days of the week (Prien et al., 1971), but 'drug holidays' for any substantial period of time are neither feasible nor fair to the patient. It is not only impossible to predict in advance which schizophrenic patient will tolerate a prolonged drug holiday, but it has not been shown that exposure to drugs can be reduced by this approach more than by trying assiduously to find the least possible maintenance dose.

Many patients take their own drug holidays, either by discontinuing the drug altogether or by taking less than the prescribed amount (Renton et al., 1963). In one study, 39 of 85 chronic schizophrenic patients took less drug than prescribed when followed over a 2-year period (Van Putten, 1974). The major reason proposed for discontinuation was the unpleasant effect of a subtle akathisia. This rate of non-compliance is not much different from that of patients taking antihypertensive drugs or those on prophylactic regimens of antituberculosis drugs.

Assuming that one has found the minimum maintenance dose, the patient should be cautioned to continue medication even though he feels well, and should be reassured about fears of becoming 'addicted'. He should be cautioned about possible drowsiness and interference with skilled movements, and warned against the concomitant use of alcoholic beverages. The patient's family should have the same instructions. Information should be provided to the family physician and pharmacist and an uninterrupted supply of medication should be assured. The ever increasing number of patients discharged from hospitals on antipsychotic drugs poses a special challenge to follow-up clinics. One should make efforts to keep patients on drugs.

Long acting depot preparations are particularly useful for maintenance therapy in outpatient treatment, especially when patients are unreliable about taking medication (Johnson, 1977). A single injection of a fluphenazine preparation (enanthate or decanoate) needs to be repeated only every 2 to 4 weeks in most patients so that drug intake is assured; provided patients are followed up to identify defaulters. Several studies have shown a decreased rate of relapse among patients so maintained, as contrasted with those asked to take daily oral medication (Johnson, 1976; Rifkin et al., 1977). Readmission rates to hospitals and days spent in the hospital are often markedly reduced, but sometimes results are less spectacular (Denham and Adamson, 1973). Estimating the dose of depot preparation needed for conversion to such a regimen has usually been empirical. One possible way to do it more accurately is suggested in table V. These preparations do not release large amounts of drug unevenly, but acute extrapyramidal reactions of the dystonic type or akinesia or akathisia may be encountered. These are likely to be maximal in the first few days following an injection and along with other side effects can be minimised by adjustment of dose size and dose interval; side effects are related to the size of the individual injection dose and if this can be reduced and the dose interval decreased some patients can tolerate an equal, or even higher, total dose (Johnson, 1973; 1978). Dose size and dose interval need to be individualised to maintain remission with the least side effects; there is no recommended maintenance dose regimen (Johnson, 1977). Other injectable compounds such as flupenthixol decanoate are also available for use every 2 to 4 weeks, as are long acting oral preparations such as penfluridol and fluspirilene, which can be

Table V. A suggested guide to calculation of initial dose of fluphenazine enanthate

1. Multiply daily dose of previous oral antipsychotic (equiv fluphenazine) by dose interval intended; assume 14 days

2. Divide by 4 — assume that a parenteral drug will be 4x more potent than one given orally (not known for fluphenazine but applicable to a few others).

3. Reduce by one-third — assume that in a day or two a slight excess of fluphenazine will be released before a steadily declining plateau occurs (this occurred in one study with perphenazine enanthate) and to avoid possible exacerbation of acute dystonias, akathisia or extrapyramidal reaction.

Example: Patient's present maintenance dose is equivalent to 10mg of fluphenazine:

Dose of fluphenazine enanthate $= \dfrac{(10 \times 14) - 1/3}{4}$

$= 35 - 1/3 = 25\text{mg approx.}$

---

given once weekly (Quitkin et al., 1978). Such oral preparations taken regularly are as effective as long acting injectable preparations and are therefore suitable for fully cooperative patients, particularly those strongly averse to injections. Long acting preparations have no place in the initial treatment of patients; not only is there lack of flexibility with dosage but the inability to withdraw treatment is potentially dangerous in cases of misdiagnosis (e.g. depression rather than schizophrenia).

The question of how long to continue maintenance treatment is one that tests good clinical judgment and cannot be answered categorically or generally. Most clinicians would assume that any patient who has gone into full remission after several months of treatment with antipsychotic drugs following an initial 'schizophrenic break' should be tried without drug. A substantial number may not require additional drug (the diagnosis may have been in error) or may require retreatment only much later in the course of their illness (so-called 'good prognosis' schizophrenia). Those patients who show relapse after such an initial period of discontinuation of drug should be placed on long term maintenance treatment. Even in this situation, one may wish from time to time to test how the patient does without drug, but after several failures one should become reconciled to a long term maintenance programme. A great many studies of drug maintenance have been summarised. Relapse rates were 65% in patients switched to a placebo (698 of 1068 patients) as compared with 30% in patients maintained on drugs (639 of 2127 patients; Davis and Casper,

1977). Considering that many patients maintained on drugs may take these agents rather irregularly, and sometimes not at all, the true relapse rate, were treatment perfectly maintained, might be still less. Further, many of these studies were short term and were therefore less likely to include the majority of chronic schizophrenics who would require indefinite maintenance treatment to avoid relapse.

3.3 Antipsychotic Drug Combinations

Little or no rationale exists for combining two antipsychotic drugs. Some justify a combination by using a less sedative drug during the daytime and a more sedative drug at bedtime. By moving daily doses to the late afternoon or bedtime period, one should get enough sedative effect; if not, a chloral derivative or a benzodiazepine such as nitrazepam or flurazepam would be more reasonable than adding more antipsychotic drug just to make the patient sleep.

Combinations of an antipsychotic such as perphenazine, and an antidepressant, such as amitriptyline, are often used. Pharmacologically, they don't make much sense, for some of their crucially important actions should oppose each other, yet when you need perphenazine for treating schizophrenia, amitriptyline doesn't seem to get in the way (Chouinard et al., 1975), and vice versa for depression. The only rational justification for using the combination is when one isn't sure of which diagnosis the patient may have, as in the differential diagnosis between a depressed schizophrenic or a psychotic depression (see also section 7). Using the combination is a way to cover both bets. Extemporaneous combinations of these drugs are preferred to fixed dose preparations, as the individual drugs (and doses) can be changed as the diagnosis becomes clearer, so that eventually a patient may receive one drug or the other. The anticholinergic effect of the tricyclic eliminates the need for any antiparkinson drug.

Anxiety in schizophrenics is part of the illness, so that antipsychotics might be expected to ameliorate it eventually. Antianxiety drugs may however, be used adjunctively, especially when single doses given at night do double duty as hypnotics. Mild akathisia may sometimes be mistaken for anxiety; diphenhydramine or hydroxyzine both having sedative and anticholinergic actions, may be a better choice than any antianxiety agent.

3.4 Combination with Anti-Parkinsonian Drugs

Anti-Parkinsonian drugs are most often used in combination with antipsychotics. Many clinicians use them routinely, even in the absence of any extrapyramidal symptoms. Such gratuitous use of anticholinergic drugs carries some hazards, as their peripheral (e.g. dry mouth etc) and central (e.g. deliria) anticholinergic effects may be additive with those of the antipsychotics or the more strongly anticholinergic tricyclic antidepressants. One would prefer to await the development of a clear indication for treatment with any drug, particularly since development of extrapyramidal side effects is an important guide to dose adjustment (see section 3.1) but even then, anti-Parkinsonian agents may not be necessary in many cases (Johnson, 1978). Practical considerations lead to some exceptions to this rule. If the patient is to be treated intensively with an initial course of parenteral medication or high doses of oral medication one may predict that extrapyramidal reactions will occur and prophylactic treatment may be warranted. Either when anti-Parkinsonian drugs are used to treat a drug induced extrapyramidal syndrome or when their use is prophylactic, one can discontinue the drug after several weeks (months in the case of long acting antipsychotics) of treatment with no return of the extrapyramidal disorders (Klett and Caffey, 1972; Johnson, 1978) in most cases. Quite possibly, this well documented clinical observation is due to the fact that drug induced extrapyramidal reactions may be self limiting. The practice of routine use of these drugs in-

definitely results in monumental overuse of these drugs.

3.5 Side Effects and Complications of Antipsychotic Drugs

Most side effects from these drugs are attributable to extensions of the known multiple pharmacological effects of antipsychotic drugs (e.g. behavioural and neurological effects; metabolic and endocrine effects). A few are idiosyncratic or allergic in origin (e.g. cholestatic jaundice), and at least one, agranulocytosis, is due to direct toxicity (Pisciotta, 1978). After so many years of clinical experience with these drugs, most important side effects are known (table VI). To be forewarned is in this case to be truly forearmed; one should always have a keen sense of anticipation for possible side effects.

Monitoring for side effects is best done by close clinical observation rather than by routine use of laboratory tests. The latter may be useful to establish baselines against which subsequent departures may be measured, and from time to time during the first several weeks of treatment these may be repeated. Excessive reliance on laboratory tests to detect complications is poor practice. Both jaundice and agranulocytosis characteristically occur early in treatment, the former usually within the first 4 weeks, the latter usually within the first 8 weeks. As both are initially manifested by fever, an accurate daily temperature record might be the best early warning device. The most problematic side effects are the syndrome of late appearing (tardive) dyskinesia and cardiac arrhythmias. The former is common, the latter is not.

3.5.1 Tardive Dyskinesia

As with all drug side effects, the frequency of tardive dyskinesia depends on how carefully one looks for the complication. In one survey, minimal to marked evidence of the syndrome was diagnosed in up to 40 % of chronic mental hospital patients (Bell and Smith, 1978). It seems to be more prevalent in women (Simpson et al., 1978) and need not be confined to the elderly (having been observed in children), nor to patients under long term treatment (some cases develop within weeks). The fact that it may occur in non-psychotic patients treated with antipsychotic drugs is warning enough against using these drugs for trivial indications. The essential feature of tardive

Table VI. Side effects of antipsychotic drugs

Effect	Reaction	Notes/action
Behavioural	Oversedation	See section 15.6
	Psychomotor impairment	
	Akathisia	Common. Add drug such as small doses of
	(uncontrollable restlessness)	diphenhydramine to curb effect
Neurological	Extrapyramidal syndrome	Manage by reduction of dose, administra-
	(akathisia, symptoms and signs of	tion of anti-Parkinsonian drug[1], or both
	Parkinsonism, acute dystonias)	
	Tardive dyskinesias	See section 3.5.1
Autonomic	Acute hypotensive crises	Elderly and debilitated patients or after large parenteral doses.
	Anticholinergic effects	Usually only bothersome (more of a prob-
	(e.g. dry mouth, blurred vision;	lem in elderly). Immediate medical atten-
	urinary retention, paralytic ileus)	tion for urinary retention, paralytic ileus.
	Inhibition of ejaculation	Thioridazine
Metabolic and endocrine	Weight gain	Often to a remarkable degree (see chapter XVI; sect. 14.4)
	Galactorrhoea, amenorrhoea	See chapter XV; sect. 23.6
	Gynaecomastia (men)	
	Loss of libido (men)	Frequent
Toxic and allergic	Agranulocytosis (direct toxicity)	Most often associated with chlorpromazine and thioridazine (see also chapter XXIII; sect. 8.7)
	Cholestatic jaundice	Not common. Do not use these drugs in
	(? allergic reaction)	patients with advanced liver failure (see also chapter XIX; sect. 1.4)
Miscellaneous	Cardiac arrhythmias	See section 3.5.2
	Ocular (phenothiazines)	See chapter XII (sect. 11.1.1)

1   Continue any anti-Parkinsonian drug for several weeks and withdraw gradually. Daily doses of some effective drugs are: procyclidine 10mg; benzhexol (trihexphenidyl) 4 to 8mg; benztropine 4mg; ethoheptazine 40 to 200mg; biperiden 2 to 6mg (see also section 3.4). Dystonic syndrome relieved by 0.5g caffeine sodium benzoate intravenously, or parenteral anti-Parkinsonian drug or barbiturate, repeated if necessary in 30 minutes. The antipsychotic drug should be discontinued briefly and an anti-Parkinsonian drug given when treatment (preferably with another compound) is resumed.

dyskinesia is repetitive involuntary movements of a choreoathetoid type involving the mouth, lips, tongue, trunk and extremities (ACNP-FDA Task Force, 1973).

The basic mechanism proposed for the onset of this syndrome is the development of dopaminergic hypersensitivity in the striatonigral system with a relative reduction in cholinergic function (Klawans, 1973). Such a formulation explains several clinical phenomena: (a) most, if not all, cases of tardive dyskinesia are preceded by the Parkinsonian syndrome, and occasionally one sees mixed syndromes; (b) anticholinergic drugs are not only ineffective, but often unmask a latent dyskinesia; (c) augmenting doses of antipsychotic drugs, either by using more of the same or adding another, often ameliorate the picture, at least temporarily; (d) sudden withdrawal from an antipsychotic drug may exacerbate a latent syndrome; (e) levodopa makes it worse and physostigmine may briefly ameliorate it. Tardive dyskinesia is a complex syndrome and it seems possible that different mechanisms, involving the dopaminergic and cholinergic systems, may have a role in different patients or with different drugs (Simpson et al., 1977).

Management of tardive dyskinesia is as a consequence difficult (Kobayashi, 1977). Firstly, if the patient is still on an anti-Parkinson drug, that should be immediately discontinued; further reduction of cholinergic activity tends to aggravate the situation. Secondly, reducing the dose of antipsychotic drug should be done gradually, trying to find an appropriate balance between maintaining the desired antipsychotic action and not making tardive dyskinesia worse. If the patient can tolerate complete withdrawal of antipsychotic drugs, a brief period without treatment may allow remission of tardive dyskinesia; treatment may later be resumed with smaller doses. Diazepam, which may act through the gamma-aminobutyric acid mediated portion of the nigrostriatal system, has occasionally been beneficial; doses of 20 to 40mg daily may be required. Use of drugs that reduce the effects of dopamine are occasionally helpful; of these, reserpine is currently the most favoured drug, given in doses of 1 to 2mg daily. Drugs that increase cholinergic transmission, such as deanol or choline, are still experimental approaches.

Although cases of tardive dyskinesia are sometimes irreversible, with appropriate management, many will reverse completely and the patient will make a complete recovery. Prevention, by judicious use of antipsychotic drugs or early detection of emerging neurological disorder, is the best means of treatment.

3.5.2 Cardiac Arrhythmias

Prolonged ventricular repolarisation can be observed almost routinely in patients on substantial doses of thioridazine, and to a lesser extent in patients on other antipsychotic drugs (Alexander et al., 1967; Backman and Elosuo, 1968). Both overnight fasting and oral supplements of 10g of combined potassium salts reverse these changes, while giving a 100g glucose load exacerbates them. It is believed that phenothiazines affect the ECG by shifting potassium to the intracellular compartment. The significance of such a reversible disorder remains controversial. Regardless of its cause, any increase in ventricular repolarisation enhances the likelihood of re-entry rhythms. Instances of sudden, unexpected deaths from such arrhythmias have occurred (Leemsta and Koenig, 1968). Other cases are probably seldom reported as the nature of the death is uncertain and the event is so rare that few single centres develop an extensive experience with this complication.

3.5.3 Overdosage in Children

Excessive doses of phenothiazines used as antiemetics can readily lead to acute poisoning in children. Although these drugs can be very useful in controlling severe vomiting in children, great care should be taken not to exceed the recommended dosage, particularly in the face of fever or dehydration, which predispose to the development of toxicity. Symptoms of overdosage are more marked in infants and young children than in adults, and frequently produce a bizarre and alarming neurological picture, which is often confused with tetanus or encephalitis (Duffy, 1971). Recovery is complete following withdrawal of the drugs, and use of an anti-Parkinsonian drug if there are painful muscle spasms (see also chapter XXV; sect. 15.5).

4. Organic Brain Syndromes

Acute brain syndromes due to withdrawal from alcohol or other drugs are best treated by replacing the abused drug with one that is pharmacologically equivalent (see section 12.3, 12.4, 13.1). Such is clearly not the case with antipsychotic drugs, which are contraindicated. Acute disorders associated with hallucinogenic drugs are usually self limiting and respond as well or better to antianxiety drugs or conventional sedatives. Antipsychotic drugs may produce more disabling effects in these otherwise normal persons than the disorder being treated. When a schizophrenic-like psychosis is precipitated by hallucinogenic drugs, then antipsychotic drugs may be indicated, but this situation is usually not evident for several days. Acute brain syndromes associated with being placed in recovery rooms, coronary care units or other strange medical surroundings seem to respond better to potent antipsychotics, such as haloperidol, than to conventional sedatives, which often aggravate the delirium.

Patients with chronic brain syndromes of any aetiology who are overactive and delusional often respond well to phenothiazine compounds, used cautiously in small doses (Prien, 1973). Though seizures may sometimes be precipitated, phenothiazines have been used in management of behavioural disturbances in chronic epileptics. However, the benzodiazepines are more logical choices as they also have anticonvulsant properties. Alternatively, carbamazepine may be used (see chapter XXV; sect. 3.4).

5. Manic-Depressive Disorder

The bizarre increase in psychomotor activity, grandiosity and emotional lability which characterise the manic state are dramatic and tragic symptoms. In its extreme guise, a manic attack is clearly recognisable as abnormal; many of those afflicted with the disorder can recognise its onset. Milder forms of mania, often called hypomania, are less easily recognised as abnormal.

Manic attacks may occur repetitively with relatively normal intervals between, or more commonly may occur in cycles alternating with depression, the so called manic-depressive psychosis. Mania may often be part of the presenting picture of schizophrenia, and some confusion between manic-depressive psychosis and schizophrenia has long existed. Patients who have initially presented as being purely manic have eventually been diagnosed as schizophrenic. Recently the opposite sequence has been described. As yet, no pathogenetic mechanism of manic disorders is known. Mania has been aggravated by treatment which increases dopaminergic activity, as with levodopa. It has been alleviated, at least temporarily, by increasing cholinergic activity, as with injections of physostigmine (Davis et al., 1978). Thus, these two neurotransmitters seem to be involved, but their relative contribution, as opposed to still other neurotransmitters, is still uncertain.

5.1 Manic Phase

Lithium is almost universally accepted as the preferred treatment, especially in the manic phase (American Psychiatric Association, 1975). Because the onset of its full therapeutic effect is slow, concomitant treatment with antipsychotic drugs or electroconvulsive therapy is desirable for severely manic patients. The choice of antipsychotic drug might be any preferred by the clinician, although haloperidol has an excellent reputation. Initial doses of the antipsychotic might be parenteral to ensure the most rapid control of the patient. Doses would depend on the clinical response, and when mania becomes manageable, the antipsychotic drug might be discontinued. For lesser degrees of mania. lithium alone is adequate. The more typical the presentation of manic-depressive disorder and the more assured the diagnosis, the better the response. With these provisos, the overall success rate for the manic phase of this

Table VII. Summary of principles of use of lithium in manic-depressive disorder

---

1. Manic phase
    a) Slow onset until therapeutic plasma concentrations of lithium have been established [0.8 to 1.0mmol(mEq)/L]
    b) May require concomitant antipsychotic drugs early
    c) Divided doses. Gradual increase to optimum dose in elderly; obtain baseline creatinine clearance
    d) Monitor plasma concentrations frequently (see section 5.3, 5.4, table VIII)

2. Prevention of recurrence
    a) Rarely requires antipsychotic drugs, may require tricyclic antidepressant for depressive episodes
    b) Plasma concentrations about 0.8 to 1.0mmol/L, adjusted to lower level or upper level of 1.2mmol/L as necessary (see section 5.2 to 5.4, table VIII)
    c) Doses need to be divided
    d) Side effects appear at over 1.5mEq/L concentrations; toxicity at 2.0 to 2.5mEq/L or more (see section 5.4)
    e) Monitor renal function periodically in all patients and investigate closely those with impaired glomerular function and/or urine concentrating ability

---

disorder is estimated to be around 80% in attaining remission. The principles of use of lithium in manic-depressive psychosis are summarised in table VII.

The initial dosage of lithium (usually as the carbonate) is of the order of 900mg, increasing to 1200 to 1800mg the next day, with adjustment thereafter in the range of 600 to 3,600mg per day depending upon the patient's course. Plasma concentrations should be monitored after the first 2 and 5 days and then regularly (weekly decreasing to monthly) thereafter. One should strive for an initial therapeutic plasma concentration ranging between 0.8 and 1.0mmol(mEq)/litre 12 hours after the previous dose (Prien et al., 1972; Amdisen, 1977). Levels less than the lower limit are not fully effective while nothing seems to be gained by exceeding the upper limit and more importantly incur the very real risk of causing incipient lithium toxicity (see section 5.4). As the patient comes under control, doses may be reduced to produce lower plasma concentrations, usually about two-thirds the level required to attain remission. The long plasma half-life of lithium makes single daily dose administration of the drug possible, but is not feasible because of gastrointestinal intolerance and particularly because excessive peak concentrations which follow single doses expose the distal nephron to unacceptably high concentrations (see section 1.5.4). Conventional tablets should therefore be given 3 or 4 times daily. Sustained release preparations are available in some countries and can be used for twice daily dose administration but an appropriately formulated tablet of suitable release rate must be used and some patients experience diarrhoea with sustained release preparations (Amdisen, 1977; Fyro et al., 1970). Precision in dosage by both doctor and patient is of paramount importance as serious toxicity occurs with plasma concentrations not far removed from the upper limit of the desired therapeutic range (see section 5.4).

5.2 Prevention of Recurrences

Lithium is also the treatment of choice in preventing recurrences of manic-depressive disorder (Baastrup et al., 1970; American Psychiatric Association, 1975). Still, this does not mean that every patient treated for an episode of this illness must be treated for the remainder of his life, nor that everyone so treated will remain well. The decision to use lithium as a prophylactic treatment depends on many factors: the frequency and severity of previous episodes, a crescendo pattern of appearance, and the degree to which the patient is willing to follow and understand a programme of indefinite maintenance therapy. If the present attack was the patient's first, one might prefer to terminate treatment after it subsided. The next attack may recur in a few months, or not for a few decades, and it might be wise to determine the pattern. Anyone with a frequency of one or more episodes of illness a year might be considered to be a prime candidate for maintenance treatment. Even so, if the patient is not reliable, efforts might be better spent to alert him or his family to the initial signs of recurrence and provision of prompt treatment when the disorder recurs. Some patients with mania voluntarily discontinue treatment, for they feel their spirits and initiative are suppressed by lithium.

In general, control with lithium is effective in about 60 to 70% of cases (Baldessarini and Lipinski, 1975). Failure of maintenance treatment is most apt to occur with the most serious forms of the disorder, that is, in those patients with multiple and severe recurrences. A poor prior res-

ponse to lithium also augurs poorly for maintenance therapy. Fortunately, patients who can maintain themselves on a programme of treatment for a year without further episodes seem to have a good long term prognosis. Some clinicians find that depressive episodes during typical bipolar illness may respond better by addition of a tricyclic antidepressant to lithium maintenance during this period (Fieve et al., 1976).

The prophylactic dose of lithium may be established by using an initial blood level of 0.8 to 1.0mmol(mEq)/litre as a guide, with subsequent dose adjustment as required to a lower level or an upper level around 1.2mmol/L; plasma concentrations should be monitored after the first week following a low starting dose, and regularly thereafter to establish and follow the desired therapeutic range (Amdisen, 1977). The daily dose may be as low as 300mg but will usually be between 600 and 1,500mg per day. In the outpatient phase of treatment, the patient should be urged to take his medication faithfully (since relapses have occurred after years when medication was interrupted) and precisely as prescribed (since toxicity can be just a few mmol/litre away — see section 5.4). An extra tablet or two when the patient feels it is advisable may prove just enough to bring on toxic symptoms.

5.3 Lithium Plasma Concentrations and Clinical Response

Monitoring of lithium therapy by plasma level estimations 12 hours after the last dose is a simple and important guide to assessing the dose required for satisfactory treatment of acute mania and as a safety monitor in long term prophylactic treatment (see Amdisen, 1975, 1977). The desirable therapeutic plasma ranges are not absolute and must be viewed in the light of what is happening clinically (Strayhorn and Nash, 1977), particularly in regard to those factors which can influence plasma levels (table VIII). It is important to realise that plasma levels of lithium can change quickly when doses are omitted or taken irregularly (Crammer et al., 1974). Thus a blood test taken at the wrong time after the expected last dose of lithium can be misleading. In practice, one should not hesitate to increase doses of lithium if the patient has not responded and shows no major toxic symptoms, even though the present plasma levels are at the upper limit. Conversely, a patient doing well, even though his plasma level was less

Table VIII. Factors which affect plasma concentrations of lithium (Amdisen, 1977; Cramer et al., 1974; Hansen and Amdisen, 1978)

Factor	Effect[1]
Renal function	Increased plasma concentration with impaired renal function (NB elderly)
Sodium balance (extremes of sodium intake or loss)	Increased plasma concentrations due to decreased renal clearance with sodium loss (e.g. excessive sweating in hot weather, persistent vomiting, persistent diarrhoea, intercurrent infection, long term diuretics, reducing diet, low sodium diet). Decreased plasma concentrations due to increased renal clearance with increased sodium intake
Patient compliance	Irregularity in taking medication (omission, or doubling of dose when not 'feeling' well or to 'catch up')
Gastric emptying rate[1]	Delayed gastric emptying slows absorption and may decrease peak levels. Increased gastric emptying hastens absorption and time of peak plasma levels
Gastrointestinal function	Individual variation in plasma concentrations and changes in plasma levels with altered gastrointestinal function (e.g. change in clinical state of patient with malabsorption syndrome)

1   Changes to plasma concentration may occur rapidly. Alteration in gastric emptying rate probably relates more to a change in plasma concentration at the time when plasma level estimations normally made than to overt risk of side effects or toxicity; most likely of importance with slow release preparations (see also section 5.3, 5.4).

than the desirable therapeutic range, is better off left alone. Whenever a question of possible toxicity arises, plasma concentrations might help settle the issue. Measurement of erythrocyte concentrations of lithium has not been widely adopted despite the fact that preliminary evidence suggests that these concentrations vary much less during a 24 hour period than the lithium concentration in the serum.

5.4 Dosage, Renal Excretion and Side Effects of Lithium

The undesired effects of lithium can be placed into two categories; one related to dose and one that is not (table IX).

Side effects can occur at any plasma concentration, but are much more apt to appear at levels above 1.5mmol(mEq)/litre. Major toxic effects of lithium are due to a decreased ability to excrete the drug as a consequence of impaired renal function or water and electrolyte loss (see section 1.5.4; Hansen and Amdisen, 1978). Under ordinary circumstances, sodium balance and urine volume are the major determinants of lithium excretion. Increased sodium intake increases lithium excretion, while sodium loss has the opposite

effect (Thomsen and Schou, 1968). Renal lesions can be a potential problem, particularly if polyuria or episodes of toxicity are allowed to occur (see section 1.5.4; table IX). All patients receiving lithium should have periodic renal function tests and those with impaired glomerular function and/or urine concentrating ability investigated closely.

Lithium intoxication may appear when the plasma level exceeds 1.5 to 2.5mmol/litre or more, particularly if exposure to such levels is prolonged. The level at which toxicity appears varies among individuals but in general, concentrations of 1.5 to 2.5mmol/L are usually accompanied by slight or moderate symptoms of intoxication while concentrations of 2.5 to 3.5mmol/L are regarded as serious and levels above 3.5mmol/L are life threatening. However, the toxic level is always close to the therapeutic range and it is particularly important not to attain excessive plasma concentrations initially or for prolonged periods, since continued lithium intake may result in accumulation and toxicity. A vicious circle may develop as a critical level of lithium *per se* in an individual patient seems to exert a nephrotoxic effect, which results in reduced renal clearance of lithium (Li^+) and despite reduction

Table IX. Side effects of lithium (see also section 5.4)

Effect	Reaction	Notes/action
Neurological and psychiatric	Tremor	Common. Can be controlled by propranolol. Occurs at usual therapeutic dose levels.
	Choreothetosis, motor hyperactivity, ataxia, dysarthria, aphasia	Occur at 'usual' therapeutic dose levels. Spread medication over full 24 hrs (i.e. change from 3 to 4 divided doses) or reduce dose
	Marked mental confusion, bizarre motor movements	
Gastrointestinal	Nausea, vomiting diarrhoea, abdominal pain	Adaptation may occur; may be due to associated gastro-intestinal disorders; fasting. Spread medication over full 24 hours if persistent problem
Thyroid	Hypothyroidism, often with goitre	May occur at low dosage, usually of late onset and reversible, or treatable with thyroxine while lithium continued (Brownlie et al., 1976; Lindstedt et al., 1977)
	Thyrotoxicosis	Less common than hypothyroidism. Late onset and reversible. Can occur in absence of goitre (Todd and Jerram, 1978; Merry, 1977)
Chronic nephropathy	Focal nephron atrophy and/or fibrosis	Prolonged treatment, especially in those with lithium in-duced nephrogenic diabetes insipidus or episodes of lithium intoxication (Hestbech et al., 1977). Lesions progress slowly and can impair the clearance of lithium
Renal tubular lesion	Mainly distal convoluted tubule and collecting ducts	Early in course of treatment (Burrows et al., 1978). All patients on lithium should have periodic renal function tests and those with impaired glomerular function and/or urine concentrating ability investigated closely
Reduced renal concentrating ability	Increased risk of water and electrolyte loss and lithium intoxication	Early in course and in association with nephropathy or renal tubular lesion. Those who become polyuric must drink plenty of fluids
Nephrogenic dia-betes insipidus	Mild intermittent thirst	Common early side effect.
	Severe persistent thirst with polyuria	Uncommon later side effect with larger doses. Symptoms of thirst and polyuria are poor indicators of reduced renal concentrating ability (Baylis and Heath, 1978) Reduce dose (patients must be advised to drink plenty of fluids); thiazide diuretic
Electrolyte and water balance	Oedema	Frequent side effect (? some effect on sodium retention).
	Weight gain	Water retention alone does not account for all of weight gain
Skin	Acneiform eruptions	Early in treatment. May or may not recur with resumption of treatment.
	Folliculitis	Asymptomatic. May recur with resumption of treatment.
Miscellaneous	T-wave abnormality	Frequent if sought carefully. ?Significance, but may be additive with other drugs (quinidine, atropine, thioridazine, tricyclic antidepressants, hydroxyzine)
	Arrhythmias	Occasional reports. Ventricular arrhythmias or sinus node abnormalities may occur or be aggravated during lithium therapy but do not contraindicate its use in those with cardiac disease in whom there are clear indications for its use (Tilkian et al., 1976)
	Erectile impotence	Uncommon

in dosage, further accumulation and toxicity (Hansen and Amdisen, 1978; table IX). Situations such as excessive sweating in hot weather, persistent vomiting or diarrhoea, intercurrent infection and long term diuretic therapy, can increase plasma concentrations by decreasing lithium clearance and may lead to toxic symptoms if dosage is not adjusted.

The central nervous system is the chief target. The initial symptoms usually present several days before more serious ones appear, and include drowsiness, muscle twitching or coarse tremors, and slurred speech. When unmodified administration of the drug has been continued, most likely in the presence of impaired renal function or water and electrolyte loss, the initial toxic manifestations have been followed by retching, tremor, cog wheel rigidity, myoclonic contractions and death from pulmonary complications. Prompt treatment will minimise problems and consists of supportive measures and attempts to remove lithium. Saline infusion with or without forced alkaline diuresis is only adequate in patients with early symptoms of lithium intoxication and normal renal function. Dialysis, particularly haemodialysis, is the most effective method of removing lithium. Prevention requires assessment of renal function and renal concentrating ability during therapy, regular monitoring of plasma lithium concentration and thorough training of staff, patient and family so that early manifestations of serious difficulties may lead promptly to further investigations. For a review of lithium intoxication, see Hansen and Amdisen (1978).

Toxic situations require special attention in patients being considered for lithium treatment. The presence of renal (especially a reduced glomerular filtrate rate) or cardiovascular diseases (especially heart failure) may so interfere with excretion or so alter electrolytes (as a result of low sodium intake) that the medication may present undue hazards. However, careful dose adjustment and regular monitoring of plasma concentrations and renal function allow lithium to be used in those patients who have clear indications for its use. Thiazide diuretics can also be used, provided dosage of lithium is reduced and plasma concentrations assessed regularly (Himmelhoch et al., 1977). Advanced age also warrants special care, since the ability to excrete lithium declines with age and an effective dose therefore may be much less in the elderly than in the younger person (see section 1.5.4). It is wise to increase the dose at a less rapid rate in searching for the optimum level in the older patient. Possible drug interactions with lithium are given in appendix C.

5.5 Lithium in Pregnancy and the Puerperium

Concern that lithium might cause dysmorphogenesis has led to the establishment of international registries of lithium babies. Some reports suggest that the prevalence of malformations noted is not appreciably higher than might be expected from such retrospective analyses (Schou, 1976). Other studies suggest the possibility of an alarming increase in the frequency of cardiac anomalies, especially the Ebstein anomaly, in lithium babies (Weinstein and Goldfield, 1975; Rane et al., 1978). At the moment one must revert to the old cover: don't use any drug in pregnancy unless it is of proven benefit and the need is essential (see chapter XV; sect. 2.1).

Renal clearance of lithium increases during pregnancy and reverts to a lower rate immediately after delivery (Schou et al., 1973; see chapter XV, sect. 1.1.4). A patient whose plasma lithium concentration is in a good therapeutic range during pregnancy may develop toxic levels following delivery if dosage is not reduced. Special care and more frequent monitoring of lithium levels is needed at these times. Lithium is transferred to breast fed infants through breast milk, and attains a concentration in serum of the infants about one-fifth to two-thirds that of maternal serum (Schou and Amdisen, 1973). The phenomenon of lithium toxicity in newborns is manifested by lethargy, cyanosis, poor suck and Moro reflexes, and possibly hepatomegaly. Rules for treating pregnant women with lithium include close monitoring of plasma levels to keep them at the low end of the therapeutic range, avoidance of salt restriction or diuretics, giving regular small doses, and discouraging breast feeding (Goldfield and Weinstein, 1973).

6. Schizoaffective Disorders

These disorders are characterised by a mixture of schizophrenic symptoms and altered affect, either in the form of depression or excitement. They are not easily distinguished from psychotic depressions or the manic phase of manic-depressive disorder. The preponderance of evidence suggests that antipsychotic drugs are the preferred treatment. Some mildly excited patients respond to lithium alone and some respond better to combined treatment. The possibility has been raised that concurrent lithium treatment may reduce the need for antipsychotic drugs.

7. Depressive Illness

Depression and anxiety are inextricable and the diagnosis of depression is difficult and often missed (Davies, 1973). Making the diagnosis of depression however, is not enough.

Firstly, one must try to classify the depression. One must rule out causes of secondary depressions, such as physical illnesses, psychiatric disorders (e.g. early stages of senile brain disease) or therapeutic drugs (see section 15.2). Reactive depressions may be precipitated by some adverse life experience, the usual key word being 'loss'. The loss may be of any type and often is idiosyncratic in its meaning to the patient. Reactive or secondary depressions are the most common and are characterised clinically by the core depression syndrome and may vary from mild to severe in degree. Tender loving care, psychotherapy, or manipulation of the patient's environment may be adequate for many such depressions. Those related directly to life experiences often resolve spontaneously (Hollister et al., 1967).

Endogenous depressions respond more specifically to drugs since they probably represent a genetic biochemical abnormality that affects the individual's ability to cope (see section 1.4.2). Such depressions may occur at any age, but most often in middle years of life. As with reactive depressions a precipitating factor in the patient's life may be identified; however, in the former, the response is appropriate, whereas in endogenous depressions it is often inappropriate. Despite remissions, endogenous depression is a relapsing disorder, so that most patients will experience multiple episodes of depression after the initial attack. Maintenance treatment to prevent recurrence is sometimes necessary.

Least common are depressions associated with manic-depressive disorder, an entity which is also believed to be a genetically determined biochemical abnormality. The depressed phase may be indistinguishable from that of endogenous depression. The presence of attacks of mania or hypomania is the key to its diagnosis. The preferred treatment is lithium (see section 5).

Secondly, one must decide on the desirable approach to treatment. Does the patient merit treatment as an inpatient under the care of a psychiatrist or as an outpatient under the care of a non-psychiatric clinician? What factors suggest that treatment should be urgent? What is the possible risk of suicide? What is the natural history of the disorder? Have there been previous episodes of depression or mania? How were they manifested? How long did they last? What method of treatment may be best right now (Ashcroft, 1975): psychotherapy, antidepressant drugs, electroconvulsive therapy, or some combination of two or more? It is likely that all depressions, even those with a strong biological basis, can benefit from the use of psychotherapy. The latter is not of much use when the patient is severely depressed but is more productive after some amelioration of the depression. Thus, where indicated initial treatment might best be pharmacological followed by appropriate psychotherapy. Electroconvulsive therapy is indicated for depressed patients who are at risk for committing suicide or for those patients who have failed to respond to drug therapy. Each of these non-drug treatments can be used advantageously combined with drug treatment.

7.1 Choice of Antidepressant

In selecting drugs for depressed patients one should be prepared to use a range of agents depending on the presenting depressive syndrome (table X). If symptoms are primarily bodily complaints, anxiety and tension, then treatment with antianxiety drugs may suffice, not only to relieve the attendant symptoms but also the depression. Accompanying symptoms of severe anxiety or agitation, as in the 'agitated' depression, may require an antipsychotic drug. Not all depressions require 'antidepressants'. Whenever the issue is in doubt about whether anxiety or depression is the primary disorder, an initial trial of treatment with an antidepressant might be the best strategy. If the patient does not really need the antidepressant the drug will be poorly tolerated at usual therapeutic doses. Then the switch can be made to an antianxiety drug.

The classical retarded or endogenous depression constitutes a clear indication for tricyclic antidepressants and is the type of depression most likely to respond well to these drugs. Controlled comparisons of the tricyclics have usually concluded that they are approximately equivalent

Table X. Choice of treatment for depression

---

1. Mild reactive or secondary depression
   a) 'Benign neglect'
   b) Supportive psychotherapy
   c) Brief course of dextroamphetamine or methylphenidate in secondary depressions (e.g. following physical illness)

2. Moderate to severe depression of known or unknown cause, with symptoms of:
   a) Anxiety — chlordiazepoxide, diazepam
   b) Severe anxiety or agitation — thioridazine, acetophenazine, thiothixene
   c) Retardation (endogenous depression) — tricyclics; MAO inhibitors in failures only
   d) Psychosis — amitriptyline-perphenazine combination

3. Severe depression with suicidal risk
   a) ECT
   b) Appropriate drug to follow

---

drugs (Rogers and Clay, 1975; Morris and Beck, 1974). While this may be the case in groups of patients, it does not necessarily hold for individual patients. Individual patients may fare better on one drug than on another, for reasons which are uncertain. Finding the right drug for the patient is accomplished empirically at the moment. Some have averred that sedative tricyclics, such as amitriptyline or doxepin, are the preferred drugs for patients with high levels of anxiety or agitation and with multiple somatic complaints including sleep disorders, while those with the least sedative action, such as desipramine and protriptyline, may be preferred in patients with psychomotor retardation. Much of this distinction is based on speculation rather than on firm clinical or experimental data.

The past history of the patient's drug experience, if available, should be used as the major guide. At times, such history may lead to the exclusion of tricyclics, as in patients who may have responded well in the past to monoamine oxidase inhibitors.

Experimental work suggests that determination of urinary excretion of 3-methoxy-4-hydroxyphenylglycol (MHPG) may prove to be an effective guide to the type of drug to use in a particular patient, since some patients may suffer endogenous depression due primarily to a deficiency of noradrenergic transmission whereas others may primarily be deficient in serotoninergic transmission (Maas, 1975). Such procedures are

not ready for clinical use (see also section 1.4.2). Failing that, one can still take advantage of some of the pharmacological differences between tricyclics to plan a logical sequence of drugs to be tried. A tertiary amine such as amitriptyline or imipramine should probably be the first drug tried for, due to the formation of an active metabolite, 2 drugs are present (see section 1.5.2). Further, it is possible that depressions based on deficiency of serotoninergic neurotransmission may be more frequent than those due to deficiency of noradrenaline (norepinephrine). Amitriptyline is the most commonly used tertiary amine and of the tricyclics is considered to be the most specific inhibitor of the amine pump for serotonin, as it is less readily converted to its secondary amine metabolite than is imipramine; the metabolite of which desipramine, more selectively blocks the noradrenaline pump mechanism (section 1.4.2). However, imipramine may substitute for amitriptyline in patients who obtain a favourable therapeutic response but who complain of excessive sedation or anticholinergic side effects (table XIIa).

Should amitriptyline not provide the desired results, one might move to a drug that is least like it. Desipramine fits these requirements. It is believed to act almost exclusively on the amine pump for noradrenaline, so that it would stand at the opposite pole from amitriptyline in terms of its effect on the presumed pathogenetic mechanisms of depression. It is also the tricyclic with the least sedative and anticholinergic effects. Drugs such as doxepin (Pinder et al., 1977) or the newer non-tricyclic compounds mianserin (Brogden et al., 1978) and nomifensine (Brogden et al., 1979) are probably better tolerated by the cardiovascular system and might be preferred in the elderly and in those with cardiovascular disease. Those drugs such as doxepin and mianserin which do not affect the noradrenaline pump mechanism are indicated in depressions associated with use of adrenergic neurone blocking antihypertensive drugs (see section 7.6).

Monoamine oxidase (MAO) inhibitors are helpful in particular patients. Such patients have been described as having 'atypical' depressions (Johnson, 1975), which scarcely helps in their identification. Depressed patients with considerable attendant anxiety, phobic features and hypochondriasis are the ones who do best on these drugs (Tyrer, 1976). Either phenelzine or tranylcypromine may be used, following the trial of tricyclic antidepressants. Clinical opinion is divided as to whether MAO inhibitors should be used in combination with tricyclics or alone. By phasing them into an ongoing programme of treatment with tricyclics, one can see if the combination works. If it does, one can phase out the tricyclic to see if the MAO inhibitor alone has produced the improvement. Such use of MAO inhibitors is risky (see section 7.6) and experimental, but is practical in treatment failures (Goldberg and Thornton, 1978), except if the patient's incapacity and suffering and risk of suicide were a cause for concern when electroconvulsive therapy is indicated.

Severe depression is one of the few psychiatric disorders with a fatality rate (Guze and Robins, 1970). Depression is often thought to represent hostility, directed inward, against oneself. Self destruction is the ultimate act of such hostility. To temporise with drug therapy and not to offer ECT that has been proven to be rapidly effective in a high percentage of patients is to risk disaster. Appropriate drug therapy can be used concurrently, there being some reason for believing that such combined treatment may reduce both the course of shock therapy required to attain a remission, as well as sustain it longer (Turek, 1973). Occasionally, one might wish to use one of the benzodiazepines in patients who are less seriously depressed, in whom tricyclic antidepressants alone do not manage the often stubborn problem of insomnia. The benzodiazepines have no discernible effects on plasma levels of nortriptyline or amitriptyline. Thus, there is no reason to fear using these drugs concurrently *when they are indicated*. The same situation applies to use of antipsychotics (see section 3.3). The principles of use of antidepressant drugs are summarised in table XI and discussed further below (see also Hollister, 1972b; 1978a,b; Shaw, 1977).

7.2 Doses and Dose Schedules of Antidepressants

Doses of tricyclics have been largely determined empirically; the patient's tolerance of the medication is often the limiting factor (Johnson, 1974). Tolerance to some of the objectionable side effects develops, so the usual pattern of treatment has been to start with small doses increasing either to a predetermined daily dose, or to one that produces relief of depression, or to the maximum tolerated dose. Effective doses of the major tricyclics range between 50 and 600mg daily, de-

Table XI. Summary of principles of use of antidepressants

---

1. Do not neglect other therapies
   a) ECT may save a life in a severe suicidal depression
   b) 'Psychotherapy' (of many different types) may be useful
   c) Environmental alteration sometimes helpful

2. Be aware of possibly limiting pharmacological actions
   a) Tricyclics have strong anticholinergic effects which may limit dose; also may be sedative for some individuals
   b) MAO inhibitors — dangerous interactions with sympathomimetic amines and foods rich in tyramine or dopamine

3. Choice of drug is largely empirical
   a) Based on depressive syndrome and pharmacological differences between drugs
   b) Past experience of patient is always the best guide

4. Doses must be individualised
   a) No set dose. Wide variations in plasma concentrations among individuals on same dose.
   b) Dose to attain therapeutic benefit or limited by side effects (side effects may limit dose but are not necessarily secure guides of adequacy of dose).
   c) Conservative doses should be used in the elderly (say a reduction from usual doses by about a half to a third)

5. Dosage schedules need not be traditional
   a) Small initially divided doses provide rapid titration and avoid intolerance, but
   b) Later, doses may be less frequent and once daily
   c) Should see some effect in 2 to 3 weeks; if not, assuming diagnosis correct, consider alternatives; 3 weeks at a reasonable dose (usually 150mg daily) is a minimum therapeutic trial

6. Duration of treatment depends on natural history of disorder
   a) Treatment may be tapered gradually and eventually discontinued after a few months in those with first episode of depression, and:
   b) Relapses may be treated episodically
   c) Treatment may need to be continued in those with history of prior attacks of depression (e.g. attack one of a series becoming more frequent, more severe or more refractory to treatment)
   d) Maintenance doses are much lower than full therapeutic doses

---

pending upon many factors (Hollister, 1977). Undertreatment has been thought to be a frequent cause for an apparent failure of drug therapy to relieve depression, with unwanted side effects limiting dosage more than might have been really necessary (Tyrer, 1978; Kline, 1974). Monitoring of plasma concentrations of tricyclics may soon become clinically feasible, and might be a guide to undertreatment, non-compliance or the elucidation of possible adverse reactions (see section 1.6.3).

A daily dose of 150mg is a reasonable goal for treatment of most patients. Most patients attain steady-state plasma concentrations of the drug that are in the presumed therapeutic range at this dose. Treatment may begin with a daily dose of 50mg with increases of 25mg daily or less often to a dose of 150mg daily by the end of 7 to 10 days. After 2 weeks of treatment with this dose, the patient should be re-evaluated. If response is less than desired and the dose is tolerable, then further gradual increments of 25mg every 2 to 3 days should be added until either a therapeutic response is seen, or side effects become intolerable, or a ceiling dose of 300mg is reached. These doses and all others mentioned in this section do not apply to protriptyline or the newer antidepressants (see table XII).

One should remember that interpatient variability in rate of biotransformation and bioavailability of these drugs is axiomatic (see section 1.5.2). One simply cannot establish any standardised scheme nor follow slavishly the recommendations of the package label. The dosage schedule outlined above represents the worst possibility; that of a patient who may require large doses to have an adequate trial of treatment. Many patients do well with less drug, while others will be unable to take such large doses safely. Some patients tolerate a tricyclic drug well at daily doses of 300mg and have no signs of toxicity (one might look at the ECG for evidence of prolonged cardiac conduction times and T-wave abnormalities), yet are refractory to treatment. In such cases, the dose may be increased to as much as 600mg daily (Schuckit and Feighner, 1972). Patients who fail to respond adequately to these very large doses should be re-evaluated and the diagnosis reconsidered before a change is made to another drug or treatment (see above). Older persons show less extensive protein binding of the drug than do young adults, as well as a slower rate of metabolism of the drug (Nies et al., 1977); both factors argue for much smaller doses than one would give a fairly robust person in the fourth decade of life. A reduction from usual doses by about a half to a third would seem reasonable in the elderly (see section 1.5.2). The dose for children should not exceed 2.5mg/kg/day under any circumstances (Robinson and Barker, 1976).

Table XII. Chemical classes and dosage guide for antidepressants

Class and drug	Total daily dosage in mg[1]	
	outpatient range	hospital range
Tricyclic derivatives		
Amitriptyline	50-150	75-300
Nortriptyline	50-150	50-200
Protriptyline	10-40	15-60
Imipramine	50-150	75-300
Desipramine	75-150	75-300
Trimipramine	50-150	75-300
Clomipramine	75-200	75-300
Doxepin	75-150	75-300
Maprotiline	75-200	150-300
Tetracyclic derivatives		
Mianserin	30-80	30-120
Modified cyclic derivatives		
Nomifensine	50-150	75-200
Viloxazine	150-300	150-400
Hydrazide MAO inhibitors		
Isocarboxazid	10-30	10-50
Nialamide	25-75	100-450
Phenelzine	15-45	45-90
Non-hydrazide MAO inhibitors		
Tranylcypromine	20-30	20-30
Stimulants		
Dextroamphetamine	5-15	10-30
Methamphetamine	2.5-10	10-20
Methylphenidate	10-30	20-60

1   Rough guide only (see section 1.5.2, 7.2).

A single daily dose may be given rather than the traditional practice of equally divided doses several times daily (Ayd, 1974). The plasma half-life of these drugs is generally in the order of 24 hours or more (table I), so that a once daily dosage schedule is feasible from that consideration alone for most antidepressants (see section 1.5.2). Doses are best given 2 or 3 hours before the patient's customary bedtime. The sedative and anticholinergic side effects will be less bothersome at this time of day. Drugs such as amitriptyline, trimipramine, doxepin and mianserin are highly sedative; imipramine is less so; the demethylated metabolites of amitriptyline and imipramine, nortriptyline and desipramine, are less sedative than the parent compounds; protriptyline is the only drug that has little apparent sedative action.

The principle of dosage with MAO inhibitors is quite different. A large loading dose is used right off, and then the optimum smaller daily dose to attain maximum therapeutic effects found, with the endpoint perhaps monitored by evidence of sympathetic inhibition such as orthostatic hypotension, slowed heart rate, increased bowel sounds. As these drugs are intrinsically very long acting, due to their irreversible inhibition of the enzyme, single daily doses given in the morning should suffice. Dosage of phenelzine should take into account its genetically determined metabolism by acetylation, since its effects are possibly dependent on acetylator status; slow acetylators in some studies showing a better response than fast acetylators given the same dose (Johnstone, 1976; see also chapter VII, sect. 4.2.1).

When sympathetic stimulants are used for treating depression, a single morning dose may suffice. These drugs are fairly long acting, so that doses later in the day may interfere with sleep. Generally, the starting dose should be the smallest possible to attain benefit, possibly no more than 5mg of dextroamphetamine or 10mg of methylphenidate. Any side effects of weight loss (unless this is desired as well) or insomnia are indications for stopping treatment or reducing the dose. Treatment might be given in a brief course of 7 to 10 days, interrupted by at least equivalent periods, if it must be continued longer.

7.3 Onset of Effect of Antidepressants

It is often averred that tricyclic antidepressants take a long time to work, which may be true if doses are conservative and increments infrequent. With close attention to regulating doses, steady-state plasma concentrations in the therapeutic ranges of tricyclics and tetracyclics such as mianserin should be reached fairly quickly.

The first symptom to show improvement may be a return to a more normal sleep pattern. Improvement in nervousness, somatic complaints, appetite and motor activity may follow. The patient is often less aware of improvement than those around him. Therefore, one should enlist the help of those in close contact with the patient as observers of his progress. Full remission of a depressed mood may be slow (Oswald et al., 1972). Nevertheless, some benefits, if they are to occur at all, should be seen within a week or two. Should none be apparent by 3 weeks, assuming that one has scrupulously attempted to find the proper dose and the diagnosis is correct, serious consideration should be given to using another tricyclic drug or another treatment. Morbidity among depressed patients, unlike schizophrenics,

is an important consideration. One should strive to reduce the time the patient is disabled, as many depressed patients have responsibilities and must return quickly to their jobs, their businesses, their professions or their families. Clinical experience with the demethylated compounds (e.g. desipramine, nortriptyline) suggests that they are not more rapid acting or superior to the parent drugs, if indeed they are not less effective.

7.4 Maintenance Treatment

Assuming that a satisfactory degree of remission is attained from drug therapy, then how long should it be continued? The best guide would seem to be the patient's past history of depression (Davis, 1976). If the attack of depression was mild, quick to respond, and the first one requiring treatment, one might be tempted to taper off treatment within several weeks after remission was attained. During this period, the clinician should be especially alert to any signs of relapse, which might then require a slower pace of discontinuing treatment. That more treatment may be required is highly probable, for relapse in depressed patients is common. The decision in this case would be to treat the illness episodically. On the other hand, if the attack of depression was one of a series which were becoming more frequent, more severe, and more refractory to treatment, maintenance therapy for months or even years, might be considered. Patients have been maintained free of depression on very small doses (usually given once daily at night) of tricyclic antidepressants, but who experience a rapid recrudescence of symptoms when attempts are made to discontinue the drug. Sometimes doses as low as 25 to 50mg of a tricyclic daily may suffice. The natural history of a disorder is the best guide to prognosis, as well as choice of treatment. Those close to the patient should be instructed in how to detect early signs of relapse since the patient himself may be a poor judge of that.

Maintenance treatment with lithium is effective in preventing recurrent depressions in patients with manic-depressive disorder (see section 5.2) as well as those with endogenous depression, but whether it is preferable to tricyclics in long term maintenance of patients with endogenous depression is not clear (Prien and Caffey, 1977). As patients with endogenous depression will have been treated with tricyclics, it would seem reasonable to let the treatment continue rather

Table XIIa. Some pharmacological action differences (relative effects) between some tricyclic antidepressants (after Hollister, 1978b)

Drug	Sedation	Anticholinergic effects	Block of amine pump	
			for serotonin	for noradrenaline
Imipramine	++	++	++	++
Amitriptyline	+++	+++	+++	+
Desipramine	+	+	0	+++
Nortriptyline	++	++	+	++
Doxepin	+++	+++	0	±
Protriptyline	0	++	?	?

than to make a switch to lithium. With manic-depressive disorder, lithium is the principal treatment regardless of which affective disturbance predominates and would be the logical choice for maintenance treatment.

7.5 Side Effects and Complications of Antidepressants

7.5.1 Therapeutic Doses

Many of the side effects of antidepressants are extensions of their pharmacological actions. The dry mouth or blurred vision produced by the peripheral anticholinergic actions of tricyclics and MAO inhibitors may be managed by such simple expedients as hard candy or magnifying lenses. Sweating, constipation and delayed ejaculation are other common unwanted effects on the autonomic nervous system. More serious side effects, such as urinary retention or paralytic ileus, require immediate medical attention and possibly treatment with a peripherally acting cholinergic drug such as bethanechol (Everett, 1975). One may often think that a formerly depressed patient is really psychotic when he merely suffers a toxic delirium due to the treatment. Toxic delirium and postural hypotension is especially a hazard in the elderly with both the tricyclics and MAO inhibitors (see section 11). Tremor occurs frequently at therapeutic doses of tricyclics; treatment with propranolol has been tried with varying success. Just as with the phenothiazines, tricyclic antidepressants have been reported to cause cholestatic jaundice and agranulocytosis. Both of these complications however, are rare. Weight gain is frequent with the tricyclics, just as it is with the phenothiazines (see chapter XVI; sect. 14.4).

The cardiac abnormalities produced by tricyclics are matters of concern (Jefferson, 1975), but have probably been overemphasised with normal therapeutic doses in patients without significant heart disease. Nonspecific T-wave changes, somewhat similar to those observed with some phenothiazines, are seen in many patients but return to normal during the course of long term (months) treatment (Burckhardt et al., 1978). Disturbances of cardiac rate, rhythm and conduction are frequent complications of overdoses and are also seen in patients with hypertension and/or a recent history of myocardial infarction. The mechanism may involve the anticholinergic and quinidine-like effects of the tricyclic drugs. They also inhibit the uptake of catecholamines by the adrenergic neuron (see section 1.4.2), leading to a high concentration of circulating catecholamines. Guanethidine-type drugs also gain access to the adrenergic neuron by this same uptake mechanism and cardiac standstill has been reported in a patient who had previously been pretreated with guanethidine (see also section 7.5). Tricyclic antidepressants should be used cautiously and in conservative doses in a patient with hypertension and/or myocardial insufficiency. The lowering of blood pressure produced by these drugs could be due to a combination of peripheral adrenergic blocking action as well as a decreased inotropic action on the heart. Newer agents such as mianserin and nomifensine appear to be better tolerated in this respect (Brogden et al., 1978; Brogden et al., 1979).

7.5.2 Toxic Doses

It would be quite fitting if drugs used for treating depressed patients, where suicide is an ever present danger, should be as safe as the antipsychotics. Unfortunately, with the tricyclic antidepressants this is not the case and self poisoning with these drugs has become frequent. Doses of imipramine or amitriptyline in excess of 1.2g are seriously toxic, with fatalities in adults fairly common after ingestion of 2.5g or more. Small doses of the range of 75 to 100mg may however, produce dangerous toxicity in infants and a fatality has been recorded with 350mg imipramine (Bickel, 1975). A decreasing level of consciousness leading to coma is regularly observed; early, this may be preceded by agitation or delirium. Some patients with tricyclic overdosage present fully alert and conscious only to lapse into coma within a few hours. All patients should probably be admitted to an intensive care unit for observation. The newer antidepressants such as mianserin and nomifensine do not cause the severe complications which characterise overdosage with tricyclic antidepressants and seem less likely to cause serious cardiotoxicity on overdosage (Brogden et al., 1978, 1979).

The diagnostic triad of coma, seizures and cardiac arrhythmias should raise the suspicion of tricyclic antidepressant overdose if a verified history of drug intake is lacking (Jefferson, 1975). Cardiac arrhythmias and conduction abnormalities are the major distinguishing feature. A trial of intravenously administered doses of physostigmine, 1 to 4mg, may suggest the diagnosis by awakening the patient, but there must be the usual preparedness for cardiac complications (Newton, 1975; Aquilonius and Hedstrand, 1978). The effects of physostigmine are transient and it is not a definitive treatment (see chapter IX; sect. 3.3). Other problems encountered in such poisonings include neuromuscular irritability, delirium, hyperpyrexia, hypotension and bladder or bowel paralysis.

The cardiac arrhythmias are life threatening so that the patient must be closely monitored with facilities available for resuscitation (Vohra et al., 1975). Drugs such as quinidine and procainamide are contraindicated, but lignocaine (lidocaine), propranolol and phenytoin have been used safely and effectively. Arterial blood gases and pH, and electrolytes should be monitored to avoid metabolic acidosis or hypokalaemia which aggravates the arrhythmias further. Electrical pacing may be required when antiarrhythmic drugs fail.

Other treatment is supportive and symptomatic. Attempts should be made to remove the drug even hours after ingestion; activated charcoal may prevent further absorption. Ventilatory support is critical. Shock should be treated only with fluids or plasma expanders; tricyclics cause potentiation of sympathomimetic drugs, which should

be avoided. Hyperpyrexia is treated by cooling. Seizures may be managed by intravenous doses of diazepam.

Determination of plasma concentrations of drug may be helpful in checking progress of treatment but are most valuable as the patient shows signs of improvement (Spiker and Biggs, 1976). Some patients have died of late complications because of relaxed vigilance. Plasma concentrations of drug may help one to assess this risk better than clinical signs, which may be misleading at this late stage. Patients should not be discharged until they have returned to their normal state for a day or two.

7.6 Drug Interactions with Antidepressants

Interaction between tricyclic antidepressants and adrenergic neurone blocking antihypertensive drugs such as guanethidine, bethanidine and debrisoquine was, until the advent of β-adrenoceptor blocking drugs for hypertension, one of the most common and predictable drug interactions encountered in clinical practice (Stafford and Fann, 1977; Simpson, 1973b). It is important because the interaction invariably leads to loss of blood pressure control or even a marked rise in blood pressure, and because it is not uncommon for hypertensive patients to be considered for antidepressant therapy, either for endogenous depression or depression induced by the antihypertensive drugs (Simpson and Waal-Manning, 1971). However, since the introduction of newer antihypertensive drugs, the interaction can be avoided (see chapter XVIII; sect. 10.1.3). The tricyclic antidepressants have an increased risk of causing paralytic ileus and CNS depressant effects when given with alcohol. The risk of excessive sedation and impaired psychomotor performance is greatest in the first few days of therapy and has particularly been noted with amitriptyline (Patman et al., 1969; Seppala, 1977). The risk of troublesome anticholinergic effects in the elderly is increased if tricyclics are given with other anticholinergic drugs (e.g. peptic ulcer therapy, some antihistamines, anti-Parkinsonian drugs etc). Although the therapeutic efficacy of tricyclics might be increased by thyroid drugs (Prange et al., 1969), the risk of cardiovascular complications may also be increased and such a combination is an experimental manoeuvre not to be widely adopted clinically.

The unexpected interactions between the MAO inhibitors and certain drugs and foods first focussed attention on the problem of multiple drug therapy (Sjoqvist, 1965), and the hazards of MAOI's in this regard, have since largely militated against their widespread use. The *extent* of the risk of interactions, particularly with tricyclic anti-depressants and foods, has however, been over-emphasised. Indeed, MAO inhibitors and tricyclic antidepressants can be effectively and safely used together (see section 7.1), provided both drugs are started simultaneously, are given orally, and the dose of each is lower than when used alone, or treatment is started with a tricyclic and an MAO inhibitor is added later, but never *vice versa*. The most important interaction is with sym-pathomimetic amines (e.g. anorexiants, common cold remedies) or foodstuffs *rich* in tyramine (e.g. yeast extracts, certain matured cheeses such as cheddar and wines such as chianti) or dopamine (e.g. pods of broad beans). The clinical picture is one of an acute adrenergic crisis, similar to attacks associated with phaeochromocytomas — and for the same reason: an increased amount of circulat-ing noradrenaline (norepinephrine). Nervous system signs include headache, stiff neck, nausea and vomiting, and sometimes subarachnoid haemorrhage. Cardiovascular signs include tachy-cardia, marked hypertension, and possibly acute pulmonary oedema. The treatment of these reac-tions is like that of attacks of phaeochromocy-tomas; phentolamine, 5mg intravenously would be the preferred drug. Chlorpromazine would be a reasonable alternative for intramuscular injection. Monoamine oxidase inhibitors can interact with a number of other drugs (see chapter VIII; sect. 3), including pethidine/meperidine (chapter X; sect. 6.2.1) and possibly oral sulphonylurea hypo-glycaemic drugs (chapter XVI; sect. 3.3.5).

8. Anxiety States

Anxiety is a subjective symptom which is clearly related to life experiences (Lader and Marks, 1972). Tension is the sign of anxiety. The quavering voice, the wet armpits, the tremulous hands, the nervous tics of patients should not escape notice; they help to confirm the presence and severity of the symptom. The major thera-peutic approaches to anxiety are psychotherapy (to learn the causes of anxiety and how to cope with them) or environmental alterations (to learn how to avoid anxiety producing situations). The goal of treatment is to alleviate symptoms to a tolerable degree. Use of drugs, at least in our present under-standing, should be considered no more than symptomatic, adjunctive treatment. Much clinical experience indicates that antianxiety drugs used for proper purposes can help patients. While popularity of drugs is not necessarily a good guide to their relative value, it seems unlikely that so many of these drugs would be prescribed if they did so little, but they are still much overused (Blackwell, 1973). Nevertheless, anxiety is not always a minor emotional disability.

Anxiety is such a ubiquitous symptom in a limited repertoire of emotional expression that it may accompany many more serious emotional disorders. One must differentiate so-called neurotic anxiety from that accompanying various depressive syndromes, especially the more serious endogenous depressions. Early on, many patients who subsequently become clearly schizophrenic, present with symptoms and signs suggesting only rather severe anxiety. Somatisation may be an early aspect of the evolving schizophrenic psy-chosis. Finally, anxiety may accompany the early symptoms of organic impairment of later life. Whether it plays a primary or secondary role in alcohol or drug abuse remains disputed, but it may also mask these disorders.

Besides being a primary symptom associated with almost all kinds of emotional disorders, anx-iety is a frequent secondary symptom of physical illnesses. It may aggravate angina pectoris, peptic ulcer disease or irritable bowel syndrome; it may complicate acute myocardial infarction and many surgical procedures. On the other hand, it may be mimicked by thyrotoxicosis, temporal lobe epilep-sy, or phaeochromocytoma. Not surprisingly, most prescriptions for drugs to treat anxiety are written by non-psychiatric clinicians (Balter et al., 1974).

Severe anxiety, whether primary or secondary, can be extremely disabling. It is never a trivial complaint, and often is the presenting symptom of a more serious emotional disorder, such as depres-sion or schizophrenia.

8.1 Treatment of Anxiety and Use of Antianxiety Drugs

Many types of drugs may be used for treating anxiety (Lader, 1975, 1976; table XIII; section 1.4.3). Most clinicians, as well as patients, prefer

Table XIII. Chemical and pharmacological classes and dosage guide for antianxiety drugs

Class and drug	Bedtime dose[1] (mg)	Daytime dose in mg (1-2 times)	Maximum total[2] (mg)
1. Sedative-hypnotic			
Barbiturates			
Phenobarbitone	32-65	16	100
Buto(a)barbitone	30-90	15-30	150
Glycerol derivatives			
Meprobamate	400-800	200-400	1600
Benzodiazepines			
Chlordiazepoxide	10-50	5-25	100
Diazepam	2-10	2-5	20
Oxazepam	15-30	10-15	60
Clorazepate	7.5-30	3.75-7.5	45
Lorazepam	1-4	1-2	10
2. Sedative-autonomic			
Diphenylmethane antihistamines			
Hydroxyzine	25-50	10-25	100
Diphenhydramine	25-50	10-25	100
Phenothiazine antipsychotics			
Trifluoperazine	5-10	2-5	20
Tricyclic antidepressant			
Doxepin	10-50	10-25	100

1   Wherever possible use single daily dose at night with doses during day only taken as required (see section 1.5.3, 8.2).
2   All doses are rough guide. Maximum doses may be less than required by some patients; they are unlikely to lead to any physical dependence.

drugs of the sedative-hypnotic type. Their sedation is more familiar to us, resembling that of alcohol. The sedative-autonomic drugs often create feelings of inner restlessness and mental fuzziness, as well as having bothersome peripheral side effects, such as dry mouth or blurred vision. These same effects make such drugs unlikely choices for drugs of abuse, but less acceptable therapeutic agents. Still, some patients tolerate the side effects and gain more therapeutic benefit from these drugs than from the other group. Although differences between sedative-hypnotic drugs are more often ones of degree than of type, they may help to determine one's choice of a drug. The various rankings in table XV for differing degrees of pharmacological effects are at best contentious estimates, but they highlight some of the possible differences between 6 possible classes of antianxiety drugs. None of the classes of drugs available meets the ideal desiderata of an antianxiety drug, each having some drawbacks. On the whole, the benzodiazepines most closely approach the ideal (Hollister, 1972b; Rickels, 1978), which may account for their vast popularity despite a substantial price differential over drugs such as phenobarbitone or meprobamate.

The choice of a specific drug for an individual patient is best made on the basis of the patient's acceptance of the drug, either from his past experience or from experience obtained in an empirical clinical trial. One would tend to try first the three types of sedative-hypnotic drugs before experimenting with any of the sedative-autonomic agents, although eventually one or another of the latter may prove to be the drug of choice for a small number of patients.

For many of the mixed anxiety-depression syndromes, antianxiety drugs continue to be used with about as much effect as the tricyclic antidepressants. From a clinical viewpoint, it might still be better strategy to start treatment in such cases with a tricyclic antidepressant. Any difference in efficacy is likely to be slight and if one has missed a patient with endogenous depression, no great harm will have been done.

When antianxiety drugs are used to treat anxiety secondary to some physical illness which requires another drug, it is better to use extemporaneous combinations, following the general principles outlined below, rather than some fixed combination. The latter do not afford the desired flexibility of dose and dose schedules. Even the benzodiazepines, which are least likely of all these drugs to produce severe respiratory depression should be used cautiously, if at all, in patients with severe bronchial asthma or chronic obstructive bronchitis (see chapter XX; sect. 3.2.2, 5.2).

It makes no sense to combine antianxiety drugs with each other. Among such combinations may be an inadvertent one in which one type of drug is used during the day, because it has been most extensively promoted as a daytime sedative, while another is used at night, because it has been labelled by advertising as a hypnotic. Whether the combination of sedative-hypnotic antianxiety drugs with β-adrenoceptor blocking drugs will ultimately prove to be an advantage awaits much further study, although such combined use often ameliorates somatic symptoms such as palpitations and tremor (Editorial, 1976).

8.2 Doses and Dose Schedules of Antianxiety Drugs

As discussed in section 1.5.3 plasma concentrations obtained from equivalent doses of antianxiety drugs in different patients vary widely. Dosage must therefore be individualised and the doses shown in table XIII are consequently to be viewed as gross approximations.

A reasonable approach to individualisation of dosage would be to establish the minimally effective hypnotic dose of the drug. Initial doses of the drug would be given 2 to 3 hours before bedtime, while the patient is still active, and patients would be instructed to look for enforced sleepiness, deeper than usual sleep and a minimally discernible degree of 'hangover'. When this dose had been found, it could be assumed to provide the desired effects of the drug. Starting, for example, with initial doses of 2mg of diazepam, one could increase the dose to 5, 10, or even 20mg on successive nights, to establish the required dose. Thus, in 3 or 4 nights one could, if necessary, explore a 10-fold range of dose. All of this dose ranging could be done with 10mg tablets, by breaking them twice. Doses used during the day would be taken as needed, usually one-third to one-fourth the night-time dose. Such an empirical approach to establishing dose may bother those who like to keep things simple and not have to

Table XIV. Summary of principles of use of antianxiety drugs

---

1. Use with restraint
   a) Severity of anxiety as a primary symptom associated with emotional disorder
   b) Need when anxiety a secondary symptom of physical illness

2. Do not neglect other therapies
   a) 'Psychotherapy' (to learn the causes of anxiety and how to cope with them)
   b) Alteration of environment (to learn how to avoid anxiety producing situations)

3. Choice of drug
   a) Past response best guide
   b) Patient preferences (sedative-hypnotic type)
   c) Pharmacological differences (table XV)

4. Doses
   a) No set dose. Plasma concentrations vary widely among individuals on the same dose
   b) Dose to attain therapeutic benefit without impairment of psychomotor function during day

5. Dosage schedules
   a) Titration to minimum effective hypnotic dose
   b) Single daily dose at night
   c) Fractional dose taken as needed for any daytime stresses

6. Duration of treatment
   a) Treatment follows course of anxiety
   b) Short (7 days) interrupted courses as episodes demand

---

worry about these matters. Such clinicians should not be prescribing drugs but should limit themselves to providing psychotherapy.

Long duration of action is a desirable attribute for antianxiety drugs. Most desirable are drugs such as chlordiazepoxide, diazepam or phenobarbitone, with plasma half-lives of 24 hours or more depending on different estimates (table I). The long acting drugs provide a means of sustaining effective plasma concentrations with relatively infrequent dosage. They are also well suited to single daily dosage. Such a dosage schedule is desirable for antianxiety drugs, as one does not wish unduly to emphasise drug taking. The most appropriate time to give the single dose would be in the evening, when one can exploit the hypnotic effects of these drugs. A patient with anxiety so severe that drug treatment is required would commonly also have some difficulty sleeping. Further, it does not make pharmacological sense to instruct a patient

Table XV. Selection of an antianxiety drug. Balance of favourable and unfavourable attributes of 6 classes of antianxiety drugs

	Pheno-barbitone	Mepro-bamate	Benzo-diazepines	Diphen-hydramine	Pheno-thiazines	Tri-cyclics
Favourable attributes [1]						
Sedative/antianxiety ratio	+	++	++	±	±	±
Muscle relaxation	±	++	+++	0	−	0
Duration of action	+++	++	+++	+	++	++
Unfavourable attributes						
Tolerance, habituation	±	+++	±	0	0	0
Physical dependence	+	+++	+	0	0	0
Disturbed sleep pattern	++	++	±	++	++	++
Potential suicide use	++	++	0	++	0	+++

1   Degree of probability: (−) opposite effect; (0) none; (±) minimal; (+) slight; (++) moderate; (+++) great.

to take a sedative right after his morning stimulant, coffee. The 'daytime hangover' which is inevitable with these long acting drugs provides precisely the degree of mild sedation compatible with unimpaired daily activities but relief of troublesome symptoms. Fractional doses of drug may be used as needed for particular daytime stresses. Flexible dosage schedules are acceptable to patients. Indeed, patients rarely take antianxiety medications on an equally divided dose schedule anyway. They take them as they need, which with this class of drug, in contrast to antipsychotic drugs (see section 3.2), may be entirely proper.

8.3 Duration of Treatment

Anxiety is often episodic, waxing and waning with changes in one's life. In such cases, treatment might follow the course, drugs being used only when symptoms are discomforting or disabling and not indefinitely. Such episodes of treatment might be limited to a week. If anxiety is relieved, it might remain so without drugs. The knowledge that relief is available may sustain the patient over subsequent episodes. By limiting treatment to short courses, problems of tolerance with loss of efficacy, or increased doses with the risk of physical dependence, are avoided.

Not all patients who complain of anxiety have it episodically. Some have it chronically, and this may simply represent an unusually high level of 'trait' anxiety. These patients often do very well with small doses of some antianxiety drug maintained indefinitely. Generally, one need not worry about physical dependence developing in such

patients, although undoubtedly they have some degree of psychological dependence to the drug.

As anxiety is so often episodic, it seems reasonable to plan its treatment with drugs around such episodes, rather than on some indefinite basis which continues treatment far beyond what might have really been required. A 5 to 7 day course of treatment should be planned, following which the drug would be discontinued if results were satisfactory. If they were not, another course of treatment of a higher dose might be required. Retreatment would be deferred until recrudescent symptoms became discomforting or disabling enough to merit it.

8.4 Side Effects and Complications of Antianxiety Drugs

Oversedation is the most common side effect. The elderly are most susceptible (see chapter V; sect. 4.7). Directing patients to take the largest dose or only dose in the evening hours converts the sedative effect from something potentially harmful to something beneficial. Patients should be warned about the possibility of sedation from any dose taken during the day. Usually it will be greatest 1 to 2 hours after it is taken. Dangerous activities, such as driving an automobile, or critical judgments, should be deferred, particularly if alcohol has been consumed (see section 8.5, 15.6) or if the antianxiety drug has been used for other purposes (e.g. intravenous diazepam in dentistry). Although it is possible in experimental situations to demonstrate impaired function, provided the dose of drug is large enough and the tests hard enough, studies of human performance during usual clinical use of these drugs are extremely rare. For all we know, the drugs may on balance actually improve performance, the benefit of relief of anxiety exceeding any mild degree of sedation.

8.4.1 Tolerance

Tolerance can come about through several possible mechanisms. In the broadest clinical sense, a reasonable assumption is that tolerance may develop to any of the sedative-hypnotic antianxiety drugs if they are used for long enough. Drugs differ in the rate at which tolerance occurs. It develops rapidly to meprobamate, laboratory evidence indicating that the rate of metabolism (hydroxylation) of the drug doubles after a week of exposure. Although phenobarbitone also stimulates hepatic microsomal enzymes for its own metabolism (Conney, 1967), clinical evidence of tolerance to this drug is less dramatic. Such tolerance as has been observed with benzodiazepines has been slow to develop (Greenblatt and Shader, 1974). Most drugs of the sedative-autonomic class do not readily produce tolerance.

Development of tolerance obliges the patient to increase his dose to continue to obtain desired clinical effects. The key to the development of tolerance is chronic uninterrupted use of the drug; thus, the fashion in which these drugs are commonly used makes tolerance scarcely avoidable. The recommendation given in section 8.3 for using these drugs in brief, interrupted courses has the potential for minimising or avoiding the development of tolerance.

The demonstration of physical dependence to barbiturates in the 1950s opened the door for a host of new, 'non-barbiturate' sedatives. Glutethimide was a modification of the phenobarbitone molecule which was all bad: the drug is much weaker; it is far more dependence producing; it is not excreted unchanged and accumulation of its active hydroxy metabolite create problems on overdosage. Meprobamate was the first successful substitute and enjoyed an enormous vogue. Early on, physical dependence was observed, often with total daily doses only 2 or 3 times greater than customary therapeutic doses. Rapid tolerance to the drug and this low margin for physical dependence has led many to abandon its use. It is a pity that phenobarbitone was tarred with the same brush as short duration of action barbiturates, such as pentobarbitone or quinalbarbitone (secobarbital) sodium. Spontaneous abuse and

physical dependence is rare with phenobarbitone. The same considerations probably apply to buto- and butabarbitone sodium as well.

The introduction of chlordiazepoxide, the first of the benzodiazepines, provided two advantages: (a) physical dependence required a much greater level of abuse (6 to 20 times the therapeutic dose) than with meprobamate, and (b) the withdrawal syndrome from this drug was markedly attenuated and milder (Hollister et al., 1961). Withdrawal reactions are of greatest severity and intensity with drugs having a rapid rate of disappearance from the plasma (provided it is not so rapid that sustained levels can hardly ever be attained, as in the case of tybamate), and those from meprobamate and the short duration of action barbiturates resemble that from alcohol. With longer acting drugs, such as chlordiazepoxide, diazepam and, very likely, phenobarbitone, the onset is gradual and the course of the whole syndrome may extend over a week or more. Thus, these drugs contain a certain degree of self protection against severe withdrawal reactions. Considering their wide use, the number of validated reports have been gratifyingly rare (Greenblatt and Shader, 1974; Maletzky and Klotter, 1976; Marks, 1978).

8.4.2 Overdoses

It is probably impossible to commit suicide with benzodiazepines taken alone; almost all reported fatalities included other drugs or were due to other causes. The rare instances in which they were not reported in association with other drugs have not been adequately documented (Greenblatt et al., 1977c; Cate and Jatlow, 1973).

In one series, no deaths were encountered in 22 instances of chlordiazepoxide overdose, even with doses up to 2.25g (Zbinden et al., 1961). In cases of poisoning with chlordiazepoxide, when the drug is used alone, symptoms are quite mild, consisting only of drowsiness or stupor. If another drug is also present, its effects usually predominate and it appears that the poisoning syndrome is largely attributable to the other drugs taken. Instances of overdose with diazepam have been equally mild, characterised by marked muscle relaxation but little fall in blood pressure or respiratory depression. Recovery is rapid, even in patients who have ingested massive overdoses, and is not related to the rate of elimination of the parent drug or active metabolites which persist for many days at high concentration (Greenblatt et al., 1978d). With the exception of drowsiness, no untoward effects were observed in one series of 27 cases of acute overdoses of nitrazepam, even when up to 80 tablets (4g) were consumed (Matthew et al., 1969). As anxious patients may often be issued large amounts of drug supplies between visits to the clinician, lethal amounts of barbiturates, meprobamate or other possible antianxiety drug may be given. The availability of such safe antianxiety drugs as the benzodiazepines is a distinct advantage.

8.5 Drug Interactions with Antianxiety Drugs

Pharmacodynamic interactions of these drugs with others with sedative effects are the most important. The greatest hazard is that some combination of drugs will produce oversedation with impairment of function, respiratory depression or even an unwitting suicide. Impaired function is especially important in regard to driving automobiles, a potentially lethal activity; particularly when drugs with sedative properties are combined with alcohol (Milner, 1972; MacLeod et al., 1977b).

Alcoholic beverages are the most widely used social sedative and can interact with many drugs (see appendix C; Seixas, 1975). The alcoholic, because of the cross tolerance of alcohol with sedative-hypnotic drugs, may require, and take, much larger doses than an ordinary person. Following acute alcohol ingestion in the presence of large amounts of ethanol, say with plasma concentrations of over 200mg per 100ml, metabolism of short duration of action barbiturates is slowed. The additive effects of the two drugs become further enhanced by the longer persistence of the barbiturate (Pirola, 1977). Such a mechanism explains some of the lethal interactions between alcohol and barbiturates. Other drugs with sedative properties may also be taken concurrently. These may include other psychotherapeutic drugs, antihistamines, and a variety of over-the-counter medications.

The ability of *chronic* alcohol ingestion to induce hepatic enzymes which metabolise drugs is well known, and explains in part the enormous tolerance for common sedatives that many alcoholics develop (Pirola, 1977). On the other hand, when high levels of blood alcohol prevail as following *acute* alcohol ingestion, the metabolising enzymes are poisoned, and metabolic clearance is inhibited (Rubin and Lieber, 1968). Thus, doses

of sedatives which are ordinarily well tolerated may, when combined with the depressant effects of alcohol itself, become lethal. The number of unwitting suicides due to combinations of quinalbarbitone (secobarbital) sodium and alcohol seems to be declining as the various benzodiazepines replace the use of quinalbarbitone sodium.

A careful drug history should be taken from all patients being treated with antianxiety drugs to rule out 'confounding' drugs. Other types of drugs than those with sedative actions should be considered. Excessive coffee intake or concurrent use of a stimulant-type appetite suppressant may negate the desired therapeutic effects of the antianxiety drug.

Phenobarbitone is rather notorious for its many pharmacokinetic interactions with other drugs, but the benzodiazepines have few that are of any major clinical importance (appendix C). For example, neither chlordiazepoxide, diazepam nor nitrazepam alter control with oral anticoagulants (see chapter XXIII; sect. 3.6). In general, the benzodiazepines produce fewer important pharmacokinetic interactions with other drugs than do most available hypnotics, sedatives or antianxiety drugs.

9. Sleep Difficulties

Sleep occupies nearly a third of our lives, but the precise needs for sleep, particularly its quality, remain an enigma. Its disorders merit a listening ear and an understanding of the person's sleep difficulty more often than a specific remedy (Oswald, 1975). Some people complain of too little sleep (insomnia), while there are a few patients in whom too much sleep is a problem (e.g. narcolepsy, hypersomnia). Some others experience peculiarities during sleep (e.g. enuresis, night terrors, sleepwalking).

9.1 Insomnia

As in constipation, another disturbance of normal function, defining 'normal' is difficult (see chapter V; sect. 4.7.6). The sleeping time needed per day varies widely among individuals, from approximately 3 hours a night to 10. Most have sleep habits between 7 and 8 hours nightly. Some people change their sleeping habits with ease while others, particularly the elderly, have a great deal of difficulty in adjusting to a change in sleeping pattern (Kales and Kales, 1974).

Insomnia is primarily the highly subjective symptom of not being able to sleep when or as well as the individual believes he should. Many patients have unreasonable expectations about their sleep, and their anxiety about not sleeping may be worse than the insomnia itself. Most agree that insomnia essentially involves taking a long time to fall asleep initially, waking up frequently and for prolonged periods during the night, or waking up too early in the morning. Often there is more than one of these manifestations of insomnia in the same subject. Another important feature of the insomniac's sleep is its variability. A few night's poor sleep tend to be followed by a much better night.

Insomnia is a real complaint. Although it may often be a symptom without a disease, the many other complaints of insomniacs should alert the clinician to look for physical (e.g. pain; sudden fearful arousals with palpitation and sweating due to angina etc; arousal accompanied by dyspnoea which may signal incipient heart failure) and emotional disorders which should be treated in their own right. Minor emotional disturbances such as worry over one's job, financial or love affairs etc are usually easily uncovered. Chronic anxiety reactions are almost always accompanied by some degree of sleep disturbance, as is depressive illness. Sleep disturbances are also seen in schizophrenia, but it is doubtful that they are pathogenic. Treatment of such sleep difficulties associated with psychiatric disorders is discussed in the relevant sections above.

Treatment of insomnia is by explanation and reassurance. Much benefit can be gained simply by determining what the patient's sleep habits actually are, and reassuring him that no serious harm will follow, for example, from the loss of some sleep. Regular times of going to bed, exercise in the early part of the day and a hot milk drink at bedtime can help to re-establish more 'normal' sleep habits. Sometimes the alcohol nightcap is more likely to produce disturbed sleep than improved sleep. The same can be said for stimulants such as coffee, which may have had little effect on a patient's sleep when he or she was 20, but may do so 20 years later. Some other drugs might also interfere with sleep (see section 15.8). Attention should also be paid to such simple things as the condition of the patient's mattress. The relaxation that follows a warm bath, a massage, or the relief of sexual tension can also be used to promote sleep. Some patients might simply have to learn to live with the fact that they will usually sleep for only about 4 hours each night, or require it in a more infantile pattern such as by frequent 'cat naps' rather than by sustained sleep.

If the insomnia does not respond to reassurance and explanation or other measures such as those outlined above, prescription of an hypnotic drug in limited quantities at any single time is justified (Johns, 1975). The agent used should above all be safe on overdosage. It should also maintain its effectiveness (Kales et al., 1977), have a low abuse potential and other desirable properties (table XVI). The drugs which come closest to fulfilling all criteria are the benzodiazepines (Greenblatt et al., 1975b) such as flurazepam (15 to 30mg), flunitrazepam (1 to 2mg) and nitrazepam (5 to 10mg), and chloral derivatives such as chloral hydrate or triclofos (0.5 to 2g) or dichloralphenazone (0.65 to 1.3g). Doses should be taken 30 minutes before retiring.

The commencing dose should be small and should be increased only if necessary. Once a good night's sleep has been attained, the drug should not be used for 2 or 3 nights. The patient should be told that the aim is to restore his normal sleep pattern and not to make him dependent on the drug (Kales et al., 1974; Clift, 1972). It should be stressed that sleep during many nights without drug will be good and that occasional imperfect sleeps will do little harm. Sometimes the knowledge that relief is ultimately attainable will tide a patient over a few bad nights. As depression may be a cause of insomnia, a trial of a tricyclic antidepressant (see section 7) may be worthwhile, but only if depression is suspected as an aetiological factor.

All possible factors that may interact subjectively with drugs should be considered in exploiting their hypnotic effect. No drug that affects the mental state works in a vacuum. All interact to some extent with the personality of the patient and the setting in which they are given (Rickels, 1968). Thus, it may be worthwhile to plan some sort of ritual for patients who seek relief from insomnia and to link this with drug therapy, to exploit the conditioned reflex aspect of the process of going to sleep (e.g. undressing, attending to various items of toilet etc). It also means working up some enthusiasm for the drug and communicating this to the patient. The special problems in treatment of insomnia in the elderly are discussed in chapter V (sect. 4.7.1).

Table XVI. Selection of an hypnotic. Balance of favourable and unfavourable attributes (adapted after Johns, 1975)

	Barbit-urates[1]	Nitra-zepam	Flura-zepam	Chloral hydrate and triclofos	Dichlor-alphen-azone	Metha-qualone	Gluteth-imide	Methy-prylone
Favourable attributes[2]								
Effectiveness in initiating and maintaining sleep:								
a) For the first few nights;	++	++	++	++	++	++	++	++
b) After 2 weeks treatment	0	++	++	0	0	0	0	0
Unfavourable attributes								
Inhibition of REM sleep, at least initially[3]	++	±	0	0	0	+	++	++
REM rebound after drug withdrawal[4]	++	+	0	0	0	+	++	++
Inhibition of delta-wave sleep[3]	±	+	++	0	0	±	+	0
Tolerance, habituation	++	±	±	±	±	++	++	++
Physical dependence	++	±	±	+	+	+	++	+
Potential suicide use	++	0	0	+	+	++	++	++
Drug interaction potential[5]	++	0	0	±	++	++	++	?

1   Excluding phenobarbitone.
2   Signs indicate degree or probability ranging from (0) insignificant; (±) slight; (+) moderate; (++) marked. The magnitude of each effect is dose dependent.
3   Affects 'quality' of sleep, although importance of these stages remains uncertain.
4   May be associated with increased frequency of disturbing dreams or nightmares.
5   Excluding enhancement of sedative effect by alcohol or other drugs with sedative properties. Ratings are applicable to pharmacokinetic interactions (see section 8.5; appendix C).

9.2 Other Sleep Disorders

9.2.1 Somnambulism and Night Terrors

Medical advice is less often sought for sleep disorders such as somnambulism and night terrors than it is for insomnia. Drug treatment of somnambulism is seldom required. Benzodiazepines (e.g. diazepam or flurazepam) may help, but this has not been clearly established. Somnambulism and night terrors in children is often outgrown as they mature and is not necessarily associated with psychological disturbances, although this may not be true in adults (Kales et al., 1966). Diazepam has been claimed to decrease the frequency of attacks of night terrors in adults (Fisher et al., 1973).

9.2.2 Hypersomnia

Hypersomnia must be considered as a possible psychological disorder, or due to the presence of cardiopulmonary disease or organic disease of the central nervous system. The patient's previous sleep habits, his age and social circumstances must be taken into account before treatment with central nervous system stimulants is begun, as these drugs are best avoided for long term use unless strongly indicated.

9.2.3 Narcolepsy

Narcolepsy can be a very disabling condition. It is a condition in which patients have irresistible sleepiness, maybe 2 or 3 times a day for periods of 10 to 15 minutes. Often they are precipitated by specific circumstances. When narcolepsy has been present for some years, cataplectic attacks may also occur. These consist of periods of sudden muscular weakness, maybe lasting a few seconds and affecting either part or the whole of the body. They are usually precipitated by emotion, either laughter or anger. Cataplectic spells can usually be controlled by tricyclic antidepressant drugs such as imipramine (75 to 100mg daily). These drugs have a specific action in preventing the attacks which is unrelated to their antidepressant properties (Oswald, 1975). However, narcolepsy is the greater problem and this usually responds to dextroamphetamine, 5mg taken as required for special occasions. Normally, patients should be encouraged to take a 15 minute nap, say in the lunch and tea breaks at work, as this will help avert attacks at other times.

9.2.4 Enuresis

Enuresis in schoolchildren who do not have organic disease of the urinary tract or elsewhere has been treated successfully with tricyclic antidepressants such as imipramine, but there is a tendency to relapse after the drug is withdrawn (Miller et al., 1968) and supplies must be packaged or stored in a way to inhibit accidental poisoning by any other young children in the household. Improvement with the drug is not related to changes which it causes in the stages of sleep. Psychological support and measures other than drug treatment such as the electric buzzer conditioning device, continue to be important in the primary management of enuresis.

10. Psychiatric Disorders in Children

The major problem in dealing with the choice of drugs for treating children is to establish an accurate diagnosis. Generally, childhood and adolescent behaviour disorders fit into four major categories:

a) Behaviour disturbances such as hyperactivity, delinquency, or sociopathic-aggressive behaviour.
b) Organic brain syndromes, such as epilepsies, brain damage from birth, trauma or disease, or so-called minimal brain damage with only borderline neurological signs and EEG abnormalities.
c) Schizophrenias of the usual types, in addition to childhood autism.
d) Affective disorders, chiefly depression, in postpubertal children.

Many young patients do not fall into these categories, so that a purely empirical approach is necessary in some, using graded ratings of symptoms and signs.

The indications and principles of use for psychotherapeutic drugs are somewhat similar in children to those which should be followed in using these drugs in adults (Werry, 1978; table

Table XVII. General principles of use of psychotherapeutic drugs in children

1. Drugs may be quite useful in children, but establishing a correct diagnosis and selection of the best possible drug is paramount, as it is with most other types of drug therapy.
2. The better one knows the pharmacological effects of the drugs, the better one can anticipate their side effects, which are most often extensions of their pharmacological effects. Warning about possible side effects is especially important when treating children, lest both parent and child become so alarmed by them that they will no longer consider drug treatment.
3. Drugs should not be used for trivial indications in children, especially not a sop to parents. One should be convinced that the situation is not due to some self limited condition, that the problem is serious enough to justify all the risks of drug therapy, and that one can provide the proper clinical controls and precautions to avoid serious complications.
4. Familiar drugs are generally preferred over the newer ones, at least until the latter have had fairly extensive trials in adults.
5. Doses are flexible and variable; there is no fixed therapeutic dose. Dosage schedules should be geared to fit the pharmacokinetics of the drug.
6. Interrupted treatment may be used in lieu of placebo control to determine that the drug is really efficacious, that it is still required, and to reduce the possibility of tolerance or some complication due to cumulative doses.
7. Drugs in children, even more than in adults, require other concomitant treatments or services if best results are to be obtained.

XVII). Results from drug therapy of childhood psychiatric disorders are however, much less dramatic than in adults. Moreover, far more than in adults, drug therapy should be accompanied by rigorous social, educational and vocational rehabilitative measures. Drugs should not be used in acute stress or adjustment reactions where the cause is clearly apparent, such as a change in home or school, an illness, or separation from a friend. These episodes are usually self limiting and it might be best for the child's future development to work through them psychologically rather than to seek help from a bottle of pills.

10.1 Hyperkinetic Children

The 'hyperkinetic' or 'minimal brain dysfunction' syndrome is characterised by short attention span, distractability, emotional lability, aggressiveness, and hyperactivity in a child who has normal intelligence but fails to learn at a normal rate (Werry, 1976). This syndrome is estimated to affect 3 to 4 % of school age children, most often becoming evident during the early school years. Boys are much more frequently diagnosed as having this disorder than girls. Minor neurological abnormalities or EEG abnormalities may be found, as well as some history of difficult birth or early injury or infection which may be viewed as a possible cause for brain damage. Although some children seem to undergo a spontaneous remission at about age 12 years, especially if they have been adequately treated, those children who are untreated have a much higher risk of later becoming delinquent, schizophrenic, or having some other psychiatric disorder (Weiss et al., 1968). Thus, proper recognition of the disorder and its early treatment are highly desirable. Because the diagnosis of borderline cases is difficult, some children are probably undiagnosed, while others may be diagnosed inappropriately. Sometimes the diagnosis is established on the basis of a therapeutic trial with stimulant drugs.

Stimulant drugs seem to be the most effective agents for the treatment of the characteristic behaviour disorders, although little is known of their effect on such aspects as poor motor integration, deficits in the perception of space form, movement and time, and disorders of language and symbol development (Council on Child Health, 1975). Those stimulants which can be used include dextroamphetamine, methylphenidate and pemoline. The dose of each agent must be carefully selected and tailored to the needs of the individual child. An empirical starting dose would be 0.1mg/kg dextroamphetamine, 0.2mg/kg methylphenidate or 0.5 to 1mg/kg pemoline. Large maintenance doses are not more effective than conservative doses (e.g. 0.3mg/kg methylphenidate) and produce more marked side effects (Sprague and Sleator, 1975; Werry and Sprague, 1974). Doses are usually divided. Some patients seem to require more frequent dosage than others, to avoid brief periods of emotional lability as the effect of the drug wears off. Thus, a single morning dose might last throughout the school day, but has probably worn off by the time the child has returned home from school.

Side effects must be looked for, although the common ones, anorexia and insomnia are usually transient and can be minimised by use of conservative doses. Growth retardation may occur and should be looked for. Suppression of growth rate persists as long as medication is given (Safer and Allen, 1975) although it does not occur until the dose of methylphenidate exceeds 20mg per day — another argument for the lower doses of 0.3 to 0.5mg/kg suggested above. Regular weight and height checks and maintaining a record of a child's progress on a height and weight percentile chart are obligatory for all children on stimulants, particularly where the daily dose must exceed 0.5mg/kg (Werry, 1976). The cause of the growth retardation is not clear (Barter and Kammer, 1978). Habituation does not seem to be a problem (Weiss, 1975) and there is no evidence that stimulants given in childhood predispose to drug abuse in later life. Antipsychotic drugs are sometimes useful but carry the risk of depressing higher CNS functions such as attention and cognition. Other drugs which have been shown to be of value include tricyclic antidepressants, although their effect is less predictable and less striking than that of the stimulants (Werry, 1976).

Fortunately, any beneficial effects from stimulant drugs are usually evident fairly soon, usually within the first 3 weeks of treatment. Courses of treatment are often geared to the school year, with vacation periods being used for testing possible withdrawal of drug. The drug programme may be resumed only if relapse occurs. Pharmacological treatment may be expected to help from one-half to two-thirds of those treated (Anders and Ciarnello, 1977). In general, it seems to be more likely to succeed in those instances in which there is more definitive evidence of some organic brain impairment. Other treatment which must be included in any reasonable total therapeutic programme includes family counselling and special teaching for any specific learning disabilities.

10.2 Schizophrenia and Depression

Childhood schizophrenia and depression are probably best treated with the same drugs used to treat these disorders in adults (Eveloff, 1966; Frommer, 1967). Just as in adults, the severity of these disorders covers a broad range. Severely autistic children, such as those unable to talk or make social contact, may show limited responses to antipsychotic drugs. Less severely schizophrenic children may respond better to drugs, along with a programme of social rehabilitation. In general, one starts with low doses of drugs, gradually increasing them until such time as side effects limit further increases, or until therapeutic effects are attained. Dystonic reactions are especially common in children being treated with antipsychotic drugs (see also sect. 3.5.3), but are often quite amenable to treatment or prevention by use of elixir of diphenhydramine, an antihistamine which has enough anticholinergic action to be effective. The latter type of drug is also a preferred sedative for children who often do not tolerate barbiturates well.

10.3 Mental Deficiency

The great hope for a drug which increases mental capacity has not yet been realised. Drugs currently available can only influence the mentally retarded by indirect actions, such as controlling motor behaviour and distractability, which in turn may lead to increased attention span and better intellectual performance. Treatment is entirely symptomatic, any gains are likely to be small ones. Antipsychotic drugs (e.g. haloperidol) may be required to control disturbed behaviour; such treatment may be prolonged.

11. Psychoses Associated with Old Age

These disorders include principally presenile, senile, arteriosclerotic and mixed types of brain syndromes. Many conditions may predispose to or mimic the mental changes of senility (e.g. onset of congestive heart failure of malignancy; undernutrition, especially if complicated by alcohol ingestion). Thus these diagnoses should not be a wastebasket in which to categorise all mental disturbances of old age, but rather a challenge to one's general medical acumen (Hollister, 1975).

Analeptic-stimulant therapy with leptazole (pentylenetetrazole) still has its proponents, but almost all adequately controlled studies have been negative. Sympathomimetic stimulants may be dangerous or even aggravate irritability or psychotic symptoms. Tricyclic antidepressants may be used, but with great caution, in such patients who have a concurrent retarded depression. The peripheral and central anticholinergic actions of these drugs may cause severe side effects, including aggravation of the confused mental state. In addition, hypotension has resulted in physical injuries due to falls (Glassman et al., 1979), or possibly has precipitated myocardial infarction.

Most symptomatic control of the psychosis of the aged has come from the judicious use of antipsychotics. Irritability, disturbed sleep and careless personal hygiene may be alleviated. As in the case with tricyclic antidepressants, doses must be very low initially and adjusted with great care. In the past, thioridazine was used, largely because it has little predilection for evoking extrapyramidal reactions. Recent apprehensions about its cardiotoxicity, as well as its greater tendency to produce orthostatic hypotension or mental confusion, have led to greater use of the more potent antipsychotics, such as haloperidol or thiothixine. An initial dose of thioridazine might be 10mg 3 times daily. No single dose should be greater than 100mg and the total daily dose should probably not exceed 200mg. As is usually the case with these drugs, the major fraction of the maintenance dose should be given at night. Initial doses of haloperidol or thiothixene might be 1mg given at night with increments of 1mg gradually until symptoms are controlled. Any emerging extrapyramidal syndrome should be treated with a modest dose of some anti-Parkinson drug, possibly diphenhydramine 25mg.

The propensity for paradoxical reactions with increased agitation from use of conventional sedatives in the elderly seems to have been somewhat exaggerated. One should not hesitate to treat an elderly patient who has marked fears and anxieties with simple drugs such as the benzodiazepines. If symptoms are controlled with these drugs, one need not use the more potentially dangerous drugs, such as antipsychotics.

Until the basic mechanisms of these disorders are better understood, treatment will be limited to a purely symptomatic approach. Whether use of vasodilator drugs such as hydrogenated ergot alkaloids, nafronyl, betahistine, papaverine, piracetam, isoxsuprine, cyclandelate, etc which augment blood flow in the microcirculation (Kugler et al., 1978; Seipel et al., 1977), can significantly improve function in cerebral arteriosclerosis to be useful clinically is open to question.

Improvement in the patient's social and occupational circumstances is more likely to reduce mental and behavioural symptoms in the elderly or senile patient.

Treatment of the common psychiatric symptoms of old age, insomnia, anxiety, confusion and behaviour disorders, is discussed in more detail in chapter V (sect. 4.7).

12. Alcoholism

Despite the concern about drugs of abuse, alcohol remains the most widely abused of all. The enormous morbidity and mortality associated with alcohol abuse make it a major contemporary public health problem (Glatt, 1974; Seixas et al., 1975).

12.1 Acute Alcoholism

Practising clinicians are frequently confronted with the treatment of acute alcoholics. Plasma concentrations of alcohol over 300mg/100ml, especially if these are accompanied by other drugs or by unsuspected illnesses or injuries, may be rapidly fatal. The principal aim of treatment is to prevent death from respiratory depression. Drugs may be required for control of disturbed behaviour, but sedatives must be used carefully in the presence of high levels of blood alcohol, lest exacerbation of respiratory depression or unexpected fatalities occur (see section 8.5). Supportive treatment often suffices, and when toxic levels of alcohol have been taken, dialysis by any technique may be life saving by rapidly removing alcohol from the body. Attempts to hasten the metabolism of alcohol, which is a fixed, zero order process, have generally been unsuccessful. There is no known substance that rapidly 'sobers up' a person (see further Sellers and Kalant, 1976).

12.2 Chronic Alcoholism

Many alcoholics, especially after reaching some crisis in their lives or after a bout of delirium tremens, become dry for a while. The odds are overwhelming that they will once again resume drinking. Many types of interval treatment have been proposed. Aversive therapy with drugs such as disulfiram has only limited application. Management and rehabilitation of the alcoholic demands the skills of a number of medical and non-medical disciplines. Provided the goals are flexible and realistically set a great deal can be achieved for alcoholics and their families. Drugs have a limited role in overall management, but are necessary adjuncts in control of alcohol withdrawal reactions.

12.3 Alcohol Withdrawal Reactions

Alcohol withdrawal syndromes vary from the 'shakes' to hyperthermic, and possibly fatal, delirium tremens. As the term implies, these syndromes appear in the presence of a declining or absent level of plasma alcohol. Consequently, many anonymous alcoholics become manifest only when some intercurrent injury puts them into a hospital and removes the source of their drug (Seixas et al., 1975).

There are two major principles of treatment: (a) replacement of alcohol with a pharmacologically or physiologically equivalent drug such as chlordiazepoxide, diazepam or chlormethiazole, and (b) gradual withdrawal of the equivalent drug.

The goal of drug treatment is to keep the patient in a state of light sleep until symptoms are controlled and gradual withdrawal of drug can be undertaken. Obviously, doses of substitutive drugs must be entirely flexible to meet the varying need of the patient, the amount given being limited only by the onset of hypotension. Exceedingly large initial doses, at least by usual standards, may be required; for example, doses of chlordiazepoxide of 600 to 800mg daily are frequently necessary, gradually tapered to make accumulation less likely (see 1.5.3). Some clinicians prefer diazepam or chlormethiazole (Hollister et al., 1972) because of their anticonvulsant properties, but chlormethiazole should be given on a rigid prescribing schedule as its use in these circumstances can readily lead to dependence (Reilly, 1976). Propranolol can be useful in patients with severe withdrawal tremor (Drew et al., 1973). Phenytoin may be used in addition to benzodiazepines in those with a previous history of withdrawal seizures. Weaning from the sedative drug should be gradual and guided by the patient's clinical state. Most patients can be brought down to somewhat conventional sedative doses within a week. These should be continued in conservative doses for a limited period in the early recovery phase as a substitute for alcohol to relieve tension, which might otherwise lead to a rapid return of drinking, or in higher dosage, to manage more severe psychiatric disorders.

The greatest value of drug therapy of milder alcohol withdrawal syndromes may be the prevention of more serious complications, such as frank delirium tremens or convulsions and arrhythmias, in a relatively few patients (Klett et al., 1971; Kaim, 1973). Even frank delirium tremens has a favourable outcome if one provides good supportive treatment. Thus drug treatment is not primary in alcoholic withdrawal states. Excellent medical supervision, with an alert eye for potentially dangerous medical and surgical complications, as well as good supportive treatment, including B complex vitamins, adequate attention to hydration, electrolyte balance, and good nursing care, is essential (see further, Sellers and Kalant, 1976).

12.4 Withdrawal Reactions to Sedatives

Dependence on sedative-hypnotics and alcohol is so similar that it is usually called 'dependence of the alcohol-barbiturate' type (Wikler, 1968). Treatment of withdrawal reactions to sedatives is based on the same general principles as that for alcohol withdrawal. When the sedative being used is short acting, such as meprobamate or quinalbarbitone (secobarbital) sodium, one substitutes a longer acting drug, such as phenobarbitone or chlordiazepoxide. If an intrinsically long acting drug such as diazepam or phenobarbitone has been abused, which is far less commonly the case, one might simply stay with that drug, but taper doses according to the usual schedules.

13. Abuse of Opiates

Opiate abuse is currently epidemic in the United States and is showing an ominous increase in other countries of the western world. Most of the abuse stems from 'street' use. Despite the fact that hundreds of thousands of doses of opiates are given daily for medical purposes, documented cases of addiction from medical use of the drugs are rare. The abuse of these drugs is a complicated social phenomenon with many possible causes. Pharmacologically, opiates possess the two major attributes of drugs of dependence, the production of both euphoria and tolerance. The most widely used drug is diacetylmorphine or diamorphine (heroin) almost exclusively of illicit manufacture. Other opiates or opioids are abused to a much lesser extent and usually create less severe problems.

13.1 Withdrawal Reactions to Opiates

The principles in treating withdrawal reactions to opiates are essentially similar to those used for alcohol withdrawal, the substitution of a physiologically equivalent drug followed by gradual weaning. Methadone is the preferred agent for such substitution, the dose generally being based on the presence of symptoms and signs of withdrawal. Symptoms tend to be greatly exaggerated, so that objective manifestations, such as gooseflesh, sneezing, vomiting, and so forth, should be used for making estimates of the need for more drug.

13.2 Maintenance Treatment During Rehabilitation of Addict

The prophylactic use of methadone for rehabilitating narcotic addicts is one of the more exciting developments in drug therapy of the past decade (Goldstein, 1972). The principle involved is the deliberate substitution of one addicting drug by another which has less euphoriant effect and is active orally. Presumably, drug seeking behaviour will be diminished, or at least, continued use of heroin will be less compulsive. Due to a half-life of about 24 hours, it is necessary to give methadone on a daily basis. Although established patients may be permitted 'take-home' privileges, clinic attendance is usually required at least 2 to 3 times a week. Some drug has been diverted and that has been cause for concern. Governmental controls limit the places where methadone maintenance can be given, creating problems for patients who may not have easy access to clinics. For a number of reasons, methadone maintenance is falling out of favour, so that the number of patients actively being treated now is less than it was several years ago (Dole and Nyswander, 1976).

A new approach to these problems has been the use of acetylmethadol (also known as methadyl acetate or LAAM), a long-acting homologue of methadone that may afford easier adherence to maintenance programmes (Jaffe and Senay, 1971). However, clinic attendance is still required 3 times weekly, unless take-home privileges are provided. A completely different approach, which requires that the patient be completely opiate free before it is begun, is to treat the patient with a long-acting narcotic antagonist and 'immunise' them against the action of opiates. Naltrexone is such a drug which can be given in doses that will block most doses of opiates commonly obtainable by addicts for periods of from 48 to 72 hours. Nonetheless, 3 clinic visits a week are required, with the same disadvantages as for methadone. More to the point, the drug has little appeal to patients, so that the number who accept treatment with it is small, and those who stay with a prolonged course of treatment seem to be limited to a relatively few patients with high motivation for overcoming the addiction (Report of the National Research Council Committee on Clinical Evaluation of Narcotic Antagonists, 1978).

Problems of treating opiate dependent persons with pharmacological methods are about as great as they are with psychosocial methods. It is somewhat disheartening that so little progress has been made towards treating these patients.

13.3 Overdoses of Narcotics

Fatal overdoses of narcotics make opiate dependence a highly dangerous practice. Effective narcotic antagonists such as naloxone or nalorphine, rapidly reverse the respiratory depression that leads to a fatal outcome. Early diagnosis is essential, for once fullblown pulmonary oedema develops, the situation becomes virtually irretrievable. In using naloxone, one must be aware of the fact that it is a comparatively short acting drug, while the large dose of narcotic may persist for many hours (see also chapter IX, sect. 6.1; X, sect. 8.4.4). Monitoring of patients must be intense, even when their initial responses seem to be quite favourable. If vigilance is relaxed, the patient may quickly revert into respiratory failure and die before treatment can be resumed. Besides overdoses of narcotics, many other medical complications constitute a threat to the life of a narcotic user.

14. Use of Drugs in the Presence of Associated Psychiatric Disorders

Certain drugs can precipitate or aggravate psychiatric disorders. Thus, oral contraceptives and corticosteroids for example, should be used carefully in patients with schizophrenia or depression or a previous history of these disorders. Levodopa seems to unmask the tendency to psychiatric illness in patients with parkinsonism, particularly depression. Some non-psychotherapeutic drugs can cause mental disturbances and these should be used carefully (some not at all) in patients with psychiatric disorders (see section 15). On the other hand, tricyclic and monoamine oxidase inhibitor type antidepressants can interact with a number of other drugs, sometimes dangerously (see section 7.5).

Interactions involving psychotherapuetic drugs have clear endpoints and oversedation due to the combined effects of drugs with sedative properties is one of the most common and readily diagnosed of all drug interactions. It can be avoided by using drug combinations only when they are needed and by employing single daily doses of psychotherapeutic drugs at night. Alcohol can enhance the sedative effects of many drugs and its additive effects can be especially dangerous with barbiturates and in those driving motor vehicles (see section 15.6).

15. Drug Induced Psychiatric Disorders

Drug induced psychiatric syndromes may be either associated with the therapeutic use of a drug or due to abuse of a drug (Hollister, 1972c; Johnson, 1972). The effects produced vary from the subtle to the dramatically obvious. The elderly are particularly susceptible to mental effects of drugs and the true cause of their psychiatric disturbance can often go unrecognised. An accurate drug history should be obtained from any patient presenting with new mental symptoms to avoid the possibility of making a diagnosis of some functional psychiatric disorder when, in fact, it may be drug induced, or of mistaking drug side effects as developments in the primary psychiatric illness (e.g. confused states due to sedatives and tricyclic antidepressants in the elderly). Some of the reactions associated with therapeutic use of drugs are simply extensions of their desired pharmacological effects; for example, psychomotor impairment due to sedatives, or delirium associated with the anticholinergic tricyclic antidepressant drugs. Some reactions may be extensions of pharmacological effects to organ systems other than the principal target; for example, depression with centrally acting antihypertensive drugs. Many reactions are idiosyncratic or have unknown mechanisms, such as delirium from digitalis.

Reactions which occur secondary to drug abuse may occur while the drug is being taken (e.g. bromides), soon after its withdrawal (e.g. alcohol) or long after its use (e.g. delayed 'turn-on' with prolonged use of hallucinogens or marihuana). Drug induced neurological disorders are discussed in chapter XXV (sect. 15).

15.1 Schizophrenic-Like Reactions

Abuse of hallucinogenic drugs such as lysergic acid diethylamide (LSD) can lead to a number of adverse mental reactions ranging from acute anxiety or panic, acute paranoia, and acting out behaviour during the period of drug effect to increasing mental depression and even suicide, 'flashbacks' or mild recrudescences of the acute hallucinogenic state; and in those so predisposed, to persistent later appearing psychoses which run the usual course of acute schizophrenia (Schwartz, 1968). Prolonged abuse of sympathomimetic drugs (e.g. ephedrine, amphetamines) can lead to symptoms which closely resemble those of paranoid schizophrenia (Kramer et al., 1967), but which can be detected by a number of tell-tale physical signs such as tachycardia, poor nutrition and hygiene, fever, cold sweats, dilated pupils etc. Levodopa has produced paranoia, hallucinations and other psychotic symptoms, primarily in patients who were also taking anticholinergic drugs or had a history of mental disorder (Brogden et al., 1971). Rarely, alcoholics while they are still drinking, rather than during the withdrawal phase, experience a psychosis which resembles schizophrenia.

Prolonged use of anticonvulsants may rarely be associated with mental symptoms which range from confusion to those of schizophrenia. Attempts have been made to link these personality changes with drug induced folate deficiency, but the evidence has not been able to be supported by controlled studies (Norris and Pratt, 1974).

15.2 Depressive Reactions

Many drugs may cause depression but only a relatively small number are associated with depressive reactions with any frequency. Drug induced depression is most likely to occur in those individuals who are genetically susceptible to depression or who have had a previous depressive illness and in the elderly (Whitlock and Evans, 1978).

Centrally acting antihypertensive drugs such as Rauwolfia, methyldopa, clonidine and β-adrenoceptor blocking agents such as propranolol can cause severe depression in a few patients (Waal, 1967; Zacharias, 1976). The drug must be stopped immediately. The depression with reserpine may be particularly severe and its appearance may be delayed. It is less likely to occur when daily dosage of reserpine does not exceed 0.25mg (Smith et al., 1969), but when it does occur with low dosage regimens may be difficult to recognise (Simpson, 1973a). Patients with a history of depression are most likely to become depressed on antihypertensive drugs. Many hypertensive patients are in the age group when endogenous depression is common. Hypertensive patients may have depression prone personalities, since according to psychoanalytical theory both depressed and hypertensive patients have difficulty expressing anger. Thus, the inter-relationships of hypertension and depression are complex and often cause management problems (Simpson and Waal-Manning, 1971; see chapter XVIII; sect. 10.1.3).

The relationship between depression and oral contraceptive use is rather obscure. A history of previous depression is held by some to be an important aetiological factor, as is the use of high dose combination preparations. A few women can be shown to have biochemical evidence of pyridoxine deficiency. Depression in these women responds to pyridoxine therapy, whereas depression in women without evidence of pyridoxine deficiency does not respond. Patients with a history of depression should be carefully observed and the preparation withdrawn if depression recurs. Problems are likely to be decreased with the advent of low dose preparations (see chapter XV; sect. 13.10). Depression may follow withdrawal of amphetamines after use of large doses or prolonged administration, and after too rapid a withdrawal of the anorexiant fenfluramine (Steel and Briggs, 1972). Corticosteroids in large doses have caused depression, particularly in patients with a past history of depressive illness.

Levodopa has been reported to cause depression with or without suicidal tendencies in many patients in some studies, but symptoms have most often occurred in patients with a history of depression or in those who were disappointed in their improvement. In other cases, depressive symptoms have diminished despite continuation of treatment at the same dosage level. Controlled studies have not provided any evidence for an effect of levodopa on mood in those with no previous history of psychiatric disorder (Brogden et al., 1971).

Indomethacin has an indole moiety similar to that in serotonin, and causes a variety of unpleasant cerebral sensations, including occasional instances of depression which may be very severe (Thompson and Percy, 1966). The sensitivity of patients varies widely but night time dosage is well tolerated (see chapter XXII; sect. 3.2.3). Although antipsychotic drugs will probably make truly endogenous depressions worse (e.g. misuse in such depressed patients diagnosed as schizophrenia), which will be a particular problem with long acting injectable preparations (de Alarcon and Carney, 1969), they can be used in the mixed anxiety-depression syndrome associated with reactive depressions (see also section 7). Drugs that cause sedation or inhibit postganglionic sympathetic function (e.g. guanethidine) may indirectly cause depression by adverse effects on sexual performance (see chapter XV; sect. 23.2).

Heavy bouts of alcohol ingestion and barbiturates are well known causes of depressive reactions.

15.3 Manic or Excited Reactions

Antidepressant drugs sometimes convert a patient with a retarded depression into one with agitation or mania. Isoniazid, which has weak monoamine oxidase inhibitor activity, has been similarly implicated on isolated occasions (Kane and Taylor, 1963). Acute transient CNS stimulation has quickly followed inadvertent intravenous administration of procaine penicillin; the reaction is probably due to acute procaine poisoning (Daneel, 1969).

Any disinhibiting agent, which would include most antianxiety drugs, is likely to unmask hostility but never to create it. Nothing approaches alcohol as a drug which unmasks hostility and violence. Consequently, it seems reasonable to assume that an occasional hostile outbreak may be encountered with antianxiety drugs. Attempts to imply that these are caused by the drug, or peculiar to certain ones, remain incredible. Large doses of hypnotics may produce release phenomena with signs of drunkenness, emotional disinhibition, or excitement in susceptible individuals.

15.4 Euphoria

Euphoria or hypomania and hyperactivity have occasionally followed use of levodopa. Amphetamines rapidly lead to a pleasant state of euphoria and if abused long term can cause psychosis (see section 15.1), with depression on withdrawal. Some patients on corticosteroids or corticotrophins appear to develop an increased sense of well being which may progress to euphoria or hypomania with depression on withdrawal (McCawley, 1965). The degree of change in mood depends on the dose and duration of treatment, the sensitivity of the patient and on the underlying personality of the individual. Patients with chronic adrenal insufficiency are particularly sensitive to corticosteroids, even to normal substitution doses, and it may be necessary to give an Addisonian patient no more than half the substitution dose to keep him mentally stable.

15.5 Deliria and Perceptual Disturbances

Confusion, disorientation, hallucinations and fluctuating levels of awareness are characteristic signs of overdosage of many centrally acting anticholinergic drugs, particularly in the elderly. These include anti-Parkinsonian and antidepressant drugs. Topical anticholinergics in the eye can also lead to deliria and psychotic reactions, especially use of excessive amounts in young children or use in hot weather or climates (see chapter XII; sect. 9.6). The antiarrhythmic drug disopyramide, which has anticholinergic properties, has been associated with delirium and psychotic reactions (Falk et al., 1977; Padfield et al., 1977). Delirium is a complication of larger doses of amantadine, especially in the elderly (Schwab et al., 1969). Sleeping preparations containing hyoscine (scopolamine) and anticholinergic antihistamines have produced delirium in susceptible individuals and in those who abuse these drugs.

The histamine (H_2) receptor antagonist drug cimetidine has been associated with mental confusion and agitation, usually in elderly patients with impaired renal function (McMillan et al., 1978; Wood et al., 1978). A delirious state may be a sign of digitalis toxicity, particularly in the elderly (see chapter V; sect. 4.7.2). Toxic doses of isoniazid may produce delirium, but in rare instances it has occurred at usual therapeutic doses in those who are genetically slow acetylators of the drug (Devadatta, 1965). Cycloserine and ethionamide may cause a disoriented confused state and even 'full blown' psychosis. Para-aminosalicylic acid (PAS) may very rarely do likewise. Pentazocine can lead to hallucinatory experiences and depersonalisation, especially at high doses (Brogden et al., 1973; Taylor et al., 1978). Barbiturates occasionally may be associated with delirium especially in the elderly in whom sensory monotony of hospitalisation and sleeplessness may be contributing factors. β-Adrenoceptor blocking drugs such as propranolol can occasionally produce confusion, vivid dreams and even auditory and visual hallucinations (Hinshelwood, 1969). Disulfiram infrequently evokes psychotic behaviour, particularly when combined with metronidazole (Goodhue, 1969).

Bromide intoxication initially presents as confusion, ataxia and vague neurological signs, but later frank delirium occurs. The onset is usually insidious and the patient may increase the dose to meet the increasing symptoms. Skin rashes, particularly acneiform eruptions and salivary gland enlargement frequently occur. Bromureides such as carbromal are less of a problem than the proprietary bromides.

Hallucinogenic drugs such as LSD, mescaline, psilocybin, 'STP' and stramonium are often the source of deliria. Large doses of marihuana may evoke similar states but sleepiness usually supervenes. Acute panic reactions or dissociative reactions precede or follow frank deliria. Treatment is by conventional sedatives such as amylobarbitone (amobarbital) or diazepam. Other drugs which may cause confusion or toxic delirium are discussed in chapter XXV (sect. 15.1).

15.6 Oversedation and Impaired Psychomotor Function

Oversedation is a common problem with antianxiety drugs and sometimes with antipsychotics and tricyclic antidepressants. It can arise from: too large a single daily dose, too frequent dosage, combinations of drugs with sedative effects, failure to adjust dosage at the extremes of life, and sometimes even by failure to recognise that a drug has sedative properties. 'Additive' effects may be especially dangerous when alcohol is combined with sedatives, particularly barbiturates, and many unwitting suicides have resulted. Sedative drug combinations with alcohol may also be particularly dangerous for the motorist. Drugs add to the effects of alcohol on driving skills in proportion to their sedative effect (Milner, 1972). It is highly advisable to warn all patients on antipsychotics, tricyclic antidepressants, antianxiety agents and certain antihistamines that they must not drive after drinking even a small amount of alcohol (see section 8.4).

15.7 Anxiety States

Sympathomimetic amines used in asthma such as parenteral adrenaline or inhaled isoprenaline (isoproterenol) and excessive dosage of any orally administered agent can produce a state of apprehension, nervousness, tremor and tachycardia. Stimulant-type anorexiants have a similar effect. A paradoxical anxiety reaction may sometimes occur with use of barbiturates in the elderly and young children. Excessive caffeine intake can cause symptoms resembling anxiety states (Greden, 1974). Enquiry into tea or coffee drinking habits of patients with anxiety is well justified.

Extrapyramidal side effects of antipsychotic drugs can be mistaken for primary psychiatric symptoms such as agitation or 'hysteria'. The onset of akathisia can be readily confused with the restlessness often associated with psychosis (although most patients recognise it as drug induced) and the dose of drug wrongly increased on the supposed basis of a deterioration of the psychiatric condition. The rapid development of an oral dyskinesia, with its marked and understandable increase in anxiety and agitation, should not be dismissed as 'hysteria'.

15.8 Sleep Disturbances

Two widely taken social drugs may interfere with sleep. Caffeine is generally recognised as having this effect, but for curious reasons, it may not do so until the middle years of life. Therefore, persons who have been able to drink their evening cup of coffee with impunity may begin to find sleep more difficult and may fail to associate the insomnia with ingestion of this drug. Although alcohol is a depressant, and often enhances the onset of sleep, for poorly understood reasons, it may interfere with sleep in some persons, particularly in heavy drinkers. Anorexiants, nasal vasoconstrictors, asthma preparations containing sympathomimetics, antidepressants of the sympathomimetic or monoamine oxidase inhibitor type and levodopa may also interfere with sleep in some individuals.

Further Reading

Barchas, J.D. and others: Psychopharmacology: From Theory to Practice (Oxford University Press, Oxford 1977).

Hollister, L.E.: Clinical Pharmacology of Psychotherapeutic Drugs (Churchill Livingstone, Edinburgh, 1978).

Jarvik, M.E.: Psychopharmacology in the Practice of Medicine (Appleton Century Crofts, New York 1977).

References

ACNP-FDA Task Force: Neurologic syndromes associated with antipsychotic-drug use. New England Journal of

Medicine 289: 20 (1973).

Alexander, S.; Shader, R. and Grinspoon, L.: Electrocardiographic effects of thioridazine hydrochloride (Mellaril). Lahey Clinic Foundation Bulletin 16: 207 (1967).

Alvan, G.; Siwers, B. and Vessman, J.: Pharmacokinetics of oxazepam in healthy volunteers. Acta Pharmacologica et Toxicologica 40: 40 (1977).

Amdisen, A.: Monitoring of lithium treatment through determination of lithium concentration. Danish Medical Bulletin 22: 277 (1975).

Amdisen, A.: Serum level monitoring and clinical pharmacokinetics of lithium. Clinical Pharmacokinetics 2: 73 (1977).

American Psychiatric Association Task Force on Lithium Therapy: The current status of lithium therapy: Report of the APA Task Force. American Journal of Psychiatry 132: 997 (1975).

Anders,T.F. and Ciarnello, R.D.: Pharmacological treatment of the minimal brain dysfunction syndrome; in Barchas et al. (Ed) Psychopharmacology. From Theory to Practice, p.425 (Oxford University Press, New York 1977).

Andreasen, P.B.; Hendel, J.; Greisen, G. and Hvidberg, E.F.: Pharmacokinetics of diazepam in disordered liver function. European Journal of Clinical Pharmacology 10: 115 (1976).

Antelman, S.M. and Caggiula, A.R.: Norepinephrine-dopamine interactions and behavior. Science 195: 646 (1977).

Aquilonius, S.-M. and Hedstrand, U.: The use of physostigmine as an antidote in tricyclic anti-depressant intoxication. Acta Anaesthesia Scandinavica 22: 40 (1978).

Asberg, Marie: Individualisation of treatment with tricyclic compounds. Medical Clinics of North America 58: 1083 (1974).

Aschcroft, G.W.: Management of depression. British Medical Journal 2: 372 (1975).

Axelrod, J.: Noradrenaline fate and control of its biosynthesis. Science 173: 598 (1971).

Axelsson, R. and Martensson, E.: Serum concentration and elimination from serum of thioridazine in psychiatric patients. Current Therapeutic Research 19: 242 (1976).

Axelsson, R. and Martensson, E.: The concentration pattern of nonconjugated thioridiazine metabolites in serum by thioridazine treatment and its relationship to physiological and clinical variables. Current Therapeutic Research 21: 561 (1977).

Ayd, F.J.: Single daily dose of antidepressants. Journal of the American Medical Association 230: 263 (1974).

Ayd, F.J.: Guidelines for using short-acting intramuscular neuroleptics for rapid neuroleptization. International Drug Therapy Newsletter 12: 5 (1977).

Baastrup, P.C.; Poulsen, J.V.; Schou, M.; Thomsen, K. and Amdisen, A.: Prophylactic lithium. Double-blind discontinuation in manic-depressive and recurrent depressive disorders. Lancet 2: 326 (1970).

Backman, H. and Elosuo, R.: The effects of neuroleptics on electrocardiograms. Acta Medica Scandinavica 183: 543 (1968).

Baldaressini, R.J.: The basis for amine hypotheses in affective disorders. Archives of General Psychiatry 32: 1087 (1975).

Baldessarini, R.J. and Lipinski, J.F.: Lithium salts: 1970-1975. Annals of Internal Medicine 83: 527 (1975).

Balter, M.B.; Levine, J. and Manheimer, D.I.: Cross-national study of the extent of anti-anxiety/sedative drug use. New England Journal of Medicine 290: 769 (1974).

Barter, M. and Kammer, H.: Methylphenidate and growth retardation. Journal of the American Medical Association 239: 1742 (1978).

Baylis, P.H. and Heath, D.A.: Water disturbances in patients treated with oral lithium carbonate. Annals of Internal Medicine 88: 607 (1978).

Beckman, H. and Goodwin, F.K.: Antidepressant response to tricyclics and urinary MHPG in unipolar patients. Archives of General Psychiatry 32: 17 (1975).

Bell, R.H. and Smith, R.C.: Tardive dyskinesia: Characterization and prevalence in a statewide system. Journal of Clinical Psychiatry 39: 39 (1978).

Berlin, A.; Siwers, B.; Agurell, S.; Hiort, A.; Sjoqvist, F. and Strom, S.: Determinations of bioavailability of diazepam in various formulations from steady-state plasma concentration data. Clinical Pharmacology and Therapeutics 13: 733 (1972).

Bertilsson, L.; Asberg, M. and Thoren, P.: Differential effect of chlorimipramine and nortriptyline on cerebrospinal fluid metabolites of serotonin and noradrenaline in depression. European Journal of Clinical Pharmacology 7: 365 (1974).

Bickel, M.H.: Poisoning by tricyclic antidepressant drugs. General and pharmacokinetic considerations. International Journal of Clinical Pharmacology 11: 145 (1975).

Blackwell, B.: Psychotropic drugs in use today. The role of diazepam in medical practice. Journal of the American Medical Association 225: 1637 (1973).

Bliding, A.: Effects of different rates of absorption of two benzodiazepines on subjective and objective parameters: Significance for clinical use and risk of abuse. European Journal of Clinical Pharmacology 7: 201 (1974).

Bond, A.J.; Hailey, D.M. and Lader, M.H.: Plasma concentrations of benzodiazepines. British Journal of Clinical Pharmacology 4: 51 (1977).

Boston Collaborative Drug Surveillance Program: Clinical depression of the central nervous system due to diazepam and chlordiazepoxide in relation to cigarette smoking and age. New England Journal of Medicine 288: 277 (1973).

Boxenbaum, H.G.; Geitner, K.A.; Jack, M.L.; Dixon, W.R. and Kaplan, S.A.: Pharmacokinetic and biopharmaceutic profile of chlordiazepoxide HCl in healthy subjects. Journal of Pharmacokinetics and Biopharmaceutics 5: 25 (1977).

Breimer, D.D.: Clinical pharmacokinetics of hypnotics. Clinical Pharmacokinetics 2: 93 (1977).

Brogden, R.N.; Speight, T.M. and Avery, G.S.: Levodopa: A review of its pharmacological properties and therapeutic uses with particular reference to parkinsonism. Drugs 2: 262 (1971).

Brogden, R.N.; Speight, T.M. and Avery, G.S.: Pentazocine: A review of its pharmacological properties, therapeutic efficacy and dependence liability. Drugs 5: 6 (1973).

Brogden, R.N.; Heel, R.C.; Speight, T.M. and Avery, G.S.: Mianserin: A review of its pharmacological properties and therapeutic efficacy in depressive illness. Drugs 16: 273 (1978).

Brogden, R.N.; Heel, R.C.; Speight, T.M. and Avery, G.S.: Nomifensine: A review of its pharmacological properties and therapeutic efficacy in depressive illness. Drugs 18: 1 (1979).

Brownlie, B.E.W.; Chambers, S.T.; Sadler, W.A. and Donald, R.A.: Lithium associated thyroid disease — a report of 14 cases of hypothyroidism and 4 cases of thyrotoxicosis.

Australian and New Zealand Journal of Medicine 6: 223 (1976).

Bruce, R.B.; Turnbull, L.B.; Newman, J.H.; Kinzie, J.M.; Morris, P.H. and Pinchbeck, F.M.: Butaperazine dimaleate metabolism. Xenobiotica 4: 197 (1974).

Burckhardt, D.; Raeder, E.; Muller, V.; Imhof, P. and Neubauer, H.: Cardiovascular effects of tricyclic and tetracyclic antidepressants. Journal of the American Medical Association 239: 213 (1978).

Burrows, G.D.; Davies, B. and Kincaid-Smith, P.: Unique tubular lesions after lithium. Lancet 1: 1310 (1978).

Buyze, G.; Egberts, P.F.C.; Muusze, R.G. and Poslavsky, A.: Blood levels of thioridazine and some of its metabolites in psychiatric patients. A preliminary report. Psychiatrie, Neurologie and Neurochirurgerie (Amsterdam) 76: 229 (1973).

Byck, R.: Drugs and the treatment of psychiatric disorders; in Goodman and Gilman (Eds) Pharmacological Basis of Therapeutics, 5th ed, p.152 (Macmillan, New York 1975).

Cade, J.F.J.: Lithium — when, why and how? Medical Journal of Australia 1: 684 (1975).

Carlsson, A.: Antipsychotic drugs, neurotransmitters, and schizophrenia. American Journal of Psychiatry 135: 164 (1978).

Carlsson, A.; Corrodi, H.; Fuxe, K. and Hokfelt, T.: Effects of some antidepressant drugs on the depletion of intraneuronal brain catecholamine stores caused by 4-alpha-dimethyl-meta-tyramine. European Journal of Pharmacology 5: 367 (1969).

Cate, J.C. and Jatlow, P.I.: Chlordiazepoxide overdose: Interpretation of serum drug concentrations. Clinical Toxicology 6: 553 (1973).

Chouinard, G.; Annable, L.; Serrano, M.; Albert, J.M. and Chorette, R.: Amitriptyline-perphenazine interaction in ambulatory schizophrenic patients. Archives of General Psychiatry 32: 1295 (1975).

Clift, A.D.: Factors leading to dependence on hypnotic drugs. British Medical Journal 3: 614 (1972).

Conney, A.H.: Pharmacological implications of microsomal enzyme induction. Pharmacological Reviews 19: 317 (1967).

Cooper, S.F.; Albert, J-M.; Hillel, J. and Caille, G.: Plasma-level studies of chlorpromazine following administration of chlorpromazine hydrochloride and chlorpromazine embonate in chronic schizophrenics. Current Therapeutic Research 15: 73 (1973).

Cooper, T.B.: Plasma level monitoring of antipsychotic drugs. Clinical Pharmacokinetics 3: 14 (1978).

Council on Child Health: Medication for hyperkinetic children. Pediatrics 55: 560 (1975).

Crammer, J.L.; Rosser, R.M. and Crane, G.: Blood levels and management of lithium treatment. British Medical Journal 3: 650 (1974).

Crane, G.E.: The prevention of tardive dyskinesia. Report: Special section on tardive dyskinesia. American Journal of Psychiatry 134: 756 (1977).

Cressman, W.A.; Bianchine, J.R.; Slotnick, V.B.; Johnson, P.C. and Plostnieks, J.: Plasma level profile of haloperidol in man following intra-muscular administration. European Journal of Clinical Pharmacology 7: 99 (1974).

Curry, S.H.; Davis, J.M.; Janowsky, D.S. and Marshall, J.H.L.: Factors affecting chlorpromazine plasma levels in psychiatric patients. Archives of General Psychiatry 22: 209 (1970).

Curry, S.H.; D'Mello, A. and Mould, G.P.: Destruction of chlorpromazine during absorption in the rat *in vivo* and *in vitro*. British Journal of Pharmacology 42: 403 (1971).

Dahl, S.G. and Strandgord, R.E.: Pharmacokinetics of chlorpromazine after single and chronic dosage. Clinical Pharmacology and Therapeutics 21: 437 (1977).

Daneel, J.A.C.G.: Procaine-penicillin reaction. South African Medical Journal 43: 192 (1969).

Davies, B.: Diagnosis and treatment of anxiety and depression in general practice. Drugs 6: 389 (1973).

Davis, J.M.: Overview: Maintenance therapy in psychiatry. I: Schizophrenia. American Journal of Psychiatry 132: 1237 (1975).

Davis, J.M.: Overview: Maintenance therapy in psychiatry: II. Affective disorders. American Journal of Psychiatry 133: 1 (1976).

Davis, J.M. and Casper, R.: Antipsychotic drugs: Clinical pharmacology and therapeutic use. Drugs 14: 260 (1977).

Davis, K.L.; Berger, P.A.; Hollister, L.E. and De Fraites, E.: Physostigmine in mania. Archives of General Psychiatry 35: 119 (1978).

de Alarcon, R. and Carney, M.W.P.: Severe depressive mood changes following slow release intramuscular fluphenazine injections. British Medical Journal 3: 564 (1969).

Denham, J. and Adamson, L.: Long-acting phenothiazines in the prevention of relapse of schizophrenic patients. Canadian Psychiatric Association Journal 18: 235 (1973).

Devadatta, S.: Isoniazid-induced encephalopathy. Lancet 2: 440 (1965).

Dixon, R.; Brooks, M.A.; Postma, E.; Hackman, M.R.; Spector, S.; Moore, J.D. and Schwartz, M.A.: N-desmethyl-diazepam: A new metabolite of chlordiazepoxide in man. Clinical Pharmacology and Therapeutics 20: 450 (1976).

Dole, V.P. and Nyswander, M.E.: Methadone maintenance treatment. A ten-year perspective. Journal of the American Medical Association 235: 2117 (1976).

Drew, L.; Moon, J. and Buchanan, F.: Propranolol in the treatment of alcoholism. Medical Journal of Australia 2: 282 (1973).

Duffy, B.: Acute phenothiazine intoxication in children. Medical Journal of Australia 1: 676 (1971).

Dundee, J.W.; Lilburn, J.K.; Toner, W. and Howard, P.J.: Plasma lorazepam levels. A study following single dose administrations of 2 and 4mg by different routes. Anaesthesia 33: 15 (1978).

Editorial: Beta-adrenergic blockade and anxiety. Lancet 2: 611 (1976).

Elonen, E.; Linnoila, M.; Lukkari, I. and Matilla, M.J.: Concentration of tricyclic antidepressants in plasma, heart and skeletal muscle after their intravenous infusion to anesthetized rabbits. Acta Pharmacologica et Toxicologica 37: 274 (1975).

Eveloff, H.H.: Psychopharmacologic agents in child psychiatry. Archives of General Psychiatry 14: 472 (1966).

Everett, H.C.: The use of bethanechol chloride with tricyclic antidepressants. American Journal of Psychiatry 132: 1202 (1975).

Falk, R.H.; Nisbet, P.A. and Gray, T.J.: Mental distress in patients on disopyramide. Lancet 1: 858 (1977).

Fieve, R.R.; Dunner, D.I. and Kumbaraci, T.: Lithium prophylaxis of depression in bipolar I, bipolar II and unipolar patients. American Journal of Psychiatry 133: 925 (1976).

Fisher, C.F.; Kahn, E.; Edwards, A. and Davis, D.M.: A pathophysiological study of nightmares and night terrors.

The suppression of stage 4 night terrors with diazepam. Archives of General Psychiatry 28: 252 (1973).

Forsman, A. and Ohman, R.: Applied pharmacokinetics of haloperidol in man. Current Therapeutic Research 21: 396 (1977).

Forsman, A.; Folsch, G.; Larsson, M. and Ohman, R.: On the metabolism of haloperidol in man. Current Therapeutic Research 21: 606 (1977).

Frommer, E.A.: Treatment of childhood depression with antidepressant drugs. British Medical Journal 1: 729 (1967).

Fyro, B.; Pettersson, U. and Sedvall, G.: Serum lithium levels and side effects during administration of lithium carbonate and two slow release lithium preparations to human volunteers. Pharmacologica Clinica 2: 236 (1970).

Gamble, J.A.S.; Dundee, J.W. and Assaft, R.A.E.: Plasma diazepam levels after single dose oral and intramuscular administration. Anaesthesia 30: 164 (1975).

Glassman, A.H.; Bigger, J.T.; Giardina, E.V.; Kantor, S.J.; Perel, J.M. and Davies, M.: Clinical characteristics of imipramine-induced orthostatic hypotension. Lancet 1: 468 (1979).

Glatt, M.M.: Alcoholism. British Journal of Hospital Medicine 11: 111 (1974).

Goldberg, R.S. and Thornton, W.E.: Combined tricyclic-MAOI therapy for refractory depression: A review with guidelines for appropriate usage. Journal of Clinical Pharmacology 18: 143 (1978).

Goldfield, M.D. and Weinstein, M.R.: Lithium carbonate in obstetrics: Guidelines for clinical use. American Journal of Obstetrics and Gynecology 116: 15 (1973).

Goldstein, A.: Heroin addiction and the role of methadone in its treatment. Archives of General Psychiatry 26: 291 (1972).

Goodhue, W.W.: Disulfiram-metronidazole (well-identified) toxicity. New England Journal of Medicine 280: 1482 (1969).

Gram, L.F.: Plasma level monitoring of tricyclic antidepressant therapy. Clinical Pharmacokinetics 2: 237 (1977).

Gram, L.F. and Christiansen, J.: First-pass metabolism of imipramine in man. Clinical Pharmacology and Therapeutics 17: 555 (1975).

Gram, L.F.; Reisby, N.; Bech, P.; Nagy, A.; Petersen, G.O.; Ortmann, J.; Ibsen, I.; Dencker, S.J.; Jacobsen, O.; Krautwald, O.; Sondergaard, I. and Christiansen, J.: Imipramine: Clinical effects and pharmacokinetic variability. Psychopharmacology 54: 263 (1977).

Greden, J.F.: Anxiety or caffeinism: A diagnostic dilemma. American Journal of Psychiatry 131: 1089 (1974).

Green, D.E.; Forrest, I.S.; Forrest, F.M. and Serra, M.T.: Interpatient variation in chlorpromazine metabolism. Experimental Medicine and Surgery 23: 278 (1965).

Greenblatt, D.J. and Allen, M.D.: Toxicity of nitrazepam in the elderly: A report from the Boston Collaborative Drug Surveillance Program. British Journal of Clinical Pharmacology 5: 407 (1978).

Greenblatt, D.J. and Koch-Weser, J.: Clinical toxicity of chlordiazepoxide and diazepam in relation to serum albumin concentration: A report from the Boston Collaborative Drug Surveillance Program. European Journal of Clinical Pharmacology 7: 259 (1974).

Greenblatt, D.J. and Shader, R.I.: Benzodiazepines in Clinical Practice (Raven Press, New York 1974).

Greenblatt, D.J.; Shader, R.I. and Koch-Weser, J.: Pharmacokinetics in clinical medicine: oxazepam versus other benzodiazepines. Diseases of the Nervous System 36: 6 (1975a).

Greenblatt, D.J.; Shader, R.I. and Koch-Weser, J.: Flurazepam hydrochloride, a benzodiazepine hypnotic. Annals of Internal Medicine 83: 237 (1975b).

Greenblatt, D.J.; Shader, R.I. and Koch-Weser, J.: Flurazepam hydrochloride. Clinical Pharmacology and Therapeutics 17: 1 (1975c).

Greenblatt, D.J.; Schillings, R.T.; Kyriakopoulos, A.A.; Shader, R.I.; Sisewine, S.F.; Knowles, J.A. and Ruelius, H.W.: Clinical pharmacokinetics of lorazepam. I. Absorption and disposition of oral ^{14}C-lorazepam. Clinical Pharmacology and Therapeutics 20: 329 (1976).

Greenblatt, D.J.; Knowles, J.A.; Comer, W.H.; Shader, R.I.; Harmatz, J.S. and Ruelius, H.W.: Clinical pharmacokinetics of lorazepam. IV. Long-term oral administration. Journal of Clinical Pharmacology 17: 495 (1977a).

Greenblatt, D.J.; Joyce, T.H.; Comer, W.H.; Knowles, J.A.; Shader, R.I.; Kyriakopoulos, A.A.; MacLaughlin, D.S. and Ruelius, H.W.: Clinical pharmacokinetics of lorazepam. II. Intramuscular injection. Clinical Pharmacology and Therapeutics 21: 222 (1977b).

Greenblatt, D.J.; Allen, M.D.; Noel, B.J. and Shader, R.I.: Acute overdosage with benzodiazepine derivatives. Clinical Pharmacology and Therapeutics 21: 497 (1977c)

Greenblatt, D.J.; Shader, R.I.; MacLeod, S.M. and Sellers, E.M.: Clinical pharmacokinetics of chlordiazepoxide. Clinical Pharmacokinetics 3: 381 (1978a).

Greenblatt, D.J.; Shader, R.I.; Weinberger, D.R.; Allen, M.D. and MacLaughlin, D.S.: Effect of a cocktail on diazepam absorption. Psychopharmacology 57: 199 (1978b).

Greenblatt, D.; Shader, R.I.; MacLeod, S.M.; Sellers, E.M.; Franke, K. and Giles, H.G.: Absorption of oral and intramuscular chlordiazepoxide. European Journal of Clinical Pharmacology 13: 267 (1978c).

Greenblatt, D.J.; Woo, E.; Allen, M.D.; Orsulak, P.J. and Shader, R.I.: Rapid recovery from massive diazepam overdose. Journal of the American Medical Association 240: 1872 (1978d).

Guze, S.B. and Robins, E.: Suicide and primary affective disorders. British Journal of Psychiatry 117: 437 (1970).

Hansen, H.E. and Amdisen, A.: Lithium intoxication. Quarterly Journal of Medicine 47: 123 (1978).

Hansen, C.E.; Christensen, T.R.; Elley, J.; Hansen, L.B.; Kragh-Sorensen, P.; Larsen, N-E.; Nestoft, J. and Hvidberg, E.F.: Clinical pharmacokinetic studies of perphenazine. British Journal of Clinical Pharmacology 3: 915 (1976).

Hestbech, J.; Hansen, H.E.; Amdisen, A. and Olsen, R.: Chronic renal lesions following long-term treatment with lithium. Kidney International 12: 205 (1977).

Hewick, D.S.; Newbury, P.; Hopwood, S.; Naylor, G. and Moody, J.: Age as a factor affecting lithium therapy. British Journal of Clinical Pharmacology 4: 201 (1977).

Hillestad, L.; Hansen, T. and Melsom, H.: Diazepam metabolism in normal man. II. Serum concentration and clinical effect after oral administration and cumulation. Clinical Pharmacology and Therapeutics 16: 485 (1974a).

Hillestad, L.; Hansen, T.; Melsom, H. and Drivenes, A.: Diazepam metabolism in normal man. I. Serum concentrations and clinical effects after intravenous, intramuscular and oral administration. Clinical Pharmacology and Therapeutics 16: 479 (1974b).

Himmelhoch, J.M.; Poust, R.I.; Mallinger, A.G.; Hanin, I. and Neil, J.F.: Adjustment of lithium dose during lithium-chlorothiazide therapy. Clinical Pharmacology and Therapeutics 22: 225 (1977).

Hinshelwood, R.D.: Hallucinations and propranolol. British Medical Journal 2: 445 (1969).

Hogarty, G.E. and Goldberg, S.C.: Drugs and sociotherapy in the aftercare of schizophrenic patients. Archives of General Psychiatry 28: 54 (1973).

Hollister, L.E.: Clinical use of psychotherapeutic drugs I: Antipsychotic and antimanic drugs. Drugs 4: 321 (1972a).

Hollister, L.E.: Clinical use of psychotherapeutic drugs II. Antidepressants and antianxiety drugs and special problems in the use of psychotherapeutic drugs. Drugs 4: 361 (1972b).

Hollister, L.E.: Psychiatric syndromes due to drugs; in Meyler and Peck (Eds) Drug-Induced Diseases, vol. 4, p.561 (Excerpta Medica, Amsterdam 1972c).

Hollister, L.E.: Clinical Use of Psychotherapeutic Drugs (Thomas, Springfield 1973).

Hollister, L.E.: Drugs for emotional disorders: Current problems. Journal of the American Medical Association 234: 942 (1975).

Hollister, L.E.: Individualised dosage of tricyclic antidepressants. Drugs 14: 161 (1977).

Hollister, L.E.: Treatment of depression with drugs. Annals of Internal Medicine 89: 78 (1978a).

Hollister, L.E.: Tricyclic antidepressants. New England Journal of Medicine 299: 1106, 1168 (1978b).

Hollister, L.; Motzenbcker, F.P. and Degan, F.O.: Withdrawal reactions from chlordiazepoxide (Librium). Psychopharmacologia 2: 63 (1961).

Hollister, L.E.; Kanter, S.L. and Wright, A.: Comparison of intramuscular and oral administration of chlorpromazine and thioridazine. Archives Internationales de Pharmacodynamie et de Therapie 144: 571 (1963).

Hollister, L.E.; Overall, J.E.; Bennett, J.L.; Kimbell, I. and Shelton, J.: Specific therapeutic actions of acetophenazine, perphenazine and benzquinamide in newly-admitted schizophrenic patients. Clinical Pharmacology and Therapeutics 8: 249 (1967).

Hollister, L.E.; Curry, S.H.; Derr, J.E. and Kanter, S.L.: Studies of delayed-action medication V. Plasma levels and urinary excretion of four different dosage forms of chlorpromazine. Clinical Pharmacology and Therapeutics 11: 49 (1970).

Hollister, L.E.; Prusmack, J.J. and Lipscomb, W.: Treatment of acute alcohol withdrawal with chlormethiazole (Heminevrin). Diseases of the Nervous System 33: 247 (1972).

Jaffe, J.H. and Senay, E.C.: Methadone and 1-methadyl acetate. Use in management of narcotics addicts. Journal of the American Medical Association 216: 1303 (1971).

Jefferson, J.W.: A review of the cardiovascular effects and toxicity of tricyclic antidepressants. Psychosomatic Medicine 37: 160 (1975).

Johns, M.W.: Sleep and hypnotic drugs. Drugs 9: 448 (1975).

Johnson, D.A.W.: The psychiatric side-effects of drugs. Practitioner 209: 320 (1972).

Johnson, D.A.W.: The side-effects of fluphenazine decanoate. British Journal of Psychiatry 123: 519 (1973).

Johnson, D.A.W.: A study of the use of antidepressant medication in general practice. British Journal of Psychiatry 125: 186 (1974).

Johnson, D.A.W.: The duration of maintenance therapy in chronic schizophrenia. Acta Psychiatrica Scandinavica 53: 298 (1976).

Johnson, D.A.W.: Treatment of chronic schizophrenia. Drugs 14: 291 (1977).

Johnson, D.A.W.: The prevalence and treatment of drug induced extrapyramidal symptoms. British Journal of Psychiatry 132: 27 (1978).

Johnson, W.C.: A neglected modality in psychiatric treatment — the monoamine oxidase inhibitors. Diseases of the Nervous System 36: 521 (1975).

Johnstone, E.: The relationship between acetylator status and inhibition of monoamine oxidase, excretion of free drug and antidepressant response in depressed patients on phenelzine. Psychopharmacologica 46: 289 (1976).

Kaim, S.C.: Benzodiazepines in the treatment of alcohol withdrawal states; in Garattini, Mussini and Randall (Eds) The Benzodiazepines, p. 571 (Raven Press, New York 1973).

Kales, A. and Kales, J.D.: Sleep disorders. New England Journal of Medicine 290: 487 (1974).

Kales, A.; Paulson, M.J.; Jacobson, A. and Kales, J.D.: Somnambulism: Psychological correlates. II. Psychiatric interviews, psychological testing and discussion. Archives of General Psychiatry 14: 595 (1966).

Kales, A.; Bixler, E.O.; Tan, T.L.; Scharf, M.B. and Kales, J.D.: Chronic hypnotic use: Ineffectiveness, drug withdrawal insomnia and hypnotic drug dependence. Journal of the American Medical Association 227: 513 (1974).

Kales, A.; Bixler, E.O.; Scharf, M. and Kales, J.D.: Sleep laboratory studies of flurazepam: A model for evaluating hypnotic drugs. Clinical Pharmacology and Therapeutics 19: 576 (1976).

Kales, A.; Bixler, E.O.; Kales, J.D. and Scharf, M.B.: Comparative effectiveness of nine hypnotic drugs: sleep laboratory studies. Journal of Clinical Pharmacology 17: 207 (1977).

Kane, F.J. and Taylor, T.W.: Mania associated with the use of INH and cocaine. American Journal of Psychiatry 119: 1098 (1963).

Kane, J.; Rifkin, A.; Quitkin, F. and Klein, D.F.: Antipsychotic drug blood levels and clinical outcome; in Klein and Gittelman-Klein (Eds) Progress in Psychiatric Drug Treatment, p.399-408 (Brunner/Mazel, New York 1976).

Kaplan, S.A.; de Silva, J.A.F.; Jack, M.L.; Alexander, K.; Strojny, N.; Weinfeld, R.E.; Puglisi, C.V. and Weissman, L.: Blood level profile in man following chronic oral administration of flurazepam hydrochloride. Journal of Pharmaceutical Sciences 62: 1932 (1973).

Karim, A.K.M.B. and Price Evans, D.A.: Polymorphic acetylation of nitrazepam. Journal of Medical Genetics 13: 17 (1976).

Klawans, H.L. Jr.: The pharmacology of tardive dyskinesias. American Journal of Psychiatry 130: 82 (1973).

Klett, C.J. and Caffey, E. Jr.: Evaluating the long-term need for antiparkinson drugs by chronic schizophrenics. Archives of General Psychiatry 26: 374 (1972).

Klett, C.J.; Hollister, L.E.; Caffey, E.M. and Kaim, S.C.: Evaluating changes in symptoms during acute alcohol withdrawal. Archives of General Psychiatry 24: 174 (1971).

Kline, N.S.: Antidepressant medications: A more effective use by general practitioners, family physicians, internists and others. Journal of the American Medical Association 227: 1158 (1974).

Klotz, U.; Avant, G.R.; Hoyumpa, A.; Schenkler, S. and Wilkinson, G.R.: The effects of age and liver disease on the disposition and elimination of diazepam in adult man. Journal of Clinical Investigation 55: 347 (1975).

Klotz, U.; Antonin, K.L. and Bieck, P.R.: Comparison of the

pharmacokinetics of diazepam after single and subchronic doses. European Journal of Clinical Pharmacology 10: 121 (1976).

Kobayashi, R.M.: Drug therapy of tardive dyskinesia. New England Journal of Medicine 296: 257 (1977).

Kragh-Sorensen, P.K.; Hansen, E.; Baastrup, P.C. and Hvidberg, E.F.: Self-inhibiting action of nortriptyline's antidepressive effect at high plasma levels. A randomized, double-blind study controlled by plasma concentrations in patients with endogenous depression. Psychopharmacologia 45: 305 (1976).

Kramer, J.C.; Fischman, V.S. and Littlefield, D.C.: Amphetamine abuse. Pattern and effects of high doses taken intravenously. Journal of the American Medical Association 205: 305 (1967).

Kraus, J.W.; Desmond, P.V.; Marshall, J.P.; Johnson, R.F.; Schenker, S. and Wilkinson, G.R.: Effects of aging and liver disease on disposition of lorazepam. Clinical Pharmacology and Therapeutics 24: 411 (1978).

Kugler, J.; Oswald, W.D.; Herzfeld, V.; Seus, R.; Pingel, J. and Welzel, D.: Long term treatment of cerebrovascular changes in the elderly. Deutsche Medizinische Wochenschrift 103: 456 (1978).

Lader, M.: Anxiolytic drugs. Practitioner 215: 468 (1975).

Lader, M.: Antianxiety drugs: Clinical pharmacology and therapeutic use. Drugs 12: 362 (1976).

Lader, M. and Marks, I.M.: Clinical Anxiety (Grune and Stratton, New York 1972).

Leemsta, J.E. and Koenig, K.L.: Sudden death and phenothiazines. A current controversy. Archives of General Psychiatry 18: 137 (1968).

Lehmann, K. and Merten, K.: Elimination of lithium dependent of age in healthy people and patients suffering from renal insufficiency. International Journal of Clinical Pharmacology, Therapy and Toxicology 10: 292 (1974).

Lindstedt, G.; Nilsson, L.A.; Waldinder, J.; Skott, A. and Ohman, R.: On the prevalence, diagnosis and management of lithium-induced hypothyroidism in psychiatric patients. British Journal of Psychiatry 130: 452 (1977).

MacLeod, S.M.; Giles, H.G.; Bengert, B.; Liu, F. and Sellers, E.M.: The influence of age and sex on diazepam pharmacokinetics. Clinical Research 25: 676A (1977a).

MacLeod, S.M.; Giles, H.G.; Patzalek, G.; Thiessen, J.J. and Sellers, E.M.: Diazepam actions and plasma concentrations following ethanol ingestion. European Journal of Clinical Pharmacology 11: 345 (1977b).

McCawley, A.: Cortisone habituation — a clinic note. New England Journal of Medicine 273: 976 (1965).

McGeer, P.L. and McGeer, E.G.: Possible changes in striatal and limbic cholinergic systems in schizophrenia. Archives of General Psychiatry 34: 1319 (1977).

McMillan, M.A.; Ambis, D. and Siegel, J.H.: Cimetidine and mental confusion. New England Journal of Medicine 298: 284 (1978).

Maas, J.W.: Biogenic amines and depression. Biochemical and pharmacological separation of two types of depression. Archives of General Psychiatry 32: 1357 (1975).

Maletzky, B.M. and Klotter, J.: Addiction to diazepam. International Journal of Addictions 11: 95 (1976).

Mallach, H.J.; Moosmayer, A.; Gottwald, K. and Staak, M.: Pharmacokinetic studies on absorption and excretion of oxazepam in combination with alcohol. Arzneimittel-Forschung 25: 1840 (1975).

Mandelli, M.; Tognoni, G. and Garattini, S.: Clinical pharmacokinetics of diazepam. Clinical Pharmacokinetics 3: 72

(1978).

Marks, J.: The Benzodiazepines. Use, Overuse, Misuse, Abuse, p.111 (MTP, Lancaster 1978).

Martin, P.R.; Billings, B.H.; Giles, H.G. et al.: Inhibition of drug biotransformation by disulfiram. Canadian Federation of Biological Societies: Proceedings 20: 125 (1977).

Mason, R.W.; McQueen, E.G.; Keary, P.J. and James, N. McL.: Pharmacokinetics of lithium: Elimination half-time, renal clearance and apparent volume of distribution in schizophrenia. Clinical Pharmacokinetics 3: 241 (1978).

Mathew, H.; Proudfoot, A.T.; Aitken, R.C.B.; Raeburn, J.A. and Wright, N.: Nitrazepam — a safe hypnotic. British Medical Journal 3: 23 (1969).

Maxwell, J.D.; Carrella, M.; Parkes, J.D.; Williams, R.; Mould, G.P. and Curry, S.H.: Plasma disappearance and cerebral effects of chlorpromazine in cirrhosis. Clinical Science 43: 143 (1972).

Melander, A.; Danielson, K.; Vessman, J. and Wahlin, E.: Bioavailability of oxazepam: Absence of influence of food intake. Acta Pharmacologica et Toxicologica 40: 584 (1977).

Merry, J.: Lithium and thyrotoxicosis. British Medical Journal 2: 765 (1977).

Miller, P.R.; Champelli, J.W. and Dinello, F.A.: Imipramine in the treatment of enuretic school children: A double-blind study. American Journal of Diseases of Children 115: 17 (1968).

Milner, G.: Drugs and Driving (ADIS Press, Sydney 1972).

Morris, J.B. and Beck, A.T.: The efficacy of antidepressant drugs: A review of research (1958 to 1972). Archives of General Psychiatry 30. 667 (1974).

Muusze, R.G.: Analysis of thioridazine and some of its metabolites in blood by liquid chromatography. University of Amsterdam: Doctoral Thesis (1975).

Nagy, A. and Treiber, L.: Quantitative determination of imipramine and desipramine in human blood plasma by direct densitometry of thin-layer chromatograms. Journal of Pharmacy and Pharmacology 25: 599 (1973).

Newton, R.W.: Physostigmine salicylate in the treatment of tricyclic antidepressant overdosage. Journal of the American Medical Association 231: 941 (1975).

Nies, A.; Robinson, D.S.; Friedman, M.J.; Green, R.; Cooper, T.B.; Ravaris, C.L. and Ives, J.O.: Relationship between age and tricyclic antidepressant plasma levels. American Journal of Psychiatry 134: 790 (1977).

Norris, J.W. and Pratt, R.F.: Folic acid deficiency and epilepsy. Drugs 8: 366 (1974).

Odar-Cederlof, I.; Vessman, J.; Alvan, G. and Sjoqvist, F.: Oxazepam disposition in uremic patients. Acta Pharmacologica et Toxicologica 40(Suppl. 1): 52 (1977).

Oswald, I.: Psychological medicine. Sleep difficulties. British Medical Journal 1: 557 (1975).

Oswald, I.; Brezinova, V. and Dunleavy, D.L.F.: On the slowness of action of tricyclic antidepressant drugs. British Journal of Psychiatry 120: 673 (1972).

Padfield, P.L.; Smith, D.A.; Fitzsimons, E.J. and McCruden, D.C.: Disopyramide and acute psychosis. Lancet 1: 1152 (1977).

Patman, J.; Landauer, A.A. and Milner, G.: The combined effects of alcohol and amitriptyline on skills similar to motor-car driving. Medical Journal of Australia 2: 946 (1969).

Petersen, V.; Hvidt, S.; Thomsen, K. and Schou, M.: Effect of prolonged thiazide treatment on renal lithium clearance. British Medical Journal 3: 143 (1974).

Piafsky, K.M. and Borga, O.: Plasma protein binding of basic drugs II. Importance of α_1-acid glycoprotein for interindividual variation. Clinical Pharmacology and Therapeutics 22: 545 (1977).

Pinder, R.M.; Brogden, R.N.; Speight, T.M. and Avery, G.S.: Doxepin Up-to-date: A review of its pharmacological properties and therapeutic efficacy with particular reference to depression. Drugs 13: 161 (1977).

Pirola, R.C.: Drug Metabolism and Alcohol (ADIS Press, Sydney 1977).

Pisciotta, V.: Drug-induced agranulocytosis. Drugs 15: 132 (1978).

Prange, A.J.; Wilson, I.C.; Rabon, A.M. and Lipton, M.A.: Enhancement of imipramine antidepressant activity by thyroid hormone. American Journal of Psychiatry 126: 457 (1969).

Prien, R.F.: Chemotherapy in chronic organic brain syndrome. A review of the literature. Psychopharmacology Bulletin 9: 5 (1973).

Prien, R.F. and Caffey, E.M.: Long-term maintenance drug therapy in recurrent affective illness: Current status and issues. Diseases of the Nervous System 38: 981 (1977).

Prien, R.F.; Levine, J. and Switalski, R.W.: Discontinuation of chemotherapy for chronic schizophrenics: results from two collaborative studies. Hospital Community Psychiatry 22: 4 (1971).

Prien, R.F.; Caffey, E.M. Jr. and Klett, C.J.: Relationship between serum lithium level and clinical response in acute mania treated with lithium. British Journal of Psychiatry 120: 409 (1972).

Quitkin, F.; Rifkin, A. and Klein, D.F.: Very high dosage vs. standard dosage fluphenazine in schizophrenia. A double-blind study of nonchronic treatment-refractory patients. Archives of General Psychiatry 32: 1276 (1975).

Quitkin, F.; Rifkin, A.; Kane, J.; Ramos-Lorenzi, J.R. and Klein, D.F.: Long-acting oral vs injectable antipsychotic drugs in schizophrenics. A one-year double-blind comparison in multiple episodic schizophrenics. Archives of General Psychiatry 35: 889 (1978).

Rane, A.; Tomson, G. and Bjarke, B.: Effects of maternal lithium therapy in a newborn infant. Journal of Pediatrics 93: 296 (1978).

Reidenberg, M.M.; Levy, M.; Warner, H.; Coutinho, C.B.; Schwartz, M.A.; Yu, G. and Cheripko, J.: Relationship between diazepam dose, plasma level, age and central nervous system depression. Clinical Pharmacology and Therapeutics 23: 371 (1978).

Reilly, T.M.: Physiological dependence on, and symptoms of withdrawal from, chlormethiazole. British Journal of Psychiatry 128: 375 (1976).

Reisby, N.; Gram, L.F.; Bech, P.; Nagy, A.; Petersen, G.O.; Ortmann, J.; Ibsen, I.; Denker, S.J.; Jacobsen, O.; Krautwald, O.; Sondergaard, I.; and Christiansen, J.: Imipramine: Clinical effects and pharmacokinetic variability. Psychopharmacology 54: 263 (1977).

Renton, C.A.; Affleck, J.W.; Carstairs, M. and Forrest, A.D.: A follow-up of schizophrenic patients in Edinburgh. Acta Psychiatrica Scandinavica 39: 548 (1963).

Report of the National Research Council Committee on Clinical Evaluation of Narcotic Antagonists: Clinical evaluation of naltrexone treatment of opiate-dependent individuals. Archives of General Psychiatry 35: 335 (1978).

Rickels, K.: Non-specific factors in drug therapy of neurotic patients; in Rickels (Ed) Non-specific Factors in Drug Therapy (Thomas, Springfield 1968).

Rickels, K.: Use of antianxiety agents in anxious outpatients. Psychopharmacology 58: 1 (1978).

Rifkin, A.; Quitkin, F.; Rabiner, C.J. and Klein, D.F.: Fluphenazine decanoate, fluphenazine hydrochloride given orally, and placebo in remitted schizophrenics. Archives of General Psychiatry 34: 43 (1977).

Rivera-Calimlim, L.; Nasrallah, H.; Strauss, J. and Lasagna, L.: Clinical response and plasma levels. Effect of dose, dosage schedules, and drug interactions on plasma chlorpromazine levels. American Journal of Psychiatry 133: 646 (1976).

Rivera-Calimlim, L.; Kerzner, B. and Karch, F.E.: Effect of lithium on plasma chlorpromazine levels. Clinical Pharmacology and Therapeutics 23: 451 (1978).

Robinson, D.S. and Barker, E.: Tricyclic antidepressant cardiotoxicity. Journal of the American Medical Association 236: 2089 (1976).

Rogers, S.C. and Clay, P.M.: A statistical review of controlled trials of imipramine and placebo in the treatment of depressive illnesses. British Journal of Psychiatry 127: 599 (1975).

Rubin, E. and Lieber, C.S.: Hepatic microsomal enzymes in man and rat: induction and inhibition by ethanol. Science 162: 690 (1968).

Safer, D. and Allen, R.: Side-effects from long-term use of stimulants in children. International Journal of Mental Health 4: 105 (1975).

Schildkraut, J.J.: Neuropharmacology of the affective disorders. Annual Review of Pharmacology 13: 427 (1973).

Schildkraut, J.J.: The current status of biological criteria for classifying the depressive disorders and predicting responses to treatment. Psychopharmacology Bulletin 10: 5 (1974).

Schou, M.: What happened later to the lithium babies? A follow-up study of children born without malformations. Acta Psychiatrica Scandinavica 54: 193 (1976).

Schou, M. and Amdisen, A.: Lithium and pregnancy — III. Lithium ingestion by children breast-fed by women on lithium treatment. British Medical Journal 2: 138 (1973).

Schou, M.; Amdisen, A. and Steenstrup, D.R.: Lithium and pregnancy II. Hazards to women given lithium during pregnancy and delivery. British Medical Journal 2: 137 (1973).

Schuckit, M.A. and Feighner, J.P.: Safety of high-dose tricyclic antidepressant therapy. American Journal of Psychiatry 128: 1456 (1972).

Schwab, R.S.; England, A.C.; Poskaner, D.C. and Young, R.R.: Amantadine in the treatment of Parkinson's disease. Journal of the American Medical Association 208: 1168 (1969).

Schwartz, C.J.: The complications of LSD: A review of the literature. Journal of Nervous and Mental Disease 146: 174 (1968).

Seipel, J.H.; Fisher, R.; Blatchley, R.J.; Floam, J.E. and Bohm, M.: Rheoencephalographic and other studies of betahistine in humans. IV Prolonged administration with improvement in arteriosclerotic dementia. Journal of Clinical Pharmacology 17: 140 (1977).

Seixas, F.A.: Alcohol and its drug interactions. Annals of Internal Medicine 83: 86 (1975).

Sellers, E.M. and Kalant, H.: Alcohol intoxication and withdrawal. New England Journal of Medicine 294: 757 (1976).

Seppala, T.: Psychomotor skills during acute and two-week

treatment with mianserin (ORG GB 94) and amitriptyline and their combined effects with alcohol. Annals of Clinical Research 9: 66 (1977).

Shader, R.; Georgotas, A; Greenblatt, D.J.; Harmatz, J.S. and Allen, M.D.: Impaired absorption of desmethyldiazepam from chlorazepate by magnesium aluminium hydroxide. Clinical Pharmacology and Therapeutics 24: 308 (1978)

Shaw, D.M.: The practical management of affective disorders. British Journal of Psychiatry 130: 432 (1977).

Shull, H.J.Jr.; Wilkinson, G.R.; Johnson, R. and Schenker, S.: Normal disposition of oxazepam in acute hepatitis and cirrhosis. Annals of Internal Medicine 84: 420 (1976).

Simpson, F.O.: Hypertension and depression and their treatment. Australian and New Zealand Journal of Psychiatry 7: 133 (1973a).

Simpson, F.O.: Antihypertensive drug therapy. Drugs 6: 333 (1973b).

Simpson, F.O. and Waal-Manning, H.J.: Hypertension and depression: Interrelated problems in therapy. Journal of the Royal College of Physicians of London 6: 14 (1971).

Simpson, G.M.; Voitashevshy, A.; Young, M.A. and Lee, J.H.: Deanol in the treatment of tardive dyskinesia. Psychopharmacology 52: 257 (1977).

Simpson, G.M.; Varga, E.; Lee, J.H. and Zoubok, B.: Tardive dyskinesia and psychotropic drug history. Psychopharmacology 58: 117 (1978).

Singer, I. and Rotenberg, D.: Mechanisms of lithium action. New England Journal of Medicine 289: 254 (1973).

Siwers, B.; Ringberger, V-A.; Tuck, J.R. and Sjoqvist, F.: Initial clinical trial based on biochemical methodology of zimelidine (a serotonin uptake inhibitor) in depressed patients. Clinical Pharmacology and Therapeutics 21: 194 (1977).

Sjoqvist, F.: Psychotropic drugs (2). Interaction between monoamine oxidase (MAO) inhibitors and other substances. Proceedings of the Royal Society of Medicine 58 (Pt 2): 967 (1965).

Sjoqvist, F.: Assessment of antidepressants — pharmacokinetic aspects; in Breckenridge (Ed) Advanced Medicine. Topics in Therapeutics 1, p.198 (Pitman, London 1975).

Smith, W.H.; Thurn, R.H. and Bromer, L.: Comparative evaluation of rauwolfia root and reserpine. Clinical Pharmacology and Therapeutics 10: 338 (1969).

Snyder, S.H. and Yamamura, H.I.: Antidepressants and the muscarinic acetylcholine receptor. Archives of General Psychiatry 34: 236 (1977).

Spiker, D.G. and Biggs, J.T.: Tricyclic antidepressants; prolonged plasma levels after overdose. Journal of the American Medical Association 236: 1711 (1976).

Sprague, R. and Sleator, E.: What is the proper dose of stimulant drugs in children? International Journal of Mental Health 4: 75 (1975).

Stafford, J.R. and Fann, W.E.: Drug interactions with guanidinium antihypertensives. Drugs 13: 57 (1977).

Steel, J.M. and Briggs, M.: Withdrawal depression in obese patients after fenfluramine treatment. British Medical Journal 3: 26 (1972).

Strayhorn, J.M. and Nash, J.L.: Severe neurotoxicity despite "therapeutic" serum lithium levels. Diseases of the Nervous System 38: 107 (1977).

Taylor, M.; Galloway, D.B.; Petrie, J.C.; Davidson, J.F.; Gallon, S.C. and Moir, D.C.: Psychomimetic effects of pentazocine and dihydrocodeine tartrate. British Medical Journal 2: 1198 (1978).

Thomson, N. and Percy, J.S.: Further experience with indomethacin in the treatment of rheumatic disorders. British Medical Journal 1: 80 (1966).

Thomsen, K. and Schou, M.: Renal lithium excretion in man. American Journal of Physiology 215: 823 (1968).

Tilkian, A.G.; Schroeder, J.S.; Kao, J. and Hultgren, H.: Effect of lithium on cardiovascular performance: Report on extended ambulatory monitoring and exercise testing before and during lithium therapy. American Journal of Cardiology 38: 701 (1976).

Todd, J. and Jerram, T.C.: Thyrotoxicosis during lithium treatment. British Journal of Clinical Practice 32: 201 (1978).

Tognoni, G.; Gomeni, R.; De Maio, D.; Alberti, G.G.; Franciosi, P. and Scieghi, G.: Pharmacokinetics of N-demethyldiazepam in patients suffering from insomnia and treated with nortriptyline. British Journal of Clinical Pharmacology 2: 227 (1975).

Turek, I.S.: Combined use of ECT and psychotropic drugs: Antidepressives and antipsychotics. Comprehensive Psychiatry 14: 495 (1973).

Tyrer, P.: Towards rational therapy with monoamine oxidase inhibitors. British Journal of Psychiatry 128: 354 (1976).

Tyrer, P.: Drug treatment of psychiatric patients in general practice. British Medical Journal 2: 1008 (1978).

Van Putten, T.: Why do schizophrenic patients refuse to take their drugs? Archives of General Psychiatry 31: 67 (1974).

Verbeeck, R.; Tjandramaga, T.B.; Verberckmoes, R. and De Schepper, P.J.: Biotransformation and excretion of lorazepam in patients with chronic renal failure. British Journal of Clinical Pharmacology 3: 1033 (1976).

Vohra, J.; Hunt, D.; Burrows, G. and Sloman, G.: Intracardiac conduction defects following overdose of tricyclic antidepressant drugs. European Journal of Cardiology 2: 443 (1975).

Waal, H.J.: Propranolol-induced depression. British Medical Journal 2: 50 (1967).

Weil-Malherbe, H. and Szara, S.I.: The Biochemistry of Functional and Experimental Psychoses, p.55 (Charles C. Thomas, Springfield, 1971).

Weinstein, M.R. and Goldfield, M.D.: Cardiovascular malformations with lithium use during pregnancy. American Journal of Psychiatry 132: 529 (1975).

Weiss, G.: The natural history of hyperactivity in childhood and treatment with stimulant medication at different ages: A summary of research findings. International Journal of Mental Health 4: 213 (1975).

Weiss, G.; Werry, J.; Minde, K.; Douglas, V. and Sykes, D.: Studies on the hyperactive child. V. The effects of dextroamphetamine and chlorpromazine on behaviour and intellectual functioning. Journal of Child Psychology and Psychiatry 9: 145 (1968).

Werry, J.S.: Medication for hyperkinetic children. Drugs 11: 81 (1976).

Werry, J.S.: Pediatric Psychopharmacology: The Use of Behaviour Modifying Drugs in Children (Brunner/Mazel, New York 1978).

Werry, J. and Sprague, R.: Methylphenidate in children - effect of dosage. Australia and New Zealand Journal of Psychiatry 8: 9 (1974).

Whitlock, F.A. and Evans, L.E.J.: Drugs and depression. Drugs 15:53 (1978).

Wikler, A.: Diagnosis and treatment of drug dependence of the barbiturate type. Amer. J. Psych. 125: 758 (1968).

Wise, C.D.; Berger, B.B. and Stein, L: Benzodiazepines: Anxiety-reducing activity by reduction of serotonin turnover in the brain. Science 177: 180 (1972).

Wood, C.A.; Isaacson, M.L. and Hibbs, M.S.: Cimetidine and mental confusion. Journal of the American Medical Association 239: 2550 (1978).

Wretlind, M.; Pilbrand, A.; Sundwall, A. and Vessman, J.: Disposition of three benzodiazepines after single oral administration in man. Acta Pharmacologica et Toxicologica 40: 28 (1977).

Zacharias, F.J.: Patient acceptability of propranolol and the occurrence of side-effects. Postgraduate Medical Journal 52 (Suppl. 4): 87 (1976).

Zbinden, G.; Bagdon, R.E.; Keith, E.F.; Phillips, R.D. and Randall, L.O.: Experimental and clinical toxicology of chlordiazepoxide (Librium). Toxicology and Applied Pharmacology 3: 619 (1961).

Zeigler, V.E.; Meyer, D.A.; Rosen, S.H.; Knesevich, J.W. and Biggs, J.T.: Amitriptyline dosage schedule, sampling time and tricyclic plasma levels. British Journal of Psychiatry 131: 168 (1977).

Chapter XXVII
Principles and Practice of Antibacterial Chemotherapy

L.P. Garrod

Synopsis of Important Principles

1) The successful chemotherapy of bacterial infections requires an accurate bacteriological as well as clinical diagnosis.

2) This alone may enable suitable treatment to be chosen, but if the causative organism is one now sometimes possessing abnormal resistance to antibiotics and other drugs, skilled laboratory guidance is required in making this choice.

3) The site of infection is an important factor to take into account: if this is in the urinary or biliary tract or the meninges a drug must be chosen which attains adequate concentrations in these areas.

4) Preference should be given to the less toxic of two drugs if both will serve the purpose.

5) A combination of two agents may be advisable either to prevent the development of bacterial resistance or to achieve a synergic effect. Some combinations, so far from achieving this, are actually antagonistic.

6) Dosage often requires reduction at the two extremes of life. It often needs to be reduced in renal disease, since otherwise drugs eliminated by this route accumulate to dangerous levels. Dosage may also require modification in severe disease of the liver.

7) A choice between different derivatives of a particular class of drug, not only needs to be assessed in terms of degree of activity against a susceptible organism, but also in terms of efficiency of absorption and extent of protein binding.

8) Sometimes, factors such as convenience or ease of administration, relative incidence of troublesome side effects and cost influence the choice.

Other chapters in this book deal with the use of antibacterial drugs in different kinds of disease, classified mainly on a regional basis. This chapter defines the general principles which should govern all such treatment, and applies them to the direction of treatment for some of the more important infections, classified not regionally, but according to the identity of the responsible micro-organism. This arrangement, which includes no systematic description of the properties of antibacterial drugs or even of those of groups to which many of them belong, requires that two of these properties should first be discussed, if only briefly.

1. Clinical Pharmacological Considerations

1.1 Modes of Action of Antibacterial Drugs

Drugs in general owe their activity to an effect on body tissues. It is a merit in any drug used to combat microbic infection that it should exert no such effect; its sole purpose is its action on the invader, with as little as possible on the body itself. Processes are involved here which have almost no parallel in other fields of medicine, and a full understanding of them is not necessary to successful therapeutics. Indeed, the earlier antibiotics had achieved a therapeutic revolution well before their mode of action was even suspected, still less elucidated. The pace and success of subsequent studies have been astonishing; chemists and bacteriologists between them have opened up a new world.

There are four main ways in which antibacterial drugs act (see Gale et al., 1972; Weinstein, 1972). The first to be discovered, by Woods in 1940, is as an *antimetabolite,* by competitive inhibition of an enzyme responsible for some stage in a vital synthetic process. Woods showed that sulphonamides prevent the utilisation of *p*-aminobenzoic acid, at a very early stage of the process leading ultimately to the synthesis of nucleic acids. That trimethoprim blocks the next stage, the conversion of folic to folinic acid, was proved by Hitchings (see Hitchings, 1969), the discoverer of this and other valuable 2:4-diaminopyrimidines. The 'sequential enzymic blockade' exerted by a sulphonamide and trimethoprim (co-trimoxazole) acting together is a unique and highly effective example of synergy. In the final stage of the same long process, nalidixic acid and rifamycin derivatives inhibit the formation of DNA and RNA respectively.

A second important mechanism is *inhibition of cell wall synthesis,* both preventing multiplication and leading, except under very favourable osmotic conditions, to lysis. This complex process, about which almost nothing was known until the study of this subject began in earnest, can be interfered with at several stages. The·earliest of these is the action of cycloserine, a structural analogue of D-alanine, in preventing the linkage of molecules of this amino acid, which is the first stage in the formation of a peptide chain. This combines with a sugar, acetylmuramic acid, and other constituents to form long chained molecules. The transport and assembly of these is interrupted in different ways by vancomycin and bacitracin, and their final binding to give cohesion, on which the integrity of the cell wall depends, is prevented by penicillins and cephalosporins.

Inhibition of protein synthesis is the mode of action of several families of antibiotics, and the processes involved are so complex and various that any attempt to describe them would be out of place here (for review, see Pestka, 1971). It is a remarkable fact, not fully understood, that the effect may be rapidly lethal (bactericidal) or only growth inhibitory (bacteristatic). Streptomycin is rapidly bactericidal in higher concentrations, unlike penicillin, the lethal effect of which is relatively slow and unimproved by raising the concentration above a low optimum. Chloramphenicol, although acting by a generally similar mechanism, is purely bacteristatic, the population of organisms remaining stationary for many hours regardless of antibiotic concentration. The bactericidal action of streptomycin is shared by other 'aminoglycosides' (kanamycin, gentamicin and others) and the bacteristatic effect of chloramphenicol by tetracyclines, macrolides (e.g. erythromycin) and lincomycin, except that some of these agents may exert a slow and partial lethal effect in higher concentrations (see appendix D).

The fourth distinct and well ascertained mode of action is *increased permeability of the cell membrane* which underlies the cell wall, leading to escape of cell constituents and death. This is the characteristic action of peptides, among which only the polymyxins are suitable for systemic use, and the polyene antifungal agents nystatin and amphotericin B.

1.2 Pharmacokinetic Properties of Antibacterial Drugs

An understanding of absorption and disposition of antibacterial drugs is of much more importance in directing treatment (for review, see Schonfeld, 1978). It must first be understood that the object of all true (i.e. systemic) chemotherapy is that the drug shall enter the blood stream and thus be carried to the site of infection, wherever situated, from within. This is far more effective than any kind of local application, although drugs with a systemic action are also sometimes applied locally.

If the drug is well absorbed from the alimentary tract, oral administration may be preferred for its convenience. There is an entire spectrum of behaviour from this point of view, from the total non-absorption of aminoglycosides, which simply remain in the lumen and exert an antibacterial effect there, to almost complete absorption, of which the best example is cephalexin. In the intermediate range, incomplete absorption may be due to destruction by gastric acid; oral benzylpenicillin is very poorly and irregularly absorbed for this reason, and some forms of erythromycin suffer from this defect. Acid stable penicillins such as ampicillin are broken down by bacterial enzymes in the bowel. The absorption of tetracyclines is always incomplete — hence their disturbing effects on bowel flora and function — owing largely to combination with divalent cations such as calcium. The behaviour of different forms of the same drug varies; sulphonamides are absorbed well or poorly according to their solubility, and phenoxypenicillins are acid stable and hence regularly although still incompletely absorbed. The absorption of ampicillin, which despite its acid stability is far from completely absorbed, can be improved by esterification. Three such esters are available: pivampicillin, bacampicillin and talampicillin, which are hydrolysed in the blood and tissues to ampicillin; these and amoxycillin, a near relative of ampicillin which is not hydrolysed to ampicillin but is absorbed and acts as such, are twice as well absorbed as ampicillin itself.

The alternative is parenteral injection, either intravenous, the full effect of which is immediate, or intramuscular, when the peak blood level may be attained within very few minutes (benzylpenicillin) or after as long as 1 to 2 hours. Whether the oral or parenteral route is used, the duration of effect from a given dose has next to be considered. This depends on the rate of elimination, which for most antibacterial drugs is mainly renal. The most rapidly excreted of all is benzylpenicillin; the Oxford workers in early days compared their efforts to sustain the blood level to 'keeping up that of water in a bath with the plug out'. This difficulty can be overcome by giving enormous doses, which is common practice, or by injecting a suspension of a much less soluble product, procaine penicillin, which is slowly dissolved at the site of injection. Alternatively, the renal excretion of penicillin may be delayed by concurrent administration of probenecid, which inhibits renal tubular secretion of penicillins; use of this is made in treatment of gonorrhoea (see chapter XXIX; sect. 3). Assuming that a continuous effect is necessary, the proper interval between given doses of any antibacterial drug can be ascertained from knowledge of its rate of renal excretion — or biotransformation, since this is also a mechanism for elimination of some antibacterial drugs (see Barza and Weinstein, 1976; appendix E).

Some other aspects of distribution and elimination are discussed elsewhere in this and other chapters (see chapter XXI; sect. 1). Among these is the degree of binding of the drug to protein while in the blood (see Craig and Welling, 1977). This is a loose combination with albumin, from which release occurs as the total concentration falls. This may have some advantage in delaying excretion and so prolonging the effect, but it has the greater disadvantage that bound drug is antibacterially inactive. Its extent varies widely in similar groups; in penicillins from 17% for amoxycillin to 98% for dicloxacillin, and in cephalosporins from 15% for cephalexin and 20% for cephaloridine to 84% for cephazolin (see appendix A). It is indeed surprising that some of the most highly bound antibiotics have the therapeutic action of which they are unquestionably capable.

2. Bacteriological Considerations

2.1 Diagnosis

However obscure the clinical condition, treatment should be based on some provisional diagnosis. In a seriously ill febrile patient immediate treatment may seem essential, but it should at least be delayed until all specimens have been obtained, which should enable the cause of the infection to be identified (including where applicable and possible, blood for culture). The patient may prove to have, say pneumonia, septicaemia or meningitis, but here the clinical diagnosis is not enough to enable the correct treatment to be chosen: each of these conditions can have several different microbic causes and usually no single drug is effective against all of them. In fact, a bacteriological diagnosis is more important for the present purpose than the clinical.

There are probably many who still treat infections by rule-of-thumb methods, no doubt often successfully when these are based on enough experience. Nevertheless, it would be an advance if everyone in clinical practice were trained to think bacteriologically, and to have, rather than a disease, a specific micro-organism in mind when prescribing. In the present crowded undergraduate curriculum, the introduction of new subjects is tending to reduce the time available for teaching various branches of pathology, and in the present context this appears a retrograde step.

Fortunately, there are many specific diseases which have only a single microbic cause and the antibacterial drugs to which they constantly respond are well known. It is with nonspecific infections that difficulties arise: for example, pneumonia, septicaemia or meningitis, and infections involving wounds and soft tissues generally and the urinary tract. There may be a double difficulty here: not only is the nature of the infection unknown, but even when it is known it remains to determine whether the strain of organism is normally sensitive to any drug which it is proposed to use.

2.2 The Contribution of the Laboratory

It is here that the laboratory must help: as Sir *James Howie* has said, 'Chemotherapy without bacteriology is guess work'. But let it not be thought that this help is automatic and unfailing. There are several stages at which it can in fact fail.

The specimen must be properly collected, free from contamination and speedily transmitted. It should be examined by an experienced worker: this is not always possible in understaffed laboratories where junior technicians make the cultures and may mistake a commensal in them for the pathogen. Finally, the method used for the sensitivity tests must be correct and properly executed and interpreted.

Unfortunately there is still a good deal of variation in the methods used, and four 'quality control surveys', two each in England and Australia, in which the same cultures were sent to many laboratories for examination and report, each produced a crop of discrepant results, particularly in tests of two bacterial species and with only a few drugs (Association of Clinical Pathologists, 1965; Beaney et al., 1970; College of Pathologists, 1968; Report, 1960). In other words, laboratory reports are not infallible, but with progress towards standardising methods, errors should become very infrequent. There is much to be said for the establishment of reference laboratories for this purpose, both to advise on and regulate work elsewhere and to undertake more difficult tests, such as those of bactericidal and combined drug action.

2.3 Bacterial Resistance

After a new antibacterial drug has been in use for some time, resistant strains of previously sensitive species may begin to appear (for review, see Garrod, 1976). Sometimes the change is rapid, and may be seen in a single patient. Streptomycin and rifampicin exemplify this, and should consequently be used only in combination. More often it is gradual, and seen only as an increase in the frequency of resistance in a population, whether of a hospital or of a larger community.

Five mechanisms may be concerned in development of resistance. One is simply selection from a small minority of originally resistant strains such that gradually a stage is reached at which the concentration of drug needed to inhibit the organism exceeds that which can be achieved in plasma and tissues of the patient by use of conventional therapeutic doses; the organism is then 'resistant' to the drug. Other mechanisms involve changes in the micro-organism itself, one being mutation and the rest involving transfer of extra-chromosomal genetic material (plasmids) from another and resistant cell; the organism changing directly from 'sensitive' to 'resistant'. These mechanisms are transformation (involving uptake of genetic material already liberated from another cell), transduction and conjugation. The last of these is transferred infectiously and occurs only between Gram-negative bacilli, but of many different species, and is often the origin of resistance in intestinal pathogens and other organisms which can cause infections elsewhere in the body. The pro-

Table I. Principles of minimising resistance to antibacterial drugs (after Garrod, 1976; Holloway and Asche, 1977)

1. Only use antibacterial drugs for clearly necessary indications.
2. Restrict use of valuable antibacterial drugs to which resistance is readily acquired, to specific indications (e.g. rifampicin for tuberculosis).
3. Other considerations being equal, use an antibacterial drug to which resistance is rarely acquired (e.g. penicillin).
4. Avoid antibacterial drugs to which resistance is already widespread; because treatment may fail (e.g. tetracycline and streptococcal infection).
5. Avoid use of valuable antibacterial drugs to an area of the body with a varied flora among which resistance may arise (e.g. do not use an oral non-absorbable drug such as gentamicin for pre-operative bowel sterilisation).
6. Choose antibacterials for topical application from those where development of resistance is uncommon.
7. In prophylaxis, use an antibacterial drug which will prevent colonisation of a specific organism or eradicate it shortly after it has been established.
8. When a combination regimen is used to prevent emergence of resistant strains, the individual drugs should be used in full dosage.
9. Information on local infection and sensitivity patterns should be regularly sought and used in the rational choice of an antibiotic drug.
10. Adequate dosage of the antibacterial drug should always be achieved. If a drug is ineffective and deemed non-therapeutic, it should be withdrawn.

---

cess of transduction occurs in Gram-positive cocci and involves transfer of plasmids by a bacteriophage particle (bacterial virus) that acts as a vector and can occur in many species (Lacey, 1973). Such transference of resistance to staphylococci is particularly likely to occur on external surfaces such as the skin (Noble and Naidoo, 1978). A given plasmid can carry resistance to a number of different antibacterial drugs; 3 to 5 being common, but even up to 9 has been known.

Every one of these five processes is favoured, if not solely determined, as in selection, by the presence of the drug. There is abundant evidence that the frequency of resistance to antibacterial drugs in any population is determined by the extent of its use. Hence, the best way to diminish resistance and so preserve the usefulness of a drug is to restrict its use. There are clear examples in past history of sensitivity to a drug being restored when for some reason it ceased to be prescribed so freely, such as the sensitivity of gonococci to sulphonamides when penicillin took their place for treating gonorrhoea, and of various species to chloramphenicol when the revelation that it can cause fatal marrow aplasia greatly reduced its consumption.

Hence the adoption of 'policies' for chemotherapy either in hospital units or on a wider scale designed to limit consumption and to promote rational choice and use (table I), particularly of drugs more vulnerable to this kind of counter attack by their intended victims. There is no doubt that much prescription is ill advised, either for trivial or insusceptible infections, or for ill considered prophylatic purposes (section 6). It is on record that in some hospitals far more antibiotics are prescribed for prophylaxis than for the treatment of existing infections, and this certainly does not mean that the first of these types of use has obviated the need for the second.

3. The Choice of Drug

This may be made with or without laboratory guidance. If without, it demands in some cases wide clinical experience and a knowledge of the applicability of different antibiotics and other drugs to particular infections.

3.1 Causative Organism and Drug Sensitivity

The experienced clinician can tell by inspection of faeces whether dysentery is amoebic or bacillary, often whether pneumonia is pneumococcal by the character of the sputum at the onset, and may even usually be right in deducing the causation of meningitis from the patient's age and other circumstances (see chapter XXV; sect. 13). In less serious conditions the initial prescription, as of a sulphonamide for urinary tract infection, can easily be replaced by another should it fail.

A knowledge of the antibacterial 'spectrum' of the principal drugs is essential (e.g. see appendix D), and not only of this but of the frequency of resistance to some of them in previously sensitive species (Finland, 1972). As an example, tetracycline at one time afforded successful treatment for pneumonia and for acute sore throat, but now that both pneumococci and haemolytic streptococci are commonly tetracycline resistant it is unwise to use them for these purposes (Dadswell, 1967; Study Group, 1977). Local knowledge of the frequency of certain resistances, i.e. in either a hospital or an entire community, may be a helpful guide. The situation can certainly vary from place to place: dysentery bacilli can be sensitive to ampicillin in two countries but almost invariably resistant in another (Nelson and Haltalin, 1967; Tong et al., 1970; Davies et al., 1970).

If laboratory guidance is available it may still afford a wide choice, since the organism may be reported sensitive to a number of drugs. The actual choice in these and indeed any circumstances should take the following further considerations into account (see also table II).

3.2 The Site of the Infection

In most parts of the body the concentrations known to be attained by a drug in the blood are an indication of what may be expected in the tissues (see chapter I; sect. 3.2.3), but there are exceptions. Some drugs diffuse well into the cerebrospinal fluid, others scarcely at all (see chapter XXV; sect.

Table II. General principles and considerations relating to choice and use of systemic antibacterial drugs

1. *Assessment*
   a) If possible determine nature of infection.
   b) Severity of infection — withhold systemic drugs in trivial infections.
   c) Obtain specimens for culture — mandatory in severe infections to confirm the provisional diagnosis. Choice of therapy may have to be made on clinical grounds, and if it is based on past comparable experience it may well be a good one, but with the help of a painstaking bacteriologist, therapy is more likely to succeed.

2. *Causative organism*
   a) Identify organism — if a specific disease with a single microbic cause, clinical diagnosis alone may suffice, but
   b) Verify susceptibility — to what drug is the strain of organism most sensitive? N.B. In absence of laboratory guidance this requires knowledge of antimicrobial 'spectrum' of *clinical* activity of drug *and* local knowledge of frequency of certain resistances to drugs.
   c) Interpretation of laboratory findings — reports are not infallible; seek specialist advice if these conflict with clinical experience.

3. *Drug characteristics*
   a) Site of infection — does drug attain adequate concentration at location of infection?
   b) Toxicity — if a choice exists between drugs, use less toxic one (see also section 7).
   c) Single drug or combination — use combination to prevent development of resistance to some drugs or attain synergy.
   d) Drug interaction or incompatability with other therapy? (see chapter VIII; appendix C and D).
   e) Cost.

4. *Patient characteristics (see also appendix D)*
   a) Age — reduce dose at both extremes of life (see also chapters IV, V).
   b) Renal disease — avoid some drugs; modify dose of others (see chapter XXI; appendix E).
   c) Liver disease — some drugs may be hepatotoxic; modify dose of some others in severe liver disease (see chapter XIX).
   d) Allergy — increased risk of sensitisation reactions; avoid some drugs (see chapter VII).
   e) Other associated diseases — may influence efficacy or increase risk of toxicity with some drugs
   f) Pregnancy — avoid some drugs (see chapters III, XV).

5. *Choice among a class of drug*
   a) Degree of antibacterial activity.
   b) Efficiency of absorption — blood or tissue concentration attained; effect of food.
   c) Degree of protein binding — does a greater degree of binding negate superior absorption or intrinsic antibacterial activity?
   d) Convenience or ease of administration — does a particular derivative simplify administration or require less frequent dosage?
   e) Relative incidence of troublesome side effects.
   f) Relative cost.

13). Some are excreted in high concentrations in the bile: these are ampicillin, amoxycillin, cephalexin and rifamide, which are useful in biliary tract infections, and erythromycin and novobiocin which are not because they lack adequate activity against biliary pathogens. On the other hand, erythromycin and novobiocin, of which only a small proportion of the dose is excreted in the urine, may therefore seem unsuitable choices for urinary tract infections, although both have in fact been so used. Some drugs such as nitrofurantoin attain therapeutic concentrations only in the urine, but inappropriate sensitivity tests have been known to lead to its prescription for pneumonia.

3.3 Toxicity

When two drugs offer an equal prospect of cure, the less toxic will naturally be preferred (see also section 7). When the more potentially toxic is also likely to be rather more effective, the choice demands balanced judgment.

Chloramphenicol is alone in being capable of causing a fatal reaction when given in ordinary doses to apparently normal patients, and there are very few conditions for which no effective alternative to it exists — some would now say none if it be accepted that co-trimoxazole (trimethoprim-sulphamethoxazole) is effective in typhoid fever.

Permanent loss of vestibular function or hearing from an aminoglycoside is also in a class by itself. This possibility should not inhibit the necessary use of kanamycin or gentamicin for a severe *Proteus* or *Pseudomonas* infection under proper safeguards. On the other hand, it strongly contraindicates the casual and usually unnecessary administration of streptomycin with penicillin as operation cover. In patients with unrecognised impairment of renal function, vestibular damage can be caused by only a few doses (see also chapter XI; sect. 7.1).

3.4 Single Drug or Combination

Of several alleged indications for prescribing antibacterial drugs in combination, only two are important.

The first is to prevent the development of bacterial resistance, particularly to antibiotics against which this can develop rapidly. This lesson was thoroughly learned in early studies of the treatment of tuberculosis with streptomycin, and what happens in this disease in a few months can happen in days or even overnight in some other infections (Garrod, 1976). Perhaps the most rapid mutation to resistance is that of ordinary bacteria such as staphylococci to rifampicin: this drug should always be combined with another to which the organism is sensitive. The same argument applies, although perhaps with less force and not in all infections, to erythromycin and fusidic acid.

The second important object is to achieve synergy. A special example of this is trimethoprim, which is available only in combination with a sulphonamide, because the two together act synergically on successive stages of the same bacterial metabolic process. Few combinations act thus and none do so invariably, but it will often be found that a combination of penicillin and streptomycin, or one of the newer aminoglycosides such as gentamicin or tobramycin, is totally bactericidal for a streptococcus when there are survivors to either antibiotic acting alone. This is of the utmost importance in treating some forms of bacterial endocarditis, the disease *par excellence* in which a total bactericidal effect is essential. Other types of combined effect are described as additive, indifferent or antagonistic. Antagonism is an undoubted reality, and may be seen when a bactericidal antibiotic, which acts only on multiplying bacteria, is combined with one which is only bacteristatic and thus prevents the necessary multiplication (Lepper and Dowling, 1951). The law on combined action propounded by Jawetz and Gunnison (1952) is still valid, but exceptions to it have come to light, some due to a peculiarity in the action of one of the components. Nevertheless, it remains a sound rule that bacteristatic and bactericidal antibiotics should not be combined unless for a well ascertained reason.

3.5 Choice Among a Class of Drugs

With some antibiotics there is a bewildering range of derivatives available for clinical use and there is no better example than the penicillins and cephalosporins (Garrod, 1974). The relative merits of the various derivatives against a susceptible organism therefore need to be assessed in terms of other factors such as degree of antibacterial activity, efficiency of absorption and extent of protein binding. Sometimes, factors such as convenience or ease of administration (particularly less frequent dosage) and relative incidence of troublesome side effects also influence the choice of drug.

Table III. Factors to take into account when making a choice between cephalosporins (after Garrod, 1974). Cephalothin, cephaloridine and cephazolin are given as examples

Property	Cephalothin	Cephaloridine	Cephazolin
Antibacterial activity	Equal against most species	Rather higher against staph, strep and pneumococci	Rather higher against coliforms
Resistance to staphylococcal penicillinase	High	Lower	Lower
Injection	May be painful	Less painful	Less painful
Protein binding	50%	20%	80%
Nephrotoxicity	Low	High	Low
Stability in body	Lower	High	High
Blood levels	Lower	Higher and better sustained	Still higher and longer sustained

These considerations are well illustrated by the penicillinase resistant isoxazole (isoxazolyl) penicillins where there is a choice from at least four derivatives — oxacillin, cloxacillin, dicloxacillin, flucloxacillin. All are given orally 6-hourly and their intrinsic antistaphylococcal activity varies little. Dicloxacillin is the best absorbed but also the most protein bound (appendix A). Flucloxacillin combines good absorption with a lower degree of protein binding — the approximate blood level ratio of unbound (i.e. active) drug for flucloxacillin being twice that of dicloxacillin and cloxacillin and four times that of oxacillin. Thus on theoretical grounds, flucloxacillin may be judged to be, dose for dose, the most therapeutically efficient of the four. A choice between the phenoxypenicillins (Bond et al., 1963) and aminopenicillins (i.e. ampicillins; Neu, 1975) is made along similar lines with the factors of intrinsic antibacterial activity (phenoxypenicillins) and frequency of administration (aminopenicillins) assisting with the choice. The choice between cephalosporin derivatives involves a few further considerations (see table III). The advantages of cephaloridine are rather higher and more sustained blood levels and a lower degree of protein binding. Its disadvantages are a lesser resistance to staphylococcal penicillinase, so that it may be ineffective in infection by a strain producing a large

amount of this enzyme, and nephrotoxicity when large doses are given — particularly in patients with otherwise impaired renal function. Cephazolin has an advantage in achieving the highest blood levels, and drawbacks in susceptibility to staphylococcal penicillinase and in diminished *in vivo* activity due to high protein binding. Consideration of these and other factors should enable a choice between the products to be made.

Newly introduced derivatives of an antibiotic can pose other considerations. No one wants to stand in the way of progress, particularly when a new derivative of an antibiotic can do something which its predecessors cannot. But this is not so if the new activity is only against a rather uncommon and not very important nonspecific infection. Thus, the very latest agent is not always the best for the purpose(s) for which it is advocated by its manufacturer. For example, if it were possible to analyse the purposes for which a new cephalosporin is being prescribed, it would probably be found that many of them would be as well or better served by ampicillin or amoxycillin. If the same exercise were undertaken for ampicillin or amoxycillin prescriptions, some of them would certainly prove to be for purposes well served by penicillin (Macaraeg et al., 1971). The large field of urinary tract infections is also served by five different types of synthetic drug, and here there may sometimes be no real need to look to any antibiotic at all (see chapter XXI; section 3).

Sometimes it is not easy to determine for what purposes a new derivative is to be preferred. Defining what these should be, depends very much on how far the factor of cost should be taken into account.

4. Dosage of Antibacterial Drugs

The appropriate dosages of the most common antibacterial drugs are well known. It should be emphasised that many of these are strictly limited to a narrow range by liability to toxic or other side effects, while that of penicillins in particular, thanks to their non-toxicity, is widely elastic. In determining correct dosage, several factors should be taken into account (for review, see Weinstein and Dalton, 1968).

4.1 Age

Usual dosages need to be reduced at both extremes of life. The newborn infant, and still more the premature, has an imperfectly developed capacity for excreting drugs (and for conjugating those such as chloramphenicol which are normally metabolised by the liver in this way). This defect is rapidly overcome (see further chapter IV; sect. 2.3), renal excretory capacity improving within a few days and reaching that of older children within 4 weeks, but while it lasts it may be a positive convenience, since for instance, a dose of penicillin which would have to be given at 4-hour intervals to an older infant needs to be given only at 12-hour intervals during the first few days of life (see McCracken, 1974).

In old people, the rate of renal elimination of drugs diminishes, even in the absence of overt renal disease (see chapter V; sect. 2.1.3). Dosage and frequency may be varied accordingly and the dose of toxic antibiotics such as the aminoglycosides (streptomycin, gentamicin, etc) should always be reduced.

4.2 Renal Disease

Much has been written in recent years about the use of antibacterial drugs in renal disease, and

only an outline of the main facts is possible here (for further information see chapter XXI; sect. 2.1, 14.1, and appendix E).

Certain drugs are better avoided: tetracyclines (except doxycycline) which because of their anti-anabolic action increase the work load on the kidney, and those which are themselves nephrotoxic. Among the latter cephaloridine and polymyxins may sometimes be safely given in restricted doses. Some antibacterial drugs can be given in normal doses, either because they are unstable and thus broken down in the body (cephalothin, oxacillin) or excreted mainly in the bile (erythromycin, rifamycins). Those of which the dose needs careful modification, are stable and excreted in the urine, and such dose modification is all the more important if they are toxic (Kunin, 1967; O'Grady, 1971). All these characteristics are possessed by the aminoglycosides, and elaborate schemes have been proposed, some even involving the use of a computer program, for determining the correct dose of kanamycin or gentamicin according to the degree of impairment of renal function (Dettli, 1976; Mawer, 1976). Lengthening the inter dose interval is preferable to reducing the dose. Blood assays are valuable in verifying the correctness of the schedule (Barza and Lauermann, 1978; Reeves, 1977; see further chapter I; sect. 4.3.4).

Penicillins can also accumulate, and although high levels are tolerated, there are limits even to these: reduced doses should therefore be given. Haemodialysis will reduce the blood levels of most but not all antibiotics: two exceptions are vancomycin and lincomycin (see Gibson and Nelson, 1977).

4.3 Liver Disease

Tetracyclines in excessive doses are hepatotoxic: so also is erythromycin estolate. Chloramphenicol is conjugated in the liver and has been shown to accumulate in patients with severe cirrhosis (Suhrland and Weisberger, 1963). Lincomycin has also been shown to persist in the blood when liver function is markedly impaired. Rifampicin can cause some derangement of function in the normal liver, particularly when combined with isoniazid in patients who are slow acetylators of this drug (Smith et al., 1972; Lal et al., 1972). Although there is little information about actual worsening of liver disease by antibacterial drugs, it is from these agents that it might be expected (see also chapter I, sect. 4.3.3; chapter XIX, sect. 1.4, 13.4).

5. Treatment of Some Individual Infections

5.1 Streptococcal Infections

5.1.1 Streptococcus pyogenes
The sole claim made for 'Prontosil', the forerunner of the sulphonamides, when it was introduced in 1935, was that it would overcome haemolytic streptococcal infection. Indeed it did, and the mortality from puerperal and other forms of streptococcal septicaemia fell steeply: erysipelas, scarlet fever and other manifestations of this infection also responded to these drugs. It was not until some years later that sulphonamide resistant streptococci began to appear, notably in populations subjected to mass sulphonamide prophylaxis of rheumatic fever. In the meantime, penicillin had come on the scene, to which these streptococci are even more sensitive and have remained so to the present day.

A known haemolytic streptococcal infection, of which the more severe forms once had a high mortality even in young and previously healthy subjects, has thus become the easiest of all acute infections to treat. It is the clearest of all indications for the use of penicillin. There is no need for large doses, but a nearly continuous effect is desirable, and most conveniently achieved by twice daily injections of procaine penicillin or 4-hourly oral doses of a phenoxypenicillin. However prompt the clinical response, treatment must be continued for 10 days: acute throat infections are otherwise liable to relapse (see chapter XI; sect. 2). In patients sensitised to penicillin, convenient alternatives are erythromycin and cephalexin (see chapter VII; sect. 4.1.3). More vigorous parenteral treatment may seem indicated in more severe infections, but it is now very rare for them to reach such a stage.

In the long term prophylaxis of rheumatic fever, monthly injections of benzathine penicillin are very effective and oral administration of ordinary penicillin (i.e. benzylpenicillin) much less so. This is not surprising in view of its acid lability and therefore poor and irregular absorption: a phenoxypenicillin is at least theoretically far preferable.

5.1.2 Streptococcus viridans
This organism is only of interest as the most common cause of bacterial endocarditis. It is usually, but not always, very penicillin sensitive and a prolonged course of penicillin alone has cured many patients, but there had for years been some doubt whether streptomycin should always be given in addition to enhance the bactericidal effect, and whether if so the course can be shortened. This question has been answered in a convincing way by the late Morton Hamburger of Cincinnati and his colleagues (Tan et al., 1971). They achieved consistent success in penicillin sensitive *Str. viridans* infections with only a 14 day course of oral phenoxypenicillin (600 to 750mg 4-hourly) and parenteral streptomycin (0.5 to 1g 12-hourly).

5.1.3 Streptococcus faecalis
This is a much more drug resistant organism, and although sometimes causing urinary tract and other infections, is again of chief interest as a cause of endocarditis. Although it is slightly more sensitive to ampicillin than to penicillin, neither is totally bactericidal: combination with an aminoglycoside, nowadays preferably gentamicin, provides the only dependable treatment. It is essential that *bactericidal* action of the combinations be tested on the patient's own strain *in vitro*, to verify that a total bactericidal effect can be achieved. I have never known treatment to fail when its efficacy has been so predicted. Resistant strains of *Str. viridans* should be subjected to the same tests.

5.1.4 Streptococcus pneumoniae
This organism was regarded for years as incapable of acquiring antibiotic resistance. The first antibiotics to fall victims to it were tetracyclines; resistance to them appeared in the early 'sixties, mainly in chronic bronchitics under prolonged treatment, and is of high degree (inhibition only by about 50µg/ml); this is now widespread. Penicillin resistance was first observed in Australia and New Guinea in 1967, and was relatively of much lower degree (inhibition usually by 0.5µg/ml, sometimes slightly more), but response to treatment is more seriously impaired than such figures would suggest. Resistant strains have been reported from elsewhere only as rarities until recent news from South Africa, reviewed by Jacobs et al. (1978), which is much more alarming. There, strains of types 6 and 19, resistant not

only to penicillin but to many other antibiotics, have been isolated in large numbers. A common cause of pneumonia in young children with measles, they have shown an exceptional capacity for colonising the throats of contacts, both patients and staff. A final policy for meeting this threat, which may have to include immunisation, has yet to be formulated. A vigilant outlook for the appearance of such strains elsewhere should be maintained.

5.2 Staphylococcal Infections

These contrast with those due to haemolytic streptococci in almost every possible way. Although it was claimed for sulphathiazole that it had an action on staphylococci exceeding that of other sulphonamides (which was almost *nil*) experience did not bear this out, and it was only when penicillin was introduced that a remedy was available. Indeed, staphylococcal infections and syphilis were the only common conditions amenable to penicillin but not to sulphonamides. For several years staphylococcal osteomyelitis, pyaemia and septicaemia, wound infections and others among the varied and less serious manifestations of this infection, responded to penicillin in what then seemed an almost miraculous way.

This happy position was not to last (see Finland, 1972). Resistant strains of staphylococcus began to appear, descendants of a very small original minority producing an enzyme, penicillinase, which destroyed the antibiotic. In environments such as hospital wards where penicillin was freely used, therapeutic selection enabled these strains to continue multiplying and to spread until they actually predominated. In the general population this change proceeded at a slower pace.

This was only the beginning of the defence of this most versatile organism against therapeutic attack. As other antibiotics were substituted for penicillin it became resistant also to them, commonly and early to streptomycin and tetracycline. Chloramphenicol, erythromycin, novobiocin and kanamycin sometimes suffered the same fate. It was only when the penicillinase resistant semisynthetic penicillins were introduced that the outlook for patients with staphylococcal infections improved again dramatically. Methicillin was followed by cloxacillin and other similar isoxazolyl derivatives which can be given by the mouth: we now also have the cephalosporins,

among which cephalothin is the most penicillinase resistant. Probably in consequence of the use of these drugs, hospital staphylococcal infections are now less frequent and less often severe.

It is difficult to be dogmatic about indications for these drugs and their use. Staphylococcal infections are of great variety and enormous range of severity, and the first decision to make is whether a given case requires an antibiotic at all. Secondly, some cases also need surgical treatment, without which an antibiotic cannot succeed, whereas with it the antibiotic may be unnecessary.

Treatment having been decided on, penicillin remains the first choice if the strain is sensitive. If not, or until this has been ascertained, cloxacillin or one of its relatives (the newest, flucloxacillin, seeming marginally superior; see section 3.5) given orally affords the most convenient treatment, but care must be taken to give each dose when the stomach is empty, or absorption may be inadequate. It is in any case never complete, and the parenteral route is preferable in the early stages of a serious infection.

In an infection which threatens life, and particularly in endocarditis, combined treatment is advisable. This is all the more necessary if the strain is resistant, even to the newer penicillins and the cephalosporins: such strains are still fortunately rare in most places, but when this resistance exists, it embraces the whole of this group of antibiotics. A full series of tests of the combined bactericidal action of penicillins and cephalosporins on the one hand and of aminoglycosides on the other, should be carried out, just as in designing treatment for endocarditis due to resistant streptococci.

5.3 Gonococcal Infections

The history of the treatment of gonorrhoea is interesting in illustrating the development of bacterial resistance by three different mechanisms. The disease also presents therapeutic difficulties peculiar to itself.

Sulphonamides were initially very successful, but then cases resistant to treatment began to be seen, whose organisms were resistant to the drug *in vitro*. A small minority of such strains were identifiable in culture collections made before the treatment was introduced. There is therefore little doubt that as with penicillin resistant staphylococci, therapeutic selection favoured the spread of the few resistant strains. During World War II these came to predominate in areas with a large population of Service personnel.

This situation was eventually relieved when penicillin became available. The gonococcus was of all bacteria the most sensitive to penicillin: a single dose would cure the disease, and repeated microscopy of pus from the male urethra showed degenerative changes and disappearance of the gonococci within no more than 3 hours. Some were encouraged to believe that a vigorous penicillin campaign might stamp out the disease altogether. No prediction could have been further from the truth: in fact its incidence has steadily increased.

Penicillin remained regularly effective for over 10 years, but in 1958 cases resistant to treatment, whose gonococci were not fully sensitive to penicillin, began to be seen, and now present a problem everywhere, although their frequency and the degree of resistance of the organism, varies in different countries. Gonococci were originally sensitive to about $0.01\mu g/ml$ of penicillin: strains of progressively diminishing sensitivity have since been found, latterly including some inhibited only by $0.5\mu g/ml$, a 50-fold increase in resistance: even higher figures than this have been reported from some areas.

In devising and assessing treatment to meet this situation the 'peculiar difficulties' referred to are the advisability of supervising administration, since these patients cannot be relied on to complete a course themselves, and the impossibility of distinguishing relapse from reinfection. One solution is to give a much larger dose of penicillin, reinforcing and prolonging its action with probenecid (Olsen and Lomholt, 1969). A mixture of ordinary and procaine penicillin is probably best, totalling several mega units. Benzathine penicillin should not be included, or indeed used in any circumstances for treating this disease: the prolonged maintenance of a low level in the blood is best calculated to promote gonococcal resistance. A single dose of 3.5g ampicillin or 3g amoxycillin reinforced with probenecid has also been successful: penicillin resistant strains are sometimes more susceptible to ampicillin or amoxycillin, although highly sensitive strains are less sensitive to them (Watts et al., 1977). Various other antibacterial agents have been used and can be considered in certain circumstances (see chapter XXIX; sect. 3).

The third mechanism, apart from selection and what may appear to be gradual habituation, by

which resistance has developed in gonococci is plasmid determined penicillinase formation. Such strains, first detected in 1976, will pose a formidable threat if they spread, since only alternative treatments to penicillin will serve for them (see chapter XXIX; sect. 3).

5.4 Salmonella and Shigella Infections

5.4.1 Typhoid Fever

It was shown soon after its discovery in 1948 that chloramphenicol is a specific for typhoid fever and this antibiotic has remained the mainstay in its treatment ever since (except in areas where the typhoid bacillus is resistant to it). Mortality was sharply reduced and haemorrhage or perforation are now rarely seen. The treatment is not without drawbacks: a shock-like state is liable to occur during its early stages, there is the ever present if remote danger of producing aplastic anaemia, and since chloramphenicol is not bactericidal, it does nothing to prevent the subsequent persistence of a carrier state.

If only for these reasons, alternatives have been sought, although with singularly little success. Tetracyclines, although almost equally active against the typhoid bacillus *in vitro,* are almost without effect. Moreover, other antibiotics, including some more recently discovered, which are not only equally or more active but possess what should be the immense advantage that their action is bactericidal, are similarly ineffective. This has been shown for polymyxin, gentamicin and cephaloridine in therapeutic studies of the experimental disease in volunteer American prisoners (Dawkins and Hornick, 1967). Typhoid fever is thus peculiar in failing to respond to antibiotics which should theoretically be well able to control it, and the reason for this is not known.

The advent of ampicillin raised high hopes. The typhoid bacillus is sensitive to it, and not only is it also bactericidal, but because of its non-toxicity it could be given in larger doses than any antibiotic previously tried. Yet numerous comparative trials have all shown that a total daily dose of 6 or 8g of ampicillin is far inferior in effect to one or 2g of chloramphenicol: indeed in some studies patients remained so ill during ampicillin treatment that chloramphenicol had to be substituted for it (De Ritis et al., 1972). It has been claimed that ampicillin may with advantage be given *in addition to* chloramphenicol (De Ritis et al., 1972), but it is doubtful whether it should ever be relied on alone.

On the other hand, ampicillin does exert its expected action in the biliary and urinary tract: vigorous (preferably parenteral) and patient treatment will usually eliminate the typhoid carrier state. Amoxycillin, a near but much better absorbed relative of ampicillin, has given better results than ampicillin in typhoid fever (Herzog, 1976; Butler et al., 1977) and promising results in the carrier state (Nolan and White, 1978). Some chloramphenicol resistant strains may also be resistant to amoxycillin. Mecillinam, an amidinopenicillin with very high activity against enterobacteria, has also given promising results in the disease itself (Geddes and Clarke, 1977) and in the carrier state (Jonsson, 1977).

Another alternative treatment for infection by chloramphenicol resistant strains which appeared first in Mexico and are now being found elsewhere, is with co-trimoxazole (trimethoprim-sulphamethoxazole). Typhoid bacilli are usually sensitive to both of its components, which exert their usual synergic action. There have been enthusiastic reports of its action in typhoid fever from India, Egypt and Italy, one unfavourable report from South Africa, and several expressing only qualified approval from elsewhere (Herzog, 1976; Butler et al., 1977). Almost all are agreed on the prompt symptomatic relief achieved: the patients soon feel better (sometimes described as the relief of 'toxaemia') and toxic crises do not occur, but there is disagreement about the duration of bacteriaemia and fever after treatment has begun, and a few examples of frank failure and of toxic effects on the marrow have been described. Factors which may possibly account for these discrepancies are racial differences in susceptibility to the infection, differences in nutritional state or coexistence of other disease, the virulence of the responsible strain of *S. typhi,* age and the dosage used.

5.4.2 Other Salmonelloses

Paratyphoid fever, although usually a milder disease, requires the same treatment as typhoid. Salmonella enteritis, as distinct from enteric fever, is a totally different condition, with a very short incubation period, a distinct clinical picture and usually a very short duration. Most cases do not require treatment with any antibacterial drug and should not receive one. The immediate effect is negligible, and the only other is sometimes to prolong the subsequent carrier state (Aserkoff and Bennett, 1969), probably by suppressing other elements in the normal intestinal flora: the causative organism itself may have been initially resistant or may acquire resistance from an R factor during such treatment.

There are two kinds of exception to this. Any *Salmonella* enteritis carries a greater risk in the very young and in the old, or in patients debilitated by other disease. Secondly, certain serotypes of *Salmonella,* notably *S. choleraesuis,* tend to produce a more typhoid-like and prolonged illness, accompanied by bacteriaemia, which is no part of the simple enteritis caused by, say, *S. typhimurium.* Each of these categories of patient may be judged to require chemotherapy. The choice of drug is as for typhoid fever, unless the strain responsible possesses any peculiar resistances: during an epidemic these should have been identified at an early stage. Here again, co-trimoxazole (trimethoprim-sulphamethoxazole) has been commended as an alternative to antibiotics, but further study of its efficacy seems advisable.

5.4.3 Shigella Infections

These again vary much in severity, and for a simple *Sh. sonnei* infection chemotherapy is not only unnecessary but actually undesirable for a reason already given, namely that it often prolongs the subsequent carrier state. For more severe forms of dysentery it is indicated, but the choice of drug presents a problem not met with in enteric fever, which is that dysentery bacilli are often drug resistant. Sulphonamides were once the mainstay of treatment, but resistance to them is now almost universal. Tetracycline resistance is also widespread. Chloramphenicol and ampicillin have both been commended, the latter very favourably in reports from areas where resistance to it has apparently not developed (Nelson and Haltalin, 1967): elsewhere it is common. This finding and that of a poor effect of amoxycillin in shigellosis (Nelson and Haltalin, 1974), suggests that efficacy in enteric fever and dysentery do not necessarily correspond. Co-trimoxazole has also been found effective (Nelson et al., 1976), despite the sulphonamide resistance of the organism (Lexomboon et al., 1972), and was particularly commended in treating a *Sh. flexneri* outbreak in an institution for mental defectives because it eliminated the organism from the faeces, whereas chloramphenicol did not (Freiberg, 1971).

It is impossible to be dogmatic about the proper treatment of this disease, except to the extent of saying that the choice of drug should be guided by

Table IV. The sensitivity of coliform bacilli to antimicrobial drugs[1]

Organism	Minimum inhibitory concentration (µg/ml)							
	ampi-cillin and amoxy-cillin	carbeni-cillin	cepha-loridine	cefu-roxime	cefox-itin	genta-micin	poly-myxin	trimetho-prim
Escherichia coli	2-8	5	2-4	1-16	4-16	1	0.25	0.03-0.12
Proteus mirabilis	2-8	2.5	8	1-4	1-4	2	R[2]	0.5-4
Proteus mirabilis (penicillinase forming)	R	R	8	1-8	1-4	2	R	0.5-4
Proteus spp. (indole forming)	16-R	5	R	R	4-16	1	R	0.5-4
Klebsiella pneumoniae	R	R	2-8	4-16	4-32	0.5-2	0.25	1
Enterobacter aerogenes	R	R	R	4-16	R	0.5-2	0.25	3
Pseudomonas aeruginosa	R	50	R	R	R	4	0.12	R
Serratia marcescens	R	4-R	R	R	16-R	0.5	R	< 2-16

1   This table is based on various publications, on observations by *Pamela M. Waterworth* and the author, and on some personal communications. The sensitivities are those normal for the species; individual strains may be more resistant.

2   R = resistant to attainable concentrations.

sensitivity tests which are likely already to have been performed on local strains.

5.5 Enterobacterial and *Pseudomonas* Infections

These form a subject of general interest for several reasons. The organisms concerned are naturally much more resistant to antibacterial drugs than most others: moreover they can acquire resistance, often multiple, from simple contact with another resistant species. The choice of a drug for treating such infections may therefore present peculiar difficulties. These infections have become more common, now that other causes of sepsis have been brought under better control, and also because more patients are submitted to drastic treatments (surgical and by antineoplastic and immunosuppressive drugs) which diminish their resistance.

These infections occur in various parts of the body. Those involving the urinary and respiratory tracts are dealt with elsewhere (see chapters XX and XXI). Other sites are the skin (e.g. otitis externa) the bowel, wounds, the meninges and the blood stream. It is not proposed to consider the treatment of infection at these sites individually, but only the merits of different antibiotics and other drugs for treating any severe infections of this nature, with special reference to septicaemia.

The sensitivities of the principal species to the more useful antibacterial drugs are given in table IV. Those listed do not include all the newer penicillins and aminoglycosides, the properties of which are noted in the following summary.

Ampicillin and amoxycillin: Possess good activity only against *E. coli* and non-penicillinase-forming *Pr. mirabilis:* resistant strains of the former are now fairly common.

Carbenicillin: Also susceptible to *Pr. mirabilis* penicillinase but active against other *Proteus* species. Its most important property is activity against *Ps. aeruginosa;* although only moderate, this can be compensated for by giving large doses (for septicaemia 30g daily is advisable), and gentamicin may be given in addition. *Ticarcillin,* more recently introduced, has substantially more activity against this organism, and other derivatives still under investigation, such as *piperacillin,* are more active still.

Cephalosporins: All cephalosporins inhibit normally sensitive strains of *E. coli, Proteus mirabilis,* even when it forms penicillinase (an important advantage over penicillins) and *Klebsiella* spp. Among those which have been longer in use, *cephazolin* is perhaps the most useful for these infections. Indole-forming *Proteus* spp., and *Enterobacter* spp. are resistant, this resistance depending on the possession of enzymes which destroy the antibiotic. Such enzymes may also be formed by resistant strains of *E. coli* and *Klebsiella*. The main advance in this field has been the introduction of two derivatives resistant to many of these enzymes, *cefuroxime* (Brogden et al., 1979b) and *cefoxitin* (Brogden et al., 1979a), the latter being not a cephalosporin but a cephamycin, which has a closely related structure. These drugs may therefore be effective in infections resistant to other cephalosporins.

Aminoglycosides: Gentamicin has almost entirely replaced streptomycin and kanamycin for this purpose. All the species hitherto named are sensitive to it, including *Ps. aeruginosa,* and another important sensitive species resistant to many other drugs is *Serratia marcescens. Tobramycin* is rather more active against *Ps. aeruginosa,* and among other additions to this group is *amikacin,* a semisynthetic derivative of kanamycin unaffected by some of the plasmid borne enzymes on which resistance to aminoglycosides may depend.

Polymyxins: All *Proteus* spp. are resistant, as is *Serratia;* otherwise the species named are sensitive, but therapeutic results have been disappointing.

Trimethoprim: Also highly active against all species except *Ps. aeruginosa* and *Serratia.* Clinical utility will also depend on degree of sensitivity to sulphamethoxazole in the combination co-trimoxazole.

These facts provide the initial basis for choice. Localised infections may respond to a single drug, but systemic respond better to combined treatment. A known *Ps. aeruginosa* septicaemia is an indication for carbenicillin (or ticarcillin) plus gentamicin (or tobramycin). For the rest of these infections, an exact bacteriological diagnosis with sensitivity tests is highly desirable. The type of combination most widely used is an aminoglycoside plus a penicillin or cephalosporin. For Gram-negative septicaemic shock this should be administered forthwith, pending the results of blood culture. Such combinations have also been extensively used for treating or preventing Gram-negative infections in neutropenic patients undergoing treatment for leukaemia or cancer.

5.6 *Haemophilus influenzae* Infections

This organism is commonly implicated in chronic bronchial infection, and capsulated type b strains are a cause of acute purulent meningitis in children under 5 years of age. It is in connection with this disease that correct chemotherapy is most important, since it can be life saving. It should first be understood, and this applies also to respiratory tract infections, that most cephalosporins have not the degree of activity against this species with which they have been credited. Much the most active is cefamandole, but there is little information about its efficacy in meningitis. The widely varying degree of activity of 8 cephalosporins is well illustrated by the studies of Yourassowsky et al. (1976). *H. influenzae* is highly sensitive to ampicillin and this has been widely used in the treatment of meningitis, but it may fail for one of two reasons.

The diffusion of all penicillins into the cerebrospinal fluid is adequate when the meninges are inflamed but only slight when they are not; hence as inflammation subsides their concentration falls and relapse may occur. Clinical improvement may thus paradoxically demand an increase in dose. The second reason is the occurrence of type b strains which are ampicillin resistant by virtue of forming penicillinase. Children with meningitis have died because this property of the strain was unrecognised; it is important to use a disc of low content, and rapid methods of detecting penicillinase formation are now available. The most dependable antibiotic is unquestionably chloramphenicol; not only is *H. influenzae* highly sensitive to it, but it diffuses into the cerebrospinal fluid better than any other antibiotic. The remote but serious risk of marrow aplasia contraindicates its use for many other purposes, but when life is endangered it should be used unhesitatingly. Although its action on most bacteria is purely bacteriostatic, that on *H. influenzae* is bactericidal. This action has been fully verified by Turk (1977), who showed in a study of many strains that chloramphenicol is actually more bactericidal than ampicillin. The role of *H. influenzae* in acute otitis media is discussed in chapter XI (sect. 3.2.1).

5.7 *Bacteroides* Infections

Bacteroides spp. and other genera of Gram-negative non-sporing anaerobes are commensals in the alimentary tract (in the colon they far outnumber all other species), and infections due to them arise there but may involve other organs. These are very common, almost all foul-smelling pus is produced by them, but have not been well studied until recent years. Some species are sensitive to penicillin and other older antibiotics such as chloramphenicol, but it seems that resistance to these is now more common. They are almost uniformly sensitive to only 2 drugs, clindamycin, which is liable to cause 'pseudomembranous' colitis, particularly in severely ill patients (see chapter XIX; sect. 14.4.3), and metronidazole, which is better tolerated and more effective. This drug, an imidazole derivative, the general properties of which are reviewed by Roe (1977), was used for some years only in trichomoniasis and amoebiasis, but was later observed to be highly active against exclusively anaerobic bacteria. It has been very successful not only in the treatment of *Bacteroides* infections in association with the alimentary tract (including the mouth, where Vincent's infection is one of them; see chapter XIII, sect. 3.4), and in those metastasising to the lungs and brain, but also in the prophylaxis of such infections after operation on the appendix or colon (Brogden et al., 1978). It is well absorbed orally or from rectal suppositories, which enable treatment to be uninterrupted during an operative period. Tinidazole, another imidazole derivative, used successfully in trichomoniasis (see chapter XXIX; sect. 6.1), amoebiasis and giardiasis (see chapter XIX; sect. 11.3, 11.4.8), is also highly active against obligate anaerobes (Applebaum and Chatterton, 1978).

5.8 Fungus Infections

Mycoses fall into three principal classes: (1) those due to dermatophytes, affecting only the skin, hair and nails; (2) local and usually superficial infections caused by *Candida albicans;* and (3) systemic infections, which may also be caused by *Candida* species, of which other examples are aspergillosis, coccidioidomycosis, cryptococcosis and histoplasmosis (for review, see Cartwright, 1978; Kobayashi and Medoff, 1977). The drugs available for their treatment are the following:

Griseofulvin: This antibiotic was discovered and characterised nearly 40 years ago, but had to be rediscovered and to survive a period when it was unjustly suspected of toxicity before it came into clinical use. It is unique in being deposited in

keratin as this is laid down, and is therefore concentrated and persists in precisely the area attacked by dermatophytes. It now provides the standard treatment for dermatomycoses (see chapter XIV; sect. 2.3.2).

Nystatin: This was the first of the polyenes to be discovered, a group of antibiotics acting on a wide range of fungi, particularly *Candida* species. Nystatin has an exceedingly low solubility — so low indeed that its therapeutic effect is surprising — and is used in the form of a suspension for application to mucous and other surfaces attacked by *Candida albicans*. These areas include the mouth and alimentary tract: bronchial lesions can be treated by inhalation, vaginal by pessary or cream and skin by various dosage forms. Other polyenes also used for some of these purposes are candicidin, natamycin (pimaricin) and hachimycin (trichomycin). See further (chapter XIII, sect. 6; chapter XIV, sect. 2.3.1; chapter XXIX; section 6.2).

Amphotericin B: This later discovered polyene is active against all fungi causing systemic infections, and can be solubilised to permit intravenous injection. It is also the most toxic of all antibiotics in clinical use: the individual dose, given at 2-day intervals, should not exceed 1mg per kg, or the total dose in the course 3g. Even so, vomiting, fever, thrombophlebitis, hypokalaemia and a raised blood urea are common effects, and some degree of permanent renal damage results from a full course. Thus, although success has often been achieved with this drug in treating all systemic mycoses, it has for long been hoped that some other better tolerated treatment may take its place. This hope is being fulfilled in some directions, although to what extent is still uncertain, by the following drugs:

5-Fluorocytosine: This synthetic compound interferes in a well ascertained way with the metabolism of yeast-like fungi. It is absorbed when given orally and large doses, which appear to be quite safe, produce high concentrations not only in the blood but also in cerebrospinal fluid. There are now fairly numerous reports of its successful use in some cases of cryptococcal meningitis, and of systemic candidiasis.

The most promising recent development has been combined treatment with fluorocytosine and amphotericin B. One effect of this combination is that amphotericin B increases the permeability of the fungal cell, thus permitting a higher concentration of fluorocytosine to be attained within it. There is evidence that it also permits a lower dose of the more toxic drug to be given, and that the development of resistance to its partner is discouraged. A synergic action has been demonstrated in several experimental mycoses in mice. Favourable clinical reports are those of Utz et al. (1975) on the treatment of cryptococcosis and of Ellard et al. (1976) on success in cases of *Candida* endophthalmitis, *Candida* septicaemia and *Torulopsis* endocarditis. Failure with fluorocytosine treatment is sometimes accompanied by a large increase in resistance of the infecting organism.

Imidazoles: Clotrimazole, introduced some years ago as a systemic antifungal agent, had serious side effects, and is now used mainly for the local treatment of candidiasis. *Miconazole,* which in addition to a wide antifungal spectrum, some action on Gram-positive bacteria, is administrable not only locally for infections due to yeasts and dermatophytes, but also both orally and parenterally and is well tolerated (Sawyer et al., 1975). At a Symposium (1977a) success with it was claimed in the treatment of various deep seated mycoses. An impressive report is that by Deresenski et al. (1977) on the treatment of meningitis due to *Coccidioides immitis*. These authors administered miconazole intrathecally by several routes including the intraventricular. It does not seem possible yet to assess the relative merits of this drug and amphotericin B, but certainly miconazole has an advantage in lower toxicity. *Econazole,* is another imidazole, which has also been successfully used locally in infections due to yeasts and dermatophytes. It has also been investigated in deep seated mycoses (Heel et al., 1978).

The use of these and other antifungal agents in mucocutaneous mycoses and vaginal candidiasis is discussed in chapter XIII (section 6), chapter XIV (section 2.3.1) and chapter XXIX (section 6.2).

6. Prophylactic Administration of Antibacterial Drugs

This type of use, reviewed by Garrod (1975) has often been carried to excess and created more problems than it solves. Absolute indications for it are few, but include two aimed at protecting the heart. These are the long term treatment, preferably with benzathine penicillin, of rheumatic subjects to prevent streptococcal throat infections and thus recurrences of rheumatic fever (see chapter XII; sect. 2), and cover for dental extractions of patients predisposed to bacterial endocarditis, either by past rheumatic fever or a congenital cardiac abnormality (see chapter XIII; sect. 12.1). This calls for adequate doses of penicillin or some other bactericidal antibiotic or combination. Another imperative indication is the prevention of gas gangrene with large doses of penicillin both for severe contaminated trauma and for amputation through the thigh in obliterative arterial disease.

A more debatable field is the prevention of postoperative infection generally (Kunin, 1977; Chodak and Plaut, 1977; Berger et al., 1978). This should be attempted only if there is a manifest risk of sepsis, and not for most clean operations, although even here there may be a case for it when infection can have disastrous consequences, as in prosthetic replacement of the hip joint. Well informed surgical opinion (Symposium, 1977b) now increasingly favours short term cover, such as three doses of an appropriate antibiotic given immediately before, during and some hours after the operation. This may be a penicillinase resistant penicillin if staphylococcal infection is mainly to be feared, or a broad spectrum antibiotic such as cephaloridine for operations on the alimentary tract. Metronidazole as a prophylactic for operations on the bowel has been mentioned (section 5.7). Here, preoperative preparation by administering orally antibacterial drugs acting mainly (sulphasuxidine or succinyl sulphathiazole) or solely (neomycin) in the bowel also has its advocates. Such treatment should be limited to 1 or 2 days and is less important than mechanical cleansing.

Prophylaxis may also be indicated in several special branches of surgery. The kind of treatment which used to be popular and should be avoided is the routine administration for several days of a broad spectrum antibiotic such as tetracycline (or combination), with the object of preventing both wound sepsis and postoperative chest infection. Not only did this often fail, but also it predisposed to infection by resistant bacteria, such as staphylococcal enterocolitis and lung infections by Gram-negative bacilli, which are much more difficult to treat than those (e.g. pneumococcal) likely to arise in patients not so treated.

7. Side Effects of Antibacterial Drugs

The choice of drug must be influenced by its liability to cause side effects, especially if these are of a serious nature (see Weinstein and Dalton, 1968).

7.1 Fatal Effects

An excessive intrathecal dose of penicillin may be fatal, as may a dose by any route in a highly sensitised individual who goes into shock from which appropriate treatment is not given to rescue him. Otherwise the only antibacterial drug which can be directly fatal is chloramphenicol, and this in two ways: (1) as a result of the 'grey syndrome' in infants or (2) of aplastic anaemia. The former results only from excessive dosage (see chapter IV; sect. 3.1) and can thus be avoided: the latter, although to some extent dose related, can occur after any course of treatment (see chapter XXIII; sect. 8.3). How seriously to take the admittedly remote risk of this disastrous effect is a matter for individual judgment.

7.2 Nephrotoxicity

All peptides are nephrotoxic, bacitracin much more so than polymyxins. The latter can be given safely in reasonable doses to patients with already damaged kidneys and renal function has been seen to improve when the infection has been overcome. Aminoglycosides are also to some extent nephrotoxic: indeed this property is believed to be at least part of the reason why two of them, paromomycin and framycetin, are not recommended for systemic use. Those which are so used are unlikely to damage a normal kidney in conventional doses, but caution is advisable in pre-existing renal disease. Cephaloridine (and to a much lesser extent cephalothin) is nephrotoxic in large doses, particularly when renal damage already exists and when diuretics are given at the same time. As already noted, amphotericin B is also nephrotoxic (see section 5.8). See further (chapter XXI; sect. 15.2).

7.3 Ototoxicity

This is a hazard with the aminoglycosides, capreomycin and vancomycin. Some limitations which this property should impose on the use of aminoglycosides are mentioned earlier (see section 3.3). Choice among them may be governed by two considerations: (1) the frequency of toxic effect; neomycin for instance, is far more liable than kanamycin to cause deafness, and (2) that auditory damage is far more disastrous than vestibular, hence the abandonment of dihydrostreptomycin. This may also be thought a reason for preferring gentamicin to kanamycin since gentamicin mainly affects vestibular function whereas kanamycin mainly affects auditory function (see chapter XI; sect. 7.1).

7.4 Effects on Haemopoiesis

That caused by chloramphenicol has been described above (section 7.1). Generally less severe effects, most often granulocytopenia, can be produced by sulphonamides, and trimethoprim can interfere with folate metabolism, but manifestations of this are rare and readily reversible (see also chapter XXIII; sect. 7.2, 8).

7.5 Gastrointestinal Effects

Nausea, vomiting, abdominal pain and diarrhoea have been reported with varying frequency as resulting from the oral administration of a great variety of antibacterial drugs and usually represent nothing more than mucosal intolerance of an unaccustomed chemical. The prolonged changes in the intestinal flora caused by tetracyclines are a different matter: a rather intractable chronic diarrhoea is common and an acute and much more serious effect, mostly confined to surgical patients, is staphylococcal enterocolitis. Lincomycin and clindamycin, and other antibacterial drugs, have been associated with a severe form of colitis with characteristic lesions visible on sigmoidoscopy. The incidence of this complication is a subject of dispute, and its relationship to forms of colitis of different causation is uncertain (see also chapter XIX; sect. 14.4.3).

7.6 Sensitisation Reactions

Urticarial reactions may occur in patients sensitised to sulphonamides, penicillin, streptomycin and novobiocin. In addition, sensitisation to penicillin may take a form in which a dose produces immediate shock. Sensitisation to other antibacterial drugs is rare and unimportant except in the case of topical neomycin (see chapter XIV; sect. 7.1, 22.3.4).

Further Reading

Ball, A.P.; Gray, J.A. and Murdoch, J.McC.: Antibacterial Drugs Today (ADIS Press, Sydney; MTP, London; University Park Press, Baltimore 1978).

Garrod, L.P.; Lambert, H.P. and O'Grady, F.: Antibiotic and Chemotherapy, 4th ed (Churchill Livingstone, Edinburgh 1973).

References

Appelbaum, P.C. and Chatterton, S.A.: Susceptibility of anaerobic bacteria to ten antimicrobial agents. Antimicrobial Agents and Chemotherapy 14: 371 (1978).

Aserkoff, B. and Bennett, J.V.: Effect of therapy in acute salmonellosis on salmonellae in feces. New England Journal of Medicine 281: 636 (1969).

Association of Clinical Pathologists: Report on antibiotic sensitivity test trial organised by the Bacteriological Committee of the Association of Clinical Pathologists. Journal of Clinical Pathology 18: 1 (1965).

Barza, M. and Weinstein, L.: Pharmacokinetics of penicillins in man. Clinical Pharmacokinetics 1: 297 (1976).

Barza, M. and Lauermann, M.: Why monitor serum levels of gentamicin. Clinical Pharmacokinetics 3: 202 (1978).

Beaney, N.; Goodwin, N.G.; Jones, R.V.; Winter, R. and Sippe, G.R.: Antibiotic sensitivity testing. Medical Journal of Australia 1: 483 (1970).

Berger, S.A.; Nagar, H. and Weitzman, S.: Prophylactic antibiotics in surgical procedures. Surgery, Gynecology and Obstetrics 146: 469 (1978).

Bond, J.M.; Lightbown, J.W.; Barber, M. and Waterworth, P.M.: A comparison of four phenoxypenicillins. British Medical Journal 2: 956 (1963).

Brodgen, R.N.; Heel, R.C.; Speight, T.M. and Avery, G.S.: Metronidazole in anaerobic infections: A review of its activity, pharmacokinetics and therapeutic use. Drugs 16: 387 (1978).

Brogden, R.N.; Heel, R.C.; Speight, T.M. and Avery, G.S.: Cefoxitin: A review of its antibacterial activity, pharmacological properties and therapeutic use. Drugs 17: 1 (1979a).

Brogden, R.N.; Heel, R.C.; Speight, T.M. and Avery, G.S.: Cefuroxime: A review of its antibacterial activity, pharmacological properties and therapeutic use. Drugs 17: 233 (1979b).

Butler, T.; Linh, N.N.; Arnold, K.; Adickman, M.D.; Chau, D.M. and Muoi, M.M.: Therapy of antimicrobial-resistant typhoid fever. Antimicrobial Agents and Chemotherapy 11: 645 (1977).

Cartwright, R.Y.: Use of antibiotics. Antifungals. British Medical Journal 2: 108 (1978).

Chodak, G.W. and Plaut, M.E.: Use of systemic antibiotics for prophylaxis in surgery: A critical review. Archives of Surgery 112: 326 (1977).

College of Pathologists of Australia: A survey of antibiotic sensitivity testing. Medical Journal of Australia 2: 171 (1968).

Craig, W.A. and Welling, P.G.: Protein binding of antimicrobials: Clinical pharmacokinetic and therapeutic implications. Clinical Pharmacokinetics 2: 252 (1977).

Dadswell, J.V.: Survey of the incidence of tetracycline-resistant haemolytic streptococci between 1958 and 1965. Journal of Clinical Pathology 20: 641 (1967).

Davies, J.R.; Farrant, W.N. and Uttley, A.H.C.: Antibiotic resistance of *Shigella sonnei*. Lancet 2: 1157 (1970).

Dawkins, A.T. and Hornick, R.B.: Evaluation of antibiotics in a typhoid model. Antimicrobial Agents and Chemotherapy 1966, p.6 (American Society for Antimicrobial Agents and Chemotherapy, Ann Arbor 1967).

Deresenski, S.C.; Lilly, R.B.; Levine, H.B.; Galgiani, J.N. and Stevens, D.A.: Treatment of fungal meningitis with miconazole. Archives of Internal Medicine 137: 1180 (1977).

De Ritis, F.; Giammanco, G. and Manzillo, G.: Chloramphenicol combined with ampicillin in treatment of typhoid. British Medical Journal 4: 17 (1972).

Dettli, L.: Drug dosage in renal disease. Clinical Pharmacokinetics 1: 126 (1976).

Ellard, T.; Beskow, D.; Norrby, R.; Wahlen, P. and Alestig, K.: Combined treatment with amphotericin B and flucytosine in severe fungal infections. Journal of Antimicrobial Chemotherapy 2: 239 (1976).

Finland, M.: Changing patterns of susceptibility of common bacterial pathogens to antimicrobial agents. Annals of Internal Medicine 76: 1009 (1972).

Freiberg, T.: Erfahrung mit der kombination sulphamethoxazol-trimethoprim bei der behandlung von shigella-flexner-erkrankungen. Arzneimittel-Forschung 21: 599 (1971).

Gale, P.F.; Cunliffe, E.; Reynolds, P.E.; Richmond, M.H. and Waring, M.J.: The molecular basis of drug action. (Wiley, London 1972).

Garrod, L.P.: Choice among penicillins and cephalosporins. British Medical Journal 3: 96 (1974).

Garrod, L.P.: Chemoprophylaxis. British Medical Journal 4: 561 (1975).

Garrod, L.P.: Defence against bacterial drug resistance. British Medical Journal 2: 933 (1976).

Geddes, A.M. and Clarke, P.D.: The treatment of enteric fever with mecillinam. Journal of Antimicrobial Chemotherapy 3 (Suppl. B): 101 (1977).

Gibson, T.P. and Nelson, H.A.: Drug kinetics and artificial kidneys. Clinical Pharmacokinetics 2: 403 (1977).

Heel, R.C.; Brodgen, R.N.; Speight, T.M. and Avery, G.S.: Econazole: A review of its antifungal activity and therapeutic efficacy. Drugs 16: 177 (1978).

Herzog, Ch.: Chemotherapy of typhoid fever: A review of literature. Infection 4: 166 (1976).

Hitchings, G.H.: Species differences among dihydrofolate reductase as a basis for chemotherapy. Postgraduate Medical Journal 45 (Suppl): 7 (Nov. 1969).

Holloway, B.W. and Asche, L.V.: Mechanisms and clinical implications of antibiotic resistance in bacteria. Drugs 14: 283 (1977).

Jacobs, M.R.; Koornhof, H.; Robins-Browne, R.M. et al.: Emergence of multiply resistant pneumococci. New England Journal of Medicine 299: 735 (1978).

Jawetz, E. and Gunnison, J.B.: Antibiotic synergism and antagonism; an assessment of the problem. Bacteriological Reviews 5: 175 (1952).

Jonsson, M.; Pivmecillinam in the treatment of *Salmonella* carriers. Journal of Antimicrobial Chemotherapy 3 (Suppl. B): 103 (1977).

Kobayashi, G.S. and Medoff, G.: Antifungal agents: Recent developments. Annual Review of Microbiology 31: 291 (1977).

Kunin, C.M.: A guide to the use of antibiotics in patients with renal disease. Annals of Internal Medicine 67: 151 (1967).

Kunin, C.M.: Antimicrobial prophylaxis in surgery. Israel Journal of Medical Sciences 13: 547 (1977).

Lacey, R.W.: Genetic basis, epidemiology, and future significance of antibiotic resistance in Staphylococcus aureus: A review. Journal of Clinical Pathology 26: 899 (1973).

Lal, S.; Singhal, S.N.; Burley, D.M. and Crossley, G.: Effect of rifampicin and isoniazid on liver function. British Medical Journal 1: 148 (1972).

Lepper, M. and Dowling, H.: Treatment of pneumococci meningitis with penicillin compared with penicillin plus aureomycin. Archives of Internal Medicine 88: 489 (1951).

Lexomboon, U.; Mansuwan, P.; Duangmani, C.; Benjadol, P. and McMinn, M.T.: Clinical evaluation of co-trimoxazole and furalozidone in treatment of shigellosis in children. British Medical Journal 3: 23 (1972).

McCracken, G.H.: Pharmacological basis for antimicrobial therapy in newborn infants. American Journal of Diseases of Childhood 128: 407 (1974).

Macaraeg, P.V.J.; Lasagna, L. and Bianchine, J.R.: A study of hospital staff attitudes concerning the comparative merits of antibiotics. Clinical Pharmacology and Therapeutics 12: 1 (1971).

Mawer, G.E.: Computer assisted prescribing of drugs. Clinical Pharmacokinetics 1: 67 (1976).

Mouton, R.P.; Glerum, J.H. and van Loenen, A.C.: Relationship between antibiotic consumption and frequency of antibiotic resistance of four pathogens — a seven-year survey. Journal of Antimicrobial Chemotherapy 2: 9 (1976).

Nelson, J.D. and Haltalin, K.C.: Broad-spectrum penicillins in enteric infections of children. Annals of the New York Academy of Sciences 145: 414 (1967).

Nelson, J.D. and Haltalin, K.C.: Amoxicillin less effective than ampicillin against Shigella in vitro and in vivo: Relationship of efficacy to activity in serum. Journal of Infectious Diseases 129(Suppl.): 123 (June 1974).

Nelson, J.D.; Kusmiesz, H. and Jackson, L.H.: Comparison of trimethoprim-sulfamethoxazole and ampicillin therapy for shigellosis in ambulatory patients. Journal of Pediatrics 89: 491 (1976).

Neu, H.C.: New broad-spectrum penicillins. Drugs 9: 81 (1975).

Noble, W.C. and Naidoo, J.: Evolution of antibiotic resistance in Staphylococcus aureus: the role of the skin. British Journal of Dermatology 98: 481 (1978).

Nolan, C.M. and White, P.C.: Treatment of typhoid carriers with amoxycillin. Journal of the American Medical Association 239: 2352 (1978).

O'Callaghan, C.H.; Sykes, R.B.; Griffiths, S.A. and Thornton, J.E.: Cefuroxime, a new cephalosporin antibiotic: activity in vitro. Antimicrobial Agents and Chemotherapy 9: 511 (1976).

O'Grady, F.: Antibiotics and renal failure. British Medical Bulletin 27: 142 (1971).

Olsen, G.A. and Lomholt, G.: Gonorrhoea treated by a combination of probenecid and sodium penicillin G. British Journal of Venereal Diseases 45: 144 (1969).

Pestka, S.: Inhibitors of ribosome functions. Annual Review of Biochemistry 40: 769 (1971).

Reeves, D.S.: Prescription of aminoglycosides by nomogram. Journal of Antimicrobial Chemotherapy 3: 533 (1977).

Report: A survey of antibiotic sensitivity tests. Journal of Medical Laboratory Technology 17: 133 (1960).

Roe, F.J.C.: Metronidazole: Review of uses and toxicity. Journal of Antimicrobial Chemotherapy 3: 205 (1977).

Sawyer, P.R.; Brogden, R.N.; Pinder, R.M.; Speight, T.M. and Avery, G.S.: Miconazole: A review of its antifungal activity and therapeutic efficacy. Drugs 9: 406 (1975).

Schonfeld, H.: Antibiotics and Chemotherapy, vol. 25, Pharmacokinetics (Karger, Basel 1978).

Smith, J.; Tyrrell, W.F.; Gow, A.; Allan, G.W. and Lees, A.W.: Hepatotoxicity in rifampicin-isoniazid treated patients related to their rate of isoniazid inactivation. Chest 61: 587 (1972).

Study Group on Antibiotic Resistance: Tetracycline resistance in pneumococci and group A streptococci. British Medical Journal 1: 131 (1977).

Suhrland, L. and Weisberger, A.: Chloramphenicol toxicity in liver and renal disease. Archives of Internal Medicine 112: 161 (1963).

Symposium: New possibilities in the treatment of systemic mycoses. Reports on the experimental and clinical evaluation of miconazole. Proceedings of the Royal Society of Medicine 70(Suppl. 1) (1977a).

Symposium: Prophylactic use of antibiotics. Southern Medical Journal 70(Suppl. 1) (1977b).

Tan, J.S.; Terhune, C.A. Jr.; Kaplan, S. and Hamburger, M.: Successful two-week treatment schedule for penicillin-sensitive Streptococcus viridans endocarditis. Lancet 2: 1340 (1971).

Tong, M.J.; Martin, D.G.; Cunningham, J.J. and Gunning, J.J.: Clinical and bacteriological evaluation of antibiotic treatment in shigellosis. Journal of the American Medical Association 214: 1841 (1970).

Turk, D.C.: A comparison of chloramphenicol and ampicillin as bacterial agents for Haemophilus influenzae type b. Journal of Medical Microbiology 10: 127 (1977).

Utz, J.P.; Garriques, I.L.; Sande, M.A. et al.: Therapy of cryptococcosis with a combination of flucytosine and amphotericin B. Journal of Infectious Diseases 132: 368 (1975).

Watts, B.A.; Phillips, I. and Stoate, M.W.: In vitro activity of 15 penicillins and mecillinam against Neisseria gonorrhoeae. Journal of Antimicrobial Chemotherapy 3: 331 (1977).

Weinstein, L.: Modes of action of antibiotics on bacteria and man. New York State Journal of Medicine 72: 2166 (1972).

Weinstein, L. and Dalton, A.C.: Host determinants of response to antimicrobial agents. New England Journal of Medicine 279: 467, 524, 580 (1968).

Williams, J.D.: Which cephalosporin? Journal of Antimicrobial Chemotherapy 4: 109 (1978).

Woods, D.D.: The relation of p-aminobenzoic acid to the mechanism of the action of sulphanilamide. British Journal of Experimental Pathology 21: 74 (1940).

Yourassowsky, E.; Schoutens, E. and Vanderlinden, M.P.: Journal of Antimicrobial Chemotherapy 2: 55 (1976).

Chapter XXVIII
Viral Diseases

A.J. Steigman†

Synopsis of Important Principles

1) Management of viral diseases chiefly involves specific preventive measures and recognition and symptomatic treatment of complications.

2) Viral vaccines are used for active immunisation of individuals prior to exposure or for epidemiological control of viral disease in a community.

3) The desirability of controlling a viral disease in a community depends on whether the disease is worth preventing and whether one attack of the natural disease confers long lasting immunity.

4) The effectiveness of mass immunisation programmes against a specific viral infection is decreased if new susceptibles born into a community are not vaccinated at the appropriate time.

5) Viruses can cross the placenta and sometimes may cause adverse pathological effects or severe viral illness in the newborn. Only rubella, varicella and cytomegalovirus have been proven to cause true congenital malformation.

6) Vaccines for prevention of poliomyelitis, measles, rubella, mumps, smallpox and yellow fever and for protection against influenza and rabies are available.

7) The multiplicity of rhinoviruses ('common cold'), the enteroviruses, and the host of respiratory viruses has precluded the development of practical vaccines for these most frequent clinical diseases.

8) Antiviral drugs are available for prevention or treatment of a few specific virus infections. They should not be used unless the aetiological diagnosis is certain.

9) For most viral diseases, treatment of established infection is symptomatic.

10) Antibacterial drugs should not be used routinely in the hope of preventing complications, but they do have a role in treating early developing or established bacterial complications.

Viral infection without accompanying illness occurs frequently. Were this not so, the hundreds of now known serotypes of respiratory viruses, to say nothing of the many other viruses, would immobilise humanity. When illness does occur, the clinical course is generally self limited and of relatively short duration, leading to long lasting immunity to the specific virus concerned. Certainly, some common virus diseases such as measles may be associated with some fatalities or sequelae; some uncommon ones such as rabies are almost universally fatal. Others will cause hepatitis or give rise to recurrent clinical troubles such as fever blisters (herpes hominis) or shingles (herpes zoster). Some viruses may lie dormant for years only to cause tragic neurological damage in later life. Still other viruses may have a role in certain human cancers (e.g. Burkitt's tumour).

This chapter concerns acute viral infections and their resulting diseases and the specific and non-specific measures to deal with prevention and treatment.

1. General Principles

At present, specific preventive measures are more widely available and understood than are specific therapeutic measures (see table I). For most viral infections, this is not only due to the problems involved in developing specific antiviral drugs, but also because of the difficulties involved in making a sufficiently prompt and accurate aetiological diagnosis (see section 4). Thus, specific preventive measures relate to use of viral vaccines for active immunisation of individuals prior to exposure or to epidemiological control of viral diseases in a community (see section 2). Non-specific preventive measures, which apply to individuals as opposed to a community, are the same as for non-viral infections and may be summarised as 'good genes and good health habits'. This is largely influenced by socioeconomic factors of which adequate nutrition is most important. For example, the mortality rate of measles was 15% in Western countries a century ago, a figure which now obtains only in deprived developing countries.

While it may appear tempting to endeavour to eradicate all viral diseases in man, this is improbable and indeed may perhaps even be undesirable. In theory it should be possible to eradicate at least some virus diseases, but in practice, for a variety

of reasons, this goal does not as yet appear attainable. Moreover, eradication of all virus disease may well expose the population to the risk of more serious infection by non-virus organisms. Control of viral disease in the community by vaccination, for example, therefore depends on whether the disease is worth preventing (incidence of complications and sequelae compared with incidence of adverse reactions to vaccination itself) and whether the natural history of the disease is such that one attack confers long lasting or permanent immunity.

In very general terms, many virus infections, if we must have them, are better contracted in childhood, particularly those that carry immunity of some duration, since complications are generally less severe than in later life. Similarly, the young adult is far more likely to have a severe primary vaccination reaction and complications than a normal child (see Juel-Jensen, 1974; Stuart-Harris, 1975).

2. Approach to Epidemiological Control of Viral Diseases

Apart from quarantine control measures, a number of methods can be used in attempts to control certain viral diseases in a community (Stevens and Merigan, 1971; Stuart-Harris, 1975):

1) Raise the degree of herd immunity (active immunisation)
2) Environmental sanitary control
3) Early warning mechanisms for detection of new virus invasions
4) Control life cycle of zoonotic viruses responsible for viral disease transmission.

2.1 Raise the Degree of Herd Immunity

When a sufficient percentage of susceptible individuals are rendered immune by virus vaccines, the quantity of wild circulating virus in a community is reduced. This operates to reduce by degrees the risk of exposure in those who are not immunised. The herd immunity principle is not always very effective. Enthusiastic campaigns to immunise large numbers of children against a specific viral infection are all too often followed by complacency; in a short time new susceptibles born into the community are not vaccinated and

Table I. Approaches available for specific management of some viral infections

Nucleic acid	Virus group	Infection	Methods available[1]
DNA	Poxviruses	Smallpox (variola)	Vaccine (L) Vaccinia immune globulin Antiviral drugs[2]
	Herpesvirus	Herpes Cytomegalovirus	Antiviral drugs[2]
		Varicella-zoster	Antiviral drugs[2] Zoster immune globulin
RNA	Myxovirus	Influenza	Vaccine (K) Antiviral drugs[2]
		Mumps	Vaccine (L)
	Paramyxovirus	Measles (rubeola)	Vaccine (L) Immune serum globulin
	Arbovirus	Rubella	Vaccine (L)
		Yellow fever	Vaccine (L)
	Enterovirus	Poliomyelitis	Vaccine (L)
	Rhabdovirus	Rabies	Vaccine (K) Rabies immune globulin (human) Antirabies serum

1   K = killed, L = live attenuated vaccine.
2   See also section 4 and table III for specific details.

diminish the effectiveness of herd immunity (see also section 3.4).

2.2 Environmental Sanitary Control

Appropriate environmental sanitary control, especially of water, food and sewage, is an effective general approach. The means for achieving this can be readily applied in developed affluent countries, but cannot be so readily applied in underdeveloped countries, where such measures are most needed. In the case of viruses spread by the oral-faecal route, one effect of improved sanitation has been that diseases such as poliomyelitis (and other enteroviruses), hepatitis, and viral diarrhoea affect more older persons than they otherwise would. This is not always advantageous, since adult response to children's virus disorders often takes on increased severity.

2.3 Early Warning Mechanisms

Establishment of early warning mechanisms to detect promptly the incursion of new viral activity provides valuable information. A global network of laboratory surveillance posts for influenza virus provides information which may be used to modify the constituents of vaccines for influenza, a virus whose antigenic components are subject to periodic changes (see section 3.2.1). Systematic trapping of animal and insect vectors of viruses which may give rise to human viral disease is another method of providing useful epidemiological information. Special centres for rapid identification of smallpox by electron microscopy, combined with contact finding, is another example of an early warning system. This can lead to control, either by vaccination, or when appropriate by passive immunisation using vaccinia immune human globulin.

2.4 Control Life Cycle of Zoonotic Viruses

Interruption in insects, birds and mammals of the normal life cycle of certain zoonotic viruses in which man becomes infected is a desirable goal in some cases.

Mosquito control, bird and bat elimination, and rabies vaccination of animals are some examples of the vector control approach.

3. Management of Viral Diseases

Management of viral infection primarily involves use of vaccines for those diseases which can be prevented in this way (see table I) and recognition and symptomatic treatment of complications for those illnesses which cannot or need not be prevented by vaccination. Antiviral chemotherapy has only a limited place in management at the present time (see section 4). Although vector control and other specific measures have been useful in preventing viral disease in a community, active immunisation has proved the most effective. With some viral diseases it is not desirable or thought necessary to provide community protection (see section 1). In such cases, vaccines are used on an individual basis — in those at special risk or in travellers to endemic areas. In unvaccinated individuals or in those who cannot be given live vaccines, human immune gamma globulin (of high titre) or specific antiviral drugs can be useful in modifying or preventing some viral illnesses (see table I), if given soon after exposure.

3.1 General Principles

3.1.1 General Principles in the Use of Viral Vaccines

Live attenuated virus vaccines are more effective than are killed vaccines. Virus combinations in a single injection or simultaneously at different sites are now available. With the exception of oral poliomyelitis vaccine, viral vaccines should not ordinarily be used in children under 1 year of age, since maternal immunity present at this time decreases the vaccine induced immune response. If a child is vaccinated before age 1 year a second dose should be given. The most frequent cause of vaccine failure is improper storage.

Best results are achieved when the viruses concerned exist in a single or only a few serotypes. Live attenuated viral vaccines carry relatively few hazards, but should not be used for individuals who are pregnant, who have conditions associated with immunodeficiency — either inherent or due to malignancy, or are receiving therapy with corticosteroids, antineoplastic or immunosuppressive drugs or irradiation.

3.1.2 General Principles of Treatment

In bacterial diseases specific chemotherapy aimed at the organism is nearly always available (see chapter XXVII). However, in the management of viral diseases, with a few exceptions, therapy is symptomatic and therefore aimed at the patients. Awareness of the severe effects and complications and an understanding of the natural history of viral disorders is essential, for it permits the clinician to:

a) Describe to the patient what is happening, i.e. prognosis
b) To anticipate and often to avoid the complications of the disease and of the use of unnecessary medication, and
c) Possibly help limit spread of illness to others, by the imposition of reasonable isolation for particularly contagious conditions such as chicken pox and mumps.

The skilled use of cheerful support and of symptomatic measures is thus the foundation of management. The following symptoms are most commonly associated with acute viral infections: fever, headache, cough, malaise, muscle pain, nausea and vomiting, diarrhoea, insomnia, itching, photophobia. Treatment of the 'standard' case therefore usually revolves around bed rest and use of analgesics and antipyretics for relief of fever and body aches and pain. A linctus may be indicated for troublesome cough, and diarrhoea at the outset may occasionally, in children, warrant specific measures for fluid replacement. A more vexing problem is the protracted convalescent asthenia and depression which may follow such viral illnesses as infectious mononucleosis, influenza and hepatitis. Encouragement, placebos and surveillance to assure oneself and the patient that a new insidious process is not developing is safer and more effective than antidepressant drugs.

The present paucity of antiviral drugs need not induce despair or nihilism. Nor should it lead to unwarranted use of antibiotics, often expected if not demanded by patients. Careful studies have established that the blind 'prophylactic' use of antibiotics in measles, for example, is associated with an increased incidence of complications (Weinstein, 1955). Thus, antibacterial drugs should not be used routinely in the expectation of preventing complications but they do have a role in treating early developing or established secondary bacterial complications. In influenza for example, the illness usually subsides in 3 to 5 days, but if the viral symptomatology is severe (e.g. persistent cough; change in character of sputum), or there is some degree of airway obstruction, supervention of bacterial infection can cause rapid aggravation and onset of pneumonia should be anticipated; in these circumstances broad spectrum antibiotic treatment (e.g. ampicillin/amoxycillin) is advisable from the early stages (Forbes, 1973).

3.2 Viral Infections of the Respiratory Tract

There are more than 150 serologically distinct viruses which infect the human respiratory tract. They include the rhinoviruses ('common cold' virus, about 100 types), respiratory-syncitial viruses, adenoviruses, para-influenza viruses, influenza viruses, certain enteroviruses and others yet to be identified.

3.2.1 Influenza

At present, killed virus influenza vaccines for subcutaneous administration, are the only ones widely available. They usually include antigens of both viral types A and B. Although recent vaccines have been improved in antigenic potency and purified (by zonal centrifugation) to decrease allergic side effects, at best they provide only moderate and short lived protection and they do not prevent the spread of influenza virus. Further shortcomings of the vaccine arise from the fact that natural infection with influenza virus is strain specific and it is very rare for the same antigenic strain of influenza virus to reinfect a normal individual. Thus, the antigenic shift in the virus and the periodic appearance of different antigenic strains of type A virus, with subsequent pandemic spread replacing the previous pandemic strains of virus, pose unique problems in vaccine development (Knight, 1976). Manufacturers must therefore keep pace with the antigenic changes that take place in the virus and must be able to produce adequate quantities of antigenically 'up-to-date' vaccines faster than epidemic spread. Potential hazards with the use of such vaccines was evident in 1976 in the USA. The nationwide vaccine campaign against 'swine-influenza' was associated with an excessive number of cases of Guillain-Barre syndrome (Editorial, 1977).

Since immunity to influenza is mainly related to the specific IgA content of respiratory mucus and local factors in the respiratory epithelium, the development of live attenuated virus vaccines for nasal instillation which aim at producing local immunity, appears in principle to be preferable to injection of killed vaccine (Lee et al., 1977). How-

ever, the duration of protection at best is only likely to persist for a few years and the problem of the periodic sudden appearance of a new antigenic strain of type A, to which the world population is susceptible, remains.

Because of the partial effectiveness of presently available killed influenza virus vaccines, immunisation is primarily recommended for the groups at greatest risk — the elderly, the young debilitated child, and those with pre-existing chronic disease, particularly cardiovascular and pulmonary disease. These are the groups in which the main mortality occurs and in which the vaccine's partial immunogenicity may have some tangible benefit (see Beare, 1975; Feery, 1978).

The antiviral drug amantadine may also be considered for prophylaxis in unvaccinated special risk patients and in patients with immunodeficiency diseases exposed to influenza A virus. It can also be considered for treatment in special risk patients if given within 48 hours of onset of symptoms (see section 4.4).

3.2.2 Other Respiratory Viruses: 'Common Cold'

Efforts to develop vaccines for the vast number of other respiratory viruses are interesting but have not yet resulted in practical application. Indeed, it is doubftul whether it is possible to produce an effective vaccine against the 'common cold' because there are too many virus types involved.

The use of large doses of vitamin C as prophylaxis or treatment of symptoms of the common cold is controversial (e.g. Dykes and Meier, 1975; Ritzel, 1976; Coulehan, 1976). Some investigators have however, demonstrated a useful prophylactic effect and a beneficial therapeutic effect if given when the cold symptoms first appear (Anderson et al., 1975; Wilson, 1975). Any beneficial therapeutic effect of vitamin C appears to be associated with its influence on ascorbic acid metabolism, which is abnormal during the early course of the cold (Wilson and Loh, 1974).

Antihistamine drugs are frequently empolyed for relief of 'common cold'-like symptoms. Their effect is variable and the mechanism when effective is unknown, Nevertheless, some patients and clinicians report an amelioration of the clinical course under the influence of antihistamines (see West et al., 1975). As with influenza, antibacterial drugs can be given for complications but are of no benefit given routinely (see chapter XI; sect. 2.2).

3.3 Measles

Prevention prior to exposure is feasible through the use of a further attenuated living strain of measles virus (Dudgeon, 1969, 1977; Krugman, 1977). Untoward reactions are uncommon and a seroconversion success rate of 95 % is expected, providing the vaccine is properly refrigerated and kept from exposure to light, Measles is a good example of the desirability of mass immunisation of children in a community since the incidence of encephalitis with natural measles is 1 in 1,000 cases and that of vaccine associated encephalitis is 1 in 1,000,000, and immunity is likely to be long lasting (Miller, 1964; Krugman, 1971). Combined viral vaccines are commercially available in some countries and appear to be equally effective as single ones injected at different sites. These include: measles and rubella, and measles, rubella and mumps combined.

Prevention or modification of disease *after* exposure (which may be desired only for very young infants or those suffering another illness at the time) can be accomplished by injecting human immune serum globulin intramuscularly; the preventive dose is 0.25ml/kg, the modifying dose is 0.05ml/kg.

The management of uncomplicated measles is symptomatic; routine 'prophylactic' antibiotics have been shown to increase the incidence of pyogenic complications, e.g. otitis media and pneumonia (see also section 3.1.2).

3.4 Rubella

An effective live attenuated virus vaccine is available for use alone or in combination with other attenuated virus vaccines (Dudgeon, 1977; Katz, 1972; Krugman, 1977). The sole aim is to prevent fetal rubella in early pregnancy and its consequent dysmorphogenic effects. There are two basic strategic approaches to accomplish this:

1) To immunise all children between the age of 1 year and puberty in the hope of achieving 'herd immunity' in the age group which may transmit rubella to a susceptible pregnant mother, and

2) To immunise *all* girls in the pre-pubertal age group (i.e. age 11 to 14).

Mass immunisation of children is the method most often used, but it may not be the preferred method since it may be more difficult to achieve success with this approach.

Immunity in one segment of the population may have no influence on the occurrence of the disease in the rest of the community (Klock and Rachelefsky, 1973), particularly if the epidemiology of rubella is different within the school, family, armed forces, suburban and rural settings. Moreover, preventing virus transmission in the community depends on the proportion of children who are immunised at any one time. For example, in the USA in one community where 70 to 100 % of children were immunised, the incidence of rubella fell by 60 % in the following year, but in communities where only 20 to 30 % were immunised, the incidence rose by 50 % (Katz, 1972). Therefore, while mass childhood immunisation remains an important method of rubella prevention, other methods such as vaccination of susceptible non-pregnant women and postpubertal girls, should supplement it; the vaccine being given on an individual basis. Women in the childbearing age can be tested (haemagglutination inhibition test) to determine whether immune. If not immune, and if pregnancy can be avoided in the following 2 to 3 months, the vaccine may be given. Since immunised children are not contagious, pregnancy, which is a contraindication to vaccination of the non-immune mother, is an indication for vaccination of her susceptible child because an unimmunised child may introduce wild rubella into the household. It seems unlikely that fetal infection will occur in association with re-infection which has been observed among persons with natural as well as vaccine induced immunity.

It is important that male and female personnel in the health care industry be immune to rubella. Instances have occurred when non-immune personnel incubating rubella have exposed patients in the early stage of unrecognised pregnancy.

As occurs in rubella itself, the vaccine may result in arthralgia and arthritis, the incidence of which increases with age and is more prominent in females than males, but is less than that which occurs following natural rubella infection. Transient neuropathies, which appear to be more common in the preschool child, have also been described (Gilmartin et al., 1972; Kilroy et al., 1970).

The management of congenital rubella depends upon which ocular, auditory, cardiac or other defects have occurred. These infants continue to excrete rubella virus for prolonged periods and may infect those taking care of them.

3.5 Smallpox

This disease is preventable by the use of vaccinia, a virus closely related to the variola virus of smallpox (Karzon, 1974). The resulting immunity is not lifelong and vaccination needs to be repeated periodically depending upon the intensity of exposure. Smallpox has virtually been eradicated but continuance of such a status requires vigilance. Indications for the use of vaccination is limited to health personnel potentially exposed to smallpox, and for travellers to such countries as continue to require it by statute. Other means of prevention depend upon prompt recognition, isolation and the vaccination of exposed persons. Vaccinia immune human globulin (0.33ml/kg) may have a beneficial effect if given soon after exposure, but vaccination is preferred.

The antiviral drug methisazone (see section 4.2) has also been tried as a means of prevention in unprotected contacts of the disease. Methisazone is of no value if infection is clinically apparent, but by limiting multiplication of the virus, it may lessen the chance of disease if taken during the incubation period. At present it is recommended that non-immune persons exposed to smallpox be vaccinated before methisazone is given (2 doses of 3g given 8 hours apart). Methisazone also appears to be effective in reducing the prevalence of alastrim (variola minor) in those exposed to this milder form of smallpox. It is also used to treat life threatening complications of smallpox vaccination (see section 4.2), but vaccinia immune globulin (0.6ml/kg/24h) is preferable for this purpose.

Treatment in unmodified cases of smallpox is directed at the many specific complications which arise. Although cytarabine (see section 4.3) gave most promising results in the treatment of smallpox in Bangladesh, its reported benefits were not confirmed in controlled trials in other countries (Dennis et al., 1974). Similarly, vidarabine is not effective in treatment of smallpox (Koplan et al., 1975).

3.6 Mumps

An effective live virus vaccine used alone or in combination is available (Editorial, 1974; Steigman, 1974). The need for such a vaccine is debated by some, but the complications of the infection, especially orchitis in the male and less commonly permanent deafness, are not negligible, and the vaccine is finding increasing favour. At present, it is mainly indicated for selective use for prevention of mumps in individuals or groups at special risk. If given soon enough, vaccination might be of use on special occasions to control outbreaks, for example in residential institutions.

The management of mumps, whether accompanied by sialadenitis, pancreatitis, encephalitis, nerve deafness or gonadal inflammation, is symptomatic. For severe orchitis the use of prednisone 20 to 40mg daily for 3 to 4 days is helpful. The use of mumps immune human globulin is not recommended.

3.7 Poliomyelitis

The proper use of trivalent oral live attenuated virus is highly effective in preventing poliomyelitis (Beale, 1969; Sabin, 1964). In addition to rendering the person immune, alimentary tract immunity results, which sharply reduces the dissemination of disease producing wild strains of poliovirus. The multiplication of the 3 serotypes of poliovirus may interfere with one another (as may other enteroviruses common in the community in summer). At least 3 doses spaced several months apart should be given in infancy. Reinforcing doses every 3 to 4 years in childhood are recommended. Those children who received the earlier killed virus vaccine should be given a full course of the live virus vaccine as this provides greater and longer lasting immunity.

The killed poliomyelitis vaccine requires a series of injections; its routine use is still preferred to oral attenuated vaccine in several countries. It is also used when there is a family history suggestive of an immunodeficiency background.

The abortive and non-paralytic forms of poliomyelitis require only symptomatic management. The paralytic forms, especially when severe, require artificial respiratory support, orthopaedic management and close attention to nutrition, fluid and electrolyte disturbance and bowel and bladder care.

Long term rehabilitation and occupational counselling are required.

3.8 Varicella (Chickenpox) and Herpes Zoster (Shingles)

These conditions are caused by the same virus, varicella-zoster or VZ virus — herpes zoster representing an endogenous reactivation of the latent virus in a partly immune individual (see Brunell, 1977; Juel-Jensen and MacCallum, 1972; Juel-Jensen, 1974).

Although chickenpox is a common disease of childhood it is infrequently associated with serious complications or sequelae in the normal child. However, chickenpox (or infection with other herpes viruses: herpes simplex, cytomegalovirus) can be very severe or even fatal in children with lymphoproliferative disorders, who are receiving immunosuppressive therapy or high doses of corticosteroids, or who have an inherent state of immunodeficiency. These high risk children can fortunately be protected by passive immunisation with zoster immune globulin (ZIG) made from plasma of convalescent herpes zoster patients, provided it is given within 72 hours of exposure to a contact (Brunell and Gershon, 1973; Gershon et al., 1974). A live attenuated varicella vaccine has also recently been developed for this purpose (Izawa et al., 1977). When an immunodeficient child does contract chickenpox the outcome is unpredictable and death is not rare. In desperate circumstances treatment with antiviral drugs or human leucocyte interferon as for generalised herpes may be tried (see section 4.3.1; 4.5).

Normal children with chickenpox require minimum management — such as local (calamine lotion; tar bath solution) and oral agents (antihistaminics) to reduce pruritus. Some adults with chickenpox become quite ill and may require prednisone therapy in addition to general supportive therapy. In exceptional cases, a severe attack may warrant specific treatment with an antiviral drug, particularly if it is associated with varicella hepatitis.

When children exhibit herpes zoster the local symptoms of pain, tingling and pruritus generally require topical antipruritics (not calamine: it cakes) or simple analgesics such as paracetamol (acetaminophen). Reactivation of the latent VZ virus is more common after the age of 50 when the immunological 'memory' begins to fade; recurrence occurs at varying intervals and is most often due to injury to the affected dermatome in the recent past. Treatment of choice consists of a 35% solution of idoxuridine in dimethylsulphoxide (Juel-Jensen et al., 1970) applied continuously for 4 days on lint cut to the shape of the dermatome, with daily rewetting of the same piece of lint. Alternatively, 5% idoxuridine in dimethylsulphoxide can be applied 3 to 4 times daily for 1 week. The patient must be treated as soon as possible after the eruption has appeared. Cortico-

steroids, if given early and in large doses, can also be used for relief of pain and motor symptoms (e.g. 45mg daily for 1st week, 30mg for 2nd and 15mg for 3rd week) and may be combined with gamma globulin (Ferrara et al., 1976). Adults, particularly the elderly, often have neuralgia for lengthy periods after the eruption has resolved and this presents other problems in management (see chapter XXV; section 6.2).

Recurrent and severe zoster can be a considerable problem in those who are immunodeficient and these patients, as with those with motor zoster or zoster encephalitis, must be managed in hospital. It should be pointed out that zoster cannot be contracted from patients with chickenpox, and while the neurological distribution of the lesions of herpes zoster may be determined by a malignant deposit at the appropriate root level, there is no evidence that malignant disease is more common in zoster patients than in the general population (see Juel-Jensen, 1974).

3.9 Virus Infections in Pregnancy and the Newborn

Virus infection in pregnancy poses two dilemmas — the extent of any adverse effect on the fetus and/or mother, and whether or not to offer immunisation to non-immune women during outbreaks and to those contemplating travel to affected areas. Not only is there sufficient evidence to indicate that viruses can cross the placenta, but also to support the concept of increased severity of, and perhaps, susceptibility to certain viral diseases during pregnancy. In addition, there is the problem of treatment of severe infection in the newborn offspring (see Dudgeon, 1968a,b; Hanshaw and Dudgeon, 1978; Menser and Forrest, 1973).

At present only rubella, varicella and cytomegalovirus have been proven to cause true congenital malformation, although there have been isolated case reports of abnormalities associated with maternal infection with other viruses (e.g. measles). Nevertheless, these and other viruses may cause prenatal infection with a variety of effects (see table II), including intrauterine growth retardation, and involvement of liver, brain and haemopoietic tissues, In some cases infection may be localised to the placenta and cause only fetal malnutrition, but infection with smallpox always increases the risk of death for both the mother and fetus and maternal infection

Table II. Effects of maternal virus infection on the fetus (after Dudgeon, 1968a)

---

1. *Fetal infection*
   a) Fetal death: abortion, stillbirth
   b) Intrauterine growth retardation
   c) Congenital malformations (rubella, varicella, cytomegalovirus)
   d) Defective tissues and organs (brain, liver, blood)

2. *Subclinical infection* (virus excretion and/or antibody response)

3. *No effect*

---

in late pregnancy with Coxsackie B virus may lead to a widely disseminated and often fatal illness in the newborn infant.

Treatment of severe virus infection in the newborn is limited (Brunell, 1975). Infants severely affected with cytomegalovirus may be treated with idoxuridine, cytarabine or vidarabine (see section 4.3). Neonatal herpes infection (a disease with severe sequelae), which is mainly acquired as a result of transmission of the virus at the time of birth, can also be treated with these antiviral drugs (see section 4.3.1). Congenital varicella in infants born within 4 days of the onset of rash in the mother, are at special risk of severe infection and should be given zoster immune globulin as soon as possible after delivery (Gershon et al., 1976).

Indications for immunisation in non-immune pregnant women are likewise limited (Levine et al., 1974). Poliomyelitis and yellow fever vaccines are indicated in pregnant women contemplating travel to affected areas or in the event of an outbreak. For rubella, mumps and smallpox, routine vaccination is contraindicated. Measles vaccination is not considered necessary in pregnancy. Antiviral drugs (see section 4) should not be used during pregnancy unless the woman suffers from a treatable, potentially life threatening infection. In some virus infections (e.g. measles, rubella, varicella-zoster) immune serum globulin preparations may be considered as a means of preventing or modifying the course of the infection if they can be given soon after exposure.

4. Antiviral Chemotherapy

Slow but steady progress is becoming evident in the development of antiviral chemotherapy.

Although there remain few situations of practical clinical pertinence, the expanded role of amantadine (see section 4.4) is itself responsible for a long awaited breath of optimism (see Merigan, 1976; Symposium, 1977).

The many candidate antiviral agents studied suffer the following problems: (1) toxicity to host cells resulting in a low therapeutic index; (2) poor response owing to the rapid multiplication cycle effect of viruses; (3) the emergence of drug resistant virus; and (4) difficulty in conclusively demonstrating clinical effectiveness in the numerous self limiting virus diseases. Exaggerated unsubstantiated claims for the utility of a host of drugs proposed as safe and effective has retarded rather than assisted the development of suitable therapeutic agents. Antiviral therapy or chemoprophylaxis should not be started unless the aetiological diagnosis is certain.

4.1 Viruses and Drug Action

Viruses are divided into two classes depending on whether their nucleic acid is deoxyribonucleic acid (DNA) or ribonucleic acid (RNA). The larger and more complex the virus, the greater the likelihood of interrupting its activity at some vulnerable phase of its replication, as can be shown with methisazone for smallpox virus, a large DNA virus (Stalder, 1977). Most of the viruses causing human disease are much smaller and less complex and most are RNA viruses, but with one exception, the use of amantadine for influenza A virus, these are not so far amenable to therapy. The possibility nevertheless exists that enzymes crucial for replication may be found which are coded in the virus (and formed in the infected cell) but whose action is sufficiently different from the corresponding host cell enzyme such that an agent could inhibit the formation of a unique enzyme carried by the virus.

There is more than mere hope for development of clinically useful antiviral drugs. Not only are a few agents already available, but also the approaches to drug inhibition of virus replication are becoming more rational, particularly now that it is appreciated that the infecting virus induces, and is completely reliant upon, several biochemical processes for which the host cell itself has no need. The 10 steps involved in the virus multiplication cycle, at any one of which an antiviral agent might be useful, are represented schematically in figure 1.

Antiviral drugs are of potential use in treatment of established infection, if given promptly, and in chemoprophylaxis, when given before or as soon as possible after exposure (Weinstein and Chang, 1973; Juel-Jensen, 1974). It may well be that chemoprophylaxis offers more hope than treatment, particularly if drugs could be developed which prevent attachment of the virus to the host cell surface. Whereas protection provided by vaccination may take some time to develop and is aimed at producing long lasting immunity against future infection, the protection given by chemoprophylaxis is immediate but only lasts while the drug is being taken. Thus vaccination may not prevent disease at the time of an outbreak (immunity may not develop quickly enough) or if the infection is already acquired, but an antiviral drug if given soon enough could modify or prevent disease by halting multiplication of the virus in the body during the incubation period.

At present, there are 3 main classes of chemical compound with antiviral activity which have been employed usefully in man — thiosemicarbazones, nucleosides and cyclic amines (table III). In addition, there are experimental drugs which induce the formation of interferon, a substance which renders cells resistant to viruses without affecting the virus directly (sect. 4.5), and drugs such as inosiplex which have both immunostimulant and antiviral activity (Hadden et al., 1977).

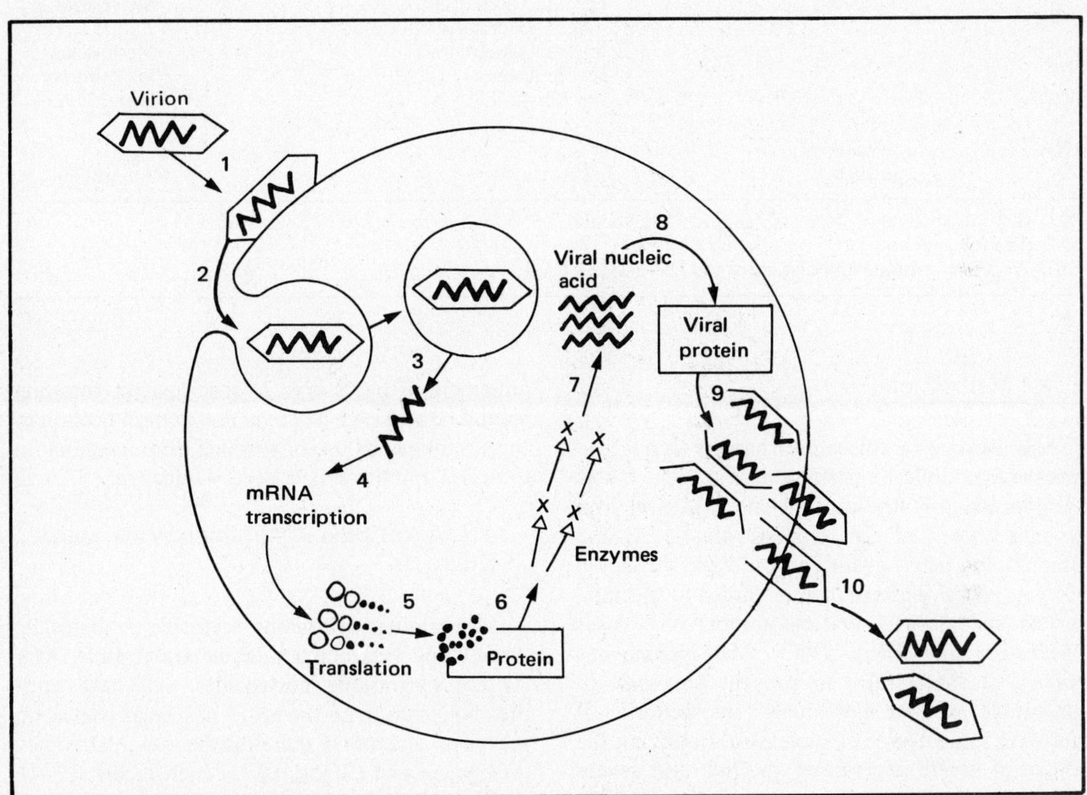

Fig. 1. Schematic representation of multiplication cycle of viruses (and inhibitory action of antiviral drugs).
1   Attachment to cell surface
2   Penetration into the cell (amantadine)
3   Uncoating of viral nucleic acid molecule (amantadine)
4   Transcription of viral messenger RNA (interferon)
5   Translation of proteins which depress synthesis of cell molecules (interferon)
6   Translation of enzymes required for viral nucleic acid replication (idoxuridine, cytarabine, vidarabine)
7   Replication of the viral nucleic acid
8   Translation of virus proteins (methisazone)
9   Assembly of new virions
10 Release of more virions; can attack more cells (photodynamic inactivation)

Table III. Uses and potential uses of antiviral drugs

Nucleic acid	Virus group	Clinical condition	Drug
DNA	*Herpesviruses*		
	Herpes simplex	Keratitis	Idoxuridine[1] (or vidarabine)
		Cutaneous herpes	Idoxuridine[1]
		Herpetic whitlow	Idoxuridine[1]
		Recurrent genital herpes	Idoxuridine[1]
		Encephalitis, generalised infection	Vidarabine
	Varicella-zoster	Severe keratitis	Vidarabine
		Severe cutaneous zoster	Idoxuridine[1]
		Severe disseminated varicella-zoster infection	Vidarabine
	Cytomegalovirus	CNS infection of newborn	Vidarabine
	Poxiviruses		
	Variola major	Smallpox	Methisazone[2]
	Variola minor	Alastrim	Methisazone[2]
	Vaccinia	Eczema vaccinatum[3] severe generalised vaccinia[3]	Methisazone
		Vaccinia gangrenosa[3]	Methisazone
		Severe lesions	Idoxuridine[1]
		Keratitis[3]	Idoxuridine[1]
RNA	*Myxoviruses*		
	Influenza	Influenza A	Amantadine

1   Topical application (see also chapter XII, section 3.6; XIV, section 2.2; XXIX, section 7.1).
2   Prophylaxis only.
3   Vaccinia immune globulin must also be used.

4.2 Methisazone

Methisazone, a thiosemicarbazone derivative, was the first clinically useful antiviral drug. It acts by suppressing synthesis of the late structural viral proteins (step 8 of the 10 steps; see fig. 1) and although it is active against a number of viruses *in vitro,* its effectiveness in man is limited to vaccinia, variola and alastrim (variola minor) poxviruses (Weinstein and Chang, 1973). Methisazone has been used successfully to prevent smallpox in susceptible exposed individuals (see section 3.5) and with some degree of success in modifying the course of severe generalised vaccinia and severe eczema vaccinatum, a life threatening complication of smallpox vaccination in those suffering from eczema (McClean, 1977). It has also been used as one of the measures in treating vaccinia gangrenosa. The dosage used in the treatment of complications of vaccinia is 200mg/kg initially, followed by 8 doses of 50mg/kg every 6 hours. Although methisazone is relatively non-toxic, nausea and vomiting are common. Vomiting may be reduced by giving the drug after meals, with an antiemetic if necessary. A dose lost by vomiting should be replaced. There is no contraindication to the simultaneous use of vaccinia immune globulin (0.6ml/kg/24h) which is very effective.

4.3 Idoxuridine, Cytarabine, Vidarabine, Ribavirin

Idoxuridine, cytarabine (cytosine arabinoside; Ara-C) and vidarabine (adenine arabinoside; Ara-A) are pyrimidine nucleosides. All have antimetabolic effects on the host's tissues as well as on the virus and must therefore be used cautiously (Weinstein and Chang, 1973; Juel-Jensen, 1974).

Idoxuridine has a number of biological actions, but it appears to act predominantly by competitive inhibition of thymidine incorporation into viral DNA. The other two pyrimidine nucleoside analogues interfere selectively with DNA synthesis and have been more widely used for this effect in leukaemia than for the treatment of primary acute viral infections. All three compounds are active *in vitro* against DNA-containing viruses, primarily the herpesvirus group, cytomegalovirus, varicella-zoster and vaccinia. Development of resistance is common to idoxuridine but has not been reported with cytarabine and vidarabine.

Ribavirin, a synthetic nucleoside, is the newest addition to this group. Laboratory studies indicate that it has antiviral activity against some RNA viruses as well as some DNA viruses. *In vitro* studies suggest that herpes virus is less likely to become drug resistant with this agent than with the use of idoxuridine. Infections in humans with influenza (types A and B) and with viral hepatitis have been treated with ribavirin but there is insufficient careful study data to assess its place in clinical therapy. Transient elevation of serum bilirubin has been noted in some studies (Magnussen et al., 1977).

4.3.1 Herpes Simplex, Varicella and Zoster, Cytomegalovirus

A number of primary or recurrent herpesvirus infections have been treated with these drugs with varying degrees of success. Local infections have in general, responded best. Thus topical idoxuridine and vidarabine applied frequently are of proven value in the early superficial phase of herpetic keratitis (see chapter XII; section 3.6) and in appropriate formulations and regimens of administration, idoxuridine can be used successfully in mucocutaneous herpes infections — including recurrent genital herpes (see chapter XXIX; section 7.1), severe and painful shingles (see section 3.8) and various cutaneous herpes simplex infections (see chapter XIV; section 2.2). Topical cytarabine and vidarabine have been effective in patients with herpes keratitis resistant to idoxuridine.

Systemic use of idoxuridine, cytarabine and vidarabine has been difficult to evaluate (Weinstein and Chang, 1973; Longson, 1977). They have been tried in cases of encephalitis and disseminated infection due to herpes simplex virus, in cytomegalovirus infection, and disseminated severe varicella-zoster infection with many claims of success and failure. Many consider that the gravity of these conditions merits the risk of toxicity from these agents (see below), but it is far from clear whether outcome of treatment is favourably affected by their addition to intensive supportive care and other nonspecific treatment, such as large doses of corticosteroids in herpes encephalitis. There is also uncertainty about the effects on the postnatal development of the brain of infants treated with these antiviral agents (Brunell, 1975).

Answers to these questions must therefore await the outcome of controlled trials by interinstitutional study groups. Such studies are now being reported with the use of these agents. Idoxuridine has been rejected as having unacceptable toxicity in the therapy of herpes simplex virus encephalitis (Boston Virus Study Group, 1975). However, vidarabine is considered acceptable therapy in herpes simplex virus encephalitis, provided the drug is given early before the onset of coma (Whitley et al., 1977). Although not all investigators are completely satisfied by the evidence (e.g. Tager; 1977; Gluckman, 1977), at the present time, vidarabine is considered to be the drug of choice in the treatment of generalised herpesvirus encephalitis (Taber et al., 1977) and can be tried in other severe generalised herpesvirus infections (Aronson et al., 1976). When disseminated varicella-zoster infection occurs in immunosuppressed persons, the use of vidarabine systemically should be strongly considered as it is much less toxic than cytarabine (Whitley et al., 1976).

Attention must also be paid to the intrinsic antiviral activity and pharmacokinetic properties of these agents.

All three compounds are eliminated rapidly in the urine, largely as metabolites. The elimination half-life of vidarabine being around 1.5 hours while that of cytarabine and idoxuridine are around 30 minutes. The metabolites of cytarabine and idoxuridine have no antiviral activity. The deaminated metabolite of vidarabine (ara-Hx) is less active than the parent drug but serum concentrations are much greater (10 to 1000-fold) than those of vidarabine (Whitley et al., 1975). Both ara-Hx and vidarabine attain high concentrations in erythrocytes, indicating that they are capable of concentrating intracellularly. This is of importance since viral replication is an intracellular phenomenon. Vidarabine readily penetrates into the cerebrospinal fluid where concentrations are about a half of those in the plasma. Cytarabine also enters the CSF and concentrations around a half of plasma concentrations can be maintained by a continuous infusion (Frei et al., 1973). Vidarabine and cytarabine retain their activity in the CSF but idoxuridine is rapidly inactivated in the brain.

Apart from the rapid elimination of idoxuridine, viruses of the herpes group are generally more sensitive to cytarabine and vidarabine, resistance has not been reported, and they are not inactivated in the brain, making them potentially more effective in management of central nervous system infections. These advantages are probably borne out by the more encouraging results with cytarabine and vidarabine in generalised herpes, herpes encephalitis and severe disseminated varicella-zoster infection. The results of cytarabine in congenital cytomegalovirus infection have not been particularly convincing. Vidarabine may be superior since it is metabolised to compounds which retain antiviral activity (see above). It has been successfully tried in adults with central nervous system cytomegalovirus disease (Phillips, 1977) and in congenital cytomegalovirus infection (Ch'ien et al., 1972). These observations need to be confirmed in controlled clinical trials.

The adverse reactions of vidarabine, cytarabine and idoxuridine differ. Whereas cytarabine and idoxuridine cause bone marrow suppression, alopecia and oral ulceration, vidarabine causes encephalopathy (usually at high dosage; i.e. 20mg/kg/day), nausea, vomiting and weight loss. Leucopenia, thrombocytopenia and megaloblastic anaemia have been reported with vidarabine but usually in patients with haematological disorders (Chang and Snydman, 1979).

4.3.2 Poxviruses

Cytarabine has been used effectively in generalised vaccinia following smallpox vaccination of patients with atopic eczema, although patients with true generalised vaccinia usually recover with little or no specific therapy. Cytarabine and vidarabine have no effect in the treatment of smallpox (see section 3.5). Topical idoxuridine in DMSO (35% soaked on lint) has hastened healing of severe vaccinia lesions without interfering with immunity (see Juel-Jensen, 1974). As an eye ointment, idoxuridine or vidarabine can be used in ocular infections involving vaccinia (see chapter XII; section 3.6).

4.4 Amantadine and Rimantadine

Amantadine is a cyclic amine which exerts its antiviral effect by preventing viral penetration into host cells.

Earlier observations with amantadine indicated its usefulness against influenza virus in a very limited way. It is now clear that this important agent is effective against all tested strains of influenza A virus (but not type B) and may be expected to be useful against new emerging strains of influenza A virus. In that regard amantadine has advantages over influenza virus vaccines in *prophylaxis* (Chanin, 1977). The drug would need to be administered for the duration of a threatened outbreak for the following circumstances: (1) elderly patients in institutions; (2) persons with severe underlying cardiac and respiratory diseases; (3) medical and community service personnel during a pandemic; and (4) family contacts of an early recognised case of influenza A virus.

Among deterrents to the widespread application of amantadine for chemoprophylaxis are the cost, the concerns about CNS side effects in the elderly and the fact that many persons who would not develop illness in any event would be receiving amantadine for extended periods of time. Nevertheless, the emergence of this drug gives encouragement for those engaged in the difficult area of developing antiviral chemotherapy (Jackson and Stanley, 1976; Jackson, 1977).

Amantadine is also effective in the treatment of uncomplicated influenza due to type A virus, provided treatment is given early after the onset of symptoms. It has produced a substantial reduction in fever, headache and respiratory symptoms when started within 48 hours of onset of symptoms and may be considered for such use in special risk cases when epidemiological data support the specific diagnosis (Jackson and Stanley, 1976; Jackson, 1977).

Amantadine is completely absorbed after oral administration. It has an elimination half-life of 9 to 37 hours. About 90% of an oral dose is excreted in the urine unchanged, mostly by tubular secretion and to a much lesser extent by glomerular filtration (Weinstein and Chang, 1973; Chang and Snydman, 1979). Dosage should be reduced in patients with impaired renal function to avoid accumulation and toxicity (Ing et al., 1974). Amantadine attains concentrations in saliva similar to those in plasma and readily penetrates the cerebrospinal fluid. It is also excreted in breast milk.

The recommended dosage for prophylaxis and treatment in adults and children over 9 years is 100mg twice daily and for children 5 to 9 years 4.5 to 9mg/kg up to a maximum daily dose of 150mg in 2 or 3 equally divided doses. Side effects are dose related, usually mild and generally occur within the first 48 hours of administration (La Montagne and Galasso, 1978). Difficulty in concentration is the most common, and less often depression, psychosis, confusion and dizziness. Orthostatic hypotension has also occurred. A lower dosage (100mg daily) may be desirable for prophylaxis in the elderly, who can experience CNS side effects at doses of 200mg daily.

Rimantadine, a congener of amantadine has similar antiviral activity and has been widely used in the USSR for prophylaxis. It is not available elsewhere (La Montagne and Galasso, 1978).

4.5 Interferon

Another approach to the prophylaxis and perhaps early therapy of virus infections is the use of chemical inducers of interferon, a naturally occurring substance which renders cells resistant to viruses without affecting the virus directly. Thus, unlike antiviral chemotherapeutic drugs, a wide variety of both DNA and RNA viruses are subject to the influence of interferon and therefore preliminary precise viral aetiological diagnosis may not be necessary before instituting prophylaxis or treatment. Interferon also inhibits cell growth (hence investigation of its possible use in malignant disease) and has an immunoregulatory activity (see Chang and Snydman, 1979; Pollard and Merigan, 1978).

The development of intrinsic interferon during recovery from viral illness has led to important studies on how to: (1) administer interferon made exogenously, either in cell cultures of human fibroblasts or human leucocytes (since mammalian interferons are species specific, human sources are necessary); and (2) to develop chemical stimulants to give to patients to induce endogenous interferon.

To manufacture, standardise and to administer to humans exogenously prepared human interferon is still a tour de force; the details of which are beyond the scope of this section. However, it can be done and is being done successfully, admittedly in unusual circumstances; for example, herpes zoster in patients with cancer (Merigan et al., 1978). The presently available supply is far exceeded by the demand; suitable clinical trials are under way in chronic active viral hepatitis, herpes simplex virus, varicella-zoster virus and respiratory virus diseases. The possibility that interferon together with vidarabine is synergistic is under consideration, for these 2 substances have been shown to be effective against the herpes family of viruses (Hirsch, 1978).

The role of using chemical inducers of interferon is also evolving. These substances include high molecular weight polyanions such as polyionosinic : polycytidylic acid (poly I:C). This material has been used topically with some success in herpetic keratitis, herpes zoster and by intranasal instillation in volunteers infected with a rhinovirus (Pollard and Merigan, 1978). Recently, a new interferon inducer has been developed, which is both more effective and less toxic, by complexing poly I:C with poly-L-lysine (poly ICLC). Studies in animals are under way to determine its potential role in human disease (Olsen et al., 1978).

Further Reading

Bedson, S.; Downie, A.W.; MacCallum, F.O. and Stuart-Harris, C.H.: Virus and Rickettsial Diseases, 4th ed (Arnold, London 1967).

Hanshaw, J.B. and Dudgeon, J.A.: Viral diseases of the fetus and newborn (Saunders, Philadelphia 1978).

Horsfall, F.L. and Tamm, I.: Viral and Rickettsial Infections in Man, 4th ed (Lippincott, Philadelphia 1965).

Merigan, T.: Antivirals with clinical potential. Journal of Infectious Diseases 133: Suppl. (June 1976).

Steigman, A.J. (Ed): Report of the Committee on Infectious Diseases, 18th ed (American Academy of Pediatrics, Evanston 1977).

Symposium: Third conference on antiviral substances. Annals of the New York Academy of Sciences 282: 1 (1977).

Weinstein, L. and Chang, T-W.: Viral infections: an overview. American Journal of the Medical Sciences 272: 301 (1976).

References

Anderson, T.W.; Beaton, G.H.; Corey, P.N. and Spero, L.: Winter illness and vitamin C.: The effect of relatively low doses. Canadian Medical Association Journal 112: 823 (1975).

Aronson, M.D.; Phillips, C.F.; Gump, D.W.; Albertini, R.J. and Phillips, A.: Vidarabine therapy for severe herpesvirus infections: An unusual syndrome for chronic varicella and transient immunologic deficiency. Journal of the American Medical Association 235: 1339 (1976).

Beale, A.J.: Immunisation against poliomyelitis. British Medical Bulletin 25: 148 (1969).

Beare, A.S.: Vaccination against influenza. Practitioner 215: 315 (1975).

Boston Interhospital Virus Study Group: Failure of high dose 5-iodo-2-deoxyuridine in the therapy of herpes simplex virus encephalitis — evidence of unacceptable toxicity. New England Journal of Medicine 292: 599 (1975).

Brunell, P.: Antiviral drugs for the neonate: The risk-benefit ledger. Journal of Pediatrics 86: 317 (1975).

Brunell, P.: Protection against varicella. Pediatrics 59: 1 (1977).

Brunell, P.A. and Gershon, Anne A.: Passive immunisation against varicella-zoster infections and other modes of therapy. Journal of Infectious Diseases 127: 415 (1973).

Chang, T-W. and Snydman, D.R.: Antiviral agents: Action and clinical use. Drugs. In press (1979).

Chanin, A.: Influenza: Vaccines or amantadine? Journal of the American Medical Association 237: 1445 (1977).

Ch'ien, L.T.; Benton, J.W.; Buchanan, R.A. and Alford, C.A.: Adenine arabinoside (Ara-A) treatment of severe pox and herpetic infections of man. Pediatric Research 6: 384/124 (1972).

Coulehan, J.L.; Eberhard, Susan; Kapner, L.; Taylor, F.; Rogers, K. and Garry, P.: Vitamin C and acute illness in Navajo schoolchildren. New England Journal of Medicine 295: 973 (1976).

Dennis, D.T.; Doberstyn, E.B.; Awoke, S.; Royer, G.L. and Renis, H.E.: Failure of cytosine arabinoside in treating smallpox. Lancet 2: 377 (1974).

Dudgeon, J.A.: Breakdown in maternal protection: Infections. Proceedings of the Royal Society of Medicine 61 (pt 2): 1236 (1968a).

Dudgeon, J.A.: Dysmorphogenesis: The role of infection. Proceedings of the Royal Society of Medicine 61 (pt 2): 1285 (1968b).

Dudgeon, J.A.: Measles vaccines. British Medical Bulletin 25: 159 (1969).

Dudgeon, J.A.: Measles and rubella vaccines. Archives of Disease in Childhood 52: 907 (1977).

Dykes, M.H.M. and Meier, P.: Ascorbic acid and the common cold. Evaluation of its efficacy and toxicity. Journal of the American Medical Association 231: 1073 (1975).

Editorial: Guillain-Barre syndrome and influenza vaccine. British Medical Journal 1: 1373 (1977).

Editorial: Mumps vaccine. Lancet 2: 326 (1974).

Feery, B.J.: Influenza: A continuing problem. Medical Journal of Australia 1: 321 (1978).

Ferrara, R.J.: Herpes zoster: A combined therapy regimen. Cutis 17: 103 (1976).

Forbes, J.A.: Complications of influenza and their management. Medical Journal of Australia 1 (Suppl.): 28 (1973).

Frei, E.; Ho, D.H.W; Bodey, G.P. and Freireich, E.: Pharmacologic and cytokinetic studies of arabinosylcytosine. Verifying concepts of leukemia. Bibliotheca Haematologica 39: 1085 (1973).

Gershon, Anne A.; Steinberg, Sharon and Brunell, P.: Zoster immune globulin: A further assessment. New England Journal of Medicine 290: 243 (1974).

Gershon, A.A.; Raker, R.; Steinberg, S.; Topf-Olstein, B. and Drusin, L.M.: Antibody to varicella-zoster virus in parturient women and their offspring during the first year of life. Pediatrics 58: 692 (1976).

Gilmartin, R.C.; Jabbour, J.T. and Duenas, D.A.: Rubella vaccine myeloradiculoneuritis. Journal of Pediatrics 80: 406 (1972).

Gluckman, J.C.: Ara-A for herpes encephalitis. New England Journal of Medicine 297: 1289 (1977).

Hadden, J.W.; Lopez, C.; O'Reilly, R.J. and Hadden, E.M.: Levamisole and inosiplex: Antiviral agents with immupotentiating action. Annals of the New York Academy of Sciences 284: 139 (1977).

Hanshaw, J.B. and Dudgeon, J.A.: Viral diseases of the fetus and newborn (Saunders, Philadelphia 1978).

Hirsch, M.S.: Interferon — it's hour come at last? New England Journal of Medicine 298: 1022 (1978).

Ing, T.S.; Rahn, A.C.; Armbruster, K.F.W.; Oyama, J.H. and Klawans, H.L.: Accumulation of amantadine hydrochloride in renal insufficiency. New England Journal of Medicine 291: 1257 (1974).

Izawa, T.; Ihara, T.; Hattori, A.; Iwasa, T.; Kamiya, H.; Sakurai, M. and Takahashi, M.: Application of a live varicella vaccine in children with acute leukemia or other malignant diseases. Pediatrics 60: 805 (1977).

Jackson, G.G.: Sensitivity of influenza A virus to amantadine. Journal of Infectious Diseases 136: 301 (1977).

Jackson, G.G. and Stanley, E.D.: Prevention and control of influenza by chemoprophylaxis and chemotherapy. Prospects from examination of recent experience. Journal of the American Medical Association 235: 2739 (1976).

Juel-Jensen, B.E.: Virus diseases. Practitioner 213: 508 (1974).

Juel-Jensen, B.E. and MacCallum, F.O.: Herpes Simplex, Varicella and Zoster (Heinemann, London 1972).

Juel-Jensen, B.E.; MacCallum, F.O.; Mackenzie, A.M.R. and Pike, M.C.: Treatment of zoster with idoxuridine in dimethyl sulphoxide. Results of two double-blind controlled trials. British Medical Journal 4: 776 (1970).

Karzon, D.T.: Smallpox vaccination: The end of an era. Acta Medica Scandinavica Suppl. 576: 29 (1974).

Katz, S.L.: Experience with rubella vaccines in the USA. Scandinavian Journal of Infectious Diseases 6 (Suppl.): 14 (1972).

Kilroy, A.W.; Schaffner, W.; Fleet, W.F.; Lefkowitz, L.B.; Karzon, D.T. and Fenichel, G.M.: Two syndromes following rubella immunization. Clinical observation and epidemiological studies. Journal of the American Medical Association 214: 2287 (1970).

Klock, L.E. and Rachelefsky, G.S.: Failure of rubella herd immunity during an epidemic. New England Journal of Medicine 288: 69 (1973).

Knight, V.: Influenza. Disease-a-Month 22: 1 (1976).

Koplan, J.P.; Monsur, K.A.; Foster, S.O.; Farida, H.; Rahaman, M.M.; Huq, S.; Buchanan, R.A. and Ward, N.A.: Treatment of variola major with adenine arabinoside. Journal of Infectious Diseases 131: 34 (1975).

Krugman, S.: Present status of measles and rubella immunization in the United States: A medical progress report. Journal of Pediatrics 78: 1 (1971).

Krugman, S.: Present status of measles and rubella immunization in the United States: A medical progress report. Journal of Pediatrics 90: 1 (1977).

La Montagne, J.R. and Galasso, G.J.: Report of a workshop on clinical studies of efficacy of amantadine and rimantadine against influenza virus. Journal of Infectious Diseases 6: 928 (1978).

Lee, J.D.; Khakoo, R.A.; Street, C.K. and Waldman, R.H.: Journal of Infectious Diseases 135: 824 (1977).

Longson, M.: The treatment of herpes encephalitis. Journal of Antimicrobial Chemotherapy 3 (Suppl. A): 115 (1977).

Levine, M.M.; Edsall, G. and Bruce-Chwatt, L.J.: Live-virus vaccines in pregnancy: Risks and recommendations. Lancet 2: 34 (1974).

McClean, D.M.: Methisazone therapy in pediatric vaccinia complications. Annals of the New York Academy of Science 284: 118 (1977).

Magnussen, C.R.; Douglas, R.G.; Betts, R.I.; Roth, Frieda K. and Meagher, Mary P.: Double-blind evaluation of oral ribovarin (virazole) in experimental influenza A virus infection in volunteers. Antimicrobial Agents and Chemotherapy 12: 498 (1977).

Menser, Margaret and Forrest, Jill, M.: Maternal infections and the developing fetus. Medical Journal of Australia 1: 448 (1973).

Merigan, T.C.; Rand, K.H.; Pollard, R.B.; Abdallah, P.S.;

Nordan, G.W. and Fried, R.P.: Human leucocyte interferon for the treatment of herpes zoster in patients with cancer. New England Journal of Medicine 298: 981 (1978).

Merigan, T.: Antivirals with clinical potential. Journal of Infectious Diseases 133: Suppl. (June 1976).

Miller, D.L.: Frequency and complications of measles. British Medical Journal 2: 75 (1964).

Olsen, G.A.; Kern, E.R.; Overall, J.C. and Glasgow, L.D.: Effect of treatment with exogenous interferon, poly I-C, and poly ICLC on herpesvirus hominis in mice. Journal of Infectious Diseases 137: 428 (1978).

Phillips, C.A.; Fanning, W.L.; Gump, D.W. and Phillips, Carol, F.: Cytomegolovirus encephalitis in immunologically normal adults; successful treatment with vidarabine. Journal of the American Medical Association 238: 2299 (1977).

Pollard, R.B. and Merigan, T.C.: Experience with clinical applications of interferon and interferon inducers. Pharmacology and Therapeutics 2: 783 (1978).

Ritzel, G.: Ascorbic acid and the common cold. Journal of the American Medical Association 235: 1108 (1976).

Sabin, A.B.: Oral poliomyelitis vaccine: History of its development and prospects for eradication of poliomyelitis. Journal of the American Medical Association 194: 49 (1964).

Stalder, H.: Antiviral therapy. Yale Journal of Biology and Medicine 50: 507 (1977).

Steigman, A.J.: Mumps vaccine. Lancet 2: 1276 (1974).

Stevens, D.A. and Merigan, T.C.: Approaches to the control of viral infections in man. Rational Drug Therapy 5: 1 (1971).

Stuart-Harris, C.: The principles and practice of immunization. Practitioner 215: 285 (1975).

Symposium: Third conference on antiviral substances. Annals of the New York Academy of Sciences 284: 1 (1977).

Taber, L.H.; Greenberg, S.B.; Perez, F.I. and Couch, R.B.: Herpes simplex encephalitis treated with vidarabine (adenine arabinoside). Archives of Neurology 34: 608 (1977).

Tager, I.B.: Ara-A for herpes encephalitis. New England Journal of Medicine 297: 1289 (1977).

Weinstein, L.: Failure of chemotherapy to prevent the bacterial complications of measles. New England Journal of Medicine 253: 679 (1955).

Weinstein, L. and Chang, T-W.: The chemotherapy of viral infections. New England Journal of Medicine 289: 725 (1973).

West, S.; Brandon, B.; Stolley, P. and Rumrill, R.: A review of antihistamines and the common cold. Pediatrics 56: 100 (1975).

Whitley, R.J.; Chien, L.T.; Buchanan, R.A. and Alford, C.A.: Studies on adenine arabinoside: a model for antiviral chemotherapeutics. Perspectives in Virology 9: 315 (1975).

Whitley, R.J.; Ch'ien, L.T.; Dolin, L.; Galasso, G.J.; Alford, C.A. and The Collaborative Study Group: Adenine arabinoside therapy of herpes zoster in the immunosuppressed. New England Journal of Medicine 294: 1193 (1976).

Whitley, R.J.; Soong, S.J.; Dolin, R.; Galasso, G.J.; Ch'ien, L.T.; Alford, C.A. and The Collaborative Study Group: Adenine arabinoside therapy of biopsy-proved herpes simplex encephalitis. New England Journal of Medicine 297: 289 (1977).

Wilson, C.W.M.: Colds, ascorbic acid metabolism, and vitamin C. Journal of Clinical Pharmacology 15: 570 (1975).

Wilson, C.W.M. and Loh, H.S.: Vitamin C metabolism and the common cold. European Journal of Clinical Pharmacology 7: 421 (1974).

Chapter XXIX
Sexually Transmissible Diseases

W.M. Platts

Synopsis of Important Principles

1) Sexually transmissible diseases have increased dramatically over the past 20 years, especially gonorrhoea and non-gonococcal urethritis and more recently, the two viral conditions genital herpes and genital warts.

2) Effective control is aimed at seeking out cases and reducing the 'silent reservoir' of infection thus preventing further spread of the disease.

3) This can only be accomplished by contact tracing, screening, education and other social awareness programmes, accurate diagnosis, specific and curative treatment schedules, and regular post-treatment surveillance.

4) The aim of routine treatment is to use a drug regimen which approaches a 100% cure rate.

5) A curative drug regimen means use of a drug highly specific for the causative organism and given in a dose schedule which avoids or minimises non-compliance by the patient. Single dose regimens, when feasible, are always to be preferred given by the parenteral rather than oral route.

6) The level of relative resistance of the gonococcus to penicillin varies in different areas. With the exception of penicillinase producing strains, it is not an indication of which drugs are needed, but rather of what doses of penicillin are necessary.

7) Routine use of a curative penicillin regimen in a community will actually result in a decrease of relative resistance of the gonococcus to penicillin, and consequently of the dosage needed to effect a cure. It will also prevent the occurrence of penicillinase producing strains.

8) Non-gonococcal urethritis is increasing at a rate faster than gonorrhoea. Patient and partner(s) should be treated with a full dose course of a tetracycline.

9) In all sexually transmissible diseases, a basic principle is identification and treatment of the sexual partner(s) who may be asymptomatic. Wherever possible, a diagnosis must be established first.

10) Effective treatment of vaginitis depends on differentiation of trichomoniasis and candidiasis and use of a highly specific agent, not a dual spectrum agent moderately effective against both.

After being nearly beaten in the early 1950s, the sexually transmitted diseases have staged a phenomenal comeback, and some are now epidemic or pandemic in most countries of the western world. The primary reasons for this are largely social, not medical. Popularisation of pre- and extramarital sex, a proportion of which is always promiscuous, and the decline in popularity of the condom as a contraceptive with the advent of the 'pill', have probably facilitated the spread of the organisms concerned, which have over-whelmed the epidemiological defences in many countries.

The five official venereal diseases comprise gonorrhoea and syphilis and the three tropical diseases chancroid, lymphogranuloma venereum and granuloma inguinale. Non-gonococcal (non-specific) urethritis is also transmitted by sexual activity. Other diseases in the sexually transmitted group are three viral infections (herpes genitalis, genital warts and molluscum contagiosum); two parasitic diseases (pubic lice and scabies) and two vaginitides (trichomoniasis and candidiasis). Recently, two other viral conditions have been found to be transmitted by intercourse — hepatitis B (for certain) and cytomegalovirus (probably) — and amongst those adopting 'alternative life styles', members of the enteric group of infections (amoebiasis, giardiasis, salmonellosis, and shigellosis; see chapter XIX, sect. 11) are also believed to be sexually transmitted (Sohn and Robilotti, 1977; Willcox, 1977).

1. Prevalence

The World Health Organisation has in numerous articles drawn attention to the extraordinary high level and seemingly increasing prevalence (many countries produce no statistics of sexually transmitted diseases) almost everywhere in the world (see Willcox, 1977). Hardest hit are the emerging countries with the striking exception of China.

Studies in Africa indicate that 20 to 40% of females of childbearing age in many areas suffer from a sexually transmitted disease, principally gonorrhoea, the resulting infertility acting as a significant agent in population control. European countries, where gonorrhoea rates are more moderate (200 to 600/100,000 of the population), have fared better. After rising continuously since the late fifties the incidence has at last fallen, first in Sweden, commencing in 1971, extending to Denmark in 1973, then Finland and East Germany (fig. 1). The USA, where 80% of cases are seen by private doctors, stands out with an estimated gonorrhoea rate stated to be 10 times that in the UK, and involving 2.5 to 3 million people per year. However, the steeply rising trend levelled in 1976 and 1977 for the first time since the early sixties (CFDC, 1977). New Zealand's clinic cases have at last also shown a fall for the years 1976 and 1977. The significance of these decreases in prevalence is uncertain and although encouraging, may not necessarily be due to success in control

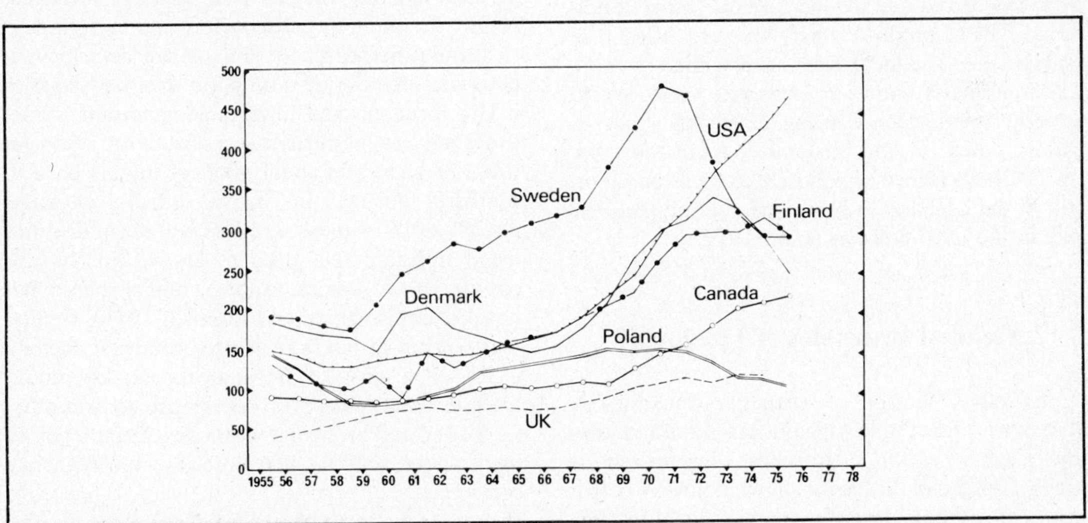

Fig. 1. Reported cases of gonorrhoea (1955-1975). Incidence per 100,000 population. 1955-1969 reported cases during financial year; 1970-1975 reported cases during calendar year.

methods or changes in sexual behaviour. A phenomenon in practically all countries except in those with established prostitution, is the youth of those involved, the majority being teenaged; the incidence of venereal disease amongst 15 to 19 year olds has increased more rapidly than in older persons.

With infectious syphilis the position is a little more encouraging. The incidence, after a marked rise in the early sixties, has been held in check in most countries from which statistics are obtainable, although in the USA the reported rate has reached a high 10 cases/100,000 population per year, giving cause for concern, although there has been a slight decrease in prevalence over the past 2 years. Reasons for the better control of this disease are thought to be the long incubation period enabling more effective contact tracing, and fortuitous use of penicillin in large dosage for all types of infections. A new and disturbing feature in syphilis epidemiology has been the influence of the homosexual who has become the principal spreader of the disease; e.g. 45% of all infectious syphilis in Britain now occurs in homosexuals (British Cooperative Clinical Group, 1973).

Apart from this classical pair which head the list of the five official venereal diseases, the biggest problem amongst the 'minor' sexually transmissible diseases, is non-gonococcal urethritis, which in most countries, has increased at a rate faster than gonorrhoea to a position where it is probably the most common sexually transmissible condition encountered in clinical practice. More recently, there has been a marked increase in 2 other conditions which produce their severest effects in females — genital herpes and genital warts. Trichomoniasis, shows an extremely varied world pattern; the incidence being extremely high in eastern countries and moderately so in the USA (twice the incidence of gonorrhoea), less common still in the UK, and in New Zealand only half the rate in the UK (Weisner et al., 1976).

2. General Principles of Treatment

Effective control of sexually transmissible diseases is aimed at seeking out cases and reducing the 'silent reservoir' of infection thus preventing further spread of the disease. This requires a major team effort and depends upon contact tracing, screening, education and other social (and medical) awareness programmes, accurate diagnosis, specific and curative treatment schedules, and regular post-treatment surveillance. It also means that the conditions should be recognised as deserving of treatment and prevention.

2.1 Why Treat?

Syphilis is a potentially lethal and crippling disease, especially to the fetus, and to those who later develop tertiary symptoms.

Gonorrhoea can cause infertility in a sizeable proportion (5 to 10%) of its female sufferers, most of whom are unaware that they have the disease until the onset of the pelvic inflammation heralding salpingitis. It can also cause septicaemia with arthritis, particularly in females, and in infants born of mothers with gonorrhoea. Complications in the male are uncommon in the developed countries.

Non-gonococcal urethritis causes an arthritis in 0.5 to 1% of treated or untreated cases. This is often mild, afflicting one or two joints only, but it can be crippling in the fully developed Reiter's syndrome. It can cause ocular infection in the neonate. However, its most damaging and frequent effect is the psychological trauma it causes. Moreover, its incidence is increasing faster than any other sexually transmissible disease.

Trichomoniasis in the female, if not diagnosed (as is frequently the case) or adequately treated, results in continuing discomfort and suffering.

Genital herpes in the female can be crippling, necessitating hospital admission. In many couples it is a recurrent and intractable condition, sometimes proscribing further sexual activity. Neonatal infection occurs in about 50% of infants born to mothers during an active attack. Approximately 60% of these neonates will die of disseminated infection (Nahmias et al., 1976). Its oncogenic role in cervical cancer is highly suspect but not proven (Roizman and Frenkel, 1976). Genital warts result in hours of treatment at the doctor's office or a visit to hospital for an operation. Despite these measures recurrence is common. Laryngeal and bronchial warts have been reported in neonates, and a severe infection in pregnancy can occasionally result in delivery by elective Caesarean section. Cytomegalovirus is not uncommon and can cause pneumonitis or severe brain damage to the fetus *in utero* (Nahmias, 1975).

2.2 Diagnosis

Accurate history taking and diagnosis (clinical and laboratory) are essential for the proper treatment and control of the major sexually transmissible diseases.

Culture sites are all important in gonorrhoea in females (Schroeter and Pazin, 1970). The endocervix yields the highest number of positives with the urethra close behind. Anal culture is next in importance. The vaginal swab is used for culture of *Trichomonas* and *Candida* spp. It should never be relied on to diagnose gonorrhoea if only one site is used. Males are diagnosed by a Gram-stained smear of the urethral discharge which should be routinely cultured, not only for confirmation but also as a laboratory efficiency control in culture technique.

Throat swabs should be taken in those who admit to orogenital contact. Pharyngeal gonorrhoea can be more difficult to cure than genital gonorrhoea (Eisenstein, 1977) and therefore the site has to be cultured during surveillance. Swabs from the throat, rectum and urethra should be routine in homosexuals.

In infectious syphilis the dark ground microscopic examination of serum squeezed from the suspected chancre, or any moist lesion, is the first effective diagnostic measure to be undertaken. Pitfalls are lack of familiarity with the technique of setting up a dark ground microscope or preparing a proper dark ground slide, and the positive identification of *Treponema pallidum* from the commensal varieties that are often present. Determinations from dark ground examination of mouth lesions are especially unreliable. Standard and treponemal antibody serological tests are essential for diagnosis.

Non-gonococcal urethritis is diagnosed by exclusion (see section 5). There are no specific serological tests for non-gonococcal urethritis. Serological tests for syphilis should be performed in all cases of sexually transmissible diseases.

2.3 Effective Treatment Regimen

The aim of treatment is to approach a 100% cure rate; not only to prevent further spread of disease but also to limit (or even decrease) the development of 'relatively resistant' organisms due to failed treatment (Willcox, 1977). This goal can only be achieved if a drug highly specific for the causative organism is used and if the treatment regimen minimises or avoids non-compliance by the patient (Anderson, 1966). Single dose curative regimens are possible in gonorrhoea and trichomoniasis and should always be used in preference to others.

Selection of the most effective drug and method of administration is the key to success. For example, use of an appropriate parenteral penicillin regimen in gonorrhoea, not only can achieve a virtually 100% cure rate, but also importantly, can when used in a community over a period of time, lead to a significant decrease in the percentage of gonococcal strains 'relatively resistant' to penicillin (Olsen and Lomholt, 1969). Selection of such a curative regimen is based on both pharmacokinetic and bacteriological considerations (see section 3). There is probably no such phenomenon as absolute drug resistance in any of the sexually transmissible diseases and if an agent is chosen which is highly specific for the causative organism any problems with 'relative resistance' should not arise. In gonorrhoea, the resistance to penicillin varies from place to place, but highly 'resistant' strains may be found in any location. These patterns, with the exception of penicillinase producing strains (see section 3.3), do not indicate which drugs are needed, but rather what doses of penicillin are necessary.

A curative drug regimen also means not using a dual spectrum agent for any infective vaginitis, without attempting differentiation of trichomoniasis and candidiasis, since such agents are not as effective as those specific for either organism.

Effective treatment also implies prevention of further spread of the disease (e.g. syphilis, gonorrhoea) or reinfection (e.g. trichomoniasis, nongonococcal urethritis) by treatment of the sexual partner(s). The partners of patients with gonorrhoea should be identified and treated as quickly as possible, since the disease has a short incubation period.

2.4 Contact Tracing

Individual contact tracing is a most important method of control. It aims at determining not only the source of infection but also secondary contacts to whom the disease may have been passed by the patient.

For success, speed is essential, particularly with the short incubation period of gonorrhoea where further spread from infected contacts occurs before effective contact tracing can be achieved.

The symptomless female consort of the male attending for treatment of gonorrhoea has traditionally been the target. However, since the comprehensive female screening programmes in the USA have been in progress, 5 to 10 % of the male consorts of positive cases have been found to have asymptomatic gonorrhoea (Handsfield et al., 1974). This means that, as well as a large female reservoir of gonorrhoea, there is also a sizeable male one which is only uncovered by taking deep (4cm) urethral cultures and smears. In the USA, with its pandemic situation, tracing of all contacts has proved impossible and reliance is being placed on routine screening for gonorrhoea of all young females gynaecologically examined for any reason.

Contact tracing in syphilis, with its long incubation period is the key to epidemiological control and must be pursued relentlessly. Contacts of a proven case of infectious syphilis should be treated prophylactically during the incubation period. If a lesion is already present a diagnosis must be made by serology and dark ground examination before treatment is given.

2.5 Surveillance

Relapse of gonorrhoea occurs most often during the week after treatment. Thus to evaluate cure, 2 or 3 repeat cultures should be made at weekly intervals. Patients who relapse or who are treatment failures should be retreated with a higher dose of penicillin augmented with probenecid (see table I).

Post-treatment surveillance is essential in infectious syphilis and consists of serological studies monthly for 6 months, 3-monthly for 6 months, and again a year later. Seroreversal takes 6 to 12 months if the case is treated in the infectious stage. In late syphilis, seropositivity usually remains despite successful treatment. Cerebrospinal fluid serology is done on all cases treated in the secondary latent and late phase, preferably at the end of surveillance. If not intended to be done an augmented dose of penicillin is advisable, using preferably the procaine penicillin G regimen.

3. Gonorrhoea

The key to gonorrhoea control is casefinding. Close to this in importance is effective treatment (for review, see Eisenstein, 1977; Willcox, 1977). Only by ensuring that the cure rate approaches 100 % can the all important relative sensitivity of the gonococcus to penicillin be kept high enough to prevent escalation of the dose needed for cure (see section 2.3; also chapter XXVII, sect. 5.3). It is paramount that penicillin, with its wide safety factor, its cheapness, and not least its treponemacidal effect be retained as the standard treatment of gonorrhoea.

No other antibacterial drug is as active as benzylpenicillin against sensitive strains of gonococci. The aim of treatment in gonorrhoea is therefore to:

a) Use a penicillin regimen which will approach a 100 % cure rate.
b) Identify and treat the sexual partner(s).
c) Routinely test for cure in all patients, especially females.

Selection of a curative penicillin regimen depends upon the following presumptive reasoning and considerations:

1) The most widely used form of penicillin today is a single intramuscular injection of the procaine salt of benzylpenicillin (penicillin G); either alone (Holmes et al., 1967a), or combined with soluble benzylpenicillin (Johnson et al., 1970; Juhlin, 1965); the aim being the attainment of a fairly short high serum concentration, the peak of which exceeds the minimum inhibitory concentration of the organism by at least a factor of five (Olsen and Lomholt, 1969). Doses used vary from 2.2 mega units to 4.8 mega units (USPHS), depending on the sensitivity of the local strains of gonococci. Soluble benzylpenicillin alone in a dose of 5 mega units dissolved in 8ml 0.5 % lignocaine solution, with probenecid given 30 minutes before the injection, has also given excellent results (Krook and Juhlin, 1965).

2) The concomitant use of probenecid, by delaying renal excretion of penicillin, has in most cases increased the serum concentration of penicillin by 50 % or more and enables a cure rate greater than that from penicillin alone (Johnson et al., 1970; Holmes et al., 1967a). Because over half the penicillin is protein bound and the intracellular penicillin concentration is half that in the extracellular fluid, high *in vivo* concentrations of penicillin are necessary (Thayer et al., 1957). Two 0.5g probenecid tablets (1g) just before the injection (except when using soluble benzylpenicillin when the interval should be 30 minutes) is probably all that is required (Kaufman et al., 1976), but

in some areas and in pharyngeal gonorrhoea, 3 further doses of 0.5g are given 6 hours apart.

3) Single dose parenteral treatment is regarded as the ideal because patient compliance can be guaranteed, and because of its greater likelihood of consistent absorption, giving an approximately predictable and reproducible serum concentration.

4) Second preference is single dose oral treatment with ampicillin or amoxycillin (together with probenecid), despite considerable individual variation in gastric absorption (Kvale et al., 1971; Johnson et al., 1970). A course of multiple dose oral treatment is not desirable because it is often defeated by failure of the patient to take the full treatment course (Anderson, 1966).

3.1 Gonococcal Infection in Adults and Adolescents

The parenteral and oral penicillin regimens which comply with the above requirements are given in table I. Procaine penicillin G with probenecid is the treatment of choice in most world clinics, although a mixture with soluble penicillin G with probenecid has its adherents. Both these regimens give the required high initial peak and serum concentration extending for up to 12 hours (Eisenstein, 1977). Soluble penicillin G in a dose of 5 mega units with probenecid, although not used widely, is a high dose regimen giving equally satisfactory results, but it needs to be dissolved in 0.5% lignocaine solution and the probenecid has to be given 30 minutes before the injection — a disadvantage in a busy surgery or clinic. Patient acceptance of all the above regimens (the larger doses of which require a double injection) is increased by the use of 0.5% lignocaine solution as the solvent. The incidence of severe hypersensitivity reactions due to penicillin allergy or of 'pseudoanaphylactic' neuropsychiatric reactions due to procaine (Kraus and Green, 1976; Dry et al., 1976) have been exceedingly low in venereal disease clinics; for example in the USA, 52 cases of anaphylaxis due to penicillin allergy but 1 death in 94,655 patients (Rudolph and Price, 1973).

Spectinomycin given as a single treatment, in an intramuscular dose of 2g gives consistent cure rates approaching 100%, but is reserved for patients infected with penicillinase producing strains of gonococci (see sect. 3.3), and their sexual contacts, penicillin or tetracycline treatment failures (table I), and less importantly those allergic to penicillin (Karney et al., 1977). Ab-

solute resistance to spectinomycin, although rare, has been reported (Reyn et al., 1973; Thornsberry et al., 1977) and over use of spectinomycin could lead to emergence of spectinomycin resistant gonococci by plasmid transfer or to an increase in spectinomycin resistance in penicillinase producing gonococci (Siegel et al., 1977, 1978). Side effects are minimal and the injection is much less painful than large doses of penicillin G.

Oral tetracyclines in a 4 or 5-day regimen provide cure rates in the mid 90%s, but gastric absorption is variable, the patient may not take the full 4 or 5-day course, and resistance develops much more quickly than to penicillin. Notwithstanding, *when the strain is sensitive to tetracycline* (tetracycline failure is correlated with resistance), it is especially useful in those allergic to penicillin, in males to reduce the rate of postgonococcal urethritis, and as an alternative to spectinomycin to treat those with penicillinase producing gonococci (section 3.3). Because of moderate intrinsic cross resistance between penicillins and tetracycline, it is not indicated for retreatment of penicillin or ampicillin/amoxycillin failed cures (Karney et al., 1977). Many other drugs have been studied as alternatives to penicillin, but they have either not been proven to provide consistently acceptable cure rates or have to be given as a multiple dose regimen (Elliott et al., 1977; Schroeter and Pazin, 1970).

The male sex partners of females with gonorrhoea must be examined, and treated if necessary, because of the high prevalence of asymptomatic gonococcal urethritis in such men. Pharyngeal gonorrhoea may require more intensive treatment than anogenital infection. Complications such as acute salpingitis (as evidenced by acute lower abdominal pain and adnexal tenderness on pelvic examination) and disseminated gonococcal infection (gonococcal arthritis), certainly require more prolonged and intensive treatment (table I; for reviews, see Eschenbach and Holmes, 1975; Handsfield et al., 1976). Urethritis which may follow cure of gonorrhoea (postgonococcal urethritis) with penicillin derivatives or spectinomycin (Oriel et al., 1977) should be treated with tetracyclines or erythromycin.

3.2 Neonatal Gonococcal Infection

In areas where the incidence of gonorrhoea is high, because of the neonatal morbidity and the risk of septicaemia with arthritis in the mother

Table I. Curative regimens for gonorrhoea in adults and adolescents in areas of low prevalence of penicillinase producing gonococci[1]

Regimen	Drug	Dose schedule
Uncomplicated gonorrhoea First choice	Penicillin G (intramuscular)	Single intramuscular dose procaine penicillin G 1.2 to 2.4[2] mega units + soluble penicillin G 1.0 to 2.0[2] mega unit, with 1g probenecid just beforehand. (In some areas and in pharyngeal gonorrhoea this is followed by 0.5g probenecid 6-hourly for 3 doses) or Single dose procaine penicillin G 2.4 to 4.8[2] mega units, with probenecid as above
Alternative	Amoxycillin	Single oral dose 3g with 1g probenecid
	Ampicillin	Single oral dose 3.5g with 1g probenecid
Regimen for treatment of cure failures[3]	Penicillin G (intramuscular)	Add 2.0 mega units soluble penicillin to soluble + procaine regimen above; with probenecid beforehand and 6-hourly for 3 further doses Increase procaine penicillin regimen above to 4.8 mega units; with probenecid beforehand and 6-hourly for 3 further doses Soluble penicillin G 5.0 mega units with 1g probenecid given 30 min beforehand and 6-hourly for 3 further doses (0.5% lignocaine necessary)
	Spectinomycin[5]	Single intramuscular dose of 2g in cure failures from oral or larger dose intramuscular penicillin or tetracycline regimens (if failure with spectinomycin, re-treat with the same dose)
Penicillin allergy	Oxytetracycline[4] Tetracycline[4] Chlortetracycline[4]	500mg 6-hourly orally for 4 or 5 (USPHS) days
	Co-trimoxazole[5]	6-9 tablets daily in 1 or 2 doses for 3 days
	Minocycline[4] Doxycycline[4]	300mg as single oral dose with milk or food to minimise nausea (use when compliance to conventional tetracycline expected to be poor)
Penicillinase producing gonococci cases and their sexual contacts	Spectinomycin[5]	Single intramuscular dose of 2g (can also be used in penicillin allergy). If failure re-treat with the same dose
	Tetracyclines[4]	As above
	Cefuroxime	Under investigation

Complicated gonorrhoea Pelvic inflammatory disease (PID)[6]	Penicillin G	Single dose intramuscular regimens as described above, followed by oral amoxycillin 0.5g 8-hourly or ampicillin 0.5g 6-hourly for 10 days
		10 to 20 mega units soluble penicillin G IV daily until improvement occurs (hospitalised cases), followed by oral amoxycillin or ampicillin as above to complete 10 days of therapy
	Tetracycline[4]	500mg 6-hourly orally for 10 days; or in hospitalised cases 250mg IV 6-hourly until improvement occurs, followed by 500mg 6-hourly orally to complete 10 days of therapy
Epididymo-orchitis	Tetracycline[4]	500mg orally 6-hourly for 10 days
Disseminated gonococcal infection (gonococcal arthritis)	Penicillin G	10 to 20 mega units soluble penicillin G IV daily until improvement occurs (hospitalised cases), followed by oral amoxycillin or ampicillin as above to complete 7 days of therapy, or
	Amoxycillin Ampicillin	3g amoxycillin or 3.5g ampicillin orally with probenecid, followed by 0.5g amoxycillin 8-hourly or 0.5g ampicillin 6-hourly for 7 days
penicillin allergy	Tetracycline[4]	500mg orally 6-hourly for 7 days
	Co-trimoxazole[5]	6-9 tablets daily in 1 or 2 doses for 7 days
	Erythromycin	500mg orally 6-hourly for 7 days in those in whom tetracycline or co-trimoxazole are contraindicated (pregnancy)
penicillinase producing gonococci cases	Spectinomycin[5]	2g intramuscularly twice a day for 3 days
	Tetracycline	As above

1 *Note:* In areas where penicillinase producing gonococci are common (> 10%):
  a) Consider discontinuing the penicillin group for primary treatment.
  b) Use tetracycline if resistance of local organisms are low.
  c) Otherwise, use spectinomycin 2g intramuscularly as drug of first choice.
2 The larger dose is required in areas with a high incidence of strains 'relatively resistant' to penicillin (see section 2.3; also chapter XXVII, sect. 5.3).
3 These augmented penicillin regimens should be used in failed cures from use of smaller doses, providing penicillinase producing gonococci are absent.
4 In pregnancy, tetracyclines are contraindicated and other non-penicillin antibiotics (except erythromycin which is less effective) should be used with care.
Tetracyclines should only be used where surveys show a low incidence of tetracycline and penicillin resistant strains (see Karney et al., 1977).
5 Does not affect *Treponema pallidum.*
6 In intractable cases, a trial of metronidazole is recommended, as the causative organisms are often anaerobes (Eschenbach et al., 1975).

during pregnancy, all women should have endocervical cultures examined as a routine part of antenatal care. Babies born to mothers with gonorrhoea should routinely have orogastric and rectal cultures taken (Handsfield et al., 1973), and blood cultures should be taken if septicaemia is suspected, especially if the membranes have ruptured prematurely. If cultures or Gram-stained smears show gonococci, soluble penicillin G, 50,000 units should be given as a single intravenous or intramuscular dose. Babies with gonococcal ophthalmia should have soluble penicillin G 50,000 units/kg/day in 2 doses intravenously for 7 days, plus frequent saline irrigations followed by instillation of penicillin, tetracycline, or chloramphenicol eye drops. Prevention of gonococcal ophthalmia neonatorum is discussed in chapter XII (section 3.4).

3.3 Penicillinase Producing Gonococci

Recently, a new strain of gonococcus, with the ability to produce a penicillinase (β-lactamase), has been reported from several areas of the world (World Health Organisation, 1977; Willcox, 1977). This strain was entirely different from any previously encountered, being completely resistant to all concentrations of penicillin (Ashford et al., 1976; Philips, 1976). The pockets of penicillinase producing strains reported from developed countries where penicillin is fully effective, have however, been fairly quickly eliminated by using effective non-penicillin drugs (i.e. spectinomycin), but large numbers of cases are continuing to appear, mainly from the Far East, with only a few from Central Africa the other birthplace of the new strain (Willcox, 1977; Siegel et al., 1978). Both these regions have in common poor gonorrhoea control, antibiotics being sold over the counter, resulting in a large proportion of strains possessing high relative penicillin resistance and thus setting the stage for the acquisition from other bacteria (probably *Haemophilus influenzae* and *Escherichia coli*) of plasmids (see chapter XXVII; sect. 2.3) which determined the absolute resistance (Elwell et al., 1977; Williams, 1978). Fortunately, areas where penicillin is fully effective (most developed countries) are not favourable for the maintenance of the new strains, and contact tracing has failed to demonstrate a chain of infection beyond 2 to 4 (patient) generations of spread. This suggests that the R plasmid is genetically unstable (World Health Organisation, 1978).

In terms of treatment, this means that providing: (1) curative penicillin regimens are used (see above); (2) there is routine bacteriological follow-up of cases; (3) contact tracing from known or suspected cases is rigid, and (4) all highly resistant strains (e.g. with an MIC of greater than 1.0u/ml) are tested for the production of penicillinase, the effective establishment of the new strains in most developed countries, where penicillin is effective, should be able to be prevented. However, the utmost vigilance is necessary as new cases will continue to appear, especially as imports from the worst afflicted areas, and some of their contacts will also harbour penicillinase producing strains.

4. Syphilis

Penicillin is still the drug of choice, and in contrast to the gonococcus no increased resistance of the treponeme has been proved (Willcox, 1974). A serum level of only 0.03 units/ml is treponemacidal (in contrast to gonorrhoea where serum levels must be up to 1000 times higher) but it must be continuous, and must extend over a period of 8 or 10 to 14 days in infectious syphilis, and 21 days in all late and latent cases. This can be achieved in two ways; either by weekly injections of 2.4 (or 3.0 in late cases) mega units of benzathine penicillin, or daily injections of 600,000 units (or 1 mega unit) of procaine penicillin G suspension. The procaine penicillin G regimen is indicated in neurosyphilis as benzathine penicillin passes the blood-brain barrier poorly.

In congenital syphilis, a total dose of 450,000 to 500,000 units of procaine penicillin/kg body weight is divided by 10 and given in 10 daily doses, or else a single injection of benzathine penicillin (in infants with normal CSF) in a dose of 100,000 units/kg body weight (McCracken and Kaplan, 1974).

In those allergic to penicillin, tetracyclines or erythromycin are given in a dose of 30 to 40g over a period of 15 to 20 days for early syphilis, and 40 to 60g over 20 to 30 days for late syphilis. Long term evaluation of both these drugs is incomplete so close follow up is essential. Tetracyclines should not be used in pregnant women because of the risk of hepatotoxicity (see chapter XV; sect. 1.1.5) and effects on the fetal skeleton (see chapter XXII; sect. 14.5) and teeth, or in children under the age of 10 years because of the risk of tooth discolouration (see chapter XIII; section 13.3)

Cephalosporins are extremely promising but not yet fully evaluated.

It must be realised that tetracyclines and erythromycin as alternatives to penicillin, are much less efficient antitreponemal drugs and should only be used where penicillin is fully contraindicated.

Increased promiscuity, particularly in tropical (yaws) areas, has changed the presentation of treponemal infection. In areas where treatment has nearly overcome the incidence of yaws, the herd immunity to syphilis, previously given by yaws has disappeared and cases of venereal syphilis (atypical primary lesions, secondary condylomata) are being reported.

5. Non-gonococcal Urethritis

Non-gonococcal urethritis is probably the most common form of sexually transmissible disease encountered in clinical practice (Melton, 1976; Oriel, 1976). It is diagnosed by exclusion of the gonococcus from a Gram-stained smear of the urethral discharge. The clinical symptoms, which occur at varying times after sexual intercourse (usually from 6 days to 3 weeks), differ from those of the gonococcal disease. The dysuria tends to be less severe and the urethral discharge is less profuse and tends to be watery or mucoid rather than purulent. If the discharge is purulent it is indistinguishable clinically from gonorrhoea. Although it is often possible to suspect clinically whether a patient has non-gonococcal or gonococcal urethritis, physical examination alone is not a satisfactory means of differentiating the two conditions.

The main problem with non-gonococcal urethritis is its tendency to recur, sometimes years later and frequently in multiple attacks. The disorder is also subject to remissions, which makes assessment of treatment difficult.

Only the parasite *Chlamydia trachomatis,* of the family which causes lymphogranuloma venereum and trachoma inclusion conjunctivitis (TRIC) has been shown to be of probable aetiological importance in the disease (Holmes et al., 1975; Oriel et al., 1976), but it appears to be responsible for only about half of the cases. The cause(s) in other cases is obscure, although *Ureaplasma urealyticum* (T strain *Mycoplasma*) could be responsible for a definite though much smaller proportion (Ford and Henderson, 1976; Bowie, 1978; Bowie et al., 1977).

Tetracyclines are considered the drugs of choice, although the optimum dose and duration of treatment have not been determined (Holmes et al., 1967b; Willcox, 1977). A minimum course should be 8 to 10 days on full dosage (e.g. tetracycline 500mg 6-hourly), the maximum being 3 weeks, but in those in whom symptoms present when intercourse is unavoidable, e.g. within a stable relationship, a long term (e.g. 1 to 2 months) maintenance course of tetracycline 250mg 3 times a day often prevents recurrences. Alternatively, doxycycline or minocycline may be given in equivalent doses — e.g. 200mg initially followed by 100mg daily (doxycycline) or 12-hourly (minocycline) in full dosage schedules. Second line drugs which have been shown to be effective in treating non-gonococcal urethritis are erythromycin in doses of 250 to 500mg 6-hourly for 8 to 10 days and spiramycin in doses of 500mg 6-hourly for 8 to 10 days. Penicillin and sulphonamide drugs are not recommended.

It appears desirable to treat both sex partners. Endocervical chlamydia can be found in the majority of sex partners of males with proven urethral chlamydial infection and also in a minority of those without urethral chlamydial infection. Moreover, chlamydia can be recovered from the endocervix of a proportion of young women with asymptomatic or minimally symptomatic genital infection (Holmes et al., 1975; Richmond and Oriel, 1978).

6. Vaginitis

A pale, cloudy or mucoid vaginal discharge with its constant discomfort is a common complaint. It is due to an overproduction of cervical mucus, i.e. mucorrhoea, and is physiological, so should be treated by reassurance and not pessaries or vaginal creams. The 'pill' is often the cause. The odd nonspecific vaginitides do not fit into these categories and are difficult to deal with, but are usually mild. They can occasionally be due to a severe cervical erosion or possibly infection with *Corynebacterium vaginale (Haemophilus vaginalis),* a sexually transmissible organism the pathogenicity of which is unknown (Dunkelberg, 1977). Metronidazole has been effective for treatment (Pheifer et al., 1978). Some cases of vaginal discharge may be due to irritation from 'vaginal deodorant' use or a 'lost' vaginal tampon; others from lack of hygiene. The few cases of female gonorrhoea presenting with a vaginal discharge show a purulent endocervicitis, not a vaginitis. A slight mucopurulent discharge in females with multiple sex partners is almost the norm and is best left untreated.

Trichomoniasis and candidiasis account for practically all the marked and mild degrees of vaginitis. Effective treatment depends on their differentiation and the use of a highly specific agent, not a broad spectrum agent moderately effective for any vaginal discharge (Dennerstein, 1972). Diagnosis is by culture, together with a wet smear if a microscope is available.

6.1 Trichomoniasis

Trichomoniasis is due to infection with the flagellate protozoan *Trichomonas vaginalis*. The condition is always sexually transmitted, but demonstration of the organism in the asymptomatic male sex partner, in whom it is thought to exist only for a transient period, is difficult. It frequently coexists with gonorrhoea. The organism tends to produce an upper vaginitis, unlike *Candida* which has a predilection for the lower vagina and vulva. The classical clinical features (a bright red vaginal mucosa and thin, yellow, frothy, malodorous discharge) are usually evident, but some merely present as a mildly inflamed vagina of nonspecific appearance.

The standard treatment has been metronidazole, 200mg orally 3 times daily for 7 to 10 days for both patient and partner, but a single dose of 2 or 2.5g is to be preferred (Fleury et al., 1977). This achieves a comparable cure rate, although not as high as that of tinidazole (see below) and the taking of tablets is assured, at least in the clinic situation, since the dose can be given under supervision. Moreover, the convenience of the single dose regimen is more likely to be accepted by the male sex partner who is often symptom free and may see no need to take a multiple dose course of treatment. The treatment of choice today is probably the newer imidazole analogue tinidazole in a 2g single oral dose for both patient and partner, cure rates being higher than attained with an equivalent single dose regimen of metronidazole (Anjaneyulu et al., 1977). Alternative regimens include 400mg metronidazole 4 times daily for 2 days, and 3 doses of 1g nimorazole or tinidazole 12 hours apart, or a single 1.5g dose of another imidazole derivative, ornidazole (Hillstrom et al.,

1977). Other imidazoles are also under study (Editorial, 1978). If possible, a follow-up smear and culture should be made a week later and after the patient's next menstrual period. In those few cases of true treatment failure one of the other agents should be tried, or alternatively double dosage of one of the multiple dose schedules. A few patients may vomit with the large single dose regimens and such patients should then be given one of the multiple dose schedules. Patients taking metronidazole should not drink any alcoholic beverages because of a possible disulfiram-like intolerance reaction. Fear of possible carcinogenicity following use of metronidazole in trichomoniasis has not been substantiated (Weltman, 1978).

Local treatment is only necessary in those who do not tolerate oral therapy, or possibly during early pregnancy. Numerous preparations are available and include di-iodohydroxyquinoline, acetarsol and hydrargaphen. These agents can also be used as an antiseptic pessary in a nonspecific vaginal discharge which is offensive.

6.2 Candidiasis (candidosis)

The fungus *Candida albicans* is often present in the female genital tract without causing infection. It can be found in the vagina in about a fifth of sexually active women, being most common in the younger age groups. Clinical infection usually occurs when a suitable environment is produced hormonally (in pregnancy, by oral contraceptive use or premenstrually), in diabetic patients or following elimination of the normal bacterial flora by antibiotic treatment. Approximately 20% of sexually active women harbour *Candida albicans* in the ano-rectum and there is a strong association between rectal and vaginal candidiasis. Treatment should therefore be based on oral anticandidal agents to prevent reinfection from the bowel in addition to intravaginal application (cream or pessary at the top of the vagina and cream at the introitus). Symptoms produced are pruritus vulvae, a vaginal discharge with or without a typical thrush vaginitis (white, 'cheesy' deposits), or a combination of these. However, many are symptomless. Diagnosis is by culture or examination of a smear obtained by a firm wipe from the area of greatest inflammation.

The yeast is found as frequently (20%) on the penis of the circumcised as the uncircumcised male, but only in the uncircumcised male is candidal balanitis common. Sexual transmission therefore does occur and the male partner should be routinely treated with an appropriate antifungal cream.

Treatment of this common and recurring infection is far from satisfactory, as shown by the large number of drugs available for treatment and the differing lengths of treatment courses recommended (Willcox, 1977). The standard treatment has been nystatin, which is specific for the condition, but imidazole derivatives are at least as effective and may be preferable (see below). Nystatin is administered vaginally, in the form of a cream, pessary or foaming vaginal tablet; the latter probably being more effective than a conventional pessary (Vellupillai and Thin, 1977). A recommended regimen is one applicatorful of cream twice daily or 2 vaginal tablets (200,000u) inserted at night for 7 to 14 days, continued regardless of menstrual periods or relief of symptoms. Oral tablets (500,000u) are prescribed 3 or 4 times daily for the same time to prevent reinfection from the bowel, and a topical cream (100,000u/g) is applied to the vulva, surrounding skin and vestibule, twice daily.

Imidazole derivatives such as miconazole and clotrimazole have given cure rates at least comparable with nystatin, and must be considered as alternative therapy, particularly because they are effective when used for a shorter course (Sawyer et al., 1975a,b). Cure rates have generally been superior to nystatin given as conventional pessaries, but adequate dosage of nystatin cream seems to be as effective as a standard regimen of miconazole cream (Svendsen et al., 1978). Miconazole cream (2%) is inserted into the vagina at night for 7 days and clotrimazole pessaries are inserted 1 at night for 6 days or 2 at night for 3 days. These very short courses apparently give acceptable results and can be extremely useful. Another imidazole derivative, econazole, is also effective as a short course regimen; one 150mg pessary being inserted at night for 3 days. It is also available as a cream, inserted at night for 7 days (Heel et al., 1978). Amphotericin B, given as for nystatin, can be used as an alternative.

Recurrent infections are common and are sometimes the result of a too short a course of treatment. They may also be associated with the predisposing factors listed above, especially high dose oestrogen containing oral contraceptives. Recurrences can also be due to reinfection from a male sex partner. In all recurrences, the full regimen described above should be repeated, or an alternative one prescribed.

7. Viral Infections

7.1 Genital Herpes

Genital ulcers in women and blisters or ulcers in men due to the herpes simplex virus are increasingly common, the *Herpesvirus hominis* (types I and II) being widespread amongst young sexually active adults (Chang et al., 1974; Chang, 1977). Diagnosis is by exclusion of *Treponema pallidum,* and where virology is available, the demonstration of *Herpesvirus hominis* from the lesion, or a rise in antibodies in the blood. It is a condition of moderate infectivity with a short incubation period of a few days. Once infected, recurrences can occur, triggered by local and systemic stimuli. Asymptomatic infected females shed virus from the cervix.

Genital herpes commences as typical vesicles and eventually, in moist areas, forms single or multiple ulcers, which can progress to deep erosive sores in the female. They are very painful and there is a tender inguinal adenitis. Lesions can be single in both sexes. There is no effective cure. All the available measures do not eradicate the disease, but merely shorten the duration of each episode. The psychological stress associated with the onset of attacks and the variation in the course of the lesions makes assessment of treatment difficult. There is a high placebo response in recurrent infections, probably because of the short-lived nature of the lesions.

A mild attack, in which the lesions can be kept dry, is best left alone. If the lesion is moist or ulcerated, lotions or creams containing a corticosteroid and an antibiotic may sometimes be helpful. Gentamicin or neomycin are first choice agents as they are not treponemacidal. The antiviral drug idoxuridine, which is active against the herpes simplex virus (see chapter XXVIII; sect. 4.3.1), as an 0.5% solution painted on at frequent intervals in the prodromal stage can help, especially in recurrent cases. 5 to 35% idoxuridine in dimethylsulphoxide, painted on 5 times daily for not more than 3 days, may be more effective, but does little to modify the natural incidence of recurrence (Parker, 1977). Other regimens, including topical ether (Corey et al., 1978), topical vidarabine (Hilton et al., 1978) and oral levamisole (Chang and Fiumara, 1978) have been disappointing in controlled trials. To be effective, therapy probably has to be given early after onset of the attack (Spruance et al., 1977).

In women with genital herpes, a 5 % lignocaine (lidocaine) ointment can be used for relief of pain. If this fails, repeated spraying of cold water (from a plastic squeeze spray bottle) onto the painful area will prevent pain from occurring throughout urination.

7.2 Genital and Anorectal Warts (condylomata acuminata)

This troublesome and increasingly common condition is sexually transmitted in about 60 % of cases. It has a long incubation period, of about 1 to 3 months. Genital warts require a careful search in the female. They are pale and moist, with a cauliflower like surface, and occur most commonly in the vestibule near the fourchette, but also around the hymen, on the inside of the labiae minores, on the cervix and in the vagina. They also occur, with a horny surface, on the dry perivulval and perianal skin. In males, warts occur on the perianal skin and penis, and in homosexual males they can also occur within the anal canal and even the lower rectum (Schlappner and Shaffer, 1978). The sexual partner should also be examined. Under certain conditions, especially during pregnancy, there is rapid growth and extension of the lesions, which can form masses several centimetres across on the vulva, in the vagina, on the cervix or around the anus. 'The pill' seems to have a milder but similar effect.

Treatment is by destruction of the lesions, and is best done chemically by the use of 25 % podophyllin in 90 % alcohol, which both penetrates the lesion and dries after a few minutes, thus preventing its being wiped off. The paint is best applied with an orange stick or the butt end of a swab, rubbing it well into the wart structure. After application to vulval warts, the area should be dried and a piece of gauze inserted to prevent apposition of the labiae. Urination should be delayed for as long as possible. Anaesthetic ointment should be given to counter pain the next day, and lesions should be retreated every 5 to 7 days. Diathermy is also effective but needs local anaesthesia and leaves ulcers in moist areas. Cryotherapy can also be successfully used, applying liquid nitrogen with a swab or a slush of acetone and carbon dioxide snow. Machines are available for point source cryotherapy. In general, cryotherapy is disappointing due to the profuse blood supply to the area, but is the treatment of choice for hard warts.

7.3 Mollusca Contagiosa

The pearly papules, with an umbilicated centre, of molluscum contagiosum on the lower abdomen or upper thighs are easy to diagnose and cure. This can be achieved by application of an orange stick dipped in phenol, by cautery, cryotherapy, or by lifting out the 'mollusc body' with a needle.

8. Parasitic Infestation

8.1 Pubic Lice

Pediculosis pubis due to the pubic or crab louse *Phthirus pubis* is usually self evident, but on occasions tends to be missed by both doctor and patient, unless a thorough search in good light is made for nits and adults which are semi-transparent and very variable in size. They lie tightly applied to the skin of the pubic area by their specially hooked claws, but can spread to leg, abdominal and axillary hairy areas. Sometimes, the nits or eggs attached to the hairs like tiny 'grains of wheat', are the only visible signs.

Treatment is by application of dicophane powder or cream, or preferably gamma benzene hexachloride lotion or cream, for 2 consecutive nights rubbing it well into the hairy areas. On the third night a *cool* bath should be taken after which only clean clothes should be worn and laundered sheets used (see chapter XIV; sect. 3.2). The patient should be examined a week later as nits take about 7 to 10 days to hatch; proper treatment should however, kill nits as well as adult lice. The treatment of head and body lice is discussed in chapter XIV (sect. 3.2).

8.2 Scabies

Scabies is an increasingly common condition caused by the mite *Sarcoptes scabiei* var. *hominis*. It should be suspected in any person without a history of allergy or eczema who complains of a persistent severe generalised itching, especially at night. The rash is nonspecific, consisting of mainly scratch marks and a few small papules. Typical scaly plaques can occur on the periareola area of the breast and on the glans penis, with papules on the shaft. It is commonly acquired through the close bodily contact associated with sexual activity, and in this context is usually seen in adolescents and young adults. As the incubation period is about a month, and the mite can be transferred by normal social contact amongst a group of people living together, all members of the household or residence, whether symptomatic or not should be treated, as well as the sexual partner.

Treatment is by a careful routine of application of benzylbenzoate emulsion or gamma benzene hexachloride cream (see chapter XIV; sect. 3.1). Disinfestation of clothing and bedding etc. should be carried out more fully than for pubic lice. Itching does not stop for a week or more, despite cure. Corticosteroid creams should be avoided as they may mask the condition.

Further Reading

Catterall, R.D. and Nicol, C.S. (Ed): Sexually Transmitted Diseases: Proceedings of a Conference Sponsored Jointly by the Royal Society of Medicine and the Royal Society of Medicine Foundation Incorporated, London, 23-25 June, 1975, p.6 (Academic Press, London 1976).

Platts, W.M.: Handbook of Venereal Diseases 2nd edition (Peryer, Christchurch 1974).

Morton, R.S. and Harris, J.R.W.: Recent Advances in Sexually Transmitted Diseases (Churchill Livingstone, Edinburgh 1975).

Willcox, R.R.: A Textbook of Venereal Diseases and Treponematoses, 2nd ed. (Thomas, Springfield Ill. 1964).

References

Anjaneyulu, R.; Gupte, S.A. and Desai, D.B.: Single-dose treatment of trichomonal vaginitis: A comparison of tinidazole and metronidazole. Journal of International Medical Research 5: 438 (1977).

Ashford, W.A.; Golash, R.G. and Hemming, V.G.: Penicillinase-producing neisseria gonorrhoeae. Lancet 2: 657 (1976).

Bowie, W.R.: Etiology and treatment of nongonococcal urethritis. Sexually Transmitted Diseases 5: 27 (1978).

Bowie, W.R.; Wang, S-P.; Alexander, E.R.; Floyd, J.; Forsyth, P.S.; Pollock, H.M.; Lin, J-S.L.; Buchanan, T.M. and Holmes, K.K.: Etiology of nongonococcal urethritis. Evidence for *Chlamydia trachomatis* and *Ureaplasma urealyticum*. Journal of Clinical Investigation 59: 735 (1977).

British Cooperative Clinical Group: Homosexuality and venereal disease in the United Kingdom. British Journal of Venereal Diseases 49: 329 (1973).

Center for Disease Control: Gonorrhoea and early syphilis cases — United States, 1976. Morbidity and Mortality Weekly Report 26: 1 (1977).

Chang, T-W.: Genital herpes and type I *herpesvirus hominis*. Journal of the American Medical Association 238: 155 (1977).

Chang, T-W. and Fiumara, N.: Treatment with levamisole of recurrent herpes genitalis. Antimicrobial Agents and Chemotherapy 13: 809 (1978).

Chang, T-W.; Fiumara, N.J. and Weinstein, L.: Genital herpes. Some clinical and laboratory observations. Journal of the American Medical Association 229: 544 (1974).

Corey, L.; Reeves, W.C.; Chiang, W.T.; Vontver, L.A.; Remington, M.; Winter, C. and Holmes, K.K.: Ineffectiveness of topical ether for the treatment of genital herpes simplex infection. New England Journal of Medicine 299: 237 (1978).

Dennerstein, G.: Vaginitis: Diagnosis and treatment. Drugs 4: 419 (1972).

Dry, J.; Leynadier, F.; Damecour, C.; Pradalier, A. and Herman, D.: Pseudo-anaphylactic reaction to procaine-penicillin G. Three cases of Hoigne's syndrome. Nouvelle Presse Medicale 5: 1401 (1976).

Dunkelberg, W.E.: *Corynebacterium vaginale.* Sexually Transmitted Diseases 4: 69 (1977).

Editorial: The nitroimidazole family of drugs. British Journal of Venereal Diseases 54: 69 (1978).

Eisenstein, B.I.: Effective treatment of gonorrhoea. Drugs 14: 57 (1977).

Elliott, W.C.; Reynolds, G.; Thornsberry, C.; Kellogg, D.S.; Jaffe, H.W.; Brown, S.T.; Armstrong, J. and Rein, M.F.: Treatment of gonorrhea with trimethoprim-sulfamethoxazole. Journal of Infectious Diseases 135: 939 (1977).

Elwell, L.P.; Roberts, M.; Mayer, L.W. and Falkow, S.: Plasmid-mediated beta-lactamase production in Neisseria gonorrhoeae. Antimicrobial Agents and Chemotherapy 11: 528 (1977).

Eschenbach, D.A. and Holmes, K.K.: Acute pelvic inflammatory disease. Current concepts of pathogenesis, etiology and management. Clinical Obstetrics and Gynecology 18: 35 (1975).

Eschenbach, D.A.; Buchanan, T.M.; Pollock, H.M.; Forsyth, P.S.; Alexander, E.R.; Lin, J.-S.; Wang, S.-P.; Wentworth, B.B.; McCormack, W.M. and Holmes, K.K.: Polymicrobial etiology of acute pelvic inflammatory disease. New England Journal of Medicine 293: 166 (1975).

Fleury, F.J.; Van Bergan, W.S.; Prentice, R.L.; Russell, J.G.; Singleton, J.A. and Standerd, J.V.: Single dose of two grams of metronidazole for *Trichomonas vaginalis* infection. American Journal of Obstetrics and Gynaecology 128: 320 (1977).

Ford, D.K. and Henderson, E.: Nongonococcal urethritis due to T-mycoplasma (*Ureaplasma urealyticum*) serotype 2 in a conjugal sexual partnership. British Journal of Venereal Diseases 52: 341 (1976).

Handsfield, H.H.; Hodson, W.A. and Holmes, K.K.: Neonatal gonococcal infection: Orogastric contamination with *Neisseria gonorrhoeae*. Journal of the American Medical Association 225: 697 (1973).

Handsfield, H.H.; Lipman, T.O.; Harnisch, J.P.; Tronca, Evelyn and Holmes, K.K.: Asymptomatic gonorrhoea in men: Diagnosis, natural course prevalence and significance. New England Journal of Medicine 290: 117 (1974).

Handsfield, H.H.; Wiesner, P.J. and Holmes, K.K.: Treatment of the gonococcal arthritis-dermatitis syndrome. Annals of Internal Medicine 84: 661 (1976).

Heel, R.C.; Brogden, R.N.; Speight, T.M. and Avery, G.S.: Econazole: A review of its antifungal activity and therapeutic efficacy. Drugs 16: 177 (1978).

Hillstrom, L.; Pettersson, L. and Palsson, E.: Comparison of ornidazole and tinidazole in single-dose treatment of trichomoniasis in women. British Journal of Venereal Diseases 53: 193 (1977).

Hilton, A.L.; Bushell, T.E.C.; Waller, D. and Blight, J.: A trial of adenine arabinoside in genital herpes. British Journal of Venereal Diseases 54: 50 (1978).

Holmes, K.K.; Johnson, D.W. and Floyd, T.M.: Studies of venereal disease. I. Probenecid-procaine penicillin G combination and tetracycline hydrochloride in the treatment of 'penicillin-resistant' gonorrhoea in men. Journal of the American Medical Association 202: 461 (1967a).

Holmes, K.K.; Johnson, D.W. and Floyd, T.M.: Tetracycline treatment of non-gonococcal urethritis. Journal of the American Medical Association 202: 474 (1967b).

Holmes, K.K.; Handsfield, H.; Wang, S.P.; Wentworth, Berttina B.; Turck, M.; Anderson, Joanne B. and Alexander, E.R.: Etiology of nongonococcal urethritis. New England Journal of Medicine 292: 1199 (1975).

Johnson, D.W.; Kvale, P.A.; Afable, V.L.; Stewart, S.D.; Halverson, C.W. and Holmes, K.K.: Single dose antibiotic treatment of asymptomatic gonorrhoea in hospitalised women. New England Journal of Medicine 283: 1 (1970).

Juhlin, I.: Problems in diagnosis, treatment and control of gonorrhoeal infections. Acta Dermatologica Venereologica 45: 231 (1965).

Karney, W.W.; Pedersen, A.H.B.; Nelson, M.; Adams, H.; Pfeifer, R.T. and Holmes, K.K.: Spectinomycin versus tetracycline for the treatment of gonorrhea. New England Journal of Medicine 296: 889 (1977).

Kaufman, R.E.; Johnson, R.E.; Yaffe, H.W.; Thornsberry, C.; Reynolds, G.H.; Wiesner, P.J. and the Cooperative Study Group: Gonorrhea therapy monitoring: Treatment results. New England Journal of Medicine 294: 1 (1976).

Kraus, S.J.and Green, R.L.: Pseudoanaphylactic reactions with procaine penicillin. Cutis 17: 765 (1976).

Krook, G. and Juhlin, L.: Problems in diagnosis, treatment and control of gonorrheal infections. Acta Dermatologica Venereologica 45: 142 (1965).

Kvale, P.A.; Keys, T.F.; Johnson, D.W. and Holmes, K.K.: Single oral dose ampicillin-probenecid treatment of gonorrhoea in the male. Journal of the American Medical Association 215: 1449 (1971).

McCracken, G.H. and Kaplan, J.M.: Penicillin treatment for congenital syphilis. A critical reappraisal. Journal of the American Medical Association 228: 855 (1974).

Melton, L.J.: Comparative incidence of gonorrhoea and non-gonococcal urethritis in the United States Navy. American Journal of Epidemiology 104: 535 (1976).

Nahmias, A.J.: Sexually transmitted diseases from the pediatrician's viewpoint. Journal of the American Venereal Diseases Association 2: 5 (1975).

Nahmias, A.J.; Josey, W.E.; Naib, Z.M. and Visintine, A.M.: Genital herpetic infection — the old and the new; in Catterall and Nicol (Ed) Sexually Transmitted Diseases: Proceedings of a Conference Sponsored Jointly by the Royal Society of Medicine and the Royal Society of Medicine Foundation Incorporated, 23-25 June, 1975, p.135 (Academic Press, London 1976).

Olsen, G.A. and Lomholt, G.: Gonorrhoea treated by a combination of probenecid and sodium penicillin G. British Journal of Venereal Diseases 45: 144 (1969).

Oriel, J.D.: Nature, diagnosis, and management of nonspecific urethritis. Bulletin of the New York Academy of Medicine 52: 877 (1976).

Oriel, J.D.; Reeve, P.; Wright, J.T. and Owen, J.: Chlamydial infection of the male urethra. British Journal of Venereal Diseases 52: 46 (1976).

Oriel, J.D.; Ridgway, G.L.; Tchamouroff, S. and Owen, J.: Spectinomycin hydrochloride in the treatment of gonorrhoea: its effect on associated *Chlamydia trachomatis* infections. British Journal of Venereal Diseases 53: 226 (1977).

Parker, J.D.: A double-blind trial of idoxuridine in recurrent genital herpes. Journal of Antimicrobial Chemotherapy 3(Suppl. A): 131 (1977).

Pheifer, T.A.; Forsyth, P.S.; Durfee, M.A.; Pollock, H.M. and Holmes, K.K.: Nonspecific vaginitis. Role of *Haemophilus vaginalis* and treatment with metronidazole. New England Journal of Medicine 298: 1429 (1978).

Phillips, I.: β-lactamase-producing, penicillin-resistant gonococcus. Lancet 2: 656 (1976).

Reyn, A.; Schmidt, H.; Trier, M. and Bentzon, M.W.: Spectinomycin hydrochloride (Trobicin) in the treatment of gonorrhoea. Observation of resistant strains of *Neisseria gonorrhoeae*. British Journal of Venereal Disease 44: 54 (1973).

Richmond, S.J. and Oriel, J.D.: Recognition and management of genital chlamydial infection. British Medical Journal 2: 480 (1978).

Roizman, B. and Frenkel, N.: Does genital herpes cause cancer? — A midway assessment; in Catterall and Nicol (Ed) Sexually Transmitted Diseases: Proceedings of a Conference Sponsored Jointly by the Royal Society of Medicine and the Royal Society of Medicine Foundation Incorporated, London, 23-25 June, 1975, p.151 (Academic Press, London 1976).

Rudolph, A.H. and Price, E.V.: Penicillin reactions among patients in venereal disease clinics. A national survey. Journal of the American Medical Association 223: 499 (1973).

Sawyer, P.R.; Brogden, R.N.; Pinder, R.M.; Speight, T.M. and Avery, G.S.: Miconazole: A review of its antifungal activity and therapeutic efficacy. Drugs 9: 406 (1975a).

Sawyer, P.R.; Brogden, R.N.; Pinder, R.M.; Speight, T.M. and Avery, G.S.: Clotrimazole: A review of its antifungal activity and therapeutic efficacy. Drugs 9: 424 (1975b).

Schlappner, O.L.A. and Shaffer, E.A.: Anorectal condylomata acuminata: a missed part of the condyloma spectrum. Canadian Medical Association Journal 118: 172 (1978).

Schroeter, A.L. and Pazin, G.J.: Gonorrhea. Annals of Internal Medicine 72: 553 (1970).

Siegel, M.S.; Thompson, S.E. and Perine, P.L.: Penicillinase-producing *Neisseria gonorrhoeae*. Sexually Transmitted Diseases 4: 32 (1977).

Siegel, M.S.; Thornsberry, C.; Biddle, J.W.; O'Mara, P.R.; Perine, P.L. and Wiesner, P.J.: Penicillinase-producing *Neisseria gonorrhoeae:* Results of surveillance in the United States. Journal of Infectious Diseases 137: 170 (1978).

Sohn, N. and Robilotti, J.G.: The gay bowel syndrome. American Journal of Gastroenterology 67: 478 (1977).

Spruance, S.L.; Overall, J.C.; Kern, E.R.; Krueger, G.G.; Pliam, V. and Miller, W.: The natural history of recurrent herpes simplex labialis. Implications for antiviral therapy. New England Journal of Medicine 297: 69 (1977).

Svendsen, E.; Lie, S.; Gunderson, Th.; Lyngstad-Vik, I. and Skuland, J.: Comparative evaluation of miconazole, clotrimazole and nystatin in the treatment of candidal vulvo-vaginitis. Current Therapeutic Research 23: 666 (1978).

Thayer, J.D.; Field, F.W.: Magnuson, H.J. et al.: The sensitivity of gonococci to penicillin and its relationship to "penicillin failures". Antimicrobial Agents and Chemotherapy, Vol. 7, p.306 (American Society for Antimicrobial Agents and Chemotherapy, Ann Arbor 1957).

Thornsberry, C.; Jaffee, H.; Brown, S.T.; Edwards, T.; Biddle, J.W. and Thompson, S.E.: Spectinomycin-resistant *neisseria gonorrhoeae*. Journal of the American Medical Association 237: 2405 (1977).

Vellupillai, S. and Thin, R.N.: Treatment of vulvovaginal yeast infection with nystatin. Practitioner 219: 897 (1977).

Weisner, P.J.; Jones, O.G. and Blount, J.H.: World trends in sexually transmitted diseases. The situation in the United States; in Catterall and Nicol (Ed) Sexually Transmitted Diseases: Proceedings of a Conference Sponsored Jointly by the Royal Society of Medicine and the Royal Society of Medicine Foundation Incorporated, London, 23-25 June, 1975, p.5 (Academic Press, London 1976).

Weltman, R.: New metronidazole study: some reassuring findings for now. Journal of the American Medical Association 239: 1371 (1978).

Willcox, R.R.: Recent advances in venerology. I. Syphilis. British Journal of Clinical Practice 27: 115 (1973).

Willcox, R.R.: Changing patterns of treponemal disease. British Journal of Venereal Diseases 50: 169 (1974).

Willcox, R.R.: How suitable are available pharmaceuticals for the treatment of sexually transmitted diseases? I. Conditions presenting as genital discharges. British Journal of Venereal Diseases 53: 314 (1977).

Williams, J.D.: Spread of R-factors outside the Enterobacteriaceal. Journal of Antimicrobial Chemotherapy 4: 6 (1978).

World Health Organisation: Weekly Epidemiologic Record 52: 357 (1977). See also Penicillinase-(β-lactamase) producing *Neisseria gonorrhoeae* — Worldwide Morbidity and Mortality Weekly Report 27: 10 (1978).

World Health Organisation: *Neisseria gonorrhoeae* and Gonococcal Infections. Report of a WHO Scientific Group. Technical Report Series 616 (World Health Organisation, Geneva 1978).

Chapter XXX
Diseases of a Tropical Environment

Kamala Krishnaswamy and P.C. Teoh

Synopsis of Important Principles

1) Although modern drugs have contributed towards improved health standards in tropical countries, because of other closely linked detrimental factors, tropical diseases and the problems associated with them still continue to pose an increasing threat to the welfare of mankind.

2) The pattern of drug consumption in tropical and developing countries will be largely determined by inter-related factors such as the existence and development of a local pharmaceutical industry, the availability and cost of drugs, their distribution between urban and rural areas, the purchasing capacity of individuals, and the health care delivery system.

3) Dosage of drugs based on a Western population are inappropriate for use in tropical countries because of differences in the genetic profile, body weight, nutritional status and the environment in which peoples of a tropical country are placed. Of all the factors which may influence drug response in a tropical environment, nutrition is probably the most important.

4) Drug dosages may have to be altered depending on the nutritional status of an individual, the type of nutrient deficiency (proteins, calories, vitamins, minerals or trace metals) and the extent of change in the pharmacokinetics of a particular drug.

5) The interplay between malnutrition and infection is of considerable importance in developing countries; one leading to the other through a vicious cycle. Malnourished children are particularly susceptible to infectious diseases; tuberculosis and pertussis for example being common and occurring at an earlier age and measles being much more severe in tropical countries, than in well nourished children living in a Western environment.

6) Better drugs are needed for treatment of tropical parasitic diseases, but control or eradication of these diseases will only result from measures such as vector control, immunisation and improvement in public health and sanitation practices.

7) Choice of an appropriate drug regimen in a tropical country for control of diseases such as tuberculosis, leprosy and malaria is not only determined by each country's financial and manpower resources, but also by study of those factors in a given population which influence drug response.

8) Glucose-6-phosphate dehydrogenase deficiency is relatively common and severe in a number of ethnic groups in tropical countries and should be excluded before certain drugs are given (e.g. primaquine, dapsone, phenacetin, sulphonamides, co-trimoxazole, nitrofurantoin). Folate deficiency is common in tropical countries and drugs which can impair folate metabolism (e.g. pyrimethamine, co-trimoxazole) should not be given in the presence of folate deficiency or where diet is inadequate without folate supplements.

The importance of geographical and environmental factors in determining the prevalence, incidence, progress, recovery and relapse of tropical diseases is well recognised. However, a multidisciplinary approach is required to tackle the health problems and lessen the burden of diseases in overpopulated, overcrowded, poorly developed and economically backward countries. The measurement of health needs in the tropics itself is beset with problems. Although sufficient knowledge exists with regard to the nature of the problem, quantitative data with respect to the extent are not always available. Health problems and diseases in the tropics are closely linked with other factors like the social and economic structure, culture and religion, food production and distribution, and other factors like lack of transportation facilities (communication), unhygienic surroundings, illiteracy and overpopulation. Health resources in these underprivileged countries are hardly comparable with other well developed countries and are certainly inadequate with respect to the health needs of the population.

Medical practice and administration of therapeutic agents in these areas to begin with comprised some crude extracts, powders and juices from animal, plant and other resources and even today the practice of traditional medicine continues in many parts. For example, in India, China, Ceylon and in Japan, institutional forms of professional education and practice have been adapted to indigenous medical traditions. However, with advances in physiology, chemistry, biochemistry and other related disciplines and with an increase in world travel and infiltration of modern medicine (Western) into the tropics, the modern age of pharmacology has come into existence. Although the flow of drugs has been large and has greatly contributed towards improved health standards, due to certain other closely linked detrimental factors, tropical diseases and the problems associated with them still continue to pose an increasing threat to the welfare of mankind.

One of the most important practical measures in management of disease is the practice of modern medicine. Trends in morbidity and mortality due to tropical diseases is on the decline in most of the countries. The marked improvement in health standards is due, to a certain extent, to the drugs made available for control of diseases both by local governmental organisations and by the support of international organisations.

1. Drugs and Developing Countries

Drug prescription in tropical and under-developed countries will be determined to a great extent by factors such as the existence and development of a local pharmaceutical industry, availability of drugs, cost of preparations, production and distribution of medicines in health centres (rural and urban), purchasing capacity of individuals, the health structure, and health care and other related programmes.

1.1 Development of Pharmaceuticals

With the advent of modern medicine, drug manufacturing facilities are being established in many countries and with the help of foreign collaborations, bulk drugs are being produced from basic stages using raw materials that are available in the country (OPPI, 1976). Research, development and available technological facilities in the drug industry have a great bearing on the cost of drugs in these countries. Despite price controls, however, certain drugs are still beyond the financial means of the common person, especially in rural areas. In certain situations, domestic production of bulk drugs may not be sufficient to meet the entire requirements, in which case bulk drugs and raw materials have to be imported. However, while 25 years ago, 90% of the requirements were met by imports, currently imports account for hardly 10% of local production in a country like India.

1.2 Production and Distribution of Drugs

The drugs which are manufactured by a local industry cover a wide therapeutic spectrum. In India, for example, antibiotics, sulphonamides, vitamins, hormones, antihistamines, tranquillisers, anaesthetics, antituberculosis, antileprotic, antimalarial, antidiarrhoeal and antidysentery drugs, analgesics, antipyretics, antidiabetic drugs and vaccines are at present being produced. All these drugs are manufactured from basic stages using mostly indigenous raw materials and chemicals. The pharmaceutical industry in India produces annually Rs 4,500 millions (about US $500 million) value of formulations for a population of 695 million. Many of the drugs produced are used in tropical diseases like malaria, tuberculosis, leprosy, diarrhoea and dysentery due to various aetiological factors, infectious diseases, parasitic and bacterial diseases and sexually transmissible diseases.

The industry in India has also built up over the years a fairly good system of distribution that ensures the ready availability of essential medicines throughout the country. The distribution of medicines is mediated through chemists, druggists and general merchants having drug licences (public and private sector). Despite these developments, the vast rural population (about 70% to 80%) does not receive the full benefits of modern medicine. The organisation of medical stores (equipment, temperature used for safeguard of shelf life, location-accessibility) will naturally have a great influence on the drug consumption pattern. Pharmacies in rural areas are rare because of their remoteness from large centres, the isolated groups of population for which a pharmacy would have to cater, the low purchasing power of the people and absence of trained personnel.

In many tropical countries, a major problem is the availability of too many different drugs and too many brands, instead of bulk supplies of a few essential drugs available throughout the country (WHO, 1977a). Often, the large urban hospitals or the patients of doctors with private practices in urban areas, receive most of the available drugs.

1.3 Consumption of Drugs

Although rapid and major advances have been made in the local drug industry, the per capita consumption of medicines in India is hardly Rs 7-8 (less than US $1) per annum as against Rs 100 to Rs 300 ($10 to 30) in developed countries. The population covered is just 20%. The drug consumption pattern is somewhat similar in other developing countries like Indonesia, Pakistan, Egypt, Korea, Thailand, Brazil and Mexico. Even a doubling of production of drugs will result only in a per capita consumption of not more than Rs 12 to 14 (less than US $2) per annum and a population coverage of not more than 40%.

Therefore, it is evident that there has to be a sustained and progressive growth in production and distribution to reach the rural population. Simultaneously, the other health facilities in terms of doctors, hospitals, dispensaries, clinics, rural health centres and allied services have to be developed. However, most of the diseases in the tropics are preventable either by chemoprophylaxis, immunisation and/or improvement in environmental sanitation. Hence, although drug produc-

tion may have to be increased in the immediate future, if prevention programmes are successful, drug requirement, consumption and production may be lessened.

1.4 Problems Associated with Drug Usage

It is evident that as the problem of tropical diseases is endemic and is confined to the developing or the 'third world', discovery of new and better drugs is at a very minimum level. The international pharmaceutical industry is geared to the needs of the well developed countries with entirely different health problems (Binns, 1976). Considerable investments are required for the development of new drugs. In industrial research in developed countries, expected financial return is one of the important goals in determining the direction of research and hence the possible risk of failure and low financial gains. Inadequate research and development facilities in tropical countries, themselves are to an extent responsible for the failure to develop promising new drugs. There is an urgent need to encourage the development and production of new drugs adapted to the real health requirements of developing countries (WHO, 1975).

The pattern of drug consumption in a developing country varies within the same country widely (Yudkin, 1978); use of antibacterial and antiparasitic drugs being maximum in district hospitals, while the national teaching hospitals spend most drug funds on tranquillisers, sedatives and antidepressants. More than 40% of drug prescriptions in teaching hospitals are for more expensive proprietary preparations. This may not be true if the teaching hospitals do not give medicines free of charge. In some countries, the pattern of drug consumption may be widely different between the high and low income groups and will also depend on the prescribing habits of general practitioners and the purchasing capacity of the individual. Delayed and at times total lack of communication, lower standards of medical care, low clinician to population ratio, availability of drugs (free of cost), marketing practices, economic status and educational level affect all phases of drug consumption in developing countries (Kaldor, 1976). Indiscriminate use of intravenous fluids and inappropriate prescribing of drugs, including excessive demands on drug supplies by medical personnel and their families, are other factors which influence the use of drugs in developing countries

(Bygbjerg, 1978). Use of local herbal medicines also contributes to the pattern of drug use, as well as to adverse drug reactions (Teoh, 1975; Wong, 1977).

A number of inter-related factors therefore determines the drug consumption pattern and there is an urgent need for constructing a proper infrastructure itself (fig. 1). The wide system of drug development, research, distribution and prescribing patterns may have to be standardised and structured to the needs of the population. Simultaneously, the health personnel and health services have to be improved and balanced between the vast rural and urban areas, since they are responsible for supplying medicines.

2. Clinical Pharmacological Considerations

2.1 Determinants of Dose and Dosage Schedules in a Tropical Environment

Drug therapy in tropical countries has a profound influence on health statistics. However, rational use of drugs based on pharmacokinetic and pharmacodynamic studies in these populations is lacking for obvious reasons. Drug dosages as recommended in textbooks and as advised by the pharmaceutical manufacturer are followed by clinicians. Most of these dosage regimens are standardised on a Western population who are genetically different and are also placed in a different environment. Populations differ widely in relation to their physiological and/or biochemical constitution. The genetic profile, body weight, nutritional status and the environment are four major factors which have a direct bearing on drug dosage (table I).

2.1.1 Genetic Profile

Literature is replete with evidence that genetic factors profoundly influence drug metabolism, efficacy and toxicity of xenobiotics (Vessell, 1974). It is estimated that about a third of known enzymes in the human system exist in a polymorphic form and two or more variants of each enzyme are recognised (WHO, 1974). These variants undoubtedly affect drug response. Polymorphic acetylation of drugs like isoniazid, dapsone, some sulphonamides, procainamide and hydrallazine may determine not only the clinical response but also greater likelihood of toxicity reactions (see chapter VII; sect. 4.2.1). Isoniazid is the most effective and widely used antituberculosis drug in Asia, Africa and South America. There are large interindividual differences in the rates of isoniazid metabolism (see chapter XX; sect. 8.1). Meticulously controlled clinical trials have indicated that the clinical response is identical between individuals with different capacities to acetylate isoniazid, provided the drug is given on a daily basis. However, twice weekly regimens and once weekly treatment in rapid acetylators is inadequate as compared with slow acetylators (Ellard, 1976). Development of toxic effects like neuropathies with isoniazid will be determined by the respective genomes for slow and fast acetylation (see chapter VII; sect. 4.2.1).

Geographic and ethnic variation in drug oxidation rates may account for significant variation in the steady-state plasma concentration of drugs

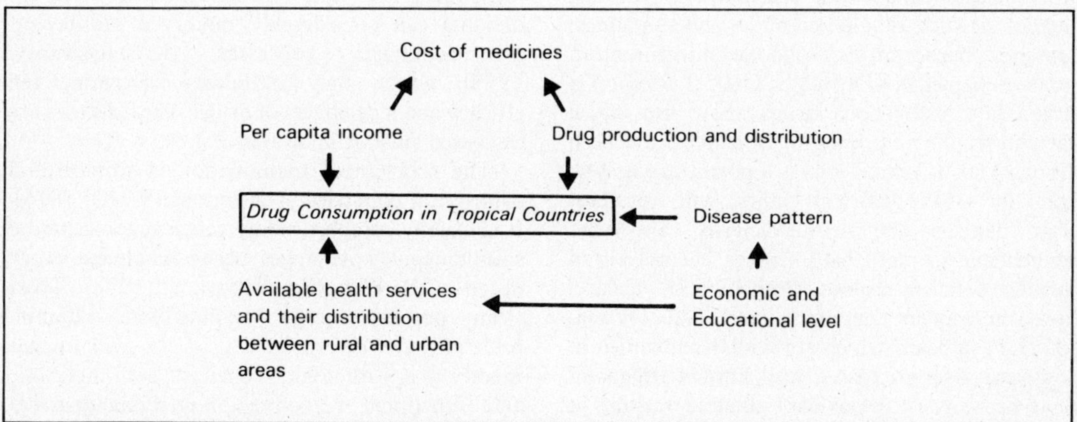

Fig. 1. Inter-related factors in drug consumption pattern in tropical countries.

Table I. Determinants of dose and dosage schedules in tropical countries

1. Genetic profile

2. Body weight

3. Nutritional status and dietary habits

4. Tropical environment
   a) Climatological factors
   b) Infections and infestations
   c) Environmental pollutants like mycotoxins and other food poisons

with dose dependent kinetics (e.g. phenytoin, dicoumarol), drugs with a narrow therapeutic ratio and drugs which bind extensively to plasma and tissue proteins (Fraser et al., 1976; see further chapter I, sect. 4).

Toxic reactions to drugs due to genetic variation may be encountered in certain populations; one of the best known, and most common examples being enzyme deficiency of glucose-6-phosphate dehydrogenase (G6PD). Different types of G6PD deficiency predominate in different ethnic groups (WHO, 1974; see chapter VII, sect. 4.2.2). The use of some antimalarials such as primaquine, even in therapeutic doses, can precipitate haematological abnormalities. In Africans, usually a mild deficiency (enzyme activity 8 to 20% of normal) is encountered, whereas in the Mediterranean regions, the deficiency is severe (0 to 4% enzyme activity). A number of variants are described in East and Southeast Asia and it is likely that at least some of these may be as severe as the Mediterranean types.

The incidence of haemolytic episodes will vary in different ethnic groups. There are a number of other drugs which can precipitate significant haemolysis such as sulphonamides and sulphones, dapsone, phenacetin, furazolidone, nitrofurantoin etc (see chapter XXIII; table XIII), if used on a large scale. Indigenous drugs may also cause haemolysis. For example, in Singapore the herb 'Chuan Lian' (Coptis Teeta) is a potent haemolytic agent for G6PD deficient babies, with resultant brain damage due to kernicterus. Similarly, naphthalene in moth balls, causes haemolysis in enzyme deficient babies clothed with apparel stored in drawers containing moth balls (Wong, 1977). Fava beans which are widely consumed in Southeast Asia are also a well known trigger of acute haemolysis; the oxidant alkaloid varying in concentration depending on the time the bean is

harvested and its mode of preparation. The use of such drugs in populations at risk will be determined by factors like sex of the patient, severity of G6PD deficiency, the need for the drug and duration of therapy, and the presence of other factors such as infections which can also precipitate haemolysis in enzyme deficient individuals. Drug induced cyanosis and hereditary methaemoglobinaemia (for methaemoglobin forming drugs such as dapsone, primaquine and chloroquine) are also one of the important genetically determined drug reactions (see further chapter VII; sect. 4.2.2).

2.1.2 Body Weight

Most of the initial studies on drugs take into consideration body weight and doses are often fixed for an average weight of 70kg. These doses are then extrapolated to other populations and it is usual practice to follow absolute doses without relevance to body weight. However, on an average, the weight of an adult in developing countries is about 55kg and consequently most Asians, for example, receive about 30% more drug/dose based on recommendations for most developed populations (Salafsky, 1976). This problem may be more acute in children since dosage of a number of drugs is based on age, and for the same age, the body weights and growth patterns are entirely different for the well developed Western and underdeveloped Eastern populations (Teoh, 1977). Thus, drug doses should be recommended on a body weight basis, rather than on the basis of age or an absolute fixed quantity.

2.1.3 Nutritional Status

Of all the environmental factors which may influence drug response, nutrition may be one of the most important. The nutritional status of an individual can considerably modify a number of pharmacokinetic processes (Krishnaswamy, 1978), which may ultimately determine the efficacy and side effects of drugs. These factors are discussed further in section 2.2.

The problem of malnutrition in tropical and subtropical countries is enormous (WHO, 1976). It is usually complex; many deficiencies occurring simultaneously. Changes occur in almost every organ of the body (Krishnaswamy, 1978). Apart from protein energy malnutrition; vitamin, mineral and trace metal deficiencies will further modify the pathological changes and metabolic and functional responses. Nutritional-pharmacological interactions will determine drug responses and therefore these have to be evaluated carefully. Drug dosages may have to be altered depending on the nutritional status, the type of nutrient deficiency and the extent of change in the pharmacokinetics of a drug.

2.1.4 Environment

Some factors which determine the metabolism of and response to drugs are related to the physical and chemical environment (Sanvordeker and Lambert, 1972). Higher altitudes have been shown to alter drug responses. For example, impairment in performance due to the antihistamine chlorpheniramine, increases as a function of increasing altitude (Higgins et al., 1968). Light has also been shown to modify metabolism and response to drugs (Nair and Casper, 1969). Relative humidity in an environment can also alter phototoxic responses to topically applied drugs (Levine and Harper, 1969). Changes in ambient temperature has a pronounced effect on toxicity of drugs; griseofulvin levels in the skin are higher in summer as compared with winter months (Epstein et al., 1972). Therefore, it seems likely that in extreme weather conditions, such as those experienced in tropical and subtropical areas, drug distribution, phototoxicity and metabolic disposition may be altered by climatological factors. Epidemiological factors like differences in disease pattern, intestinal microflora, atmospheric contamination amd mycotoxins may further modify drug response. Systematic studies of drug response in relation to the physical and chemical environment, particularly in tropical countries, have yet to be undertaken.

2.2 Drug Pharmacokinetic Processes as Influenced by a Tropical Environment

It is a well recognised fact that drug pharmacokinetics can be influenced by a number of internal and external variables (see chapter I). Apart from intrinsic factors like age, sex and species, environmental factors like temperature, altitude, light exposure, atmospheric pollution and other climatological factors play an important role in determining many biological processes. In a tropical environment, there are a number of factors such as malnutrition, infectious diseases, parasitic infections, naturally occurring toxins and contaminants and food habits, which may have a profound influence on the way in which a drug is handled by individuals (Krishnaswamy, 1978).

Table II. Processes likely to be altered by malnutrition, infection and the environment

1. Absorption of drugs

2. Binding and distribution of drugs

3. Biotransformation of drugs

4. Excretion of drugs — biliary, renal

5. Tissue uptake, localisation and response to drugs (drug-receptor interactions)

Very little information is available on this aspect in tropical countries and it appears to be an area open for research activity.

The environment around a subject or a patient prior to, during and after drug administration may have an important influence on drug response in terms of both clinical efficacy and adverse drug reactions. It is possible that extremes of environmental temperature and other co-existent epidemiological and socio-cultural factors may alter significantly some of the important pharmacokinetic processes of drug absorption, distribution, protein binding, biotransformation and excretion (table II).

Infectious diseases constitute the main cause of morbidity and mortality in the tropics. Nutritional disorders are predominant in these areas, particularly in Latin and South America, Africa and Asian countries. Standards of environmental hygiene are quite low due to overpopulation and inadequate sanitary facilities, which further contribute to spread of infections and infestations. The triad of malnutrition, infection and unhygienic environmental background have to be considered equally when any drug response is to be discussed in relation to diseases.

2.2.1 Drug Absorption and Bioavailability

The extent of absorption of an orally administered drug is modified by a number of factors like the pH in the intestinal lumen, gastric emptying rate, intestinal transit time, surface area of the gastrointestinal tract and mesenteric blood flow. In addition, drug metabolism by gut bacteria and by enzymes in the gut wall and presence of infections and infestations may influence the amount of active drug passing across the mucous membrane (see chapter I; sect. 3.1). In tropical countries, the effect of malnutrition and malabsorption syndromes coupled with worm infestation and bacterial infection, can modify the extent of absorption and availability of orally administered drugs (see section 11). The gastrointestinal tract, both histologically and functionally, is said to be different in a tropical environment (see Rosenberg and Scrimshaw, 1972). These alterations have been used to explain malabsorption of nutrients. However, in a tropical environment, there are very few investigations on drug absorption in general and of the effect of malnutrition in particular. Absorption studies need to be undertaken, particularly in the presence of parasitic and bacterial infections.

In addition, different diets *per se* may modify drug absorption. Populations in different parts of the world and individuals within the same population differ widely in their diets. Therefore, it is not possible to extrapolate data from one country to another. Hence, apart from nutritional status, food habits may profoundly influence drug absorption and the steady-state concentration of drug. Absorption of drugs with a marked first-pass effect due to gut or hepatic metabolism (see chapter I; sect. 2.1.4, 3.3.3) and absorption of drugs which are administered parenterally, also needs to be studied.

2.2.2 Drug Protein Binding and Distribution

Drug protein binding has many clinical implications (see chapter I; sect. 3.2). Such interactions frequently determine the rate at which drugs are absorbed from the gastrointestinal tract, transported to tissues and eliminated from the body. Drug protein interactions are usually reversible, with the free drug in plasma being in equilibrium with that in tissue fluids. Protein energy malnutrition alters plasma and tissue proteins quantitatively and probably also qualitatively. Association (binding) of drugs with proteins, particularly albumin and tissue proteins, is of importance in drug distribution and influences drug delivery to receptor sites of action and to metabolic sites of elimination. Albumin is the main binding protein in plasma and hypoalbuminaemia is a characteristic finding in malnutrition. The rate of albumin synthesis is directly related to the level of protein intake and amino acid supply (Waterlow, 1975). The profile of plasma proteins (albumin, globulins and other carrier proteins) is altered in protein energy malnutrition. Glycoproteins, particularly α_1-acid glycoproteins which transport basic drugs, are also likely to be altered in malnutrition. The relationship of concentration of free drug to total drug may vary as a function of drug concentration, total protein concentration and albumin concentration. However, other physicochemical and pharmacokinetic properties also influence disposition of the drug and the magnitude of its pharmacological activity (see chapter I; sect. 3.2.3). Almost every drug exerts its pharmacological effect by interacting with some kind of protein in the body.

Since infectious diseases are very common in tropical countries and a number of antibiotics are commonly employed in their treatment, it is important to discuss the clinical relevance of antimicrobial therapy in relation to plasma protein binding. The effect of protein binding on the *in vitro* activity of antimicrobial agents in serum has been extensively studied (Craig and Kunin, 1976 ; Craig and Welling, 1977). It is reasonably clear from many observations, that only the free drug in serum is available for antimicrobial action. Therefore, changes in binding of antimicrobial agents to serum proteins would be expected to influence the therapeutic effect *in vivo*. It is difficult to generalise on the influence of changes in binding on drug disposition and response. It will be determined by a number of other factors like the physicochemical properties of the drug, ability of the drug to bind to tissue proteins and cellular membranes which will determine cellular transport, elimination and toxicity, and importantly on inter-related kinetic processes of clearance (see chapter I; sect. 3.2.3, 4.3.2).

Recent work by Buchanan (1977) has indicated that protein binding *in vitro* of a number of drugs such as salicylate, warfarin, digoxin, thiopentone is altered in malnourished children. However, the clinical implications, particularly in actual clinical use situations, have yet to be evaluated in most cases.

2.2.3 Drug Biotransformation

Drugs and other compounds which are foreign to the body (xenobiotics) have to be eliminated from the body. Most drugs are metabolised in the liver by metabolising enzymes present in the microsomal, mitochondrial and soluble fractions (see chapter I; sect. 3.3). Therapeutic efficacy and toxicity of such drugs are directly related to their rate of metabolism by the liver.

The implications of liver disease in relation to drug therapy are obvious and need not be elaborated here (see chapter XIX; sect. 1.3, 1.4, 13.4). However, it is important to discuss the common liver diseases or conditions with liver involvement which are encountered in tropical countries. These may be broadly divided into four groups; (a) malnutrition; (b) parasitic infestation; (c) liver injury due to mycotoxins; and (d) cirrhosis and/or malignancy. Malnutrition, as already discussed, is a major public health problem in tropical countries and fatty infiltration with impaired synthesis of lipoproteins is a characteristic feature in severe protein calorie malnutrition (Krishnaswamy, 1978). More commonly, however, one encounters only vacuolation in the liver. Involvement of the endoplasmic reticulum is also one of the features in protein energy malnutrition (Bhamarapravati, 1975). Therefore, it is important to evaluate whether such changes impair the mixed function oxidases involved in drug metabolism. The literature is replete with evidence that nutritional constraints in experimental animals impair drug metabolising enzymes (Campbell, 1977). However, studies in experimental animals cannot be directly extrapolated to man because of large species variation in drug metabolising enzymes. Nevertheless, studies in human subjects (Krishnaswamy and Naidu, 1977) with varying grades of malnutrition do indicate that the mixed function oxidase system may be affected in severe malnutrition. Vitamin C and iron deficiency have been shown to result in altered antipyrine kinetics in human subjects; iron deficiency anaemia resulting in accelerated metabolism and vitamin C deficiency resulting in a decreased rate of metabolism (Langman and Smithard, 1977; Smithard and Langman, 1978; see also chapter XXIII, sect. 1.4). However, administration of vitamin C which is sulphated in the body, has been shown to prolong the half-life of paracetamol in man by competing for available sulphate (Houston and Levy, 1976).

Nutritional-pharmacological interaction is a relatively young field of science and only very recently have nutritionists become aware of such interactions (Hathcock and Coon, 1978). The long term sequelae, particularly the possible development of cirrhosis consequent to severe malnutrition, has long been debated. The relationship between malnutrition and liver diseases has been overemphasised (Rubin and Lieber, 1968). Several studies show that there is in fact no cause and effect relationship (Ramalingaswami and Nayak, 1970; Keet et al., 1971). However, cirrhosis of the liver is commonly encountered in adults in the tropics. In addition, Indian childhood cirrhosis and idiopathic portal hypertension predominate in cer-

tain areas. Naturally occuring hepatotoxins especially aflatoxin as well as viral hepatitis and probably a host of other unknown factors may be aetiologically related. Liver function, particularly in relation to drug biotransformation in such situations, may be impaired. Hepatic blood flow and hepatic extraction of drugs may also be different in such conditions (see also chapter XIX; sect. 1.4).

Haemochromatosis, parasitic diseases with liver involvement (amoebiasis, leishmaniasis, schistosomiasis) and yellow fever may considerably modify drug metabolism, depending on the duration and degree of infection and concomitant pathological changes. In *Schistosoma mansoni* infection portal systemic vascular shunts can develop through which drugs can initially bypass the liver. In such cases, oral bioavailability of highly extracted drugs such as niridazole will be markedly increased (section 6.3.3; chapter XIX, sect. 1.4). The prevalence of hepatic carcinoma (primary) is highest in African countries. Mycotoxins, particularly aflatoxin and its association with malignancy, has been repeatedly stressed. Aflatoxin itself is metabolised by the liver enzymes and has an inhibitory effect on carcinogen metabolism (Gurtoo et al., 1968). The effects on drug and xenobiotic metabolism will obviously be determined by factors such as the quantum and the duration of exposure and the inherent capacity to eliminate the toxin.

It is obvious that in tropical countries, a number of factors can modify the mixed function oxidase drug metabolising enzyme system and therefore drug response. Only future studies can clarify the nature of and the mechanisms involved and establish a basis for rational use of drugs.

2.2.4 Excretion of Drugs

The two most important organs involved in the excretion of foreign compounds are the liver and the kidney. As mentioned in section 2.2.3, liver involvement can modify hepatobiliary excretion and enterohepatic circulation of drugs, particularly in cases with obstructive pathology. Similarly, tropical diseases can result in kidney involvement (renal lithiasis) and have the potential to interfere with glomerular filtration, tubular secretion and reabsorption of drugs eliminated by renal mechanisms; depending on the protein binding of the drug, renal plasma flow, urinary pH and the extent of tubular involvement (reabsorption). *Schistosoma haematobium* infection for example,

Table III. Consequences of altered pharmacokinetics in a tropical environment

1. Altered drug plasma concentration
2. Alteration in clinical response
3. Changes in incidence of toxic and adverse drug reactions, including drug interactions
4. Increased susceptibility to organ damage

is often complicated by abnormal kidney function and some of the drugs used for treatment such as antimonials are largely eliminated unchanged in the urine, necessitating assessment of renal function and great care with dosage. See further chapter I (sect. 3.4) and XXI (sect. 1.4).

2.2.5 Consequences of Altered Pharmacokinetics

Changes in pharmacokinetics of drugs will ultimately be reflected in altered blood concentrations and clinical response. Associated with these, the incidence of adverse reactions and drug interaction with some drugs and susceptibility to organ damage due to genetic variation and nutritional influences for example, may all be expected to be different in a tropical environment (table III).

Drug response in a tropical environment will ultimately be the net result of a number of influencing factors including malnutrition and the type and degree of malnutrition; co-existing disorders; the genetic constitution and age of the patient; the environment in terms of exposure to chemicals and other pollutants; and the physicochemical properties and pharmacokinetic characteristics of the particular drug (fig. 2). The extent of change in pharmacokinetics will certainly determine the drug dosage regimen. Tissue response to the drug may also be altered in a tropical environment.

2.3 Altered Tissue Responsiveness to Drugs as Influenced by a Tropical Environment

One of the most difficult areas of study in clinical pharmacology is to quantitate the effect of drugs in relation to plasma concentrations so as to indicate tissue uptake and response to the therapeutic agent. Apart from clinical response, there are very few pharmacodynamic studies in human subjects. Clinical response is determined by a number of factors and hence objective methods of

evaluation have to be developed for each drug before one can talk about tissue response. However, a few studies indicate that disposition of drugs can be altered by factors such as infection and pyrexia.

In acute falciparum malaria, the hepatic metabolism of quinine is impaired leading to higher plasma concentrations and more frequent side effects, probably as a consequence of higher tissue uptake of the drug (Trenholme et al., 1976). Influenza A and adenovirus infection have been shown to prolong theophylline half-life during the acute stage of the infection and increase the risk of toxicity (Chang et al., 1978). In undernutrition, tissue uptake of tetracycline has been shown to be poor (Shastri and Krishnaswamy, 1976). In febrile conditions, due to cardiovascular changes associated with fever, gentamicin blood levels are lower due to a shift of the drug from plasma to other body fluid compartments (Pennigton et al., 1975), which may result in therapeutic failure. The hypotensive response to propranolol seems to be less in Kenyan subjects, particularly in the presence of severe undernutrition (Obel and Vere, 1978). Similarly, some Negro patients require a higher dose of prazosin to control blood pressure than Caucasian hypertensives (Falase et al., 1976; Mroczek et al., 1974), probably indicating a higher tissue requirement. Such isolated studies indicate an altered tissue response which may not necessarily be accompanied by changes in kinetics.

3. Protein Calorie Deficiency

Protein calorie or protein energy malnutrition (PCM, PEM) is one of the most important and widespread nutritional disorders, accounting for high child mortality and morbidity (for review, see Gopalan and Srikantia, 1973; Olson, 1977). It includes many different clinical syndromes all of which are accompanied by retardation of growth and development, with protean manifestations. As the name implies, it is due to inadequate food intake. Both calories and proteins are inadequate and chronic dietary inadequacy over a period of time results in the extreme forms of malnutrition in children — kwashiorkor and marasmus. The interplay between malnutrition and infection is of considerable importance in developing countries; one leading to the other through a vicious cycle.

The other accompanying features like anaemia, dehydration due to gastrointestinal disorders, concomitant infections and infestation and co-existing deficiencies will determine the morbidity and mortality pattern. Apart from protein energy malnutrition in children, famine oedema or war oedema is frequently seen in the same population in adults due to chronic starvation.

The main aim in management of protein energy malnutrition is to feed the child a high calorie, high protein diet. Co-existent electrolyte, mineral and vitamin deficiencies also require appropriate therapy. Acute infections, respiratory and gastrointestinal, need to be treated. Chronic infections like pulmonary tuberculosis need prolonged therapy. The following measures are usually adopted in hospital based therapy.

1) The calorie requirement of children suffering from protein calorie malnutrition is twice that recommended for normal children of the same age. Each child should be given about 200kcal/kg body weight/day. About 40% of calories can be derived from fat, so that the bulk of food to be consumed will be small.

2) Protein intake should be around 4g/kg bodyweight/day. Skimmed milk and whole milk will be a very good source of protein. However, the availability and the cost are the limiting factors. Hence diets based on locally available food materials (cereals and food legumes) are the best sources of protein and calories, although recovery may be slightly delayed on a vegetable protein combination. The advantages of these sources of protein are that they are inexpensive, locally available and also find ready cultural acceptance. On a long term basis, diets based on vegetable foods are essentially as satisfactory as diets based on animal proteins.

3) Almost all patients recover on oral feeding with a few exceptions. Parenteral feeding is indicated only in very severe cases of gastrointestinal disorder. In fact, large infusions are dangerous in a wasted child and man, since there is evidence to suggest that the myocardium may be damaged in protein energy malnutrition (Smythe et al., 1962). One of the most important complications of rapid refeeding, particularly in adults on parenteral therapy, is congestive cardiac failure and pulmonary oedema.

4) In severe cases of dehydration due to diarrhoea, electrolyte and intravenous fluids are indicated. Potassium and magnesium depletion is a frequent occurrence among such patients. Therefore, potassium and also magnesium, should be administered in appropriate amounts.

5) Vitamin supplements, particularly vitamin A and B complex vitamins, are necessary since children with protein energy malnutrition manifest signs and symptoms of vitamin deficiencies. All these nutrients are required for proper func-

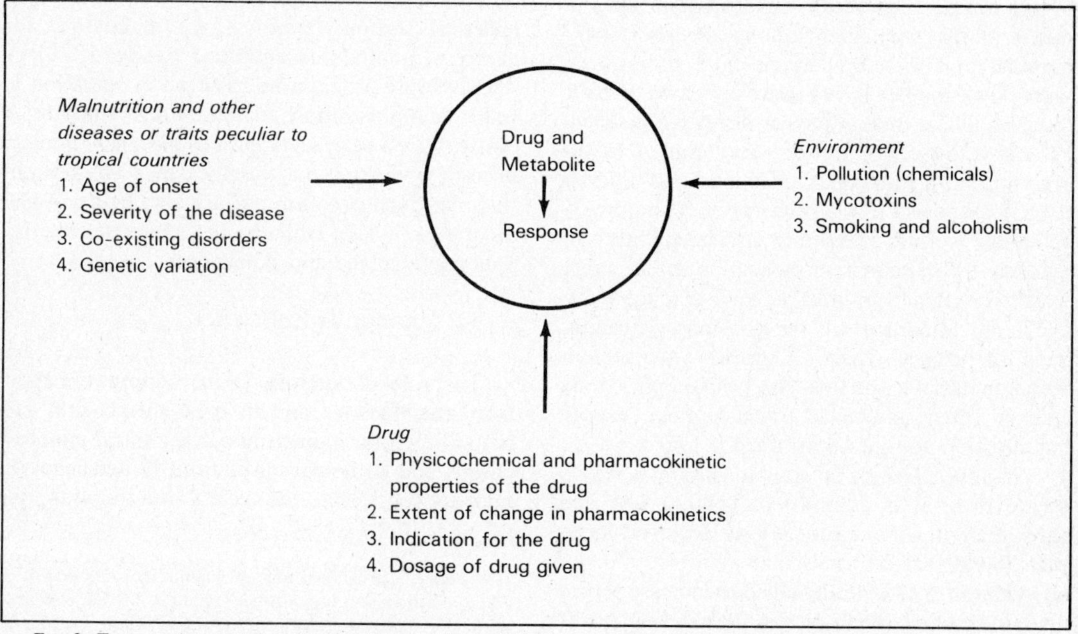

Fig. 2. Factors determining drug response (therapeutic and toxic) in a tropical environment.

tion of new tissue generated during recovery and subsequent growth.

6) Anaemias accompanying protein deficiency deserve special mention. Apart from proteins *per se,* iron, folic acid, vitamin E and recently vitamin A have all been shown to be related to haemoglobin regeneration in protein energy malnutrition.

7) Administration of antibiotics and/or other drugs depends on the type of infection/infestation as well as the severity of infection. There is a close relationship between recovery from infection and nutritional rehabilitation.

8) Use of drugs in general in patients with protein energy malnutrition and the potential for altered pharmacokinetics or tissue response are discussed in section 2.

4. Vitamin Deficiencies

4.1 Vitamin A Deficiency

4.1.1 Clinical Pharmacological Aspects

Human vitamin A deficiency has a global distribution and is one of the most important aetiological factors contributing towards 'preventable blindness', particularly in young children in all developing countries. Inadequate intake of vitamin A is the primary cause for the widespread prevalence of vitamin A deficiency. Dietary intake of vitamin A in general is inadequate in all segments of the population among the poor communities and therefore infants born to mothers with low intake have relatively low hepatic reserves. These infants further develop a deficiency due to low concentration of vitamin A in the breast milk. In addition, infections and infestations impair vitamin A absorption. Vitamin A deficiency is more commonly associated with protein calorie malnutrition, which is much more widely prevalent. Conjunctival xerosis, bitot spots, and night blindness are the commonly encountered deficiency signs. Corneal involvement (keratomalacia) is the final stage of xerophthalmia and is often associated with protein energy malnutrition and infection (Reddy, 1978).

Vitamin A being a fat soluble vitamin is stored in the liver. It is administered both orally and parenterally for therapeutic effect. However, it has been found that intramuscular administration of oily vitamin A (30,000µg) failed to increase serum vitamin A levels in children suffering from PEM (Reddy and Srikantia, 1966). In contrast, in tramuscular injections of water miscible vitamin A resulted in a rapid and striking increase in serum vitamin A levels[1].

A single injection of 30,000µg of water miscible vitamin A will result in rapid clinical improvement; corneal xerosis improves and vision is normalised within a few days after the dose. Conjunctival lesions and night blindness respond to a dose of 1000µg daily for a week. However, in severe cases involving the cornea, parenteral preparations (water misible) are indicated, since a number of children have associated gastroenteritis. Corneal involvement further requires local treatment with antibiotics for prevention and control of secondary infection.

4.1.2 Prevention and Prophylaxis

Since inadequate dietary intake of vitamin A (both pre-formed and provitamin) is the major aetiological factor, the most rational approach for the control and prevention would be to improve the diet. Consumption of inexpensive and rich sources of β-carotene like green leaf vegetables, should be encouraged in the population. This, however, involves nutrition education and at present may be considered as a long term approach.

Since vitamin A can be stored in the body, massive doses (60,000µg) can be administered at infrequent intervals for a prolonged effect. With such doses, more than 50 % is retained in the body (Reddy and Sivakumar, 1972) and significant levels of serum vitamin A are maintained for nearly 6 months (Srikantia and Reddy, 1970). A massive dose programme has been in operation in India (administration of 60,000µg vitamin A orally twice a year) and indicates that there is a significant reduction in the incidence of xerophthalmia. Such programmes are also being implemented on a large scale in other countries like Indonesia, Thailand and Bangladesh.

4.2 Vitamin D Deficiency

The role of vitamin D in calcium transport from the intestine and in bone metabolism has been known for a long time. The clinical manifestations and pathology of vitamin D deficiency in man are confined to the skeletal and the muscular

---

1 One international unit of vitamin A is equivalent to 0.3µg of retinol, 0.344µg of retinyl acetate, 0.55µg of retinyl palmitate, 0.6µg of β-carotene or 1.2µg of provitamin A carotenoids other than β-carotene.

system. Rickets and osteomalacia are disorders of phosphorus and calcium metabolism, characterised by defective mineralisation and resulting in bending and distortion of bones, skeletal deformities and tetanic spasms of muscles. Dietary deficiency, defective absorption, liver abnormalities and renal defects can lead to vitamin D deficiency. Vitamin D resistant rickets due to a genetically determined metabolic abnormality have also been described.

Recent research has shown that cholecalciferol (vitamin D_3), synthesised in the skin, is converted to 25-hydroxycholecalciferol (calcifediol) in the liver, which is then further hydroxylated in the kidney to the active hormone $1\alpha,25$ dihydroxycholecalciferol (1,25 DHCC or calcitriol). Calciferol (vitamin D_2) from the diet is also metabolised in an identical manner. $1\alpha,25$ dihydroxycholecalciferol is necessary for the synthesis of a (binding) protein in the intestine which is responsible for calcium absorption (Deluca, 1975).

Vitamin D may be administered orally or parenterally. Oral administration has been found to be quite effective as a cure of rickets. Daily administration of 1500 to 5000IU of vitamin D_2 (calciferol) will produce healing, demonstrable on x-ray, within 2 to 4 weeks. Parenteral administration is indicated in cases of malabsorption. Massive doses of calciferol (600,000 IU) in 2 or 3 divided doses at fortnightly intervals have also been tried in cure of rickets.

Although vitamin D is a good therapeutic agent for dietary deficiency, in cases of chronic liver disease and renal failure, it is obvious that the biologically active metabolites of vitamin D will be more beneficial. Direct administration of the metabolites of vitamin D, 25-hydroxycholecalciferol or $1\alpha,25$ dihydroxycholecalciferol, will also help in the treatment of rickets and osteomalacia resistant to calciferol. The more readily synthesised 1α-hydroxycholecalciferol or alfacalcidol (1 to $2\mu g/day$), an analogue of $1\alpha,25$ dihydroxycholecalciferol (calcitriol), and calcitriol itself (1 to $1.5\mu g/day$) are being increasingly used to promote calcium absorption, particularly in the osteodystrophy of chronic renal failure (Chalmer et al., 1973; Madsen et al., 1978; see chapter XXI, sect. 9.6)

4.3 Vitamin B Complex Deficiencies

Vitamin B complex deficiency diseases such as beri beri, pellagra, orolingual lesions, peripheral neuropathy and central nervous system manifestations contribute significantly towards morbidity among the poorer segments of the population in developing countries. The prevalence of clinical and subclinical deficiency of these vitamins is very high, particularly in the vulnerable segment of the population such as pregnant and lactating women, children of growing age and during adolescence. Certain clinical symptoms such as the neurological manifestations, with or without oral lesions, are often encountered in the adult segment of the population. The main aetiological factors of vitamin B complex deficiency disorders are inadequate intake, malabsorption due to a number of aetiopathological factors (malabsorption syndromes), excessive requirement during certain physiological stress situations (pregnancy, fever), increased excretion due to tissue depletion as a result of diseases and drugs, and rarely due to defective utilisation of the vitamin.

4.3.1 Thiamine Deficiency

The severe forms of thiamine (aneurine or vitamin B_1) deficiency leads to the disease beri beri, which has diverse manifestations. It may present as cardiac beri beri (acute and chronic forms), atrophic beri beri or polyneuritis, infantile beri beri, Wernicke's encephalopathy and/or Korsakoff's psychosis. The disease is encountered, either in rice eating populations of Southeast Asian countires, or in chronic alcoholics.

Thiamine is absorbed from the upper small intestine by a specialised saturable transport process. Oral doses above 2.5mg appear to be largely unabsorbed (Campbell and Morrison, 1963). The capacity to retain thiamine is also low. Alcoholism and concomitant folate deficiency decrease thiamine absorption. Although both riboflavine and thiamine are absorbed by saturable intestinal transport mechanisms, the two vitamins do not share a common specialised absorption pathway (Levy and Hewitt, 1971). Certain thiamine derivatives, like thiamine allyl disulphide, thiamine propyl disulphide, S-diacetyl thiamine and O,S-dibenzoyl thiamine, are absorbed more easily than thiamine hydrochloride (Thompson et al., 1971) and are useful in the treatment of thiamine deficiency where a rapid and sustained response is needed.

Thiamine in doses of 5 to 10mg is curative for most manifestations. Larger doses by the oral or parenteral route may be wasted. Treatment may be necessary for 4 to 6 weeks, depending on the deficiency and the type of clinical manifestation.

4.3.2 Riboflavine Deficiency

The clinical manifestations of ariboflavinosis are the orolingual lesions, seborrhoeic dermatitis and scrotal dermatitis. Riboflavine (vitamin B_2) is absorbed from the proximal part of the intestine, which is again a capacity limited process. The absorption of riboflavine is increased in the presence of food (Jusko and Levy, 1968). The transport, distribution and elimination are determined by the extent of its binding to plasma proteins. If a large dose is administered, nearly all of it is recovered in the urine. The renal clearance of riboflavine exceeds the glomerular filtration rate, suggesting that renal tubular secretion of riboflavine occurs.

Clinical recovery is complete with doses of 5 to 10mg/day over a period of 14 to 21 days. Derivatives such as riboflavine tetrabutyrate and riboflavine tetranicotinate appear as promising agents in therapy, since blood levels are better maintained and urinary excretion is slower as compared with free riboflavine (Yagi, 1972).

4.3.3 Vitamin B_6 Deficiency

The prevalence of vitamin B_6 deficiency in humans is not well documented. Oral lesions, convulsions in infants (pyridoxine dependent), peripheral neuropathy and sideroblastic anaemias (pyridoxine dependent), dermatitis and behavioural changes have been reported to occur in pyridoxine deficiency (natural or induced).

Pyridoxine, pyridoxal and pyridoxamine are equally utilised and are rapidly absorbed by passive diffusion from the jejunum. More than 30% of vitamin B_6 in plasma is in the form of pyridoxal phosphate and is bound to albumin. The tissue content of pyridoxal phosphate is regulated by the binding of this coenzyme with the protein moiety (Lakshmi and Bamji, 1975). Riboflavine and pyridoxine are closely inter-related and clinical signs and response are identical, irrespective of whether pyridoxine or riboflavine is administered in cases of oral lesions (Krishnaswamy, 1971). The biochemical basis for these deficiencies has been recently reviewed by Bamji and Faizy (1978).

Although clinical signs of pyridoxine deficiency are not clearly delineated, pyridoxine has been used for treating a number of clinical disorders like hyperemesis in pregnancy, myoclonic epilepsy, muscular dystrophy, depression induced by oral contraceptives, homocystinuria and cystathioninuria.

Pyridoxine in doses of 20 to 50mg by the oral or parenteral route has been used to treat various clinical conditions. Conditions, which are pyridoxine dependent, however, require larger amounts (100 to 200mg).

4.3.4 Nicotinic Acid Deficiency

Nicotinic acid (niacin) deficiency results in a clinical disorder called pellagra which is characterised by bilateral symmetrical dermatitis on the exposed extensor surfaces, orolingual manifestations, gastrointestinal disturbances and dementia. Nicotinic acid is absorbed readily from the intestinal tract. Storage in the body is not large. It is metabolised in the body and the metabolites are excreted in urine. Nicotinic acid is present in tissues, largely as coenzymes nicotinamide-adenine dinucleotide (NAD) and nicotinamide-adenine dinucleotide phosphate (NADP). It is administered in doses of 50 to 300mg for treating pellagra. All the manifestations respond to therapy and 4 to 6 weeks therapy is required for complete clinical cure.

4.4 Vitamin C Deficiency

Severe vitamin C (ascorbic acid) deficiency leads to scurvy in man and is characterised by weakness, anaemia, spongy gums, mucocutaneous and subperiosteal haemorrhages, pseudoparalysis and marked irritability. Repeated infections are common in vitamin C deficiency.

In man, absorption of ascorbic acid occurs mainly from the proximal part of the small intestine by a non-passive saturable process (Hornig, 1975). In the blood, ascorbic acid is almost exclusively present in its reduced form. It is excreted as oxalic acid, unchanged ascorbic acid and very little as dehydroascorbic acid.

Oral administration gives satisfactory results. Scurvy responds to as little as 10mg of ascorbic acid daily. However, in infants, 100 to 200mg daily in divided doses will produce clinical response much faster. Vitamin C in large doses has been used for a variety of diseases like the common cold (see chapter XXVIII; sect. 3.2.2), atherosclerosis, infections and fluorosis, with doubtful clinical efficacy.

4.5 Toxic Reactions Associated with Excessive Intake of Vitamins

Although vitamin deficiency states are of prime concern, it is also important to consider the possible effects of excessive vitamin intake within the body. Toxic manifestations are more often encountered with fat soluble vitamins (e.g. A,D,E), since water soluble vitamins (e.g. B,C) have a renal threshold and consequently excess results in urinary elimination. The following toxic manifestations have been described (see Dipalma and Ritchie, 1977).

Vitamin A: Increased intracranial pressure associated with headache, vomiting, drowsiness, bulging of fontanelles, diplopia and papilloedema occur in acute hypervitaminosis A (dose $>$ 300,000IU). Chronic hypervitaminosis A manifests as anorexia, pruritus increased irritability, swelling of bones, seborrhoeic cutaneous lesions and hepatomegaly. X-rays reveal hyperosteosis (after ingestion of excessive doses for several weeks or months).

Vitamin D: Symptoms develop after 1 to 3 months of large intakes of vitamin D (e.g. $>$ 4000IU daily). They include hypotonia, anorexia, irritability, constipation, polydipsia and polyuria. Hypercalcaemia and hypercalciuria are characteristic features. Aortic valvular stenosis may occur. X-rays reveal metastatic calcification and generalised osteoporosis.

Thiamine: Anaphylactic reactions have been described due to sensitisation to the vitamin. Toxic doses of thiamine affect the cardiovascular system, producing symptoms of peripheral circulatory failure (Haley and Flesher, 1946).

Nicotinic acid in doses of 50 and 100mg produces flushing and pruritus, whereas nicotinamide is free from such reactions. The most common serious toxicities reported for nicotinic acid are abnormal liver function and jaundice with doses of 3g daily for at least a year.

Ascorbic acid: Excess vitamin C (1 to 3g daily) may result in acidosis, gastrointestinal complaints, glycosuria, oxaluria, renal stones (particularly in subjects prone to develop oxalosis, hyperuricaemia and cystinuria) and a state of conditioned need.

5. Anaemias

Nutritional anaemias are highly prevalent almost all over the world. Iron deficiency anaemia is one of the important public health problems facing many developing countries. Anaemias due to deficiency of folate/vitamin B_{12} are also common in underdeveloped or developing countries, as well as in some well developed countries.

5.1 Iron Deficiency Anaemias

Dietary inadequacy, poor absorption of iron from diets primarily based on plant foods, hookworm infestation and repeated pregnancies are common causes of iron deficiency in the tropics and subtropics. As in developed countries, the majority of patients can be treated with oral iron. Most will respond readily to the cheapest preparation, ferrous sulphate. If side effects are troublesome, ferrous gluconate may be tried. Ferrous fumarate and ferrous succinate are alternative choices. The properties and dosage of the various oral iron preparations and the limited indications for parenteral iron are discussed in chapter XXIII (sect. 6.1.1.).

In view of the widespread nature of iron deficiency, in tropical countries, it is important that major public health measures are undertaken to prevent anaemias. Routine iron supplementation to pregnant women and preschool children, in whom anaemia is a serious problem, has been advocated. Yet another practical measure to combat anaemia is fortification of foods with iron. A number of vehicles have been proposed and used for iron fortification in several countries. In India, common salt appears to be a suitable vehicle since it is universally consumed and centrally processed and produced in bulk quantities. Iron salts selected for this purpose have to be stable, colourless and availability should be satisfactory when ingested with food. Recent studies indicate that ferric orthophosphate, together with a promotor of absorption like sodium sulphate, is ideal for salt fortification (Narasinga Rao, 1978). Preliminary community trials have revealed satisfactory results.

5.2 Folate Deficiency Anaemia

Deficiency of folic acid leads to megaloblastic anaemia, which is quite often seen in pregnant women and in infants and children in tropical countries (due to dietary deficiency or increased requirements of folate as a consequence of malarial haemolysis or haemoglobinopathies), in malabsorption syndromes and in patients on anticonvulsant drugs. Megaloblastic anaemia may also occur in association with poverty, malnutrition and infection/infestations. Folic acid is rapidly absorbed from the upper part of the small intestine (jejunum) by active transport. About 65% of folic acid in plasma is protein bound and the free folate is cleared by the kidney by glomerular filtration. There is a tubular reabsorption of folate at plasma concentrations less than 10ng/ml.

Folic acid in large doses is cleared at a fast rate and is excreted. A dose of 5mg of folate by mouth once daily is more than adequate, even in patients with malabsorption. The duration of folate therapy depends on the nature of the underlying disorder. Long term folic acid administration is indicated only in sickle cell anaemias and thalassaemias. In tropical countries, prophylactic doses of folic acid (300µg) are required for prevention of pregnancy anaemias (Iyengar and Rajalakshmi, 1975).

Although folic acid is relatively non-toxic, a few examples of sensitivity reactions to folic acid in man have been recorded. Long term folate therapy may increase fit frequency in some epileptics and precipitate vitamin B_{12} neuropathy in some cases of megaloblastic anaemias (see chapter XXIII; sect. 6.1.3, 8.5).

5.3 Vitamin B_{12} Deficiency Anaemia

Vitamin B_{12} deficiency in man is either due to dietary inadequacy, malabsorption or to pernicious anaemia, which is the main form of megaloblastic anaemia in Western populations. Dietary inadequacy of vitamin B_{12} occurs only among vegetarian populations, since there are absolutely no plant sources of vitamin B_{12}. However, vitamin B_{12} deficiency is not as common as other vitamin B complex deficiencies in those living in a tropical environment; possibly due to poor hygiene vitamin B_{12} synthesised by bacteria may be available to this population. Pernicious anaemia on the other hand is a genetically determined disorder, characterised by failure to absorb vitamin B_{12}. Other aetiological factors include gastrectomy and ile-ectomy anaemias, intestinal disorders like tropical sprue, blind loop syndromes, fish tape worm infestation, and some drugs which interfere with absorption (chapter XXIII; sect. 8.5). In addition to anaemias, neurological manifestations are encountered in vitamin B_{12} deficiency. Treatment is discussed in chapter XXIII (sect. 6.1.2)

6. Tropical Parasitic Infections

Parasitic infestation is usually taken to imply infection caused by protozoa and helminths. They are prevalent under conditions of overcrowding, poverty and poor sanitation. Although parasitic infestations usually are not responsible for producing a fulminant, life threatening situation, the potential hazards of such infections lie in their marked and chronic effects on nutrition, growth and mental acuity. The chronic disability may have far reaching effects on society in hyperendemic areas where there is substantial undernutrition as well. Treatment of tropical parasitic diseases is complicated by a number of factors. Firstly, the size of the population infected with parasites is enormous. Secondly, the possibility of frequent reinfection is always present as long as the environmental conditions permit repeated exposure. Mass treatment and control measures must, as far as possible, run in parallel. However, treatment is not always successful because patients are often not sufficiently well educated to understand the need for prolonged therapy. Non-compliance with the treatment programme is the rule rather than the exception.

Since there are still no effective immunisation procedures for protection against protozoa and helminthic diseases, clinicians must rely on drugs for treatment. Unfortunately, many of the drugs used are toxic both to the parasite and the host and their mechanisms of action are little known in most cases. With some drugs, such as antimonials and arsenicals, the toxic dose for man is near the therapeutic dose. Since many patients with parasitic infestations also suffer from malnutrition, the use of toxic antiparasitic drugs becomes more hazardous as these patients are more liable to suffer from severe adverse drug reactions as a result of alteration of drug response (see section 2.2). It is clear that many of the existing toxic antiparasitic drugs should be replaced by better and safer remedies. Although drugs available for amoebiasis and most intestinal helminthic infestations are relatively effective and safe (see chapter XIX; sect. 11.3, 11.4), unfortunately, despite the claim that many new, less toxic and more selective antiparasitic drugs have recently been produced (Van den Bossche, 1978), progress in chemotherapy of the tropical parasitic diseases is not as yet encouraging. Such pessimism was first voiced by the World Health Organisation in 1976 that 'No major new drugs for the treatment of any of the tropical diseases have been produced within the past three decades' (WHO, 1976). This lack of interest in the chemotherapy of tropical parasitic diseases is well illustrated by the fact that US $800 million were allocated for cancer research in the

amounts of the drug can penetrate the cerebrospinal fluid. The mechanism of action is still unknown but its ability to interact with sulphydryl groups in the cells of the parasites may explain its trypanocidal action. Integrity of sulphydryl groups is essential in maintaining the appropriate structure and consequently the functions of a number of enzymes.

Melarsoprol is usually administered slowly by intravenous infusion. It should be given through a fine needle and extravasation avoided since it is intensely irritating. The drug is excreted rapidly and this limits its use in prophylaxis.

Melarsoprol therapy is often accompanied by a number of side effects which include hypertension, abdominal pain, vomiting, proteinuria, peripheral neuropathy, arthralgia, angioneurotic oedema and rashes. Toxic encephalopathy is the most common and it occurred in about 12.5% of patients in one large study (Robertson, 1963). This condition may be fatal in severe cases. In view of the many and sometimes fatal complications, patients should be hospitalised and remain in bed while on treatment and the condition of the patient should be closely monitored.

6.3.10 Suramin

Suramin, a benzidine derivative, has been used in the treatment of both types of African trypanosomiasis in the early stages of the disease. It is also effective in the treatment of onchocerciasis when used together with diethylcarbamazine (section 6.4.3). The mechanism of action of suramin is unknown. However, it does inhibit a variety of enzyme systems forming firm complexes with the protein (Rollo, 1975).

Suramin is not absorbed following oral administration and it must be administered intravenously. It binds firmly with plasma proteins and it, therefore, can persist for as long as 3 months in the blood. The drug is excreted very slowly in unchanged form by the kidney. The slow release from plasma proteins and slow renal excretion permit the drug to be administered on a bimonthly basis which is valuable in the prophylaxis of trypanosomiasis. It is usually given by slow intravenous injection in a 10% aqueous solution. It does not cross the blood-brain barrier, therefore it is of no value in treating trypanosomiasis when the central nervous system is affected.

Suramin is a very toxic drug and adverse reactions are many and often serious in patients who are malnourished. Nausea, vomiting and serious reactions like hypotension or even shock can occur immediately after too rapid an intravenous injection. Therefore, it is wise to give a 100 to 200mg test dose to assess the patient's tolerance. Later reactions include skin eruptions, paraesthesiae, photophobia, lacrimation, haematuria and proteinuria. If heavy proteinuria or casts appear during treatment, suramin should be discontinued. It is nephrotoxic and should therefore be used with great caution in patients with impaired renal function.

6.4 Treatment of Filariasis

Filariasis is a group of disorders produced by infection with the threadlike nematodes of the *Filarioidea* family. Lymphatic filariasis is caused by *Wuchereria bancrofti* and *Brugia malayi*, the organism responsible for lymphatic blockade and elephantiasis. *Loa loa* causes loiasis, a disease characterised by transient subcutaneous swellings (calabar) and *Onchocerca volvulus* produces blindness and pruritic skin rashes.

6.4.1 Lymphatic Filariasis

Treatment aims to eliminate the adult worms and to alleviate any lymphoedema which may have resulted from their presence in the lymph nodes. Diethylcarbamazine is the most effective drug. It has a rapid destructive effect on microfilariae and a slower action on adult filariae. The initial dose is 50mg orally, which is increased to 9 to 12mg/kg body weight daily in 3 divided doses for 21 days. This course may be repeated twice at intervals of 4 to 6 weeks. Hypersensitivity reactions caused by diethylcarbamazine treatment sometimes occur (see section 6.3.1) and can be prevented by the administration of antihistamines or corticosteroids. Such reactions are more frequent and more severe in *B. malayi* infections than in those caused by *W. bancrofti* (Ramachandran and Dondero, 1976). Treatment with diethylcarbamazine, given early in the disease, produces cure and may lead to some improvement in recently established cases of elephantiasis. But long standing elephantiasis with fibrotic obliterative changes in the lymphatics will not be reversed, and in such cases plastic surgery is indicated.

6.4.2 Filariasis Due to Loa loa

Diethylcarbamazine gradually increased to a dose of 9 to 12mg/kg body weight daily and continued at that dosage for 21 days is curative. It leads to the death of microfilariae and adult *Loa loa* but unfortunately severe febrile reactions, joint and muscle pain, and toxic encephalopathy may occur. These reactions are poorly controlled by corticosteroids and antihistamines. Therefore, the initial dose should be small; i.e. 50mg and increased to the full dose very gradually over a period of 2 weeks.

6.4.3. Onchocerciasis

Any cutaneous and subcutaneous nodules detected should be removed by excision — this is especially important should any occur under the scalp, since the local liberation of microfilaria is likely to cause eye damage. Diethylcarbamazine rapidly kills the microfilariae which leads to an allergic reaction for the first few days of treatment (see section 6.3.1). Marked exacerbation of skin and eye lesions always accompanies early treatment, and hydrocortisone eye drops may be required to stop the eye irritation. Antihistamines, aspirin and occasionally topical corticosteroids may help to control pruritus and pain during this phase of treatment (Connor, 1978). Only a small dose of diethylcarbamazine should be given initially; 0.5mg/kg body weight on the first day, gradually increased as the drug is tolerated until, if possible, a dose of 12mg/kg body weight is reached. This dose should be continued for 21 days.

Since the adult worms are only moderately susceptible to diethylcarbamazine, some may survive one or more courses of therapy and recurrence of skin lesions occur. Suramin given intravenously may be necessary to prevent recurrence, as adult worms are killed effectively by this drug. The course of treatment consists of a weekly intravenous injection of 1g of suramin for a total of 6 or 7 injections. Alternatively, to avoid the potential toxicity of suramin (see section 6.3.10) which should be given only at centres experienced in its use, diethylcarbamazine may be administered at regular intervals to suppress the number of microfilariae sufficiently that no further serious or irreversible lesions will develop. In endemic areas where reinfection is inevitable, long term suppression with 100mg of diethylcarbamazine weekly may be undertaken.

6.5 Treatment of Schistosomiasis

Schistosomiasis is a geographically widely distributed worm infestation caused by three closely related species of trematodes — *Schistosoma haematobium, Schistosoma mansoni* and *Schistosoma japonicum.*

S. haematobium occurs primarily in Africa and the Middle East; *S. mansoni* in Africa, the Middle East, South America and the Carribbean and *S. japonicum* mainly in Japan, China and Southeast Asia. These parasites lodge themselves in the vesical plexus *(S. haematobium),* inferior mesenteric veins *(S. mansoni)* and superior mesenteric veins *(S. japonicum),* producing tissue injury and scarring as a result of the large numbers of eggs (and possibly other metabolic products) retained in the host tissues. The enzymatic, antigenic secretions of the eggs induce a marked granulomatous response of lymphocytes, eosinophils and macrophages; these large granulomatous lesions becoming permanent as they fibrose, thus obstructing blood flow (Mahmoud, 1977). In the liver, the block to the portal circulation may result in the formation of portal systemic shunts (see section 6.3.3).

Some of the eggs are excreted from the host in the urine (primarily *S. haematobium*) and faeces *(S. mansoni* and *S. japonicum),* but the majority are retained in the intestines, urinary tract and liver, and these are the tissues usually most severely damaged.

Since adult schistosomes do not multiply within man, but constantly produce eggs, quantitation of the infection through excreta egg counts is useful. Minimal infestations are often asymptomatic, and the object of treatment is therefore to markedly reduce the worm load. Treatment of asymptomatic patients with minimal egg counts (e.g. in *S. mansoni* infections less than 50 eggs per gram of faeces) may involve a higher risk from the therapeutic measures than that expected from the infestation (Mahmoud, 1977). In severe or advanced stages of schistosomiasis the best time for treatment should be determined by the general condition of the patient (Omer, 1978b). A high intensity infection is an indication for treatment, while in a patient with a low intensity infection whose general condition is poor the initial emphasis should be on improving the general condition before treating the infection. Intermediate situations require careful individual consideration before instituting a treatment programme. At present, drug treatment of schistosomiasis is aimed at the specific infecting species; there is no schistosomicide yet available which is satisfactory against all species.

6.5.1 Schistosoma mansoni

Antimonial drugs, emetine derivatives, lucanthone and niridazole are active against *S. mansoni,* but they are not as effective, convenient or as well tolerated as other newer agents, and have largely been replaced.

Oxamniquine is the preferred drug for treating *S. mansoni* infections (Omer, 1978a,b). It may be given as a single oral dose or in 2 divided doses on consecutive days, or may be given intramuscularly. The usual adult dosage in most areas is 15mg/kg while children should receive 20mg/kg; however, in Africa a much higher dose has often been required, some workers considering 60mg/kg to be the effective dose (Omer, 1978b). Since convulsions may follow oxamniquine administration, particularly in patients with a history of epilepsy, such patients should remain under supervision for several hours after a dose.

Hycanthone also has the advantage of being effective in a single dose; it should be given as an intramuscular injection of 3mg/kg of body weight which may be repeated after 3 months. Hycanthone may be less effective in young children than in adults (Prata, 1978). Since advanced stages of *S. mansoni* infections are usually characterised by hepatosplenic involvement, hycanthone which may be hepatotoxic (sect. 6.3.4) is better avoided in such cases. Vomiting induced by hycanthone should not be treated with phenothiazine drugs for fear of synergistic toxic effects on the liver.

Niridazole is also effective in *S. mansoni* infections provided the patient can be relied upon to complete a 7 to 10 day course of treatment. An oral dose of 25mg/kg of body weight daily in 3 divided doses for 7 days may be used, but 20mg/kg daily in 3 doses for 10 days may be more effective. Niridazole may produce central nervous system disturbances, such as psychoses or convulsions, particularly in patients with hepatic complications in whom portal systemic shunts have developed and it should thus be avoided in such patients (see section 6.3.3).

If economic or other practical considerations require the use of an antimonial drug rather than a newer agent, antimony dimercaptosuccinate (stibocaptate) may be given intramuscularly in a dosage of 6 to 8mg/kg (to a maximum of 500mg) once weekly for 5 to 7 weeks; 7 injections being preferable. Since antimonial drugs induce a very rapid hepatic 'drift' of the worms, more liver damage may occur in patients who already have hepatic involvement. The lower dosage range should be used in such patients. Although inclusion of dimercaprol in this drug has reduced the toxic effect of antimony, cardiotoxicity may nevertheless occur, and bed rest with medical supervision is thus advisable for 3 days after administration.

6.5.2 Schistosoma haematobium

Metrifonate is an effective and relatively safe drug for all stages of *S. haematobium* infections, and has the advantage of being very inexpensive. It is the preferred drug when *S. haematobium* is the primary contributing factor to the illness (Omer, 1978b). However, it has the disadvantage of requiring a month to complete a course of treatment; the dosage schedule being 7.5 to 10mg/kg orally once every 2 weeks for 3 doses. Metrifonate markedly depresses cholinesterase activity and may prolong the effect of the muscle relaxant drug suxamethonium (see section 6.3.5).

Hycanthone, niridazole or antimony dimercaptosuccinate are also effective when administered as above. Hycanthone has the important advantage of being a single dose treatment but should not be used in seriously ill patients with liver involvement (see section 6.3.4). Since abnormalities of the bladder, ureter and kidneys are often involved in *S. haematobium* infections and renal function may already be decreased, the use of antimonial drugs such as antimony dimercaptosuccinate, which are largely excreted unchanged by the kidneys, requires assessment of renal function and adjustment of dosage if renal function is impaired.

Niridazole may have an anti-inflammatory effect which is useful in resolving advanced granulomas. It is therefore recommended in patients with advanced lesions, especially when there is oedema or fibrosis of the lower ureter and associated urological complications.

6.5.3 Mixed Advanced Infections

The most appropriate treatment in patients with advanced disease infected with both *S. mansoni* and *S. haematobium* is less obvious, since the preferred drug in each individual infection is not usefully active against the other trematode. Other drugs with activity against both infecting agents are usually used (Omer, 1978b). If liver involvement is marked, hycanthone and niridazole are best avoided and an antimony drug used. If *S. haematobium* is the predominant infection, and complications of the urinary tract are primarily involved, niridazole should be used.

6.5.4 Schistosoma japonicum

None of the schistosomicides discussed in section 6.3 are entirely satisfactory in treating *S. japonicum* infections. Antimonial drugs in relatively high doses are effective in some cases, but adverse effects may be troublesome at the dosage required, resulting in a large proportion of patients defaulting from treatment (Yokogawa, 1976). *S. japonicum* is less sensitive to more complex trivalent antimonials, and antimony tartrate compounds are thus the preferred antimony drugs, despite their greater toxicity. An initial dose of 30mg of sodium antimony tartrate by slow intravenous injection followed by 60mg every other day for a total of at least 1.2g is used in Japan (Yokogawa, 1976). Alternatively, an initial dose of 15mg increased by 20mg increments to 140mg per dose may be given on alternate days, to a total dose of 1.8g (Katz, 1977). A more intensive course of treatment (a total of 6g given intramuscularly over 14 days) has been used in American military personnel with *S. japonicum* infections, with a cure rate of about 80% (Rollo, 1975).

Niridazole has been used in various dosage schedules in an attempt to find a satisfactory regimen in *S. japonicum* infections, but results have usually been disappointing, negative stools being achieved in about 40 to 50% of patients (Sy, 1977; Yokogawa, 1976).

As in *S. mansoni* infections, niridazole should not be used in patients with *S. japonicum* infections with hepatic complications (see section 6.3.3).

6.6 Treatment of Leishmaniasis

Leishmaniasis is a group of diseases caused by the protozoa of the genus *Leishmania* which are transmitted by the bite of sandflies (see Marsden, 1979). It has different forms. It can either be visceral or cutaneous. The former, also known as Kala-azar, is characterised by chronic recurrent fever, splenomegaly, weight loss and high mortality.

Cutaneous leishmaniasis may present as single or multiple skin ulcers, mucocutaneous lesions or a disseminated infection.

6.6.1 Visceral Leishmaniasis

Two groups of drugs, pentavalent antimonial compounds and aromatic diamidines, are effective in the treatment of visceral leishmaniasis. However, the response to treatment varies with the geographical area in which the disease has been acquired. In Asia, the disease is readily cured, but in East Africa and the Mediterranean area, it is more resistant to therapy. Sodium stibogluconate, a pentavalent antimony compound (see section 6.3.7), gives good results and is the drug of choice. The dose is 20mg/kg of body weight daily. A suitable course of treatment for an adult is 10 daily intravenous injections of 600mg of sodium stibogluconate.

This is normally adequate to control the Indian kala-azar, but elsewhere, particularly in Africa and the Mediterranean countries, the course needs to be repeated (and in some cases pentamidine or amphotericin B added; see below) once or twice after intervals of 14 days up to a total dosage of 12 or even 18g. Toxic effects are rare but vomiting, collapse and cardiac arrhythmias may occur.

Antimony resistance is occasionally encountered and it is in these resistant cases that the diamidine compounds pentamidine isethionate (see section 6.3.8) and 2-hydroxystilbamidine isethionate, or possibly amphotercin B, have been found useful. Hydroxystilbamidine isethionate is given by slow intravenous injection of 250mg daily for an adult and each course comprises 10 daily injections; the course may be repeated after an interval of 14 days up to a total of 7.5g given over a period of 2 months. Serious side effects like hypotension and hypoglycaemia can occur but the more common side effects of fever, rigors and headache can be relieved by the concurrent administration of oral antihistamines. The dose of pentamidine is 3 to 5mg/kg body weight by intramuscular injection every 3 to 4 days for 10 doses, or less frequently if side effects develop. Cumulative side effects include fatigue, anorexia, nausea, abdominal pain, and in around 2% of cases, prolonged hypoglycaemia. Amphotericin B has been given in several dosage schedules, such as 0.25mg/kg infused intravenously on the first day, followed by an increment of 0.25mg/kg each day to a maximum of 1mg/kg (or 1.5mg/kg in very severe infections). Amphotericin B can cause a number of adverse effects, the most important of which is dose related nephrotoxicity (see chapter XXVII; sect. 5.8).

With these drugs, the untreated mortality of 95% can be reduced to between 2 to 5%. Complete cure usually takes about 6 months, but 2 to 15% of patients relapse within the next two years.

6.6.2 Cutaneous Leishmaniasis of the Old World (oriental sore)

Treatment remains unsatisfactory and depends upon the site and number of the lesions. A single lesion may be treated with unipolar coagulation diathermy. This has replaced earlier methods of inducing an inflammatory reaction to expedite cure. Multiple lesions and lesions on the face require a course of injections of sodium stibogluconate or hydroxylstilbamidine, as for visceral leishmaniasis. However, some lesions are more resistant and therefore more prolonged therapy will be necessary. Very chronic and resistant lesions, such as those of the recidiva type, may eventually respond to Grenz rays, which heat the tissues to 40ºC, a temperature which is lethal to the parasite. Failure to respond to antimony is usually due to inadequate treatment, but some strains of *Leishmania* may be resistant, in which case pentamidine or amphotericin B may be indicated.

Preliminary results using rifampicin at 600mg daily for 1 to 4 months have seemed encouraging (Iskandar, 1978), but further studies of such treatment are needed. Follow-up is especially important in mucocutaneous leishmaniasis since relapses do occur; clinical healing can occur with live organisms present in the lesion (Marsden, 1979).

6.7 Treatment of Trypanosomiasis

Trypanosomiasis is a disease of tropical Africa, both of men and of cattle, due to the protozoa *Trypanosoma brucei rhodesiense* and *gambiense* (in man) and *T. brucei congolense* and *vivax* (in cattle), and of tropical Central and South America where *T. cruzi* is the intractable agent of human trypanosomiasis (Chagas' disease). In man, African trypanosomiasis begins with an irregular fever and lymphadenopathy; it is only after a few weeks or months that the invasion of the central nervous system takes place with the characteristic headaches, cramps, lethargy, melancholia and terminal coma. The *T. gambiense* and *T. rhodesiense* forms of trypanosomiasis differ somewhat in symptoms, severity and duration. *T. rhodesiense* trypanosomiasis is the more acute and severe of the two forms, usually terminating fatally within a year without treatment, while the *T. gambiense* form usually runs a more chronic course with typical clinical manifestations of the sleeping sickness syndrome.

If treatment is begun early, before the brain has been invaded, it will be curative. At this early stage, either suramin (section 6.3.10) or pentamidine (section 6.3.8) may be used, the latter being employed only for the *T. gambiense* form of trypanosomiasis. Since these drugs do not penetrate the blood-brain barrier, they become ineffective once the brain has been invaded; consequently, examination of the cerebrospinal fluid is of importance in deciding which drug to use. To eliminate infection from the central nervous system, an arsenical, melarsoprol (see section 6.3.9), is required as it alone penetrates into the brain.

Suramin is given intravenously after a test dose of 0.1 to 0.2g, in case the patient has an idiosyncratic reaction to the drug. If there is no reaction, the course of 20mg/kg body weight is started 24 hours later and given on days 1, 3, 7, 14 and 21; weekly doses may then be given for an additional 5 weeks. Toxic effects include dermatitis, nausea, vomiting, peripheral neuritis and nephritis. Since suramin can produce serious renal damage, the urine must be examined before each injection. If heavy albuminuria, casts and red blood cells are seen, suramin should be discontinued and pentamidine given instead. Pentamidine is less toxic than suramin. The intramuscular dose is 3 to 5mg/kg of body weight daily for 10 injections. Side effects include hypotension and hypoglycaemia which may require appropriate intravenous fluid infusion. Severe hypotension and collapse can occur if the drug is given intravenously; therefore, this route is not recommended.

Patients who show evidence of central nervous system involvement should be treated with intravenous melarsoprol, a trivalent organic arsenical chelated to dimercaprol for slow release (see section 6.3.9.). It is effective in all stages of the disease and it is highly efficacious in advanced *T. brucei rhodesiense* infections, and in other resistant cases. However, it is also highly toxic and its real danger is encephalopathy which may occur in the early stages of melarsoprol therapy. Melarsoprol has been given in various dosage schedules which are basically similar, involving gradually increasing doses, with repeated administration at intervals. For example, the initial dose for an adult is 1.0mg/kg of body weight, but a smaller dose may be given if the patient's general condition is poor. This is followed by 2mg, 3mg and 3.6mg/kg of body weight on the second, third and fourth days (maximum individual dose 200mg). These 3 day courses are given on 3 or 4 occasions 1 week apart. The patient's general condition can be improved first by giving the patient a preliminary course of suramin to kill the trypanosomes outside the central nervous system before the commencement of melarsoprol therapy. Being a highly toxic drug (see section 6.3.9), melarsoprol must be given under strict medical supervision and there is no justification in its use in conditions other than proven cerebral trypansomiasis. A less toxic water soluble derivative of melarsoprol, melarsonyl potassium, is available but unfortunately, it is not as effective. Good results have been obtained in *T. brucei gambiense* infections but it is not a reliable drug for *T. brucei rhodesiense* infections.

South American trypanosomiasis is due to infection with *T. cruzi* (Chagas' disease). Unlike the African form which primarily affects the central nervous system, it is characterised by some degree of cardiac involvement in all cases (Marsden, 1974). The initial acute phase, which 90% of patients survive, is followed by an asymptomatic period of 10 to 20 years, but it is doubtful that the infection is eradicated during this period; however, the role of reinfection in the course of the disease is unclear. The common presentation in the subsequent chronic phase is congestive heart failure, often involving both ventricles. Drug treatment of Chagas' disease has been unsatisfactory; although several drugs including primaquine, nitrofurans and trivalent arsenical compounds show some activity against the blood forms, these drugs do not show marked activity against the intracellular forms of the trypanosome. The nitrofurazone drug, nifurtimox (15 to 20mg/kg daily for 90 days in children 10 years of age or less; 12.5 to 15mg/kg daily for 90 days 11 to 16 years; 8 to 10mg/kg daily for 120 days in adults), is effective in the acute phase (Wegner and Rohwedder, 1972), but its useful effectiveness against intracellular parasites in the chronic phase is probably less (Gutteridge, 1976). Side effects, especially gastrointestinal effects, may be severe and the drug should be used under medical supervision.

6.8 Amoebiasis and Intestinal Helminthiasis

Treatment of these parasitic infestations, which have a global distribution, is discussed in chapter XIX (sect. 11.3, 11.4) and is the same in a tropical environment, although economic factors will in-

fluence selection of drugs. Nevertheless, the expression of some of these diseases may differ between countries or even in different population groups in the same geographical environment. For example, although intestinal amoebiasis appears to be a less serious disease in Southeast Asia than in Africa, it still causes a significant amount of morbidity. Among the Caucasian citizens of the city of Durban in South Africa, intestinal amoebiasis tends to be a 'nuisance' rather than a 'disease', whereas in the Bantu community in the same city, amoebic dysentery is often an acute, devastating illness which ranks as a major cause of morbidity and mortality in the African population (Elsdon-Dew, 1949). The reasons for this marked variability in expression of infection by the same parasite are not clear, but host factors are implicated; of these, malnutrition is probably a major determinant of morbidity. Differences in the predominant types of gut microbial flora may also influence pathogenicity.

7. Leprosy

Dapsone, a sulphone derivative, is still the drug of choice for the treatment of leprosy. It is safe and cheap. In full dosage (50 to 100mg daily) it is slowly bactericidal, but in low dosage it is only bacteriostatic, suppressing the growth of *Mycobacterium leprae*. The minimum inhibitory concentration (MIC) for many wild strains of *M. leprae* is as low as 3ng/ml. Therefore *M. leprae* is exquisitely sensitive to dapsone. Peak plasma concentrations achieved with 100mg dapsone are 500 to 600 times the MIC. Therefore, although its mechanism of action is probably similar to that of sulphonamides, as some antagonism is produced by para aminobenzoic acid, it is possible that it also acts as its own dihydrofolate reductase inhibitor.

Dapsone is slowly but completely absorbed following oral administration and peak plasma concentrations are reached in 1 to 3 hours after oral administration. About 50% of the drug is protein bound in the plasma but it is well distributed in total body water and is present in all tissues of the body, especially the liver, muscle, kidney and skin. Dapsone is metabolised in the liver by acetylation (individuals may be fast or slow acetylators; see chapter VII, sect. 4.2.1) and the metabolites excreted in the urine. Because enterohepatic circulation follows biliary excretion of the free drug, a single dose of dapsone may be detected in the plasma for up to 12 days.

Dapsone can cause a variety of adverse reactions. Some of them are dose dependent and these include nausea, vomiting, anorexia, abdominal pain and constipation or diarrhoea; these gastrointestinal upsets are uncommon, provided that the dose does not exceed 100mg daily. Use of dapsone in high doses (200 to 300mg per day), especially in slow acetylators of the drug, can lead to methaemoglobinaemia, sulphaemoglobinaemia and Heinz-body formation. Haemolysis of varying degree can occur, especially in patients with glucose-6-phosphate dehydrogenase deficient red cells (see further chapter VII; sect. 4.2.2; XXIII, sect. 8.4).

Dapsone allergy occurs in perhaps 1 in 400 to 1 in 500 patients suffering from any kind of leprosy. The allergy usually appears 3 to 6 weeks after the start of treatment with pruritus, dermatitis and fever. If the dapsone therapy is not discontinued immediately, then the patient may develop exfoliative dermatitis, jaundice and mental symptoms. In addition to stopping dapsone immediately, corticosteroid therapy should be instituted. Patients with a known history of sulphone allergy should not be treated with sulphonamides, as cross allergy frequently occurs.

7.1 Treatment of Leprosy

Tuberculoid leprosy can be successfully treated with dapsone alone, in a dosage of 50mg daily for a period of 3 to 7 years. This dosage will not normally cause any untoward side effects such as haemolytic anaemia or sulphaemoglobinaemia, although sulphone allergy with fever and dermatitis may rarely occur. In addition, patients should be educated to prevent the complications of anaesthesia, physiotherapy may be needed to prevent muscle contractures and deformities will require surgical correction.

The treatment of bacilliferous leprosy must be more prolonged; borderline leprosy requires a minimum of 10 years and lepromatous leprosy should be treated for 20 years or preferably for life. Dapsone remains the basic drug, although dapsone resistant strains of *M. leprae* are being recognised more and more frequently around the world. To prevent the emergence of dapsone resistance, it is essential to give the drug regularly and the recommended dose is 100mg daily throughout life for full sized healthy adults. This dose produces a peak blood concentration of about 500 times the minimal inhibitory concentration of dapsone for *M. leprae*. Clinical improvement may be detected after 6 to 8 weeks, and the patient is rendered non-infectious in about 3 months. Complete resolution, however, takes many years and small numbers of persisting drug sensitive bacilli may survive for 10 to 20 years, causing relapse if the drug is stopped prematurely. Spot urine tests for dapsone are of great help to ensure that the patient is taking the prescribed treatment.

To avoid the increasing problem of dapsone resistance, it is recommended that lepromatous leprosy should be treated with an initial intensive course of two or more drugs. These drugs include rifampicin, and the phenazine derivative clofazimine.

Dosages for an adult of 50kg or more are: rifampicin 600mg daily for 2 to 4 weeks; clofazimine 100mg 3 times weekly for 6 months; ethionamide 375mg daily for 3 months; each combined with dapsone 50 to 100mg daily given for life. Unfortunately, the cost and possible increased toxicity of the combined therapy regimens have prevented their widespread use. Ideally, all lepromatous patients should receive initial treatment in hospital for 2 to 4 weeks while the infection is brought under control and while the patient is taught about his disease. Rifampicin is the most rapidly bactericidal drug available for the treatment of leprosy. It will kill the great majority of the *M. leprae* in the skin and upper respiratory tract within 3 to 4 days, thus rendering the patient virtually non-infectious within 2 weeks (Waters et al., 1978).

Rifampicin however, should not be given alone otherwise rifampicin resistant *M. leprae* might emerge. Rifampicin increases the rate of elimination of dapsone (Gelber and Rees, 1975) and in regimens employing these drugs, dosage of dapsone should be 100mg daily given regularly. The high cost of rifampicin limits its use in most tropical countries. Clofazimine is, like dapsone in full dosage, slowly bactericidal and in addition, it has marked anti-inflammatory properties. It is relatively non-toxic but has the important disadvantage that it causes a reddish discolouration of the skin with hyperpigmentation. Brown coloured retinal or corneal opacification can also occur with daily dose regimens of clofazimine (Ohman and Wahlberg, 1975). Ethionamide is also bactericidal, but it has been little studied in leprosy and frequently causes gastrointestinal side effects.

7.2 Management of Lepromatous Reactions

Acute reactions during drug therapy require immunosuppressive drugs. Reversal (type I) reaction, which causes pain or tenderness in the nerves and inflammation and oedema of the skin lesions, should be treated with prednisolone 40mg initially, followed by 20mg daily for a few weeks until the inflammation has settled, and the drug is finally tailed off over several months. Milder reactions may be controlled with a smaller dose of prednisolone.

Erythema nodosum leprosum (type II) reactions in lepromatous leprosy respond dramatically to thalidomide in an initial dosage of 100mg 4 times a day, which can usually be reduced within a few weeks to a maintenance dose of 100 to 200mg every evening. However, the drug must not be given to premenopausal women because of its dysmorphogenic effect. In those countries in which thalidomide is not available or in patients where the drug is contraindicated, it may be necessary to use prednisolone 20 to 40mg daily, or clofazimine 100mg 3 times daily for up to 3 months and then 100mg daily. Since the local complication of iritis can be dangerous, it should also be treated locally with 1% atropine drops daily and 1% hydrocortisone drops 4-hourly. For a review on leprosy and its treatment, see Shepard et al., (1976) and World Health Organisation (1977b).

8. Tuberculosis in a Tropical Environment

Tuberculosis in many tropical countries differs from that generally seen in Western countries in the severity of the infections, which often present at a much more advanced stage. The large populations of bacilli result in haematological spread to a wider spectrum of organs causing for example, meningitis, osteitis or lymphadenitis. Extensive tissue damage is more common during both the infective and healing phases. Children under 5 years are more frequently involved. Malnourished children seem to have a deficient cellular immune system which makes them susceptible to infectious diseases, particularly tuberculosis.

Factors such as malnutrition, isolation and bed rest are no longer thought to be significant in determining the outcome of treatment (Ramakrishnan et al., 1966) in comparison with the strength and duration of the chemotherapy regimens and the regularity with which these are taken (Fox, 1977). Considerations which apply in the choice of a regimen for pulmonary disease in a tropical country are illustrated by the following three examples:

1) Rifampicin and isoniazid daily for 9 months with an initial supplement of streptomycin is a powerful bactericidal regimen, highly effective but expensive and hence beyond the financial resources of many of the poorer tropical countries.

2) Streptomycin, isoniazid and para-aminosalicylic acid (PAS) for at least 12 to 18 months is also effective, but the longer duration of therapy (as it is a weaker combination) and the unpleasant side effects of PAS reduce patient compliance. Moreover, in many developing countries the daily administration of streptomycin almost invariably requires hospital admission for the duration of treatment.

3) Thiacetazone and isoniazid eliminate the bacilli from the sputum after 12 months treatment in over 80% of cases. The addition of streptomycin during the first 2 months improves the rate of sputum conversion to 90%. Relapse, however, is frequent. Thiacetazone is a weak, bacteriostatic drug whose main action is to prevent isoniazid resistance. The combination is, however, very cheap, compact and stable in tropical conditions and on these grounds is widely used; but in some populations (e.g. Filipinos), it is very poorly tolerated and is unacceptable for use.

The overall success of antituberculosis compaigns depends on the best use of resources and the organisation of personnel. Money should be spent on the purchase of effective drug regimens which can be dispensed by relatively untrained staff from general purpose dispensaries or clinics rather than on building hospitals. Intermittent regimens given 2 or 3 times a week, which are as effective as daily treatment (see chapter XX; sect. 8), often allow the best use of manpower and are to be recommended. However twice weekly regimens based on isoniazid may possibly be less effective than daily regimens in patients who are rapid acetylators of the drug if a short period of initial chemotherapy is given and the companion drug used in the continuation phase is relatively weak (Ellard, 1976). Three times weekly regimens based on isoniazid are therefore preferable in Asian populations, of whom 80 to 90% or more can be classified as rapid acetylators (see chapter

VII; sect. 4.2.1). Choice of an appropriate regimen in a tropical country is therefore not only determined by each country's financial and manpower resources, but also by study of those factors in a given population which influence drug response (Stott, 1978).

Priority in treatment should be given to 'open cases'. The vast majority of these will present at a clinic with symptoms and the diagnosis is easily confirmed by microscopic examination. The provision of an adequate health infrastructure is basic to an efficient programme and it is vital that the patient can obtain medication as near to his or her home as possible. The widespread use of BCG immunisation as a preventive measure, is of course, now accepted practice in areas with a high incidence of tuberculosis.

Dosages and side effects of drugs used in pulmonary disease and general considerations in treatment are discussed in chapter XX (section 8) and regimens for tuberculous meningitis in chapter XXV (section 13).

9. Whooping Cough in a Tropical Environment

Whooping cough (pertussis) is a highly infectious disease spread by droplet infection. It may be very debilitating to the child because of the long duration of illness. The incidence of whooping cough in most tropical countries is high and infection occurs at an earlier age than in developed countries due to earlier exposure. Since morbidity and mortality in whooping cough is closely related to the age at which the child is infected, the lower age incidence found in the developing countries is of considerable significance.

Although the malnourished child will clearly not withstand so well a severe attack of whooping cough, the disease does not seem to be that much more severe in the undernourished child compared with his well nourished counterpart with whooping cough. However, there is considerable evidence that whooping cough may cause malnutrition because of its long duration of debility. While antibiotics are useful in the first week of the disease, and when bronchopneumonia develops, management of the disease and its successful outcome will largely depend on the standard of nursing and maternal care, which may be lacking in tropical countries (see further chapter IV; sect. 5.1.4).

10. Measles in a Tropical Environment

Measles is a very severe disease in many tropical countries and has a high mortality rate (Morley, 1969a,b). It is an excellent example of the interaction of nutrition and infection in the child. In the malnourished child, measles is much more severe and may have a mortality 400 times higher than his well nourished counterpart with measles (Morley, 1973). Often malnourished children die of giant cell pneumonia without classical skin lesions. In addition, measles has a deleterious effect on the nutritional status of the child to a far greater extent than any other common childhood infection (Axton, 1979). The age incidence of measles in developing countries is unlike that of developed countries. It occurs in younger children. Around 75 % of the children in tropical countries are likely to have become infected before 3 years of age.

The possible explanation for the greater severity of the disease in the malnourished child is that children with kwashiorkor show a depression of the cell mediated immunity which is necessary to deal successfully with viruses invading the body.

As the severity of measles depends on the state of nutrition, and the disease is so likely to precipitate the child into malnutrition, maintenance of adequate intake of food and fluid must be a priority in treatment. Because of its severity, many doctors will find it difficult not to give the child with measles routine antibiotics. The few controlled studies available suggest that prophylactic antibiotics do not prevent bacterial complications but rather increase the incidence of complications (Weinstein, 1955). However, when the child's condition suggests secondary bacterial invasion, antibiotic therapy is essential (see further chapter XXVIII; sect. 3.3).

11. Use of Drugs in a Tropical Environment

Problems in the use and availability of drugs in tropical countries are many and complex (see sections 1 and 2). In terms of prescribing, these problems relate in particular to dosage and administration of drugs and use of drugs in the presence of diseases and co-existing conditions encountered in a tropical environment.

11.1 Dosage and Administration of Drugs

The first problem is the danger of toxicity from overdosage if the same dose schedules used in Western countries are followed (see section 2.1). On the basis of body weight alone, Asians in Southeast Asia for example would receive about 30% more drug/dose than their heavier body weight Western counterparts. This is of most significance if a drug of low therapeutic ratio is administered or when drugs are given on a long term basis. Signs of overdosage will soon develop. This problem is more acute in children as the dosage of many drugs is recommended on an age basis. But their body weight, compared with European or North American children of the same age, may differ by as much as 40%. Malnutrition contributes further to low body weight. Hence, overdosage may result from failure to consider body weight whenever a drug is prescribed and is particularly likely in children.

Although it would be expected that malnutrition and other tropical diseases would have a major effect on the response to drugs due to alteration in absorption, distribution or elimination, or tissue sensitivity, knowledge in this field is still small (see section 2.2). Nevertheless, prescribers should be aware that protein deficiency may lead to a decreased rate of metabolism of drugs eliminated mainly by hepatic metabolism. Similarly, many parasitic infections are associated with liver or kidney complications which may affect clearance of drugs eliminated by these routes. Alteration of response may become a major problem of treatment with some drugs; for example, in mansoni schistosomiasis with niridazole and hycanthone (see section 6.3.3; 6.5). Protein energy malnutrition may have a profound influence on binding and distribution of drugs.

Malnutrition can also lead to problems of drug administration and absorption (Buchanan, 1978). Children with kwashiorkor often have oedema of the lower limbs and this makes intramuscular injections of drugs into the quadriceps a problem and may also affect the absorption of some drugs. Children with kwashiorkor and marasmus have a diminished muscle mass making recurrent intramuscular injections difficult. Oral administration of drugs can also be affected by vomiting and diarrhoea which occur not infrequently in protein calorie malnutrition. Drugs are poorly retained and absorption may be impaired due to the short intestinal transit time. Mucosal atrophy of the bowel, which occurs in severe cases, may also impair drug absorption.

Many diseases in a tropical environment other than malnutrition can give rise to difficulty of absorption of drugs after oral administration. This can occur in patients with a primary malabsorption syndrome of unknown aetiology such as tropical sprue or in patients with infections caused by *Giardia lamblia, Capillaria philippinensis* or by *Strongyloides stercoralis*. These parasitic infections can give rise to similar events as in tropical sprue. Such difficulties must be borne in mind when oral administration of drugs is considered in these conditions.

11.2 Use of Drugs in the Presence of Folate Deficiency

Folate deficiency is a common problem in a tropical environment and the small body store of folate can easily be depleted during growth, in pregnancy, or in the presence of infections or increased production of red blood cells as in haemolytic anaemia. In addition, many drugs can adversely affect folate metabolism (see chapter XXIII; sect. 8.5) and in combination with these factors may eventually precipitate folate deficiency into frank megaloblastic anaemia. Drugs which affect folate metabolism include pyrimethamine and co-trimoxazole.

Pyrimethamine (see section 6.1.3) inhibits the enzyme dihydrofolate reductase which converts dihydrofolate to tetrahydrofolate. Co-trimoxazole consists of sulphamethoxazole and trimethoprim. Sulphamethoxazole inhibits the formation of para aminobenzoic acid and trimethoprim, like pyrimethamine, blocks the enzyme dihydrofolate reductase leading to impaired folate formation in bacterial cells. Pyrimethamine and co-trimoxazole are frequently used drugs in tropical areas where malnutrition is common. Use of either pyrimethamine or co-trimoxazole alone in usual doses is unlikely to lead to impaired folate metabolism, except in those actually or potentially folate deficient (Chanarin and England, 1972). Clearly, simultaneous use of co-trimoxazole for the treatment of a bacterial infection in a patient receiving pyrimethamine for malaria prophylaxis would further impair a folate deficiency state and even lead to frank megaloblastic anaemia (Ansdell et al., 1976).

Where diet is inadequate, these drugs should be given with folate supplements.

11.3 Use of Drugs in Populations with G6PD Deficiency

A number of ethnic groups in tropical countries have a deficiency of the enzyme glucose-6-phosphate dehydrogenase (G6PD) which makes their red blood cells susceptible to haemolysis by a variety of oxidant drugs such as primaquine, dapsone, phenacetin, many sulphonamides and nitrofurantoin. The deficiency is severe in North West Indian, East and Southeast Asian peoples. Any patient with haemolytic episodes (haemoglobinuria is the usual presentation), particularly following use of an oxidant drug (see chapter XXIII; table XIII), should be suspected of G6PD deficiency. Affected individuals should be given advice about medication to avoid (see section 2.1.1; chapter VII, sect. 4.2.2). In some situations, the greater likelihood of acute haemolysis may influence the choice of drug or the need to exclude G6PD deficiency before a drug is given. For example, co-trimoxazole (trimethoprim-sulphamethoxazole) is more likely than chloramphenicol to induce haemolysis when used in typhoid fever in Hong Kong Chinese with G6PD deficiency (Chan and McFadzean, 1974; Chan et al., 1976) and phenacetin is best avoided in Southeast Asians because of the severe haemolysis it commonly causes in enzyme deficient individuals (Wong, 1977).

11.4 Use of Corticosteroids

Corticosteroids have many therapeutic uses and indications for their use are on the increase. However, indiscriminate administration of corticosteroids to patients in a tropical environment can be hazardous, especially in patients with occult *Strongyloides* infestation or amoebic infection. In the case of *Strongyloides* infestation, a massive autoinfection with widespread dissemination of larvae to intestinal organs may occur (Plorde et al., 1971). This hyperinfection is often associated with severe enterocolitis and Gram-negative septicaemia. Unrecognised, it may lead to death.

Amoebiasis is often unrecognised and corticosteroids prescribed for other disorders may provoke exacerbation of amoebiasis, acute amoebic dysentery and even fulminating progression of hepatic amoebiasis. Since amoebiasis can mimic almost any abdominal or hepatic disorder but especially ulcerative colitis, administration of corticosteroids for the treatment of misdiagnosed ulcerative colitis is likely to have a disastrous effect. This is a real problem since patients with 'colitis', rightly or wrongly, are often treated with corticosteroids at some stage. Apparently, the amoebae become more 'aggressive' and invasive after corticosteroid administration. A possible explanation is that suppression of the inflammatory and immunological response interferes with the host-parasite equilibrium (Stuiver and Goud, 1978). It is prudent, therefore, to investigate a patient who has lived in the tropics for amoebiasis, whenever corticosteroid therapy is considered. The best laboratory procedure is serological investigation together with repeated stool examination.

12. Drug Induced Nutritional Deficiencies

The risk of drug induced nutritional deficiencies varies, depending on the chemistry and pharmacological action of the drugs concerned. Drugs can affect protein, carbohydrate, fat, vitamin and mineral requirements (Roe, 1976). The variables which determine the incidence of drug induced deficiencies are the nutrient intake and storage, genetic variability in handling the drug, the dose and duration of drug therapy, the combinations of drugs used, the disease states, certain physiological situations (pregnancy, growth) and other environmental factors.

Many of these changes are not often clinically significant under circumstances of normal nutrition, but clearly may become important in states of malnutrition or undernutrition as exist in a tropical environment. This is as yet a poorly studied area.

The common symptoms due to drug induced malnutrition are weight loss, growth retardation, diarrhoea, dermatitis, paraesthesiae, bone pains, bleeding gums, anorexia and anaemia. Such side effects are induced because drugs can interfere with intake, absorption, binding, excretion and metabolism of nutrients. Some of the more important aspects of nutrient-drug interactions are summarised in table IV.

Anorectic drugs (e.g. amphetamines) suppress appetite and food intake. Many antibiotics also decrease appetite by precipitating gastrointestinal disturbances. A variety of compounds decrease absorption of nutrients like amino acids, vitamins and minerals — through their effect on intestinal

Table IV. Drug induced nutritional deficiencies

1. Effects on intake
   a) Anorectic drugs (e.g. amphetamines)
   b) Gastrointestinal disturbances (e.g. antibiotics)

2. Effects on absorption
   a) Intestinal hurry (e.g. laxatives)
   b) Mucosal alterations (e.g. colchicine, neomycin)
   c) Sequestration of bile salts leading to malabsorption of fat and fat soluble vitamins (e.g. cholestyramine, neomycin)
   d) Inhibition of specific absorption of nutrients like vitamin B_{12}, folate (biguanides, PAS, phenytoin, sulphasalazine, chlorpromazine and chloramphenicol
   e) Nutritional drug interaction in the gut lumen (e.g. tetracycline and iron)

3. Effects on metabolism
   a) Drugs altering metabolism of nutrients
      i) Affecting many nutrients like vitamin A, B complex vitamins and ascorbic acid (oral contraceptives)
      ii) Affecting vitamin K metabolism (antibiotics, analgesics, steroids, anticonvulsants)
      iii) Induction of enzymes increasing vitamin D metabolism (e.g. anticonvulsants)
   b) Drugs interfering with the metabolic function of nutrients (antimetabolites)
      i) Antifolates (e.g. cytostatic drugs, antimalarials, trimethoprim, triamterene, anticonvulsants)
      ii) Vitamin B_6 antagonists (e.g. antituberculosis agents)

4. Hyperexcretion and tissue depletion
   a) Phosphates (antacids)
   b) Calcium and magnesium (diuretics)
   c) Zinc and copper (D-penicillamine)
   d) Vitamin B_6 and flavins (isoniazid, borates)
   e) Increased urinary excretion of vitamin C (aspirin, barbiturates, tetracyclines)

motility, intestinal mucosal changes, specific inhibition of active transport mechanisms, suppression of bacterial growth and intraluminal interactions (see chapter XIX; sect. 14.3.1). Malabsorption (primary or secondary) can lead to deficiencies of vitamins A, D, K, folate and vitamin B_{12}. A number of drugs (e.g. phenytoin, phenobarbitone, primidone, glutethimide, prednisone, diphosphonates) may result in vitamin D mediated hypocalcaemia. Metabolic antagonists like purine or folic acid antagonists, antimalarials, isoniazid and the hydrazine group of compounds (e.g. hydrallazine) are known antivitamins, resulting in folic acid or vitamin B_6 deficiency (see chapter XXIII; sect. 8.5, 8.6). Oral contraceptives produce a number of metabolic alterations, particularly involving

B complex vitamins and vitamin A and C (Faizy et al., 1975; Briggs, 1976; see chapter XV, sect. 13.4, 13.10). Hepatic enzyme inducing drugs such as anticonvulsants can lead to faster metabolism of nutrients like vitamin A and vitamin D (see chapter XXII; sect. 14.5). A number of drugs interfere with vitamin K and its action. Broad spectrum antibiotics, analgesics, anticonvulsants and corticosteroids for example, may interfere either with absorption, binding or synthesis of vitamin K dependent clotting factors (Koch-Weser and Sellers, 1971).

Hyperexcretion and tissue depletion of nutrients can lead to mineral and trace nutrient deficiencies. It is usually seen with chronic usage of antacids, diuretics, chelating agents etc. In addition, a number of agents (steroids, antibiotics, contraceptives, phenothiazines, thiazides) interfere with amino acid absorption, nitrogen balance, or carbohydrate and fat metabolism.

Acknowledgements

The assistance and comments of the following specialists is gratefully acknowledged in the preparation of various sections of the chapter: Sister Mary Aquinas (Hong Kong), Dr B. Cabrera (Manila), Dr T. Dyson (Hong Kong), Prof. Tranakchit Harinasuta (Bangkok), Dr S.G. Srikantia (Hyderabad), Dr Priscilla J. Tablan (Manila), Prof. D. Todd (Hong Kong), Dr M.F.R. Waters (Selangor), Prof. Wong Hock Boon (Singapore) and Prof. V. Zaman (Singapore).

Further Reading

Dijukanovic, V. and Mach, E.P.: Alternative Approaches to Meeting Basic Health Needs in Developing Countries. A Joint UNICEF/WHO study (WHO Geneva 1975).

Indian Council of Medical Research (ICMR): Alternative Approaches to Health Care. Report of a symposium organised jointly by ICMR and Indian Council of Social Science Research (1976).

Shaper, A.G.; Kibukamusoke, J.W. and Hutt, M.S.R.: Medicine in a Tropical Environment (British Medical Association, London 1972).

Wilcocks, C. and Manson-Bahr, P.E.C.: Manson's Tropical Diseases, 17th ed (Cassell, London 1972).

Woodruff, A.W.: Medicine in the Tropics (Churchill Livingstone, Edinburgh 1974).

References

Ansdell, V.E.; Wright, S.G. and Hutchinson, D.B.A.: Megaloblastic anaemia after pyrimethamine and co-trimoxazole. Lancet 2: 1257 (1976).

Arnold, K.: Trends in the development of chemotherapy for parasitic diseases. Southeast Asian Journal of Tropical Medicine and Public Health 9: 177 (1978).

Axton, J.H.M.: Measles and the state of nutrition. South African Medical Journal 55: 125 (1979).

Bamji, M.S. and Faizy, A.: Vitamin deficiency in man — recent studies on fat soluble vitamins, thiamin, riboflavin pyridoxine and vitamin C. Journal of Scientific and Industrial Research 37: 42 (1978).

Bhamarapravati, N.: The liver in protein-calorie malnutrition; in Olson (Ed) Protein-Calorie Malnutrition, p. 299 (Academic Press, New York 1975).

Binns, T.B.: Drugs for the third world. British Journal of Clinical Pharmacology 3: 975 (1976).

Briggs, M.: Biochemical effects of oral contraceptives. Advances in Steroid Biochemistry and Pharmacology 5: 65 (1976).

Bryceson, A.D.M.; Warrell, D.A. and Pope, H.M.: Dangerous reactions to treatment of onchocerciasis with diethylcarbamazine. British Medical Journal 1: 742 (1977).

Buchanan, N.: Drug-protein binding and protein-energy malnutrition. South African Medical Journal 52: 733 (1977).

Buchanan, N.: Drug kinetics in protein energy malnutrition. South African Medical Journal 53: 327 (1978).

Bueding, E. and Mansour, J.M.: The relationship between inhibition of phosphofructokinase activity and the mode of action of trivalent organic antimonials on Schistosoma mansoni. British Journal of Pharmacology 12: 159 (1957).

Bueding, E. and Fisher, J.: Biochemical effects of niridazole on Schistosoma mansoni. Molecular Pharmacology 6: 532 (1970).

Bygbjerg, I.C.: Use of drugs in developing countries. Tropical Doctor 8: 174 (1978).

Campbell, T.C.: Nutrition and drug metabolising enzymes. Clinical Pharmacology and Therapeutics 22: 699 (1977).

Campbell, J.A. and Morrison, A.B.: Some factors affecting the absorption of vitamins. American Journal of Clinical Nutrition 12: 162 (1963).

Chalmer, T.M.; Darie, M.W.; Hunter, J.O.; Szaz, K.F.; Pelc, B. and Kodicek, E.: 1-alphahydroxy cholecalciferol as a substitute for the kidney hormone, 1,25 dihydrocholecalciferol in chronic renal failure. Lancet 2: 696 (1973).

Chan, T.K. and McFadzean, A.J.S.: Haemolytic effect of trimethoprim-sulphamethoxazole in G-6-PD deficiency. Transactions of the Royal Society of Tropical Medicine and Hygiene 68: 61 (1974).

Chan, T.K.; Todd, D. and Tso, S.C.: Drug-induced haemolysis in glucose-6-phosphate dehydrogenase deficiency. British Medical Journal 2: 1227 (1976).

Chanarin, I. and England, J.M.: Toxicity of trimethoprim-sulphamethoxazole in patients with megaloblastic haemopoiesis. British Medical Journal 1: 651 (1972).

Chang, K.C.; Bell, T.D.; Lauer, B.A. and Chai, H.: Altered theophylline pharmacokinetics during acute respiratory viral illness. Lancet 1: 1132 (1978).

Clyde, D.F.; McCarthy, V.C.; Miller, R.M. and Hornick, R.B.: Suppressive activity of mefloquine in sporozoite-induced human malaria. Antimicrobial Agents and Chemotherapy 9: 384 (1976).

Connor, D.H.: Current concepts in parasitology. Onchocerciasis. New England Journal of Medicine 298: 379 (1978).

Coutinho, A. and Barreto, F.T.: Treatment of hepatosplenic Schistosomiasis mansoni with niridazole: relationships among liver function, effective dose and side effects. Annals of the New York Academy of Sciences 160: 612 (1969).

Craig, W.A. and Kunin, C.M.: Significance of serum protein and tissue binding of antimicrobial agents. Annual Review of Medicine 27: 287 (1976).

Craig, W.A. and Welling, P.G.: Protein binding of antimicrobials: clinical pharmacokinetic and therapeutic implications. Clinical Pharmacokinetics 2: 252 (1977).

Deluca, H.F.: The kidney as an endocrine organ involved in the function of vitamin D. American Journal of Medicine 58: 39 (1975).

DiPalma, J.R. and Ritchi, D.M.: Vitamin toxicity. Annual Review of Pharmacology and Toxicology 17: 133 (1977).

Doberstyn, E.B.; Hall, A.P.; Vetvutanapibul, K. and Sonkom, P.: Single-dose therapy of falciparum malaria using pyrimethamine in combination with diformyldapsone or sulfadoxine. American Journal of Tropical Medicine and Hygiene 25: 14 (1976).

Edgcomb, J.H.; Arnold, J.; Yount, E.H.; Alving, A.S. and Eichelberger, L.: Primaquine, SN 13272, a new curative agent in vivax malaria: a preliminary report. Journal of the National Malaria Society 9: 285 (1950).

Ellard, G.A.: Variations between individuals and populations in the acetylation of isoniazid and its significance for the treatment of pulmonary tuberculosis. Clinical Pharmacology and Therapeutics 19: 610 (1976).

Elsdon-Dew, R.: Endemic fulminating amebic dysentery. American Journal of Tropical Medicine 29: 337 (1949).

Epstein, W.L.; Shah, V.P. and Riegelman, S.: Griseofulvin levels in stratum corneum. Study after oral administration in man. Archives of Dermatology 106: 344 (1972).

Fabre, J.; de Freudenreich, J.; Duckert, A.; Pitton, J.S.; Rudhardt, M. and Virieux, C.: Influence of renal insufficiency on the excretion of chloroquine, phenobarbital, phenothiazine and methacycline. Helvetica Medica Acta 303: 307 (1967).

Faigle, J.W.: Blood levels of a schistomicide in relation to liver function and side effects. Acta Pharmacologica et Toxicologica 29(Suppl. 3): 233 (1971).

Faigle, J.W. and Keberle, H.: Metabolism of niridazole in various species, including man. Annals of the New York Academy of Sciences 160: 544 (1969).

Faizy, A.; Bamji, M.S. and Iyengar, L.: Effect of oral contraceptive agents on vitamin nutrition status. American Journal of Clinical Nutrition 28: 606 (1975).

Falase, A.O.; Salako, L.A. and Aminee, J.M.: Lack of effect of low doses of prazosin in hypertensive Nigerians. Current Therapeutic Research 19: 603 (1976).

Fox, W.: Modern management and therapy of pulmonary tuberculosis. Proceedings of the Royal Society of Medicine 70: 4 (1977).

Fraser, H.S.; Bulpitt, C.J.; Khan, C.; Mould, G.; Mucklow, J.C. and Dollery, C.T.: Factors affecting antipyrine metabolism in West African villagers. Clinical Pharmacology and Therapeutics 20: 369 (1976).

Frisk-Holmberg, M.; Bergkvist, Y.; Nyberg-Domeij, B.; Hellstrom, L. and Jansson, F.: Chloroquine serum concentration and side effects: Evidence for dose-dependent kinetics. Clinical Pharmacology and Therapeutics 25: 345 (1979).

Gaudette, L.E. and Coatney, G.R.: A possible mechanism of prolonged antimalarial activity. American Journal of Tropical Medicine and Hygiene 10: 321 (1961).

Gelber, R.H. and Rees, R.J.W.: Dapsone metabolism in patients with dapsone-resistant leprosy. American Journal of Tropical Medicine and Hygiene 24: 963 (1975).

Gopalan, C. and Srikantia, S.G.: Nutrition and disease. World Review of Nutrition and Dietetics 16: 97 (1973).

Gurtoo, G.M.; Campbell, T.C.; Webb, R.E. and Plowman, K.M.: Effect of aflatoxin and benzpyrene pretreatment upon the kinetics of benzpyrene hydroxylase. Biochemical and Biophysical Research Communication 31: 588 (1968).

Gutteridge, W.E.: Chemotherapy of Chagas' disease. Transactions of the Royal Society of Tropical Medicine and Hygiene 70: 123 (1976).

Haley, J.J. and Flesha, A.M.: A toxicity study of thiamine hydrochloride. Science 104: 567 (1946).

Hall, A.P.: The treatment of malaria. British Medical Journal 1: 323 (1976).

Hall, A.P.; Doberstyn, E.B.; Karnchanachetanee, C.; Samransamruajkit, S.; Laixuthai, B.; Pearlman, E.J.; Lampe, R.M.; Miller, C.F. and Phintuyothin, P.: Sequential treatment with quinine and mefloquine or quinine and pyrimethamine-sulfoxadine for falciparum malaria. British Medical Journal 1: 1626 (1977).

Hathcock, J.N. and Coon, J.: Nutrition and Drug Interrelations (Academic Press, New York 1978).

Higgins, E.A.; Davis, Jr, A.W.; Fiorica, V.; Iampietro, P.F. and Vaughan, J.A.: Effects of two antihistamine containing compounds upon performance at three altitudes. Aerospace Medicine 19: 1167 (1968).

Holmstedt, B.; Nordgren, I.; Sandoz, M. and Sundwall, A.: Metrifonate. Summary of toxicological and pharmacological information available. Archives of Toxicology 41: 3 (1978).

Hornig, D.: Metabolism of ascorbic acid. World Review of Nutrition and Dietetics 23: 225 (1975).

Houstan, J.B. and Levy, D.G.: Drug biotransformation interaction in man: IV. Acetaminophen and ascorbic acid. Journal of Pharmaceutical Sciences 65: 1219 (1976).

Iskandar, I.O.: Rifampicin in cutaneous leishmaniasis. Journal of International Medical Research 6: 280 (1978).

Iyengar, L. and Rajalakshmi, K.: Effect of folic acid supplement on birth weights of infants. American Journal of Obstetrics and Gynaecology 122: 332 (1975).

James, M.F.M. and Jewsbury, J.M.: Schistosomiasis, metriphonate, cholinesterase, and suxamethonium. British Medical Journal 1: 442 (1978).

Jewsbury, J.M.; Cooke, M. and Weber, M.C.: Field trial of metrifonate in the treatment and prevention of schistosomiasis infection in man. Annals of Tropical Medicine and Parasitology 71: 67 (1977).

Jusko, W.J. and Levy, G.: Plasma protein binding of riboflavin and riboflavin-5'-phosphate in man. Journal of Pharmaceutical Science 56: 58 (1968).

Kaldor, A.: Patterns and problems of drug consumption in a developing country. Clinical Pharmacology and Therapeutics 19: 657 (1976).

Katz, M.: Anthelmintics. Drugs 13: 124 (1977).

Keet, M.P.; Hansen, J.D.L.; Moddie, A.D. and Wittman, W.: Kwashiorkor: A ten years follow up study. Proceedings of the Twelfth International Congress of Pediatrics. Vol. 2, p.387 (Vienna 1971).

Koch-Weser, J. and Sellers, E.M.: Drug interactions with coumarin anticoagulants. New England Journal of Medicine 285: 487, 545 (1971).

Krishnaswamy, K.: Erythrocyte glutamic oxalo acetic tranaminase activity in patients with oral lesions. International Journal of Vitamin and Nutrition Research 41: 247 (1971).

Krishnaswamy, K.: Drug metabolism and pharmacokinetics in malnutrition. Clinical Pharmacokinetics 3: 216 (1978).

Krishnaswamy, K. and Naidu, A.N.: Microsomal enzymes in malnutrition as determined by plasma half-life of antipyrine. British Medical Journal 1: 538 (1977).

Kuroda, K.: Detection and distribution of chloroquine metabolites in human tissues. Journal of Pharmacology and Experimental Therapeutics 137: 156 (1962).

Lakshmi, A.V. and Bamji, M.S.: Pyridoxal 5'-phosphate dependent enzymes in riboflavin deficiency. Indian Journal of Biochemistry and Biophysics 12: 136 (1975).

Langman, M.J.S. and Smithard, D.J.: Antipyrine metabolism in iron deficiency. British Journal of Clinical Pharmacology 4: 631P (1977).

Larter, W.E.; John, J.; Sieber, O.F.; Johnson, H.; Corrigan, J. and Fulginiti, V.A.: Trimethoprim-sulfamethoxazole treatment of *Pneumocystis carinii* pneumonitis. Journal of Pediatrics 92: 826 (1978).

Levine, G.M. and Harber, L.C.: The effect of humidity on the phototoxic response to 8-methoxy psoralen in guinea pigs. Acta Dermato-Venerologica 49: 82 (1969).

Levy, G. and Hewitt, R.R.: Evidence in man for different specialized intestinal transport mechanisms for riboflavin and thiamine. American Journal of Clinical Nutrition 24: 401 (1971).

Lubran, M.: Determination of hetrazan in biological fluids. British Journal of Pharmacology 5: 210 (1950).

McChesney, E.M.; Fasco, M.I. and Banks, W.F.: The metabolism of chloroquine in man during and after repeated oral dosage. Journal of Pharmacology and Experimental Therapeutics 158: 323 (1967).

Macomber, P.B.; O'Brien, R.L. and Hahn, F.E.: Chloroquine: Physiological basis of drug resistance in Plasmodium berghei. Science 152: 1374 (1966).

Madsen, S.; Olgaard, K. and Ladefoged, J.: Bone mineral content in chronic renal failure during long-term treatment of l-alphahydroxy cholecalciferol. Acta Medica Scandinavica 203: 385 (1978).

Mahmoud, A.A.: Current concepts in parasitology. Schistosomiasis. New England Journal of Medicine 297: 1329 (1977).

Marks, P.A. and Banks, J.: Drug-induced haemolytic anaemia associated with glucose-6-phosphate dehydrogenase deficiency: a genetically heterogenous trait. Annals of the New York Academy of Science 123: 198 (1965).

Marsden, P.D.: South American trypanosomiasis; in Woodruff (Ed) Medicine in the Tropics, p.91 (Churchill Livingstone, Edinburgh 1974).

Marsden, P.D.: Current concepts in parasitology. Leishmaniasis. New England Journal of Medicine 300: 350 (1979).

Morley, D.C.: Severe measles in the tropics — I. British Medical Journal 1: 297 (1969a).

Morley, D.C.: Severe measles in the tropics — II. British Medical Journal 1: 363 (1969b).

Morley, D.C.: Severe measles; in Paediatric Priorities in the Developing World, p.207 (Butterworths, London 1973).

Mroczek, W.J.; Fotiu, S.; Davidov, M.E. and Finnerty, Jr., F.A.: Prazosin in hypertension: A double-blind evaluation with methyldopa and placebo. Current Therapeutic Research 16: 769 (1974).

Nair, V. and Casper, R.: The influence of light on daily rhythm in hepatic drug metabolizing enzymes in rat. Life Sciences 8: 1291 (1969).

Narasinga Rao, B.S.: Studies on iron deficiency anaemia. Indian Journal of Medical Research 68: 58 (1978).

Obel, A.O.K. and Vere, D.W.: Antipyrine and propranolol disposition in malnutrition. East African Medical Journal 55: 20 (1978).

Ohman, L. and Wahlberg, I.: Ocular side-effects of clofazimine. Lancet 2: 933 (1975).

Olson, R.E.: Protein-calorie malnutrition (Academic Press, New York 1975).

Omer, A.H.S.: Oxamniquine for treating schistosoma mansoni infection in the Sudan. British Medical Journal 2: 163 (1978).

Omer, A.H.S.: Treatment of severe forms of schistosomiasis. Tropical Doctor 8: 3 (1978b).

Omer, A.H.S. and Teesdale, C.H.: Metrifonate trial in the treatment of various presentations of *Schistosoma haematobium* and *S. mansoni* infections in the Sudan. Annals of Tropical Medicine and Parasitology 72: 145 (1978).

OPPI (Organisation of pharmaceutical producers of India): The Nation's health and the pharmaceutical industry (1976).

Pennigton, J.E.; Dale, D.C.; Reynolds, H.Y. and MacLowry, J.D.: Gentamycin sulfate pharmacokinetics: lower levels of gentamycin in blood during fever. Journal of Infectious Diseases 132: 270 (1975).

Plorde, J.J.; Ivan, L.B. and Petersdorf, R.G.: Other intestinal nematodes: Strongyloidiasis; in Harrison's Principles of Internal Medicine, p.1050, 6th ed (McGraw-Hill, New York 1971).

Peters, W.: Current concepts in parasitology. Malaria. New England Journal of Medicine 297: 1261 (1977).

Ponnampalam, J.T.; Seow, C.L. and Roy, O.S.: A comparative study of the efficacy of chloroquine and a combination of dapsone and pyrimethamine in the prophylaxis of malaria in peninsular Malaysia. Journal of Tropical Medicine and Hygiene 79: 220 (1976).

Prata, A.: *Schistosomiasis mansoni.* Clinics in Gastroenterology 7: 49 (1978).

Ramachandran, C.P. and Dondero, T.J.: The epidemiology and immunology of Malayan filariasis in Southeast Asia: A review. Modern Medicine of Asia 12: 41 (1976).

Ramakrishnan, C.V.; Rajendran, K.; Mohan, K.; Fox, W. and Radhakdrishnan, S.: The diet, physical activity and accommodation of patients with quiescent pulmonary tuberculosis in a poor South Indian community. A four-year follow-up study. Bulletin of the World Health Organisation 34: 553 (1966).

Ramalingaswami, V. and Nayak, N.C.: Liver disease in India; in Popper and Schaffner (Eds) Progress in Liver Diseases, Vol. III, p.222 (Grune and Stratton, New York 1970).

Reddy, V.: Vitamin A deficiency and blindness in Indian children. Indian Journal of Medical Research 68: 48 (1978).

Reddy, V. and Sivakumar, B.: Studies on vitamin A absorption in children. Indian Pediatrics 9: 307 (1972).

Reddy, V. and Srikantia, S.G.: Serum vitamin A in kwashiorkor. American Journal of Clinical Nutrition 18: 105 (1966).

Robertson, D.H.H.: The treatment of sleeping sickness with melarsoprol. I. Reactions observed during treatment. Transactions of the Royal Society of Tropical Medicine and Hygiene 57: 122 (1963).

Roe, D.A.: Drug Induced Nutritional Deficiencies. (The AVI Publishing Co. Inc., Connecticut 1976).

Rollo, I.M.: Chemotherapy of parasitic diseases; in Goodman and Gilman (Ed) The Pharmacological Basis of Therapeutics, p.1018 (MacMillan, New York 1975).

Rosenberg, I.H. and Scrimshaw, N.S.: Workshop on malabsorption and malnutrition. American Journal of Clinical Nutrition 25: 1046, 1225 (1972).

Rubin, E. and Lieber, C.S.: Malnutrition and liver diseases — an overemphasised relationship. American Journal of Medicine 45: 1 (1968).

Salafsky, B.: Dangers of drug toxicity due to over dosage in Southeast Asia. Journal of Tropical Medicine and Hygiene 79: 49 (1976).

Sanvordekar, D.R. and Lambert, H.J.: Environmental modification of mammalian drug metabolism and biological response. Drug Metabolism Reviews 3: 201 (1972).

Schulert, A.R.; Browna, H.G. and Salem, H.H.: Human disposition of antimony sodium dimercaptosuccinate: With analysis of antimony concentration in excreted Schistosoma haemotobium ova. Transactions of the Royal Society of Tropical Medicine and Hygiene 58: 48 (1964).

Schultz, M.G.: Current concepts in parasitology. The New England Journal of Medicine 297: 1259 (1977).

Shastri, R.A. and Krishnaswamy, K.: Undernutrition and tetracycline half life. Clinica Chimica Acta 66: 157 (1976).

Shepard, C.C.; Ellard, G.A.; Levy, L.; de AraujoOpromolla, V.; Pattyn, S.R.; Peters, J.H.; Rees, R.J.W. and Waters, M.F.R.: Experimental chemotherapy in leprosy. Bulletin of the World Health Organisation 53: 425 (1976).

Smithard, D.J. and Langman, M.J.S.: The effect of vitamin supplementation upon antipyrine metabolism in the elderly. British Journal of Clinical Pharmacology 5: 181 (1978).

Smythe, P.M.; Swanepoel, A. and Campbell, A.H.: The heart in kwashiorkor. British Medical Journal 1: 67 (1962).

Srikantia, S.G. and Reddy, V.: Effect of a single massive dose of vitamin A on serum and liver levels of the vitamin. American Journal of Clinical Nutrition 23: 114 (1970).

Stott, H.: The treatment of pulmonary tuberculosis in the developing countries. Transactions of the Royal Society of Tropical Medicine and Hygiene 72: 564 (1978).

Stuiver, P.C. and Goud, Th. J.L.M.: Corticosteroids and liver amoebiasis. British Medical Journal 2: 394 (1978).

Sy, F.S.: Niridazole in the treatment of *Schistosomiasis japonica.* Journal of the Phillipine Medical Association 53: 151 (1977).

Teoh, P.C.: Hospital admissions due to adverse reactions to drug therapy. Australian Family Physician 4: 191 (1975).

Teoh, P.C.: Drug dosage for Southeast Asian patients. Medical Progress 4: 11 (Feb 1977).

Thompson, A.D.; Frank, O.; Baker, H. and Leevy, C.M.: Thiamine propyl disulfide: absorption and utilisation. Annals of Internal Medicine 74: 529 (1971).

Trenholme, G.M.; Williams, R.L.; Rieckman, K.H.; Frischer, H. and Carson, P.E.: Quinine disposition during malaria and induced fever. Clin. Pharm. Ther. 19: 459 (1976).

Van den Bossche, H.: Chemotherapy of parasitic infections. Nature 272: 626 (1978).

Vesell, E.: Relationship between drug distribution and therapeutic effects in man. Annual Review of Pharmacology 14: 249 (1974).

Waterlow, J.C.: Adaptation to low-protein intakes; in Olson (Ed) Protein Calorie Malnutrition, p.23 (Academic Press, New York 1975).

Waters, M.F.R.; Rees, R.J.W.; Pearson, J.M.H.; Laing, A.B.G.; Helmy, H.S. and Gelber, R.H.: Rifampicin for lepromatous leprosy: nine years' experience. British Medical Journal 1: 133 (1978).

Wegner, D.H.G. and Rohwedder, R.W.: The effect of nifurtimox in acute Chagas' infection. Arzneimittel-Forschung 22: 1624 (1972).

Weinstein, L.: Failure of chemotherapy to prevent the bacterial complications of measles. New England Journal of Medicine 253: 679 (1955).

Western, K.A.; Perera, D.R. and Schultz, M.G.: Pentamidine isethionate in the treatment of pneumocystic carinii pneumonia. Annals of Internal Medicine 73: 695 (1970).

Wong, H.B.: Acute haemolysis in Southeast Asia. Medical Progress 4(3): 12 (March 1977).

World Health Organisation: Pharmacogenetics — the influence of heredity on the response to drugs. World Health Chronicle 28: 25 (1974).

World Health Organisation: National drug policies. World Health Chronicle 29: 337 (1975).

World Health Organisation: Food and Nutrition Strategies in National Development. Technical Report Series No. 584 (World Health Organisation, Geneva 1976).

World Health Organisation: The Selection of Essential Drugs. Technical Report Series 615 (World Health Organisation, Geneva 1977a).

World Health Organisation Expert Committee on Leprosy, 5th Report. Technical Report Series 607 (World Health Organisation, Geneva 1977b).

Yagi, K.: Studies on riboflavin. Proceedings of the First Asian Congress of Nutrition, p.157 (Nutrition Society of India, Hyderabad 1972).

Yokogawa, M.: Current chemotherapy of schistosomiasis in Japan. Southeast Asian Journal of Tropical Medicine and Public Health 7: 310 (1976).

Yudkin, J.S.: Provision of medicines in a developing country. Lancet 1: 810 (1978).

Zvaifler, N.J.; Rubin, M. and Bernstein, H.: Chloroquine metabolism — drug excretion and tissue deposition. Arthritis and Rheumatism 6: 799 (1963).

Appendix A
Drug Data Information

R.C. Heel and G.S. Avery

Drugs, besides being remedies for a particular disease, are molecules with characteristic physico-chemical and pharmacokinetic properties. As discussed in chapter I, these properties govern the behaviour of a drug in the body and are of fundamental importance in determining the time course of drug effects. Knowledge of these properties is an important guide to selection of appropriate doses and dosage intervals.

The table which follows is intended to provide ready access to some of the basic physicochemical and pharmacokinetic properties of individual drugs *in man* so that the general principles discussed in chapter I and elsewhere in the book can be applied for many different drugs commonly used in therapeutics. The data provided are not intended for precise drug dosage calculation, but rather to indicate which drugs are weak acids or bases, are highly protein bound, have a small apparent volume of distribution, a long, intermediate or short plasma half-life and so on. It is hoped that by classifying the drugs according to their predominant pharmacological action or therapeutic use, differences and similarities between individual drugs within a class of drug can be readily seen. Drugs in the same therapeutic or pharmacological class are not necessarily the same in terms of their pharmacokinetic behaviour.

It is important to realise that the values given for the elimination half-life from plasma (β-phase; i.e. after distribution of the drug into the tissues of the body), the apparent volume of distribution and extent of protein binding, are those which apply in normal adult subjects. For many drugs these values can be profoundly changed by disease or altered pathophysiological states such as in the very young and the elderly.

Knowledge of the route of elimination is also of importance in the selection of a drug and in adjustment of drug dosage in the presence of associated diseases such as severe renal and liver disease, and in the context of multiple drug therapy. Information on elimination of drugs is given in many tables throughout this book, and because of its special importance, as a separate appendix on drug dosage in renal failure (appendix E).

The data included in the table have been obtained from a multitude of sources, including general reviews and compilations and original articles; many specific references for which are given in the relevant chapters in section 2 of the book. Much of the data are scattered diffusely throughout the published literature. For many drugs, particularly older ones, the basic data are simply not available. In some cases, the pharmacokinetic properties of the drug have not even been studied in man! Although great care has been taken in compiling the many values, some 'incorrect' data may have been included. The editor would be very grateful to readers who advise him of those values missing and also of any incorrect values noted in this and other compilations in the appendices and elsewhere in the book.

General References

Anton, A.H. and Solomon, H.M.: Proceedings of conference on drug-protein binding. Annals of New York Academy of Sciences 226: 5 (1973).

Ritschel, W.A.: Biological half-lives and their clinical application; pK_a values and some clinical applications; in Francke and Whitney Perspectives in Clinical Pharmacy, p.286, 325 (Drug Intelligence, Hamilton Ill. 1972).

Pagliaro, L.A. and Benet, L.Z.: Critical compilation of terminal half-lives, percent excreted unchanged, and changes in half-life in renal and hepatic dysfunction for studies in humans with references. Journal of Pharmacokinetics and Biopharmaceutics 3: 333 (1975).

Schonfeld, G.: Antibiotics and Chemotherapy, Vol. 25 Pharmacokinetics (Karger, Basel 1978).

SingSum Chow, M. and Ronfield, R.A.: Pharmacokinetic data and drug monitoring: I. Antibiotics and antiarrhythmics. Journal of Clinical Pharmacology 15: 405 (1975).

Smith, S.E. and Rawlins, M.D.: Variability in Human Drug Response (Butterworth, London 1973).

Various Authors: Clinical Pharmacokinetics (ADIS Press, Sydney 1976-1979).

Vesell, E.: Proceedings of conference on drug metabolism in man. Annals of the New York Academy of Sciences 179: 9 (1971).

Appendix A. Drug data information (see also appendix E)

Drug	Nature[1]	pK$_a$[2]	T$_{1/2}$[3] (hours)	V$_d$[4] (L/kg)	Protein[5] binding	Notes[6]
β-Adrenoceptor Blocking Drugs						
Acebutolol	B	9.4	~8	1.2	84	
Alprenolol	B	9.63	2-3	3-3.3	83-88	
Atenolol	B	9.6	6-9	0.7	< 5	
Metoprolol	B	9.68	3-4	5.6	10-13	
Nadolol			9.6-14.2	1.4-3.4		
Oxprenolol	B		2-3	1.5		
Pindolol	B	8.8	3-4	2*	57**	*136L **to albumin (total unknown)
Practolol	B	9.5	5-13	1.6	32*	*to albumin (total unknown)
Propranolol	B	9.45	2-6*	3-4.3	90-96**	*2-4 (iv), 3.5-6 (po) **62% to albumin
Sotalol	B		5-13	0.7	54*	*to albumin (total unknown)
Timolol	B		4-5	1.3-1.7		
Tolamolol	B		~2.5	3.2	91	
Anaesthetics, intravenous						
Alphaxalone	S		0.17	0.64*	46	*45L
Droperidol	B	7.6	~2		85-90	
Etomidate		4.24	3.9	4.6	75	
Fentanyl			1-4*		~95	*dose dependent
Flunitrazepam	B	1.84	9.5-25*	3.4-5.5*		*oral administration
Ketamine		7.5	~3-4			
Thiopentone	A	7.6	3-8		72-86	
Anaesthetics, local						
Bupivacaine	B	8.1	2.7	1.04*	96	*73L
Etidocaine	B	7.7	2.7	1.9*	94	*133L
Lignocaine (lidocaine)	B	7.9	1.6	1.3*	64	*91L
Mepivacaine	B	7.6	1.9	1.2*	77	*84L
Prilocaine	B	7.9			50	

1   A = acid; Aac = amino acid; Alc = alcohol; Amp = ampholyte; B = base; B$_4$ = base with quaternary ammonium group; Gly = glycoside; Pep = peptide; S = steroid; Sa = substituted amide.

2   The pH at which the drug is 50% ionised. For clinical application of this value see chapter I (sect. 1.1).

3   Elimination (plasma; t$_{1/2β}$) half-life (normal value in adults). Plasma half-lives of many drugs show much interindividual variability due to differences in rates of metabolism. A single value reflects the mean plasma half-life and does not necessarily indicate that interindividual variability does not exist. See further chapter I (sect. 2.1.1; 4.2).

4   Apparent volume of distribution (normal value in adults). See further chapter I (sect. 2.1.2). In most cases these are approximate average values for the β-phase or steady-state volume of distribution. Values indicated by an asterisk have been obtained by assuming the body weight as 70kg.

5   Normal values. See further chapter I (sect. 3.2).

6   See introductory notes and acknowledgements for source data.

Appendix A. (continued)

Drug	Nature[1]	pK$_a$	T$_{1/2}$[3] (hours)	V$_d$[4] (L/kg)	Protein[5] binding	Notes[6]
Analgesics — anti-inflammatory agents						
Alclofenac	A	4.6	1.5-5.5	0.07-0.1*	90-99	*5-7L
Aspirin	A	3.5	2-4.5* 16-19*	0.10-0.20*	50-90*	*salicylate: dose- and pH-dependent; t$_{1/2}$ 2-4.5 (<3g), 16-19 (large dose)
Azapropazone	A		4.0-16.5	0.08*	~95	*5.6L, dose dependent
Diclofenac	A				99.7	
Fenbufen	A		~15			
Fenclofenac	A	5.5	~21	0.18*	~96	*12.5L
Fenoprofen	A	4.5	1.5-3	0.08-0.1*	>99	*5.4-7.5L
Flurbiprofen	A		3.8	0.1*	>99.5	*7.3L
Ibuprofen	A	4.4; 5.2	2	0.14*	99	*10L
Indomethacin	A	4.5	4-12	0.34-1.57	92-99	
Ketoprofen	A		1.6-1.9		<94	
Naproxen	A	5	10-17	0.09	98-99.5	
Oxyphenbutazone	A	4.7	27-64	0.14*	99	*10L, estimated from figure
Phenylbutazone	A	4.5	29-175*	0.02-0.15	98-99	*dose dependent
Sulindac	A		~7*		93	*~18h for active metabolite
Tolmetin	A	3.5	5.3*	0.04*	>90	*assuming non-linear kinetics
— strong analgesics						
Buprenorphine	B	8.49, 10.03			~96	
Butorphanol			2.4-3.5		80	
Methadone	B	8.6	18-97	~5	71-87*	*70% to albumin
Morphine	B	8.05	1.9-3.1	≤3-4	35	
Nefopam		9.2	~4			
Pentazocine	B	9.0	2	4.89*	60-70	*342L
Pethidine (meperidine)	B	8.7	2.4-4	3.84*	65-75	*269L
— simple analgesics						
Codeine	B	8.2	3-4		~7	
Dextropropoxyphene	B	6.3	12		78	
Diflunisal	A		5-6, 10-11*	0.1	98-99	*dose dependent; 50mg, 500mg
Paracetamol (acetaminophen)	Alc	9.5	2-2.4	~0.7*	25	*48L
Phenacetin	Sa		0.7-1.25	1-2.1	33	
Aminopyrine (amidopyrine)	B	5.0	2-7		15-20	
Anorexiants						
Chlorphentermine	B	9.6	~120	3.04*		*213L
Fenfluramine	B	9.9	13-30	12-16	34	
Mazindol		8.6	33-55			
Phentermine	B	10.1	19-24			
*Antianginal Agents**						*see also β-blockers
Glyceryl trinitrate			≤0.5			
Nifedipine			4-5		>90	
Perhexiline			~72-288			
Verapamil			3-7	6.5	90	

Appendix A. (continued)

Drug	Nature[1]	pK_a	$T_{1/2}$[3] (hours)	V_d[4] (L/kg)	Protein[5] binding	Notes[6]
*Antianxiety Drugs**						**see also Hypnosedatives*
Bromazepam	B	2.9, 11.0	8-19	—*	70	*90% of body weight
Chlordiazepoxide	B	~4.8	5-30	~0.3-0.5	94-97	
Clobazam			~50		87-90	
Desmethyldiazepam			~51-120	1.11		
Diazepam	B	3.3	24-48*	0.7-2.6	94-98	*can range 9-53h; ~51-120h active metabolite
Ketazolam			1.5*			*parent drug; active metabolites have longer half-lives
Lorazepam	Amp	1.3, 11.5	9-16	0.9	>90	
Medazepam			1-2*			*parent drug; active metabolites have longer half-lives
Meprobamate			6-17			
Oxazepam	Amp	1.7, 11.6	6-25	1.6	~90	
Prazepam			~78		~85	
Triazolam			~5			
Antiarrhythmic Drugs						
Aprindine			30	3.7	85-95	
Bretylium	B₄		4-17			
Disopyramide	B	9.6	4.4-8.2	0.6-1.3	35-95*	*dose dependent
Lignocaine	B	7.9	1-2*	0.7-2.2	45-80*	*dose dependent
Lorcainide	B		5.1	6.4	85	
Mexiletine		9.05	~10	9.5*	70	*663L
N-Acetylprocainamide			6-11	1.5	11	
Phenytoin (diphenylhydantoin)	B	8.3	8-60*	0.5-0.8	89-91	*dose dependent
Practolol			9-12	~1.6	<10	
Procainamide	B	9.2	2.2-4	1.7-2.2	15	
Propranolol	B	9.45	2-6*	3.6; 4.6	90-96**	*2-4 (iv), 3.5-6 (po) **62% to albumin
Quinidine	B	4.3, 8.4	3-16	2.1-2.6	80-90	
Tocainide	B		12-15	~1.4-1.6	50	
Verapamil	B		3-7	6.5	90	
Antibacterial Agents — *aminoglycosides*						
Amikacin	B		2-3	0.2-0.3	<10	
Gentamicin	B	8.2	2-3	0.28	<10	
Kanamycin	B	7.2	2-5	0.2-0.3	0-3	
Lividomycin	B		2.01-2.5		20-30	
Netilmicin	B		2.2	0.25		
Sisomicin	B		3.5	0.2		
Streptomycin	B		2-3	0.26	20-30	
Tobramycin	B	6.7, 8.3, 9.9	2-3	0.31	<10	

Appendix A. (continued)

Drug	Nature[1]	pK_a[2]	$T_{1/2}$[3] (hours)	V_d[4] (L/kg)	Protein[5] binding	Notes[6]
— cephalosporins						
Cefoxitin	A		1	0.1-0.2*	65-80	*8-12L
Cefuroxime	A	~2.5	1.1-1.4	0.2-0.3*	~40	*12-18L
Cephacetrile	A	1.97	~1	0.27-0.32*	23-26	*18.7-22.5L
Cephalexin	A	2.5, 7.3	0.5-1	0.23	15	
Cephaloglycin	A	4.7	1.5-2.2		0-30	
Cephaloridine	A	3.4	1-1.5	0.23	20	
Cephalothin	A	2.5	0.5-1	0.26	70	
Cephamandole	A		~1	~0.145	67-80	
Cephanone	A		~2.5-3	0.17-0.19*	88	*12-13.6L
Cephapirin	A		0.6	0.14*	44-50	*10L
Cephatrizin	A		1.4		58	
Cephazolin	A	2.3	1.75-2	0.13	84	
Cephradine	A	2.6, 7.3	0.7	0.29	10	
Chloramphenicol	Alc	5.5	1.6-3.3	0.57*	60-80	*40L
Clindamycin	B	7.45	2-4	1.14*	94	*80L
Colistimethate	B		4.5	0.54*	50	*38L
Erythromycin	B	8.8	1.4	0.57	73*	*base; 93% propionate salt
Fusidic acid		5.35	4.8-16.5	0.08-0.24*	97	*6-17L
Lincomycin	B	7.6	4.6-5.6	0.41-0.57	72	
Metronidazole			6-12	0.6-0.8	<20	
Nalidixic acid	A	6.7	1.1-2.5	0.26-0.45	93-97	
Nitrofurantoin	A	7.2	0.3-0.6		25-60	
— penicillins						
Amoxycillin	A	2.4, 7.4, 9.6	1	0.2*	17	*14L
Ampicillin	A	2.5, 7.2	1-1.5	0.4-0.7	15-29	
Bacampicillin	A		0.7-1.0	0.36*		*25.5L
Benzylpenicillin	A	2.8	0.5	~0.5	65	
Carbenicillin	A	3.3	1-1.5	0.14*	50	*10L
Cloxacillin	A	2.7	0.5	0.15*	95	*10.8L
Dicloxacillin	A	2.7	0.7	~0.1-0.2	98	
Flucloxacillin (floxacillin)	A	2.7	0.8	0.12*	95	*8.2L
Hetacillin	A		~1	0.37		
Mecillinam	A	3.4, 8.9	1.0		~10-25	
Methicillin	A	3	0.5	0.31*	30-50	*22L
Nafcillin	A	2.7	0.5	0.6-0.7	87-90	
Oxacillin	A	2.9	0.5	0.41*	94	*29L
Phenoxymethylpenicillin	A	2.7	0.5	0.73*	79	*51L
Pivmecillinam		8.9	~1.0		15-25	
Propicillin	A	2.7	0.57	0.41*		*29.1L
Ticarcillin	A	2.5, 3.42	1.2	0.21*	65	*15L
Polymyxin B		8.9	3-6			
Spectinomycin	B	7, 8.7	1.7	0.16*	not sig	*11.5L
Spiramycin	B	8.0	5-6			

Appendix A. (continued)

Drug	Nature[1]	pK_a[2]	$T_{1/2}$[3] (hours)	V_d[4] (L/kg)	Protein[5] binding	Notes[6]
— sulphonamides						
Sulphadiazine	A	6.4	10	0.36	60	
Sulphadimethoxine	A	5.9	20-40	0.15	97	
Sulphadimidine (sulphamethazine)	A	7.4	7.6	0.61*	80	*43L
Sulphafurazole (sulfisoxazole)	A	4.9	3-7	0.16	84	
Sulphamerazine	A	6.7	23-35	0.36	85	
Sulphamethizole	A	5.4	1-2	0.35	90	
Sulphamethoxazole	A	5.7	7-12*	0.17**	62	*pH-dependent **11.7L
Sulphamethoxydiazine	A	7	36	0.25	87	
Sulphamethoxypyridazine	A	6.1	35-60	0.18-0.20	60-70	
Sulphaphenazole	A	6.5	8-12	0.29	>99	
Sulphasalazine	A		5.7, 7.6*			*single dose, multiple dose
— tetracyclines						
Chlortetracycline	B	3.3, 7.4, 9.3	5-6	0.9-1.5	~50-60	
Demethylchlortetracycline	B	3.3, 7.2, 9.4	10-13	1.79	~40-50	
Doxycycline	Amp	3.4, 7.7, 9.7	~15-24		25-31	
Methacycline		3.5, 7.6, 9.2	8-14	0.97	~80	
Minocycline		2.8, 5.0, 9.5, 7.8,	12-16	0.14*	65-75	*9.5L
Oxytetracycline	B	3.3, 7.3, 9.1	9-10	0.9-1.9	20-30	
Rolitetracycline		7.4	6-12	0.8	20	
Tetracycline	B	3.3, 7.7, 9.7	6-10	1.3-1.6	~20-40	
Thiamphenicol			4.2			
Trimethoprim	B	6.4	9-13*	1.2	70	*pH-dependent
Vancomycin	B		6-11	0.47*	<10	*33L
Anticholinergics						
Atropine	B	9.8	13-38	~2-4	50	
Hyoscine N-butyl-bromide	B₄		7.6		10	
Propantheline	B₄		9	1.54*		*108L
Anticoagulants						
Nicoumalone (acenocoumarol)	A		8.2-8.7*; 20-30**		98.7	*radiochemical assay **photometric assay
Dicoumarol (bishydroxycoumarin)	A	5.7	60-100*	0.14**	>99	*dose dependent. In some $t_{1/2}$ may be as low as 7h. **9.8L
Ethylbiscoumacetate	A	3.1	2-5*		~90	*dose dependent
Heparin	A		~1-2*	0.05-0.2	95**	*iv bolus, dose dependent **to lipoproteins
Phenindione	A		5-10			
Phenprocoumon	A		65-170	~0.1-0.2	>99	
Warfarin	A	5.05	35-45*	~0.1	⩾99	*Can range 15-70h

Appendix A. (continued)

Drug	Nature[1]	pKa[2]	T$_{1/2}$[3] (hours)	Vd[4] (L/kg)	Protein[5] binding	Notes[6]
Anticonvulsants						
Carbamazepine	Sa		18-65, 10-20*	0.8-1.8	70-80**	*single dose, multiple dose **active metabolite 50%
Chlormethiazole	B	3.2	3-6	5.4	63	
Clonazepam	B	1.5, 10.5	20-60	~2-5	~80	
Dantrolene	A	7.5	~8.7			
Diazepam	B	3.3	24-48*	0.7-2.6	98	*can range 9-53h; active metabolite ~51-120h
Ethosuximide	A	9.3	~60*	0.9	0	*~30h in children
Methsuximide			2.6*		~0	*active metabolite 36-45h
Nitrazepam	B	3.2, 10.8	21-28	2.1	85	
Phenobarbitone	A	7.2	48-144	0.5-0.6	50-60	
Phensuximide			5-12		~0	
Phenytoin	A	8.3	8-60*	0.5-0.8	87-93	*dose dependent
Primidone	A		3.3-12.5*	~1	~0	*parent drug; metabolised to phenobarbitone and another active compound PEMA (t$_{1/2}$ = 29-36h)
Sulthiame		9.97	~30		29	
Trimethadione (troxidone)			12-24*		0	*t$_{1/2}$ of active metabolite ~240h
Valproate sodium	A	4.8	13-21	0.13-0.18	~80-90	
Antidepressants						
Amitriptyline	B	9.4	32-40		82-96	
Clomipramine	B		11.6-35.8			
Desipramine	B	9.5	12-54	22-59	~70-90	
Doxepin	B	8	8-25	9.1-33		
Imipramine	B	9.5	6-20	20-40	80-95	
Maprotiline			27-58	22.6	88	
Mianserin			7.7-19.2	47.1*	~90	*3300L
Nomifensine			3-5	5.4-8.4	60-75	
Nortriptyline	B	9.73	15-90	20-57	90-95	
Protriptyline	B		53.6-91.7*	15.0-31.2	92	*may range up to 198h
Viloxazine	B	8.13	2-3	1.5	85-90	
Antidiarrhoeals						
Diphenoxylate	B	7.07	2.5	4.6		
Loperamide	B	8.60	7-15		97	
Antifungal Agents						
Amphotericin B	Amp	5.5, 10.0	24-48 (360*)	~4	>90	*Following slow release from tissues
Clotrimazole			~4		~98	
Fluorocytosine (flucytosine)			3-8	~0.7	2-4	
Griseofulvin			10-24	1-2		
Miconazole		6.65	~24	21*	~98	*1474L
Antihistamines						
Chlorpheniramine	B	9.2	30		72	
Diphenhydramine	B	8.3	4-10	3-4	98-99	
Diphenylpyraline	B		24-40			
Mebhydroline		6.7	4		~4	

Appendix A. (continued)

Drug	Nature[1]	pK_a[2]	$T_{1/2}$[3] (hours)	V_d[4] (L/kg)	Protein[5] binding	Notes[6]
*Antihypertensive Drugs**						*see also β-blockers and diuretics
Bethanidine	B		17-20	7*	< 8	*1 patient
Clonidine	B	8.25	12.7*		20	*oral
Debrisoquine			13-26			
Diazoxide	A	8.74	21-36	0.19-0.24	90-93	
Guanethidine	B	9.0, 12.0	~120-240			
Hydrallazine	B	7.1	2-4, 1-3*	1.63	88-90	*slow, fast acetylators
Labetalol		7.38	3.5-4.5	~11.5	~50	
Methyldopa	Aac	2.2, 9.2, 10.6, 12	8	0.29*	< 20	*20L
Prazosin			1.77-4.55	1.07*	97	*75L
Reserpine	B	6.1	46-168			
Minoxidil			3.6	2.77*		*194L
Antimalarials						
Chloroquine	B	8.4, 10.8	70-120*		55	*dose dependent
Mepacrine (quinacrine)	B	7.7, 10.3	120		90	
Pyrimethamine	B	7.2	96			
Quinine	B	4.3, 8.4	8.5		90	
Sulfadoxone			200			
Antineoplastic Drugs						
Actinomycin D	Pep		~36			
l-Asparaginase			8-30		30	
5-Azacytidine			3-6	< 1		
Azathioprine			3			
Bleomycin	Pep		~1.5*, 8.9**	~0.4*		*single dose **following continuous IV infusion
Carmustine (BCNU)			~5	3.25		
Chlorambucil	B	8.0				
Cisplatin			59-73			
Cyclophosphamide	B		3-11	0.4-0.6	0-10*	*active metabolites ~60%
Cytarabine	B	4.3	0.5-3.3			
Dacarbazine		4.42	~3-4			
Daunorubicin	A		~50			
Doxorubicin	Gly		~30			
5-Fluorouracil	B	8.1	14-29	0.38		
Melphalan	B		~3-4	0.63*	50-60	*44L
Methotrexate	A	4.3, 5.5	3.5, 6-69*		~50	*two terminal phases
Tamoxifen			>168			
Vinblastine			~3			
Vincristine		5, 7.4	~3			
VM-26 (teniposide)			11-39		>90	
VP-16 213 (etoposide)			~14			
Anti-Parkinsonian Drugs						
Amantadine	B		9-37	~6		
Bromocriptine		4.9	~3	~3.4*	~96**	*240L **to albumin
Levodopa	Aac	2.3, 8.7, 9.9	2.5			

Appendix A. (continued)

Drug	Nature[1]	pK$_a$[2]	T$_{1/2}$[3] (hours)	V$_d$[4] (L/kg)	Protein[5] binding	Notes[6]
Antipsychotic Drugs						
Butaperazine			~12-18			
Chlorpromazine	B	9.3	16-30	10-35, 32-150*	98-99	*im, oral
Haloperidol	B	8.7	13-35	18-30	92	
Lithium		6.8*	8-35**	0.4-1.4	0	*lithium carbonate **may range up to 41h
Loxapine		6.6	3-4			
Mesoridazine			~2.6-6			
Perphenazine	B	7.8	~21	10-35		
Pimozide		8.6	~29		97	
Prochlorperazine	B	8.1	~23			
Thioridazine			26-36	18	96-99	
Thiothixene			~34			
Antituberculosis Drugs						
Capreomycin	Peptide	6.2, 8.2, 10.1	3			
Cycloserine			12-20			
Ethambutol	B	6.9, 9.5	6-8	0.8	8-40	
Ethionamide	B		2.2		10	
Isoniazid	B		0.7-2, 2-4*	0.6	low	*rapid acetylators, slow acetylators
PAS	A	3.2	0.5-1.5	0.23	50-70	
Pyrazinamide	B	0.5	10-16		50	
Rifampicin	Amp		1.5-5	0.93*	~70-90	*65L
Streptomycin	B		2-3	0.26	20-30	
Antitrichomonal Drugs						
Metronidazole			6-12	0.6-0.8	<20	
Ornidazole			14.4	—*	<15	*85-91% of body weight
Secnidazole			20.2, 14.3*			*males, females
Tinidazole			9.4, 12-13*			*males, females
Antiulcer Drugs						
Carbenoxolone	A	6.7, 7.1	16.3	~0.1	99-100*	*83% to albumin
Cimetidine	B	7.09	2	0.75*	18-26	*52.3L
Antiviral Drugs						
Amantadine	B		9-37			
Cytarabine	B	4.3	0.5-3.3			
Idoxuridine			<0.5			
Vidarabine			~1.5			
Bronchodilators						
Fenoterol	B		6.6, 8*			*oral, iv
Ipratropium bromide	B$_4$		3.2-3.8			
Isoprenaline	B	8.6	2.5	~0.5	65	
Orciprenaline (metaproterenol)	B	8.8, 11.8	~6		10	
Salbutamol (albuterol)	B	9.3, 10.3	2.7-5, 1.7-7.1*			*oral, inhaled
Terbutaline	B	10.1	3-4		25	
Theophylline	A	8.75	3-13	0.3-0.7	53-65	

Appendix A. (continued)

Drug	Nature[1]	pK$_a$[2]	T$_{1/2}$[3] (hours)	V$_d$[4] (L/kg)	Protein[5] binding	Notes[6]
Cardiac Glycosides						
β-Acetyldigoxin	Gly		24; 56*	4.74**		*multiple doses **patients
Deslanoside	Gly		~36		25	
Digitalis leaf	Gly		96-144			
Digitoxin	Gly		168-192	40.9	90-97	
Digoxin	Gly		30-40	5.1-7.4	20-40	
Lanatoside C	Gly		33-36		23-25	
β-Methyldigoxin	Gly		~40-70	10.5*	~10-20	*735L
Ouabain	Gly		21	20.4*	42	*1430L
Proscillaridin	Gly		28-68			
Corticosteroids						
Betamethasone	S		⩾5			
Cortisone	S		0.5-2			
Dexamethasone	S		3-4.5		77	
Fludrocortisone	S		0.5		70-79	
Hydrocortisone	S		1.5-2	0.3	90-95	
Methylprednisolone	S		⩾3.5	1.5*		*105L
Prednisolone	S		2.1-3.5	0.43-0.67*	65, 91	*30-47L, dose dependent
Prednisone	S		3.4-3.8			
Triamcinolone	S		3->5			
Diuretics						
Acetazolamide	A	7.2	2.4-5.8		90-95	
Amiloride	B	8.7	6-9.5	5*		*350L
Bendrofluazide	A	8.5	~4*	1.5	1.18*	*patients
Bumetanide	A		3.5	0.18	95-97	
Chlorthalidone		9.4	51-89	3-13	76*	*98% bound to red blood cells
Chlorothiazide	A	6.7, 9.5	~13		20-80	
Ethacrynic acid	A	3.5	0.5-1			
Frusemide (furosemide)	A	3.8	0.3-1.6	0.07-1.8	91-99	
Hydrochlorothiazide	A	7.9, 9.2	2-15			
Hydroflumethiazide	A	8.9, 10.7	12-27	6.2-6.6		
Metolazone		9.7	~20	1.6*	~95	*113L
Polythiazide	A		26	~4	84	
Spironolactone	S		10-35*	0.05	98**	*active metabolite **parent drug + metabolite
Tienilic acid	A		2-3.3		99.5	
Triamterene	B	6.2	1.5-2.5		~80	
Gout Drugs						
Allopurinol	B	9.4	2-8*		0-4.5	*active metabolite 18-30h
Colchicine		1.7, 12.4	20	2.19	31	
Probenecid	A	3.4	4-12*	0.12-0.18	85-95	*3-8 (0.5g); 6-12 (2g)
Sulphinpyrazone	A	2.8	3-5	~0.15	98-99	

Appendix A. (continued)

Drug	Nature[1]	pK$_a$[2]	T$_{1/2}$[3] (hours)	V$_d$[4] (L/kg)	Protein[5] binding	Notes[6]
Hypnosedatives						
Amylobarbitone	A	7.7	12-27	0.5-1.2	61	
Butobarbitone	A	7.9	37.5	0.78	26	
Chloral hydrate		10.04	7-10*	~0.6	70-80*	*trichloroethanol
Chlormethiazole	B	3.2	3-9			
Ethchlorvynol			19-32	2.36-3.19*		*165-223L
Flunitrazepam	B	1.84	9.5-25	3.4-5.5		
Flurazepam	B	1.9, 8.16	47-100*			*active metabolite
Glutethimide	Amp	9.2	5-22	2.7	54	
Hexobarbitone	A	8.2	3-7	1.1		
Lorazepam	Amp	1.3, 11.5	9-16	0.9	80	
Meprobamate			6-17			
Methaqualone	Sa	2.4	20-60	6*	80	*420L
Nitrazepam	B	3.2, 10.8	18-34	2.1	~90	
Oxazepam	Amp	1.7, 11.6	6-25	1.6	~90	
Paraldehyde			3.4-9.8			
Pentobarbitone	A	7.85-8.03	23-30	0.9-1	60-70	
Phenobarbitone	A	7.2	48-144	0.5-0.6	50-60	
Quinalbarbitone (secobarbitone)	A	7.9	20-28	1.52	46-70	
Temazepam			5-8			
Triazolam			5			
Hypoglycaemic Agents						
Acetohexamide	A		3.5-11*			*drug + active metabolite
Buformin			4-6	3.11*		*218L
Chlorpropamide	A	4.8	24-42	0.09-0.27	88-96	
Glibenclamide (glyburide)	A	5.3	10-16	0.3	~99	
Glibornuride	A		5-12	0.25*	95	*17.6L
Gliclazide	A	5.8	~12		94	
Glipizide	A		3-7	0.16*	92-99	*11.1L
Glisoxepide	A		1.4-5.3		93*	*69% to albumin
Glymidine	A		2.6-5.6			
Insulin (regular)			1.5-2	0.66*	1-10	*46L
Metformin			1-2	~1*	~0	*69L
Phenformin			5-15	5-10	~20	
Tolazamide	A	3.5, 5.7	7			
Tolbutamide	A	5.3	3-25	0.1-0.15	95-97	
Thyroid and Antithyroid Drugs						
Carbimazole			~7*			*active metabolite
Methimazole			6-7			
Propylthiouracil		7.8	1-2		~75	
Thyroxine			144-168	0.1-0.2	>99	
Tri-iodothyronine (liothyronine)			35-60	0.6	>99	

Appendix A. (continued)

Drug	Nature[1]	pK$_a$[2]	T$_{1/2}$[3] (hours)	V$_d$[4] (L/kg)	Protein[5] binding	Notes[6]
Miscellaneous Drugs						
Amphetamine	B	9.9	10-30*			*urinary pH dependent
Aurothiomalate sodium			~144	0.1	95	
Baclofen	A	3.9, 9.6	3-4		30	
Bromocriptine			~48			
Clofibrate	A	2.95	6-25*	0.09-0.17	96	*single dose; 54h multiple
Cromoglycate sodium (cromolyn)	A	2.0	0.6-0.9	0.13*	63-76	*9.2L
Dapsone	A	1.2	17-21		72-80	
Dextrothyroxine			144-168		>99	
Ergotamine			~21			
Isoxsuprine	B	8.0, 9.8	1.25			
Levamisole	B	8.00	~4			
Metoclopramide		7.32	2-4.3	1.7-2.9		
Naloxone		7.94	1-1.7	3		
Orphenadrine	B	8.4	14		20	
Oxytocin			0.08-0.17	0.2	30	
Pizotifen		6.95	22	6.9*	89	*485L
Probucol			>500			
Pseudoephedrine	B		9-16, 5-8*			*pH dependent; 9-16 at pH 8, 5-8 at pH 5.5-6
d-Tubocurarine	B$_4$	8.0, 9.3	0.1	0.07	⩾40-50	

Appendix B
Guide to Adverse Drug Reactions

G.S. Avery, R.C. Heel and T.M. Speight

It is widely accepted that if the benefits of modern drug therapy are to be exploited, the occurrence of adverse reactions to drugs has to be accepted. With most drugs the risk is generally small and the reaction of little consequence to the prescriber or his patient, but every now and then something goes wrong, particularly in the hospitalised patient where the risk of an adverse drug reaction is higher and of much greater consequence. That is not to say that serious or life threatening reactions do not occur in domiciliary practice. Reactions are however, more difficult to detect. In some such cases the symptoms are trivial but nevertheless may be sufficient to discourage the patient from taking further medication, so he should be warned to expect certain side effects. More likely, he will continue treatment ignorant or unaware of the warning symptoms, so he should be asked to report any unusual or premonitory symptoms. Occasionally he will complain and receive substitute treatment or an additional drug to control his symptoms, perhaps from another doctor.

As discussed in chapter VII, many adverse drug reactions are predictable and may be avoided, particularly if the mechanisms and predisposing factors are understood. It is not uncommon for adverse reactions to occur early in the course of treatment, although a number of important reactions can develop insidiously over a period of time. An excessive amount of the drug, resulting from non-individualised dosage and/or prolonged therapy, is a common predisposing factor. Reactions are much more likely to occur in the elderly and newborn, in those with a previous history of allergy or reaction to drugs, in those taking a number of different drugs at the one time, and with some drugs in the presence of associated diseases such as renal or liver disease. Ethnic and genetic factors can also lead to an increased risk of adverse drug reactions.

Although many adverse drug reactions can be predicted on the basis of the known pharmacological action of a drug, the prescriber cannot be expected to memorise all the likely possibilities. Yet, he should be aware of the risks involved and instruct the patient accordingly, particularly to report any unusual or premonitory symptoms and to modify his daily activities to overcome certain drug side effects (e.g. alcohol intake, driving).

Since the incidence of important adverse drug reactions or interactions is in general low, prescribers should always report serious, unusual or unexpected reactions to drugs to the appropriate committee or registry. Any adverse reaction to a new drug should be reported, however trivial, for it may be the first of its kind. When in doubt report, even if you only suspect that the reaction or interaction may have been caused by a drug.

Use of Tables

The tables have been arranged according to the predominant pharmacological action or therapeutic use classifications, although in some cases where the 'anti' classification is not appropriate the drugs are listed under chemical groups, or the diseases for which they are used. Such an arrangement makes it easy to see at a glance the similarities and differences between the individual drugs.

The tables list the commonly occurring effects of the drugs which may influence the patient in his taking of medication, through to the rare but serious or life threatening reactions. 'Safety factors' and determinants of certain reactions are given in many cases and identify those types of patient who are more likely to react to certain drugs. Further information can be found elsewhere in the book by use of the relevant cross reference provided.

General References

Cluff, L.E.; Caranasos, G.J. and Stewart, R.B.: Clinical Problems with Drugs (Saunders, Philadelphia 1975).

Davies, D.M.: Textbook of Adverse Drug Reactions (Oxford University Press, Oxford 1977).

Gross, F.H. and Inman, W.H.W.: Drug Monitoring (Academic Press, London 1977).

Miller, R.R. and Greenblatt, D.J.: Drug Effects in Hospitalized Patients (Wiley, New York 1976).

Smith, S.E. and Rawlins, M.D.: Variability in Human Drug Response (Butterworths, London 1973).

Wade, O.L.: Adverse Reactions to Drugs (Heinemann, London 1970).

Wolstenholme, G. and Porter, Ruth: Drug Responses in Man (Churchill, London 1967).

Reference Texts

Cluff, L.E.; Caranasos, G.J. and Stewart, R.B.: Clinical Problems with Drugs (Saunders, Philadelphia 1975).

Davies, D.M.: Textbook of Adverse Drug Reactions (Oxford University Press, Oxford 1977).

Dukes, M.N.G.: Meylers Side Effects of Drugs, vol. 8 and Annual Supplements (Excerpta Medica, Amsterdam 1976).

Meyler, L. and Peck, H.M.: Drug-Induced Diseases, vol. 4 (Excerpta Medica, Amsterdam 1972).

Appendix B. Guide to adverse reactions of drugs

Drug class	Drug	Clinically important reactions
Adrenoceptor Blocking Drugs Alpha receptor blocking	Phenoxybenzamine	Postural hypotension and reflex tachycardia; miosis; nasal stuffiness; inhibition of ejaculation; nausea and vomiting; sedation, tiredness and weakness (may disappear)
	Phentolamine	Postural hypotension; nasal stuffiness; cardiac (tachycardia, arrhythmias, anginal pain) and gastrointestinal stimulation (abdominal pain, nausea, vomiting, diarrhoea, exacerbation peptic ulcer)
	Tolazoline	Cardiac and gastrointestinal stimulation (as for phentolamine); piloerection; chilliness, apprehension. Effects may decrease with chronic administration
	Dihydrogenated ergot alkaloids ('Hydergine')	Nausea, vomiting, flushing, headache, faintness, urinary urgency
Beta receptor blocking (see also chapter XVII, sect. 6.1.5, 10.2, 11.1; XVIII, sect. 5.6.8)	Acebutolol Alprenolol Atenolol Metoprolol Nadolol Oxprenolol Pindolol Practolol Propranolol Sotalol Timolol Tolamolol	Heart failure (give digitalis to all patients with mild or latent cardiac insufficiency); bradycardia, aggravation of heart block; hypotension (i.v.); exacerbation of asthma (less risk with atenolol, metoprolol); gastrointestinal disturbances, headache, dreams, lightheadedness, visual disturbances (infrequent); depression (propranolol; infrequent but stop drug); rash, fever, purpura (infrequent, but stop drug); peripheral arterial insufficiency (rare); hypoglycaemia; precipitation angina and acute myocardial infarction (abrupt withdrawal in patients with severe coronary artery disease); psoriasiform rash, dry eyes, corneal ulceration, LE cells, peritoneal reaction, pericarditis (practolol)
Amoebicides	Chloroquines	See under Antimalarials
	Emetine	Gastrointestinal disturbances; cardiotoxicity; skeletal muscle weakness
	Hydroxyquinolines	See under this entry
	Metronidazole Tinidazole	Nausea; skin rash. See also under Trichomonacides
	Paromomycin	Gastrointestinal disturbances; headache, vertigo; skin rash
Amphetamines		Nervousness, restlessness, sleeplessness; confusional and paranoid states (prolonged abuse and especially in mentally ill); cardiovascular stimulation; gastrointestinal disturbances; dryness of the mouth; chills, collapse and syncope (overdosage); dependence
Anabolic Hormones		Hepatic dysfunction and jaundice (not seen with nandrolone); oedema; virilising effects in women (acne, hirsutism, change of voice, menstrual irregularities); precocious sex development in boys; accelerated bone growth in children

Appendix B. (continued)

Drug class	Drug	Clinically important reactions
Anaesthetics, General (see also chapter X; sect. 2.1, 3, 4, 5)	Alphaxolone + alphadolone	Relaxes jaw muscles; flushing of skin around neck, upper chest; muscle twitching (espec. hyoscine premedication); generalised clonic muscular contractions (rare); short periods cough, hiccoughing (recovery); laryngospasm (extremely rare); respiratory depression; tachycardia; hypersensitivity (rare)
	Cyclopropane	Explosive
	Diethyl ether	Tracheobronchial irritation, convulsions
	Enflurane	Convulsions, other muscle movements
	Halothane	Hepatotoxicity (appears most likely after multiple exposure within short time); predisposes to uterine haemorrhage (relaxes uterus); increases intracranial pressure; bradycardia; may trigger malignant hyperthermia
	Isoflurane	Marked respiratory depression
	Ketamine	Raised blood pressure and increase in heart rate; psychotomimetic effects during recovery (except in children and the aged); tonic and clonic movements; diplopia and blurred vision (elderly); respiratory depression (rapid administration or overdosage); raises intracranial pressure
	Methohexitone	Respiratory disturbances (apnoea, coughing, chest-wall spasm, laryngospasm, bronchospasm); tachycardia; precipitates acute attacks in porphyria; causes hepatic microsomal enzyme induction; hypersensitivity (rare)
	Methoxyflurane	Polyuric renal failure (risk increased if surgery > 2 hours duration)
	Nitrous oxide	Bone marrow depression (prolonged administration)
	Propanidid	Hypotension (administer slowly); tachycardia; ? possibility of 'anaphylactic shock'; venous thrombosis at injection site; 'quinidine-like' effect may lead to dysrhythmias in those with heart disease; initial respiratory stimulation followed by respiratory depression
	Thiopentone	Tissue necrosis (extravenous injection); respiratory disturbances (marked respiratory depression, laryngospasm, bronchospasm); increases intracranial pressure; precipitates acute attacks in porphyria; causes hepatic microsomal enzyme induction; hypersensitivity (rare)
	Trichloroethylene	Tachypnoea, bradycardia
Anaesthetics, Local (see also chapter X, sect. 2.5; XII, sect. 4)	Systemic use	Convulsions, cardiovascular and respiratory collapse (high blood levels); sleepiness (lignocaine); hypotension; methaemoglobinaemia (large doses prilocaine; 800mg); allergic reactions (rare)
	Topical use	Skin sensitivity reactions (amethocaine, butacaine, benzocaine, cinchocaine, procaine); transient local irritation (stinging, burning in ocular use; keratitis — needs frequent application for days or weeks)
Analeptics and Narcotic Antagonists (nonspecific) (see also chapter X, sect. 8.4.4; XX, sect. 5.2.2)		CNS stimulation (large doses); cardiovascular stimulation (doxapram); skin irritation, gastrointestinal upset (nikethamide, ethamivan)

Appendix B. (continued)

Drug class	Drug	Clinically important reactions
Analgesics (see also chapter X, sect. 8.4, 8.5, XXII; sect. 3) Anti-inflammatory	Alclofenac	Gastrointestinal disturbances (rare); headache; dizziness; drowsiness; skin rashes (may be severe)
	Aspirin and salicylates	Tinnitus, nausea, gastrointestinal irritation, haematemesis and melaena, anaemia; acute bronchospasm (aspirin sensitive asthmatics); hypoprothrombinaemia; rashes, urticaria, eczematous dermatitis, hyperventilation, respiratory alkalosis (overdosage); metabolic acidosis (children; particularly those with fever and dehydration); nephropathy (prolonged abuse)
	Azapropazone	Gastrointestinal disturbances; skin rash
	Diclofenac	Gastrointestinal disturbances; headache; dizziness
	Diflunisal	Gastrointestinal disturbances (less than salicylates); skin rashes
	Fenoprofen	Gastrointestinal disturbances; headache; giddiness; tinnitus; skin rash
	Flufenamic and Mefenamic acid	Diarrhoea, indigestion, exacerbation of peptic ulcer; haemolytic anaemia (mefenamic acid); rash (stop drug); acute bronchospasm (aspirin sensitive asthmatics)
	Flurbiprofen	Gastrointestinal disturbances; headache; skin rash
	Ibuprofen	Gastrointestinal disturbances, exacerbation of peptic ulcer; headache, giddiness, drowsiness; skin rash (uncommon); ?toxic amblyopia (rare); acute bronchospasm (aspirin sensitive asthmatics)
	Indomethacin	Headaches and unpleasant cerebral sensations (dose related); gastrointestinal disturbances, anaemia, exacerbation of peptic ulcer; skin reactions (uncommon), oral ulceration; haematological complications (rare); psychotic disturbances including depression (rare); visual disturbances (rare; but sensitivity to glare in some cases night driving); acute bronchospasm (aspirin sensitive asthmatics)
	Ketoprofen	Gastrointestinal disturbances; headache, giddiness, drowsiness; skin rash (rare)
	Naproxen	Gastrointestinal disturbances; tinnitus; giddiness; skin rashes and angio-oedema (rare)
	Phenylbutazone and oxyphenbutazone	Gastrointestinal disturbances, exacerbation of peptic ulcer; salt retention and oedema (may precipitate congestive heart failure in the elderly); acute interstitial nephritis; skin reactions; ulcerative stomatitis (stop drug if sore throat or other oral lesions); haematological complications including aplastic anaemia (rare if dose below 400mg daily); goitre and myxoedema (occasionally seen); acute bronchospasm (aspirin sensitive asthmatics); salivary gland enlargement (rare)
	Sulindac	Gastrointestinal disturbances; giddiness; headache; tinnitus; skin rashes (rare)
	Tolmetin	Gastrointestinal disturbances; headache; dizziness
Antipyretic (mild or simple analgesics)	Aspirin	See above this entry
	Paracetamol (acetaminophen)	Gastrointestinal disturbances (much less common than with aspirin); anaemia, skin rash (rare); hepatic necrosis (overdosage); ?nephropathy (prolonged abuse); acute bronchospasm (aspirin-sensitive asthmatics)
	Phenacetin	Nephropathy, methaemoglobinaemia, haemolytic anaemia (prolonged abuse)

Appendix B. (continued)

Drug class	Drug	Clinically important reactions
Analgesics (continued) Narcotic (strong analgesics)		Respiratory depression; dependence; nausea, vomiting, dizziness, mental clouding; dysphoria; constipation; increased biliary tract pressure; hypotension (IV morphine); skin rashes (uncommon); dental caries (abuse); precipitate encephalopathy in liver disease (morphine)
Non-narcotic	Codeine and Dextropropoxyphene	Nausea, vomiting, constipation (codeine), dizziness; drowsiness (large doses); skin rashes; blurred vision; abuse potential (low)
	Pentazocine	Sedation, sweating, dizziness or lightheadedness; nausea; psychotomimetic effects and depersonalisation (uncommon with therapeutic doses); respiratory depression, increased blood pressure, tachycardia (high doses); abuse potential (low)
Androgens (see also chapter XVI; sect. 10)		Hepatic dysfunction and jaundice (not seen with testosterone, calusterone); oedema; virilising effects in women; See also anabolic hormones
Anorexiants (see also chapter XVI; sect. 7)		CNS and cardiovascular stimulation (generally less than amphetamine compounds; not seen with fenfluramine except in overdosage); dryness of the mouth; drowsiness, diarrhoea (fenfluramine); mood depression (abrupt withdrawal of fenfluramine); dependence (risk much less with fenfluramine)
Antacids (see also chapter XIX; sect. 4.3.1)	Aluminium hydroxide gels	Constipation; phosphorus depletion syndrome (chronic use)
	Sodium preparations	Milk alkali syndrome (prolonged use in conjunction with large amounts of calcium, particularly in presence of renal disease); sodium toxicity in those on restricted sodium intake
	Calcium carbonate	Constipation or diarrhoea; hypercalcaemia (rare); milk alkali syndrome (prolonged use, particularly in presence of renal disease); renal calculi (prolonged ingestion)
	Magnesium preparations	Diarrhoea; hypermagnesaemia (in presence of renal disease); phosphorus depletion syndrome (prolonged use)
Anthelmintics (see also chapter XIX; sect. 11.4)		Gastrointestinal disturbances (usually nausea, vomiting; uncommon with most drugs; more common with thiabendazole); headache (pyrantel, diethylcarbamazine); dizziness (pyrantel, thiabendazole); neurological effects (piperazine; rare)
Antianginal Drugs (see also chapter XVII; sect. 4.2)	β-Adrenoceptor blocking drugs	See under this entry
	Nifedipine	Flushing, headache, postural hypotension; gastrointestinal upset; tiredness; dizziness; ischaemic cardiac pain (after first dose or increased dose)
	Perhexilene	Dizziness, headache, nausea, vomiting (most common early reactions); tremors; gait disorders; raised intracranial pressure; hypoglycaemia; marked weight loss; paraesthesiae; peripheral neuropathy (reversible); hepatitis; rash (occasionally)
	Vasodilators, coronary	See under this entry
	Verapamil	Bradycardia, hypotension (esp. in those who have received β-blockers prior to verapamil); aggravation of heart block; risk of heart failure (digitalise patients with mild or latent cardiac insufficiency); avoid in those with sick sinus syndrome

Appendix B. (continued)

Drug class	Drug	Clinically important reactions
Antianxiety Agents (see also chapter XXVI; sect. 8.4)	Benzodiazepines (e.g. chlordiazepoxide, diazepam, oxazepam, etc)	Drowsiness, fatigue, ataxia (larger doses and in elderly or debilitated); confusional states (elderly); nausea, headache, blurred vision, skin rash, increased frequency vivid dreams (uncommon); difficult urination (elderly); dependence (extremes of dose and prolonged use)
	Butyrophenones and Phenothiazines (low doses)	Drowsiness, extrapyramidal reactions (restlessness with piperazine phenothiazines; seen to a much lesser extent than with doses used in psychoses); skin reactions (phenothiazines)
	Hydroxyzine	Drowsiness, dryness of mouth; tremor and convulsions (rare, high doses)
	Meprobamate	Drowsiness; allergic skin reactions; hypotension (elderly); blood dyscrasias (rare); dependence, withdrawal syndrome, convulsions (prolonged use higher doses)
Antiarrhythmic Drugs (see chapter XVII; sect. 6, 10.2, 11.1)	β-Adrenoceptor blocking drugs	See under this entry
	Digitalis glycosides	See under Cardiac glycosides
	Disopyramide	Aggravate heart block; risk of heart failure (digitalise those with severe cardiomyopathy associated with cardiac insufficiency); dry mouth, blurred vision, urinary hesitancy (?use in narrow angle glaucoma, urinary retention); gastrointestinal irritation
	Lignocaine (lidocaine)	Drowsiness; bradycardia (give atropine); conduction delays, depressed myocardial function, paraesthesias, twitching, disorientation and convulsions (large doses); respiratory arrest (rare). Toxicity more likely in presence of hepatic disease, congestive heart failure (modify dose)
	Mexiletine	Bradycardia, hypotension, AV block (rapid IV injection); hand tremor; dizziness; blurred vision, drowsiness, nystagmus; toxic confusion state (usually with IV doses or oral loading doses)
	Phenytoin	Conduction delay and depressed myocardial function (large doses); neurological symptoms (large doses); skin rash; hypotension (excessive dosage or too rapid administration, or presence severe cardiac decompensation). See also under anticonvulsants (these effects not likely in usual short term antiarrhythmic use)
	Procainamide	Hypotension, conduction defect, widening of QRS complex, ventricular arrhythmias; gastrointestinal irritation; systemic lupus-like syndrome (more rapid onset in slow acetylators); blood dyscrasias. Modify dose in renal failure
	Quinidine	Cardiac disturbances (similar to procainamide); gastrointestinal irritation; skin rash; drug fever; tinnitus, neurological symptoms; thrombocytopenia; syncope (may be fatal); respiratory distress or cyanosis (due to curare-like activity)
	Tocainide	Paraesthesia, dizziness, sweating, tremor
	Verapamil	Aggravation of heart block; risk of heart failure (digitalise patients with mild or latent cardiac insufficiency); bradycardia, hypotension

Appendix B. (continued)

Drug class	Drug	Clinically important reactions
Antibacterial Agents (see also chapter XXVII, sect. 7; XXI, sect. 14.1)	Aminoglycosides	Systemic hypersensitivity reactions (kanamycin, streptomycin); gastrointestinal disturbances; skin reactions (sensitivity with topical use); neuromuscular blockade and respiratory paralysis (all members espec. presence renal impairment); paraesthesiae (kanamycin, amikacin), headache (gentamicin, kanamycin, amikacin), peripheral neuropathy (streptomycin, kanamycin); nephrotoxicity; ototoxicity (gentamicin, tobramycin and streptomycin mainly affect vestibular function; framycetin, neomycin, kanamycin and amikacin mainly auditory function — see chapt. XI; sect. 7.1.1); pain at injection site (kanamycin, streptomycin); blood dyscrasias and visual disturbances (streptomycin); intestinal malabsorption (continued use oral framycetin, neomycin). Modify dose in renal failure
	Amoxycillin	See penicillins in this entry
	Ampicillin	See penicillins in this entry
	Cephalosporins	Hypersensitivity reactions; gastrointestinal disturbances; skin reactions; nephrotoxicity (large doses cephaloridine, cephazolin, cephalothin); + ve direct Coombs test (rarely assoc. haemolytic anaemia; cephalothin); convulsions (moderate doses in impaired renal function); pain, local reaction at injection site (cephalothin, cephazolin, cephapirin, cefoxitin). Modify dose in renal failure
	Chloramphenicol	Hypersensitivity reactions (uncommon); gastrointestinal disturbances; skin reactions; haematological complications, incl. irreversible marrow aplasia; hyperbilirubinaemia (newborn); circulatory collapse (excessive dosage newborn); optic neuritis, toxic amblyopia (long term or high dose, esp. children); peripheral neuropathy. ?Avoid in renal failure
	Clindamycin	See lincomycin in this entry
	Cloxacillin	See penicillins in this entry
	Colistin	See polymyxins in this entry
	Co-trimoxazole (trimethoprim + sulphamethoxazole)	Gastrointestinal disturbances; skin reactions; headache, dizziness; haematological complications incl. megaloblastic anaemia (folate metabolism may be impaired; N.B. elderly); avoid in pregnancy and newborn. Modify dose in renal failure
	Cycloserine	Neurotoxicity, including mood change, convulsions (do not exceed 1g daily). Avoid in renal failure
	Epicillin	See penicillins in this entry
	Erythromycins	Hypersensitivity reactions (rare); gastrointestinal disturbances; skin reactions (uncommon); reversible jaundice (erythromycin estolate or triacetyloleandomycin given for more than 10-14 days); pain, local reaction at injection site (1g doses)
	Framycetin	See aminoglycosides in this entry
	Fusidic acid	Gastrointestinal disturbances; skin reactions
	Gentamicin	See aminoglycosides in this entry
	Hexamine (methenamine)	Gastrointestinal and skin reactions. Avoid in renal failure
	Kanamycin	See aminoglycosides in this entry

Appendix B. (continued)

Drug class	Drug	Clinically important reactions
Antibacterial Agents (continued)	Lincomycin and Clindamycin	Hypersensitivity reactions (uncommon); gastrointestinal disturbances (diarrhoea); skin reactions; cardiopulmonary arrest after rapid IV infusion lincomycin
	Metronidazole	Nausea, diarrhoea; metallic taste; headache; vertigo; urticaria; transient leucopenia; colours urine dark brown; peripheral neuropathy (high doses)
	Nalidixic acid	Gastrointestinal disturbances; skin reactions, incl. photosensitivity; headache; precipitates convulsions in those predisposed (renal impairment may make this more likely); psychic and visual disturbances (uncommon). Care in renal failure
	Neomycin	See aminoglycosides in this entry
	Nitrofurantoin	Hypersensitivity reactions; gastrointestinal disturbances; skin reactions; peripheral neuropathy (high blood levels or presence renal failure); haemolytic anaemia (mainly in those with G6PD deficiency); pulmonary reactions. Avoid in renal failure
	Novobiocin	Hypersensitivity reactions; gastrointestinal disturbances; skin reactions; pain at injection site; blood dyscrasias; haemolytic anaemia (mainly in those with G6PD deficiency) hyperbilirubinaemia (newborn); yellow discolouration of skin and sclera
	Oxolinic acid	Gastrointestinal disturbances; headache, insomnia, restlessness. Care in those with convulsive disorders, renal failure
	Paromomycin	Gastrointestinal disturbances; ?nephro- and ototoxicity
	Penicillins	Hypersensitivity reactions; gastrointestinal disturbances with oral administration; skin reactions (espec. ampicillin in glandular fever); convulsions precipitated (very large parenteral doses carbenicillin, benzylpenicillin; especially in presence of renal failure); + ve direct Coomb's test (assoc. haemolytic anaemia, usually after very large doses benzylpenicillin especially in presence of renal failure); pain at injection site (benzylpenicillin, carbenicillin); increased haemorrhagic tendency, acidosis, hypernatraemia (large doses carbenicillin in renal failure); interstitial nephritis (rarely, notably methicillin); immune granulocytopenia
	Pivampicillin	See penicillins in this entry
	Polymyxins	Hypersensitivity reactions; gastrointestinal disturbances; skin reactions; dizziness; paraesthesiae, peripheral neuropathy; neuromuscular blockade and respiratory paralysis; nephrotoxicity; pain at injection site; visual disturbances; neuropsychiatric reactions in chronic renal failure. Modify dose in renal failure

Appendix B. (continued)

Drug class	Drug	Clinically important reactions
Antibacterial Agents (continued)	Rifamide	Hypersensitivity reactions; gastrointestinal disturbances; skin reactions; pain at injection site; yellow discolouration of skin, darkens urine. See also rifampicin under antituberculosis drugs
	Spectinomycin	Gastrointestinal disturbances; skin reactions; pain at injection site
	Spiramycin	Hypersensitivity and skin reactions (uncommon); gastrointestinal disturbances
	Streptomycin	See aminoglycosides in this entry
	Sulphonamides	Hypersensitivity reactions incl. acute renal failure and hepatic dysfunction, skin and mucous membrane eruptions (Stevens-Johnson syndrome); gastrointestinal disturbances; photosensitivity; headache, malaise, dizziness, paraesthesiae; peripheral neuropathy; possible crystalluria (depends on solubility and urinary concentration); haematological complications; haemolytic anaemia (espec. those with G6PD deficiency); neonatal kernicterus (if given to newborn and to mother in late pregnancy); ? precipitates polyarteritis nodosa
	Tetracyclines	Hypersensitivity reactions; gastrointestinal disturbances incl. intractable chronic diarrhoea, but also rarely staphylococcal enterocolitis (mostly in surgical patients); skin reactions, incl. photosensitivity; raised blood urea; hepatotoxicity (pregnancy; large doses, espec. parenterally); pain, local reaction at injection site; discolour teeth and nails in children; intracranial hypertension in newborn; outdated products have caused Fanconi-like syndrome; avoid in renal failure (except minocycline and doxycycline) and avoid in pregnancy; reversible nephrogenic diabetes insipidus (demethylchlortetracycline)
	Thiamphenicol	As for chloramphenicol but stated not to, or to only rarely cause irreversible aplasia
	Triacetyloleandomycin	As for erythromycin estolate in this entry
	Trimethoprim	See co-trimoxazole in this entry
	Vancomycin	Hypersensitivity reactions; skin reactions; nephrotoxicity; ototoxicity (auditory function); pain, local reaction at injection site. Modify dose in renal failure
Anticholinergics (see also chapter XIX; sect. 4.3.2)		Retrosternal pain; dry mouth, blurred vision, difficulty in micturition; impotence, aggravation constipation, palpitations, postural hypotension (large doses); skin rash (some compounds); toxic delirium (elderly)
Anticholinesterases (see also chapter XII; sect. 5; XXV, sect. 9)	Systemic use	Miosis, sweating, excessive salivation, urinary urgency, gastrointestinal distress, hypotension, bradycardia; bronchospasm; cholinergic crisis (excessive dosage in myasthenic patients); severe polyneuritis — skeletal muscle fatigue, weakness and fasciculations, may be followed by paralysis (overdosage or cumulative amount in non-myasthenic patients)
	Topical ophthalmological use	Cataract (prolonged use in glaucoma); follicular hypertrophy; headache, brow pain, blurred vision, intense photophobia, conjunctival and various allergic reactions; systemic reactions with ecothiopate; retinal detachment (dyflos; rare)

Appendix B. (continued)

Drug class	Drug	Clinically important reactions
Anticoagulants (see also chapter XXIII; sect. 3.2)	Heparin	Haemorrhagic phenomena (overdosage; risk greatest in females over 60 and with intermittent IV administration); osteoporosis (prolonged use); hypersensitivity reactions, transient alopecia (rare); thrombocytopenia
	Indanediones (e.g. phenindione)	Red colouration of urine; sensitivity reactions (fever, blood dyscrasias, diarrhoea and steatorrhoea, hepatitis, renal lesions, dermatitis); haemorrhagic phenomena (risk greatest in elderly and patients in poor condition); transient alopecia
	Coumarins (e.g. dicoumarol; warfarin)	Rash and transient alopecia (uncommon); necrosis of skin (rare); haemorrhagic phenomena (risk greatest in elderly and patients in poor condition); increased risk of congenital abnormalities with warfarin (see chapter III; sect. 6)
Anticonvulsants (see also chapter XXV; sect. 3)	Barbiturates (phenobarbitone, methylphenobar- bitone)	Nystagmus, drowsiness, incoordination and gait ataxia, diplopia, blurred vision (excessive dosage); skin eruptions; megaloblastic anaemia (rare); lupus erythematosus, polyarteritis nodosa, Stevens-Johnson syndrome (very rare); coagulation defect in newborn (responds vitamin K)
	Carbamazepine	Nystagmus, gait ataxia, diplopia, blurred vision (excessive dosage); gastrointestinal disturbances; skin rash (stop drug); bone marrow depression (rare), pulmonary eosinophilia; water intoxication (hyponatraemia); bradycardia, conduction disturbances (excessive dosage in elderly)
	Chlormethiazole	Headache; coughing; gastrointestinal disturbances; deep coma, respiratory depression (overdosage)
	Clonazepam	Drowsiness, fatigue, muscular hypotonia and coordination disturbances; salivary or bronchial hypersecretion (mainly in infants and children); behavioural disturbances
	Diazepam and Nitrazepam	Drowsiness, dizziness, fatigue, ataxia; respiratory depression, hypotension (IV diazepam in status epilepticus; rare, but avoid too rapid administration)
	Hydantoins (phenytoin, ethotoin, methoin)	Nystagmus, incoordination and gait ataxia, drowsiness and lethargy, diplopia, blurred vision (excessive dosage); gum hypertrophy; hirsutism (young patients), coarse facies, mild polyneuritis, hypocalcaemia with or without rickets or osteomalacia (long term use, esp. institutionalised children); gastrointestinal disturbances; skin eruptions; bone marrow depression, megaloblastic anaemia, hepatic necrosis, systemic lupus erythematosus-like syndrome, polyarteritis nodosa, reversible lymphadenopathy resembling lymphoma, Stevens-Johnson syndrome (very rare); hyperglycaemia, hyperosmolarity (IV administration; esp. diabetics); coagulation defect in newborn (responds vitamin K); ? impaired glucose metabolism (care in those at risk diabetes); increased risk of congenital abnormalities (see chapter III, sect. 3.10.2) Incidence of reactions less with ethotoin (but less effective than phenytoin). Methoin causes fewer minor reactions than phenytoin, but serious reactions much more common
	Oxazolidines (paramethadione, troxidone i.e. trimethadione)	Incoordination of gait (excessive dosage); photophobia; persistent hiccups (troxidone); skin eruptions, exfoliative dermatitis (stop drug); bone marrow depression, nephrotic syndrome (rare); systemic lupus-like syndrome, polyarteritis nodosa (very rare); Stevens-Johnson syndrome (troxidone, very rare); alopecia (troxidone)

Appendix B. (continued)

Drug class	Drug	Clinically important reactions
Anticonvulsants (continued)	Primidone	Nystagmus, drowsiness, mild incoordination, diplopia, blurred vision (excessive dosage); skin eruptions; megaloblastic anaemia (rare)
	Sodium valproate (valproic acid)	Nausea, vomiting, abdominal cramps, diarrhoea; drowsiness, sedation; changes in appetite; hair loss (rare); worsened behaviour (some children also receiving barbiturates); prolonged bleeding times (high doses, espec. children), thrombocytopenia
	Succinimides (ethosuximide, phensuximide, methsuximide)	Incoordination of gait (excessive dosage); gastrointestinal disturbances; skin eruptions; persistent hiccups, haematuria (ethosuximide)
	Sulthiame	Drowsiness, headache, ataxia; paraesthesiae, hyperpnoea
Antidepressants (see also chapter XXVI; sect. 7.5)	Central stimulants	See under this entry
	Monoamine oxidase inhibitors	Tremors, insomnia, hyperhydrosis; postural hypotension; dizziness, headache; constipation; inhibition of ejaculation, urinary retention, dry mouth, blurred vision; hepatitis and leucopenia (uncommon; not seen with tranylcypromine); hypomania, rarely toxic psychosis (espec. elderly), lowered seizure threshold; skin rashes; peripheral neuropathy (not seen with tranylcypromine)
	Tricyclics (imipramine, amitriptyline etc)	Dry mouth, blurred vision, constipation, dizziness; urinary retention; paralytic ileus (rare; stop drug); excessive sweating; headache; epigastric distress; postural hypotension, muscle tremors (espec. elderly); disturbances of cardiac rhythm and conduction (caution in cardiac disease); severe confusional states and toxic psychosis, mania (elderly and in those with previous or latent psychoses); lowered seizure threshold; reversible cholestatic jaundice, agranulocytosis (rare); skin rashes, incl. photosensitivity; excess weight gain
Antidiarrhoeal Drugs (see also chapter XIX; sect. 7.2, 8.1.2)	Adsorbents with anti-infective agents (neomycin, strepto-mycin; poorly absorb-ed sulphonamides)	Systemic reactions rare (do not use in those with extensive intestinal lesions); avitaminosis B_1 or K (prolonged use)
	Codeine	Infrequent: nausea, vomiting, dizziness, drowsiness; skin rashes; blurred vision
	Diphenoxylate (with atropine)	Infrequent: nausea, abdominal distension, rash, drowsiness, dizziness, restlessness; respiratory depression (overdosage in children)
	Furazolidone	Nausea, vomiting; arthralgia, fever, skin sensitivity (uncommon); haemolysis (in patients with G6PD deficiency); colours urine brown
	Loperamide	Infrequent: nausea, abdominal cramps, dizziness, rash, dry mouth
	Opium tincture	Undesirable effects of narcotic analgesics (large doses only)
	Sulphasalazine (used in ulcerative colitis)	Anorexia, nausea, vomiting; headache, malaise; arthritis, pulmonary and neurotoxicity, lymphadenopathy, drug fever, skin reactions, photosensitivity (less common); haemolytic anaemia (those with G6PD deficiency); agranulocytosis, leucopenia (rare)
Antidiuretic Drugs (see also chapter XVI; sect. 12)	Pituitary snuff	Nasal irritation; sneezing, bronchospasm; fluid retention (overdosage); myocardial ischaemia; abdominal cramps
	Desmopressin	Headaches, abdominal cramps, flushing; rhinitis, irritation of nasal mucosa; hyponatraemia
	Vasopressin	Fluid retention (excessive dosage); facial pallor (large parenteral doses); nasal irritation (topical use); myocardial ischaemia; abdominal cramps, diarrhoea; uterine contractions; skin rash, bronchospasm

Appendix B. (continued)

Drug class	Drug	Clinically important reactions
Antiemetics (see also chapter XIX; sect. 5.2)		Drowsiness; dry mouth (less with non-phenothiazines); acute dystonia (phenothiazines and metoclopramide, espec. children); postural hypotension (phenothiazines)
Antifibrinolytic Drugs (see also chapter XXIII; XXIII; sect. 5.4)	Aminocaproic acid Tranexamic acid	Possibility of vascular occlusion; hypotension, dizziness, nausea, diarrhoea, abdominal discomfort, rash, conjunctival suffusion, nasal stuffiness (usually mild)
	Aprotinin	Sensitivity reactions (rare)
Antifungal Agents (see also chapter XXVII; sect. 5.8)	Amphotericin B	Intravenous — Chills, fever, nausea, vomiting, headache (minimised by aspirin plus antihistamine or corticosteroid); local thrombophlebitis; anaemia; jaundice and hepatocellular dysfunction; nephrotoxicity; hypersensitivty reactions; hypokalaemia; hypomagnesaemia
		Intrathecal — Pain along distribution lumbar nerves, headache, paraesthesiae, nerve palsies (incl. foot drop), chemical meningitis, urinary retention, ?impaired vision
		Topical — Pruritus, burning (intertriginous areas); sensitisation (rare)
		Oral — Diarrhoea
	Miconazole (intravenous)	Phlebitis, pruritus; nausea, vomiting, anorexia, diarrhoea; fever, rash, flushing; haematological changes (reversible, may be due to drug vehicle); ?cardiotoxicity, arrhythmias (rapid injection of large doses)
	Flucytosine	Nausea, vomiting, diarrhoea; rashes; haematological abnormalities (leucopenia, thrombocytopenia)
	Griseofulvin	Headache; dry mouth, gastrointestinal disturbances; neuritic pains, arthralgia; mental confusion, diminished motor coordination (doses > 1g daily); skin sensitivity reactions, incl. photosensitivity; ? precipitates acute attacks in porphyria; gynaecomastia (large doses in children)
	Hachimycin (trichomycin)	Nausea, diarrhoea
	Natamycin (pimaricin)	Nausea, diarrhoea
	Nystatin	Nausea, diarrhoea
	Miscellaneous Topical	Photosensitivity (buclosamide, fenticlor, halogenated salicylanilides); irritation and sensitisation (diamthazole, hydroxyquinolines, undecenoates); irritation (clotrimazole, econazole, miconazole); yellow staining of fabrics (hydroxyquinolines)
Antihistamines (see also chapter XI; sect. 1.2, 2.4)		Sedation (dizziness, inability to concentrate, slowed reflex activity may occur with some compounds — phenindamine may cause stimulant effects); dry mouth; gastrointestinal disturbances; skin sensitisation (topical use); photosensitivity (promethazine, diphenhydramine); weight gain (cyproheptadine); nervousness (phenindamine); cardiac stimulation (parenteral diphenhydramine); hallucinations (abuse, high doses)

Appendix B. (continued)

Drug class	Drug	Clinically important reactions
Antihypertensive Drugs (see also chapter XVIII; sect. 5, 6.2)	β-Adrenoceptor blocking agents	See under this entry
	Adrenergic neurone blocking drugs (bethanidine, debrisoquine, guanethidine)	Postural hypotension; diarrhoea (guanethidine); fluid retention; failure of ejaculation; depression (very rare; stop drug); parotid tenderness (bethanidine and guanethidine); pressor response with tyramine-containing foodstuffs such as matured cheese (debrisoquine)
	Clonidine	Drowsiness; depression (must stop drug); dry mouth, parotid pain; constipation; fluid retention; Raynaud's phenomenon; dreams; irritability, hallucinations; impotence, postural hypotension (uncommon); blood pressure crisis may occur following abrupt withdrawal
	Diazoxide (IM)	Burning sensation along route of injection; gastrointestinal disturbances; hypotension; hyperglycaemia (repeated doses; use insulin or sulphonylurea drugs); fluid retention; substernal chest pain; interruption of labour (use oxytocics)
	Diuretics	See under this entry
	Ganglion blocking agents (mecamylamine, pempidine, pentolinium, trimetaphan)	Postural hypotension; urinary retention, constipation, paralytic ileus; blurred vision, dry mouth; impotence; precipitate anginal pain; syncope; tremors, mental aberrations (mecamylamine, pempidine)
	Hydrallazine	Headache (reduce dose temporarily); tachycardia (prevent by use of a β-blocker); dyspnoea on exertion; dizziness, nausea, vomiting, flushing; fluid retention; skin rash; drug fever (stop drug); lupus erythematosus syndrome (more likely in slow acetylators, esp. with high dose; stop drug); myocardial stimulation (caution in coronary artery disease)
	Labetalol	Postural hypotension (more apparent with high initial doses or if dose increased too rapidly); nasal stuffiness; vivid dreams; failure of ejaculation; epigastric pain (high doses); headache; nausea; tiredness; cramps; scalp tingling
	Methyldopa	Drowsiness; depression (stop drug); dry mouth, nightmares, myalgia, fluid retention; drug fever (must stop drug); + ve direct Coombs test (no need to stop drug); haemolytic anaemia (rare; must stop drug); impotence; postural hypotension (uncommon); lactation (uncommon, stop drug); hepatitis (rare)
	Pargyline	Postural hypotension; fluid retention, weight gain; insomnia, nightmares, psychotic reactions; muscle cramps, nausea, diarrhoea or constipation. See also under Antidepressants, monoamine oxidase inhibitors
	Prazosin	Postural dizziness (first dose must be small and preferably given at bedtime); oedema; drowsiness, headache; gastrointestinal disturbances, dry mouth, blurred vision, rash, pruritus
	Rauwolfia alkaloids	Drowsiness; dreams, nightmares, nasal stuffiness, weight gain (stop drug); depression (mandatory to stop drug); mild diarrhoea; bradycardia. Troublesome central side effects minimised if dose kept below 0.5mg reserpine daily
	Sodium nitroprusside	Metabolic acidosis, accumulation of cyanide (excessive rate of infusion or total dosage). See also chapter X (sect. 2.6)

Appendix B. (continued)

Drug class	Drug	Clinically important reactions
Antileprotics (see also chapter XXX; sect. 7)	Clofazimine	Red-brown pigmentation of skin (lesser degree discolouration conjunctiva, urine, sweat, sputum); nausea, diarrhoea (high dosage)
	Dapsone	Gastrointestinal disturbances; skin rashes, headache, giddiness; tachycardia; haemolytic anaemia (more severe in those with G6PD deficiency), agranulocytosis, leucopenia; hepatitis. Dosage should be kept to a minimum
	Thiambutosine	Skin rashes; antithyroid action (very high doses)
Antimalarial Drugs see also chapter XXX; (sect. 6.1)	Amodiaquine	Gastrointestinal disturbances; tiredness, vertigo; pigmentation of palate, nail beds, skin
	Chloroquine derivatives	Headache, gastrointestinal upset; pruritus, lichenoid skin eruption, skin or hair discolouration; visual disturbances, reversible corneal deposits; retinopathy; optic neuritis (rare); peripheral neuropathy; myopathy; rarely ototoxicity (long term use in discoid lupus and rheumatoid arthritis); photosensitivity; exacerbation symptoms of porphyria. See also chapter XXII (sect. 3.3.2), XII (sect. 11.1.3)
	Mepacrine (quinacrine)	Yellow pigmentation tissues; gastrointestinal disturbances; headache; allergic skin reactions (uncommon); corneal oedema; blood dyscrasias; toxic psychoses
	Quinine	Gastrointestinal disturbances (nausea); ototoxicity (tinnitus, auditory); visual impairment, generalised cutaneous erythema and pruritus, headache, confusion (idiosyncrasy or excessive dosage); thrombocytopenia, haemolytic anaemia
	Primaquine	Abdominal cramps, epigastric distress; methaemoglobinaemia and cyanosis, leucopenia, haemolytic anaemia (large doses and in those with G6PD deficiency)
	Proguanil	Vomiting, abdominal pain, diarrhoea (large doses only); red cells, casts in urine (excessive amounts)
	Pyrimethamine	Anorexia, vomiting; megaloblastic anaemia (reversible by folinic acid)
Antineoplastic Drugs (see also chapter XXIV; sect. 4, 9)		Haematological complications (except bleomycin); megaloblastic anaemia (6-mercaptopurine, thioguanine, azathioprine, methotrexate); nausea and vomiting; renal complications (due to raised serum uric acid); alopecia; local inflammatory reactions at injection site; skin rashes (rare); pulmonary fibrosis (busulphan, bleomycin, chlorambucil, cyclophosphamide, methotrexate); pneumonitis (methotrexate); neurotoxicity (vincristine, less commonly vinblastine, methotrexate, asparaginase, fluorouracil, procarbazine); oral ulceration (methotrexate, 5-fluorouracil, actinomycin D, daunorubicin); haemorrhagic cystitis (cyclophosphamide); cardiotoxicity (doxorubicin, daunorubicin); hepatocellular toxicity (methotrexate, 6-mercaptopurine, azathioprine, l-asparaginase or colaspase); ovarian and testicular toxicity; mutagenic and dysmorphogenic effects, malignant tumours (following therapeutic immunosuppression); dilutional hyponatraemia (vincristine, cyclophosphamide); bladder cancer (prolonged use cyclophosphamide); malabsorption syndrome (reversible).

Appendix B. (continued)

Drug class	Drug	Clinically important reactions
Antiparasitic Drugs (see also chapter XXX; sect. 6)	Anthelmintics	See under this entry
	Antimalarial drugs	See under this entry
	Antimony sodium dimercaptosuccinate	Cardiotoxicity; anorexia, nausea, vomiting, abdominal pain; headache; pain at injection site
	Diethylcarbamazine	Headache, malaise, weakness, joint pain, anorexia, nausea, vomiting; oedema, enlargement of lymph nodes, rash, pyrexia, cough, syncope (reaction to substances released from killed parasites; esp. in onchocerciasis)
	Lucanthone and Hycanthone	Nausea, vomiting; urine coloured orange-yellow (hycanthone); jaundice and hepatic coma (do not use if liver enlarged or history jaundice)
	Melarsoprol	Tissue irritation (extravasation); hypertension; abdominal pain, vomiting; proteinuria, peripheral neuropathy; arthralgia; angioneurotic oedema; rashes
	Metrifonate	Abdominal pain, diarrhoea
	Niridazole	Urine colour darkens; gastrointestinal upset; headache, dizziness; haemolysis (G6PD deficiency), ECG changes (rare); psychosis, convulsions, EEG changes (high plasma concentrations, as in presence of portal-systemic shunts; see also chapter XXX, sect. 6.3.3)
	Oxamniquine	Dizziness, drowsiness; hallucinations and convulsions (usually in patients with history of epilepsy); pain at injection site
	Pentamidine	Hypotension, tachycardia; vomiting; reversible renal and hepatic dysfunction; hypoglycaemia, hyperglycaemia; breathlessness, dizziness, fainting
	Suramin	Nausea, vomiting; hypotension, shock (too rapid IV injection); skin eruptions, paraesthesiae, photophobia, lacrimation; haematuria, proteinuria, nephrotoxicity
Anti-Parkinsonian Drugs (see also chapter XXV; sect. 5)	Amantadine	Intermittent confusion, nightmares, hallucinations (especially elderly), restlessness, giddiness; nausea, dry mouth, defective near vision, difficulties with micturition; palpitations; abnormal involuntary movements (uncommon)
	Anticholinergic drugs	Defective near vision, difficulty with micturition, constipation, dry mouth; excitement, agitation, mental confusion, hallucinations precipitated (especially elderly); drowsiness
	Levodopa	Abnormal involuntary movements (reduce dose); anorexia, nausea, vomiting (reduce dose temporarily); hypotension (stop dose increases or reduce dose); psychiatric disturbances (reduce dose or stop drug); 'on/off' effect (benefit with abnormal movements changes rapidly to akinesia many times in a day); cardiac arrhythmias, ocular disturbances, effects on micturition (occasionally); increased libido; haemolytic anaemia (rare)
	Levodopa + Carbidopa/Benserazide (decarboxylase inhibitor)	Abnormal involuntary movements, dyskinesia; psychiatric disturbances (reduce dose). Other side effects associated with levodopa alone (e.g. anorexia, nausea, vomiting, hypotension, cardiac arrhythmias, dizziness) are reduced in incidence or eliminated

Appendix B. (continued)

Drug class	Drug	Clinically important reactions
Antiplatelet Agents (see also chapter XXIII; sect. 3.1)	Dipyridamole	Headache; gastrointestinal upset, nausea, facial flushing (tend to be transient)
	Aspirin Indomethacin	See under analgesics
	Sulphinpyrazone	See under gout drugs
Antipsychotic Drugs (see also chapter XXVI; sect. 3.5, 5.4)	Butyrophenones (e.g. haloperidol)	Drowsiness; psychomotor impairment; extrapyramidal reactions (particularly akathisia); anorexia, sweating, excess salivation; hypotension (uncommon); skin reactions, jaundice, blood dyscrasias (rare)
	Lithium	Gastrointestinal disturbances, muscle weakness, sluggish dazed feeling (tend to disappear); thirst, polyuria, fine hand tremor (persist); drowsiness, muscle twitching, coarse tremors, ataxia, dysarthria, slurred speech, mental confusion (excess blood levels; must modify dosage immediately); convulsions, coma (overdosage; treat as for barbiturate poisoning); hypothyroidism, hyperthyroidism (long term use); nephrogenic diabetes insipidus; renal tubular damage (long term or intoxication); leucocytosis; excessive weight gain; acne, folliculitis; erectile impotence Risk of toxicity increased in presence of renal or cardiovascular disease and in presence of sodium loss; avoid in pregnancy if possible
	Phenothiazines	Drowsiness; psychomotor impairment; constipation, dry mouth, blurred vision, urinary retention, paralytic ileus (usually only a problem in elderly); postural hypotension (early in course; less common with piperazines); mental confusion (elderly); ventricular tachycardia (high dosage); skin reactions, photosensitivity; extrapyramidal reactions (more common with piperazines; akathisia, dystonia, tardive dyskinesia); pigmentation skin (purple hue), anterior lens and cornea (high doses); retinal pigmentation (high doses over prolonged period; thioridazine, chlorpromazine, prochlorperazine), optic atrophy (prolonged high doses thioridazine, chlorpromazine, perphenazine), anterior cortical lens opacities (thioridazine, trifluoperazine), posterior corneal opacities (trifluoperazine); myopia (esp. prochlorperazine); fever, jaundice, blood dyscrasias (rare); metabolic effects (weight gain, diabetes mellitus precipitated); endocrine effects (menstrual irregularities, lactation, gynaecomastia and loss of libido in men); precipitation convulsions (epileptics); failure of ejaculation (thioridazine)
	Pimozide	Drowsiness, extrapyramidal reactions (akathisia, tremor; more common at high doses); skin rash, hypotension (rare)
	Thioxanthenes (e.g. chlorprothixene, thiothixene)	Similar to the phenothiazines
Antiseptics		Possible irritation of skin and mucous membranes, sensitivity; photosensitivity (hexachlorophane, bithionol, halogenated salicylanilides); systemic absorption (prolonged contact, burns, denuded areas; NB metabolic acidosis with mafenide). See also Antifungal agents, topical
Antispasmodic Drugs	Anticholinergic drugs	See under this entry
	Mebeverine	Lacks anticholinergic effects; ? any other reactions

Appendix B. (continued)

Drug class	Drug	Clinically important reactions
Antispasticity Agents (see also chapter XXV; sect. 10)	Baclofen	Muscle hypotonia, fatigue (espec. excessive dosage); nausea, vomiting; sedation; convulsions (rare, mainly in those with history of epilepsy)
	Dantrolene	Diarrhoea (may be severe); muscle weakness (esp. those with pre-existing weakness), general malaise, fatigue; drowsiness, dizziness; nausea, vomiting, dysphagia, sialorrhoea; rash, visual disturbances; respiratory depression (caution where pulmonary function already impaired); liver dysfunction (a few cases fatal hepatitis; monitor hepatic function in long term therapy)
	Diazepam	See under Antianxiety drugs
Antithyroid Drugs (see also chapter XVI; sect. 5.2)		Skin rash; agranulocytosis (rare); arthralgia, drug fever (very rare); alopecia, ocular effects; systemic lupus-like syndrome (very rare)
Antituberculosis Drugs (see also chapter XIX, sect. 14.6.4; XX, sect. 8)	Capreomycin	Ototoxicity; nephrotoxicity; pain on injection; symptomless eosinophilia; drug fever, skin rash
	Cycloserine	CNS reactions (headache, somnolence, mental disturbances, convulsions); Seizures controlled by 100mg pyridoxine daily
	Ethambutol	Decreased visual acuity and red-green colour discrimination (uncommon at 25mg/kg/day); peripheral neuritis with numbness and tingling of extremities; joint pain; gastrointestinal disturbances; malaise, headache; allergic reactions, incl. anaphylaxis (rare)
	Ethionamide and Prothionamide	Anorexia, nausea, vomiting; metallic taste, ganglionic blockade reactions (postural hypotension, depression); hepatotoxicity (espec. diabetics); severe allergic skin rash, purpura; gynaecomastia, impotence, amenorrhoea; neurotoxicity (rare); confused state, psychosis (ethionamide)
	Isoniazid	Peripheral neuritis (pyridoxine-responsive, more likely in slow acetylators); optic neuritis; hepatotoxicity; pellagra-like syndrome; ataxia, euphoria, convulsions, restlessness, insomnia, muscle twitching (higher doses); mental abnormalities (psychosis, delirium), convulsions; epigastric distress; hypersensitivity (rare); systemic lupus-like syndrome (more likely in slow acetylators); gynaecomastia; dry mouth, urinary retention
	PAS (p-amino-salicylic acid)	Gastrointestinal disturbances (nausea, gastric irritation, diarrhoea); hypersensitivity (fever, rash, headache, sore throat); hepatotoxicity; blood dyscrasias, haemolytic anaemia, allergic pulmonary reactions, bleeding tendencies, goitre, hypokalaemia (rare); glandular fever-like syndrome
	Pyrazinamide	Hepatotoxicity; hyperuricaemia, acute gout; arthralgias; photosensitivity, anorexia, nausea, vomiting; dysuria; malaise, fever
	Rifampicin	Gastrointestinal disturbances; hepatotoxicity (more likely combined with isoniazid, in elderly and those with high alcohol intake); dizziness, blurred vision, skin rashes; immune thrombocytopenia (usually high dosage intermittent therapy); febrile illness, acute renal failure, hepatitis, asthmatic reaction (intermittent regimen or intake); haemolytic anaemia; discolours urine, sputum, tears and occasionally sweat reddish-orange
	Streptomycin	See under Antibacterial agents
	Viomycin	Allergic reactions; nephrotoxicity; ototoxicity; hypokalaemia, muscle weakness; hypocalcaemia, tetany (rare)

Appendix B. (continued)

Drug class	Drug	Clinically important reactions
Antiviral Agents see also chapter XXVIII; sect. 4)	Amantadine	Nausea; abdominal pain; insomnia; restlessness, psychiatric disturbances (more likely in the elderly); blurred vision, dizziness, convulsions (large doses)
	Cytarabine	Hepatotoxicity; bone marrow depression; alopecia; oral ulceration
	Idoxuridine	Stinging, pruritus, oedema of eye or lids, photophobia (rare) on topical use; gastrointestinal disturbances, bone marrow depression, hepatotoxicity, alopecia, oral ulceration (systemic use)
	Methisazone	Nausea, vomiting
	Vidarabine	Gastrointestinal disturbances, bone marrow depression; encephalopathy (high doses)
Asthma Drugs (see also chapter XX; sect. 2.3)	Bronchodilators	See under this entry
	Corticosteroids	See under this entry
	Sodium cromoglycate	Irritation of throat and trachea (espec. following acute infections); transient bronchospasm (uncommon)
β-Adrenoceptor Blocking Drugs		See under Adrenoceptor blocking drugs
Blood Lipid Lowering Drugs (see chapter XVII; sect. 3.2.4)	Cholestyramine	Gastrointestinal distress; constipation (espec. elderly, those with angina); hyperchloraemic acidosis (children on large dosage); aggravation malabsorption states; biliary tract calcification (prolonged use those with primary biliary cirrhosis)
	Clofibrate	Gastrointestinal disturbances; weakness, giddiness, fatigue; weight gain; skin rash, alopecia (rare); muscle pain, cramps (espec. nephrotic patients); increased incidence cholelithiasis
	Colestipol	As for cholestyramine
	Nicotinic acid	Flushing, pruritus; gastrointestinal irritation; liver function abnormalities (?discontinue); hyperuricaemia; impaired glucose metabolism; skin hyperpigmentation, dry skin (extended use)
	Probucol	Diarrhoea, gastrointestinal distress; headache, dizziness; paraesthesia; transient eosinophilia
Bronchodilator Drugs (see also chapter XX; sect. 2.3.1)	Sympathomimetic amines	Palpitation, tachycardia (more likely with oral preparations, inhaled isoprenaline, SC or IM adrenaline); headache, dizziness; nausea, muscle tremor (oral); nervousness (ephedrine; SC or IM adrenaline), urinary retention (ephedrine); serious cardiac arrhythmias (excessive dosage)
		N.B. If lack of usual response from usual inhaled dose, other therapy is indicated as non-responsive state may be developing
	Theophylline derivatives	Gastrointestinal disturbances; palpitation, restlessness, (uncommon); arrhythmias; sudden hypotension (IV aminophylline; give slowly); nightmares; convulsions
Carbonic Anhydrase Inhibitors (see also chapter XII; sect. 5)		Drowsiness, facial paraesthesiae; drug fever, skin rash, bone marrow depression, ureteral colic with calculus formation (rare)

Appendix B. (continued)

Drug class	Drug	Clinically important reactions
Cardiac Glycosides (see also chapter XVII; sect. 8)		*Non-cardiac effects:* Anorexia, nausea, vomiting, diarrhoea, abdominal pain; fatigue, dizziness, headache, muscular weakness; confusion, disorientation, delirium, overt psychosis (espec. elderly); paraesthesiae, blurred vision, difficulty in reading, altered colour vision, visual hallucinations; skin rash, gynaecomastia (rare)
		Cardiac effects: Increasing congestive heart failure; disturbances of rhythm and conduction, leading to fast and slow rates, and all types of cardiac irregularity (e.g. bradycardia, extrasystoles, bigeminal rhythm, runs of ventricular tachycardia, marked change in previously stable rhythm, paroxysmal atrial tachycardia with heart block)
		Risk of toxicity increased: Elderly; renal impairment (digoxin); low body weight; large loading dosage or loading doses after maintenance courses; certain types of heart disease (e.g. acute myocardial infarction, chronic coronary artery disease, advanced ventricular failure); chronic pulmonary heart disease (hypoxaemia); hypothyroidism; electrolyte (Na, K, Mg, Ca) or acid-base imbalance
		N.B. Digoxin dosage should in general be based on lean body weight and renal function. The smallest possible dose of digitalis to produce the desired effect should be used. Loading dose not indicated if the inotropic effect of digitalis is not immediately needed, as only maintenance doses are necessary to achieve therapeutic concentrations within a few days
Central Stimulants	Methylphenidate	Nervousness, dizziness, palpitation; headache, anorexia, nausea; elevated blood pressure (parenteral), atrial fibrillation (parenteral); dependence risk See also under Amphetamines
Chelating Agents	Desferrioxamine	Hypotension (IV); skin rash; gastrointestinal irritation (oral); flushing, tachycardia
	Dimercaprol	Rise in blood pressure, tachycardia; gastrointestinal disturbances; headache; burning sensations (particularly mouth and throat); conjunctivitis; lacrimation, rhinorrhoea, salivation, sweating; painful sterile abscess; fever (children)
	D-Penicillamine	Acute hypersensitivity — rash, fever, leucopenia, thrombo-cytopenia, mucosal injection and/or lymphadenopathy; breast enlargement; oral ulceration; proteinuria, haematuria; nephrotic syndrome; abnormal taste perception; extravasation of blood into skin over pressure points (prolonged high doses); LE cells, ANF; anorexia, nausea, vomiting; muscle weakness, myasthenic signs (long term use). See also chapter XXII (sect. 3.3.3)
	Sodium edetate	Nephrosis; thrombophlebitis (IV too concentrated); systemic febrile reaction, sneezing, nasal congestion, lacrimation, glycosuria; pyridoxine-like deficiency dermatitis
Contraceptives (see also chapter XV; sect. 13; XXV, sect. 15.2)	Progestagen-oestrogen combinations	Small risk of thromboembolic phenomena (stop if cramps, pain or oedema of legs, sudden severe chest pain, changing pattern migraine or unusual headache, any ocular symptoms, unusual and atypical abdominal pain; stop 6 weeks before planned surgery); augment risk of acute myocardial infarction in women over 40; increase risk of stroke; exacerbation of varicosities; hypertension, impairment of glucose tolerance (susceptible individuals, e.g. parental or pregnancy history); liver dysfunction (avoid in those with previous cholestatic hepatobiliary

Appendix B. (continued)

Drug class	Drug	Clinically important reactions
Contraceptives (continued)		disease); benign hepatic tumours; increased incidence of cholelithiasis; serious depression (stop drug); ?loss of libido; chorea (especially pregnancy history); corneal oedema and contact lens difficulties; menstrual cycle irregularities (breakthrough bleeding and spotting, altered menstrual flow, amenorrhoea with or without galactorrhoea); nausea (mestranol); weight gain, breast discomfort ('high dose' 19-norsteroids); chloasma and various skin reactions; acne (some preparations); folate deficiency anaemia (prolonged use); cervical epithelial aberrations (?prognostic significance); failure of lactation ('high dose' preparations); hair loss (male pattern alopecia or diffuse loss on withdrawal of agent), haemolytic uraemic syndrome, acute pancreatitis (very rare)
	Progestagens alone	Menstrual cycle irregularities (erratic bleeding, amenorrhoea); headache, bloating, nervousness, diminished libido, acne, greasy hair, breast discomfort, chloasma; impairment of glucose tolerance (IM medroxyprogesterone acetate; susceptible individuals)
Corticosteroids Glucocorticoids (see also chapter XII, sect. 11.1.2; XIV, sect. 6, 7; XVI, sect. 9.1, 14.3; XX, sect. 2.3.3; XXII, sect. 3.4)	Systemic use	Related to dose and duration of treatment. Some complications can arise following small maintenance doses. Serious reactions usually seen only with long term therapy. Effects include electrolyte disturbances (sodium and fluid retention, hypotension, potassium loss); gastrointestinal irritation (gastric upset, peptic ulcer exacerbation); skin atrophy, 'moon' facies; acne; metabolic disturbances (hyperglycaemia, redistribution body fat), myopathy (triamcinolone, usually high dose prolonged therapy); bone and joint complications (osteoporosis, aseptic necrosis, arthropathy); infection (spread, increased susceptibility); ocular complications (increase in intraocular pressure in susceptible individuals, posterior subcapsular cataracts, papilloedema); CNS effects (headache, intracranial hypertension, mental changes, may aggravate schizophrenia); adrenocortical suppression (keep maintenance dosage to lowest possible; if withdrawing, do so carefully and gradually); growth retardation (children)
	Local use (e.g. intra-articular, rectal, etc)	In general *precautions* as for systemic use (some absorption occurs); ?instability of joint (repeated IA use); subcutaneous fat atrophy (SC use)
	Inhalation (aerosol)	Irritation, hoarseness; fungal infection mouth, throat; care needed when gradually transferring from systemic steroids to aerosol; supply oral steroids in case of stress, infection, episodes severe airways obstruction
	Topical use (eye)	Increase in intraocular pressure (susceptible individuals); spread viral disease, increased susceptibility to fungal infection, retard wound healing; corneal or scleral perforation (prolonged use); corneal thinning (high dosage); rarely, posterior subcapsular cataract with prolonged use); ptosis; mydriasis
	Topical use (skin)	Dermal atrophy (prolonged use, especially stronger steroids on intertriginous areas or under occlusive dressings) leading to chronic erythema, telangiectasia, purpura, striae; systemic absorption with adrenocortical suppression (prolonged use of large dosage or over large occluded area; risk greatest in infants); spread of untreated infection; rosacea-like dermatitis (strong steroids on face); delay healing, especially ulcers; local hypertrichosis (prolonged use)
Mineralocorticoids (see also chapter XVI sect 9.2)		Sodium and fluid retention, hypertension, potassium loss; cardiac enlargement, failure

Appendix B. (continued)

Drug class	Drug	Clinically important reactions
Corticotrophin see also chapter XXII; sect. 3.4)	ACTH Tetracosactrin	Hypersensitivity reactions (sometimes with an acute onset after injection; less risk with tetracosactrin); pain at injection site; as for systemic corticosteroids (adrenal suppression probably less marked; osteoporosis not marked; smaller incidence gastrointestinal irritation, bruising, myopathy; but higher incidence electrolyte disturbances, and cause acne, hirsutism, amenorrhoea)
Decongestants, Nasal (see also chapter XI; sect. 1.4)		Temporary stinging, burning, dry mucosa (topical use); rebound hyperaemia (continued or excessive use); palpitation (more likely oral agents)
Digitalis		See under Cardiac Glycosides
Diuretics (see also chapter V, sect. 4.1.2; XVI, sect. 14.1; XVII, sect. 8.1.8, 8.3.3; XVIII, sect. 5.1)	Amiloride	Gastrointestinal disturbances; dry mouth, thirst; paraesthesiae; hyperkalaemia (do not use in renal failure); dizziness; skin rashes
	Aminophylline	Headache, dizziness; nausea; palpitation, hypotension
	Bumetanide	Hypokalaemia and hypochloraemic acidosis; hyperuricaemia; skin rashes; muscle cramps or pain (intensive therapy); ? impaired glucose metabolism (diabetics)
	Carbonic anhydrase inhibitors (e.g. acetazolamide)	Facial paraesthesia; drowsiness; gastrointestinal disturbances; hypokalaemia; hyperuricaemia; drug fever, rash, bone marrow depression, renal and ureteral colic with calculus formation (rare); renal tubular acidosis
	Ethacrynic acid	Hypokalaemia; hyponatraemia and hypochloremic alkalosis (large doses); hyperuricaemia; gastrointestinal disturbances; skin rashes; acute hypovolaemia (IV); ototoxicity (IV or large oral doses in renal failure); impaired glucose metabolism (rare)
	Frusemide (furosemide)	Hypokalaemia; hypochloraemia, hyponatraemia (large doses) hyperuricaemia; nausea; skin rashes; photosensitivity (high doses in chronic renal failure); acute transient circulatory disturbances (excessive doses); ototoxicity (rapid and large IV doses in renal failure); impaired glucose metabolism (rare); haematological reactions (rare)
	Mannitol	Withdrawal of intracellular fluid and circulatory overload (caution in those with cerebral or pulmonary oedema)
	Mefruside	Hypokalaemia; hyperuricaemia; gastrointestinal disturbances; impaired glucose metabolism (rare)
	Mercurials	Hypokalaemia; hypersensitivity (rare); risks of ventricular fibrillation (IV); renal tubular necrosis (prolonged use; avoid in renal failure)
	Spironolactone	Headache, dizziness, drowsiness; nausea, vomiting; hyperkalaemia (do not use in renal failure); skin rashes; gynaecomastia (esp. > 200mg daily); menstrual irregularities
	Thiazides and thiazide-like (e.g. chlorthalidone, clorexolone)	Hypokalaemia; hyponatraemia (rare); hyperuricaemia; gastrointestinal distrubances; impaired glucose metabolism; skin rash (incl. photo-sensitivity); paraesthesiae; weakness, fatigue; thrombocytopenic purpura, jaundice; pancreatitis, necrotising vasculitis (rare)
	Tienilic acid (ticrynafen)	Hyponatraemia, hypokalaemia; intratubular uric acid precipitation, acute gout (esp. in 'at risk' patients on initiation of therapy; maintain high fluid intake initially)
	Triamterene	Headache, dizziness; dry mouth; nausea; hyperkalaemia (do not use in renal failure); skin rashes; reversible azotaemia; hyperuricaemia; megaloblastic anaemia

Appendix B. (continued)

Drug class	Drug	Clinically important reactions
Enzymes	Proteolytic enzymes	Local hyperaemia (use on skin); tingling sensation in cheek (buccal use); aphthous stomatitis (streptokinase-streptodornase buccal); hypersensitivity, reactions at injection site (IM chymotrypsin); loss of vitreous humour (intra-ocular chymotrypsin); burning sensation, hypersensitivity reactions (topical trypsin)
	Hyaluronidase	Hypersensitivity (infrequent)
	Pancreatic	Nausea, diarrhoea, vomiting (excessive dosage); sensitivity (stop drug; unlikely with pancrelipase)
	Thrombolytic	See under Thrombolytic Drugs
Glaucoma Drugs (see also chapter XII, sect. 5)	Adrenaline	Brow ache, headache, blurred vision, ocular irritation, tearing; reactive hyperaemia, allergic conjunctivitis, dermatitis (prolonged use); pigment deposits on lids, conjunctiva, cornea (long term use); macular damage (aphakic patients); systemic reactions (in those with damaged or increased permeability of corneal epithelium)
	β-Adrenoceptor blocking drugs, topical (e.g. timolol)	Rarely bradycardia, hypotension (esp. in those with predisposing conditions, e.g. congestive heart failure)
	Anticholinesterases	See under this entry
	Carbachol and Pilocarpine	See under Miotics
	Carbonic anhydrase inhibitors	See under this entry
Gold Preparations (see also chapter XXII; sect. 3.3.1)		Pruritus, cutaneous reactions; (exfoliative dermatitis, lichenoid eruptions — stop drug); lesions of mucous membranes (stomatitis — stop drug); aplastic anaemia, leucopenia, thrombocytopenia, eosinophilia; albuminuria, haematuria; nitritoid crises (sudden nausea, vomiting, weakness following injection); pulmonary reactions. Discontinue gold as soon as toxic symptoms are reported or as soon as abnormalities appear in blood count
Gout Drugs (see also chapter XXII; sect. 12)	Allopurinol	Gastrointestinal irritation; rash, pruritus, fever; leucopenia, reversible hepatotoxicity (rare)
	Benzbromarone	Gastrointestinal irritation (diarrhoea)
	Colchicine	Gastrointestinal disturbances (nausea, vomiting, diarrhoea abdominal discomfort); haematological abnormalities, myopathy, alopecia (chronic use; infrequent); reversible malabsorption syndrome (high doses). Reduce dose in presence severe renal failure (if chronic use) or severe liver disease
	Indomethacin Oxyphenbutazone Phenylbutazone	See under Analgesics, anti-inflammatory
	Probenecid	Gastrointestinal irritation (dose related); skin rash; fever (rare)
	Sulphinpyrazone	Gastrointestinal irritation; skin rash, fever (rare)

Appendix B. (continued)

Drug class	Drug	Clinically important reactions
Haematinics (see also chapter XXIII, sect. 6.1; XXX, sect. 5)	Folic acid	Sensitivity reactions (rare)
	Iron	Oral — Nausea, diarrhoea, and/or constipation
		Intravenous — Venous spasm; systemic chills; fever; nausea; chest, lumbar and loin pain
		Intramuscular — Local pain and inflammation; skin staining (if admin. not correct); systemic reactions; metallic taste
	Vitamin B_{12}	Allergic reactions (rare)
Hydroxyquinoline Drugs	Broxyquinoline Clioquinol Halquinol Diiodohydroxy-quinoline	Gastrointestinal disturbances, pruritus ani, mild iodism (oral); optic neuropathy (prolonged high dose oral use); irritation, sensitisation, yellow staining of fabrics (topical use)
Hypnosedatives (see chapter XXVI; sect. 9.1)		Drowsiness; skin reactions; gastrointestinal disturbances; confusional states (elderly); dependence, withdrawal syndrome, convulsions (prolonged use higher doses); precipitate acute attacks in porphyria (barbiturates); acroparaesthesiae (methaqualone); respiratory depression in those with respiratory failure. See also antianxiety agents
Hypoglycaemic Agents (see also chapter XVI; sect. 3.2, 3.3)		
Insulin		Allergic response (usually at injection site); fat atrophy and insulin hypertrophy (vary site of injection, or try monocomponent preparation); insulin resistance; hypoglycaemia (particularly in patient with unstable diabetes); parotid swelling
Oral	Biguanides	Gastrointestinal intolerance (anorexia, nausea, epigastric discomfort, diarrhoea, metallic taste); 'late side effects' (weight loss, anorexia, weakness and lethargy despite good biochemical diabetic control); lactic acidosis (seen with phenformin and usually in association with severe renal, hepatic or cardiovascular diseases; other predisposing factors include tissue hypoxia, coma, pancreatitis and excessive alcohol intake. Instruct patient to report early symptoms of lactic acidosis, i.e. vomiting, malaise, abdominal pain, diarrhoea; megaloblastic anaemia (metformin)
	Sulphonylureas and sulphapyrimidines	Gastrointestinal disturbances; allergic skin rashes (incl. photosensitivity); jaundice and haematological reactions (rare); symptomatic hypoglycaemia (due to overdosage or in those not on an adequate diet); dilutional hyponatraemia, corneal opacities (chlorpropamide)
Laxatives (see also chapter XIX; sect. 7.1)		Excessive use may cause dehydration, muscular weakness and hypokalaemia
	Bisacodyl	Mild abdominal cramping (oral); tenesmus (rectal)
	Bulk-forming preparations	Intestinal obstruction (avoid by giving the granules with generous amounts water)
	Cascara preparations	Colic; rectal pigmentation
	Castor oil	Pelvic congestion
	Dioctylsodium sulphosuccinate	Anorexia, vomiting, diarrhoea

Appendix B. (continued)

Drug class	Drug	Clinically important reactions
Laxatives (continued)	Lactulose	Abdominal cramps; sweet taste, nausea; diarrhoea (excessive dosage)
	Magnesium sulphate	Hypermagnesaemia (in impaired renal function)
	Oxyphenisatin	Jaundice, hepatic fibrosis (prolonged use)
	Paraffin liquid (mineral oil)	Lipid pneumonitis, reduced absorption fat soluble vitamins (extended use); anal oil leak
	Phenolphthalein	Allergic skin reactions, pruritus (sensitive patients; stop drug); syncope
	Senna preparations	Colic; skin eruptions
Migraine Drugs (see also chapter XXV; sect. 7)	Clonidine	Drowsiness, dry mouth, gastrointestinal disturbances (nausea, constipation); mild depression, dizziness, irritability, skin rashes (rare)
	Cyproheptadine Pizotifen	Drowsiness; increased appetite and weight gain; blurred vision, dry mouth, dizziness, nausea, skin rash (infrequent)
	Ergotamine preparations	Nausea, vomiting; circulatory disturbances (paraesthesiae of extremities, leg cramps, muscle pains, anginal pain, transient tachycardia or bradycardia); oedema and itching (sensitive patient); gangrene (prolonged use, increased sensitivity in febrile and septic states, liver dysfunction; not seen with hydrogenated alkaloids); habituation (vicious circle of continued use after daily rebound headache when effect drug ceases)
	Methysergide	Gastrointestinal disturbances; dizziness; nervousness, confusion; circulatory disturbances (paraesthesiae extremities, leg cramps, muscle pain, anginal pain, tachycardia); retroperitoneal fibrosis, ureteric obstruction, pleural pulmonary fibrosis, endocardial fibrosis (long term use; withdraw drug for 1 to 2 months every 6 months)
Miotics (see also chapter XII; sect. 5)	Anticholinesterases	See under this entry
	Carbachol and Pilocarpine	Accommodative spasm, headache
Monoamine Oxidase Inhibitors		See under Antidepressants and Antihypertensive drugs (pargyline)
Mucolytic Drugs	Acetylcysteine	Bronchospasm (espec. asthmatics); rhinorrhoea; stomatitis; nausea
	Bromhexine	Gastrointestinal disturbances (espec. those with peptic ulcer)
	Detergents (tyloxapol)	Respiratory tract irritation (prolonged use)
	Trypsin	Respiratory tract irritation; transient hoarseness, dyspnoea (avoid by premedication with antihistamines)

Appendix B. (continued)

Drug class	Drug	Clinically important reactions
Muscle Relaxants, Skeletal Neuromuscular Blocking (see also chapter X; sect. 2.2, 3)		Prolonged apnoea (espec. suxamethonium); histamine release (not seen with pancuronium); hypotension (tubocurarine, alcuronium); bradycardia (suxamethonium, decamethonium; give atropine); muscle pain and stiffness, rise in intraocular pressure (suxamethonium); hyperkalaemia (suxamethonium use following trauma, wounds, burns, muscular disorders); myoglobinaemia (suxamethonium), risk malignant hyperpyrexia in those with muscular disorders (suxamethonium); hypersensitivity (esp. gallamine)
Centrally Acting	Orphenadrine	Blurred vision, dry mouth etc (usually with higher doses)
	Antispasticity drugs	See under this entry
Mydriatics (see also chapter XII; sect. 9.6, 9.7)		Irritative conjunctivitis (atropine); rise in intraocular pressure; toxic psychosis (high strength atropine or cyclopentolate in children); systemic atropine-like poisoning (children with fever)
Oestrogens (see also chapter XV; sect. 13, 16, 23.3)		Risk of thromboembolism, hypertension, impairment glucose metabolism (see under Contraceptives); nausea; malaise, irritability, depression; oedema, weight gain; breast fullness; irregular bleeding (menopausal use); liver function abnormalities; loss of libido, gynaecomastia, increased risk cardiovascular mortality (used in men); ?endometrial carcinoma (prolonged use high doses); vaginal cancer (prenatal exposure)
Oxytocic Drugs (see also chapter XV; sect. 10)	Ergometrine Methylergometrine	Nausea, vomiting (espec. IV admin.); unusual elevations blood pressure (enhanced pressor response; hypertensive or toxaemic patient)
	Oxytocin	Hypotension (very large doses); water intoxication (large doses); prolonged or frequent contractions, fetal heart changes (overdosage); ?increase in neonatal hyperbilirubinaemia
Peptic Ulcer Drugs (see also chapter XIX; sect. 4.3)	Antacids	See under this entry
	Anticholinergics	See under this entry
	Carbenoxolone	Hypertension; fluid retention; hypokalaemia (in long term therapy give potassium supplements routinely and estimate serum potassium regularly); myositis with or without hypokalaemia; headache, heartburn
	Cimetidine	Diarrhoea, muscle pains, dizziness, rashes; breast changes with long term therapy (incl. pain and gynaecomastia in males, galactorrhoea in women); mental confusion (esp. elderly and patients with renal dysfunction; reduce dose if renal function impaired); impotence in males; increased serum transaminases and plasma creatinine (caution patients with hepatic or renal dysfunction)
	Colloidal bismuth (tripotassium dicitrato bismuthate)	Stools and tongue (occasionally) darkened
	Deglycyrrhizinised liquorice	Diarrhoea

Appendix B. (continued)

Drug class	Drug	Clinically important reactions
Potassium Supplements (see also chapter XIX; sect. 14.3.2; XXI, 7.1)		Nausea (uncommon); hyperkalaemia (renal failure); small bowel lesions (enteric coated tablets; slow release tablets in patients with oesophageal stasis or delayed gastrointestinal transit)
Progestagens		Nausea, dyspepsia; weight gain (19-norsteroids) masculinisation urogenital sinus of female fetus (certain compounds in threatened abortion). See also under Contraceptives
Radiographic Contrast Media		Gastrointestinal disturbances, mild dysuria (oral); hypotension, tachycardia; feeling of warmth (IV); renal failure (more likely with biliary contrast media in jaundiced patient); hypersensitivity, shock reactions, neurological reactions (rare); parotid swelling (excessive doses iodinated agents)
Thrombolytic Drugs (see also chapter XXIII; sect. 3.3)	Streptokinase	Pyrogenic and allergic reactions (usually tolerable and controllable, ? anaphylaxis — give corticosteroid before start of infusion); danger of haemorrhage in those with generalised haemorrhagic diathesis, proven peptic ulcer or severe hypertension; haemorrhagic complications (avoid large doses in early stage infusion).
Thyroid Drugs (see also chapter XVI; sect. 5.1)		Cardiac pain, palpitation, tachycardia (excessive dosage; reduce or increase more slowly); may precipitate angina and possibly myocardial infarction (patients with ischaemic heart disease); agranulocytosis (thiouracils)
Trichomonacides	Hachimycin and Natamycin	Nausea, diarrhoea
	Metronidazole	Nausea, diarrhoea; metallic taste; headache, vertigo, urticaria, vaginal and urethral discomfort (uncommon); transient leucopenia; colours urine dark brown
	Nifuratel	Nausea; breathlessness; skin rash
	Nimorazole	Nausea, heartburn
	Tinidazole	Nausea, vomiting, metallic taste, mild vertigo, headache, colours urine dark brown
	Local preparations	Hypersensitivity (iodophors and iodohydroxyquinolines; arsenicals); burning, itching
Vasodilator Drugs (see also chapter XVII, sect. 4.2.1, 8.3.4)	'Coronary' (i.e. antianginal drugs)	Headache, facial flushing; dizziness; postural hypotension (nitrates); gastrointestinal disturbances; skin rash (nitrates)
	Peripheral	Flushing, tingling; dizziness, headache; nausea; postural hypotension (large doses); sweating (cyclandelate); piloerection, gastrointestinal stimulation (tolazoline); metabolic acidosis, accumulation of cyanide (sodium nitroprusside, excessive rate of infusion or total dosage). See also under α-Adrenoceptor Blocking Drugs and Antihypertensive Drugs (diazoxide, hydrallazine, prazosin)
	Oxpentifylline (pentoxifylline)	Nausea, gastrointestinal fullness; skin reactions (rare)

Appendix B. (continued)

Drug class	Drug	Clinically important reactions
Vasopressor Agents (see also chapter XVII; sect. 5.4)		Headache, dizziness; respiratory distress; local tissue necrosis (levonoradrenaline); tingling extremities, piloerection (methoxamine); cardiac arrhythmias (myocardial infarct cases, or in conjunction with halothane, cyclopropane anaesthesia; phenylephrine, methoxamine or angiotensin amide preferred in such cases); convulsions, cerebral haemorrhage (overdosage); profound bradycardia (overdosage angiotensin); severe metabolic acidosis, decreased plasma volume (prolonged use); peripheral vasoconstriction and digital gangrene (dopamine, elderly patients with peripheral vascular disease)
Vitamins (see also chapter XXX; sect. 4.5)	Vitamin A	Fatigue, anorexia, neurological symptoms, skin and bone complaints, alopecia, menstrual irregularities (excessive doses; 40,000 units or more daily in adults, 18,500 units or more daily in children)
	Vitamin B_6 (pyridoxine)	Headache (high doses); allergic reactions (very rare)
	Vitamin B_{12} (cobalamins)	See under Haematinics
	Vitamin D	Renal calcification, hypercalcaemia (high doses; usually 100,000 units or more daily)
	Vitamin K	Haemolysis, kernicterus (overdosage of aqueous preparations in prematures), flushing, sweating, tachycardia, peripheral vascular collapse (IV; given slowly)

Appendix C
Guide to the Clinically More Important Drug Interactions

G.S. Avery and R.C. Heel

Chapters VII and VIII discuss the pharmacological basis and mechanisms, as well as general considerations, of drug interactions. From these discussions it will be realised that predicted interactions often fail to manifest themselves in clinical practice. Thus, it does not necessarily follow that an interaction will in fact always occur with a given combination of potentially interacting drugs in every patient. Moreover, not all interactions are harmful. While some may be serious or even life threatening, others are only a nuisance or may even be beneficial; e.g. modest increase in a previously low plasma phenytoin concentration may actually improve seizure control whereas marked elevation of a previously high or low plasma phenytoin level may lead to toxicity (see chapter XXV; sect. 3.1). Some others may nevertheless lead to ineffective therapy.

The tables which follow must be used intelligently and with a knowledge of the principles of drug interaction. Because a significant interaction does not necessarily follow in every patient with a given combination of drugs listed, the tables are only intended to be a guide to the more important interactions which can be significant in some patients under certain circumstances of administration or use of the drugs involved. At present there is relatively little definitive information on the determinants and incidence of clinically important interactions involving any specific drug, or on the wider question of the frequency with which drug interaction is responsible for adverse drug effects or ineffective treatment.

Which Drug Interactions Are of Most Importance?

Interactions involving commonly used drugs or potentially interacting drugs which are often likely to be given together are of more importance than those involving drugs that are infrequently used. The table which follows is therefore not intended to be a complete list of potential clinically significant drug interactions. Rather, it is a list of those interactions of known significance which are of potential major importance — because the interacting drugs are commonly used and likely to be prescribed together and can lead to either harmful effects or ineffective therapy. The list therefore represents those interactions which all clinicians should know about. It is important to appreciate that some of the major importance interactions listed might not always occur in a particular patient and that others can be avoided by careful monitoring of therapy, modification of dosage, timing of interval between administration of the drugs, or substitution of an alternative agent.

What Factors Make Drug Interactions More Likely to Occur?

In theory at least, and depending on the pharmacological properties of the individual drugs, clinically significant interactions would in general appear more likely to occur if large doses of the potentially interacting drugs are used, if they are ingested simultaneously or close together, or if they are given in the presence of associated renal or liver dysfunction, and when therapy is continued for several days or more. Genetic differences affecting drug metabolism and other acquired differences between patients may also influence the occurrence or intensity of interactions in individual patients.

A few studies have followed up patients taking potentially interacting drugs and indicate that in general actual interaction is not as frequent or as important as publicity given the subject would suggest (see chapter VIII; sect. 1.1). Interference with therapeutic control (e.g. oral anticoagulants, sulphonylurea hypoglycaemic drugs) is much more common than interaction resulting in adverse effects. A few drugs can however, predictably cause an adverse reaction due to interaction. Phenylbutazone, for example, can affect protein binding and drug metabolism as well as renal excretion mechanisms and should be avoided in regimens involving oral coumarin anticoagulants or oral sulphonylurea hypoglycaemic drugs.

When an interaction predictably affects dosage requirements and one of the interacting drugs is withdrawn, modification of dosage may be necessary, as with oral coumarin anticoagulant dosage when barbiturates or other potent hepatic microsomal enzyme inducing agents are withdrawn or reduced in dosage. Interactions between monoamine oxidase inhibitors and indirect acting sympathomimetic amines (e.g. appetite suppressants, common cold remedies) or foodstuffs rich in tyramine (e.g. matured cheeses such as cheddar, wines such as chianti, protein extracts) or dopamine (e.g. broad beans) are important because of their alarming nature.

Minimising the Occurrence of Drug Interactions

As discussed in chapters VII and VIII, an awareness of the more important interactions and knowledge of the mechanisms of drug interactions, can help to avoid, or at least minimise, adverse drug effects or ineffective treatment resulting from multiple drug therapy.

The following guidelines would also seem to be especially important:

1) *Take a careful history from the patient* — but when asking the patient about what drugs he is taking, whether prescribed or self-administered, use terms which he understands; e.g. pain, fever or 'flu reliever for aspirin, 'flu or cough remedy for common cold preparation, blood pressure tablets for antihypertensive drugs, heart tablets for digoxin, and so on. Do not neglect useful information which can be obtained from a history of the patient's past experiences with drugs.

2) *Avoid multiple drug therapy whenever possible* — or at least limit the number of drugs prescribed for concurrent use by a patient; the incidence of adverse drug reactions increases with the number of drugs prescribed.

3) *If multiple drug therapy is required* — avoid those drugs which predictably cause clinically important interactions or make control of therapy difficult. Some drug combinations are best avoided. Substitute drugs which can be more safely given; e.g. with oral coumarin anticoagulants substitute indomethacin, naproxen or ibuprofen for phenylbutazone; paracetamol (acetaminophen) for aspirin; diazepam for a bar-

biturate sedative and flurazepam or nitrazepam for a barbiturate hypnotic. Certainly, drug combinations which can cause serious reactions should be avoided wherever possible (e.g. monoamine oxidase inhibitors).

Some other interactions, such as those involving cholestyramine or tetracyclines, can be avoided where feasible by spacing doses of the drugs a few hours apart; e.g. an hour or more in the case of cholestyramine and acidic drugs (e.g. warfarin), 1 to 2 hours with antacids and tetracyclines, 3 hours with iron salts and tetracyclines and 8 hours with digoxin or digitoxin.

If fixed combination drugs are indicated, the composition of the product must be known.

Always keep in mind genetic factors and associated diseases or pathophysiological conditions which may make an interaction more likely to occur. For example, phenytoin in patients who are slow acetylators of isoniazid (see chapter XXV; section 3.1) and certain sulphonamides (e.g. sulphafurazole/sulfisoxazole) with oral sulphonylurea hypoglycaemics in patients with impaired renal function (see chapter XVI; sect. 3.3.5).

4) *Changes of drug therapy should be kept to a minimum* — if changes are necessary and involve known interacting drugs, some alteration in dosage can be anticipated, but the time course and extent of interaction varies with the drugs and the individual patient. Any dose adjustment should only be made on the basis of results derived from close observation of therapy over a period of time after the change. This is especially important with oral coumarin anticoagulants (see chapter XXIII; sect. 3.2.5).

5) *Use special care with problem drugs* — therapy of patients receiving drugs such as oral coumarin anticoagulants, oral sulphonylurea hypoglycaemics, digitalis, cytotoxic drugs, antiepileptic drugs, antihypertensive drugs or CNS depressant drugs should be supervised properly because of the known risks of interactions leading to unwanted toxicity or interference with therapeutic control.

6) *Educate and instruct the patient* — warn the patient of the possible dangers which may arise if he changes (stops taking or alters dosage) or adds to his intake of medication, whether prescribed or self-administered, without first consulting his clinician. This applies to patients discharged from hospital as well as to outpatients and in particular with the problem drugs listed in item 5 above.

Specific instructions may be desirable in some cases (e.g. monoamine oxidase inhibitors and foodstuffs, common cold remedies). Provision of printed material might also help. The patient should also be warned of the interactions which can occur between prescribed drugs and alcohol, particularly in the first few days of therapy with antianxiety and antidepressant drugs (see chapter XXVI; sect. 8.5). A number of drugs can cause an unpleasant disulfiram-like reaction with alcohol (e.g. chlorpropamide, metronidazole).

Use of Tables

As with appendix B, the tables have been arranged according to pharmacological action or therapeutic use classifications. The listings have been organised so that the description of the effects produced is given under the drug classification where a change in the activity of the drug can lead to an increased risk of side effects or reduced therapeutic efficacy. For example, the effect of antacids in markedly reducing serum concentrations of simultaneously administered tetracyclines is described under antibacterial agents (tetracyclines) and not under antacids. In this way the prescriber can become aware of the consequences of adding (or withdrawing) other drugs to the important primary agent. Cross references to all the drugs involved are, however, provided in the main index of the book.

In many cases, the potentially interacting drugs can be given concurrently, provided the possibility of interaction is kept in mind and appropriate modification of dosage or therapy is anticipated or instituted promptly. In some cases, the interacting drugs should usually not be given concurrently.

General References

Baker, S.B. de C. and Neuhaus, G.A.: Toxicological Problems of Drug Combinations: Proceedings of the European Society for the Study of Drug Toxicity, vol. 13 (Excerpta Medica, Amsterdam 1972).

Cluff, L.E. and Petrie, J.C.: Clinical Effects of Interaction Between Drugs (Excerpta Medica, Amsterdam 1975).

Grahame-Smith, D.G.: Drug Interactions (Macmillan, London 1977).

Morselli, P.L.; Cohen, S.N. and Garattini, S.: Drug Interactions (Raven Press, New York 1974).

Reference Texts

American Pharmaceutical Association: Evaluations of Drug Interactions, 2nd ed and supplements (American Pharmaceutical Association, Washington 1976).

Cohen, S.T. and Armstrong, Marsha, F.: Drug Interactions: A Handbook for Clinical Use (Williams and Wilkins, Baltimore 1974).

Hansten, P.D.: Drug Interactions, 4th ed (Lea and Febiger, Philadelphia 1979).

Interactions Involving Specific Drug Groups

Bender, R.A.; Zwelling, L.A.; Doroshow, J.H.; Gershon, Y.L.; Hande, K.R.; Murinson, D.S.; Cohen, M.; Myers, C.E. and Chabner, B.A.: Antineoplastic drugs: Clinical Pharmacology and Therapeutic Use. Drugs 16: 46 (1978).

Binnion, P.F.: Drug interactions with digitalis glycosides. Drugs 15: 369 (1978).

Crook, J.E. and Nies, A.S.: Drug interactions with antihypertensive drugs. Drugs 15: 72 (1978).

Davie, I.T.: Specific drug interactions in anaesthesia. Anaesthesia 32: 1000 (1977).

Hansen, J.M. and Christensen, L.K.: Drug interactions with oral sulphonylurea hypoglycaemic drugs. Drugs 13: 24 (1977).

Hempel, E. and Klinger, W.: Drug stimulated biotransformation of hormonal steroid contraceptives. Clinical implications. Drugs 12: 442 (1976).

Hurwitz, A.: Antacid therapy and drug kinetics. Clinical Pharmacokinetics 2: 269 (1977).

Kabins, S.A.: Interactions among antibiotics and other drugs. Journal of the American Medical Association 219: 206 (1972).

Koch-Weser, J.: Drug interactions in cardiovascular therapy. American Heart Journal 90: 93 (1975).

Koch-Weser, J. and Sellers, E.M.: Drug interactions with coumarin anticoagulants. New England Journal of Medicine 285: 487, 547 (1971).

Kutt, H.: Interactions of antiepileptic drugs. Epilepsia 16: 393 (1975).

MacLeod, S.M. and Sellers, E.M.: Pharmacodynamic and pharmacokinetic drug interactions with coumarin anticoagulants. Drugs 11: 461 (1976).

Neuvonen, P.J.: Interactions with the absorption of tetracyclines. Drugs 11: 45 (1976).

Nies, A.A.: Adverse reactions and interactions limiting the use of antihypertensive drugs. American Journal of Medicine 58: 495 (1975).

Richens, A.: Interactions with antiepileptic drugs. Drugs 13: 266 (1977).

Roberton, Y.R. and Johnson, E.S.: Interactions between oral contraceptives and other drugs: A review. Current Medical Research and Opinion 3: 647 (1976).

Seixas, F.A.: Alcohol and its drug interactions. Annals of Internal Medicine 83: 86 (1975).

Sellers, E.M. and Holloway, M.R.: Drug kinetics and alcohol ingestion. Clinical Pharmacokinetics 3: 440 (1978).

Sjoqvist, F.: Interaction between monoamine oxidase (MAO) inhibitors and other drugs. Proceedings of the Royal Society of Medicine 58 (2): 967 (1965).

Stafford, J.R. and Fann, W.E.: Drug interactions with guanidinium antihypertensives. Drugs 13: 57 (1977).

Udall, J.A.: Clinical implications of warfarin interactions with five sedatives. American Journal of Cardiology 35: 67 (1975).

Appendix C. Guide to the clinically more important drug interactions

Primary drug	May interact with	Potential result (see introductory notes)	Management and how to avoid
Alcohol (see also chapter XXVI; sect. 8.5)			
	Analgesics, narcotic Antianxiety drugs Antidepressants Antihistamines (some compounds) Antipsychotics Hypnosedatives	Enhanced CNS depressant effects with acute alcohol ingestion	Instruct the patient. Warn about possible adverse effect on driving skills, especially with first few days of therapy
	Monoamine oxidase inhibitors	Enhanced CNS depressant effects with acute alcohol ingestion. Hypertensive crisis with high tyramine content wines (e.g. Chianti, Alicante type) and some beers	Advisable to avoid all alcoholic beverages since tyramine content not likely to be known to the patient
	Biguanide oral hypo-glycaemic drugs (e.g. phenformin, metformin)	Risk of hyperlacticacidaemia	Instruct the patient to avoid excessive quantities (moderate to large) of alcohol and to be aware of and to report *early* symptoms of lactic acidosis (vomiting and malaise, abdominal pain, diarrhoea)
	Sulphonylurea oral hypoglycaemic drugs (e.g. chlorpropamide, tolbutamide, etc)	Disulfiram-like intolerance (facial flushing, headache) of alcohol in some cases (particularly chlorpropamide). Hypoglycaemic activity may be increased with acute alcohol ingestion if food intake is restricted (e.g. malnutrition, prolonged fasting)	Instruct the patient about possibility of intolerance of alcohol and to avoid moderate to large quantities of alcohol. Intolerance of small quantities of alcohol more likely with chlorpropamide (see chapter XVI; sect. 3.3.5). Educate patient to maintain adequate nutrition
	Metronidazole Nifuratel	Disulfiram-like intolerance of alcohol in some cases	Instruct the patient about possibility of reaction and to avoid excessive alcohol consumption
Anaesthetics, general (see also chapter X; sect. 2.1.6)			
Cyclopropane Enflurane Halothane	Adrenaline	Anaesthetic sensitises myocardium to catecholamines with risk of severe ventricular arrhythmias	Avoid intravenous use of adrenaline. Dilute adrenaline solutions may be given intramuscularly or subcutaneously with appropriate precautions
Ketamine	Quinalbarbitone Diazepam Hydroxyzine	Prolonged recovery time (by around 30 to 40 %) with use of these drugs as premedicants	Be aware of extended recovery when used for short surgical procedures
	Thyroid drugs	Severe hypertension and tachycardia	Try control with propranolol
Methoxyflurane	Tetracycline	Risk of renal failure increased	Avoid this combination Substitute another antibacterial agent

Propanidid	Suxamethonium (succinylcholine)	Activity of suxamethonium markedly prolonged (by about 50%)	Prepare for prolonged artificial ventilation and ensure that patient is asleep
	Anticholinesterases (ecothiopate eye drops, pesticides) Cyclophosphamide Phenelzine	Serum pseudocholinesterase levels decreased and prolonged duration of anaesthesia	Desirable to test serum pseudocholinesterase activity prior to use of propanidid. Be aware of extended recovery time
Thiopentone	Pancuronium Suxamethonium	Chemically incompatible	Mix in separate syringes
Trichlorethylene	Adrenaline	See above	See above
	Soda lime	Neurotoxic products may be formed	Avoid soda lime

Analgesics (see also chapter XXII; table IV, sect. 3.2.1; X, sect. 6.2, 8.4)

Aspirin and salicylates	Antacids	Therapeutic serum salicylate levels not maintained in rheumatoid arthritis and rheumatic fever by concurrent use of aluminium and magnesium hydroxide, calcium carbonate, magnesium hydroxide, sodium bicarbonate	Avoid this combination in treatment of rheumatoid arthritis and rheumatic fever. The combination product of aluminium hydroxide and dihydroxyaluminium amino-acetate apparently has no real effect on serum salicylate. Alternatively, substitute another anti-inflammatory analgesic in RA patients
	Corticosteroids	Reduced plasma salicylate concentrations (therapeutic concentrations may not be attained). Accumulation of salicylate with risk of toxicity when corticosteroid dosage reduced and dose of salicylate not altered	There should be no need to use two anti-inflammatory agents in rheumatic diseases
Narcotic (strong analgesics)	Alcohol Butyrophenones Hypnosedatives Phenothiazines	Enhanced CNS depressant effects	Instruct patient. Modify dosage of antipsychotic if necessary. Warn about possible effect on driving skills
	Monoamine oxidase inhibitors	Severe reactions with pethidine in some patients	Avoid pethidine. Substitute (with caution) another strong analgesic
Methadone	Rifampicin Phenytoin (presumably other enzyme inducing agents)	Decreased plasma concentrations of methadone and symptoms of narcotic withdrawal in those addicts receiving drug in maintenance programmes	Dosage of methadone in maintenance programmes will need to be increased if enzyme inducing agents are given concurrently
Pethidine (meperidine)	Phenobarbitone	Enhanced CNS depressant effects with doses of 120mg phenobarbitone daily	Avoid pethidine-phenobarbitone (and other enzyme inducing agents) combination

Appendix C. (continued)

Primary drug	May interact with	Potential result (see introductory notes)	Management and how to avoid
Antianxiety Drugs (see also chapter XXVI; sect. 8.5)			
Barbiturates Benzodiazepines	Alcohol Other CNS depressants	Enhanced CNS depressant effects	Instruct patient. Modify dosage if necessary. Warn about possible effect on driving skills
Antiarrhythmic Drugs (see also chapter XVII; sect. 6, 10.3)			
Quinidine	Antacids (magnesium-aluminium hydroxide)	Quinidine intoxication (case report)	Administer antacids cautiously. Monitor urine pH (not alkaline) and serum quinidine levels if any evidence of toxicity is suspected
	Phenobarbitone Phenytoin	Serum levels of quinidine decreased by around 50%	Avoid use of barbiturates as occasional hypnotics. Substitute a benzodiazepine. Monitor serum concentrations of quinidine with use of phenytoin and phenobarbitone as anticonvulsants and adjust dose accordingly
Antibacterial Agents (see also chapter VIII, sect. 4; appendix D)			
Amino-glycosides (amikacin, gentamicin, kanamycin, streptomycin, tobramycin)	Ethacrynic acid Frusemide	Increased risk of ototoxicity when combined with ethacrynic acid, or frusemide in renal failure	If possible, avoid this combination; or reduce the aminoglycoside dosage to the minimum effective level (monitored by serum assay) and regularly check renal function
	Penicillins	Most penicillins can inactivate aminoglycosides if mixed together	Do not mix together and hang in a slow intravenous infusion bottle. Administer by different routes
Cephaloridine Cephalothin	Amikacin Gentamicin Kanamycin Streptomycin Tobramycin Ethacrynic acid (large doses) Frusemide (large doses)	Increased risk of nephrotoxicity particularly in the elderly	If possible, avoid this combination; or reduce dosage of one or both agents and regularly check renal function
Chloramphenicol	Phenobarbitone	Serum levels of chloramphenicol decreased to subtherapeutic amounts	Avoid use of phenobarbitone as an anticonvulsant or monitor serum concentrations of chloramphenicol and adjust dose accordingly

Tetracyclines	Antacids	Serum level of tetracycline markedly decreased by simultaneous administration of aluminium, calcium and magnesium containing liquid antacids	Give drugs 1 to 2 hours apart if possible
	Bismuth complex	Serum level of tetracyclines decreased by tri-potassium di-citrato bismuthate	Unknown whether a dose time-related absorption mechanism involved. In meantime, avoid this combination
	Iron haematinics	Serum levels of tetracycline and absorption of iron markedly decreased	Give conventional iron tablets 3 hours apart if possible. ? May not be a problem with slow release iron preparations
	Zinc sulphate	Serum levels of tetracycline markedly decreased	Not a problem with doxycycline
Anticholinergics	Antidepressants Antihistamines Anti-Parkinsonian drugs (anticholinergic drugs) Antipsychotics	Anticholinergic side effects increased by monoamine oxidase inhibitors, tricyclic antidepressants, some antihistamines (e.g. diphenhydramine, phenidamine, promethazine), anti-Parkinsonian drugs (e.g. orphenadrine, benzhexol, procyclidine) and antipsychotics, particularly in the elderly	Modify dosage if necessary, particularly in the elderly

Primary drug	May interact with	Potential result (see introductory notes)	Management and how to avoid
Anticoagulants (see also chapter XXIII; sect. 3.2.5)			
1. *Drugs which increase anticoagulant action*			
Coumarins (warfarin)	Anabolic steroids	Marked potentiation of coumarin anticoagulant (warfarin, dicoumarol)	Modify dose of coumarin. ? Avoid by use of non C-17 alkylated anabolic steroid such as nandrolone
	Clofibrate	In many patients markedly potentiates effect of anticoagulant (warfarin, ethylbiscoumacetate)	Reduce dose of coumarin (e.g. by 25 to 30 % with warfarin) when clofibrate added. Monitor degree of hypoprothrombinaemia daily for a few days
	Dextropropoxyphene + paracetamol	Case reports of potentiation of effect of warfarin	Avoid this combination. Substitute paracetamol alone
	Glucagon	Doses greater than 24mg daily markedly potentiate effect of warfarin	Avoid this combination. Use other treatment for refractory heart failure
	Metronidazole	Marked potentiation of warfarin (case report and a careful study in volunteers)	Reduce dose of warfarin. Monitor degree of hypoprothrombinaemia daily for a few days or more or substitute alternative agent (effect of other imidazole derivatives on warfarin metabolism unknown).
	Oxyphenbutazone Phenylbutazone	Predictably and markedly potentiates effect of warfarin (by 50 to 75 %) and other coumarins (phenprocoumon, dicoumarol, ethylbiscoumacetate)	Avoid this combination. Substitute indomethacin (does not affect warfarin kinetics or anticoagulant control but may still increase risk of bleeding due to antiplatelet aggregating activity or risk of gastrointestinal bleeding in those with ulcer symptoms)
	Phenyramidol	Markedly potentiates effect of warfarin and dicoumarol (and also phenindione)	Avoid this combination. Substitute paracetamol (analgesic effect) or diazepam (if muscle relaxation desired)
	Quinidine	Markedly potentiates effect of warfarin in some patients	Avoid this combination. Substitute procainamide
	Salicylates	Increased risk of bleeding due to effect on platelet function and haemorrhagic action on gastric mucosa. No effect on anticoagulant control	Avoid this combination. Substitute paracetamol (analgesic effect) or indomethacin (anti-inflammatory analgesic). See also above under oxyphenbutazone
	Sulphaphenazole	Potentiation of effect of warfarin likely	Avoid this combination. Substitute another antibacterial agent. Other sulphonamides are not likely to lead to significant effect on anticoagulant control except perhaps sulphafurazole, particularly in presence of impaired renal function. Co-trimoxazole (trimethoprim-sulphamethoxazole) can also potentiate the effect of warfarin
	d-Thyroxine	In virtually all patients markedly potentiates effect of warfarin and dicoumarol	Reduce dose of coumarin (e.g. by one third with warfarin) when d-thyroxine added. Monitor degree of hypoprothrombinaemia daily for a few days or more

Anticoagulants (continued)

2. *Drugs which decrease anticoagulant action*

	Barbiturates	A marked decrease in effect of coumarins (warfarin, dicoumarol, nicoumalone/acenocoumarol, ethylbiscoumacetate, phenprocoumon) in many patients. Dose requirement may increase many fold (even up to 10x)	Avoid use of barbiturates as occasional hypnotics. Substitute a benzodiazepine. Barbiturates taken regularly as anticonvulsants (i.e. in a steady state) do not affect anticoagulant control, unless the barbiturate is withdrawn or reduced in dosage without modifying the dose of the anticoagulant
	Cholestyramine	Markedly reduces absorption of warfarin when given with cholestyramine or 3 hours after it	Give warfarin 2 or more hours before cholestyramine if possible
	Dichloralphenazone Ethchlorvynol Glutethimide	Can antagonise effect of warfarin	Avoid this combination. Substitute a benzodiazepine
	Griseofulvin	Can in some patients decrease effect of warfarin	Monitor closely and adjust dose of anticoagulant carefully
	Rifampicin	Marked decrease in effect of warfarin and also nicoumalone and phenprocoumon	Monitor anticoagulant control and adjust dose of warfarin carefully, or avoid rifampicin in antituberculosis regimen (e.g. if compliance cannot be guaranteed) **Note:** Any adjustment of coumarin dosage should only be made on the basis of results derived from close observation of therapy over a period of time after the change
Indanediones (phenindione)	Salicylates	Increased risk of bleeding due to effect on platelet function and haemorrhagic action on gastric mucosa. No effect on anticoagulant control	Avoid this combination. Substitute paracetamol (analgesic use) or indomethacin (anti-inflammatory analgesic)

Primary drug	May interact with	Potential result (see introductory notes)	Management and how to avoid
Anticonvulsants (see also chapter XXV; sect. 2.3; 3)			
Carbamazepine	Dextropropoxyphene (propoxyphene)	Marked increase in serum level of carbamazepine and toxicity	Avoid use of dextropropoxyphene for pain relief of more than 1 day. Substitute aspirin and codeine
	Triacetyloleandomycin (troleandomycin)	Marked and rapid increase in serum level of carbamazepine and toxicity	Avoid use of triacetyloleandomycin. Substitute penicillin V
Phenobarbitone Primidone	Sulthiame	Marked increase in serum level of phenobarbitone in many patients	Monitor serum levels of phenobarbitone when sulthiame added to stable regimen and reduce dose of phenobarbitone or primidone if necessary
	Sodium valproate	Marked sedation	Reduce dose of phenobarbitone or primidone when sodium valproate added
Phenytoin	Chloramphenicol	Marked increase in serum level of phenytoin	Avoid use of chloramphenicol, or if essential monitor serum levels of phenytoin and adjust dose accordingly
	Diazoxide (oral)	Mutual antagonism. Marked decrease in serum level of phenytoin. Hyperglycaemic effect of diazoxide antagonised	Avoid this combination
	Dicoumarol	Marked increase in serum level of phenytoin when dicoumarol added	Avoid this combination. Substitute warfarin
	Disulfiram	Marked increase in serum level of phenytoin in many patients	If possible, avoid this combination; or monitor serum levels of phenytoin and reduce dose if necessary
	Isoniazid	Marked increase in serum level of phenytoin in some patients who are slow acetylators of isoniazid	Monitor serum levels of phenytoin when isoniazid added to stable phenytoin regimen and reduce dose if necessary
	Phenobarbitone	Variable effect on serum phenytoin level and also dependent on dosage; occasionally a marked increase may occur on adding phenobarbitone or after its withdrawal (substrate competition for metabolism occurs immediately phenobarbitone is started but a more slowly developing enzyme induction reverses this effect)	Monitor serum levels of phenytoin whenever phenobarbitone is added to stable regimen or if phenobarbitone is withdrawn
	Phenylbutazone	Marked increase in serum level of phenytoin in a few patients	Avoid this combination. Substitute indomethacin

Sodium valproate	Marked but temporary increase in serum level and drug effects	Monitor serum levels of phenytoin when sodium valproate added to stable regimen. Free phenytoin concentration will be higher than expected for a given total serum phenytoin concentration. Initial temporary reduction in phenytoin dosage may be necessary (see chapter I; sect. 3.2.3)
Sulphaphenazole	Marked increase in serum level of phenytoin in a few patients	Avoid this combination. Substitute another agent (except sulpha-methiazole or chloramphenicol which may inhibit phenytoin metabolism)
Sulthiame	Marked increase in serum level of phenytoin in many patients	Monitor serum levels of phenytoin when sulthiame added to stable phenytoin regimen and reduce dose if necessary
		Note: Most clinically significant interactions with phenytoin become manifest within 1 to 6 weeks after addition of the other drug. Interactions with phenytoin may not always be detrimental. Thus, modest elevation of a low serum level of phenytoin may actually improve seizure control. A marked increase in serum concentration increases risk of intoxication

Antidepressants (see also chapter X, sect. 6.2; XXVI, sect. 7.6)

Monoamine oxidase inhibitors (iproniazid, isocarboxazid, phenelzine, tranylcypromine)	Amphetamines Ephedrine Fenfluramine Phenylpropanolamine Phenylephrine Pseudoephedrine Levodopa Foodstuffs containing tyramine (Chianti and Alicante-type wines, some beers, matured cheese, yoghurt, pickled herrings, chicken liver, vegetable, yeast and meat extracts) or dopamine (broad bean pods)	Acute adrenergic crisis (marked headache, severe hypertension, subarachnoid haemorrhage) if MAOI given with these agents (N.B. anorexiants and common cold remedies)	Avoid these combinations. Treat crises with phentolamine 5mg IV
	Tricyclic antidepres-sants (imipramine, amitriptyline etc)	Agitation, tremor, hyperpyrexia and coma if given *inadvertently* with tricyclic antidepressants	Allow space of 2 to 3 weeks after withdrawal of MAOI. These agents can be given together if order of administration and dosage of each is carefully tailored (see chapter XXVI; sect. 7.1, 7.6)
	Pethidine	Severe reaction (excitation, sweating, rigidity, hyper- or hypotension, coma) in some patients	Avoid this combination. Cautious use of another strong analgesic
	Alcohol Analgesics, strong Hypnosedatives	CNS depressants effects increased	Instruct patient. Warn about possible adverse effect on driving skills, especially with first few days of therapy. Advisable to avoid alcoholic beverages since tyramine content not likely to be known by patient

Appendix C. (continued)

Primary drug	May interact with	Potential result (see introductory notes)	Management and how to avoid
Antidepressants (continued)			
Tricyclic (amitriptyline, imipramine etc)	Anticholinergics Antihistamines Antiparkinsonian drugs	Increased risk of troublesome atropine-like side effects in the elderly if given with anticholinergics, antiparkinsonian drugs or some antihistamines (e.g. diphenhydramine, phenidamine, promethazine)	Use conservative doses of tricyclics in the elderly
	Alcohol	Increased risk of paralytic ileus and CNS depressant effects when given with alcohol	Instruct patient to limit consumption of alcohol. Warn about possible adverse effects on driving skills, especially with first few days of therapy on amitriptyline
	Monoamine oxidase inhibitors	Agitation, tremor, hyperpyrexia and coma if given *inadvertently* with monoamine oxidase inhibitors	Allow space of 2 to 3 weeks after withdrawal of MAOI. These agents can be given together if order of administration and dosage of each is carefully tailored (see chapter XXVI: sect. 7.1, 7.6)
Antifungal Agents			
Griseofulvin	Phenobarbitone	Absorption of griseofulvin impaired	Give griseofulvin in 3 divided doses or avoid phenobarbitone
Antihistamines			
	Alcohol Sedatives	CNS depressant effects of some compounds increased with alcohol, other sedatives	Instruct patient. Warn about possible adverse effect on driving skills, especially with first few days of therapy
Antihypertensive Drugs (see also chapter XVIII; sect. 10)			
Adrenergic neurone blocking drugs (bethanidine, debrisoquine, guanethidine)	Amphetamines Ephedrine Phenylephrine Phenylpropanolamine Pizotifen Pseudoephedrine (N.B. anorexiants, except fenfluramine; common cold remedies) Tricyclic antidepressants (imipramine, amitriptyline and derivatives) Chlorpromazine	Antihypertensive effect antagonised and control of blood pressure may be lost	Avoid these combinations, especially oral common cold remedies. Substitute a β-adrenoceptor blocking drug, or use an antidepressant with little or no effect on the noradrenaline (norepinephrine) uptake pump such as mianserin or doxepin at a daily dose not exceeding 200mg

Methyldopa	Amphetamines etc Tricyclic antidepressants	Antihypertensive effect may be antagonised and control of blood pressure may be lost	Interaction not as predictable or as well documented as with adrenergic neurone blocking drugs. See above
	Pargyline (MAOI)	Likely to be dangerous (headache, severe hypertension, hallucination)	Avoid this combination. Substitute another agent for pargyline
All agents	Antimigraine drugs	Some patients are more sensitive to vasoconstrictors	Avoid ergotamine
	Antihistamines	Some compounds may cause rise in blood pressure	Monitor blood pressure regularly
	Oral contraceptives	Increased risk of vascular damage	Preferable to avoid oestrogen-progestagen oral contraceptives in any patient needing antihypertensive therapy
	Bronchodilators Carbenoxolone Indomethacin Phenylbutazone	Can sometimes make antihypertensive therapy more difficult	Monitor blood pressure regularly. Modify therapy if necessary
	Fenfluramine Glyceryl trinitrate Phenothiazines	Can lower blood pressure considerably (fenfluramine with Rauwolfia and methyldopa)	Monitor blood pressure regularly. Modify therapy if necessary

Antineoplastic and Immunosuppressive Drugs (see also chapter XXIV, sect. 2.3.1, 8)

Azathioprine Mercaptopurine	Allopurinol	Activity of azathioprine increased	Decrease dose of azathioprine to 33 % of usual
Methotrexate	Phenylbutazone	Activity of methotrexate may be increased	Avoid this combination. Substitute indomethacin
	Salicylates	Activity of methotrexate may be increased	Avoid this combination. Substitute paracetamol

Anti-Parkinsonian Drugs (see also chapter XXV; sect. 5.1.1)

Levodopa	Monoamine oxidase inhibitor antidepressants	Acute adrenergic crisis	Avoid this combination
	Papaverine	Therapeutic efficacy of levodopa gradually reduced over some weeks	Avoid this combination
	Pyridoxine	Therapeutic efficacy of levodopa reduced (except when given with a decarboxylase inhibitor)	Avoid this combination or use levodopa plus a decarboxylase inhibitor

Appendix C. (continued)

Primary drug	May interact with	Potential result (see introductory notes)	Management and how to avoid
Antipsychotic and Antimanic Drugs (see also chapter XXVI; sect. 1.5.1, 5.4, 12)			
Butyrophenones (haloperidol)	Alcohol Analgesics, narcotic Hypnosedatives	Increased CNS depressant effects	Instruct patient. Warn re possible adverse effect on driving skills, especially with first few days of therapy
Lithium	Diuretics	With loss of sodium, lithium retention and toxicity may occur	Use reduced doses of lithium and monitor serum lithium levels regularly (probably more frequently than usual)
	Methyldopa	Toxicity at relatively low serum lithium levels may occur	Avoid this combination
	Sodium chloride	The lower the sodium intake, the greater the lithium retention; the higher the sodium intake, the greater the lithium excretion	Instruct the patient. Warn about conditions leading to sodium loss and hence lithium retention (e.g. excessive sweating in hot weather, vomiting, intercurrent infection, low sodium diet, long term diuretics)
Phenothiazines	Alcohol Analgesics, narcotic Hypnosedatives	Increased CNS depressant effects	Instruct patient. Modify dosage of antipsychotic if necessary. Warn about possible effect on driving skills
	Antacids	Absorption of chlorpromazine may be impaired by concurrent aluminium hydroxide or aluminium hydroxide plus magnesium trisilicate gel antacids	Give drugs a few hours apart if possible
	Lithium	Decreased bioavailability of chlorpromazine	Increased dosage of chlorpromazine should be anticipated or reduction of dosage when lithium withdrawn
Antituberculosis Drugs (see also chapter XX; sect. 8.1)			
Isoniazid	Aluminium hydroxide gel	Decreased absorption of isoniazid	Only likely to be significant with intermittent isoniazid regimens. Give isoniazid 1 hour before antacid if possible
Rifampicin (rifampin)	PAS (bentonite as excipient)	Serum levels of rifampicin markedly decreased	Give PAS preparations containing bentonite 8 to 12 hours apart from rifampicin
	Phenobarbitone (? other enzyme inducing drugs)	Serum levels of rifampicin markedly decreased by phenobarbitone	Avoid occasional use of barbiturates. Substitute a benzodiazepine for occasional hypnotic use. Modify dosage of rifampicin (or phenobarbitone) in long term antituberculosis/antiepileptic therapy if necessary

Antiulcer Drugs (see also chapter XIX; sect. 4)

Carbenoxolone	Spironolactone	Ulcer healing properties of carbenoxolone abolished (thiazides do not interfere with ulcer healing)	Avoid this combination. Substitute a thiazide diuretic *but* monitor serum potassium regularly

Bronchodilators (see also chapter XX; sect. 2.3.1)

Theophylline	Erythromycin Triacetyloleandomycin (troleandomycin)	Increase in serum theophylline levels; toxicity may result if concentrations already in upper therapeutic range	Avoid this combination. Substitute penicillin
	Phenobarbitone	Decreased serum theophylline levels	Larger than normal doses of theophylline may be needed in epileptics on long term phenobarbitone.

Cardiac Glycosides (see also chapter XVII; sect. 8.1.3; 8.1.4)

Digoxin Digitoxin Lanatocide C and so on	Diuretics	Risk of digitalis toxicity increased in presence of hypokalaemia	Ensure adequate intake of potassium
	Suxamethonium	Risk of dangerous arrhythmias due to sudden release of potassium	More likely to be a problem in presence of trauma, burns, wounds, muscular disorders. Avoid suxamethonium in such cases
Digoxin	Antacid gel liquids (aluminium hydroxide or magnesium-containing)	Decreased bioavailability of digoxin with concomitant administration of aluminium hydroxide or magnesium salts	Give drugs about 6 hours apart if possible. More likely to be a problem with slowly dissolving digoxin tablets
	Antidiarrhoeals (adsorbent type)	Decreased bioavailability of digoxin with concomitant administration of kaolin-pectin suspension	Give drugs about 6 hours apart if possible. More likely to be a problem with slowly dissolving digoxin tablets
	Cholestyramine Colestipol	Decreased bioavailability of digoxin possible	Give drugs about 8 hours after digoxin
	Quinidine	Marked increase in serum levels of digoxin with real risk of toxicity	Anticipate need to reduce digoxin dosage if quinidine added and monitor serum digoxin levels closely
Digitoxin	Cholestyramine Colestipol	Decreased bioavailability of digitoxin possible	Give drugs about 8 hours after digitoxin

Cholestyramine (see also chapter XVII; sect. 3.2.4)

	Acidic drugs (e.g. digoxin, warfarin)	Because it is an anion exchange resin, cholestyramine may bind acidic drugs in the gut, delaying or impairing their absorption	Give other drugs an hour or more before cholestyramine if possible

Appendix C. (continued)

Primary drug	May interact with	Potential result (see introductory notes)	Management and how to avoid
Contraceptives, Oral (see also chapter XV; sect. 13.5)			
	Ampicillin	? Interference in enterohepatic circulation of oestrogen (see chapter I; sect. 3.5). Pregnancy and high incidence of menstrual irregularities has resulted	Advise additional use of condom and/or spermicidal foam during a course of ampicillin therapy
	Carbamazepine Rifampicin Phenobarbitone Phenytoin	Increased metabolism of oestrogen. A high incidence of menstrual irregularities has resulted and pregnancy with rifampicin and anticonvulsants	Advise use of an intrauterine contraceptive device. Avoid occasional use of barbiturates. Substitute diazepam **Note:** Bleeding disturbances in a previously regular contraceptive cycle indicate that the method is no longer reliable. Increasing the dose or a change of contraceptive does not eliminate the risk of bleeding disturbances or pregnancy. The offending drug should be withdrawn, the disturbed contraceptive table cycle terminated and a new one started along with an additional method of contraception for the first new course. When the offending drug cannot be withdrawn, an alternative method of contraception is advised. Any enzyme inducing drug is a potential source of risk to contraceptive efficacy in users of oral contraceptives
Corticosteroids, Systemic (see also chapter XVI; sect. 9.1.2)			
Dexamethasone Hydrocortisone Methylpred- nisolone Prednisone Prednisolone	Barbiturates (phenobarbitone)	Dexamethasone, hydrocortisone, methylprednisolone, prednisolone and prednisone metabolism enhanced by phenobarbitone (and other barbiturates). Efficacy of steroid reduced	A need for increase in steroid dosage, particularly if large doses of barbiturate used (e.g 120mg phenobarbitone daily) and with the longer acting steroids (e.g. dexamethasone). Doubling of usual steroid dosage may be necessary, but careful follow up and with further adjustments according to clinical response is essential. Avoid occasional use of barbiturates. Substitute a benzodiazepine. Interpret dexamethasone suppression tests cautiously
Dexamethasone	Ephedrine	Dexamethasone metabolism enhanced	Avoid this combination. Substitute a β_2-adrenoceptor agonist bronchodilator or theophylline
Dexamethasone Hydrocortisone Methylpred- nisolone Prednisolone	Phenytoin	Dexamethasone, hydrocortisone, prednisolone and methylprednisolone metabolism enhanced by phenytoin. Reduced efficacy of steroid	A need for increase in steroid dosage, particularly with the longer acting steroids (e.g. dexamethasone). A doubling of the usual steroid dosage may be necessary, but careful follow up with further adjustments according to clinical response is essential. Interpret dexamethasone suppression tests cautiously
Cortisone Dexamethasone Prednisone Prednisolone	Rifampicin (rifampin)	Increased steroid dose requirements due to enhanced steroid metabolism by rifampicin	Increase steroid dosage but adjust dosage when rifampicin withdrawn (e.g. in patients with tuberculosis as a consequence of long term immunosuppressive therapy with corticosteroids). A doubling of usual steroid dosage may be necessary, but careful follow up with further adjustments according to clinical response is essential. In Addison's disease, consider alternative agent to rifampicin

Diuretics (see also chapter XXI; sect. 7)

Amiloride Spironolactone Triamterene	Potassium supplements	Risk of hyperkalaemia	In general, avoid this combination and certainly in presence of impaired renal function
Ethacrynic acid Frusemide (furosemide)	Amikacin Gentamicin Kanamycin Streptomycin Tobramycin	Increased risk of ototoxicity when combined with ethacrynic acid, or frusemide in renal failure	If possible, avoid this combination; or reduce the aminoglycoside dosage to the minimum effective level (monitored by serum assay) and regularly check renal function
	Cephaloridine Cephalothin	Increased risk of nephrotoxicity with large doses of ethacrynic acid or frusemide	If possible, avoid this combination; or reduce dosage of one or both agents and regularly check renal function
Frusemide	Indomethacin	Therapeutic efficacy of frusemide may be reduced	Increased dose requirements of frusemide should be anticipated

Gout Drugs (see also chapter XXII; table IV, sect. 12.2.1)

Probenecid Sulphinpyrazone	Salicylates (low doses)	Therapeutic efficacy of probenecid and sulphinpyrazone markedly inhibited	Avoid low doses of salicylates. Occasional small analgesic doses seem to be without significant effect on uricosuric action
	Thiazide diuretics	Therapeutic efficacy of urate altering drug may be inhibited	An increase in dosage of the uricosuric agent may be needed

Hypnosedatives

Barbiturates Chloral hydrate Dichloral- phenazone Glutethimide Methaqualone Nitrazepam Flurazepam	Alcohol (acute ingestion) Analgesics, narcotic Antihistamines Antidepressants Antipsychotics	Increased CNS depressant effects	Instruct the patient. Warn about possible adverse effects on driving skills, especially with first few days of therapy, and to avoid excessive quantities of alcohol

Hypoglycaemic Agents (see also chapter XVI; sect. 3.3.5)

Biguanides (metformin, phenformin)	Alcohol	Risk of hyperlacticacidaemia	Instruct the patient to avoid excessive quantities (moderate to large) of alcohol and to be aware of and to report *early* symptoms of lactic acidosis (vomiting and malaise, abdominal pain, diarrhoea)

Primary drug	May interact with	Potential result (see introductory notes)	Management and how to avoid
Hypoglycaemic Agents (continued) Sulphonylureas	Alcohol	Disulfiram-like intolerance (facial flushing, headache) of alcohol in some cases, particularly with chlorpropamide. Hypoglycaemic activity may be increased with acute alcohol ingestion if food intake is restricted (e.g. malnutrition, prolonged fasting)	Instruct the patient about possibility of intolerance of alcohol and to avoid moderate to large quantities of alcohol. Intolerance of small quantities of alcohol more likely with chlorpropamide (see chapter XVI; sect. 3.3.5). Educate patient to maintain adequate nutrition
	β-Adrenoreceptor blocking drugs	Hypoglycaemic activity may be increased in some patients	Reduced dose requirement of sulphonylureas may be needed in some patients. β-Adrenoreceptor blocking drugs prevent the release of lactate from muscle which is normally subsequently converted in the liver to glucose. In the absence of lactate, hypoglycaemia may result, particularly when the liver contains little or no glycogen (e.g. as after prolonged fasting, in ketosis, in any patient with liver disease, or in alcoholics)
	Barbiturates Rifampicin (rifampin)	May make diabetic control more difficult	Likely to be a problem with compounds extensively metabolised in the liver (e.g. tolazamide, tolbutamide, glibenclamide, acetohexamide). Avoid occasional use of barbiturates. Substitute a benzodiazepine
	Clofibrate	Severe hypoglycaemia has been reported with tolbutamide and clofibrate	A reduced dose of tolbutamide may be needed in some patients
	Corticosteroids Diuretics (e.g. thiazides)	May make diabetic control more difficult	Modify dose of sulphonylurea if necessary
	Oxyphenbutazone Phenylbutazone	Hypoglycaemic coma has been reported on many occasions with phenylbutazone and chlorpropamide, acetohexamide, carbutamide, glibenclamide or tolbutamide	Avoid this combination. Substitute indomethacin or naproxen
	Sulphaphenazole Sulphadimidine (sulphamethazine)	Hypoglycaemic coma has been reported with sulphadimidine and chlorpropamide and with sulphaphenazole and tolbutamide	Avoid this combination. Substitute another antibacterial agent (except sulphafurazole or chloramphenicol, both of which under certain circumstances can increase the activity of the sulphonylureas) **Note:** The risk of drug-induced hypoglycaemic reactions is increased in the presence of associated renal impairment or liver dysfunction, with restricted food intake and in the elderly

Iron Haematinics (see also chapter VIII; sect. 2.3.1)

	Antacid liquids	Absorption of oral iron impaired by magnesium- or carbonate-containing antacids	Give drugs as far apart as possible
	Tetracyclines	Serum levels of tetracycline and absorption of iron markedly decreased	Give conventional iron tablets 3 hours apart if possible. ? May not be a problem with slow release iron preparations

Migraine Drugs

Ergotamine	Triacetyloleandomycin	Real risk of peripheral ischaemia	Avoid this combination. Substitute penicillin V

Monoamine Oxidase Inhibitors
    See: Antidepressants

Muscle Relaxants, Skeletal (see also chapter X, sect. 2.2, 6)

Depolarising (e.g. suxamethonium)	Amikacin Gentamicin Kanamycin Streptomycin Tobramycin Polymyxin	Neuromuscular blocking activity may be increased. Also danger of respiratory arrest	Give these antibiotics with extreme caution during surgery or postoperative period. Anticipate prolongation of block. Interaction has most often followed streptomycin and neomycin and appears most predictable if antibiotics are given intraperitoneally or if usual doses are used in a patient with impaired renal function or muscle weakness. The block can often be antagonised by neostigmine and calcium, or by germine diacetate
	Propanidid Procaine (large doses)	Neuromuscular blocking activity may be increased	Give these combinations with caution and anticipate prolongation of block. Large doses of procaine seem necessary to enhance block
	Lithium	Neuromuscular blocking activity may be prolonged	Anticipate prolongation of block
	Anticholinesterases (ecothiopate eye drops, pesticides) Cyclophosphamide Phenelzine	Serum pseudocholinesterase levels decreased and neuromuscular blocking activity may be prolonged	Desirable to assess pseudocholinesterase activity prior to use of suxamethonium. Avoid suxamethonium if levels of pseudocholinesterase significantly decreased (as likely in case with ecothiopate eye drops). If suxamethonium is necessary, use with extreme caution
Non-depolarising (e.g. tubocurarine, pancuronium)	Amikacin etc (see above)	Neuromuscular blocking activity may be increased. Also danger of respiratory arrest	See above under these antibiotics
	Hypokalaemia	Neuromuscular blocking activity may be increased	Correct potassium deficit
	Anticholinesterases Immunosuppressives	Neuromuscular blocking activity may be decreased in some patients	Anticipate need to modify dose of relaxant
Pancuronium	Lithium	Neuromuscular blocking activity may be increased	Anticipate prolongation of block
	Corticosteroids	Rapid termination of action by large doses of steroids	Careful monitoring of neuromuscular transmission if this combination is used

Appendix C. (continued)

Primary drug	May interact with	Potential result (see introductory notes)	Management and how to avoid
Potassium Supplements (see also chapter XXI; sect. 7)			
	Amiloride Spironolactone Triamterene	Risk of hyperkalaemia	In general, avoid this combination and certainly in presence of impaired renal function
Thyroid Drugs			
	Cholestyramine	Absorption of thyroid impaired	Give drugs 4 to 5 hours apart if possible
	Ketamine	Severe hypertension and tachycardia	Try control with propranolol
Trichomonacides			
Metronidazole Nifuratel	Alcohol	Disulfiram-like intolerance of alcohol (facial flushing, headache) may occur in some cases	Instruct the patient about possibility of reaction and to avoid excessive alcohol consumption
Vasopressor Agents (see also chapter X; sect. 6.2)			
Levo-noradrenaline (levarterenol)	Amitriptyline Imipramine Guanethidine Methyldopa	Marked increase in pressor response (N.B. not with MAOI)	Give noradrenaline only with caution; beginning with very small doses
Metaraminol Methoxamine	Monoamine oxidase inhibitors	Marked increase in pressor response	Avoid this combination. Noradrenaline may be preferable
Mephentermine	Tricyclic antidepressants	Circulatory effect enhanced	Give such indirect acting vasopressors only with caution
Phenylephrine	Guanethidine	Marked increase in pressor response, even from eye drops of either agent	Give such combinations only with caution
	Monoamine oxidase inhibitors	Slight to moderate increase in pressor response (only real problem with oral phenylephrine)	Avoid oral and probably also nasal phenylephrine. Give parenteral phenylephrine with caution
	Tricyclic antidepressants	Circulatory effect enhanced	Give phenylephrine only with caution

Appendix D
Guide to Selection of a Systemic Antibacterial Agent

G.S. Avery, R.N. Brogden and R.C. Heel

The choice of the most appropriate antibacterial agent is largely dependent upon:

1) The causative organism — diagnosis and susceptibility
2) The patient — host factors which may lead to adverse reactions or altered responsiveness
3) The drug — pharmacokinetic properties; cost
4) Nature of the illness — parenteral or oral therapy; multiple or single agents.

In any given situation there may be a number of suitable treatments to choose from, and thus there are bound to be individual preferences in some cases. Nevertheless, when all factors are considered there is generally one agent, or sometimes a combination of agents, that is likely to be a better choice than other agents, or combinations. The tables which follow are intended to complement the principles enunciated in chapter XXVII, to which readers are referred. They are not intended to be dogmatic statements, but rather an attempt to reflect the current consensus of informed opinion on a worldwide basis. Individual clinicians may however, disagree with some of the recommendations. With the passage of time, new studies and the introduction of new agents will undoubtedly necessitate revision of the tables. When referring to the tables it is very important to take cognisance of the footnotes and the principles discussed in chapter XXVII and elsewhere in the book. *In particular, it must be stressed that the sensitivity patterns of a number of organisms can vary with the hospital, clinic or community in which they are isolated.*

Before prescribing an antibacterial drug, a diagnosis should be formed which is strongly suggestive of the presence of a given bacterial infection. To a large extent *initiation* of treatment is based on intelligent clinical or bacteriological guesswork. On the basis of such a tentative diagnosis, the clinician can select an agent which is most likely to be effective (and safe) against the suspected causative organism(s) or disease (see tables I and II).

Where appropriate, specimens for laboratory examination should be obtained before commencing treatment with the chosen agent. At a later stage, a change in therapy may be necessary on the basis of the laboratory results and patient response. A bacteriological diagnosis is mandatory in life threatening infections such as meningitis, suspected septicaemia or severe pneumonia.

Clinical judgement should always be used when interpreting laboratory findings, particularly when they appear to conflict with sound clinical evidence. In such cases specialist advice should be sought.

A Gram stain may not always suffice, and in cases where organisms are known to have varying sensitivities or local differences in sensitivity (see table I), the sensitivity pattern to a number of agents should be ascertained — for there is no guarantee that the causative organism(s) will be sensitive to the agent of obvious first or alternate choice.

Susceptibility to an appropriate agent implies that the concentration in the blood or urine, or at the site of infection, exceeds by several-fold the minimum concentration of the drug necessary to inhibit or kill the causative organism(s). Such considerations should always be taken into account and have dictated for the most part the guide to the *normal* preferred choices in tables I and II.

If adverse drug reactions are to be avoided, bacteriological investigation must not outweigh careful consideration of the individual who is being treated. Certain host factors can also be of great consequence in determining the response to therapy. Thus the choice of an appropriate agent is sometimes influenced by important considerations set out in tables III and IV.

Multiple drug therapy may occasionally influence the choice of an antibacterial agent or dictate the most appropriate manner of administration of doses (see table V). Physical or chemical incompatibilities occurring when an antibacterial agent is given concurrently with another drug or antibacterial agent have not been included in the table. The hospital microbiologist or pharmacist should always be consulted for relevant compatibility information.

General References

Anon: Handbook of Antimicrobial Therapy (Medical Letter, New Rochelle 1972).

Ball, A.P.; Gray, J.A. and Murdoch, J.McC.: Antibacterial Drugs Today (ADIS Press, Sydney; MTP, London; University Park Press, Baltimore 1978).

Eichenwald, H.F. and McCracken, G.H.: Antimicrobial therapy in infants and children. Part I. Review of antimicrobial agents. Journal of Pediatrics 93: 337 (1978).

Garrod, L.P.; Lambert, H.P. and O'Grady, F.: Antibiotic and Chemotherapy, 4th ed (Churchill Livingstone, Edinburgh 1973).

McCracken, G.H. and Eichenwald, H.F.: Antimicrobial therapy in infants and children. Part II. Therapy of infectious conditions. Journal of Pediatrics 93: 357 (1978).

Marks, M.I.: Common Bacterial Infections in Infancy and Childhood (ADIS Press, Sydney; MTP, London; University Park Press, Baltimore 1979).

Weinstein, L.: Chemotherapy of microbial diseases; in Goodman and Gilman The Pharmacological Basis of Therapeutics, 5th ed, p.1090, 1113, 1130, 1167, 1183 (Macmillan, New York 1975).

Weinstein, L. and Dalton, A.C.: Host determinants of response to antimicrobial agents. New England Journal of Medicine 279: 467, 524, 580 (1968).

Table I. Range of bacteriological activity and clinical usefulness of systemically administered antibacterial agents

Symbols: ● = highly active; ⊕ = active; ○ = limited / variable activity; ± = intermediate. Action: C = bactericidal, S = bacteriostatic.

Agent	Amikacin	Amoxycillin	Ampicillin[17]	Benzylpenicillin[18]	Carbenicillin[19]	Cefoxitin	Cefuroxime	Cephalexin[20]	Cephaloridine[20]	Cephalothin[20]	Cephamandole
Bacteroides fragilis[16]					○	⊕					
Br. abortus[15]		○	○								
Ps. aeruginosa[14]	⊕[a]				●						
Shigella spp[13]	○		●		○	○	○	○	○	○	○
Salmonella spp[12]		●[a] ⊕[b]	●[a]		○	○	○	○	○	○	○
Pr. morgani	⊕				●	⊕	⊕			⊕	
Pr. rettgeri	⊕				●	○	○			⊕	
Pr. vulgaris	⊕				●	⊕				○	
Pr. mirabilis (PP3)[11]	⊕					⊕	○				
Pr. mirabilis[11]	⊕	●[b]	●[b]		⊕	⊕	⊕	○	○		⊕
Kl. Enterobacter spp[10]	⊕	±[a]	±[a]		⊕[b,c]	○[a]	⊕	○[a] ⊕[c]	○[a]		
Esch. coli[9]	⊕[e]	●[b,e] ⊕[a]	●[b,e] ⊕[a]		⊕[b]	⊕[e]	⊕[e]	⊕[b]	○[e]	○[e]	⊕[e]
Bord. pertussis	○	⊕	⊕	○	○			○		○	
H. influenzae[8]	○	●	●		○	○	⊕	±	±	±	○
N. meningitidis[7]		⊕	⊕	●	○	○	⊕	○	○	○	○
N. gonorrhoeae[6]		⊕	⊕	●	±	○	⊕	○	○	○	○
Str. pneumoniae[4]		○	○	●	○	○	⊕	○	⊕	⊕	⊕
Str. faecalis[5]		●[a]	●[a]	●[a,b]	○[c]			±			
Str. pyogenes[4]		○	○	●	○		⊕	⊕	⊕	⊕	⊕
Staph. aureus (PP)[3]	○					±	○	⊕	⊕	⊕	○
Staph. aureus[2]	○	○	○	●	○	±	○	⊕	⊕	○	⊕
Action[1]	C	C	C	C	C	C	C	C	C	C	C

Agent	Cephazolin[20]	Chloramphenicol[21]	Clindamycin[22]	Cloxacillin[23]	Colistin	Co-trimoxazole[24]	Erythromycin	Framycetin	Fusidic acid	Gentamicin	Kanamycin
Bacteroides fragilis[16]		●	●								
Br. abortus[15]		⊕[a]				⊕		○	○	○	
Ps. aeruginosa[14]					⊕					●[a]	
Shigella spp[13]	○	⊕			⊕	⊕		○		○	○
Salmonella spp[12]	○	●[b]			○	⊕[b]		○		○	○
Pr. morgani		○				○		○		●	⊕
Pr. rettgeri						○				●	⊕
Pr. vulgaris		⊕								●	⊕
Pr. mirabilis (PP3)[11]	○	○				⊕		○		●	●
Pr. mirabilis[11]	○					⊕		○		⊕	○
Kl. Enterobacter spp[10]	⊕	⊕			⊕	⊕		○		●	⊕
Esch. coli[9]	⊕[e]	○			⊕[d,e]	●[b] ⊕[a,c,e]		⊕[d]		●[d,e]	⊕[c]
Bord. pertussis		○			○	○	●	○		○	○
H. influenzae[8]	±	⊕		±	○	⊕	○			○	○
N. meningitidis[7]		⊕		○	⊕	○	○				
N. gonorrhoeae[6]	○	±		±	○	⊕	○		±		
Str. pneumoniae[4]	⊕	⊕		⊕	○	⊕	⊕		±		
Str. faecalis[5]		○			○	⊕				±[b]	
Str. pyogenes[4]	○	⊕		⊕	⊕		⊕		±		
Staph. aureus (PP)[3]	⊕	⊕	⊕	●	⊕	○	⊕	⊕	⊕	⊕	○
Staph. aureus[2]		⊕	⊕	○	⊕	⊕	○	○	⊕	○	
Action[1]	C	S	S/C	C	C	C	S/C	C	C	C	C

Key

* Strains of these species show large variations in sensitivity; *in vitro* susceptibility test should be performed.
● Drug(s) of first choice. Organism highly sensitive or usually sensitive to concentrations readily attained in blood, urine or tissues. Therapeutic efficacy well established.
⊕ Drug(s) of second choice; or alternative first choice in cases of known penicillin allergy. Organism sensitive or usually sensitive to concentrations attained in blood, urine or tissues. Therapeutic efficacy also established.
○ Organism sensitive or usually sensitive to concentrations attained in blood, urine or tissues. Other agents preferred because of higher degree of sensitivity, lower order of toxicity, or wider therapeutic experience.
± Organism less sensitive, or high concentrations of antibacterial agent required, or desired therapeutic response may not be consistently obtained.

1 C = Bactericidal; S = Bacteristatic; S/C = Bacteristatic in low concentrations, bactericidal at high concentrations.
2 Non-penicillinase producing strains of *Staphylococcus aureus*. Certain strains may be resistant to methicillin and also to all other penicillins and many other antibacterial drugs. In the USA where this has been a problem, vancomycin is the most consistently effective agent against such organisms.
3 Penicillinase (β-lactamase) producing strains.
4 Occasional strains may be resistant to erythromycin.
5 In endocarditis, the disc sensitivity test may not be sufficiently reliable and tube dilution studies should be performed to establish bactericidal as well as minimal inhibitory concentrations. The bactericidal activity of the patient's serum against his own organism should be estimated — peak activity should be adequate at a serum dilution of at least 1:8.
  a In endocarditis, first choice in combination with streptomycin, kanamycin or gentamicin.
  b In combination with streptomycin.
  c Urinary tract infections only.
6 Essential that a curative dosage regimen is used (see chapter XXIX).
7 a Preferred choice only for control of carriers (minocycline is tetracycline of choice, preferably in combination with rifampicin).
  b Sulphonamides to be used only when causative strains proven sensitive.
8 Ampicillin-resistant strains have been reported in some areas.
  a Preferred choice for acute otitis media in young children.
  b Preferred choice except meningitis.
9 a Preferred choice for uncomplicated urinary infection primary treatment (domiciliary acquired).
  b Preferred choice for urinary infection retreatment.
  c Preferred choice for urinary infection prophylaxis.
  d Preferred choice for diarrhoea due to invasive enteropathogenic strains (give orally).
  e Preferred choice for sepsis and other infections. Ampicillin resistant strains of *Esch. coli* are fairly common.
10 a *Klebsiella* spp. only.
  b *Enterobacter* spp. only.
  c *Kl. aerogenes* urinary tract infections.
  d *Kl. pneumoniae* lobar pneumonia.

11 a Preferred choice for uncomplicated urinary infection primary treatment (domiciliary acquired).
  b Large doses may be necessary (e.g. 6g daily).
12 a Preferred choice for carrier state and in meningitis.
  b Preferred choice for typhoid (enteric) fever and when indicated in severe enteritis.
13 Some strains are resistant to ampicillin. Chloramphenicol, tetracyclines and sulphonamides should only be used if the causative strain is proven sensitive.
14 Some gentamicin-resistant strains are sensitive to tobramycin. All tobramycin-resistant strains are resistant to gentamicin. Colistin and polymyxin B are effective in urinary tract infections, but systemic therapy of tissue infections is of limited efficacy and probably ineffective in pulmonary infections.
  a Many clinicians prefer to use gentamicin, tobramycin or amikacin in combination with carbenicillin or ticarcillin (not in same infusion solution).
15 a Chloramphenicol and tetracyclines can be used with streptomycin in severe infections.
16 Metronidazole is highly active against *Bacteroides fragilis* and is considered the drug of first choice by some.
17 Other ampicillins include bacampicillin, pivampicillin, hetacillin and talampicillin which are hydrolysed in the body to ampicillin.
18 For initial therapy of severe infections, parenteral administration of soluble benzylpenicillin (penicillin G) is first choice penicillin. Phenoxymethylpenicillin (penicillin V) or phenethicillin can be used as an alternative to benzylpenicillin in oral treatment of infections caused by susceptible Gram-positive cocci. Oral penicillins should be given 1 hour before meals.
19 Carindacillin is oral dosage form; ticarcillin has a similar spectrum of activity and may be used in place of carbenicillin.
20 Use with caution in penicillin allergic patients. Other cephalosporins include cephradine, cephapirin, cephaloglycin, cephacetrile etc.
21 Should only be used when clearly drug of first choice (i.e. ●) and as an alternative antibacterial agent in severe infections when these are resistant or much less sensitive to other agents (e.g. ⊕).
22 Most workers rate clindamycin at least the equal of oral lincomycin.
23 Other cloxacillins include oxacillin, dicloxacillin, flucloxacillin (floxacillin) and nafcillin (see chapter XXVII; sect. 3.5).
24 Trimethoprim-sulphamethoxazole in ratio of 1:5.

Table I. (continued)

Agent	Action[1]	*Staph. aureus*[2]	**Staph. aureus* (PP)[3]	*Str. pyogenes*[4]	**Str. faecalis*[5]	*Str. pneumoniae*[4]	*N. gonorrhoeae*[6]	*N. meningitidis*[7]	*H. influenzae*[8]	*Bord. pertussis*	**Esch. coli*[9]	**Kl. Enterobacter* spp[10]	**Pr. mirabilis*[11]	**Pr. mirabilis* (PP[3])[11]	**Pr. vulgaris*	**Pr. rettgeri*	**Pr. morgani*	**Salmonella* spp[12]	**Shigella* spp[13]	**Ps. aeruginosa*[14]	*Br. abortus*[15]	*Bacteroides fragilis*[16]
Lincomycin	S/C	⊕	⊕	⊕		⊕																⊕
Mecillinam[25]	C	±	±	○		○	±				○	○	○	±	±			○	○			
Methenamine[26] (UTI)	S	○	○								⊕[c]	±			±							
Methicillin	C	○	●	○		○	±	○														
Nalidixic acid (UTI)	C										⊕[a,c]	○	○	○	○	○	○					
Neomycin	C	○	○								●[d]	○	○	○	○	○	○	○	○			
Nitrofurantoin (UTI)	C	○	○		○						●[c] ⊕[a]	○[b]	○									
Novobiocin	S/C	○	○			○	±	○	○	○					○							
Paromomycin	C	○	○								⊕[d]	○	○	○	○	○	○	○	○			
Phenoxymethyl-penicillin[18]	C	●		●	○	●	±	○														
Polymyxin B	C								○	○	⊕[e]	⊕						○	○	⊕		
Rifamide[27]	S/C	○	○	○	±	○	±	○			○		○	○								
Spectinomycin	?						⊕															
Spiramycin	S/C	○	○	○	○	○	○	○	±													
Streptomycin	C	○	○						○	○	⊕	⊕	○	○	⊕	⊕	⊕	○	○		○	
Sulphonamides	S			○		○		⊕[b]	⊕[a]		●[a]	○[d]	●[a]	●[a]					○		○	
Tetracyclines[28]	S	○	○	○	○	○	⊕	●[a]	⊕[b]	⊕	⊕[b,e]	⊕			○		○	○	⊕		●[a]	⊕
Thiamphenicol[29]	S	○	○	○	○	○	○	○	○	○	○	○	○	○	○		○	○	○		○	
Tobramycin	C	⊕	⊕								●[e]	●	⊕	⊕	⊕	⊕	⊕	±	±	●[a]	○	
Triacetyl-oleandomycin	S/C	○	○	○	○	○			±													
Vancomycin	C	⊕	⊕	○	⊕	○																

25 Pivmecillinam is the pivaloyloxymethyl ester which is hydrolysed in the body to mecillinam. Results of sensitivity studies vary between centres.

26 Also known as hexamine.

27 In the case of *Str. faecalis, Esch. coli* and *Pr. mirabilis*, adequate concentrations of rifamide are only attained in the bile. Not now available in some countries.

28 Some organisms which are resistant to the older tetracyclines may be sensitive to the newer derivatives, particularly doxycycline and minocycline.

29 Further studies are needed to compare with chloramphenicol.

Table II. Principal therapeutic usefulness of systemically administered antibacterial agents

Agent	Pharyngitis, acute sinusitis	Acute otitis media	Chronic bronchitis	Pneumonias[3]	Urinary tract infections	Gonorrhoea	Nonspecific urethritis[6]	Osteomyelitis[7]	Septicaemias	Other Uses[8]
Amikacin				⊕	⊕			○	⊕	Of use in *Pseudomonas* and *Serratia marcescens* infections
Amoxycillin and ampicillin		●[1]	●[2]	⊕	⊕	⊕[5]		⊕	⊕	Meningitis; endocarditis; typhoid carriers; *Shigella* enteritis (ampicillin); enteric fever, invasive *Salmonella* enteritis (amoxycillin); pertussis; biliary infections; *H. influenzae* cellulitis, arthritis; croup; acute epiglottitis (after tracheostomy)
Benzylpenicillin	●			●	⊕[4]	●[5]		⊕	⊕	Meningitis; endocarditis; syphilis (procaine salt); cellulitis; abscesses; erysipelas; septic arthritis; rheumatic fever prophylaxis, scarlet fever (benzathine salt); diphtheria (large doses); erythema serpens; tetanus and gas gangrene (plus antitoxin)
Carbenicillin (ticarcillin)				⊕	⊕				⊕	Endocarditis; meningitis
Cefoxitin				⊕	⊕			○	⊕	*Bacteroides fragilis* and *Serratia marcescens* infections
Cefuroxime				⊕	⊕	⊕*		○	⊕	*Penicillinase producing strains of gonococci
Cephalexin	⊕			⊕	⊕			⊕		Biliary infections
Cephaloridine				⊕				⊕	⊕	Endocarditis; septic arthritis (penicillin allergic patient)
Cephalothin				⊕				⊕	⊕	Endocarditis; septic arthritis (penicillin allergic patient)
Cephamandole				○	○			○	○	Meningitis
Cephazolin				⊕				⊕	⊕	Endocarditis; septic arthritis (penicillin allergic patient)
Chloramphenicol									⊕	*Haemophilus influenzae* meningitis; enteric fever; invasive *Salmonella* enteritis; *Bacteroides, Serratia marcescens* infections; brucellosis
Clindamycin				⊕				⊕	⊕	Of use in *Bacteroides* infections, severe infections in penicillin allergic patients
Cloxacillins				●				⊕	⊕	Meningitis; endocarditis; septic arthritis; acute furunculosis (severe); abscesses; skin infections; scalded skin syndrome

Table II. (continued)

Agent	Pharyngitis, acute sinusitis	Acute otitis media	Chronic bronchitis	Pneumonias[3]	Urinary tract infections	Gonorrhoea	Nonspecific urethritis[6]	Osteomyelitis[7]	Septicaemias	Other Uses[8]
Colistin	⊕	⊕		⊕					⊕	Acute *Esch. coli* infantile gastroenteritis (orally)
Co-trimoxazole (trimethoprim + sulphamethoxazole)	⊕	⊕	⊕	○	●[4]	⊕		○	⊕	Enteric fever; *Shigella* and invasive *Salmonella* enteritis; prostatic infection; brucellosis; meningitis; endocarditis
Erythromycin	⊕	⊕[1]		⊕			⊕			Impetigo; erythrasma; diphtheria and carriers; pertussis; syphilis (penicillin allergic patient); skin infections; acute furunculosis; Legionnaire's disease
Framycetin										Bowel sterilisation; acute infantile gastroenteritis (orally)
Fusidic acid								⊕	⊕	Used in penicillin resistant staphylococcal infections
Gentamicin				⊕	⊕			⊕	⊕	Meningitis; endocarditis; septic arthritis; *Serratia marcescens* infections
Kanamycin				⊕	⊕	○			⊕	Meningitis; endocarditis; bowel sterilisation; acute *Esch. coli* infantile gastroenteritis (orally)
Lincomycin				⊕	⊕			⊕	⊕	Of use in *Bacteroides* infections, severe infections in penicillin allergic patients
Mecillinam					⊕					Enteric fever, typhoid carriers
Methenamine (hexamine)					⊕[4]					
Methicillin				●				⊕	⊕	Endocarditis; septic arthritis
Metronidazole				○				○	⊕	Of use in *Bacteroides* infections; prevention of postoperative anaerobic infection (e.g. operation on the appendix or colon)
Nalidixic acid					⊕[4]					
Neomycin										Bowel sterilisation; hepatic coma, chronic portal systemic encephalopathy; acute *Esch. coli* infantile gastroenteritis (orally)
Nitrofurantoin					⊕[4]					
Novobiocin				⊕						

Agent	1	2	3	4	5	6	7	8	9	Indications
Paromomycin										Amoebiasis; bowel sterilisation
Phenoxymethylpenicillin	●	⊕		⊕						Endocarditis; rheumatic fever prophylaxis; impetigo; erysipelas
Polymyxin B					⊕				⊕	Meningitis
Rifamide										Biliary infections
Spectinomycin						⊕				
Spiramycin						⊕	⊕			
Streptomycin				⊕	⊕					Meningitis; endocarditis; brucellosis
Sulphonamides		⊕[1]		⊕	●[4]					Meningococcal meningitis (sensitive organisms); bowel sterilisation (non-absorbable compounds)
Tetracyclines			●	⊕	⊕	⊕	●			Acne vulgaris; meningococcal carriers (minocycline); cholera; brucellosis; lymphogranuloma venereum; chancroid; granuloma inguinale; syphilis, tetanus (penicillin allergic patients); psittacosis; leptospirosis; relapsing fever; erythema serpens; peritonitis; ?*Shigella* enteritis
Thiamphenicol										As for chloramphenicol. Claimed that irreversible marrow aplasia has not or only very rarely occurred
Tobramycin				⊕	⊕			○	⊕	Of use in *Pseudomonas* infections
Triacetyloleandomycin (troleandomycin)										Substitute for erythromycin
Vancomycin				⊕					⊕	Endocarditis; enterococcal enterocolitis (oral solution)

● Drug of first choice for empirical therapy.
⊕ Effective agent (where appropriate, chosen on basis of bacteriological examination) and/or in cases of known penicillin allergy.
○ Should be effective, but experience limited.

1 Ampicillin or amoxycillin first choice in acute otitis media, particularly in under 6-year-olds (greater predominance of *Haemophilus influenzae*).
2 Ampicillin or amoxycillin first choice in children (see chapt. XX; sect. 4.2).
3 Bacteriological examination highly desirable. In most pneumonias, penicillin can be used first while awaiting laboratory results. In staphylococcal pneumonia, cloxacillin or methicillin should be used initially if a penicillinase-producing organism is likely to be implicated.
4 Sulphonamide first choice as primary treatment of uncomplicated urinary infections in domiciliary practice. Co-trimoxazole (trimethoprim-sulphamethoxazole) is probably first choice as primary treatment of uncomplicated hospital acquired urinary infections (see chapter XXI; sect. 3.1). If primary therapy fails and diagnosis correct, other agents should be chosen, after assessing the sensitivity of the causative organism (see table I; chapter XXI, sect. 3.1). Low doses of nitrofurantoin (50mg nightly) first choice for prophylactic therapy in recurrent episodes of urinary infection. Benzylpenicillin (250mg orally at night) and a number of other agents can be used as an alternative prophylactic agent (see chapter XXI; sect. 3.2).
5 Single dose administration in conjunction with probenecid.
6 6-10 day courses (or longer, particularly in persistent recurrences) with all agents.
7 In acute osteomyelitis, a combination of benzylpenicillin plus one of other agents listed should be used initially; while awaiting results of sensitivity test. Agent for chronic osteomyelitis should be chosen on basis of bacteriological findings.
8 Boils and aerobic wound infections can generally be adequately managed by local treatment. Systemic treatment necessary with spread of boil or boil on face (use antistaphylococcal agent such as erythromycin, cloxacillin), or in cases of deep seated or generalised wound infection [select agent after assessing sensitivity of causative organism(s)].

Table III. Profile of the principal types of adverse reactions to systemically administered antibacterial agents (see also table IV and appendix E)

Agent	Injection site[1]	Hypersensitivity[2]	Gastrointestinal[3]	Dermatological[4]	Neurological[5]	Nephrotoxicity[6]	Ototoxicity[7]	Haematological[8]	Hepatotoxicity[9]	Other
Amikacin					●[d]	●	●			
Amoxycillin/ampicillin		●	●	●						
Benzylpenicillin	●[a]	●	●	●	●[b]			●[c]		
Carbenicillin/ticarcillin	●[a]	●		●						
Cefoxitin	●	●		●				●[c]		
Cefuroxime		●		●				●[c]		
Cephalexin		●	●	●				●[c]		
Cephaloridine		●		●		●[a]		●[c]		
Cephalothin	●	●		●		●[a]		●[c]		
Cephamandole		●		●				●[c]		
Cephazolin		●		●				●[c]		
Chloramphenicol		●	●	●				●[a,b,d]	●[b]	Circulatory failure in newborn; optic neuritis
Clindamycin			●	●						
Cloxacillin		●	●	●						
Colistin	●	●	●	●	●[a,d,e]	●				Visual disturbances
Co-trimoxazole		?	●	●	●[a,e]			●[a,b]		Avoid in pregnancy, in newborn, and in those with megaloblastic anaemia
Erythromycins	●	●	●	●					●[a]	
Framycetin				●	●[d]	●	●			Intestinal malabsorption following prolonged oral therapy
Fusidic acid			●	●						
Gentamicin			●	●	●[a,d]	●	●			
Hexamine			●	●						
Kanamycin	●	●	●	●	●[a,d,e]	●	●			
Lincomycin		●	●	●						Cardiopulmonary arrest after rapid IV infusion
Mecillinam		●	●	●						
Methicillin		●		●				? ●[a]		Allergic interstitial nephritis (large doses)
Metronidazole			●		●[c]					Dark colouration of urine
Nalidixic acid			●	●	●[a,b]					Visual disturbances (glare reaction)

	1	2	3	4	5	6	7	8	9	
Neomycin				•	•[d]	•	•			Intestinal malabsorption following prolonged oral therapy
Nitrofurantoin		•	•	•	•[c]			•[d]		Pulmonary reactions
Novobiocin	•	•	•	•				•[a,d]	•[b]	Yellow discolouration of skin and sclera
Paromomycin			•	•						
Phenoxymethylpenicillin		•	•	•						
Polymyxin B	•	•	•	•	•[a,d,e]	•				Visual disturbances
Rifamide	•	•	•	•					?•[c]	Yellow discolouration of skin and mucosae; darkens urine
Spectinomycin	•		•	•						
Spiramycin		?	•	•						
Streptomycin	•	•		•	•[c,d]	•	•	•[a]		Visual disturbances
Sulphonamides		•	•	•	•[a,e]	•[b]		•[a,b,d]	•[d]	?Polyarteritis nodosa
Tetracyclines	•	•	•	•		•[c]			•[e]	Discolour teeth and nails in children; intracranial hypertension in newborn; avoid in pregnancy and renal failure[6c]; outdated tetracycline has caused Fanconi-like syndrome
Thiamphenicol		•	•	•				•[a,b]		?Circulatory failure in newborns; ?optic neuritis
Tobramycin			•	•	•[a,d]	•	•			
Triacetyloleandomycin		•	•	•					•[a]	
Vancomycin	•	•		•		•	•			

1   Moderate or severe pain on intramuscular injection (a = large doses); as well as thrombophlebitis or phlebitis following intravenous injection of cephalothin, cefoxitin, 1g doses erythromycin, repeated doses of penicillin to same vessel, tetracyclines, vancomycin.

2   Hypersensitivity reactions in a susceptible individual: including eosinophilia, angioneurotic oedema, 'serum sickness', anaphylaxis. Reactions most likely to occur with penicillins, cephalosporins, sulphonamides and novobiocin (see chapter VII; sect. 4.1).

3   Nausea, vomiting, epigastric and abdominal discomfort or diarrhoea.

4   Mucocutaneous rashes and eruptions, including hypersensitivity reactions.
N.B. Stevens-Johnson syndrome with sulphonamides and photosensitivity with nalidixic acid, sulphonamides and tetracyclines.

5   a   Headache, malaise, dizziness.
    b   Convulsions precipitated (penicillin in very large doses; nalidixic acid in those predisposed); intracranial hypertension in infants (nalidixic acid, tetracyclines).
    c   Peripheral neuropathy (metronidazole; usually with high doses).
    d   Neuromuscular blockade and respiratory paralysis. With exception of colistin and polymyxin B, can generally be reversed by neostigmine or calcium gluconate.
    e   Paraesthesiae.

6   a   Cephaloridine causes most often at daily doses of 4 to 6g or more. Much less frequently reported with cephalothin. More likely when used in combination with aminoglycosides or potent diuretics such as frusemide (furosemide) or ethacrynic acid.
    b   Sulphonamide crystalluria depends on urinary concentration and solubility of drug.
    c   Tetracyclines raise blood urea and aggravate renal impairment (doxycycline and minocycline can be used in renal failure with caution).

7   In clinical practice gentamicin, tobramycin and streptomycin *mainly* affect vestibular function; framycetin, neomycin, amikacin and kanamycin *mainly* auditory function and vancomycin only auditory function.

8   a   Agranulocytosis, leucopenia, neutropenia or thrombocytopenia.
    b   Marrow aplasia (can be irreversible with chloramphenicol).
    c   Positive direct Coombs test; uncommonly associated with haemolytic anaemia following benzylpenicillin (usually large doses in renal failure) and cephalothin.
    d   Haemolytic anaemia; mainly in those with glucose 6-phosphate dehydrogenase deficiency (see chapter XXIII; sect. 8.4).

9   a   Erythromycin estolate and triacetyloleandomycin only; reversible jaundice if given for more than 10 to 14 days.
    b   Jaundice associated with high serum levels of unconjugated bilirubin; mainly a problem in the newborn.
    c   Rifamycins are extensively handled by hepatobiliary system.
    d   Neonatal kernicterus if sulphonamides given to newborn (espec. prematures) and mother late in pregnancy.
    e   Large doses (e.g. 2g or more daily) and in pregnancy; more likely with parenteral administration.

Table IV. Host determinants of response to antibacterial agents

Host factor	Relevant in	Antibacterial agent	Potential effect	Due to
Age (see also chapter IV, V) Renal function	Neonates, particularly prematures Aged	Penicillins Cephalosporins Streptomycin Kanamycin Gentamicin Tobramycin Amikacin Tetracycline	High serum levels Toxicity	Impaired renal excretion of antibacterial agent with high and sustained serum levels (modify dosage)
Hepatic function	Neonates	Chloramphenicol	Grey syndrome: vasomotor collapse and death	Impaired hepatic conjugation and urinary excretion of free drug
		Nalidixic acid	Intracranial hypertension	Impaired hepatic metabolism
		Sulphonamides Co-trimoxazole	Kernicterus	Displacement of bilirubin from plasma albumin
Tissue incorporation of drug	Fetal development Neonates Infants and Children	Tetracyclines	Discolouration of teeth ?Retardation of bone growth	Concentration and accumulation in growing tissues
Allergy	Aged	Penicillins Cephalosporins Other antigenic antibacterial agents	Hypersensitivity reaction	With age there is probably an increasing chance of prior exposure to antigenic drug
Neurological (see also chapter X, sect. 6.2.5; XXV, sect. 14.1, 15.3) Brain disease (localised lesion, generalised organic brain disease)		Penicillin G Nalidixic acid	Convulsions	Very large doses of penicillin: aggravated by renal dysfunction, concurrent probenecid
Hydrocephalus		Chloramphenicol	Suboptimal CSF levels	Impaired drug penetration into CSF

Neurological (continued)

Anaesthesia, especially with muscle relaxants	Bowel surgery	Streptomycin Kanamycin Neomycin Framycetin	Respiratory paralysis	Curare-like effect; aggravated by renal dysfunction
Muscle weakness	Myasthenia gravis	Gentamicin Tobramycin Amikacin Colistin Polymyxin Clindamycin ?Lincomycin Tetracyclines (rolitetracycline)	Aggravate muscle weakness, respiratory paralysis	

Hepatic Dysfunction (see also chapter XIX; sect. 13.4)

	Cirrhosis, chronic hepatitis, biliary obstruction	Chloramphenicol	High serum level of free drug; depression of erythropoiesis	Impaired hepatic metabolism
		Tetracyclines Streptomycin Erythromycin (espec. estolate, triacetyloleandomycin) Lincomycin Novobiocin Semisynthetic penicillins Rifamycins	High serum drug levels. Increased risk of hepatic as well as generalised toxicity	Impaired hepatic metabolism and biliary excretion

Renal Dysfunction (see also appendix E; chapter XXI, sect. 1, 14)

	Kidney disease Aged (see also above under age)	Gentamicin Streptomycin Tobramycin Kanamycin Amikacin Neomycin and Framycetin (orally) Vancomycin	Ototoxicity Risk nephrotoxicity increased	Impaired renal excretion, high serum levels
		Colistin Polymyxin	Neurotoxicity Renal insufficiency aggravated	Impaired renal excretion, high serum levels

Table IV. (continued)

Host factor	Relevant in	Antibacterial agent	Potential effect	Due to
Renal Dysfunction (continued)				
		Tetracyclines	Raise blood urea Renal insufficiency aggravated (except doxycycline, minocycline)	Impaired renal excretion, high serum levels Disturbed tissue metabolism
		Penicillins	Convulsions, haemolytic anaemia with very high dosage	Impaired renal excretion, high serum levels
		Penicillin-K salts Penicillin-Na salts	High serum potassium or sodium levels	Accumulation of the potassium or sodium component
		Carbenicillin	Increased haemorrhagic tendency, acidosis, hypernatraemia	Impaired renal excretion, high serum levels
		Methicillin	Very rare allergic interstitial nephritis	Impaired renal excretion
		Cephaloridine Cephalothin	Risk nephrotoxicity increased, + ve Coombs test and haemolytic anaemia (cephalothin)	Impaired renal excretion
		Chloramphenicol	?Risk of bone marrow toxicity from metabolites	Impaired renal excretion, high serum levels of metabolites
		Nitrofurantoin	Adequate urine levels fail to appear Peripheral neuropathy Pulmonary toxicity	
		Nalidixic acid	?Neurotoxicity	
		Sulphonamides	Risk crystalluria increased with some compounds	
		Co-trimoxazole	Severe renal insufficiency may be aggravated	?Hypersensitivity to sulphonamide component

Table V. Potential clinically significant drug interactions of systemically administered antibacterial agents (see also chapter VIII and appendix C)

Agent	Interacting Drug	Potential effect and Mechanism[1]
Amikacin *Gentamicin* *Kanamycin* *Streptomycin* *Tobramycin*	Neuromuscular blocking agents	Increase in activity of depolarising and non-depolarising relaxants [2.1]
	Cephaloridine Cephalothin	Increased risk of nephrotoxicity [2]
	Cyclopropane	Apnoea with intraperitoneal administration of aminoglycosides [2]
	Ethacrynic acid (E) Frusemide (F)	Increased risk of ototoxicity when combined with E, or F in renal failure [2]
Cephaloridine *Cephalothin*	Gentamicin Kanamycin Amikacin Streptomycin Tobramycin Ethacrynic acid (large doses) Frusemide (large doses)	Increased risk of nephrotoxicity [2]
Chloramphenicol	Dicoumarol (D)	Marked increase in serum levels and half-life of D [1.3.1]
	Phenobarbitone	Serum levels of chloramphenicol decreased to subtherapeutic amounts [1.3.2]
	Phenytoin (P)	Marked increase in serum levels and half-life of P [1.3.1]
	Tolbutamide (T)	Hypoglycaemic reaction with T. Marked increase in serum half-life of T [1.3.1]
	Tricyclic antidepressants	Increase in serum levels and side effects of nortriptyline and imipramine [1.3.1]
	Penicillins	Theoretical decrease in therapeutic efficacy of penicillins [3]
Colistin	Neuromuscular blocking agents	Increase in activity of depolarising and non-depolarising relaxants [2.1]
Co-trimoxazole	Methotrexate	?Additive antifolate effect [2]
	Warfarin	Activity of warfarin increased [?1.2 + 1.3.1]
Lincomycin	Kaolin-pectin suspension	Marked decrease in serum levels of lincomycin [1.1]. Give drug 2 hours apart
?Lincomycin *Clindamycin*	Neuromuscular blocking agents	Increase in activity of depolarising and non-depolarising relaxants [2.1]

Table V. (continued)

Agent	Interacting Drug	Potential effect and Mechanism[1]
Neomycin *Framycetin*	Warfarin	Slight increase in hypoprothrombinaemic action in some patients [2.2]
	Neuromuscular blocking agents	Increase in activity of depolarising and non-depolarising relaxants [2.1]
	Cyclopropane	Apnoea with intraperitoneal administration of aminoglycosides [2]
Penicillins	Chloramphenicol Erythromycin Tetracyclines	Therapeutic efficacy of penicillins theoretically decreased [3]
	Neomycin Framycetin	Marked decrease in serum levels of penicillin V by oral neomycin therapy [1.1]
	Allopurinol	Increased incidence of ampicillin rash
Polymyxin B	Neuromuscular blocking agents	Increase in activity of depolarising and non-depolarising relaxants [2.1]
Sulphonamides Sulphaphenazole	Tolbutamide (T)	Hypoglycaemic reaction. Marked increase in serum levels and half-life of T [?1.2 + 1.3.1]
	Chlorpropamide (C)	Marked increase in plasma half-life of C [?1.2 + ?1.4]. No clinical reports of hypoglycaemia
Sulphadiazine Sulphadimethoxine Sulphadoxine (sulformethoxine) Sulphafurazole (sulfisoxazole) Sulphamethizole Sulphamethoxazole	Tolbutamide (T)	No significant increase in half-life or hypoglycaemic action of T, except perhaps in the presence of associated renal impairment
Sulphaphenazole Sulphamethizole	Phenytoin (P) Phenytoin (P)	Increase in serum levels of P in a few cases [1.3.1] Increase in serum levels of P in rare cases [1.3.1]
Sulphaphenazole	Warfarin Phenprocoumon	No clinical reports of increased hypoprothrombinaemic action of coumarins, despite *in vitro* evidence of decrease in coumarin albumin binding. Sulphaphenazole may also inhibit metabolism of coumarin
Sulphaphenazole	Methotrexate (M)	Increase in antifolate activity and toxicity of M [1.2]

Sulphonamides (continued)		
Sulphafurazole (sulfisoxazole)	Methotrexate (M)	No clinical reports of increased antifolate activity of methotrexate despite *in vitro* evidence of decrease in methotrexate albumin binding and minor impairment of renal tubular secretion of M
Tetracycline	Iron haematinics	Marked decrease in serum levels of tetracycline and of iron [1.1]. Give drugs 3 hours apart
	Antacids	Preparations containing aluminium, calcium, magnesium markedly decrease serum levels of tetracycline [1.1]. Give drugs 1-2 hours apart
	Penicillins	Theoretical decrease in therapeutic efficacy of penicillins [3]
	Methoxyflurane	Increased risk of polyuric renal failure [2]
	Warfarin	Slight increase in hypoprothrombinaemic action in some patients [2.2]
Triacetyloleandomycin (troleandomycin)	Carbamazepine (C)	Marked and rapid increase in serum levels of C [1.3.1]
	Ergotamine (E)	Real risk of peripheral ischaemia [1.3.1]
	Theophylline (T)	Marked increase in serum levels of T [1.3.1]

1   Mechanism of interaction (see further chapter VIII)
   1. *Pharmacokinetic*
      1.1 Impaired gastrointestinal absorption
      1.2 Displacement from plasma protein binding site
      1.3 Altered hepatic drug metabolising activity
         1.3.1 Inhibition of hepatic microsomal enzyme activity
         1.3.2 Induction of hepatic microsomal enzyme activity
      1.4 Inhibition of renal excretion

2. *Pharmacodynamic*
2.1 Aminoglycosides inhibit prejunctional release of acetylcholine, and depress post-junctional sensitivity to the humoral agent; by competition with calcium ions for receptor sites on the nerve terminal. Mechanism of interaction of polymyxins and lincomycin not known.
2.2 Impaired vitamin K absorption
3. *Bacteriological antagonism*
There are very few conclusive clinical examples of antibacterial antagonism. *In vitro*, combinations of a bactericidal and a bacteriostatic drug (see table I) may be antagonistic, but in practice may not be significant. In general, antagonism is likely to be serious only when both agents are near their minimum effective level.

Appendix E
Guide to Drug Dosage in Renal Failure

R.C. Heel and G.S. Avery

As discussed in chapter I (section 4.3.4) and XXI (section 1.4), the dosage of many drugs largely excreted unchanged or as active metabolites by the kidneys must be modified in the patient with renal failure if toxicity to the kidney or other organs is to be avoided. Moreover, in uraemia, there is an abnormal response to a number of drugs not primarily eliminated by the kidneys.

The basis of dose adjustment and rational therapy in renal failure is discussed in the chapters indicated above. While therapy should ideally be monitored by estimation of drug plasma concentrations, such precise blood level services are not as yet widely available for most drugs. The guide which follows is therefore intended to provide *rough guidelines* on dosage in renal failure in the absence of plasma concentration monitoring services, and has been compiled on the basis of presently available clinical information. The dosage guidelines given must not be interpreted as absolute but it is hoped that they are better than no starting point at all. The dosage schedules suggested are a compromise between excessive plasma concentrations and toxicity on the one hand and inadequate concentrations and therapeutic failure on the other. For many of the drugs, precise guidelines cannot be given because definitive information derived from actual therapeutic use of the drugs in renal failure is not available.

An alternative approach to estimation of drug dosage in renal failure, by use of a nomogram, is given on page 1292.

Use of the Tables

The drugs are listed in alphabetical order according to their predominant pharmacological action or therapeutic use. An 'anti' classification has been used in most cases. The maintenance dosage recommendations are based on the excretion or metabolism of the drug or active metabolite, as well as the normal elimination (plasma) half-life of the parent drug and/or active metabolite and its prolongation with various degrees of renal failure. Where data were available, an indication is given of the plasma half-life of the drug in the anuric patient and of the percentage excreted unchanged in the urine.

1) *Loading dose:* In general, all patients are given a loading dose which is the same as the 'usual' initial dose for a patient with normal renal function.

2) *Maintenance dose:* The table is prepared on the basis of two methods of dose modification: (a) the 'usual' maintenance dose given at various increased intervals according to the estimated prolongation in plasma half-life with renal insufficiency and (b) reduction of the size of the maintenance dose leaving the dose interval unchanged. The dose reduction method is used in particular for drugs for which a relatively constant plasma concentration is desired. With antimicrobial drugs in particular, a commonly used method is to give half the initial dose (i.e. half the 'usual' loading dose) as the maintenance dose each calculated half-life. This method is probably most applicable in very ill patients with severe renal failure.

Limitations of Table

When using the dosage guidelines the following points must be considered:

1) *The status of renal function must be determined not only before but also during the entire period of treatment* — the appropriate maintenance dose for a patient is not a stable characteristic if the kidney function is not stable. It can change as dramatically as kidney function; a dose which was carefully calculated yesterday may have become excessive overnight, because in the meantime the patient has stopped secreting urine.

2) *The dosage guidelines do not necessarily apply to elderly patients* — even when blood urea

nitrogen and creatinine concentrations are normal, since elderly patients with low muscle mass can have 'normal' serum urea or creatinine in the presence of reduced renal function. A particular drug largely eliminated by the kidney may therefore accumulate in an elderly patient for this reason. Other changes in drug disposition in the elderly patient may also be important, such as decreased protein binding capacity and change in apparent volume of distribution (see further chapter V; sect. 2.1.2).

3) *Many aspects of patient variation influence drug response in uraemia* — the complexity of clinical status in individual uraemic patients, as well as variables such as possible altered absorption, protein binding or metabolism, liver function, other drug therapy etc, makes any fixed approach to drug dosage subject to error (see chapter I, sect. 4; XXI, sect. 1). *Individual patients must always be followed for clinical evidence of drug toxicity or lack of efficacy.* The dosage guidelines given may therefore require frequent reappraisal to ensure effective and safe therapy.

4) *Monitoring of drug plasma concentrations is ideal* — particularly with drugs with a low therapeutic ratio such as aminoglycoside antibacterials (see chapter I, sect. 4.3.4; 5).

5) *Uraemic patients should always be observed carefully for unexpected drug toxicity* (see chapter VII, sect. 5.3; XXI, sect. 1.5).

General References

Bennett, W.M.; Singer, I.; Golper, T.; Feig, P. and Coggins, C.J.: Guidelines for drug therapy in renal failure. Annals of Internal Medicine 86: 754 (1977).

Fabre, J.: Comment prescrire les medicaments en presence de fonctions renales deficientes? Tables d'adaptation posologique. Schweizerische Medizinische Wochenschrift 102: 251 (1972).

Fabre, J. and Balant, L.: Renal failure, drug pharmacokinetics and drug action. Clinical Pharmacokinetics 1: 99 (1976).

Jackson, E.A. and McLeod, D.C.: Pharmacokinetics and dosing of antimicrobial agents in renal impairment. American Journal of Hospital Pharmacy 31: 36, 137 (1974).

Kunin, C.M.: A guide to the use of antibiotics in patients with renal disease. A table of recommended doses and factors governing serum levels. Annals of Internal Medicine 67: 151 (1967).

O'Grady, F.: Antibiotics and renal failure. British Medical Bulletin 27: 142 (1971).

Pagliaro, L.A. and Benet, L.Z.: Critical compilation of terminal half-lives, percent excreted unchanged, and changes of half-life in renal and hepatic dysfunction for studies in humans with references. Journal of Pharmacokinetics and Biopharmaceutics 3: 333 (1975).

Reubi, F.: Posologie des medicamentes dans l'insuffisance renale. Schweizerische Medizinische Wochenschrift 104: 968 (1974).

Richet, G.; de Novales, E.L. and Verroust, P.: Drug intoxication and neurological episodes in chronic renal failure. British Medical Journal 2: 394 (1970).

Weinstein, L.: Chemotherapy of microbial diseases; in Goodman and Gilman The Pharmacological Basis of Therapeutics, 5th ed, p.1090 (Macmillan, New York 1975).

Whelton, A.: Antibacterial chemotherapy in renal insufficiency; in Schonfeld, Brockman, Hahn (Eds) Antibiotics and Chemotherapy, vol. 18, p.1 (Karger, Basel 1974).

Nomogram Method of Dose Estimation in Renal Failure

For drugs excreted entirely or partly unchanged by the kidneys, the nomogram method for calculating dosage in renal failure is based on the linear relationship which exists between the overall drug elimination rate constant and glomerular filtration rate, as determined by the endogenous creatinine clearance. This relationship allows the elimination rate of certain drugs in an individual patient with renal failure to be estimated from the patient's creatinine clearance or serum creatinine concentration. By means of a simple nomogram, the elimination rate fraction is determined which describes the elimination rate of the drug as a fraction of its normal elimination rate. Based on the estimated elimination rate fraction, the dosage regimen in the patient with renal failure is individually modified according to the dosage rules described below. The method is applicable for the drugs indicated in table I.

Graphical Estimation of Individual Drug Elimination Parameters

The individual value of the elimination rate fraction of a drug in any patient with renal failure $(\hat{Q})$ may be estimated in the following way by means of table I and the nomogram depicted in figure 1.

The value Q_O for the minimal elimination rate fraction of the drug in an anuric patient, is read off from table I and is plotted on the left ordinate of the nomogram and connected by a straight line — the so-called *dosing line* — with the upper right corner of the nomogram. The point of intersection between the patient's endogenous creatinine clearance, Cl (lower abscissa) or serum creatinine concentration, C_{cr} (upper abscissa) with the dosing line indicates at the left ordinate the individual elimination rate fraction $(\hat{Q})$ in the patient.

Dosage Rules

1) *Continuous drug administration* (i.e. continuous IV infusion)

The 'usual' loading dose (D*) is administered to all patients and the modified maintenance dose in the individual patient with renal failure $(\hat{D}/T)$ is found by multiplying the 'usual' maintenance dose (D/T) by the patient's individual elimination rate fraction $(\hat{Q})$.

$$\hat{D}^* = D^*; \hat{D}/T = \hat{Q} \cdot D/T \qquad \text{(Rule 1)}$$

Example: Administration of erythromycin by continuous intravenous infusion to an anuric patient. It is assumed that D = 3000mg/24 hours represents the 'usual' maintenance dose in patients with normal renal function. In table I, one finds the value $Q_O = 0.25$ for the elimination rate fraction of erythromycin in an anuric patient. Rule 1 results in:

$$\hat{D} = D \cdot Q_O = 3000 \cdot 0.25 = 750\text{mg}/24\text{h}$$

With the 'normal' elimination half-life $t_{1/2N} = 1.4$ (see table I) the correct loading dose $(\hat{D}^*)$ is calculated according to the following equation:

$$\hat{D}^* = \frac{D/T}{0.7/t_{1/2N}} = \frac{3000/24}{0.7/1.4} = 250\text{mg}$$

Thus in an anuric patient the loading dose of erythromycin is 250mg and the modified maintenance dose is 750mg per 24 hours.

2) *Intermittent drug administration*

The 'usual' loading dose (D*) is administered to all patients. The maintenance dose $(\hat{D})$ is half the loading dose, and the dosage interval $(\hat{T})$ is equal to the estimated individual half-life of the drug in the patient with renal failure $(\hat{t}_{1/2})$. The dosage schedule is derived from the following equation:

$$\hat{D}^* = D^*; \hat{D} = {}_{1/2}\hat{D}^*; \hat{T} = \hat{t}_{1/2} = \frac{t_{1/2N}}{\hat{Q}}$$

$$\text{(Rule 2)}$$

Example: Intermittent administration of gentamicin to a patient with a creatinine clearance (Cl) of 8ml/min. It is assumed that D* = 80mg, D = 80mg and T = 8 hours represents the 'usual' dosage regimen. In table I, one finds for gentamicin the estimating parameters $Q_O = 0.02$ and $t_{1/2N} = 2.4$. The value $Q_O = 0.02$ is plotted on the left ordinate of the nomogram (fig. 1) and connected by the straight dosing line with the right upper corner of the nomogram. The point of intersection of the dosing line with Cl = 8ml/min corresponds to $\hat{Q} = 0.1$ at the left ordinate. Based on these values rule 2 results in the following modified dosage regimen:

$$\hat{D}^* = D^* = 80mg$$

$$\hat{D} = {}_{1/2}\hat{D}^* = {}_{1/2} \cdot 80 = 40mg$$

$$\hat{T} = \hat{t}_{1/2} = \frac{t_{1/2N}}{\hat{Q}} = \frac{2.4}{0.1} = 24 \text{ hours}$$

Thus in a patient with a creatinine clearance of 8ml/min, the loading dose of gentamicin is 80mg and the modified maintenance dose equals 40mg every 24 hours.

The above rule is not applicable in *slight* renal impairment *for drugs whose half-life is normally much shorter than the usual dosage* interval (e.g. aminoglycosides), since the calculated dose interval in *slight* renal impairment may be less than the usual dose interval. In this situation the following rule may be used.

$$\hat{D}^* = D^*; \hat{D} = D; \hat{T} = T/\hat{Q} \qquad \text{(Rule 3)}$$

The loading dose and the maintenance dose remain unchanged and the dosage interval $(\hat{T})$ is increased in proportion to the increased elimination rate fraction $(\hat{Q})$. This rule is not however, applicable in severe renal failure for drugs such as the aminoglycosides, since the calculated dosage interval in an anuric patient for gentamicin would be 400 hours.

Limitations of Nomogram

1) Serum creatinine (C_{cr}) should *never* be used as an estimating parameter in patients with acute renal failure or changing kidney function, or in patients undergoing haemodialysis, until the steady-state serum concentration of creatinine is reached again. In patients with severe acute renal failure, it may take several weeks before the steady-state concentration of creatinine corresponding to the functional state of the kidneys is eventually reached. Serum creatinine is also inaccurate as an estimating parameter of the individual drug elimination rate in elderly patients, in the presence of severe uraemia $(C_{cr} > 8mg/100ml)$ or muscular abnormalities (e.g. cachexia, systemic muscular disease).

2) For reasons discussed in chapter I (sect. 4.3.4) and XXI (sect. 1.4.1, 2.1), a dosage schedule calculated by the nomogram method does not obviate the need to monitor therapy by plasma concentration estimations whenever possible. Dose adjustments should be made if indicated.

3) All uraemic patients should always be carefully observed for signs of unexpected drug toxicity (chapter VII, section 5.3; XXI, section 1.5, 14).

References

Basis of Nomogram
Spring, P.: Calculation of drug dosage regimens in patients with renal disease: A new nomographic method. International Journal of Clinical Pharmacology and Biopharmacy 11: 76 (1975).

Background Theory
Dettli, L.: Individualization of drug dosage in patients with renal disease. Medical Clinics of North America 58: 977 (1974).
Dettli, L.: Drug dosage in renal disease. Clinical Pharmacology and Therapeutics 16: 274 (1974).
Dettli, L.: Drug dosage in renal disease. Clinical Pharmacokinetics 1: 126 (1976).
Dettli, L.: Elimination kinetics and dosage adjustment of drugs in patients with kidney disease. Progress in Pharmacology, volume 1, number 4 (Fischer, Stuttgart 1977).
Dettli, L.; Spring, P. and Habersang, R.: Drug dosage in patients with impaired renal function. Postgraduate Medical Journal 46: (Suppl.): 32 (1970).

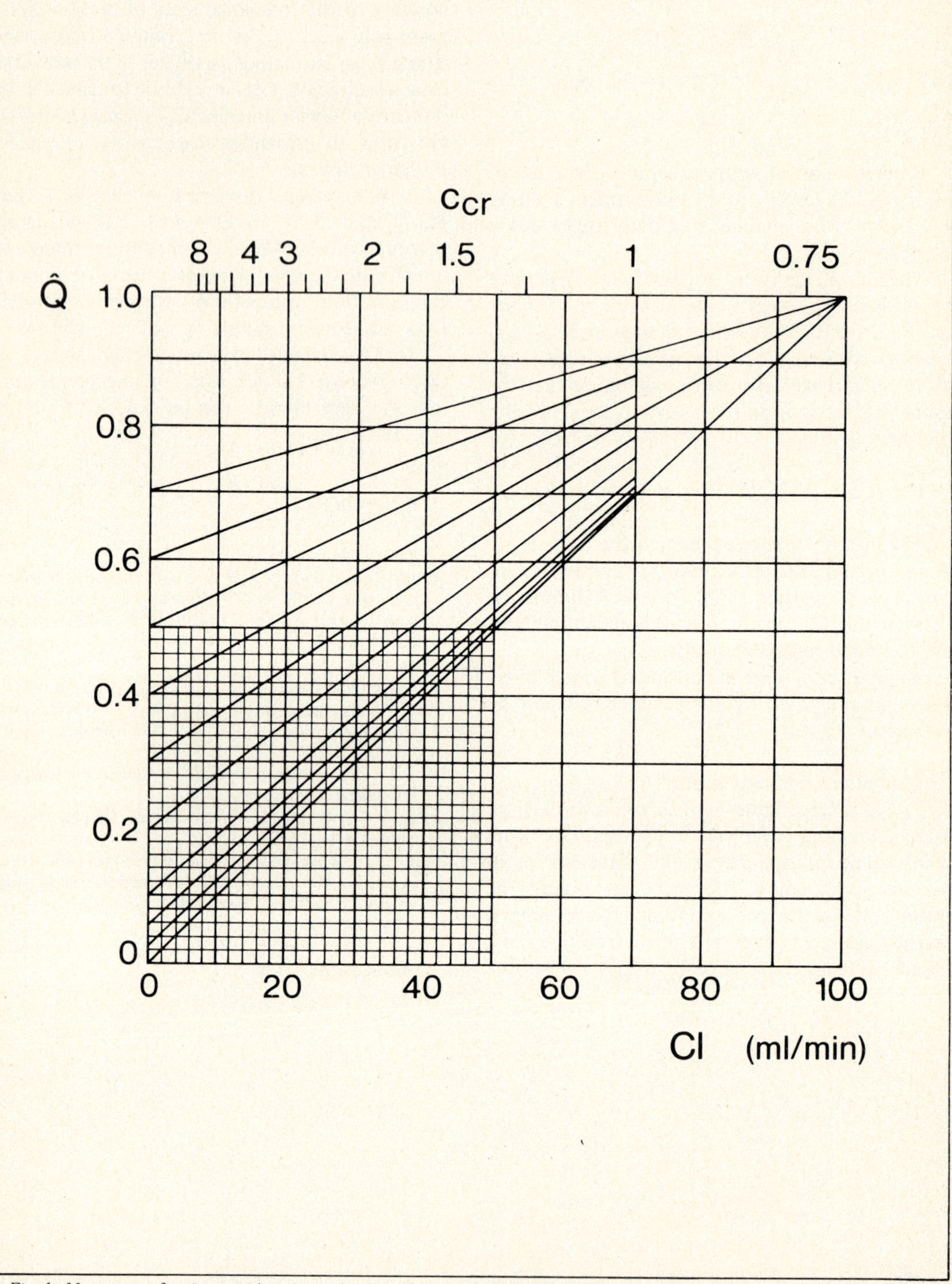

Fig. 1. Nomogram for the graphical determination of the individual elimination rate fraction of drug in a patient with renal failure, Q̂ (left ordinate) from the endogenous creatinine clearance, Cl (lower abscissa) or from the serum creatinine concentration, C_{cr} (upper abscissa). Use of the nomogram is explained in the text (simplified after Spring: J. Clin. Pharm. Biopharm. 11: 76, 1975; by permission of author and editor).

Table I. Mean overall elimination half-lives in subjects with normal renal function ($t_{1/2N}$) and elimination rate fractions in anuric patients (Q_O) [after Dettli, L.: Arzneimitteldosierung bei Niereninsuffizienz, 1979]

Drug	Q_O	$t_{1/2N}$ (h)
Acebutolol	0.6!!	2.6
Acetohexamide	0.6!!	1.3
Acetyldigoxin	0.3!!	24
Allopurinol	0.9!!	3 (20)
Alprenolol	1.0!!	1.7
Amantadine	0.15!	10
Amikacin	0.01	1.7
Amiloride	0.5!	6.0
Amoxycillin	0.1	1.0
Amphetamine	0.5!	12
Amphotericin B	0.95!	34
Ampicillin	0.12	0.9
Atenolol	0.06	5.5
Azlocillin	0.4	1.0
Bacampicillin	0.12	0.9
Barbitone	0.2!	70
Bleomycin	0.45	?
Carbenicillin	0.1	1.2
Cefoxitin	0.04	0.8
Cefuroxime	0.07	1.1
Cephacetrile	0.04!!	1.0
Cephalexin	0.04	1.0
Cephaloridine	0.08	1.7
Cephalothin	0.04!!	0.5
Cephamandole	0.04	1.2
Cephapirin	0.4!!	0.8
Cephazolin	0.06	2.0
Chlorphentermine	0.8!	120
Chlorpropamide	0.8!	36
Chlorthalidone	0.5!	48
Ciclacillin	0.1	0.7
Cimetidine	0.25!	1.8
Clofibrate	0.1!!	16
Clonidine	0.4!	8
Cloxacillin	0.25	0.6
Colistin	0.1	3
Cortisone	1.0	0.5
Cyclophosphamide	0.7!!	5
Cycloserine	0.4!	10
Cytarabine	0.9!	2
Dapsone	0.9!	20
Dextropropoxyphene	0.5!!	12
Dicloxacillin	0.3	0.7
Digitoxin	0.7!!	170
Digoxin	0.3	36
Diphenoxylate	1.0!	2.5
Disopyramide	0.5!	5
Doxycycline	0.7	20
Epicillin	0.1	1.4
Erythromycin	0.25	1.4
Ethambutol	0.4!	4
Flucloxacillin	0.3	2
Fluorocytosine	0.03	3
Fosfomycin	0.06	2
Gentamicin	0.02	2.4
Hydrallazine	0.9!!	2.5
Hydrochlorothiazide	0.5	10
Indapamide	0.9!	18
Isoniazid		
Rapid acetylators	0.8	1.3
Slow acetylators	0.5	3.3
Isosorbide dinitrate	0.95	8
Kanamycin	0.03	2.0
Lignocaine (lidocaine)	0.95!!	2.3
Lincomycin	0.4!	5
Lithium	0.02	20
Mercaptopurine	0.8!	0.5
Methadone	0.8	55
Methotrexate	0.2!!	12
β-Methyldigoxin	0.5!!	70
α-Methyldopa	0.4!	8
Methicillin	0.12	0.5
Mexiletine	0.9!	12
Mezlocillin	0.25	0.8
Minocycline	0.9	18
Minoxidil	0.9!	4
Nalidixic acid	0.8	1.0
Netilmicin	0.01	2.2
Nicoumalone (acenocoumarol)	1.0!!	9(24)
Nitrofurantoin	0.5	0.3
Oxacillin	0.25	0.5
Oxprenolol	0.95!!	1.5
Pancuronium	0.4	2.0
Penicillin G	0.1	0.5
Pentazocine	0.8	2.5
Pethidine (meperidine)	0.95!!	4
Phenobarbitone	0.8	80
Pindolol	0.3!	3
Pivampicillin	0.12	0.9
Polymyxin B	0.12	4.5
Pralidoxime	0.8	1.3
Procainamide	0.5!!	3.5
Propranolol	1.0!	5
Quinidine	0.8!!	7.0
Rolitetracycline	0.3	12
Salbutamol	0.8	4
Salicylic acid	0.8	3
Sisomicin	0.01	2.8
Sotalol	0.4!	6
Spectinomycin	0.25	1.7
Streptomycin	0.04	2.8
Sulphadiazine	0.45	10
Sulphafurazole (sulfisoxazole)	0.5	6
Sulphamethoxazole	0.85	10
Sulphamethoxypyridazine	0.5	36
Sulphinpyrazone	0.55!!	2.3
Sulphisomidine	0.08	4.6
Talampicillin	0.12	0.9
Tetrahydrouridine	0.1	7
Thiamphenicol	0.1	3
Ticarcillin	0.1	1.2
Timolol	0.8!	3
Tobramycin	0.02	2.0
Trimethoprim	0.45	12
Valproic acid	0.45	12
Vancomycin	0.03	6

For drugs denoted by an exclamation mark, formation of active metabolites may occur (!) or has been shown to occur (!!). Figures in parentheses are the half-lives of active metabolites.

Appendix E. Guide to drug dosage in renal failure[1]

1296

Appendix E

Drug	Elimination half-life (adults)		Excreted unchanged (%)	Extra renal excretion[2] (normal)	Normal dose interval (hours)	Dose adjustment for renal failure[3]				Dialysis[5]	Toxic effects in renal failure/Notes[6]
	normal (hours)	anuria (hours)				method[4]	creatinine clearance (ml/min)				
							> 50	10-50	< 10		
β-*Adrenoceptor Blocking Drugs* (see chapter XVIII, sect. 5.6.6; XXI, sect. 14.2.4)											
Acebutolol	~8; 13*	~40*	56	H	12	D	?Unch	?RD**	?RD**	-H	Accumulation of drug + *active metabolite
Alprenolol	2-3		<1	H	6	D	Unch	?RD*	?RD*		*?Accumulation active metabolite
Atenolol	6-9	⩾22	most	—	24	D	Unch	50-100	50*		*Increase interval to 48h
Pindolol	3-4	slight ↑	~40	H	12	D	Unch	Unch	Unch		Bioavailability decreased but renal clearance reduced
Practolol	5-13	40-120	85-100	—	8-12	I	8-12	RD*	RD*	+ H	*Reduce dose approx. proportional to decrease in creatinine clearance
Propranolol	2-6	1.1-6.2	negligib	H	6-12	D	Unch	Unch*	50**	-H	*?Dose reduction (oral bioavailability increased; active metabolites may accum.). **May reduce renal blood flow
Sotalol	5-13	56	~60	H	12	I	?Unch	RD	RD	? + H	
Analgesics (see chapter XXI; sect. 14.4.6)											
Aspirin	2-19*	same	10*	H	4	I	4	4-6	Avoid	+ HP	*Salicylate. May add bleeding, gi distress
Dextropropoxyphene	12		⩽20	H	4	D	Unch	Unch	RD*	-HP	May add sedation; * toxic metabolite accum.
Diflunisal	10.8	114.9	<5	H	12	I	12	?24*	Avoid	-H	*?Reduce dose size
Ibuprofen	2		10	—	6	I	6	8	12		May add gi distress
Indomethacin	4-12	same	10-20	H	8-12	D	Unch	Unch	Unch	?	May add gi distress, sedation
Methadone	18-97	13-55	5-22; 58	G	6-8	I	6-8	?8**	?8-12**	-HP	Excessive depressant effects; **may not be needed due to faecal elimination
Pethidine (meperidine)	2.4-4		~5	—	4	D	Unch	Unch	RD*		*Toxic metabolite accumulates
Phenylbutazone	29-175		1	H	8	D	Unch	Unch	Avoid		May add gi distress; renal cortical necrosis, sodium retention
Antiarrhythmic Drugs (see also β-blocking drugs above; chapter XVII, sect. 6.1; XXI, sect. 14.2)											
Bretylium	4-17	16-32	~90	—	6-8	I	RD	RD	RD	+ H	Hypotension
Lignocaine (lidocaine)	1-2		<10-20	—		D	Unch	RD*	RD*		*Toxic metabolite accum. prolonged infusion
Phenytoin	8-60	↓	⩽5	H	8	D	Unch	Unch	Unch	? + H	Decreased protein binding in uraemia. Monitor plasma levels (bound + unbound)
Procainamide	2.2-4	↑	45-65	H	3-4	I	4	6-12	8-24	+ H	Arrhythmias. Active metabolite persists. Monitor plasma levels parent drug + metabolite
Quinidine	3-16	same	10-50	H	6-12	I	6-12	6-12	6-12	+ HP	Arrhythmias, lupus nephritis. Monitor plasma levels. Active metabolites

Antibacterial Drugs (see chapter XXI, sect. 14.1; XXVII, sect. 4.2)

— *aminoglycosides**

Drug											*Monitor serum levels
Amikacin	2-3	30	94	—	8-12	I	12-18	24-36	36-48	+ H-P	Ototoxicity, nephrotoxicity
Gentamicin	2-3	35-67	86-100	—	8	D	75-100	50-75	25-50	+ H-P	Ototoxicity, nephrotoxicity
						I	8-12	12-24	24-48		
Kanamycin	2-5	72-96	52-90	—	8	D	75	50	25	+ HP	Ototoxicity, nephrotoxicity
						I	24	24-72	72-96		
Netilmicin	2.2	42			8-12	D	50-100	10-50	10	+ H	Ototoxicity, nephrotoxicity
Streptomycin	2-3	52-100	30-90	—	12	I	24	24-72	72-96	+ HP	Ototoxicity
Tobramycin	2-3	45-70	80-90	—	8	I	8-12	12-36	48-72	?H + P	Ototoxicity, nephrotoxicity

— *cephalosporins*

Drug											
Cefaclor	~1	3	most	—	8	D	100	50	25		
Cefoxitin	1	~13-20	>90	—	6-8	I	8	8-24	12-48	+ H	
Cefuroxime	1.1-1.4	~15	>90	—	6-8	I	8	8*	12*	+ H	*Reduce dose size to 500mg
Cephacetrile	0.5-1.4	16	~75	H		?	?RD	RD	RD		
Cephalexin	0.5-1	5-30	90-96	—	6	I	6	6-12	18-24*	+ HP	*6h for urinary tract infection
Cephaloridine	1-1.5	20-23	70-85	—	6	I	6	Avoid	Avoid	+ HP	Nephrotoxicity, convulsions
Cephalothin	0.5-1	12-18*	60-90	H	6	I	6	6	8-12	+ HP	Nephrotoxicity; haemolytic anaemia; convulsions (large doses). *Much less active desacetyl derivative 3h
Cephamandole	0.5-0.9	9-11	100	—	4-6	D	100	50-75	50	-HP	
						I	6	6-9	9		
Cephapirin	0.6	2.4	~50	H	6	I	6	6	12	+ H	
Cephazolin	1.75-2	42-69	90-96	—	8	I	8	12	24-48	+ H-P	Convulsions
						D	100	50	25		
Cephradine	0.7	8-15	100	—	6	D	100	50	25	+ HP	

1   See introduction for acknowledgement of source data.
2   H = hepatic; G = gastrointestinal; N = non-renal (precise route unknown or not clear). Although some antibacterial agents may not require any dosage modification because of extrarenal excretion, adequate urinary concentrations may not be obtained when treating urinary infections (e.g. erythromycin, doxycycline).
3   *See also introduction. Plasma concentrations should always be used to monitor therapy whenever feasible, especially when the agent is potentially toxic and/or when lengthy intervals are required between doses* These intervals, which reflect the 'usual' maintenance dose, are based on typical dosage regimens and should only be considered as a representative *rough* guide. Other dosage regimens for an individual drug can be modified in proportion to the dose adjustments shown. Associated liver disease for most drugs with an hepatic route of elimination, would generally have to be severe to alter dosage schedules further.
4   I = increase in dosage interval, and figures indicate the dose interval in hours; D = reduction in dose size, and figures indicate the dose size as percentage of usual dose; Unch = unchanged; RD = reduce dose according to indicated method.
5   Denotes significant dialysis such that a supplemental dose is necessary during, or following dialysis. A lack of requirement for additional medication in therapeutic situations does not necessarily imply a lack of utility of dialysis in cases of poisoning. H = haemodialysis; P = peritoneal dialysis; (+) = significant; (-) = insignificant.
6   See also discussion in chapter I (sect. 4.3.2, 4.3.4), VII (sect. 5.3), XXI (sect. 1, 14), and specifically for the drugs listed in the chapter given by the cross-reference beside the drug class heading.

Appendix E. (continued)

Drug	Elimination half-life (adults)		Excreted unchang- ed (%)	Extra renal excre- tion[2] (nor- mal)	Normal dose interval (hours)	Dose adjustment for renal failure[3]				Dia- lysis[5]	Toxic effects in renal failure/Notes[6]
	normal (hours)	anuria (hours)				meth- od[4]	creatinine clearance (ml/min)				
							> 50	10-50	< 10		
Antibacterial Drugs (continued)											
Chloramphenicol	1.6-3.3	3-7	5-15	H	6	D	Unch	Unch*	Unch*	-HP	Added myelosuppression, particularly hepato- renal disease. *Some avoid, especially if therapy > 10 days
Clindamycin	2-4	4.5-6	5-15	H	6	D	Unch	Unch	Unch	-HP	?Increased incidence diarrhoea
Colistimethate	4.5	20-35	40-80	—	6-12	D	75	50	25	-H + P	Nephrotoxicity, neurotoxicity
Erythromycin	1.4	5-6	15*	H	6	D	Unch	Unch	Unch	-HP	Hepatotoxicity (rare). *Glucoheptonate
Lincomycin	4.6-5.6	10-13	10-15	H	6	I	6	12	12-24	-HP	Slight increase incidence diarrhoea
Metronidazole	6-12*	?↑	< 10	H	8	I	8	12	24	+ H	Neurotoxicity, gastrointestinal symptoms. *Some active metabolites
Nalidixic acid	1.1-2.5	21	20	?H	6	D	Unch	Unch	Avoid*		May add gi distress; ?convulsions. *Metabolites accumulate
Nitrofurantoin	0.3-0.6	slight↑	30-40	—	8	D	Unch	Avoid*	Avoid*	+ H	Peripheral neuropathy, pulmonary toxicity. *Ineffective
— *penicillins*											
Amoxycillin	1	5-15	45-80	H	8	I	8	8(12*)	8(16*)	+ H	?Skin rash. *Large doses (convulsions)
Ampicillin	1-1.5	12-20	50-90	H	6	I	6	6(9*)	6(12*)	+ H-P	Skin rash. *Large doses (convulsions)
Benzylpenicillin	0.5	6-20	58-85	H	6-8	D	100	100	50*	+ H-P	*Large doses (convulsions, haemolytic anaemia, hyperkalaemia, hypernatraemia)
						I	6-8	6-8	8-12*		
Carbenicillin	1-1.5	12-15	80-84	H	4-6	I	4-6	6-12	12-16	+ H-P	Increased bleeding tendency; hypernatraemia, hypokalaemic alkalosis; convulsions (large doses)
						D	100	75	25-50		
Cloxacillin	0.5	1	35-62	H	6	I	6	6	6	-H	
Dicloxacillin	0.7	1-2	36-73	H	6	I	6	6	6	-H	
Flucloxacillin	0.8	2.25	22-52	H	6	I	6	6	6	-H	
Methicillin	0.5	4	25-82	H	4-6	I	4-6	4-6	8-12	-HP	Interstitial nephritis (also with others), neurotoxic
Nafcillin	0.5	1.2-1.5	38	H	6	I	6	6(8)	6(12)	-H	
Oxacillin	0.4	0.5-1	40-55	H	6	I	6	6	6(8-12)	-HP	Hypernatraemia, hypokalaemic alkalosis
Ticarcillin	1.2	16	most	—	4-6	D	100	50-75	50	+ HP	Hypernatraemia, hypokalaemic alkalosis; increased bleeding tendency
						I	4-6	8	12		
Thiamphenicol	4.2	30			6	I	6-12	24-36	36-48		
Polymyxin B	3-6	20-35	60-90	—	12	I	24	36-60	60-96*	? + HP	Nephrotoxicity, neurotoxicity; *?avoid

— sulphonamides											
Sulphafurazole	3-7	6-12	50-70	—	6	I	6	8-12	12-24*	+ HP	?Crystalluria, interstitial nephritis. *6h if high urine levels required
Sulphamethizole	1-2	58	90	—	6	I	Unch	RD	Avoid*		?Crystalluria. *No urine levels
Sulphamethoxazole	7-12	28	30-50	—	12	I	12	24	24*	+ H	?Crystalluria; *?deterioration renal function
— tetracyclines											
Chlortetracycline	5-6	7-11	18	H	6	—	Avoid	Avoid	Avoid	-HP	Acidosis, BUN↑, aggravate renal insuffic.
Demethylchlor-tetracycline	10-13	↑	42	H	12	—	Avoid	Avoid	Avoid	-HP	As chlortetracycline
Doxycycline	15-24	18-25	33-45	H	24	I	24	24*	24*	-HP	*No important accum, but may BUN↑ (see text)
Methacycline	8-14	44	50-60	H	12	—	Avoid	Avoid	Avoid	-HP	As chlortetracycline
Minocycline	12-16	12-18	6-10	G	12	I	12	12*	12*	-HP	*No accum, but may BUN↑ (see text)
Oxytetracycline	9-10	47-66	70	H	6	—	Avoid	Avoid	Avoid	-HP	As chlortetracycline
Rolitetracycline	6-12	30-54	60	H	12	—	Avoid	Avoid	Avoid		As chlortetracycline
Tetracycline	6-10	57-108	48-60	H	6	I	8-12	12-24	Avoid	-HP	As chlortetracycline and doxycycline
Trimethoprim	9-13	20-49	40-70	H	12	I	12	18	24*	+ H	*?Deterioration renal function; haematol. effects (antifolate action)
Vancomycin	6-11	144-240	90-100	—	6	I	24-72	72-240	240	-HP	Ototoxicity
Anticholinergics											
Hyoscine N-butyl bromide	7.6		69-77	?	6	?	6	Care	Care		Potential for accumulation
Propantheline	9		50	?	6	?	6	Care	Care		Acute urinary retention (elderly)
Anticoagulants (see chapter XXIII; sect. 3.2)											
Heparin	1-2	↑	?	H	4-6	D	Unch*	Unch*	Unch*	-H	*Adds bleeding tendency; ?start with lower dose
Warfarin	35-45		negligib	H	24	D	Unch*	Unch*	Unch*		*Adds bleeding tendency
Anticonvulsants (see chapter I, sect. 4.3.2; XXI, sect. 14.4.5; XXV, sect. 3)											
Phenobarbitone	48-144		27-50	H	8	I	8	8	8-16	+ HP	Excessive sedation
Phenytoin	8-60	↓	≤ 5	H	8	D	Unch	Unch	Unch	? + H	See Antiarrhythmic Drugs
Primidone	3.3-12.5		?*	?	8-12	I	12	12-18	18-24	+ H	Excessive sedation (*active metabolites, unchanged drug), folate deficiency
Sulthiame	~30		60-70	H	8	?		?	?		Neurotoxicity
Trimethadione	12-24*		~1	H	8	I	8	8-12	12-24		Neurotoxicity; ?nephrotic syndrome; *active metabolite ~240h

Appendix E. (continued)

| Drug | Elimination half-life (adults) | | Excreted unchang-ed (%) | Extra renal excre-tion[2] (nor-mal) | Normal dose interval (hours) | Dose adjustment for renal failure[3] | | | | Dia-lysis[5] | Toxic effects in renal failure/Notes[6] |
| | normal (hours) | anuria (hours) | | | | meth-od[4] | creatinine clearance (ml/min) | | | | |
							> 50	10-50	< 10		
Antidepressants (see chapter XXI, sect. 14.4.3; XXVI, sect. 1.5.2)											
Amitriptyline	32-40		5	H	8	D	Unch	Unch*	Unch*	-HP	*Sedation, acute urinary retention (elderly)
Desipramine	12-54		< 5	H	8	D	Unch	Unch*	Unch*	-HP	*As above
Imipramine	6-20		< 1	H	8	D	Unch	Unch*	Unch*	-HP	*As above
Nomifensine	2-4	46	15-22*	H	8-12	D	?RD	RD	?Avoid	-H	Active metabolite; *of total drug in plasma
Nortriptyline	15-90		5	H	8	D	Unch	Unch*	Unch*	-HP	*As above
Antifungal Agents											
Amphotericin B	18-24	40	5-40	N*	24	I	24	24	36**	-H	Nephrotoxicity; *important; **ineffective renal parenchyma infections
Fluorocytosine	3-8	28-430	90	—	6	I	6	12-24	24-48	+ HP	?Leucopenia, thrombocytopenia
Antihistamines											
Chlorpheniramine	~30		13-30	N	4-6	D	Unch	Unch	Unch		?Sedation
Diphenhydramine	4-10		< 4	H	6	I	6	6-9	9-12	? + H	?Sedation; acute urinary retention (elderly)
Promethazine			?	?	12	I	12	12-18	18-24		As above (also anticholinergic activity)
Antihypertensive Drugs (see also β-blocking drugs above; chapter XVII, sect. 5; XXI; sect. 6.1)											Blood pressure response best guide
Bethanidine	17-20		48-61*	G	8	I	8	?RD	?RD		*Hypertensives. ?Reduction renal blood flow
Clonidine	12.7		41-47	?	6-8	D	Unch	Unch	Unch		?Excessive sedation
Debrisoquine	13-26		~20-70*	H	8-12	I	?RD	?RD	?RD		*Wide interpatient variation
Diazoxide	21-36	20-53	~50	N		D	Unch	Unch*	Unch*	+ HP	*Decrease dose size if given repeatedly
Guanethidine	~120-240		25-50	N	24	I	24	24*	24-36*		May decrease renal blood flow. Orthostatic hypotension. *Non-renal excretion increases
Hexamethonium			signific	—	4-6	?	?	Avoid	Avoid		May decrease renal blood flow
Hydrallazine	2-4, 1-3*	↑	2-14; 7-58**	H,G	8, 12***	I	8, 12***	8, 12***	8-16, 12-24***	-HP	*Slow, fast acetylators; **nonspecific assay. Headache. Accumulates but no > incidence toxic side effects. ***Fast, slow acetylators
Mecamylamine			signific	—	8	?	?	Avoid	Avoid		May decrease renal blood flow
Methyldopa	8	↑	20-55	H	6	I	6	9-18**	12-24**	+ HP	?Sedation; hepatitis; **?active metabs accum.
Pentolinium			signific	—	8	?	?	Avoid	Avoid		May decrease renal blood flow
Reserpine	46-168	87-323	< 1	H	24	D	Unch	Unch*	Unch*	-HP	Excessive sedation, gi bleed; *some avoid unless acute use
Prazosin	1.8-4.6		?negligib	H	8-12	D	Unch*	RD*	RD*		*Lower dose especially initially

Antineoplastic Drugs (see chapter XXIV; sect. 2.3)											
Actinomycin D	36		< 20	H	24	I	24	?24-36	?24-48		?Enhanced myelosuppression, hyperuricaemia
Azathioprine	3		50*	N	24	I	24	24	24-36	+ H	As above; *converted to 6-mercaptopurine
Bleomycin			60	H	2x/wk	D	100	100	50-75		Hyperuricaemia
Cyclophosphamide	3-11	↑	< 25	N	12	I	12	12	18-24	+ H	?Enhanced myelosuppression, hyperuricaemia
Dacarbazine	~3-4		50	H	24	I	24	?24-36	?24-48		As above; active metabolite
Dibromomannitol			~25	H	24	I	24	?24-36	?24-48		As above
Daunorubicin	~50		~25*	H	—	D	Unch	?RD	?RD		*Unchanged drug + active metabolite; cardiotoxicity may add to uraemic cardiomyopathy
6-Mercaptopurine	1.5		20	N	24	I	24	?24-36	?24-48		As above
Methotrexate	3.5, 6-69	↑	~90	H	—	D	Unch	75	50	+ H	As above, hepatotoxicity, nephrotoxic.
Mitomycin C			~30	?	24	I	24	?24-36	?24-48		?Enhanced myelosuppression
Vincristine	~3		signific	H	1x/wk	D	Unch	Unch	Unch		Neurotoxicity may add to uraemic neuropathy
Antipsychotic Drugs (see chapter XXI, sect. 14.4.2; XXVI, sect. 1.5.1, 1.5.4)											
Chlorpromazine	16-30		1-6	H		D	Unch	Unch	Unch*	-HP	Excessive sedation; acute urinary retention (elderly); skin pigmentation; galactorrhoea. *Reduce dose if excess sedation
Lithium	8-41	↑	100	—	8	D	Unch*	Avoid*	Avoid*	+ HP	CNS toxicity, nephrogenic diabetes insipidus; *monitor plasma levels if use essential
Antituberculosis Drugs (see chapter XX; sect. 8.1)											
Capreomycin	3	↑	50-70	—	12	I	24	24-72	72-96		Ototoxicity, nephrotoxicity
Cycloserine	12-20	↑	65	H	12	I	?24	Avoid	Avoid	+ H	Mood disturbances
Ethambutol	6-8	↑	75-90	—	24	I	24	24-36	48	+ HP	Ocular toxicity, peripheral neuropathy
Isoniazid	0.7-4	17	5-27*	H	8	I	8	8	8(12**)	+ HP	Peripheral neuropathy; *slow acetylators 27%, rapid 5%; **slow acetylators
PAS	1.5	23	40	H	8	I	8	12	Avoid	+ H	Adds gi distress, acidosis
Rifampicin	1.5-5	1.8-3.1	15-30	H	24	I	24	24	24		Dose reduction in hepatorenal failure
Streptomycin	2-3	52-100	30-90	—	12	I	24	24-72	72-96	+ HP	Ototoxicity
Cardiac Glycosides (see chapter XVII, sect. 8.1.3, 8.1.5; XXI, sect. 14.2.1)											*Monitor plasma levels
β-Acetyldigoxin	24	66			24	D	?Unch	RD	RD		See digoxin
Digitoxin	168-192	240	< 30	H	24	D	Unch	Unch	50-75	-HP	Active metabolite digoxin — ?importance
Digoxin	30-40	87-100	76-85	G	24	D	100*	25-75*	10-25*	-HP	Digitalis toxicity. Decrease size of
						I	24-36*	36-48*	48-72*		dose (loading dose reduced to 1/2 to 2/3 normal in severe renal failure if used for inotropic use).
Lanatoside C	33-36	↑	signific	G	24	I	24-36*	36-48*	48-72*		Digitalis toxicity.
β-Methyldigoxin	43	100			24	D	?Unch	RD	RD		See digoxin
Ouabain	21	60-70	37-50	G	12-24	I	24*	24-36*	36-48*	-HP	Digitalis toxicity.

Appendix E. (continued)

| Drug | Elimination half-life (adults) | | Excreted unchang-ed (%) | Extra renal excre-tion[2] (nor-mal) | Normal dose interval (hours) | Dose adjustment for renal failure[3] | | | | Dia-lysis[5] | Toxic effects in renal failure/Notes[6] |
| | normal (hours) | anuria (hours) | | | | meth-od[4] | creatinine clearance (ml/min) | | | | |
							> 50	10-50	< 10		
Diuretics (see chapter XXI; sect. 7.1, 14.2.5)											
Acetazolamide	2.4-5.8		100	—	6	I	6	12	Avoid*		*Ineffective; potentiate acidosis
Amiloride	6-9.5		50	H	12-24	I	24	24*	Avoid*		*Hyperkalaemia (monitor K⁺)
Bumetanide	3.5		33	N	6	D	Unch	Unch	Unch		Cramps with high doses
Chlorothiazide	~13		100	—	12	I	12	12	Avoid*		*Ineffective
Chlorthalidone	51-89		~50	N	24	I	24	24	48		
Ethacrynic acid	0.5-1		20	H	6	I	6	6	Avoid*		*Risk ototoxicity (more likely lge doses)
Frusemide (furosemide)	0.3-1.6	1.3-14	67	H	6	D	Unch	Unch	Unch*	-H	*Risk ototoxicity (more likely lge doses)
Mercurials	2-3*	> 16*	100	—	24	I	24	Avoid**	Avoid**		**Nephrotoxicity, accum. Hg; *excretion $T_{1/2}$
Spironolactone	10-35*			H	6	I	6	6**	Avoid**		*Active metabolite. **Hyperkalaemia (monitor K⁺); gynaecomastia
Triamterene	1.5-2.5			H	12	I	12	12*	Avoid*		*Hyperkalaemia (monitor K⁺)
Gout Drugs (see chapter XXII; sect. 12.2)											
Allopurinol	2-8*	↑	30	N	8	I	8	8-12	12-24		Rash, gi distress; *active metabolite 18-30h
Colchicine	20	↑	5-17	H	12	I	12	12*	18*		Gi distress; *unchanged acute use
Probenecid	4-12		1-5	N	12	D	Unch	Avoid*	Avoid*		*Ineffective
Sulphinpyrazone	3-5	↑	50	N	6-8	I	8	Avoid*	Avoid*		*Ineffective
Hypnosedatives (see chapter XXI; sect. 13.4; XXVI, sect. 1.5.3, 1.5.5)											
Meprobamate	6-17		8-19	H	6	I	6	9-12	12-18	+ HP	Excessive sedation
Pentobarbitone	23-30	same	20	H	8-24	D	Unch	Unch	Unch	-HP	Excessive sedation
Phenobarbitone	48-144		27-50	H	8	I	8	8	8-16	+ HP	Excessive sedation
Hypoglycaemic Drugs (see chapter XVI, sect. 3.3.3; XXI, 14.3)											
Acetohexamide	3.5-11	31	47*	H	12	I	12-24	Avoid	Avoid		Hypoglycaemia, accum. active metabolite; insulin preferred
Chlorpropamide	24-42	50- > 200	6-60	N	24	I	24-36	Avoid	Avoid	-P	Hypoglycaemia; insulin preferred
Glibornuride	5-12	30		H	24	I	?RD	?RD	?RD		Hypoglycaemia; insulin preferred
Metformin	1-2	⩾ 5	66	N	8-12	I	12	Avoid*	Avoid*		*Lactic acidosis, accumulation
Phenformin	5-15		33-66**	H	8	D	Unch	Avoid*	Avoid*		*Lactic acidosis; **of amount absorbed
Tolbutamide	3-25	same	negligib	N	8	D	Unch	Unch	Unch*	-H	*Insulin preferred

Muscle Relaxants (see chapter X, sect. 2.2, 4.5; XXI, sect. 14.5.3)

Decamethonium			signific	—		?	?	Avoid	Avoid		Prolonged apnoea
Gallamine		↑	signific	—		D	Unch	Avoid	Avoid	+ HP	Prolonged apnoea
Pancuronium	2.2	4.3	~40	H		D	Unch	Unch*	50*		Duration of action prolonged. *Accumulation especially likely after large or repeated doses
Suxamethonium		↑		H		—	Unch	Unch*	Unch*		?Prolonged apnoea (decreased pseudo-cholinesterase activity with some dialysis membranes) *hyperkalaemia with large or repeated dosage
Tubocurarine	0.1		33	H		D	Unch	Unch	Unch*		*Duration of action prolonged with large or repeated doses
Miscellaneous Drugs											
Amantadine	9-37		90	?	12	D	?Unch	?RD	?RD		Neurotoxicity
Aminocaproic acid			>95	?							?Kidney blockade
Amphetamine	10-30*		70-90	?							*Urinary pH dependent
Baclofen	3-4		>75	—	8	?	?RD	?RD	?RD		Muscle hypotonia, fatigue
Chloroquine	72	↑	50-70	N	24	D	Unch	Unch	Unch*		Skin, ocular, ECG toxicity (long term); *reduce if treatment prolonged
Cimetidine	2	5	40-70	H	6	I	6	8-12	12*	? + H	Mental confusion, convulsions; gynaecomastia. *?Reduce dose size
Clofibrate	6-25	110	18-32	—	6	I	6-12	12-18	24-48		Myopathy; decreased protein binding and clearance of active metabolite
						D	50	25-50	10-25		
Emepronium	2		70	?	8	D	?Unch	?RD	?RD		Acute urinary retention
Metronidazole	6-12		60-70	?	8	D	?Unch	?RD	?RD		?Neurotoxicity
Penicillamine	>7		signif	—	6	I	6	9-12	12-24		Nephrotic syndrome
Propylthiouracil	1-2	8.5		—	8	D	100	75	50		Cardiotoxicity
Salbutamol	2.7-7.1		40-50	?	6-8	D	?Unch	?RD	?RD		Tachycardia
Thiopentone	3-8		<1			D	Unch	RD*	RD*		*Enhanced activity (decreased protein binding)
Tranexamic acid	2.3		>95		6-12	I	12	24	48		?Kidney blockade

Subject Index

dry: treatment principles 366

F

Fanconi syndrome
  treatment 824
Fatty acids
  drug binding displacement 17
Fava beans
  breast feeding 119
  haemolytic anaemia from 1178
Favism
  genetically determined reaction 31
Fazadinium
  elimination 293
  pharmacology 293, 295
Febrile seizures
  treatment 147, 148
Felypressin
  drug interactions 314
Fenbufen
  half-life 1213
Fenclofenac
  distribution volume 1213
  half-life 1213
  pKa 1213
  protein binding 1213
  rheumatoid arthritis: use in 861
Fenfluramine
  distribution volume
  drug interactions 245, 670, 671, 1263,
    1265
  half-life 1213
  obesity: use in 524
  overdosage 257
  pharmacology 524
  pKa 1213
  protein binding 1213
  side effects 524
  withdrawal depression 524, 1111
Fenoprofen
  adverse reactions 853, 1228
  anti-inflammatory efficacy 859
  distribution volume 1213
  dosage 853
  elderly: use in 174
  elimination 853
  half-life 1213
  pKa 1213
  properties 853
  protein binding 1213
  rheumatoid arthritis: use in 861, 864
Fenoterol
  adverse effects 765
  dysmenorrhoea: use in 478
  elimination 765
  half-life 1219
  labour, premature: use in 467
  pharmacology 765
Fentanyl
  clinical use 325
  half-life 296, 1212
  metabolism 296
  neuroleptanalgisa: use in 296
  pharmacology 296, 325
  protein binding 1212
Fenticlor
  adverse reactions 1236
Feprazone
  drug interactions 244
  rheumatoid arthritis: use in 861
Ferric orthophosphate
  iron deficiency: use in 1187

Ferrous aminoacetosulphate
  dosage 934
  iron content 934
  side effects 934
Ferrous carbonate
  dosage 934
  iron content 934
  side effects 934
Ferrous fumarate
  dosage 934
  iron content 934
  iron deficiency: use in 1187
  side effects 934
Ferrous gluconate
  children: use in 150
  dosage 934
  iron content 934
  iron deficiency: use in 1187
  side effects 934
Ferrous succinate
  dosage 934
  iron content 934
  iron deficiency: use in 1187
  side effects 934
Ferrous sulphate
  children 150
  constipation from 741
  dosage 933, 934
  drug interactions 251, 938
  iron content 934
  iron deficiency: use in 1187
  nausea and vomiting from 738
  side effects 934
Fertility control
  methods 469-470
  steroids, hormonal: use in 469-475
Fetogenesis
  dysmorphogenicity and 72
Fetus
  clinical pharmacology 76-96
  drug disposition 456
  drug metabolism 79
  drug transfer 77-80
  drugs: effects 80-92, 460
  viral infection 1150
Fever
  children: treatment 147
  drug allergy and 213, 217
  gentamicin: blood levels and 1182
  theophylline clearance and 769
Fever, relapsing
  tetracycline: use in 1281
Fibre, dietary
  constipation: use in 711
  diverticular disease: use in 714
  irritable bowel: use in 714
Fibrillation, atrial
  treatment 602
Fibrillation, ventricular
  treatment 604
Fibrinolysis inhibitors
  anaemia, aplastic: use in 937
  bleeding disorders: use in 938
Fibrinolytic enzyme system 891, 892
Fibrinolytic stimulants
  mode of action 893
  properties 916
Fibrocystic disease, pancreas
  see cystic fibrosis
Fibrositic pains
  treatment 867
Filariasis
  treatment 1195

First-pass metabolism
  see metabolism, first pass
Flatulence
  treatment 706
Floctafenine
  clinical use 328
  pharmacology 328
Floxacillin
  see flucloxacillin
Fluclorolone acetonide
  potency, topical 425
Flucloxacillin
  distribution volume 1215
  absorption: newborns 99
  antibacterial activity 135
  children: properties and uses in 135
  half-life 1215
    renal failure 1298
  impetigo: use in 419
  otolaryngology: use in 339
  pKa 1215
  pneumonia: use in 782
  properties 1129
  protein binding 1215
  pulmonary infections: use in 778
  renal failure: use in 1295, 1298
Flucytosine
  see fluorocytosine
Fludrocortisone
  adrenal insufficiency: use in 534
  dosage 530
  half-life 530, 1220
  potency 530
  protein binding 1220
Flufenamic acid
  adverse reactions 853, 1228
  asthma: use in 795
  breast milk 114
  dosage 853
  drug interactions 252
  haemorrhage, uterine dysfunctional: use
    in 477
  elimination 853
  properties 853
  protein binding 17
  rheumatoid arthritis: use in 861
Fluid balance
  drug interactions and 247
Fluid retention
  drugs causing 834
Flumethasone pivalate
  potency, topical 425
Flunisolide
  rhinitis, allergic: use in 343
Flunitrazepam
  anaesthesia: use in 292
  distribution volume 1212, 1221
  elimination 1064
  half-life 1064, 1212
  insomnia: use in 1103
  pKa 1212
    sedation, preoperative: use in 298
  thrombosis from 298
Fluocinolone acetonide
  potency, topical 425
  psoriasis: use in 428
Fluocinonide
  potency, topical 425
Fluocortin butylester
  potency, topical 425
Fluocortolone
  potency, topical 425
Fluorescein